Amato and Russell's Neuromuscular Disorders

Notice

Medicine is an ever-changing science. As new research and clinical experience broaden our knowledge, changes in treatment and drug therapy are required. The authors and the publisher of this work have checked with sources believed to be reliable in their efforts to provide information that is complete and generally in accord with the standards accepted at the time of publication. However, in view of the possibility of human error or changes in medical sciences, neither the authors nor the publisher nor any other party who has been involved in the preparation or publication of this work warrants that the information contained herein is in every respect accurate or complete, and they disclaim all responsibility for any errors or omissions or for the results obtained from use of the information contained in this work. Readers are encouraged to confirm the information contained herein with other sources. For example and in particular, readers are advised to check the product information sheet included in the package of each drug they plan to administer to be certain that the information contained in this work is accurate and that changes have not been made in the recommended dose or in the contraindications for administration. This recommendation is of particular importance in connection with new or infrequently used drugs.

Amato and Russell's Neuromuscular Disorders

THIRD EDITION

Anthony A. Amato, MD
BWH Distinguished Chair in Neurology
Chief, Neuromuscular Division
Brigham and Women's Hospital
Professor of Neurology
Harvard Medical School
Boston, Massachusetts

Christopher T. Doughty, MD
Clinical Director, Neuromuscular Division
Brigham and Women's Hospital
Program Director, Mass General Brigham Neuromuscular Fellowship Program
Assistant Professor of Neurology
Harvard Medical School
Boston, Massachusetts

Sabrina Paganoni, MD, PhD
Department of Physical Medicine and Rehabilitation
Spaulding Rehabilitation Hospital
Co-Director, Neurological Clinical Research Institute
Sean M. Healey & AMG Center for ALS
Department of Neurology
Massachusetts General Hospital
Associate Professor of Physical Medicine and Rehabilitation
Harvard Medical School
Boston, Massachusetts

Amanda C. Guidon, MD, MPH
Chief, Division of Neuromuscular Medicine
Director, EMG Laboratory
Massachusetts General Hospital
Director, MGH Myasthenia Gravis Program
Assistant Professor
Harvard Medical School
Boston, Massachusetts

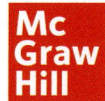

Amato and Russell's Neuromuscular Disorders, Third Edition

Copyright © 2025 by McGraw Hill LLC. All rights reserved. Printed in Hong Kong. Except as permitted under the United States Copyright Act of 1976, no part of this publication may be reproduced or distributed in any form or by any means, or stored in a data base or retrieval system, without the prior written permission of the publisher.

1 2 3 4 5 6 7 8 9   DSS   29 28 27 26 25 24

ISBN 978-1-264-62190-3
MHID 1-264-62190-6

This book was set in Minion Pro by Aptara, Inc.
The editor was Sydney Keen Vitale.
The production supervisor was Catherine H. Saggese.
Some illustrations were created by Renee L. Cannon, MA, CMI.
Project management was provided by Dinesh Pokhriyal, Aptara, Inc.

Library of Congress Cataloging-in-Publication Data

Names: Amato, Anthony A., 1960- author. | Doughty, Christopher, author. | Paganoni, Sabrina, author. | Guidon, Amanda, author.
Title: Amato and Russell's neuromuscular disorders / Anthony A. Amato, Christopher Doughty, Sabrina Paganoni, Amanda Guidon.
Other titles: Neuromuscular disorders
Description: Third edition. | New York, NY : McGraw Hill, [2025] | Preceded by Neuromuscular disorders / Anthony A. Amato, James A. Russell. Second edition. [2016] | Includes bibliographical references and index. | Summary: "This text provides information to understand and diagnose many neuromuscular disorders and attempts to bridge the gap between translational science and practical application at the bedside"– Provided by publisher.
Identifiers: LCCN 2024020065 (print) | LCCN 2024020066 (ebook) | ISBN 9781264621903 (hardcover) | ISBN 1264621906 (hardcover) | ISBN 9781264622429 (ebook) | ISBN 1264622422 (ebook)
Subjects: MESH: Neuromuscular Diseases–diagnosis | Medical History Taking | Diagnostic Techniques, Neurological
Classification: LCC RC346 (print) | LCC RC346 (ebook) | NLM WE 550 | DDC 616.8–dc23/eng/20240517
LC record available at https://lccn.loc.gov/2024020065
LC ebook record available at https://lccn.loc.gov/2024020066

McGraw Hill books are available at special quantity discounts to use as premiums and sales promotions or for use in corporate training programs. To contact a representative, please visit the Contact Us pages at www.mhprofessional.com.

I want to express my gratitude to my good friend, Dr. James Russell, who co-wrote the first and second editions of this textbook with me. He is enjoying retirement now with his wife, Michele, but he graciously took time to review and comment on chapters in this third edition. I was so lucky to enlist my excellent colleagues, Drs. Doughty, Paganoni, and Guidon, all amazing neuromuscular clinicians and teachers, to co-author this third edition with me. Most of all I would like to thank and dedicate this book to my wife, Mary, and our children, Joseph, Erin, Michael, and Katie, for their unconditional love and support over the years and the newest editions to our growing family, our grandchildren, Lily, Calvin, Colby, and Anthony.
— **Anthony A. Amato, MD** —

I would first like to thank my mentors who jump-started my career in neuromuscular medicine: Dr. Amato and Dr. David, who laid the foundation for everything I know about neuromuscular medicine; Dr. Milligan, for first fostering my love of the neurologic examination, sparking my initial interest; and Dr. Guidon and Dr. Bowley who showed me how to teach about neuromuscular disorders and EMG with passion and precision. A career in neuromuscular medicine means a career of lifelong learning—I am especially grateful for my colleagues and all of the neuromuscular fellows who have trained at Mass General Brigham, for keeping me sharp and honest and teaching me new things every day. Finally, a special thanks to my friends and family for their unwavering support and inspiration.
— **Christopher T. Doughty, MD** —

To my mentors, whose guidance has shaped my journey as a physician scientist. Dr. Amato and Dr. David, training as a fellow in neuromuscular medicine with you laid the foundation for my career. Meeting the late Dr. Krivickas gave it direction and purpose, as her passion for ALS ignited my own. Dr. Cudkowicz, I will forever be grateful for the opportunity to learn from you: your vision, leadership, wisdom, and generosity are transformative. Dr. Zafonte, your unwavering support since residency has been invaluable. I would be remiss if I didn't thank my colleagues, whose camaraderie makes each workday fulfilling, and our patients, whose resilience inspires us endlessly. My deepest gratitude also goes to my family, especially my husband, and cherished friends, whose love and companionship sustain me through every endeavor.
— **Sabrina Paganoni, MD, PhD** —

I am privileged to have had the opportunity to contribute to this 3rd Edition of Neuromuscular Disorders with my close colleagues and to learn neuromuscular and electrodiagnostic medicine from some of the best teachers. I am particularly grateful to Dr. Amato for the opportunity to collaborate on this text book and for sharing so much of his neuromuscular know-how over the years and showing me the ropes of the editorial process. Mostly, I would like to express my extreme appreciation for and dedicate this work to my husband, Arnaud Guidon, my greatest supporter and co-pilot, and my son Matthias, who I hope I can inspire to pursue his own passions with rigor, commitment, and joy. I would also like to thank my parents and in-laws, without whom I would not have had the space and time for this project. Finally, I humbly acknowledge the patients we treat, the privilege to be involved in their lives, and the many lessons they have offered.
— **Amanda C. Guidon, MD, MPH** —

CONTENTS

Contributor .... *ix*

Foreword .... *xi*

Preface .... *xii*

SECTION I: EVALUATION AND MANAGEMENT OF PATIENTS WITH NEUROMUSCULAR DISEASE

Chapter 1. Approach to Patients with Neuromuscular Disease 2

Chapter 2. Testing in Neuromuscular Disease 23

Chapter 3. Muscle and Nerve Histopathology 83

Chapter 4. Principles of Immunotherapy 112

Chapter 5. Rehabilitation for People with Neuromuscular Disease 131

SECTION II: SPECIFIC DISORDERS

Chapter 6. Motor Neuron Diseases and Amyotrophic Lateral Sclerosis 166

Chapter 7. Hereditary Spastic Paraplegia 193

Chapter 8. Spinal Muscular Atrophies 202

Chapter 9. Other Motor Neuron Diseases 219

Chapter 10. Disorders of Motor Nerve Hyperactivity 233

Chapter 11. Charcot–Marie–Tooth Disease and Related Disorders 256

Chapter 12. Other Hereditary Neuropathies 297

Chapter 13. Guillain–Barré Syndrome and Related Disorders 326

Chapter 14. Chronic Inflammatory Demyelinating Polyradiculoneuropathy and Related Neuropathies 346

Chapter 15. Vasculitic Neuropathies 383

Chapter 16. Neuropathies Associated with Systemic Disease 397

Chapter 17. Neuropathies Associated with Infections 411

Chapter 18.	Neuropathies Related to Nutritional Deficiencies 430
Chapter 19.	Neuropathies Associated with Malignancy 440
Chapter 20.	Toxic Neuropathies 472
Chapter 21.	Neuropathies Associated with Endocrinopathies 491
Chapter 22.	Idiopathic Polyneuropathy 504
Chapter 23.	Focal Processes Affecting the Upper Extremity and Trunk: Radiculopathies, Brachial Plexopathies, and Mononeuropathies 517
Chapter 24.	Focal Neuropathies of the Lower Extremities: Radiculopathies, Plexopathies, and Mononeuropathies 563
Chapter 25.	Autoimmune Myasthenia Gravis 607
Chapter 26.	Other Disorders of Neuromuscular Transmission 660
Chapter 27.	Muscular Dystrophies 701
Chapter 28.	Congenital Myopathies 773
Chapter 29.	Metabolic Myopathies 798
Chapter 30.	Mitochondrial Disorders 831
Chapter 31.	Myotonic Dystrophies 857
Chapter 32.	Nondystrophic Myotonias and Periodic Paralysis 864
Chapter 33.	Inflammatory Myopathies 887
Chapter 34.	Myopathies Associated with Systemic Disease 940
Chapter 35.	Toxic Myopathies 957
Chapter 36.	Neuromuscular Mimics 983
Index	 999

CONTRIBUTOR

Erik Ensrud, MD
Professor, Neurology
Professor, Physical Medicine and Rehabilitation
Director, M.D.A. Clinic and ALSA Center of Excellence
University of Missouri
Columbia, Missouri

FOREWORD

To quote the late US historian, David McCullough, likely paraphrased from the 33rd President of the United States Harry S. Truman "There is nothing new but the history we have forgotten".[1] Despite the relevance of this insight to most aspects of life, it does not fully apply to the evolving nature of medical practice.

In this, the third edition of *Neuromuscular Disorders*, doctors Amato, Doughty, Guidon, and Paganoni remain committed to this historical principle. They continue to promote that optimal patient care in Neuromuscular Medicine begins and ends with an accurate diagnosis, provided by master clinicians, and centered at the bedside. These individuals are skilled in listening to and examining the patient, thus providing the foundation for diagnostic problem solving. They are then positioned to guide their patient in a shared decision-making process, integrating optimal evaluation and management decisions aligned with patient values and goals.

At the same time, in contrast to McCullough's valued principle, the authors have applied their considerable knowledge regarding the notable advances in neuroscience that have occurred since the last edition of this book. By doing so, they have skillfully and pragmatically blended the art and science of medicine. They have provided a template to aid their readers in the judicious application of serological, genetic and imaging tools serving to confirm or refute the clinically established working diagnosis. This strategy is particularly evident in Dr. Doughty's chapter on CIDP where the nuanced distinction of the various subtypes is determined largely by phenotype, not the supporting laboratory profile. It is also notably evident by the detailed consideration of the rapidly increasing and also nuanced role of neuromuscular genetic testing incorporated into individual chapters when relevant.

The third edition of *Neuromuscular Disorders* also provides a measured and experienced perspective on when and how to apply a slowly but nevertheless expanding armamentarium of therapeutic interventions. This is particularly true in the chapter on autoimmune myasthenia gravis where Dr. Guidon provides valuable guidance regarding how to judiciously integrate new, effective treatments with novel mechanisms of action with established effective therapies. In contrast, Dr. Paganoni reviews new treatments in ALS that provide hope. She uses her considerable experience and judgment to help the clinician to guide their patient in deciding when and how long these treatments should be utilized.

Finally, the authorship of this book, like the practice of medicine, has also evolved in contrast to McCullough's principle. One of the original authors has moved into the history book, succeeded by three more contemporary colleagues whose contributions to this edition far surpass anything their predecessor could have offered. In his foreword to the second edition of this text, Dr. Barohn spoke of the potential longevity of this book. Whatever success this book has had, or may have in the future is largely attributable to the historical tie that binds. Tony Amato is the person who first conceived of *Neuromuscular Disorders* and has catalyzed it through its three editions. He represents what this book attempts to develop, a master clinician skilled at blending the art and science of medicine.

James A. Russell, DO, FAAN
Emeritus Clinical Professor of Neurology
Tufts University School of Medicine
Boston, Massachusetts

---

[1]McCullough David. *Truman*. 1992. Simon and Schuster.

PREFACE

It has been eight years since the publication of the second edition of this book. Much has changed, particularly in our knowledge of the imaging, genetic, and immunologic tools at our disposal that aid in our ability to understand and diagnose many neuromuscular disorders. Most importantly, there have been incredible advances in the treatment of various neuromuscular disorders with new gene therapies and immunotherapies now available. Dr. James Russell retired, but I was grateful to enlist my close neuromuscular colleagues, Drs. Chris Doughty, Sabrina Paganoni, and Amanda Guidon to co-author this third edition with me. In addition, Dr. Erik Ensrud kindly contributed again to this edition helping on chapters regarding the rehabilitation of neuromuscular diseases and on other disorders that may confound the clinician as neuromuscular mimics. All chapters in the book have been rewritten, in many cases extensively with the assimilation of contemporary citations. We have attempted to read and consider as much of this information as possible and translate it into a text that attempts to bridge the gap between translational science and practical application at the bedside. Once again, we attempt to blend our understanding of evidence-based medicine with our personal experiences as "seasoned" clinicians to provide a resource that is of pragmatic value to others.

What remains unchanged, however, is the fundamental principle that optimal patient care depends on accurate diagnosis. Judicious use of tests, prescription of effective treatment(s) and avoidance of potentially harmful ones, recognition of potential comorbidities, and accurate patient counseling are all dependent on this principle. For the foreseeable future, the focal point of accurate diagnosis will be at the bedside and will depend on the skills of the master clinician who recognizes and formulates information. This book is written in respect of and support for this time-honored and effective clinical approach.

SECTION I

EVALUATION AND MANAGEMENT OF PATIENTS WITH NEUROMUSCULAR DISEASE

CHAPTER 1

Approach to Patients with Neuromuscular Disease

▶ GENERAL PRINCIPLES

The evaluation of patients with suspected neuromuscular disease remains first and foremost a bedside exercise. Accurate diagnosis requires consideration of individual patient and disease differences. Despite the benefits of evidence-based medicine, its conclusions are more relevant to populations than to individuals. Confounding variables that are part of the human experience may be overlooked or overemphasized by testing algorithms. This textbook will repeatedly endorse the strongly held philosophy of its authors, that is, patient management flows from an accurate diagnosis. An accurate diagnosis is most likely to be obtained based on a differential diagnosis driven by clinical assessment and hypotheses. These hypotheses should be formulated based on the principles of neurologic localization, the correlation of the chronologic course of symptom development with the behaviors of differing disease conditions, and the application of risk factor analysis. Ideally, the tests described in the subsequent two chapters and throughout the text would be utilized with the primary intent of resolving a clinically established differential diagnosis to confirm a working diagnosis. As all tests are potentially fallible, the credibility of their results diminishes when they are used as screening procedures. A laboratory abnormality, occurring without the context of clinical correlation, fails to establish the desired confidence in a cause-and-effect relationship with the patient's complaint(s). Metaphorically, laboratory tests are analogous to a carpenter's tools. They are of great value when placed in the hands of a skillful artisan but are potentially damaging if used injudiciously.

In this book, a neuromuscular disorder will refer to any condition that affects the structure and/or function of any component of the neuromuscular system, beginning and working centrifugally from the cell bodies of the anterior horn and dorsal root ganglion. This will include disorders of nerve root, plexus, nerve, neuromuscular junction, and muscle. The clinician has three main goals in evaluating a patient with a neuromuscular disorder: (1) identify where the lesion is, (2) identify the cause, and (3) determine the proper management. The first goal is accomplished by obtaining a thorough history, neurologic examination, and other testing as necessary (laboratory studies, electrophysiology, genetic testing, muscle, or nerve biopsy). This chapter focuses on the important details of the history and physical examination which is structured based on eight key questions. The goal of these questions is to define the pattern of involvement in order to condense the differential diagnosis (Table 1-1).

The differential diagnosis of disorders of the neuromuscular system is in part age dependent. The differential diagnosis of neuromuscular conditions in infants, children, and adolescents is both overlapping and unique in comparison to their adult counterparts (Tables 1-2 to 1-4). The applied diagnostic principles are similar although both the examination and review of symptoms may be hampered in infants. In the pediatric population, parents must be questioned with great care and sensitivity. The heightened concern of the parents may cause them to unconsciously omit important details of the patient's condition or history or assume a benign attribution as the cause of the symptom. Parents may also bring a considerable amount of guilt to the evaluation, which may limit their willingness to share information. The parents' fears and associated guilt and professional counseling should be considered if warranted. Childhood illness can have profound repercussions on the entire family.

Clinicians frequently evaluate patients with symptoms that are subjective and nonspecific which may or may not be attributable to an underlying neuromuscular disorder. For example, a complaint of weakness may represent either asthenia due to a myriad of causes, or an actual loss of muscle strength or endurance. Confidence in the ability to exclude neuromuscular disorders from consideration is enhanced by a thorough knowledge of how these conditions behave. The strategies outlined in this chapter are based on the general principle that diagnostic accuracy is enhanced by correlation of the patient's signs and symptoms, with knowledge of the natural history and behavior of the ever-expanding menu of neuromuscular diseases. In our opinion, adherence to these principles will improve diagnostic accuracy. This chapter will attempt to provide an organizational framework, utilizing information that is important to elicit, to allow accurate interpretation of these frequent subjective and nonspecific complaints.

▶ TABLE 1-1. APPROACH TO NEUROMUSCULAR DISORDERS: EIGHT KEY QUESTIONS

1. **When did the symptoms begin?**
   - Birth/infancy
   - Early childhood
   - Late childhood
   - Early or mid-adulthood
   - Late adulthood
2. **What is the temporal evolution?**
   - Acute (days to 4 weeks)
   - Subacute (4–8 weeks)
   - Chronic (>8 weeks)
   - Monophasic, progressive, or relapsing-remitting
3. **What systems are involved?**
   - Motor, sensory, autonomic, or combinations
4. **Is there weakness and what is the distribution?**
   - Only distal vs. proximal and distal
   - Focal/asymmetric vs. symmetric
5. **Is there sensory involvement and what is the distribution?**
   - Temperature loss or burning or stabbing pain (e.g., small fiber)
   - Vibratory or proprioceptive loss or sensory ataxia (e.g., large fiber)
6. **Is there evidence of upper motor neuron involvement?**
   - Without sensory loss
   - With sensory loss
7. **Is there evidence for a hereditary neuromuscular disorder?**
   - Family history
   - Clinical examination findings (e.g., scapular winging, pseudohypertrophy, myotonia, pes cavus, hammer toes, lack of sensory symptoms despite sensory signs)
8. **Are there any associated medical conditions?**
   - Cancer, diabetes mellitus, connective tissue disease or other autoimmune diseases, infection (e.g., HIV, COVID-19, Lyme disease, leprosy)
   - Medications including over-the-counter drugs that may cause a toxic neuropathy
   - Preceding events, drugs, toxins

Modified from: Amato AA, Barohn RJ. Peripheral neuropathies. In: Fauci AS, Braunwald E, Kasper DJ, Hauser SL, Longo DL, Jamesion JL, Loscalzo J, eds. *Harrison's Principles of Internal Medicine.* McGraw Hill, 2022 (in-press).

▶ TABLE 1-2. DIFFERENTIAL DIAGNOSIS OF THE FLOPPY INFANT

Central nervous system disorders (most common etiology)
Anterior horn cell
    Spinal muscular atrophy types I and II
Peripheral neuropathy
    CMT III (Dejerine–Sottas, congenital hypomyelinating/amyelinating neuropathy)
    CMT I and CMT II—rare
    Giant axonal neuropathy
Neuromuscular junction
    Infantile botulism
    Transient neonatal myasthenia gravis
    Congenital myasthenic syndromes
Myopathy
    Congenital myopathies
    Muscular dystrophies
        Congenital muscular dystrophies
        Other limb-girdle muscular dystrophies (e.g., dystrophinopathy/sarcoglycanopathy—rare)
        Congenital myotonic dystrophy
    Metabolic myopathies
        Glycogen storage defects
            Acid maltase deficiency
            Debrancher deficiency
            Branching enzyme deficiency
            Myophosphorylase deficiency (rare)
        Disorders of lipid metabolism
            Carnitine deficiency
            Other fatty acid/acyl-CoA dehydrogenase deficiencies
    Mitochondrial myopathies
        Benign and fatal infantile myopathy
        Leigh's syndrome
    Endocrine myopathies (e.g., hypothyroidism)

Modified with permission from Dumitru D, Amato AA. Introduction to myopathies and muscle tissue's reaction to injury. In: Dumitru D, Amato AA, Swartz MJ, eds. *Electrodiagnostic Medicine.* 2nd ed. Hanley & Belfus; 2002.

▶ DOES THE PATIENT HAVE A NEUROMUSCULAR PROBLEM?

HISTORY TAKING

Neuromuscular diseases manifest themselves through some symptoms or combination of symptoms attributable directly or indirectly to the dysfunction of peripheral motor, sensory, and autonomic nerves, neuromuscular junction, or muscle (Table 1-1). Motor symptoms are typically expressed in a "negative" fashion (weakness or atrophy). Occasionally, "positive" symptoms referable to overactivity [e.g., muscle cramps and fasciculations with LMN involvement and stiffness or flexor spasms in upper motor neuron (UMN) involvement] may dominate the clinical presentation. Sensory symptoms may also manifest with either a positive (e.g., paresthesia) or a negative (e.g., numbness or sensory ataxia) manner. Although pain may be considered a positive sensory symptom, it will be considered as an independent symptom in this text as it is neither a common nor dominant feature in many neuromuscular conditions.

Neuromuscular disorders which manifest themselves solely within the domain of the motor system typically originate from anterior horn cells, the neuromuscular junction, muscle, or rarely motor nerve fibers. Sensory symptoms typically imply a disorder of nerve root, dorsal root ganglion, plexus, or one or more peripheral nerve trunks. During history acquisition, there is considerable value in identifying both the location and the nature of the initial symptom(s), including the context in which that symptom developed. The

TABLE 1-3. NEUROMUSCULAR CAUSES OF WEAKNESS PRESENTING IN CHILDHOOD OR EARLY ADULTHOOD

Anterior horn cell
  Spinal muscular atrophy type III
  Poliomyelitis
  Amyotrophic lateral sclerosis

Peripheral neuropathy
  Acute or chronic inflammatory demyelinating polyneuropathy
  Hereditary neuropathies

Neuromuscular junction
  Botulism
  Myasthenia gravis
  Congenital myasthenic syndromes
  Lambert–Eaton syndrome

Myopathy
  Congenital myopathies
    Central core
    Multicore
    Centronuclear
    Nemaline
  Muscular dystrophies
    Dystrophinopathy (Duchenne or Becker)
    Limb-girdle muscular dystrophies
    Myofibrillar myopathy
    Myotonic dystrophy
    Other dystrophies (e.g., FSHD and EDMD)
  Metabolic myopathies
    Glycogen storage defects
      Acid maltase deficiency
      Debrancher and branching enzyme deficiency
    Disorders of lipid metabolism
      Carnitine deficiency
      Other fatty acid/acyl-CoA dehydrogenase deficiencies
  Mitochondrial myopathies
  Periodic paralysis
  Electrolyte imbalance
    Hyperkalemia
    Hypokalemia
    Hypophosphatemia
    Hypercalcemia
  Endocrine myopathies
  Toxic myopathies
  Inflammatory myopathies
    Dermatomyositis
    Antisynthetase syndrome
    Immune-mediated necrotizing myopathy
    Overlap syndromes
    Polymyositis (after the age of 20 years)
    Infectious myositis

EDMD, Emery–Dreifuss muscular dystrophy; FSHD, facioscapulohumeral muscular dystrophy.
Modified with permission from Dumitru D, Amato AA. Introduction to myopathies and muscle tissue's reaction to injury. In Dumitru D, Amato AA, Swartz MJ. eds. *Electrodiagnostic Medicine*. 2nd ed. Hanley & Belfus; 2002.

TABLE 1-4. NEUROMUSCULAR CAUSES OF WEAKNESS PRESENTING IN MIDDLE TO LATE ADULTHOOD

Anterior horn cell
  Spinal muscular atrophy type III
  Kennedy disease
  Poliomyelitis
  Amyotrophic lateral sclerosis

Peripheral neuropathy
  Hereditary neuropathies
  Acute or chronic inflammatory demyelinating polyneuropathy
  Drug-induced or toxic neuropathies
  Diabetic neuropathy
  Amyloid
  Vasculitis

Neuromuscular junction
  Botulism
  Myasthenia gravis
  Lambert–Eaton syndrome

Myopathy
  Muscular dystrophies
    Dystrophinopathy (Becker)
    Limb-girdle muscular dystrophies
    Myofibrillar myopathy
    Oculopharyngeal dystrophy
    Bent spine/dropped head syndrome
  Metabolic myopathies
    Glycogen storage defects
      Acid maltase deficiency
      Debrancher deficiency
    Disorders of lipid metabolism (rare)
    Congenital myopathies
    Sporadic late-onset nemaline myopathy
  Mitochondrial myopathies
  Periodic paralysis
    Familial hypo-KPP manifests within the first three decades
    Familial hyper-KPP usually manifests in the first decade
  Electrolyte imbalance
    Hyperkalemia
    Hypokalemia
    Hypophosphatemia
    Hypercalcemia
  Endocrine myopathies
  Toxic myopathies
  Myopathy associated with systemic disease (e.g., cancer), poor nutrition, and disuse
  Amyloid myopathy
  Inflammatory myopathies
    Inclusion body myositis (most common inflammatory myopathy after the age of 50 years)
    Dermatomyositis
    Antisynthetase syndrome
    Immune-mediated necrotizing myopathy
    Overlap syndromes
    Polymyositis (after the age of 20 years)
    Infectious myositis

hyper-KPP, hyperkalemic periodic paralysis; hypo-KPP, hypokalemic periodic paralysis.
Modified with permission from Dumitru D, Amato AA. Introduction to myopathies and muscle tissue's reaction to injury. In: Dumitru D, Amato AA, Swartz MJ, eds. *Electrodiagnostic Medicine*. 2nd ed. Hanley & Belfus; 2002.

subsequent evolution of symptoms should then be developed in a chronologic fashion with particular attention to the topographical distribution. The value of this approach may be illustrated with the example of multifocal neuropathy. At the time of their initial neurologic assessment, the patient's deficits may have become confluent and indistinguishable from a length-dependent neuropathy and its far more extensive differential diagnosis. Identifying that the initial symptom occurred in a focal nerve distribution narrows the differential diagnosis and improves diagnostic accuracy. The benefit of defining the chronologic course is that the differential diagnosis of acute neuromuscular disorders is notably disparate from that of its chronic counterparts (Tables 1-5 to 1-7).

When acquiring a history, it is imperative not to accept words at face value and to explore what that word means to a patient. For example, it is not uncommon for patients to say "numb" when they mean weak, and "weak" when they mean numb. The mechanism of impaired function should be explored. For example, questions should be formulated to determine whether a fall is due to proximal weakness resulting in failure of antigravity muscles, tripping due to a foot drop, or loss of balance due to impaired proprioception, vestibular function, or disordered postural reflexes originating at the central nervous system (CNS) level. Detailed questioning may be required to determine whether the inability to get out of the chair is due to proximal weakness or impaired central nervous initiation.

It is important to identify symptoms not only referable to the peripheral neuromuscular system but also to symptoms relating to impairment of higher cortical or cranial nerve

▶ **TABLE 1-5. NEUROMUSCULAR DISORDERS PRESENTING WITH ACUTE OR SUBACUTE PROXIMAL OR GENERALIZED WEAKNESS**

Anterior horn cell
   Poliomyelitis
Peripheral neuropathy
   Guillain–Barré syndrome
   Porphyria
   Diphtheria
   Tick paralysis
   Toxic neuropathies
   Diabetic amyotrophy
   Vasculitis
   Carcinomatous infiltration (e.g., leukemia and lymphoma)
   Paraneoplastic neuropathy
Neuromuscular junction
   Botulism
   Lambert–Eaton syndrome
   Myasthenia gravis
Myopathy
   Periodic paralysis
   Electrolyte imbalance
   Endocrinopathies
   Inflammatory myopathies
      Dermatomyositis
      Antisynthetase syndrome
      Immune-mediated necrotizing myopathy (e.g., anti-HMGCR and anti-SRP)
      Overlap syndromes
      Polymyositis
      Infectious myositis
   Toxic myopathies
   Metabolic myopathies
      Glycogen and lipid disorders
Neuromyopathy
   Critical illness neuromyopathy

Modified with permission from Dumitru D, Amato AA. Introduction to myopathies and muscle tissue's reaction to injury. In: Dumitru D, Amato AA, Swartz MJ, eds. *Electrodiagnostic Medicine*. 2nd ed. Hanley & Belfus; 2002.

▶ **TABLE 1-6. DIFFERENTIAL DIAGNOSIS OF CHRONIC PROGRESSIVE PROXIMAL WEAKNESS**

Anterior horn cell
   Amyotrophic lateral sclerosis
   Spinal muscular atrophy type III
   Kennedy disease
Peripheral neuropathy
   Chronic inflammatory demyelinating polyneuropathy
   Multifocal motor neuropathy
   Toxic neuropathies
   Neuropathy associated with systemic disorders
      Connective tissue disease (e.g., vasculitis)
      Diabetes mellitus
      Amyloidosis
   Paraneoplastic
   Carcinomatous infiltration (e.g., leukemia and lymphoma)
Neuromuscular junction
   Lambert–Eaton syndrome
   Myasthenia gravis
Myopathy
   Limb-girdle muscular dystrophy
   Periodic paralysis
   Electrolyte imbalance
   Endocrinopathies
   Inflammatory myopathies
      Inclusion body myositis (proximal legs, but distal arms)
      Dermatomyositis
      Antisynthetase syndrome
      Immune-mediated necrotizing myopathy (e.g., anti-HMGCR and anti-SRP)
      Overlap syndromes
      Polymyositis
      Infectious myositis
   Toxic myopathies
   Sporadic late-onset nemaline myopathy
   Metabolic myopathies
      Glycogen and lipid disorders
Miscellaneous: Tick paralysis, hypophosphatemia; hypokalemia

Modified with permission from Dumitru D, Amato AA. Introduction to myopathies and muscle tissue's reaction to injury. In: Dumitru D, Amato AA, Swartz MJ, eds. *Electrodiagnostic Medicine*. 2nd ed. Hanley & Belfus; 2002.

▶ **TABLE 1-7. NEUROMUSCULAR CAUSES OF CHRONIC DISTAL WEAKNESS CAUSING BILATERAL FOOT AND/OR HEEL DROP**

Anterior horn cell
  ALS[a]

Distal spinal muscular atrophy
  Polio and other enterovirus[a]
  Conus medullaris syndrome—e.g., myelodysplasia, ependymoma, syringomyelia
  Scapuloperoneal form of SMA

Nerve
  Charcot–Marie–Tooth disease and similar hereditary polyneuropathies
  Multifocal neuropathies[a]—infiltrative (neoplastic, amyloid, sarcoid, neurofibromatosis), vasculitic, immune mediated (DADS, MADSAM, MMN, nodal/paranodal myopathies)

NMJ
  Myasthenia gravis (rare)
  Congenital myasthenia

Muscle
  Distal myopathies—Myofibrillar myopathy, Udd, Welander, Laing, GNE
  Muscular dystrophies—Miyoshi type (ANO-5, Dysferlin), calveolinopathy, scapuloperoneal, facioscapulohumeral, Emery–Dreifuss, oculopharyngeal distal myopathy
  Congenital myopathies—nemaline, central core, nemaline
  Glycogen storage diseases—brancher, debrancher/polyglucosan body disease, Pompe, phosphorylase B kinase deficiency
  Lipid storage disorders—neutral lipid storage myopathy, multiple acyl-coA dehydrogenase deficiency
  Inflammatory—inclusion body myositis, granulomatous myositis

[a]Usual notable asymmetries.

function. In addition, a major discriminator in the development of a differential diagnosis is the presence or absence of symptoms referable to involvement of other organ systems. A careful system review is important in an attempt not only to achieve a diagnosis but also to fully anticipate the scope of its potential morbidity. For example, the recognition of orthostasis either by history or examination can provide insight that an evolving, otherwise nonspecific neuropathy pattern may be attributable to amyloidosis. Symptoms referable to cardiomyopathy or cardiac conduction defects, impaired gastrointestinal motility, cutaneous change, and contractures may clarify the differential diagnosis in the heritable myopathies.

As muscle weakness is usually the most objective manifestation of neuromuscular disease, emphasis is placed not only on its existence but on its characteristics (e.g., upper or lower motor neuron) and on the pattern of involvement (Tables 1-5 to 1-8). The existence of weakness may be apparent either through history taking or, more commonly, by examination. Even though muscle weakness is the hallmark of neuromuscular disease, patients frequently identify and validate true weakness by its functional consequences.

The complaint of weakness is more commonly used by patients as a synonym for asthenia—a more pervasive, generalized complaint due to several different conditions. History taking pertaining to muscle weakness has numerous benefits. It should focus on the identification of specific functions or activities that the patient finds difficult. If a patient who claims to be weak cannot describe a specific activity that is problematic for them, the existence of true muscle weakness remains suspect unless subsequently corroborated by the physical examination. Conversely, it is not rare for a disorder such as Lambert–Eaton myasthenic syndrome to produce credible functional impairments due to muscle weakness that appears disproportionate to actual weakness found on bedside examination.

In addition, correlating specific actions and activities of living with weakness in specific muscles and muscle groups can be very beneficial when direct patient examination is not possible. This situation is increasingly prevalent, due to the expansion of telehealth practice and the contact restrictions imposed by the COVID-19 pandemic. Although not as accurate as direct examination, identifying patterns of weakness integral to accurate bedside neuromuscular diagnosis can be accomplished at times with precise and informed history taking.

At times, weakness may present with pain rather than with symptoms directly attributable to weakness. For example, patients with trapezius weakness commonly present with shoulder pain, presumably due to traction on pain-sensitive structures resulting from their "shoulder drop." Pain originating from strain on joints or soft tissues, as a secondary consequence of neuromuscular disease and the weakness it produces, is not uncommon, even in disorders such as amyotrophic lateral sclerosis (ALS) and muscular dystrophy which do not involve sensory nerves.

UMN involvement needs to be considered in patients with potential neuromuscular disease, either as an alternative explanation for symptoms or as a component of their neuromuscular condition. UMN pathology interferes with the synergistic functions of multiple muscle groups. As a result, functional activities highly dependent on coordinated muscle actions are commonly impaired early in the disease course. Impaired running and hand dexterity are notable examples. In addition, positive motor symptoms that occur commonly in UMN disease such as limb stiffness or spasms are readily recognized. Patients may complain of a tendency to drag one or both lower extremities. If the corticobulbar tracts are affected, swallowing and articulation are affected early and prominently, as these functions are dependent on the coordinated interplay of multiple muscle groups. The resulting speech pattern is often halting, effortful, and "strangled" in its characteristics. Patients may lose their ability to effectively sniff or blow their nose. Patients with corticobulbar tract involvement may also develop forced yawning, or lability of affect known as pseudobulbar palsy.

In contrast, as the final common pathway, lower motor neuron disorders express themselves in a limited number of ways, typically as a direct effect of loss of specific functions

▶ **TABLE 1-8. PATTERNS OF MUSCLE WEAKNESS AND CORRELATIONS WITH NEUROMUSCULAR LOCALIZATION**

Patterns of Weakness	Localization
• Weakness of extensor muscles in the upper extremities, flexors in the lower extremities	UMN
• Hemiparesis	UMN
• Multifocal, asymmetric weakness without sensory involvement	MND
	Multifocal motor neuropathy
	MG (uncommon)
• Multifocal, asymmetric weakness with sensory involvement	Polyradiculopathy; multifocal CIDP (Lewis–Sumner syndrome or MADSAM)
	Multifocal neuropathy
• Multifocal sensory loss	Dorsal root ganglionopathy
• Symmetric weakness, proximal or generalized without sensory involvement	Myopathy
	MND
	DNMT
• Generalized motor > sensory	Polyradiculoneuropathy
• Asymmetric cranial nerve ± limbs	MG
• Distal symmetric—motor only	Distal myopathies
	Distal spinal muscular atrophy
• Distal symmetric—sensory > motor	LDPN
• Multiple nerve—asymmetric	Multifocal neuropathy
• Multiple root—asymmetric	Polyradiculopathy
• Multiple nerves and roots, single extremity	Plexopathy
• Single root	Monoradiculopathy
• Single nerve	Mononeuropathy

DNMT, disorders of neuromuscular transmission; LDPN, length-dependent polyneuropathy; MG, myasthenia gravis; MND, motor neuron disease; PN, polyneuropathy; UMN, upper motor neuron.

due to weakness. Depending on a patient's handedness, vocation, or hobbies, this may not be noticed until the weakness is substantial. Less commonly, the patient's initial complaints pertaining to lower motor neuron loss may reflect awareness of atrophy, fasciculations, or cramps.

Patients with weakness of hip flexion will have difficulty getting in and out of a car without manually lifting their thighs. Unless there is concomitant knee extensor weakness, patients will have more difficulty going upstairs than down as the former requires active hip flexion against gravity. Patients with weakness of hip abductors will waddle as a compensatory maneuver to maintain their center of gravity and balance. Patients with chronic weakness of hip extension will have difficulty rising from a chair and a tendency to have exaggerated lumbar lordosis as well, the latter resulting from posterior displacement of the shoulders for the same compensatory reasons. Knee extension weakness will result in difficulty getting up from a squat or out of deep chairs and commonly results in falls due to buckling of one or both knees. These patients may hyperextend their knees to prevent this (i.e., genu recurvatum). Ankle dorsiflexion weakness often results in tripping or audible foot slapping while walking. Ankle plantar flexion weakness affects the efficiency of walking and deprives individuals from the ability to stand on their toes and run effectively.

In the upper extremity, people with weakness of the shoulder girdle will have difficulty with antigravity movements such as washing their hair, lifting heavy pans, inserting arms into coat sleeves, or retrieving objects from shelves. Weakness of elbow flexion and extension often goes unnoticed until severe but may be recognized while attempting to open doors that require pull and push, respectively. Wrist and digit weaknesses interfere with grip and dexterity, which may impair multiple ADLs, including opening bottles and cans, grasping zipper tabs, turning ignition keys, or buttoning buttons.

Neuromuscular disorders often affect the motor and, to a lesser extent, sensory function of the cranial nerves. Extraocular muscle involvement is a key discriminating factor in working through the differential diagnosis of neuromuscular disorders. For example, the extraocular muscles are rarely affected in motor neuron disease (MND), most axonal polyneuropathies, or acquired inflammatory myopathies. Conversely, they may represent prominent manifestations of the inflammatory demyelinating polyneuropathies, disorders of neuromuscular transmission, and a finite list of muscle diseases, typically heritable in nature.

Patients typically become aware of ptosis by personal or family observation (Table 1-9). Occasionally, they first become aware when their vision is impaired by the drooping eyelid. Extraocular muscle involvement is typically expressed as diplopia, although patients with slowly progressive, symmetric involvement of the extraocular muscles such as in chronic progressive external ophthalmoplegia may have limited awareness of their deficit.

Patients with acute onset of unilateral facial weakness are usually very aware of the existence and nature of their

TABLE 1-9. NEUROMUSCULAR CAUSES OF PTOSIS OR OPHTHALMOPLEGIA/OPHTHALMOPARESIS

Peripheral neuropathy
    Guillain–Barré syndrome
    Miller Fisher syndrome
    CANVAS
    CANOMAD
    Mitochondrial

Neuromuscular junction
    Botulism
    Lambert–Eaton syndrome (ptosis only)
    Myasthenia gravis (pupil sparing)
    Congenital myasthenia

Myopathy
    Mitochondrial myopathies
        Kearn–Sayres syndrome
        Progressive external ophthalmoplegia
    Oculopharyngeal and oculopharyngodistal muscular dystrophy
    Myotonic dystrophy (ptosis only)
    Congenital myopathy
        Myotubular
        Nemaline (ptosis only)
        Congenital fiber-type disproportion
        Multiminicore disease
    Hyperthyroidism/Graves disease (ophthalmoplegia without ptosis)
    Hereditary inclusion body myopathy type III
    Inflammatory myopathies (e.g., check-point inhibitor myositis, giant cell/granulomatous myositis, IgG4 disease)

CANOMAD, chronic ataxic neuropathy ophthalmology IgM paraprotein cold agglutinins disialosyl antibodies; CANVAS, chronic ataxic neuropathy, vestibular areflexia syndrome; SANDO, sensory ataxic neuropathy, dysarthria, ophthalmoplegia.
Modified with permission from Dumitru D, Amato AA. Introduction to myopathies and muscle tissue's reaction to injury. In: Dumitru D, Amato AA, Swartz MJ, eds. *Electrodiagnostic Medicine*. 2nd ed. Hanley & Belfus; 2002.

TABLE 1-10. NEUROMUSCULAR DISORDERS ASSOCIATED WITH FACIAL WEAKNESS

Anterior horn cell
    Amyotrophic lateral sclerosis
    Facial-onset sensory and motor neuronopathy (FOSMN)
    Spinal muscular atrophy
    Kennedy disease

Polycranialradiculoneuropathy
    Lyme
    Sarcoidosis
    Neoplastic meningitis
    Chronic meningitis
    GBS
    CIDP

Neuromuscular junction
    Myasthenia gravis
    Congenital myasthenia gravis
    Lambert–Eaton myasthenia gravis
    Botulism

Muscle
    Facioscapulohumeral muscular dystrophy
    Congenital myopathies
    Myotonic muscular dystrophy
    Inclusion body myositis
    Oculopharyngeal myopathy

problem. In many neuromuscular disorders, facial weakness is often chronic and symmetric, and as a result, the patient may not be aware of their deficit (Table 1-10). It is not rare for chronic bifacial weakness to be recognized for the first time on a routine neurologic examination. Questions pertaining to a tendency to sleep with eyes incompletely closed, the ability to blow up balloons or whistle may help to estimate the duration of a problem in situations such as these.

Symptomatic jaw weakness, manifesting as difficulties with jaw opening or jaw closing, is an infrequent neuromuscular complaint. When present, it is often overshadowed by symptoms referable to muscles concomitantly affecting speech, swallowing, and breathing. Difficulty with chewing should nonetheless be inquired about, as it may sometimes be the initial or key symptom in a limited number of disorders such as myasthenia or Kennedy disease.

Symptoms referable to tongue weakness are common in many neuromuscular disorders. Patients typically become aware of tongue weakness manifesting as dysarthria. Other issues may include the inability to manipulate food properly within their mouth. This kind of detail is uncommonly volunteered by the patient and is more frequently elucidated by detailed questioning.

Weakness of the neck muscles may be noticed by patients or their families when the neck extensors can no longer support the weight of the head and head drop develops (Table 1-11). This is often accompanied by nuchal discomfort, presumably due to the constant and unaccustomed traction on posterior cervical ligamentous structures. Neck discomfort from head drop may be distinguished from other, more common causes of neck pain, by the relief allowed by neck support. Head drop may contribute to dysphagia as well. Trapezius weakness is most commonly symptomatic when acute and unilateral and is usually a result of a mononeuropathy of the accessory nerve. As discussed above, patients with trapezius weakness usually present with shoulder pain as the index symptom. Shoulder drop can be easily missed unless the patient is viewed from the rear, with the back exposed.

Neuromuscular causes of scapular displacement can result from weakness of the trapezius, serratus anterior, or to a lesser extent, rhomboid muscles (Table 1-12). Scapular winging interferes with both shoulder-girdle positioning, strength, and mobility. Patients may note either difficulty in raising an arm above the head or an inability to push with the accustomed force, for example, while doing push-ups.

The symptoms of ventilatory muscle weakness represent an ominous, occasionally initial manifestation of a

▶ TABLE 1-11. NEUROMUSCULAR DISORDERS ASSOCIATED WITH HEAD DROP OR AXIAL WEAKNESS (CAMPTOCORMIA)

Anterior horn cell
  Amyotrophic lateral sclerosis
  Radiation myelopathy
  Syringomyelia

Neuromuscular junction
  Myasthenia gravis

Neuropathy
  Guillain–Barré syndrome
  CIDP

Muscle
  Isolated neck extensor myopathy
  Inclusion body myositis
  Focal myositis
  Sporadic late-onset nemaline myopathy (SLONM)
  Hereditary inclusion body myopathy
  Laminopathy
  Selenoproteinopathy
  Facioscapulohumeral muscular dystrophy
  Myofibrillar myopathy
  Proximal myotonic myopathy
  McArdle disease
  Pompe disease
  Carnitine deficiency
  Mitochondrial myopathy
  Hyperparathyroidism
  Hypokalemia

▶ TABLE 1-12. NEUROMUSCULAR DISORDERS ASSOCIATED WITH SCAPULAR WINGING

Anterior horn cell
  Scapuloperoneal spinal muscular atrophy

Nerve
  Accessory nerve palsy
  Long thoracic nerve palsy
  Scapuloperoneal neuropathy (Davidenkow syndrome)

Muscle
  Facioscapulohumeral muscular dystrophy
  Scapuloperoneal muscular dystrophy
  Limb-girdle muscular dystrophy (e.g., calpainopathy)
  Pompe disease
  Sporadic late-onset nemaline myopathy

Neuromuscular diseases where scapular winging occurs uncommonly
  Myotonic muscular dystrophy
  Emery–Dreifuss muscular dystrophy
  Myotubular myopathy
  Nemaline rod myopathy
  Central core myopathy
  Phosphofructokinase deficiency
  Inclusion body myositis
  Immune-mediated necrotizing myopathy

▶ TABLE 1-13. NEUROMUSCULAR DISORDERS ASSOCIATED WITH VENTILATORY MUSCLE WEAKNESS

Anterior horn cell
  Motor neuron disease/amyotrophic lateral sclerosis
  Poliomyelitis including West Nile virus

Nerve
  Bilateral phrenic neuropathies (brachial plexus neuritis)
  Critical illness neuropathy
  Guillain–Barré syndrome
  CIDP (consider POEMS)
  CMT (particularly CMT2C)
  Multifocal motor neuropathy with phrenic neuropathy (rare)
  Amyloidosis
  Porphyria
  Toxins (thallium, lead, arsenic, organophosphates, vincristine)

Neuromuscular junction
  Myasthenia gravis
  Congenital myasthenia
  Botulism
  Lambert–Eaton myasthenic syndrome
  Envenomations (reptile, insect, marine)
  Tick paralysis

Muscle
  Myotonic muscular dystrophy
  Dystrophinopathies
  Limb-girdle muscular dystrophy
  Emery–Dreifuss muscular dystrophy
  Pompe disease
  Phosphofructokinase deficiency (rare)
  Carnitine deficiency
  Myotubular myopathy
  Multiminicore disease with rigid spine (SEPN-1)
  Nemaline rod myopathy (Hereditary forms)
  Sporadic late-onset nemaline myopathy
  Congenital fiber-type disproportion
  Carnitine deficiency
  Mitochondrial myopathy (rare)
  Myofibrillar myopathy
  Inflammatory myositis including immune-mediated necrotizing myopathies
  Electrolyte disturbance (hypokalemia, hypophosphatemia)
  Critical illness myopathy

select group of neuromuscular disorders (Table 1-13). In this textbook, ventilation will refer to the mechanical act of air exchange from atmosphere to alveoli as opposed to respiration, the act of gas exchange between alveoli and the circulation. Dyspnea on exertion is the typical symptom of hypoventilation but may not become evident in this population due to the limited ability of patients to exert themselves. Diaphragmatic weakness is more symptomatic in the supine position leading to orthopnea. Symptomatic hypoventilation in neuromuscular disorders often presents in a protean fashion with nonspecific, frequently nocturnal symptoms, the significance of which can be easily overlooked. The nocturnal predilection may be multifactorial. In addition to orthopnea from diaphragmatic weakness, the supine position also places more of the surface area of the chest wall against surfaces that add further resistance to chest wall expansion. Weakness of pharyngeal musculature may diminish the support of the upper airway, further compromising the upper airway integrity during inspiration. As a result, sleep-disordered breathing is common in neuromuscular disorders. Patients who are dependent on accessory muscles, paralyzed during REM sleep, will experience further compromise of ventilation during this stage of sleep. Resulting nocturnal hypercarbia may interrupt normal sleep cycling and promote nocturnal restlessness and diurnal fatigue. Early morning headache and confusion due to carbon dioxide retention are usually late symptoms that clearly warrant the provision of positive pressure airway support.

With the sensory history, there is great value in allowing the patient to identify the topographic area of involvement which is frequently more accurately identified by the patient than by the examining physician. For example, paresthesia confined to one or two contiguous digits would, in the vast majority of cases, indicate a disorder of the neuromuscular system that may be difficult to corroborate even by a detailed sensory examination conducted by an experienced physician. With the sensory history, it is also important to identify any associated loss of function, for example, loss of balance or ability to identify a coin in a pocket due to proprioceptive loss.

Disorders that affect sensory neurons may lead to a variety of perceived sensations that may in part be related to the size of the sensory axons affected and the duration of the illness. Paresthesia (a positive or abnormal spontaneous sensation) may be described as tingling, prickly, burning, shooting, or electrical sensations, often with an unpleasant or painful characteristic. The latter three sensations are thought to indicate preferential involvement of small unmyelinated sensory nerve endings. Other abnormal, although probably less specific perceptions, include coldness as well as itching. If large myelinated sensory fibers are affected, the patient may describe a band-like, wrapped, swollen, "shrink-wrapped," "pad-like," or wooden sensation. They may feel as though they have cotton stuffed between their toes or that their body parts are encased in plastic, dried glue, or that their skin is foreign to them. Pain associated with large-diameter nerve fibers is often deep, dull, and aching in characteristic.

Numbness can be conceptualized as a loss of sensation, that is, a negative sensory symptom. It is often a sign in that it may not be recognized by the patient until the affected body region is touched. It is largely held that unrecognized loss of sensation unaccompanied by paresthesia is indicative of a very chronic, slowly progressive process. As an example, unrecognized sensory loss without paresthesia is one of the characteristic features of Charcot–Marie–Tooth disease.

As with the motor history, it is important to explore the functional consequences of sensory loss although these may be less specific. In the authors' experience, the complaint of "dropping things" from the hands has poor discriminating value in the separation of definable from nondefinable neurologic disease. Conversely, impaired balance from large fiber sensory loss, that is, sensory ataxia, is an important symptom associated with significant morbidity. Inquiries should be made regarding nocturnal balance, the use of a night-light, and balance in the shower while hair washing.

Impaired autonomic system function occurs in certain causes of peripheral neuropathy as well as in presynaptic disorders of neuromuscular transmission. Identification of dysautonomia may aid greatly in focusing the differential diagnosis. Common symptoms include orthostatic intolerance with faintness and nuchal discomfort, constipation, diarrhea, or early satiety, urinary retention, incontinence, erectile dysfunction, sweating abnormalities including dry cracked feet, blurred vision, dry eyes, or dry mouth.

Perception of pain is dependent on nerve transmission but typically originates from injury to other tissues. Pain caused by direct nerve injury or dysfunction is referred to as neuropathic pain. Neuropathic pain is recognized by its characteristics or by its association with objective evidence of relevant nerve injury. It is often linear in its orientation and often, but not always, has burning, lancinating, deep boring, or electrical characteristics. Allodynia, or cutaneous pain triggered by a normally innocuous stimulus, for example, the touch of bedclothes may occur in patterns not typically recognized as typical nerve or nerve root distributions. The truncal neuropathy of diabetes is a notable example of this. Muscle pain is also a common complaint brought to the attention of the neuromuscular clinician. Along similar lines, myalgia without a definable trigger, associated weakness, or some other objective finding is unlikely to be of neuromuscular causation. As mentioned previously, pain commonly occurs as a consequence of neuromuscular disease, frequently mechanical in nature and related to imbalanced forces on joints and other connective tissues promoted by muscle weakness or impaired sensation.

Many neuromuscular disorders are the result of or are influenced by single gene or complex genetic mutations. Many of these patients will not recognize the hereditary nature of their disease. This may be due to a recessive inheritance pattern, spontaneous mutation, false paternity, or incomplete or delayed penetrance. Frequently, it is due to a lack of familiarity with the medical issues of other family members. In suspected hereditary disease, acquisition of family history, particularly if done in a cursory fashion, may be insufficient. Examination of other family members, even if only briefly, is strongly recommended when heritable diseases are considered.

THE EXAMINATION

Time constraints are a medical reality. Examining clothed patients represents an understandable but unfortunate response to this inconvenience. In neuromuscular medicine, this shortcut is not a viable option. As emphasized later in this section, there are numerous observations that can be made only by direct observation of exposed body parts that provide clues integral to accurate diagnosis.

The strategy of the neuromuscular examination is to identify patterns of weakness and sensory loss and correlate them with typical patterns of specific disorders. In certain cases, such as multifocal neuropathy, the patterns are more readily identifiable early in the disease, whereas in others, for example, ALS, some degree of disease evolution may be required for the diagnosis to become apparent. Either by history or examination but ideally by both, involvement of motor, sensory, and/or autonomic systems should be sought. Recognized patterns such as distal symmetric (length-dependent), proximal symmetric, UMN, single or multiple peripheral nerve patterns, and single or multiple nerve root patterns should be sought for and ideally recognized. In an analogous manner, sensory loss should be characterized as small fiber, large fiber, or both. When possible, the recognition of length-dependent, multifocal, single nerve and single nerve root distribution of sensory signs and symptoms will provide an invaluable diagnostic clue.

The motor examination of cranial nerves begins with observation. In childhood spinal muscular atrophy, the upper lip may have a tented configuration. Several myopathies are associated with "myopathic facies" in which there is a transverse smile with little or no elevation of the corners of the mouth. With severe weakness of muscles of mastication, the jaw may be slack and hang open. Patients with facial weakness affecting the orbicularis oculi may have ptosis of the lower lid resulting in visible sclera between the lower limbus of the cornea and the margin of the lower eyelid. These same patients may be observed not to oppose their eyelids completely while blinking. More subtle facial weakness may be noticeable when the eyelids are not completely "buried" when the patient is asked to squeeze their eyes shut as hard as they can.

Atrophy in muscles innervated by cranial nerves may be evident in the temporalis, sternocleidomastoid, and particularly in the tongue. The former two are common features of myotonic muscular dystrophy. Tongue atrophy can be seen in several neuromuscular disorders most notably the MNDs where it is usually bilateral. Unilateral tongue atrophy suggests a less common hypoglossal mononeuropathy. The presence of fasciculations of the face and tongue are key diagnostic features, particularly in the evaluation of bulbar syndromes, and should be actively sought for in suspected ALS and the spinal muscular atrophies. Their presence offers strong support for a neurogenic as opposed to myopathic cause of atrophy or weakness. As with any other muscle, it is important to examine the muscle in a relaxed rather than partially contracted state as muscle movement in the latter situation may be readily misinterpreted as fasciculations. It is also important to distinguish a generalized tremulousness of the tongue, which occurs frequently in normal patients from the random twitching of individual motor units that represent fasciculations.

Manual muscle testing in cranial innervated muscle is an integral part of the neuromuscular examination. Facial weakness can be assessed by attempting to pry the tightly closed eyes and/or lips apart. We grade facial weakness on a mild, moderate, and severe scale. Mild weakness means that the eyelids oppose and generate some but inadequate strength with an attempt to open them. Moderate weakness means that the eyelids oppose but offer minimal resistance whereas severe weakness means that the eyelids cannot completely oppose. With the lips, mild weakness is determined by the ability to blow up the cheeks with air but the inability to prevent air leakage when the cheeks are compressed. Moderate weakness is the ability to oppose the lips but not puff out the cheeks whereas severe weakness is the inability to oppose the lips.

Jaw strength can be tested by looking for lateral chin deviation upon opening or by trying to pry open the fully closed jaw by placing the fingers on the back of the neck and applying downward pressure on the chin with the thumbs. Attempting to assess jaw opening strength should be done with caution as inadvertent trauma to the teeth may occur if the jaw snaps shut forcefully.

Tongue strength is best tested by having the patient "pocket" each cheek with manual pressure being placed on the cheek and indirectly on the tongue attempting to force it back to the midline. Again, we use a mild, moderate, and severe scale. Mild weakness is a retained ability to pocket but an inability to resist pressure. Moderate weakness is the ability to pocket the cheek in a limited fashion with little or no resistance to pressure. Severe weakness refers to little or no tongue movement. Neck flexion and extension strength is tested in the customary isometric manner by having the patient resist full neck flexion and extension, respectively, with or without the use of a dynamometer.

Myotonia and paramyotonia of eyelid opening and closing, as well as in limb muscles, may be sought for in the appropriate context, particularly in suspected paramyotonia congenita and myotonia congenita. In assessing for eyelid myotonia or paramyotonia, the patient is asked to repetitively close their eyes tightly and open them quickly. With myotonia, the delay in opening is most apparent with the first attempt whereas in paramyotonia, it gets worse with subsequent efforts. The examiner can also ask the patient to look up for several seconds and then rapidly look back down to the primary position. If the eyelid does not return to the primary position as fast as the globe, myotonia of the eyelid elevators may be considered along with other causes of lid lag. Myotonia can also be sought for by percussing the tongue with the assistance of gauze and two tongue blades, but this is cumbersome procedure that probably adds little to the assessment of myotonia through grip or percussion of limb muscles. An additional eyelid sign of potential use in neuromuscular disease is the Cogan eyelid twitch. The patient is asked to look down, and then rapidly saccade to midposition. A positive result is identified by an overshoot of the upper lid followed by a few oscillatory movements of the upper lid until it settles back to its normal relationship with the globe.

Relevant to this is our belief that ptosis, proptosis, and to a certain extent facial weakness are best recognized by understanding the normal anatomic relationship between the eyelids and the globe. Typically, the lower margin of the upper lid covers the upper 2–3 mm of the limbus whereas the upper margin of the lower lid typically intersects the lower limbus. The observation of sclera between the upper lid and the limbus indicates eyelid retraction or proptosis. The observation of sclera between the lower lid and the limbus represents orbicularis oculi weakness or proptosis. A narrowed palpebral fissure represents squinting, blepharospasm, atrophy, or retraction of the globe.

Observation of the eyebrow position is also helpful in the interpretation of abnormal eyelid positioning. If the lower margin of the upper lid is lower than it should be due to ptosis, the eyebrow is typically elevated in a compensatory attempt of the frontalis muscle to elevate it unless the frontalis is weak as well, for example, myasthenia. Conversely, if the upper lid position is lowered by squinting from blepharospasm, the eyebrow is usually lower than the opposite side if uninvolved. At the same time, the upper margin of the lower lid is typically elevated as well resulting in narrowing of the ocular aperture.

The pupils should be examined, preferably, at least initially, in a dimly lit room to assess for the possibility of Horner's syndrome. The lack of pupillary reactivity may represent an autonomic component of the patient's disorder. Perhaps, the greatest value of the pupil examination in neuromuscular disease is to distinguish neuromuscular disorders causing ophthalmoparesis that spare the autonomic nervous system and the pupil from those that do not. Myasthenia, most diabetic third nerve palsies, and myopathic causes of ophthalmoparesis fit into the former category. Ophthalmoparesis with pupillary involvement may occur in Guillain–Barré syndrome and its variants, presynaptic disorders of neuromuscular transmission such as botulism. Pupil involvement (mydriasis) may also occur from injury of parasympathetic fibers in third nerve palsies or from sympathetic injury (miosis) in their course anywhere between the first thoracic nerve root and the supraorbital fissure.

Examination of limb and trunk muscles also begins with observation. Again, it is our strongly held belief that although the patient should be gowned with appropriate undergarments, every part of the body should be available to direct observation. There are many potential clues that can be obtained in this manner. Muscle atrophy, focal or generalized, and muscle hypertrophy should be sought for. Viewing the shoulder girdles from the back may identify shoulder drop from trapezius weakness or overt scapular winging. Viewing the chest in males may disclose gynecomastia. Viewing the shoulder girdles from the front may disclose a crease in the pectoralis, an elevated scapula producing a pseudohypertrophic appearance of the trapezius, or a horizontally oriented clavicle, all resulting from weakness of periscapular muscles. In a similar vein, abnormal scapular positioning may affect the positioning of the arms which may be internally rotated so that back of the hand rather than the thumb is anteriorly oriented producing a simian posture. Arm movement during conversation, that is, gesticulation may identify diminished spontaneous movements of one or both upper extremities due to proximal weakness, limitation of joint movement, or CNS disease. Conversely, the physician may notice completely normal spontaneous movement under these conditions which is subsequently found to be incongruous with the patient's inability (or unwillingness) to use the limb properly during the examination, implicating decreased effort from pain, apraxia, or psychogenic etiology.

Muscles should be closely observed for adventitious movements such as tremor, fasciculations, myokymia, or rippling. In our experience, benign fasciculations tend to be felt by the patient more frequently than they are seen, are most commonly evident in the calves, and occur briefly and repetitively in a single spot before disappearing. Fasciculations that occur in multiple locations in multiple muscles simultaneously are more ominous and suggest excessive cholinesterase inhibitor effect, a nerve hyperexcitability disorder, or most commonly, a motor system disease. Postural tremor is not rare in neuromuscular disease and may be a notable feature of Charcot–Marie–Tooth disease, chronic inflammatory demyelination polyneuropathy, or spinal muscular atrophy. Muscle contractures (nonphysiologic) or other dysmorphic features may be noted either by observation or during passive movement of limbs. Contractures may be seen in a number of neuromuscular conditions as listed in Table 1-14 and may provide key diagnostic clues. Dysmorphic features such as long thin facies, high-arched palates, kyphoscoliosis, exaggerated lumbar lordosis, cavus foot deformities, and hammer toes are also key diagnostic clues. Cavus foot deformities are usually indicative of long-standing disorders dating to childhood and are frequent accompaniments of Charcot–Marie–Tooth disease,

▶ **TABLE 1-14. NEUROMUSCULAR DISORDERS ASSOCIATED WITH EARLY JOINT CONTRACTURES**

Anterior horn cell
  Arthrogryposis multiplex congenita
  SMA

Nerve
  CMT3

Neuromuscular junction
  Congenital myasthenia

Muscle
  Central core disease

Nemaline myopathy
  Congenital fiber type disproportion
  Bethlem myopathy
  Ullrich congenital muscular dystrophy
  Dystrophinopathy
  Emery–Dreifuss muscular dystrophy
  Juvenile dermatomyositis

distal forms of spinal muscular atrophy, hereditary spastic paraparesis, and Friedreich ataxia. There are many neuromuscular conditions with accompanying dermal or epidermal changes. These include the ecchymoses of Cushing disease, the angiokeratomas of Fabry disease, stigma of neurocutaneous diseases that may affect the neuromuscular system such as café-au-lait patches in neurofibromatosis, hyperpigmentation in adrenal insufficiency, the skin changes of POEMS syndrome, the skin and nail bed changes of dermatomyositis, Mee's lines in finger and toenails representing growth arrest in response to arsenic or lead intoxication among others.

The identification of scapular winging may require provocative posturing as well as observation. It is an important and easily overlooked diagnostic clue in the assessment of neuromuscular disease. Affected patients will be unable to raise their hand over their head effectively. Scapular winging may be evident by simply looking at the patient from the rear. It may be accentuated by several maneuvers depending on which muscles are weak. Scapular winging due to weakness of the serratus anterior results in the inferior medial angle of the scapula being elevated more off the ribcage and migrating further away from the midline than its superior medial counterpart. It can be accentuated by having the patient push against a wall or by putting downward pressure on the humerus when the arm is flexed at the shoulder. With scapular winging resulting from trapezius weakness, the entire medial border is elevated. Winging is accentuated by attempted external rotation or abduction of the arm at the shoulder against resistance. The dynamics of scapular winging resulting from the more diffuse myopathic and motor neuron disorders affecting multiple muscles are more complex.

Provocative muscle testing should also be performed when relevant. Percussion myotonia is most commonly tested in the extensor digitorum communis (EDC) and thenar eminence. In the former, the forearm is supported by the examiner in a pronated position, allowing the wrist and fingers to hang limply. The EDC is percussed just distal to the head of the radius. A normal response is no movement or a minimal brief flicker of digit extension. The presence of myotonia is suggested when one or more of the digits extends at the metacarpophalangeal joints and sustains this posture for a second or so. Percussion of the thenar eminence is performed in a similar manner with the wrist and forearm supported while the forearm is fully supinated. The thumb should be maintained limply in the same plane as the palm. Myotonia is identified when the thumb abducts notably in response to a brief percussive strike to the abductor pollicis brevis muscle. Grip myotonia is sought for by having the patient tightly grip an object, for example, the examiners index and middle finger for a few seconds, then rapidly release the grip. A slow and deliberate extension of the fingers indicates myotonia. Typical myotonia improves with repeated trials. Paradoxical myotonia worsens with repeated trials. Myoedema refers to a mounding of muscle in response to percussion of a muscle belly that represents an uncommon finding in some muscle diseases.

The foundation of the neuromuscular examination is the assessment for the presence and pattern of muscle weakness. Two strategies are typically employed: isometric manual muscle resistance and functional testing. Ideally, suspected weakness identified by the first method, for example, reduced resistance of foot dorsiflexors, would be confirmed by the latter, that is, the inability to walk on the heels. There is an art to manual muscle testing, which is undoubtedly improved upon by experience, particularly in the distinction of true weakness as opposed to that due to impaired effort. Muscles are typically tested in an isometric fashion that is a contracted position with the patient asked to resist the force applied by the examiner. For example, elbow flexors are tested with the patient's fist resting against their shoulder. The patient is held by the examiner in such a way that the muscle(s) tested are isolated to the extent possible. Again, in the case of the elbow flexors, the examiner would place the hand that delivers the force just proximal to the wrist to produce the greatest mechanical advantage, while at the same time removing wrist movement from consideration. The other hand, which serves to stabilize, is placed on the biceps just proximal to the elbow.

To obtain full patient effort, the patient must have confidence that the examiner will not harm them. The examiner should sustain full effort long enough to detect either true weakness with its smooth characteristics or "give way" weakness with its "ratchety" and inconsistent character. It is important, however, to relinquish effort before the full range of motion is exhausted to avoid injury. Along similar lines, great caution should be exercised to avoid pathologic fracture in any patient with cancer potentially metastatic to bone.

Mild degrees of weakness may easily go unrecognized by both patient and examiner alike. This is particularly true in strong muscles like the quadriceps and the gastrocnemius, or when the strength or effort of the examiner is limited. It is imperative that the examiner places themselves at the greatest mechanical advantage and makes an appropriate effort to avoid a false-negative result. For ideal examination of neck flexion, elbow flexion, knee extension, and trunk flexion, the patient should be tested in the supine position, where the patient must move against gravity and resistance. Testing a patient on their side is ideal for testing hip abduction and the prone position optimal for elbow, hip, and neck extension as well as knee flexion and foot plantarflexion.

It is in these same strong muscles where functional testing is particularly useful. For example, hip and knee extension strength can be assessed by the patient's ability to get up from a deep chair or their ability to perform a partial squat or hop on one leg. Foot plantar flexion strength can be assessed by having the patient elevate their heel while standing on one leg.

Once weakness is recognized, two characteristics are of paramount importance: its pattern and its severity. The primary importance of the pattern of weakness is in the formulation of the initial diagnosis. Pattern recognition as a diagnostic tool is addressed in Tables 1-5 to 1-8 and will be elaborated on repeatedly in this and subsequent chapters.

The importance of the degree of weakness may also contribute to the diagnosis, for example, demonstrating progression both within and between different muscle groups is a key in the diagnosis of ALS. In addition, and perhaps more importantly, establishing the degree of weakness is also key in establishing treatment responsiveness.

To this end, accurate quantitative measurements of strength are paramount. Historically, the Medical Research Council (MRC) scale has been used by most institutions for this purpose. This is a 0–5 scale, with 5 representing normal strength and 0 representing no discernible muscle movement. By definition, the MRC scale requires muscles to be examined against gravity. An MRC grade of 3 preserves ability to move the joint through a full range of motion against gravity but with negligible resistance to the examiner. An MRC grade of 2 represents movement through a complete range of motion with gravity eliminated. An MRC grade of 1 represents observed muscle contraction with little or no limb or digit movement. With the MRC scale, most weak muscles will fall into the 4 (modest weakness) range. For this reason, the MRC scale has been modified to include a 4− and 4+ category to expand this largest group of weak muscles.

The MRC scale is problematic, as it may be insensitive, qualitative, and subjective. The potential exists for considerable interexaminer variability. It has been documented that patients lose 80% or more of their motor units in a given muscle before they receive a 3 or less MRC rating. In the opinion of the authors, it is a poor tool to measure motor deficits in UMN disease where functional impairment may be more on the basis of altered coordination and tone rather than loss of strength. In some clinical trials and to some extent in clinical practice, tools such as hand-held dynamometry are used in an attempt to measure strength in a more objective, linear, and reproducible manner. As an example, in the experience of the authors, most men can generate 40 or more kilograms of force in the majority of upper extremity muscles. An MRC grade of 3 approximates a force of 10 kg, implying that a modified MRC grade between 4− and 4+ represents approximately 75% of the weakness spectrum in these muscle groups.

Ventilation can be assessed at the bedside by several techniques. There is value in asking the patient to generate a forceful sniff or cough. Use of accessory muscles should be noted as well as a tendency for the patient to interrupt sentences to catch their breath. Shallow breathing can be detected by auscultation. The vital capacity can be roughly estimated in the cooperative patients by having them inspire fully and then count out loud at the rate of 1 per second until that single breath is exhausted. That number multiplied by a hundred will estimate their vital capacity measured in cubic centimeters. There may be value as well in examining the patient in the supine position to assess for paradoxical abdominal movements (outward abdominal movement in response to inspiration) as an indicator of diaphragmatic weakness.

UMN signs in the cranial nerve distribution are limited in number and in specificity. An enhanced jaw jerk or gag reflex, the presence of a snout reflex, forced yawning, and a pseudobulbar affect are all accepted UMN signs. Reduction in the speed in which a patient can repetitively blink or wiggle their tongue back and forth, in the absence of weakness or mechanical restriction of the respective muscles probably represents CNS dysfunction but is unlikely to specify corticobulbar tract pathology. The same is likely true for synkinesis of two muscles innervated by different cranial nerves, for example, the inability to keep the jaw from moving side to side when the requested task is wiggling the tongue back and forth in the horizontal plane.

Impaired motor function of corticospinal tract origin may include weakness, particularly if acute in onset, but tends to be dominated by impaired coordination and function. Clumsiness disproportionate to the degree of weakness is a sensitive, albeit nonspecific indicator of UMN disease. UMN weakness may also be suspected based on the topographic pattern of involvement. A hemiparetic pattern, even in ALS (also known as the Mill's variant) is rarely LMN in nature. A paraparetic or quadriparetic pattern often occurs because of corticospinal involvement of the spinal cord but may just as easily occur in a neuromuscular disorder as well. UMN weakness when limited in distribution is often more distal than proximal, particularly in the upper extremity. Often, UMN weakness can be implicated when flexors are stronger than extensors in the upper limbs and the opposite in the lower extremities. For example, preferential weakness of hip flexion, knee flexion, and foot dorsiflexion in combination strongly suggests UMN disease. Impaired motor function of CNS origin can often be deduced by observation, that is, the reduced spontaneous use of a body part such as diminished gesturing of an arm during talking.

UMN disease is also implicated when deep tendon reflexes are exaggerated, particularly in a focal or asymmetric fashion, with or without the existence of pathologic reflexes or spastic tone. The detection of hyperactive deep tendon reflexes can be somewhat subjective. Sustained clonus is undoubtedly pathologic in all cases. Deep tendon reflexes that persist in a limb that is weak and atrophic, unsustained clonus, and reflex spread are all suggestive of UMN pathology but are probably not pathognomonic. Babinski signs are universally accepted as a marker of UMN pathology, but bilateral Hoffman's signs and absent abdominal reflexes need to be interpreted with some caution.

Like its motor counterpart, the results of the sensory examination are most credible when they are concordant with both the history and available functional tests of sensation. There are many sensory examination strategies. In the authors' experience, the application of sensory stimuli in a random fashion with subsequent attempts to identify the boundaries of the sensory loss is often difficult to interpret and may produce false-positive results. An alternative technique is a hypothesis-driven approach in which the examiner attempts to prove or disprove a specified pattern of sensory loss, for example, a length-dependent pattern in a patient with numb feet. As examiners can apply stimuli with different intensities inadvertently and as patients have different thresholds for what they consider reduced (or increased), it is important to perform sensory testing in a reproducible and as unbiased manner as is possible. For this reason, there is a benefit from testing with the patient's eyes closed and with the addition of random null stimuli. This is particularly true with vibration when patients commonly confuse the touch of the tuning fork with vibration as the sensation in question. Using the tip of the examiner's finger as a random substitute for the tuning fork is a means to ensure that the patient is responding positively to vibration and not simply to pressure.

There are a few important points to recognize in performing the sensory examination. As already emphasized, it is not uncommon to be unable to convincingly demonstrate sensory loss in a symptomatic region in a person with credible sensory complaints. Conversely and somewhat paradoxically, it is not uncommon to find patients in the setting of a partial nerve injury who claim to react to a stimulus in a hypersensitive manner in an area that they claim to be numb. Finally, it is important to realize that the topographical area where sensory symptoms are perceived, and sensory loss is found is often far smaller than published anatomical charts would suggest for any nerve or dermatomal distribution. As an example, patients with a C6 monoradiculopathy typically describe altered sensation in their thumb, not the entire length of the dermatome as depicted in dermatomal charts. Presumably, this is the result of the considerable overlap between contiguous nerve territories.

There are a limited number of functional sensory tests to corroborate the findings on the direct sensory examination. The best known of these is the Romberg test, which assesses proprioceptive (or less likely bilateral vestibular) dysfunction in the lower extremities arising from either the peripheral or the CNS. The finger–nose test, also done with the eyes closed, is an analogous test for proprioceptive loss in the upper extremities. Stereognosis testing can be helpful at times. Even with severe nerve injuries, absolute anesthesia is rare. Patients who claim to feel absolutely nothing in their hands yet can readily manipulate an object in that hand with their eyes closed are unlikely to have the degree of sensory loss that is claimed.

Common bedside screening tests of autonomic function include observation of pupillary responses as described above. The feet should be observed for the presence of dry, cracked skin suggesting the possibility of anhidrosis. Pulse variation in response to deep breathing is a test of parasympathetic function. Arguably, the most commonly performed and valuable bedside autonomic test is orthostatic blood pressure and pulse measurements. They should be done after a few minutes in the supine position. Both blood pressure and pulse should be measured immediately on standing (or sitting) and at 1-minute intervals for at least 3 minutes, depending on the index of suspicion and the result.

Examination of young children, particularly infants, can be a challenge. Infants can be placed in a prone position to observe if they can extend their head. An inability to do so suggests weakness of the neck extensor muscles. Most infants have considerable subcutaneous fat that makes muscle palpation quite difficult. Palpating neck extensor muscles is a good place to attempt this evaluation as little subcutaneous fat overlies this muscle group. Neck flexion strength can be assessed as the child is pulled by the arms from a supine to a sitting position. Crying during the examination allows the opportunity to assess the child's vocalization (e.g., presence of a weak cry) and fatigability to the physical examination. Muscle weakness in infants is usually manifested by an overall decrease in muscle tone and many children with profound weakness are characterized as "floppy." This terminology does not necessarily imply a neuromuscular disorder. In fact, most floppy infants result from a CNS problem. In view of prominent subcutaneous tissue, fasciculations may be visible only in the tongue. Observation of tremor is important as it may be a feature of spinal muscular atrophy and some hereditary neuropathies. It is important to examine the parents of floppy infants for the possibility of a neuromuscular disorder. This is particularly important in children suspected of having myotonic dystrophy when the myotonia characteristic of the condition may not be initially detectable. In addition, weakness can transiently develop in infants born to mothers with myasthenia gravis.

▶ WHAT IS THE NEUROMUSCULAR PROBLEM?

The following section will attempt to summarize the patterns of motor and sensory involvement that typify the diseases described in this text to facilitate the localization process. Further formulation of the differential diagnosis will require knowledge of the epidemiology, typical patterns of weakness, and time course of the disorders that are described in detail in subsequent chapters of this book.

MOTOR NEURON DISEASES

The hallmark of the MND, also known as anterior horn cell diseases or motor neuronopathies, is painless weakness and atrophy frequently accompanied by the positive symptoms of cramps and fasciculations. Although cramps and fasciculations may occur in apparent absence of disease, and can be seen with any peripheral nerve disorder, they are far more prevalent in disorders of the anterior horn. As mentioned above, benign fasciculations are commonly evanescent and confined to a singular area at any given time. Conversely, fasciculations seen in numerous locations on a continuous or near-continuous basis are almost always the result of a motor neuron disorder. The absence of fasciculations does not preclude a motor neuron localization, particularly where there is considerable subcutaneous tissue that may obscure their observation, infants and those with an elevated body mass index being the most notable examples. Sensory symptoms and sensory loss do not typically occur in MND except in Kennedy disease and facial-onset sensory and motor neuronopathy (FOSMN). Nonetheless, it may occasionally occur in ALS due to other unrelated problems.

Most motor neuron disorders are hereditary/degenerative in nature associated with a customary insidiously progressive course. The rate of progression varies both with and between different MND; ALS and spinal muscular atrophy type I having the most virulent courses. The pattern of weakness varies with the disorder. With ALS, onset is typically focal and asymmetric, for example, foot drop. Even early in the course, however, weakness can be recognized as being multisegmental and outside of a single nerve or nerve root distribution. Poliomyelitis and other neurotropic viruses may present focally as well with marked asymmetry or with a more generalized presentation. The spinal muscular atrophies tend to have a symmetric presentation that is generalized or proximally predominant in both the X-linked bulbospinal (Kennedy disease) and infantile forms. The more uncommon distal spinal muscular atrophies have a distal, symmetric pattern of weakness that may mimic neuropathies or distal myopathies. Juvenile segmental spinal muscular atrophy (Hirayama disease) presents focally in the distal aspect of first one and at times the other upper extremity.

The recognition of MND is also aided by the identification of functions that are spared. Most notably, patients with MND virtually never experience ptosis or ophthalmoparesis except in the rare cases of ALS that behave more like a multisystem disorder. Impaired bulbar function (i.e., speech and swallowing) is common in many MND. Facial and jaw weakness may occur but are typically less prominent than the weakness of the tongue and throat muscles. Deep tendon reflexes tend to be lost unless there is concomitant UMN involvement in ALS.

DORSAL ROOT GANGLIONOPATHIES

These disorders, also known as sensory neuronopathies, are characterized by non–length-dependent, multifocal sensory signs and symptoms. Like many nerve diseases, distal aspects of limbs tend to be more afflicted than proximal, thus potentially mimicking the far more common length-dependent polyneuropathy pattern. Careful history taking may be required to identify the non–length-dependent or asymmetric features. Both the resulting chronologic course and the presence or absence of pain is variable and in large part dependent on etiology. Electrodiagnosis is useful to demonstrate that sensory fibers alone are affected. In polyneuropathies, there is almost always some indication of motor involvement, even when not apparent clinically, particularly if fibrillation potentials within intrinsic foot muscles are sought for with needle electromyography. Sensory ataxia is a common manifestation of these disorders. Dorsal root ganglionopathies may be autoimmune, toxic, infectious, or at times hereditary in etiology.

MONORADICULOPATHIES

Monoradiculopathies are among the most common neurologic problems, typically caused by some manner of mechanical nerve root compression associated with degenerative spine and disc disease. Their phenotype is in turn dependent on the mechanism and acuity of nerve root compression. The prototypical symptom of an acute monoradiculopathy, usually related to disc herniation is pain, limited to one extremity, and following the course of the involved dermatome. The pain may not affect the entire dermatome simultaneously, for example, buttock and anterolateral leg pain sparing the thigh in an L5 radiculopathy. Contrary to common belief, the pain usually begins in the scapular and the buttock area rather than the neck or back. Sensory and motor deficits are not universal, but when present, should be confined to a single segment. Weakness should be confined to a single myotome but involve more than one peripheral nerve distribution. For example, in a C7 monoradiculopathy, both elbow extension (C7/radial) and wrist flexion (C7/median) are often involved. Conversely, weakness may not be detectable in all muscles innervated by that particular myotome. For example, demonstrating weakness only in the extensor hallucis longus is not uncommon in an L5 monoradiculopathy. A helpful caveat is the recognition that a given muscle is virtually never completely paralyzed from a single nerve root lesion as virtually all muscles are innervated by multiple segments. In a similar fashion, sensory symptoms and deficits virtually always involve a smaller region than is predicted from dermatomal maps due to overlap of territories from contiguous dermatomes. Again, patients with L5 radiculopathies may describe their numbness or paraesthesia as affecting only their big toe.

A deep tendon reflex may be diminished if appropriate to the involved root. The pain of an acute monoradiculopathy in the lower extremity may be reproduced by the straight-leg or reverse straight-leg raising signs or by lateral bending toward the affected extremity. In the cervical region, it may be reproduced by extending and laterally bending the head and neck toward the symptomatic side in an attempt to promote foraminal compression.

In chronic radiculopathies, pain may be intermittent and position/activity dependent such as in lumbar spinal stenosis or may be minimal or nonexistent. Chronic radiculopathies typically occur from some component of spondylotic spine disease resulting from bone spurs or hypertrophied ligaments. Multiple rather than single nerve roots are more commonly affected by this process and motor and sensory deficits may be less dramatic in their manifestations.

POLYRADICULOPATHY

The typical phenotype of polyradiculopathy is the sequential development of motor and sensory signs and symptoms involving more than one spinal segment in one or more extremities. These disorders are typically painful, and with certain etiologies, involve cranial nerves as well.

The etiologies are heterogeneous and often involve diseases with a predilection for cerebrospinal fluid, the meninges, or neural foramen. Nerve roots and cranial nerves are compromised as they pass through one or more sites on their journey from spinal cord to limbs, head, and trunk. The most common cause of polyradiculopathy is lumbosacral spinal stenosis typically presenting with back and lower extremity pain provoked by standing and walking. Diabetic radiculoplexopathy can be another common cause of what may be considered a polyradiculoneuropathy. This typically presents as an acute painful disorder preferentially affecting the L2–L4 innervated muscles in one leg. Some patients will have their other leg affected on a delayed basis. Other causes of polyradiculopathy are relatively uncommon and are typically related to inflammatory, infectious, or neoplastic disorders that produce a chronic meningitis. Cranial nerves, both motor and sensory, are commonly affected in these disorders.

PLEXOPATHY

A plexopathy is suspected when sensory and motor deficits are restricted to a single limb, the deficits being more widespread than can be explained on the basis of a single nerve or nerve root dysfunction. Pain is the rule rather than the exception, as the causes of plexopathy are most commonly traumatic, inflammatory, or neoplastic which either compress, infiltrate or inflame nerve. Occasionally, most notably with acute brachial plexus neuritis, or diabetic radiculoplexopathy, sensory signs and symptoms may be modest or nonexistent. The reasons for this may be multifactorial. Acute brachial plexus neuritis has a predilection affecting purely motor nerves, for example, the long thoracic or anterior interosseous nerves. In fact, it is this multifocal nerve pattern confined to one upper extremity or adjacent cranial or upper cervical nerves that often serves as a diagnostic clue. The motor predominant nature of acute brachial plexopathy may be related to a demyelinating pathophysiology that may preferentially affect motor function in a manner similar to the Guillain–Barré syndrome.

MONONEUROPATHY

Mononeuropathy syndromes are usually readily recognizable due to their frequency and relative homogeneity of presentation for a particular compression or entrapment syndrome. They most commonly result from the anatomic vulnerability to compression (external forces—e.g., Saturday night palsy) or entrapment (internal forces—e.g., carpal tunnel syndrome) of particular nerves at specific locations. The mode of presentation between different mononeuropathies is variable, in part due to the constituency of the nerve. For example, weakness will not occur in lesions affecting purely sensory nerves such as the lateral femoral cutaneous nerve. More commonly, the mode of presentation varies due to pathophysiology which may be primarily axonal or the result of differing mechanisms of demyelination. In the case of carpal tunnel syndrome and ulnar neuropathies at the elbow, sensory symptoms tend to initially predominate. Common peroneal or radial neuropathies at the spiral groove tend to have more of a motor predominance. Pain may or may not be an issue. Pain without motor, sensory, or reflex signs or symptoms is uncommonly due to a definable mononeuropathy despite descriptions of alleged mononeuropathy syndromes such as the piriformis and pronator syndromes.

In any event, signs and symptoms should be restricted to the distribution of a single peripheral nerve, distal to the site of nerve injury. The converse is not always true. For example, it may be very difficult to demonstrate weakness of ulnar forearm muscles, which are at risk from ulnar neuropathies at the elbow. This phenomenon has been attributed to selective fascicular involvement. As nerve fibers destined for the same muscle tend to sequester themselves in the same fascicle even in proximal locations, these fascicles may be relatively spared from a compression or entrapment process that may affect certain fascicles more than others. Alternatively, weakness of ulnar wrist flexion may be obscured by the preservation of median wrist flexion.

LENGTH-DEPENDENT POLYNEUROPATHY

Length-dependent polyneuropathy is one of the most common neuromuscular problems encountered both by neurologists and other physicians. Long, narrow axons are presumably vulnerable to disruption of the axonal transport mechanisms on which axonal viability and function is dependent. There are more than 200 recognized etiologies for length-dependent polyneuropathy. Despite a common initial phenotype that usually begins with symmetric motor and/or sensory involvement of the toes and feet, there is considerable heterogeneity in clinical evolution. Conceptually, most of these disorders result from toxic, metabolic, or hereditary disturbances of cell body metabolism or myelin growth resulting in impaired axon transport or disrupted nerve impulse transmission. This provides a cogent explanation for preferential involvement of most distal aspects of the longest nerves in the body affected in a symmetric, "length-dependent" fashion. Usually, sensory, motor, and reflex functions are all impaired in this length-dependent pattern although sensory signs and symptoms typically predominate. The best explanation for this phenomenon is that sensory nerve endings of the feet have no backup system. Denervation of intrinsic foot muscles that flex and extend the toes, however, is clinically masked by leg muscles providing the same function. The inability to spread the toes provides a nonspecific but sensitive means of clinically suspecting motor involvement in length-dependent neuropathies.

Identifying fibrillation potentials or low-amplitude compound muscle action potentials in intrinsic foot muscles may be the only reliable way to detect early motor involvement in many length-dependent polyneuropathies. Again, it is important to plot the evolution of sensory symptoms to ensure that they are not asymmetric or non–length dependent in pattern suggesting a different anatomic localization such as multifocal neuropathy, polyradiculopathy, or sensory neuronopathy.

SMALL FIBER SENSORY NEUROPATHY/NEURONOPATHY

Most patients recognized as having small fiber neuropathies present with insidious, slowly progressive burning pain and paresthesia in a length-dependent fashion beginning in the toes and feet. Most are idiopathic in nature, but maybe associated with diabetes, amyloidosis, Sjögren syndrome, and hereditary sensory and autonomic neuropathy. A suspected but unproven relationship between small fiber neuropathy and impaired glucose tolerance absent overt diabetes remains. Additionally, some individuals present with symptoms suggestive of a small fiber neuropathy that are not length dependent. These are felt to be more likely autoimmune in nature. Affected individuals often describe numbness, tingling, burning pain, or an itching discomfort in the face, trunk, or arms before or more severe than in the distal lower extremities. Neurologic examination discloses normal muscle strength and a non–length-dependent sensory loss for pain or temperature. Proprioception, vibratory perception, and reflexes are normal.

POLYRADICULONEUROPATHY

Polyradiculoneuropathy refers to a disorder that affects multiple nerves both at the nerve and nerve root level. The most commonly encountered polyradiculoneuropathies are acquired, inflammatory, and demyelinating in nature, for example, the Guillain–Barré syndrome and chronic inflammatory demyelinating polyneuropathy (CIDP). Uncommonly, this pattern may occur as an axon loss process secondary to a disorder such as acute intermittent porphyria or Lyme disease.

Polyradiculoneuropathies are usually readily distinguished from length-dependent polyneuropathy. They tend to be motor rather than sensory predominant. The pattern of involvement is typically symmetric but is usually more generalized and non–length dependent. There may be cranial nerve involvement, which would be an extremely rare occurrence in most causes of length-dependent polyneuropathy. Reflex loss is typically generalized rather than length dependent. This is a consequence of the predominantly demyelinating pathophysiology that commonly dominates this phenotype. This results in differential slowing in different fibers within the same nerve. In turn, desynchronization of impulse transmission occurs, rendering functions particularly dependent on synchronous impulse transmission such as deep tendon reflexes and vibration perception impaired.

▶ MULTIFOCAL NEUROPATHY

Multifocal neuropathy has been historically referred to as mononeuritis multiplex or multiple mononeuropathies. It is not a universally accepted term but will be the preferred term in this chapter for the following reasons. Multiple mononeuropathy is an equally accurate descriptor but may imply to some a more benign multifocal compressive syndrome in contrast to many causes of multifocal neuropathy which tend to be systemic in nature. Mononeuritis multiplex is a frequently used designation but is unsatisfactory to us in that it implies an inflammatory pathology that may not exist or may go unproven. For this reason, we have chosen to avoid it.

The deficits of multifocal neuropathy are often abrupt and painful, particularly when ischemically mediated, occurring haphazardly (although usually distally) and asymmetrically. Weakness and sensory loss can be mapped to individual peripheral nerve distributions in more than one extremity. As described above, clinical recognition may depend on examination of the patient early in the disease, or obtaining an accurate history of early disease evolution, prior to the inevitable confluence of deficits. Multifocal neuropathy is often the result of disorders that infiltrate (sarcoidosis, lymphoma, amyloidosis) or infarct (vasculitis, diabetes) nerve or provide susceptibility to compressive and/or demyelinating nerve injury (multifocal motor neuropathy, multifocal acquired demyelinating sensory and motor neuropathy, hereditary liability to pressure palsy).

▶ NEUROMUSCULAR TRANSMISSION DISORDERS

These disorders are difficult to lump together from a clinical perspective, as there is phenotypic variability. Like MND and myopathy, the signs and symptoms are attributable exclusively to the motor domain. As the neuromuscular junction is a more physiologically dynamic structure than nerve or muscle, fluctuations in strength and stamina are hallmarks of these disorders. In acquired disorders of neuromuscular transmission, muscle atrophy is notable for its absence.

In postsynaptic disorders of neuromuscular transmission like myasthenia, for reasons not clearly understood, there is a predilection for cranial innervated musculature. Ptosis, diplopia, dysarthria, dysphagia, and chewing difficulties are common complaints. The deficits can be quite asymmetric and at times remarkably focal. Rarely, myasthenia may present with limb weakness with little, if any, oculobulbar involvement. This can also be either symmetric in nature mimicking a myopathy or focal such as a finger or foot drop, thus potentially mimicking an MND. Postsynaptic disorders of neuromuscular transmission do not affect the cholinergic receptors of the autonomic nervous system. Pupils should be spared even with complete ophthalmoparesis. Deep tendon reflexes are commonly spared in myasthenia gravis unless involved muscles are significantly weak.

Signs and symptoms of cholinergic dysautonomia are commonplace in presynaptic disorders of neuromuscular transmission such as botulism and the Lambert–Eaton myasthenic syndrome. Weakness in these two disorders tends to be symmetric and is often proximally predominant and generalized. Cranial nerve involvement is very common in botulism. It does occur in the Lambert–Eaton myasthenic syndrome, although not as prominently as in botulism or myasthenia gravis. Deep tendon reflexes are commonly lost in a generalized pattern in any presynaptic disorder of neuromuscular transmission. Presynaptic disorders of neuromuscular transmission should be strongly suspected, however, when reflexes are briefly restored after exercise as a manifestation of posttetanic facilitation. If a presynaptic disorder is suspected from the history, eliciting deep tendon reflexes both prior to and following manual muscle testing is a potentially revealing strategy.

▶ MYOPATHIES

Myopathy is suspected in three different clinical settings: (1) fixed, typically painless, and symmetric weakness, (2) periodic weakness due to disorders of ion channels, and (3) exercise-induced muscle pain, fatigue, stiffness, and myoglobinuria due to disorders of muscle energy metabolism. With fixed weakness, symmetry is a relative term. Minor asymmetries are common in disorders such as facioscapulohumeral muscular dystrophy and inclusion body myositis (IBM). The distribution of weakness is often proximal, but there are many notable exceptions. Myopathies presenting with symmetric, distally predominant weakness are not rare. These usually begin in the lower extremities but may begin in the hands as well. Myopathies, particularly those of a hereditary nature (e.g., facioscapulohumeral or oculopharyngeal dystrophy) and IBM, may also be recognized by regional patterns of weakness. Weakness in neck flexors and extensors should be sought in all neuromuscular disease but are particularly common in myopathy in addition to disorders of neuromuscular transmission and anterior horn cells. Cranial muscle involvement is variable. Dysphagia, ptosis, ophthalmoparesis, facial, jaw, and tongue weakness may occur and aid in the differential diagnosis of myopathic disorders. Reflexes may be lost or preserved, depending on the pattern and severity of muscle involvement.

Attention to other elements of the examination may aid in the identification of the existence, type, and potential complications of muscle disease. Percussion, grip, or electrical myotonia will serve to identify a select group of myopathies (see Chapter 2). Several myopathies may be associated with joint contractures or skeletal abnormalities.

Muscle hypertrophy is a constant feature of the dystrophinopathies and may occur with certain limb-girdle dystrophy phenotypes as well as infiltrative disorders of muscle such as amyloid myopathy. Involvement of ventilatory and cardiac muscle as well as other organ systems may aid in diagnosis and allow anticipation of future morbidity (Table 1-13).

RHABDOMYOLYSIS/MYOGLOBINURIA

The clinical phenotypes related to ion channel disorders and metabolic muscle diseases, like the majority of myopathies, typically present as fixed weakness. At times, however, these myopathies may express themselves as rhabdomyolysis and myoglobinuria (RHB/MGU). RHB/MGU, although conceptually different, are terms that are often used interchangeably. In this book, they will be discussed as a singular clinical and laboratory entity. They are addressed here in order to provide an overview and strategic approach to the problem.

Rhabdomyolysis refers to an acute, large-scale breakdown of striated muscle fibers whereas myoglobinuria implicates the urinary excretion of the pigment myoglobin released into the bloodstream as a consequence. Attempts have been made to define these terms quantitatively. Myoglobin is visible in the urine when its concentration exceeds 100 μg/dL or when plasma levels exceed 1.5 mg/dL but is an insensitive means to detect small or chronic CK elevations and usually becomes undetectable within hours, long before serum CK normalizes. Rhabdomyolysis has been defined by serum CK levels exceeding five times the upper limits of normal. As there are many patients with chronic CK levels in excess of this, often asymptomatically, this quantitative definition fails to conceptually capture the acute and potentially catastrophic nature of the RHB/MGU syndrome. Those experiencing the RHB/MGU syndrome typically have serum CK levels in tens of thousands.

There are numerous potential causes of RHB/MGU. Episodes are typically monophasic and result from toxic, traumatic, or infectious insults (Table 1-15). In addition, several heritable metabolic myopathies pose a risk for recurrent episodes. There is some evidence that there may be genetic susceptibility underlying some individuals who experience RHB/MGU in apparent response to an environmental provocation. Unfortunately, many cases remained undiagnosed despite intensive evaluation.

The symptoms of RHB/MGU are often nonspecific. There is often a nonspecific fever and malaise, usually accompanied by the more specific myalgias, muscle swelling, tenderness, and a generalized sense of weakness (asthenia). In the author's experience, it can be difficult to discern the cause of diminished patient movement. Both muscle pain and actual weakness may play a role, the former seemingly being the primary mechanism in most cases. The release of myofiber contents into the bloodstream can lead to nausea and vomiting, cardiac arrhythmia (hyperkalemia), and even CNS side effects such as confusion and coma.

▶ **TABLE 1-15. CAUSES OF RHABDOMYOLYSIS/MYOGLOBINURIA**

Toxic
  Envenomation—specific species of snake, bees, spiders
  Ingestion—(1) animals who have ingested toxins—e.g., Haff disease (fish), quail that have eaten hemlock, (2) certain mushroom species
  Recreational drugs—cocaine, heroin, alcohol, amphetamines, LSD, loxapine, hemlock, mercuric chloride, phencyclidine, strychnine, terbutaline
  Environmental exposure—monensin, chlorophenoxy herbicides, toluene, pentaborane
  Medications—cholesterol-lowering agents (statins), amiodarone, emetine, epsilon amino caproic acid, isoniazid, lamotrigine, pentamidine, propofol, proton pump inhibitors, valproate, zidovudine, neuroleptic malignant syndrome, checkpoint inhibitors

Metabolic
  Hypokalemia
  Hyperthermia
  Hyperosmolality (hyperglycemia)
  Hypophosphatemia

Infectious
  Bacteria (tetanus, salmonella, Legionella, group A beta-hemolytic strep)
  Virus (influenza, EBV, CMV, HIV, coronaviruses)
  Parasites (malaria)
  Rickettsial

Ischemic—acute peripheral arterial occlusion

Traumatic
  Crush injury
  Compartment syndrome

Miscellaneous
  Status epilepticus
  Delirium tremens
  High voltage electrical shock
  Excessive exercise in the deconditioned

Heritable
  Mitochondrial (many forms)
  Glycogen storage disease—myophosphorylase, phosphofructokinase, phosphoglycerate mutase and kinase, LDH deficiency, phosphorylase B kinase deficiency
  Lipid storage disease—carnitine palmitoyl transferase deficiency, carnitine translocase, acyl-CoA dehydrogenase deficiency
  Channelopathies—malignant hyperthermia types I–VI, hypokalemic periodic paralysis
  Congenital myopathies—King–Denborough syndrome, central core disease
  Muscular dystrophy—dysferlinopathy, anoctaminopathy, dystrophinopathy, and other LGMDs (much less common)

Autoimmune—dermatomyositis, immune mediated necrotizing myopathy (rare)

Rhabdomyolysis, if severe enough, can lead to enough movement of fluid into muscle to cause intravascular volume depletion and hypotension. Rhabdomyolysis can trigger the coagulation cascade and lead to disseminated intravascular coagulation. The most notorious complication is the development of acute tubular necrosis secondary accumulation of myoglobin with formation of cases within renal tubules. Ventilatory failure due to involvement of diaphragm and chest wall muscles is a rare complication of rhabdomyolysis.

The pathophysiology of RHB/MGU is not fully understood. The intracellular migration of sodium and water may lead to a secondary exchange of intracellular sodium with extracellular calcium in muscle fibers that remain viable. This in turn may lead to persistent activation of the myofiber contractile apparatus that may perpetuate muscle injury. The need to pump sodium out of cells may deplete ATP as an additional adverse effect of this cascade. Furthermore, injury may occur as a consequence of the ischemia created by increased compartmental pressure, even in the absence of crush injury, by the fluid migration described above. The biochemical milieu created by muscle breakdown may in itself be toxic either through the release of the normally sequestered contents of the muscle fibers, from calcium-dependent proteases and phospholipases, or from the cytokines release by the customary inflammatory response to injury.

Recognition of RHB/MGU may or may not be obvious. A high index of suspicion should be maintained with predisposing conditions such as crush injury, prolonged immobilization, or introduction of potentially myotoxic drugs. Myoglobinuria and acute, diffuse myalgias are obvious clues but are not always readily evident, particularly when detailed history is not readily available. Patients typically have leukocytosis. The measurement of serum CK is the most efficient and direct diagnostic tool. A positive urine dipstick for (which detects both myoglobin and hemoglobin) in the absence of red blood cells on microscopic examination of the urine strongly suggests myoglobinuria.

Diagnosis of the underlying cause may also be obvious or remain enigmatic despite extensive evaluation. In most series, drugs and metabolic disturbances are the most common identified cause of RHB/MGU. It is estimated that approximately a third to a half of patients who do not have an obvious cause of their RHB/MGU, will be found to have an identifiable enzymatic deficiency or underlying muscle disease as a cause of their syndrome. The yield is higher in patients who have had recurrent episodes.

In RHB/MGU, CK levels typically peak in 12–24 hours and remain at peak levels for a few days. In response to minor muscle injury such as EMG examinations, CK levels typically normalize in a week. In more protracted causes of muscle injury such as infection or with very high CK elevations, it would be prudent to wait a few weeks to determine if CK has normalized. Once the CK peaks, it can be anticipated that it will drop by 50% every 48 hours. This is a potentially valuable diagnostic tool as normalization of CK should suggest a monophasic cause of RHB/MGU or carnitine palmitoyl transferase deficiency. Persistent elevations, although not universally found, would be more in keeping with glycogen storage disease or other pre-existing and persistent myopathic disorders.

The forearm exercise test is a valuable screening tool for those glycogen storage disorders characterized by exercise-induced symptomatology and the potential for RHB/MGU. Its yield will be greatest in those individuals whose RHB/MGU is provoked by brief periods of intense exercise. Its yield will be less in individuals whose RHB/MGU appears to occur sporadically, on a delayed basis after more protracted exertion, or following fasting. In these circumstances, CPT deficiency will be the most common hereditary etiology. Forearm exercise testing will be described in detail in the section on glycogen storage disease. In summary, baseline determinations of venous lactate and ammonia were obtained. Forearm muscles are then repetitively and forcefully exercised, typically with a grip dynamometer. Using a blood pressure cuff to render the forearm ischemic is no longer done by most neuromuscular specialists as the risk of patient injury is felt to exceed any additional diagnostic yield. Serial measurements of venous lactate and ammonia are obtained from the ipsilateral basilic or cephalic veins in the antecubital fossa. In patients with glycogen storage disease, these measurements are often superfluous as the affected patient will develop a sustained painful "contracture" of the forearm muscles often leading to a dystonic posture with forearm pronation, wrist flexion with ulnar deviation, and finger flexion. A threefold elevation or more above baseline of either lactate or ammonia signifies adequate effort. With the glycogen storage disease associated with RHB/MGU, ammonia will elevate but lactate will not. Genetic testing is done to confirm the exact cause. In young adults experiencing RHB/MGU during or after protracted exercise, particularly if recurrent or with normalization of CK following the acute episode, we commonly obtain genetic testing for CPT deficiency and other disorders of fatty acid oxidation.

Muscle biopsy in the acute setting is to be avoided. Random myofiber necrosis in similar stages of degeneration, affecting both type I and type II fibers, without any specific diagnostic features is the anticipated outcome. Whether muscle biopsy should be performed subsequent to the RHB/MGU episode is a more difficult question to answer. The yield in identifying the exact cause of RHB/MGU is extremely low, and the cost of providing a comprehensive analysis of the muscle biopsy can be substantial. In our opinion, muscle biopsy in RHB/MGU should be reserved for those individuals with recurrent episodes of RHB/MGU of indeterminate cause with negative exercise forearm testing and genetic analysis for hereditary causes of myoglobinuria.

Hydration is the most important therapeutic intervention. Six to twelve liters of intravenous fluids in the first 24 hours are recommended in the absence of comorbidities. Urine output should ideally be in the 200–300 mL/h range. The fluid should not be hypotonic. Mannitol and sodium bicarbonate are frequently added although there is limited evidence to support their efficacy. Vigorous diuresis with furosemide represents a mainstay of treatment as well. A high index of suspicion for compartment syndrome should be maintained and fasciotomy considered when clinically appropriate. Hypokalemia, hypocalcemia, and hypophosphatemia should be screened for and treated if necessary. Awareness of adult respiratory distress syndrome, ischemic bowel, and the possibility of hemorrhage secondary to DIC should be maintained. Alkalinization should be utilized where appropriate.

▶ SUMMARY

Diagnostic accuracy is in large part dependent on a clinician's ability to elicit and formulate pertinent information from three domains of the patient's history and examination, these being anatomic localization, definition of the disease course, and relevant risk factors. The astute clinician will learn to discard information that is not germane to the patient's current problem and formulate a differential diagnosis by accurately matching the information from the three domains mentioned above to the known behaviors of different diseases. An accurate diagnosis may be evident solely from this clinical process or may require further testing to confirm or refute the differential diagnosis generated by this process. This chapter has addressed the strategies that serve as the foundation for this problem-solving approach. Subsequent chapters will discuss the features of the neuromuscular diseases in an attempt to complete this diagnostic and hopefully therapeutic endeavor.

FURTHER READING

Amato AA. Neuromuscular junction disorders. In: Fauci AS, Braunwald E, Kasper DJ, et al., eds. *Harrison's Principles of Internal Medicine*. McGraw Hill; 2022.

Amato AA, Barohn RJ. Peripheral neuropathies. In: Fauci AS, Braunwald E, Kasper DJ, et al., eds. *Harrison's Principles of Internal Medicine*. McGraw Hill; 2022.

Amato AA, Brown RJ. Muscular dystrophies and other muscle diseases. In: Fauci AS, Braunwald E, Kasper DJ, et al., eds. *Harrison's Principles of Internal Medicine*. McGraw Hill; 2021.

Amato AA, Hauser SL. Guillain-Barre syndrome and autoimmune neuropathies. In: Fauci AS, Braunwald E, Kasper DJ, et al., eds. *Harrison's Principles of Internal Medicine*. McGraw Hill; 2022.

Amato AA, Ropper AH. Sensory ganglionopathies. *New Eng J Med*. 2020;383:1657–1662.

Barohn RH, Amato AA. Pattern-recognition approach to neuropathy and neuronopathy. *Neurol Clin*. 2013;31:343.

Dumitru D, Amato AA, Swartz MJ, eds. *Electrodiagnostic Medicine*. 2nd ed. Hanley & Belfus; 2002.

Freeman R, Gewandter JS, Faber CG, et al. Idiopathic distal sensory polyneuropathy: ACTTION diagnostic criteria. *Neurology*. 2020;95(22):1005–1014.

Gemignani F, Bellanova MF, Saccani E, Pavesi G. Non-length-dependent small fiber neuropathy: not a matter of stockings and gloves. *Muscle Nerve.* 2022;65(1):10–28.

Hobson-Webb LD, Juel CV. Common entrapment neuropathies. *Continuum (Minneap Minn).* 2017;23:487–511.

Lamotte G, Sandroni P. A practical approach to peripheral autonomic neuropathies. *Curr Opin Neurol.* 2021;34:638–647.

Oaklander AL, Nolano M. Scientific advances in and clinical approaches to small-fiber polyneuropathy: a review. *JAMA Neurol.* 2019;76:1240–1251.

Pasnoor M, Dimachkie MM. Approach to muscle and neuromuscular junction disorders. *Continuum (Minneap Minn).* 2019;25(6):1536–1563.

Savarese M, Sarparanta J, Vihola A, et al. Panarama of the distal myopathies. *Acta Myol.* 2020;39(4):245–265.

Siao P, Kaku M. A clinician's approach to peripheral neuropathy. *Semin Neurol.* 2019;39(5):519–530.

Witting N, Andersen LK, Vissing J. Axial myopathy: an overlooked feature of muscle diseases. *Brain.* 2016;139(Pt 1):13–22.

CHAPTER 2

Testing in Neuromuscular Disease

The role of laboratory testing in the diagnosis of neuromuscular disease is described in the first chapter. Tests are ideally used to support a clinically established working diagnosis, not in a random search process. False-positive test results occur with some frequency and can easily lead to unnecessary testing and interventions as well as potential harm if not measured against pensive clinical analysis.

This chapter will focus on nonhistologic tests that are readily available to most clinicians and potentially useful to the neuromuscular physicians in their assessment of patients. There are many approaches and algorithms used to diagnose patients with different neuromuscular disorders.[1-17] In keeping with the philosophy of this text, emphasis will be placed on tests that have pragmatic application. The science behind the testing will be provided only to the extent necessary to understand the utility, performance, interpretation, and limitations of a test within a given clinical context. The following topics will be addressed:

- Electromyography (EMG) and nerve conduction studies (NCS), collectively known as electrodiagnosis (EDX)
- Quantitative sensory testing (QST)
- Autonomic nervous system testing (ANST)
- Routine laboratory (blood) testing
- Serologic testing
- Cerebrospinal fluid (CSF) analysis
- Genetic testing
- Nerve and muscle imaging

▶ EMG AND NCS (EDX)

BASIC PRINCIPLES

Physician Skill and Knowledge

Like all tests, EDX has limitations, as do the people who order, perform, and interpret them.[6-11] The most satisfactory results occur when the requesting physician understands the tests' value and limitations and posits specific questions to the electromyographer that the test can answer. A satisfactory result is also dependent on an electromyographer who examines the patient, understands the differential diagnosis of the clinical problem, and tailors the electrodiagnostic examination to adequately explore those possibilities. In keeping with this philosophy, it is readily understandable that the nerves tested during the NCS, and the muscles selected for EMG, although often guided by algorithm, are frequently modified on a case-by-case basis both prior to and during its performance.

Temperature Considerations

Attention to detail is important in EDX. One notable example is attention to limb temperature. As a rule, hand temperatures of >33°C and foot temperatures of >31°C are desirable. Although warm water baths and heating lamps may be used, in our experience, reusable microwaveable heating pads applied to the limbs are the most effective technique for obtaining and maintaining this thermal environment.

With cold limbs, the amplitudes of both compound motor action potentials (CMAPs) and sensory nerve action potentials (SNAPs) are increased. Abnormally low CMAP and SNAP amplitudes could be potentially normalized. Conversely, conduction speeds are reduced, including slowing of conduction velocities and prolongation of distal, F wave, and H reflex latencies (Fig. 2-1). Repetitive stimulation techniques are also affected by limb temperature. Limb cooling diminishes the degree of the decremental response in patients with disorders of neuromuscular transmission (DNMT). Failure to maintain adequate limb or facial temperature could readily lead to a false-negative result. Although it would be unusual for fibrillation potentials to disappear with limb cooling, their prevalence and therefore their detection may be hampered by cool body temperatures as well. Except for cold-induced myotonic discharges in paramyotonia congenita (PMC) and repetitive stimulation techniques in certain muscle channelopathies described below, the accuracy of EDX is improved upon by establishing and maintaining adequate limb warmth of at least 32°C.

Safety Considerations

Patients and their physicians are concerned about the potential EDX risks in patients who have pacemakers, defibrillators, central lines, and altered hemostasis. Although testing under these circumstances is not risk free, available published data suggests that the risk is limited if appropriate precautions are taken. Like most medical decisions, the potential benefits of EDX testing in a patient with any of these situations should be balanced against the risks.

The risk of performing NCS in patients with external wires leading to the heart is unknown but is considered a relative if not absolute contraindication. There is a paucity of information as well regarding the risk to patients with central

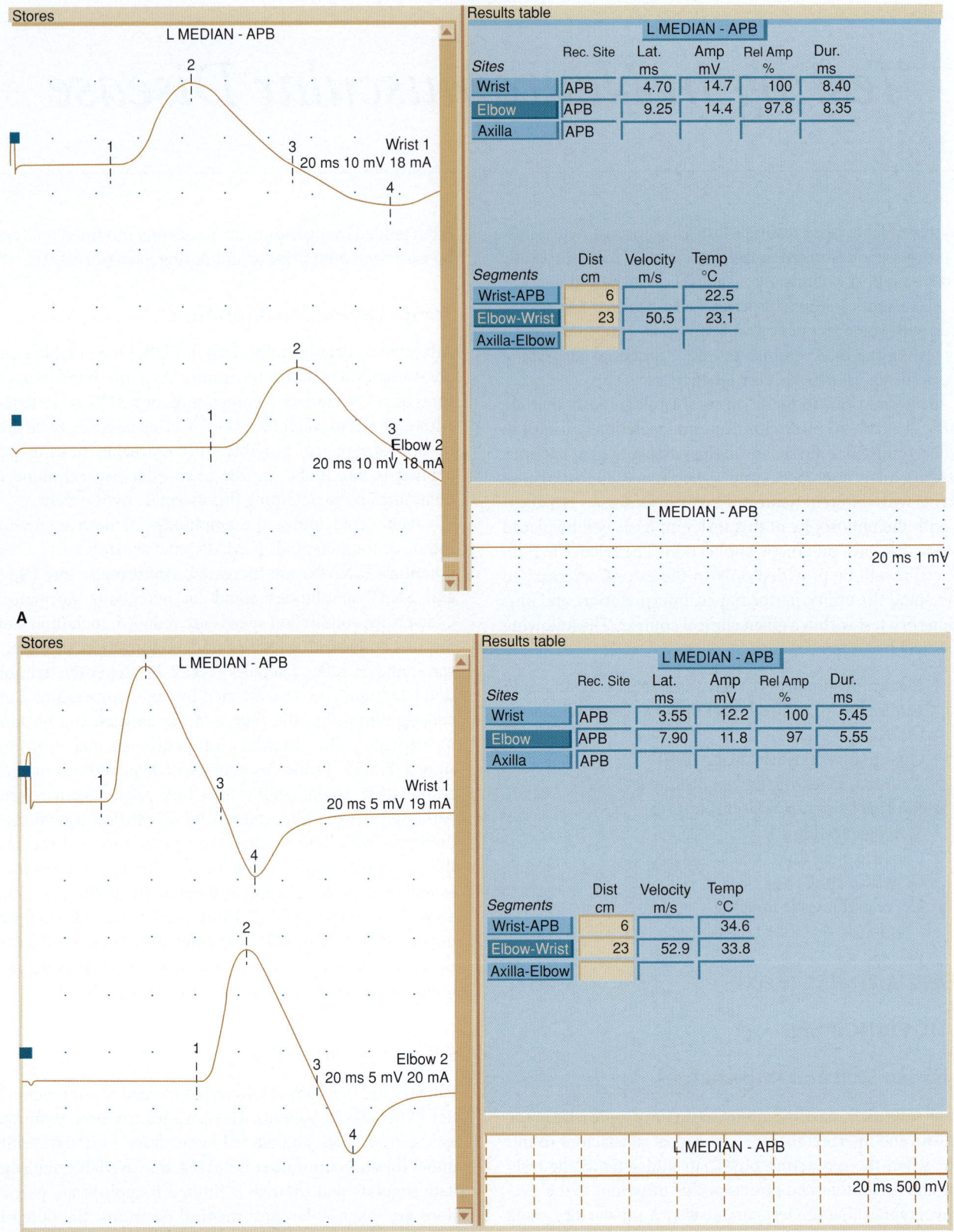

Figure 2-1. Effect of cool limb temperature on motor nerve conduction studies—median CMAPs (compound muscle action potentials) demonstrating factitiously significant increase in distal latency, slightly decreased conduction velocity, prolonged CMAP duration, and increased amplitude (note different gain settings) following cooling (**A**) and corrected by limb warming (**B**).

lines, pacemakers, and defibrillators. Both experience and theory suggest the risk is small and nerve conductions appear safe if the stimulus is not delivered in topographical proximity (within 6 cm) to the tubing or wire and a stimulation of 0.2 ms or less is used.[18–20] Even less is known about the safety of repetitive nerve stimulation (RNS) techniques in this setting. A study to address this issue is underway.

Regarding the needle examination and hemostasis, the risk of bleeding or hematoma formation in patients taking anticoagulants or antiplatelet drugs also appears small and is estimated to be approximately 1.5%.[21] When present, the risk of clinically significant bleeding also appears to be small. On the other hand, compartment syndrome has been reported in patients with normal hemostasis although its risk is generally considered minimal.[22] Available, albeit limited, evidence would support the performance of needle examination in patients who are therapeutically anticoagulated. Caution should be exercised when the international normalized ratio (INR) is supratherapeutic (i.e., >3), platelet count is less than 20,000, or in deep muscles where hematoma formation may not be readily evident or easily compressible. If needle examination is to be done, the smallest diameter that is feasible should be utilized. Needle EMG also poses the risk of pneumothorax, particularly when studying the serratus anterior and diaphragm.[20] These muscles should be studied by those well versed in anatomy, who are well experienced in the technique, and then only when clinical circumstances warrant. EMG poses a risk to electromyographers as well, largely in the form of the potential transmission of infectious agents through inadvertent needle sticks. The most common preventable reason for these accidents appears to be a hurried and harried examiner who is not adequately attentive.[23]

Test Construction and Reporting

Opinions differ regarding the role of clinical assessment in the construction and reporting of the EDX evaluation. Purists believe that EDX conclusions should be based solely on the results of the study and should not be influenced by clinical bias. The argument in support of this philosophy is the potential risk that meaningful EDX observations will be ignored if they do not conform to a pre-existing clinical belief. This potential bias is valid and should be considered and avoided by introspective electromyographers. Having said that, it is the strongly held belief of the authors that clinical perspective in the EDX evaluation is integral to the efficient construction and accurate interpretation of the study. There are several lines of reasoning to support this perspective.

For example, there are disorders that share identical electrodiagnostic signatures but have differing etiologies, natural histories, and treatment potentials. Early amyotrophic lateral sclerosis (ALS) affecting the lower extremities, polyradiculopathy of severe lumbosacral spinal stenosis, or a dural arteriovenous malformation may be electrodiagnostically indistinguishable.[24,25] The EDX conclusions, in this case, should be appropriately weighted by clinical insight. In addition, patients may have more than one disorder affecting the same components of the neuromuscular system. If this is the case, accurate EDX conclusions will be confounded without the clinical insights necessary to determine if abnormal EDX parameters are germane to the problem at hand. A third argument in support of coupling EDX impressions with clinical insight is the realization that in some cases, pathology may be subclinical. It is not uncommon to find mild median nerve conduction slowing across the wrist in individuals with a vocation that involves repetitive hand use whose complaints bear no resemblance to the clinical phenotype of carpal tunnel syndrome (CTS). Reporting based solely on EDX result risks unnecessary surgery in patients whose morbidity rests primarily on tendon or joint injury.

Normative Data

With the improvements and uniformity provided by contemporary electrodiagnostic equipment, it can be argued that it is no longer necessary for each laboratory to establish its own normative data. Assuming that attention is paid to accurate measurement, adequate temperature maintenance, and standardized distances for distal latency measurements, normative data are provided by several reliable published sources. It is important, however, to recognize the potential pitfalls of population-based "normal" values. Normative data are influenced by age. EDX in infants must be interpreted by a completely different set of norms than are used in adults. By the same token, conduction studies must be more cautiously interpreted in the elderly, particularly lower extremity sensory conductions. Although sural and superficial peroneal SNAPs are elicitable in many older patients, they can be absent in otherwise normal patients 60 years of age and older. This may confound the distinction between two common problems in this age group, peripheral neuropathy and lumbosacral polyradiculopathy due to spinal stenosis, the distinction of which relies heavily on evaluation of SNAPs.

Another age-related finding is that larger motor unit potentials (MUPs) can be seen in seemingly normal elderly individuals, particularly in intrinsic hand and foot muscles. This has been attributed to reinnervation resulting from (1) the wear and tear of the process in intrinsic hand or foot muscles, (2) motor unit loss resulting as a normal component of aging, or (3) in response to remotely symptomatic or asymptomatic spondylosis of the lumbar or cervical spine.

There is considerable heterogeneity in normative values for NCS within healthy populations. Any parameter measured may be normal within population-based norms but may differ from the patient's frequently unknown baseline values. For this reason, focal or unilateral problems are best studied by comparing results with the analogous nerve of the opposite extremity rather than utilizing population norms. In most laboratories, a side-to-side amplitude difference of more than 50% is considered abnormal. Even this represents a potentially insensitive means to detect subtle nerve pathology.

Timing

Timing considerations in EDX are critical. In general, it is estimated that complete Wallerian degeneration requires 3–5 days to produce a noticeable decline in CMAP amplitudes, with the nadir occurring between days 7 and 9. Wallerian degeneration in sensory nerves lags slightly behind with amplitude loss becoming apparent between the fifth and seventh days. The SNAP amplitude reaches its lowest point in a monophasic nerve injury by the 10th or 11th day.[26] For this reason, an interval of 10 days to 2 weeks between injury and the performance of NCS is ideal in most instances. There is a risk of false interpretation if NCS are preformed prematurely.

This is particularly true with conduction block. In most circumstances, a significant CMAP amplitude above but not below a focal nerve lesion suggests a demyelinating conduction block. This conclusion would implicate a limited number of peripheral nerve disorders with the potential for full and relatively rapid recovery in many cases. If motor conductions are performed hyperacutely within the aforementioned 9-day window before Wallerian degeneration is complete, an axon loss lesion may be falsely interpreted as demyelinating conduction block resulting in erroneous differential diagnostic and prognostic considerations.

The interpretation of the needle portion of the EDX examination is also subject to timing considerations. Fibrillation potentials and positive waves occurring in a muscle at rest, the most sensitive indicator of ongoing denervation on EMG, may develop within days in muscles that are in close anatomic proximity to the site of nerve injury. Three weeks may be required, however, for these to develop within all muscles at risk. As many patients may be reluctant to undergo multiple examinations, the EDX should be ideally postponed for 3 weeks after disease onset in most circumstances.

There are at least two circumstances in which it may be preferable to perform EDX earlier than the normal 3-week recommendation. One of these occurs when there is the suspicion or knowledge of a pre-existing nerve injury. It may be important for either legal or medical reasons to identify pre-existing abnormalities before new ones develop. Performing two examinations, one as early as possible and then a second examination a month or more later, would be best suited to address this issue. A second scenario would be a suspected Guillain–Barré syndrome (GBS) where rapid EDX support for the diagnosis is desired. As in other neuromuscular disorders, it may require days or weeks for the complete EDX signature of GBS to fully develop. Nonetheless, the rapid evolution of NCS abnormalities, even if not diagnostic, in the absence of findings characteristic of other potential causes of acute generalized weakness, can be reassuring to the clinician and guide management decisions in the critical first week of the illness.

Additional Considerations

EMG is often performed in the evaluation of patients who may eventually undergo muscle biopsy. To avoid the potentially confounding variable of needle artifact, it is our practice to restrict the needle examination to one side of the body if muscle biopsy is a consideration. The most appropriate muscle on the opposite side is then recommended to the referring physician. Needle EMG can also elevate serum CK values and potentially introduce another confounding variable in the evaluation of the patient with neuromuscular disease. For this reason, blood should be ideally drawn prior to, immediately after, or greater than 72 hours after EMG performance.[27]

PERFORMANCE OF THE ELECTRODIAGNOSTIC EXAMINATION

The routine EMG/NCS examination traditionally consists of motor NCS, sensory NCS, and the needle electromyographic examination.[6–11] F waves and H reflexes are also commonly tested although in most cases provide complementary rather than novel information. As previously mentioned, nerves and muscles should be selected on a case-by-case basis. Initial selection is based on the diagnostic question posed, the clinical information available, and may be modified as the test unfolds. It is appropriate to emphasize that techniques used to detect DNMT such as RNS testing and single fiber EMG (SFEMG) are not part of the routine evaluation of all patients in most laboratories. Once again, the importance of clinical surveillance in test construction is emphasized.

NERVE CONDUCTION STUDIES

Motor Nerve Conductions

Motor nerve conductions are performed by applying an active surface recording electrode to the midportion of a muscle belly and stimulating the nerve innervating it at one or more locations. The active electrode position is chosen to overly the motor point, that is, the confluence of neuromuscular junctions. This allows for a biphasic waveform known as the compound muscle action potential (CMAP) with a well-defined takeoff point for accurate measure of latency, waveform amplitude, and area. In addition, a reference electrode is used, placed off the muscle belly and usually on the over the tendon or bone. The CMAP is obtained by stimulating the nerve in question at anatomically accessible points. To elicit the desired response, the intensity of the electrical stimuli applied to the nerve is increased until all involved axons and muscle fibers are activated and the maximal response is obtained. This is referred to as the supramaximal stimulus and is the desired effect in all routine motor and sensory conduction studies. Each nerve tested may be stimulated at one or more locations, limited only by anatomical accessibility and patient tolerance.

Readily testable motor nerves are the median, ulnar, radial, accessory, facial, tibial, and common peroneal. The phrenic, femoral, axillary, and musculocutaneous nerves can be tested, although in each case technical issues may make reliable and reproducible information more difficult to obtain. The CMAP waveform that is obtained represents the sum of all the individual single muscle fiber action potentials (SFMAPs) within that muscle activated by the nerve stimulus. Because different fibers within a nerve have different conduction velocities, the waveform is shaped like a dome rather than spiked in its configuration. The proximal or left-hand side of the waveform represents the action potentials of the fibers innervated by the fastest conducting axons. The trailing aspect of the dome represents the action potentials of the muscle fibers innervated by the slowest conducting motor axons (Fig. 2-1). As stimuli are delivered at increasing distances from the target muscle, that is, more proximal locations, the distance between the initial and terminal aspects of the CMAP waveform widens. This results in an increasing duration of the CMAP waveform without a reduction in the area under the curve, the number of activated nerve and muscle fibers being identical. This is the basis of the normal physiologic waveform dispersion described below.

Typically, three parameters are measured with an additional parameter assessed more subjectively. The baseline to peak amplitude and the area under the curve of the CMAP waveform are proportionate to the number of viable muscle fibers that are activated within the recording radius of the active recording electrode. These parameters represent an indirect measure of the number of viable and excitable axons that innervate them. Reduction in CMAP amplitude results from axon loss anywhere between anterior horn cell and neuromuscular junction, impaired neuromuscular transmission (particularly presynaptic), or of loss of muscle. In some instances, the CMAP amplitude may be adversely affected by diseases that preferentially affect the integrity of the myelin sheath producing conduction block or temporal dispersion. This will be described subsequently.

The other two parameters routinely measured are distal latency (time between stimulus delivery and lead edge of CMAP) and conduction velocity. These parameters are measures of conduction speed and therefore primarily reflect myelin integrity. Conduction velocity and distal latency are reported separately in motor conduction studies for several reasons. The distal latency reflects conduction along different segments of nerve (wrist to hand or ankle to foot) than the conduction velocity (elbow to wrist or knee to ankle). In certain pathologic conditions, one parameter may be abnormal whereas the other remains unaffected. Distal latency and conduction velocity are also reported differently for purposes of technical accuracy. Distal latency measures not only nerve conduction but neuromuscular transmission time as well. In addition, terminal nerve twigs attenuate in diameter and have a conduction velocity that does not accurately reflect conduction speed in the more proximal nerve.

The last parameter to be assessed on a more subjective basis is CMAP appearance. Although morphologic changes can be measured by comparing ratios of CMAP duration to amplitude, these are usually made on a qualitative rather than quantitative basis. Subtle changes may occur in normal individuals when CMAPs are obtained from stimulation at different points along the course of a nerve. As previously described, this is referred to as physiologic dispersion. With physiologic dispersion, it is estimated and modeled that the CMAP amplitude with proximal stimulation should never drop below 80% of that obtained from the most distal stimulus site. Nerve root stimulation sites provide the notable exception to this rule.[13] More dramatic reductions of CMAP amplitude, particularly over short segments of nerve, suggest demyelinating pathology due to conduction block or temporal dispersion, anatomic variants such as a median to ulnar crossover, or alternatively technical error (Figs. 2-2A,B and 2-3).

CMAP afterdischarges represent one other potential alteration of CMAP morphology. When present, these repetitive CMAPs follow single or repetitive supramaximal nerve stimuli. They appear as one or more additional negative peaks in the immediate aftermath of initial CMAP detectable either with routine motor conductions, with repetitive stimulation, or with F wave assessment. The afterdischarges may interfere with F wave identification. Afterdischarges are not uniform with consecutive stimuli and have much smaller amplitudes than the initial supramaximal response (Figs. 2-4 and 2-5). They are uncommon, typically identified in disorders of nerve hyperexcitability in which nerve or muscle depolarization persists or repolarization is delayed **(Chapter 10).** They are commonly associated with continuous motor unit activity at rest with needle EMG. There is a spectrum of these spontaneous discharges ranging from single random MUP discharges (i.e., fasciculation potentials), to doublets or other multiplets which when discharging rhythmically or semirhythmically appear as myokymic discharges. At the extreme of these spontaneous discharges are high-frequency decrescendo waveforms known as neuromyotonic discharges. The generators of these discharges are believed to reside within motor nerve, probably within terminal twigs.

The clinical value of afterdischarge identification is derived from their specificity. They are associated with a limited number of disorders that may affect nerve, neuromuscular transmission, or muscle. Neuromyotonia, also known as Isaacs syndrome or the syndrome of continuous muscle fiber activity is the most notable form of nerve hyperexcitability.[28-31] Our current understanding implicates malfunction of nerve potassium channels by antibodies directed against contactin-associated protein-like 2 (Caspr2) or to leucine-rich glioma-inactivated 1 (LGI1). Presumptively, the afterdischarges result from prolonged nerve depolarization due to impaired potassium channel function resulting in the inability of nerves to rapidly repolarize.

In addition, afterdischarges may occur in disorders in which there is prolonged cholinergic activity at neuromuscular junctions such as toxic exposures to organophosphates, anticholinesterases or congenital acetylcholinesterase deficiency, and

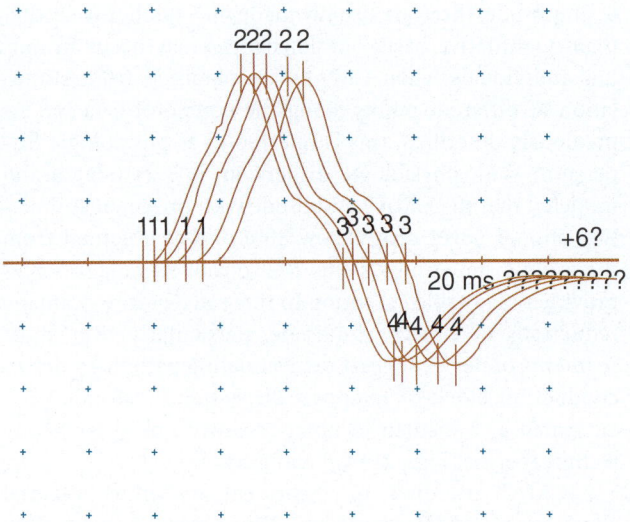

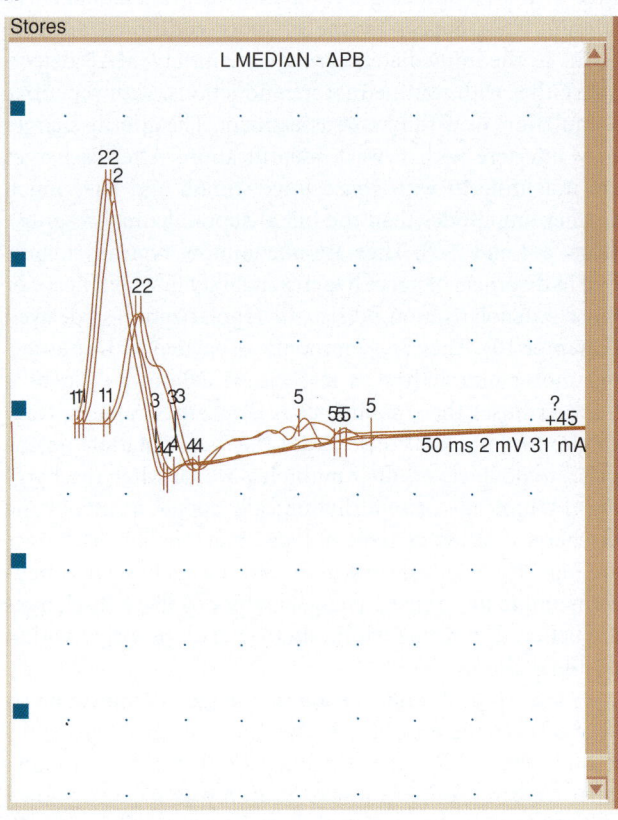

Figure 2-2. (**A**) Short segmental incremental stimulation in normal individual demonstrating identical CMAP (compound muscle action potential) waveforms with equivalent spacing between consecutive waveforms and (**B**) ulnar neuropathy at the elbow with focal demyelination with conduction block (amplitude reduction between responses 3 and 4), focal slowing (widening baseline interval between responses 3 and 4), and mild temporal dispersion (increased CMAP duration between responses 3 and 4).

slow channel syndrome.[32] These afterdischarges appear similar to those that occur in disorders of nerve hyperexcitability in that they occur following a single supramaximal stimulus delivered to a motor or mixed nerve. The physiologic basis for these afterdischarges appears to be prolongation of the end-plate potential (EPP) at the neuromuscular junction, unrelated to the delayed neurotoxic effects that frequently occur with toxic organophosphate exposure.

A different type of afterdischarge of muscle rather than nerve origin referred to as postexercise myotonic potentials (PEMPs) may occur with myopathy associated with impaired sodium channel, particularly PMC, and to a lesser extent chloride channel function, that is, myotonia congenita (MC).[33-35] PEMPs are not seen in sodium or calcium ion channel disorders that produce periodic paralysis phenotypes.[33] These afterdischarges can be differentiated from those of neural origin as they do not occur after a single supramaximal motor stimulation but only in the context of the short exercise testing that is described below. They persist if repetitive stimulation is delivered immediately postexercise but dissipate as the interval between exercise and stimuli evolves, whether the stimuli are repetitive or individual.

Sensory Nerve Conductions

Sensory conduction studies are also performed with surface electrodes in most instances. Unlike motor conductions, the recording electrodes are placed over nerve not muscle. Nerve rather than muscle action potentials are measured, with maximal amplitudes measured in micro- rather than millivolts: making them more technically difficult to obtain. The resulting wave form is the SNAP. The same disc recording electrodes, or in the case of the median and ulnar nerves, ring electrodes on digits are utilized. The reference electrode is also placed over the nerve. To maximize the amplitude of the sensory potential, the recording and reference electrodes should be placed at least 3–4 cm apart. This of course is not possible in everyone, particularly in children.[7] The tested nerve is then stimulated at either a more proximal or a distal location than the recording site. The former technique is described as antidromic, as the impulse travels in the direction opposite to that of normal centripetal physiologic conduction in sensory nerve fibers. With stimuli delivered distal to the recording site in sensory or mixed nerves, conduction is considered orthodromic. Nerves routinely studied include the median, ulnar, dorsal cutaneous ulnar, radial, medial antebrachial cutaneous, lateral antebrachial cutaneous, sural, and superficial peroneal. The lateral femoral cutaneous, saphenous, posterior cutaneous nerve of the forearm, medial and lateral plantar nerves, and median and ulnar studies with less commonly used digits are less frequently tested. Many of these latter studies are easy to obtain in the young, healthy, slender, and nonedematous but can be technically difficult in those with the opposite characteristics.

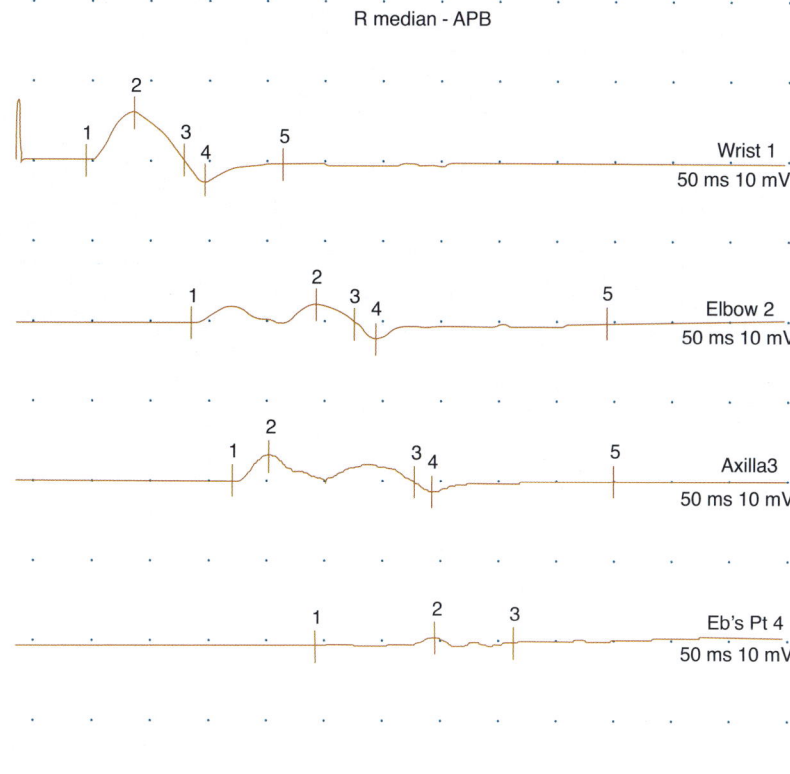

Figure 2-3. Median motor nerve conduction at four different points of stimulation demonstrating differential slowing (temporal dispersion) in patient with multifocal motor neuropathy.

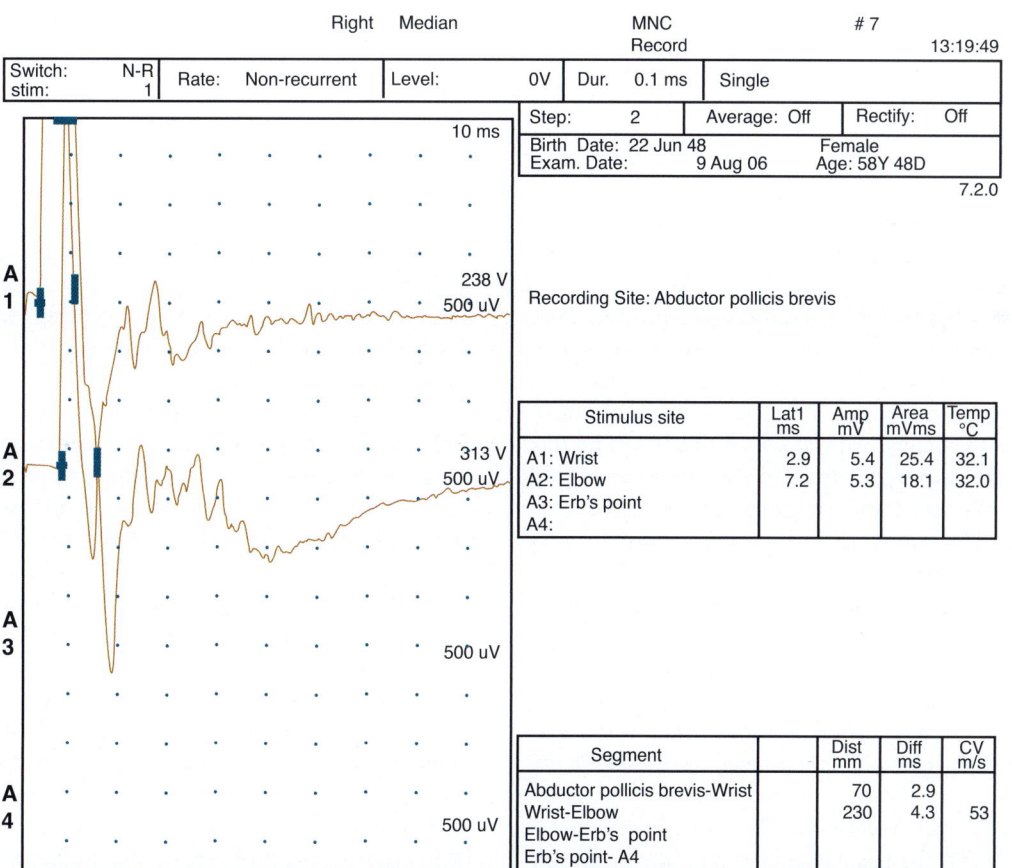

Figure 2-4. Afterdischarges in neuromyotonia with routine motor conduction studies. (Used with permission of Dr. Steven Vernino, University of Texas Southwestern.)

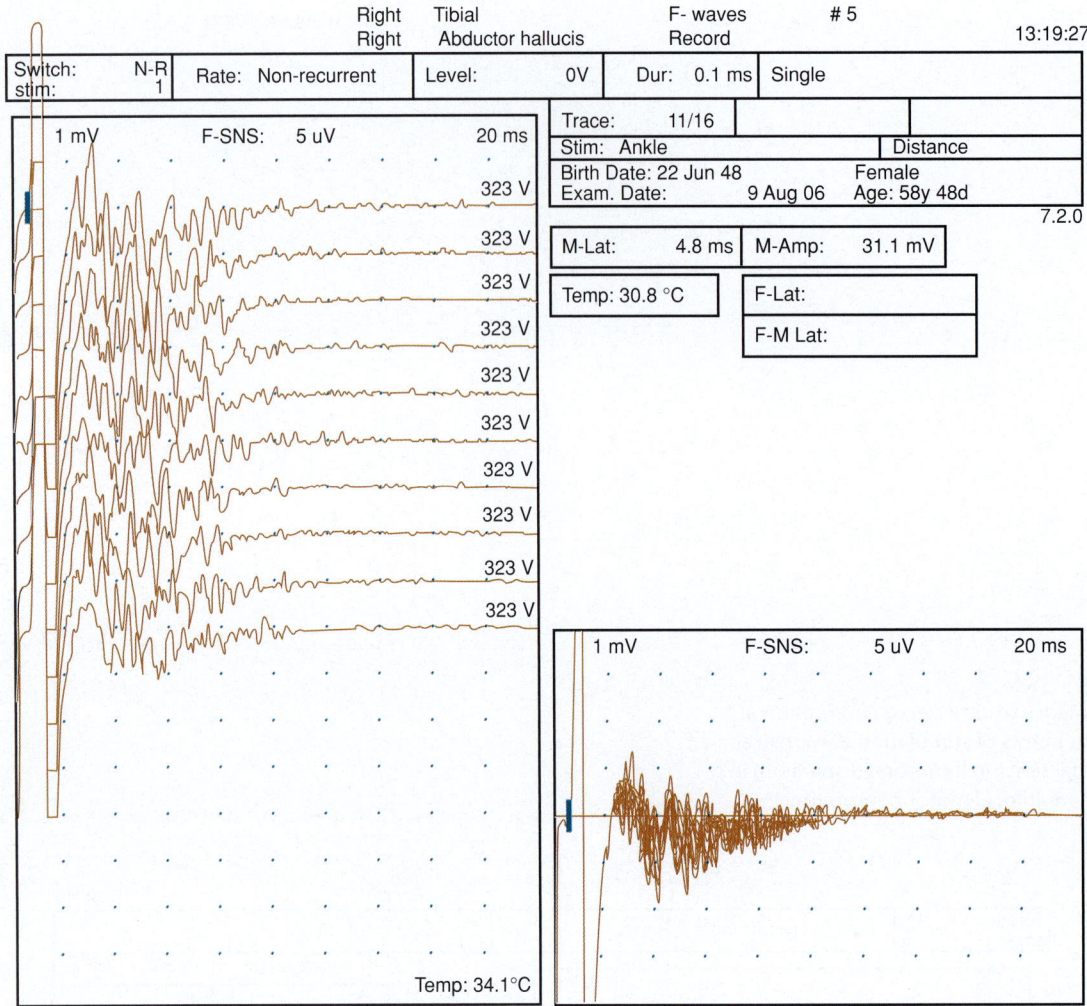

Figure 2-5. Afterdischarges in neuromyotonia with F wave determinations. (Used with permission of Dr. Steven Vernino, University of Texas Southwestern.)

The SNAP amplitude and the distal latency and conduction velocity should be measured (Fig. 2-6). Conduction velocity can also be assessed between distal and proximal stimulation sites, if performed. As there are no neuromuscular junctions to contend with in sensory nerves, both the distal latency and the conduction velocity are measures of nerve conduction speed, differing only in the segment of nerve tested and the units with which it is reported. With motor conductions, there are some disorders in which distal latencies are prolonged disproportionate to forearm or leg conduction velocities. As there are few, if any, recognized conditions in which conduction speed is consistently more affected in one segment of sensory nerves than another, it can be argued that the reporting of distal latency as the sole measurement of sensory conduction speed is adequate. With motor distal latencies, the onset of the waveform is used for measurement, thereby identifying the fastest conducting axons. With SNAPs, the distal latency is typically measured from the waveform peak rather than the onset. This is done for technical reasons, as the onset of the SNAP waveform may be difficult to reproducibly identify. Sensory conduction velocities are, however, measured utilizing the SNAP takeoff from baseline rather than peak.

The second, and in most situations, more important SNAP parameter is amplitude. As SNAPs are nerve rather than muscle action potentials, amplitude reduction does not occur on the basis of impaired neuromuscular transmission or myofiber loss. Except for certain types of demyelinating pathology described below, reduced SNAP amplitude indicates either advanced age, excessive subcutaneous tissue or fluid, poor technique, or, most commonly, loss of peripheral sensory axons. The pathology in the sensory nerve can occur anywhere at or distal to the dorsal root ganglia.

Detecting morphologic change of SNAP waveforms is of limited value. Waveforms obtained with proximal stimuli are typically significantly reduced in amplitude and prolonged in duration in comparison to their distally obtained counterparts (Fig. 2-6). This is due to the same principle of physiologic dispersion described above. This phenomenon is more pronounced than its motor counterpart due to the far

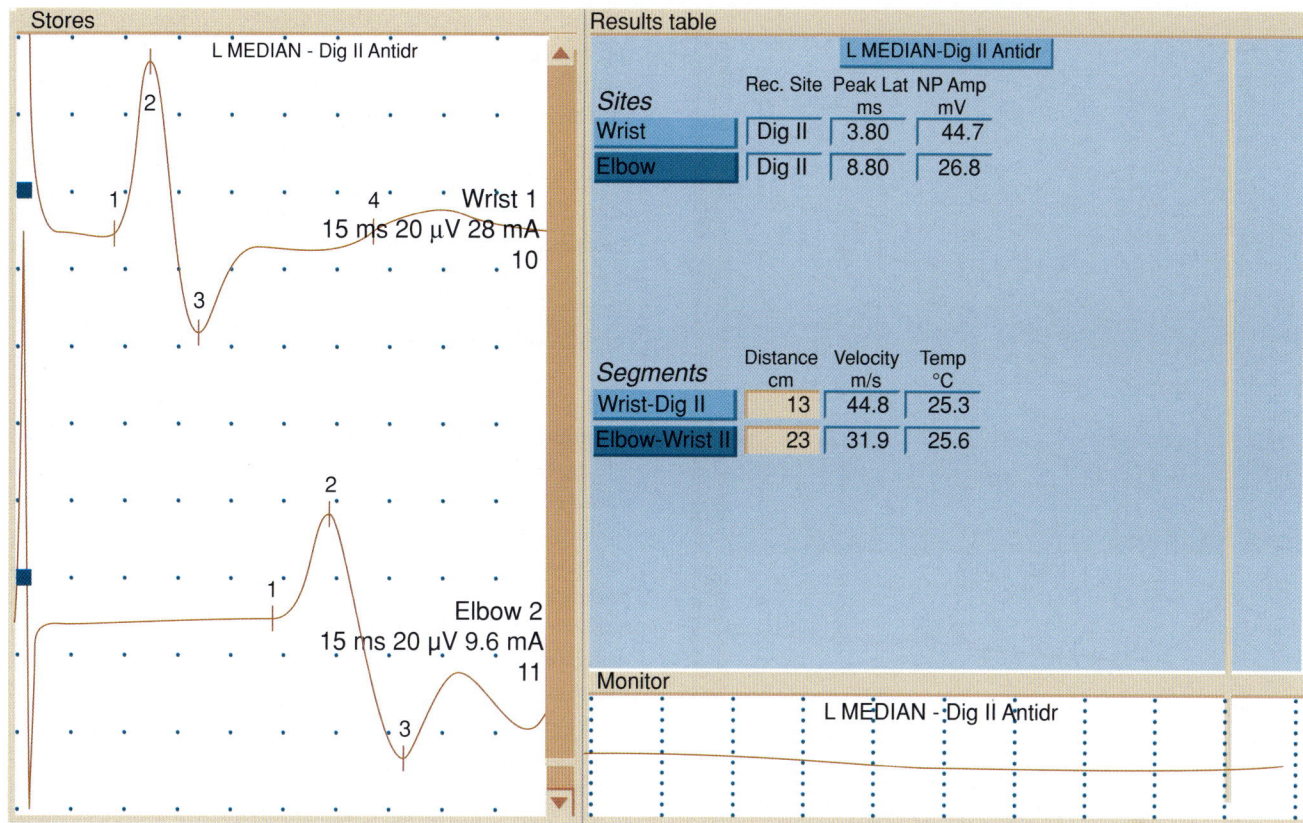

Figure 2-6. Sensory nerve action potentials in a normal individual demonstrating normal physiologic dispersion over distance with decreased amplitude and prolonged duration of median SNAP (sensory nerve action potential) waveform stimulating at elbow (bottom) as compared to stimulating at the wrist (top).

wider range of conduction velocities in sensory nerves. As a result, attempts to identify demyelinating conduction block or significant morphologic differences in SNAP waveforms are not routinely attempted, particularly with stimuli delivered at wide interval distances.

F Waves and H Reflexes

Motor and sensory conduction studies are typically performed in the below elbow and knee segments where nerves are more anatomically accessible. F waves and H reflexes have potential value because of their ability to assess conduction in more proximally located nerve segments. F waves can be obtained by delivering supramaximal stimulation to any motor or mixed nerve in a normal individual, in most instances. F waves can be difficult to obtain in certain nerves, for example, common peroneal, with increased age even in the apparent absence of pathology. For that reason, it can be perilous to suggest the existence of nerve injury based solely on the absence of an F response from a single nerve. In normal adults less than 60 years of age, H reflexes can be elicited from the soleus muscle while stimulating the tibial nerve and, on occasion, from the flexor carpi radialis. Identification of H reflexes in other nerve/muscle pairs implies the existence of upper motor neuron disease due to decreased central nervous system (CNS) inhibition on the reflex arc, analogous to a hyperactive deep tendon reflex.

The relevant anatomy and physiology of an F response can be described in the following manner. When a supramaximal stimulus is delivered to a nerve, the primary orthodromic response is the CMAP (M wave) as previously described. In addition, the initial nerve depolarization also produces an antidromic action potential traveling centripetally toward the spinal cord. At the level of the corresponding anterior cell(s), this antidromic action potential establishes a persistent or second action potential at the level of either the perikaryon or its axon hillock. This supplemental action potential is carried in a centrifugal or orthodromic direction along the entire length of one or more of the same motor axon(s) back to the original target muscle. As a result, the muscle is depolarized twice in response to a single stimulus, the second muscle action potential (F wave) having understandably a much longer latency and smaller amplitude. Unlike the initial CMAP, which represents the action potentials of all the responsive muscle fibers, each (F) response represents the action potentials of muscle fibers belonging to a single motor unit. With each sequential stimulus, different motor units are typically activated. As a result, sequential F wave responses have varying latencies and morphologies in comparison to those occurring with the previous or subsequent stimuli.

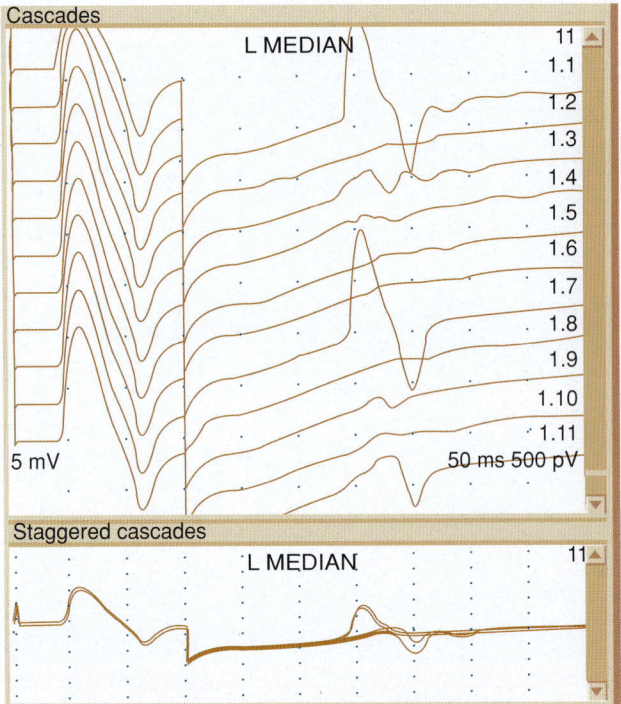

Figure 2-7. F waves—11 consecutive supramaximal stimuli delivered to the median nerve at the wrist in a normal individual while recording from the abductor pollicis brevis muscle demonstrating uniform CMAPs (compound muscle action potentials) but typical F wave behavior, that is, waveforms that are variable in occurrence, latency, and morphology.

F waves have significant limitations. Even in a normal nerve/muscle pair, F waves do not result from each stimulus. Amplitude measurements are of no particular value, as these represent the action potentials of only a small and varying proportion of single muscle fibers. There is heterogeneity of F wave latencies as sequential responses rarely arise from motor axons with identical conduction velocities (Fig. 2-7). We usually record 10 F waves reported the earliest latency along with the percentage of times out of 10 maximal stimulations that an F wave was recorded. We only "count" an F wave if we see more than one response. The persistence of F waves is useful in the arms as we typically get an F wave 80% or more in the arms (less so in the legs), and if say we see a normal minimum median F wave with normal distal amplitude of the CMAP, we wonder if there is proximal demyelination or conduction block but there are at least some motor units unblocked. In this regard, one can also look at increased disparity between the earliest F wave latency and the longest. Generally, we do not see greater than a 10–15 ms difference. Again, a large disparity can suggest proximal demyelination with some axons being spared while others are demyelinated. The potential value of F waves is their ability to detect conduction slowing over the segments of nerve not tested by routine conduction velocity measurements, that is, the proximal to elbow and knee segments. This value is most apparent early in the course of acquired demyelinating neuropathies, where prolonged F wave latencies may occur because of disease predilection for nerve roots, prior to slowing of conduction velocity or prolongation of distal latency in more distal nerve segments. In most cases, however, F waves are either absent, or prolonged in the setting of slowed conduction velocities. Simultaneous slowing of conduction velocities and F waves has no localizing value, as the slowing of the F latency in this circumstance may represent slowing in the same distal aspect of the nerve where the conduction velocity is measured.

The H reflex represents the electrophysiologic analog of the Achilles deep tendon reflex. As in the F wave, the stimulus applied to the tibial nerve in the popliteal fossa will travel in two directions. Unlike F waves, the H reflex is obtained with submaximal stimulus intensity. With delivery of stimuli of low intensity and long duration (1 ms), the lower-threshold 1 A sensory fibers within the tibial nerve are preferentially activated. As a result, the initial action potentials are propagated solely within thickly myelinated sensory nerve fibers. These impulses travel both centrifugally, where they have no known clinical or diagnostic consequence, and centripetally (orthodromically) along tibial and sciatic sensory fibers. Impulse transmission through the dorsal root of the S1 segment allows completion of a monosynaptic reflex to S1 anterior horn cells. Activation of these produces the H reflex representing a long-latency CMAP originating from the soleus muscle. Typically, the H reflex has a latency in the high 20 to mid-30 μs range, depending on patient height.

As the intensity of the stimulus delivered to the tibial nerve increases, characteristic H reflex behavior is demonstrable. Action potentials will develop within the higher-threshold tibial motor fibers in addition to the 1 A sensory fibers already activated. These motor nerve action potentials also travel bidirectionally. The orthodromic impulses will activate the soleus muscle producing a typical CMAP. This has a far shorter latency than the H reflex and does not typically make its appearance until the H reflex is well established. The antidromic action potentials created in tibial motor fibers have a different effect. These will collide in a proximal location with the action potentials responsible for the H reflex. As the stimulus intensity increases, more tibial motor axons are depolarized resulting in increasing soleus CMAP amplitude but declining H reflex amplitude. Eventually, the H reflex will disappear while the CMAP will become supramaximal.

In summary, in response to sequential stimuli of 0.5–1-ms duration delivered to the tibial nerve in the popliteal fossa with increasing intensities, the H reflex appears first. Subsequently, the CMAP or M wave appears and enlarges to its supramaximal amplitude while the H reflex declines in amplitude and disappears. The tibial motor fibers distal to the stimulus site are depolarized twice, whereas both the tibial sensory fibers and the tibial motor fibers proximal to the stimulation site are depolarized once in response to a single stimulus (Fig. 2-8).

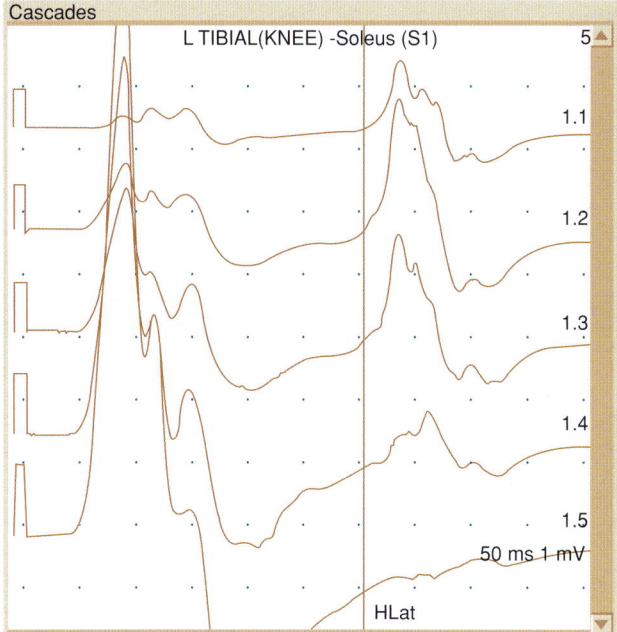

Figure 2-8. H reflex—five consecutive and increasing stimuli to the tibial nerve in the popliteal fossa in a normal individual, recording from the soleus demonstrating a typical H reflex pattern, that is, H reflex amplitude initially > M response amplitude, subsequent peaking than decline, and eventual absence of H reflex, associated with gradual increase to supramaximal M response. Note uniform H reflex latency.

Both the maximal amplitude and the latency of the H reflex can be measured. The former estimates the number of viable motor units and muscle fibers within the S1 segment/soleus muscle complex and is typically greater than 1 mV in size. The latter provides at least an estimate of conduction speed within the motor and sensory fibers of the S1 segment. As in the case of F waves, H reflexes have greatest utility and localization value when these are abnormal in the setting of normal routine conduction parameters. This applies most frequently early in the course of acquired demyelinating polyneuropathies. In addition, H reflex amplitudes have value in the assessment of S1 radiculopathies. If an H reflex is absent more than a week after symptom onset in the setting of normal routine conduction parameters and reduced recruitment in S1 innervated muscles, proximal conduction block in the tibial nerve, sciatic nerve, sacral plexus, or S1 nerve root can be inferred. Focal slowing of nerve conduction in a proximal location is theoretically detectable by H reflex assessment. This slowing is usually obscured by normal conduction speed in the other normal and more extensive parts of the S1 reflex arc. Attempts to provide an anatomic diagnosis of a focal neuropathy or radiculopathy based on by F and H responses alone are discouraged.

Repetitive Nerve Stimulation

Performance and interpretation of RNS techniques evolves from an understanding of the normal physiology of neuromuscular transmission. Muscle EPPs are the precursors of muscle fiber action potentials. Unlike nerve or muscle action potentials that are all or none events that precede and follow EPPs respectively, EPPs are graded. Their amplitudes are proportional to the number of successful interactions between acetylcholine (ACh) molecules and muscle end-plate receptor sites. Quantal release of ACh decreases with successive stimuli delivered in intervals of greater than 200 μs (e.g., <5 Hz). Under normal circumstances, this quantal and resultant EPP decline is of no practical importance, as there is a considerable physiologic reserve. With disease states that alter either the presynaptic release of ACh or postsynaptic receptor responsiveness, this reserve becomes inadequate. The EPP at individual neuromuscular junctions may fall below the threshold for myofiber action potential generation, and both CMAP amplitude and muscle strength may decline. As a result, slow (2–5 Hz) repetitive stimulation may produce a successive decline or decrement in CMAP amplitude in both pre- and postsynaptic DNMT (Fig. 2-9). To avoid false-positive results based on technical factors, a decrement of at least 10% is required to be considered abnormal although a smaller decrement in a technically pristine study is suspicious. This decremental response has both clinical and single fiber analogs, that is, fatigable weakness and blocking of single fiber action potentials, respectively.

The recording and stimulating electrode placement in RNS are identical to routine motor conductions. Only the manner of stimulus delivery is altered. As mentioned above, the diagnostic yield of RNS will improve by ensuring that the tested muscle is warm and by removing drugs that augment neuromuscular transmission such as pyridostigmine prior to testing. RNS often produces unwanted movement artifact, which may require limb immobilization to secure a technically reliable study. Unfortunately, the muscles with the highest diagnostic yield are also those most prone to movement and technical artifact.

False-positive decremental responses due to technical error are commonplace. For a decremental response to be considered pathologic, it must be reproducible and conform to the typical pattern. This pattern is best understood by understanding its physiologic basis. Pathologic decrements are not linear. Typically, the CMAP decline between two consecutive responses is greatest between the first and second stimuli and reaches its nadir by the fourth response. The reason for this latter phenomenon is the mobilization of ACh stores in the presynaptic neuron that allows delayed restoration of the immediate release pool. This allows for partial augmentation of the EPP after the fourth or fifth consecutive stimulus. With subsequent stimuli, the CMAP amplitude then begins to increase slightly although it never reaches the size of the initial response. If a train of 8–10 stimuli are delivered, the resulting configuration will have an asymmetric saucer-like appearance, with the left edge being higher. This configuration is of particular importance in distinguishing variation in CMAP amplitude due to disease from that due to technical considerations which are commonplace and easily misinterpreted by the unwary.

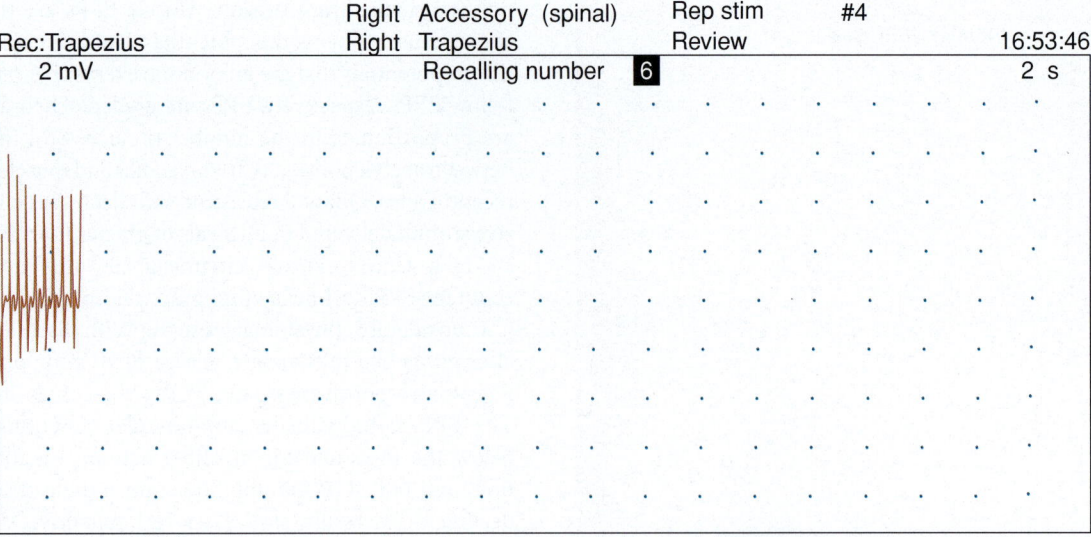
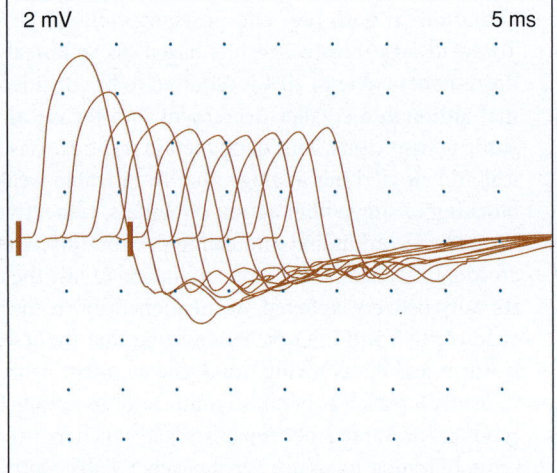

Figure 2-9. Decremental response to slow (3 Hz) repetitive stimulation with typical pattern in myasthenia gravis (note normal initial CMAP amplitude of 7.61 mV).

The electrophysiologic basis of the incremental response is closely related to calcium's role in the presynaptic release of ACh. When presynaptic ACh release is impaired by disease, it can be enhanced by augmenting the concentration of calcium in the presynaptic terminal. In a seemingly paradoxical manner, this can be accomplished by the delivery of repetitive stimuli at a frequency of greater than 5 Hz. Stated in a different way, this is accomplished with stimuli delivered at intervals shorter than 200 μs. In presynaptic DNMTs, the baseline CMAP is typically reduced, at times dramatically. This is the most notable difference between pre- and postsynaptic disorders and sets the stage for the ability to demonstrate an incremental response. The initial low-amplitude CMAP can be increased by a factor of 100% or more by either "fast" repetitive stimulation (5–50 Hz) or more humanely by brief exercise of the muscle being studied (Fig. 2-10A and B). With the brief exercise technique, a supramaximal stimulus is followed by 10 seconds of isometric exercise to the muscle being studied, and then immediately by a second postexercise supramaximal stimulus. Trains of fast repetitive stimulation are typically reserved for those who cannot perform or cooperate with the postexercise technique.

An incremental response is defined by a >100% increase in CMAP amplitude comparing the postexercise response to the baseline. The degree of increment cannot exceed the difference between the baseline and premorbid CMAP amplitude for that muscle. A physiologic increment (i.e., higher amplitude, shorter duration, identical area under the curve) may occur in normal patients but typically does not exceed 40% of the baseline. It implies a more synchronous discharge of the component SFMAPs that constitute that CMAP waveform.

The electrodiagnostic approach to a patient with a suspected DNMT is dependent on the clinical context and on the initial, supramaximal CMAP amplitude. To overly simplify the concept, if it is small, try to make it bigger, and if it is big, try to make it smaller. In other words, in the case of either a reduced initial CMAP amplitude or a decrement in response to

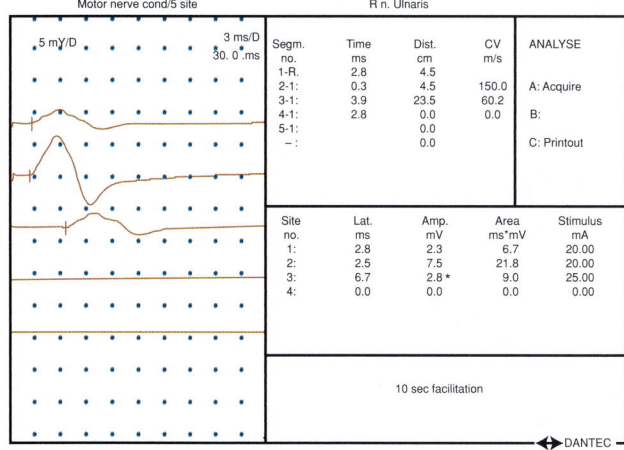

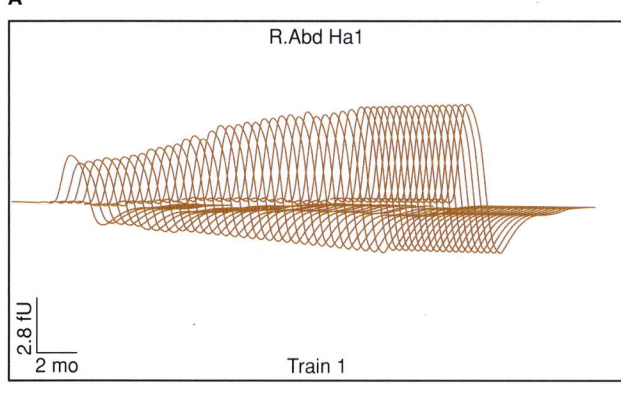

Figure 2-10. Incremental response to brief (10 seconds) exercise in patient with Lambert–Eaton myasthenic syndrome (LEMS) (**A**) [trace 1 ulnar compound muscle action potential (CMAP) at baseline stimulating at wrist, trace 2 ulnar CMAP immediately after 10 seconds of isometrically resisted finger abduction stimulating at wrist, trace 3 ulnar CMAP 1 minute later stimulating at elbow]. Incremental response to 20 Hz fast repetitive stimulation (**B**).

slow repetitive stimulation, an attempt to increase the CMAP amplitude is made. This can be accomplished by 10 seconds of brief exercise, fast repetitive stimulation (10–50 Hz), or by administration of an anticholinesterase medication. Conversely, when faced with a normal initial CMAP amplitude and a suspected DNMT, the electrodiagnostician should seek to produce a decrement by slow repetitive stimulation without, or if necessary, with 1 minute of isometric exercise.

To elaborate, presynaptic DNMT have electrophysiologic properties that are both shared and distinctive in comparison to their postsynaptic counterparts. In suspected myasthenia gravis (MG), the initial CMAP amplitude is typically normal. The first step is to try and demonstrate a decremental response to slow repetitive stimulation. Ideally, for the sake of efficiency, RNS would be performed on a clinically weak muscle that has been warmed. The absence of decremental response to slow repetitive stimulation in a weak muscle would effectively preclude the diagnosis of autoimmune MG as the cause of that weakness. If a decrement is demonstrated, the train of stimulation can be repeated following 10 seconds of exercise to look for postexercise facilitation or decrement repair. If a decrement is not demonstrable at baseline, repeating the train once a minute for 5 minutes following 1 minute of exercise applied to that muscle may improve diagnostic yield. This phenomenon is referred to as postexercise exhaustion.

Presynaptic DNMT also decrement with low rates of repetitive stimulation. Early in the course, this may be the only abnormality found with nerve conductions. Presynaptic DNMT is usually distinguished from MG electrodiagnostically because of low baseline CMAP amplitudes. In this case, the initial response from the electrodiagnostician should be to attempt to elicit an incremental response. This is easily done in a cooperative patient by exercising the appropriate muscle for 10 seconds and then immediately delivering a second supramaximal stimulus as described above. If the patient is not cooperative, a train of fast repetitive stimuli (10–50 Hz) may be used as a surrogate. If an increment is demonstrated, a subsequent train of stimuli delivered at 2–3 Hz will produce a characteristic decrement and further solidify the diagnosis of a neuromuscular transmission defect.

Short- and Long-Exercise Tests

The nondystrophic muscle channelopathies constitute a complex, overlapping group of disorders related to gene mutations of chloride, calcium, sodium, and potassium (Andersen–Tawil syndrome) channels in muscle. They will be described in detail in Chapter 29. As a result of their pathophysiologies, the phenotypes are typically dominated at least initially by episodic symptoms, either stiffness related to myotonia, weakness related to periodic paralysis, or a combination of both. Stiffness is felt to result from persistent muscle fiber depolarization and contraction whereas periodic weakness is felt to represent a more severe degree of depolarization rendering the muscle inexcitable. In chronic stages, particularly in the periodic paralyses, persistent weakness may develop.

Electrophysiologic testing of the nondystrophic myotonias involves detection of afterdischarges known as PEMPs as previously described in both routine motor conductions and F wave determinations, the presence or absence of myotonic discharges on needle EMG, response to RNS, and in particular, responses to short- and long-exercise testing which will be the focus of this section. Short- and long-exercise tests offer diagnostic support for both the existence and type of muscle channelopathy.[33–35] The tests are variations of standard motor NCS which utilize the ulnar or common peroneal nerves recording from the abductor digiti minimi or extensor digitorum brevis muscles, respectively. Both forms of exercise testing require careful attention to uniform patient positioning, limb temperature, muscle relaxation, and stimulus intensity.

Both short- and long-exercise tests are performed by maintaining limb temperature at 32–34°C and establishing a stable baseline, supramaximal CMAP amplitude. With the

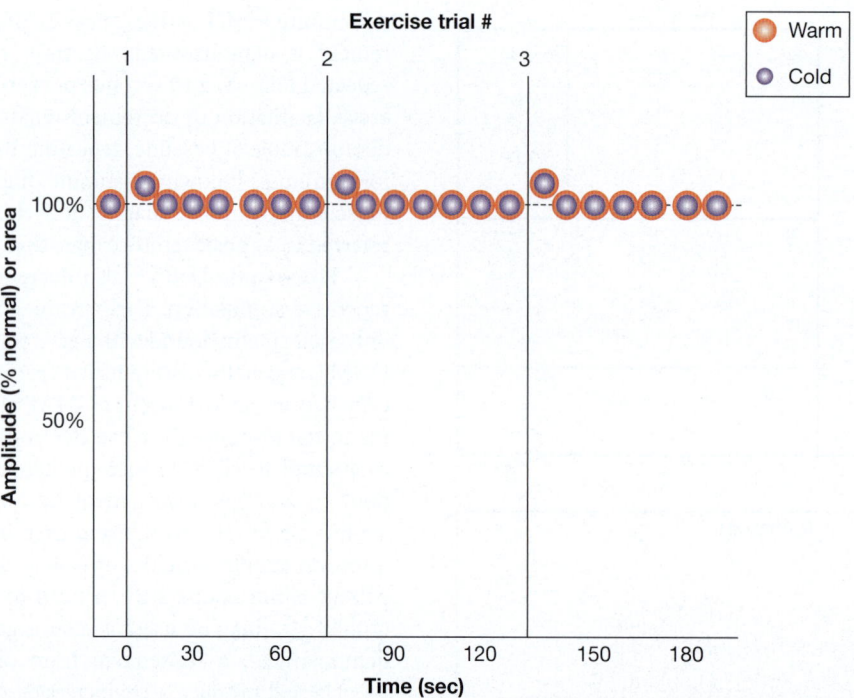

Figure 2-11. Short-exercise test—normal.

short-exercise test, a single supramaximal stimulus is delivered, the tested muscle is isometrically exercised for 10 seconds, followed by an immediate postexercise supramaximal stimulus and six additional single stimuli every 8 seconds are delivered over the course of the next 50 seconds. After a 10-second rest period between trials, two subsequent, identical trials are performed, each preceded by 10 seconds of isometric exercise. Five patterns of abnormality have been described, the first three of which utilize the short-exercise test alone.[33–35] The other two patterns are defined by a combination of the long- and short-exercise tests.

In normal individuals, there is a slight CMAP amplitude and/or area increment immediately following exercise that rapidly returns to baseline during the first trial and does not differ with the second and third trials.[33] The CMAP amplitude rapidly returns to baseline by the second or third stimulus of the first trial (Fig. 2-11).[33,35] The mean increment in immediate postexercise CMAP amplitude is 4% (range −28 to +27) and the mean increment of CMAP area is +3% (range −58 to +84).[35] An increment of <10% or decrement <20% in CMAP amplitude and/or area compared to baseline is considered normal.[35] The short-exercise test has been further refined by using the same algorithm following limb cooling and rewarming, utilizing a combination of both amplitude and area to improve both the sensitivity and specificity of increment or decrement measurements.[35] Cooling is typically delivered for 7 minutes with a target cutaneous temperature of 15°C. In normal individuals, cooling with or without rewarming the limb does not alter the normal pattern.[34,35]

The long-exercise test is performed with identical electrode application.[35] The muscle to be studied is isometrically exercised for 5 minutes. During the period of exercise, single supramaximal stimuli are delivered at 1-minute intervals. After the exercise, single supramaximal stimuli are then delivered immediately, every minute for 5–6 minutes, and then every 2–5 minutes for 40–50 minutes. The long-exercise test is of the greatest utility in the identification of the periodic paralyses. Normal patients may demonstrate a minimal initial decrement in CMAP amplitude and/or area with a rapid return to baseline (Fig. 2-12). In African-Caribbean controls, the mean decrement may be slightly greater. Authorities recommend that an abnormal decrement on long-exercise testing for amplitude and area exceeds 40%.[35]

The response patterns with repetitive stimulation seen in the dystrophic or nondystrophic myotonic disorders differ from those seen in pre- and postsynaptic DNMT. Because of discomfort, repetitive stimulation is performed in suspected nondystrophic myotonia cases only when the remainder of the electrodiagnostic assessment is inconclusive. The major value of repetitive stimulation in this setting is increased sensitivity, particularly in recessively inherited MC.[36] In the nondystrophic myotonias, there is typically no decremental response prior to exercise. Depending on the specific disorder and the frequency of repetitive stimulation, there may be either a decrescendo pattern in which the CMAP amplitude continuously declines (10-Hz stimulation in a warm limb in MC, or 10-Hz stimulation following limb cooling in PMC) or a pattern in which there is an initial dramatic reduction in CMAP amplitude following exercise which then declines further and then gradually increases with 3-Hz stimulation in PMC (Fig. 2-13).[33,35,36]

The following is a summary of the typical patterns of abnormalities seen in MC phenotype associated with chloride

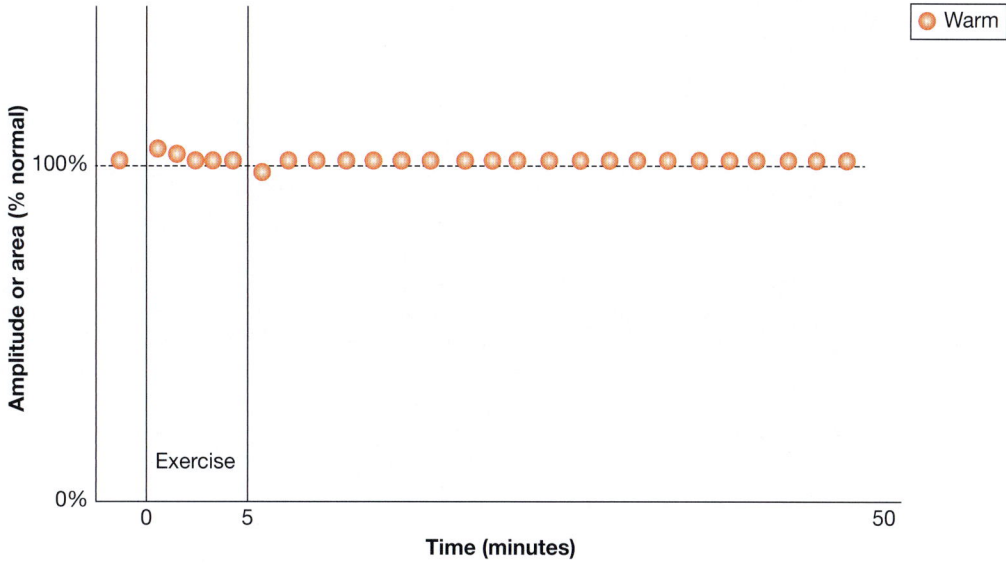

Figure 2-12. Long-exercise test—normal.

channel mutations, PMC, potassium-aggravated myotonia (PAM), sodium channel myotonia (SCM), and hyperkalemic periodic paralysis (hyperKPP) associated with sodium channel mutations, and hypokalemic periodic paralysis associated with both calcium (hypoKPP1) and sodium channel (hypoKPP2) mutations. The reader is referred to Table 2-1 and Chapter 29 for summary and complete description of these disorders.

In MC with short-exercise testing, CMAP amplitude and area decrement is the greatest in the initial response following exercise (Figs. 2-14 and 2-15). If it exceeds 40% of baseline, it is considered pathognomonic of a chloride channel disorder.[35] With the next six stimuli delivered over the ensuing 50 seconds, the decrement lessens and the CMAP amplitudes and areas gradually approach baseline, thus rendering a curve with an ascending positive slope. With the subsequent two trials, the magnitude of the decrement lessens but the trajectory of the curves remains the same. With cooling, the magnitude of the decrement increases slightly, particularly in dominantly inherited disease. Although this *type 2* pattern is seen with both recessively and dominantly inherited forms of MC, the decrement is far more dramatic in the former (Fig. 2-14).[34] This pattern is seen in approximately 83% of patients with confirmed chloride channel mutations with traditional amplitude comparisons but improves to 100% if amplitude and area comparisons are done concordantly.[33,35] PEMPs in the short-exercise test in response to single or repetitive stimuli are found in approximately one-third

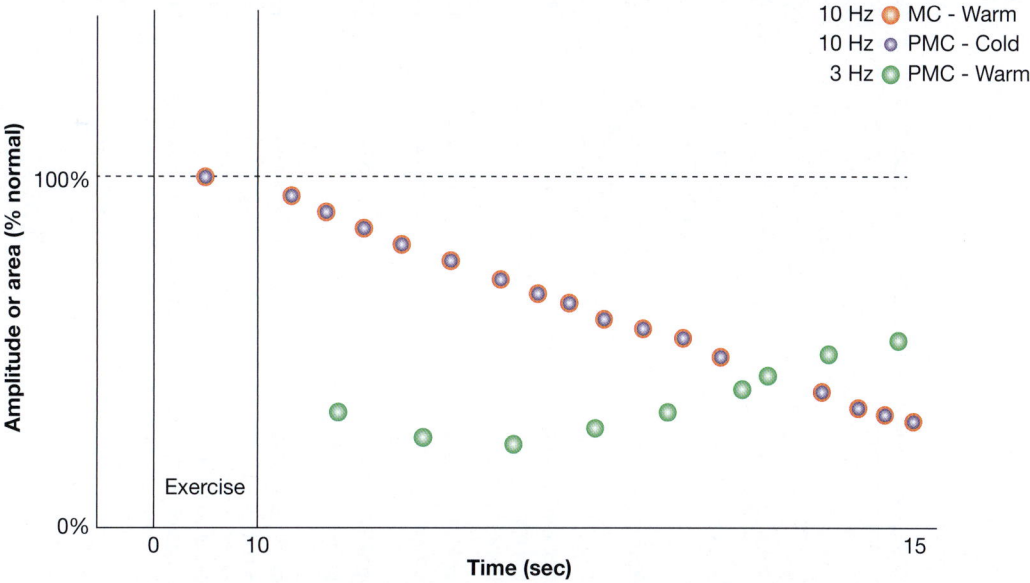

Figure 2-13. Repetitive stimulation in nondystrophic myotonia.

TABLE 2-1. SHORT- AND LONG-EXERCISE TESTS IN THE NONDYSTROPHIC MYOTONIAS AND PERIODIC PARALYSES

Phenotype	Channel	Short-Exercise Effect on CMAP Amplitude	Postexercise Myotonic Potentials	Response to Repeat Short Exercise	Response to Cooling and Repeat Short Exercise	Long-Exercise Effect on CMAP Amplitude	Myotonic Discharges on EMG	Other Disorders in Which This Pattern Can Be Identified
MC (type 2 pattern)	Cl⁻	Immediate ↓ with subsequent repair	Yes	Less prominent CMAP ↓	AR—no change AD—exaggerated ↓ CMAP amplitude	No change	Yes	PAM MD 1 and 2
PMC (type 1 pattern)	Na⁺	Immediate ↓ but less than type 2 but with longer effect[a]	Yes	More prominent ↓ CMAP amplitude	Even further ↓ CMAP amplitude	Prolonged and significant ↓ amplitude	Yes	None to date
Other sodium channel myotonias (type 3 pattern)	Na⁺	No change	No	No change	Variable	No change	Yes	None to date
HyperKPP (type 4 pattern)	Na⁺	Immediate ↑ that persists	No	Further ↑ CMAP amplitude	Unknown	↑ amplitude immediately that ↓ over time	Yes (not universal)	HypoKK-2
HypoPP-1 (type 5 pattern)	Ca⁺⁺	No change	No	No change	Unknown	↓ amplitude immediately that ↓ further over time	No	HypoKK-2
HypoPP-2 (type 4 or 5 patterns)	Na⁺	Type 4 or 5	No	Type 4 or 5	Unknown	Type 4 or 5	No	HyperKPP HypoPP-1

[a]Exceptions with Q270 K⁺ mutation.

MC, myotonia congenita; PMC, paramyotonia congenita; HypoPP, hypokalemic periodic paralysis; HyperKPP, hyperkalemic periodic paralysis; DM, myotonic dystrophy; EMG, electromyography; CMAP, compound muscle action potential.

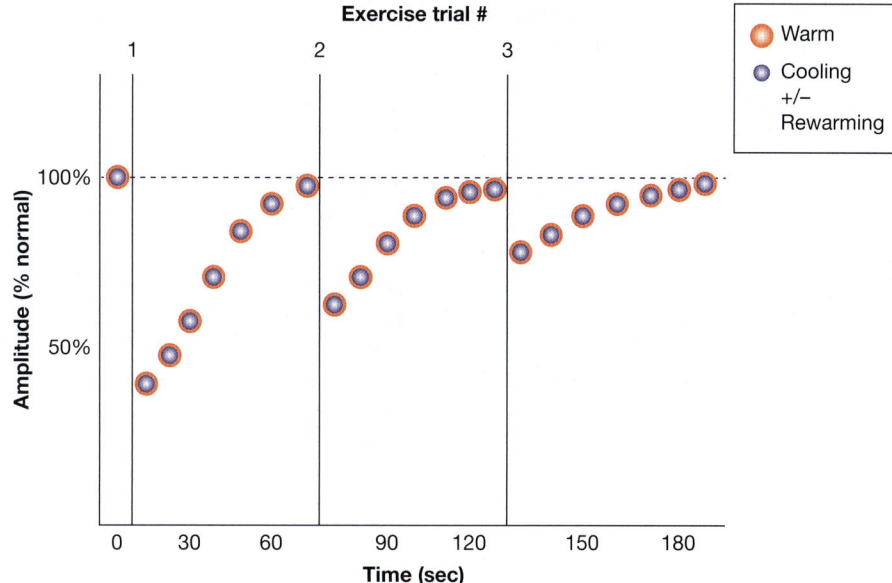

Figure 2-14. Short-exercise test—type 2 pattern—recessive inheritance.

of individuals with MC. Myotonic discharges with EMG are found in essentially all patients with MC.

The *type 2* pattern is seen predominantly in patients with MC but has been identified in sodium channel mutations associated with PAM, hyperKPP with myotonia, and both myotonic muscular dystrophy types 1 and 2.[33,35] In myotonic muscular dystrophy, the short-exercise testing with and without cooling produces a similar pattern of lesser magnitude than recessively inherited MC. Long-exercise testing in MC patients produces a pattern indistinguishable from controls.

Short-exercise testing in PMC produces a different configuration. There is little or no decrement in CMAP amplitude and area immediately following exercise. With the subsequent six stimuli, however, the amplitude increasingly declines, providing a curve with a negative rather than positive slope. The magnitude of this response becomes more dramatic in the second and third trials. In this *type 1* pattern, the most dramatic effect occurs following limb cooling, or rewarming following cooling.[33,35] Although the configuration of the curves remains the same, the magnitude of CMAP amplitude and/or area decrement is even more dramatic. A CMAP amplitude and area decrement of >20% in response to cooling with or without rewarming is thought to be pathognomonic of PMC (Fig. 2-16).[35]

PEMPs in response to single or repetitive stimuli following brief exercise are found in essentially all PMC patients.

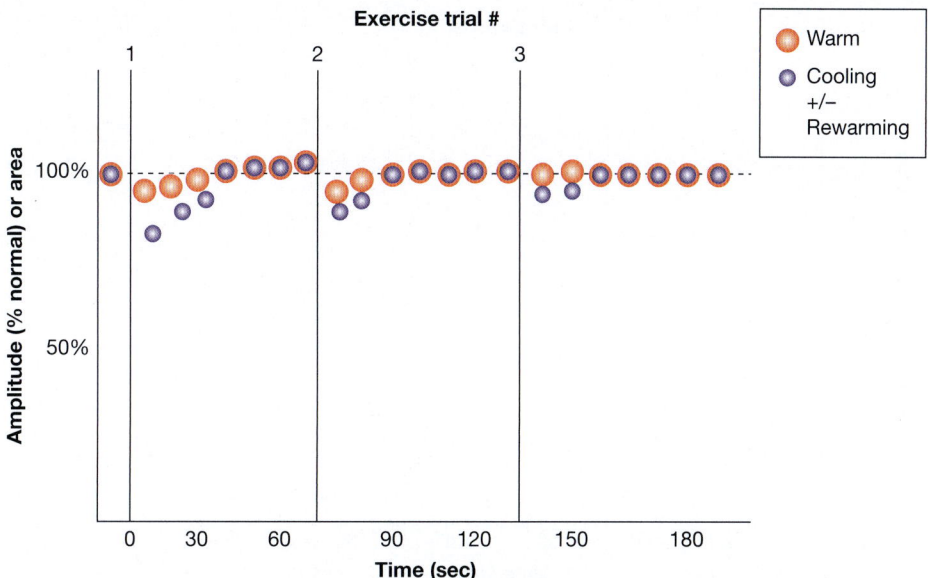

Figure 2-15. Short-exercise test—type 2 pattern—dominant inheritance.

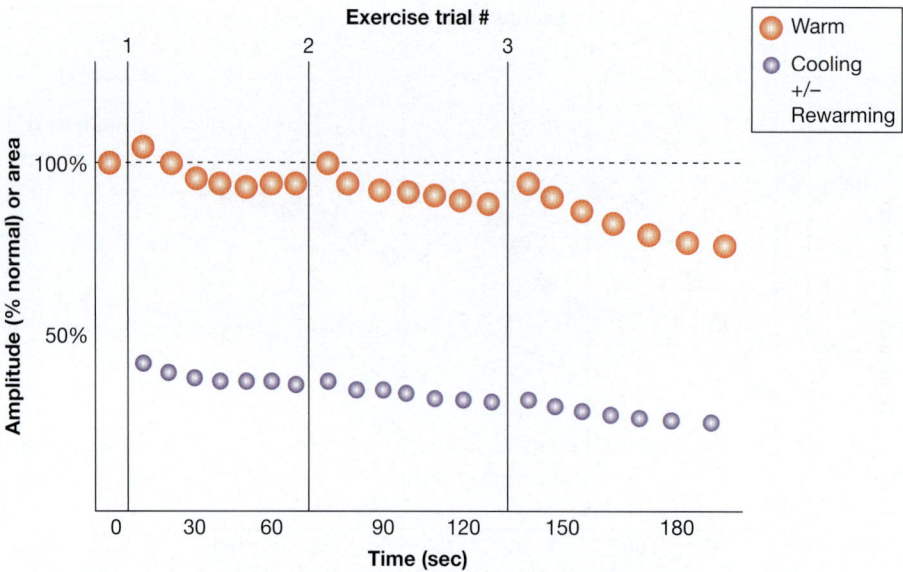

Figure 2-16. Short-exercise test—type 1 pattern.

They dissipate both within an individual trial and between subsequent short-exercise trials. Pattern 1 has been exclusively associated with the PMC phenotypes/genotypes to date. The result of long-exercise testing in PMC also differs considerably from MC. A significant and persistent CMAP amplitude and area decrement occurs averaging a 66% reduction in comparison to baseline. The clinical weakness associated with the long-exercise test may preclude its completion. Myotonic discharges with EMG are anticipated in patients with PMC.

One specific sodium channel gene mutation resulting in the PMC phenotype (Q270 K) has an apparent unique short-exercise test signature.[34] Short-exercise testing without cooling demonstrates a *type 2* pattern essentially identical to that seen in MC, that is, an initial CMAP amplitude and/or area decrement immediately postexercise that improves within the first trial and then between subsequent trials. After limb cooling, the pattern reverts to approximate the type 1 pattern typically seen in PMC, that is CMAP amplitudes and/or areas decrement with a downward slope within the first trial that worsens with each of the subsequent two trials.

In most PAM and other myotonia/periodic paralysis syndromes associated with other sodium channel mutations, short-exercise testing is essentially normal although cold-induced reduction in CMAP amplitudes has been described in at least two genotypes.[34] PEMPs are rarely described in PAM and the SCMs, disorders that clinically overlap PMC and MC.[33-35] There is no significant CMAP amplitude and area decrement with short exercise, either prior to or subsequent to limb cooling. This has been referred to as the *type 3* pattern (Fig. 2-17). No significant change in CMAP amplitude or area

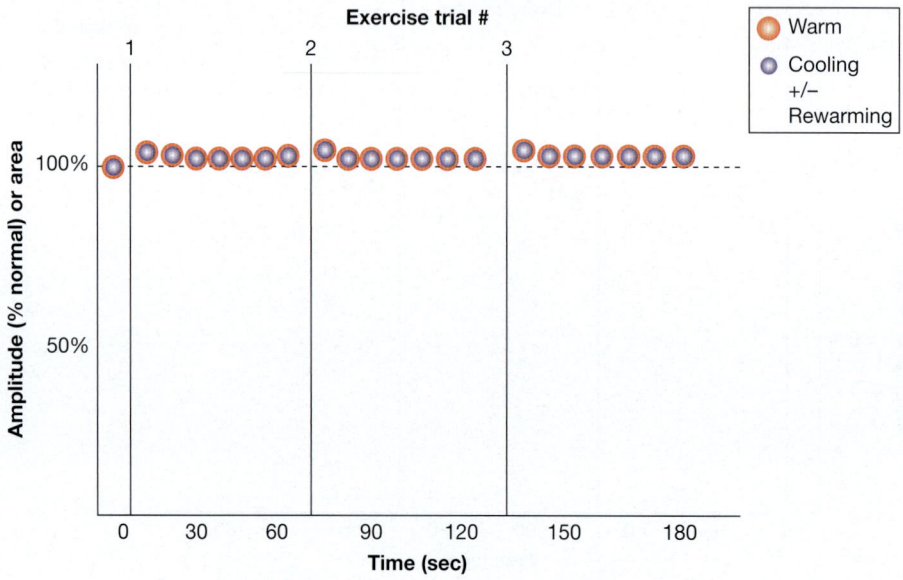

Figure 2-17. Short-exercise test—type 3 pattern.

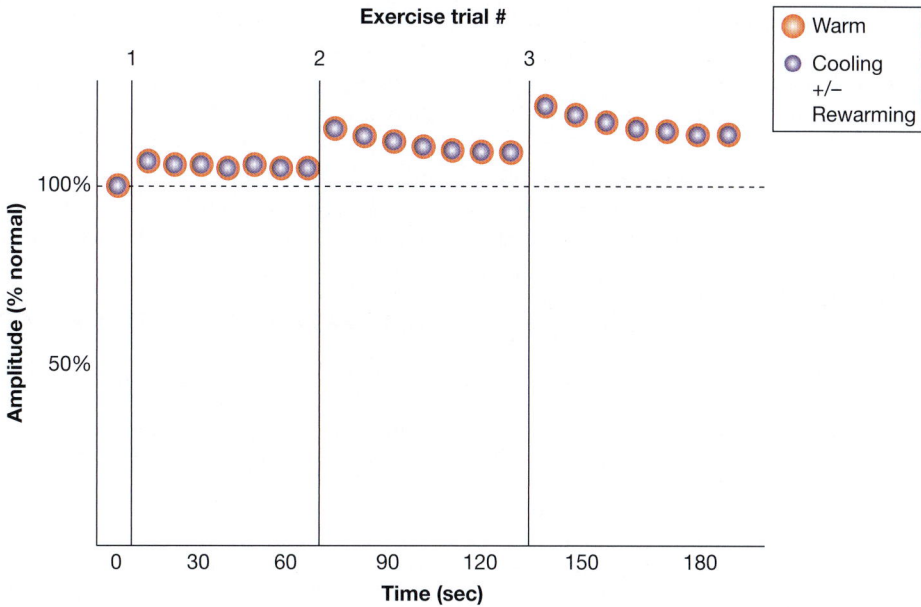

Figure 2-18. Short-exercise testing—type 4 pattern.

is seen in response to long-exercise testing in PAM. Myotonic discharges with EMG are anticipated in these disorders.

In hyperKPP, different authors describe different short-exercise test results. Fournier et al. describe an immediate CMAP amplitude and area increment that exceeds that seen in controls both in amplitude and in duration of effect (Fig. 2-18).[33] It persists throughout the entire minute of the study. With repetitive trials of short exercise, the CMAP amplitude and area increments in comparison to baseline by an average of 64%.[33] According to Tan et al., however, short-exercise testing does not differ from normal in either hyper-KPP or hypoKPP-1 patients.[35]

Distinguishing between hyperKPP and hypoKPP electrophysiologically may be either relatively easy or hard depending on the response to short-exercise testing and the presence or absence of myotonic discharges. According to Fournier and colleagues, the *type 4* pattern is characteristic of hyperKPP or some hypoKPP-2 patients (Fig. 2-19). It is defined by occasional myotonic discharges in some hyper-KPP patients, an absence of PEMPs, an incremental CMAP amplitude pattern in short-exercise testing as described in the previous paragraph, and the long slow decrement in response to long-exercise testing.[33] A decrement of at least 40% of CMAP amplitude and area with long-exercise testing is found

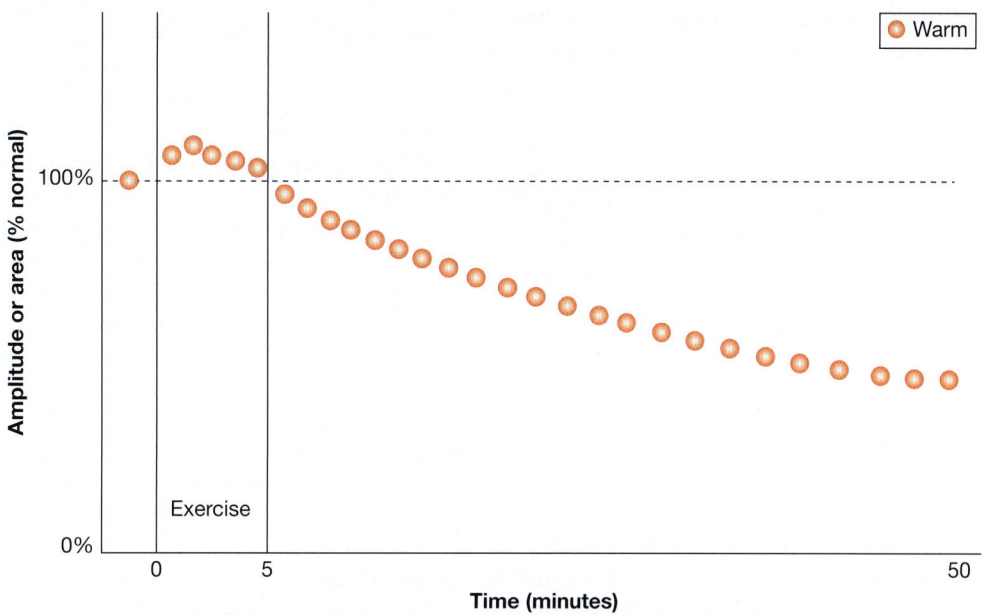

Figure 2-19. Long-exercise testing—type 4 or 5 pattern.

in a majority of periodic paralysis patients and may be seen in Andersen–Tawil syndrome patients as well.[21] The mean time to reach an abnormal decrement in periodic paralysis is approximately 25 minutes but may take the full 50 minutes of the test to appear, or perhaps even longer in hypoKPP-2.[35] The *type 5* pattern is the typical signature of hypoKPP-1 or occasional hypoKPP-2 patients (Fig. 2-19).[33] Neither myotonic discharges nor PEMPs are seen. The short-exercise test is normal, and the long-exercise test demonstrates the same slowly developing decremental pattern that is seen in the type 4 pattern.[33]

Motor Unit Number Estimates

Considerable loss of motor units may occur without clinically evident weakness. This is particularly true in slowly progressive disorders where collateral sprouting and reinnervation are at least partially compensatory. In patients with ALS, it has been shown that the CMAP amplitude may not reliably decline until the estimated number of motor units drops below 10% of normal.[37] Numerous motor unit number estimation (MUNE) techniques have been developed in an attempt to count the number of viable motor units in a given muscle.[38] This has been done with the belief that MUNE would represent a more accurate means to monitor disease course or to detect a response to treatment than measurements of strength. All techniques attempt to estimate motor unit number by estimating the average size of the amplitude generated by a single motor unit and then dividing this number into the maximal CMAP amplitude for the entire muscle.

MUNE is, in large part, a research technique, with limited application in the daily practice of neuromuscular disease. It can be time-consuming and, with some techniques, technically challenging due to unstable neuromuscular transmission that may occur with reinnervation. Unlike standard EDX techniques, which can offer a panoramic perspective on multiple nerves and multiple muscles, MUNE is typically done on one or at most a limited number of nerves in a single setting. In addition, individual techniques have their limitations including the nerve/muscle pairs that are accessible to them.[38] MUNE has probably been most frequently used in the ALS population and has been successfully utilized in at least two clinical trials.[39–41] Multiple authors have demonstrated that MUNE declines and the size of individual MUPs increases sequentially in patients with ALS, consistent with our understanding of the denervating/reinnervating process.[37,40–44]

NEEDLE EMG

Needle EMG is performed by inserting a recording electrode into muscle and assessing the electrical waveforms both at rest and with voluntary muscle activation. EMG is interpreted by determining the type of abnormality within a specific muscle, identifying the pattern of muscles in which those abnormalities occur, and then correlating these results with those of NCS as well as the clinical context. Muscles are typically evaluated under three conditions: at rest assessing insertional and spontaneous activity, with minimal voluntary activation assessing motor unit action potential (MUAP) morphology and stability, and with a gradual increase in muscle activation assessing MUAP recruitment.

Insertional and Spontaneous Activity

Spontaneous activity and insertional activity are similar but not synonymous concepts. Insertional activity refers to the immediate response to needle movement. A brief burst of insertional activity occurring with each needle movement within viable muscle is how the examiner is certain that they are in muscle. Increased insertion can refer to a protracted and nonspecific response to needle movement seen immediately after axon loss as a harbinger of the abnormal spontaneous activity in the form of positive waves and fibrillation potentials in muscles tested early after nerve injury. Abnormal spontaneous activity such as complex repetitive and myotonic discharges are often triggered by needle insertion. In disease, and in numerous other situations, increased insertional and abnormal spontaneous activities occur together.

Spontaneous activity refers to activity that occurs independently of needle movement. It may occur with or without a provoking needle movement but is sustained long after any provoking stimulus ceases. To further emphasize the subtle, but meaningful differences in the terminology, it is possible to have a situation in which there is increased spontaneous activity in the setting of decreased insertional activity, a concept that at first glance may seem counterintuitive. For example, it is not uncommon to experience this scenario while studying intrinsic foot muscles in patients with chronic polyneuropathies. There is often reduced insertional activity, presumably due to replacement of viable muscle by connective tissue. By the same token, there are isolated areas in that muscle where fibrillation potentials can be found, presumably representing isolated, viable, and nonreinnervated muscle fibers.

Some forms of spontaneous activity are normal. End-plate spikes and end-plate noise represent miniature EPPs and are seen in normal muscles at rest when the needle is in proximity to the motor endplate. In contrast, there are several abnormal waveforms that may occur in an abnormal muscle at rest. These include fibrillation potentials, positive sharp waves, cramp potentials, myokymic discharges, myotonic discharges, complex repetitive discharges, and neuromyotonic discharges (Figs. 2-20 to 2-24). Of these, fibrillation potentials and positive sharp waves are the most prevalent (Fig. 2-20). They are recognized by their metronomic and regular firing pattern. When present, these suggest that anatomic continuity has been lost between a muscle fiber and its innervating axon. Fibrillation potentials and positive waves

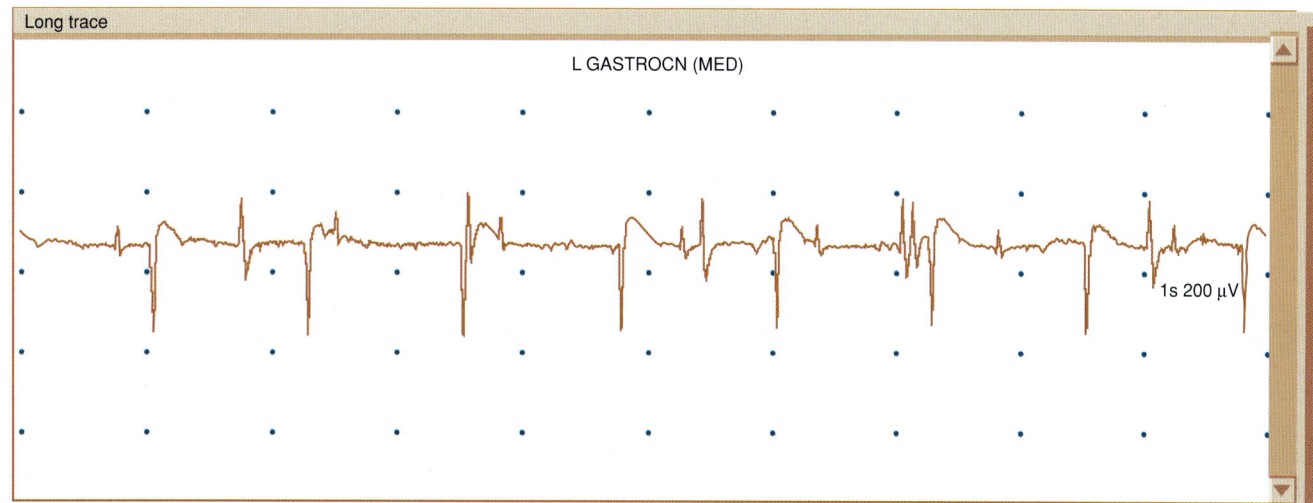

Figure 2-20. Fibrillation potentials and positive waves—single action potentials that usually fire with metronomic frequency; fibrillation potentials have short duration, positive waves with characteristic configuration, and longer duration. The sound produced by fibrillations can be described as a "ticking." Positive waves have a more nonspecific, duller sound than fibrillation potentials, with recognition based more on their firing pattern and characteristic shape. These waveforms may occur in isolation or concurrently as in this figure.

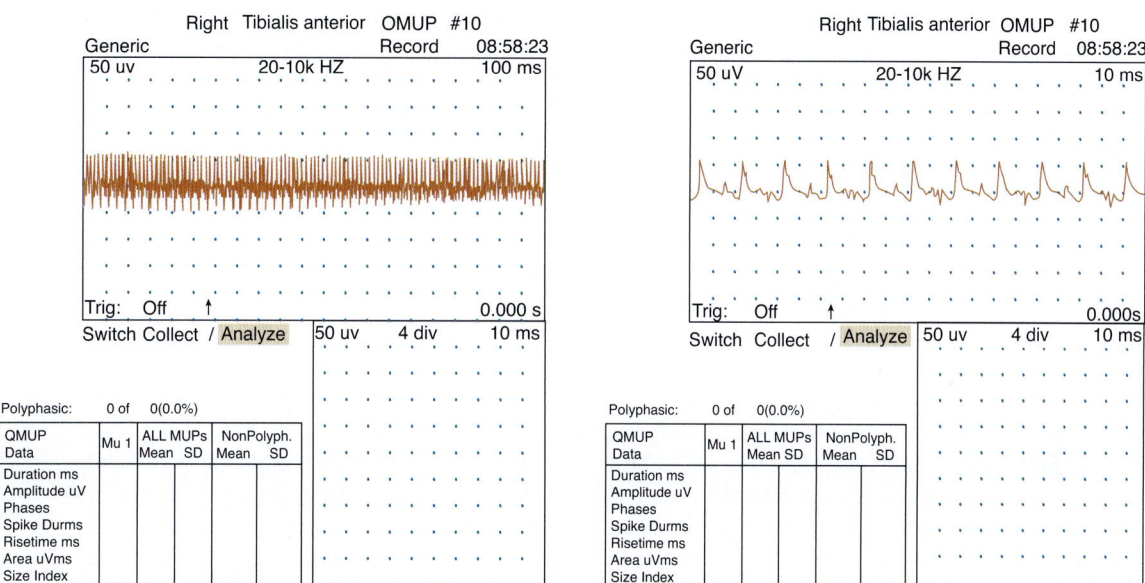

Figure 2-21. Complex repetitive discharges—a discharge with abrupt onset and cessation, the sound produced frequently described as "machinery like."

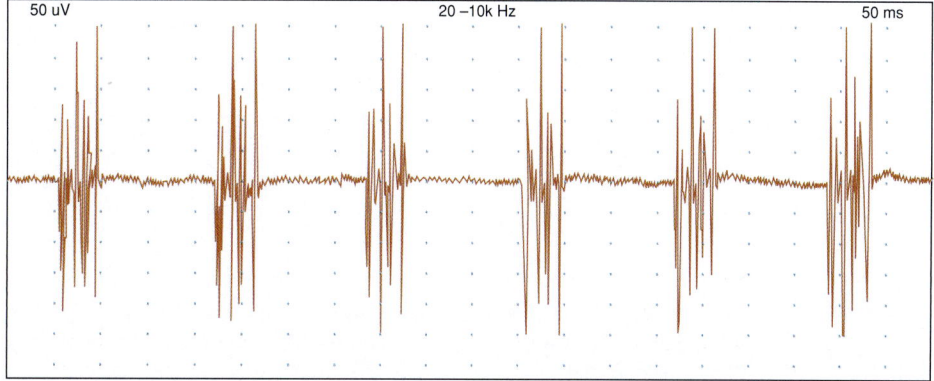

Figure 2-22. Myokymic discharges—semirhythmic grouped discharges, the sound produced frequently likened to the troops marching. (Used with permission of Dr. Devon Rubin, Mayo Clinic, Jacksonville.)

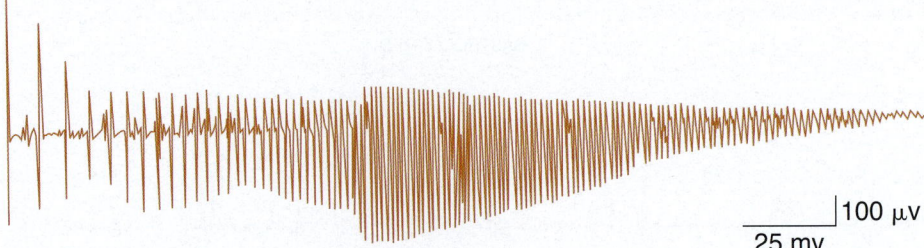

Figure 2-23. Myotonic discharges—with variable waveform amplitude and frequency, producing a waxing and waning discharge likened to an accelerating and decelerating chain saw or motorbike motor.

occur most commonly from denervation in association with axon loss at any location from anterior horn cell to terminal twig (Table 2-2). They do not occur in demyelinating neuropathies in the absence of axon loss.

Fibrillation potentials and positive waves are not, however, specific for axon loss (Table 2-2). They may be observed in both DNMT and certain muscle diseases. In the former, the axon may be effectively separated from its target muscle by ablation of the neuromuscular junction. In myopathy, particularly those associated with the pathologic features of segmental necrosis of muscle or fiber splitting, viable segments of muscle may be separated from segment of muscle containing the neuromuscular junction. By doing so, the myopathic process has effectively denervated segments of viable muscle. There are several myopathies, notably the channelopathies, and some of the congenital and mitochondrial myopathies, where these forms of abnormal spontaneous activity occur without clear explanation of the denervating mechanism. Presumably, muscle membrane instability provides an alternative explanation for this form of waveform generation.

Other forms of abnormal spontaneous activity are less common. As some of these discharges have clinical concomitants that go by the same name, this text will follow the convention used by others. The clinical observation will be referred to by the name alone, for example, fasciculation whereas the waveform will be referred to as a potential or discharge, for example, fasciculation potential. Complex repetitive discharges are nonspecific and occur in both chronic nerve and muscle disorders (Fig. 2-22). Although usually considered an indication of nerve or muscle pathology, current thinking suggests that they may be occasionally identified as a normal finding in both the biceps and more commonly, the iliopsoas muscles. Complex repetitive discharges have a machinery-like sound that typically starts and stops abruptly. Whether related to nerve or muscle disease, they are thought to originate from a reverberating circuit that develops within contiguous myofibers. Complex repetitive discharges are typically unassociated with any observable clinical concomitant.

Myotonic discharges also appear to originate from muscle and are primarily associated with heritable muscle disease (Fig. 2-23). These produce a waxing and waning sound historically likened to a dive bomber. From a more contemporary perspective, a revving chain saw or motor bike may represent a more apt simile. Myotonic discharges do not sustain themselves and typically dissipate until such time that they are provoked by the next needle movement or muscle contraction. Their presence often obscures the ability to adequately study MUAPs or assess other forms of abnormal spontaneous activity. Myotonic discharges are the major EDX signature of myotonic muscular dystrophies, (particularly DM1) the nondystrophic myotonias associated with chloride and certain sodium channel disorders, and in some patients with hyperKPP. These are also seen in certain glycogen storage disorders, most notably Pompe disease, branching and debranching enzyme deficiencies, myofibrillar myopathy,

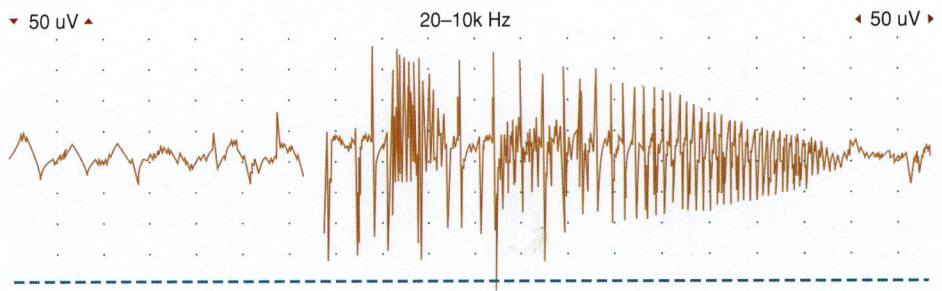

Figure 2-24. Neuromyotonic discharges—very high-pitched discharges with sound likened to "screaming Formula One race car" engine. (Used with permission of Dr. Devon Rubin, Mayo Clinic, Jacksonville.)

TABLE 2-2. DISORDERS ASSOCIATED WITH POSITIVE WAVES AND FIBRILLATION POTENTIALS

Site	Type	Examples
Anterior horn	Axon loss	ALS, SMA, poliomyelitis, syringomyelia, spinal cord infarction
Ventral root	Axon loss	Spinal stenosis, neoplastic meningitis
Plexus	Axon loss	Trauma, tumor, plexitis, diabetic radiculoplexopathy
Peripheral Nerve	Axon loss	Toxic, metabolic, hereditary, entrapment, and compression
NMJ	Presynaptic	Botulism, LEMS[a]
	Postsynaptic	Autoimmune myasthenia gravis
Muscle	Inflammatory	Dermatomyositis, necrotizing, polymyositis, antisynthetase syndrome, inclusion body myositis
	Infiltrative	Amyloidosis, sarcoidosis
	Dystrophic	Dystrophinopathy, limb-girdle, myotonic dystrophy and other channelopathies
	Toxic	Cholesterol-lowering agents, chloroquine
	Sporadic late-onset nemaline myopathy	Antisignal recognizing protein, anti-HMCCR m
	Inherited metabolic	Some glycogen and lipid storage myopathies
	Congenital myopathies (certain)	Myotubular myopathy, Nemaline
	Infectious	HIV, other viral, trichinosis

Fournier E, Arzel M, Sternberg D, et al. Electromyography guides toward subgroups of mutations in muscle channelopathies. *Ann Neurol.* 2004;56(5):650–661.

and occasionally in toxic and inflammatory myopathies (Table 2-3). Myotonic discharges are not clinically observable but are commonly associated with muscle stiffness.

Other forms of abnormal spontaneous activity appear to be generated by nerve such as fasciculations potentials and myokymic and neuromyotonic discharges. All of them can be conceptualized as part of nerve hyperexcitability spectrum disorders. Fasciculation potentials are singular, spontaneous discharges of single MUPs that represent the electrophysiologic correlate of the fasciculations that can often be seen while observing the muscle with the naked eye. They can be seemingly benign (or at least associated with subclinical pathology) or associated with any one of several

TABLE 2-3. DISORDERS ASSOCIATED WITH MYOTONIC DISCHARGES

Myotonic muscular dystrophy types 1 and 2
Myotonia congenita
Paramyotonia congenita
Other nondystrophic myotonias, e.g., potassium-aggravated myotonia
Hyperkalemic periodic paralysis
Azacholesterol
Monocarboxylic acids
Colchicine myopathy
Cholesterol-lowering agent myopathy
Hypothyroidism
Inflammatory myopathies
Pompe disease
Branching enzyme deficiency myopathy
Debranching enzyme deficiency myopathy
Hereditary vacuolar myopathies (Danon disease and X-linked myopathy with excessive autophagy)
Myofibrillar myopathy and other distal myopathies with rimmed vacuoles

nerve diseases. They are most closely linked and probably most seen in anterior horn cell diseases. Numerous authors have attempted to identify the morphologic or behavioral characteristics of fasciculation potentials that would distinguish benign from more ominous forms. There have been recent publications that promote the concept that complex and unstable fasciculation potentials correlate with pathology and can be used as a surrogate marker for fibrillation potentials and positive waves in the electrodiagnostic evaluation of ALS patients.[45–47] Ironically, a contributing author to one of these papers has studied fasciculation potentials and has concluded that there are no characteristics that confidently allow the distinction of benign from pathologic fasciculations.[48] The ability to observe clinical fasciculations, in association with fasciculation potentials, is undoubtedly related to the thickness of subcutaneous tissue, the depth of the muscle, and whether the fasciculations arise from superficially placed motor units within that muscle.

Cramp potentials are groups of spontaneously firing, otherwise normal MUPs that discharge in a sputtering pattern, typically with abrupt onset and cessation. Like fasciculations, they are typically neurogenic in origin and may have either a benign or pathologic significance. They are commonly found in chronic neuropathic conditions such as motor neuron diseases, radiculopathy, or polyneuropathy but can occur in any of the nerve hyperexcitability syndromes discussed subsequently in the following paragraphs on myokymic and neuromyotonic discharges or in some metabolic disturbances including uremia and hypothyroidism. Cramp potentials are typically associated with clinical cramping.

Myokymic discharges are grouped discharges of two or more MUPs that fire repeatedly in a semirhythmic manner with interval gaps of electrical silence. The intraburst frequency is between 40 and 150 Hz. The sound produced has been likened to troops marching. These probably result

TABLE 2-4. DISORDERS ASSOCIATED WITH MYOKYMIC DISCHARGES

Location	Disorder
Facial muscles	Multiple sclerosis Brainstem glioma Guillain–Barré syndrome Bells palsy Head and neck radiation
Limb muscles	Radiation Chronic nerve compression, e.g., CTS Isaacs syndrome and its differential diagnosis (see Table 2-5)

Fournier E, Arzel M, Sternberg D, et al. Electromyography guides toward subgroups of mutations in muscle channelopathies. *Ann Neurol.* 2004;56(5):650–661.

TABLE 2-5. DISORDERS ASSOCIATED WITH NEUROMYOTONIC DISCHARGES

Acquired	Isaacs or Morvan syndrome Cramp-fasciculation syndrome Paraneoplastic (thymoma, thyroid carcinoma) Multifocal motor neuropathy IgM kappa paraproteinemic neuropathy Diabetic neuropathy Copper deficiency Creutzfeld–Jakob disease Intraoperative nerve irritation Anticholinesterase poisoning Timber rattlesnake envenomation Radiation
Hereditary	Charcot–Marie–Tooth disease (e.g., HINT1 mutations) ALS (rare) Spinal muscular atrophy (rare)

Oaklander AL, Nolano M. Scientific advances in and clinical approaches to small-fiber polyneuropathy: A review. *JAMA Neurol.* 2019;76:1240–1251; Gruis KL, Little AA, Zebarah V, Albers JW. Survey of electrodiagnostic laboratories regarding hemorrhagic complications from needle electromyography. *Muscle Nerve.* 2006;34(3):356–358.

from ephaptic transmission between injured, contiguous axons. Myokymic discharges can be seen in several disorders (Fig. 2-21 and Table 2-4). These may be associated with disorders as mundane as CTS or as unusual as rattlesnake envenomation. Myokymic discharges involving cranial musculature can be seen in multiple sclerosis, GBS, and brainstem neoplasms. These are common in disorders of neural overactivity such as the cramp-fasciculation syndrome and Isaacs syndrome. Myokymic discharges are most commonly associated with radiation-induced nerve injury. Myokymic discharges may or may not be associated with the recognition of clinical myokymia.

Neuromyotonic discharges are infrequently seen (Fig. 2-24). They are commonly associated with other waveforms such as myokymic discharges, cramp discharges, and fasciculation potentials that occur in disorders of neural hyperexcitability. Their duration is brief as their high frequency (150–300 Hz) precludes them from sustaining themselves for protracted periods. Their sound has been likened to the scream of a formula-one race car engine. These are most closely linked to the disorder known by the names neuromyotonia, Isaacs syndrome, or the syndrome of continuous muscle fiber activity. Neuromyotonic discharges are nonspecific and may be associated with a number of neurogenic disorders, some of which are paraneoplastic (Table 2-5). Although initially some of these cases were attributed to antibodies directed against voltage-gated potassium channels (VGKCs), subsequent studies have revealed that these antibodies actually are specifically directed against Caspr2 and LGL1.[29–31] An analogous discharge, the neurotonic discharge, may be recorded from muscles during intraoperative monitoring, particularly with acoustic nerve surgery, as a means of detecting potential injury to the facial nerve.

Motor Unit Action Potential Analysis

The purpose of examining the muscle with minimal levels of voluntary activation is to assess the morphology and stability of individual MUAPs. The motor unit consists of an anterior horn cell, its axon, and all the muscle fibers it innervates. The MUAP refers to the collection of all single fiber action potentials arising from the muscle fibers of that motor unit that are within the recording radius of the needle. MUAPs become smaller when there is a loss or physiologic nonparticipation of muscle fibers within the motor unit. This typically occurs in disorders of muscle and neuromuscular transmission. In the former, the number of fibers within the motor unit decreases because of myofiber degeneration. Additionally, the size of the action potential that each fiber generates decreases because of myofiber atrophy. In DNMT, the amplitude and/or duration of the MUAP may decrease from blockade of neuromuscular transmission, physiologically reducing the number of SFMAPs contributing to that MUAP.

Conversely, MUAPs typically become larger following chronic denervation and reinnervation typically occurring between 3 and 6 months after disease onset. An orphaned muscle fiber deprived of its axon supply may be reinnervated by a collateral nerve twig belonging to a neighboring viable motor unit. As a result, surviving motor units in the aftermath of axon loss will typically grow both in amplitude and in duration.

Normal values for both amplitude and duration are available but vary depending on patient age and the muscle studied. In general, most MUAPs in most limb muscles are between 8 and 15 μs in duration and less than 2 mV in amplitude. MUAP morphology does not change in a substantive manner in a purely demyelinating nerve disorder, although both increased duration and polyphasia may result from variable conduction slowing in terminal nerve twigs.

MUAPs typically have triphasic configurations, although occasional MUAPs with a few extra turns or phases are common. Polyphasic or serrated MUAP morphology implies that the individual SFMAP components of that MUAP have become desynchronized. Satellite potentials, that is, waveforms that are separate from but time-locked to the primary

MUAP waveform, are considered as a subtype of polyphasia. An abundance of polyphasic MUAPs implies that the process, if monophasic is subacute, that is, of weeks to months duration. Polyphasic MUAPs have no etiologic specificity and can be seen in myopathies, axon loss, and demyelinating nerve disease. Polyphasic motor units will eventually reconfigure themselves into a triphasic configuration, even in those MUAPs that have been exceptionally enlarged in remote denervating and reinnervating disease such as polio.

The concepts outlined in the preceding three paragraphs are generally accurate but have exceptions. Large motor units reminiscent of reinnervation following denervation occur in chronic myopathies, particularly inclusion body myositis.[49,50] Long-duration MUAPs in myopathy are possibly related to muscle fiber splitting and increased separation of muscle fibers due to endomysial fibrosis. Conversely, small MUAPs, referred to as nascent units, are seen in complete axonopathies in which there is subsequent sprouting from the site of the injured nerve to previously denervated atrophic muscle fibers.[51] Small MUAPs also be seen in rapidly evolving denervating disorders in which degeneration of terminal twigs occurs early in the disease course effective reinnervation does not occur. The familial form of ALS associated with the A4V mutation of the SOD1 gene is perhaps the most notable example of this latter mechanism. In either case, small motor units from nerve and muscle diseases are most readily distinguished from one another by their characteristic decreased and increased recruitment patterns respectively as described below.

MUAP variability or instability refers to the alteration of MUAP morphology on consecutive discharges (Fig. 2-25). Under normal circumstances, every single fiber action potential within a given motor unit discharge in a near-concordant fashion. Thus, as long as the needle position is stable, the MUAP will have an identical configuration each time it discharges. With disordered neuromuscular transmission of any cause, transmission at one or more individual neuromuscular junctions may be delayed or fail. As this is a physiologic rather than a direct structural effect, this provides a dynamic process affecting different neuromuscular junctions variably with consecutive discharges. As a result, the configuration of the MUAP may change quite dramatically with consecutive discharges. Variability of amplitude is best demonstrated by having the patient minimally activate the muscle being tested in order to isolate an individual MUAP, while using slow sweep speeds (50–100 ms/division) and high settings on low-frequency filters, similar to what is deployed in SFEMG. This allows the examiner to visualize the same MUAP multiple times on the same screen. MUAP variability is most closely associated with DNMT. It can often be seen, however, in early reinnervation where neuromuscular junctions are immature. Traumatic nerve injury and ALS are notable examples.[51]

Motor Unit Action Potential Recruitment

MUAP recruitment is the last component of the needle examination and perhaps the most difficult to understand and a major reason for misinterpretation of EMG studies. Assessment of MUAP recruitment is not just based on determining how many MUAPs are firing but more importantly how fast individual MUAPs fire when additional units are activated.[7] This is done by having the patient gradually increase the amount of isometric resistance in the muscle being tested. Under normal circumstances, an increasing number of MUAPs will be recruited, which is seen and heard on the EMG machine display. There is a "rule of 5s" by which MUAPs are normally recruited. The "onset frequency" is how fast the first MUAP starts firing and is generally around 5 Hz (in reality closer to 7 Hz). When the patient is asked to activate their muscle a little more, the first unit fires faster and generally around 10 Hz, what is termed the "recruitment onset," a second unit begins firing (again at around 5–7 Hz). As patient activates more and the first unit fires at 15 Hz, the second at 10 Hz, the third unit kicks in at 5–7 Hz. "Reduced recruitment" is when the recruitment onset is >15 (i.e., an individual MUAP is firing at >15 Hz before a second unit is activated). Another way to quantify recruitment is by the recruitment ratio: the mean firing rate of the individual MUAPs divided by the number of MUAPs. So, if one unit is firing at 15 Hz, the second at 10 Hz, and the third at 5 Hz, the mean firing rate is 5 and that divided by 3 would give a recruitment ratio of 3.3. The recruitment ratio is clearly abnormal when >10.

In neurogenic disorders including motor neuron disease, axonal neuropathies, and demyelinating neuropathies with conduction block, there are a reduced number of MUAPs that can be recruited. As a result, the remaining activatable MUAPs that fire do so with a greater frequency than normal to compensate for MUAP loss leading to reduced recruitment. Reduced recruitment is one cause of a reduced

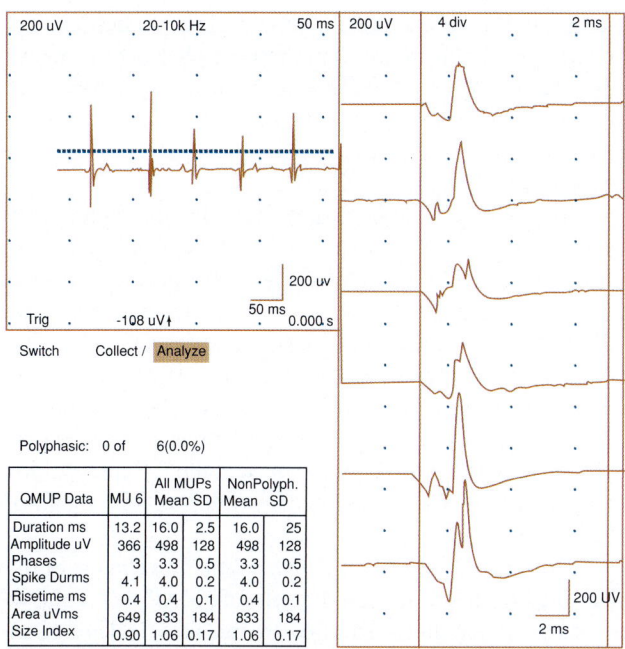

Figure 2-25. Motor unit potential (MUP) variability.

interference pattern. Again, these are two terms that are related, but not synonymous. A reduced interference pattern may also occur because of a patient's inability or unwillingness to fully activate all MUAPs at their disposal due to disorders of the CNS, pain, or malingering. In this case, there may only be a few MUAPs firing, but they are firing at a normal rate. This is not reduced recruitment, but rather reduced or central activation. This is again a common source of erroneous interpretation of EMG findings when a few units are activity but fire at a normal rate but are wrongly interpreted as reduced recruitment.

Many strategies are utilized to quantitate MUAP loss. Reduced recruitment can be estimated by training one's ear to detect MUAPs firing at rates that are excessive. The ear is quite sensitive in its ability to detect rapidly firing MUAPs in response to motor unit loss. Many electromyographers can accurately estimate the firing frequency of an MUAP to within 2 Hz, certainly within 5 Hz. With full recruitment resulting in a full interference pattern, there will be an amorphous blending of the sound created by all activated motor units. With reduced recruitment, rapidly firing individual MUAPs can be detected by hearing the distinctive sound that each MUAP firing at an accelerated pace produces. This effect has been likened to the sound produced by a baseball card placed in the spokes of a child's moving bicycle wheel. This can be done at very low levels of recruitment by estimating the firing frequency of the first MUAP when the second MUAP is recruited, and the firing frequency of the second MUAP when the third MUAP is recruited and so on. Hearing MUAP firing faster than this is an accurate indicator of axon loss or demyelinating conduction block.

In myopathies or DNMT, the problem is not a reduced number of motor units but reduced MUAP size. As the amount of force generated by individual MUAPs is often reduced, more motor units need to be recruited earlier than normal to generate the same amount of force. The firing rates of these MUAPs remain normal. This effect has been termed as early or increased recruitment. As determination of early recruitment is somewhat subjective and depends on an experienced examiner estimating in their own minds how many MUAPs should be firing at any given sense of the power generated by the muscle movement by the patient, it is less reliable and is usually not recognized until other EDX features of muscle disease or DNMT are evident.

Single Fiber Electromyography and Other Specialized Techniques of Motor Unit Analysis

Single fiber electromyography (SFEMG) is primarily used to enhance the sensitivity of DNMT testing. Unfortunately, what is gained in sensitivity is often lost in specificity. For this reason, its greatest utility lies in its ability to discriminate between subtle presentations of DNMT from nonneuromuscular diseases. It is limited in its ability to distinguish one neuromuscular disorder from another. However, large jitter values associated with frequent neuromuscular blocking is more likely to represent a DNMT than in diseases of the anterior horn cell, nerve, or muscle.

The basic goal of SFEMG is to capture and analyze two or more SFMAP belonging to the same MUAP. To do so, it is necessary to limit MUAP recruitment to be able to see, hear, and cleanly record these SFMAPs. In cooperative patients, this can be accomplished on a voluntary basis. In patients who are unable to activate a limited number of MUAPs and maintain a stable level of recruitment for any reason, stimulated SFEMG, as described below, may well represent a better option. Historically, there are two significant technical differences between SFEMG and standard EMG recordings. Both involve limiting the recording radius of the needle to facilitate SFMAP acquisition and analysis. Limiting the recording radius involves increasing the low-frequency (high-pass) filter setting to 500 Hz. The second means to limit the recording radius is to use a special SFEMG needle whose recording radius is smaller than its concentric or monopolar counterparts. In part due to the cost and inconvenience involved in the use of SFEMG needles, that require both repeated sterilization and sharpening, electromyographers are now utilizing standard, disposable concentric EMG needles. Normative jitter data for concentric needles are approximately 5 µs less at any given age for any given muscle, in comparison to published norms using SFEMG needles.

The primary parameter measured by SFEMG is jitter which represents the variation in the interval between two SFMAPs belonging to the same MUAP. Jitter is a property of normal neuromuscular transmission. Its physiologic basis is derived from the variable nature of the EPP as was described in the section on RNS. The key to understanding the origin of jitter is the knowledge that the slope of the rise in membrane potential that occurs between the resting membrane potential and action potential threshold is proportionate to the amplitude of the EPP. In other words, the higher the EPP, the steeper the slope and the shorter the interval between the inciting nerve and the resulting muscle fiber action potential. As a result, the interval between consecutive discharges of two SFMAPs belonging to the same motor unit will fluctuate with the normal variation in quantal ACH release and resultant EPP amplitude and slope.

In practice, two (or more) SFMAPs are captured by using a triggered delay line. To do so, the electrodiagnostician will carefully manipulate the EMG needle until it is within an acceptable recording distance from at least one SFMAP. The optimal needle position is determined by listening for generation of the sharp, crisp sound that is generated by this proximity and then confirming the proximity by assuring that the rise time of the waveform is less than 300 µs with an amplitude that is greater than 200 µV. Typically, this is done with a sweep speed of 1 ms/division and a gain of 100–200 µV/division.

Once this SFMAP is isolated, subtle movements of the electrode are made to find a second SFMAP belonging to the same motor unit, identified by its "time-locked" characteristics. The interval between the two (or more) spikes should be far enough apart to be measurable but not farther than 4 ms, for purposes of measurement accuracy. Ideally, a steady, low level of contraction will allow the recording of a 100 consecutive discharges of this fiber pair. At least 50 of these 100 discharges must be captured to allow for accurate statistical analysis. Under normal circumstances, the waveforms representing the second of the two SFMAP waveforms will be nearly overlapping with each other but will not be perfectly superimposed. This variation between the first and fluctuating second single muscle fiber action potentials is the basis of normal jitter (Fig. 2-26). This variation in interpotential interval is usually expressed as the mean consecutive difference (MCD), a calculation readily computed by most contemporary EMG machines. The mean sorted difference (MSD) is also calculated and is a more accurate measure of jitter if the MCD/MSD ratio exceeds 1.25.

Assuming constant positioning of the needle in relation to the muscle fiber pair, there are five normal physiologic and anatomical factors that contribute to the interpotential interval: (1) the length of the terminal twigs, (2) the conduction velocity of the terminal twigs, (3) neuromuscular transmission time, (4) the distance between muscle fiber and recording needle, and (5) the velocity of muscle fiber action potential propagation. Of these, only three are physiologic and therefore potentially capable of varying from discharge to discharge. As long as the firing rate is kept relatively constant, and the interpotential interval does not exceed 4 ms, jitter occurs almost exclusively because of variable neuromuscular transmission time.

Normal values for jitter vary with patient age and the muscle selected but are typically in the 15–45-μs range. Twenty fiber pairs are usually acquired and analyzed to

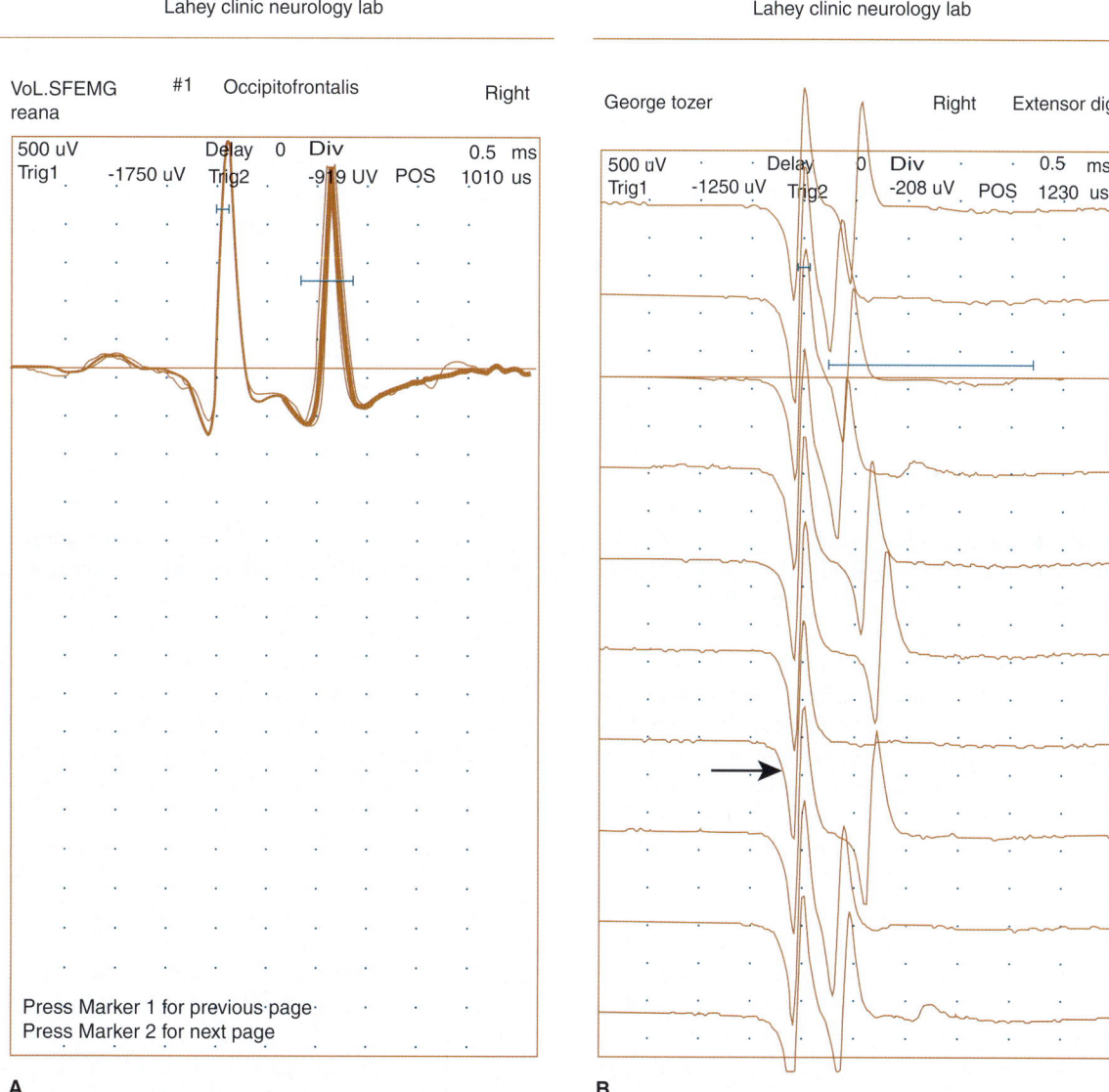

Figure 2-26. Single fiber electromyography demonstrating a normal recording (**A**) and increased jitter and blocking (seventh pair from top—*arrow*) (**B**).

provide adequate statistical significance. The need to acquire this amount of data stems from the observation that MG can be as patchy electrophysiologically as it is clinically. Abnormally high jitter values can also be declared if more than 10% or 2 of the 20 fiber pairs have jitter values that exceed a second higher set of normative values that are also age and muscle specific. The benefit of this second set of norms is that it allows this sometimes labor-intensive test to be terminated early when strikingly abnormal. Abnormally low jitter values are also potentially pathologic. For example, reduced jitter has been in disorders associated with myofiber splitting. Reduced jitter is uncommonly recognized, as disorders with reduced jitter values are uncommonly tested with this methodology.

The second parameter that is typically sought after is neuromuscular blocking. Blocking does not typically occur until jitter values are high, typically with MCD values in excess of 100 μs. Blocking is recognized when a triggering potential, identical in morphology to previous and successive triggering potentials, is unaccompanied by a second, time-locked SFMAP (Fig. 2-26). It is of course possible that the triggering potential itself is blocked, but it is likely that this occurrence would go unrecognized. Blocking rarely occurs in seemingly normal, older individuals.

Another parameter that can be measured by the SFEMG needle is fiber density, the electrophysiologic analog of reinnervation and type grouping seen on muscle biopsy. Fiber density is not as commonly used as a clinical tool as are assessments of jitter and blocking. Under normal circumstances, a random placement of the SFEMG needle will reveal only a single fiber action potential from a given motor unit 60% of the time. A couplet, that is, two SFMAPs belonging to the same motor unit will be identified in 35% of insertions and a triplet only 5% of the time. The technique for fiber density determination differs slightly from jitter measurements. The SFEMG needle is manipulated to obtain maximal amplitude from the first single fiber action potential that is obtained. Once that is accomplished, the number of single fiber potentials, regardless of size, that are time linked to the index potential are counted. This is done for at least an additional 19 potentials. The total number of fiber potentials is then divided by the number of test sites. For example, if 30 potentials are identified at 20 sites, the fiber density will be 1.5. Fiber density is considered an index of successful reinnervation and differs from jitter, which in denervating diseases is considered an index of immature reinnervation. Contrasting jitter values with fiber density values is one way to estimate how complete the reinnervation process is. High fiber density values with normal jitter are an indication that the reinnervation process has matured. Normative values for fiber density again vary with patient age and muscle selected and are based on measurements made with SFEMG needles.

Another form of SFEMG referred to as stimulated SFEMG. In this technique, small electrical stimuli are delivered by a needle electrode to a nearby nerve fiber within the tested muscle. Jitter is then recorded from a single muscle fiber innervated by the same nerve. There are both advantages and disadvantages of this technique. As it does not depend on voluntary muscle activation, it is more readily performed on those who cannot (or will not) cooperate. As the stimulus rate does not vary as opposed to voluntary activation, a spurious MCD value secondary to varying firing rates will not occur. The time-consuming effort of finding a fiber pair is removed from consideration. Drawbacks include the recognition that normal values for jitter are less than those with voluntary SFEMG. The optimal frequency of stimulation must be adjusted to ensure accurate jitter measurements; too low a rate of stimulation will produce falsely high MCD values. There is also the possibility of falsely reduced jitter values if the muscle fiber is stimulated directly, eliminating neuromuscular transmission from the equation.

The primary value of SFEMG is its enhanced sensitivity and its ability to detect delays rather than overt failure of neuromuscular transmission through the identification of increased jitter values, prior to the development of actual muscle weakness. Once a DNMT is severe enough to produce weakness, a decremental response to RNS will be found in that muscle. As SFEMG is typically more labor intensive than RNS, SFEMG becomes superfluous unless the muscle is not readily accessible by RNS techniques. SFEMG, in a weak muscle, will demonstrate not only increased jitter (delayed neuromuscular transmission) but actual blocking or failure of neuromuscular transmission at multiple neuromuscular junctions within that muscle. Blocking is typically seen only when jitter values exceed 100 μs. As implied above, the other advantage of SFEMG other than its increased sensitivity in identifying abnormalities in muscles that are not weak is that it is a needle rather than nerve conduction technique. Accordingly, the anatomic limitations imposed by RNS are not as relevant to SFEMG where numerous muscles are readily available for study.

There are other EMG techniques that are uncommonly used in clinical settings. Macro EMG involves the use of a specialized needle with multiple recording ports. This allows waveform acquisition over a far wider recording radius than with conventional concentric or monopolar EMG needles. Macro EMG is used primarily in research settings to assess the size and distribution of SFMAP components of MUAPs.

MUAPs of increased duration and amplitude are often so strikingly different from normal MUAPs that these may be readily identified by subjective means. The distinction between normal MUAPs that are small and pathologic MUAPs that are reduced in amplitude and duration is more difficult to assess subjectively. MUAP analysis or quantitation is a technique that has been used to objectively measure the average amplitude and duration of a population of MUAPs. An abnormal result is determined by comparison of the average size of an MUAP in a studied muscle to normative data. These norms account for MUAP size variability based on patient age and muscle selected. MUAP quantitation may be used as both a clinical and, more commonly, a research tool in laboratories that offer it.

THE PATHOPHYSIOLOGY OF NERVE INJURY—ELECTRODIAGNOSTIC AND CLINICAL CORRELATES

The pathophysiology of peripheral nerve lesions can be inferred from EDX data, as can the clinical symptoms that the pathophysiologic process produces. Four different pathophysiologies can be considered from an EDX perspective, axon loss, and three forms of demyelination. The latter have been referred to as focal or uniform slowing, differential slowing also known as temporal dispersion, and conduction block. More than one of these mechanisms may coexist with any given disease or injury. There is a fifth pathophysiology of nerve to consider from at least a theoretical if not a practical basis, that being disordered function of ion channels. Neuropathies due to certain marine toxins, drugs, and autoantibodies are hypothesized to produce symptoms by impaired ion channel function.

Loss of CMAP and SNAP amplitudes are the primary nerve conduction manifestations of axon loss. With axon loss, conduction slowing may occur if the largest, fastest conducting axons degenerate. Conduction slowing tends to be modest with axon loss alone unless severe. In pure axon loss, focal conduction abnormalities do not typically occur unless conduction studies are done hyperacutely before axonal degeneration takes place. The needle examination in axon loss is characterized by abnormal spontaneous activity within 1–3 weeks of disease onset, reduced motor unit recruitment immediately, and enlarged, reinnervated MUPs within a matter of months. Axon loss leads to muscle atrophy and weakness, loss of all sensory modalities, and loss of deep tendon reflexes within the territories of nerves that are affected.

Demyelination may cause uniform slowing of nerve conduction. Conceptually, in uniform slowing, conduction is slowed equally in all fibers within the affected segment(s) of nerve. As all impulses traverse the affected portion of nerve synchronously, the only clinical consequence of such a lesion is paresthesia, with or without pain. Uniform slowing may occur in a focal segment of nerve as a consequence of mechanical injury. It is a common EDX signature of CTS, ulnar neuropathies at the elbow, and peroneal neuropathy across the fibular head. It may occur along the entire course of multiple nerves in the hereditary demyelinating and dysmyelinating disorders. It may occur because of disordered ion channel function as well.

Differential slowing and demyelinating conduction block are almost always associated with acquired nerve disease and may occur in either a focal or a multifocal distribution. Conceptually, differential slowing results from different degrees of slowing within different nerve fibers within the same segment of nerve. As a result, the CMAP waveform broadens and becomes dispersed with a resulting loss of amplitude and increased CMAP duration. Typically, the waveform takes on a serrated rather than smooth contour (Fig. 2-3). Theoretically, as all axons are conducting and all muscle fibers activated, the area under the curve remains the same. Differential slowing may occur either from mechanical nerve injury in a mononeuropathy or in a multifocal fashion in the acquired demyelinating polyradiculoneuropathies such as GBS and chronic inflammatory demyelinating polyradiculoneuropathy (CIDP). Clinically, differential slowing primarily affects clinical modalities that require synchronous impulse transmission, notably deep tendon reflexes and vibratory perception.

Conduction block usually implies demyelination affecting consecutive myelin internodes precluding effective action potential transmission in affected fibers. It is most accurately recognized when stimuli can be delivered sequentially over short segments of nerve. When a nerve is stimulated distal to the affected area, the CMAP amplitude is normal as demyelinating lesions have no upstream or downstream effect on axon viability and nerve conduction. Stimulation above the block results in a drop in CMAP amplitude and area proportionate to the number of fibers affected (Fig. 2-2B). This same phenomenon may also occur without overt demyelination, presumably because of immune-mediated ion channel dysfunction.

Clinically, conduction block produces neither significant muscle atrophy, loss of the so-called small fiber modalities including autonomic functions, nor perception of pain and temperature. Significant atrophy does not occur as the trophic influence of preserved axons remains. The latter functions are preserved as small poorly myelinated or unmyelinated fibers remain relatively unscathed, as demyelinating lesions have little or no influence on these fiber types. Conduction block is the only type of demyelinating pathology that results in muscle weakness.

THE VALUE AND LIMITATIONS OF EDX

EDX studies are very helpful in certain circumstances and of limited utility in others. In essence, these can, with varying degrees of confidence, determine the following:

- The existence of a problem within the neuromuscular system.
- Where within an individual nerve the problem lies.
- The topographic pattern of that problem, for example, single nerve, single root, length dependent, etc.
- The pathophysiology of the problem and the expected clinical consequences.
- Insight into the severity and, to a lesser extent, the prognosis of the problem.
- Guidance on the role of nerve transfers, nerve repair, and grafting in focal nerve injuries.

Although disease etiology may be implied by the electrodiagnostic findings, it is rarely, if ever, defined as a direct result of EDX interpreted in isolation. Although the EDX examination is fairly sensitive and can provide support for the existence of most neuromuscular disorders, there are notable exceptions. One of these is small fiber polyneuropathy/neuronopathy. Conventional EDX techniques exclusively test large myelinated fibers. They do not adequately assess disorders that exclusively affect small myelinated or unmyelinated fibers producing distortions in perception of pain and thermal sense with or without impaired autonomic function. Other tests, described later in this chapter, in the subsequent chapter on histologic testing, and in the chapter on distal symmetric polyneuropathy (DSPN) have been used in attempts to assess small fiber integrity.

Another arena in which EDX is insensitive is in muscle disorders where both the existence and classification of myopathy may be challenging. Myopathies in which the pathology consists solely of myofiber atrophy or nondestructive internal changes of myofiber architecture can be particularly difficult. Certain endocrine, congenital, and mitochondrial myopathies are examples of this. In the myopathy of excessive corticosteroid use characterized by type II myofiber atrophy, the abnormal type II MUAPs are not detectable, as these are obscured by their initially recruited type I counterparts.

As previously mentioned, an additional drawback of EDX is the time required for the full complement of EDX abnormalities to develop following nerve injury. In addition, with traumatic injuries, EDX cannot adequately distinguish between complete severance of axons with preservation of the connective tissue sheath and complete nerve transaction. This is of pragmatic importance as the current standard of care would be to attempt primary nerve reanastomosis acutely if complete nerve transaction had occurred. Another potential problem related to timing and prognosis is falsely identifying a lesion as demyelinating conduction block, when it is actually due to axon loss, a phenomenon known as pseudoconduction block. This may occur if motor nerve conductions are performed within 5 days of injury, prior to Wallerian degeneration. In this situation, the amplitude below the lesion may be initially preserved but reduced above the lesion, thus mimicking conduction block and suggesting an inappropriately optimistic prognosis.

ELECTRODIAGNOSTIC LOCALIZATION WITHIN THE NEUROMUSCULAR SYSTEM

EDX is capable, in many cases, of clarifying or reinforcing the localization of the pathologic process within the neuromuscular system (Table 2-6). The strategy is similar to the same pattern recognition methods used clinically at the bedside. Differential diagnosis is greatly facilitated in nerve disease by anatomic categorization, that is, identifying the problem as a mononeuropathy, a monoradiculopathy, a polyradiculopathy, a polyradiculoneuropathy, a plexopathy, a multifocal neuropathy, a DSPN (length-dependent polyneuropathy—LDPN), or a motor or sensory neuronopathy. Neuronopathy refers to a disorder affecting the cell bodies (i.e., the anterior horn cells or dorsal root ganglia). Myopathies and DNMT have distinctive EDX signatures in most cases that allow localization to these structures as well.

▶ TABLE 2-6. ELECTRODIAGNOSTIC LOCALIZATION (TYPICAL PRESENTATIONS)

Diagnosis	CMAP Amp	Cond Slow	Disp/CB	SNAP Amp	Fibs/PW	Other Abnl Spon Act	Prsp dnrv	MUP Size	MUP No.	Pattern
Mononeuropathy	↓	+/−	+/−	↓	Yes	+/−	No	↑	↓	Single nerve
Multifocal neuropathy	↓	No	+/−	+/−	Yes	+/−	No	+/−	↓	Multiple nerves
LD polyneuropathy	+/−	+/−	No	↓↓	Yes	No	No	↑	↓	LD symmetric LE > UE
Polyradiculoneuropathy (demyelinating)	↓	No	Yes	↓	+/−	No	+/−	+/−	↓	Diffuse non-LD
Monoradiculopathy	+/−	No	No	NL	Yes	+/−	Yes	↑	↓	Monosegmental
Polyradiculopathy	↓	No	No	NL	Yes	+/−	Yes	↑↑	↓	Polysegmental
Plexopathy	↓	No	No	↓↓	Yes	Occ Myk	No	↑↑	↓	Multiple nerves and roots in single extremity
Sensory neuronopathy	NL	No	No	↓↓	No	No	No	NL	NL	Diffuse non-LD
Motor neuron disease	↓↓	+/−	No	NL	No	+/−	Yes	↑↑	↓↓	Diffuse non-LD
Presynaptic DNMT	↓↓	No	No	NL	+/−	No	+/−		NL	Diffuse
Postsynaptic DNMT	NL	No	No	NL	+/−	No	+/−	↓	NL	Diffuse
Myopathy without abnormal spont act	+/−	No	No	NL	No	No	No	↓	NL	Diffuse or proximally predominant
Myopathy with fibs and positive waves	+/−	No	No	NL	Yes	No	Yes	↓	NL	Diffuse or proximally predominant
Myopathy with myotonia	+/−	No	No	NL	+/−	Myt	+/−	↓	NL	Diffuse, may affect facial and distal muscles

Amp, amplitude; Slow, slowing; Disp, dispersion; CB, conduction block; Abnl spon act, abnormal spontaneous activity; Prsp dnrv, paraspinal denervation; LD, length dependent; LE, lower extremity; Myt, myotonic potentials; Myk, myokymic potentials; Occ, occasional; UE, upper extremity; +/−, may or may not occur depending on severity or pathophysiology (e.g., axonal or demyelinating) of disorder.

There are essentially three means to predict pathologic localization in focal nerve disease. The first involves identification of CMAP and SNAP amplitude abnormalities and understanding their localization significance. Sensory nerve conductions are abnormal in axon loss lesions affecting the dorsal root ganglion, the plexus, or the peripheral nerve. They are normal in disorders of the anterior horn, the neuromuscular junction, and muscle. They are usually normal as well in disorders affecting nerve roots, despite clinical sensory symptoms. The reason for this is not intuitive. An axon separated from its nucleus will degenerate. In disorders of the dorsal root proximal to the sensory ganglia (e.g., a severe radiculopathy), Wallerian degeneration takes place in a centripetal fashion, that is, toward and within the posterior column of the spinal cord. The more peripheral sensory axons remain viable and capable of conducting externally applied impulses in a normal fashion, even within symptomatic regions. A normal SNAP in a clinically affected territory implies that the patient's sensory symptoms are attributable to small fiber involvement, which cannot be detected by standard NCS techniques, that the patient is feigning symptoms, or that the pathology is proximal to the dorsal root ganglia. Abnormal SNAP amplitudes in both upper and lower extremities with normal CMAP amplitudes imply disorders of the dorsal root ganglia.

Conversely, abnormal CMAP amplitudes with spared SNAPs imply a localization to anterior horn, ventral root, neuromuscular junction, muscle, or those uncommon disorders that exclusively affect motor nerve fibers within the peripheral nerve trunk. The latter possibility is most readily defined by the identification of demyelinating features confined to motor nerves. Reduced CMAP and SNAP amplitudes together imply disorders of peripheral nerve or plexus, which are in turn distinguished by the pattern of involvement within and between limbs.

The second and most precise means of localization occurs when a focal demyelinating lesion exists and is detectable. Detection requires the ability to stimulate both above and below the site of the nerve lesion. Specifically, an abrupt change in waveform latency, amplitude, or configuration occurring over a short segment of nerve implies demyelinating pathology as long as it is identified more than 7 days following symptom onset. The ability to identify these changes is, however, limited by anatomy and nerve accessibility. Deeply situated nerves in proximal locations are in large part inaccessible, or if accessible, cannot be stimulated comfortably or in isolation. If the lesion is purely axonal or if the lesion is in an area that is difficult to access with NCS, nerve conductions will be able to localize the problem to the nerve but not within the nerve.

There are situations in which demyelinating pathology can be implied but not proven. If a muscle is clinically weak but has a normal CMAP from all accessible points of stimulation of the nerve that innervates it, an absent F wave from that nerve and muscle suggests proximal conduction block. In a similar context, if the conduction velocity and distal latencies of a motor conduction study are normal but the F latency is prolonged, a demyelinating lesion with focal slowing at a proximal location is suggested. The third scenario arises when needle EMG is performed in a weak muscle that has a normal CMAP amplitude. Reduced recruitment with fast-firing MUAPs occurring in the absence of abnormal spontaneous activity or morphologic changes in MUAPs implies a demyelinating conduction block pathophysiology as well. To implicate predominantly demyelinating pathophysiology in each of these situations, testing would have to occur at an interval after potential Wallerian degeneration and the development of fibrillation potentials would have had a chance to occur.

The third localization opportunity occurs in axon loss lesions in which localization can be inferred by the pattern of denervation. Here, the electromyographer is hampered by at least three aspects of anatomy. Localization is limited by the anatomical location and distribution of branch points to individual muscles and their location along the course of a given nerve. In the ulnar nerve, for example, branches occur only in the hand and at the elbow, with none in the arm and forearm segments. Localization in this manner is also hindered by the tendency for fibers designated for certain muscles to be sequestered in selected fascicles. For example, it is common for ulnar forearm muscles to be spared with ulnar neuropathies occurring at the elbow. The presumption is that the fascicles containing the fibers supplying forearm muscles are rendered less vulnerable to nerve entrapment or compression by their position within the nerve, a concept referred to as selective fascicular involvement. Finally, most muscles are innervated by multiple roots. This benefits the patient but potentially confounds the electromyographer. This overlap may make it difficult to provide single root localization. As an example, most muscles innervated by the C5 myotome are also innervated by the C6 myotome and vice versa, making discrimination between these two monoradiculopathies potentially challenging.

A mononeuropathy is defined by NCS and/or EMG abnormalities confined to a single nerve distribution. Mononeuropathies are most frequently caused by external nerve compression or by entrapment within a normally existing anatomical structure rendered abnormal from mechanical or other factors. Mononeuropathies may be associated with all the pathophysiologic processes defined above, with the possible exception of ion channel dysfunction, often in combination. Prognosis is determined by etiology as well as by the type and relative degree of pathophysiology.

A monoradiculopathy is defined when sensory conductions are normal, and denervation exists in a myotomal or segmental pattern. In other words, all affected muscles should share the same root innervation but include innervations from more than one peripheral nerve. For example, in a C7 radiculopathy, denervation would be expected in both the triceps and the flexor carpi radialis muscles. Both have singular root but different nerve innervation. CMAP amplitudes are usually spared in monoradiculopathies for the following reasons. Many of the commonly affected nerve roots, particularly in the upper extremities, do not correspond to the same segments as the routinely performed conduction studies. In addition, most muscles have multiple root innervations. Even if there is significant axon loss within a given segment, potential loss of CMAP amplitude is buffered by the contribution(s) of other unaffected segments. Finally, if root pathophysiology is predominantly demyelinating, it will not alter routine motor nerve conduction parameters.

Conceptually, all mono- or polyradiculopathies, that have some degree of axon loss and affect ventral roots, should manifest paraspinal denervation. In reality, this may not always be demonstrable. It is not uncommon to identify a segmental (myotomal) pattern of denervation with normal SNAPs in the same segment in the apparent absence of paraspinal denervation. In this situation, the electrodiagnostician should not be dissuaded from rendering an anatomic diagnosis of radiculopathy, particularly in the appropriate clinical context. For example, ALS can have an identical electrodiagnostic signature, which can be falsely localized to root disease if clinical context is not considered, and a more extensive needle examination not performed.

For the most part, monoradiculopathies are most readily recognized when there is axon loss. For the reasons described above, demyelinating radiculopathies can only be inferred, may only have subtle electrodiagnostic findings, and therefore may go unrecognized.

Polyradiculopathy is defined by denervation in the distribution of multiple segments and their corresponding paraspinal musculature. Again, sensory potentials should be spared. CMAP amplitudes are more likely to be affected than monoradiculopathies, as the buffering provided by multiple root innervations is not as pronounced. As already mentioned, polyradiculopathies may be electrodiagnostically indistinguishable from early motor neuron disease, as in both cases, the pattern of denervation is polysegmental with paraspinal involvement, occurring with sparing of sensory conduction parameters.

Rarely, a purely sensory polyradiculopathy affecting dorsal roots exists that can present with multifocal sensory symptoms, including sensory ataxia.[52] In these cases, localization is postulated based on imaging, somatosensory-evoked potential abnormalities, and/or dorsal rootlet biopsy result. SNAPs are normal in the symptomatic regions. H reflexes are typically absent if the S1 segments are affected. In reported cases, motor conduction studies and needle examination were normal in most patients in keeping with the proposed dorsal root localization.[52]

Polyradiculoneuropathy differs conceptually from polyradiculopathy, involving nerve trunk as well as nerve root. This distinction is usually made electrodiagnostically although maybe confirmed by gadolinium-enhanced magnetic resonance imaging (MRI). The electrodiagnostic signature of polyradiculopathy is the concomitant involvement of SNAPs and paraspinal denervation. Although there are several potential etiologies, the most readily recognized causes of polyradiculoneuropathies are the acquired inflammatory demyelinating polyradiculoneuropathies, that is, GBS and CIDP. In these disorders, motor conduction studies are commonly replete with demyelinating features, including uniform and differential slowing (temporal dispersion) and conduction block. Some degree of axon loss is common in most cases, although pure axon loss variants of GBS exist making EDX more complicated. In addition, there are axonal forms of polyradiculoneuropathy (e.g., severe porphyria, diabetes, carcinomatous infiltration, infections such as Lyme and CMV). In the acquired demyelinating polyradiculoneuropathies (e.g., GBS, CIDP), sensory conductions are affected although "sural sparing" may occur. Sural sparing refers to a non–length-dependent pattern of SNAP abnormalities where upper extremity SNAP abnormalities occur with preservation, or relative preservation of the sural, and/or superficial peroneal sensory responses. Denervation, when present in polyradiculoneuropathies, occurs on a generalized basis without length dependency and by definition effects the paraspinal muscles.

Plexopathies are typically defined when both sensory and motor abnormalities affect more than one nerve and nerve root distribution confined to a single limb, both clinically and electrodiagnostically. There are exceptions. Specific etiologies of plexopathy such as acute brachial plexus neuritis may affect more than one limb, in either a clinically evident or an occult basis. Plexopathies affect both SNAP and CMAP amplitudes. In most cases, SNAPs are affected to a greater degree than CMAPs although brachial plexus neuritis with a predilection toward pure motor nerves such as the long thoracic or anterior interosseous provides a notable exception to this generalization. In this disorder, the pattern may conform more to multifocal neuropathy confined to the upper limb, rather than to an anatomically defined plexopathy. In acute brachial plexus neuritis, the pathology may extend beyond the boundaries of the brachial plexus to involve other nerves such as the recurrent laryngeal and phrenic. When the CMAP amplitudes are affected disproportionately to the SNAPs, concomitant involvement of the ventral roots should be considered. The pattern of denervation in plexopathy varies with etiology. A plexopathy is best defined electrodiagnostically when the pattern of abnormalities is identified and is only explained by pathology in a distinct plexus element, for example, the upper trunk of the brachial plexus. In traumatic and inflammatory plexopathies, localization to a single plexus component is the exception rather than the rule. In a true anatomic plexopathy, sparing of paraspinal musculature is expected.

Polyneuropathies will be discussed next in four categorical domains: multifocal neuropathy or multiple mononeuropathies, distal symmetric sensory polyneuropathy (DSPN), sensory neuronopathy, and motor neuronopathy (i.e., motor neuron disease). Although it is unusual to discuss motor neuron diseases in the context of polyneuropathies, it is done so here as it is conceptually difficult to discuss disorders affecting dorsal root ganglia (which can phenotypically resemble polyneuropathy) without discussing disorders of their anterior horn cell counterparts.

The recognition of multiple mononeuropathies is that it implies a readily recognizable pattern of neuropathy affecting multiple nerves in multiple locations. Multiple mononeuropathies typically result from disorders that are capable of either infarcting or infiltrating peripheral nerve, often occurring in the context of an associated systemic disease. It is diagnosed when EDX abnormalities occur in multiple nerve distributions, typically in an asymmetric fashion. Typically, there is both sensory and motor involvement, although both pure motor and perhaps pure sensory variants exist. When multifocal neuropathies are either pure motor or sensory, distinction from the neuronopathies may be difficult. The pathophysiology is usually axonal. If the pattern is demyelinating, hereditary neuropathy with liability to pressure palsy (HNPP), multifocal-acquired demyelinating sensory and motor neuropathy (MADSAM or the Lewis–Sumner syndrome), or if purely motor, multifocal motor neuropathy (MMN) should be considered. Electrodiagnostic definition of multifocal neuropathy often requires a careful historical review as well as an extensive electrodiagnostic examination with fastidious attention to detail.

DSPN is the most common polyneuropathy phenotype. Signs and symptoms first occur in the most distal aspects of the longest nerves in a symmetric or near-symmetric fashion. DSPN is defined electrodiagnostically when both sensory and motor abnormalities are identified in a symmetric, length-dependent fashion. Potential reason for this is that many axonopathies are associated with impaired axoplasmic flow of regenerated proteins that are made in the cell bodies that are needed for maintenance and repair of axon function distally. The longer the axon, the more likely these proteins are not transported all the way. One way to demonstrate this is by showing that muscles innervated by the L5 and S1 myotomes in the foot and distal lower leg are affected to a greater extent L5–S1 innervated muscles in the thigh or hip region. As the etiologies of DSPN are usually toxic, metabolic, or hereditary, an axonal pathophysiology usually predominates. A predominantly demyelinating DSPN pattern is most commonly seen in hereditary neuropathies and in a few acquired neuropathies such as those associated with IgM monoclonal proteins (MCPs). Other acquired demyelinating neuropathies such as AIDP and CIDP are more correctly categorized as polyradiculoneuropathies and may be distinguished from length-dependent DSPN through features such as sural sparing.

Many DSPNs appear to be predominantly sensory in nature, both from a clinical and NCS basis. There are at least three potential reasons for this. SNAPs are typically affected earlier and to a greater extent than their CMAP counterparts. The second potential explanation is anatomical. At onset, involvement of sensory nerve endings in the toes commonly produces symptoms that are typically positive (pain and paraesthesia) and are therefore easily recognized. Conversely, clinical detection of motor abnormalities in the intrinsic foot muscles is rendered difficult by the duplicate function of leg muscles which also contribute to toe flexion and extension. Only toe abduction/adduction, a function difficult to clinically assess, is controlled solely by intrinsic foot muscles. Finally, the detection of motor involvement in DSPN may be obscured by an electromyographic bias. In the authors' experience, many patients with normal CMAP amplitudes in intrinsic foot muscles and no detectable weakness will be found to have fibrillation potentials and/or positive wave in intrinsic foot muscles. As the intrinsic foot muscles are frequently avoided by many electromyographers, the opportunity to identify subclinical motor involvement may be overlooked.

Sensory neuronopathies or dorsal root ganglionopathies are typically caused by toxic, inflammatory, or infectious mechanisms. They may have a length-dependent appearance but are often asymmetric and non–length dependent, either by clinical or by EDX means. From a clinical standpoint, a non–length-dependent sensory neuropathy should be considered when sensory symptoms appear in the face, trunk, or upper extremities before or at the same time as they begin in the distal feet. Multifocal reductions in SNAP amplitudes are the hallmark of these disorders. The most readily definable pattern of sensory neuronopathy is when upper extremity SNAPs are reduced to the same extent or more than their lower extremity counterparts, without involvement of lower extremity CMAPs. This pattern of sensory nerve conduction abnormalities is analogous to the pattern of sural sparing described above. In sensory neuronopathies, however, unlike the inflammatory myelinating polyradiculoneuropathies, both motor conduction and needle EMG abnormalities are by definition abnormal.

Motor neuronopathies or motor neuron disorders are commonly degenerative, hereditary, or infectious. The pattern of weakness varies with cause. Sensory conductions are usually normal except in Kennedy disease, facial-onset motor and sensory neuropathy (FOSMN), or when there is a second, potentially confounding disorder. The pathophysiology appears to be that of axon loss, occurring in a polysegmental pattern early in the disease or diffusely when the disease is more established. Denervation occurring in a nerve or length-dependent distribution pattern should suggest an uncommon motor neuropathy. Once again, except for the potential of prolonged H reflex latencies in polyradiculopathy, the NCS and EMG pattern of motor neuronopathies and polyradiculopathy may be electrodiagnostically indistinguishable.

Presynaptic DNMTs are usually multifocal if not diffuse in their topographic distribution, both clinically and electrodiagnostically. They are more likely to be symmetric in manifestation than their postsynaptic counterparts. Their hallmark is CMAP amplitude reduction of >10% with SNAP sparing. As described above, the hallmark of presynaptic DNMTs is low CMAP amplitudes that increment after brief exercise or in response to repetitive stimulation at rates of 20 Hz or more. A decremental response to slow repetitive stimulation (2–3 Hz) may also be demonstrated. Fibrillation potentials occur in botulism but are infrequent in the Lambert–Eaton myasthenic syndrome (LEMS). MUAPs may be normal or reduced in size, that is, small in amplitude, short in duration, and polyphasic in configuration. Like all DNMT, motor unit variability will be demonstrable in a clinically affected muscle if sought for. Recruitment may be concomitantly increased.

Postsynaptic DNMTs have an electrodiagnostic signature that overlaps with its presynaptic counterpart. As a rule, abnormalities may be more focal and therefore more difficult to identify in postsynaptic disorders. The major discriminator is that CMAP amplitudes are typically normal at rest in postsynaptic disorders except in the most severe cases. The typical EDX strategy in postsynaptic disorders is to perform routine conductions and needle examination first to potentially identify other pure motor disorders. In postsynaptic DNMT, routine conductions are typically normal. Decremental responses are first sought for at rest with slow repetitive stimulation (2–3 Hz). If decrement is demonstrated, we see if the decrement can be repaired by 10 seconds of brief exercise (postexercise repair/facilitation) followed again by slow repetitive stimulation to see if the baseline observed decrement worsens (postexercise exhaustion). If no decrement is found on slow repetitive stimulation at rest, we have patients isometrically exercise the muscle for a minute. We then repeat slow repetitive stimulation once a minute for 5 minutes to see if a decrement now appears (again, postexercise exhaustion).

A clinically weak muscle in MG should demonstrate a decremental response to 2–3 Hz repetitive stimulation in all cases, as the decrement is the EDX analog of clinical weakness. This may be easy to accomplish in generalized MG but elusive in patients whose signs and symptoms are restricted to the oculomotor system. As in the case of presynaptic DNMT, MG spares sensory potentials and may be associated with small MUPs. Fibrillation potentials are uncommon but may occur when receptor sites are damaged sufficiently to essentially denervate muscle fibers.

EDX AS A PROGNOSTIC TOOL

The extent to which EDX is used as a prognostic tool undoubtedly varies from laboratory to laboratory and can be ascertained in several ways.[53] In general, demyelinating lesions are likely to resolve quickly (weeks to months) and completely if their cause is eliminated. There are certain disorders such as radiation injury and MMN in which conduction block may persist. The prognosis for axon loss lesions is more uncertain and depends on the degree and location of the injury, as well as the age and comorbidities of the patient. The severity of the lesion is best judged by the amplitudes of the SNAP and CMAP responses. Severely reduced CMAP amplitudes, in the absence of demyelinating conduction block, imply that a limited number of residual axons are available for collateral sprouting, and many orphaned muscle fibers are in need of reinnervation. Prognosis for significant recovery in these situations is guarded. Prognosis is also determined in axon loss lesions by the distance between the injury and the target. For example, in brachial plexus injuries, improvement in biceps and deltoid function occurs far more frequently than return of hand function. Although fibrillation potentials in neurogenic disease indicate axon loss, grading systems for fibrillation potentials are not adequately linear or quantitative enough to utilize in disease prognostication.

In ALS, rapid disease progression correlates with at least three recognized electrodiagnostic patterns. These are an abundance of fibrillation potentials associated with modest changes of chronic denervation and reinnervation, prominent MUAP variability, and rapid MUNE decline.[41,54]

Prognosis in the GBS had been linked to a composite of CMAP amplitudes. In some cases, the reduced CMAP amplitudes represent distal demyelination with partial conduction block in terminal nerve twigs. In such cases, the low amplitudes are usually accompanied by prolonged distal latencies. Low amplitudes with normal distal latencies and conduction velocities can be seen in "pure" conduction block, which can recover quickly. Finally, low amplitudes with normal distal latencies and conduction velocities can be seen in pure axonal forms of GBS that are associated with a longer recovery time.[55] The identification of conduction block at the elbow in combination with a normal CMAP when stimulating distally suggests an 86% likelihood of full subjective recovery from an ulnar neuropathy at the elbow.[56]

EDX TO GUIDE REPAIR OF NERVE INJURIES

EDX is also used to help guide the role of nerve transfers, nerve repair, and grafting in focal nerve injuries.[51] In such cases, EDX is instrumental in localizing the lesion, defining the pathophysiology (e.g., neuropraxia, demyelination, axonal degeneration), the severity, and prognosis. Neuropraxia and demyelination indicate the axons are intact with good potential for recovery within days to 3 months. When there is severe weakness, markedly reduced CMAP and SNAP amplitudes and needle EMG showing abundant fibrillation potentials and no or few recruitable MUAPs, the prognosis for recover is poor. It is important for the electromyographer to assess the continuity of the axons and if there is evidence of distal axonal sprouting and regeneration as reflected by increasing CMAP amplitude, appearance of small nascent MUAPs, and large polyphasic MUAPs. The trajectory of improvement over time can help guide prognosis and when surgery may be indicated.

Presurgical evaluation should also ensure that the transferred nerve itself is not also injured and that there are redundant counterparts that are intact to compensate for loss of function associated with transferring that specific distal nerve branch. For example, with a severe ulnar nerve injury, the branch of the anterior interosseous nerve (AIN) innervating the pronator quadratus could serve as the donor to the ulnar nerve provided there is no evidence of denervation of the pronator quadratus (suggesting branch of AIN is also injured here) and that there is preserved forearm pronation by the pronator teres. Additionally, in this setting, the electrodiagnotician needs to make sure there is not a Martin–Gruber anastomosis (a normal anatomic variant in which branches to the interossei, abductor digiti minimi, or flexor pollicis brevis travel with the median nerve or AIN before transversing over to the ulnar nerve in the forearm). In such cases, sacrificing the AIN can lead to worsening function of these muscles. (More regarding the role of surgery in repair of nerve injuries is discussed in Chapter 23.)

Quantitative Sensory Testing

QST is used in both clinical and research settings, to provide measurements of small myelinated and unmyelinated nerve functions.[57–61] Peripheral neuropathies, in most cases, are thought to be pathologically indiscriminate and affect peripheral nerve fibers of all sizes. The concept of small fiber neuropathy (SFN) recognizes the existence of a select group of neuropathy patients in whom the signs and symptoms suggest preferential injury to small, poorly myelinated (A-delta) or unmyelinated (C) peripheral nerve fibers less than 7 µm in diameter. As mentioned previously, conventional EDX does not assess small fiber viability and function and is therefore of limited utility in pure SFN. QST represents an attempt to fill this diagnostic gap as well as to provide a potential tool for epidemiologic studies and therapeutic trials. It also provides a potential means to screen for subclinical neuropathy in industries where the potential for neurotoxic exposure exists.[57,58,61] Two other techniques that may also be used in SFN assessment, autonomic testing and the assessment of intraepidermal nerve fiber density (IENFD) via skin biopsy, will be discussed in the next section and next chapter, respectively. The various test results may not be concordant, implying the potential benefit of using multiple testing modalities in SFN suspects.[62–64]

SFNs, as discussed in detail in Chapter 22, are often length-dependent and represent 5% of the DSPN population.[62,65] The natural history of SFN may include evolution into a more typical DSPN phenotype with both small and large fiber involvement. Non–length-dependent SFNs also occur and are suspected of being ganglionopathies or neuronopathies.

QST is a psychophysical test whose accuracy is dependent on optimal control of multiple environmental variables including patient understanding and cooperation.[58] Understandably there are certain patient populations in whom testing is unlikely to succeed. Although the stimuli delivered are quantified, the patient responses are largely subjective. There are numerous testing algorithms used by different commercial vendors that have been developed to make QST as accurate, reproducible, and efficient as possible.[66] It is unclear which existing algorithm achieves these goals with the most success. Results are very much dependent on the patient population studied, the environment in which they are studied, as well as the equipment and testing algorithm used.[58,67] QST should not be used as the sole means to detect nerve pathology.

It is beyond the scope of this chapter to provide a detailed discussion of QST algorithms. There are several paradigms used in terms of both stimulus threshold and reproducibility of result. Threshold algorithms attempt to identify the smallest stimulus intensity perceived, the smallest difference in stimulus intensity perceived, or the lowest stimulus intensity that provides a given magnitude of response, for example, pain. Reproducibility algorithms are dynamic paradigms, which involve ramping stimulus intensity up or down until identical thresholds are identified. Results are considered abnormal when these exceed 95% of age-matched norms. In contrast to threshold testing algorithms, static stimuli are delivered as individual stimuli of set duration and intensity. Either flanking or forced choice algorithms can be used. The 4–2–1 paradigm is the most frequently used flanking algorithm. If a stimulus is perceived, the stimulus is reduced by four orders of magnitudes at a time until no longer perceived, then increased by two levels of magnitude until recognized, and then reduced by one order of magnitude. In a sense, the process "zeros in" on the threshold. The forced choice paradigm provides paired stimuli, one of which is null. The true stimulus varies in intensity, and the null stimulus varies randomly in its order of delivery.

The most common QST testing algorithms assess thresholds for cooling and vibration, particularly in a diabetic population.[68] In SFN, the expectation is that thermal thresholds would be affected disproportionately to those for vibration. Although QST is used predominantly for suspected peripheral neuropathy, one of its limitations is that it tests the entirety of the somatosensory system. Accordingly, abnormal test results have no localizing value. One potentially beneficial, although unvalidated, application of QST is its use in topographical areas not readily accessible to conventional EDX. For example, it provides a theoretical means to evaluate sensory complaints of the trunk or genitalia.

QST has been studied in several clinical applications. Thermal testing may be abnormal in diabetic patients before the onset of symptoms or abnormal EDX.[61,69–71] In uremic patients, altered vibratory thresholds seem to be more prevalent than their thermal counterparts in presumed neuropathy.[72] Conversely, impaired thermal threshold may be the first abnormality to occur, and the paradoxical heat perception resulting from a cold stimulus may also occur in the uremic population.[73,74] QST has been applied in the evaluation of painful distal sensory neuropathy in the HIV population.[75,76]

In studies conducted to date, QST sensitivity for the detection of SFN has ranged from 60% to 85%. The sensitivity in the detection of small fiber pathology is similar to both quantitative sudomotor axon reflex testing (QSART) discussed below and IENF density on skin biopsy discussed in the following chapter. At least one study has suggested that IENFD provides a more sensitive means to confirm small fiber involvement.[62] In general, however, the information derived from different testing modalities utilized in an attempt to identify SFN is universally more complementary than overlapping. Accordingly, multiple modalities may be required both to identify small fiber dysfunction and to convince the physician that an abnormal result is valid.[67] As QST abnormalities may reflect either peripheral or CNS pathology, and in consideration of their apparently similar thresholds for detection of abnormalities within the peripheral nervous system, abnormal QST coupled with normal epidermal nerve fiber density should provoke consideration of CNS pathology.[54]

Autonomic Nervous System Testing

Symptoms that implicate dysautonomia can be classified as either cholinergic, adrenergic, or as sudomotor in nature. Orthostatic intolerance manifested as light-headedness or fainting, fading of visual or auditory perception, and fatigue or nuchal discomfort are all symptoms that may result from impaired sympathetic vasomotor tone. In an older population, orthostatic intolerance may manifest as cognitive change without the perception of lightheadedness. Other symptoms of impaired sympathetic function include ptosis and impaired ejaculation. Symptoms of cholinergic dysautonomia include blurred vision and photophobia from impaired pupillary constriction, impotence, resting tachycardia, the sicca complex of dry eyes and dry mouth, urinary retention, gastroparesis, and intestinal pseudo-obstruction. Symptoms of sudomotor dysfunction relate to disordered sweating. The latter may manifest as dry feet or somewhat paradoxically by hyperhidrosis in unaffected areas to compensate for hypohidrosis in other topographic distributions.

Detecting pathologic involvement of the autonomic nervous system provides at least three potential applications in the evaluation of patients with neuromuscular disease. In patients with suspected neuropathic pain without signs of large fiber neuropathy, for example, burning feet and suspected SFN, autonomic testing provides a means to document small myelinated (A-delta) or unmyelinated (C) nerve fiber involvement. In patients with large fiber, sensory motor neuropathies, autonomic testing may allow documentation of autonomic involvement. By doing so, it may limit differential diagnostic considerations and focus evaluation. As there are a limited number of diseases that have combined somatic and autonomic neuropathy, autonomic testing can facilitate this strategic approach (Table 2-7).[78–82] Finally, the coexistence of dysautonomia with somatic peripheral neuropathy provides potential prognostic insight. In this regard, diabetic autonomic neuropathy is associated with increased morbidity and mortality.[83]

The pharmacology of the autonomic nervous system is complex but integral to the understanding of autonomic testing. In way of brief and simplified review, all preganglionic neurons of both the parasympathetic and the sympathetic

▶ **TABLE 2-7. PERIPHERAL NEUROPATHY ASSOCIATED WITH DYSAUTONOMIA**

Idiopathic
Immune mediated
- Paraneoplastic
- Guillain–Barré syndrome
- Idiopathic

Infiltrative
- Light chain amyloidosis

Metabolic
- Porphyria
- Diabetes mellitus

Toxic
- *cis*-Platinum
- Vinca alkaloids
- Perhexilene
- Hexacarbons
- Thallium
- Arsenic
- Acrylamide
- Taxol
- Lead
- Pesticides
- Pyridoxine toxicity

Hereditary
- Familial amyloidosis
- Hereditary sensory and autonomic neuropathy
- Fabry disease
- Tangier disease
- Mitochondrial disorders

nervous systems are thinly myelinated and use ACh as their primary neurotransmitter. The postganglionic ACh receptors (AChRs) are populated by nicotinic receptors whose activation is blocked by hexamethonium. These ganglionic receptors are thought to represent the targets for circulating autoantibodies found in the serum of approximately half of autoimmune autonomic neuropathy patients. Although nonautonomic cholinergic receptors on skeletal muscle are also nicotinic, they differ pharmacologically. These receptors are blocked by curare and are the target of different antibodies, particularly the AChR antibodies of MG.

The postganglionic parasympathetic fibers synapse with muscarinic cholinergic receptors on the end organs that they innervate. There are at least three types of muscarinic receptors in the body. M1 receptors are found in the cerebral cortex and 5% of sympathetic ganglia, M2 receptors are found primarily in the heart, and M3 receptors populate secretory glands.[84] Atropine is the primary antagonist at these receptors.

The majority of postganglionic sympathetic neurons release norepinephrine as their primary neurotransmitter. The notable exceptions to this rule are sweat glands, smooth muscle fibers within the walls of blood vessels populating skeletal muscle that promote vasodilatation, and some of the chromaffin cells of the adrenal medulla. All of these are cholinergic in nature. There are four currently recognized types of adrenergic receptors, two alpha and two beta. Alpha-1 receptors mediate vasoconstriction, intestinal relaxation, and pupillary dilation, components of the primordial flight response. Alpha-2 receptors are presynaptic in location and inhibit norepinephrine release. Activation of beta-1 receptors, which may be induced by both epinephrine and norepinephrine, increases both heart rate and contractility. Beta-2 receptors are primarily receptive to the effects of epinephrine and are most prevalent in the smooth muscle of blood vessels within muscle. Stimulation of beta-2 receptors results in vasodilatation.

Autonomic testing provides a means by which to detect cardiovagal, adrenergic, and postganglionic sudomotor dysfunction.[85] Autonomic testing encompasses an extensive list of testing modalities that are capable of assessing autonomic nervous system function, most of which are beyond the scope of this chapter. The most commonly utilized tests assess cardiovagal function through heart rate responses to deep breathing, the Valsalva maneuver, and tilt table testing, adrenergic function through blood pressure responses to the Valsalva maneuver and tilt table testing, and sudomotor function through QSART. Illustrations of normal and abnormal responses to these tests are provided in Figures 2-27 to 2-29.

In normal individuals, the heart rate will accelerate in response to inspiration and the associated increased venous return to the right heart and will decelerate in response to expiration (sinus arrhythmia). This response will diminish as a normal consequence of aging. The afferent receptors for this reflex include pulmonary stretch receptors, cardiac mechanoreceptors, and possibly baroreceptors. Sinus arrhythmia is a consequence of normal, parasympathetic, cardiovagal tone. There are numerous protocols that address both the performance and the measurement of heart rate variability. Typically, the patient is positioned with the head up 30 degrees from supine. The patient is asked to breath slowly and steadily at a rate of 6/min (5-second inspirations and 5-second expirations), usually for a period of 1 minute. Heart rate response to deep breathing can be measured either by the greatest difference between the fastest and slowest rate that occur during this interval or by the calculation of an E (expiration) to I (inspiration) ratio. As in our illustrations, the average of the greatest difference between the fastest and slowest rate for the six trials is utilized. The E:I ratio is calculated by measuring the shortest (I) and longest (E) intervals between QRS complexes (R–R interval) as a singular, summed, or averaged value. As the heart rate is the slowest during expiration, the R–R interval increases accordingly resulting in an $E:I$ ratio of >1. There are published, age-matched normative data for both the R–R interval and E:I ratio. The mean heart rate variation in heart rate in a teenager is 30 beats per minute (bpm) with the 5th to 95th percentile range being 14–41 bpm. Between 60 and 69 years of age, the mean heart rate variation is closer to 18 with the 90% of normal being in the 7–27 bpm range.

The physiology of the Valsalva maneuver is more complex. The patient is asked to sustain a constant expiratory pressure of 40 mm Hg for approximately 15 seconds by exhaling into a mouthpiece attached to a manometer. A slow leak in the system is provided. Both heart rate and blood pressure responses are monitored during and in the immediate aftermath of this maneuver. Four distinct phases are discernible, the first and third and the first part of the second phase (IIA) are mechanical in nature and phase IIB and IV result from autonomic nervous system response to these mechanical events. During the first phase, there is a transient increase in blood pressure resulting from direct mechanical compression of the aorta to increased intrathoracic pressure. Phase IIA also results from increased intrathoracic pressure and is defined by a drop in blood pressure occurring from reduced venous return to the heart. Phase III is initiated with glottic release and a resultant decline in intrathoracic pressures. Blood pressure transiently declines as relatively collapsed intrathoracic venous structures can now readily refill and temporarily limit venous return.

Phase IIB is normally identified by rising blood pressure that approaches baseline. This is promoted by increased vasomotor tone mediated by the increased alpha-adrenergic output of the sympathetic nervous system. During the entirety of phase II, heart rate increases as a consequence of cardiovagal withdrawal. During phase IV, blood pressure rises and pulse declines under normal circumstances, with over- and undershoots of their respective baseline values. Increasing blood pressure is due to increased venous return and cardiac output coupled with the persistent effects of increased, sympathetically mediated vasomotor tone. The cardiovagal effects that are measured during the Valsalva maneuver can be quantitated by calculating the Valsalva ratio, the fastest heart rate during phase II divided by the slowest rate recorded during phase IV. The ratio does not change as dramatically with age and gender as do other autonomic parameters. A normal ratio averages 1.6 for males and 1.5 for females during their teenage years. Abnormal sympathetic responses are best identified by a failure of both blood pressure rise during phase IIB and blood pressure overshoot during phase IV to occur.

Tilt table testing is used to assess heart rate and blood pressure in response to standing in a controlled but somewhat artificial environment. The primary utility is to explore potential mechanisms of syncope or near syncope. Normally, despite a 25%–30% shift in venous blood from central to peripheral compartments with assumption of the upright position, rapid compensatory responses from the autonomic nervous system preclude major changes in either pulse or blood pressure. Orthostatic hypotension is frequently defined as a drop in either systolic blood pressure of ≥ 20 or diastolic blood pressure of ≥ 10 mm Hg. Typically, symptoms do not develop until systolic blood pressure drops of 30 or diastolic pressures of 15 mm Hg occur. Orthostatic hypotension usually occurs either immediately or within a few minutes of standing. A drop in blood pressure with an associated tachycardia suggests hypovolemia of whatever cause. A drop in blood pressure without compensatory tachycardia implicates dysautonomia due to disease or drug effect. Symptomatic tachycardia with a heart rate ≥ 30 bpm above baseline without a significant drop in blood pressure is the signature

Test Results

Analysis type : HRDB **Analysis ID** : 423
Analysis date : 08/25/2006 **Analyst** : HRDB
Analysis comments:

Max rate	Min rate	Rate difference
75.0	58.0	17.0
78.0	57.0	21.0
76.0	58.0	18.0
76.0	65.0	11.0
76.0	62.0	14.0
77.0	63.0	14.0
	Avarage HR difference:	15.8

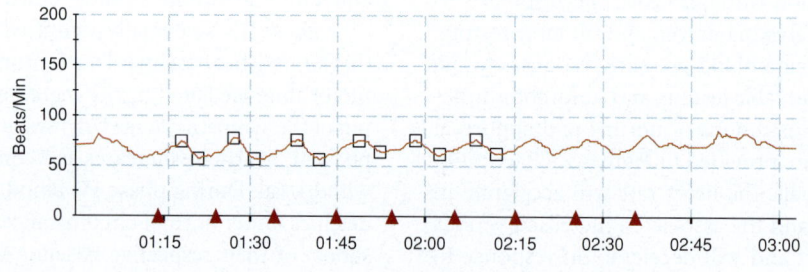

A

Test Results

Analysis type : HRDB **Analysis ID** : 63
Analysis date : 01/31/2007 **Analyst** : HRDB
Analysis comments :

Max rate	Min rate	Rate difference
61.0	52.0	9.0
62.0	54.0	8.0
59.0	55.0	4.0
60.0	56.0	4.0
60.0	57.0	3.0
59.0	57.0	2.0
	Average HR difference:	5.0

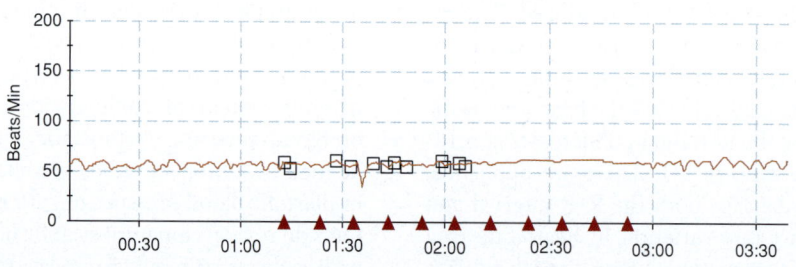

B

Figure 2-27. Normal (average heart rate difference 15.8) (**A**) and abnormal (average heart rate difference 5.0) (**B**) heart rate responses to deep breathing.

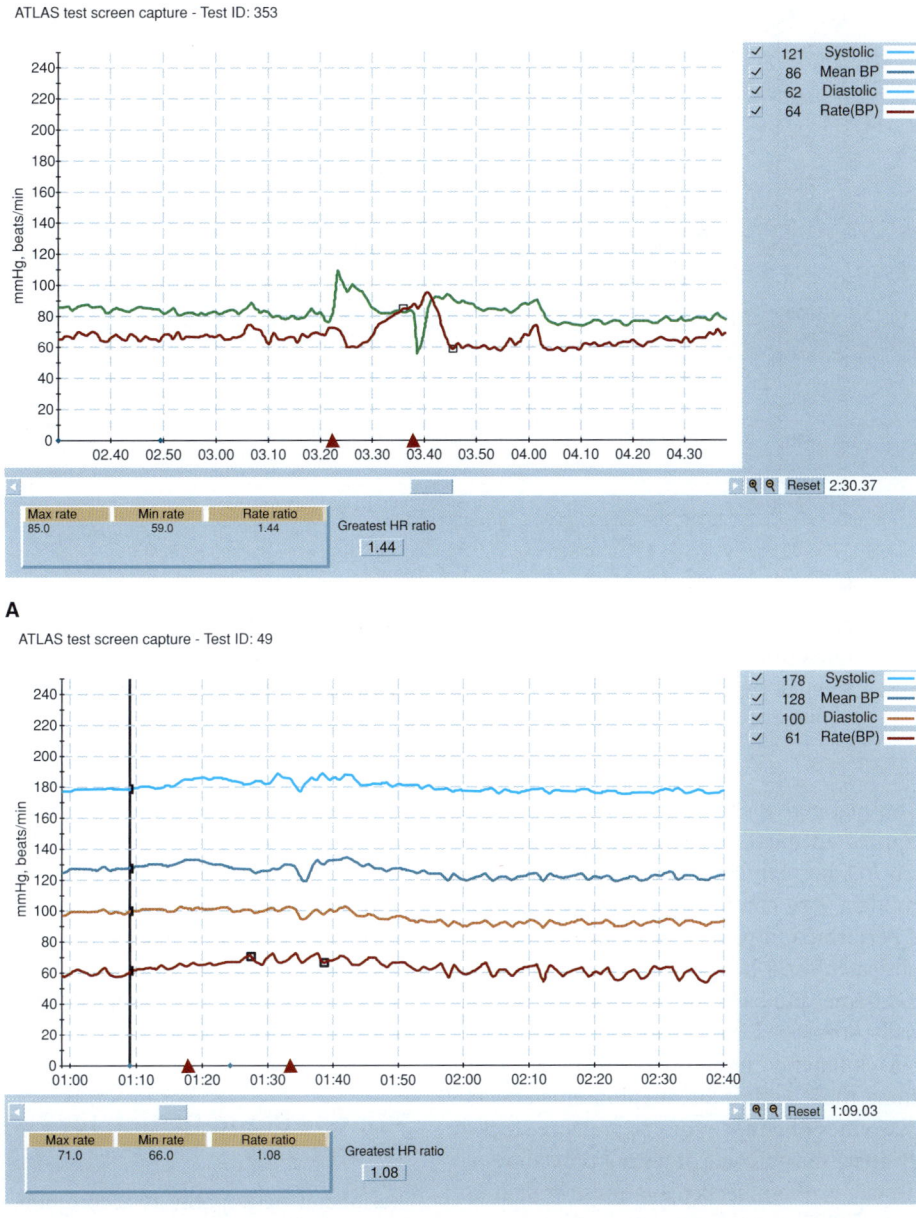

Figure 2-28. Normal (**A**) and abnormal (**B**) responses to the Valsalva maneuver. *Red line*, heart rate; *green line*, mean arterial blood pressure. First *red arrowhead*, glottic closure; second *red arrowhead*, glottic release.

of the postural orthostatic tachycardia syndrome. Finally, prolonged tilt table monitoring may be utilized to reproduce symptoms in patients believed to suffer from neurocardiogenic syncope (vasovagal syncope). In these patients, symptoms of impaired CNS blood flow are accompanied by hypotension and paradoxical bradycardia.

QSART is a means to assess cholinergic, postganglionic sympathetic sudomotor function.[86-88] It is particularly attractive as a test for SFN and other DSPNs with dysautonomic components. It can be applied in numerous topographical locations and is therefore potentially capable of identifying a length-dependent pattern of hypohydrosis.

Typically, QSART is performed by placing sweat capsules in four standardized locations: the dorsum of the foot, shin, thigh, and forearm. These capsules measure the humidity produced by sweat production emanating from the tested skin surface in response to an injected intradermal cholinergic stimulus. The sensitivity of QSART in the detection of SFN ranges between 60% and 80%, similar to QST. In diabetic patients, there are similar rates of both sensitivity and concordance regarding results of the heart rate response to deep breathing, the Valsalva maneuver, and QSART.[89] Normative data for QSART also varies by gender, age, and area tested. Mean values range between 1 and 3 μL/cm squared.

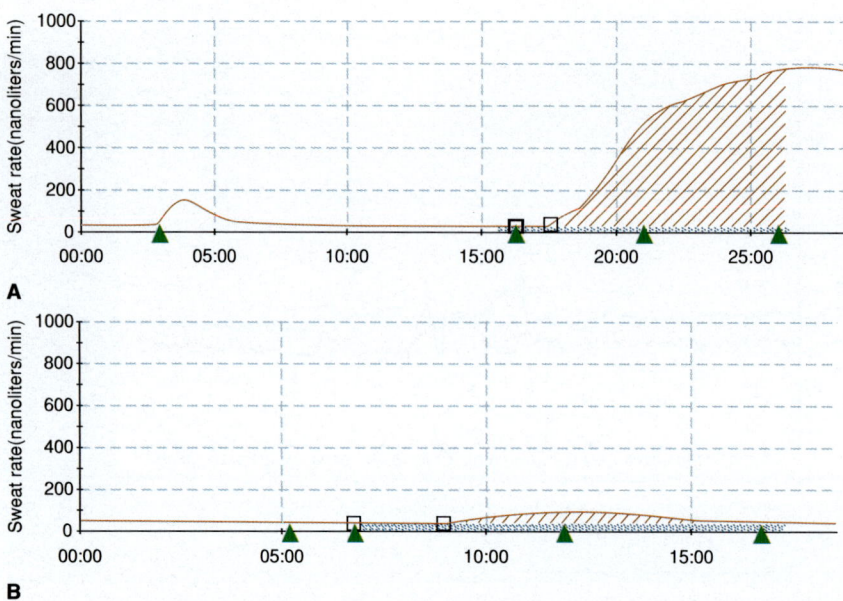

Figure 2-29. Normal (**A**) and abnormal (**B**) responses to quantitative sudomotor axon reflex testing. First *green arrowhead*, ACh injection; second *green arrowhead*, 2 mA stimulus begins; third *green arrowhead*, stimulus ceases; fourth *green arrowhead*, 5 minutes post stimulus cessation.

Autonomic testing, perhaps more than any other testing modality, requires adequate control of environmental variables that may readily confound the accuracy of test results. Normative data vary considerably with patient age. Ideally, testing is performed in patients who are adequately hydrated, have not eaten for 8 hours, nor smoked tobacco, drank ethanol or caffeine, and have not been recently physically or emotionally stressed. Drugs that potentially react with adrenergic or cholinergic receptors are to be avoided if possible, including those with indirect autonomic effects such as insulin. Extremes of temperature or pressure stockings can adversely affect the outcome of testing procedure.

Autonomic testing is recommended as a consideration in patients with suspected SFN or autonomic neuropathy phenotypes.[85] Neither the American Academy of Neurology nor the authors recommend ANST as part of the routine evaluation of patients with DSPN without clinical suggestion of autonomic nervous system involvement. Heart rate variability to deep breathing is felt to have a greater than 90% sensitivity and greater than 97% specificity for the identification of dysautonomia in a diabetic neuropathy cohort, in the absence of confounding cardiac disease.[85] QSART is reported to have a sensitivity exceeding 75% in detecting sudomotor abnormalities in a population with an SFN phenotype.[85] Like QST, it is felt that both the sensitivity and specificity of ANST are improved upon either performance of a battery of tests rather than a single test.[85]

Blood Testing

There is limited evidence to identify a sensitive, specific, and cost-effective laboratory evaluation strategy for most neuromuscular syndromes. As evaluations for specific neuromuscular syndromes will be addressed in detail in subsequent chapters of this book, they will be mentioned here only in summary terms. An ideal blood test would be cost effective, and accurate in identifying or excluding a specific disorder in a tested population. There are few tests that conform to this description, with ACh receptor (AChR) binding antibodies being arguably the best example.

Routine Blood Testing for Peripheral Neuropathy

Peripheral neuropathy is a common neuromuscular problem, often associated with a nonspecific phenotype, and associated with an extensive list of potential causes. The etiology, however, is undiscovered in approximately 50% of patients despite extensive evaluation. Understandably, there is an incentive to test extensively to fill in this gap. There are many published algorithms that attempt to provide clinicians with an ideal battery of screening tests for peripheral neuropathy.[65,85,90–94] Practice parameters constructed by the American Academy of Neurology recommends fasting blood sugar, vitamin B12 levels and serum protein electrophoresis in a patient with a typical, sensory predominant, axonal DSPN.[85,94] A more extensive evaluation is justified when there are atypical phenotypic features. Specifically, a neuropathy with acute–subacute onset, a multifocal or non–length-dependent pattern, associated with significant sensory ataxia or with associated systemic symptoms is worthy of a more aggressive diagnostic approach that could include more extensive blood work, CSF analysis, and imaging or histologic analysis of nerve or other relevant tissues.[91,92] As the selection of additional tests is dependent on both the neuropathy phenotype, as well as in the context in which the neuropathy occurs, recommendations concerning selection of other tests will be provided in the following paragraphs, rather than in an algorithmic format.

Deficiency of vitamins B1, B6, B12, E, and folic acid are potentially causally related to peripheral neuropathy. In addition, a sensory neuropathy/neuronopathy may occur with vitamin B6 toxicity in daily doses that are estimated to exceed 200 mg. Other than for B12, testing for vitamin deficiency is generally not recommended on a routine basis and is generally reserved for those patients perceived to be at higher risk.[93] This group would include patients with a sensory predominant neuropathy who are at risk of nutritional deficiency due to alcoholism, dietary anomalies, isoniazid exposure, and malabsorption from bariatric surgery or enteral disease such as celiac sprue. Symptom onset in the hands may indicate a myeloneuropathy, a common presentation of vitamin B12 deficiency. Measurements of serum levels of methylmalonic acid may improve detection of this latter disorder when B12 levels are in the borderline 200–300 ng/L range. As copper deficiency produces a phenotype in many ways identical to B12 deficiency, determination of serum copper and ceruloplasmin levels are recommended with any evaluation for myeloneuropathy.

Serum MCPs have been recognized to occur with an increased prevalence in patients with polyneuropathy for decades. Most MCPs associated with peripheral neuropathy will initially be designated as being of unknown significance (MGUS). The neuropathy associated with MGUS may vary depending on MCP type but is typically a nonspecific, sensory great than motor, and length-dependent phenotype. Both the clinical and EDX features implicate a primarily axonal, DSPN phenotype in neuropathies associated with IgG and IgA MCPs.[95,96] In these cases, the association between the neuropathy and MGUS is statistical; a causal relationship remains unproven.

The best evidence for a causal relationship for MGUS exists in patients with an IgM kappa MCP. IgM kappa-related neuropathy has a very distinctive demyelinating sensory-predominant phenotype, frequently with sensory ataxia. This is in turn often associated with antibodies directed toward myelin-associated glycoprotein (MAG) in a significant percentage of cases. These antibodies will be discussed further in the following section.

A few patients with an MCP at the time of initial evaluation and a larger percentage subsequently will have a secondary cause.[104] Multiple myeloma, amyloidosis, lymphoma, cryoglobulinemia, or POEMS syndrome are noteworthy examples. A lambda, rather than a kappa, light chain increases the probability of a secondary cause of an MCP. Secondary causes of MCP-related neuropathy often have more distinctive phenotypes. For example, polyneuropathy, organomegaly, endocrinopathy, MCP, and skin changes (POEMS) syndrome is often associated with a motor-predominant, demyelinating, non–length-dependent CIDP phenotype. Serum measurements of vascular endothelial growth factor (VEGF) may represent a serum marker for this disease and may aid discriminating POEMS from other disorders associated with neuropathy, an MCP, and multiorgan involvement.[97,98] Amyloidosis may manifest with a number of phenotypes such as a small fiber phenotype with prominent dysautonomia or as a severe multifocal, axonal, sensorimotor neuropathy. MCPs or light chains can be detected in these disorders in serum and/or urine by immunoelectrophoresis (SIEP, UIEP) or preferably by immunofixation (IFE). The latter is more sensitive but is also more labor intensive. For these reasons, it is not used as a default screening procedure by many laboratories.

Diabetic neuropathy is common and is associated with multiple phenotypes. The diagnosis of diabetic neuropathy is dependent on the fulfillment of criteria outlined by the American Diabetes Association and by the association with one or more of the characteristic clinical and EDX diabetic neuropathy phenotypes.[99] Although thickening of the basal membranes of the vasa nervorum demonstrable by nerve biopsy is characteristic of diabetes, the role of basement membrane thickening in the pathogenesis of diabetic nerve injury remains uncertain. A direct causal relationship between diabetes and neuropathy is only suggested pathologically. Alternative causes of peripheral neuropathy should always be considered in diabetic patients, particularly if the phenotype is atypical. The American Diabetes Association indicate that an elevated fasting blood sugar ($\geq$124 mg/dL), an abnormal 2-hour glucose tolerance test ($\geq$200 mg/dL), or an elevated hemoglobin A1C ($\geq$6.5%) are diagnostic of diabetes mellitus.[94] Traditionally, neuropathy was not readily attributed to diabetes unless the diagnosis of diabetes was well established. More recently, a statistical association has been demonstrated between impaired glucose tolerance (FBS 110–125 mg/dL, GTT 140–199 mg/dL, hemoglobin A1C between 5.7% and 6.4%) and an SFN phenotype.[100-103]

In patients with a multiple mononeuropathy pattern, particularly those of acute to subacute onset, screening blood tests relevant to this pattern of neuropathy are recommended. The odds of identifying an underlying cause, particularly a systemic disease, is much higher in this phenotype than in DSPN. Notable considerations include serum and urine IFE, sedimentation rate and/or c-reactive protein, eosinophil count and tests for anticytoplasmic neutrophilic antibodies, rheumatoid factor, SS-A and SS-B antibodies, angiotensin converting enzyme, cryoglobulins, hepatitis B and C, and Lyme and HIV serology.[104] In these patients, relevant imaging, CSF evaluation for potential neoplastic meningitis which may mimic a multifocal neuropathy, and potential nerve biopsy should be additional considerations.

Sensory ataxia is usually the result of a neuronopathy/ganglionopathy and often autoimmune in nature. The possible causes include an underlying inflammatory condition (e.g., Sjögren syndrome, systemic lupus erythematosus, celiac disease), a paraneoplastic process (e.g., anti-Hu syndrome), toxin (e.g., platin, B6 toxicity), and infections (e.g., HIV), but in at least half of cases are idiopathic despite extensive workup.[92] It is most important to evaluate for an underlying tumor. We order paraneoplastic antibodies (e.g., anti-Hu, anti-CRMP5, antiamphiphysin) as well as an SPEP/IFE as well as a whole-body PET/CT to search for malignancy. To assess for Sjögren syndrome, we check for antinuclear antibodies (ANAs), anti-Ro/La antibodies, perform a Schirmer or Rose-Bengal tests, and minor salivary gland biopsy. Sensory ataxia can also occur in GBS and related disorders [e.g., Miller Fisher syndrome (MFS)], chronic demyelinating neuropathies as seen in classic CIDP or variants (chronic inflammatory sensory polyradiculopathy or CISP and distal acquired demyelinating sensorimotor polyneuropathy or DADS), anti-MAG antibodies, as well as the newer antinodal or paranodal antibody-associated polyradiculoneuropathies. More is discussed below under **Serologic Testing** and in the disease-specific chapters in this textbook.

Blood testing for heavy metals known to cause peripheral neuropathy (arsenic, lead, mercury and thallium) has a limited role in the evaluation of patients with peripheral neuropathy. The reasons are both the rarity of the conditions and the short circulating half-life of the toxic substances. Neuropathies resulting from heavy metal exposure are frequently motor predominant and commonly coexist with CNS and systemic symptoms such as abdominal pain, hair, skin, and nail changes. Blood testing is most likely to be helpful in the setting of an acute monophasic exposure. Urine, nail, and hair assessments are more likely to be positive with chronic low-level exposures. A particular pitfall is the possibility of false-positive urine arsenic testing resulting from seafood ingestion. Many seafood species contain significant amounts of the relatively innocuous pentavalent forms of arsenate as opposed to the more toxic trivalent arsenate species.

Routine Blood Testing for Myopathy

Measurement of serum creatine kinase (CK) is a valuable adjunct in the evaluation of patients with neuromuscular disease.[105] Although considered to be primarily a marker of muscle disease, increased serum CK levels commonly occur in ALS and other neurogenic disorders. Conversely, elevated CK levels do not occur in all myopathies. In normal individuals, levels may reach 5× the upper limits of normal following EDX or other invasive medical procedures and perhaps as high as 50× the upper limits of normal in extreme, protracted exercise. Levels increased by any of these provocations should return to normal by 1 week after the event but have been reported to remain elevated for 3 weeks following eccentric exercise involving protracted muscle contraction.[106] The level of CK does not typically correlate with the degree of muscle destruction or weakness.

Elevations of serum CK may occur in asymptomatic individuals. Normal CK levels vary with race, sex, age, muscle mass, and physical activity. A population study demonstrated that 13% of Whites, 23% of South Asians, and 49% Blacks had CK measurements at rest that exceeded manufacturer's upper limits of normal.[107] At the extreme, the upper limits of normal (97.5th percentile) for serum CK in their Black male population was 801 IU.[107] What may appear to be an abnormality may not be so in an individual when normative data for race and sex are considered. As neuromuscular specialists commonly evaluate patients with elevated CK levels, both with and without statin exposure, knowledge of this variability in normal populations becomes quite important.

Recognizing that a certain percentage of patients with hyperCKemia are likely to be normal, there are undoubtedly inherited neuromuscular conditions in which elevated serum CK levels may be prepenetrant, that is, exist in individuals with disease-causing mutations who have yet to develop recognizable signs or symptoms. It is equally plausible that many of these patients with "idiopathic hyperCKemia" harbor sequence alterations in various muscle proteins that are not "disease causing" but capable of causing CK "leak."

There are other blood tests that may be helpful in the identification of specific muscle diseases. Growth differentiation factor 15 (GDF-15) and fibroblast growth factor 21 (FGF-21) are elevated in many mitochondrial disorders, particularly in those with muscle involvement.[108–111] Some studies suggest GDF-15 are more sensitive,[108–110] while others have noted that FGF-21 levels are more sensitive and specific.[111] Measurement of serum lactate, although neither sensitive nor specific, provides a screening test for certain mitochondrial myopathies. A nonischemic exercise forearm test to measure if there is a normal rise in lactic acid with ammonia level serving as a control is a useful test when looking for glycogen storage diseases associated with recurrent myoglobinuria (e.g., McArdle disease)[112] as mentioned in Chapter 1 and discussed in greater detail in Chapter 29 (Metabolic Myopathies). A dried blood spot for alpha-glucosidase activity is useful screening test for Pompe disease.[113] Serum carnitine levels may be extremely low (<5% of normal) in primary carnitine deficiency but slightly reduced levels are not helpful as secondary carnitine deficiency is evident in many different myopathies. A plasma acylcarnitine profile may be helpful in suspected disorders of lipid metabolism, particularly multiple acyl-dehydrogenase deficiency. A peripheral blood smear may be helpful in identifying lipid-containing vacuoles within leukocytes known as Jordan bodies which may be found in neutral lipid storage disorders.

Serologic Testing

There is a wide spectrum in the value of serologic tests available in the evaluation of neuromuscular disease. At one end of the spectrum are AChR-binding antibodies that are sensitive, specific, and undoubtedly of pathophysiologic relevance. On the other hand, there are commercially available antibodies that have at best a tenuous relationship to disease causation and any phenotype. Like all testing, the specificity of antibody testing is increased when a hypothesis-driven approach is used. Ideally, a specific test is ordered to support or confirm a clinically suspected diagnosis. When large panels are ordered indiscriminately, an opportunity facilitated by industry marketing practices, the probability of a false-positive result increases.

This section will address those antibody tests that are commercially available, that appear to represent legitimate markers of specific neuromuscular phenotypes, and have adequate sensitivity to warrant their use when clinically indicated. Tests with limited sensitivity and/or specificity are purposefully omitted. In the patients with peripheral neuropathy, the yield of antibody tests will increase in patients with subacute courses, demyelinating pathophysiology, multifocal distributions, and phenotypes restricted to either a motor, sensory, or autonomic domain.[75] Chronic neuropathies that are length dependent, predominantly axonal, and sensorimotor in their characteristics are less likely to associate with abnormal serologic tests of diagnostic significance.

Paraneoplastic Antibodies

Approximately 5% of patients with peripheral neuropathy may be found to have cancer with aggressive investigation.[114] In most cases, the neuropathy will conform to a nonspecific DSPN phenotype. Accordingly, there is uncertainty as to whether the relationship is causal or coincidental. A subacute course, recognition of a suspicious phenotype such as sensory neuronopathy, and, identification of a "paraneoplastic antibody" increases the likelihood that the cancer and neuropathy are related. Paraneoplastic antibodies associated with peripheral neuropathy include those directed against the antineuronal nuclear type 1 (ANNA-1 or anti-Hu), the antineuronal nuclear types 2 and 3, the collapsing response-mediator protein 5 (CRMP-5), amphiphysin, and N-type calcium channel antigens.[75] In general, "paraneoplastic" antibodies are a marker of the existence and type of cancer, and do not specifically correlate with a singular phenotype.[115]

Anti-Hu (ANNA-1) has a clearly defined phenotype and is the most common paraneoplastic antibody in disorders of the peripheral nervous system. Hu refers to an antigen found within the nuclei of dorsal root ganglia, the CNS, the myenteric plexus, and in certain cancers, most notably small cell carcinoma of the lung (SCCL).[115–117] Although many of the phenotypes associated with Hu antibody correlate with the locations of Hu antigen, the weight of existing evidence does not provide a direct pathogenetic role for these antibodies. Detecting anti-Hu antibodies in the serum will lead to the detection of an underlying malignancy in greater than 90% of cases. Some of these may not be initially detectable by conventional imaging methods.

Anti-Hu antibodies are most closely correlated with a sensory neuronopathy phenotype, that is, a non–length-dependent, multifocal syndrome of sensory loss that frequently includes pain and sensory ataxia. In a cohort of patients with anti-Hu antibodies in the serum, neuropathy represents 70%–80% of all neurologic complications. Having said that, only 1% of patients with SCCL will develop a sensory neuronopathy. Conversely, it is estimated that 20% of patients presenting with a sensory neuronopathy will be found to have an underlying malignancy. Not all neuropathies associated with anti-Hu antibodies, however, conform to a sensory neuronopathy phenotype. Some will be found to have a DSPN, a motor predominant phenotype, or an acute autonomic neuropathy/neuronopathy.[117] The latter may approximate the clinical features of the nonparaneoplastic, immune-mediated autonomic neuropathy/neuronopathy associated with antibodies directed against the ganglionic ACh receptor as described below. Impaired enteric motility is the most common manifestation of the paraneoplastic form of acute autonomic neuropathy, frequently presenting as constipation, vomiting, early satiety, or abdominal pain. Cerebellar degeneration, and limbic and brainstem encephalitis are other notable Hu-related syndromes. Testing for anti-Hu antibodies is recommended in the appropriate clinical context, that is, a subacute sensory syndrome occurring in a smoker, with or without other symptoms suggesting neoplasia or other concomitant paraneoplastic syndromes. Antibodies directed against the collapsing response-mediator protein 5 (CRMP5), initially calledanti-CV2, have an even more diverse association with neurologic and nonneurologic syndromes.[118,119] Patients with CRMP5 antibodies most often manifest with an asymmetric, painful axonal polyradiculoneuropathy that is usually asymmetric onset and precedes the diagnosis of cancer by approximately 6 months (range 60–540 days).[119] Patients with anti-CRMP5 antibodies also can present with a painful axonal, sensory polyneuropathy in which the sensory axons appear to be the target of the suspected immune-mediated injury. Other manifestations include cerebellar degeneration, MG, uveitis, optic neuropathy, chorea, and dysgeusia/dysosmia. Again, the presence of these antibodies correlates best with small cell lung cancer.

Patients with antiamphiphysin–IgG antibodies also most commonly present with a painful polyradiculoneuropathy but can manifest as a sensory neuronopathy, or autonomic neuropathy (gastroparesis). It can overlap with stiff-person syndrome, the most common CNS presentation. These antibodies are most commonly associated with breast cancer.[120]

Nicotinic ganglionic ACh receptor autoantibodies (α3-AChR) target the receptors that mediate synaptic transmission in autonomic ganglion.[121] As mentioned above, their presence in the serum often correlates with a syndrome of subacute dysautonomia. The phenotype may include orthostatic hypotension, erectile dysfunction in men, sicca symptoms, heat intolerance secondary to anhidrosis, abnormal pupillary responses, impaired gastrointestinal motility with gastroparesis and constipation, and urinary retention secondary to neurogenic bladder. Other neurologic manifestations associated with these antibodies may include peripheral neuropathy in approximately 36% of individuals and encephalopathy in 13%. Like LEMS, these autoantibodies may be either paraneoplastic or nonparaneoplastic. They are identified in approximately 50% of patients with an acute or subacute autonomic neuropathy. When paraneoplastic, they are often associated with adenocarcinoma of the breast, prostate, lung, or GI tract.

Antibodies Directed Toward Components of Peripheral Nerves

An increasing number of antibodies have been discovered that target components of peripheral nerve, including the myelin sheath and axonal proteins in the nodal and paranodal regions (Fig. 2-30). As they are exclusively found in peripheral nerve, and are frequently superficially positioned, they provide an exposed and potentially specific antigenic target for an autoimmune attack. In addition, some of these antigens share epitopes with bacterial species that may be relevant to the pathogenesis of neuropathies such as GBS.

Antibodies directed against MAG, first described in 1980, have a very well-defined phenotype and are the most likely of all currently available peripheral neuropathy antibody tests to have a direct pathogenic role.[122,123] Typically, MAG-associated neuropathy, referred to by the DADS acronym (distal acquired demyelinating sensory neuropathy), is a slowly progressive disorder that affects males more than females. Middle-aged and older individuals are at risk. It is characterized by large fiber sensory loss and sensory ataxia, global areflexia, demyelinating neurophysiology, and often by tremor. Distal weakness, when present, develops later in the course.

In nerve biopsies from patients with this disorder, immunofluorescent staining has detected radiolabeled antibody bound to peripheral nerve myelin. This is associated with the distinctive pathologic feature of myelin membrane separation. MAG antibodies are found in 50%–70% of patients with the characteristic phenotype associated with an IgM kappa MCP.[124–126] Conversely, approximately 85% of patients with this phenotype and anti-MAG antibodies will have a detectable IgM MCP.[127] The presence or absence of an anti-MAG antibody in patients with the DADS phenotype and an IgM MCP does not appear to change either natural history or the lack of responsiveness to immunotherapy. In light of this, it can be argued that testing for anti-MAG antibodies is superfluous in patients who have the characteristic clinical syndrome, EDX pattern, and presence of an IgM kappa MCP. If anti-MAG activity is sought, it is important to be aware of the potential for false-positive test results for the enzyme-linked immunosorbent assay (ELISA) screening technique. Conversely, the specificity for the Western Blot confirmatory test has been reported to be as high as 80%–90%. Furthermore, not all patients with anti-MAG antibodies have the characteristic DADS clinical phenotype and EDX findings; some have a large fiber axonal sensory or sensorimotor polyneuropathy or SFN and the pathogenic relevance of the antibody to the neuropathy is unclear.

IgM antibodies directed against the GM1 ganglioside, first described in 1984, correlate with the syndrome of MMN, with or without detectable demyelinating conduction block.[128–135] Although the GM1 glycolipid exists in motor nerves, there is no convincing evidence to date that these antibodies are pathogenic. In high titer, IgM-anti-GM1 antibodies appear to be fairly specific for MMN. Their specificity declines in low titer, being detectable in motor neuron disease, inflammatory demyelinating neuropathy, and normal individuals. The utility of anti-IgM-GM1 antibody testing is greatest in the clinical setting of a lower motor neuron syndrome in which

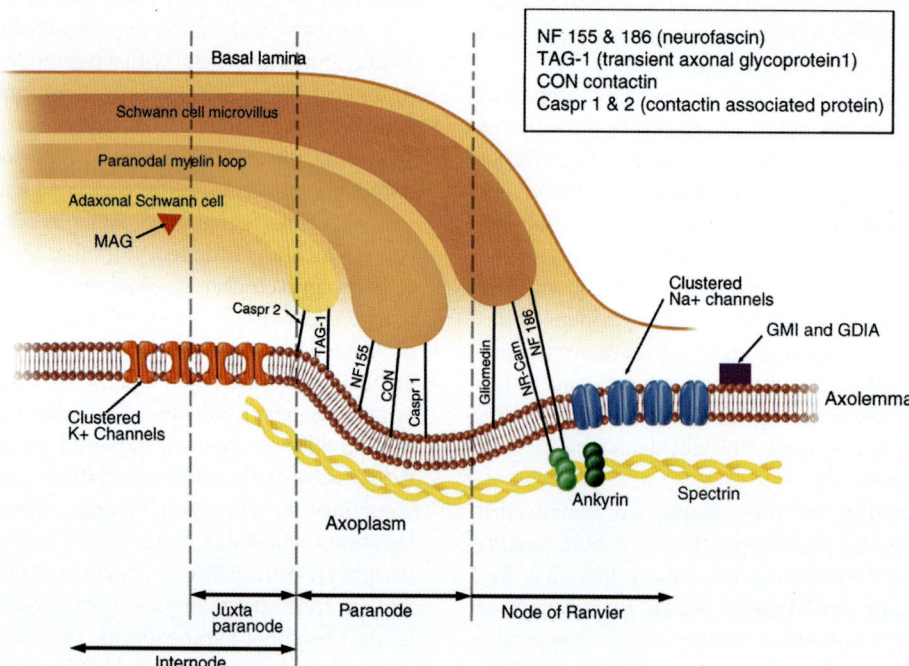

Figure 2-30. Simplified schematic of a peripheral nerve fiber (motor) nodal/paranodal junction with locations of proteins and ion channels potentially relevant to the pathogenesis of antibody-associated polyneuropathies.

demyelinating conduction block cannot be demonstrated. Identification of high titers of IgM anti-GM1 antibodies in this population support the diagnosis of a treatable motor neuropathy and distinguish it from a treatment-resistant, degenerative, or hereditary motor neuron disease. Although the sensitivity of this test has been quoted to be as high as 85%, their absence does not preclude treatment responsiveness as their sensitivity is a more modest 40%–60%. Testing for anti-GM1 antibodies in lower motor neuron syndromes accompanied by definite upper motor neuron and/or bulbar features has a low yield and is not generally recommended.

Anti-IgG-GM1 antibodies are linked to the classic demyelinating form of GBS may also have serologic evidence of *Campylobacter jejuni* infection, thus providing a potential antigenic link between these two entities. Anti-IgG-GD1 autoantibodies have been specifically linked to the acute motor axonal neuropathy (AMAN) variant of GBS but not to *C. jejuni* infection. In general, testing for either of these antibodies adds little to the traditional clinical, EDX and CSF diagnostic evaluation for GBS.

Testing for antibodies directed against the GQ1b ganglioside is helpful in the appropriate clinical setting as a marker for GBS and its Miller Fisher variant in patients presenting with acute ophthalmoparesis, providing high levels of sensitivity and specificity.[136–138] They are found in the serum of 80%–100% of patients with the MFS.[137,138] The apparent relevance of anti-GQ1b antibodies is made even more attractive by the demonstration that this antigen is abundantly expressed in the paranodes of the cranial nerves affecting oculomotor function. The GQ1b antigen can be found in certain strains of *C. jejuni*. That said, the clinical phenotype suffices in making the diagnosis and treatment decisions not hinge upon waiting for the results of the antibody testing that can take days or weeks. Therefore, we do not typically order in clear cases of MFS.

IgG4 antibodies directed against contactin-1 (CNTN1), previously known as contactin-associated protein-1 (Caspr1), and neurofascin 155 (NF155) are found in 10% of patients who were previously deemed to have a form of chronic inflammatory polyneuropathy (CIDP) (Fig. 2-30).[139–141] However, although EDX suggests a demyelinating polyneuropathy, the clinical phenotype and histopathology suggest these are distinct from classic CIDP. They are often associated with distal weakness, sensory ataxia, pain, and tremor in young adults and associated with early nodal and paranodal damage and refractoriness to intravenous immunoglobulin. Furthermore, some cases of chronic immune sensory polyradiculopathy have been associated with IgG4-contactin-1 and to a lesser extent IgG4-NF155 antibodies.[142] IgM and non-IgG4 IgG directed against NF155 as well as antibodies directed against NF140/186 do not have a specific clinical or EDX phenotype.

IgM antibodies directed against the sulfatide moiety of peripheral nerve correlates with a chronic, axonal, sensory predominant phenotype that may be painful. These antibodies, however, are found in less than 1% of patients with typical DPSN.[143] Approximately half of patients with antisulfatide activity will be found to have an associated MCP. Furthermore, trisulfated heparin disaccharide (TS-HDS) and fibroblast growth factor-3 (FGFR-3) autoantibodies have been found in some patients with SFN and ganglionopathy.[144–147] As these antibodies occur infrequently, are of uncertain pathophysiologic significance, and do not define an apparent treatable condition, they have limited clinical utility in the author's estimation.

Antibody Testing for DNMT

The basis for antibody testing in MG has evolved from the initial pathogenetic observations of Patrick and Lindstrom in 1973.[148] Testing for the presence of antibodies directed at various components of the nicotinic, postsynaptic anti-AChR remains the most accurate of neuromuscular antibody tests. Anti-AChR antibodies are present in approximately 50% of patients with ocular myasthenia and 80%–90% of patients with generalized MG.[3,149–151] There are binding, blocking, and modulating antibodies of which the antibinding antibodies are most common. ACh-modulating antibodies may be detected in a significant titer in approximately 5% of patients who lack AChR-binding antibodies. Blocking antibodies alone are even less informative. False-positive AChR antibodies tests are uncommon but have been reported to occur. These may be found in LEMS, graft-versus-host disease, autoimmune hepatitis, patients with thymoma (but no symptoms or signs of myasthenia), and rare patients with lung cancer and motor neuron disease. A recent study from the Mayo Clinic found that specificity improved (95%) by first testing for AChR-binding antibodies and if positive then reflex testing for AChR-modulating antibodies.[151] This resulted in a 45% reduction of false positives while maintaining AChR-Bi 90% sensitivity. There is no correlation between antibody titer and the severity of MG. AChR antibodies have no utility in monitoring treatment response, as titers do not reliably decline coincident with successful treatment and as antibodies may remain in patients who enjoy clinical remission. Occasionally, patients with MG will seroconvert so that repeating the test in someone who is initially seronegative may be of potential value.

Autoantibodies targeting muscle-specific kinase (MuSK), a protein involved in AChR clustering at the NMJ, occur in ~10% of patients (~40% of AChR antibody–negative patients)[152–157] and 1%–3% have antibodies to low-density lipoprotein receptor-related protein 4 (LRP4) or agrin, which are also important for clustering of AChRs.[158–160] More detail regarding the differences in clinical phenotype, and importantly response to treatment, are discussed in detail in Chapter 25.

Autoantibodies targeting striational proteins (including titin, myosin, actin, α-and actinin, as well as the ryanodine receptors) have been linked to thymoma; however, a recent study from the Mayo Clinic reported that these antistriational antibodies are neither specific nor sensitive in predicting malignancy or neurologic phenotypes and proposed eliminating test for this specific in the evaluation of myasthenia.[161] Antibodies targeting glutamic acid decarboxylase-65 (GAD65), voltage-gated Kv1 potassium channel (VGKC) complex, collapsin response mediator protein-5 (CRMP5), and the ganglionic AChR (α3) have also been detected in myasthenics with thymoma.[161] However, we do not routinely assess for these either- in part because all patients with MG are imaged for thymoma.

Rippling muscle syndrome is a rare disorder found in the limb-girdle dystrophy muscular dystrophy type 1C associated with caveolin-3 mutations. It may also occur as an acquired disorder in association with MG, thymoma, and AChR antibodies. Recently, antibodies have been found to be directed against autoantibody specific to caveolae-associated protein 4 (cavin-4) that localizes to T-tubules where it interacts with cavelin-3.[162]

The LEMS is an immune-mediated, presynaptic disorder neuromuscular transmission. It may occur as an isolated disorder in young women but most frequently occurs as a paraneoplastic condition in older individuals. The most common associated neoplasm is SCCL. Detection of an underlying malignancy has been reported to occur at a frequency between 43% and 69% of individuals with the LEMS phenotype.[3,163] Autoantibodies directed against the P/Q type of voltage-gated calcium channels are pathogenetic and represent a highly sensitive and specific marker for this disease. These antibodies do not block calcium channels but rather bind to them, resulting in downregulation through endocytosis. This in turn reduces the number of active zones in the presynaptic region and results in diminished quantal release. These antibodies were originally estimated to occur in high titer in virtually 100% of paraneoplastic LEMS and in greater than 90% of LEMS occurring independent of any underlying malignancy.[163] As in seronegative MG, seronegative LEMS appears to be an antibody-mediated autoimmune disorder. False-positive test results are rare and usually occur in low titer. Anti-glial nuclear antibodies (SOX-1) directed against the Bergmann glia of the cerebellum have been identified as a marker of neoplasia in LEMS. In one study, SOX-1 autoantibodies have been found in 64% of LEMS patients with small cell lung cancer, but in none of the patients with apparent idiopathic LEMS.[164]

Serologic Testing for Muscle Disease

Myositis-specific (MSA) or myositis-associated (MAA) antibodies are detected in 60%–80% of patients with idiopathic inflammatory myopathy.[164–168] The MSAs have been increasingly found to be helpful as they are often associated with characteristic clinical and histopathological features, different prognoses, and response to treatments. For example, anti-TIF1-gamma antibodies are associated with dermatomyositis and cancer; antisynthetase antibodies are associated with interstitial fibrosis, arthritis, Raynaud phenomena, and mechanic hands; anti-3-hydroxy-3-methylglutaryl-coenzyme A reductase (HMGCR) and signal recognition particle (SRP) antibodies are found in patients with autoimmune necrotizing myopathies; anti-NT5C1A antibodies have a high specificity for inclusion body myositis. A problem is that there are a variety of commercial laboratories using different methods to detect these antibodies (immunoprecipitation, ELISA, dot blot, Western blot) that can lead to false positive results, particularly at low levels.

MAA (e.g., antinuclear and extractable nuclear antibodies) typically occur in individuals with other connective tissue diseases, with or without an associated myositis (e.g., overlap syndromes). These antibodies and associations are discussed in greater detail in Chapter 33 (Inflammatory Myopathies).

Serologic Testing for Infectious Causes of Neuromuscular Disease

Lyme disease can cause cranial neuropathy and polyradiculopathy. Serology is the primary testing method for confirmation because of the difficulties inherent in the culture of the *Borrelia burgdorferi* spirochete. There are several controversies. In most laboratories, initial screening is performed on serum by ELISA methodology, a test with high sensitivity but limited specificity.[169–171] ELISA is estimated to have a 5% false-positive rate. False negatives are typically due to early testing, delayed seroconversion that requires 2–8 weeks to occur, or early antimicrobial exposure. By the time neurologic manifestations occur in the early disseminated phase of the disease, false-negative results are unexpected. If the ELISA screen is positive, confirmation is achieved by Western blot detection of IgM and IgG antibodies directed at specific Lyme antigens.[172] There is no recognized role for Western blotting in the setting of a negative ELISA screen. Despite its specificity, the use of Western blotting alone without ELISA screening provides some risk of a false-negative result. Polymerase chain reaction, C6 ELISA antigen detection in urine, detection of immune complex disruption, and B lymphocyte chemoattractant have either not been adequately tested or not achieved adequate levels of sensitivity and/or specificity to be routinely applied to either serum or CSF.[173] In the CSF, demonstrating IgG and IgM Lyme antibodies in concentrations greater than those found in serum is currently the recommended means to confirm CNS involvement. The detection of Lyme antibodies in the spinal fluid may lack sensitivity, and CSF pleocytosis and/or elevation of protein levels in the appropriate clinical context is considered sufficient by some to identify CNS Lyme disease.[174–177]

HIV is a neurotropic virus that is associated with several neuromuscular disorders.[178–180] Serologic testing is based on the detection of IgG antibodies directed against the p24 nucleocapsid and gp41 and 120 envelope proteins. These antibodies appear within 6 weeks in most infected individuals and within 6 months in 95%. A positive test requires detection of two of these three antigens and has a detected sensitivity and specificity of over 99%. As in Lyme disease, serologic testing for HIV typically consists of an ELISA screen followed by Western blot confirmation. HIV antigens can be detected in the CSF in patients with CNS involvement.

Other Serologic Tests in Neuromuscular Disease

Neuropathy is estimated to occur in approximately 10% of patients with Sjögren and/or the sicca syndrome. There are several neuropathy phenotypes that occur with this condition.[181,182] A sensory neuronopathy syndrome, with or without an associated trigeminal neuropathy, is the most distinctive of these. As trigeminal neuropathy is infrequent in paraneoplastic sensory neuropathy, its identification serves as a potentially helpful clue in distinguishing between these two disorders. An SFN phenotype may be the most common neuromuscular condition associated with Sjögren syndrome. Multiple mononeuropathies and cranial neuropathies may occur as well. Anti-Ro (SS-A) and anti-LA (SS-B) antibodies represent a reasonable screening test in patients with a neuropathy with sicca symptomatology or a typical Sjögren phenotype. These are detectable in approximately 60% of patients. Detection of ANAs or the rheumatoid factor provides less specific support for a Sjögren diagnosis. The diagnosis of seronegative Sjögren or sicca-related neuropathy is dependent on tissue analysis, usually provided by lip biopsy that will reveal an inflammatory response directed against minor salivary glands.

Celiac disease has been reported by some in as many as 2.5% of individuals with an apparent idiopathic polyneuropathy, but the association between celiac sprue and polyneuropathy is controversial.[182–185] The neuropathy pattern is typically DSPN, that is, sensory predominant, axonal, and length dependent. The neuropathy is reported to occur at times in the absence of gastrointestinal symptoms. Gliadin, transglutaminase, and endomysial antibody tests are all potential screening tests for this disorder, the former having the least specificity. IgA rather than IgG gliadin antibodies are felt to be more specific for celiac disease. When these are detected in neuropathy patients, it is usually in individuals with known sprue, thus limiting the utility as a screening tool in idiopathic neuropathy patients. At best, these antibodies represent screening tools, and the diagnosis is ultimately dependent upon the demonstration of malabsorption and typical small bowel pathology. Neuropathy response to dietary and immunomodulating treatment has been disappointing to date, suggesting that the neuropathy is due to alternative mechanism, or that nerves are irreparably damaged.

Vasculitic neuropathy may occur in either a multifocal or DSPN pattern. The latter may represent the confluence of a multifocal neuropathy syndrome. Neuropathy occurs in approximately half of the patients with systemic necrotizing vasculitis with the greatest prevalence in polyarteritis nodosa, eosinophilic granulomatosis with polyangiitis (EGPA), and granulomatosis with polyangiitis (GPA). It is often the initial organ-specific manifestation of these disorders. Antineutrophilic cytoplasmic antibodies (ANCAs) are markers for these disorders.[186,187] P-ANCA directed against myeloperoxidase represents a marker for the former two disorders. C-ANCA directed against antiproteinase 3 is highly specific for GPA. Neuropathy also occurs as a rare consequence of vasculitis in association with rheumatoid arthritis and other connective tissue disorders. Titers of rheumatoid factor tend to be high in with rheumatoid arthritis. Typically, patients have long-standing rheumatoid arthritis, usually with associated signs and symptoms of systemic disease including palpable purpura. Predictably, the yield and accuracy of ANCA and rheumatoid factor testing will be greatest in patients with acute to subacute painful multiple mononeuropathies patterns who have signs and symptoms of an underlying systemic disease.

Some patients with disorders of peripheral nerve hyperexcitability (e.g., Isaacs syndrome or acquired neuromyotonia, cramp-fasciculation syndrome) have antibodies both in serum and CSF that were initially attributed to VGKC antibodies. As previously discussed, subsequent studies demonstrated these antibodies actually are specifically directed against Caspr2 and LGL1.[29–31] These antibodies are also associated with limbic encephalitis/Morvan syndrome. The classic peripheral phenotype associated with these disorders is known as Isaacs syndrome that can be conceptualized as part of the spectrum of a peripheral nerve hyperexcitability syndrome. As in LEMS, Isaacs syndrome is an autoimmune disorder that can occur in isolation, in association with other autoimmune diseases, or as a paraneoplastic syndrome. When Isaacs syndrome is associated with concomitant CNS pathology, usually a behavioral syndrome, it has been historically referred to as Morvan syndrome.

CSF Analysis

CSF analysis is a helpful evaluation in a very select groups of patients with neuromuscular disease. From an anatomic perspective, an abnormal CSF result implies the existence of pathology in the CNS or within the nerve roots. As such, these are diagnostically helpful from several different perspectives. An elevated CSF protein level without a cellular response is the hallmark of the acute and chronic inflammatory demyelinating polyneuropathies (AIDP and CIDP). This profile can also be seen in structural disorders of nerve root such as disc herniations and spinal stenosis, mitochondrial disorders, paraneoplastic disorders, spinal cord infarction, and a third to half of ALS cases.[124] A CSF pleocytosis is expected in infectious disorders affecting nerve roots and/or spinal cord such as Lyme, syphilis, poliomyelitis, West Nile virus, enterovirus, CMV, and HIV infections. Serologic and genetic tests for these organisms can provide a specific diagnosis. A CSF pleocytosis is also seen in most cases of neoplastic meningitis, which can be confirmed through cytologic or flow cytometric evaluations. Paraneoplastic disorders affecting both the peripheral and/or CNS are frequently associated with some combination of pleocytosis, elevated CSF protein, or oligoclonal bands.[124] It is hoped that the emerging field of proteomics will allow for identification of a specific biomarker(s) within spinal fluid that will allow for early diagnosis in disorders such as ALS where there is currently no confirmatory test. Detection of a reliable biomarker also holds promise of identifying an effective response to treatment.

Genetic Testing

Genetic testing is constantly evolving and complex diagnostic tool for neuromuscular disease.[187–194] There are many nuances associated with genetic testing that the neuromuscular clinician should be familiar with before ordering DNA testing; this is particularly true with an asymptomatic patient at perceived risk. This is also true when attempting to counsel a patient regarding the implications of their genetic test result, whether it be positive or negative. Many of the heritable disorders discussed in this book are Mendelian in nature, that is, a single gene mutation is sufficient to cause disease. Increasingly, the cryptic world of complex genetics is coming slowly into focus. There are probably far more mutations that confer increased risk for disease development in concert with some other genetic or environmental influence (epigenetic factors) than cause disease independently in a Mendelian fashion. A specific example of genetic complexity, even within the domain of Mendelian genetics, is the recognition that specific mutations may behave differently in those with different ethnic origins. For example, the G90A mutation of the SOD1 gene causes an ALS phenotype in Scandinavians only in the homozygotes. In non-Scandinavians, it behaves as a dominantly inherited disease.

Genotype–phenotype correlations are also complex. As mentioned above, differing phenotypes may evolve from mutations of a single gene. For example, mutations of the lamin A/C gene may cause distinctive phenotypes including Charcot–Marie–Tooth disease (CMT), Emery–Dreifuss muscular dystrophy, congenital muscular dystrophy, and an adult-onset limb-girdle muscular dystrophy phenotype. Conversely, many similar, if not identical, phenotypes arise from mutations arising from different genes on multiple chromosomes. For example, there are numerous genes associated with different forms of CMT and limb-girdle muscular dystrophy. Both the identification and exclusion of pathologic mutations may be rendered difficult for several reasons. We do not know all the pathologic mutations for most diseases. Even with known genotypes, there are multiple mutation mechanisms, not all of which may be identified by the technology used by the laboratory called upon to detect it.

DNA mutational analysis is mostly used to diagnose symptomatic individuals. These tests may also be applied to individuals who are understandably concerned about future risk. When used in these latter situations, it is incumbent upon the ordering physician to be fully cognizant of all potential ramifications of the testing result and to provide fully informed consent. This would include the implications of both positive and negative results. It must also consider the potential impact on other family members whose genotype may be inadvertently illuminated. Both patient and physician should be aware that these costly tests may not be reimbursed by third-party payers in presymptomatic individuals.

Physicians, institutions, payers, and patients have struggled to identify the appropriate paradigm for genetic testing, one that balances the considerable cost with the value to patient, physician, and society as a whole. Ideally, precise phenotyping would allow for genetic confirmation or exclusion by utilizing a single test or rational algorithm, making cost considerations more manageable. Next-generation sequencing panels are now available for many hereditary myopathies, neuropathies and motor neuron syndromes that are cost effective.[94,188,189] There are clear benefits provided by confirming a disorder to have a genetic etiology. These include diagnostic closure, thus eliminating the need for further diagnostic and for the most part therapeutic intervention. In addition, the opportunity for more accurate genetic counseling is provided. Genotype identification often does not alter patient management or the natural history of the patient's disease. There are increasing examples in which identifying the gene does open up options for important new treatments though (e.g., SMN mutations in spinal muscular atrophy, transthyretin mutations for familial amyloid polyneuropathy, alpha-glucosidase mutations for Pompe disease, specific dystrophin mutations in Duchenne muscular dystrophy). Identifying a specific mutation may allow for enrolment in specific gene therapy trials or approved gene therapy (e.g., SOD1 associated familial ALS).

Mutational analysis is available for many specific hereditary neuromuscular disorders and there are several modes of genetic testing.[193] Traditional Sanger sequencing allows for sequencing of an entire gene but is time consuming and expensive. Next-generation sequencing (NGS) allows for less expensive sequencing of panel of many genes that might be responsible for a similar clinical phenotype when mutated and have become increasingly less expensive. NGS can be cost effective when the clinical phenotype (e.g., limb-girdle muscular dystrophy or CMT type 2) can be caused by many genes and not dominated by a specific genetic mutation. The drawback of NGS is the clinician needs to make sure that the gene(s) of interest are on the specific panel that is ordered, different commercial laboratories have different coverages that assess for mutations in specific genes, NGS often misses large deletions and duplications as seen in many disorders (e.g., myotonic dystrophy, facioscapulohumeral dystrophy), and does assess the introns well in which mutations can affecting splicing.

If these standard techniques do not turn up a known pathogenic mutation, whole exome sequencing (WES) or whole genome sequencing (WGS) can be done but these take more time, are more costly, and may uncover only "novel" sequence alterations of unclear pathogenic bases. However, the diagnostic rate across the wide variety of these disorders even with currently commercially available techniques still only ranges from approximately 25%–50%.[193]

Another complexity is the recognition that not all sequence alterations within known disease-related genes are pathogenic mutations that will cause disease. Such sequence alterations may represent benign polymorphisms or variations of unclear significance (VOUS), and some occur so infrequently that we are not yet aware of whether they are pathogenic or not. In suspected myopathies in which a VOUS is identified, a muscle biopsy may be helpful. For example, if a patient has an LGMD and genetic testing reveals a VOUS in the alpha-sarcoglycan gene, a biopsy can be performed along with immunostaining and immunoblot (Western blot) for alpha-sarcoglycan. Research studies evaluated the role of transcriptome sequencing [RNA sequencing (RNA-seq)] on muscle tissue to identify expression outliers, cryptic splice alterations, and expression profiling analysis to look for genetic pathway disruptions.[194]

Ongoing research to increase the diagnostic yield of genetic testing includes manual curation of whole genome data using the latest computational genomics pipelines to perform short-tandem repeat (STR) expansion analysis and structural variation (SV) detection. Additionally, long-read sequencing from whole blood to improve the diagnostic yield of complex SV that can be missed from short-read WGS performed that are most commonly performed at this time.

Mitochondrial disorders have an added degree of complexity as they can be inherited through mutations in nuclear DNA with a Mendelian inheritance pattern (AD, AR, or X-linked) or might be caused by mutations in mitochondrial DNA (mtDNA). The overwhelming mitochondrial proteins are encoded by nuclear DNA. That said, the mutations in these nuclear genes often lead to secondary deletions of large segments and depletion of mtDNA. Furthermore, the degree or absence of a specific tissue being affected by a mtDNA mutation depends on the degree of mutant homoplasmy in that tissue. So, patients with a mtDNA mutation with a high degree of mutant homoplasmy is muscle tissue, but not in white blood cells, may have normal mtDNA testing of blood, and require testing in muscle tissue. We go into more detail on Mitochondrial Disorders (see Chapter 30).

Nerve and Muscle Imaging

Imaging of nerve and muscle is being used with increased frequency in the evaluation of patients with neuromuscular disorders.[195–204] Arguably, this role will continue to evolve as resolution of the images and clinician's familiarity with the benefits of imaging expand. The advantages provided by MRI over CT include increased resolution, the ability to easily image in multiple planes, and the availability of a noniodinated contrast agent. In addition, MRI has the potential advantage over CT in terms of timing of injury. For example, chronic nerve and muscle diseases are both associated with fatty replacement of muscle manifesting as increased signal in T1-weighted images. Acutely denervated muscle will demonstrate little if any signal change with T1 sequencing. T2-weighted images accentuate the signal produced by water and fat. Increased (bright) T2 signal occurs within acutely denervated muscle and necrotic fibers (due to inflammation, rhabdomyolysis) related to associated edema or inflammation but is also related to fatty replacement as seen in muscular dystrophy or other chronic destructive process of muscle.[195–197] Short-TI Inversion Recovery (STIR) is typically used to null the signal from fat to help distinguish this from edema and inflammatory processes affecting muscle (Fig. 2-31).

For these reasons, MRI has supplanted CT as the imaging modality of choice in most cases of suspected nerve or

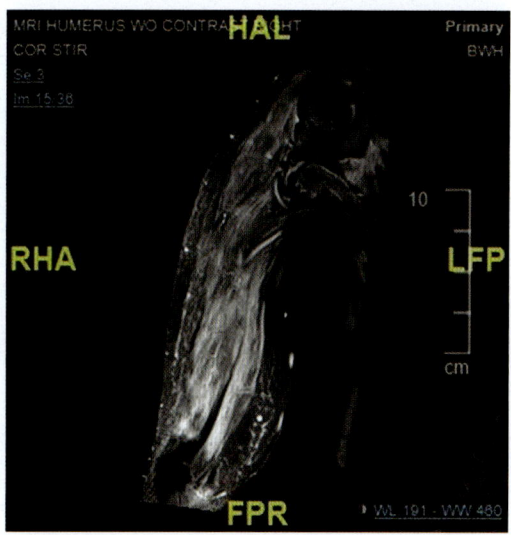

Figure 2-31. Short-TI Inversion Recovery (STIR) of the right upper arm in a patient with a necrotizing myopathy demonstrated increased (bright) signal in the biceps brachii and deltoid muscles.

muscle pathology except in those who cannot receive or tolerate MR due to financial considerations, their size, MRI availability, claustrophobic tendencies, or contraindications such as pacemakers. Nonetheless, CT is not without value in neuromuscular disease. It can differentiate nerve from muscle disease, not only based on the pattern of muscular involvement but based on the basis of x-ray attenuation changes within individual muscles as well. CT has been demonstrated to be 85% sensitive in detecting neuromuscular pathology in general, using muscle histology as the comparative gold standard.[202] Traditional roles of imaging, for example, detection of a herniated disc, a Pancoast tumor, or a retroperitoneal hematoma will not be addressed in this chapter. Ideally, future imaging techniques will provide a means to track axonal regrowth following injury or intervention, as well as development of specific imaging markers that would allow detection of substances such as amyloid within nerve or muscle.

Imaging of muscle has numerous potential applications. For example, in the dropped head or bent spine syndromes, fatty replacement of paraspinal muscles readily detectable on MRI can define a neuromuscular as opposed to an extrapyramidal or orthopedic cause of the patient's abnormal posture (Fig. 2-32). Uncommonly, MRI of the spine may demonstrate unexpected abnormalities within paraspinal muscles identifying a neuromuscular rather than etiology as the cause of the patient's back or neck pain. MRI is useful in detecting edema associated with the inflammatory myopathies but is not specific, particularly to subtypes. Signal changes have also been documented to occur coincident with treatment responsiveness in these disorders.[205] MRI can be used to distinguish increased muscle weakness due to steroids from increased weakness due to a flare

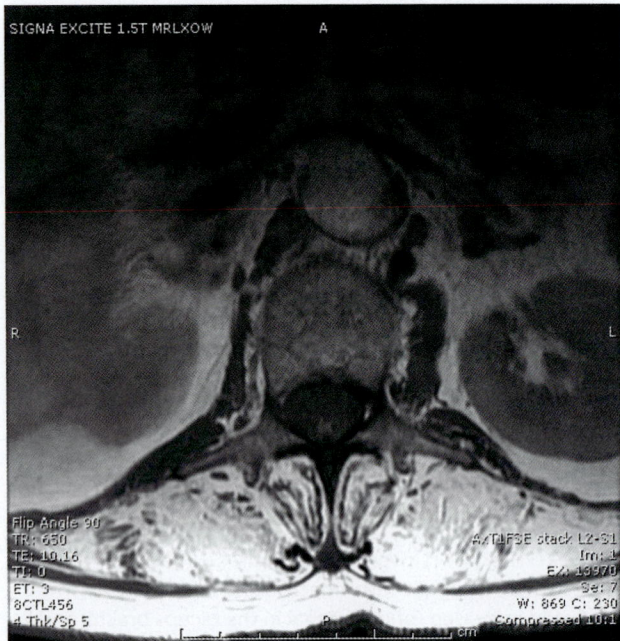

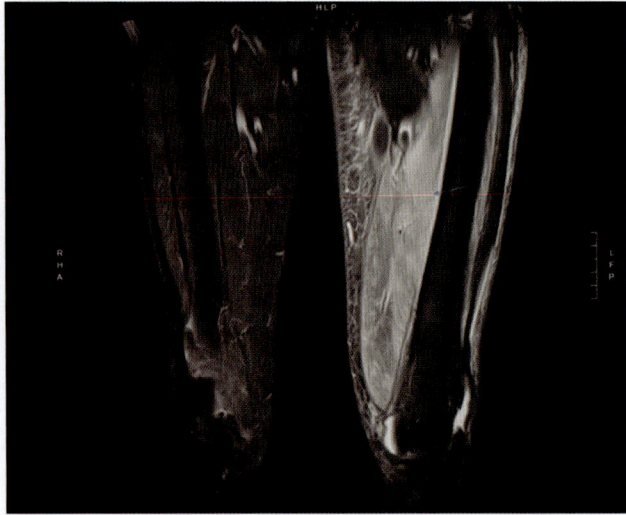

Figure 2-33. Short-TI Inversion Recovery (STIR) of the left thing in a patient with diabetic muscle infarct demonstrated increased (bright) signal in the medial thigh muscles (*arrow*).

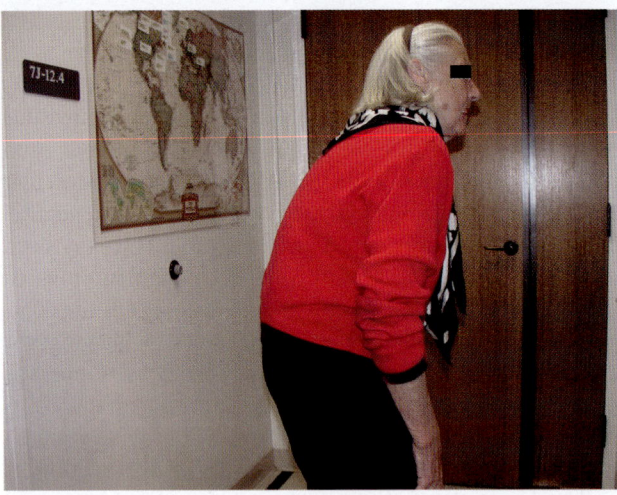

Figure 2-32. (**A**) MRI (T1 sequence) demonstrating fatty replacement and atrophy of the lumbar paraspinal musculature in (**B**) a woman with bent spine syndrome.

of myositis as no signal abnormalities (edema) is seen with steroid myopathy. The pattern of muscle involvement may also be helpful in the identification of certain muscle diseases such as the muscular dystrophies and inclusion body myositis where specific patterns of muscle involvement are known to occur. Although the authors do not routinely use MRI in the selection of an appropriate muscle to biopsy, it can be a very helpful tool in the appropriate clinical context. For example, certain patients with neuromuscular disease may have muscles that are at the extremes of the spectrum, that is, either end stage or normal. In this context, MRI may allow detection of a modestly affected muscle suitable for biopsy.

Although of limited pragmatic benefit, rhabdomyolysis is associated with a diffuse pattern of increased signal on STIR sequences. Gadolinium has a limited role in MRI of muscle but can highlight fasciitis. MRI can be helpful as well in the detection of the relatively rare conditions of muscle infarction (Fig. 2-33) and rhabdomyosarcoma.

MRI has beneficial applications in nerve disease as well.[200,201,207–213] MRI imaging may identify a pattern of muscle involvement that defines a specific nerve lesion while at the same time implicating the site of lesion within the nerve. Normal nerve is isointense to muscle on both T1- and T2-weighted sequences. An axonal injury will have increased signal characteristics within nerve on cross-sectional images using STIR and T2 fast spin echo sequences both at and distal to the injury site, which will also enhance with gadolinium. STIR enjoys the benefit of more intense signal characteristics and fat signal suppression but does not provide the image resolution of its T2 fast spin echo counterpart. Acutely denervated muscle will also have increased signal characteristics on STIR and T2 fast spin echo sequences that may precede the development of acute denervation on the EDX examination. Chronic denervation produces fatty infiltration of denervated muscle. Signal changes do not take place in muscles associated with purely demyelinating nerve injuries. Ideally, MRI could accurately identify nerve transaction or avulsion in traumatic injury to expedite surgical intervention in these cases. Unfortunately, current imaging resolution and evolution of signal changes within nerve and muscle do not provide this capability.

MRI imaging can detect focal nerve entrapment or compression syndromes. One potential benefit of MRI imaging in this context is its potential ability to identify a secondary pathology as a contributor to the syndrome, for example, a ganglion cyst within Guyon canal (Fig. 2-34). In the case of CTS, MRI has not usurped the traditional role

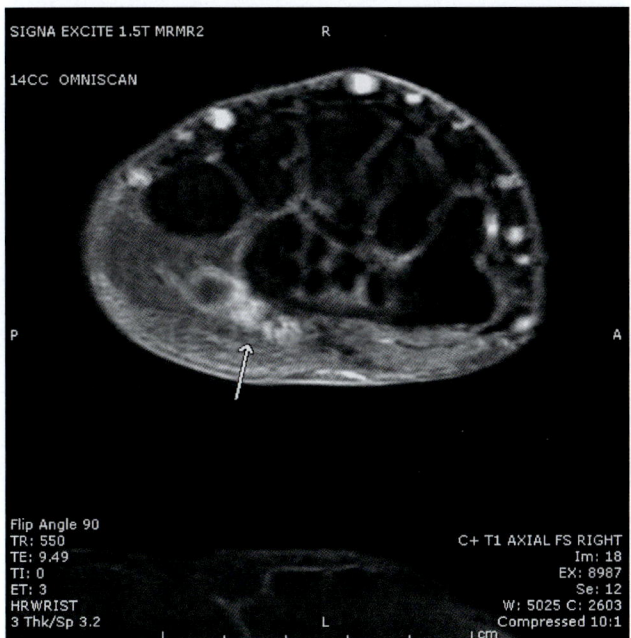

Figure 2-34. MRI (T1 sequence with gadolinium) demonstrating enhancing mass (*arrow*) in Guyon canal (ganglion cyst) in a young woman presenting with painless weakness and atrophy restricted to intrinsic right-hand muscles innervated exclusively by the ulnar nerve.

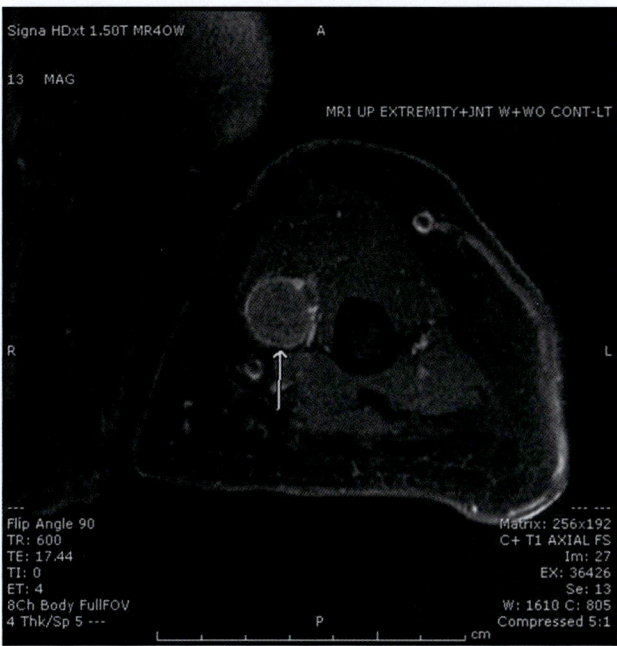

Figure 2-35. MRI (T1 sequence with fat saturation and gadolinium) axial image of the humerus demonstrating an enlarged and enhancing median nerve due to biopsy-proven metastatic lymphoma.

of EDX in most institutions as CTS has a demyelinating pathophysiology in most if not all cases and is therefore readily detectable. There is the potential for a greater role for MRI in the evaluation of ulnar neuropathy at the elbow. It has been estimated that up to one-half of ulnar neuropathies have a predominantly axonal pathophysiology, which usually precludes precise EDX localization. MRI has been shown to identify increased signal in areas consistent with ulnar nerve injury at least in some cases and may do so when EDX is normal. MRI has been reported to be occasionally beneficial in other less frequent and at times controversial mononeuropathies including thoracic outlet, piriformis syndromes, and tarsal tunnel syndromes, as well as posterior interosseous and peroneal neuropathies. It would be prudent to interpret subtle imaging abnormalities cautiously in these aforementioned contexts and to accept their validity only when congruent with clinical and EDX data.

MRI is the current diagnostic modality of choice to identify peripheral nerve tumors (Fig. 2-35). Virtually all of these, regardless of histology, demonstrate gadolinium enhancement. Benign histology cannot reliably be distinguished from its malignant counterpart by MRI, although positron emission tomography may be helpful in this regard. A potentially vexing clinical problem, the separation of recurrent tumor versus radiation-induced plexus injury, may be solved in some cases by different MR characteristics. Recurrent tumor tends to be focal, irregular, and enhancing. Radiation-induced nerve injury tends to produce either uniform enlargement or focal atrophy.

MRI is useful in detecting areas of presumed inflammation, edema, and demyelination in the acquired inflammatory demyelinating neuropathies, including MMN, GBS, and CIDP,[208–210] and in brachial plexus neuritis.[212] In some cases, nerve roots are preferentially involved in keeping with known pathologic data.[208] T2 signal abnormalities in brachial plexus elements may be seen in both CIDP and MMN. Other than for symmetry, these changes are identical. These may be of considerable utility, however, allowing for the discrimination of MMN and other, presumed degenerative and untreatable lower motor neuron syndromes. This latter application may be particularly helpful as it can detect abnormalities of peripheral nerve in locations proximal to where NCS are easily applied. Although insightful in the appropriate clinical context, neither the location, signal characteristics, nor the morphology of imaging abnormality predicts pathology in these disorders. Similar changes, particularly in nerve roots, may be seen in infectious, neoplastic, or other inflammatory diseases (e.g., sarcoidosis) with affinity for peripheral nerve.[200] MRI may be capable of identifying hypertrophic nerves seen in conditions such as CMT disease and CIDP,[213] particularly within the spinal canal where these may lead to the clinical syndrome of neurogenic claudication.

MRI can also provide valuable insight into the cause of intramedullary disorders of the spinal cord whose phenotypes may overlap with neuromuscular syndromes (Figs. 2-36A,B and 2-37A,B). Syringomyelia, spinal cord infarction, intramedullary neoplasms, vitamin B12, and copper deficiency are notable examples.[214–216]

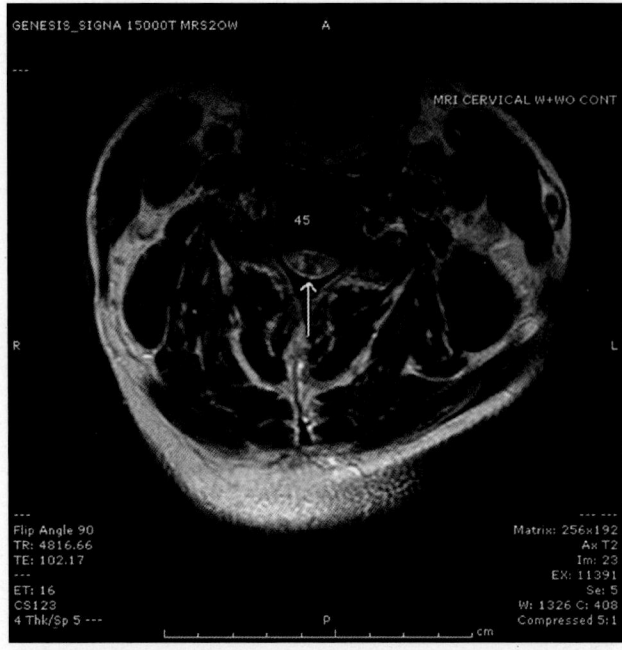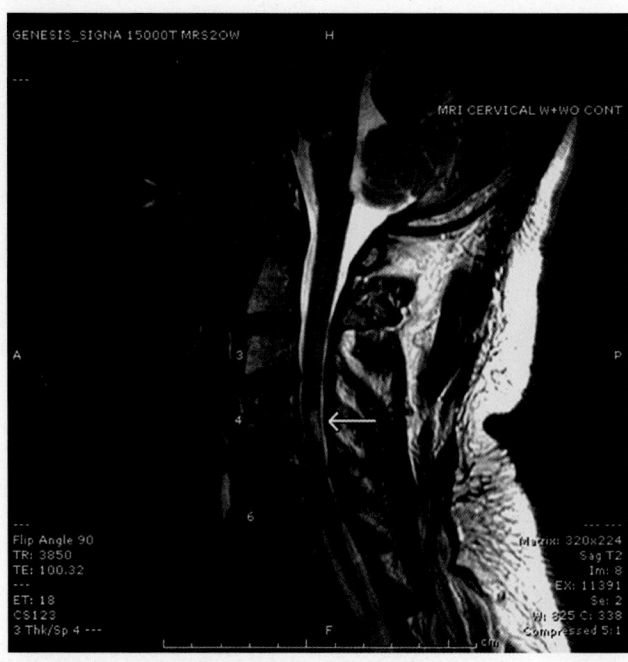

Figure 2-36. T2 sequence axial plane (**A**) and T2 image sagittal plane (**B**) demonstrating increased signal of the gray matter at the C4–C5 interspace in a man with painless weakness and atrophy of the shoulder girdle.

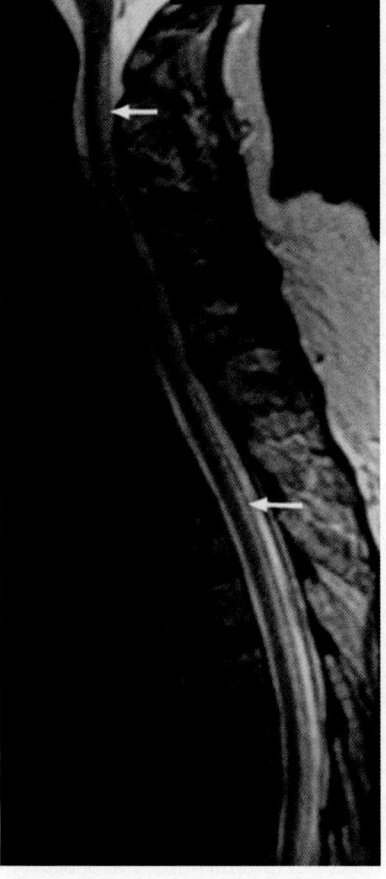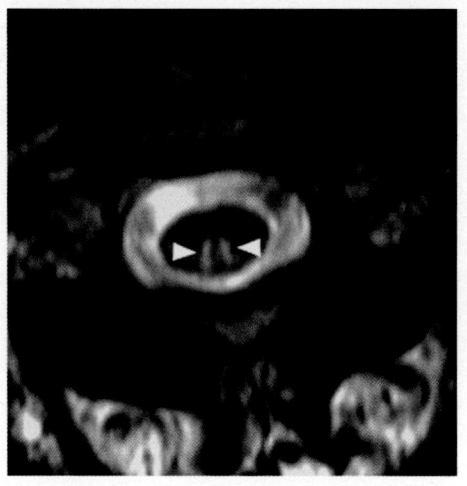

Figure 2-37. T2 sequence axial (**A**) and sagittal planes (**B**) demonstrating increased signal within the posterior columns in an individual with cyanocobalamin deficiency.

Ultrasonography is an increasingly used diagnostic tool that is readily available, relatively inexpensive, quick, and painless.[198,199,217,218] It is limited by specificity and its ability to visualize deep structures, particularly in individuals with a large body habitus. Measured parameters include the cross-sectional area of nerve in comparison to normative values and in comparison to unaffected nerve segments. In general, the cross-sectional area of the nerve will normally increase at proximal sites, in taller individuals, and at sites of nerve entrapment. Ultrasound can identify nerve transaction and has demonstrated an 89% sensitivity and 95% specificity under experimental conditions.[219] Nerve ultrasound is frequently utilized in the evaluation of patients with known or suspected entrapment/compression mononeuropathies, including CTS and ulnar neuropathy at the elbow (Fig. 2-38).[220–225] Ultrasound can be used to demonstrate an increase in nerve cross-sectional area as a common feature in either inherited or acquired demyelinating neuropathy whereas this same parameter is commonly reduced in axonal neuropathies.[226] Ultrasound has been utilized to detect nerve root hypertrophy in CIDP.[227]

Muscle ultrasound has been used as a potential diagnostic tool in muscular dystrophies and inflammatory myopathies.[228–230] It is capable of detecting altered echogenicity within muscle indicative of pathology as well as defining the existence and pattern of muscle atrophy or hypertrophy, edema from inflammation, or fatty replacement (Fig. 2-39). Like MRI, it can be applied to identify an ideal muscle to biopsy. This may be particularly relevant with young children where the identification of a moderately involved muscle may be problematic either through clinical or electrodiagnostic assessment.

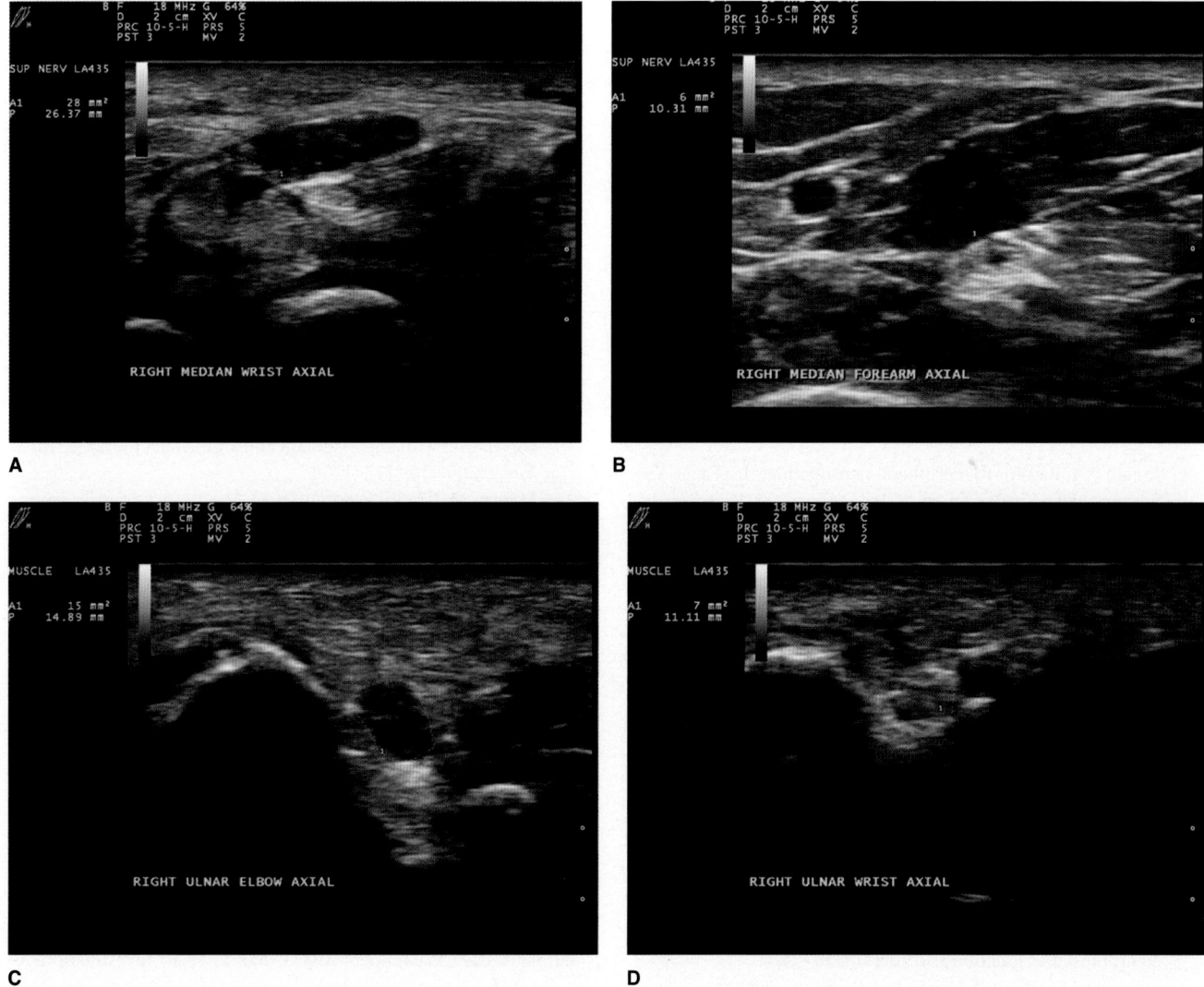

Figure 2-38. Ultrasound of nerve median nerve at wrist (**A**) showed marked swelling (cross-sectional area 28 m^2; normal <12 m^2) with normal area in distal forearm (**B**) supportive of diagnosis of carpal tunnel syndrome. Ultrasound of ulnar nerve at the elbow (**C**) shows swelling (cross-sectional area 15 m^2; normal <10 m^2) with normal area at the wrist (**D**) that supports the diagnosis of an ulnar neuropathy at the elbow.

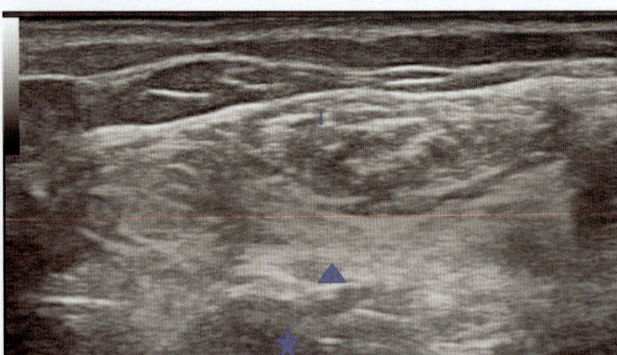

Figure 2-39. Ultrasound of forearm in patient with inclusion body myositis. Mild increased echogenicity (*brightness*) is apparent in the flexor digitorum superficialis muscles (*arrow*). There is increased echogenicity in the deeper flexor digitorum profundus muscles from severe fibrotic replacement (*arrowhead*) that obscures the outline of the bones in the forearm (*star*).

▶ SUMMARY

This chapter has attempted to provide an even and practical description of many of the ancillary tests available to the neuromuscular clinician. It has attempted to fairly emphasize both the strengths and the weaknesses of each modality. Again, these tests represent a proverbial double-edged sword that may achieve either a desired or an undesired effect dependent on the skill, knowledge, and particularly judgment of the individual that utilizes them.

REFERENCES

1. Amato AA, Barohn RJ. Peripheral neuropathies. In: Fauci AS, Braunwald E, Kasper DJ, et al., eds. *Harrison's Principles of Internal Medicine*. McGraw Hill; 2022:3480–3501.
2. Amato AA, Hauser SL. Guillain-Barre syndrome and autoimmune neuropathies. In: Fauci AS, Braunwald E, Kasper DJ, et al., eds. *Harrison's Principles of Internal Medicine*. McGraw Hill; 2022:3501–3508.
3. Amato AA. Neuromuscular junction disorders. In: Fauci AS, Braunwald E, Kasper DJ, et al., eds. *Harrison's Principles of Internal Medicine*. McGraw Hill; 2022:3509–2516.
4. Amato AA, Brown RJ. Muscular dystrophies and other muscle diseases. In: Fauci AS, Braunwald E, Kasper DJ, et al., eds. *Harrison's Principles of Internal Medicine*. McGraw Hill; 2022:3516–3532.
5. Amato AA, Ropper AH. Sensory ganglionopathies. *New Eng J Med*. 2020;383:1657–1662.
6. Rosow LK, Amato AA. The role of electrodiagnostic testing, imaging, and muscle biopsy in the investigation of muscle disease. *Continuum (Minneap Minn)*. 2016;22(6, Muscle and Neuromuscular Junction Disorders):1787–1802.
7. Dumitru D, Amato AA, Swartz MJ. *Electrodiagnostic Medicine*. 2nd ed. Hanley & Belfus, Inc; 2002.
8. Preston DC, Shapiro BE. *Electromyography and Neuromuscular Disorders: Clinical-Electrophysiologic-Ultrasound Correlations*. 4th ed. Elsevier; 2020.
9. Rubin DI. Needle electromyography: basic concepts. *Handb Clin Neurol*. 2019;160:243–256.
10. Martinez-Thompson JM. Electrodiagnostic assessment of myopathy. *Neurol Clin*. 2021;39:1035–1049.
11. Lamb CJ, Rubin DI. Electromyography case examples: practical approaches to neuromuscular symptoms. *Neurol Clin*. 2021;39:1097–1111.
12. Siao P, Kaku M. A clinician's approach to peripheral neuropathy. *Semin Neurol*. 2019;39:519–530.
13. Freeman R, Gewandter JS, Faber CG, et al. Idiopathic distal sensory polyneuropathy: ACTTION diagnostic criteria. *Neurology*. 2020;95:1005–1014.
14. Gwathmey KG, Smith AG. Immune-mediated neuropathies. *Neurol Clin*. 2020;38:711–735.
15. Oaklander AL, Nolano M. Scientific advances in and clinical approaches to small-fiber polyneuropathy: a review. *JAMA Neurol*. 2019;76:1240–1251.
16. Lamotte G, Sandroni P. A practical approach to peripheral autonomic neuropathies. *Curr Opin Neurol*. 2021;34:638–647.
17. Pasnoor M, Dimachkie MM. Approach to muscle and neuromuscular junction disorders. *Continuum (Minneap Minn)*. 2019;25:1536–1563.
18. Mellion ML, Buxton AE, Iyer V, Almahameed S, Lorvidhaya P, Gilchrist JM. Safety of nerve conduction studies in patients with peripheral intravenous lines. *Muscle Nerve*. 2010;42(2):189–191.
19. Schoeck AP, Mellion ML, Gilchrist JM, Christian FV. Safety of nerve conduction studies in patients with implanted cardiac devices. *Muscle Nerve*. 2007;35(4):521–524.
20. Al-Shekhlee A, Shapiro BE, Preston DC. Iatrogenic complications and risks of nerve conduction studies and needle electromyography. *Muscle Nerve*. 2003;27(5):517–526.
21. Caress JB, Little AA, Zaebarah V, Albers JW. Survey of electrodiagnostic laboratories regarding hemorrhagic complications from needle electromyography. *Muscle Nerve*. 2006;34:356–358.
22. Lynch SL, Boon AJ, Smith J, Harper CM Jr, Tanaka EM. Complications of needle electromyography: hematoma risk and correlation with anticoagulant and antiplatelet therapy. *Muscle Nerve*. 2008;38:1225–1230.
23. Mateen FJ, Grant IA, Sorenson EJ. Needlestick injuries among electromyographers. *Muscle Nerve*. 2008;38:1541–1545.
24. Daube JR, Armon C. Electrophysiological signs of arteriovenous malformations of the spinal cord. *J Neurol Neurosurg Psychiatry*. 1989;52:1176–1181.
25. Linden D, Berlit P. Spinal arteriovenous malformations: clinical and neurophysiologic findings. *J Neurol*. 1996;243:9–12.
26. Chaudhry V, Cornblath DR. Wallerian degeneration in human nerves: serial electrophysiological studies. *Muscle Nerve*. 1992;15:687–693.
27. Levin R, Pascuzzi RM, Bruns DE, Boyd JC, Toly TM, Phillips LH 2nd. The time course of creatine kinase elevation following concentric needle EMG. *Muscle Nerve*. 1987;10:242–245.
28. Auger RG, Daube JR, Gomez MR, Lambert EH. Hereditary form of sustained muscle activity of peripheral nerve origin causing generalized myokymia and muscle stiffness. *Ann Neurol*. 1985;15:13–21.
29. Lancaster E, Huijbers MGM, Bar V, et al. Investigations of Caspr2, an autoantigen of encephalitis and neuromyotonia. *Ann Neurol*. 2011;69:303–311.
30. Michael S, Waters P, Irani SR. Stop testing for autoantibodies to the VGKC-complex: only request LGI1 and CASPR2. *Pract Neurol*. 2020;20:377–384.

31. Hutto SK, Harrison TB. Electrodiagnostic assessment of hyperexcitable nerve disorders. *Neurol Clin.* 2021;39:1083–1096.
32. Maselli RA, Soliven BC. Analysis of the organophosphate-induced electromyographic response to repetitive nerve stimulation: paradoxical response to edrophonium and D-tubocurarine. *Muscle Nerve.* 1991;14:1182–1188.
33. Fournier E, Arzel M, Sternberg D, et al. Electromyography guides toward subgroups of mutations in muscle channelopathies. *Ann Neurol.* 2004;56(5):650–661.
34. Fournier E, Viala K, Gervais H, et al. Cold extends electromyography distinction between ion channel mutations causing myotonia. *Ann Neurol.* 2006;60:356–365.
35. Tan SV, Matthews E, Barber M, et al. Refined exercise testing and a DNA-based diagnosis in muscle channelopathies. *Ann Neurol.* 2011;69(2):328–340.
36. Michel P, Sternberg D, Jeannet PY, et al. Comparative efficacy of repetitive nerve stimulation, exercise, and cold in differentiating myotonic disorders. *Muscle Nerve.* 2007;36:643–650.
37. Cudkowicz M, Qureshi M, Shefner J. Measures and markers in amyotrophic lateral sclerosis. *NeuroRx.* 2004;1(2):273–283.
38. Gooch CL, Shefner JM. ALS surrogate markers. MUNE. *Amyotroph Lateral Scler Other Motor Neuron Disord.* 2004;5(Suppl 1):104–107.
39. Cudkowicz ME, Shefner JM, Schoenfeld DA, et al. Trial of celecoxib in amyotrophic lateral sclerosis. *Ann Neurol.* 2006;60(1):22–31.
40. Shefner JM, Cudkowicz ME, Zhang H, Schoenfeld D, Jillapalli D; Northeast ALS Consortium. The use of statistical MUNE in a multicenter clinical trial. *Muscle Nerve.* 2004;30:463–469.
41. Armon C, Brandstater ME. Motor unit number estimate-based rates of progression of ALS predict patient survival. *Muscle Nerve.* 1999;22(11):1571–1575.
42. Bromberg MB, Larson WL. Relationships between motor-unit number estimates and isometric strength in distal muscles in ALS/MND. *J Neurol Sci.* 1996;139(Suppl):38–42.
43. Felice KJ. A longitudinal study comparing thenar motor unit number estimates to other quantitative tests in patients with amyotrophic lateral sclerosis. *Muscle Nerve.* 1997;20(2):179–185.
44. Yuen EC, Olney RK. Longitudinal study of fiber density and motor unit number estimate in patients with amyotrophic lateral sclerosis. *Neurology.* 1997;49:573–578.
45. de Carvalho M, Dengler R, Eisen A, et al. Electrodiagnostic criteria for ALS. *Clin Neurophysiol.* 2008;119:497–503.
46. de Carvalho M, Swash M. Awaji diagnostic algorithm increases sensitivity of El Escorial criteria for ALS diagnosis. *Amyotroph Lateral Scler.* 2009;10:53–57.
47. Douglass CP, Kandler RH, Shaw PJ, McDermott CJ. An evaluation of neurophysiological criteria used in the diagnosis of motor neuron disease. *J Neurol Neurosurg Psychiatry.* 2010;81:646–649.
48. Mills KR. Characteristics of fasciculations in amyotrophic lateral sclerosis and the benign fasciculation syndrome. *Brain.* 2010;133:3458–3469.
49. Dabby R, Lange DJ, Trojaborg W, et al. Inclusion body myositis mimicking motor neuron disease. *Arch Neurol.* 2001;58:1253–1256.
50. Uncini A, Lange DJ, Lovelace RE, Solomon M, Hays AP. Long-duration polyphasic motor unit potentials in myopathies: a quantitative study with pathological correlation. *Muscle Nerve.* 1990;13:263–267.
51. Robinson LR, Bihammer P. Role of electrodiagnosis in nerve transfers for focal neuropathies and brachial plexopathies. *Muscle Nerve.* 2022;65:137–146.
52. Sinnreich M, Klein CJ, Daube JR, Engelstad J, Spinner RJ, Dyck PJB. Chronic immune sensory polyradiculopathy. *Neurology.* 2004;63:1662–1669.
53. Gilchrist JM, Sachs GM. Electrodiagnostic studies in the management and prognosis of neuromuscular disorders. *Muscle Nerve.* 2004;29:165–190.
54. Daube JR. Electrophysiologic studies in diagnosis and prognosis of motor neuron diseases. *Neurol Clin.* 1985;3:473–493.
55. Cornblath DR, Mellits ED, Griffin JW, et al. Motor conduction studies in Guillain–Barré syndrome: description and prognostic value. *Ann Neurol.* 1988;23:354–359.
56. Friedrich JM, Robinson LR. Prognostic indicators from electrodiagnostic studies for ulnar neuropathy at the elbow. *Muscle Nerve.* 2011;43:596–600.
57. Dyck PJ, Zimmerman IR, O'Brien PC, et al. Introduction of automated systems to evaluate touch-pressure, vibration, and thermal cutaneous sensation in man. *Ann Neurol.* 1978;4:502–510.
58. Dyck PJ, O'Brien PC. Quantitative sensation testing in epidemiological studies of peripheral neuropathy. *Muscle Nerve.* 1999;22:659–662.
59. Shy ME, Frohman EM, So YT, et al; Therapeutics and Technology Assessment Subcommittee of the American Academy of Neurology. Quantitative sensory testing: report of the Therapeutics and Technology Assessment Subcommittee of the American Academy of Neurology. *Neurology.* 2003;60:898–904.
60. Quantitative sensory testing: a consensus report from the Peripheral Neuropathy Association. *Neurology.* 1993;43:1050–1052.
61. Bird SJ, Brown MJ, Spino C, Watling S, Foyt HL. Value of repeated measures of nerve conduction and quantitative sensory testing in a diabetic neuropathy trial. *Muscle Nerve.* 2006;34:214–224.
62. Periquet MI, Novak V, Collins MP, et al. Painful sensory neuropathy: prospective evaluation using skin biopsy. *Neurology.* 1999;53:1641–1647.
63. Singer W, Spies JM, McArthur J, et al. Prospective evaluation of somatic and autonomic small fibers in selected neuropathies. *Neurology.* 2004;62:612–618.
64. Walk D, Wendelschafer-Crabb G, Davey C, Kennedy WR. Concordance between epidermal nerve fiber density and sensory examination in patients with symptoms of idiopathic small fiber neuropathy. *J Neurol Sci.* 2007;255(1–2):23–26.
65. Wolfe GI, Baker NS, Amato AA, et al. Chronic cryptogenic sensory polyneuropathy: clinical and laboratory characteristics. *Arch Neurol.* 1999;56(5):540–547.
66. Yarnitsky D. Quantitative sensory testing. *Muscle Nerve.* 1997;20:198–204.
67. Gibbons C, Freeman R. The evaluation of small fiber function—autonomic and quantitative sensory testing. *Neurol Clin.* 2004;22:683–702.
68. Dyck PJ, Kratz KM, Lehman KA, et al. The Rochester diabetic neuropathy study: design, criteria for types of neuropathy, selection bias, and reproducibility of neuropathic tests. *Neurology.* 1991;41:799–807.
69. Jensen TS, Bach FW, Kastrup J, Dejgaard A, Brennum J. Vibratory and thermal thresholds in diabetes with and without clinical neuropathy. *Acta Neurol Scand.* 1991;84:326–333.
70. Ziegler D, Mayer P, Gries FA. Evaluation of thermal, pain, and vibration sensation thresholds in newly diagnosed type 1 diabetic patients. *J Neurol Neurosurg Psychiatry.* 1998;51:1420–1424.

71. Bravenboer B, Van Dam PS, Hop J, Steenhoven J, Erkelens DW. Thermal threshold testing for the assessment of small fibre dysfunction: normal values and reproducibility. *Diabetic Med*. 1992;9:546–549.
72. Lindblom U, Tegnér R. Thermal sensitivity in uremic neuropathy. *Acta Neurol Scand*. 1985;71:290–294.
73. Angus-Lepman H, Burke D. The function of large and small nerve fibers in renal failure. *Muscle Nerve*. 1992;15:288–294.
74. Yosipovitch G, Yarnitsky D, Reiss J, et al. Paradoxical heat sensation in uremic polyneuropathy. *Muscle Nerve*. 1995;16:768–771.
75. Simpson DM, Kitch D, Evans SR, et al; The ACTG A5117 Study Group. HIV neuropathy natural history cohort study: assessment measures and risk factors. *Neurology*. 2006;66(11):1679–1687.
76. Winer JB, Bang B, Clarke JR, et al. A study of neuropathy in HIV infection. *Q J Med*. 1992;302:473–488.
77. Gibbons CH, Freeman R, Veves A. Diabetic neuropathy: a cross-sectional study of the relationships among tests of neurophysiology. *Diabetes Care*. 2010;33:2629–2634.
78. Freeman R. Autonomic peripheral neuropathy. *Continuum (Minneap Minn)*. 2020;26:58–71.
79. Novak P. Autonomic testing. *J Clin Neurophysiol*. 2021;38:251.
80. Cheshire WP, Freeman R, Gibbons CH, et al. Electrodiagnostic assessment of the autonomic nervous system: a consensus statement endorsed by the American Autonomic Society, American Academy of Neurology, and the International Federation of Clinical Neurophysiology. *Clin Neurophysiol*. 2021;132:666–682.
81. Low PA, Vernino S, Suarez G. Autonomic dysfunction in peripheral nerve disease. *Muscle Nerve*. 2003;27:646–661.
82. Sandroni P, Vernino S, Klein CM, et al. Idiopathic autonomic neuropathy; comparison of cases seropositive and seronegative for ganglionic acetylcholine receptor antibodies. *Arch Neurol*. 2004;61:44–48.
83. Ewing DJ, Campbell IW, Clarke BI. Mortality in diabetic autonomic neuropathy. *Lancet*. 1976;1:601–603.
84. Goyal RK. Muscarinic receptor subtypes. Physiology and clinical implications. *N Engl J Med*. 1989;321:1022–1029.
85. England JD, Gronseth GS, Franklin G, et al; American Academy of Neurology. Practice parameter: evaluation of distal symmetric polyneuropathy: role of autonomic testing, nerve biopsy, and skin biopsy (an evidence-based review). Report of the American Academy of Neurology, American Association of Neuromuscular and Electrodiagnostic Medicine, and American Academy of Physical Medicine and Rehabilitation. *Neurology*. 2009;72:177–184.
86. Kennedy WR, Sakuta M, Sutherland D, Goetz FC. Quantitation of the sweating deficiency in diabetes mellitus. *Ann Neurol*. 1984;15:482–488.
87. Low PA, Caskey PE, Tuck RR, Fealey RD, Dyck PJ. Quantitative sudomotor axon reflex test in normal and neuropathic subjects. *Ann Neurol*. 1983;14:573–580.
88. Stewart KD, Low PA, Fealey RD. Distal small-fiber neuropathy: results of tests of sweating and autonomic cardiovascular reflexes. *Muscle Nerve*. 1992;15:661–665.
89. Tobin K, Giuliani MJ, Lacomis D. Comparison of different modalities for detection of small-fiber neuropathy. *Clin Neurophys*. 1999;110:1909–1912.
90. Burns TM, Bauermann ML. The evaluation of polyneuropathies. *Neurology*. 2011;76:S6–S13.
91. Gemignani F, Bellanova MF, Saccani E, Pavesi G. Non-length-dependent small fiber neuropathy: not a matter of stockings and gloves. *Muscle Nerve*. 2022;65:10–28.
92. Amato AA, Ropper AH. Sensory Ganglionopathy. *N Engl J Med*. 2020;383:1657–1662.
93. Lubec D, Mülbacher W, Finsterer J, Mamoli B. Diagnostic work-up in peripheral neuropathy: an analysis of 171 cases. *Postgrad Med J*. 1999;75:723–727.
94. England JD, Gronseth GS, Franklin G, et al; American Academy of Neurology. Practice parameter: evaluation of distal symmetric polyneuropathy: role of laboratory and genetic testing (an evidence-based review). Report of the American Academy of Neurology, American Association of Neuromuscular and Electrodiagnostic Medicine, and American Academy of Physical Medicine and Rehabilitation. *Neurology*. 2009;72:185–192.
95. Schaumburg H, Kaplan J, Windebank A, et al. Sensory neuropathy from pyridoxine abuse. A new megavitamin syndrome. *N Engl J Med*. 1983;309(8):445–448.
96. Kelly JJ Jr, Kyle RA, O'Brien PC, Dyck PJ. Prevalence of monoclonal protein in peripheral neuropathy. *Neurology*. 1981;31:1480–1483.
97. Nobile-Orazio E, Terenghi F, Giannotta C, Gallia F, Nozza A. Serum VEGF levels in POEMS syndrome and in immune-mediated neuropathies. *Neurology*. 2009;72(11):1024–1026.
98. Briani C, Fabrizi GM, Ruggero S, et al. Vascular endothelial growth factor helps differentiate neuropathies in rare plasma cell dyscrasias. *Muscle Nerve*. 2011;43:164–167.
99. Kahn R. Proceedings of a consensus development conference on standardized measures in diabetic neuropathy. Clinical measures. *Diabetes Care*. 1992;15:1081.
100. Novella SP, Inzucchi SE, Goldstein JM. The frequency of undiagnosed diabetes and impaired glucose tolerance in patients with idiopathic sensory neuropathy. *Muscle Nerve*. 2001;24:1229–1231.
101. Russell JW, Feldman EL. Impaired glucose tolerance—does it cause neuropathy? *Muscle Nerve*. 2001;24(9):1109–1112.
102. Sumner CJ, Sheth S, Griffin JW, Cornblath DR, Polydefkis M. The spectrum of neuropathy in diabetes and impaired glucose tolerance. *Neurology*. 2003;60:108–111.
103. Singleton JR, Smith AG, Bromberg MB. Painful sensory polyneuropathy associated with impaired glucose tolerance. *Muscle Nerve*. 2001;24:1225–1228.
104. Hansen K, Legech A-M. The clinical and epidemiological profile of Lyme neuroborreliosis in Denmark 1985–1990. A prospective study of 187 patients with Borrelia burgdorferi specific intrathecal antibody production. *Brain*. 1992;115:399–423.
105. Katirji B, Al-Jaberi MM. Creatine kinase revisited. *J Clin Neuromusc Dis*. 2001;2:158–163.
106. Nicholson GA, McLeod JG, Morgan G, et al. Variable distributions of serum creatine kinase reference values. Relationship to exercise activity. *J Neurol Sci*. 1985;71:233–245.
107. Brewster LM, Mairuhu G, Sturk A, van Montfrans GA. Distribution of creatine kinase in the general population: implications for statin therapy. *Am Heart J*. 2007;154:655–661.
108. Davis RL, Liang C, Sue CM. A comparison of current serum biomarkers as diagnostic indicators of mitochondrial diseases. *Neurology*. 2016;86:2010–2015.
109. Formichi P, Cardone N, Taglia I, et al. Fibroblast growth factor 21 and grow differentiation factor 15 are sensitive biomarkers of mitochondrial diseases due to mitochondrial transfer-RNA

109. ...mutations and mitochondrial DNA deletions. *Neurol Sci.* 2020;41:3653–366.
110. Poulsen NS, Madsen KL, Hornsyld TM, et al. Growth and differentiation factor 15 as a biomarker for mitochondrial myopathy. *Mitochondrion.* 2020;50:35–41.
111. Riley LG, Nafisinia M, Menezes MJ, et al. FGF21 outperforms GDF15 as a diagnostic biomarker of mitochondrial disease in children. *Mol Genet Metab.* 2022;135:63–71.
112. Kazemi-Esfarjani P, Skomorowska E, Jensen TD, Haller RG, Vissing J. A nonischemic forearm exercise test for McArdle disease. *Ann Neurol.* 2002;52:153–159.
113. American Association of Neuromuscular and Electrodiagnostic Medicine. Diagnostic criteria for late-onset (childhood and adult) Pompe disease. *Muscle Nerve.* 2009;40:149–160.
114. Antoine JC, Mosnier JF, Absi L, Convers P, Honnorat J, Michel D. Carcinoma associated paraneoplastic peripheral neuropathies in patients with and without anti-onconeural antibodies. *J Neurol Neurosurg Psychiatry.* 1999;67:7–14.
115. Dalmau J, Furneaux HM, Rosenblum MK, Graus F, Posner JB. Detection of anti-Hu antibody in specific regions of the nervous system and tumor from patients with paraneoplastic encephalomyelitis/sensory neuropathy. *Neurology.* 1991;41:1757–1764.
116. Camdessanche JP, Antoine JC, Honnorat J, et al. Paraneoplastic peripheral neuropathy associated with anti-Hu antibodies. A clinical and electrophysiological study of 20 patients. *Brain.* 2002;125:166–175.
117. Dalmau J, Graus F, Rosenblum MK, Posner JB. Anti-Hu-associated paraneoplastic encephalomyelitis/sensory neuronopathy. A clinical study of 71 patients. *Medicine (Baltimore).* 1992;71:59–72.
118. Yu Z, Kryzer TJ, Griesmann GE, Kim K, Benarroch EE, Lennon VA. CRMP-5 neuronal autoantibody: marker of lung cancer and thymoma-related autoimmunity. *Ann Neurol.* 2001;49:146–154.
119. Dubey D, Lennon VA, Gadoth A, et al. Autoimmune CRMP5 neuropathy phenotype and outcome defined from 105 cases. *Neurology.* 2018;90:e103–e110.
120. Dubey D, Jitprapaikulsan J, Bi H, et al. Amphiphysin-IgG autoimmune neuropathy: a recognizable clinicopathologic syndrome. *Neurology.* 2019;93:e1873–e1880.
121. McKeon A., Lennon VA, Lachance DH, Fealey RD, Pittock SJ. Ganglionic acetylcholine receptor autoantibody: oncologic, neurological, and serological accompaniments. *Arch Neurol.* 2009;66(6):735–741.
122. Yuki N, Sato S, Tsuji S, Ohsawa T, Miyatake T. Frequent presence of anti-GQ1b antibody in Fisher's syndrome. *Neurology.* 1993;43:414–417.
123. Nobile-Orazio E, Francomano E, Daverio R, et al. Anti-myelin-associated glycoprotein IgM antibody titers in neuropathy associated with macroglobulinemia. *Ann Neurol.* 1989;26:543–550.
124. Latov N, Sherman WH, Nemni R, et al. Plasma-cell dyscrasia and peripheral neuropathy with a monoclonal antibody to peripheral-nerve myelin. *N Engl J Med.* 1980;303:618–621.
125. Gosselin S, Kyle RA, Dyck PJ. Neuropathy associated with monoclonal gammopathy of undetermined significance. *Ann Neurol.* 1991;30:54–61.
126. Katz JS, Saperstein DS, Gronseth G, Amato AA, Barohn RJ. Distal acquired demyelinating symmetric neuropathy. *Neurology.* 2000;54:615–620.
127. Nobile-Orazio E, Manfredini E, Carpo M, et al. Frequency and clinical correlates of anti-neural IgM antibodies in neuropathy associated with IgM monoclonal gammopathy. *Ann Neurol.* 1994;36:416–424.
128. Freddo L, Yu RK, Latov N, et al. Gangliosides GM1 and GD1b are antigens for IgM M-protein in a patient with motor neuron disease. *Neurology.* 1986;36:454–458.
129. Kinsella LJ, Lange DJ, Trojaborg W, Sadiq SA, Younger DS, Latov N. Clinical and electrophysiologic correlates of elevated anti-GM-1 antibody titers. *Neurology.* 1994;44:1278–1282.
130. Nobile-Orazio E, Cappellari A, Priori A. Multifocal motor neuropathy: current concepts and controversies. *Muscle Nerve.* 2005;31:663–680.
131. Pestronk A, Chaudhry V, Feldman EL, et al. Lower motor neuron syndromes defined by patterns of weakness, nerve conduction abnormalities, and high titres of antiglycolipid antibodies. *Ann Neurol.* 1990;27:316–326.
132. Taylor BV, Gross L, Windebank AJ. The sensitivity and specificity of anti-GM1 antibody testing. *Neurology.* 1996;47:951–955.
133. Gooch CL, Amato AA. Are anti-ganglioside antibodies of clinical value in multifocal motor neuropathy? *Neurology.* 2010;75:1950–1951.
134. Cats EA, Jacobs BC, Yuki N, et al. Multifocal motor neuropathy: association of anti-GM1 IgM antibodies with clinical features. *Neurology.* 2010;75:1961–1967.
135. von Schaik IN, Bossuyt PM, Brand A, Vermeulen M. Diagnostic value of GM1 antibodies in motor neuron disorders and neuropathies: a meta-analysis. *Neurology.* 1995;45:1570–1577.
136. Carpo M, Pedotti R, Allaria S, et al. Clinical presentation and outcome of Guillain–Barré and related syndromes in relation to anti-ganglioside antibodies. *J Neurol Sci.* 1999;168:78–84.
137. Chiba A, Kusunoki S, Obata H, Machinami R, Kanazawa I. Serum anti-GQ1b IgG antibody is associated with ophthalmoplegia in Miller Fisher syndrome and Guillain–Barré syndrome: clinical and immunohistochemical studies. *Neurology.* 1993;43.
138. Willison HJ, Veitch J, Paterson G, Kennedy PG. Miller Fisher syndrome is associated with serum antibodies to GQ1b ganglioside. *J Neurol Neurosurg Psychiatry.* 1993;56:204–206.
139. Cortese A, Lombardi R, Briani C, et al. Antibodies to neurofascin, contactin-1, and contactin-associated protein 1 in CIDP. Clinical relevance of IgG isotype. *Neurol Neuroimmunol Neuroinflamm.* 2020;7:e639.
140. Shelly S, Klein CJ, Dyck PJB, et al. Neurofascin-155 immunoglobulin subtypes: clinicopathologic associations and neurologic outcomes. *Neurology.* 2021;97:e2392–e2403.
141. Dubey D, Honorat JA, Shelly S, et al. Contactin-1 autoimmunity. Serologic, neurologic, and pathologic correlates. *Neurol Neuroimmunol Neuroinflamm.* 2020;7:e771.
142. Shelly S, Shouman K, Paul P, et al. Expanding the spectrum of chronic immune sensory polyradiculopathy CISP-Plus. *Neurology.* 2021;96:e2078–e2089.
143. Lopate G, Parks BJ, Goldstein JM, Yee WC, Friesenhahn GM, Pestronk A. Polyneuropathies associated with high titre antisulfatide antibodies: characteristics of patients with and without serum monoclonal proteins. *J Neurol Neurosurg Psychiatry.* 1997;62:581–585.
144. Antoine JC, Boutahar N, Lassablière F, et al. Antifibroblast growth factor receptor 3 antibodies identify a subgroup of patients with sensory neuropathy. *J Neurol Neurosurg Psychiatry.* 2015;86:1347–1355.

145. Samara V, Sampson J, Muppidi S. FGFR3 antibodies in neuropathy: what to do with them? *J Clin Neuromuscul Dis*. 2018;20:35–40.
146. Levine TD, Kafaie J, Zeidman LA, et al. Crytogenic small-fiber neuropathies: serum autoantibody binding to trisulfated heparin disaccharide and fibroblast growth factor receptor-3. *Muscle Nerve*. 2020;61:512–515.
147. Pestronk AM, Schmidt RE, Choksi RM, Sommerville RB, Al-Lozi MT. Clinical and laboratory features of neuropathies with serum IgM binding to TS-HDS. *Muscle Nerve*. 2012;45:866–872.
148. Patrick J, Lindstrom J. Autoimmune response to acetylcholine receptor. *Science*. 1973;180:871–872.
149. Lindstrom JM, Seybold ME, Lennon VA, Whittingham S, Duane DD. Antibody to acetylcholine receptor in myasthenia gravis. Prevalence, clinical correlates, and diagnostic value. *Neurology*. 1976;26:1054–1059.
150. Vincent A, Newsom-Davis J. Acetylcholine receptor antibody as a diagnostic test for myasthenia gravis: results in 153 validated cases and 2967 diagnostic assays. *J Neurol Neurosurg Psychiatry*. 1985;48:1246–1252.
151. Shelly S, Paul P, Bi H, et al. Improving accuracy of myasthenia gravis autoantibody testing by reflex algorithm. *Neurology*. 2020 Dec 1;95(22):e3002–e3011.
152. Hoch W, McConville J, Helms S, Newsom-Davis J, Melms A, Vincent A. Autoantibodies to the receptor tyrosine kinase MuSK in patients with myasthenia gravis without acetylcholine receptor antibodies. *Nat Med*. 2001;7:365–368.
153. Deymeer F, Gungor-Tuncer O, Yilmaz V, et al. Clinical comparison of anti-MuSK- vs anti-AchR-positive and seronegative myasthenia gravis. *Neurology*. 2007;68:609–611.
154. Evoli A, Padua L, Monaco ML, et al. Clinical correlates with anti-MuSK antibodies in generalized seronegative myasthenia gravis. *Brain*. 2003;126:2304–2311.
155. Sanders DB, El-Salem K, Massey JM, McConville J, Vincent A. Clinical aspects of MuSK antibody positive seronegative MG. *Neurology*. 2003;60:1978–1980.
156. Bartoccioni E, Scuderi F, Minicuci GM, Marion M, Ciaraffa F, Evoli A. Anti-MuSK antibodies: correlation with myasthenia gravis severity. *Neurology*. 2006;67:505–507.
157. Ohta K, Shigemoto K, Kubo S, et al. MuSK antibodies in AchR AB-seropositive MG vs. Ach R Ab-seronegative MG. *Neurology*. 2004;62:2132–2133.
158. Rivner MH, Quarles BM, Pan JX, et al. Clinical features of LRP4/agrin-antibody-positive myasthenia gravis: a multicenter study. *Muscle Nerve*. 2020;62:333–343.
159. Yu Z, Zhang M, Jing H, et al. Characterization of LRP4/Agrin Antibodies from a patient with myasthenia gravis. *Neurology*. 2021;97(10):e975–e987.
160. Lisak RP. Antibodies to LRP4 and agrin are pathogenic in myasthenia gravis: at the junction where it happens. *Neurology*. 2021;97(10):463–464.
161. Shelly S, Mills JR, Dubey D, et al. Clinical utility of striational antibodies in paraneoplastic and myasthenia gravis paraneoplastic panels. *Neurology*. 2021;96(24):e2966–e2976.
162. Dubey D, Beecher G, Bakri Hammami M, et al. Identification of caveolae-associated Protein 4 autoantibodies as a biomarker of immune-mediated rippling muscle disease in adults. *JAMA Neurol*. 2022;79(8):808–816.
163. Lennon VA, Kryzer TJ, Griesmann GE, et al. Calcium-channel antibodies in the Lambert–Eaton syndrome and other paraneoplastic syndromes. *N Engl J Med*. 1995;332:1467–1474.
164. Sabater L, Titulaer M, Saiz A, Verschururen J, Güre AO, Graus F. SOX1 antibodies are markers of paraneoplastic Lambert-Eaton myasthenic syndrome. *Neurology*. 2008;70:924–928.
165. McHugh NJ, Tansley SL. Autoantibodies in myositis. *Nat Rev Rheumatol*. 2018;14:290–302.
166. Mammen AL, Chung T, Christopher-Stine L, et al. Autoantibodies against 3-hydroxy-3-methylglutaryl-coenzyme A reductase in patients with statin-associated autoimmune myopathy. *Arthritis Rheum*. 2011;63:713–721.
167. Larman HB, Salajegheh M, Nazareno R, et al. Cytosolic 5′-nucleotidase 1A autoimmunity in sporadic inclusion body myositis. *Ann Neurol*. 2013;73:408–418.
168. Lundberg IE, Tjärnlund A, Bottai M, et al; International Myositis Classification Criteria Project consortium, The Euromyositis register and The Juvenile Dermatomyositis Cohort Biomarker Study and Repository (JDRG) (UK and Ireland). 2017 European League Against Rheumatism/American College of Rheumatology classification criteria for adult and juvenile idiopathic inflammatory myopathies and their major subgroups. *Ann Rheum Dis*. 2017;76:1955–1964.
169. Halperin JJ. Lyme disease and the peripheral nervous system. *Muscle Nerve*. 2003;28(2):133–143.
170. Halperin JJ, Logigian EL, Finkel MF, Pearl RA. Practice parameters for the diagnosis of patients with nervous system Lyme borreliosis (Lyme disease). *Neurology*. 1996;46:619–627.
171. Tugwell P, Dennis DT, Weinstein A, et al. Laboratory evaluation in the diagnosis of Lyme disease. *Ann Intern Med*. 1997;127:1109.
172. Wormser GP, Dattwyler RJ, Shapiro ED, et al. The clinical assessment, treatment and prevention of Lyme disease, human granulocytic anaplasmosis, and babesiosis: Clinical practice guidelines by the Infectious Diseases Society of America. *Clin Infect Dis*. 2006;43:1089.
173. Dressler F, Whalen JA, Reinhardt BN, Steere AC. Western blotting in the serodiagnosis of Lyme disease. *J Infect Dis*. 1993;167(2):392–400.
174. Nocton JJ, Bloom BJ, Rutledge BJ, et al. Detection of Borrelia burgdorferi DNA by polymerase chain reaction in cerebrospinal fluid in Lyme neuroborreliosis. *J Infect Dis*. 1996;174:623–627.
175. Coyle PK, Schutzer SE, Deng Z, et al. Detection of Borrelia burgdorferi-specific antigen in antibody-negative cerebrospinal fluid in neurologic Lyme disease. *Neurology*. 1995;45(11):2010–2015.
176. Halperin JJ, Luft BJ, Anand AK, et al. Lyme neuroborreliosis: central nervous system manifestations. *Neurology*. 1989;39(6):753–759.
177. Logigian EL, Kaplan RF, Steere AC. Chronic neurologic manifestations of Lyme disease. *N Engl J Med*. 1990;323(21):1438–1444.
178. Brew BJ. The peripheral nerve complications of human immunodeficiency virus (HIV) infection. *Muscle Nerve*. 2003;28:542–552.
179. Robinson-Papp J, Simpson DM. Neuromuscular diseases associated with HIV-infection. *Muscle Nerve*. 2009;40:1043–1053.
180. Lange DJ, Britton CB, Younger DS, Hays AP. The neuromuscular manifestations of human immunodeficiency virus infections. *Arch Neurol*. 1988;45:1084–1048.
181. Sène D, Jallouli M, Lefaucheur JP, et al. Peripheral neuropathies associated with primary Sjögren syndrome immunologic profiles of nonataxic sensory neuropathy and sensorimotor neuropathy. *Medicine (Baltimore)*. 2011;90:133–138.

182. Chai J, Hermman D, Stanton M, Barbano RL, Logigian EL. Painful small-fiber neuropathy in Sjögren syndrome. *Neurology*. 2005;65:925–927.
183. Chin RL, Sander HW, Brannagan TH, et al. Celiac neuropathy. *Neurology*. 2003;60:1581–1585.
184. Cross AH, Golumbek PT. Neurologic manifestations of celiac disease: proven, or just a gut feeling? *Neurology*. 2003;60:1566–1568.
185. Hadjivassiliou M, Grünewald RA, Davies-Jones GA. Gluten sensitivity as a neurological illness. *J Neurol Neurosurg Psychiatry*. 2002;72:560–563.
186. Guchelaar NAD, Waling MM, Adhin AA, van Daele PLA, Schreurs MWJ, Rombach SM. The value of anti neutrophil cytoplasmic antibodies (ANCA) testing for the diagnosis of ANCA-associated vasculitis, a systematic review and meta-analysis. *Autoimmun Rev*. 2021;20:102716.
187. Chalk CH, Homburger HA, Dyck PJ. Anti-neutrophil cytoplasmic antibodies in vasculitic peripheral neuropathy. *Neurology*. 1993;43:1826–1827.
188. Saporta ASD, Sottilel SL, Miller LJ, Feely SME, Siskind SE, Shy ME. Charcot-Marie-Tooth disease uptight and genetic testing strategies. *Ann Neurol*. 2011;69:22–33.
189. Klein CJ. Charcot-Marie-Tooth disease and other hereditary neuropathies. *Continuum (Minneap Minn)*. 2020;26:1224–1256.
190. Narayanaswami P, Weiss M, Selcen D, et al; Guideline Development Subcommittee of the American Academy of Neurology, Practice Issues Review Panel of the American Association of Neuromuscular & Electrodiagnostic Medicine. Evidence-based guideline summary: diagnosis and treatment of limb-girdle and distal dystrophies: report of the guideline development subcommittee of the American Academy of Neurology and the practice issues review panel of the American Association of Neuromuscular & Electrodiagnostic Medicine. *Neurology*. 2014; 83:1453–1463.
191. Kassardjian CD, Amato AA, Boon AJ, Childers MK, Klein CJ; AANEM Professional Practice Committee. The utility of genetic testing in neuromuscular disease: A consensus statement from the AANEM on the clinical utility of genetic testing in diagnosis of neuromuscular disease. *Muscle Nerve*. 2016;54:1007–1009.
192. Ramchandren S. Charcot-Marie-Tooth disease and other genetic polyneuropathies. *Continuum (Minneap Minn)* 2017;23 (Peripheral Nerve and Motor Neuron Disorders):1360–1377.
193. Nicolau S, Milone M, Liewluck T. Guidelines for genetic testing of muscle and neuromuscular junction disorders. *Muscle Nerve*. 2021;64:255–269.
194. Cummings BB, Marshall JL, Tukiainen T. et al. Improving genetic diagnosis in Mendelian disease with transcriptome sequencing. *Sci Transl Med*. 2017;9:eaal5209.
195. Pilania K, Jankharia B. Role of MRI in idiopathic inflammatory myopathies: a review article. *Acta Radiol*. 2022;63:200–213.
196. Leung DG. Advancements in magnetic resonance imaging-based biomarkers for muscular dystrophy. *Muscle Nerve*. 2019;60:347–360.
197. Warman Chardon J, Díaz-Manera J, Tasca G, et al; MYO-MRI Working Group. MYO-MRI diagnostic protocols in genetic myopathies. *Neuromuscul Disord*. 2019;29:827–841.
198. Mah JK, van Alfen N. Neuromuscular ultrasound: clinical applications and diagnostic values. *Can J Neurol Sci*. 2018;45:605–619.
199. Wijntjes J, van Alfen N. Muscle ultrasound: present state and future opportunities. *Muscle Nerve*. 2021;63:455–466.
200. Grant GA, Britz GW, Goodkin R, Jarvik JG, Maravilla K, Kliot M. The utility of magnetic resonance imaging in evaluating peripheral nerve lesions. *Muscle Nerve*. 2002;25:314–331.
201. Filler AG, Maravilla KR, Tsuruda JS. MR neurography and muscle MR imaging for image diagnosis of disorders affecting the peripheral nerves and musculature. *Neurol Clin*. 2004;22:643–682.
202. vd Vliet AM, Thijsssen HO, Joosten E, Merx JL. CAT in neuromuscular disorders as comparison of CT and histology. *Neuroradiology*. 1988;30:421–425.
203. Olsen NJ, Qi J, Park JH. Imaging and skeletal muscle disease. *Curr Rheumatol Rep*. 2005;7:106–114.
204. Scott DL, Kingsley GH. Use of imaging to assess patients with muscle disease. *Curr Opin Rheumatol*. 2004;16:678–683.
205. Chapman S, Sopiuthwood TR, Fowler J, Ryder CA. Rapid changes in magnetic resonance imaging of muscle during the treatment of juvenile dermatomyositis. *Br J Rheumatol*. 1994;33:184–186.
206. Fleckenstein JL, Archer BT, Barker BA, Vaughan JT, Parkey RW, Peshock RM. Fast short-tau inversion-recovery MR imaging. *Radiology*. 1991;179:499–504.
207. Britz GW, Haynor DR, Kuntz C, et al. Ulnar nerve entrapment at the elbow: correlation of magnetic resonance imaging, clinical, electrodiagnostic, and intraoperative findings. *Neurosurgery*. 1996;38:458–465.
208. Bertorini T, Halford G, Lawrence J, Vo D, Wassef M. Contrast-enhanced magnetic resonance imaging of the lumbosacral roots in the dysimmune inflammatory polyneuropathies. *J Neuroimaging*. 1995;5:9–15.
209. Kuwabara SK, Nakajima M, Matsuda S, Hattori T. Magnetic resonance imaging at the demyelinative foci in chronic inflammatory demyelinating polyneuropathy. *Neurology*. 1997;48:874–877.
210. Midroni G, de Tilly LN, Gray B, Vajsar J. MRI of the cauda equina in CIDP: Clinical correlations. *J Neurol Sci*. 1999;170:36–44.
211. Cosgrove JC. Magnetic resonance imaging in the evaluation of carpal tunnel syndrome: a literature review. *J Clin Neuromusc Dis*. 2000;1:175–183.
212. Zhou L, Yousem DM, Chaudhry V. Role of magnetic resonance neurography in brachial plexus lesions. *Muscle Nerve*. 2004;30:305–309.
213. Ellegala DB, Lankerovich L, Haynor D, Bird T, Goodkin R, Kliot M. Characterization of genetically defined types of Charcot–Marie–Tooth neuropathies using magnetic resonance neurography. *Neurosurgery*. 1998;43:655–721.
214. Jaiser SR, Winston GP. Copper deficiency myelopathy (review). *J Neurol*. 2010;257(6):869–881.
215. Kumar N, Ahlskog JE, Klein CJ, Port JD. Imaging features of copper deficiency myelopathy: a study of 25 cases. *Neuroradiology*. 2006;48(2):78–83.
216. Locatelli ER, Laureno R, Ballard P, Mark AS. MRI in vitamin B12 deficiency myelopathy. *Can J Neurol Sci*. 1999;26(1):60–63.
217. Halford H, Graves A, Bertorinie T. Muscle and nerve imaging techniques in neuromuscular diseases. *J Clin Neuromusc Dis*. 2000;2:41–51.
218. Walker FO, Alter KE, Boon AJ, et al. Qualifications for practitioners of neuromuscular ultrasound: position statement of the American Association of Neuromuscular and Electrodiagnostic Medicine. *Muscle Nerve*. 2010;42(3):442–444.

219. Walker FO, Cartwright MS, Wiesler ER, Caress J. Ultrasound of nerve and muscle. *Clin Neurophysiol.* 2004;115:495–507.
220. Hobson-Webb LD, Massey JM, Juel VC, Sanders DB. The ultrasonographic wrist-to-forearm median nerve area ratio in carpal tunnel syndrome. *Clin Neurophysiol.* 2008;119:1353–1357.
221. Claes F, Meulstee J, Claessen-Oude Luttikhuis TTM, Huygen PLM, Verhagen WIM. Usefulness of additional measurements of the median nerve with ultrasonography. *Neurol Sci.* 2010;31(6):721–725.
222. Yoon JS, Walker FO, Cartwright MS. Ultrasonographic swelling ratio in the diagnosis of ulnar neuropathy at the elbow. *Muscle Nerve.* 2008;38:1231–1235.
223. Visser LH. High-resolution sonography of the common peroneal nerve: detection of intraneural ganglia. *Neurology.* 2006;167:1473–1475.
224. Beekman R, Visser LH. Sonography in the diagnosis of carpal tunnel syndrome: a critical review of the literature. *Muscle Nerve.* 2003; 27:26–33.
225. Beekman R, Wokke JH, Schoemaker MC, Lee ML, Visser LH. Ulnar neuropathy at the elbow: followup in prognostic factors determining outcome. *Neurology.* 2004;63:1675–1680.
226. Zaidman CM, Al-Lozi M, Pestronk A. Peripheral nerve size in normals and patients with polyneuropathy: an ultrasound study. *Muscle Nerve.* 2009;40(6):960–966.
227. Matsuoka N, Kohriyama T, Ochi K, et al. Detection of cervical nerve root hypertrophy by ultrasonography and chronic inflammatory demyelinating polyradiculoneuropathy. *J Neurol Sci.* 2004;219:15–21.
228. Heckmatt JZ, Dubowitz V, Leeman S. Detection of pathological change in dystrophic muscle with B-scan ultrasound imaging. *Lancet.* 1980;1:1389–1390.
229. Reimers CD, Fleckenstein JL, Wiltt TN, Muller-Felber W, Pongratz DE. Muscular ultrasound in idiopathic inflammatory myopathies of adults. *J Neurol Sci.* 1993;116:82–92.
230. Reimers CD, Schlotter B, Eicke BM, Witt TN. Enlargement in neuromuscular diseases: a quantitative ultrasound study in 350 patients and review of the literature. *J Neurol Sci.* 1996;143:46–56.

CHAPTER 3

Muscle and Nerve Histopathology

Muscle and nerve biopsies can be extremely useful in the evaluation of patients with myopathies and neuropathies. That said, not everyone suspected of having a muscle or nerve disorder needs a biopsy. In this chapter, we discuss the indications and limitations for muscle and nerve biopsies, how specific muscle or nerves are selected for biopsy, and various aspects of specimen handling. Further, we review the routine stains that are performed on muscle and nerve tissue, other stains or studies that can be performed on the tissue, and when to order them. We also mention the role of skin biopsy to assess epidermal nerve fibers in the evaluation of patients with peripheral neuropathy. This chapter is not designed to make the reader a neuropathologist. However, clinicians who take care of patients with neuromuscular disease and order biopsies should have at least a working knowledge of muscle and nerve histopathology.

▶ MUSCLE BIOPSIES

Muscle biopsies are studied through a combination of various histochemistry stains on frozen sections and paraffin-embedded tissue, electron microscopy (EM), and molecular studies [e.g., enzyme assay, protein analysis by Western blot, mitochondrial deoxyribonucleic acid (DNA) mutations, ribonucleic acid (RNA) sequencing].[1–7] It is important to correlate the histopathologic findings with clinical history, neuromuscular examination, and electrodiagnostic findings.

▶ INDICATIONS FOR MUSCLE BIOPSY

A muscle biopsy may be helpful when the patient has objective muscle weakness, abnormal muscle enzymes [e.g., elevated serum creatine kinase (CK) levels], abnormal skeletal muscle magnetic resonance imaging, or myopathic electromyography (EMG) findings. These findings may point to a myopathy but not the exact etiology, and therefore a muscle biopsy may be indicated. That said, if the diagnosis is suspected based on the clinical phenotype and can be made by less invasive means, we generally opt for this first. For example, in a young boy with proximal weakness and large calves, we would first do genetic testing for a dystrophinopathy. Muscle biopsies are less helpful in evaluating patients with only myalgias, subjective weakness, or just slight elevations of CK in the absence of objective abnormalities.[8]

▶ TECHNIQUES

Muscle tissue can be obtained through an open (minor surgical procedure) or needle biopsy. A larger sample of tissue can be biopsied by the open surgery technique, and we prefer this method in patients who may have patchy pathology (e.g., inflammatory myopathies) or myopathies that require metabolic analysis (e.g., mitochondrial disorders or glycogen storage diseases), molecular studies (e.g., Western blotting, RNA sequencing, and mitochondrial DNA mutations), or EM. Needle biopsy can also be technically difficult in patients with substantial subcutaneous tissue or in end-stage muscles in which there is marked atrophy and fibrofatty replacement. However, the yield of a needle biopsy can be quite high in laboratories that are experienced in handling the small amount of tissue obtained by this technique.[9–12] The advantage of a needle biopsy is that it allows for the examination of multiple sites within the muscle, and it is a less invasive procedure than an open muscle biopsy.

We select the specific muscle to biopsy mainly based on the clinical examination, and occasionally aided by skeletal muscle magnetic resonance imaging or EMG guidance. If the requesting physician is not the person who performs the surgery (the usual situation), communication between the two is essential to ensure that the proper site is chosen. Preferably, one should biopsy a mildly weak muscle in the Medical Research Council (MRC) grade 4 out of 5 range to increase the yield. If the muscle is too weak (i.e., MRC grade 3 or less), the tissue typically has end-stage damage. It is often impossible to discern a myopathic process from severe neurogenic atrophy under these conditions. In patients with little, if any, weakness on examination, or those who might only have weakness in muscles that are not easily accessible to biopsy (e.g., iliopsoas muscle in a patient with only hip flexor weakness), needle EMG or skeletal muscle magnetic resonance imaging are used to select the muscle to biopsy. However, it is important to biopsy the contralateral muscle to the needle examination to avoid artifact from needle EMG.

We find that the easiest muscle to biopsy with open surgery is the biceps brachii and is our first choice if clinically affected. Other muscles that are commonly biopsied are the deltoid, triceps, and quadriceps. We occasionally biopsy the cervical paraspinals/upper trapezius muscles in patients with isolated neck extensor weakness or bent spine syndrome. The peroneus brevis muscle is useful to biopsy along with the overlying superficial peroneal nerve in patients suspected of having vasculitis. In patients with suspected distal myopathies,

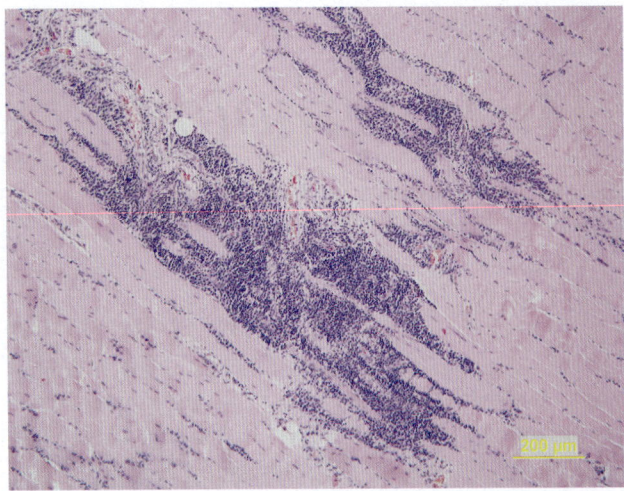 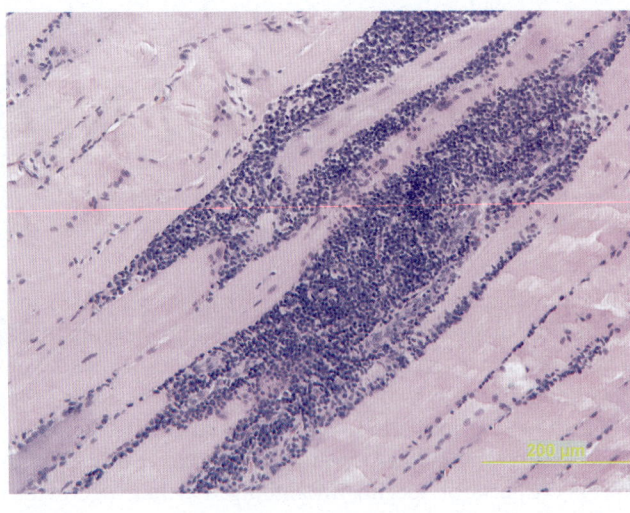

Figure 3-1. Paraffin sections are useful because large, longitudinal segments of muscle fibers can be cut and stained compared to frozen sections. Marked endomysial inflammatory cell infiltrate in this biopsy of a patient with polymyositis (**A**). On higher-power, inflammatory cell infiltrates can be seen to invade the necrotic segments (**B**). Paraffin sections, hematoxylin and eosin (H&E).

we have found the tibialis anterior, gastrocnemius, and forearm extensor muscles (e.g., extensor digitorum communis) easy to biopsy. Otherwise, we tend to avoid the gastrocnemius or tibialis anterior muscle, because asymptomatic radiculopathies or unrelated axonal polyneuropathies may give a false impression that the primary abnormality is a neurogenic process and therefore overshadow an underlying myopathy.

In adults, muscle biopsies are performed under local anesthesia, but young children require sedation or general anesthesia. The biopsies are taken from the belly of the muscle, and it is important to avoid the region of the tendon. Each specimen should be about 1–2 cm in length and 0.5 cm in width. The specimens should be wrapped in slightly moist gauze and placed in separate labeled sterile containers until they reach the laboratory. It is important not to place the specimens in a container of saline else this will lead to artifact. Nor should the entire specimen be placed in fixative else the important histochemistry stains, protein/enzyme analysis, and mutation analysis cannot be performed. Again, this information needs to be communicated with the surgeon and the pathology laboratory. Because muscle disorders can be multifocal (e.g., inflammatory myopathies), we obtain at least two separate specimens that are mounted on a cork and then snap frozen in isopentane cooled in liquid nitrogen. The frozen tissue is then sectioned and stained for routine histochemistry. If the specimen is not snap frozen and placed in ice or freezer, then ice crystal artifact can develop within muscle fibers, rendering the tissue uninterpretable. The frozen tissue can be wrapped in precooled foil and placed in labeled container for freezer storage at 80°C until ready to cut in a cryostat and then stain. In patients with prominent myalgias and tenderness, we may biopsy a piece of the overlying fascia to assess for fasciitis. Separate specimens may also be taken and again frozen immediately for biochemical analysis (e.g., for glycogen or lipid storage disorders and mitochondrial myopathies), mitochondrial DNA analysis, or for Western blot or RNA sequencing (e.g., for various forms of muscular dystrophy or other suspected hereditary myopathies).

In addition, a separate piece of muscle tissue is fixed in formalin or Bouin's fluid for paraffin sections. Paraffin sections can be particularly useful in inflammatory myopathies, vasculitis, and amyloidosis as they allow for the examination of a somewhat larger piece of tissue than that used for histochemistry in cross-section and longitudinal section and assess inflammatory cells and vasculature more effectively (Fig. 3-1). However, due to shrinkage of the muscle tissue associated with the processing, the muscle fibers in paraffin sections often appear cracked and are not ideal for the evaluation of histochemical abnormalities. Finally, an additional piece of muscle is usually taken for possible ultrastructural examination by EM. This small piece of muscle tissue is secured on a clamp or stretched out by suturing the muscle over a tongue blade, to prevent hypercontraction artifact. This tissue is fixed in glutaraldehyde for plastic (epoxy resin or epon) embedding for EM.

A standard battery of histochemical stains is used for light-microscopic evaluation of frozen sections.[1-7] Hematoxylin and eosin (H&E) and modified Gomori trichrome stains assess the size, shape, and cytoarchitecture of the muscle fibers, presence of internalized nuclei, destruction of fibers (e.g., necrosis) and regeneration, as well as the supporting connective tissue (e.g., increased endomysial connective tissue as seen in dystrophies) and vasculature (vasculitis) (Figs. 3-2 and 3-3). Inflammatory cell infiltration is easily appreciated with these stains. In addition, some specific abnormalities are well demonstrated with modified Gomori trichrome stain: ragged red fibers associated with mitochondrial myopathies (Fig. 3-4A), nemaline rods (Fig. 3-4B), tubular aggregates (Fig. 3-4C),

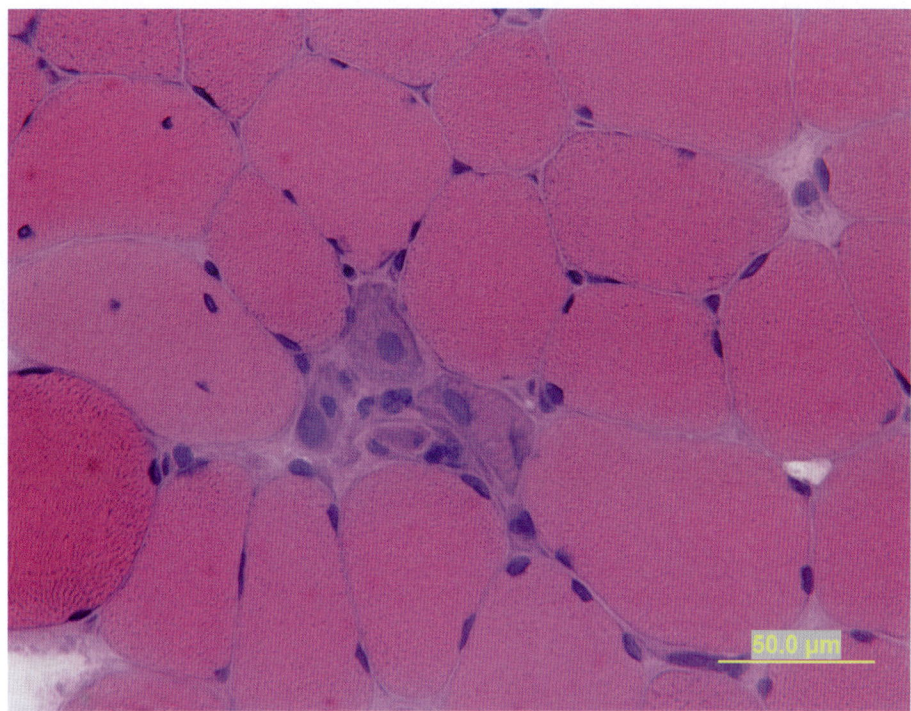

Figure 3-2. A cluster of regenerating muscle fibers are apparent on this H&E stain.

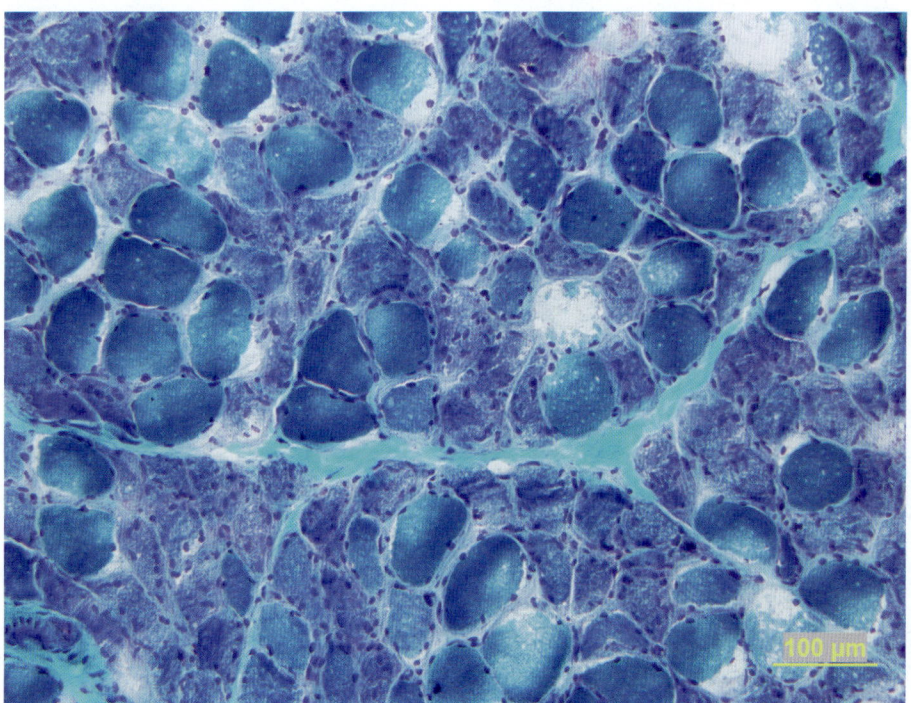

Figure 3-3. Muscle biopsy in a patient with acute quadriplegic myopathy reveals marked atrophy and degeneration of muscle fibers on this modified Gomori trichrome stain.

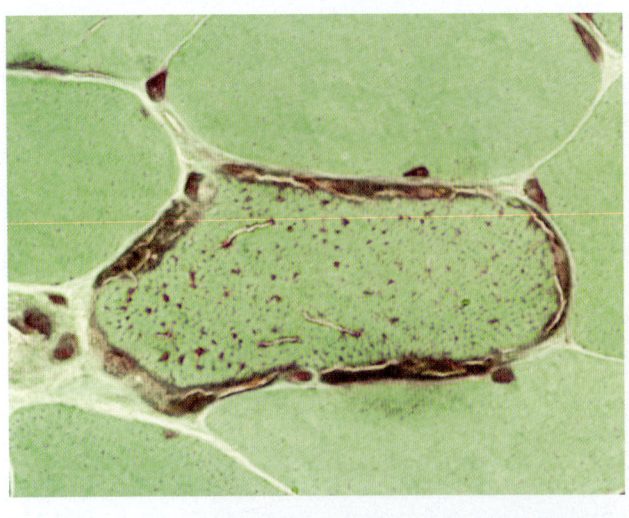
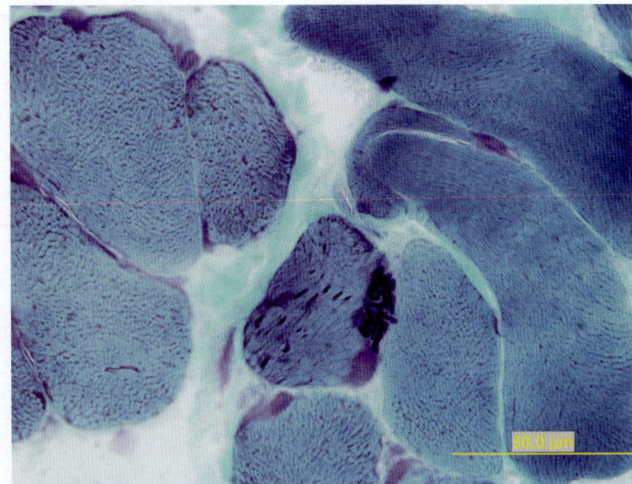
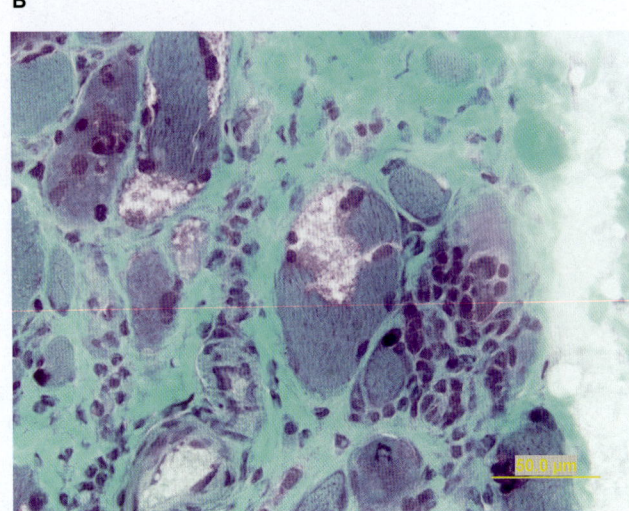
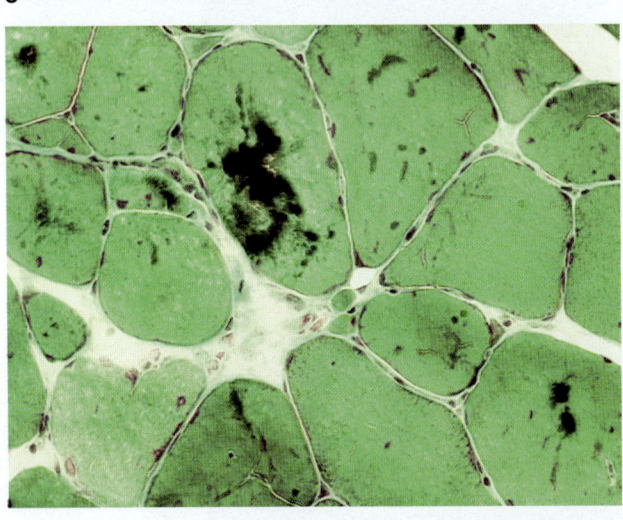

Figure 3-4. Modified Gomori trichrome stain reveals a ragged red fiber in a patient with a mitochondrial myopathy (**A**), nemaline rods in a patient with congenital myopathy (**B**), tubular aggregates in a patient with myalgias (**C**), and rimmed vacuoles filled with debri in a patient with IBM (**D**). Myofibrillar myopathy is best recognized on the modified Gomori trichrome stain as amorphous accumulation of dark green or bluish-purple debri and more distinct, denser cytoplasmic inclusions (**E**).

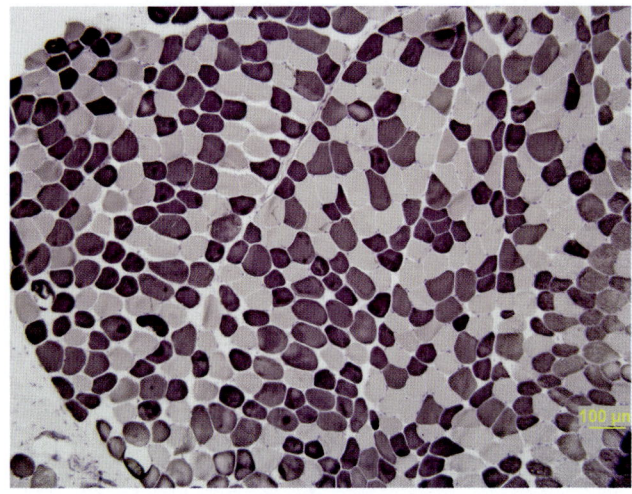

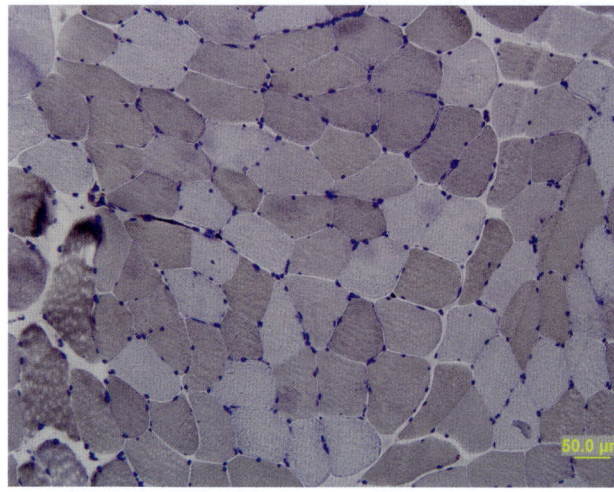

Figure 3-5. The myofibrillar adenosine triphosphatase (ATPase) is typically performed at three pHs: 4.3, 4.6, and 9.4. Type 1 fibers are lightly stained, whereas type 2 fibers are dark on ATPase 9.4 stain (**A**). Type 1 fibers are dark, whereas type 2 fibers are light on ATPase 4.3 stain (**B**). The ATPase 4.6 stains type 1 fibers dark, type 2A fibers light, and type 2B fibers in between (**C**).

rimmed vacuoles (Fig. 3-4D), and features of myofibrillar myopathy (Fig. 3-4E).

The myofibrillar adenosine triphosphatase (ATPase) is typically performed at three pHs, 4.3, 4.6, and 9.4, in order to assess the size and distribution of different muscle fiber types (Fig. 3-5). Individual muscle fibers can be classified into four different fibers based on their staining characteristics and physiologic properties: types 1 (slow twitch, fatigue resistant, and oxidative metabolism), 2A (fast twitch, intermediate fatigue resistance, and oxidative and glycolytic metabolism), 2B (fast twitch, poor fatigue resistance, and glycolytic metabolism), and 2C (undifferentiated and embryonic). In adults, only about 1%–2% of muscle fibers are the undifferentiated type 2C fibers.[13] The specific muscle fiber type is determined by the innervating motor neuron. The different muscle fiber types are normally distributed randomly, forming a so-called checkerboard pattern. Alterations in the random distribution of fiber such as seen with fiber-type grouping are a sign of denervation with subsequent reinnervation. Some myopathies are associated with a predominance or atrophy of a specific fiber type. For example, some congenital myopathies are associated with a predominance of type 1 fibers, which are also smaller in diameter than normal. Disuse and steroid myopathy are associated with preferential atrophy of type 2B fibers.

Periodic acid–Schiff (PAS) stain is used to assess glycogen content, which may be increased in the glycogen storage disorders (Fig. 3-6). If there is abnormal PAS staining, then a PAS with diastase should be performed, as glycogen is removed with diastase, but more complex carbohydrates (such as polyglucosan bodies) are resistant to digestion with diastase. Sometimes, in polyglucosan body neuropathy, PAS-positive inclusions are evident in small intramuscular nerves on muscle biopsies (Fig. 3-6C). Loss of some enzyme activities associated with some metabolic myopathies can be detected by specific staining protocols (e.g., myophosphorylase and phosphofructokinase) (Fig. 3-7). Acid phosphatase stains can highlight lysosomes that are increased in certain disorders (e.g., Pompe disease) as well as macrophages that may be present in muscle tissue (Fig. 3-8). In addition, oil red O or Sudan black can evaluate lipid content, which may be increased in patients with lipid

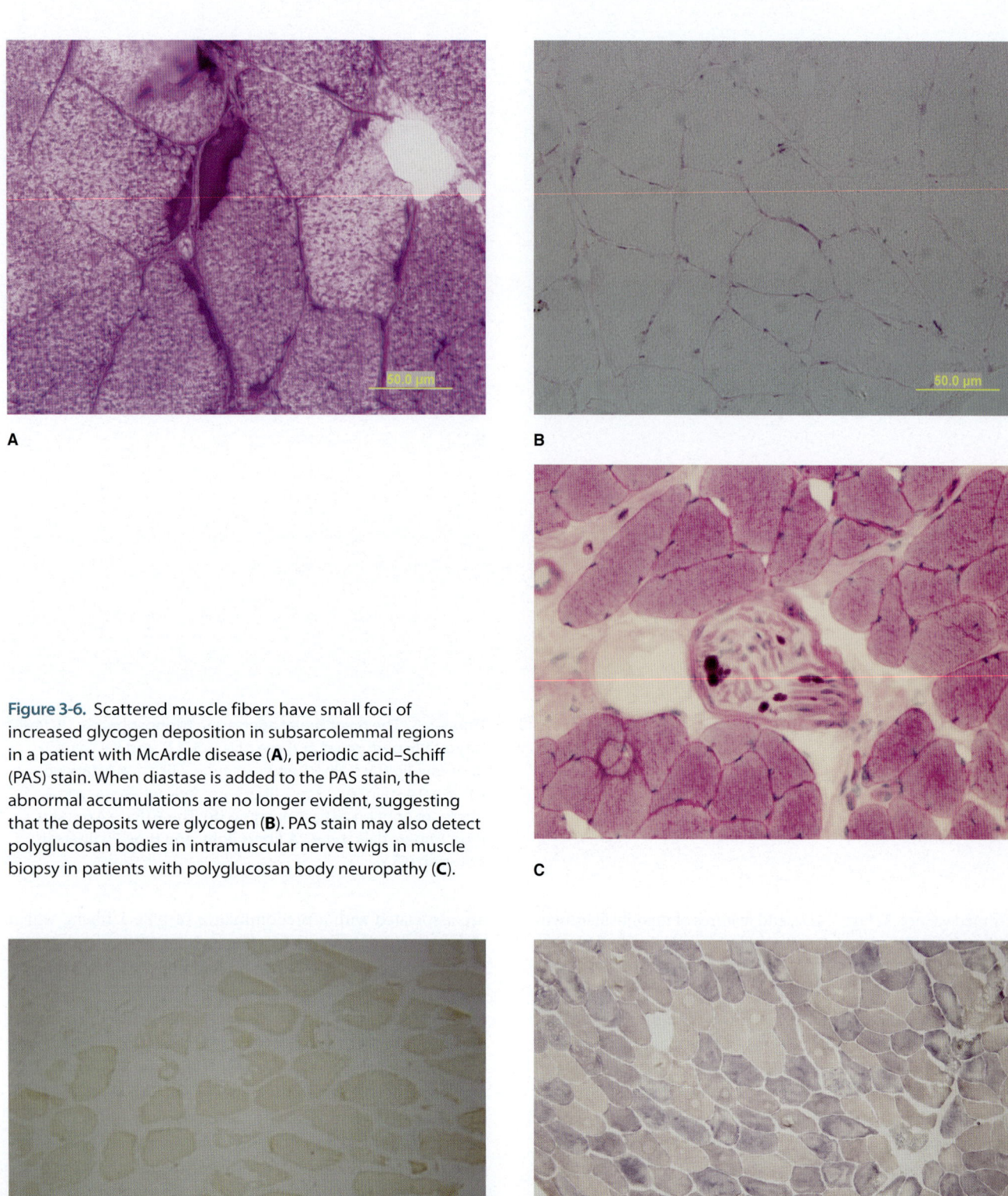

Figure 3-6. Scattered muscle fibers have small foci of increased glycogen deposition in subsarcolemmal regions in a patient with McArdle disease (**A**), periodic acid–Schiff (PAS) stain. When diastase is added to the PAS stain, the abnormal accumulations are no longer evident, suggesting that the deposits were glycogen (**B**). PAS stain may also detect polyglucosan bodies in intramuscular nerve twigs in muscle biopsy in patients with polyglucosan body neuropathy (**C**).

Figure 3-7. Myophosphorylase stain demonstrates absent myophosphorylase activity in a patient with McArdle disease (**A**). Myophosphorylase activity in a healthy control biopsy (**B**). Type 2 fibers that contain more myophosphorylase stain are darker than type 1 fibers.

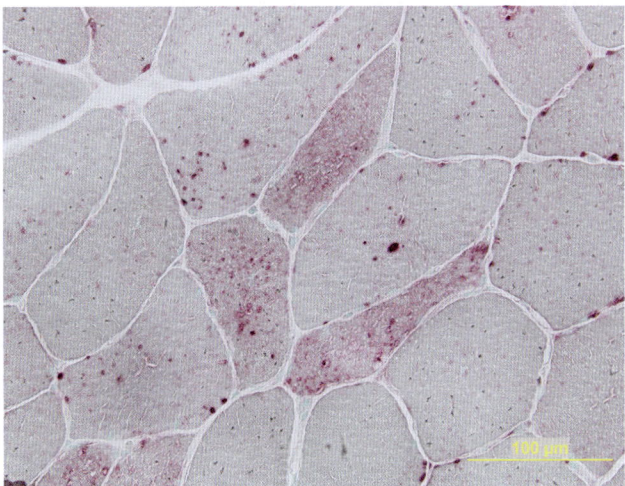

Figure 3-8. Acid phosphatase stains macrophages and muscle fibers lysosomes. In patients with Pompe disease, a lysosomal glycogen storage disorder, increased lysosomes are evident and brought out by acid phosphatase stain even when vacuoles may be difficult to appreciate on other routine stains such as H&E and modified Gomori trichrome.

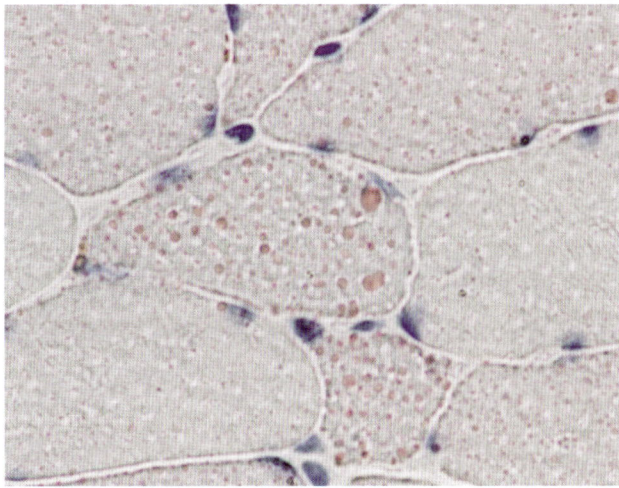

Figure 3-9. Increased lipid droplets in muscle fibers are evident on this oil red O stain in a case of a lipid storage myopathy.

storage myopathies (Fig. 3-9). Oxidative enzyme stains (nicotinamide adenine dinucleotide tetrazolium reductase or NADH-TR, succinate dehydrogenase or SDH, cytochrome-C oxidase or COX) are useful for identifying mitochondrial and intermyofibrillar network abnormalities (Fig. 3-10A and B). The SDH and COX stains can be combined to highly SDH-positive, COX-negative fibers characteristic of disorders associated with mitochondrial DNA mutations (Fig. 3-10C). Target fibers and central cores are also particularly well seen with the NADH-TR stain (discussed later). In addition, a so-called trabeculated or lobulated staining pattern is seen on NADH-TR in some dystrophies as well as sporadic late-onset nemaline myopathy, although this is not a disease-specific abnormality (Fig. 3-10D). Various stains (Congo red, crystal violet, cresyl violet, and Alcian blue) can be performed to assess for amyloid deposition (Fig. 3-11).

Immunohistochemistry is important in evaluating specific types of muscular dystrophies (e.g., dystrophin staining for Duchenne and Becker muscular dystrophy; merosin and alpha-dystroglycan staining for congenital muscular dystrophy; sarcoglycans, caveolin, and dysferlin for limb girdle muscular dystrophies; and emerin for X-linked Emery–Dreifuss muscular dystrophy) (Fig. 3-12). Immunohistochemistry can also be valuable in inflammatory myopathies and vasculitis [e.g., stains for major histocompatibility antigens, MHC1 and MHC2 (HLA-DR2), complement, membrane attack complex (MAC), immunoglobulins, and appropriate inflammatory cell

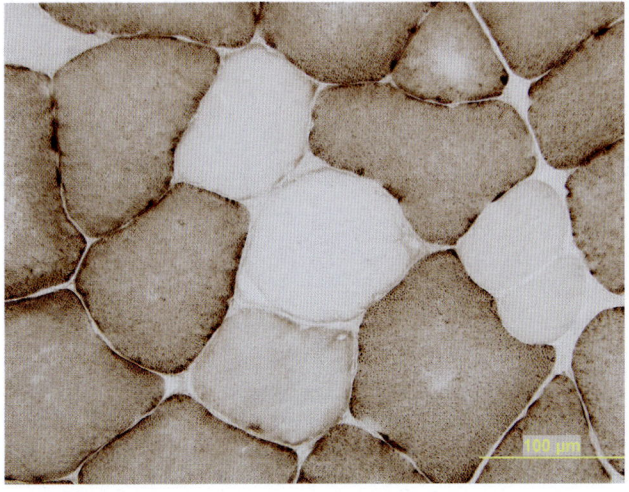

A

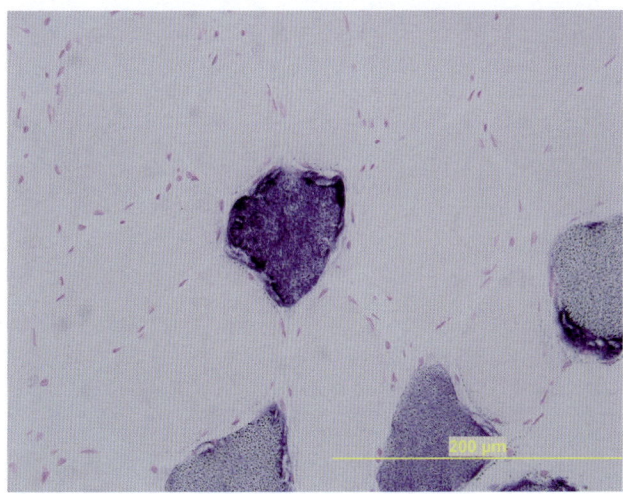

B

Figure 3-10. In addition to ragged red fibers seen on modified Gomori trichrome stain (Fig. 3-4A), mitochondrial myopathies may demonstrate muscle fibers with absent or reduced cytochrome oxidase staining (COX) (**A**) or increased succinic dehydrogenase staining (SDH) (**B**). (*continued*)

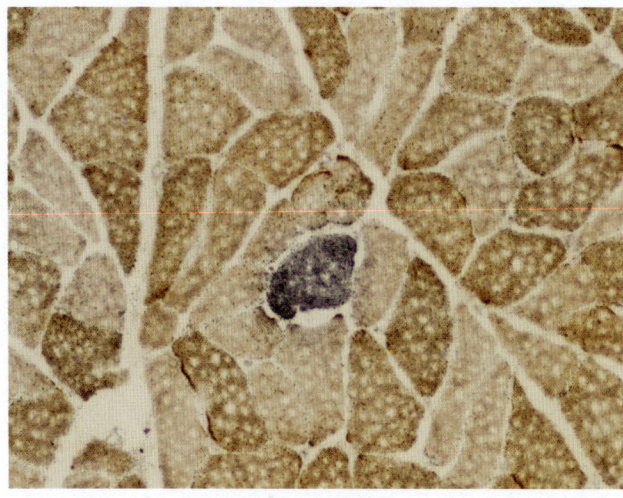
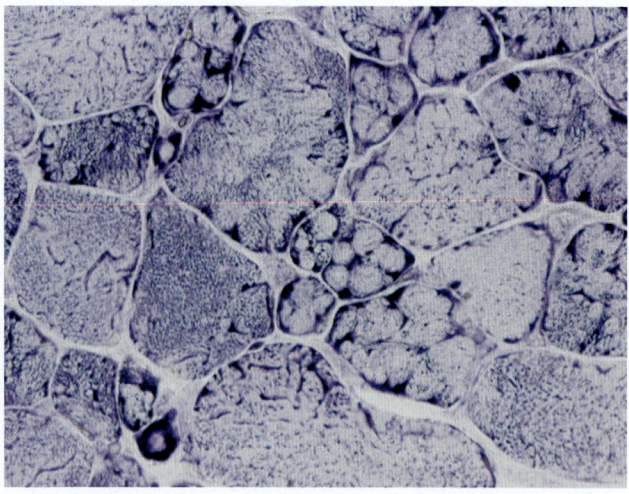

C

D

Figure 3-10. (*Continued*) The COX and SDH stains can be combined such that COX-negative fibers that are SDH-positive show up intensely blue (**C**). These stains are useful because ragged red fibers that are COX negative but SDH positive are usually associated with mitochondrial DNA mutations—though the primary mutation may still involve nuclear-encoded genes that govern mitochondrial DNA. NADH-TR stain also highlights trabeculated or lobulated fibers as seen in this biopsy in a patient with muscular dystrophy (**D**).

markers in order to differentiate macrophages, B-lymphocytes, different T-lymphocytes, and plasma cells] (Fig. 3-13).

EM is used to assess the ultrastructural components of muscle fibers (e.g., the sarcolemma, sarcomeres, nuclei, and mitochondria) and vasculature (e.g., tubulofilaments in capillaries in dermatomyositis).[14] Various myopathies have specific ultrastructural abnormalities that are more readily characterized by EM (e.g., nemaline rods, central cores, proliferation of abnormal appearing mitochondria, myofibrillar disarray, tubular aggregates, vacuoles, and inclusions in nuclei and sarcoplasm) (Fig. 3-14).

▶ STRUCTURE OF NORMAL SKELETAL MUSCLE

Skeletal muscle is a syncytial tissue composed of sheets of individual muscle fibers with multiple nuclei. The connective tissue within muscles includes the endomysium that surrounds individual muscle fibers, the perimysium that groups muscle fibers into primary and secondary bundles (fasciculi), and the epimysium that envelops single muscles or large groups of fibers. Normally, myonuclei are located adjacent to the muscle membrane (sarcolemma)

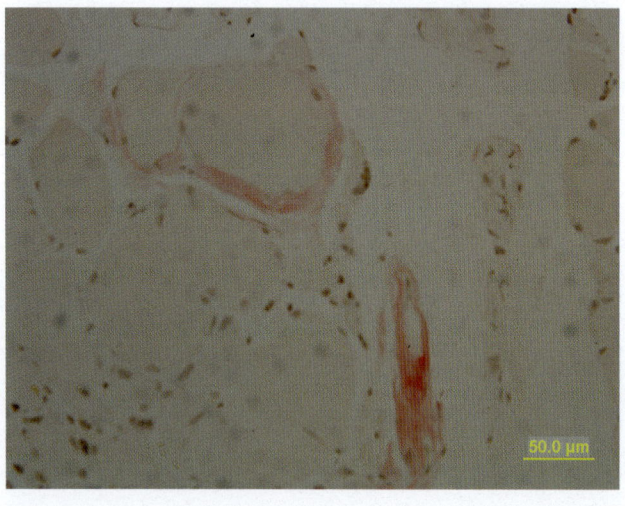
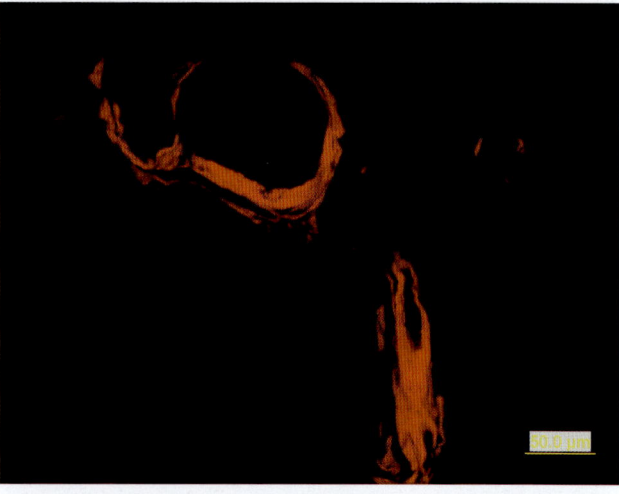

A

B

Figure 3-11. Congo red stain demonstrates amyloid deposition surrounding muscle fibers and blood vessels. Under routine light microscopy, the amyloid deposition is pinkish red staining (**A**), apple green under polarized light, but is most easily appreciated as bright red using rhodamine optics (**B**).

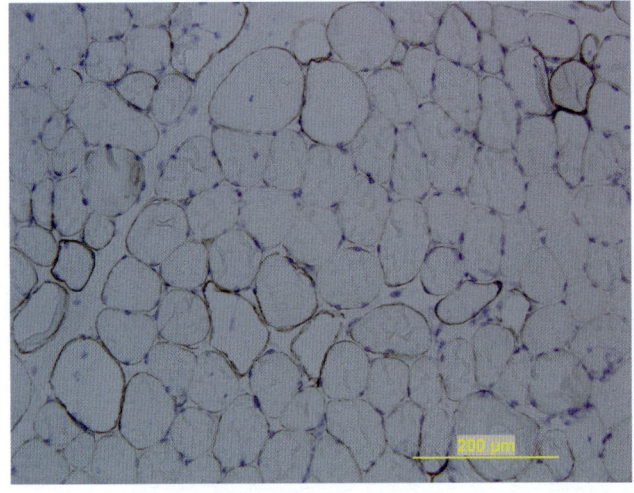
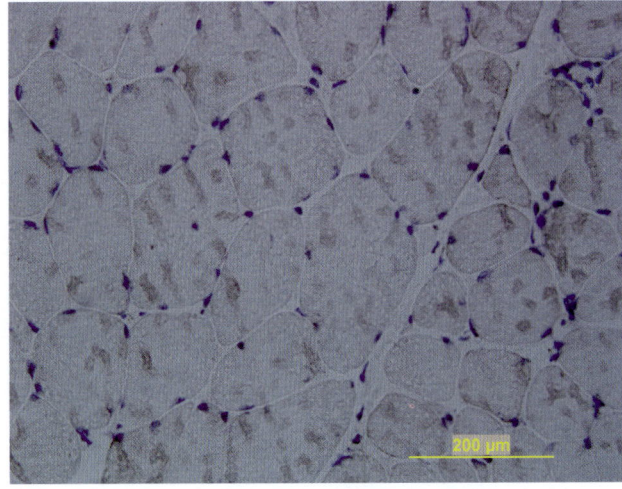
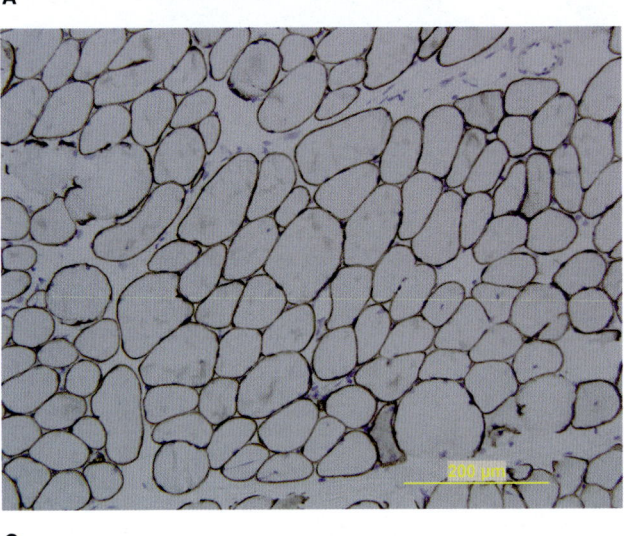

Figure 3-12. LGMD 2I. Muscle biopsies demonstrate reduced or patchy merosin staining (**A**), absent alpha-dystroglycan staining (**B**), but normal dystrophin staining (**C**) around the sarcolemma. Immunoperoxidase stains.

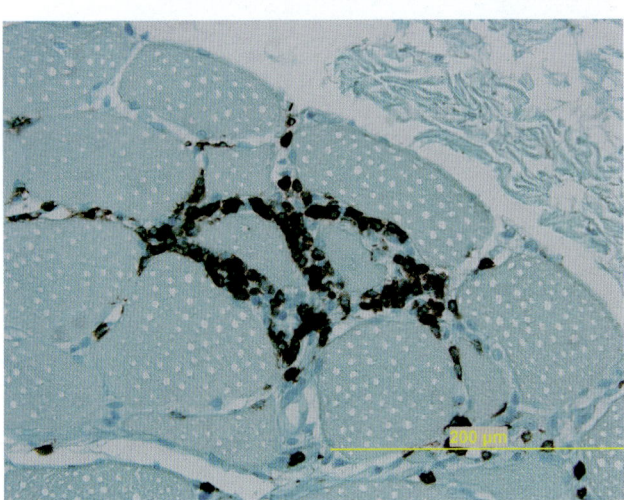

Figure 3-13. Specific types of inflammatory cells, in this case, CD8+ T lymphocytes can be seen in the endomysium surrounding muscle fibers in polymyositis. Immunoperoxidase stain.

and are oriented parallel to the length of the fiber. These are oval in shape and contain evenly distributed chromatin and inconspicuous nucleoli. In approximately 3% of normal adult fibers, the myonuclei lie more internal within the cytoplasm (sarcoplasm). Increased internalized nuclei are a nonspecific abnormality, as these are seen in different types of myopathies as well as in neurogenic disorders. Satellite cells are present next to the sarcolemma and are enveloped by basement membrane that surrounds the muscle fibers. Most of the sarcoplasm of the muscle fiber contains myofilaments, which form the contractile apparatus and supporting structures. Individual muscle fibers contain repeating units (sarcomeres) of interlaced, longitudinally directed thin filaments and thick filaments and perpendicularly oriented Z-bands to which the thin filaments are connected (Fig. 3-14A). The sarcomere is connected to the sarcolemma via filamentous actin. The sarcolemma is composed of various protein complexes and is connected to the extracellular matrix. Greater detail of the sarcolemmal proteins and extracellular matrix is discussed in Chapter 27 (Muscular Dystrophies).

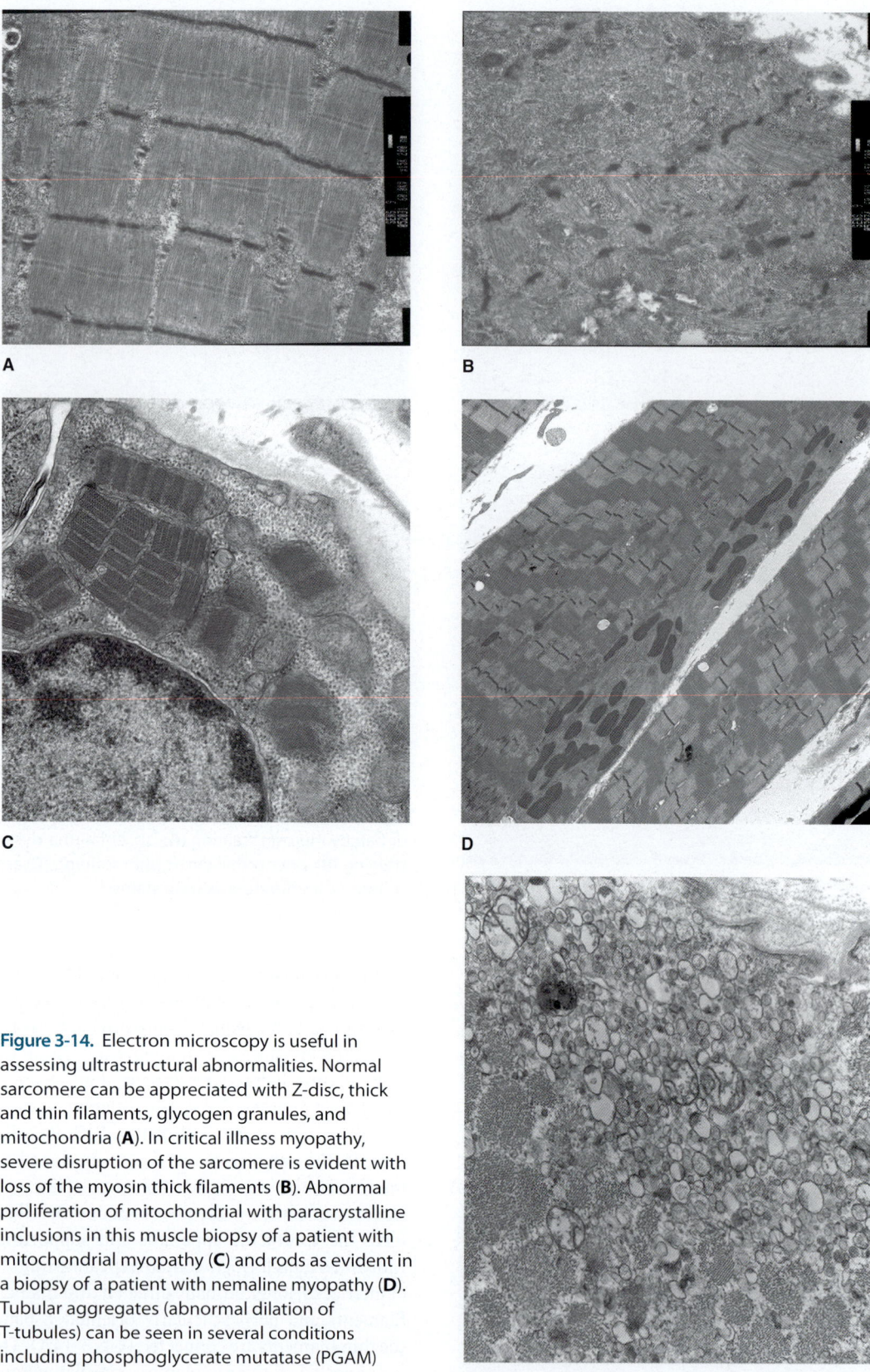

Figure 3-14. Electron microscopy is useful in assessing ultrastructural abnormalities. Normal sarcomere can be appreciated with Z-disc, thick and thin filaments, glycogen granules, and mitochondria (**A**). In critical illness myopathy, severe disruption of the sarcomere is evident with loss of the myosin thick filaments (**B**). Abnormal proliferation of mitochondrial with paracrystalline inclusions in this muscle biopsy of a patient with mitochondrial myopathy (**C**) and rods as evident in a biopsy of a patient with nemaline myopathy (**D**). Tubular aggregates (abnormal dilation of T-tubules) can be seen in several conditions including phosphoglycerate mutatase (PGAM) deficiency (**E**).

The T-tubules are composed of invaginations of the sarcolemmal membrane into the interior of the muscle fibers. Their course is parallel to the Z-bands, and they are surrounded on each site by the sarcoplasmic reticulum. The T-tubules allow for rapid depolarization of muscle membrane deep within muscle fiber cells and the accelerated release of calcium from the sarcoplasmic reticulum during excitation.

Adult muscle fibers are polygonal in appearance but are more rounded in shape in infancy and early childhood. The cross-sectional diameter of individual fibers varies depending on the specific muscle, fiber type, and age of the individual. The motor unit comprises the motor neuron and the muscle fibers it innervates. The individual muscle fibers of a motor unit are normally randomly distributed as previously mentioned, within a sector approximating 30% of the muscle's cross-sectional diameter.

The percentages of type 1, 2A, and 2B fibers differ in various muscle groups, and it is important to be aware of the normal percentages of these fibers in the biopsied muscle for accurate assessment.[15] The most commonly biopsied muscles (i.e., biceps brachii, triceps, and quadriceps) have approximately equal amounts of the three major fiber types, although the deltoid muscle has more type 1 fibers than type 2A and 2B. Because muscle fibers from a single motor unit are randomly distributed among muscle fibers of different motor units and fiber types, a checkerboard or mosaic pattern is appreciated on ATPase stains (Fig. 3-5).

Although ATPase stain is primarily used to assess fiber type, we can often ascertain the fiber types from other standard stains. For example, type 1 fibers stain more intensely with modified Gomori trichrome, lipid, and oxidative enzyme stains than type 2 fibers because of the increased number of mitochondria and oxidative metabolism associated with type 1 fibers. In contrast, type 2 fibers, which are involved with glycolytic metabolism, stain more intensely with PAS, as these contain more glycogen but are lighter staining on modified Gomori trichrome, lipid, and oxidative enzyme stains.

The diameters of individual muscle fibers are assessed to characterize their size. Quantitative analysis is performed by measuring the mean and range of the diameters for each different fiber type.[16–19] Importantly, the diameters of muscle fibers increase to a point during childhood until the early teens. At 1 year of age, the mean muscle fiber diameter is approximately 16 µm. The size increases by about 2 µm/year until the age of 5 years and subsequently by 3 µm/year until 9 years of age. By 10 years of age, mean muscle diameters range from 38 to 42 µm. Normal adult size is reached between the ages of 12 and 15 years.[19] There is usually less than 12% difference in the largest mean fiber diameters between the major fiber types. Both types 1 and 2 adult muscle fibers are larger in men than in women. Type 2 fibers are usually larger than type 1 fibers in men; type 1 fibers are larger than type 2 fibers in women. The diameter of muscle fibers is also dependent on the specific muscle biopsied. For example, in adults, the diameters of muscle fibers in the biceps brachii are as follows: type 1 fibers 64.3 +/− 3.7 µm and type 2 fibers 72.7 +/− 5.3 µm in men and type 1 fibers 56.8 +/− 4.8 µm and type 2 fibers 54.6 +/− 7.0 µm in women. In the vastus lateralis, the diameters of muscle fibers are slightly different: type 1 fibers 59.5 +/− 6.4 µm and type 2 fibers 64.8 +/− 8.1 µm in men and type 1 fibers 58.8 +/− 6.1 µm and type 2 fibers 49.9 +/− 6.2 µm in women.[16]

▶ REACTIONS TO INJURY

Muscle abnormalities may be classified on histopathologic and etiologic grounds into three major categories: (1) neurogenic atrophy: a pattern of muscle pathology consequent to denervation, and if present, reinnervation; (2) myopathies: inherited and acquired diseases characterized by abnormalities in the muscle fiber itself; these include dystrophies, congenital, inflammatory, metabolic (abnormal glycogen or lipid), mitochondrial disturbance, amyloid deposition, and toxic myopathies; and (3) disorders of the neuromuscular junction. Patients with neuromuscular junction defects usually have only slight and nonspecific alterations apparent on routine light microscopy and are rarely biopsied except at very specialized centers.[1–7]

Upon review of muscle biopsy slides, specific features on various stains are important to note. It is essential to assess the size and variability of muscle fibers, the distribution of fiber types, the size and location of the myonuclei, the presence of necrotic and regenerating muscle fibers, other alterations in the cytoarchitecture and organelles (e.g., the presence of target fibers, cores, vacuoles, tubular aggregates, and ragged red fibers), and any abnormal accumulation of glycogen or lipid. Besides the muscle fibers, we evaluate the surrounding vasculature (is there evidence of vasculitis and thickened basement membranes?) and the supportive tissue (is there increased endomysial connective tissue, edema, or amyloidosis?). One should characterize any inflammatory cell infiltrate making note of the type (lymphocytes, plasma cells, eosinophils, and macrophages), the location (endomysial, perimysial, and perivascular), and if there is cellular invasion of nonnecrotic or just necrotic appearing fibers. We discuss some of the common abnormalities seen on muscle biopsy in the following section, but in more detail in the subsequent chapters where specific disorders and their characteristic histologic features are described.

In the setting of axonal degeneration, the muscle fibers within that motor unit lose their neural input and undergo denervation atrophy. This leads to decreased synthesis of myofilaments, degeneration of myofibrils, and a reduction in the size of the muscle fiber.[20] The atrophic fibers lose their polygonal appearance, become more angulated in shape, and may just appear as a clump of nuclei with a small wisp of sarcoplasmic (pyknotic nuclear clumps) (Fig. 3-15). Neurogenic disorders affect motor nerves that innervate both type 1 and 2 fibers. Therefore, in early denervation, muscle biopsies reveal scattered, atrophic angulated muscle fibers of

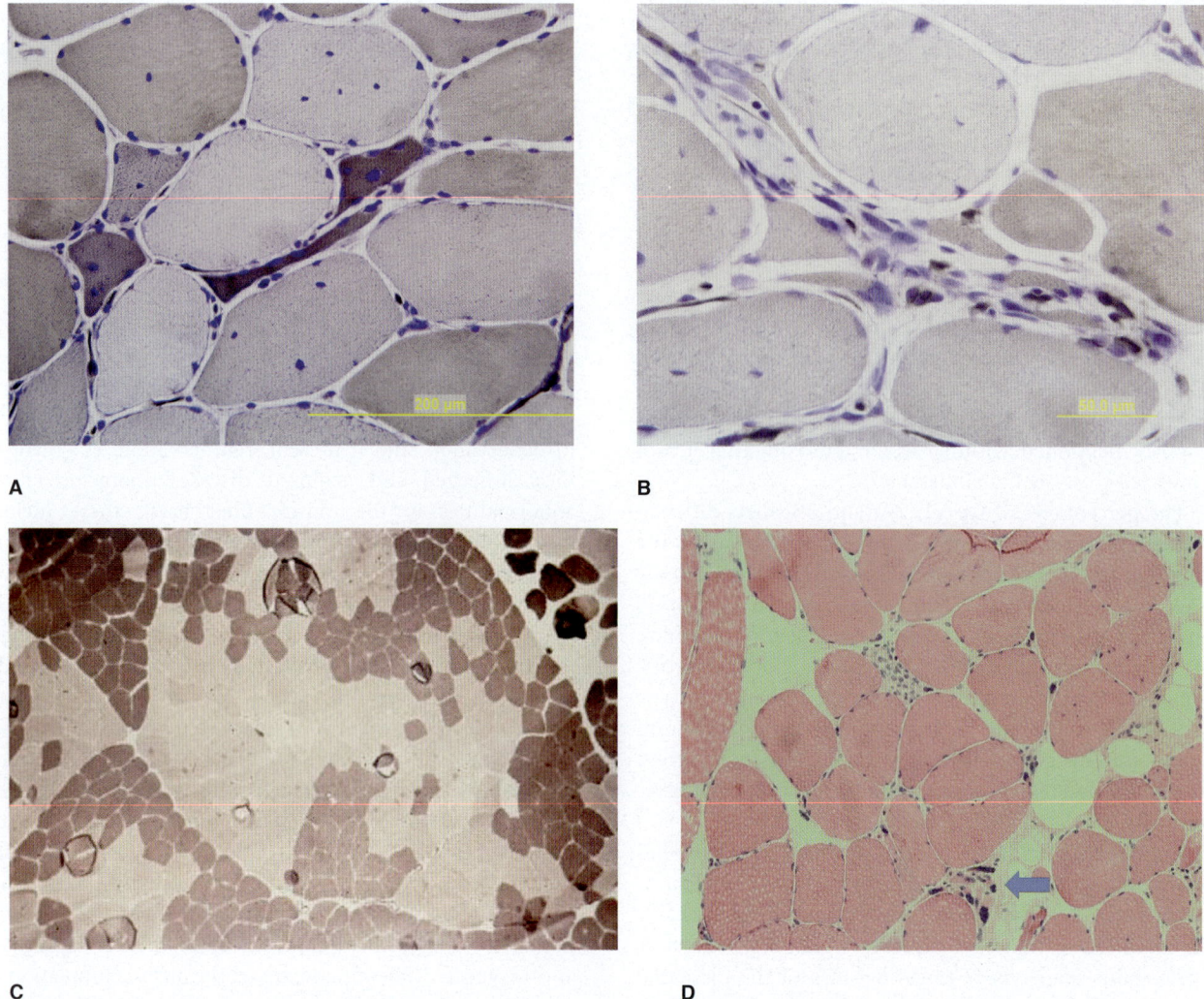

Figure 3-15. Neurogenic atrophy. Denervation results in muscle fibers becoming atrophic and angulated in appearance (**A**), ATPase 4.3. Several atrophic and angulated fibers clustered together are referred to as group atrophy (**B**), ATPase 4.3. If surrounding nerve fibers sprout and reinnervate nearby denervated muscle fibers, the newly reinnervated fibers assume the fiber type of the motor nerve that now innervates them. This leads to the loss of the mosaic pattern on ATPase stains and the appearance of fiber-type grouping (**C**, ATPase 4.3). The atrophic fibers may just appear as a clump of nuclei with a small wisp of sarcoplasmic (*blue arrow*) the so-called pyknotic nuclear clumps (**D**), Paraffin, H&E stain.

both fiber types. As more motor nerves degenerate, rather than seeing isolated atrophic angulated fibers, there are groups of adjacent muscle fibers that are atrophic (grouped atrophy). A feature of denervation is the presence of the so-called target fibers. Reorganization of the cytoarchitecture within muscle cells results in a rounded central zone of disorganized filaments that contain fewer mitochondrial and glycogen. Target fibers have three zones that are circumferentially oriented, which are best seen on NADH-TR staining (Fig. 3-16A and B). The innermost zone is devoid of mitochondrial, glycogen, phosphorylase, and ATPase enzymatic activity; the second zone has increased enzymatic activity, whereas the third zone exhibits intermediate enzymatic activity. Target fibers occur in neurogenic disorders during reinnervation and need to be distinguished from central cores in which there are just two zones of staining (Fig. 3-16C). Central cores are specific for the congenital myopathy central core disease. The so-called moth-eaten or targetoid fibers resemble targets and cores on the NADH-TR stain but have less circumscribed patches of reduced oxidative enzyme staining again without a distinct intermediate zone of enzyme activity. Moth-eaten targetoid fibers (Fig. 3-16D) are nonspecific and can be seen in myopathic and neurogenic disorders. Both central cores and target fibers preferentially affect type 1 fibers. In contrast to central core myopathy in which the cores are present in most of the type 1 fibers, the percentages of fibers with target and targetoid abnormalities are less abundant. Target fibers and central cores can also be appreciated on other stains such as the ATPase, PAS, and modified Gomori trichrome stains (Fig. 3-16E).

Denervated muscle fibers send out trophic signals that lead nearby unaffected axons to sprout collateral branches

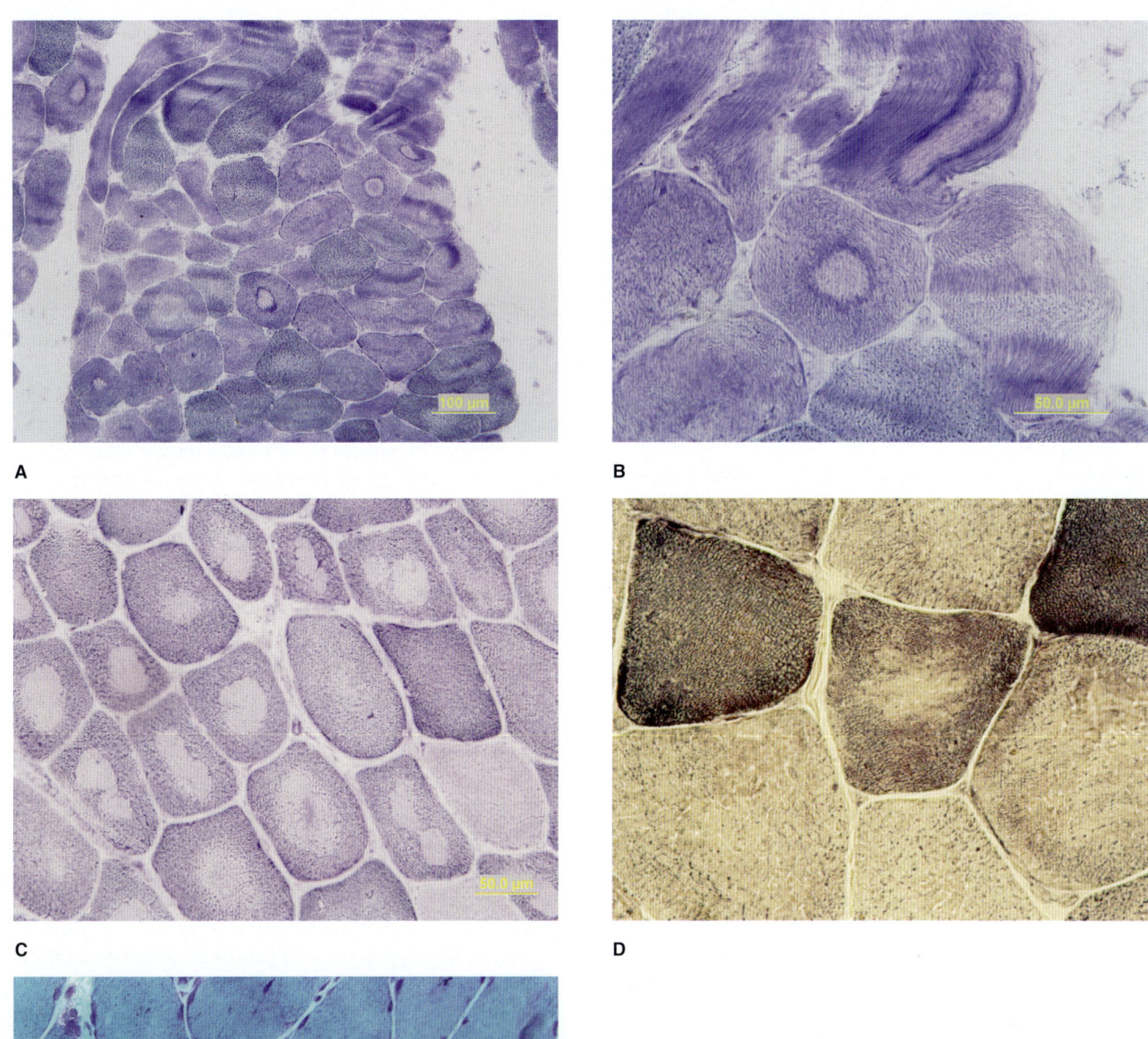

Figure 3-16. In the course of reinnervation, target fibers may develop. True target fibers have three zones in the center of the muscle fibers that are best seen on NADH-TR staining, at low power (**A**), and at higher power (**B**). The innermost zone is pale; the second zone has increased enzymatic activity, whereas the third zone exhibits intermediate enzymatic activity. Central cores resemble targets, but there is no second zone with increased enzyme activity (**C**). In targetoid or the so-called moth-eaten fibers, the zones of reduced activity are even less distinct (**D**). Target fibers and cores can also be appreciated on other stains such as the modified Gomori trichrome stain (**E**). On the Gomori trichrome stain, the center of the target fibers stain dark and are surrounded by pale staining zone.

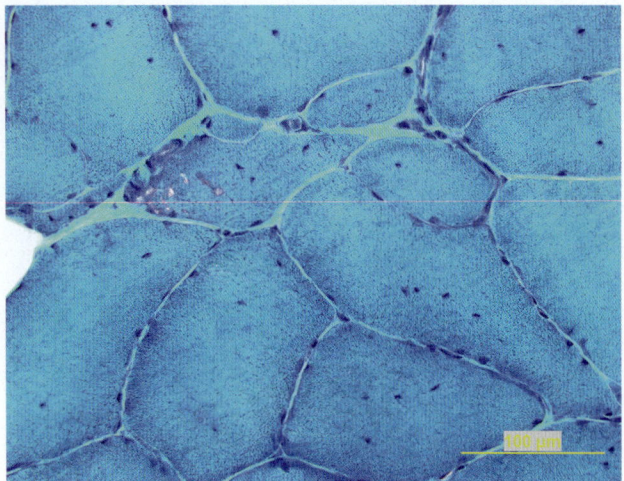

Figure 3-17. Variability in muscle fiber size, increased internalized nuclei, muscle fiber splitting, and small intracytoplasmic vacuoles are nonspecific myopathy features appreciated on this modified Gomori trichrome stain.

to reinnervate the newly denervated muscle fibers. Once successful reinnervation is accomplished, the newly reinnervated muscle fiber assumes the physiologic properties of the reinnervating neuron. This may lead a type 1 fiber to become a type 2A fiber or a type 2B fiber to become a type 1 fiber. Consequently, the normal checkerboard appearance of muscle tissue is replaced by large groups of single muscle fibers, all with the same fiber type (e.g., fiber-type grouping) (Fig. 3-15C). If these larger motor nerves subsequently degenerate, large areas of atrophic fibers of the same fiber type are seen—a different type of grouped atrophy.

In contrast to neurogenic atrophy, myopathic disorders are associated with a wider spectrum of histopathologic alterations (Fig. 3-17). Remember that muscle is a syncytium formed from the fusion of thousands of myoblasts. Because of its syncytial nature, histopathologic abnormalities may be focal rather than occurring along the entire length of a muscle fiber (e.g., segmental necrosis). Genetic disorders can manifest discrete abnormalities, with other regions of the single fiber appearing relatively normal. An example of this can be seen in mitochondrial myopathies in which the histopathologic alterations are dependent on the degree of abnormal mitochondria, which in turn reflects the percentage of mutated mitochondrial DNA in the region. Thus, when cut longitudinally, one may appreciate segments of the muscle fiber with a ragged red appearance, which do not stain with cytochrome oxidase, whereas other nearby segments of the same fiber may be normal. In dystrophies, one often sees scattered necrotic muscle fibers on the cross-section. However, if the tissue is cut longitudinally, one sees that necrosis is segmental in nature. Likewise, inflammatory myopathies are multifocal, resulting in infiltrates surrounding and invading segments of muscle fibers along their length.

Myopathies are usually associated with a random loss of muscle fibers belonging to different motor units. Atrophy of muscle fibers is a common histopathologic feature in myopathies, but rather than fibers becoming angular as in neurogenic atrophy, these usually become more rounded in appearance in myopathic disorders. Small groups of atrophic fibers of similar type may be observed in myopathies due to muscle fiber splitting, degeneration, and regeneration; however, large areas of group atrophy or fiber-type grouping are more typical of neurogenic atrophy. Preferential atrophy or hypotrophy of type 1 fibers is seen in certain myopathic disorders (e.g., myotonic dystrophy and various congenital myopathies). On the other hand, preferential type 2 fiber atrophy can be seen in certain endocrine disorders (e.g., steroid myopathy), as well as a complication of disuse.

Besides atrophy of muscle fibers, hypertrophy can develop in response to increased load, either in the setting of exercise or in pathologic conditions where other muscle fibers are injured. Large fibers may divide along a segment (muscle fiber splitting) so that, in cross-section, a single large fiber contains a cell membrane traversing its diameter. Because both chronic myopathic and neurogenic disorders can be associated with a mixture of atrophic and hypertrophic fibers, increased variability of muscle fiber size is a nonspecific abnormality.

Necrosis is a feature more common in myopathies, but it can also rarely occur in denervated muscle fibers (Fig. 3-18). A single muscle fiber can undergo either total necrosis or segmental necrosis, but again, given the syncytial nature of muscle, atrophy along the entire fiber length is rare. The more common form of muscle tissue loss is referred to as segmental necrosis in which a relatively small segment of the single muscle fiber is affected. The site of necrosis may be focal at first, but it extends longitudinally along the muscle fiber with disease progression. Segmental necrosis is best appreciated on paraffin or semithin sections of muscle fibers cut longitudinally. With segmental necrosis, the affected portion of the single muscle fiber becomes more rounded and the sarcoplasm begins to have a featureless ground-glass appearance. Semithin and EM sections reveal degeneration of the Z-disc and myofibrillar network as well as abnormal mitochondria. Macrophages are recruited into the area and infiltrate the necrotic segments in order to digest the disintegrating muscle tissue and damaged tissue. In certain diseases [inclusion body myositis (IBM)], macrophages and lymphocytes may invade nonnecrotic tissue such that a muscle fiber can be "severed" into distinct segments.

Repair of necrotic segments can occur and begins with the proliferation of adjacent satellite cells in the region of the destroyed portion of the fiber.[21] The satellite cells align next to each other to form myotubes. Several myotubes form per segment and adhere to the surrounding basal lamina. The expansion of myotubes occurs laterally and longitudinally, eventually reaching and fusing with the healthy muscle tissue stumps. The regenerating muscle fibers can be appreciated by their large, internalized nuclei with prominent nucleoli and their basophilic cytoplasm that is laden with RNA

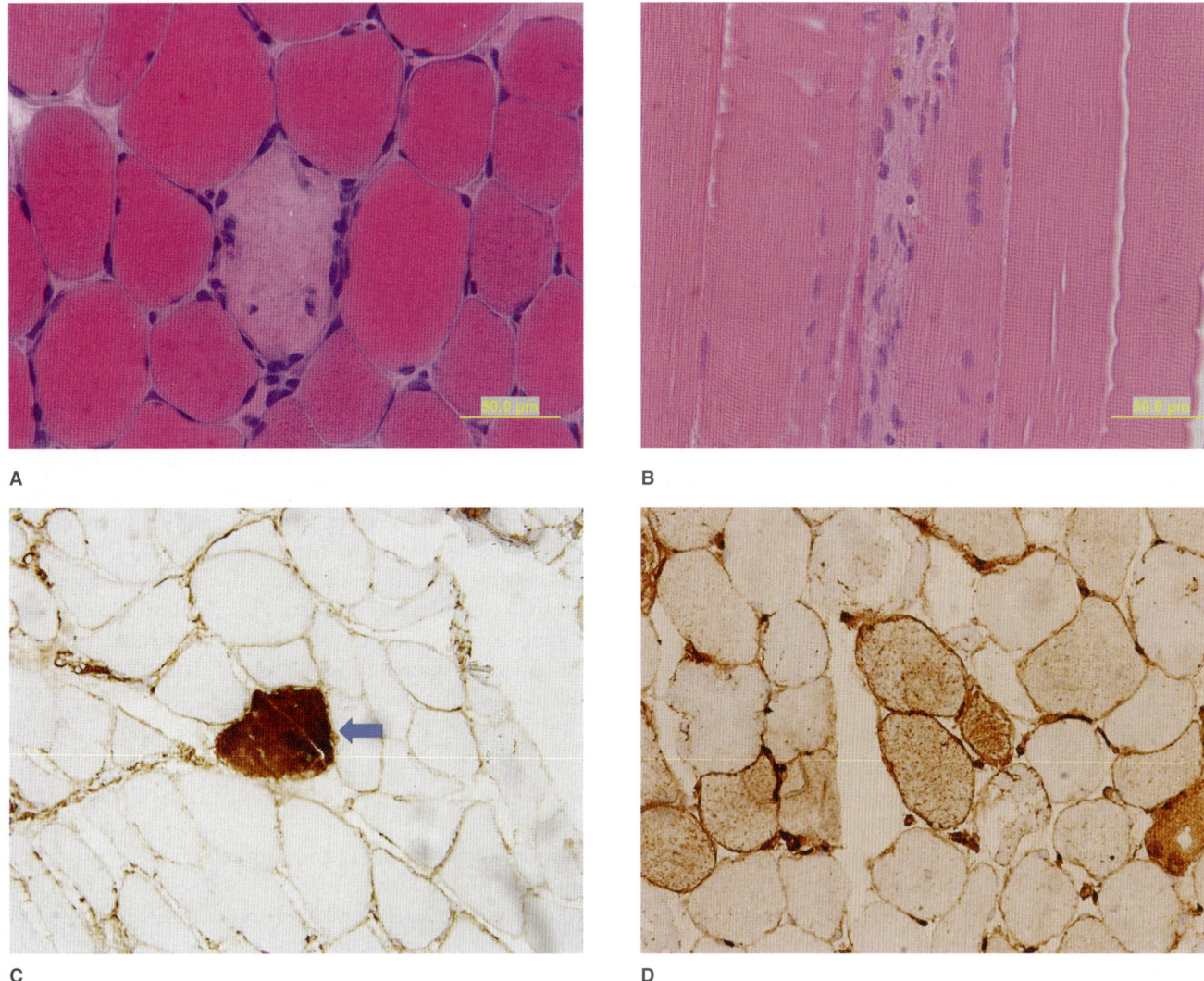

Figure 3-18. A necrotic muscle fiber is pale staining in comparison to surrounding muscle fibers in cross-section, H&E stain. (**A**) Segmental necrosis is often well appreciated on paraffin sections in which large, longitudinal segments can be visualized. The striations of the sarcomeres can be appreciated in normal fibers, whereas the necrotic segment of an adjacent fiber loses the striations. The necrotic segment is invaded by macrophages (**B**), Paraffin section, H&E stain. Immunoperoxidase stain demonstrated membrane attack complex (MAC) deposition throughout the sarcoplasm of a necrotic muscle fibers (*blue arrow*), but with autoimmune necrotizing myopathy, there is also deposition of MAC on the sarcolemma of nonnecrotic muscle fiber (**C**). Major histocompatibility antigen type 1 (MHC1) is not normally expressed on muscle fibers, but it is expressed on the sarcolemma of nonnecrotic fibers in immune-mediated myopathies (**D**). Immunoperoxidase.

(Fig. 3-19). Old damage can be ascertained by the increase in the number of internalized nuclei (Fig. 3-17). Myonuclei, which usually lie along the subsarcolemmal membrane, are more internalized in regenerated segments.

Other characteristics of myopathic injury include alterations in structural proteins or organelles, formation of vacuoles, and accumulation of intracytoplasmic deposits. Increased endomysial connective tissue is a common feature of muscular dystrophies but is also seen in chronic inflammatory myopathies and severe end-stage neurogenic atrophy. One of the most common reasons for a muscle biopsy in adults is to assist in diagnosis of a primary inflammatory myopathy. The characteristic histopathologic features on muscle biopsies in dermatomyositis are perifascicular atrophy and perivascular, perimysial inflammatory cell infiltrate with many plasmacytoid dendritic cells (Fig. 3-20A). On the other hand, polymyositis is associated with endomysial T cells that surround and often appear to invade nonnecrotic muscle fibers (Fig. 3-20B). These features are actually more common in IBM than polymyositis, and in addition, there are often rimmed vacuoles and various inclusions apparent on light microscopy, immunostaining, and EM (Fig. 3-20C). It is important to note that rimmed vacuoles and inclusions are not seen in at least 20% of any given IBM biopsy, so the diagnosis of IBM cannot be excluded in the absence of these findings. Furthermore, one will not see rimmed vacuoles on paraffin

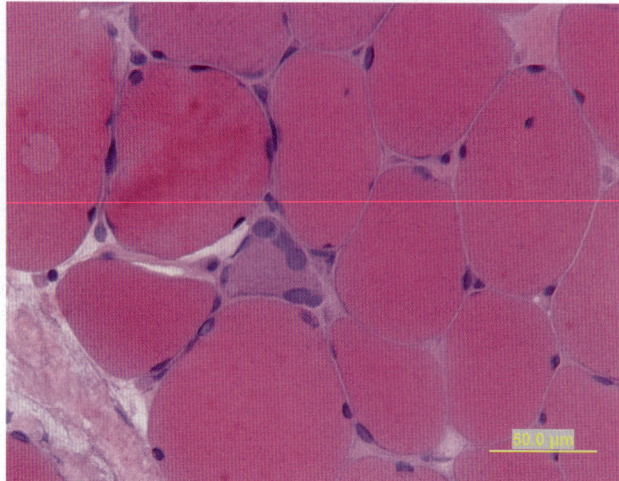

Figure 3-19. Regenerating muscle fibers are smaller and more basophilic than normal fibers and contain enlarged nuclei sometimes with nucleoli, as these are very active in trying to replenish necessary muscle proteins. H&E stain.

sections, only on frozen sections—so it is imperative to do histochemistry staining of frozen section and not just paraffin sections. Immune-mediated necrotizing myopathy (IMNM) is associated with scattered necrotic and regenerating muscle fibers in the absence of significant inflammatory cell infiltrate (Fig. 3-18A and B). A helpful feature to distinguish IMNM from toxic causes of necrotizing myopathy is to assess for MAC and major histocompatibility antigen type 1 (MHC1) on the sarcolemma of nonnecrotic, nonregenerating muscle fibers (Fig. 3-18C and D). Less common forms of inflammatory myopathy include granulomatous or giant cell myositis (Fig. 3-20D) and eosinophilic myositis (Fig. 3-20E).

A precautionary note is that inflammatory cell infiltrates are seen in dystrophies and other types of myopathy and thus are not specific for an immune-mediated process.

▶ NERVE BIOPSIES

As is true for muscle biopsies, the interpretation of a nerve biopsy requires correlation of histologic changes, with clinical information including the results of electrophysiologic investigations. Nerve biopsies are generally less useful than muscle biopsies because the pathologic abnormalities are often nonspecific and frequently do not help distinguish one form of peripheral neuropathy from the other.[5,22–29] In addition, there is increased morbidity associated with the removal of a segment of sensory nerve, which leads to permanent numbness in the corresponding cutaneous distribution. Also, nerve biopsies can be complicated by significant neuropathic pain in the distribution of the nerve for several months and the potential for growth of painful neuromas. Therefore, we do not recommend nerve biopsies just because the patient has a generalized neuropathy of undetermined etiology despite an extensive laboratory evaluation. This situation is quite common, as discussed in Chapter 22.

▶ INDICATIONS FOR NERVE BIOPSY

Suspected amyloidosis and vasculitis are the major indications for nerve biopsy. Amyloidosis should be considered in patients with a monoclonal gammopathy, autonomic neuropathy, systemic signs of amyloidosis (e.g., renal insufficiency or cardiomyopathy), or a family history

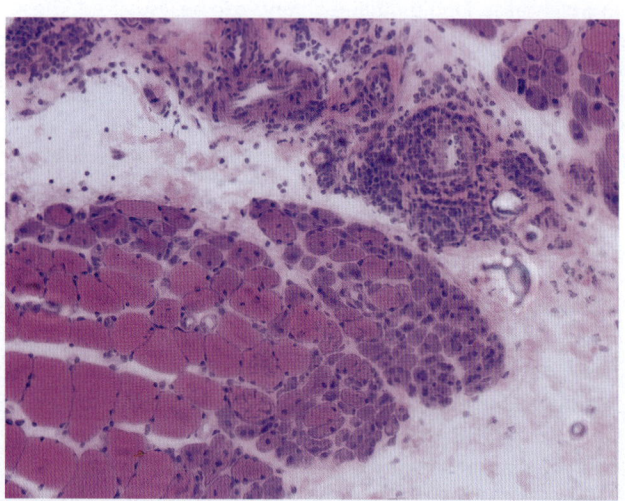
A

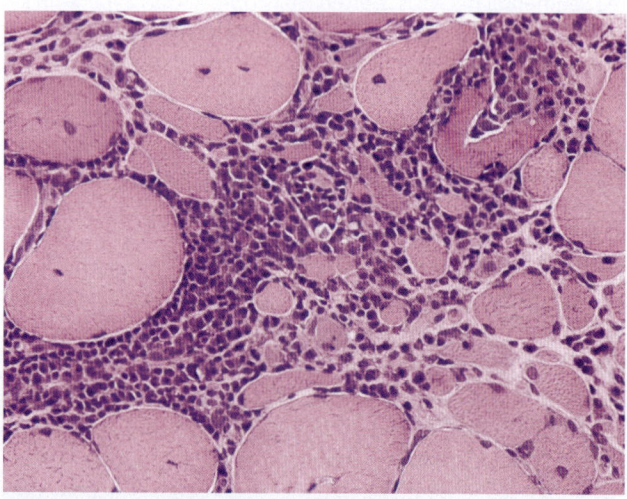
B

Figure 3-20. The characteristic feature of dermatomyositis is perifascicular atrophy and perivascular, perimysial inflammation (**A**), H&E stain. Polymyositis is associated with endomysial inflammatory cell infiltrates surrounding and often appearing to invade nonnecrotic muscle fibers but this pathological feature is far more common in inclusion body myositis. (**B**), H&E stain. (*continued*)

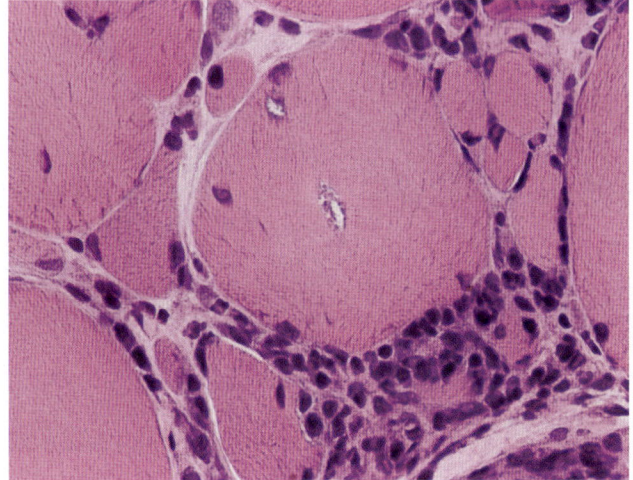
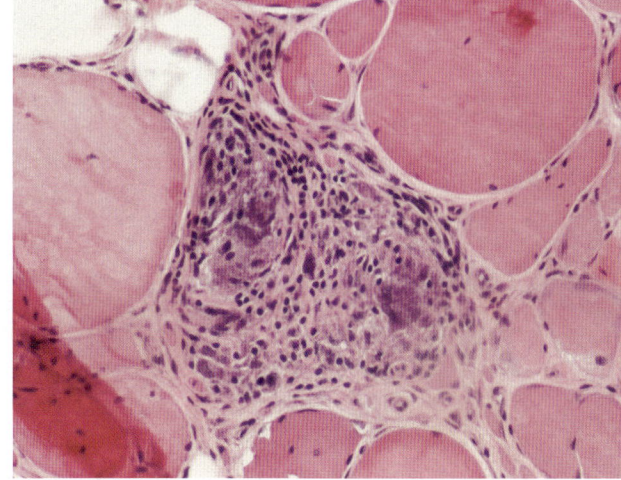
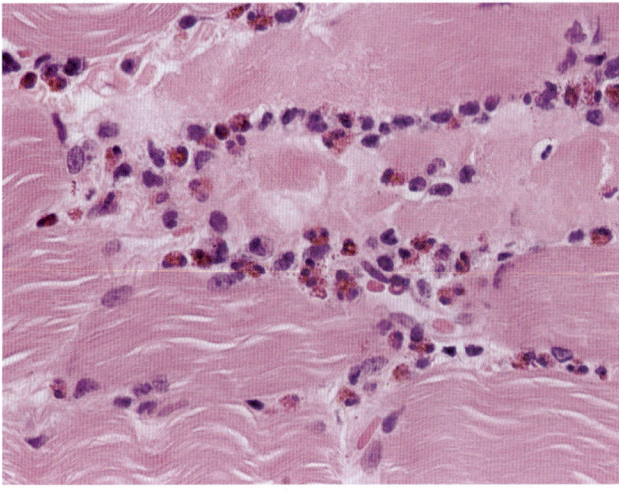

Figure 3-20. (*Continued*) Inclusion body myositis likewise has features of polymyositis but rimmed vacuoles are often apparent (**C**), H&E stain. Importantly, rimmed vacuoles are not appreciated in 20-30% of any given muscle biopsy of patients with IBM. In sarcoidosis and granulomatous myositis, the biopsies reveal granulomas (**D**), H&E stain. Eosinophils are prominent among the inflammatory cells in eosinophilic myositis, but these cells may rarely also be seen in certain inflammatory dystrophies (**E**), H&E stain.

of amyloidosis. Vasculitic neuropathy is in the differential diagnosis in people presenting with a history of multiple mononeuropathies, particularly when of acute onset and painful, and when there is an underlying connective tissue disease (e.g., systemic lupus erythematosus and rheumatoid arthritis), eosinophilia or late-onset asthma (Churg–Strauss syndrome), renal failure or chronic sinusitis, hepatitis B or C, an elevated erythrocyte sedimentation rate or C-reactive protein, or antinuclear cytoplasmic antibody. Additional indications for nerve biopsy include other autoimmune inflammatory conditions (e.g., sarcoidosis), IgG4 disease, light chain deposition not in the form of amyloid, possible infectious processes (e.g., leprosy), and tumor infiltration (e.g., lymphoma and leukemia). Also, a nerve biopsy may be required for the diagnosis of a tumor of the peripheral nerve (e.g., perineurioma). Less commonly, nerve biopsy may be warranted to diagnose uncommon forms of hereditary neuropathy when DNA testing is not available or inconclusive (e.g., giant axonal neuropathy and polyglucosan body neuropathy).

▶ TECHNIQUES

We usually biopsy a superficial sensory nerve that is clinically affected and also abnormal on sensory nerve conduction studies. The most common nerve biopsied is the sural nerve. We prefer to biopsy the sural nerve in the midshin approximately one-third to one-fourth of the distance from ankle to knee, as opposed to the lateral ankle itself where the nerve may be more prone to trauma and healing may not be as good (Fig. 3-21). Patients should be warned that following the sural nerve biopsy, there is often pain for several months as well as permanent loss of sensation on the lateral aspect of the ankle and foot.[26] A superficial peroneal nerve biopsy is particularly useful when vasculitic neuropathy is suspected and there is foot drop because the underlying peroneus brevis muscle can also be biopsied through the same incision site, thereby increasing the diagnostic yield (Fig. 3-22). Biopsy of the superficial peroneal nerve will lead to numbness of the dorsum of the foot and again often neuropathic pain for several months. If only the upper extremities are involved, the

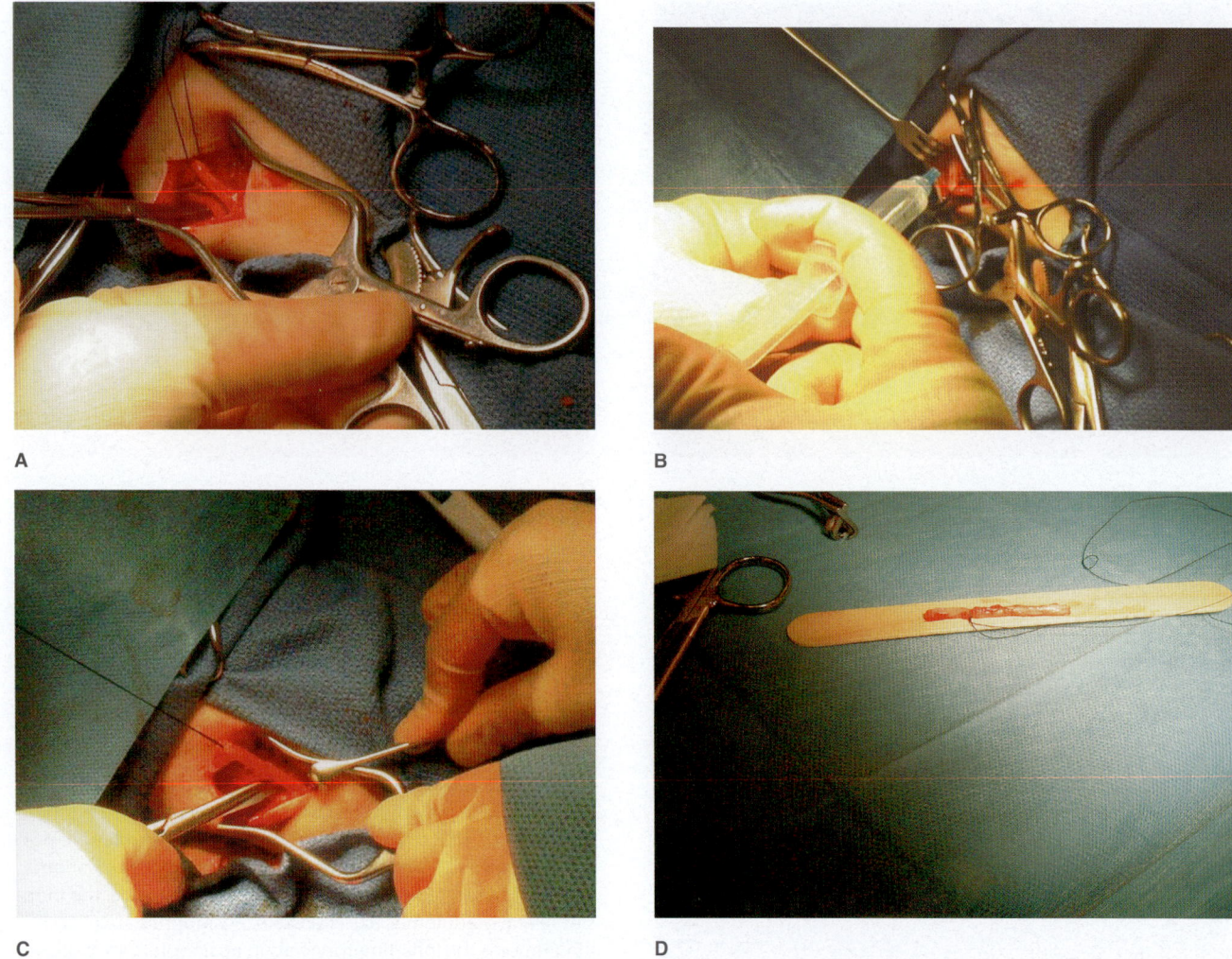

Figure 3-21. The sural nerve is usually biopsied approximately one-third up from the ankle just lateral to the midline in the grove made by the Achilles tendon. It is important for the surgeon to isolate and distinguish the saphenous vein from the sural nerve as they lie next to each other. The saphenous vein can look nearly identical to the sural nerve, often leading to an erroneous "nerve biopsy" with a lumen if care is not taken. A silk suture is gently lifting the sural nerve away from the saphenous vein (**A**). The nerve is injected proximally with lidocaine (**B**) and then is dissected away from the surrounding tissue (**C**). A 4-cm segment is biopsied and divided into separate specimens for frozen section, paraffin embedding, semithin, EM, and teased fiber preparations (**D**).

superficial radial nerve can be biopsied; however, this leads to numbness of the dorsum of the hand, which is problematic for most patients. Importantly, because of sampling error, the single small segment of distal sensory nerve may not be representative of focal disease processes elsewhere in the peripheral nervous system, especially in processes with predominant motor involvement. On rare occasions when a patient has a multifocal process and the lesion appears proximal (e.g., amyloidomas, inflammatory process, and tumors), a fascicular nerve biopsy of a lesion in the root, plexus, or proximal nerve may be required. This procedure should only be performed, however, by neurosurgeons experienced in the technique and where the tissue can be processed appropriately in the neuropathology laboratory.

Nerve biopsies are performed under local anesthesia in adults; general anesthesia is often required to obtain an adequate specimen from children or when a proximal nerve segment needs to be biopsied (e.g., root, plexus, or proximal nerve). The pathology laboratory should be contacted in advance of the surgery so that the tissue can be picked up directly from the operating room and processed immediately. Local anesthetic should be injected into the nerve just proximal to the site of transection in awake patients to reduce pain associated with sectioning the nerve (Fig. 3-21B). A 4- to 5-cm long section of nerve should be excised. The specimen can be wrapped in a saline-moistened gauze (not drenching wet).

The nerve biopsy is divided into several portions so that different types of studies can be performed. We generally take a small piece at the most proximal end for the frozen section. This piece is rapidly frozen in mounting medium for immunofluorescence studies. These studies can reveal the deposition of immunoglobulins or other inflammatory markers,

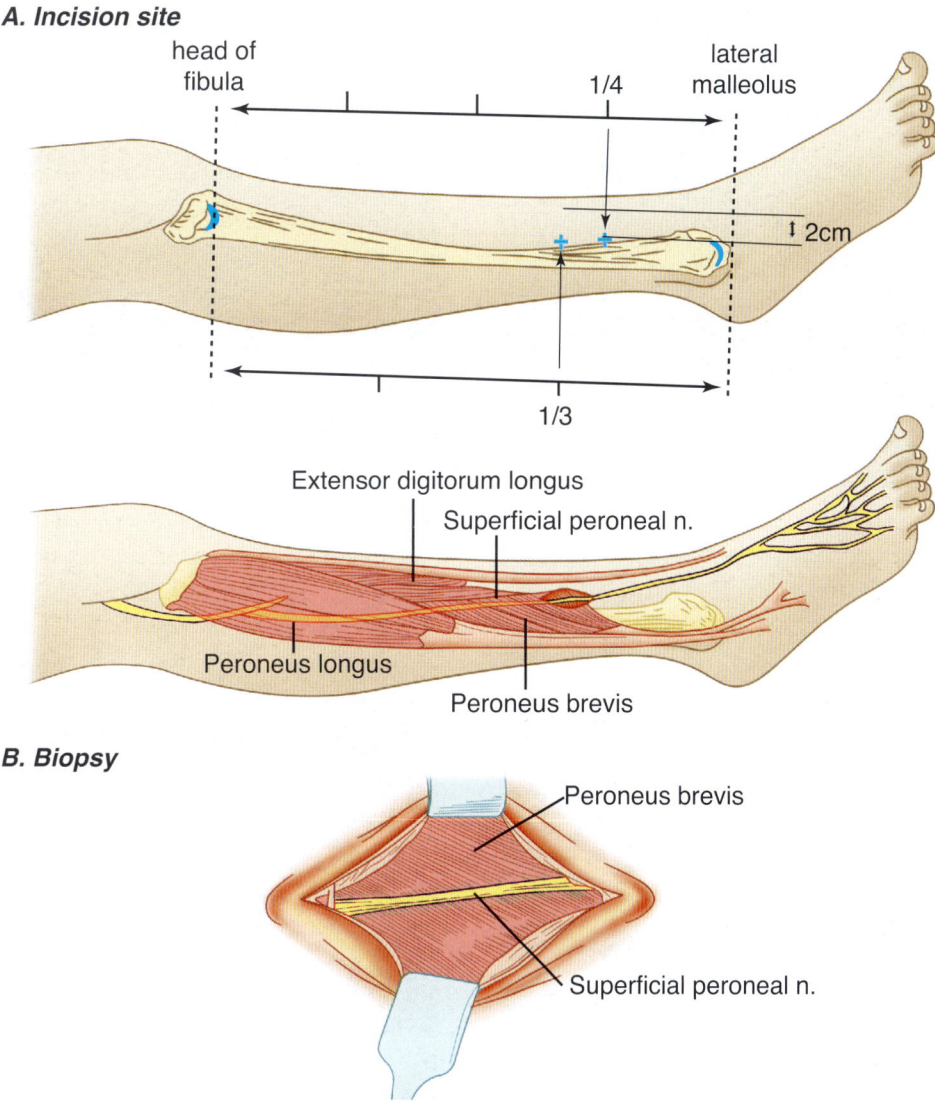

Figure 3-22. A combined superficial peroneal nerve and muscle biopsy is useful when looking for vasculitis. The nerve is typically found between one-third and one-fourth up from the lateral malleolus and approximately 1–1.5 cm anterior to the fibula. The nerve in this position can lie above or beneath the fascia overlying the peroneus brevis muscle, so both can be taken from a single incision. (Modified from Mendell JR, Erdem S, Agamonolis DR. Peripheral nerve and skin biopsies. In: Mendell JR, Kissel JT, Cornblath DR, eds. *Diagnosis and Management of Peripheral Nerve Disorders*. Oxford University Press; 2001.)

such as complement or fibrinogen, cell markers as well as for mutation analysis in cases of suspected tumor infiltration (i.e., lymphomatous polyneuropathy). Routine paraffin embedding (following fixation in formalin) is performed on a portion of tissue taken from the proximal and distal segments of the nerve biopsy (approximately 1 cm in length at both ends). The paraffin sections can be stained with H&E, trichrome, Luxol fast blue (stains myelin blue), Bodian stain, or neurofilament stains for axons (Fig. 3-23).[5,22–25,30–33] Congo red, Alcian blue, or cresyl violet should be done to look for amyloid (Fig. 3-24). A PAS stain is useful when polyglucosan body neuropathy is a consideration (Fig. 3-25), and a Fite stain can be done to look for the acid-fast bacilli if lepromatous neuropathy is possible (Fig. 3-26). Immunohistochemistry studies can be done to better assess inflammatory cell infiltrates (Fig. 3-27), and other specific stains can be done to better evaluate Schwann cells and perineurial cells when indicated. For example, immunoreactivity against the Schwann cell marker S-100 is useful for schwannomas and neurofibromas (Fig. 3-28), whereas immunoreactivity to epithelial membrane antigen (EMA), which is present on perineurial cells, is helpful in diagnosing perineuriomas. The paraffin-embedded tissue is most useful for evaluating signs of vasculitis, other inflammatory cell infiltrates including granulomas and lymphoma, infection (e.g., leprosy), and amyloidosis. Because the pathology can be multifocal, we like to take sections for paraffin embedding at the

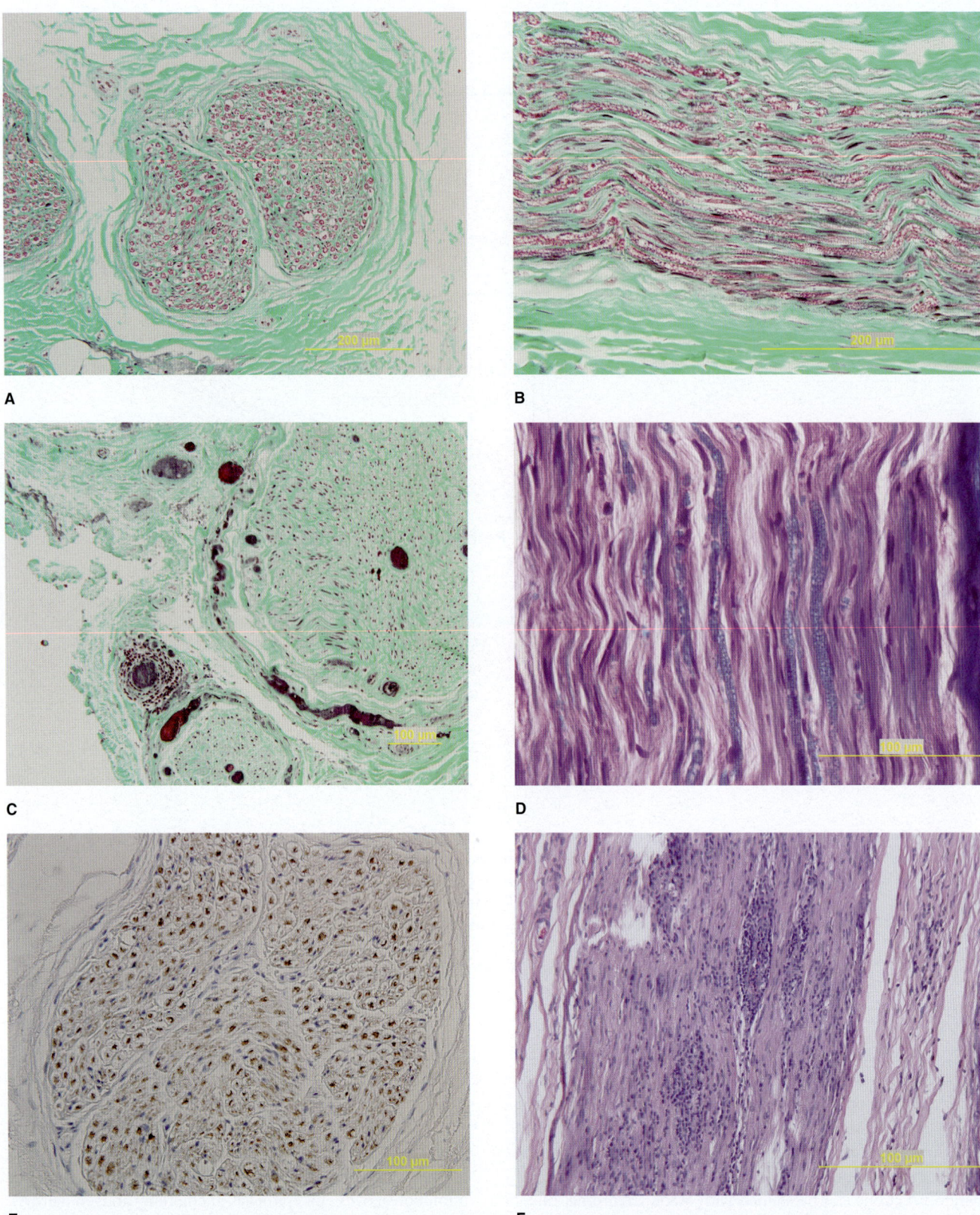

Figure 3-23. Paraffin sections of nerve biopsy. Myelin stains pink on modified Gomori trichrome in this normal nerve seen in cross-section (**A**) and longitudinally (**B**). A reduction in myelinated fibers is apparent by the loss of pink stain on this modified Gomori trichrome stain (**C**) and as blue staining myelinated nerve fibers on a Luxal fast blue stain (**D**); however, it is not possible to tell if this is due to primary demyelinating neuropathy or secondary demyelination from a primary axonopathy. SMI-31 stains phosphorylated neurofilaments that are abundant in normal axons, as seen in this normal nerve (**E**). H&E stain does not distinguish myelinated axons very well but is useful to look for vasculitis and other inflammatory cell infiltrates, as seen in this biopsy of a patient with lymphoma (**F**).

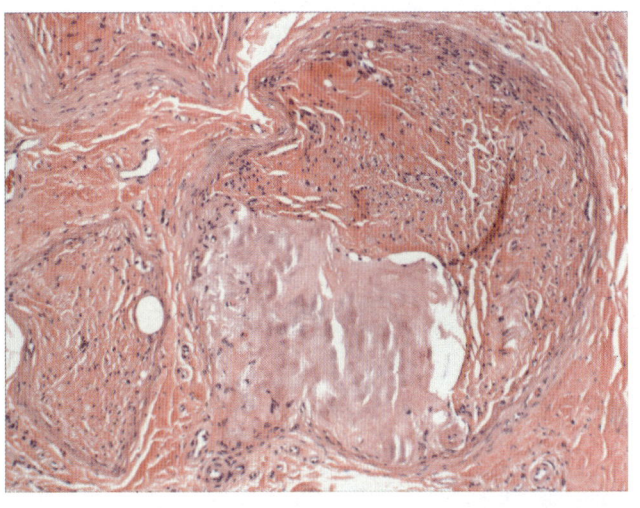

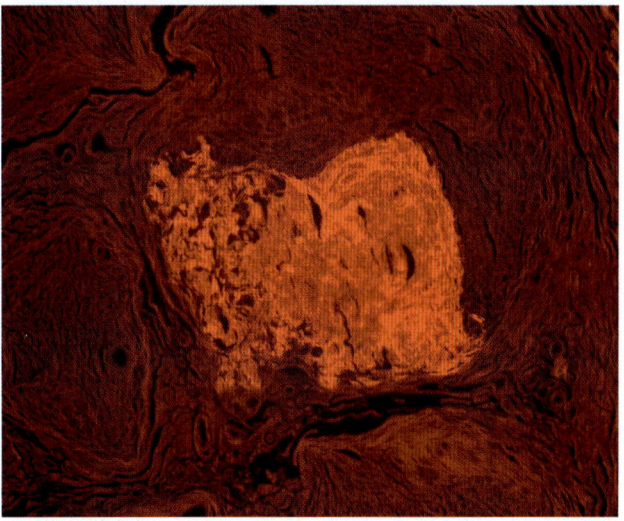

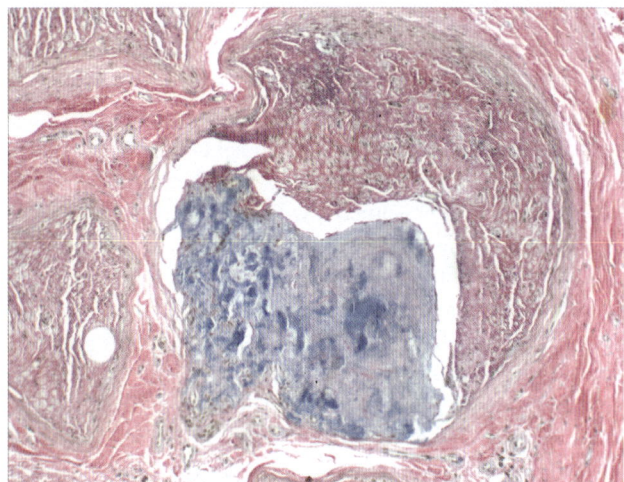

Figure 3-24. Familial amyloid polyneuropathy. Nerve biopsy demonstrates abnormal accumulation of amyloidogenic material in the endoneurium in the biopsy of a patient with a transthyretin mutation. The material stains faintly pink on H&E (**A**). With Congo red under routine light microscopy, amyloid stains intensely red when viewed under rhodamine optics (**B**). Amyloid stains blue with Alcian blue stain (**C**).

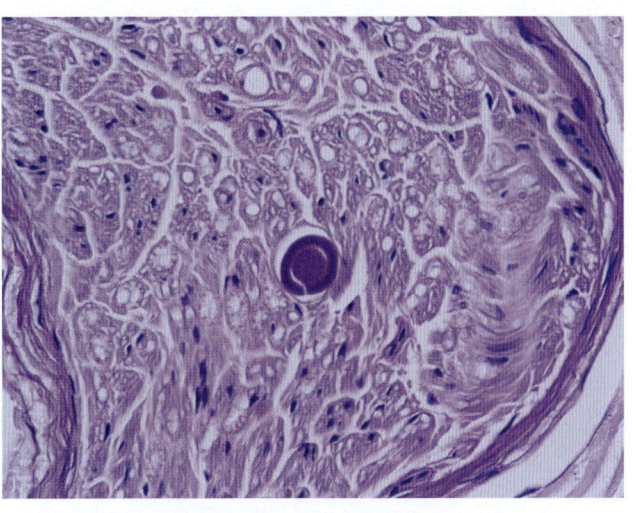

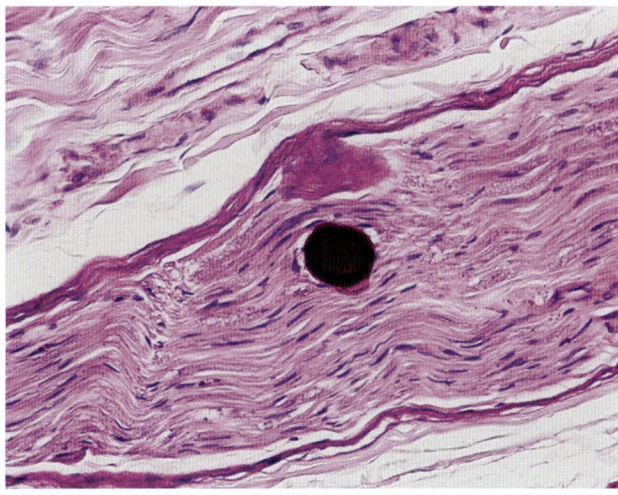

Figure 3-25. PAS stain demonstrates polyglucosan bodies within the axons in polyglucosan body neuropathy, as seen in cross-section (**A**) and longitudinal section (**B**).

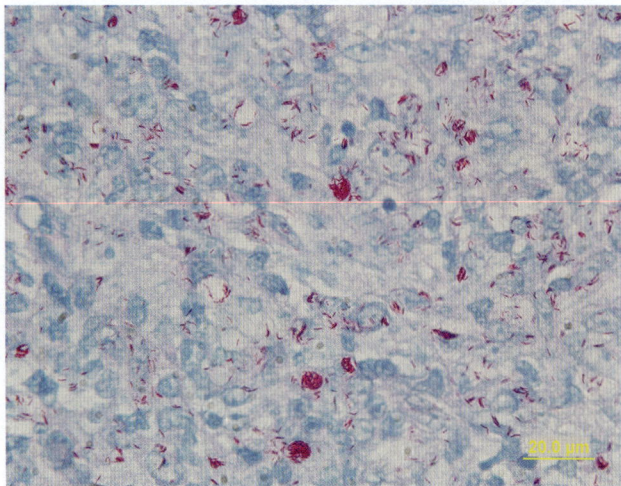

Figure 3-26. Borderline leprosy. Nerve biopsy in a patient with leprosy reveals red staining bacilli using the Fite stain on paraffin sections.

proximal and distal ends of the biopsy segment (Fig. 3-21E). In addition, loss of myelinated nerve fibers can be appreciated with various stains of paraffin-embedded tissue.

The remainder of the tissue is stretched delicately on a tongue blade or kept isometric with sutures and fixed in glutaraldehyde or other fixatives (e.g., Karnovsky's fixative). Some of this tissue will then be embedded in plastic and processed for toluidine blue-stained semithin sections (10 μm) and thin sections (1 μm) for EM.[5,22–24,27,30–34] The semithin and EM analyses are most important in assessing the axons, Schwann cells, and myelin sheath of myelinated nerve fibers as well as in looking at abnormalities in small unmyelinated nerve fibers (Fig. 3-29). Quantitative morphometric methods can be employed to assess numbers of individual large or small myelinated and unmyelinated fibers in the biopsy, as certain

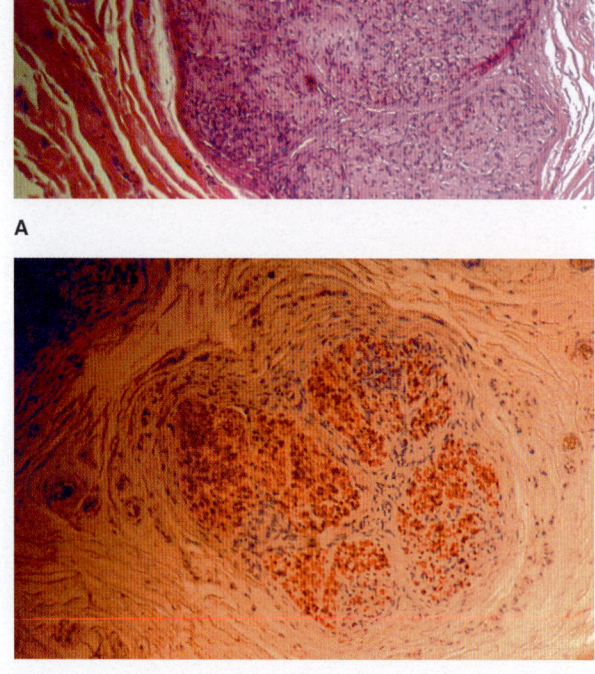

Figure 3-28. Neurofibroma. The nerve fascicle has a lobulated appearance, H&E stain (**A**). The cells have wavy, elongated nuclei, and the background material is loosely arranged and myxoid. Bands of thick collagen are apparent in the center of the tumor. Some of the proliferating tumor cells are immunoreactive for S-100, suggesting Schwann cell origin (**B**).

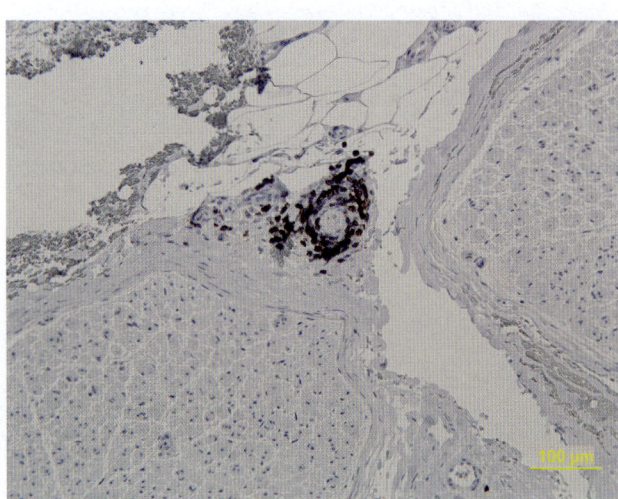

Figure 3-27. Immunoperoxidase stain reveals perivascular CD3+ T lymphocytes in a nerve biopsy in a patient with chronic inflammatory demyelinating polyneuropathy (CIDP).

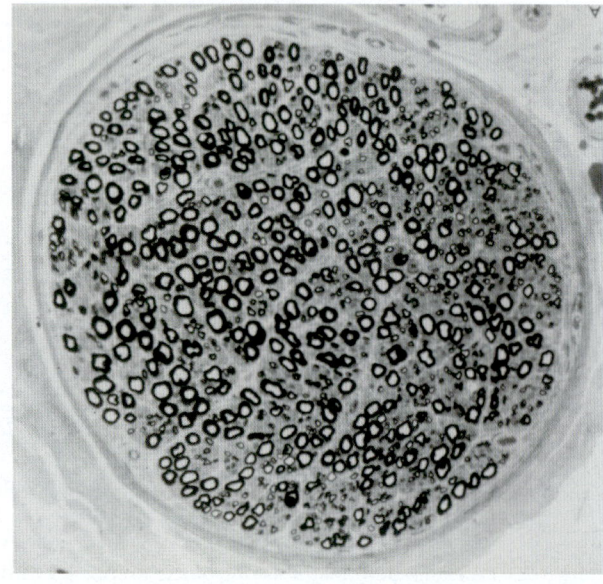

Figure 3-29. Semithin section reveals a normal nerve fascicle.

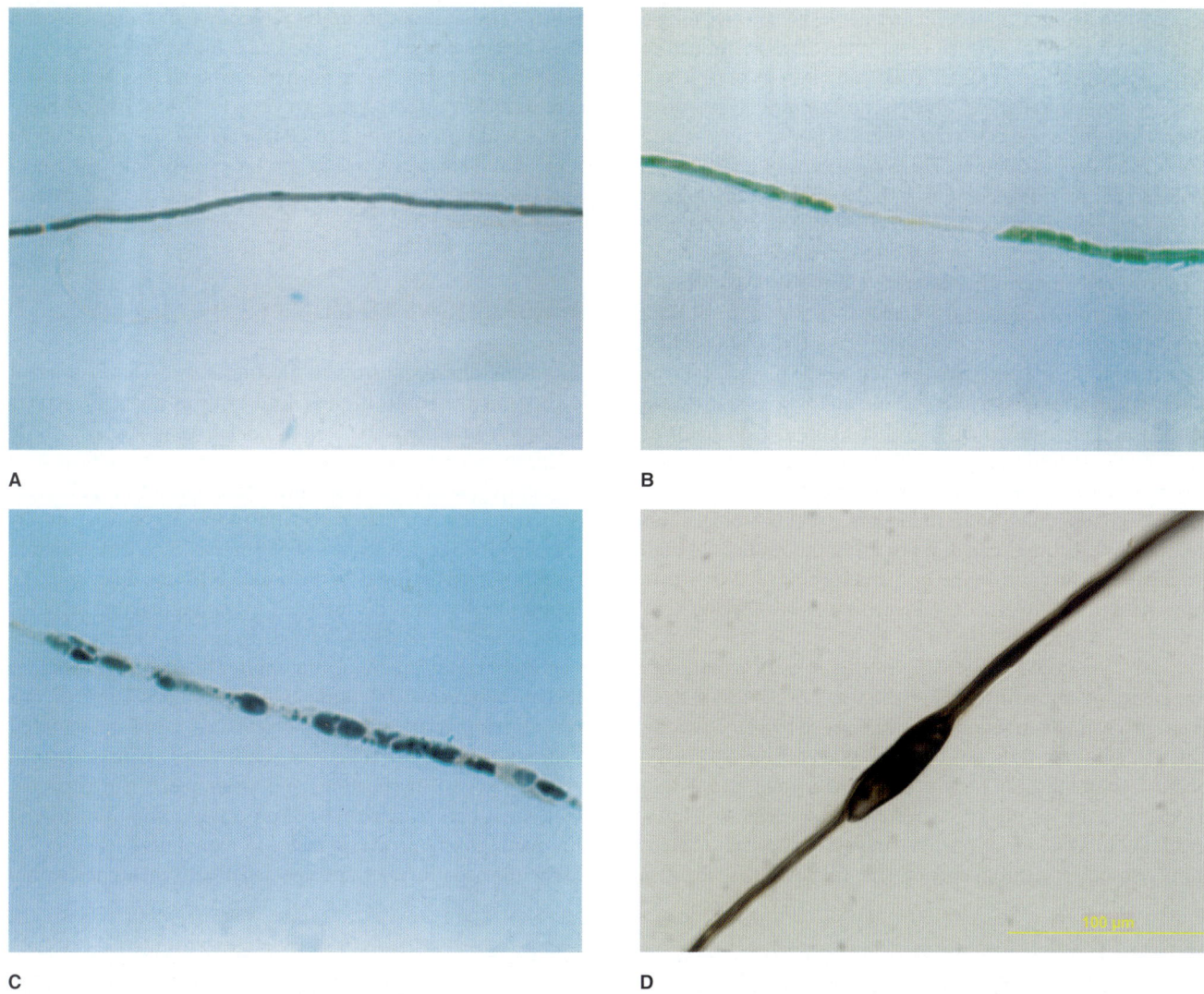

Figure 3-30. Teased nerve fibers. A normal teased fiber internode is seen (**A**) as well as a short, demyelinated internode (**B**). A teased nerve fiber segment undergoing Wallerian degeneration with myelin ovoids is appreciated in **C**. Redundant folds of myelin lead to formation of tomacula (Latin for sausage) that are best appreciated on teased fiber preparations (**D**) and are commonly seen in hereditary neuropathy with liability to pressure palsies and occasionally in other forms of Charcot–Marie–Tooth disease.

neuropathies have a predilection for certain nerve fiber types. However, this is not routinely done as it is time consuming and often of limited value. Other portions of this fixed material may be used for teased nerve fiber analysis (Fig. 3-30). With this method, individual myelinated fibers are separated from the nerve fascicles and lightly stained, allowing examination of the integrity and thickness of the myelin sheath as well as revealing alterations in internode length. Thus, one can better quantify the degree of demyelinated or thinly myelinated axon, axons with increased or redundant myelin, and axons undergoing active Wallerian degeneration. Teased fiber preparation, however, is very labor intensive and often does not add much to what can be assessed from the semithin and EM sections; thus, it is reserved for more difficult cases (e.g., the question of CIDP in biopsy with mild or nonspecific abnormalities on semithin or EM).

▶ STRUCTURE OF NORMAL NERVE

Peripheral nerves are composed of axons, Schwann cells, myelin sheaths, and supporting tissue. Individual nerve fibers are surrounded by endoneurial connective tissue and grouped into fascicles encased by perineurial sheaths. All the fascicles within a nerve in turn are surrounded by epineurial connective tissue. A blood–nerve barrier is created between the perineurial cells and endoneurial capillaries derived from the vasa nervorum, both of which form tight junctions. The blood–nerve barrier appears to be relatively less competent within nerve roots, dorsal root ganglia, autonomic ganglia, and terminal twigs. The nerve–cerebral spinal fluid (CSF) barrier is formed by the tight junctions between the cells that form the outer layer of the arachnoid membrane. These cells fuse with the perineurium of the roots and cranial nerves as these leave the subarachnoid space.

Myelinated and unmyelinated nerve fibers intermingle within each fascicle. Further, along the course of the entire nerve, individual nerve fibers course in and out of different fascicles. In the sural nerve, which is most commonly biopsied, myelinated fibers range between 2 and 15 μm in diameter and have a bimodal distribution. There are approximately twice as many small, myelinated axons as there are large myelinated fibers. Segments of myelinated fibers (internodes) are separated by nodes of Ranvier. A single Schwann cell supplies the myelin sheath for each internode. The thickness of the myelin sheath is directly proportional to the diameter of the axon, and the larger the axon diameter, the longer the internodal distance. The ratio of the diameter of the axon to the diameter of the entire nerve fiber (axon plus its surrounding myelin) or G ratio is approximately 0.6. A higher-than-normal diameter ratio implies that the axons are thinly myelinated. In contrast, lower G ratios are seen in axonopathies with axonal atrophy or rare conductions with redundant myelin (tomaculous neuropathy). Unmyelinated axons are more numerous than myelinated axons and range in diameter from 0.2 to 3 μm. Anywhere from 5 to 20 unmyelinated axons are enveloped by a single Schwann cell.

Schwann cells, regardless of their association with myelinated or unmyelinated fibers, have pale oval nuclei with an even chromatin distribution and an elongated bipolar cell body. On EM, Schwann cells can be differentiated from fibroblasts because Schwann cells have a basement membrane. Within axons, there are various organelles and cytoskeletal structures, including mitochondria, vesicles, smooth endoplasmic reticulum, lysosomes, neurofilaments, and microtubules. Because protein synthesis occurs in the cell body rather than the axon itself, essential proteins and other substances synthesized in the perikaryon are transported down the axon via axoplasmic flow. A retrograde transport system serves as feedback to the cell body. These transport systems are dependent on the microtubules and neurofilaments as well as specific proteins such as dynein and dynactin within the axons. At the distal nerve terminal, dense-cored and coated vesicles are found.

▶ REACTIONS TO INJURY

Although disease processes affecting nerves have different pathogenic mechanisms, these lead to two principal reactions to injury: demyelination and axonal degeneration.[5,22–25,30–34] Damage to Schwann cells or the myelin sheath itself can lead to demyelination. Because these diseases affect individual Schwann cells to varying degrees, the process is characteristically segmental along the length of the nerve. The disintegrating myelin is phagocytosed by Schwann cells and macrophages. Schwann cells are also stimulated to remyelinate the denuded axon. These newly remyelinated axons are thinner in total diameter and the internodes are shorter than normal—features that are best seen with teased nerve preparations. However, one can also appreciate the thinly myelinated axons on semithin sections and on EM (diameter ratio >0.6). With sequential episodes of demyelination and attempted remyelination, concentric tiers of Schwann cell processes accumulate around the axons forming the so-called "onion bulbs" (Fig. 3-31). Some disease processes are associated with inclusions within

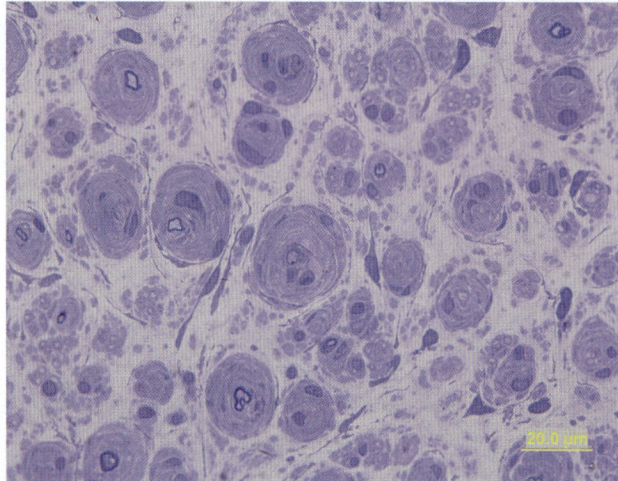

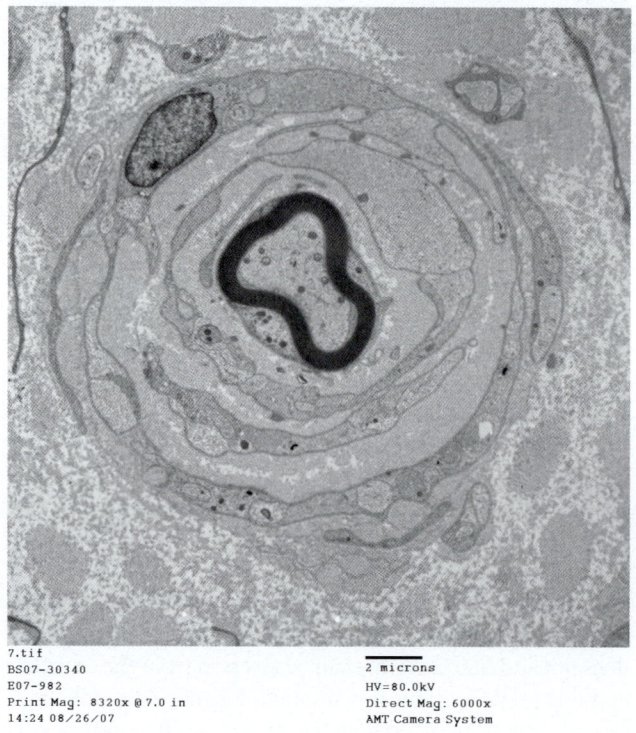

Figure 3-31. Onion bulb formation. With recurrent bouts of demyelination and remyelination, concentric layers of Schwann cell processes accumulate around the axons forming onion bulbs. Prominent onion bulbs can be seen in chronic inflammatory demyelinating neuropathy as in this case but are more typical of hereditary demyelinating neuropathies (i.e., Charcot–Marie–Tooth disease types 1, 3, and 4) on semi-thin section (**A**) and on electron microscopy (**B**).

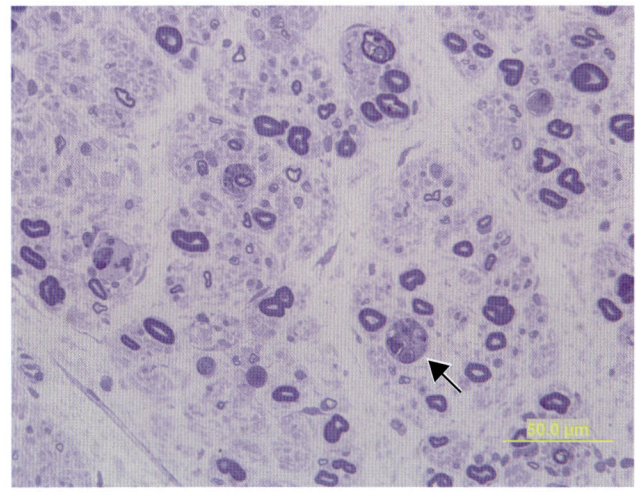
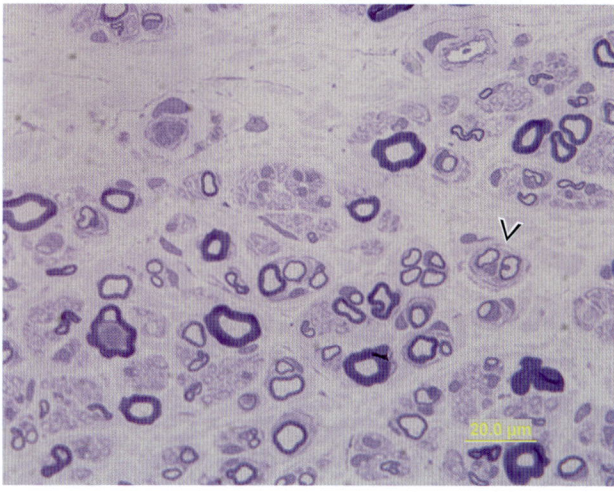
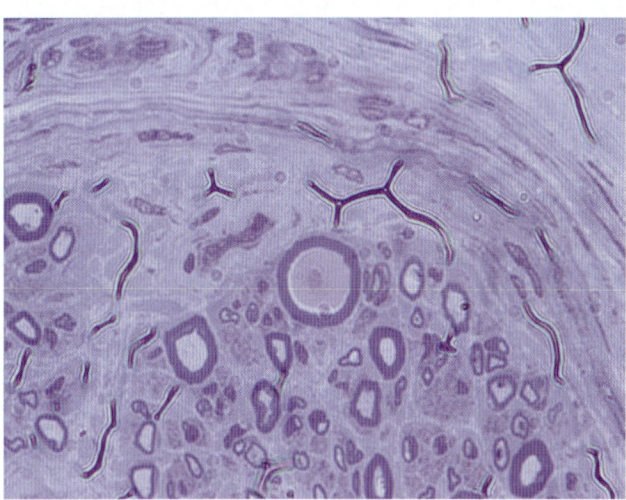

Figure 3-32. A semithin section reveals several fibers undergoing active axonal degeneration (Wallerian degeneration) (**A**). As nerve fibers attempt to regenerate, they send out nerve sprouts. These can be appreciated as groups of thinly myelinated nerve fibers surrounded by the same basement membrane (**B**). Polyglucosan bodies are abundant in nerve biopsies in patients with adult polyglucosan body disease. They appear as round, thinly lamellated inclusions within axons (**C**).

Schwann cells (e.g., metachromatic leukodystrophy and certain toxic neuropathies). Other abnormalities in the myelin sheath include tomaculae (redundant folds of myelin characteristic of hereditary neuropathy with liability to pressure palsies or HNPP) and widened periodicity of compacted myelin (seen in neuropathy associated with myelin-associated glycoprotein antibodies).

Primary damage to the axon may either be due to a discrete, localized event (trauma, ischemia, etc.) or be due to an underlying abnormality of the neuronal cell body or ganglion (neuronopathy) or its axon (axonopathy). These processes lead to axonal degeneration with secondary disintegration of its myelin sheath (Fig. 3-32A). If a nerve is transected, the distal portion of the nerve undergoes an acute disintegration (i.e., Wallerian degeneration) characterized by breakdown of the axon and its myelin sheath into fragments forming small oval compartments (i.e., myelin ovoids). These breakdown products undergo phagocytosis by macrophages and Schwann cells. Most neuronopathies or axonopathies evolve more slowly; therefore, evidence of active axon and myelin breakdown is scant because only a few fibers are degenerating at any given time. The proximal stumps of axons that have degenerated may sprout new axons that attempt to grow along the course of the degenerated axon. Small clusters of these regenerated axons, which are small in diameter and thinly myelinated, can be recognized in cross-section on semithin and EM sections (Fig. 3-32B). Also, as axonal transport of essential proteins and other substances synthesized in the perikaryon is often impaired in axonopathies, axonal atrophy becomes apparent on the semithin and EM sections (G ratio <0.6). In contrast, enlarged axons are seen in giant axonal neuropathy and hexacarbon toxicity. Polyglucosan bodies are appreciated on semithin sections (Fig. 3-32C). These are nonspecific, and although rare polyglucosan bodies may be seen on nerve biopsies in elderly and in diabetics, they are much more abundant in patients with adult polyglucosan body disease.

In addition, nerve biopsies can reveal evidence of disease processes like those found in other organ systems. Amyloid deposition around blood vessels or within the endoneurium

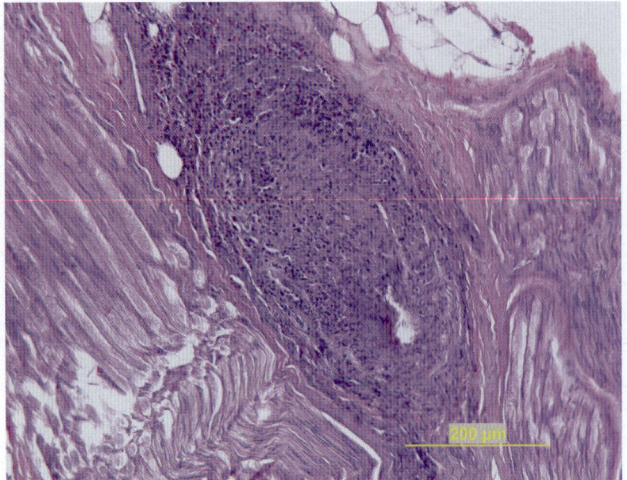

Figure 3-33. Nerve biopsy in a patient with Churg–Strauss syndrome reveals necrotizing vasculitis. Paraffin section, H&E stain.

▶ SKIN BIOPSY

Skin biopsies are increasingly being performed to evaluate patients with peripheral neuropathy.[25,35–52] These are most useful in patients with small fiber neuropathies in which other testing modalities provide normal or inconclusive results. Because nerve conduction studies only assess the conduction of large, myelinated nerve fiber, patients with pure small fiber neuropathies will have normal nerve conduction studies. Some studies have reported intraepidermal nerve fibers (IENF) density on skin biopsies represent the only objective abnormality present in at least a third of people with painful sensory neuropathies following extensive evaluation.[41]

The rationale behind performing most skin biopsies is to measure the density and assess the morphology of IENF. These fibers represent the terminals of Aδ and C nociceptors, and these may be decreased in patients with small fiber neuropathies in whom nerve conduction studies and routine nerve biopsies are often normal. Skin biopsies are relatively easy to perform and are associated with a much lower risk than standard nerve biopsies. However, there are several drawbacks to skin biopsies. Importantly, these usually just confirm what you already know about the patient. That is, if a person complains of symmetric burning or tingling pain in the distal lower extremities, has normal strength and deep tendon reflexes, and has normal nerve conduction studies, then they likely have a small fiber neuropathy. Skin biopsies are often not useful in identifying the etiology of the neuropathy. An exception is biopsy of skin lesions in suspected cases of lepromatous neuropathy (Fig. 3-34). Amyloid can be detected on skin biopsy as well in cases of suspected familial amyloid polyneuropathy and AL amyloidisis.[53,54] As stated in the previous section on nerve biopsies, we generally do not do a biopsy to prove that a patient has a neuropathy;

can be seen in systemic amyloidosis or in a familial amyloidotic polyneuropathy (Fig. 3-24). In systemic or isolated peripheral nerve vasculitis, there is transmural infiltration of vessel walls by inflammatory cells associated with fibrinoid necrosis of the vessel walls (Fig. 3-33). Because nerve fibers course between different fascicles along the length of the nerve, patchy asymmetric loss of axons within and between fascicles is a characteristic finding of ischemic nerve injury as seen in vasculitis. Infiltration of the nerve by neoplastic or inflammatory cells can also be recognized. Leprosy is one of the most common etiologies of polyneuropathy in the world. When granulomas or diffuse inflammation of the nerve is seen, a Fite stain can be done to look for the acid-fast bacilli (Fig. 3-26).

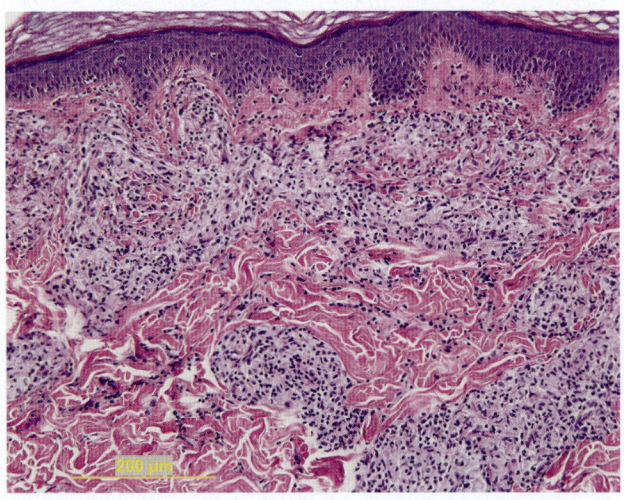

A

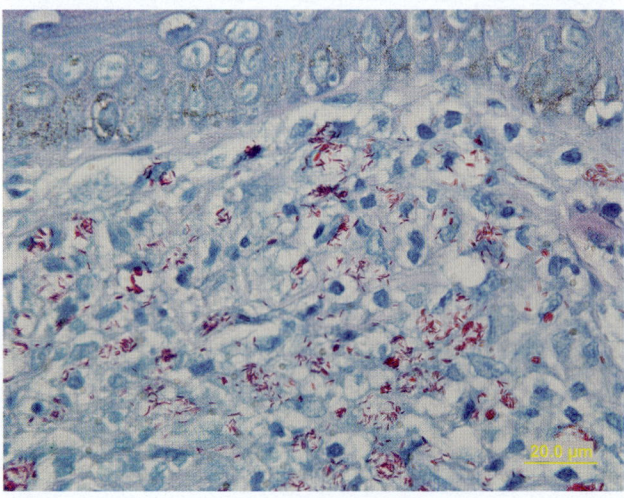

B

Figure 3-34. Borderline leprosy. Skin biopsy demonstrates marked inflammatory cell infiltrate, H&E (**A**). Red staining bacilli are evident on higher power with a Fite stain (**B**).

rather we do so in order to identify the etiology, hopefully a treatable one. Nevertheless, measurement of IENF is increasingly used to diagnose small fiber neuropathies as it provided an objective measure. Additionally, assessment of IENF density and morphology may play a role in the future by defining the natural history of various neuropathies, monitoring response of the neuropathy to various therapies, and screening for the development of toxic neuropathies (e.g., during chemotherapy). In addition, skin biopsies may be done to confirm a diagnosis of dermatomyositis.

Skin biopsies are usually done by performing a 3-mm punch biopsy of the skin under local anesthesia in the lower leg in an affected region. Other regions can be sampled to assess if there is a length-dependent loss of IENF (e.g., in the dorsum of the foot, thigh, or forearm). The tissue is fixed in formalin, and then immunostaining protein gene product 9.5 (PGP 9.5) is applied to demonstrate the small intraepidermal fibers either by indirect immunofluorescence with and without confocal analysis or by bright-field immunohistochemistry (Fig. 3-35). Importantly, normal IENF density measured by both methods differs according to patient's age, sex, height, weight, and location of biopsy. Morphometric methods are used to assess the number and complexity of these nerves, through parameters such as the linear density (number of fibers per millimeter of biopsy) or total length of IENF. The morphology of the IENF can also be assessed. Axonal swellings may be an early marker of small fiber neuropathy and may be appreciated before a

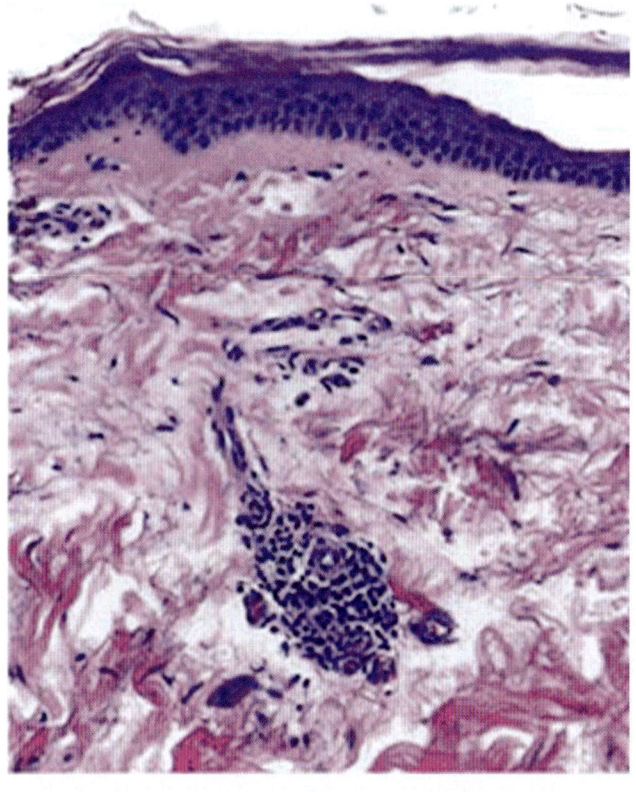

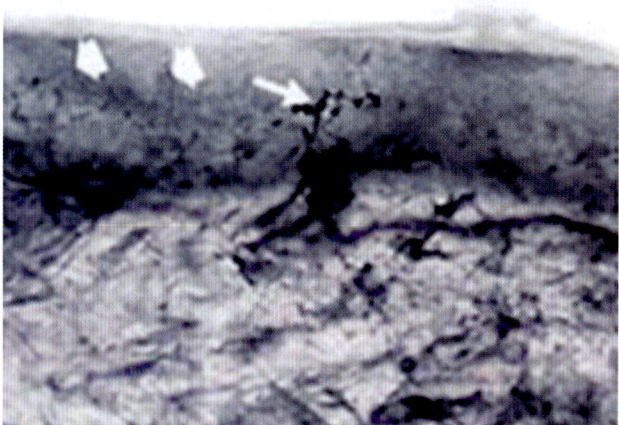

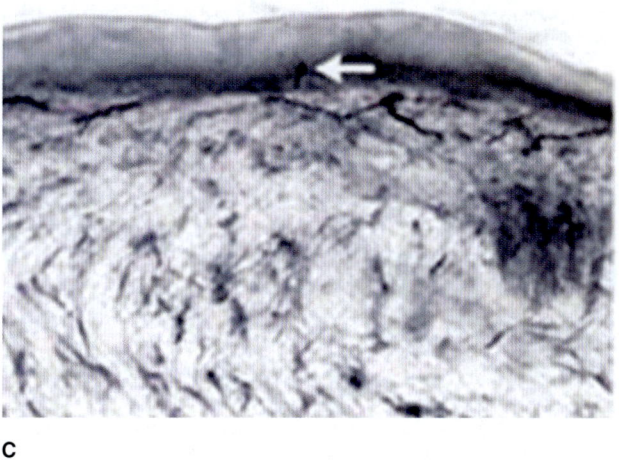

Figure 3-35. Skin biopsy in small fiber neuropathy. A specimen obtained at the time of the patient's first evaluation (**A**) shows a focal perivascular lymphocytic infiltrate (H&E, ×125). A section immunolabeled against protein gene product 9.5 reveals neural processes or axons (*thick arrows*) (**B**) showing an epidermal neurite with axonal swellings, which are abnormal (*thin arrow*). The density of nerve fibers is greater than normal (immunoperoxidase, ×500). A specimen obtained 11 months later (**C**) shows marked reduction in neurite density and axonal swelling (*arrow*) in a remaining neurite (×300). (Reproduced with permission from Drs. Thomas Smith and Lawrence Hayward, from Amato AA, Oaklander AL. Case 16 2004: A 76-year-old woman with numbness and pain in the feet and legs. *N Engl J Med*. 2004;350:2181–2189.)

reduction in density. However, axonal swellings can also be seen in normal individuals. Immunostaining for vasoactive intestinal polypeptide, substance P, or calcitonin gene-related proteins can be used to measure the density of sudomotor axons innervating sweat glands, piloerector nerves to hair follicles, and nerves to small arterioles. Myelin can be immunolabeled with antibodies directed against peripheral myelin protein 22 and myelin-associated glycoprotein. Additionally, Congo red can be used to assess for evidence of amyloid deposition.

▶ SUMMARY

Muscle, nerve, and skin biopsies for IENF analysis can be useful in diagnosis of various neuromuscular conditions. The various histopathologic abnormalities that we mentioned are discussed in more detail in subsequent chapters with the diseases in which these appear. As with electrodiagnostic and other laboratory testing, these are only helpful in conjunction with a good *clinical* assessment and cogent differential diagnosis. Further, it is imperative that just as neuromuscular clinicians must be able to independently review and interpret results of electrodiagnostic testing, the same holds true for at least understanding biopsy reports. Whenever possible, we would urge clinicians to review biopsy slides with their pathologists so that they can become more familiar with various disease processes and correlate the clinical and electrodiagnostic findings with the histopathology.

REFERENCES

1. Nix JS, Moore SA. What every neuropathologist needs to know: the muscle biopsy. *J Neuropathol Exp Neurol.* 2020;79(7):719–733.
2. Gherardi G, Amato AA, Lidov HG, De Girolami U. Pathology of skeletal muscle. In: Gray F, Duyckaerts C, De Gerolami, eds. *Escourplle and Poirier's Manual of Basic Neuropathology.* 6th ed. Oxford University Press; 2019:299–340.
3. Banker BQ, Engel AG. Basic reactions of muscle. In: Engel AG, Franzini-Armstrong C, eds. *Myology.* 3rd ed. McGraw-Hill; 2004: 691–747.
4. Carpenter S, Karpati G. *Pathology of Skeletal Muscle.* 2nd ed. Oxford; 2001.
5. De Girolami U, Frosch M, Amato AA. Biopsy of nerve and muscle. In: Samuels M, Feske S, eds. *Office Practice of Neurology.* 2nd ed. Harcourt Health Sciences; 2003:217–225.
6. Dumitru D, Amato AA. Introduction to myopathies and muscle tissue's reaction to injury. In: Dumitru D, Amato AA, Swartz MJ, eds. *Electrodiagnostic Medicine.* 2nd ed. Hanley & Belfus; 2002:1229–1264.
7. Engel AG. The muscle biopsy. In: Engel AG, Franzini-Armstrong C, eds. *Myology.* 3rd ed. McGraw-Hill; 2004:681–690.
8. Filosto M, Tonin P, Vattemi G, et al. The role of muscle biopsy in investigating isolated muscle pain. *Neurology.* 2007;68(3):181–186.
9. Coté AM, Jiménez L, Adelman LS, Munsat TL. Needle biopsy with the automatic Biopsy instrument. *Neurology.* 1992; 42(11):2212–2213.
10. Edwards RH, Round JM, Jones DA. Needle biopsy of skeletal muscle: a review of 10 years experience. *Muscle Nerve.* 1983; 6(9):676–683.
11. Heckmatt JZ, Moosa A, Hutson C, Maunder-Sewry CA, Dubowitz V. Diagnostic needle muscle biopsy: a practical and reliable alternative to open biopsy. *Arch Dis Child.* 1994;59(6): 528–532.
12. Magistris MR, Kohler A, Pizzolato G, et al. Needle muscle biopsy in the investigation of neuromuscular disorders. *Muscle Nerve.* 1988;21(2):194–200.
13. Colling-Saltin AS. Enzyme histochemistry on skeletal muscle of the human foetus. *J Neurol Sci.* 1978;39(2-3):169–185.
14. Engel AG, Banker BQ. Ultrastructural changes in diseased muscle. In: Engel AG, Franzini-Armstrong C, eds. *Myology.* 3rd ed. McGraw-Hill; 2004:749–887.
15. Johnson MA, Polgar J, Weightman D, Appleton D. Data on the distribution of fiber types in thirty-six human muscles. An autopsy study. *J Neurol Sci.* 1973;18(1):111–129.
16. Brooke MH, Engel WK. The histographic analysis of human muscle biopsies with regard to fiber types. 1. Adult male and female. *Neurology.* 1969;19(3):221–233.
17. Brooke MH, Engel WK. The histographic analysis of human muscle biopsies with regard to fiber types. 2. Diseases of the upper and lower motor neuron. *Neurology.* 1969;19(4):378–393.
18. Brooke MH, Engel WK. The histographic analysis of human muscle biopsies with regard to fiber types. 3. Myotonias, myasthenia gravis, and hypokalemic periodic paralysis. *Neurology.* 1969;19(5):469–477.
19. Brooke MH, Engel WK. The histographic analysis of human muscle biopsies with regard to fiber types. 4. Children's biopsies. *Neurology.* 1969;19(6):591–605.
20. Metafora S, Felsani A, Cotrufo R, et al. Neural control of gene expression in skeletal muscle fibers: the nature of the lesion in the muscular protein-synthesis machinery following denervation. *Proc R Soc Lond B Biol Sci.* 1980;209(1175): 239–255.
21. Bischoff R. Control of satellite cell proliferation. *Adv Exp Med Biol.* 1990;280:147–158.
22. Chkheidze R, Pytel P. What every neuropathologist needs to know: peripheral nerve biopsy. *J Neuropathol Exp Neurol.* 2020;79(4):355–364.
23. Nathani D, Spies J, Barnett MH, et al. Nerve biopsy: current indications and decision tools. *Muscle Nerve.* 2021;64(2): 125–139.
24. Luigetti M, Di Paolantonio A, Bisogni G, et al. Sural nerve biopsy in peripheral neuropathies: 30-year experience from a single center. *Neurol Sci.* 2020;41(2):341–346.
25. Sommer C. Nerve and skin biopsy in neuropathies. *Curr Opin Neurol.* 2018;31(5):534–540.
26. Hilton DA, Jacob J, Househam L, Tengah C. Complications following sural and peroneal nerve biopsies. *J Neurol Neurosurg Psychiatry.* 2007;78(11):1271–1272.
27. Lacomis D. Clinical utility of peripheral nerve biopsy. *Curr Neurol Neurosci Rep.* 2005;5(1):41–47.
28. Ruth A, Schulmeyer FJ, Roesch M, Woertgen C, Brawanski A. Diagnostic and therapeutic value due to suspected diagnosis, longterm complications, and indication for sural nerve biopsy. *Clin Neurol Neurosurg.* 2005;107(3):214–217.
29. Schweikert K, Fuhr P, Probst A, Tolnay M, Renaud S, Steck AJ. Contribution of nerve biopsy to unclassified neuropathy. *Eur Neurol.* 2007;57(2):86–90.

30. Bouche P, Vallat JM. *Neuropathies Périphériques*. Doin; 1992.
31. Dyck PJ, Dyck PJB, Engelstad J. Pathologic alterations of nerves. In: Dyck PJ, Thomas PK, eds. *Peripheral Neuropathy*. 4th ed. WB Saunders; 2005:733–829.
32. Midroni G, Bilbao JM. *Biopsy Diagnosis of Peripheral Neuropathy*. Butterworth-Heinemann; 1995.
33. Richardson EP Jr, De Girolami U. *Pathology of the Peripheral Nerve*. WB Saunders; 1995.
34. Ferreire G, Denef JF, Rodriguez J, Guzzetta F. Morphometric studies of normal sural nerves in children. *Muscle Nerve*. 1985;8(8):697–704.
35. Amato AA, Oaklander AL. Case records of the Massachusetts General Hospital. Weekly clinicopathological exercises. Case 16-2004. A 76-year-old woman with numbness and pain in the feet and legs. *N Engl J Med*. 2004;350(21):2181–2189.
36. Herrman DN, Griffin JW, Hauer P, Cornblath DR, McArthur JC. Intraepidermal nerve fiber density, sural nerve morphometry and electrodiagnosis in peripheral neuropathies. *Neurology*. 1999;53(8):1634–1640.
37. Holland NR, Stocks NR, Hauer P, Cornblath DR, Griffin JW, McArthur JC. Intraepidermal nerve fiber density in patients with painful sensory neuropathy. *Neurology*. 1997;48(3):708–711.
38. Holland NR, Crawford TO, Hauer P, Cornblath DR, Griffin JW, McArthur JC. Small-fiber sensory neuropathies: clinical course and neuropathology of idiopathic cases. *Ann Neurol*. 1998;44(1):47–59.
39. McArthur JC, Stocks EA, Hauer P, Cornblath DR, Griffin JW. Intraepidermal nerve fiber density: normative reference range and diagnostic efficiency. *Arch Neurol*. 1998;55(12):1513–1520.
40. McCarthy BG, Hseih ST, Stocks A, et al. Cutaneous innervation in sensory neuropathies: valuation by skin biopsy. *Neurology*. 1995;45(10):1845–1855.
41. Periquet MI, Novak V, Collins MP, et al. Painful sensory neuropathy: prospective evaluation of painful feet using electrodiagnosis and skin biopsy. *Neurology*. 1999;53(8):1641–1647.
42. Smith AG, Ramchandran P, Tripp S, Singleton JR. Epidermal nerve innervation in impaired glucose tolerance and diabetes-associated neuropathy. *Neurology*. 2001;57(9);1701–1704.
43. Sommer C, Lauria G. Skin biopsy in the management of peripheral neuropathy. *Lancet Neurol*. 2007;6(7):632–642.
44. Tobkin K, Guiliani MJ, Lacomis D. Comparison of different modalities for detection of small-fiber neuropathy. *Clin Neurophys*. 1999;110(11):1909–1912.
45. Walk D, Wendelschafer-Crabb G, Davey C, Kennedy WR. Concordance between epidermal nerve fiber density and sensory examination in patients with symptoms of idiopathic small fiber neuropathy. *J Neurol Sci*. 2007;255(1–2):23–26.
46. Wendelschafer-Crabb G, Kennedy WR, Walk D. Morphological features of nerves in skin biopsies. *J Neurol Sci*. 2006;242(1–2):15–21.
47. England JD, Gronseth GS, Franklin G, et al; American Academy of Neurology, American Association of Neuromuscular and Electrodiagnostic Medicine, American Academy of Physical Medicine and Rehabilitation. Evaluation of distal symmetric polyneuropathy: the role of autonomic testing, nerve biopsy, and skin biopsy (an evidence-based review). *Muscle Nerve*. 2009;39(1):106–115.
48. Oaklander AL, Nolano M. Scientific advances in and clinical approaches to small-fiber polyneuropathy: a review. *JAMA Neurol*. 2019;76(10):1240–1251.
49. Devigili G, Rinaldo S, Lombardi R, et al. Diagnostic criteria for small fibre neuropathy in clinical practice and research. *Brain*. 2019;142(12):3728–3736.
50. Freeman R, Gewandter JS, Faber CG, et al. Idiopathic distal sensory polyneuropathy: ACTTION diagnostic criteria. *Neurology*. 2020;95(22):1005–1014.
51. Gemignani F, Bellanova MF, Saccani E, Pavesi G. Non-length-dependent small fiber neuropathy: not a matter of stockings and gloves. *Muscle Nerve*. 2022;65(1):10–28.
52. Nolano M, Tozza S, Caporaso G, Provitera V. Contribution of skin biopsy in peripheral neuropathies. *Brain Sci*. 2020;10(12):989.
53. Chao CC, Hsueh HW, Kan HW, et al. Skin nerve pathology: biomarkers of premanifest and manifest amyloid neuropathy. *Ann Neurol*. 2019;85(4):560–573.
54. Wu B, Pak DM, Smith KD, Shinohara MM. Utility of abdominal skin punch biopsy for detecting systemic amyloidosis. *J Cutan Pathol*. 2021;48(11):1342–1346.

CHAPTER 4
Principles of Immunotherapy

▶ **INTRODUCTION**

The ideal of every patient and physician is to identify a diagnosis whose natural history is self-limited, or if not, a diagnosis for which an effective treatment can be administered. Autoimmunity is believed to be the contributing, if not causal, mechanism of many forms of neuromuscular disorders.[1-3] Accordingly, patients with various proven or suspected autoimmune neuromuscular disorders are candidates for immunotherapy. Familiarity with drugs or other interventions that suppress or modulate the patient's immune system is therefore a prerequisite for anyone practicing neuromuscular medicine.

This chapter will discuss the most common immunotherapies used in autoimmune neuromuscular diseases with emphasis on mechanisms of action, diseases in which they are most commonly employed, side effects, and associated management decisions that need to be considered with their use. Details of specific dosing regimens which can differ with various neuromuscular disorders are discussed in later chapters devoted to these diseases and in many nice reviews.[1-13] A summary of the most commonly used immunotherapies and details regarding dosing, side effect profiles, and recommended screening procedures are reviewed in Table 5-1.

In this book, we define immunosuppression as a subcategory of immunotherapy in which a patient's immunologic response is impaired by one of the three recognized mechanisms. One mechanism, as occurs with drugs such as azathioprine, cyclophosphamide, mycophenolate, and methotrexate, curtails B-cell and T-cell proliferation by cell cycle interruption. Another mechanism, as exemplified by drugs such as the calcineurin inhibitors (e.g., cyclosporine and tacrolimus) and corticosteroids, is impairment of T-cell or B-cell activation. Another mechanism of immunosuppression is accomplished by monoclonal antibodies–directed cell surface antigens (e.g., rituximab) and thise that block complement activation (e.g., eculizumab). We will consider interventions such as intravenous or subcutaneous immunoglobulin (IVIg or SCIg), neonatal Fc receptor (FcRn) blockade, and plasma exchange (PLEX) that are considered to be more immunomodulating than immunosuppressing.

The authors strongly endorse the concept of evidence-based medicine. At the same time, we recognize that evidence-based medicine applies to populations and that strict adherence to evidence guidance is not always in the best interests of the individual patients we are responsible for. In neuromuscular medicine, there are numerous examples of treatments that are universally considered to be efficacious yet remain of unproven benefit by "evidence-based" standards. Corticosteroids in treating inflammatory myopathies and myasthenia gravis (MG) are notable examples, discovered by innovative efforts by individual clinicians. Because of the accepted efficacy of this and other historically identified empiric treatments, it is unlikely that a number of currently accepted treatments will ever be validated by large prospective studies.

Our position is also supported by personal witnesses of unequivocal benefit to individual patients, such as rituximab in MuSK-positive MG. Accordingly, this chapter will describe, and in some cases endorse, the off-label uses of immunotherapies for various neuromuscular diseases even in the absence of evidence-based support. We do so cautiously as we recognize that these idiosyncratic responses may be harmful as well as helpful. Ultimately, each physician needs, along with their patient, to determine whether the potential benefits of immunotherapy, of proven or unproven benefit, exceed the probability and magnitude of potential risk.

▶ **GENERAL CONSIDERATIONS**

Before initiating immunotherapy, it is critical to consider the probability and magnitude of both the potential risk to an individual patient, as well as the potential benefit. Some forms of immunotherapy increase risk for both infection and malignancy. These risks are probably dependent on numerous variables including the genetics and comorbidities of the individual patient, the agent or agents used, as well as cumulative dose and duration of treatment. The following section will review some of these considerations facing clinicians and their patients who are contemplating immunotherapy.

In consideration of immunotherapy, it is important to be armed with knowledge relevant to a number of key issues in order to make rational treatment decisions. Of primary importance is the identification of an objective parameter to measure. A pretreatment baseline should be established in order to determine whether treatment is effective or not in the future. The ideal parameter(s) chosen should be not only quantifiable and reproducible, but it (they) should correlate with meaningful clinical improvements in patient comfort and function.

In neuromuscular disease, measurements of strength are the most commonly utilized. We have found manual muscle

▶ TABLE 4-1. COMMON IMMUNOTHERAPIES FOR AUTOIMMUNE NEUROMUSCULAR DISORDERS

Therapy	Route	Dose	Side Effects	Monitor
Prednisone	Oral	0.75–1.5 mg/kg to start	Hypertension, fluid and weight gain, hyperglycemia, hypokalemia, cataracts, gastric irritation, osteoporosis, infection, aseptic femoral necrosis	Weight, blood pressure, serum glucose/potassium, bone density, cataract formation; glaucoma
Methylprednisone	Intravenous	1 g in 100 mL/normal saline over 1–2 hours, daily or every other day for 3–6 doses	Arrhythmia, flushing, dysgeusia, anxiety, insomnia, fluid and weight gain, hyperglycemia, hypokalemia, infection	Heart rate, blood pressure, serum glucose/potassium
Azathioprine	Oral	2–3 mg/kg per day; single AM dose	Flu-like illness, hepatotoxicity, pancreatitis, leukopenia, macrocytosis, neoplasia, infection, teratogenicity	Blood count, liver enzymes
Methotrexate	Oral	7.5–20 mg weekly, single or divided doses; 1 day a week dosing	Hepatotoxicity, pulmonary fibrosis, infection, neoplasia, infertility, leukopenia, alopecia, gastric irritation, stomatitis, teratogenicity	Liver enzymes, blood count
Cyclophosphamide	Subcutaneously Oral Intravenous	20–50 mg weekly; 1 day a week dosing 1.5–2 mg/kg per day; single AM dose 0.5–1.0 g/m² per month ˆ6–12 months	Same as oral Bone marrow suppression, infertility, hemorrhagic cystitis, alopecia, infections, neoplasia, teratogenicity	Same as p.o. Blood count, urinalysis
Cyclosporine	Oral	4–6 mg/kg per day, split into two daily doses	Nephrotoxicity, hypertension, PRES, infection, hepatotoxicity, hirsutism, tremor, gum hyperplasia, teratogenicity	Blood pressure, creatinine/BUN, liver enzymes, cyclosporine levels
Tacrolimus	Oral	0.1–0.2 mg/kg per day in two divided doses	Nephrotoxicity, hypertension, PRES, infection, hepatotoxicity, hirsutism, tremor, gum hyperplasia, teratogenicity	Blood pressure, creatinine/BUN, liver enzymes, tacrolimus levels
Mycophenolate mofetil	Oral	Adults (1–1.5 g BID) Children (600 mg/m² per dose BID) (no >1 g/d in patients with renal failure)	Bone marrow suppression, hypertension, tremor, diarrhea, nausea, vomiting, headache, sinusitis, confusion, amblyopia, cough, teratogenicity, infection, neoplasia; reduced efficacy of COVID-19 vaccinations	Blood count
Immunoglobulin	Intravenous Subcutaneous	2 g/kg over 2–5 days; then 1 g/kg every 2–8 weeks as needed Initial dosage is 0.2–0.4 g/kg followed by 0.1–0.2 g/kg 2–3 × weekly (1:1 dosage in convert from IVIG dosing)	Hypotension, arrhythmia, diaphoresis, flushing, nephrotoxicity, headache, aseptic meningitis, anaphylaxis, stroke	Heart rate, blood pressure, creatinine/BUN
Rituximab	Intravenous	A course is typically 750 mg/m² (up to 1 g) and repeated in 2 weeks Courses are then repeated usually every 6–18 months	Infusion reactions (as per IVIG), infection, progressive multifocal leukoencephalopathy; Reduced efficacy of vaccinations	Hepatitis B serology, CBC with differential, Some check B-cell count prior to subsequent courses (but this may not be warranted); heart rate, blood pressure

(continued)

▶ TABLE 4-1. (CONTINUED)

Therapy	Route	Dose	Side Effects	Monitor
Eculizumab	Intravenous	900 mg weekly × 4 weeks, then 1,200 mg at week 5, followed by 1,200 mg every 2 weeks	Infusion reactions, nausea, back pain, renal insufficiency, anemia, leukopenia, dyspepsia, nausea, diarrhea, peripheral edema, fatigue, and both hypo- and hypertension, meningococcal meningitis	Vaccination immunized with both the MenACYW and MenB meningococcal vaccines at least two weeks prior to administering the first dose of eculizumab; Consider prophylactic antibiotics (e.g., penicillin) even after vaccination; heart rate, blood pressure
Efgartigmod	Intravenous	Initiated at 10 mg/kg weekly × 4 weeks (1,200 mg per infusion in patients weighing 120 kg or more) with maintenance courses as necessary (at least 50 days between courses in pivotal trial)	Leukopenia, infection (UR, UTI), headache, hypersensitivity reaction (g rash, angioedema, and dyspnea)	Blood count, heart rate, blood pressure
Plasma exchange		Exchange a volume of 200–250 mL/kg/day (2–3 L) for 5 days typically spread out over a 7–10 days	Often requires a central line and associated complications including thrombosis, phlebitis, air embolism, pneumothorax; hypotension, electrolyte disturbance	Blood count, comprehensive metabolic profile, coagulation profile, heart rate, blood pressure

BUN, blood urea nitrogen; CBC, complete blood count; Cr, creatinine; ECG, electrocardiogram; GI, gastrointestinal; IgA, immunoglobulin A; IVIG, intravenous immunoglobulin; LFT, liver function test; m², body surface area; PFT, pulmonary function test; PRES, posterior reversible encephalopathy syndrome; URI, upper respiratory infection; UTI, urinary tract infection.

strength testing or handheld dynamometry to be helpful in this regard, along with quantitative bedside assessments of sensation (e.g., timed vibration or the Rydel-Seiffer® tuning fork). There are many functional or quality of life scales that have been developed for specific neuromuscular diseases which facilitate determination of treatment response. For example, in MG there are the myasthenia gravis Activity of Daily Living and Quality of Life (MG-ADL and MG-QOL) scales; and in CIDP there are the Inflammatory Rasch Built Overall Disability scale (IRODS) and Inflammatory Neuropathy Cause and Treatment (INCAT) score. Unfortunately, in neuromuscular disease, other biomarkers such as imaging, electromyography and nerve conduction study data, and measurement of serologic markers are not always accurate or practical means of monitoring treatment response.

A master clinician understands the natural history of the disease they are treating as well as the properties of the agents they are using. The latency between treatment and response is dependent on at least two parameters, the pharmacology of the immunotherapy used and the pathophysiology of the disease. For example, morbidity created by disorders that impede ion channel function, demyelinate axons without otherwise injuring them, or that injure relatively easily repairable components of the neuromuscular system such as ACh receptors may be expected to respond to an effective treatment relatively rapidly, within days to weeks in many cases. Conversely, disorders that require axon regrowth may require months before return of function becomes evident depending on the number of axons injured and the distance between the site of injury and the muscle(s) that require(s) reinnervation. Finally, disorders that lead to significant destruction of motor or sensory cell bodies are limited in their ability to recover as their regeneration is unlikely, even if an effective treatment is initiated.

Furthermore, it is important to be familiar with the duration of treatment benefit as well as the latency between therapeutic intervention and clinical response. Without an appreciation of both, at least three potential risks may be encountered. A clinician may give up on a treatment before it has had a chance to work, and by doing so, initiate a second, potentially unnecessary and harmful agent. Conversely, a clinician may be overly optimistic, waiting too long for an ineffective agent to work, thus delaying exposure to an additional, potentially beneficial treatment. In addition, a clinician may unnecessarily procrastinate by waiting too long to initiate subsequent maintenance doses, allowing potentially avoidable relapses to occur and by doing so, eroding a patient's confidence in their physician.

A particularly vexing problem in this age of evidence-based medicine is the patient with a suspected or proven autoimmune disorder for which no known proven treatments exist. In these cases, a diagnostic and potentially therapeutic trial may be undertaken. IVIg is frequently used for this purpose both for its relatively rapid onset of action, its efficacy in many autoimmune diseases, and in consideration of its relative safety. We usually give a 3-month therapeutic trial of IVIg in suspected cases of an autoimmune neuromuscular disorder before we consider the treatment a failure.

Immunotherapic strategies vary in consideration with the treatment modality employed, individual disease characteristics, and individual patient context. There are general principles, however, that include the recognition of maximal achievable benefit with the goal of avoiding excessive treatment. If disease remission can be achieved with the potential in that particular disorder for a durable, treatment-free response, an attempt should be made to wean by reducing the amount and/or frequency of administration. For example, it is not uncommon for patients with vasculitic neuropathies who respond to immunotherapy to eventually be successfully weaned from treatment after 2–3 years and enjoy years of subsequent treatment-free stability. The goal with any patient is to ensure, through clinical or when relevant other means, continued patient improvement or stabilization. At the same time, the goal is to also limit potential adverse effects and costs of chronic treatment while at the same time achieve and sustain the best potential outcome.

These differing treatment strategies are illustrated in the following examples. Corticosteroids in MG or inflammatory myopathies or IVIg in multifocal motor neuropathy are often initiated at high "induction" doses and then gradually weaned in an attempt to identify the smallest dose or longest interval between treatments that will achieve remission or maintain an acceptable level of morbidity. Conversely, in Guillain–Barré syndrome (GBS), a singular prescribed course of IVIg or plasma exchange is given.

▶ RISK CONSIDERATIONS WITH IMMUNOTHERAPIES

INFECTIOUS DISEASE

Pneumocystis Jirovecii

Pneumocystis pneumonia is caused by the fungus, *Pneumocystis jurevicius* (PJP), formerly known as *Pneumocystis carinii* (PCP), that occurs predominantly in individuals who are immunosuppressed as a result of their disease or its treatment.[14] Approximately 70%–90% of patients who acquire PJP have received corticosteroid treatment. PCP prophylaxis advocates justify its use in immunosuppressed individuals in order to reduce the risk of infection. The onset of PJP may be subacute or indolent. Typical symptoms are dyspnea on exertion, nonproductive cough, fever, and tachycardia. Diagnosis is supported by imaging evidence of bilateral pulmonary infiltrates extending outward from the perihilar regions. Confirmation typically requires bronchoalveolar lavage. The mortality risk may be as high as 30%–50%, even if recognized and treated.

Trimethoprim–sulfamethoxazole, 160–800 mg/day or double strength three times a week, is often prescribed for PJP prophylaxis. Atovaquone, dapsone, and pentamidine represent alternatives for patients who are intolerant to sulfa drugs. However, it is debatable if PCJ prophylaxis in neuromuscular patients is universally required.[14] The evidence basis for PCJ prophylaxis is largely derived from cancer and pulmonary patient populations. In addition, there is a paucity of information to guide clinicians regarding adjusted risk based on the number and types of agents utilized, their doses, and the duration of exposure. Although the severity of PCJ infection is unquestioned, its frequency in neuromuscular patients treated with immunomodulating agents is less well known. Although many disciplines such as rheumatology and infectious disease seem to favor its use, neurologists appear to be in general less sanguine about prophylactic necessity. For example, a poll neuromuscular specialist posted on Rick's Real Neuromuscular Friends indicated that 53% of 45 respondents do not provide routine PCJ prophylaxis in this population. We follow the recent guidelines of other neuromuscular specialists who advocate routine prophylaxis against PJP be given to patients who require prolonged use of corticosteroid therapy and/or other immunosuppressive agents, or in those with comorbidities (e.g., intestinal lung disease, prolonged lymphopenia, low CD4 count, organ failure, and active cancer status) that appear to increase the risk for PJP infection.[14]

Tuberculosis

The risk of tuberculosis (TB) reactivation is considered to be approximately three to six times greater in patients receiving tumor necrosis factor (TNF) inhibitors and corticosteroids.[15] It becomes prudent therefore to ascertain the risk of latent tuberculosis infection (LTBI) in any individual in whom immunosuppressive treatment is considered. Screening would include determining risk of prior chest x-ray, and in those who are at risk, either tuberculin skin testing (TST) or an interferon (IFN) gamma release assay (IGRA). TST is thought to be 98% sensitive in detecting LTBI. Its limitations are that it may not detect infection in the first 8 weeks following exposure, may be falsely negative in individuals already immunocompromised, or may be falsely positive in individuals who have received prior BCG vaccination.

IGRAs are complementary in vitro blood tests of cell-mediated immune response to *Mycobacterium tuberculosis* and measure T-cell release of IFN-gamma following stimulation by antigens specific to *M. tuberculosis*. The two available IGRAs are QuantiFERON-TB Gold In-Tube and the T-SPOT.TB. They are the preferred means to confirm LTBI in individuals with prior BCG exposure. The IGRAs appear to be somewhat more specific and less sensitive for predicting future active TB than the tuberculin skin test but the differences are modest. Like TST, IGRA false negatives are more likely to occur in immunosuppressed individuals. Both IGRAs and the TST have high negative predictive values for development of future infection.[15]

Like all clinical decisions, prophylactic treatment of patients suspected of LBTI needs to consider the relative benefits and risks. Currently, someone with suspected LBTI who is going to receive immunosuppressant treatment is recommended to receive prophylactic treatment with isoniazid (with pyridoxine), rifampin, or a combination of both. Isoniazid is typically prescribed as 300 mg daily for 9 months or 900 mg twice a week for 6 months. Rifampin alone is dosed at 600 mg/day for 4 months. When both drugs are used together, 600 mg of rifampin and 300 mg of isoniazid are given daily for 3 months.[15] Other considerations are the risk of isoniazid hepatotoxicity which increases with age and exposure to other hepatotoxic agents and the numerous drug interactions that occur with rifampin use.

Progressive Multifocal Leukoencephalopathy

Progressive multifocal leukoencephalopathy (PML) is a demyelinating central nervous system disorder caused by infection with the John Cunningham (JC) virus. The JC virus is ubiquitous, found in 50%–60% of the normal population and is typically sequestered in peripheral organs. PML is a disorder seen almost exclusively in the immunosuppressed. Even in this population, the virus rarely gains access to the central nervous system.

PML has been associated with two agents commonly employed in immune-mediated neuromuscular disorders, rituximab and mycophenolate mofetil (MMF).[16,17] Undoubtedly, it will be described in association with other immunotherapeutic agents relevant to neuromuscular disease in the future. The risk for PML appears to be predominantly in those who harbor the JC virus prior to the introduction of immunosuppressant treatment. Surveillance and treatment paradigms have been developed for PML in multiple sclerosis patients exposed to natalizumab. Presumably as the risk of developing PML with the immunosuppressant drugs described in this chapter is thought to be very rare, we are unaware of any recommendations for JC virus surveillance and prophylaxis for any agents described in this chapter. As anticipated, recognition of PML in any patient receiving immunosuppressant drugs warrants drug discontinuation in virtually any clinical context.

Hepatitis B

The presence of positive hepatitis B core antibodies suggest acute, resolved, or chronic hepatitis B infection, while hepatitis B surface antibodies indicate resolved infection or immunity after immunization. Reactivation with sudden viral replication can develop in individuals with previously resolved infection, sometimes spontaneously but more often triggered by immunosuppressive therapy. There is a particular increased risk of hepatitis B reactivation (HBVr) following treatment with B-cell depleting agents, such as rituximab, leading to an FDA black box warning.[18-20] Therefore, it is important to assess hepatitis B serologies prior to treatment with rituximab and prophylactically treat with antiviral therapy to minimize the risk of HBVr. An important caveat is that false-positive hepatitis B serology can occur in patients with recent intravenous and likely subcutaneous immunoglobulin (IVIg and SQIGg) exposure due to passive transfer of these antibodies that came from many donors.[21] These passively transferred antibodies can persist for 12–16 weeks. Many patients whom we treat with rituximab have previously been treated with IVIg or SCIg. In such situations, we treat patients with prophylactic antiviral until false positive is confirmed with repeat serologic assessment 3–4 months after last IVIg or SCIg infusion.[21]

Strongyloidiasis

Stongyloidiasis is a parasite that is endemic in warm moist tropical and subtropical climates such as Eastern Europe, South and Southeast Asia, Central America, South America, and sub-Saharan Africa.[22–24] It is transmitted via skin penetration by infective filariform larvae following exposure to water or soil contaminated by human or canine fecal material. The larvae are hematogenously carried to the lungs, regurgitated, and then swallowed where they mature into adults in the intestines. The reproductive cycle of the nematode and resultant reinfection may continue indefinitely. The autoinfected human host frequently remains asymptomatic or experiences mild nonspecific skin and gastrointestinal symptoms. This equilibrium may persist indefinitely.

Immunosuppression, however, particularly with corticosteroids, may result in multiorgan dissemination and hyperinfection.[22,23] Control of parasitic infections requires Th2 cytokine, eosinophilic, and IgE influence, all of which are suppressed by steroids and other immunomodulating agents. With hyperinfection, mortality is estimated to be 60%–85%.[24] For this reason, parasitic and serologic surveillance is recommended for anyone at increased risk prior to treatment with immunosuppressive agents. The absence of hypereosinophilia occurs frequently in infected individuals and does not represent a sensitive screening test. Ideally, patients at risk should undergo three negative surveillance stool specimens and an ELISA screening test for IgG *Strongyloides stercoralis* antibodies available through the Centers for Disease Control before treatment is begun. The ELISA test is thought to be 80%–100% sensitive and highly specific in immunocompetent individuals. Its sensitivity drops significantly in immunosuppressed individuals. A negative test needs to be interpreted cautiously in individuals already exposed to immunosuppressive medications. If infected, ivermectin, thiabendazole, and albendazole are the most commonly used therapeutic agents. One suggested regimen for strongyloidiasis prophylaxis would be ivermectin 200 μg/kg/day for 2 days, repeated within 2 weeks.[23]

VACCINES

Ideally, patients should be vaccinated against COVID-19, influenza, pneumococcus, tetanus, and hepatitis A and perhaps B prior to initiation of immunosuppression whenever possible. Once immunosuppression has commenced, there appears to be a consensus that vaccines containing dead virus can be utilized without undue risk but that live-virus vaccines should be avoided.[25] Specific immunotherapies, notably B-cell depleters (e.g., rituximab) and mycophenolate virus, have been shown to reduce antibody production with various COVID-19 vaccinations.[26,27] Generally, we try to give vaccines about 3–4 weeks prior to an infusion of rituximab so as to give the body a chance to form antibodies. Also, we try to give vaccines 4–6 months after a dose of rituximab. Some studies suggest if the CD20 count is at 1/μL, an antibody response can be mounted.[28] Also, B-cell depleters do not appear to diminish a T-cell response against the virus.[27,28]

PREGNANCY AND CHILDREN

Management of immunotherapy in women of childbearing age can be challenging. Corticosteroids and IVIg provide minimal additional risk for mother or child during pregnancy. We are very reticent to use other immunotherapies agents in childhood unless patient morbidity provides no other options. If corticosteroids are used before full growth is achieved, it is recommended that linear growth be tested regularly, and growth hormone treatment considered if necessary.

CANCER

Patients who receive immunosuppressive therapy have an increased risk of developing malignancy.[29] This risk is attributed to oncogenic infectious agents, reduced immune surveillance of cells having undergone mutation in relationship to age or environmental factors, or direct effects on oncogenes. Notable oncogenic organisms whose proliferation may be aided by immunosuppression include Epstein–Barr virus, human herpesvirus 8, human papillomavirus, hepatitis B and C, and helicobacter. The malignancies most commonly associated with immunosuppression include lymphoproliferative disorders, Kaposi sarcoma, as well as anogenital, liver, and stomach cancer. Data pertaining to the relative risk of developing these malignancies, indexed to the numbers, types, and length of exposure to immunosuppressant medications are lacking, although it is widely accepted that both increased dose and duration of exposure are relevant. Of interest, available data suggests that cancer risk rapidly dissipates following discontinuation of immunosuppressive treatment. The pragmatic benefit of this knowledge is uncertain given the presumption that discontinuation of an effective immunosuppressive agent is unlikely unless cancer develops. Recommendations regarding rational, evidence-based cancer surveillance protocols for patients on immunosuppressive treatments are elusive and are beyond the scope of this text. Discussion of this risk should nonetheless be part of the informed consent process. Consideration of dose reduction and potentially discontinuation is recommended in those who achieve complete disease remission.

There also appears to be an increased risk of skin cancers in patients receiving immunosuppressant drugs. The incidence of squamous cell carcinoma is believed to be increased by 14–82-fold and malignant melanoma increased by a factor of 2.4 in the solid organ transplant population.[30] We routinely advise patients on immunosuppressant drugs of the increased skin cancer risk and recommend limiting sun exposure, ample use of sun-blocking agents, and routine skin surveillance.

▶ SPECIFIC IMMUNOTHERAPIES

In the following section, specific forms of immunotherapy commonly used in neuromuscular disease will be discussed.[1-13] Consideration of mechanisms of action, specific disorders in which individual agents are often used, adverse effects and management strategies will be addressed for each modality. For more detailed management strategies, the reader is referred to the relevant chapter on the disease in question.

CORTICOSTEROIDS

Mechanism of Action

Glucocorticoid effects are mediated through both genomic, nuclear glucocorticoid receptors as well as nongenomic cell surface receptors. They are one of the most versatile immunomodulating agents available in that they affect both cell-mediated and antibody-mediated autoimmunity.[1] Corticosteroids largely affect T-cell function by producing T-cell apoptosis, suppressing the transcription of proinflammatory cytokines and impairing dendritic cell maturation. Specifically, glucocorticoids increase the rate of lipocortin synthesis which promotes anti-inflammatory effects by inhibition of phospholipase A2 as well as the proinflammatory cytokines IL-1, IL-2, the IL-2 receptor, INF gamma, and TNF.

Uses

We commonly use prednisone as our oral corticosteroid agent of choice. In most autoimmune neuromuscular disorders, we start at a high dosage (0.75–1.0 mg/kg daily).[1-3,11,31] The use of corticosteroids in autoimmune MG deserves special consideration because initial disease may occur in approximately 15% or so of patients started on high-dose corticosteroids, typically beginning between weeks 1 and 3 and lasting approximately 1 week.[32,33] The mechanism of the worsening appears to be unique to disorders of neuromuscular transmission, apparently secondary to weak neuromuscular blocking properties of the drug supported by the demonstration of decremental responses to slow repetitive stimulation. In myasthenics who are severely weak and are hospitalized, we often start high-dose prednisone as we can watch them closely for deterioration. However, we opt with the "start low–go slow" approach in patients with less severe disease that we manage as outpatients. Our experience and others show that many patients can improve with a low dose of prednisone (10–20 mg daily) that is slowly increased as tolerated (by 5 mg every 5–7 days) as needed.

Corticosteroids are used in numerous other presumed immune-mediated neuromuscular disorders including a number of neuropathy syndromes.[1,4-8] The best evidence for efficacy exists for CIDP with a phenotype of generalized symmetric weakness, sensory signs and symptoms, and areflexia and its presumed variant, multifocal acquired demyelinating sensory and motor neuropathy (MADSAM also known as Lewis–Sumner syndrome).[34-38] Although prednisone is the most commonly used glucocorticoid for CIDP, successful intravenous methylprednisolone and oral dexamethasone regimens have been reported as well.[39] The weight of existing evidence suggests that steroids provide no benefit and may be harmful in the aggregate in GBS, MMN, and DADS associated with IgM monoclonal proteins. Corticosteroids are also commonly used as a first-line treatment based on expert opinion in dermatomyositis, polymyositis, antisynthetase syndrome, and immune-mediated necrotizing myopathy/myositis but are considered ineffective in inclusion body myositis.[2,3,9-13,40]

There is little doubt that use of immunosuppressive agents favorably alters the natural history of the systemic vasculitides. Corticosteroids, often with concomitant cyclophosphamide or rituximab, are the backbones of treatment for these disorders.[1,6,7,41-43] There is support for the use of corticosteroids in the treatment of sarcoidosis and sarcoid neuropathy but no evidence-based confirmation.[44] There is a dearth of evidence in support of corticosteroid use in cervical/brachial and lumbosacral radiculoplexitis.[45] In our experience, corticosteroids may benefit the painful aspects of this disorder, if prescribed early, but they appear to have a limited, if any, benefit in improving strength. We have used corticosteroids to treat stiff person and Isaacs syndrome.

Adverse Effects

Adverse effects of corticosteroids are largely dose dependent and include diabetes, hypertension, peptic ulcer disease, osteopenia, cataracts, glaucoma, opportunistic infections, dyslipidemia, hypokalemia, increased appetite and weight gain, insomnia, and myopathy. Steroid psychosis and aseptic necrosis appear to be adverse effects that are idiosyncratic in nature. Interventions intended to prophylaxis against these complications will be addressed in the Management Considerations section below.

Management Considerations

Corticosteroids are frequently administered in a single daily morning dose to parallel the normal circadian peak of endogenous cortisol production. Once maximal efficacy has been achieved, we attempt to wean to the smallest effective maintenance dose. The speed of weaning proceeds based on individual patient context. For example, development of significant steroid side effects such as myopathy will accelerate the weaning pace whereas any indication of disease exacerbation may put the weaning process on hold. As a general guideline, we reduce the dose by 10 mg every 4 weeks. Once a dose of 20 mg daily is reached, we taper more slowly, typically in increments of 2.5–5 mg every 4 weeks down until down to 10 mg daily, and then no faster than 2.5 mg daily based on clinical response.

We routinely question patients for potential exposure to TB and when in doubt perform PPD, chest x-ray, and IGRA testing. If there is suggestion for indolent tuberculosis infection, and immunomodulating treatment is medically necessary, we initiate isoniazid and pyridoxine treatment concomitantly unless otherwise contraindicated. If the patient comes from an area where strongyloidiasis is endemic, we consider baseline serologic testing and stool analysis.

Patients on long-term corticosteroids should receive baseline screening and periodic monitoring of intraocular pressure, blood pressure, blood sugar, lipids, and bone density. In particular, glucocorticoids facilitate osteopenia by interfering with bone formation through apoptosis of osteocytes and enhancing bone resorption through inhibition of osteoprotegerin, an endogenous antiresorptive cytokine.[46] In any patient who will be receiving corticosteroids for more than 3 months, it is prudent to obtain a bone density and initiate daily treatment with 2,000 IU of vitamin D3 and 1,000 mg of calcium, promote exercise, and suggest no more than modest alcohol intake. In men over the age of 50 years, postmenopausal women, or anyone with a T score of –1.5 or below, we initiate bisphosphonate such as alendronate at a 35 mg a week for prophylaxis and 70 mg a week if they already have osteoporosis.

We do not routinely recommend gastric protection in patients using chronic corticosteroids unless they are symptomatic or at increased risk for gastritis because of concomitant use of nonsteroidal anti-inflammatory agents. In these situations, prophylactic treatment with a proton pump inhibitor, misoprostol, or a cyclooxygenase 2 inhibitor is utilized. In addition, patients are instructed to start a low-sodium, low-carbohydrate, high-protein diet to prevent excessive weight gain and in the case of a high-protein diet, to theoretically reduce the risk of steroid myopathy. Patients are also encouraged to slowly begin an aerobic exercise program as it is hypothesized that both osteopenia and steroid myopathy are enhanced by immobility. Finally, augmentation of corticosteroid dosing should be considered perioperatively or when they have a severe infection in order to avoid risk of adrenal insufficiency.[7]

AZATHIOPRINE

Mechanism of Action

Azathioprine is a purine analog that acts as a cytotoxic immunosuppressive agent. Its main active metabolite, 6-mercaptopurine, is a purine antagonist. It is a cell-cycle–specific inhibitor, exerting its actions mainly in the resting (G1) and DNA synthesis (S) phases of the cell cycle through suppression of GTPase Rac1 activation.[2] Although its primary effects are directed at T cells, it is efficacious in T-cell–dependent antibody-mediated disorders such as MG. In addition to reducing numbers of circulating T cells, it also reduces levels of B-cell–derived immunoglobulins and interleukin-2 (IL-2).

Uses

Azathioprine is a commonly used maintenance, "steroid-sparing" therapy in various autoimmune neuromuscular disorders.[1–3,11–13,47–52] We commonly initiate azathioprine (or other corticosteroid-sparing agent) along with corticosteroids in any myasthenic patient with generalized disease in whom we anticipate the need for long-term immunotherapy. We do so in the hope of facilitating corticosteroid weaning, thereby limiting risk of long-term steroid side effects. By starting early, we take advantage of the short-term benefits of corticosteroids, recognizing the delayed therapeutic latency (3–15 months) of azathioprine which may require up to 2 years to achieve full effect.

Several trials have demonstrated the efficacy of azathioprine alone or in combination with prednisone in MG.[48–51] For the most part, the use of azathioprine in nonmyasthenic NM diseases is based on case series and expert opinion. It has been used in Lambert–Eaton myasthenic syndrome (LEMS), inflammatory myopathies, CIDP, MMN, and other inflammatory neuropathies.[1–13,52]

Adverse Effects

Side effects typically, although not invariably, develop within days to weeks of drug exposure. A systemic reaction characterized by fever, abdominal pain, nausea, vomiting, and anorexia occurs in 12% of patients requiring discontinuation of the drug.[47] This reaction generally resolves within a few days of discontinuing the azathioprine. Rechallenge with azathioprine may be successful but usually results in the recurrence of the systemic reaction. Other uncommon but major complications of azathioprine are bone marrow suppression, hepatic toxicity, pancreatitis, teratogenicity, risk of opportunistic infection, and oncogenicity including increased risk of skin cancer.[48]

Management Considerations

Azathioprine is available in 50-mg tablets without a parenteral analog. We typically begin with one tablet a day and escalate slowly to a maintenance dose of 2–3 mg/kg/day, typically 2.5 mg/kg/day. Prior to beginning azathioprine, some advocate enzyme analysis or genotype to screen for thiopurine methyltransferase (TPMT) deficiency.[53] Patients who are heterozygous for the TPMT mutation may be able to tolerate azathioprine at lower dosages, but those who are homozygous should not receive drug. They cannot metabolize it and may experience severe bone marrow toxicity. Fortunately, the majority of patients who develop adverse hematologic responses in response to azathioprine recover fully once the drug is discontinued.

In patients receiving azathioprine, complete blood count (CBC) and liver function tests are monitored monthly until the patient is on a stable dose of azathioprine and then every 3–6 months for 2 years. After that, with stable blood counts, yearly surveillance is likely to be sufficient. If the white blood count falls below 4,000/mm^3, the dose should be decreased. Azathioprine is held if the white blood count declines to 2,500/mm^3 or the absolute neutrophil count falls to 1,000/mm^3. Leukopenia can develop as early as 1 week or as late as 2 years after initiating azathioprine. As in most drugs with potential hepatotoxic effects, azathioprine should be discontinued if transaminases increase more than two to three times the baseline values. In the treatment of patients with myositis, it is important to determine whether transaminase elevation is due to liver damage from drug or muscle injury from disease. Accordingly, in these situations, we follow glutamyl transpeptidase (GGT) levels, an enzyme present in liver but not muscle, in addition to aspartate aminotransferase (AST) and alanine aminotransferase (ALT) for this reason. Liver toxicity from azathioprine generally develops within the first several months of treatment or increase in dosage. Leukopenia generally reverses in 1 month and hepatotoxicity can take several months to resolve. An elevated mean corpuscular volume is an anticipated effect of azathioprine therapy and is used by some clinicians as an indicator of a biologic response. Allopurinol should be avoided in patients who require azathioprine because it interferes with azathioprine metabolism, increasing drug levels, and increasing the risk of bone marrow and liver toxicity.

METHOTREXATE

Mechanism of Action

Methotrexate, which also mainly affects the G1 and S phases of the cell cycle, is a folate antagonist that can inhibit de novo synthesis of both purines and pyrimidines. It is a selective inhibitor of both dihydrofolate reductase and lymphocyte proliferation. As a structural analog of folic acid, it affects adenosine-mediated inflammatory mediators, resulting in apoptosis and clonal deletion of T-cell lines. It also acts to decreases the production of proinflammatory cytokines IL-1 and IL-6.

Uses

Within neuromuscular disorders, methotrexate is most commonly used in the treatment of inflammatory myopathies.[3,11–13,54–57] It is our suspicion that this is based on the frequency with which these disorders are treated by rheumatologists who are perhaps more comfortable with its use than neurologists. Furthermore, rheumatologists are not as frequently involved in the treatment of other neuromuscular conditions.

Adverse Effects

Potential side effects of methotrexate therapy include hepatotoxicity which is relatively uncommon, interstitial pneumonitis, which presents with dyspnea, fever, and dry cough and potentially leads to pulmonary fibrosis, infection, neoplasia, infertility, bone marrow suppression with leukopenia, alopecia, gastric irritation with nausea, vomiting and diarrhea, fatigue, rash, dizziness, ulcerative stomatitis, and teratogenicity.[58] Like most immunosuppressant medications, the exact incidence of neoplasia and its causal relationship to methotrexate is difficult to quantitate.

Management Considerations

Methotrexate is typically initiated orally at 7.5 mg/week or lower in the context of renal insufficiency. It can be given in a single dose or in divided doses. One regimen is three divided doses administered 12 hours apart, often Saturday morning and evening and Sunday morning so that any side effects might have a chance to dissipate before the work week begins. The total dose may be gradually escalated dependent on the development of beneficial or adverse effect to a maximal dose of 25 mg/week. All patients are concomitantly treated with folate, at least 5 mg/week. Methotrexate can also be delivered subcutaneously once weekly at a dose of 20–50 mg.

Hepatic enzymes, platelet, and white blood cell counts should be monitored closely. In patients with pulmonary symptoms, methotrexate should be held until an infectious cause and pulmonary fibrosis can be excluded. Chest imaging, pulmonary function testing, and pulmonary consultation are recommended in symptomatic patients.

MYCOPHENOLATE MOFETIL

Mechanism of Action

Mycophenolate mofetil (MMF) inhibits lymphocytic purine synthesis by selectively inhibiting the enzyme inosine-5′-monophosphate dehydrogenase. Like azathioprine, it acts predominantly on the G1 and S phases of the cell cycle and results in T-cell and B-cell depletion.

Uses

Within the spectrum of neuromuscular disorders, mycophenolate has been most diligently studied in MG. Initial open-label studies suggested notable benefit in an estimated 75% of treated individuals, primarily as an adjunctive therapy.[59–62] However, randomized, placebo-controlled studies have not been as supportive.[63,64] There is a perception that the negative studies were flawed due to their relatively short periods of observation.[62] We and other authorities feel that MMF is an effective agent in some myasthenics. MMF has also been studied in the treatment of CIDP.[65–67] Interpretation of these studies is confounded by the numerous other treatment variables that many of these patients were exposed to. Case reports and small series also suggest a benefit of MMF in systemic and nonsystemic vasculitic neuropathy, sarcoid neuropathy and myositis, immune-mediated necrotizing myopathy, and Isaacs syndrome.[3,6,11]

Adverse Effects

MMF is usually well tolerated and has little or no renal or liver toxicity. The major side effect is diarrhea. Starting slowly and increasing the dose slowly may diminish the risk and severity of this troublesome side effect. Less common side effects include abdominal discomfort, nausea, peripheral edema, fever, and leukopenia. Measurement of drug levels is not done routinely. Adverse hematologic effects may be more common in doses of greater than 2,000 mg/day. In view of the relatively short experience with this agent, long-term safety for mycophenolate is still in question. Malignancy rates do not appear higher in the transplant population; however, there are rare reports of lymphoma or lymphoproliferative disorders developing in MG patients.[68] Progressive multifocal encephalopathy is a rare, but serious, complication.

Management Considerations

MMF, available in 500-mg tablets, is typically dosed at 1,000 mg twice a day. Starting at 500 mg daily or twice a day and gradually increasing the dose may diminish the incidence and severity of diarrhea. The maximal recommended dose is 1,500 mg BID. Patients who do not respond to a daily dose of 2,000 mg but respond to higher doses are relatively uncommon in our experience. Improvement may take 6 to 12 months. MMF is excreted through the kidneys; therefore, the dose should be decreased (no more than 1 g/day total dose) in patients with renal insufficiency.

Mycophenolic acid or mycophenolate sodium (Myfortic®) is an alternative preparation that comes in 180 and 360 mg enteric-coated tablets. As a result, it has the potential for less gastrointestinal side effects. Unlike MMF, it is not available for parenteral use. The daily dose is 720–1,440 mg/day in two divided doses.

CYCLOSPORINE

Mechanism of Action

In the cytoplasm, cyclosporine binds to its immunophilin, cyclophilin. The cyclosporine–cyclophilin complex binds to and blocks the function of the enzyme calcineurin, eventually inhibiting T-cell activation and reducing production of the proinflammatory cytokine IL-2.

Uses

Cyclosporine appears to be effective in the treatment of patients with MG.[2,69–72] The therapeutic latency is typically 1–3 months following treatment initiation. Mean time to maximum improvement is approximately 7 months. Cyclosporine also appears to have a steroid-sparing effect. As many as 95% of patients are able to discontinue or decrease their corticosteroid dose. There are a number of reports that describe cyclosporine as beneficial in CIDP patients.[73–76] Cyclosporine may benefit patients with vasculitic neuropathy, sarcoid neuropathy, LEMS, and inflammatory myopathies.[3,77–79] It is used by most clinicians as a third-line drug in patients unresponsive to other modalities.

Adverse Effects

Renal toxicity occurs in approximately a quarter of patients. The need to monitor creatinine and trough cyclosporine levels frequently has limited the enthusiasm of some clinicians for its use. Patients receiving cyclosporine or any calcineurin inhibitor may also develop a calcineurin inhibition syndrome that includes prominent and at times debilitating tremor requiring dose reduction. Cyclosporine is used in MG primarily in patients who are refractory to prednisone and azathioprine.

Management Considerations

Initially, a total dose of 3.0–4.0 mg/kg/day in two divided doses is used and gradually increased to a maximum dose of 6.0 mg/kg/day as necessary. The cyclosporine dose is initially being titrated to maintain trough serum cyclosporine levels of 100–200 ng/mL. Blood pressure, electrolytes and renal function, and trough cyclosporine levels need to be monitored on a monthly basis. The dose is lowered as necessary to keep the creatinine level stable while maintaining the trough level within therapeutic range. Any upward trend of creatinine levels should promote a dose reduction. After patients achieve maximum improvement, the dose is reduced over several months to the minimum dose necessary to maintain the therapeutic response. Patients need to be informed of the numerous drugs that can aggravate renal toxicity including nonsteroidal anti-inflammatory agents and drugs that may raise blood pressure or affect serum potassium levels.

TACROLIMUS

Mechanism of Action

Tacrolimus binds to the FK506-binding protein (FKB), forming the tacrolimus–FKB complex, which also binds to and blocks calcineurin. Although cyclosporine and tacrolimus bind to different target molecules, both drugs inhibit T-cell activation in the same manner and as calcineurin inhibitors, reduce production of the proinflammatory cytokine IL-2. As is the case with cyclosporine, these are two immunomodulating drugs developed for and used by the organ transplant community.

Uses

Tacrolimus, like cyclosporine, has been undoubtedly used most frequently in MG within the spectrum of neuromuscular disease.[72,80–85] It has been used either as monotherapy or more commonly in conjunction with thymectomy or other therapies. Both favorable and equivocal results are reported. There are rare reports of benefit with LEMS, dermatomyositis/polymyositis, and inflammatory neuropathies.

Adverse Effects

Tacrolimus has similar toxicities to cyclosporine. It tends to be less nephrotoxic but more inclined to cause hyperglycemia. We generally use this before cyclosporine.

Management Considerations

Tacrolimus has been prescribed for myasthenic patients at a dosage of 0.1 mg/kg/day in two divided doses, and subsequently adjusted for plasma drug concentrations between 7 and 8 mg/mL.

CYCLOPHOSPHAMIDE

Mechanism of Action

Cyclophosphamide is a DNA-alkylating drug and nonspecific cell cycle inhibitor, with more pronounced effects on B cells than on T cells.

Uses

Cyclophosphamide is most widely used and best established for treatment of vasculitic neuropathy.[1,6,41,86,87] It may be effective treatment in patients with refractory CIDP, DADs, and MMN patients.[88–92] Cyclophosphamide may benefit patients with MG, including those with MuSK autoantibodies.[93–95] A protocol that utilizes high-dose cyclophosphamide to "reboot" the bone marrow has been suggested in individuals who have failed attempts at other less-toxic regimens.[93] We have used it in refractory cases of myositis as well.

Adverse Effects

Cyclophosphamide has a substantial side-effect profile that includes frequent nausea and vomiting with administration. Serious side effects include opportunistic infection, hemorrhagic cystitis, bone marrow depression, sterility, teratogenicity, alopecia, and late development of malignancy, particularly lymphoma and bladder cancer. The incidence of malignancy associated with cyclophosphamide use appears to increase when the cumulative dose exceeds 85 g.

Management Considerations

Cyclophosphamide may be administered either orally or intravenously. The oral dose is 2–2.5 mg/kg/day typically administered as single dose each morning. The intravenous dose is 1 g/m^2 monthly for 6 consecutive months. The latter is preferred as it is thought to be less toxic and as the adverse hematologic effects are easier to time and monitor. The therapeutic latency between administration and manifest benefit is relatively short and is estimated to be 2–6 months, dependent on both drug effect and end-organ healing.

Patients receiving intravenous cyclophosphamide should have a baseline CBC and platelet count and urinalysis done and at minimum, a repeat CBC prior to each subsequent infusion to ensure a safe neutrophil level. Like azathioprine, repeat cyclosporine infusions are held if the WBC count and absolute neutrophil count which typically nadirs between 1 and 2 weeks postinfusion do not re-establish itself to >2,500/mm^3 or >1,000/mm^3, respectively prior to the next dose. It is frequently recommended that cyclophosphamide recipients have yearly urine cytologic surveillance.

INTRAVENOUS AND SUBCUTANEOUS IMMUNOGLOBULIN

Mechanism of Action

Various preparations of exogenous human immunoglobulins, either intravenous (IVIg) or subcutaneous (SCIg), are used to treat many types of autoimmune neuromuscular disorders.[1–13,96,97] There are multiple proposed mechanisms of action for IVIg and SCIg, one or more of which may be relevant depending on the pathophysiology of the treated disease. Anti-idiotype antibodies contained within immunoglobulin preparations may react with the Fc or antigen-binding regions of pathologic autoantibodies and neutralize their effects. The nonimmunoglobulin components may beneficially interfere with T-cell function in a number of ways. It may restore the balance between T cells releasing proinflammatory Th1 and anti-inflammatory Th2 cytokines. It may cause T-cell apoptosis, interfere with T-cell interaction with antigen-presenting cells, and interrupt T-cell migration through the blood–nerve barrier. Interference with B-cell function including production of autoantibodies, activation of complement, formation of membrane attack complex, and macrophage function are other proposed mechanisms of action.

Uses

IVIg is beneficial in GBS, CIDP, multifocal motor neuropathy (MMN), MG, and certain inflammatory myopathies (dermatomyositis).[1–6,8,9,11–13,96–125] Although no large, randomized trials have yet to be done for anti-HMGCR myopathy (a form of immune-mediated necrotizing myositis), IVIg has become a standard first-line treatment for the disorder by many experts in the field based on experience and small published series.[121,122]

SCIg is also of proven benefit and approved for maintenance treatment of adults with CIDP.[126–131] Studies suggest that IVIg and SCIg have comparable long-term efficacy in CIDP. SCIg also appears to be effective in MMN, MG, and in some inflammatory myopathies.[132–141] SCIg can provide added benefits for some patients, including no requirement for venous access, the ability to self-administer at home at a convenient time or even when traveling, and reduced frequency of systemic adverse events. Local-site reactions are more common with SCIg than IVIg.

Adverse Effects

Minor infusion-related symptoms such as chills, nausea, myalgia, headache, and vasomotor disturbances are fairly common with IVIg infusion. In an attempt to avoid this reaction, we typically pretreat our patients with 650 mg of acetaminophen and 25 mg of diphenhydramine or 10 mg of loratadine orally. If an allergic reaction is experienced, we add 100 mg of intravenous hydrocortisone to the pretreatment regimen prior to every infusion.

Serious side effects from IVIg are rare and include thromboembolic diseases such as stroke and myocardial infarction, renal failure, aseptic meningitis, congestive heart failure, and anaphylactic reactions. Thromboembolic risk may be higher in those with atherosclerotic cardiovascular risk factors. Headaches seem to occur more frequently in migraineurs and do not appear to be preventable with steroid pretreatment. Rechallenging patients who have previously experienced IVIg-induced aseptic meningitis should probably be avoided unless there are particularly strong indications for its use. Rechallenge appears to have a greater success in patients without a history of migraine.

Anaphylaxis has been reported in patients deficient in IgA. The initial suggestion that this risk exists from IgG autoantibodies directed at IgA autoantibodies has been refuted by safe infusion in IgA-deficient, IgG versus IgA autoantibody-carrying patients. Recent evidence suggests that IgE versus IgA is the more likely causative pathophysiology of this reaction. As the incidence of anaphylaxis in patients receiving IVIg is extremely uncommon, screening for IgA deficiency is not recommended as a routine practice prior to IVIg exposure.

Other consequences of IVIg treatment of note include elevation of serum inflammatory markers such as erythrocyte sedimentation rates which may exceed 100 mm/h which may confound patient management. Following IVIg infusion, determination of a patient's actual immunity toward certain diseases may also be confounded. As previously mentioned, antibodies detected in a patient's serum may represent those passively transferred rather than ones generated by the patient's own immune system.

Systemic adverse events are less common with SCIg but can occur. We generally do not prophylaxis patients getting SCIg—unlike IVIg. However, local-site reactions are more common with SCIg than IVIg.

Management Considerations

IVIg is typically initiated at a dose of 2 mg/kg of ideal body weight over 2–5 days. In disorders other than GBS that require maintenance dosing, we give 1 g/kg every 3–4 weeks to start. Over time, we try to spread out the interval slowly, but some patients may need more frequent infusions (e.g., every 2 weeks). Alternatively, one can keep the same dosing interval (e.g., every 3–4 weeks) but reduce the total dosage. Most patients find it more convenient to spread out the interval and it is also less expensive.

SCIg is given 2–3 times a week. When transitioning from IVIG, we calculate what the "weekly dosage" of IVIG would be and convert 1:1 to SCIg. For example, if a patient was receiving IVIg 1 g/kg a month (averaging 0.25 g/kg a week), we would start SCIg at 0.125 g/kg twice a week. In IVIg-naive patients started on SCIg, the recommended initial dosage is 0.2–0.4 g/kg.

RITUXIMAB

Mechanism of Action

Rituximab is a monoclonal antibody directed against CD20+ B cells, developed for the treatment of B-cell lymphomas. It produces B-cell depletion, postulated to occur via complement-mediated cytotoxicity, antibody-dependent cell-mediated cytotoxicity, and induction of apoptosis. It also reduces T-lymphocyte activation and decreases cytokine production.

Uses

Early anecdotal reports suggested that rituximab may be beneficial in MG.[142,143] One randomized, double-blind, placebo-controlled trial of rituximab in patients with anti-AChR antibody-positive generalized MG failed to demonstrate efficacy, however a more recent study of newly diagnosed patients with myasthenia did demonstrate efficacy at a dose of 500 mg IV.[144,145] Our opinion and that of many authorities is the rituximab appears to be quite effective in anti–MuSK-positive MG[146–149]; we have had some patients go 2 or 3 years between infusions before developing signs of a relapse.

In consideration of rituximab's efficacy in lymphoproliferative disorders, it is rational to consider its use in polyneuropathies associated with paraproteinemia. Although initial reports of rituximab in patients with demyelination polyneuropathy associated with anti–myelin-associated (anti-MAG) antibodies were optimistic, subsequent, randomized, placebo-controlled trials found no benefit.[150,151] Our experience is that most patients do not respond, with rare patients responding dramatically in a manner that contrasts significantly with the natural history of this disorder. Whether the response is durable in these uncommon patients is uncertain. There are a handful of case reports and small case series describing a benefit of rituximab in CIDP and CIDP-like neuropathies with IgG4 antibodies directed against nodal and paranodal antigens (see Chapter 14).[152–154] Rituximab may be helpful in

MMN. The use of rituximab has become a standard treatment of choice in forms of vasculitic neuropathy, particularly this with antineutrophil cytoplasmic antibodies (ANCA).[1,6,41–43]

Although a large randomized, placebo-controlled trial of rituximab showed no benefit in adults and children with polymyositis and dermatomyositis, there were many methodologic issues in regard to trial design that may have impeded the detection of efficacy.[155] We and others have used rituximab in myositis patients (non-IBM) and have found it useful in some patients with antisynthetase syndrome and immune-mediated necrotizing myopathy (anti-signal recognition particle antibody positive).[123,156] It has also been used to treat stiff-person syndrome.[157,158]

Adverse Effects

Rituximab is well tolerated by the majority of patients. Pruritus, nausea, vomiting, dizziness, headache, angina, cardiac dysrhythmia, anemia, leukopenia, and thrombocytopenia have been reported. Myelosuppression, PML, and lymphoma are uncommon but potential risks.

Management Considerations

There are a number of dosing regimens utilized for rituximab. We usually dose at 750 mg/m^2 (up to 1 g in adults) with a repeat infusion in 2 weeks. Pretreatment with 650 mg of acetaminophen and 25 mg of diphenhydramine by mouth is suggested although the drug is well tolerated by most individuals. Our approach has been to wait at least 6 months before reinfusing and then only if initial improvement and then subsequent clinical deterioration takes place. Once we have a baseline of when relapses seem to occur, we dose at intervals to prevent relapse.

ECULIZUMAB

Mechanism of Action

Eculizumab is a humanized monoclonal antibody that acts by blocking the formation of terminal complement complex by specifically preventing the enzymatic cleavage of complement 5 (C5).[159,160]

Uses

Eculizumab has been demonstrated to be effective in myasthenic patients refractory to other agents.[159,160]

Adverse Effects

The most common adverse effects reported in clinical trials of eculizumab include nausea, back pain, nasopharyngitis, and headache. Renal insufficiency, anemia, leukopenia, dyspepsia, diarrhea, tachycardia, peripheral edema, fatigue, and both hypo- and hypertension have been reported. There is also an increased risk of meningococcal meningitis.

Management Considerations

Induction is started with eculizumab infusions at 900 mg weekly × 4 weeks, then 1,200 mg at week 5, followed by 1,200 mg every 2 weeks. Improvement is usually noted within 3 months, often within a month. If there is no improvement after 4–6 months, we discontinue. Patients need to be reduced if they undergo plasmapheresis or plasma exchange as this will eliminate the eculizumab.

Because of the risk of meningococcal meningitis, patients should be immunized with both the MenACYW and MenB meningococcal vaccines at least 2 weeks prior to administering the first dose of eculizumab. If the patient cannot wait 2 weeks for vaccination because of severe refractory disease, then prophylactic antibiotics (penicillin, azithromycin ciprofloxacin, amoxicillin, trimethoprim–sulfamethoxazole, or rifampin) can be given and continued for least 2 weeks after vaccination. We usually treat all patients with eculizumab with prophylactic antibiotics as there still remains a risk of meningococcus meningitis even in those vaccinated. In patients who discontinue eculizumab, we continue antibiotic prophylaxis 4 weeks from the last dose of eculizumab. Booster doses of MenACWY vaccine are given every 5 years in patients who received their previous dose at age 7 years or older, for the duration of complement inhibitor therapy. Depending on the brand, the full series of MenB vaccine requires 2 or 3 doses; there are no current recommendations about if or when to administer booster doses of MenB vaccine.

EFGARTIGIMOD

Mechanism of Action

Efgartigimod is a human IgG1 antibody Fc fragment that blocks the anti-FcRn.[161,162] This action increases the rate at which IgG antibodies are broken down within cells.

Uses

Efgartigimod has been demonstrated to be effective in anti-AChR antibody-positive myasthenia and was recently FDA approved for this indication.[161,162] It is being studied in other presumed antibody-mediated autoimmune neuromuscular disorders.

Adverse Effects

Hypersensitivity reaction including rash, angioedema, and dyspnea were observed in clinical trials.

Management Considerations

Efgartigimod is initiated at 10 mg/kg weekly × 4 weeks (1,200 mg per infusion in patients weighing 120 kg or more). Drug safety has been studied with administration of subsequent cycles no sooner than 50 days from the start of the previous treatment cycle based on clinical evaluation. The average time needed for a second course in clinical trials was 72 days. The optimal dosing regimen in practice is unknown and wearing off of drug effect will not be desired in many cases. We start by administering for 1–2 cycles then re-evaluate magnitude and duration of benefit and then adjust dosing so as to readminister subsequent cycles before there are relapses. Improvement is often noted within a few months. If there is no improvement (a decrease in the MG-ADL total score from baseline or an improved MGFA postintervention status) by 6 months, we discontinue. Because efgartigimod causes reduction in IgG levels, immunization with live-attenuated or live vaccines is not recommended during treatment.

PLASMA EXCHANGE

Mechanism of Action

Therapeutic PLEX reduces the titer of circulating antibodies within the bloodstream through filtration.

Uses

The most established uses for PLEX in NM disease are in GBS, CIDP, and MG.[1,2,4–6,9,112,124,125,163–169] Once again, because of cost, safety, and logistical considerations, PLEX is used primarily in initial induction treatment, not in chronic maintenance therapy. In MG, it is used primarily in patients in crisis or in those with moderate weakness prior to thymectomy in order to maximize their perioperative strength and minimize risk of postoperative complications. There are individual or small case series that suggest potential benefit in diabetic radiculoplexus neuropathy, systemic and nonsystemic vasculitic neuropathy, as well as Miller Fisher, stiff-person and Isaacs syndromes.

Adverse Effects

PLEX is associated with various complications.[170] It has limited availability and like IVIg, cost is an issue. Many of the risks related to PLEX are related to the need for large bore catheters that need to be placed in central veins in a significant portion of individuals. Potential complications include symptoms related to alkalosis, pneumothorax, and hypotension, particularly in GBS patients prone to dysautonomia, sepsis, and pulmonary embolism.

Management Considerations

The standard PLEX protocol is to exchange a volume of 200–250 mL/kg/day (2–3 L) for 5 days typically spread out over a 7–10-day period of time. The durability of the effect is usually a few weeks.

EMERGING THERAPIES

Other Complement Inhibitors and FcRn Antagonists

Aside from eculizumab and efgartigimod, other complement inhibitors and FcRn antagonists have been recently FDA and EU approved, and more that are being developed and are studied in MG (see Chapter 25 for up-to-date list) and other autoimmune neuromuscular conditions (i.e., myositis, inflammatory neuropathies). If shown to be efficacious, they will also be likely added to our therapeutic armamentarium.

Janus Kinase (JAK) Inhibitors

Although not as yet standard of care, we do want to mention there is increasing evidence suggesting that JAK inhibitors (e.g., tofacitinib) may be beneficial in dermatomyositis, particularly cases associated with rapidly progressive interstitial lung disease.[171–174] Tofacitinib is an oral JAK inhibitor approved for the treatment of rheumatoid arthritis, psoriatic arthritis, and juvenile idiopathic arthritis. Dermatomyositis is believed to be a type 1 interferonopathy. JAK inhibitors block type 1 interferon pathways that are mediated by members of the Janus kinase family (JAK1, JAK2, JAK3, TYK2). Clinical trials are underway in this and with other monoclonal antibodies that block type 1 interferons in dermatomyositis.

REFERENCES

1. Amato AA, Hauser SL. Guillain-Barre syndrome and autoimmune neuropathies. In: Fauci AS, Braunwald E, Kasper DJ, et al., eds. *Harrison's Principles of Internal Medicine*. McGraw Hill; 2022.
2. Amato AA. Neuromuscular junction disorders. In: Fauci AS, Braunwald E, Kasper DJ, et al., eds. *Harrison's Principles of Internal Medicine*. McGraw Hill; 2022.
3. Greenberg SA, Amato AA. Inflammatory myopathies. In: Fauci AS, Braunwald E, Kasper DJ, et al., eds. *Harrison's Principles of Internal Medicine*. McGraw Hill; 2022.
4. Van den Bergh PYK, van Doorn PA, Hadden RDM, et al. European Academy of Neurology/Peripheral Nerve Society guideline on diagnosis and treatment of chronic inflammatory demyelinating polyradiculoneuropathy: report of a joint Task Force-Second revision. *J Peripher Nerv Syst*. 2021;26: 242–268.
5. Stino AM, Naddaf E, Dyck PJ, Dyck PJB. Chronic inflammatory demyelinating polyradiculoneuropathy—Diagnostic pitfalls and treatment approach. *Muscle Nerve*. 2021;63:157–169.
6. Gwathmey KG, Smith AG. Immune-mediated neuropathies. *Neurol Clin*. 2020;38(3):711–735.
7. Koike H, Nishi R, Ohyama K, et al. ANCA-associated vasculitic neuropathies: a review. *Neurol Ther*. 2022;11:21–38.
8. Oaklander AL, Lunn MP, Hughes RA, van Schaik IN, Frost C, Chalk CH. Treatments for chronic inflammatory demyelinating polyradiculoneuropathy (CIDP): an overview of systematic reviews. *Cochrane Database Syst Rev*. 2017;1:CD010369.

9. Narayanaswami P, Sanders DB, Wolfe G, et al. International Consensus Guidance for Management of Myasthenia Gravis: 2020 Update. *Neurology*. 2021;96(3):114–122.
10. Tannemaat MR, Verschuuren JJGM. Emerging therapies for autoimmune myasthenia gravis: towards treatment without corticosteroids. *Neuromuscul Disord*. 2020;30(2):111–119.
11. McGrath EM, Doughty CT, Amato AA. Autoimmune myopathies: an update on classification and treatment modalities. *Neurotherapeutics*. 2018;15:976–994.
12. Oddis CV, Aggarwal R. Treatment in myositis. *Nat Rev Rheumatol*. 2018;14:279–289.
13. Pipitone N, Salvarani C. Up-to-date treatment and management of myositis. *Curr Opin Rheumatol*. 2020;32(6):523–527.
14. Claytor B, Li Y. Opinions on Pneumocystis jirovecii prophylaxis in autoimmune neuromuscular disorders. *Muscle Nerve*. 2022;65:278–283.
15. Horsburgh CR Jr, Rubin EJ. Latent tuberculosis infection in the United States. *N Engl J Med*. 2011;364:1441–1448.
16. Zaheer F, Berger JR. Treatment-related progressive multifocal leukoencephalopathy: current understanding and future steps. *Ther Adv Drug Safe*. 2012;3:227–239.
17. Takao M. Targeted therapy and progressive multifocal leukoencephalopathy (PML): PML in the era of monoclonal antibody therapies. *Brain Nerve*. 2013;65:1363–1374.
18. Mitka M. FDA: increased HBV reactivation risk with ofatumumab or rituximab. *JAMA*. 2013;16;1664.
19. Smalls DJ, Kiger RE, Norris LB, Bennett CL, Love BL. Hepatitis B virus reactivation: risk factors and current management strategies. *Pharmacotherapy*. 2019;39(12):1190–1203.
20. Dysart C, Rozenberg-Ben-Dror K, Sales M. Assessing Hepatitis B reactivation risk with rituximab and recent intravenous immunoglobulin therapy. *Open Forum Infect Dis*. 2020;7(3):ofaa080.
21. Lu H, Lok AS, Warneke CL, et al. Passive transfer of anti-HBc after intravenous immunoglobulin administration in patients with cancer: a retrospective chart review. *Lancet Haematol*. 2018;5(10):e474–e478.
22. Basile A, Simzar S, Bentow J, et al. Disseminated Strongyloides stercoralis: hyperinfection during medical immunosuppression. *J Am Acad Derm*. 2010;63:896–902.
23. Santiago M, Leitão B. Prevention of strongyloides hyperinfection syndrome: a rheumatological point of view. *Eur J Intern Med*. 2009;20:744–788.
24. Iriemenam NC, Sanyaolu AO, Oyibo WA, Fagbenro-Beyioku AF. Strongyloides stercoralis and the immune response. *Parasitol Int*. 2010;59:9–14.
25. Rahier KF, Moutschen M, Van Gompel A, et al. Vaccinations in patients with immune-mediated inflammatory diseases. *Rheumatology (Oxford)*. 2010;49:1815–1827.
26. Furer V, Eviatar T, Zisman D, et al. Immunogenicity and safety of the BNT162b2 mRNA COVID-19 vaccine in adult patients with autoimmune inflammatory rheumatic diseases and in the general population: a multicentre study. *Ann Rheum Dis*. 2021;80:1330–1338.
27. Bitoun S, Henry J, Desjardins D, et al. Rituximab impairs B-cell response but not T-cell response to COVID-19 vaccine in auto-immune diseases. *Arthritis Rheumatol*. 2022;74(6):927–933.
28. Kornek B, Leutmezer F, Rommer PS, et al. B cell depletion and SARS-CoV-2 vaccine responses in neuroimmunologic patients. *Ann Neurol*. 2022;91:342–352.
29. Gutierrez-Dalmau A, Campistol JM. Immunosuppressive therapy and malignancy in organ transplant recipients: a systematic review. *Drugs*. 2007;67(8):1167–1198.
30. Dahlke E, Murray CA, Kitchen J, Chan AW. Systematic review of melanoma incidence and prognosis in solid organ transplant recipients. *Transplant Res*. 2014;3:10.
31. Bromberg MB, Carter O. Corticosteroid use in the treatment of neuromuscular disorders: empirical and evidence-based data. *Muscle Nerve*. 2004;30:20–37.
32. Miller RG, Milner-Brown HS, Mirka A. Prednisone-induced worsening of neuromuscular function in myasthenia gravis. *Neurology*. 1986;36:729–732.
33. Panegyres PK, Squire M, Mills KR, Newsom-Davis J. Acute myopathy associated with large parenteral dose of corticosteroid in myasthenia gravis. *J Neurol Neurosurg Psychiatry*. 1993;56:702–704.
34. Hughes RA, Mehndiratta MM. Corticosteroids for chronic inflammatory demyelinating polyradiculoneuropathy. *Cochrane Database Syst Rev*. 2012;8:CD002062.
35. Mahdi-Rogers M, van Doorn PA, Hughes RA. Immunomodulatory treatment other than corticosteroids, immunoglobulin and plasma exchange for chronic inflammatory demyelinating polyradiculoneuropathy. *Cochrane Database Syst Rev*. 2013;6:CD003280.
36. Nobile-Orazio E. Chronic inflammatory demyelinating polyradiculoneuropathy and variants: where we are and where we should go. *J Peripher Nerve Syst*. 2014;19(1):2–13.
37. Viala K, Renié L, Maisonobe T, et al. Follow-up study and response to treatment in 23 patients with Lewis-Sumner syndrome. *Brain*. 2004;127:2010–2017.
38. Katz JS, Saperstein DS, Gronseth G, Amato AA, Barohn RJ. Distal acquired demyelinating symmetric neuropathy. *Neurology*. 2000;54:615–620.
39. van Schaik IN, Eftimov F, van Doorn PA, et al. Pulsed high-dose dexamethasone versus standard prednisolone treatment for chronic inflammatory demyelinating polyradiculoneuropathy (PREDICT study): a double-blind, randomised, controlled trial. *Lancet Neurol*. 2010;9(3):245–253.
40. Joffe MM, Love LA, Leff RL, et al. Drug therapy of the idiopathic inflammatory myopathies: predictors of response to prednisone, azathioprine, and methotrexate and a comparison of their efficacy. *Am J Med*. 1993;94:379–387.
41. Collins MP, Dyck PJB, Gronseth GS, et al; Peripheral Nerve Society. Peripheral Nerve Society guideline on the classification, diagnosis, investigation, and immunosuppressive therapy of non-systemic vasculitic neuropathy: executive summary. *J Periph Nerv Syst*. 2010;15:176–184.
42. Jones RB, Tervaert JWC, Hauser T, et al; European Vasculitis Study Group. Rituximab versus cyclophosphamide in ANCA-associated renal vasculitis. *N Engl J Med*. 2010;363(3):211–220.
43. Stone JH, Merkel PA, Spiera R, et al; RAVE-ITN Research Group. Rituximab versus cyclophosphamide for ANCA-associated vasculitis. *N Engl J Med*. 2010;363:221–232.
44. Burns TM, Dyck PJB, Aksamit AJ, Dyck PJ. The natural history and long-term outcome of 57 limb sarcoidosis neuropathy cases. *J Neurol Sci*. 2006;244:77–87.
45. van Eijk JJ, van Alfen N, Berrevoets M, van der Wilt GJ, Pillen S, van Engelen BGM. Evaluation of prednisolone treatment in the acute phase of neuralgic amyotrophy: an observational study. *J Neurol Neurosurg Psychiatry*. 2009;80:1120–1124.

46. Rothman MS, West SG, McDermott MT. Osteoporosis for the practicing neurologists. *Neurol Clin Pract.* 2014;4:34–43.
47. Kissel JT, Levy RJ, Mendell JR, Griggs RC. Azathioprine toxicity in neuromuscular disease. *Neurology.* 1986;36:35–39.
48. Hohlfeld R, Michels M, Heininger K, Besinger U, Toyka KV. Azathioprine toxicity during long-term immunosuppression of generalized myasthenia gravis. *Neurology.* 1988;38:258–261.
49. A randomized clinical trial comparing prednisone and azathioprine in myasthenia gravis. Results of the second interim analysis. Myasthenia Gravis Clinical Study Group. *J Neurol Neurosurg Psychiatry.* 1993;56:1157–1163.
50. Bromberg MB, Wald JJ, Forshew DA, Feldman EL, Albers JW. Randomized trial of azathioprine or prednisone for initial immunosuppressive treatment of myasthenia. *J Neurol Sci.* 1997; 150:59–62.
51. Palace J, Newsom-Davis J, Lecky B. A randomized double-blind trial of prednisolone alone or with azathioprine in myasthenia gravis. *Neurology.* 1998;50:1778–1783.
52. Bunch TW, Worthington JW, Combs JJ, Ilstrup DM, Engel AG. Azathioprine with prednisone for polymyositis. A controlled, clinical trial. *Ann Intern Med.* 1980;92(3):365–369.
53. Casajús A, Zubiaur P, Méndez M, Campodónico D, et al. Genotype-guided prescription of azathioprine reduces the incidence of adverse drug reactions in TPMT intermediate metabolizers to a similar incidence as normal metabolizers. *Adv Ther.* 2022;39(4):1743–1753.
54. Metzger AL, Bohan A, Goldberg LS, Bluestone R, Pearson CM. Polymyositis and dermatomyositis: combined methotrexate and corticosteroid therapy. *Ann Intern Med.* 1974;81:182–189.
55. Miller LC, Sisson BA, Tucker LB, DeNardo BA, Schaller JG. Methotrexate treatment of recalcitrant childhood dermatomyositis. *Arthritis Rheum.* 1992; 35:1143–1149.
56. Villalba L, Hicks JE, Adams EM, et al. Treatment of refractory myositis: a randomized crossover study of two new cytotoxic regimens. *Arthritis Rheum.* 1998;41:392–399.
57. Grable-Esposito P, Katzberg HD, Greenberg SA, Srinivasan J, Katz J, Amato AA. Immune-mediated necrotizing myopathy associated with statins. *Muscle Nerve.* 2010;41:185–190.
58. Visser K, van der Heijde DMFM. Risk and management of liver toxicity during methotrexate treatment in rheumatoid and psoriatic arthritis: a systematic review of the literature. *Clin Exp Rheumatol.* 2009;27:1017–1025.
59. Meriggioli MN, Rowin J, Richman JG, Leurgans S. Mycophenolate mofetil for myasthenia gravis: a double-blind, placebo-controlled pilot study. *Ann N Y Acad Sci.* 2003;998:494–499.
60. Meriggioli MN, Ciafaloni E, Al-Hayk KA, et al. Mycophenolate mofetil for myasthenia gravis: an analysis of efficacy, safety, and tolerability. *Neurology.* 2003;61:1438–1440.
61. Salari N, Fatahi B, Bartina Y, et al. Global prevalence of myasthenia gravis and the effectiveness of common drugs in its treatment: a systematic review and meta-analysis. *J Transl Med.* 2021;19:516.
62. Hehir MK, Burns TM, Alpers J, Conaway MR, Sawa M, Sanders DB. Mycophenolate mofetil in AChR-antibody-positive myasthenia gravis: outcomes in 102 patients. *Muscle Nerve.* 2010; 41:593–598.
63. The Muscle Study Group. A trial of mycophenolate mofetil with prednisone as initial immunotherapy in myasthenia gravis. *Neurology.* 2008;71:394–399.
64. Sanders DB, Hart IK, Mantegazza R, et al. An international, phase III, randomized trial of mycophenolate mofetil in myasthenia gravis. *Neurology.* 2008;71:400–406.
65. Gorson KC, Amato AA, Ropper AH. Efficacy of mycophenolate mofetil in patients with chronic immune demyelinating polyneuropathy. *Neurology.* 2004;63:715–717.
66. Radziwill AJ, Schweikert K, Kuntzer T, Fuhr P, Steck AJ. Mycophenolate mofetil for chronic inflammatory demyelinating polyradiculoneuropathy: an open label study. *Eur J Neurol.* 2006;56:37–38.
67. Bedi G, Brown A, Tong T, Sharma KR. Chronic inflammatory demyelinating polyneuropathy responsive to mycophenolate mofetil therapy. *J Neurol Neurosurg Psychiatry.* 2010;81:634–636.
68. Dubal DB, Mueller S, Ruben BS, Engstrom JW, Josephson SA. T-cell lymphoproliferative disorder following mycophenolate treatment for myasthenia gravis. *Muscle Nerve.* 2009;39:849–850.
69. Ciafaloni E, Nikhar NK, Massey JM, Sanders DB. Retrospective analysis of the use of cyclosporine in myasthenia gravis. *Neurology.* 2000;55:448–450.
70. Tindall RS, Rollins JA, Phillips JT, Greenlee RG, Wells L, Belendiuk G. Preliminary results of a double-blind, randomized, placebo-controlled trial of cyclosporine in myasthenia gravis. *N Engl J Med.* 1987;316:719–724.
71. Tindall RS, Phillips JT, Rollins JA, Wells L, Hall K. A clinical therapeutic trial of cyclosporine in myasthenia gravis. *Ann N Y Acad Sci.* 1993;681:539–551.
72. Ponseti JM, Azem J, Fort JM, et al. Long-term results of tacrolimus in cyclosporine- and prednisone-dependent myasthenia gravis. *Neurology.* 2005;64:1641–1643.
73. Barnett MH, Pollard JD, Davies L, McLeod JG. Cyclosporin A in resistant chronic inflammatory demyelinating polyradiculoneuropathy. *Muscle Nerve.* 1998;21:454–460.
74. Mahattanakul W, Crawford TO, Griffin JW, Goldstein JM, Cornblath DR. Treatment of chronic inflammatory demyelinating polyneuropathy with cyclosporin-A. *J Neurol Neurosurg Psychiatry.* 1996;60:185–187.
75. Matsuda M, Hoshi K, Gono T, Morita H, Ikeda S. Cyclosporin A in treatment of refractory patients with chronic inflammatory demyelinating polyradiculoneuropathy. *J Neurol Sci.* 2004;224:29–35.
76. Odaka M, Tatsumoto M, Susuki K, Hirata K, Yuki N. Intractable chronic inflammatory demyelinating polyneuropathy treated successfully with ciclosporin. *J Neurol Neurosurg Psychiatry.* 2005;76:1115–1120.
77. Heckmatt J, Hasson N, Saunders C, et al. Cyclosporin in juvenile dermatomyositis. *Lancet.* 1989;1:1063–1066.
78. Lueck CJ, Trend P, Swash M. Cyclosporin in the management of polymyositis and dermatomyositis. *J Neurol Neurosurg Psychiatry.* 1991;54:1007–1008.
79. Pistoia V, Buoncompagni A, Scribanis R, et al. Cyclosporin A in the treatment of juvenile chronic arthritis and childhood polymyositis-dermatomyositis. Results of a preliminary study. *Clin Exp Rheumatol.* 1993;11:203–208.
80. Schneider-Gold C, Hartung HP, Gold R. Mycophenolate mofetil and tacrolimus: new therapeutic options in neuroimmunological diseases. *Muscle Nerve.* 2006;34:284–291.
81. Yoshikawa H, Kiuchi T, Saida T, Takamori M. Randomised double blind, placebo controlled study of tacrolimus in myasthenia gravis. *J Neurol Neurosurg Psychiatry.* 2011;82:970–977.
82. Ponseti JM, Gamez J, Azem J, et al. Post-thymectomy combined treatment of prednisone and tacrolimus versus prednisone alone for the consolidation of complete stable remission in patients with myasthenia gravis: a non-randomized, non-controlled study. *Curr Med Res Opin.* 2007;23:1269–1278.

83. Ponseti JM, Gamez J, Azem J, López-Cano M, Vilallonga R, Armengol M. Tacrolimus for myasthenia gravis: a clinical study of 212 patients. *Ann N Y Acad Sci.* 2008;1132:254–263.
84. Evoli A, Di Schino C, Marsili F, Punzi C. Successful treatment of myasthenia gravis with tacrolimus. *Muscle Nerve.* 2002;25:111–114.
85. Tada M, Shimohata T, Tada M, et al. Long-term therapeutic efficacy and safety of low-dose tacrolimus (FK506) for myasthenia gravis. *J Neurol Sci.* 2006;247:17–20.
86. Adu D, Pall A, Luqmani RA, et al. Controlled trial of pulse versus continuous prednisolone and cyclophosphamide in the treatment of vasculitis. *QJM.* 1997;90:401–409.
87. Guillevin L, Cordier JF, Lhote F, et al. A prospective, multicenter, randomized trial comparing steroids and pulse cyclophosphamide versus steroids and oral cyclophosphamide in the treatment of generalized Wegener's granulomatosis. *Arthritis Rheum.* 1997;40(12):2187–2198.
88. Brannagan TH 3rd, Pradhan A, Heiman-Patterson T, et al. High-dose cyclophosphamide without stem-cell rescue for refractory CIDP. *Neurology.* 2002;58:1856–1858.
89. Good JL, Chehrenama M, Mayer RF, Koski CL. Pulse cyclophosphamide therapy in chronic inflammatory demyelinating polyneuropathy. *Neurology.* 1998;51:1735–1738.
90. Gladstone DE, Prestrud AA, Brannagan TH 3rd. High-dose cyclophosphamide results in long-term disease remission with restoration of a normal quality of life in patients with severe refractory chronic inflammatory demyelinating polyneuropathy. *J Peripher Nerv Syst.* 2005;10:11–16.
91. Leitch MM, Sherman WH, Brannagan TH 3rd. Distal acquired demyelinating symmetric polyneuropathy progressing to classic chronic inflammatory demyelinating polyneuropathy and response to fludarabine and cyclophosphamide. *Muscle Nerve.* 2013;47:292–296.
92. Pestronk A, Cornblath DR, Ilyas A, et al. A treatable multifocal motor neuropathy with antibodies to GM1 ganglioside. *Ann Neurol.* 1988;24:73–78.
93. Drachman DB, Jones RJ, Brodsky RA. Treatment of refractory myasthenia: "Rebooting" with high-dose cyclophosphamide. *Ann Neurol.* 2003;53:29–34.
94. Lin PT, Martin BA, Winacker AB, So YT. High-dose cyclophosphamide in refractory myasthenia with MuSK antibodies. *Muscle Nerve.* 2006;33:433–435.
95. Nagappa M, Netravathi M, Taly AB, Sinha S, Bindu PS, Mahadevan A. Long-term efficacy and limitations of cyclophosphamide in myasthenia gravis. *J Clin Neurosci.* 2014;21:1909–1914.
96. Lünemann JD, Quast I, Dalakas MC. Efficacy of intravenous immunoglobulin in neurological diseases. *Neurotherapeutics.* 2016;13:34–46.
97. Patwa HS, Chaudhry H. Katzberg H, Rae-Grant AD, So YT. Evidence-based guideline: Intravenous immunoglobulin in the treatment of neuromuscular disorders: report of the Therapeutics and Technology Assessment Subcommittee of the American Academy of Neurology. *Neurology.* 2012;78:1009–1015.
98. Hughes RA, Swan AV, van Doorn PA. Intravenous immunoglobulin for Guillain-Barré syndrome. *Cochrane Database Syst Rev.* 2012;(7):CD002063.
99. Hughes RA, Donofrio P, Bril V, et al; ICE Study Group. Intravenous immune globulin (10% caprylate-chromatography purified) for the treatment of chronic inflammatory demyelinating polyradiculoneuropathy (ICE study): a randomized placebo-controlled trial. *Lancet Neurol.* 2008;7.
100. Hahn AF, Bolton CF, Zochodne DW, Feasby TE. Intravenous immunoglobulin treatment in chronic inflammatory demyelinating polyneuropathy. A double blind, placebo controlled, cross-over study. *Brain.* 1996;119:1067–1077.
101. Hughes RA, Bensa S, Willison H, et al; Inflammatory Neuropathy Cause and Treatment (INCAT) Group. Randomized controlled trial of intravenous gammaglobulin vs oral prednisolone in chronic inflammatory demyelinating polyradiculoneuropathy. *Ann Neurol.* 2001;50:195–201.
102. Mendell JR, Barohn RJ, Freimer ML, et al; Working Group on Peripheral Neuropathy. Randomized controlled trial of IVIG in untreated chronic inflammatory demyelinating polyradiculoneuropathy. *Neurology.* 2001;56:445–449.
103. Van Schaik I, Winer JB, De Haan R, Vermeulen M. Intravenous immunoglobulins for chronic inflammatory demyelinating polyradiculoneuropathy. *Cochrane Database Syst Rev.* 2002;(2):CD001797.
104. Eftimov F, Winer JB, Vermeulen M, de Haan R, van Schaik IN. Intravenous immunoglobulin for chronic inflammatory demyelinating polyradiculoneuropathy. *Cochrane Database Syst Rev.* 2013;(12):CD001797.
105. Federico P, Zochodne DW, Hahn AF, Brown WF, Feasby TE. Multifocal motor neuropathy improved by IVIG: randomized, double-blind, placebo-controlled study. *Neurology.* 2000;55:1256–1262.
106. Leger JM, Chassande B, Musset L, Meininger V, Bouche P, Baumann N. Intravenous immunoglobulin therapy in multifocal motor neuropathy: a double-blind, placebo-controlled study. *Brain.* 2001;124:145–153.
107. van Schaik IN, van den Berg LH, de Haan R, Vermeulen M. Intravenous immunoglobulin for multifocal motor neuropathy. *Cochrane Database Syst Rev.* 2005;18:CD004429.
108. Joint Task Force of the EFNS and the PNS. European Federation of Neurological Societies/Peripheral Nerve Society Guideline on management of multifocal motor neuropathy. Report of a Joint Task Force of the European Federation of Neurological Societies and the Peripheral Nerve Society—first revision. *J Peripher Nerv Syst.* 2010;15:295–301.
109. Nobile-Orazio E, Meucci N, Barbieri S, Carpo M, Scarlato G. High-dose intravenous immunoglobulin therapy in multifocal motor neuropathy. *Neurology.* 1993;43:537–544.
110. Keddie S, Eftimov F, van den Berg LH, Brassington R, de Haan RJ, van Schaik IN. Immunoglobulin for multifocal motor neuropathy. *Cochrane Database Syst Rev.* 2022;1:CD004429.
111. Zinman L, Ng E, Bril V. IV Immunoglobulin in patients with myasthenia gravis: a randomized controlled trial. *Neurology.* 2007;68:837–841.
112. Gajdos P, Chevret S, Clair B, Tranchant C, Chastang C. Clinical trial of plasma exchange and high-dose intravenous immunoglobulin in myasthenia gravis. Myasthenia Gravis Clinical Study Group. *Ann Neurol.* 1997;41:789–796.
113. Gajdos P, Tranchant C, Clair B, et al; Myasthenia Gravis Clinical Study Group. Treatment of myasthenia gravis exacerbation with intravenous immunoglobulin: a randomized double-blind clinical trial. *Arch Neurol.* 2005;62:1689–1693.
114. Bain PG, Motomura M, Newsom-Davis J, et al. Effects of intravenous immunoglobulin on muscle weakness and calcium-channel autoantibodies in the Lambert-Eaton myasthenic syndrome. *Neurology.* 1996;47:678–683.

115. Wang DX, Shu XM, Tian XL, et al. Intravenous immunoglobulin therapy in adult patients with polymyositis/dermatomyositis: a systematic literature review. *Clin Rheumatol.* 2012;31:801–806.
116. Dalakas MC, Fujii M, Li M, Lufti B, Kyhos J, McElroy B. High-dose intravenous immune globulin for stiff-person syndrome. *N Engl J Med.* 2001;345:1870–1876.
117. Takahashi Y, Takata T, Hoshino M, Sakurai M, Kanazawa I. Benefit of IVIG for long-standing ataxic sensory neuronopathy with Sjögren's syndrome. IV immunoglobulin. *Neurology.* 2003;60:503–505.
118. Wolfe GI, Nations SP, Burns DK, Herbelin LL, Barohn RJ. Benefit of IVIG for long-standing ataxic sensory neuronopathy with Sjögren's syndrome. *Neurology.* 2003;61:873.
119. Burns TM, Quijano-Roy S, Jones HR. Benefit of IVIG for long-standing ataxic sensory neuronopathy with Sjögren's syndrome. *Neurology.* 2003;61:873.
120. Dalakas M, Illa I, Dambrosia J, et al. A controlled trial of high-dose intravenous immune globulin infusions as treatment for dermatomyositis. *N Engl J Med.* 1993;329:1993–2000.
121. Aggarwal R, Charles-Schoeman C, Schessl J, Dimachkie MM, Beckmann I, Levine T. Prospective, double-blind, randomized, placebo-controlled phase III study evaluating efficacy and safety of octagam 10% in patients with dermatomyositis ("ProDERM Study"). *Medicine (Baltimore).* 2021;100:e2367.
122. Mammen AL, Tiniakou E. Intravenous immune globulin for statin-triggered autoimmune myopathy. *N Engl J Med.* 2015;373:1680–1682.
123. Allenbach Y, Mammen AL, Benveniste O, Stenzel W; Immune-Mediated Necrotizing Myopathies Working Group. 224th ENMC International Workshop: Clinico-sero-pathological classification of immune-mediated necrotizing myopathies Zandvoort, The Netherlands, 14–16 October 2016. *Neuromuscul Disord.* 2018;28:87–99.
124. Barth D, Nabavi NM, Ng E, New P, Bril V. Comparison of IVIg and PLEX in patients with myasthenia gravis. *Neurology.* 2011;76:2017–2023.
125. Qureshi AI, Choudhry MA, Akbar MS, et al. Plasma exchange versus intravenous immunoglobulin treatment in myasthenic crisis. *Neurology.* 1999;52:629–632.
126. Markvardsen LH, Debost JC, Harbo T, et al; Danish CIDP and MMN Study Group. Subcutaneous immunoglobulin in responders to intravenous therapy with chronic inflammatory demyelinating polyradiculoneuropathy. *Eur J Neurol.* 2013;20:836–842.
127. Markvardsen LH, Harbo T, Sindrup SH, Christiansen I, Andersen H, Jakobsen J; The Danish CIDP and MMN Study Group. Subcutaneous immunoglobulin preserves muscle strength in chronic inflammatory demyelinating polyneuropathy. *Eur J Neurol.* 2014;21:1465–1470.
128. Markvardsen LH, Sindrup SH, Christiansen I, Olsen NK, Jakobsen J, Andersen H; Danish CIDP and MMN Study Group. Subcutaneous immunoglobulin as first-line therapy in treatment-naive patients with chronic inflammatory demyelinating polyneuropathy: randomized controlled trial study. *Eur J Neurol.* 2017;24:412–418.
129. van Schaik IN, Bril V, van Geloven N, et al; PATH Study Group. Subcutaneous immunoglobulin for maintenance treatment in chronic inflammatory demyelinating polyneuropathy (PATH): a randomised, double-blind, placebocontrolled, phase 3 trial. *Lancet Neurol.* 2018;17:35–46.
130. van Schaik IN, Mielke O, Bril V, et al; PATH Study Group. Long-term safety and efficacy of subcutaneous immunoglobulin IgPro20 in CIDP: PATH extension study. *Neurol Neuroimmunol Neuroinflammation.* 2019;6(5):e590.
131. Goyal NA, Karam C, Sheikh KA, Dimachkie MM. Subcutaneous immunoglobulin treatment for chronic inflammatory demyelinating polyneuropathy. *Muscle Nerve.* 2021;64:243–254.
132. Al-Zuhairy A, Jakobsen J, Andersen H, Sindrup SH, Markvardsen LK. Randomized trial of facilitated subcutaneous immunoglobulin in multifocal motor neuropathy. *Eur J Neurol.* 2019;26:1289–e82.
133. Al-Zuhairy A, Sindrup SH, Jakobsen J. Long-term follow-up of facilitated subcutaneous immunoglobulin therapy in multifocal motor neuropathy. *J Neurol Sci.* 2021;427:117495.
134. Adiao KJB, Espiritu AI, Roque VLA, Reyes JPBT. Efficacy and tolerability of subcutaneously administered immunoglobulin in myasthenia gravis: a systematic review. *J Clin Neurosci.* 2020;72:316–321.
135. Kovács E, Dankó K, Nagy-Vince M, Csiba L, Boczán J. Long-term treatment of refractory myasthenia gravis with subcutaneous immunoglobulin. *Ther Adv Neurol Disord.* 2017;10:363–366.
136. Yoon MS, Gold R, Kerasnoudis A. Subcutaneous immunoglobulin in treating inflammatory neuromuscular disorders. *Ther Adv Neurol Disord.* 2015;8:153–159.
137. Beecher G, Anderson D, Siddiqi ZA. Subcutaneous immunoglobulin in myasthenia gravis exacerbation: a prospective, open-label trial. *Neurology.* 2017;89:1135–1141.
138. Bourque PR, Pringle CE, Cameron W, Cowan J, Chardon JW. Subcutaneous immunoglobulin therapy in the chronic management of myasthenia gravis: a retrospective cohort study. *PLoS One.* 2016;11:e0159993.
139. Garnero M, Fabbri S, Gemelli C, et al. Subcutaneous immunoglobulins are a valuable treatment option in myasthenia gravis. *J Clin Neurol.* 2018;14:98–99.
140. Zuppa A, De Michelis C, Meo G, et al. Maintenance treatment with subcutaneous immunoglobulins in the long-term management of anti-HMCGR myopathy. *Neuromuscul Disord.* 2021;31:134–138.
141. Goswami RP, Haldar SN, Chatterjee M, et al. Efficacy and safety of intravenous and subcutaneous immunoglobulin therapy in idiopathic inflammatory myopathy: a systematic review and meta-analysis. *Autoimmun Rev.* 2022;21:102997.
142. Collongues N, Casez O, Lacour A, et al. Rituximab in refractory and non-refractory myasthenia: a retrospective multicenter study. *Muscle Nerve.* 2012;46:687–691.
143. Steiglbauer K, Topakian R, Schäffer G, Aichner FT. Rituximab for myasthenia gravis: three case reports and review of the literature. *J Neurol Sci.* 2009;280:120–122.
144. Nowak RJ, Coffey CS, Goldstein JM, et al; NeuroNEXT NN103 BeatMG Study Team. Phase 2 trial of rituximab in acetylcholine receptor antibody-positive generalized myasthenia gravis: the BeatMG study. *Neurology.* 2021;98:e376–e389.
145. Piehl F, Eriksson-Dufva A, Budzianowska A, et al. Efficacy and Safety of Rituximab for New-Onset Generalized Myasthenia Gravis: The RINOMAX Randomized Clinical Trial. *JAMA Neurol.* 2022;79(11):1105–1112.
146. Baek WS, Bashey A, Sheean GL. Complete remission induced by rituximab in refractory, seronegative, muscle-specific kinase positive myasthenia gravis. *J Neurol Neurosurg Psychiatry.* 2007;78(7):771.

147. Díaz-Manera J, Martínez-Hernández E, Querol L, et al. Long-lasting treatment effect of rituximab in MuSK myasthenia. *Neurology*. 2012;78:189–193.
148. Hain B, Jordan K, Deschauer M, Zierz S. Successful treatment of MuSK antibody-positive myasthenia gravis with rituximab. *Muscle Nerve*. 2006;33(4):575–580.
149. Hehir MK, Hobson-Webb LD, Benatar M, et al. Rituximab as treatment for anti-MuSK myasthenia gravis: multicenter blinded prospective review. *Neurology*. 2017;89:1069–1077.
150. Dalakas MC, Rakocevic G, Salagegheh M, et al. Placebo-controlled trial of rituximab in IgM anti-myelin associated glycoprotein antibody demyelinating neuropathy. *Ann Neurol*. 2009;65:286–293.
151. Léger JM, Viala K, Nicolas G, et al; RIMAG Study Group (France and Switzerland). Placebo-controlled trial of rituximab in IgM anti-myelin associated glycoprotein neuropathy. *Neurology*. 2013;80(24):2217–2225.
152. Gorson KC, Natarajan N, Ropper AH, Weinstein R. Rituximab treatment in patients with IVIg-dependent immune polyneuropathy: a prospective pilot trial. *Muscle Nerve*. 2007;35:66–69.
153. Hu J, Sun C, Lu J, Zhao C, Lin J. Efficacy of ritixmab treatment in chronic inflammatory demyelinating polyradiculoneuropathy: a systematic review and meta-analysis. *J Neurol*. 2022;269:1250–1263.
154. Benedetti L, Briani C, Franciotta D, et al. Rituximab in patients with chronic inflammatory demyelinating polyradiculoneuropathy: a report of 13 cases and review of the literature. *J Neurol Neurosurg Psychiatry*. 2011;82:306–308.
155. Oddis CV, Reed AM, Aggarwal R, et al; RIM Study Group. Rituximab in the treatment of refractory adult and juvenile dermatomyositis and adult polymyositis: a randomized, placebo-phase trial. *Arthritis Rheum*. 2013;65:314–324.
156. Valiyil R, Casciola-Rosen L, Hong G, Mammen A, Christopher-Stine L. Rituximab therapy for myopathy associated with anti-signal recognition particle antibodies: a case series. *Arthritis Care Res (Hoboken)*. 2010;62(9):1328–1334.
157. Baker MR, Das M, Isaacs J, Fawcett PRW, Bates D. Treatment of stiff person syndrome with rituximab. *J Neurol Neurosurg Psychiatry*. 2005;76:999–1001.
158. Dupond JL, Essalmi L, Gil H, Meaux-Ruault N, Hafsaoui C. Rituximab treatment of stiff-person syndrome in a patient with thymoma, diabetes mellitus and autoimmune thyroiditis. *J Clin Neurosci*. 2010;17:389–391.
159. Howard JF Jr, Barohn RJ, Cutter GR, et al; MG Study Group. A randomized, double-blind, placebo-controlled phase II study of eculizumab in patients with refractory generalized myasthenia gravis. *Muscle Nerve*. 2013;48:76–84.
160. Mantegazza R, Wolfe GI, Muppidi S, et al; REGAIN Study Group. Post-intervention status in patients with refractory myasthenia gravis treated with eculizumab during REGAIN and its open-label extension. *Neurology*. 2021;96:e610–e618.
161. Howard JF Jr, Bril V, Vu T, et al, ADAPT Investigator Study Group. Safety, efficacy, and tolerability of efgartigimod in patients with generalised myasthenia gravis (ADAPT): a multicentre, randomised, placebo-controlled, phase 3 trial. *Lancet Neurol*. 2021;20:526–536.
162. Howard JF Jr, Bril V, Burns TM, et al; Efgartigimod MG Study Group. Randomized phase 2 study of FcRn antagonist efgartigimod in generalized myasthenia gravis. *Neurology*. 2019;92:e2661–e2673.
163. Sorgun MH, Erdogan S, Bay M, et al. Therapeutic plasma exchange in treatment of neuroimmunologic disorders: review of 92 cases. *Transfus Apher Sci*. 2013;49:174–180.
164. Cortese I, Chaudhry V, So YT, Cantor F, Cornblath DR, Rae-Grant A. Evidence-based guideline update: plasmapheresis in neurologic disorders: report of the Therapeutics and Technology Assessment Subcommittee of the American Academy of Neurology. *Neurology*. 2011;76:294–300.
165. Plasma Exchange/Sandoglobulin Guillain-Barre Syndrome Trial Group. Randomized trial of plasma exchange, intravenous immunoglobulin, and combined treatments in Guillain-Barré syndrome. *Lancet*. 1997;349:225–230.
166. Chevret S, Hughes RA, Annane D. Plasma exchange for Guillain-Barré syndrome. *Cochrane Database Syst Rev*. 2017;2: CD001798.
167. Dyck PJ, Litchy WJ, Kratz KM, et al. A plasma exchange versus immune globulin infusion trial in chronic inflammatory demyelinating polyradiculoneuropathy. *Ann Neurol*. 1994; 36:838–845.
168. Mehndiratta MM, Hughes RAC. Plasma exchange for chronic inflammatory demyelinating polyradiculoneuropathy. *Cochrane Database Syst Rev*. 2012;9:CD003906.
169. Dau PC, Lindstrom JM, Cassel CK, Denys EH, Shev EE, Spitler LE. Plasmapheresis and immunosuppressive drug therapy in myasthenia gravis. *N Engl J Med*. 1977;297:1134–1140.
170. Guptill JT, Oakley D, Kuchibhatla M, et al. A retrospective study of complications of therapeutic plasma exchange in myasthenia. *Muscle Nerve*. 2013;47:170–176.
171. Moghadam-Kia S, Charlton D, Aggarwal R, Oddis CV. Management of refractory cutaneous dermatomyositis: potential role of Janus kinase inhibition with tofacitinib. *Rheumatology (Oxford)*. 2019;58:1011–1015.
172. Sabbagh S, Almeida de Jesus A, Hwang S, et al. Treatment of anti-MDA5 autoantibody-positive juvenile dermatomyositis using tofacitinib. *Brain*. 2019;142:e59.
173. Le Voyer T, Gitiaux C, Authier FJ, et al. JAK inhibitors are effective in a subset of patients with juvenile dermatomyositis: a monocentric retrospective study. *Rheumatology (Oxford)*. 2021;60:5801–5808.
174. Ladislau L, Suárez-Calvet X, Toquet S, et al. JAK inhibitor improves type I interferon induced damage: proof of concept in dermatomyositis. *Brain*. 2018;141:1609–1621.

CHAPTER 5

Rehabilitation for People with Neuromuscular Disease

Sabrina Paganoni and Erik Ensrud

Rehabilitation is the process of assisting a person to maximize function and quality of life. Therefore, rehabilitation matters to people with neuromuscular diseases because it enables them to reach their fullest potential despite the presence of a disability. Too often, patients are told "there is nothing we can do" for their neuromuscular conditions. At times, this judgment is not expressed explicitly but transpires from nonverbal cues during patient encounters. Such attitudes cast a dark shadow on the therapeutic alliance between the physician and the patient and lead to disengagement and lower quality of care. On the contrary, here we will argue that "there is always something we can do" for our patients. While there are no life-prolonging treatments for many neuromuscular disorders, interventions are often available that can assist people in continuing to function independently and safely, both in their vocational and personal lives, manage their symptoms, and live fulfilling lives despite the presence of a physical impairment. In this chapter, we will look at neuromuscular diseases from a rehabilitation perspective. We will first review the role of exercise, orthoses, mobility aids, adaptive equipment, and environmental modifications with respect to their impact on function and quality of life. We will then develop a rehabilitation framework to address common neuromuscular problems such as axial weakness, spinal deformities, proximal upper and lower limb weakness, hand weakness, foot drop, falls, foot abnormalities, joint contractures, spasticity, pain, ptosis, dysphagia, and dysarthria.

Rehabilitation is sometimes overlooked because it is not clear who is in charge of it and when it should begin. It is commonly accepted that the multifaceted rehabilitation needs of patients with neuromuscular diseases are best served by a multidisciplinary team that may include neurologists, physiatrists, nurses, physical therapists (PTs), orthotists, occupational therapists (OTs), speech and language pathologists (SLPs), nutritionists, respiratory therapists, psychologists, palliative care experts, pain medicine specialists, vocational consultants, recreational therapists, and social workers. Receiving care in a multidisciplinary clinic has been suggested to benefit people with certain neuromuscular diseases [i.e., amyotrophic lateral sclerosis (ALS)] by optimizing health care delivery and, possibly, prolonging survival and enhancing quality of life.[1] But what is the role of each member of the multidisciplinary team and who is responsible for advocating for the patient and for coordinating care among the different rehabilitation professionals? Neuromuscular specialists periodically assess the patients' functional status in a neuromuscular clinic. We therefore argue that the neuromuscular specialist, most often a neurologist or a physiatrist, is ideally positioned to lead the rehabilitation efforts while leveraging the expertise of the different team members. This may seem like a daunting and time-consuming task. However, most of what is required is simply adequate knowledge of the available tools and effective communication. A clear understanding of the role and capabilities of each team member is essential for proper referrals and results in higher quality of care and a time-efficient practice.

Neuromuscular specialists most commonly refer patients to PTs, OTs, and SLPs. While there is some overlap between the skill sets of PTs and OTs, PTs specialize in gait assessment and training, biomechanics, core stability, balance, and functional mobility such as transfers.[2] PTs also specialize in teaching stretching techniques and developing aerobic conditioning and strengthening exercise programs. OTs assist people to participate in the everyday activities (occupations) they need and want to do. They focus on proper posture and ergonomics related to upper limb functional activities such as feeding, grooming, dressing, and using a telephone or a computer. Both types of therapists utilize active and passive therapeutic exercises, physical modalities (such as heat, cold, and electrical stimulation), and manual techniques (such as massage, joint mobilization, and myofascial release techniques) to address pain and impairments in strength, flexibility, balance, posture, and endurance. They may work in close contact with orthotists if orthoses (i.e., braces) are indicated and they may recommend splints, assistive devices, adaptive equipment, and/or home modifications. Some PTs and OTs specialize in assistive technology, such as systems to allow access to computers and environmental controls (e.g., lights, television, etc.) for people with motor impairment.

SLPs manage disorders of speech, language, cognition, communication, and swallowing. In the setting of degenerative disease, the speech pathologist conducts serial assessments of these domains to support changes in function over time. These assessments guide interventions to maximize functional communication and to support patient and caregiver education focused on effective use of compensations when restorative efforts are not possible. Some SLPs specialize in augmentative and alternative communication (AAC) to provide systems to supplement or replace natural speech. These systems range from very high tech (e.g., computers controlled by eye gaze) to low tech (e.g., picture boards). In preparation for future AAC use, people with ALS may utilize voice banking to digitally record words and phrases while still able to do so, for later inclusion in a communication device. Some AAC systems incorporate computer access capabilities and options for environmental controls, both of which can generally be mounted on a wheelchair. When dysphagia is suspected, SLPs utilize clinical oral motor and swallowing assessments as well as instrumental measures [i.e., fiberoptic endoscopic evaluation of swallowing (FEES) and modified barium swallow (MBS) study] for proper assessment of the swallowing impairment and to guide recommendations for diet modifications and compensatory strategy use (e.g., postural maneuvers). They may also work with dieticians to optimize meal planning. In the presence of severe dysphagia, some patients move from oral nutrition to the relative ease of a feeding tube.

Depending on the individual patient's needs, additional health care professionals such as respiratory therapists, psychologists, palliative care experts, pain medicine specialists, vocational consultants, recreational therapists, and social workers can provide additional expertise to address specific rehabilitation needs.

While diagnostic procedures are often complex and energy consuming in neuromuscular medicine, it is best to start thinking "functionally" early on. The International Classification of Functioning, Disability and Health (ICF) model defines impairments as deficits within the performance of an organ or body system. For example, foot drop is an impairment caused by the weakness of a group of muscles that can result from neurogenic causes or, less frequently, other neuromuscular disorders such as myopathy or disorders of the central nervous system. Activity limitation in the ICF model refers to deficient performance of basic functional tasks, such as slowed walking speed, whereas participation restriction refers to the inability to fulfill a role within the home or community environment, such as self-care activities and shopping.[3] Rehabilitative interventions might target impairments, activity limitations, and/or participation restrictions.[4] Different strategies (and different outcome measures) need to be considered, depending on the goal of therapy. As an example, the therapy directed toward an impairment, such as exercise and bracing to target impaired range of motion (ROM) in a weak hand, might have great functional impact even if the actual degree of improvement in ROM is small. In this example, after intervention, the person might be able to perform a previously limited activity, such as typing on a computer, and as a result be able to participate in social activities which were previously restricted. Of note, similar rehabilitation strategies can often be utilized regardless of the exact etiology.

Rehabilitation should ideally start at the first patient encounter. Certainly, rehabilitation should begin before maladaptive patterns develop. As an example, it is common experience that it is much easier to prevent, rather than treat, contractures. This notion becomes especially important in rapidly progressive diseases such as ALS and requires forward thinking on the part of the rehabilitation team. We cannot emphasize enough how crucial early intervention is for people with progressive neuromuscular weakness. For instance, even in the early stages of the disease, before the onset of severe weakness, therapists can educate patients on energy conservation techniques such as pacing, taking rest breaks, and using bracing and adaptive equipment when performing demanding activities, perhaps on an intermittent basis. Such interventions might help reduce fatigue, a highly prevalent symptom in many neuromuscular diseases.[5-7] Further, early focus on biomechanics, ergonomics, stretching, and bracing helps people to remain as functional as possible and can help to delay or even prevent many of the negative sequelae of impaired strength. This framework applies to communication and cognitive abilities as well. Planning for, and exposing a family system to technologies, supportive techniques, and environmental modifications will make transition into loss of function easier to adapt to and will facilitate maximal patient participation and autonomy in care across the disease trajectory.

Rehabilitation should be approached in a problem-oriented fashion, focusing on what the person needs most at any particular time in the course of their disease in order to maintain maximal function and quality of life. Thus, rehabilitation may include management of one or more impairments (e.g., impairment in strength, ROM, tone, and cognitive–linguistic status), activity limitations (limitations with walking, standing, transferring, self-feeding, swallowing, toileting, dressing, grooming, bathing and communicating), and participation restrictions (such as participation in sports and leisure activities). Importantly, rehabilitation needs may change over time. Clinicians need to be aware of the disease's natural history and resource availability in order to anticipate needs and recommend interventions at appropriate times. In addition, rehabilitation strategies should be attentive to the person's environment and their family and support systems. Environmental modifications and family training are therefore integral to the rehabilitation process.

Given the multitude of functional challenges that many people with neuromuscular diseases may experience, it is best to approach them systematically by making a list of issues or a "rehabilitation assessment and plan" (rehabilitation A&P) that should be included in clinic notes alongside the medical A&P and reviewed at every follow-up visit. Developing a rehabilitation A&P requires consideration of the person's disease in relation to the changes in functional status that it creates. An individual with a generalized neuromuscular condition such as ALS or muscular dystrophy may present with weakness in multiple muscle groups which the clinician carefully records with periodic manual muscle testing performed at every follow-up visit. But what is the resulting activity limitation, and what can we do about it? If a person with ALS develops hand weakness, how does this impact their ability to carry out desired activities of daily living (ADLs), such as dressing and grooming, or instrumental ADLs (more complex tasks such as care of children or use of telephones and other communication devices)? Can we suggest any strategies to compensate for or adapt to the hand weakness? Can the work environment be modified to allow them to continue to work despite the hand weakness? Is abnormal muscle tone a limitation at this time? Is the patient at risk of developing finger contractures? Can the caregivers be trained to help with ROM exercises? Which health care professionals might provide optimal expertise to address this problem at this time (OTs, vocational consultants, and so on)? Can the person benefit from assistive devices to maintain independence with feeding, dressing, and toileting? If the hand weakness prevents them from comfortably using telephones and computers, which assistive technology system can we recommend? Clearly, the extent and treatment goals of the rehabilitation A&P may differ substantially depending on the underlying pathologic process. Impairments may be limited to one domain or involve multiple systems, may be static or progressive, and may be impacted by comorbidities, such as pre-existing musculoskeletal abnormalities, and environmental limitations. Rehabilitation goals may include restoration of function for some patients. When restoration of neurologic function is not achievable, teaching adaptive or compensatory techniques may allow the person to maintain independence and prevent negative sequelae of muscle weakness such as contractures and pain. Palliative care might be needed in some neuromuscular diseases and might be viewed as the end of the rehabilitation spectrum, although there is increasing acknowledgment of the role of physical therapy as a key component of both palliative and hospice care.[8]

In people with progressive disorders such as ALS, hereditary neuropathies, and muscular dystrophies, it is crucial to frequently reassess rehabilitation strategies and modify them with changes in disease status. As an example, if a person with ALS, Charcot–Marie–Tooth (CMT), or a distal myopathy develops ankle dorsiflexion weakness, an ankle–foot orthosis (AFO) may be prescribed to improve gait efficiency, conserve energy, and reduce fall risk. A few gait training sessions with a PT are important to successfully learn to ambulate with a brace. Later in the course of the disease, when the individual loses the ability to ambulate, a PT or OT should provide recommendations for a customized wheelchair. A few therapy sessions may be required for wheelchair mobility training. A few therapy sessions might also be indicated for the patient and their caregiver to provide training on stretching and ROM exercises to prevent contracture formation. If the person then develops pain or is uncomfortable when sitting in the wheelchair, wheelchair evaluation should be performed and adjustments made accordingly.

Rather than writing generic therapy prescriptions, it is best to address specific problems (e.g., gait training, transfer training, wheelchair evaluation, etc.) and periodically reassess needs. Working in close contact with therapists who are familiar with neuromuscular diseases will help ensure that therapy sessions are focused on what the individual really needs at that specific time. Of note, insurance carriers limit the number of therapy sessions for which people are eligible in a given period of time. Continued skilled therapy services (i.e., performed by a skilled health care professional such as a PT) to maintain current functional status have traditionally been denied in chronic conditions because there was no expectation for the person to "improve" (a concept known as "improvement standard"). A 2013 settlement in the class action "Improvement Standard" lawsuit (*Jimmo vs. Kathleen Sebelius*) upheld the right of patients to continue to receive reasonable and necessary care to maintain their condition and prevent or slow decline. The type of care covered under this settlement, however, refers only to skilled care and not to maintenance programs that can be performed by the patient or with the assistance of nontherapists, including unskilled caregivers. At this time of significant changes in the American health care system, the practical impact of this settlement on the rehabilitation of people with progressive neuromuscular diseases remains to be determined. Coverage for ongoing therapy and durable medical equipment (DME) may be limited. Loaner programs and support from patient advocacy organizations might help ease the financial burden and allow people to try different models of the same type of device before buying expensive material that they might not want or be able to use effectively. Of note, once patients are enrolled in hospice, there are significant restrictions for DME coverage. Hospice may cover a hospital bed and lift, but will not cover a customized power wheelchair or a device to support nonverbal communication. It is important to understand what will be covered and what will not be covered so that uncovered items can be ordered in advance if possible. This can be discussed with the hospice agency prior to enrolment. Nonprofit equipment loan programs or grants may be utilized to help cover equipment, but this can be time consuming and of limited availability, so patients or families may opt to purchase items out of pocket.

We will now review the tools that the rehabilitation team can use to assist people to maximize function and quality of life. We will then suggest a practical approach to address the rehabilitation problems that are most frequently encountered in neuromuscular medicine. However, one should keep in mind that rehabilitation science is in constant development and the clinical problems posed by particular patients might be unique and require creative thinking on the therapists' part. Therefore, the approach suggested here should not be viewed as a "fix-all recipe" but rather as a platform for discussion. Most importantly, with this chapter, we want to draw attention to the importance of periodic functional assessments and the need to think of rehabilitation as a fundamental part of neuromuscular medicine practice.

▶ REHABILITATION TOOLS AND STRATEGIES FOR THEIR USE

EXERCISE

It is not infrequent for people with neuromuscular diseases to inquire about exercise. Physical activity and exercise are an integral part of the premorbid lifestyle for many neuromuscular patients. Therefore, patients often ask whether exercise is safe, whether it can help slow down their disease, and what type of exercise is recommended for their particular condition. It is not easy to answer these questions. Strictly speaking, these are questions that cannot be answered based on the currently available evidence. Unfortunately, there is a paucity of literature on the topic of exercise in neuromuscular disorders.[9]

Exercise studies in neuromuscular medicine are limited in both quantity and quality. Limitations in the available studies include small sample size, heterogeneous patient population, uncontrolled and nonrandomized design, short-term training, variable exercise protocols, and outcome measures. Some investigators have attempted to circumvent difficulties in recruiting a nonexercising control group with similar disease characteristics by asking the subjects to exercise only one side of the body, with the contralateral side serving as control. A nonexercised limb, however, is not an appropriate control due to the phenomenon of cross-education. Unilateral training induces strength gains not only in the trained limb but also in the homologous muscles of the contralateral limb.[10] Therefore, comparisons should be made between training and nontraining patients. A recent Cochrane review on exercise training for myopathies identified only three high-quality randomized clinical trials.[9] Additional evidence mostly comes from observational or uncontrolled trials and recommendations have been primarily based on the consensus of an expert review panel.[11] The types of exercise that are relevant to people with neuromuscular disorders are flexibility, resistance, aerobic, and balance exercises (Table 5-1).

FLEXIBILITY TRAINING

Flexibility training involves stretching and ROM exercises. The potential benefits of this type of exercise include prevention and treatment of spasticity and contractures, as well as the pain that often accompanies them. Because many people with neuromuscular diseases are at risk for the development of these complications, flexibility training is often incorporated into the standard of care.[12]

Neuromuscular specialists are ideally positioned to advocate the early initiation of flexibility training. Supervision from a PT is often needed to initiate a correct stretching program. PTs may then periodically reassess progress, guide program modifications, or suggest further treatment modalities such as positioning, splinting, bracing, orthoses, and standing devices. Stretching, however, should not be limited to therapy sessions and should be done daily for any specific joint or muscle group that is at risk for contracture development. Stretching can be done at home, school, or work, as well as in the clinic.[12] It is important for people to understand that stretching can be safely performed outside of the clinic environment either independently or with caregiver assistance, and that consistency produces the best results. In this respect, caregiver involvement is essential. When individuals cannot perform active stretching due to significant weakness, active-assisted and/or passive techniques may be implemented with caregiver's help.

AEROBIC AND STRENGTHENING EXERCISE

In comparison with data from people with neuromuscular diseases, the quality of the evidence on the beneficial effects of aerobic and strengthening exercise in the able-bodied population is excellent. In healthy individuals, moderate-intensity physical activity significantly improves overall health. In addition, it is related to improving the outcomes of several chronic diseases, such as heart disease, stroke, and type 2 diabetes. Based on this evidence, the American College of Sports Medicine (ACSM) declared that "Exercise is

▶ **TABLE 5-1. TYPES OF EXERCISE RELEVANT TO PATIENTS WITH NEUROMUSCULAR DISEASES**

Type of Exercise	Description	Benefits
Flexibility	Stretching Range of motion (ROM)	Part of the standard of care for the prevention and management of contractures Might help to manage pain and spasticity
Resistance/strengthening	Repeated muscle actions against resistance: • isometric • concentric • *avoid* eccentric	*Potential* role in: • strengthening weak muscles • reversing disuse weakness • delaying onset of functional impairment More disease-specific research needed
Aerobic	Dynamic activity using large muscle groups	*Potential* role in: • improving aerobic capacity • *improving mood, quality of life, sleep, functional independence* • preventing chronic diseases and maintaining bone density More disease-specific research needed
Balance	Balance training using different modalities	*Potential* role in: • fall risk reduction More disease-specific research needed

medicine™" inviting physicians to write exercise prescriptions to promote physical activity and exercise as standard parts of disease prevention and medical treatment.[13]

Here we define aerobic exercise training, or cardiorespiratory fitness training, as an activity that uses large muscle groups that can be maintained continuously and that is rhythmical and aerobic in nature, such as walking, hiking, running, cycling, and swimming. Guidelines for aerobic training for the general population were published in 2018 by the US Department of Health and Human Services.[14] The Physical Activity Guidelines for Americans state that adults aged 18–64 years should do at least 150 minutes a week of moderate-intensity, 75 minutes a week of vigorous-intensity aerobic physical activity, or an equivalent combination of moderate- and vigorous-intensity aerobic activity in bouts of at least 10 minutes and preferably spread throughout the week. The same guidelines state that older adults (aged 65 and older) and individuals with disabilities should follow the same guidelines, but, if this is not possible due to limiting health conditions, they should be as physically active as their abilities allow and avoid inactivity.

The same guidelines also recommend performing muscle-strengthening activities that involve all major muscle groups 2 or more days per week. Strength training is defined as an activity performed to improve muscle strength and endurance and is typically carried out by making repeated muscle actions against resistance.[15] Strength training includes different types of muscle actions: isometric (i.e., performed at a constant muscle length with no joint movement, as in wall squat hold and plank exercises), concentric (i.e., the muscle generates force while shortening, as when lifting a dumbbell toward the body), and eccentric (i.e., the muscle generates force while lengthening, as when lowering a weight away from the body or landing back on the ground after jumping). For healthy adults, the ACSM recommends one set of about 10 exercises to condition all major muscle groups, 2–3 days per week. Healthy adults should complete at least one set of 8 to 12 repetitions per exercise at loads of at least 45%–50% of the one-repetition maximum (1RM) (which is the maximal load that can be lifted throughout the full ROM once).[15,16]

How can we translate these general guidelines into exercise recommendations for people with neuromuscular diseases? We will first review the available studies and then offer some general recommendations, always being mindful of the overarching principle of *primum non nocere*. When evaluating studies of the outcome of exercise in different patient populations, one should keep in mind that slowing the rate of functional impairment is a positive result in progressive neuromuscular diseases, while actual gain of strength or aerobic capacity might be a goal only in selected conditions. Additional factors that need to be considered are the presence of comorbidities (such as heart and restrictive lung disease in certain neuromuscular conditions), nutritional status and weight maintenance, the specific disorder, rate of progression, and expected natural history.

In the available studies, primary outcome measures have mostly been limited to effects at the impairment level: aerobic capacity and measures of muscle strength. Ideally, the primary outcomes of exercise studies should also include measures of function such as improvement in the ability to walk, perform ADLs, and participate in work, sports, and recreational activities, as these are the outcomes that really matter to patients. Secondary outcomes for exercise training have included measures of pain or fatigue, quality of life, and mood. These secondary outcome measures are very important to consider as well, given the high prevalence of these problems in many neuromuscular diseases.[5–7,17,18]

Exercise Studies in ALS

Preclinical evidence gathered in the transgenic mutant SOD1 mouse model of ALS has suggested a potential benefit from moderate endurance exercise with delay in disease onset and survival.[19–21] In these mice, however, high-intensity endurance training was shown to hasten the decrease in motor performance and death.[21,22] In humans, a study by Drory et al. suggested that a regular moderate exercise program (30 minutes or less daily) might have a positive effect on disability in people with ALS.[23] The study included 25 ALS participants who were randomized to perform a moderate daily program of activities as opposed to avoiding any physical activity beyond their usual daily requirements. At 3 months from the initiation of the study, participants who performed regular exercise showed less deterioration on the ALS Functional Rating Scale (ALS-FRS) and the Ashworth spasticity scale.[23] At 6 months, there was no significant difference between the groups, although a trend toward less deterioration was observed in the treated group.[23] Bello-Haas et al. have analyzed strength training in a randomized trial that included 27 ALS participants.[24] The study involved 6 months of training, three times a week, following an individualized program. The resistance exercise group had significantly better function, as measured by total ALS-FRS scores, and quality of life, without adverse effects as compared with subjects receiving usual care.[24] These studies suggest that moderate exercise might be safe for people with ALS but are too small to draw definitive conclusions. Clawson et al. completed a 6-month study in 59 people with ALS comparing three exercise programs: stretching and ROM, resistance training, and aerobic conditioning or endurance training.[25] The resistance exercises were completed at 40%–70% of their one rep maximum, and the endurance training at 40%–70% of their target heart rate. While they found that all three programs were tolerated at 12 and 24 weeks, the endurance program was less well tolerated than the stretching and ROM program. The small sample size limited their ability to assess treatment efficacy, but there was not an exacerbation of symptoms reported in any of the exercise groups.[25,26] Additional research is ongoing to confirm these findings and determine whether exercise might actually improve function in this population.

There is evidence to support expiratory muscle strength training (EMST) in people with early-stage ALS.[27,28] Plowman et al. found improvements in maximum expiratory pressures (MEP) and cough spirometry across two small studies of ALS patients with early-stage disease that utilized this mild–moderate intensity training regimen. The initial 8-week expiratory strength training regimen utilized a 50% max effort training load with ALS patients and trained expiratory functions. A subsequent study included both inspiratory and expiratory muscle training targets and utilized a reduced training load of 30% in attempt to avoid fatigue and overtraining given increased number of exercises and higher repetitions. In the initial study, expiratory strength training led to an average increase in MEP ranging from 25% to 30%. The subsequent group that trained at 30% training load demonstrated improvements in MEP of 20%, with no observed improvement in maximum inspiratory pressures (MIP). Across the two studies, the findings suggest that an expiratory strength-based program is feasible, well tolerated, and can increase physiologic capacity of specific breathing and airway clearance functions. Further investigations are warranted to examine specificity of training, and training intensity as well.

Exercise Studies in People with Charcot–Marie–Tooth Disease

There are a few randomized clinical trials on the effect of strength training in CMT disease. In one study, 29 CMT participants were randomized to 24 weeks of progressive resistance exercise of their lower limbs which was performed three times a week.[26] Participants in the training arm reported a moderate increase in knee torque without adverse effects.[26] Other small studies reported moderate strength gains in patients with CMT compared to their baseline values.[29,30] In a study of 55 children with CMT, a 6-month progressive resistance program targeting ankle dorsiflexors reduced progression of ankle dorsiflexion weakness compared to the sham exercise group.[31] Positive effects of aerobic exercise on fatigue and peak VO2 have also been reported in this patient population.[32]

Exercise Studies in the Dystrophinopathies

Preclinical studies in the *mdx* mouse model of Duchenne muscular dystrophy have led clinicians to advise against exercise in the dystrophinopathies. Dystrophin is an important structural protein and animal studies have demonstrated contraction-induced muscle injury in dystrophinopathy, especially after eccentric exercise.[33–36] In humans, the few available studies have been small and have provided conflicting results precluding any definitive conclusions.[35,37,38] High-resistance strength training and eccentric exercise are universally considered inappropriate across the lifespan owing to concerns about contraction-induced muscle-fiber injury.[12] However, submaximum aerobic exercise is recommended by some clinicians, especially early in the course of the disease, in order to avoid disuse atrophy and other secondary complications of inactivity.[12] This recommendation has been supported by a few trials demonstrating the benefits of upper and lower extremity bicycle training to delay functional deterioration in children with Duchenne muscular dystrophy.[39,40] Most clinicians advise boys with dystrophinopathy who are ambulatory or in the early nonambulatory stage to participate in regular gentle functional strengthening and recreation-based activities in the community. In this respect, low-impact activities such as swimming and assisted cycling appear most beneficial.[12,39–43] The optimal level of exercise for people with dystrophinopathy is still to be determined.

Exercise Studies in FSHD

There have been a few randomized clinical trials of strength training versus no training in adults with facioscapulohumeral muscular dystrophy (FSHD). One trial involved 65 participants and lasted 52 weeks.[44,45] The strength program in this study appeared to be safe, with only limited positive effects on muscle strength and volume. There have been a few small studies demonstrating the benefits of aerobic cycling in participants with FSHD. In two separate 12-week programs, improvements were noted in aerobic capacity, and endurance, walking speed, and self-assessed health, respectively, without any signs of muscle damage.[46,47] A 6-month home cycling program in 24 individuals with FSHD that combined moderative-intensity aerobic training and high-intensity interval training was found to improve aerobic capacity, function, and perceived fatigue, without any observed signs of muscle damage.[48] Altogether, these studies suggest that "normal" participation in sports and work appears not to be harmful.[9] One small study looked at an 8-week high-intensity interval cycling program in people with FSHD and found the program was well tolerated with only low fluctuations in plasma-CK levels and improvement in maximum oxygen uptake, but no significant improvements in strength or function.[49] Current research aims to evaluate the feasibility of interventions to improve physical activity and further work is necessary to prescribe appropriate exercise programs for patients with FSHD.[9,50,51]

Exercise Studies in Myotonic Dystrophy

One randomized clinical trial compared the effect of 24 weeks of strength training versus no training in adults with myotonic dystrophy.[26] Neither strength gains nor muscle damage was demonstrated in the exercise group compared to controls. A study of 12 weeks of hand strengthening with putty in people with myotonic dystrophy type 1 found improvements in wrist flexor strength and perceived function.[52] A study of 12 weeks of aerobic training showed that participants with myotonic dystrophy type I improved their aerobic capacity compared to their baseline without any adverse effects.[53] Based on the available evidence, it may be inferred that moderate resistance and endurance exercise is probably safe in individuals with myotonic dystrophy, but there is still insufficient evidence of benefit.[9]

Exercise Studies in the Inflammatory Myopathies

Until the early 1990s, patients with polymyositis (PM) and dermatomyositis (DM) were discouraged from exercising out of concern that it might exacerbate muscle inflammation. More recent work, however, suggests that moderate-intensity aerobic exercise does not result in worsening muscle damage, at least as assessed by creatine kinase (CK) levels, and might in fact improve aerobic capacity.[54–57] The first randomized controlled study of aerobic exercise in adult PM/DM included 14 patients with chronic disease, defined as participants with proximal muscle weakness due to PM/DM for at least 6 months and stable drug therapy over the 3 months prior to initiation of the program. After 6 weeks of training (bicycle exercise and step aerobics), there was an increase in oxygen uptake in the exercise group compared with the sedentary controls.[54] The same training paradigm was later reported to be safe and to result in improved aerobic capacity in a longer prospective nonrandomized study of 6 months of exercise.[58] A multicenter randomized controlled trial found improvements in muscle performance, aerobic capacity, and function with reduced disease activity in people with PM/DM after 12 weeks of moderate-intensity cycling and strength training.[59] A few open-label studies also supported the safety of resistance training in recent-onset disease, reporting unchanged CK levels after short-term exercise periods.[60,61] Analysis of CK levels is the most commonly used marker for muscle inflammation in exercise studies in patients with myositis. However, CK levels do not always correspond to muscle function or disease activity. Alexanderson et al. investigated MRI scans of the thighs in 7 out of 11 patients with recent-onset myositis participating in a 12-week resistance exercise program.[60] In the follow-up MRI scans, after 12 weeks of exercise, none of the cases had additional areas of increased signal as compared to the first scan, supporting the safety of the exercise protocol.[60]

Little is known about the role of exercise in inclusion body myositis (IBM). A home exercise program consisting of 15 minutes of progressive strength training and a 15-minute walk performed 5 days a week for 12 weeks did not result in adverse effects on histopathology or significant change in serum CK level but did not improve muscle strength.[62] Johnson et al. showed that a combined 12-week resistance and aerobic exercise program resulted in improved aerobic capacity in seven patients with IBM compared to their baseline.[63]

More recent work by Wallace et al. showed that a 12-week aerobic training program using a recumbent exercise bicycle improved peak VO2 in 17 people with IBM.[32]

Exercise Studies in the Mitochondrial Myopathies

People with mitochondrial myopathies suffer from exercise intolerance due to their impaired oxidative capacity and physical deconditioning. Cejudo et al. reported a randomized clinical trial of combined aerobic and resistance exercise analyzing the effects of 12 weeks of training in 20 people with mitochondrial myopathy (cycle exercise and upper-body weight lifting performed 3 days a week).[64] Training increased aerobic capacity and resulted in improved muscle strength.[64] These results are in agreement with numerous other studies supporting the notion that moderate endurance exercise increases aerobic capacity in patients with mitochondrial myopathies.[65–69] A study of 12 weeks of resistance exercise strength training in a group of patients with mitochondrial myopathy carrying a single, large-scale deletion of mtDNA resulted in strength gains.[70] Whether or not these results are applicable to other types of mitochondrial myopathy remains to be determined.

AEROBIC TRAINING IN McARDLE DISEASE

Patients with McArdle disease are susceptible to exertional cramps and rhabdomyolysis. In the past, because of the risk of rhabdomyolysis, many people with McArdle disease have been advised to avoid exercise. However, physical inactivity may worsen exercise intolerance by further reducing the limited oxidative capacity caused by blocked glycogenolysis.[71] Haller et al. examined the effect of a 14-week regimen of aerobic training on a cycle ergometer (30–40 minutes a day, 4 days a week) in eight participants with McArdle disease.[71] They reported significant increases in exercise capacity with no adverse effects, in agreement with other small, nonrandomized studies supporting the use of moderate-intensity aerobic exercise for these patients.[66,72,73] The consensus is to advise individuals with McArdle disease to engage in regular, moderate aerobic activities to prevent deconditioning.[74,75] On the other hand, intense aerobic exercise is contraindicated. Furthermore, any bout of moderate exercise should be preceded by 5–15 minutes of low-level "warm-up" exercise. This promotes the transition to a "second wind" in which exercise capacity is increased because of increased mobilization and delivery of extramuscular fuels.[73] There is limited evidence suggesting resistance training has the potential to improve muscle strength, mass, and clinical status of patients with McArdle disease; however, small sample sizes limit the ability to determine appropriate guidelines for resistance training.[76–79]

BALANCE TRAINING

Many patients with neuromuscular diseases exhibit impaired balance due to a combination of sensory neuropathy, muscle weakness, and/or spasticity and are therefore at risk for falls. Whether balance training reduces this risk has not been well studied. A few small recent studies performed in patients with diabetic neuropathy suggest that balance training might result in improved balance and trunk proprioception.[80–85] One study found improvements in balance with stretching and proprioceptive exercises with and without treadmill training in adults with CMT1A.[86] Further research is needed to determine whether these early promising results are applicable to other patient populations and whether training might result in increased independence and lower risk of falls.

ADAPTIVE SPORTS

Physical activity should be viewed as a way of improving quality of life and not just a tedious set of exercises. Many people enjoy participation in sports and other recreational activities more than individual training. Previously, it had been thought that having a disability would preclude people from sports participation. Fortunately, over the last several decades, many different groups and organizations have developed adaptive sports for a variety of patient populations. Virtually any sport can be adapted to different levels of disability (Fig. 5-1). It is important to work with organizations and therapists who have extensive experience in adaptive sports to ensure that the level of modification is safe and appropriate for the individual patient's diagnosis

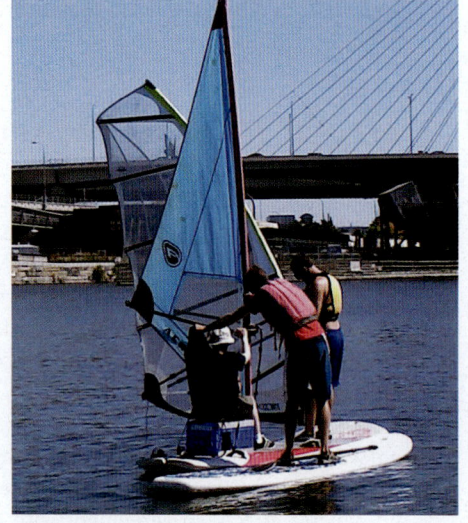

A

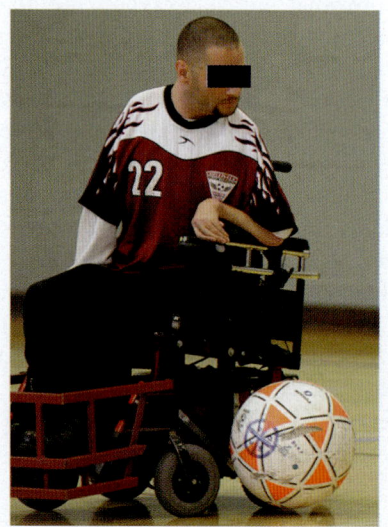

B

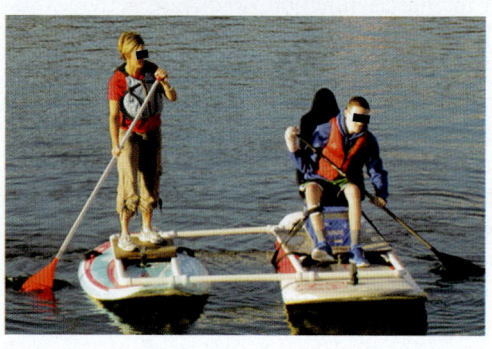

C
D

Figure 5-1. Adaptive sports. **(A)** Windsurfing can be adapted to athletes with different disabilities, including wheelchair users. The athlete sits in a high back chair and controls the back sail on a tandem board that can plane at speeds over 32.19 km/h (20 mph). Athletic trainers control the front sail and help keep the board balanced. (Used with permission of Ross Lilley, AccesSportAmerica.) **(B)** Power soccer: athletes who use power wheelchairs for mobility can participate in power soccer. A footguard is attached to the front of their power chair. This guard is for protection and is also used by the athletes to kick, dribble, and block the ball. In competition, chairs are restricted to a top speed of 10 km/h (6.2 mph). (Used with permission of Scot Goodman, Scot Goodman Photography.) **(C)** Adaptive skiing: skiing can be performed with a variety of adaptive equipment to be suitable for athletes with different disabilities. In this photo, a power wheelchair user sits in a chair on a bi-ski and is guided down the slope by a trainer. (Used with permission of Paul Martino, Adaptive Ski Program, New Mexico.) **(D)** Paddling: this setup enables athletes to stand up or sit down paddle with the direction and support of a trainer next to them. (Used with permission of Ross Lilley, AccesSportAmerica.)

and clinical status. The benefits of participation in adaptive sports include engagement with peers, accomplishment of goals that were thought to be out of reach, and improved mood, confidence, and self-esteem. In addition, sports can offer opportunities for people to maintain mobility in an integrated environment. Participation in adaptive sports may be especially important in the pediatric population, as kids enjoy learning through play and recreation.

GENERAL RECOMMENDATIONS FOR EXERCISE IN NEUROMUSCULAR DISEASES

While research is limited as reviewed above, recommendations for general exercise programs for people with neuromuscular diseases have been developed by several consensus panels and are summarized in Table 5-2.[11,12,87,88] Obviously, the level of training and expected outcomes depend on the diagnosis, disease severity, and rate of progression. As an example, people who are recovering from a single episode of a monophasic nerve disease such as neuralgic amyotrophy or Guillain–Barré syndrome are expected to improve their strength over time and exercise can potentially help their recovery, although this assumption is based solely on the known benefits of exercise in the healthy population rather than patients with disease. For patients with slowly progressive disease, exercise might help avoid secondary disuse or deconditioning weakness. On the other hand, some patients with rapidly progressive neuromuscular diseases might already be using their muscles at a maximal level while performing their daily activities. One should keep in mind that there is great variability in muscle strength among different muscle groups in individuals with different types and stages of neuromuscular disorders. Depending on the degree of weakness, some muscles may already be overworked. These specific muscles may need to rest and not perform additional resistance exercises. The oral, facial, and pharyngeal musculature serves as a good example here. These small muscle groups are greatly taxed with daily speech and swallow functions and may not tolerate the additional workload of targeted exercise without further impacting function. It should be noted, however, that additional research is needed before clearly defined exercise protocols can be prescribed in any specific disease population. Until then, one can be guided by the important principle of safety while drawing from the currently available studies. With regards to safety, the consensus is to allow submaximum aerobic training (either structured exercise or as part of recreational activities) for most patients in order to avoid deconditioning that would compound the existing weakness. In addition, when leg weakness is present, it is important to choose a mode of exercise with minimal risk of injury from falling such as recumbent stationary bike as opposed to treadmill.

Resistance exercise programs might be added as long as one is careful to avoid overwork weakness due to exercise-induced muscle injury. Muscles that do not have antigravity

▶ **TABLE 5-2. GENERAL EXERCISE RECOMMENDATIONS FOR PATIENTS WITH NEUROMUSCULAR DISEASES**

Type of Exercise and Potential Benefits	Practical Considerations
Flexibility training is safe and helps prevent contracture formation; it might help with pain and spasticity management	1. Encourage regular stretching and ROM exercises early on in the course of disease. 2. May need periodic supervision and training by a physical therapist (PT). 3. Caregiver participation is essential when muscle weakness prevents the patient from performing program independently.
Moderate, submaximum aerobic exercise is *probably* safe for most patients and *might* help prevent deconditioning and loss of cardiopulmonary fitness	1. Select a mode of exercise with minimal risk of injury from falling (e.g., recumbent stationary bike as opposed to treadmill). 2. Be aware of exercise contraindications such as associated cardiopulmonary disease. 3. A practical approach is to begin with bouts of 10 minutes of exercise 2–3 times a week and progress as tolerated. 4. A practical way to determine if the exercise intensity is appropriate is to ask the patient to talk while exercising. If the patient cannot talk comfortably during exercise, the program is too vigorous.
Moderate resistance exercise *may* help maintain or improve strength in muscles with an initial Medical Research Council (MRC) grade 3/5 or better	1. Avoid high-resistance exercise. Choose loads that correspond to 20–40% of a one-repetition maximum. A practical approach is to find a weight that the patient can lift comfortably 20 times. Then ask the patient to perform 2–3 sets of 10 repetitions each with that weight. Progression to heavier loads depends on the patient's diagnosis and severity of disease. 2. Do not exercise muscles that do not have antigravity strength. A PT might help identify what muscles can be safely exercised. 3. Avoid eccentric exercise.
For all types of exercise, the level of training depends on the diagnosis, stage, and severity of disease	1. Monitor for signs of overexertion. Excessive postexercise fatigue, muscle pain, or myoglobinuria are indicators that the patient is overworking and that the exercise program needs to be modified. 2. Postexercise fatigue should not interfere with daily activities. If a patient has fatigue or pain that lasts longer than 30 minutes after exercise, they are probably overworking.

strength should not be exercised. Eccentric muscle actions should be avoided. Eccentric muscle actions result in high force production. In healthy adults, they provide an important training stimulus leading to muscle hypertrophy.[15,89] However, eccentric muscle activities are more likely to result in microdamage at the muscle level. The concern is that, in individuals with underlying muscle disease, this may result in long-lasting or irreversible muscle damage, as suggested by some preclinical studies in the mouse model of Duchenne muscular dystrophy.[36]

With any type of exercise program, it is important to pay attention to clinical signs of overwork such as excessive post-exercise fatigue, pain, weakness, and excessive delayed-onset muscle soreness, and modify physical activity accordingly.

ORTHOSES

Orthoses (braces) are devices worn on a person's body to improve function, provide comfort, conserve energy, and prevent deformity. Orthoses can be prefabricated or custom made. Therapists and orthotists with experience with neuromuscular diseases can provide invaluable input as to the best orthosis to suit the individual patient's needs. Importantly, they can help adjust the orthosis as the status of a patient's functional needs change with time. Patient tolerability varies greatly; therefore, patient feedback on the comfort and fit of the device is paramount.

Cervical Orthoses

Several types of cervical orthoses, or collars, are available to support the neck (Fig. 5-2). For mild weakness, a soft foam collar may be tried first as it is usually comfortable to wear and well tolerated. Some people with head drop use a baseball cap attached to straps around the trunk (or "baseball-cap orthosis"[90]). For moderate to severe weakness, collars with an open-air design such as the Headmaster™ or similar models are generally well accepted and provide more support than soft collars. Other types of collars, such as the traditional Philadelphia, Aspen, or Miami-J collars, provide more stability. However, these collars are often poorly tolerated due to discomfort at points of contact and a sense of warmth and confinement. The HeadUp collar was designed in the United Kingdom for people living with motor neuron disease.[91,92] Its design is intended to offer support while also allowing for movement. It has support struts that can be heated and molded to fit the contours of the individual's neck and to provide the support where it is needed around the neck.[91,92] Its acceptance, tolerability, and use for people with motor neuron diseases outside of research trials is still to be determined. Adherence to cervical collar use can be impacted by patient perceptions and preferences around image as well as impact on other functions such as limiting jaw mobility needed for maximal speech and swallow function. These are additional considerations for selection of a best fit collar.

Thoracolumbosacral Orthoses

The primary goal of thoracolumbosacral orthoses (TLSOs) or lumbosacral orthoses (LSOs) in patients with neuromuscular diseases is comfort. In prepubertal children at risk for neuromuscular scoliosis, TLSOs may be utilized to provide support to the spinal column during growth, although the brace cannot prevent curve progression. Molded seating supports can also be used to provide additional comfort and

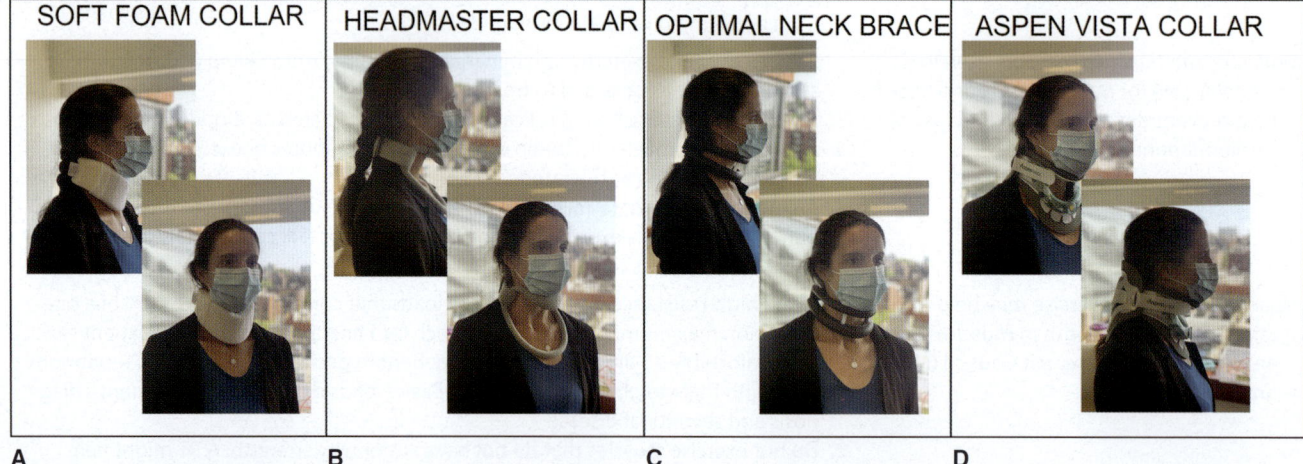

Figure 5-2. Cervical collars (A) soft foam collar—can provide some support for mild cervical weakness and is not as restrictive as other options. (B) Headmaster collar—provides anterior support under the jaw to support the head. The tubular design reduces heat retention and can improve comfort. (C) Optimal neck brace—similar to the headmaster collar with increased padding. The design also relieves pressure from the clavicle which can be bothersome for some patients wearing the headmaster collar. This collar is also waterproof. (D) Aspen Vista Collar—provides a good amount of support but is also very restrictive. This is a lighter, lower-profile version of the "traditional" Aspen collar. (Used with permission of Katherine M. Burke, DPT, Sean M. Healey & AMG Center for ALS, Massachusetts General Hospital, Boston, MA.)

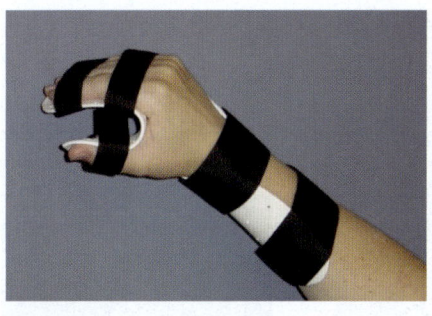 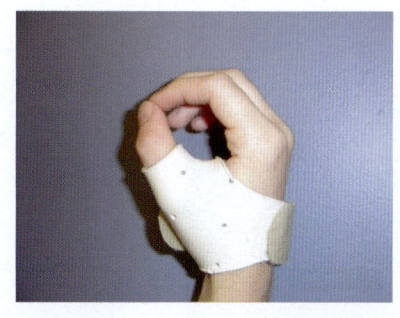 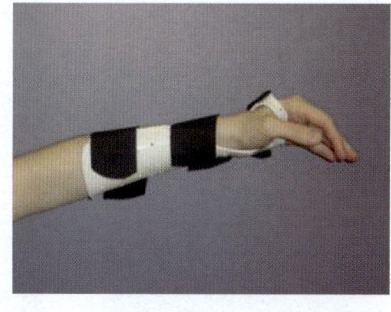

Figure 5-3. Hand splints. **(A)** Resting hand splint. **(B)** Opponens splint. **(C)** Cock-up splint. (Used with permission of Julie MacLean, Occupational Therapy Department, Massachusetts General Hospital, Boston, MA.)

stability when seating. TLSO/LSOs might be helpful in adult patients as well to provide proprioceptive input, improve alignment, and ease back pain, especially in patients with abdominal weakness.

Upper Limb Orthoses

Many different upper limb orthoses exist. Some orthoses are used to compensate for weakness and improve function, whereas others are prescribed to allow for proper positioning, provide comfort, and prevent or treat joint contractures.

Shoulder support systems are used in neuromuscular patients with proximal weakness who experience shoulder subluxation and/or pain, as can be seen in some muscular dystrophies and motor neuron disorders. Support systems are used to approximate the head of the humerus in the glenoid fossa, with the goal of providing comfort and pain relief. It is important, however, to choose an appropriate orthosis. Single-strap hemislings position the arm close to the body in adduction, internal rotation, and elbow flexion and, with prolonged use, might promote contracture development. On the other hand, axilla roll slings ("Bobath" slings), the GivMohr® sling, and humeral cuff slings help to reduce shoulder subluxation without immobilizing the arm in flexion.[93] Therapists can also recommend adjustments to seating systems and arm rests for individuals who use wheelchairs for further arm support.

The balanced forearm orthosis is a functional orthosis for people with shoulder abduction weakness designed to increase independence in performing daily activities. The orthosis supports the weight of the arm against gravity while allowing for independent horizontal movement. It can be placed on a desk or mounted on a wheelchair and is used for tasks such as self-feeding and grooming.

Splints are hand orthoses for people with intrinsic hand muscle weakness (Fig. 5-3). They can be purchased off the shelf or can be custom made by orthotists and OTs. Resting hand splints are used during the day or at night to maintain muscle length in patients at risk of finger flexion contractures (Fig. 5-3A). Anticlaw splints can reduce claw hand deformity and improve grasp by limiting metacarpophalangeal (MCP) extension. Dynamic finger extension splints are used in individuals with finger extension weakness who still have adequate finger flexor strength. This splint extends the MCP joints so that extended fingers can flex and grasp objects. The opponens splint helps patients with prehension difficulties due to thumb weakness by keeping the thumb in an abducted and opposed position (Fig. 5-3B). The volar cock-up splint supports the wrist in 20–30 degrees of extension and is used in people whose wrist extension weakness prevents them from grasping (Fig. 5-3C). The tenodesis orthosis (wrist-driven prehension orthosis) allows an individual with finger flexor weakness to create a three-jaw chuck pinch using wrist extension. Splints to correct single-digit deformities are also available.

Lower Limb Orthoses

The most common type of orthotic device prescribed by neuromuscular specialists is the AFO (Fig. 5-4). AFOs are used by patients with ankle dorsiflexion weakness to promote clearing of the toes and foot during the swing phase of gait, thus leading to a safer and more efficient ambulation. They are also used to prevent the development of ankle plantar flexion contractures. It is important, however, to carefully select candidates for bracing as an inappropriate brace might actually impair function. When patients need AFOs, it is best for them to be evaluated in brace clinics where PTs and orthotists work in close contact to provide customized AFOs and modify them as needed. Brace customization and modification can be helpful to ensure the best possible fit, patient comfort and compliance, as well as maximize functional outcomes. A few sessions of gait training with a skilled therapist are also needed to optimize braced gait. Last but not the least, patients should be instructed to perform skin checks on a regular basis and skin evaluation should be part of routine follow-up care. If skin redness, pain, or callouses develop, the brace should be promptly examined and adjusted by the orthotist. AFOs must be used with shoes that are deep and wide enough to accommodate them. They fit quite well in sneakers although they might be used with other types of shoes as well. It is best to always use shoes with the same heel height in order not to alter gait biomechanics while wearing a brace. Shoes should be in good condition as worn-out shoes may affect the gait pattern and lead to reduced brace

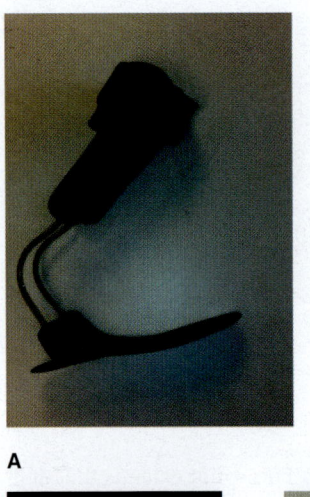
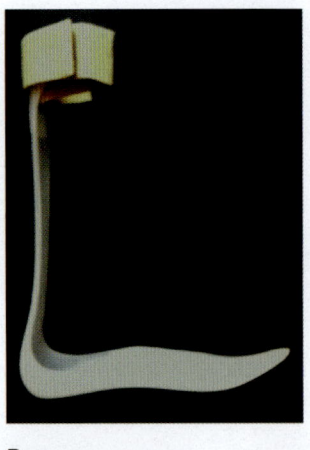
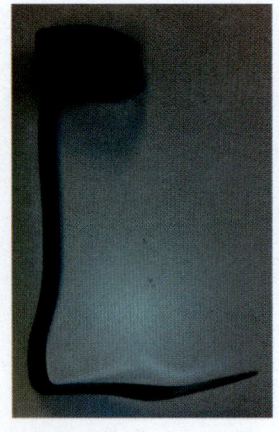
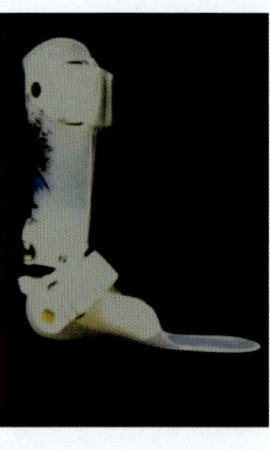
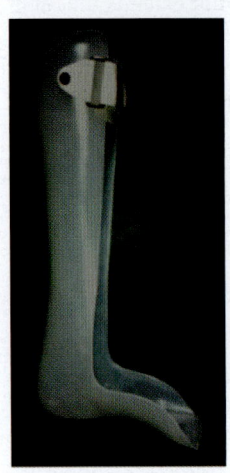
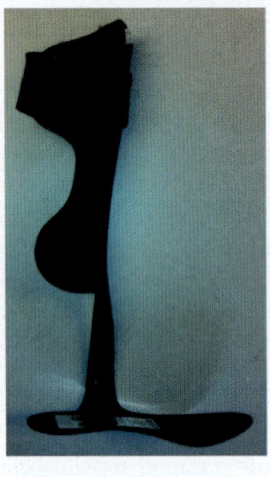
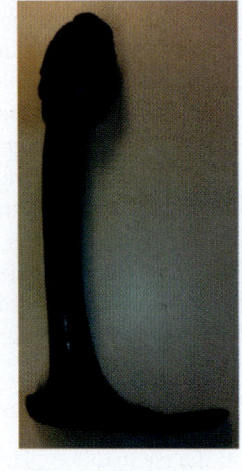

Figure 5-4. Ankle–foot–orthoses (AFOs). **(A)** Carbon fiber dorsiflexion assist orthosis. **(B)** Plastic posterior leaf spring (PLS) AFO. **(C)** Carbon fiber PLS AFO. **(D)** Plastic hinged AFO (pediatric). **(E)** Plastic solid AFO. **(F and G)** Two different models of floor reaction orthoses (FROs). (Sabrina Paganoni, MD.)

effectiveness. Some people do not want to wear ankle braces despite medical recommendation. In these circumstances, the use of footwear that crosses the ankle and is snug, such as lace-up boots, high-top sneakers, or even cowboy boots, can help provide at least some support to the ankle.

AFOs come in many different models and can be modified to suit different clinical needs (Fig. 5-4). They are generally made of either plastic or carbon fiber, with the latter being a lighter-weight option. For people with mild foot drop, dorsiflexion assist orthoses may suffice (Fig. 5-4A). These braces are lightweight and incorporate a spring that generates a dorsiflexion assist moment. Another option for mild foot drop is the posterior leaf spring (PLS) AFO (Fig. 5-4B and C). This is an orthosis with medial and lateral trim lines placed posterior to the malleoli. These braces are somewhat flexible and allow some plantar flexion to occur during heel strike. Because of their flexibility, they might not be the best choice for patients with increased tone. Hinged (articulated) AFOs include an ankle joint and are appropriate for patients with moderate weakness of ankle dorsiflexion (Fig. 5-4D). Transferring from sit to stand and negotiating stairs is easier with a hinged AFO than with a solid model, but good quadriceps strength is needed to use them. A plantar flexion stop can be incorporated into the design of a hinged AFO to prevent plantar flexion beyond a certain angle, which might be useful when spasticity is a problem. Solid AFOs provide immobilization of the ankle–foot complex and are therefore used for people with significant distal weakness and resulting medial and lateral instability of the ankle (Fig. 5-4E). However, because of the fixed ankle position, sit-to-stand transfers and climbing stairs and inclines are difficult. The angle at the ankle of a solid AFO can be set in a few degrees of plantar flexion. This modification enhances knee stability and may be useful in patients with quadriceps weakness and knee buckling. Addition of an anterior (pretibial shell) might also help to counter the tendency to knee buckling. On the other hand, setting the angle in a few degrees of dorsiflexion can help limit hyperextension at the knee (genu recurvatum). If the AFO is set in dorsiflexion, the patient must have sufficient quadriceps control to compensate for the increased knee flexion moment during the loading phase of gait. Another option for people with foot drop and/or mild quadriceps weakness is to use floor reaction orthoses (FROs) (such as the ToeOFF® braces) (Fig. 5-4F and G). FROs use ground reaction forces to offer a "push" at toe off as the orthosis dynamically unloads stored energy to assist with propulsion. This action assists with impaired ankle plantar flexion strength, which is often underdiagnosed. In addition,

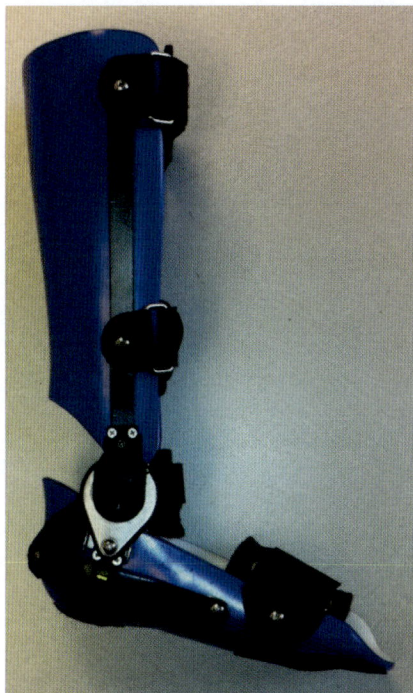

Figure 5-5. Nonambulatory AFO. This AFO provides low-load prolonged-duration stretch to the gastrocnemius–soleus complex. It might be used, especially at night, to help prevent or treat ankle plantar flexion contractures. (Sabrina Paganoni, MD.)

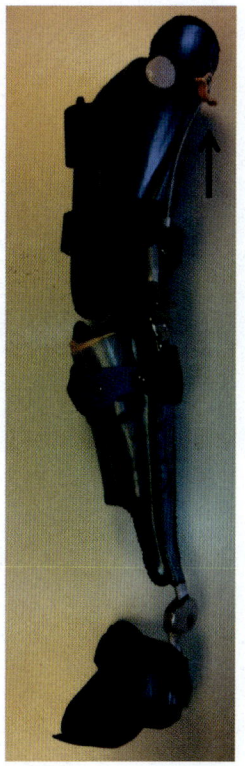 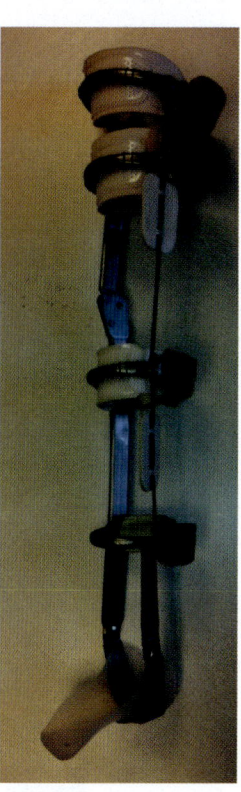

A   **B**

Figure 5-6. Knee–ankle–foot orthoses (KAFOs). **(A)** Trigger lock KAFO. **(B)** Stance control KAFO. With traditional KAFOs, the user needs to manually lock the knee joint and walk with a straight leg. Different systems are available to lock the knee such as a trigger (*arrow* in Panel A) or drop lock mechanism. Stance control KAFOs **(B)** allow for free knee flexion during swing phase while also providing knee stability in stance phase with no need to manually lock the knee joint. (Sabrina Paganoni, MD.)

FROs help create a knee extension moment which may help people with weak quadriceps and a tendency to knee buckling. For patients with spasticity, additional features might be built into the AFOs including a tone-reducing foot plate, toe extensor pads, foam toe separators, metatarsal pads, sustentaculum tali lift, or a plantar flexion stop.

In addition to improving gait efficiency, AFOs can also be used at night to help to prevent or minimize progressive equinus contractures in patients with significant ankle dorsiflexion weakness or increased lower extremity tone. Nighttime AFOs can be either resting AFOs (static braces that keep the ankle aligned in a neutral position) or dynamic AFOs (which provide a low-load prolonged-duration stretch to the gastrocnemius–soleus complex) (Fig. 5-5).

In individuals with quadriceps weakness, a different type of brace that might be tried to provide knee stability is the knee–ankle–foot orthosis (KAFO) (Fig. 5-6). Many KAFOs are too heavy for practical use by individuals with progressive neuromuscular weakness. However, they have been successfully used in patients with polio and may assist with ambulation in selected patients with other neuromuscular conditions such as IBM.

MOBILITY AIDS

In people with gait impairment, mobility aids are prescribed to maximize function and promote independence to the highest level possible. One should aim to prescribe the least restrictive device or piece of equipment without compromising safety. If the individual has a progressive disorder, it is important to address current problems as well as anticipate and plan for future needs. Most aids, particularly those classified as DME, require a written prescription, and often a letter of medical necessity, signed by the physician. Reimbursement coverage varies greatly. Therefore, it is important to work with therapists and social workers who have experience with neuromuscular disorders to allow for proper planning.

Canes, Crutches, and Walkers

Mobility aids such as canes, crutches, and walkers are prescribed to patients with neuromuscular diagnoses and lower limb weakness and/or balance problems to increase patient safety and promote independent ambulation (Fig. 5-7). These assistive devices widen the base of support and offload a weak limb. The decision as to what walking aid to prescribe depends on the degree of weakness/imbalance in the lower

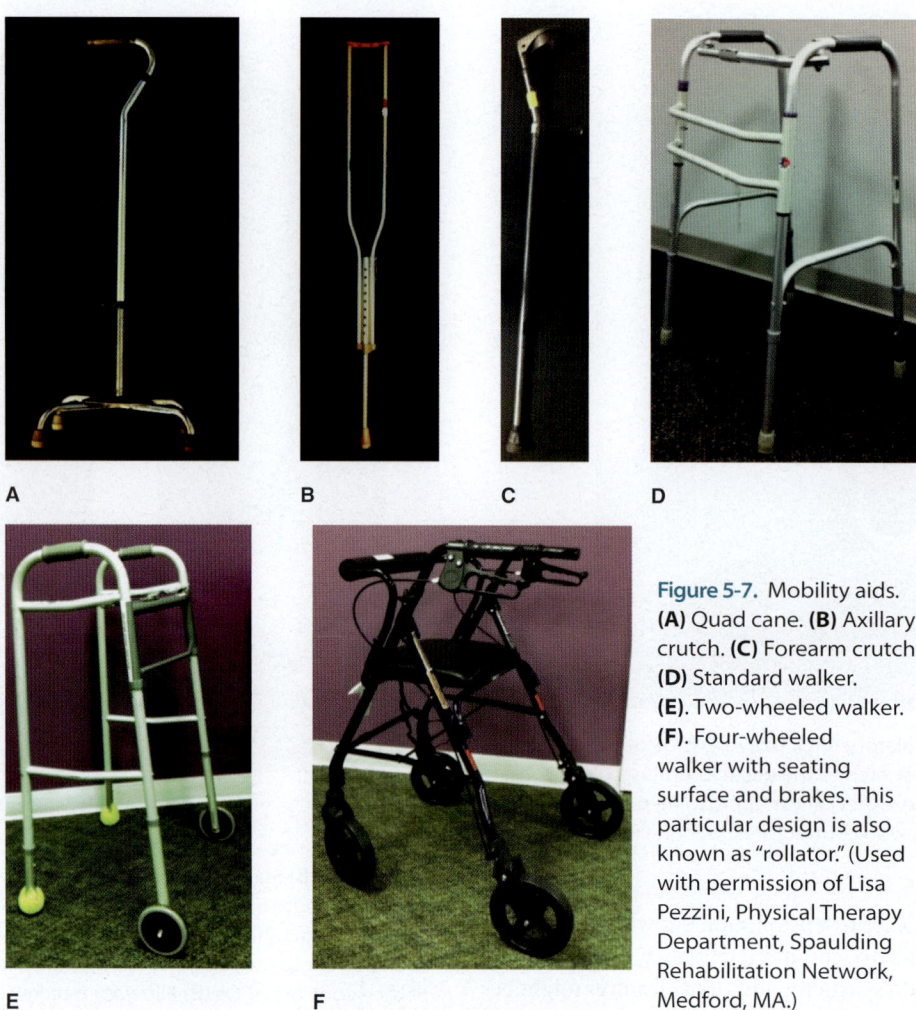

Figure 5-7. Mobility aids. **(A)** Quad cane. **(B)** Axillary crutch. **(C)** Forearm crutch. **(D)** Standard walker. **(E).** Two-wheeled walker. **(F).** Four-wheeled walker with seating surface and brakes. This particular design is also known as "rollator." (Used with permission of Lisa Pezzini, Physical Therapy Department, Spaulding Rehabilitation Network, Medford, MA.)

limbs, as well as strength in the trunk and upper extremities, grip strength, tone and ROM, and sensory problems. Patients are best served when they work with a PT to choose the most appropriate walking aid. A few sessions of gait training with the new device are recommended in order to maximize its use.

Canes provide the least amount of support and are usually recommended for people with only mild lower extremity impairment. The use of a cane also requires good upper limb strength. The total length of a cane should equal the distance from the upper border of the greater trochanter to the bottom of the heel of the shoe. The patient should be able to stand with the cane with the elbow flexed at 20 degrees and both shoulders level. A cane is generally carried in the hand opposite to the most affected leg. They can be used on stairs. One should lead with the stronger limb on flat ground and when ascending stairs, and with the more affected limb when descending stairs ("up with the good and down with the bad"). Patients might need to negotiate stairs on an angle and one step at a time depending on the degree of leg weakness. Canes come in a variety of styles and sizes of hand grips. Offset canes have a flat handle which can be built up allowing for better grip. This is beneficial for people with hand muscle weakness. Quad canes provide greater stability than traditional straight canes, but are heavier to lift, which limits their use in individuals with generalized progressive weakness (Fig. 5-7A).

There are three types of crutches: axillary (Fig. 5-7B), forearm (also known as Canadian or Lofstrand crutches) (Fig. 5-7C), and platform. Their use requires a high degree of upper body strength, coordination, and energy. Lofstrand crutches have a forearm cuff, which can free hands for use during standing. Platform crutches are useful when clinical conditions of the forearm, wrist, or hand prevent safe or comfortable weight bearing, such as in the presence of a wrist fracture or weakness of grasp. Some patients may choose to use walking sticks or trekking poles since they don't look as "medical" as crutches and tend to promote a more upright standing posture.

Walkers provide the maximum stability because of their wide base of support. However, they are bulky and may be cumbersome in confined spaces. Various types of walkers are available: standard (Fig. 5-7D), two wheeled (Fig. 5-7E), four wheeled (Fig. 5-7F), and with seating surfaces (Fig. 5-7F). Having a seat surface available increases the patient's independence if endurance is a problem. They may also be fitted with a shopping basket or a food tray. Standard walkers need to be lifted which can fatigue the upper limbs. Wheeled walkers do not need to be lifted and are preferred in people with generalized weakness if they can safely maneuver them. Four-wheeled walkers should be equipped with brakes for safety. Push-down brakes secure a walker when the patient loads their weight on the walker and are preferred over squeeze brakes for patients with hand weakness. There are three-wheeled walkers that can be easier to navigate in small spaces, but they are also less stable than the four-wheeled options, so caution should be made when recommending such devices.

Wheelchairs

In people with significant lower limb weakness and/or imbalance, the use of a wheelchair maybe indicated in order to maximize functional independence. A face-to-face mobility examination by a physician documenting inability to maintain functional ambulation and mobility-related ADLs in the home environment is required for patients to have wheelchairs, either manual or power depending on whichever is appropriate, reimbursed by Medicare. Coverage by private insurance companies is based on their policy for DME and requires a letter of medical necessity and a prescription from the treating physician. Some insurance companies cover equipment used only with adequate justification for mobility in the community. There is a wide range of choices in wheelchairs. PTs with a special expertise in wheelchairs often practice at wheelchair clinics. It is important to work with therapists who have experience with neuromuscular disorders to ensure that the optimal wheelchair is chosen for the individual patient's current and anticipated future needs. When making decisions about wheelchairs, one should keep in mind that, at present, Medicare and most private insurers limit reimbursement to only one wheelchair every few years (generally every 5 years). Therefore, expected disease progression and future needs must be kept in mind. This may be less restrictive with government-run health care such as the Veterans' Administration. Of note, some patient organizations maintain loaner closets that are available to patients so that they may try and borrow different pieces of equipment.

Power scooters should be recommended with caution to people with neuromuscular diseases. Good upper limb and trunk strength are needed to drive them. In addition, they cannot be modified for disease progression or to accommodate other equipment such as mounted trays or electronic equipment. Power scooters are considered power mobility devices. Therefore, reimbursement for a scooter precludes reimbursement for a power wheelchair, which the patient might need later in the course of their disease. However, they might be an option for those who can borrow or afford to purchase them. In these circumstances, they may be useful for outdoor use and energy conservation when one needs to walk long distances. Because of their long wheelbase and wide turning radius, it may be difficult to use them indoors.

Standard manual wheelchairs can be operated by the user alone if they have sufficient upper body function and stamina. These chairs are customized to best fit the person's needs. Multiple features of the chair need to be chosen correctly such as the weight as well as the seating characteristics. Upper body strength and endurance are impaired for many people with neuromuscular diseases. Therefore, manual wheelchairs should be of the lightweight or ultralightweight variety in order to enable the individual to propel the wheelchair independently. Additional chair features such as the type of cushion, type of armrest, and back and footrest height need to be individualized to allow for optimal comfort, support, safety, and function. If significant disease progression is expected, manual wheelchairs are not a long-term solution. However, having a backup manual wheelchair is important as it might be needed if the power chair needs repairs or when traveling if transport of the power chair is not an option. The need to accommodate growth is an additional consideration when prescribing wheelchairs for pediatric patients.

Transport or companion wheelchairs are lightweight chairs that are designed for ease of use and transport. They must be pushed by a caregiver. They fold to fit into a car's trunk and are generally used for traveling. Since they are relatively inexpensive, many families purchase one as a backup chair.

Power-assist wheelchairs are sometimes used by individuals who have a slowly progressive disease to reduce the effort required to self-propel a manual wheelchair. Power-assist wheels have an electrical motor attached to the hub which aids manually propelled use. However, they are rather heavy and are not indicated for people with rapidly progressing weakness.

When manual wheelchair use is no longer possible due to generalized weakness, respiratory compromise, or the need to use a ventilator or other equipment, power wheelchairs are prescribed. Transitioning to a power wheelchair is often challenging, both psychologically and logistically. The patient and caregivers need to adjust to disease progression and might need to have additional home and vehicle modifications as power wheelchairs do not fit into narrow doorways and standard cars, and cannot easily be carried up and down stairs. It is paramount to work closely with a wheelchair clinic with experience with neuromuscular disorders to ensure that the power wheelchair components are suitable for the individual's current and expected future needs. Proper seating and positioning are essential to ensure a comfortable and functional sitting posture and to prevent secondary injuries such as skin breakdown and back pain. Of note, wheelchair assessment and adjustment may be necessary as disease progresses if pain, skin problems, or poor posture are noted. Simple wheelchair modifications may significantly improve comfort and skincare management. One can choose among multiple options for head and neck support, trunk support, pressure relief, seatbelts, trays, BiPAP or vent holder, and drive controls. Pressure relief allows periodic redistribution of body mass to prevent skin breakdown and is accomplished

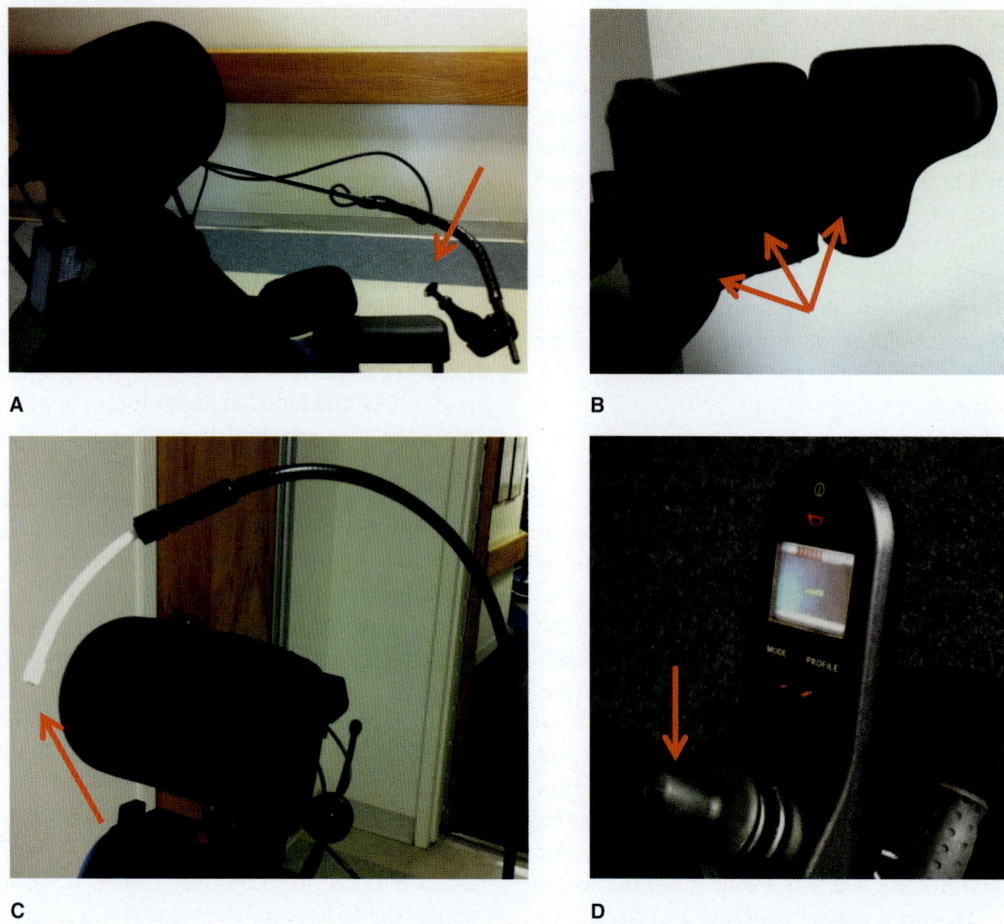

Figure 5-8. Power wheelchair drive controls. (A) The mini joystick (*arrow*) allows the individual to drive the wheelchair by using the lips or the tongue. (B) The head array is operated by coming in contact with proximity sensors located in each panel of the head array (*arrows*). (C) Sip and puff: this device allows wheelchair control by sipping and puffing on a straw located near the mouth (*arrow*). (D) The joystick (*arrow*) is used by people with at least some preserved hand/finger movements. (Used with permission of Michelle Kerr, Physical Therapy Department, Spaulding Rehabilitation Hospital, Boston, MA.)

using the tilt-in-space and recline functionalities. These functions are also beneficial in minimizing dependent edema that is commonplace in these patients and for improved comfort for those who choose to sleep in their chairs. Pressure mapping might be offered to supplement clinical impression when assessing the appropriateness of the seating system. Mapping is accomplished by using a thin mat with pressure sensors that can be placed over the chair cushion to analyze interface pressures. This can also be helpful to verify if pressure relief maneuvers are performed adequately. Multiple drive controls are available to allow users with different degrees of weakness to control the power wheelchair (Fig. 5-8). Most people use a joystick to control the wheelchair, at least initially, but may then need to progress to alternative control modes such as using a head array, lip/tongue mini joystick, foot joystick, sip and puff, single switch scanning, or other methods (Fig. 5-8). The wheelchair drive control can be adapted to integrate access to AAC devices, environmental systems, and computers within a single control interface.

Some power wheelchairs have a seat elevator that raises and lowers the seat vertically. This feature can help facilitate transfers and can provide an individual access to their environment for ADLs and instrumental ADLs (IADLs). Some power chairs have standing capabilities. An alternative option to allow periodic standing is the use of static standing frames. Potential benefits of standing include improved bone health through weight bearing, prevention of lower body contractures, and facilitation of social interactions and activities located on high counters and desks.

ADAPTIVE EQUIPMENT AND ENVIRONMENTAL MODIFICATIONS FOR DAILY LIVING

ADLs include basic ADLs (such as eating, grooming, bathing, dressing, and toileting) and IADLs which consist of more complex tasks such as working, driving, shopping, homemaking, and childcare. A diverse array of devices and equipment is available to enhance the independence of people with muscle weakness in their daily living. However, not all devices fit an individual person's needs and preferences, which may change over time. Therefore, the expertise of PTs and OTs is often needed to help patients navigate through the different options. One should also be mindful that the cost of many of these devices is not covered by insurance.

Self-Feeding and Meal Preparation

Eating utensils can be modified to facilitate grasp in the presence of hand weakness. Increasing the diameter of the handle on spoons, forks, and knives (as well as other daily tools such as writing instruments and grooming tools) improves grip (Fig. 5-9A). One can either purchase large-handled tools or cover regular utensil handles with cylindrical foam (Fig. 5-9A). Bendable utensils are also available. A spoon can be bent so that it faces the user to compensate for weakness of wrist flexion and supination. Rocker knives (or using a pizza cutter instead of a knife) make it easier to cut food (Fig. 5-9A). One can also use a cutting board with nails driven through it to hold food for chopping. When the patient's grip strength is severe enough to prevent them from holding any eating utensils, one can use a "universal" cuff which is a strap that one wears around the palm of the hand (Fig. 5-9B–D). The cuff has a pocket that can hold a variety of tools (Fig. 5-9B–D). Lightweight drinking cups, straw holders, and long straws can help to decrease the distance between hand and mouth assist with drinking (Fig. 5-9A). Using scoop dishes and plate guards helps prevent the food from falling off the side of a plate (Fig. 5-9A). Nonslip matting or using plates with suction bottoms keeps the plates from moving around on a table. Adaptive tools to open jars and cans are available. Reachers and grabbers help people get

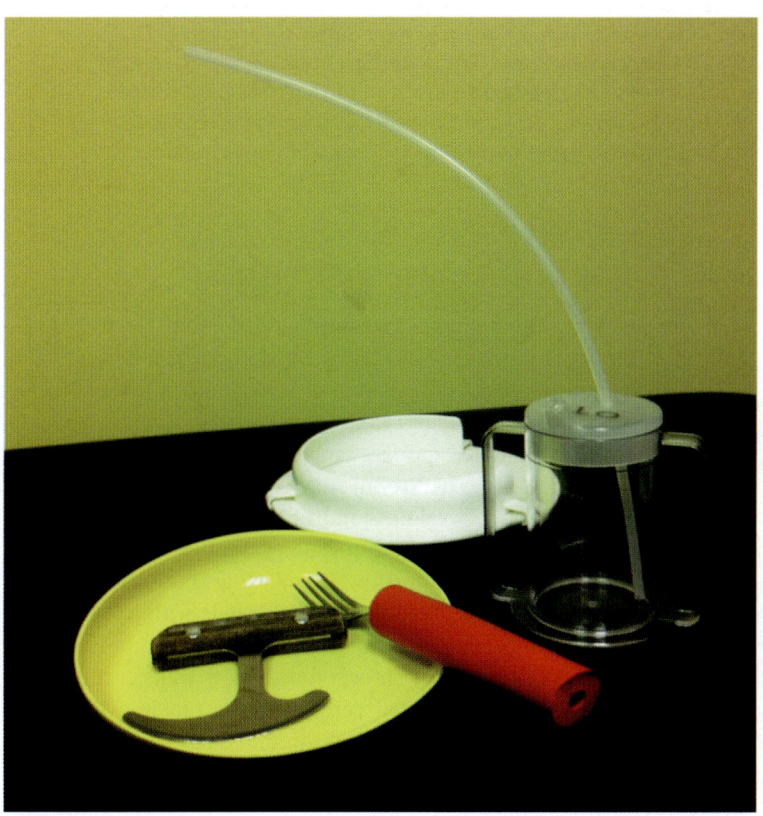

A

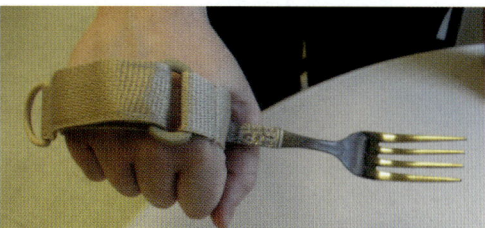

B

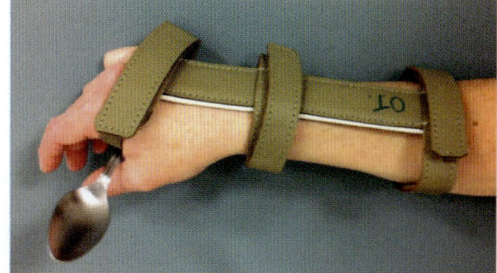

C

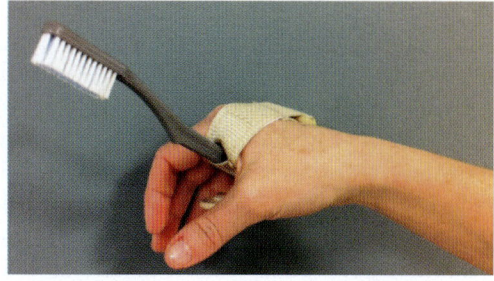

D

Figure 5-9. Adaptive equipment for eating and self-care. **(A)** Multiple adaptive tools are available to aid individuals with feeding themselves. Pictured here are a scoop plate (*yellow*), a rocker knife, a fork whose handle has been enlarged by soft foam tubing, a plate guard that has been attached to a regular plate (*white*), and a long straw. **(B–D)** The universal cuff is designed to provide individuals with little to no finger control and the ability to hold objects. Once centered over the palm, the device contains a pocket that can hold different types of tools including silverware, toothbrushes, brushes, and writing tools. In **(C)**, the universal cuff has been modified to provide support to a weak wrist. (Used with permission of Julie MacLean, Occupational Therapy Department, Massachusetts General Hospital, Boston, MA.)

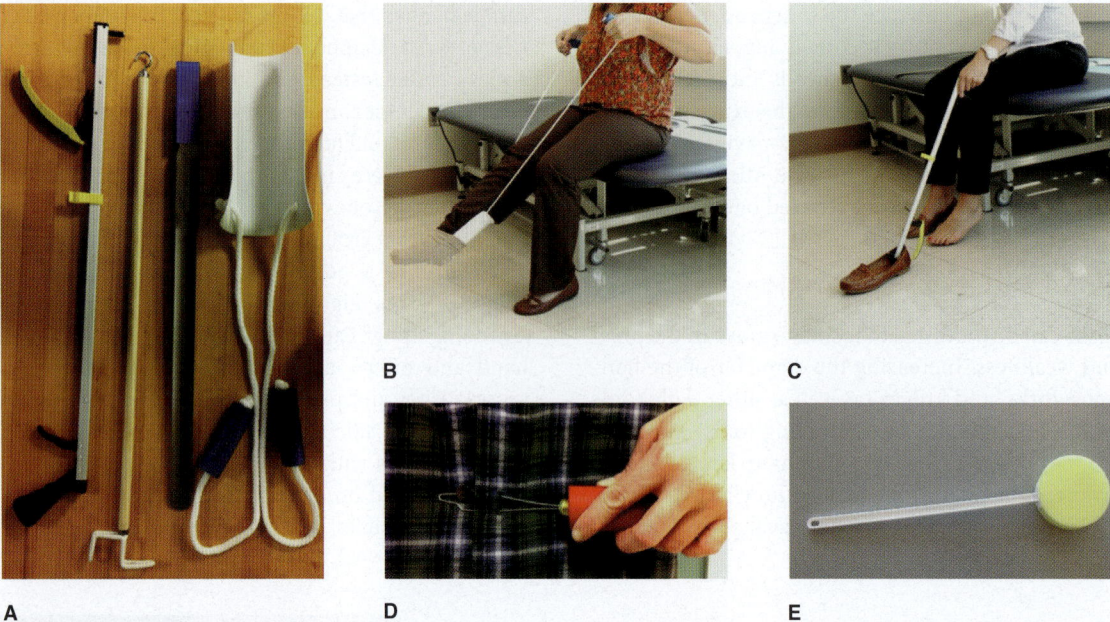

Figure 5-10. Adaptive equipment for dressing and bathing. Panel (A) shows, from the left, a reacher, a dressing stick, a long-handled shoe horn, and a sock aid. Panel (B) shows how to use a sock aid: after pulling the sock over the form and inserting the foot into the form, the individual pulls the loop handle to bring the sock up over the foot. In panel (C), the reacher is used for picking up out-of-reach items. It includes a magnetic tip to pick up metal objects, and a clip for storing the reacher on a walker or wheelchair. (D) The button hook is a tool used to facilitate the closing of apparel that uses buttons as fasteners. The hook end is inserted through the buttonhole to capture the button by the shank and draw it through the opening. (E) Long-handled sponge for bathing. (Used with permission of Julie MacLean, Occupational Therapy Department, Massachusetts General Hospital, Boston, MA.)

items from an upper cupboard and pick up objects from the floor (Fig. 5-10A and C). A mobile arm support, attached to either a table or a wheelchair, can compensate for proximal arm weakness: it will hold up the arm against gravity and help bring food to the mouth. This setup can also be used for other activities such as turning the pages of a book and grooming.

Dressing

Buttons, zippers, snaps, and shoelaces are notoriously difficult for people with hand weakness and impaired dexterity. One can try button and snap hooks (Fig. 5-10D), zipper pulls, and shoes with either Velcro® closure or elastic shoelaces. Velcro® can also be sewn behind buttons for easier fastening. Using sock aids and long-handled shoehorns reduces the need for bending forward when donning and doffing socks and shoes (Fig. 5-10A and B). Dressing sticks with mechanical graspers allow patients to compensate for upper limb weakness when putting on a sweater or shirt (Fig. 5-10A). There are adaptive clothing options that utilize magnets or Velcro®, rather than buttons or zippers. In addition to adaptive tools, OTs can suggest compensatory strategies for dressing and undressing. As an example, it is easier to don over-the-head shirts with the weaker side first, then the head, and finally the stronger side (the reverse sequence is used when doffing the shirt).

Self-Care, Bathing, and Toileting

A strap-fitted hairbrush, long-handled comb, electric toothbrush, and shaver can facilitate grooming. Cylindrical foam can be applied to the handle of multiple bath tools to facilitate grip. Pump soaps are easier to use than slippery bar soap and long-handled sponges can help with bathing (Fig. 5-10E). Transfers in the bathroom may be difficult for people with neuromuscular weakness and may pose a great danger with regards to risk of falling. Installing nonskid surfaces on the floor or in the bathtub/shower and using appropriate transfer equipment may help prevent falls. People with leg weakness or imbalance may find it hard to step over the tub. They may also need to sit in the shower for safety. A transfer tub bench is a padded seat placed across the tub that provides level transfer surface and a seat within the tub. A shower seat and a handheld shower head make showering easier. Grab bars are used for safe entering and exiting but need to be installed appropriately. It is important to educate patients on the fact that regular towel racks are not safe alternatives to grab bars as they cannot support body weight. Suction grab bars are not a viable alternative either for similar reasons. For people who use wheelchairs for mobility, a roll-in shower stall and rolling shower chair are ideal. Some shower chairs can also be used as a commode or over the toilet. People who have problems with sit-to-stand transfers might benefit from a raised toilet seat.

For people with balance problems or leg weakness, use of the bathroom at night can be especially dangerous. Having night lights and, if needed, a bedside commode may help minimize fall risk. Handheld urinals and external catheters may also be appropriate to help with nighttime urination.

Transfers

The ability to transfer allows the transition from one position or surface to another, such as from sitting to standing, from the bed to a chair, and so forth. Transfers are taken for granted by able-bodied individuals as they are an effortless activity that is performed every day countless of times. Transfers, however, are often burdensome for patients with neuromuscular conditions and their caregivers and yet they are a necessary part of daily living. Difficulties with transfers may prevent patients from getting out of bed or leaving their homes and may hamper their ability to participate in social events, attend doctor appointments, and enjoy outdoor activities. Therefore, transfer training and prescription of proper transfer aids are an essential component of the rehabilitation process. Importantly, transfer training must focus not only on efficiency but also on safety.

Bed mobility includes both repositioning while in bed and getting in and out of the bed. This can be facilitated by step stools, powered hospital beds, commercial adjustable beds, bedrails, and overhead trapezes. To get up from a chair, one can place firm cushions or blocks under the seat so that the hips are higher than the knees to facilitate sit-to-stand transfers. Swivel cushions are lightweight seats that swivel in both directions and make getting in and out of a car easier. A gait (transfer) belt allows the caregiver to provide safe lifting assistance to the patient. These belts are positioned around the patient's waist and hips and prevent traction on the patient's shoulders which may be painful. They also ease caregiver burden and potential musculoskeletal strain when assisting the patient, which are important considerations as a caregiver's ability to function is often integral to a patient's ability to continue to live in their home. There are also self-powered hydropneumatics lifting cushions (which are portable and relatively inexpensive), as well as powered recliner lift chairs that enable a person to rise to a standing position by activating an electric control. Lift chairs can also be installed in cars or vans for ease of transfer in and out of vehicles. As lower limb weakness progresses, different techniques can be used to transfer patients, such as stand pivot and squat pivot transfers with caregiver's assistance. A pivot disc can be used to assist with stand pivot transfers if the patient is able to stand but cannot step and turn. The patient's feet are placed on the disc. The patient stands and the disc is rotated. The patient is then lowered to the new surface (such as a chair or the bed). A slide board can be used for patients who are unable to stand. The patient can use the board independently if they have preserved upper body strength. Otherwise, the board can be used with the assistance of a caregiver. Finally, mechanical lifts allow for safe lifting of people who do not have the preserved strength to transfer independently. For individuals with intact cognition, the ability to direct a caregiver and provide instruction through the transfer enables a sense of autonomy despite requiring physical assistance with care.

Leisure Activities

The inability to enjoy leisure activities such as reading and writing can greatly lower quality of life. For book management, placing a book on an easel and using a page-turning device that clips to the hand allows independence with reading for some patients. Automatic page-turners that are activated by a switch are also commercially available. To facilitate grip, foam cylinders can be placed around writing instruments. There are also pen holders that hold the pen and allow writing as the patient moves the device. For television, telephone, and computer use, numerous options are available (reviewed below). Many adaptations exist for other leisure activities such as gardening, golfing, and fishing.

Driving

Driving is an activity symbolic of independence and control for many people, and one that is difficult to give up simply due to disability. However, it might be difficult for some patients with neuromuscular conditions to drive, especially for those with progressive weakness. Adaptive driving agencies and OTs can perform driving safety assessments to test the motor and cognitive skills necessary for driving. The results of the assessments are then used to make recommendations for vehicle modifications. Available modifications include left-foot accelerators for patients with right leg weakness and hand controls for patients with preserved upper body strength. Once the proper vehicle modifications have been identified, it is necessary to take adaptive driving lessons and a road test before the adaptations can be installed. This process is generally not covered by insurance and can be quite expensive; however, some nonprofit organizations offer grant support to defray the costs of modifications. In some states, vocational rehabilitation programs may also be available to provide this type of support. It can take several months to complete vehicle modifications for adaptive driving. This should be taken into consideration for patients with a more rapid disease progression who are considering this option.

Environmental Modifications

Environmental modifications at home, at school, and in the workplace may be necessary to optimize the independence and safety of some individuals. Such modifications can range from simple changes such as furniture rearrangement to extensive (and expensive) remodeling. PTs and OTs can provide home, workplace, and school evaluations and formulate recommendations for improved accessibility, function, and safety. Regional ADA centers can also provide guidance regarding how to make both private and public facilities compliant with specifications under the Americans with Disabilities Act (www.adata.org).

For wheelchair users, ramps may be needed to enter the home if there are steps. Ramps can be portable or permanent and can be rented or purchased. Narrow doorways often require widening to accommodate a wheelchair or a walker. The height of counters, sinks, light switches, and other reachable items may require modifications for accessibility from a seated position. If an individual has difficulties negotiating stairs or is a wheelchair user and their bedroom is on an upper floor, it may be necessary to accommodate for ground floor living space unless one can install an elevator or stair lift. When considering a stair lift for a wheelchair user, one must keep in mind that the individual will need to transfer in and out of the stair lift and leave a second wheelchair on the upper floor. Bedroom modifications are often needed to address problems with sleeping which are common among people with neuromuscular diseases. Hospital beds are used to elevate the head to reduce aspiration risk and help manage orthopnea. In addition, they allow repositioning and, in conjunction with special mattresses or mattress overlays, they can help alleviate the discomfort and risk of skin breakdown associated with limited mobility. Bathrooms are generally the smallest room in the home and often require the most modifications to accommodate patients with neuromuscular weakness. Walk-in or roll-in shower stalls, grab bars, and other adaptive equipment for toileting and bathing (described above) are examples of bathroom modifications.

Environmental control systems can be used to control appliances, lighting and heating systems, televisions, and telephones via a portable handheld keypad or the computer, even for individuals with very severe motor weakness. Keyboards can be modified depending on the person's motor control. As an example, the keys can be expanded to accommodate excessive movements for people with ataxia or can be reduced in size for those with minimal active finger movements. Eye gaze sensing technology enables people with severe limb weakness to access computers and environmental control systems by sensing movement from the reflection of the eye. Head movement tracking and voice-activated systems are also available.

Power wheelchairs frequently do not fit into standard vehicles and may require a modified van for transportation. Many individuals do not have the financial means to purchase a modified van and thus utilize a backup transport wheelchair to visit friends or travel to doctor appointments, for example. Alternatively, many power wheelchair users prefer to utilize accessible public transportation if it is available in their community.

A REHABILITATION APPROACH FOR COMMON NEUROMUSCULAR COMPLAINTS

After reviewing the basics of a variety of rehabilitation strategies such as exercise and the use of assistive devices, we will now suggest how to approach some of the most commonly encountered clinical problems in neuromuscular medicine from a rehabilitation perspective. Our goal is to describe how to leverage the expertise of multiple team members and integrate the different tools described above with the overarching goal of promoting patient safety, independent function, comfort, and quality of life. As each patient's set of needs, expectations, environment, and support systems are unique, the approach suggested here will need to be tailored to suit each individual and modified to adapt to changes in disease status. Thus, rather than suggesting a fixed and exhaustive solution for each clinical problem, we will propose a framework that can be used as a reference to design a customized rehabilitation plan.

AXIAL WEAKNESS AND SPINAL DEFORMITIES

Axial weakness may result in different clinical presentations including head drop (head ptosis), bent spine (camptocormia), and neuromuscular scoliosis, depending on the underlying process.

Head drop and bent spine are caused by neck extensor and paraspinal muscle weakness, respectively. In contrast with other skeletal disorders of the spine such as kyphosis, the deformity is not fixed (unless secondary contractures occur) and is corrected by passive extension or lying in the supine position. Functional consequences of these conditions might include difficulty walking, maintaining balance, conversing eye to eye, reading, and even difficulties swallowing, speaking, and breathing. Patients commonly experience pain in the nuchal region with head drop, and back pain from camptocormia, presumably due to protracted stretching of pain-sensitive spinal or paraspinal tissues. Typically, this pain is relieved by support.

Treatment is directed toward the primary pathology, if possible, as in cases of head drop due to myasthenia gravis. In progressive diseases such as ALS, one can offer supportive measures to promote good postural alignment and partially correct the deformity. Early implementation of supportive measures is important to prevent secondary complications such as contractures of the neck/back in a fixed flexed posture. We have seen individuals with ALS whose dysphagia or dyspnea improved when proper neck alignment was obtained by using an appropriate cervical orthosis. Orthoses that can be used include neck collars and baseball cap orthoses. It is important for the orthosis to provide enough support, which may require customization by an experienced PT/orthotist. These braces may be used intermittently even early in the disease for energy conservation purposes when performing certain demanding activities. Thoracic–lumbar–sacral orthoses (TLSOs) may be used to support the spine in cases of camptocormia but are often poorly tolerated. Orthotists may be able to adapt and customize TLSOs for improved comfort.[94] Stretching, physical modalities, and medications may be needed to prevent/treat neck and back pain.

Neuromuscular scoliosis is a sagittal deformity of the spine due to either neurogenic or myogenic disorders. It is especially common in progressive neuromuscular diseases that begin in childhood such as spinal muscular atrophy (SMA) and Duchenne muscular dystrophy.[95-97] Weakness in the trunk and paraspinal muscles leads to collapse of the developing spine into what is generally a long C-shaped curve with the apex in the thoracolumbar region.[96] Scoliosis causes discomfort and pain and, if severe, creates difficulties with seating, positioning, and breathing. TLSOs and molded seating systems may be utilized to provide support to the spinal column, but these interventions cannot prevent curve progression.[98] Spine development needs to be monitored periodically in consultation with orthopedic surgery.[12,97] In Duchenne muscular dystrophy, prolonged ambulation is associated with a reduced risk of developing scoliosis while steroid use slows curve progression.[99,100] The decision to perform surgical correction, generally spine fusion with instrumentation, depends on many factors including the patient's age, curvature progression, mobility status, and pulmonary function.[101] Oftentimes, spine fusion is performed around the onset of puberty in anticipation of curve progression. Careful preoperative evaluation is needed due to the increased operative risks in neuromuscular patients. Benefits of spine surgery include improved sitting balance and quality of life as well as prevention of back pain.[102] Whether the correction of spinal deformities slows the rate of ventilatory decline remains controversial.[12]

PROXIMAL UPPER LIMB WEAKNESS

Proximal upper limb weakness can be seen in multiple neuromuscular disorders and can cause difficulties with a variety of activities such as carrying objects, reaching overhead, and washing one's hair. As described above, adaptive equipment is available to help with many ADLs including reachers, dressing sticks with mechanical graspers, and long-handled combs and brushes. A mobile arm support, attached to either a table or a wheelchair, can compensate for impaired shoulder abduction by holding up the arm against gravity. This setup enables self-feeding for many patients and provides support for other activities such as grooming.

It is important to remember that chronic weakness of the shoulder girdle may lead to decreased ROM and pain. Other factors that are implicated in shoulder pain in neuromuscular patients are compensatory abnormal movement patterns, static positioning, spasticity, traction during inappropriately performed transfers, and contractures.[103] In a recent retrospective study of 193 patients with ALS, 23% reported experiencing shoulder pain at some time during the course of their illness.[104] Thus, attention to complaints of shoulder stiffness and pain should be part of routine ALS care.

While very little evidence is available to guide management of shoulder problems in neuromuscular patients, experience suggests that a proactive ROM program can often prevent the development of shoulder pain. We generally recommend beginning a daily shoulder stretching program early in the course of progressive neuromuscular disease that is likely to affect the shoulder girdle. Patients and their caregivers can be instructed on a simple, small set of ROM exercises that can be performed independently at home. If the individual is too weak to lift the shoulder overhead, stretching can be performed while lying down or with the assistance of a caregiver.

Once shoulder pain develops, a careful examination can identify the pain generator and guide treatment. Treatment strategies are highly individualized and include activity modification, stretching, physical modalities [heat, cold, massage, transcutaneous electrical nerve stimulation (TENS)], nonsteroidal anti-inflammatory and analgesic medications, and, in selected cases, steroid injections.[105-109] Surgical intervention is rarely indicated in progressive neuromuscular conditions. Individuals with significant shoulder weakness are also at risk of developing shoulder subluxation. Early use of shoulder support slings can help approximate the head of the humerus in the glenoid fossa, thus preventing/treating shoulder subluxation and resulting pain.[93] Simple modifications such as adjusting the seating system or the arm rests of the wheelchair provide additional comfort and pain relief. Positioning in bed should also be evaluated to ensure pressure on the shoulder is minimized. Pillows may be added to help support the arms and shoulders to provide pain relief.

Weakness of the thoracoscapular muscles may result in winging of the scapula. This may be seen within the context of nerve injury as in trauma to the long thoracic or the spinal accessory nerves. In these circumstances, clinical observation is generally attempted first for most patients, but bracing and surgical treatment may be considered.[110] Several myopathies can also result in scapular winging due to generalized weakness of the shoulder girdle musculature. In some patients, particularly in FSHD, the specific pattern of weakness may result in impaired shoulder ROM. Specifically, in FSHD, there is early selective weakness of the thoracoscapular muscles with relative preservation of the deltoid. When shoulder abduction is attempted using the deltoid, the scapula rotates and lifts off the chest wall impeding the movement. Scapular retraction orthoses may be tried to stabilize the shoulder blade, but they are generally considered too uncomfortable for prolonged use. Surgical scapular fixation techniques have also been proposed for people with FSHD with the goals of both improving the ability to elevate the arm at the shoulder and to improve arm strength by allowing improved scapular fixation. There have been no randomized trials of surgical versus nonsurgical treatment in patients with muscular dystrophy with scapular winging. Nevertheless, case reports and case series suggest that operative interventions can produce functional benefits in selected patients with FSHD.[111] However, these potential benefits have to be balanced against the need for postoperative immobilization, rehabilitation, and complications. Therefore, the decision to perform surgery is highly individualized. Surgical expertise is probably a critical factor in the success of these operations.[111]

HAND WEAKNESS

Hand weakness is seen in many neuromuscular diseases. Early symptoms of hand weakness include difficulties in opening jars and cans, turning doorknobs, and manipulating buttons. In more severe cases, handwriting, cutting food, using a telephone, and a multitude of other ADLs become affected.

OTs have special expertise in managing problems with upper limb functional activities secondary to hand weakness. In a cohort of 102 consecutive patients with neuromuscular diseases attending an outpatient clinic, 43% of patients were considered to potentially benefit from occupational therapy.[112] The type of OT intervention, though, was entirely based on the clinical expertise of the therapist, given the lack of research on occupational therapy specifically designed for neuromuscular disorders.

Two small studies reported some functional benefits in terms of performance and satisfaction with ADLs after 12 weeks of a hand exercise program using a silicone-based putty in 5 subjects with myotonic dystrophy and 12 subjects with Welander distal myopathy, respectively.[113] OTs can recommend adaptive equipment and braces to assist with many of the functional tasks described above. Some neuromuscular conditions are characterized by specific patterns of hand weakness. As an example, IBM typically affects the flexors of the distal phalanges, while radial neuropathy may affect finger extension. Therefore, hand orthoses most often need to be custom made to be tailored to the specific pattern of muscle weakness. Other OT interventions that might be indicated for individuals with hand weakness include ROM programs and resting hand splints to prevent contracture formation, ergonomic evaluation, and environmental modifications to maximize function at home, at school, or in the workplace, as well as driving safety assessment. Hand massage, positioning, and compression gloves may be used to manage edema secondary to limited hand function.

PROXIMAL LOWER LIMB WEAKNESS

Hip girdle and proximal leg weakness are seen in a variety of neuromuscular conditions, especially in myogenic disorders. Proximal lower limb weakness results in difficulties with transfers and gait, impaired ADLs, and increased risk of falling. It may also result in musculoskeletal pain when muscles are abnormally activated and overworked to compensate for the impaired posture and gait.

Proximal weakness makes it difficult to stand from sitting, negotiate stairs, and get in and out of a car. Adaptive equipment such as lifting cushions, stair lifts, and swivel seats have been described above. A variety of assistive devices are also available to enhance people's independence with lower body dressing, toileting, bathing, etc. For people with mild quadriceps weakness, FROs provide a knee extension moment which might help to stabilize the knee (Fig. 5-4). KAFOs have been used in some patients with polio and Duchenne to stabilize the knee in the setting of quadriceps weakness (Fig. 5-6).[114–116] With traditional KAFOs, however, the patient needs to walk with a locked knee which is difficult when significant hip girdle weakness is present. In addition, the weight of the KAFO often limits its practical application in neuromuscular patients. Newer stance control orthoses allow for free knee flexion during swing phase while also providing knee stability in stance phase. These braces have been trialed in patients with IBM and might have a role early in the course of the disease.[117] Further research is needed to clarify their role in patients with muscle disorders.

Lower limb muscle imbalance and abnormal gait may lead to low back and hip pain. Weakness of the hip girdle extensors results in hyperlordosis as a compensatory posture to maintain hip extension during ambulation. While this posture has an effective function during gait, it may also exacerbate low back pain. It is important to pay attention to symptoms of pain which may become quite disabling for the patient. Depending on the underlying neuromuscular disorder and pain generator, different interventions might be appropriate. In the absence of evidence-based guidelines, the treatment depends on the experience of the PT, physiatrist, and pain specialist. LSOs might be used for support in cases of back pain. Physical modalities such as cold, heat, massage, and TENS might be tried for comfort. An ergonomic evaluation might reveal a number of problems with the patient's workstation and biomechanics that can be fixed with simple environmental and behavioral modifications. As an example, using a footrest under one foot while standing at the kitchen counter may help ease low back pain. Gentle stretching and physical activity such as aquatic therapy might be indicated in some circumstances. If greater trochanteric pain syndrome is present, anti-inflammatory medications or steroid injections may be considered.

As weakness progresses, patients may lose the ability to ambulate. People who spend many hours a day in a wheelchair or in bed are at risk for developing hip and knee flexion contractures. These contractures are associated with further functional decline, pain, and difficulties with dressing, personal hygiene, and transfers. It is important to be mindful of this potential complication and to be proactive in recommending proper positioning, braces, and ROM exercises to prevent contracture formation.

FOOT DROP

Foot drop results from weakness of the tibialis anterior and/or weakness of the long extensors of the toes (extensor hallucis longus and extensor digitorum longus) and is due to a variety of etiologies. As a consequence, either the front of the foot or the whole foot contacts or scuffs the ground during swing-through of the leg, which can have a profound effect on gait. Tripping and falling are a major associated risk. Patients may use compensatory movement patterns, such as vaulting, circumduction, hip hiking, or a steppage gait, which result in increased energy expenditure and overwork of other muscles utilized to support the abnormal pattern.[118] Further, chronic weakness of dorsiflexion may result in reduced ankle ROM and shortening and contracture of the Achilles tendon. Many of the conditions which cause weakness of the ankle dorsiflexors also weaken muscles of eversion and inversion leading to further risk of contracture development, as well as increased risk of injury due to ankle instability. The exact contribution and severity may differ among conditions.

Traditional rehabilitation interventions for foot drop and its sequelae include stretching and strengthening exercises, orthotic and assistive devices, and surgery. Unfortunately, there is very limited evidence to aid in the clinical decision-making process.[119] Thus, the rehabilitation of foot drop is generally guided by clinician's experience. While evidence-based recommendations cannot be made due to the lack of research, the following commonly accepted interventions should be considered based on the limited available evidence and knowledge derived from other patient populations.

Stretching is used to maintain passive ROM and prevent contracture formation. One should aim at stretching both the gastrocnemius and the soleus muscles. The former is best stretched when the knee is in an extended position while the latter can be isolated with the knee in flexion.

Gait analysis of people with CMT showed that the hip flexors compensated for distal weakness and that hip flexor fatigue was a limiting factor in walking duration in these subjects.[120,121] This study suggests that strengthening proximal muscles might be used as a rehabilitation tool to improve gait function in people with foot drop.

Energy expenditure during gait increases in many patients with neuromuscular diseases.[122,123] Orthoses are used to splint the joint in a functional position with the goal of promoting a more efficient and safer gait. Studies in polio survivors showed that the energy cost of walking was decreased by wearing an orthosis.[114,115] Studies in people with CMT and FSHD suggested that use of an orthotic device resulted in improvement of walking performance and balance.[121,124,125] Gait evaluation in a brace clinic and gait training by a PT are helpful when an orthosis is being considered to ensure that the appropriate device is selected and to educate patients on its optimal use.

There has been some debate as to whether prolonged use of an orthotic device might lead to disuse atrophy. In a nonrandomized trial of 26 people with recent-onset foot drop secondary to peroneal neuropathy or L5 radiculopathy, ankle dorsiflexion strength was measured at baseline and after 6 weeks of either AFO use or no intervention.[126] All subjects had significant recovery of strength with no difference between the group that used the AFO and the group that did not, suggesting that the orthosis did not influence restoration of strength.[126] However, research on this topic is lacking in people with progressive neuromuscular diseases. In practice, we monitor gait and fall risk periodically and recommend orthoses based on clinical grounds. In cases of mild foot drop and when recovery is eventually expected, as in Guillain–Barré syndrome, one can use the AFO when walking in the community and "practice" ambulation without the brace at home as long as it is safe to do so. In rapidly progressive disease such as ALS, on the other hand, diurnal use of the brace for safety might be more appropriate.

As weakness progresses, ambulation might become unsafe even with the use of a brace, and assistive devices such as a cane, a walker, or eventually a wheelchair become necessary. Prevention and treatment of contractures resulting from chronic foot drop are described below.

FALLS

People with neuromuscular diseases may be at risk of falling due to weakness, abnormal tone, and impaired sensation and balance. Early in the course of the disease, simple strategies such as behavior modification and energy conservation techniques may suffice. As an example, people can be instructed to take rest breaks to avoid fatigue, use carts instead of carrying luggage or other objects, and negotiate stairs on an angle and one step at a time.

Oftentimes patients do not realize that some of their usual activities might be unsafe. Simple modifications may allow them to continue to function independently. A home safety evaluation by a PT can identify areas for improvement such as removing carpeting, sharp edges, and using appropriate footwear and night lights. Additional environmental modifications such as installing grab bars might be indicated. PTs and OTs can also educate patients and their caregivers on safe transfer techniques.

There is insufficient evidence that exercise results in lower fall rate in neuromuscular patients.[80–85] On the other hand, the benefits of exercise for fall prevention have been well documented in other patient populations.[127–130] If indicated, lower limb orthoses (AFOs) and spasticity management may make ambulation more efficient, although evidence is lacking on the exact impact of these interventions on the risk of falling in neuromuscular patients.

As the disease progresses, mobility aids such as canes, walkers, and wheelchairs may become necessary. Some patients choose to delay the use of mobility aids as long as possible because these tools are often perceived to signify loss of independence. It is important to remember, however, that the primary objective of using assistive devices is to actually preserve independent function. Thus, as an example, the use of a cane, perhaps on an intermittent basis even early on in the disease, may enable people to enjoy activities that would otherwise be restricted. Developing a strong therapeutic alliance with therapists and orthotists who have experience with neuromuscular diseases may assist patients to learn about and become familiar with different pieces of equipment that are available to enhance their independence. Mobility aids also help minimize falls. Falling and the potential occurrence of a bone fracture do have a significant and potentially long-lasting impact on independence in people with neuromuscular diseases. This problem is compounded by the loss of bone mass seen in many of these patients.[131] The prevalence of fractures in a cohort of boys with Duchenne muscular dystrophy attending four neuromuscular clinics was 20%, with some individuals experiencing permanent loss of independent ambulation after the fracture.[132] Falling was the most frequent cause of fractures in this study. Therefore, attention to safety and fall prevention is a crucial component of any rehabilitation program.

FOOT ABNORMALITIES

Peripheral neuropathies leading to intrinsic foot muscle weakness, such as CMT, are associated with bony and soft tissue abnormalities of the feet. These deformities include pes cavus (high-arched feet), pes equinus (excessive plantar flexion), and hammer toes (when the small toes have fixed flexion of the proximal interphalangeal joints with hyperextension of the metatarsophalangeal and distal interphalangeal joints). Functional consequences include pain, callous formation, skin breakdown, and difficulty walking. Many patients complain of and may present with frequent ankle sprains as a result of the foot deformity and underlying muscle weakness. Nonoperative treatment includes shoe modifications to improve comfort (such as using low-heeled shoes with a deep toe box, cushioned footwear, custom-molded shoe inserts, and pads to protect the toes) as well as braces (which can range from a simple Velcro-strap ankle brace for active patients with mild ankle instability to an AFO for people with foot drop). Surgical intervention may ultimately be required in some people to correct the deformities and promote ankle stability.

JOINT CONTRACTURES

Many people with neuromuscular diseases are at risk for the development of contractures defined as limitations of full passive ROM in a joint. Causes of contractures in neuromuscular diseases include decreased ability to actively move a limb, static positioning for prolonged periods of time, agonist–antagonist muscle imbalance, spasticity, and fibrotic muscle changes. Contractures are especially common in patients with progressive diseases such as muscular dystrophies. Importantly, contractures compound existing muscle weakness and can lead to pain, limit mobility, positioning, and hygiene and further hamper the quality of life.

Neuromuscular specialists play an important role in identifying the joints at risk for each particular patient. A commonly seen contracture site in neuromuscular diseases is the ankle in people with an imbalance between dorsiflexion and plantar flexion strength and/or tone (ankle plantar flexion contracture). Hips and knees are also at significant risk of contractures, especially in patients who spend most of their days in wheelchairs. People with hand weakness may experience wrist and finger flexion contractures. When patients are unable to raise their arms overhead, shoulder contractures may develop. Some neuromuscular diseases such as Emery–Dreifuss muscular dystrophy (EDMD) are characterized by early contracture formation, even at a stage of relatively preserved muscle strength. In EDMD, contractures of the elbow flexors and limitation of neck and trunk flexion are typical.

While the evidence supporting interventions to improve ROM in neuromuscular diseases is limited, generally accepted approaches for the prevention and treatment of contractures include stretching exercises, splinting, serial casting, and surgical correction for advanced fixed deformities.[119,133,134]

Daily standing and walking is important to prevent lower limb contracture formation.[133] As weakness progresses, daily upright weight bearing can be accomplished using standing frames or power wheelchairs with standing features.[133] While daily periods of standing are recommended by some practitioners, especially in the pediatric neuromuscular population, equipment cost and poor tolerance by some patients limit the implementation of standing programs.[12] In addition, further research is needed to determine the exact benefits of standing programs and to develop evidence-based guidelines for their use.

Early initiation of stretching and ROM programs is universally recommended for contracture prevention.[133,135,136] The optimal stretching regimen for people with neuromuscular diseases, however, has not been studied. One can draw from the available evidence in other populations and adjust the program to the individual patient. In healthy subjects, stretching is generally recommended one to two times per day, on most days of the week, and preferably after warm-up of the involved muscle through heat or gentle exercise. The muscle is taken to its maximal length across the affected joint until resistance is felt while stabilizing the joints that are not being moved.[2] This position is held for at least 10 seconds and then repeated several times.[2] Heat and ultrasound may enhance the effect of stretching and positioning. Patients and their caregivers can be instructed on a simple set of ROM exercises that can be performed independently at home. Ideally, such program can become part of a regular morning and evening routine. Positioning can be a useful adjunct for preventing contracture formation. As an example, lying in the prone position when possible provides an effective stretch to the hip flexors.

Bracing is another commonly used modality to prevent and manage contractures. Resting splints allow the joint to rest in a neutral position and can be used throughout the day or at night depending on the clinical scenario. In addition, one can use dynamic splints which provide low-load prolonged-duration stretch. Dynamic splinting in neuromuscular patients is most often used at the level of the ankle and at night. Unfortunately, there is no evidence to guide the timing to initiate splinting, the wear time, or the type of device.[134]

A study in Duchenne muscular dystrophy showed a decrease in ankle contractures with the use of a night splint compared to intermittent stretching.[137]

When a contracture is present, one method to improve ROM is to perform serial casting. With this approach, a series of casts with incrementally increasing angles of stretch is applied over a few weeks to gradually improve ROM. At the end of the program, the final cast can be bivalved to create a night splint for long-term maintenance of the ROM. Studies in Duchenne muscular dystrophy and CMT have shown that this approach results in increased ankle ROM, although this needs to be weighed against the possibility of worsening weakness due to cast immobility.[134,138,139]

Finally, surgical procedures for correction of fixed contractures can be considered. In some conditions, surgery may improve function. As an example, surgical procedures such as tendon lengthening, tendon transfer, and tenotomy have been used in Duchenne muscular dystrophy in an attempt to prolong ambulation. At present, however, there is no consensus on whether surgery to correct contractures results in prolonged ability to walk in patients with Duchennes. Therefore, the decision to perform surgery and its timing are strictly individualized.[12] Corrective surgery might also be performed in some patients as a palliative measure for comfort and positioning.[12]

SPASTICITY

Spasticity is a velocity-dependent increase in muscle tone. From a patient's perspective, spasticity is experienced as an inability to run or walk normally, often associated with leg dragging, loss of control or coordination, stiffness, spasms, pain, loss of fine dexterity, and fatigability. Spasticity generally has a negative impact on a variety of activities. However, in some cases, it may actually be of some functional benefit. As an example, increased tone in lower limb extensor muscles can assist weakened legs, allow standing during transfers, and facilitate bed mobility. Treatment, therefore, must be highly individualized.

Nonpharmacologic treatment options for spasticity are limited but can be offered as an adjunct. A regular stretching and ROM program is important as part of a contracture prevention program. Antispasticity features can be incorporated into AFOs as described above. Physical modalities that have been tried to reduce spasticity include the application of superficial heat and cold, massage, TENS, ultrasound, and acupuncture. The effects of these interventions, however, are generally short lived.[140] One randomized controlled trial of moderate intensity, endurance-type exercise in 25 participants with ALS showed promising positive effects on spasticity as measured by the Ashworth scale, but the trial was too small to draw definitive conclusions.[23,141] Pharmacologic agents for spasticity include oral medications, intrathecal baclofen, and botulinum toxin injections. The option of botulinum toxin needs to be weighed against its mechanism of action of causing weakness of muscles injected. These have been described in Chapter 7, Table 7-3. Finally, surgical interventions such as tendon release may be considered as a palliative measure in nonambulatory individuals to facilitate hygiene or relieve discomfort.

PAIN

Some neuromuscular diseases, such as small fiber neuropathy, directly involve pain pathways. Many others, such as ALS, are traditionally considered "painless" conditions. However, this could not be further from the truth as secondary painful musculoskeletal syndromes often arise in people with neuromuscular weakness. High prevalence of pain has been documented in multiple neuromuscular populations, including postpolio syndrome, FSHD, and myotonic dystrophy.[142-144] Pain can be reported by patients with ALS even in the early stages of their disease.[145] In a study by Engel et al., the prevalence of chronic pain among youths with a variety of muscular dystrophies was a staggering 55%.[144,146] Thus, a comprehensive rehabilitation plan for people with neuromuscular disorders must address pain.

The etiology of chronic pain in neuromuscular diseases is generally multifactorial, with contribution from both neuropathic and musculoskeletal pain generators. Primary sites of pain are the lower limbs and the back.[117,119] The first step in managing pain is to obtain a careful history and perform thorough neurologic and musculoskeletal examinations because treatment strategies vary depending on the main pain source. Importantly, soft tissue and bone problems can "mimic" neurogenic causes of pain (as further reviewed in Chapter 36). As an example, hip and thigh pain may be due to radiculopathy, hip osteoarthritis, or trochanteric bursitis, conditions that obviously warrant completely different therapeutic approaches. Foot pain can be due to neuropathy or radiculopathy, but also due to contractures, joint deformities, plantar fasciitis, and Morton's neuromas. Hand pain may be caused by median neuropathy at the wrist, osteoarthritis, or De Quervain tenosynovitis, just to name a few. We have seen patients with ALS and finger flexor tenosynovitis whose pain was greatly relieved by simple local steroid injections. A careful examination can help differentiate among these conditions. If needed, referral to physiatrists or orthopedic surgeons might help assess the cause of pain and institute proper treatment. PTs having experience with neuromuscular diseases can help manage these and additional sources of pain such as trigger points, brace problems, improper transfer techniques, and poor positioning in bed or in the wheelchair. In wheelchair users, back pain can often be relieved by providing adequate lumbar support and good cushioning. Some features of power wheelchairs can help with pain management. Power elevation leg rests can help maintain hamstring length and ease back pain, while tilting the wheelchair relieves pain from gluteal pressure. Leg discomfort can also be associated with dependent edema secondary to limited mobility. Leg elevation, massage, and use of compression stockings may provide some relief. For people with advanced weakness, positioning in bed is an important issue that should not be overlooked. Bed should be fitted with pressure relief over bony prominences to avoid pain and pressure ulcers. Foam wedges, pillows, and mattress overlays can be used to facilitate proper positioning and pressure relief.

Medications to treat neuropathic pain have been described in Chapter 22. Musculoskeletal pain typically responds to nonsteroidal anti-inflammatory medications (NSAIDs), particularly if there is evidence of an inflammatory process such as arthritis or bursitis. As needed or standing doses of acetaminophen may be used along with an NSAID or if NSAIDs are contraindicated. Physiatrists and PTs can help recommend other strategies to alleviate pain such as stretching, bracing, manual therapy, topical heat and ice (given alone or sequentially, as in contrast therapy), TENS, ultrasound, and iontophoresis. These physical modalities can be effective either alone or as an adjunct to pharmacologic treatment. Involvement of specialists from a pain clinic might be needed in more severe cases.

PTOSIS

Neuromuscular causes of ptosis (specifically, blepharoptosis) include Guillain–Barré and Miller Fisher syndromes, neuromuscular junction diseases, and certain myopathies, for example, oculopharyngeal muscular dystrophy (OPMD), mitochondrial myopathies, and myotonic dystrophy (Table 1-9). In addition to cosmetic concerns, ptosis may limit vision and interfere with driving, working, reading, and other ADLs. It may also result in neck discomfort because patients tend to compensate for ptosis by keeping a chin-up head posture. Treatment of ptosis revolves around management of the underlying disorder when disease-modifying treatments are available. In the case of the myopathies causing ptosis, no such therapies exist. Unfortunately, rehabilitation options for ptosis are very limited. Eyelid taping or eyelid prostheses (crutches) may be tried.[147] Eyelid crutches consist of attachments to glasses that hold the eyes open. Surgery is another option and different surgical techniques have been used, including silicone sling surgery which allows for adjustments for progressive ptosis. However, candidate selection is crucial. People with weak orbicularis oculi preventing complete closure of the eyelids are at risk for exposure keratopathy postoperatively.[148–150] In addition, ptosis may recur (recurrence rate among patients with OPMD was 13% in a surgical series from Quebec).[151]

DYSPHAGIA

Dysphagia refers to difficulty swallowing as a result of disruption in bulbar and respiratory function. The act of swallowing is complex; it requires adequate strength of the bulbar musculature, intact sensory, esophageal, respiratory, and cortical functions. Many neuromuscular diseases with bulbar and respiratory weakness can cause dysphagia including motor neuron disorders, neuromuscular junction diseases, Guillain–Barré syndrome, and certain myopathies (most commonly, inflammatory myopathies, OPMD, myofibrillar myopathies, some mitochondrial disorders, myotonic dystrophy, and late stages of Duchenne and other muscular dystrophies). The presence of dysphagia places patients at risk for medical complications including inadequate nutrition and hydration, pneumonia, and respiratory failure. These consequences can result in hospitalizations and reduce life expectancy. Dysphagia further impacts patients' ability to participate in daily and social activities and can significantly impact an individual's overall quality of life.[152]

Symptoms of dysphagia can include coughing and/or difficulty breathing during or after meals, episodes of choking, multiple swallows per bolus, increased secretions, frequent throat clearing, wet vocal quality (suggesting pooling of secretions), difficulty clearing food from the oral cavity, and feeling that food is "stuck" in the throat. If palatal weakness is present, the patient may also experience nasal regurgitation.

Dysphagia can be classified as either oropharyngeal or esophageal. Neuromuscular disorders generally cause the former, due to disruption of oral and/or pharyngeal processes. In the oral and pharyngeal phases of swallowing, lips are sealed, mastication occurs, a bolus is formed, the oral tongue moves the bolus to the posterior portion of the oral cavity, and propels the bolus into the pharynx. The soft palate elevates and makes contact with the superior pharyngeal constrictor to prevent food from entering the nasopharynx. In concert, airway closure occurs as the pharyngeal constrictors contract and the tongue base retracts to move the bolus toward the esophagus. Relaxation of the cricopharyngeus muscle allows the bolus to move into the cervical esophagus and toward the stomach. Achieving adequate airway protection (laryngeal vestibule closure) is complex and reliant on precise timing and completeness of movement of the tongue, pharynx, larynx, and hyoid bone. Disruption in the sensory or motor function of any of these structures places the patient with neuromuscular disease at risk for aspiration and its significant health consequences.

In the esophageal phase of swallowing, peristalsis moves the bolus through the esophagus and then into the stomach. Esophageal dysphagia is most commonly caused by mechanical causes or motility disorders, although some neuromuscular conditions such as the inflammatory myopathies can affect the esophagus as well.[153,154]

In oropharyngeal dysphagia, the type most commonly seen in neuromuscular disorders, swallowing can be impacted in terms of both safety and efficiency. Lip and tongue weakness impact bolus acceptance, preparation, propulsion, and clearance. This may result in solid food dysphagia and impact the range of foods and individual is able to consume, as well as the effectiveness and efficiency in which they are able to take a meal. Weakness of the pharyngeal musculature further impacts a patient's ability to complete the process of moving a bolus from the oral cavity into the esophagus. Difficulty swallowing liquids can also be an early symptom of dysphagia for individuals with neuromuscular conditions. Weakness impacts rate of bulbar muscle movement and coordination.

This impacts timing and completeness of laryngeal vestibule closure. The process is outpaced by the rapidity of the liquid bolus which tends to reach the laryngeal vestibule before laryngeal protection mechanisms can be fully activated, resulting in aspiration before or during the primary swallow event. In the presence of dysphagia, meals may require a longer time to complete and become a fatiguing and stressful, rather than pleasant, experience for patients and caregivers alike. The sialorrhea (drooling) seen in some neuromuscular diseases such as ALS is usually the result of decreased swallow frequency and effectiveness due to muscle weakness rather than an increase in salivation.[155–157]

Speech pathologists can provide an objective measurement of dysphagia by using clinical assessments as well as instrumental measures (i.e., MBS or FEES). Clinical bedside assessment consists of observing the swallowing function using a variety of food consistencies [liquid (thin and thick) and various solid food consistencies]. In the bedside assessment, particular attention is paid to the oral phase of swallow and signs/symptoms of pharyngeal/laryngeal dysfunction. Time to consume meals, patient-initiated diet modifications, and unintentional weight loss may increase index of suspicion for changes in swallowing function, especially the oral phase. MBS utilizes videofluoroscopy to visualize a contrast substance, barium sulfate, which is mixed with different food consistencies and swallowed. MBS is a sensitive technique for identifying oropharyngeal dysphagia as it allows tracing each bolus through the oral and pharyngeal phases as the person swallows.[158] The presence of penetration or aspiration into the larynx can be detected by MBS, thus helping gauge the risk of aspiration pneumonia. During the MBS examination, the clinician is able to isolate physiologic components of swallow and trial compensatory strategies (postural and bolus modifications) in attempt to improve airway protection and reduce postswallow residue in the oral cavity and pharyngeal recesses (residue impacts efficiency). This instrumental examination is currently considered the "gold standard" in dysphagia evaluation. Swallowing function can also be assessed endoscopically by FEES. This technique involves feeding an endoscope into the pharynx and positioning it just above the epiglottis to allow visualization of the pharyngeal phase of swallowing only. This type of swallowing examination is limited in that a whiteout period occurs when the swallow starts because the endoscope will be in contact with the base of tongue, epiglottis, and bolus. FEES is an effective way to evaluate presence of premature spillage, aspiration, and pharyngeal residue. Its portable nature makes it an accessible option in come clinical settings. However, this type of assessment may be poorly tolerated due to discomfort related to spasticity or positioning constraints in many patient populations.[159]

When dysphagia is present within the context of a treatable condition such as Guillain–Barré syndrome, myasthenia gravis, or PM/DM, treatment is directed toward the underlying pathologic process. From a rehabilitation perspective, there is no evidence that exercise improves swallowing function in patients with neuromuscular conditions. While waiting for dysphagia to improve or resolve, or in progressive diseases such as ALS and most myopathies, dysphagia management revolves around supportive care. Diet modifications, compensatory strategies, and intensive patient/caregiver education are the key features of dysphagia management in these patient populations. As an example, soft, moist foods are easier to swallow than dry, crumbly, or chewy foods. Foods that are smooth, single consistency (like pudding) are easier to manipulate in the mouth than mixed textured foods, such as dry cereal with milk. Thicker liquids (fruit nectar, smoothies) may be easier to handle than water. Commercial thickeners are available to modify the consistency of liquids to the desired level. Thickening a liquid can help to slow a bolus down enough for the pharyngeal responses to occur in a timely fashion, helping to prevent aspiration for some patients. Conversely, depending on the specific physiologic deficit of an individual's swallow, thickening liquids may further reduce swallow efficiency and/or increase aspiration risks. Thicker liquids can require more strength to propel and clear. Weakness, particularly of the pharyngeal musculature results in a pooling of postswallow residue in the pharyngeal recesses, more pronounced with thicker consistencies, that may migrate into the open airway after the initial swallow attempt. Furthermore, the chin tuck technique, a common recommendation to patients experiencing difficulty swallowing liquids, may exacerbate aspiration of bolus collections in the pharynx resulting in aspiration. A skilled clinical swallowing evaluation is essential to determine the specific type of swallowing disorder a patient is experiencing. Chilling liquids or adding carbonation may provide sensory stimulation during swallowing or improve swallowing in myasthenia by rendering neuromuscular transmission more efficient. As an example, chilled, carbonated water may be easier to swallow than room-temperature plain water. A modified diet can be recommended, ranging from soft diet (tender and moist foods), to mechanical diet (ground meats, well-cooked veggies, and soft fruits that require very little chewing), to pureed (when all foods are blended to a smooth liquid consistency). Behavioral strategies that may help to prolong people's ability to continue to eat in spite of dysphagia include taking small bites and sips, alternating bites of solid food with sips of liquid to ensure adequate clearing, sitting upright, avoid talking, and paying increased attention to each individual swallow. All strategies need to be carefully considered, there is not a prescribed regimen that is appropriate for all patients with dysphagia. If malnutrition is a concern, one can try eating smaller meals with high-calorie snacks at scheduled times, choosing calorie-dense foods or high-calorie liquid nutrition supplements. Because of difficulties managing liquids, special attention must be paid to the individual's hydration status. Gelatin, ice pops, and electrolyte supplements can help boost hydration status.

Effective management of dysphagia spans beyond diet modifications and safe swallow strategies. Patients are best served by a multidisciplinary approach to address secretion management, airway clearance, ability to self-feed, head and neck control, cultural considerations, and focus on patient autonomy. Periodic monitoring of swallowing function and nutritional status by a speech pathologist and/or dietitian helps to determine when oral intake becomes inadequate, too effortful or fatiguing, and/or compromises safety.

Alternative routes for nutrition include nasogastric tubes (generally utilized short-term) and percutaneous endoscopic gastrostomy (PEG) or radiologically inserted gastrostomy (RIG) tubes for long-term use. Enteral nutrition using either one of these methods is considered in the presence of severe bulbar symptoms, aspiration, weight loss >10%, dehydration, declining respiratory function, and diminished quality of life due to difficulties with eating/choking. In ALS, the risk of PEG placement increases when functional vital capacity falls below 50% and PEG is probably effective in prolonging survival.[160] Therefore, early intervention is advocated by many, although there is no evidence to support specific timing of PEG insertion in ALS.[160,161] Some people with progressive neuromuscular disorders choose to continue to consume limited amounts of preferred foods orally for pleasure. One should discuss the associated aspiration risks to enable the patient to make informed decisions regarding this approach.

In selected neuromuscular conditions, cricopharyngeal myotomy has been tried to alleviate dysphagia symptoms. With this procedure, the cricopharyngeal muscle, which is the major contributor to the upper esophageal sphincter (UES), is severed. This procedure might be considered in people with abnormal pharyngoesophageal junction, but adequate laryngeal/pharyngeal function, to ease the transfer of the swallowed bolus to the esophagus. Case series have reported benefits in patients with OPMD and IBM, although potential benefits have to be weighed against surgical risks.[162–167] In a series of 139 patients treated for dysphagia secondary to myopathy, complications were recorded in 16 patients, which ultimately resulted in four deaths.[163] Another method to target dysfunction at the UES is to inject the cricopharyngeal muscle with botulinum toxin. This technique was recently reported to improve dysphagia symptoms in a subset of people with motor neuron disease. Selection of appropriate candidates for the procedure was crucial as improvement was seen only in people with isolated UES hyperactivity based on videofluoroscopic or EMG assessment.[168] No improvement was seen in patients with concurrent lower motor neuron involvement of oropharyngeal muscles.[168]

DYSARTHRIA

Dysarthria is a collective name for speech disorders that impact the speed, strength, range, timing, and/or accuracy of speech movements and thus may impact the overall intelligibility of speech. Neuromuscular disorders affecting the motor neurons, the neuromuscular junction, and some myopathies can result in dysarthria. Upper motor neuron disease causes spastic dysarthria which is characterized by slow rate, harshness, and a strained-strangled vocal quality. There may be bursts of loudness and unanticipated stops. Lower motor neuron disease results in flaccid dysarthria, which presents as a weak, breathy, monopitch, and hypernasal voice. There may be imprecise articulation, but rate is generally normal. Motor neuron diseases such as ALS often present with mixed spastic–flaccid dysarthria. Dysarthria resulting from neuromuscular junction or muscle pathology typically resembles flaccid dysarthria.

When dysarthria is seen within the context of a treatable neuromuscular condition such as myasthenia gravis, treatment is directed toward the underlying pathology. On the other hand, when disease-modifying treatments are not available, referral to speech pathologists is very valuable in the evaluation and management of dysarthria. Many clinicians use intelligibility and listener effort to track changes in functional speech as disease progresses. Speaking rate is another useful means of evaluating speech production as changes in speaking rate precede reduction in intelligibility in progressive neuromuscular diseases such as ALS.[169,170] These factors should be taken into account when deciding the optimal timing for referral to an SLP and when considering introduction of AAC devices. Early introduction to SLP can provide essential counseling for patients and families so that they may have agency over monitoring for subtle changes in both speech and swallow function. This also provides an opportunity to introduce energy conservation techniques and voice/message banking; both of which are particularly important in patients with ALS before the onset of motor speech changes.[171]

Oral motor exercises are not likely to help in progressive neuromuscular disorders. A possible exception is myotonic dystrophy. In myotonic dystrophy, both muscle weakness and myotonia may contribute to impaired articulation. Warm-up exercises may improve fluency of speech and decrease the myotonic component of dysarthria without producing fatigue.[172]

In most chronic neuromuscular conditions, speech interventions revolve around techniques for compensation and adaptation to promote independence with communication. Reducing ambient noise, minimizing the distance between patient and listeners, and speaking face to face in a well-lit room are the first steps to make communication as easy and effortless as possible. In restaurants, choosing a table near a wall can help reduce distractions. Compensatory techniques to prolong verbal communication include slowing speech rate, using alternative words, spelling, and repeating and overarticulating. It is also important to develop personalized communication strategies between patient and caregivers such as shared strategies for establishing context, understanding gestures, and a system for confirming understanding. These techniques significantly reduce frustrations experienced in living with dysarthria.

A fatiguing aspect of speech production for people with concurrent weakness of the muscles of breathing is the need to develop sufficient respiratory support to speak loudly. As an example, people with ALS may have difficulties calling their caregiver in an adjacent room. Voice amplification is effective to improve vocal volume and facilitate energy conservation in these patients. The use of alerting systems such as buzzers and baby monitors can help. Similarly, it is important for people with severe dysarthria to have a plan to call for help in case of emergency.

As dysarthria progresses, AAC devices may be needed to enhance the person's ability to communicate. Such systems may be used to augment natural speech or to replace it. There is a wide range of options in devices for communication. One should keep in mind that more complex technology is not necessarily better. The choice of device is affected not only by the current degree of impairment but also by the expected disease progression, cognitive–linguistic abilities of the patient, comfort with technology, and patient/family preferences. Low-technology devices include communication boards with manual writing and letter/word/picture boards which can be used with a trained communication partner if the patient does not have functional hand use. High-technology options (defined here as anything that needs a plug or a battery) include portable voice amplifiers and speech-generating devices (SGDs). Message banking allows patients to record words and phrases while still intelligible and play them back when they are no longer able to say the messages themselves. These messages can be a helpful addition to a high-tech system that has voice output capability. Voice and message banking allows a patient to convey emotion through prosody, intonation, and quips that are not available when using preprogrammed synthetic voice outputs. SGDs allow messages to be created using selection of letters (typing), whole words, phrases, or pictures that populate to a screen and are output through a speech synthesizer. For people who are unable to use a keyboard, some speech-generating devices have the option of an on-screen keyboard with selection made by a switch using a scanning technique. Many people use computerized voice synthesizers on personal computers and tablets. Selection of information can be manual, by eye gaze, or by head movement tracking technology. Many of these assistive technology devices can be mounted on the person's wheelchair. Advances in technology continue to improve the dysarthric/anarthric patients' ability to engage meaningfully in home and work settings. SLP, PT, and OT work together to determine best access for patients and to predict evolving needs. Insurance restrictions can limit access to AAC, specifically higher tech options; a multidisciplinary approach is most effective to ensure best fit for long-term patient needs. Finally, brain–computer interfaces (BCIs) are an active area of research with promise for use in severe dysarthria or anarthria in people who also have severe motor impairment. BCIs transform signals originating in the brain into commands that translate into the movement of a cursor or a switch. Brain activity is captured by using either scalp recordings of electroencephalographic changes or direct recordings from the motor cortex.[173–175]

ADVANCES IN TECHNOLOGY

Advances in rehabilitation technology are likely to have a large impact on the function and quality of life of people living with neuromuscular diseases. Robotic assistance systems, like robotic arms or exoskeletons, have started to emerge as medical devices intended to help compensate for weakness and restore some amount of function, including basic ADLs. While they are not widely available, they should be considered as a potential tool. Considerations include the patient's experience with technology and desire to use technology, the weight of the device, the cost of device, how it is operated, and how long the person may be able to use the device. Is the device intended to be worn by the individual, and if so, can they safely don and doff it? Does it attach to a wheelchair, and can it be operated by alternative drive systems? If using an exoskeleton, it is important to monitor for, and avoid, overfatigue. Maier et al. recently showed that people with ALS have high technological commitment, and are interested in robotic devices to help promote individual autonomy and reduce caregiver burden.[176]

FINAL CONSIDERATIONS

For many neuromuscular conditions, these are exciting times for individuals, families, clinicians, and researchers. Enhanced understanding of many conditions and diseases has ushered in more effective treatments. Notably, the emergence of effective disease-modifying therapies for people living with SMA is changing the prognosis for these patients. As a result, there has been a consequent shift in rehabilitation practice for people living with SMA. The rehabilitation team is uniquely positioned to support this shifting rehabilitation paradigm by developing and validating outcome measures and appropriate exercise interventions to continue to maximize the functional potential and quality of life of these patients. This shifting paradigm will further inform the rehabilitation practices for all patients living with neuromuscular diseases.

It is critical to consider both functional potential and quality of life separately, given that the degree of weakness and physical impairment does not directly correlate with satisfaction with life.[177–180] Interestingly, both caregivers and health care professionals tend to underestimate the quality of life of neuromuscular patients based on their physical limitations.[177] Rather, in individuals with neuromuscular diseases, quality of life correlates with social interactions, ability to direct care, feelings of hope, and alleviation of manageable disease-related symptoms, all of which are factors that can benefit from a comprehensive rehabilitation plan.[181]

▶ ACKNOWLEDGMENTS

This chapter is dedicated to the memory of Lisa Krivickas, MD, exceptional mentor, ALS clinician, and researcher. We would also like to thank the following colleagues for their helpful comments and suggestions during the drafting of this chapter: Patricia Andres, DPT, MS; Jonathan Bean, MD, MS, MPH; Cheri Blauwet, MD; Katherine M. Burke, PT, DPT; Amy Swartz Ellrodt, PT, DPT; Elizabeth Hansen, PT, DPT; Max P. Higgins;

Michelle Kerr, PT/ATP; Claire MacAdam, PT; Julie MacLean, OTR/L; Paige Nalipinski, MA, CCC, SLP; Aaron Norell, CO, BOCP; Lisa Pezzini, PT; Stacey Sullivan, MS, CCC, SLP.

REFERENCES

1. Miller RG, Jackson CE, Kasarskis EJ, et al; Quality Standards Subcommittee of the American Academy of Neurology. Practice parameter update: the care of the patient with amyotrophic lateral sclerosis: multidisciplinary care, symptom management, and cognitive/behavioral impairment (an evidence-based review): report of the Quality Standards Subcommittee of the American Academy of Neurology. *Neurology*. 2009;73(15):1227–1233.
2. Johnson LB, Florence JM, Abresch RT. Physical therapy evaluation and management in neuromuscular diseases. *Phys Med Rehabil Clin N Am*. 2012;23(3):633–651.
3. Jette AM. Toward a common language for function, disability, and health. *Phys Ther*. 2006;86(5):726–734.
4. Holt NE, Percac-Lima S, Kurlinski LA, et al. The boston rehabilitative impairment study of the elderly: a description of methods. *Arch Phys Med Rehabil*. 2013;94(2):347–355.
5. Boentert M, Dziewas R, Heidbreder A, et al. Fatigue, reduced sleep quality and restless legs syndrome in Charcot-Marie-Tooth disease: a web-based survey. *J Neurol*. 2010;257(4):646–652.
6. Atassi N, Cook A, Pineda CME, Yerramilli-Rao P, Pulley D, Cudkowicz M. Depression in amyotrophic lateral sclerosis. *Amyotroph Lateral Scler*. 2011;12(2):109–112.
7. Heatwole C, Bode R, Johnson N, et al. Patient-reported impact of symptoms in myotonic dystrophy type 1 (PRISM-1). *Neurology*. 2012;79(4):348–357.
8. Patton BE, Wilson CM. Palliative care physical therapy: the challenges and the opportunities. *Rehabil Oncol*. 2021;39(3):E70–E72.
9. Voet NB, van der Kooi EL, van Engelen BG, Geurts AC. Strength training and aerobic exercise training for muscle disease. *Cochrane Database Syst Rev*. 2019;12(12):CD003907.
10. Zhou S. Chronic neural adaptations to unilateral exercise: mechanisms of cross education. *Exerc Sport Sci Rev*. 2000;28(4):177–184.
11. Fowler WM Jr. Role of physical activity and exercise training in neuromuscular diseases. *Am J Phys Med Rehabil*. 2002;81(11 Suppl):S187–S195.
12. Bushby K, Finkel R, Birnkrant DJ, et al; DMD Care Considerations Working Group. Diagnosis and management of Duchenne muscular dystrophy, part 2: implementation of multidisciplinary care. *Lancet Neurol*. 2010;9(2):177–189.
13. Phillips EM, Kennedy MA. The exercise prescription: a tool to improve physical activity. *PM R*. 2012;4(11):818–825.
14. Piercy KL, Troiano RP, Ballard RM, et al. The physical activity guidelines for Americans. *JAMA*. 2018;320(19):2020–2028.
15. Micheo W, Baerga L, Miranda G. Basic principles regarding strength, flexibility, and stability exercises. *PM R*. 2012;4(11):805–811.
16. Kraemer WJ, Ratamess NA, French DN. Resistance training for health and performance. *Curr Sports Med Rep*. 2002;1(3):165–171.
17. Mancuso M, Angelini C, Bertini E, et al; Nation-wide Italian Collaborative Network of Mitochondrial Diseases. Fatigue and exercise intolerance in mitochondrial diseases. Literature revision and experience of the Italian Network of mitochondrial diseases. *Neuromuscul Disord*. 2012;22 Suppl 3(3-3):S226–S229.
18. Angelini C, Tasca E. Fatigue in muscular dystrophies. *Neuromuscul Disord*. 2012;22 Suppl 3(3-3):S214–S220.
19. Kirkinezos IG, Hernandez D, Bradley WG, Moraes CT. Regular exercise is beneficial to a mouse model of amyotrophic lateral sclerosis. *Ann Neurol*. 2003;53(6):804–807.
20. Veldink JH, Bär PR, Joosten EA, Otten M, Wokke JH, van den Berg LH. Sexual differences in onset of disease and response to exercise in a transgenic model of ALS. *Neuromuscul Disord*. 2003;13(9):737–743.
21. Carreras I, Yuruker S, Aytan N, et al. Moderate exercise delays the motor performance decline in a transgenic model of ALS. *Brain Res*. 2010;1313:192–201.
22. Mahoney DJ, Rodriguez C, Devries M, Yasuda N, Tarnopolsky MA. Effects of high-intensity endurance exercise training in the G93A mouse model of amyotrophic lateral sclerosis. *Muscle Nerve*. 2004;29(5):656–662.
23. Drory VE, Goltsman E, Reznik JG, Mosek A, Korczyn AD. The value of muscle exercise in patients with amyotrophic lateral sclerosis. *J Neurol Sci*. 2001;191(1-2):133–137.
24. Bello-Haas VD, Florence JM, Kloos AD, et al. A randomized controlled trial of resistance exercise in individuals with ALS. *Neurology*. 2007;68(23):2003–2007.
25. Clawson LL, Cudkowicz M, Krivickas L, et al; Neals Consortium. A randomized controlled trial of resistance and endurance exercise in amyotrophic lateral sclerosis. *Amyotroph Lateral Scler Frontotemporal Degener*. 2018;19(3-4):250–258.
26. Lindeman E, Leffers P, Spaans F, et al. Strength training in patients with myotonic dystrophy and hereditary motor and sensory neuropathy: a randomized clinical trial. *Arch Phys Med Rehabil*. 1995;76(7):612–620.
27. Plowman EK, Tabor-Gray L, Rosado KM, et al. Impact of expiratory strength training in amyotrophic lateral sclerosis: results of a randomized, sham-controlled trial. *Muscle Nerve*. 2019;59(1):40–46.
28. Plowman EK, Gray LT, Chapin J, et al. Respiratory strength training in amyotrophic lateral sclerosis: a double-blind, randomized, multicenter, sham-controlled trial. *Neurology*. 2023;100(15):e1634–e1642.
29. El Mhandi L, Millet GY, Calmels P, et al. Benefits of interval-training on fatigue and functional capacities in Charcot-Marie-Tooth disease. *Muscle Nerve*. 2008;37(5):601–610.
30. Chetlin RD, Gutmann L, Tarnopolsky M, Ullrich IH, Yeater RA. Resistance training effectiveness in patients with Charcot-Marie-Tooth disease: recommendations for exercise prescription. *Arch Phys Med Rehabil*. 2004;85(8):1217–1223.
31. Burns J, Sman AD, Cornett KMD, et al; FAST Study Group. Safety and efficacy of progressive resistance exercise for Charcot-Marie-Tooth disease in children: a randomised, double-blind, sham-controlled trial. *Lancet Child Adolesc Health*. 2017;1(2):106–113.
32. Wallace A, Pietrusz A, Dewar E, et al. Community exercise is feasible for neuromuscular diseases and can improve aerobic capacity. *Neurology*. 2019;92(15):e1773–e1785.
33. Petrof BJ. The molecular basis of activity-induced muscle injury in Duchenne muscular dystrophy. *Mol Cell Biochem*. 1998;179(1-2):111–123.
34. Allen DG, Zhang BT, Whitehead NP. Stretch-induced membrane damage in muscle: comparison of wild-type and mdx mice. *Adv Exp Med Biol*. 2010;682:297–313.

35. Markert CD, Case LE, Carter GT, Furlong PA, Grange RW. Exercise and Duchenne muscular dystrophy: where we have been and where we need to go. *Muscle Nerve.* 2012;45(5):746–751.
36. Moens P, Baatsen PH, Maréchal G. Increased susceptibility of EDL muscles from mdx mice to damage induced by contractions with stretch. *J Muscle Res Cell Motil.* 1993;14(4):446–451.
37. Markert CD, Ambrosio F, Call JA, Grange RW. Exercise and Duchenne muscular dystrophy: toward evidence-based exercise prescription. *Muscle Nerve.* 2011;43(4):464–478.
38. Hammer S, Toussaint M, Vollsæter M, et al. Exercise training in Duchenne muscular dystrophy: a systematic review and meta-analysis. *J Rehabil Med.* 2022;54:jrm00250.
39. Jansen M, van Alfen N, Geurts ACH, de Groot IJM. Assisted bicycle training delays functional deterioration in boys with Duchenne muscular dystrophy: the randomized controlled trial "no use is disuse." *Neurorehabil Neural Repair.* 2013;27(9):816–827.
40. Alemdaroğlu I, Karaduman A, Yilmaz ÖT, Topaloğlu H. Different types of upper extremity exercise training in Duchenne muscular dystrophy: effects on functional performance, strength, endurance, and ambulation. *Muscle Nerve.* 2015;51(5):697–705.
41. Sveen ML, Jeppesen TD, Hauerslev S, Køber L, Krag TO, Vissing J. Endurance training improves fitness and strength in patients with Becker muscular dystrophy. *Brain.* 2008;131(Pt 11):2824–2831.
42. Sveen ML, Andersen SP, Ingelsrud LH, et al. Resistance training in patients with limb-girdle and Becker muscular dystrophies. *Muscle Nerve.* 2013;47(2):163–169.
43. Bartels B, Takken T, Blank AC, van Moorsel H, van der Pol WL, de Groot JF. Cardiopulmonary exercise testing in children and adolescents with dystrophinopathies: a pilot study. *Pediatr Phys Ther.* 2015;27(3):227–234.
44. van der Kooi EL, Vogels OJ, van Asseldonk RJ, et al. Strength training and albuterol in facioscapulohumeral muscular dystrophy. *Neurology.* 2004;63(4):702–708.
45. van der Kooi EL, Kalkman JS, Lindeman E, et al. Effects of training and albuterol on pain and fatigue in facioscapulohumeral muscular dystrophy. *J Neurol.* 2007;254(7):931–940.
46. Olsen DB, Ørngreen MC, Vissing J. Aerobic training improves exercise performance in facioscapulohumeral muscular dystrophy. *Neurology.* 2005;64(6):1064–1066.
47. Andersen G, Prahm KP, Dahlqvist JR, Citirak G, Vissing J. Aerobic training and postexercise protein in facioscapulohumeral muscular dystrophy: RCT study. *Neurology.* 2015;85(5):396–403.
48. Bankolé LC, Millet GY, Temesi J, et al. Safety and efficacy of a 6-month home-based exercise program in patients with facioscapulohumeral muscular dystrophy: a randomized controlled trial. *Medicine (Baltimore).* 2016;95(31):e4497.
49. Andersen G, Heje K, Buch AE, Vissing J. High-intensity interval training in facioscapulohumeral muscular dystrophy type 1: a randomized clinical trial. *J Neurol.* 2017;264(6):1099–1106.
50. Philp F, Kulshrestha R, Emery N, Arkesteijn M, Pandyan A, Willis T. A pilot study of a single intermittent arm cycling exercise programme on people affected by facioscapulohumeral dystrophy (FSHD). *PLoS One.* 2022;17(6):e0268990.
51. Pandya S, King WM, Tawil R. Facioscapulohumeral dystrophy. *Phys Ther.* 2008;88(1):105–113.
52. Aldehag A, Jonsson H, Lindblad J, Kottorp A, Ansved T, Kierkegaard M. Effects of hand-training in persons with myotonic dystrophy type 1—a randomised controlled cross-over pilot study. *Disabil Rehabil.* 2013;35(21):1798–1807.
53. Orngreen MC, Olsen DB, Vissing J. Aerobic training in patients with myotonic dystrophy type 1. *Ann Neurol.* 2005;57(5):754–757.
54. Wiesinger GF, Quittan M, Aringer M, et al. Improvement of physical fitness and muscle strength in polymyositis/dermatomyositis patients by a training programme. *Br J Rheumatol.* 1998;37(2):196–200.
55. Habers GEA, Takken T. Safety and efficacy of exercise training in patients with an idiopathic inflammatory myopathy–a systematic review. *Rheumatology (Oxford).* 2011;50(11):2113–2124.
56. Alexanderson H. Exercise in inflammatory myopathies, including inclusion body myositis. *Curr Rheumatol Rep.* 2012;14(3):244–251.
57. Alexanderson H, Lundberg IE. Exercise as a therapeutic modality in patients with idiopathic inflammatory myopathies. *Curr Opin Rheumatol.* 2012;24(2):201–207.
58. Wiesinger GF, Quittan M, Graninger M, et al. Benefit of 6 months long-term physical training in polymyositis/dermatomyositis patients. *Br J Rheumatol.* 1998;37(12):1338–1342.
59. Alemo Munters L, Dastmalchi M, Katz A, et al. Improved exercise performance and increased aerobic capacity after endurance training of patients with stable polymyositis and dermatomyositis. *Arthritis Res Ther.* 2013;15(4):R83.
60. Alexanderson H, Stenström CH, Jenner G, Lundberg I. The safety of a resistive home exercise program in patients with recent onset active polymyositis or dermatomyositis. *Scand J Rheumatol.* 2000;29(5):295–301.
61. Alexanderson H, Dastmalchi M, Esbjörnsson-Liljedahl M, Opava CH, Lundberg IE. Benefits of intensive resistance training in patients with chronic polymyositis or dermatomyositis. *Arthritis Rheum.* 2007;57(5):768–777.
62. Arnardottir S, Alexanderson H, Lundberg IE, Borg K. Sporadic inclusion body myositis: pilot study on the effects of a home exercise program on muscle function, histopathology and inflammatory reaction. *J Rehabil Med.* 2003;35(1):31–35.
63. Johnson LG, Collier KE, Edwards DJ, et al. Improvement in aerobic capacity after an exercise program in sporadic inclusion body myositis. *J Clin Neuromuscul Dis.* 2009;10(4):178–184.
64. Cejudo P, Bautista J, Montemayor T, et al. Exercise training in mitochondrial myopathy: a randomized controlled trial. *Muscle Nerve.* 2005;32(3):342–350.
65. Taivassalo T, De Stefano N, Argov Z, et al. Effects of aerobic training in patients with mitochondrial myopathies. *Neurology.* 1998;50(4):1055–1060.
66. Porcelli S, Marzorati M, Morandi L, Grassi B. Home-based aerobic exercise training improves skeletal muscle oxidative metabolism in patients with metabolic myopathies. *J Appl Physiol (1985).* 2016;121(3):699–708.
67. Taivassalo T, Gardner JL, Taylor RW, et al. Endurance training and detraining in mitochondrial myopathies due to single large-scale mtDNA deletions. *Brain.* 2006;129(Pt 12):3391–3401.
68. Taivassalo T, Shoubridge EA, Chen J, et al. Aerobic conditioning in patients with mitochondrial myopathies: physiological, biochemical, and genetic effects. *Ann Neurol.* 2001;50(2):133–141.
69. Siciliano G, Simoncini C, Lo Gerfo A, Orsucci D, Ricci G, Mancuso M. Effects of aerobic training on exercise-related oxidative stress in mitochondrial myopathies. *Neuromuscul Disord.* 2012;22 Suppl 3(3-3):S172–S177.
70. Murphy JL, Blakely EL, Schaefer AM, et al. Resistance training in patients with single, large-scale deletions of mitochondrial DNA. *Brain.* 2008;131(Pt 11):2832–2840.

71. Haller RG, Wyrick P, Taivassalo T, Vissing J. Aerobic conditioning: an effective therapy in McArdle's disease. *Ann Neurol.* 2006;59(6):922–928.
72. Maté-Muñoz JL, Moran M, Pérez M, et al. Favorable responses to acute and chronic exercise in McArdle patients. *Clin J Sport Med.* 2007;17(4):297–303.
73. Quinlivan R, Vissing J, Hilton-Jones D, Buckley J. Physical training for McArdle disease. *Cochrane Database Syst Rev.* 2011;(12):CD007931.
74. Lucia A, Quinlivan R, Wakelin A, Martín MA, Andreu AL. The 'McArdle paradox': exercise is a good advice for the exercise intolerant. *Br J Sports Med.* 2013;12:728–729.
75. Nogales-Gadea G, Santalla A, Ballester-Lopez A, et al. Exercise and preexercise nutrition as treatment for McArdle disease. *Med Sci Sports Exerc.* 2016;48(4):673–679.
76. Haller RG. Treatment of McArdle disease. *Arch Neurol.* 2000;7:923–924.
77. García-Benítez S, Fleck SJ, Naclerio F, Martín MA, Lucia A. Resistance (weight lifting) training in an adolescent with McArdle disease. *J Child Neurol.* 2013;28(6):805–808.
78. Santalla A, Valenzuela PL, Rodriguez-Lopez C, et al. Long-term exercise intervention in patients with McArdle disease: clinical and aerobic fitness benefits. *Med Sci Sports Exerc.* 2022;54(8):1231–1241.
79. Santalla A, Munguía-Izquierdo D, Brea-Alejo L, et al. Feasibility of resistance training in adult McArdle patients: clinical outcomes and muscle strength and mass benefits. *Front Aging Neurosci.* 2014;6:334.
80. Nardone A, Godi M, Artuso A, Schieppati M. Balance rehabilitation by moving platform and exercises in patients with neuropathy or vestibular deficit. *Arch Phys Med Rehabil.* 2010;91(12):1869–1877.
81. Kruse RL, Lemaster JW, Madsen RW. Fall and balance outcomes after an intervention to promote leg strength, balance, and walking in people with diabetic peripheral neuropathy: "feet first" randomized controlled trial. *Phys Ther.* 2010;90(11):1568–1579.
82. Song CH, Petrofsky JS, Lee SW, Lee KJ, Yim JE. Effects of an exercise program on balance and trunk proprioception in older adults with diabetic neuropathies. *Diabetes Technol Ther.* 2011;13(8):803–811.
83. Richardson JK, Sandman D, Vela S. A focused exercise regimen improves clinical measures of balance in patients with peripheral neuropathy. *Arch Phys Med Rehabil.* 2001;82(2):205–209.
84. Akbari M, Jafari H, Moshashaee A, Forugh B. Do diabetic neuropathy patients benefit from balance training? *J Rehabil Res Dev.* 2012;49(2):333–338.
85. Tofthagen C, Visovsky C, Berry DL. Strength and balance training for adults with peripheral neuropathy and high risk of fall: current evidence and implications for future research. *Oncol Nurs Forum.* 2012;39(5):E416–E424.
86. Mori L, Signori A, Prada V, et al; TreSPE study group. Treadmill training in patients affected by Charcot–Marie–Tooth neuropathy: results of a multicenter, prospective, randomized, single-blind, controlled study. *Eur J Neurol.* 2020;27(2):280–287.
87. Cup EH, Pieterse AJ, Ten Broek-Pastoor JM, et al. Exercise therapy and other types of physical therapy for patients with neuromuscular diseases: a systematic review. *Arch Phys Med Rehabil.* 2007;88(11):1452–1464.
88. Abresch RT, Carter GT, Han JJ, McDonald CM. Exercise in neuromuscular diseases. *Phys Med Rehabil Clin N Am.* 2012;23(3):653–673.
89. Rivera-Brown AM, Frontera WR. Principles of exercise physiology: responses to acute exercise and long-term adaptations to training. *PM R.* 2012;4(11):797–804.
90. Fast A, Thomas MA. The "baseball cap orthosis": a simple solution for dropped head syndrome. *Am J Phys Med Rehabil.* 2008;87(1):71–73.
91. Pancani S, Tindale W, Shaw PJ, Mazzà C, McDermott CJ. Efficacy of the head up collar in facilitating functional head movements in patients with amyotrophic lateral sclerosis. *Clin Biomech (Bristol, Avon).* 2018;57:114–120.
92. Sproson L, Lanfranchi V, Collins A, et al. Fit for purpose? A cross-sectional study to evaluate the acceptability and usability of HeadUp, a novel neck support collar for neurological neck weakness. *Amyotroph Lateral Scler Frontotemporal Degener.* 2021;22(1–2):38–45.
93. Zorowitz RD, Idank D, Ikai T, Hughes MB, Johnston MV. Shoulder subluxation after stroke: a comparison of four supports. *Arch Phys Med Rehabil.* 1995;76(8):763–771.
94. de Sèze MP, Creuzé A, de Sèze M, Mazaux JM. An orthosis and physiotherapy programme for camptocormia: a prospective case study. *J Rehabil Med.* 2008;40(9):761–765.
95. Wilkins KE, Gibson DA. The patterns of spinal deformity in Duchenne muscular dystrophy. *J Bone Joint Surg Am.* 1976;58(1):24–32.
96. Kouwenhoven JWM, Van Ommeren PM, Pruijs HEJ, Castelein RM. Spinal decompensation in neuromuscular disease. *Spine (Phila Pa 1976).* 2006;31(7):E188–E191.
97. Sucato DJ. Spine deformity in spinal muscular atrophy. *J Bone Joint Surg Am.* 2007;89(Suppl 1):148–154.
98. Colbert AP, Craig C. Scoliosis management in Duchenne muscular dystrophy: prospective study of modified Jewett hyperextension brace. *Arch Phys Med Rehabil.* 1987;68(5 Pt 1):302–304.
99. Kinali M, Messina S, Mercuri E, et al. Management of scoliosis in Duchenne muscular dystrophy: a large 10-year retrospective study. *Dev Med Child Neurol.* 2006;48(6):513–518.
100. Alman BA, Raza SN, Biggar WD. Steroid treatment and the development of scoliosis in males with Duchenne muscular dystrophy. *J Bone Joint Surg Am.* 2004;86(3):519–524.
101. Archer JE, Gardner AC, Roper HP, Chikermane AA, Tatman AJ. Duchenne muscular dystrophy: the management of scoliosis. *J Spine Surg.* 2016;2(3):185–194.
102. Granata C, Merlini L, Cervellati S, et al. Long-term results of spine surgery in Duchenne muscular dystrophy. *Neuromuscul Disord.* 1996;6(1):61–68.
103. Robinson CM, Seah KTM, Chee YH, Hindle P, Murray IR. Frozen shoulder. *J Bone Joint Surg Br.* 2012;94(1):1–9.
104. Ho DT, Ruthazer R, Russell JA. Shoulder pain in amyotrophic lateral sclerosis. *J Clin Neuromuscul Dis.* 2011;13(1):53–55.
105. Green S, Buchbinder R, Hetrick S. Acupuncture for shoulder pain. *Cochrane Database Syst Rev.* 2005;(2):CD005319.
106. Burke KM, Ellrodt AS, Joslin BC, et al. Ultrasound-guided glenohumeral joint injections for shoulder pain in ALS: a case series. *Front Neurol.* 2023;13:1067418.
107. Green S, Buchbinder R, Hetrick S. Physiotherapy interventions for shoulder pain. *Cochrane Database Syst Rev.* 2003;2003(2):CD004258.
108. Gaujoux-Viala C, Dougados M, Gossec L. Efficacy and safety of steroid injections for shoulder and elbow tendonitis: a meta-analysis of randomised controlled trials. *Ann Rheum Dis.* 2009;68(12):1843–1849.

109. Bloom JE, Rischin A, Johnston RV, Buchbinder R. Image-guided versus blind glucocorticoid injection for shoulder pain. *Cochrane Database Syst Rev*. 2012;(8):CD009147.
110. Meininger AK, Figuerres BF, Goldberg BA. Scapular winging: an update. *J Am Acad Orthop Surg*. 2011;19(8):453–462.
111. Orrell RW, Copeland S, Rose MR. Scapular fixation in muscular dystrophy. *Cochrane Database Syst Rev*. 2010;2010(1):CD003278.
112. Cup EH, Pieterse AJ, Knuijt S, et al. Referral of patients with neuromuscular disease to occupational therapy, physical therapy and speech therapy: usual practice versus multidisciplinary advice. *Disabil Rehabil*. 2007;29(9):717–726.
113. Aldehag AS, Jonsson H, Ansved T. Effects of a hand training programme in five patients with myotonic dystrophy type 1. *Occup Ther Int*. 2005;12(1):14–27.
114. Brehm MA, Beelen A, Doorenbosch CA, Harlaar J, Nollet F. Effect of carbon-composite knee-ankle-foot orthoses on walking efficiency and gait in former polio patients. *J Rehabil Med*. 2007;39(8):651–657.
115. Hachisuka K, Makino K, Wada F, Saeki S, Yoshimoto N. Oxygen consumption, oxygen cost and physiological cost index in polio survivors: a comparison of walking without orthosis, with an ordinary or a carbon-fibre reinforced plastic knee-ankle-foot orthosis. *J Rehabil Med*. 2007;39(8):646–650.
116. Bakker JP, De Groot IJ, De Jong BA, Van Tol-De Jager MA, Lankhorst GJ. Prescription pattern for orthoses in The Netherlands: use and experience in the ambulatory phase of Duchenne muscular dystrophy. *Disabil Rehabil*. 1997;19(8):318–325.
117. Bernhardt K, Oh T, Kaufman K. Stance control orthosis trial in patients with inclusion body myositis. *Prosthet Orthot Int*. 2011;35(1):39–44.
118. Waters RL, Mulroy S. The energy expenditure of normal and pathologic gait. *Gait Posture*. 1999;9(3):207–231.
119. Sackley C, Disler PB, Turner-Stokes L, Wade DT, Brittle N, Hoppitt T. Rehabilitation interventions for foot drop in neuromuscular disease. *Cochrane Database Syst Rev*. 2009;(3):CD003908.
120. Ramdharry GM, Day BL, Reilly MM, Marsden JF. Hip flexor fatigue limits walking in Charcot-Marie-Tooth disease. *Muscle Nerve*. 2009;40(1):103–111.
121. Ramdharry GM, Day BL, Reilly MM, Marsden JF. Foot drop splints improve proximal as well as distal leg control during gait in Charcot-Marie-Tooth disease. *Muscle Nerve*. 2012;46(4):512–519.
122. Menotti F, Felici F, Damiani A, Mangiola F, Vannicelli R, Macaluso A. Charcot-Marie-Tooth 1A patients with low level of impairment have a higher energy cost of walking than healthy individuals. *Neuromuscul Disord*. 2011;21(1):52–57.
123. McCrory MA, Kim HR, Wright NC, Lovelady CA, Aitkens S, Kilmer DD. Energy expenditure, physical activity, and body composition of ambulatory adults with hereditary neuromuscular disease. *Am J Clin Nutr*. 1998;67(6):1162–1169.
124. Aprile I, Bordieri C, Gilardi A, et al. Balance and walking involvement in facioscapulohumeral dystrophy: a pilot study on the effects of custom lower limb orthoses. *Eur J Phys Rehabil Med*. 2013;49(2):169–178.
125. Bean J, Walsh A, Frontera W. Brace modification improves aerobic performance in Charcot-Marie-Tooth disease: a single-subject design. *Am J Phys Med Rehabil*. 2001;80(8):578–582.
126. Geboers JF, Janssen-Potten YJ, Seelen HA, Spaans F, Drost MR. Evaluation of effect of ankle-foot orthosis use on strength restoration of paretic dorsiflexors. *Arch Phys Med Rehabil*. 2001;82(6):856–860.
127. Sinaki M, Brey RH, Hughes CA, Larson DR, Kaufman KR. Significant reduction in risk of falls and back pain in osteoporotic-kyphotic women through a Spinal Proprioceptive Extension Exercise Dynamic (SPEED) program. *Mayo Clin Proc*. 2005;80(7):849–855.
128. Sinaki M. Exercise for patients with osteoporosis: management of vertebral compression fractures and trunk strengthening for fall prevention. *PM R*. 2012;4(11):882–888.
129. Cameron ID, Gillespie LD, Robertson MC, et al. Interventions for preventing falls in older people in care facilities and hospitals. *Cochrane Database Syst Rev*. 2012;12:CD005465.
130. Moyer VA; U.S. Preventive Services Task Force. Prevention of falls in community-dwelling older adults: U.S. Preventive Services Task Force recommendation statement. *Ann Intern Med*. 2012;157(3):197–204.
131. Joyce NC, Hache LP, Clemens PR. Bone health and associated metabolic complications in neuromuscular diseases. *Phys Med Rehabil Clin N Am*. 2012;23(4):773–799.
132. McDonald DG, Kinali M, Gallagher AC, et al. Fracture prevalence in Duchenne muscular dystrophy. *Dev Med Child Neurol*. 2002;44(10):695–698.
133. Skalsky AJ, McDonald CM. Prevention and management of limb contractures in neuromuscular diseases. *Phys Med Rehabil Clin N Am*. 2012;23(3):675–687.
134. Rose KJ, Burns J, Wheeler DM, North KN. Interventions for increasing ankle range of motion in patients with neuromuscular disease. *Cochrane Database Syst Rev*. 2010;(2):CD006973.
135. Scott OM, Hyde SA, Goddard C, Dubowitz V. Prevention of deformity in Duchenne muscular dystrophy. A prospective study of passive stretching and splintage. *Physiotherapy*. 1981;67(6):177–180.
136. Burke K, DE Marchi F, Swartz Ellrodt A, et al. Exploring the use of educational materials for increasing participation in a stretching program: a quality improvement project in people with motor neuron disease. *Eur J Phys Rehabil Med*. 2021;57(1):78–84.
137. Hyde SA, FLłytrup I, Glent S, et al. A randomized comparative study of two methods for controlling Tendo Achilles contracture in Duchenne muscular dystrophy. *Neuromuscul Disord*. 2000;10(4-5):257–263.
138. Main M, Mercuri E, Haliloglu G, Baker R, Kinali M, Muntoni F. Serial casting of the ankles in Duchenne muscular dystrophy: can it be an alternative to surgery? *Neuromuscul Disord*. 2007;17(3):227–230.
139. Glanzman AM, Flickinger JM, Dholakia KH, Bönnemann CG, Finkel RS. Serial casting for the management of ankle contracture in Duchenne muscular dystrophy. *Pediatr Phys Ther*. 2011;23(3):275–279.
140. Gracies JM. Physical modalities other than stretch in spastic hypertonia. *Phys Med Rehabil Clin N Am*. 2001;12(4):769–792, vi.
141. Ashworth NL, Satkunam LE, Deforge D. Treatment for spasticity in amyotrophic lateral sclerosis/motor neuron disease. *Cochrane Database Syst Rev*. 2012;(2):CD004156.
142. Carter GT, Jensen MP, Hoffman AJ, Stoelb BL, Abresch RT, McDonald CM. Pain in myotonic muscular dystrophy, type 1. *Arch Phys Med Rehabil*. 2008;12:2382.
143. Stoelb BL, Carter GT, Abresch RT, Purekal S, McDonald CM, Jensen MP. Pain in persons with postpolio syndrome: frequency, intensity, and impact. *Arch Phys Med Rehabil*. 2008;89(10):1933–1940.
144. Jensen MP, Hoffman AJ, Stoelb BL, Abresch RT, Carter GT, McDonald CM. Chronic pain in persons with myotonic

dystrophy and facioscapulohumeral dystrophy. *Arch Phys Med Rehabil.* 2008;89(2):320–328.
145. Rivera I, Ajroud-Driss S, Casey P, et al. Prevalence and characteristics of pain in early and late stages of ALS. *Amyotroph Lateral Scler Frontotemporal Degener.* 2013;14(5-6):369–372.
146. Engel JM, Kartin D, Carter GT, Jensen MP, Jaffe KM. Pain in youths with neuromuscular disease. *Am J Hosp Palliat Care.* 2009;26(5):405–412.
147. Moss HL. Prosthesis for blepharoptosis and blepharospasm. *J Am Optom Assoc.* 1982;53(8):661–667.
148. Wong VA, Beckingsale PS, Oley CA, Sullivan TJ. Management of myogenic ptosis. *Ophthalmology.* 2002;109(5):1023–1031.
149. van Sorge AJ, Devogelaere T, Sotodeh M, Wubbels R, Paridaens D. Exposure keratopathy following silicone frontalis suspension in adult neuro- and myogenic ptosis. *Acta Ophthalmol.* 2012;90(2):188–192.
150. Kang DH, Koo SH, Ahn DS, Park SH, Yoon ES. Correction of blepharoptosis in oculopharyngeal muscular dystrophy. *Ann Plast Surg.* 2002;49(4):419–423.
151. Rodrigue D, Molgat YM. Surgical correction of blepharoptosis in oculopharyngeal muscular dystrophy. *Neuromuscul Disord.* 1997;7(Suppl 1):S82–S84.
152. Britton D, Karam C, Schindler JS. Swallowing and secretion management in neuromuscular disease. *Clin Chest Med.* 2018;39(2):449–457.
153. Vose A, Humbert I. "Hidden in plain sight": a descriptive review of laryngeal vestibule closure. *Dysphagia.* 2019;34(3):281–289.
154. Kruger D. Assessing esophageal dysphagia. *JAAPA.* 2014;27(5):23–30.
155. Marin B, Desport JC, Kajeu P, et al. Alteration of nutritional status at diagnosis is a prognostic factor for survival of amyotrophic lateral sclerosis patients. *J Neurol Neurosurg Psychiatry.* 2011;82(6):628–634.
156. Paganoni S, Deng J, Jaffa M, Cudkowicz ME, Wills AM. Body mass index, not dyslipidemia, is an independent predictor of survival in amyotrophic lateral sclerosis. *Muscle Nerve.* 2011;44(1):20–24.
157. Desport JC, Preux PM, Truong TC, Vallat JM, Sautereau D, Couratier P. Nutritional status is a prognostic factor for survival in ALS patients. *Neurology.* 1999;53(5):1059–1063.
158. Briani C, Marcon M, Ermani M, et al. Radiological evidence of subclinical dysphagia in motor neuron disease. *J Neurol.* 1998;245(4):211–216.
159. Triggs J, Pandolfino J. Recent advances in dysphagia management. *F1000Res.* 2019;8:F1000.
160. Miller RG, Jackson CE, Kasarskis EJ, et al; Quality Standards Subcommittee of the American Academy of Neurology. Practice parameter update: the care of the patient with amyotrophic lateral sclerosis: drug, nutritional, and respiratory therapies (an evidence-based review): report of the Quality Standards Subcommittee of the American Academy of Neurology. *Neurology.* 2009;73(15):1218–1226.
161. Braun MM, Osecheck M, Joyce NC. Nutrition assessment and management in amyotrophic lateral sclerosis. *Phys Med Rehabil Clin N Am.* 2012;23(4):751–771.
162. Brouillette D, Martel E, Chen LQ, Duranceau A. Pitfalls and complications of cricopharyngeal myotomy. *Chest Surg Clin N Am.* 1997;7(3):457–475; discussion 476.
163. Brigand C, Ferraro P, Martin J, Duranceau A. Risk factors in patients undergoing cricopharyngeal myotomy. *Br J Surg.* 2007;94(8):978–983.
164. Oh TH, Brumfield KA, Hoskin TL, Stolp KA, Murray JA, Bassford JR. Dysphagia in inflammatory myopathy: clinical characteristics, treatment strategies, and outcome in 62 patients. *Mayo Clin Proc.* 2007;82(4):441–447.
165. Oh TH, Brumfield KA, Hoskin TL, Kasperbauer JL, Basford JR. Dysphagia in inclusion body myositis: clinical features, management, and clinical outcome. *Am J Phys Med Rehabil.* 2008;87(11):883–889.
166. Pellerin HG, Nicole PC, Trépanier CA, Lessard MR. Postoperative complications in patients with oculopharyngeal muscular dystrophy: a retrospective study. *Can J Anaesth.* 2007;54(5):361–365.
167. Gómez-Torres A, Abrante Jiménez A, Rivas Infante E, Menoyo Bueno A, Tirado Zamora I, Esteban Ortega F. Cricopharyngeal myotomy in the treatment of oculopharyngeal muscular dystrophy. *Acta Otorrinolaringol Esp.* 2012;63(6):465–469.
168. Restivo DA, Casabona A, Nicotra A, et al. ALS dysphagia pathophysiology: differential botulinum toxin response. *Neurology.* 2013;80(7):616–620.
169. Yunusova Y, Green JR, Greenwood L, Wang J, Pattee GL, Zinman L. Tongue movements and their acoustic consequences in amyotrophic lateral sclerosis. *Folia Phoniatr Logop.* 2012;64(2):94–102.
170. Yunusova Y, Green JR, Lindstrom MJ, Ball LJ, Pattee GL, Zinman L. Kinematics of disease progression in bulbar ALS. *J Commun Disord.* 2010;43(1):6–20.
171. Rowe HP, Shellikeri S, Yunusova Y, Chenausky KV, Green JR. Quantifying articulatory impairments in neurodegenerative motor diseases: a scoping review and meta-analysis of interpretable acoustic features. *Int J Speech Lang Pathol.* 2022;25(4):486–499.
172. de Swart BJM, van Engelen BGM, Maassen BAM. Warming up improves speech production in patients with adult onset myotonic dystrophy. *J Commun Disord.* 2007;40(3):185–195.
173. Simeral JD, Kim SP, Black MJ, Donoghue JP, Hochberg LR. Neural control of cursor trajectory and click by a human with tetraplegia 1000 days after implant of an intracortical microelectrode array. *J Neural Eng.* 2011;8(2):025027.
174. Hochberg LR, Bacher D, Jarosiewicz B, et al. Reach and grasp by people with tetraplegia using a neurally controlled robotic arm. *Nature.* 2012;485(7398):372–375.
175. Collinger JL, Wodlinger B, Downey JE, et al. High-performance neuroprosthetic control by an individual with tetraplegia. *Lancet.* 2013;381(9866):557–564.
176. Maier A, Eicher C, Kiselev J, et al. Acceptance of enhanced robotic assistance systems in people with amyotrophic lateral sclerosis-associated motor impairment: observational online study. *JMIR Rehabil Assist Technol.* 2021;8(4):e18972.
177. Bach JR, Campagnolo DI, Hoeman S. Life satisfaction of individuals with Duchenne muscular dystrophy using long-term mechanical ventilatory support. *Am J Phys Med Rehabil.* 1991;70(3):129–135.
178. Paul RH, Nash JM, Cohen RA, Gilchrist JM, Goldstein JM. Quality of life and well-being of patients with myasthenia gravis. *Muscle Nerve.* 2001;24(4):512–516.
179. Simmons Z, Bremer BA, Robbins RA, Walsh SM, Fischer S. Quality of life in ALS depends on factors other than strength and physical function. *Neurology.* 2000;55(3):388–392.
180. Robbins RA, Simmons Z, Bremer BA, Walsh SM, Fischer S. Quality of life in ALS is maintained as physical function declines. *Neurology.* 2001;56(4):442–444.
181. Bromberg MB. Quality of life in amyotrophic lateral sclerosis. *Phys Med Rehabil Clin N Am.* 2008;19(3):591–605, x–xi.

SECTION II

SPECIFIC DISORDERS

CHAPTER 6

Motor Neuron Diseases and Amyotrophic Lateral Sclerosis

The motor neuron diseases (MNDs) are categorized by their pathological affinity for the voluntary motor system including anterior horn cells, certain motor cranial nerve nuclei, and corticospinal/bulbar tracts. Amyotrophic lateral sclerosis (ALS), also known as Lou Gehrig disease in the United States, is the most notorious of these disorders. The boundaries of what is and what is not ALS, particularly in the context of early diagnosis of individual patients, remain imprecise. In this chapter, in an attempt to distinguish ALS from other MNDs, we consider ALS to be a disorder that has the following characteristics: (1) the clinical manifestations are dominated by signs attributable to voluntary motor system dysfunction, (2) the disease progresses rapidly both within and between different body regions, (3) that life expectancy is less than 5 years from clinical onset in the vast majority of cases, and (4) that no other etiology can be identified.

Despite its characterization as a motor system degeneration, ALS is best conceptualized as a multisystem disorder.[1-3] This perspective is reinforced by both a clinical and pathological overlap between ALS and frontotemporal lobar degeneration (FTLD) (pathological) and frontotemporal dementia (FTD) (clinical).[4,5] Consequently, ALS is more correctly considered as a disorder in which dysfunction of the voluntary motor system involvement is the dominant source of morbidity (in the majority of cases) but in which involvement of other neurological systems at times clinically, and more commonly pathologically, develops.

The uncertain etiology of sporadic ALS (sALS) and the increasingly complex biology of ALS contribute to a lack of coherence in ALS nosology. This confusion applies to both historical and contemporary perspectives. In 1849 and 1850, respectively, Duchenne and Aran described progressive muscular atrophy (PMA), a disorder they believed to be of muscular origin. PMA has been long recognized; however, to result from anterior horn cell degeneration.[6] In 1860, Duchenne first described a syndrome of progressive dysphagia and dysarthria and coined the term progressive bulbar palsy (PBP).[6] In 1874, Charcot and Cruveilhier recognized that corticospinal tracts and anterior horn cells were often affected concomitantly. Their description serves as the basis for our current construct of ALS.[6] In the next year, Erb described primary lateral sclerosis (PLS), a progressive disorder of corticospinal tracts, without (at least initially) evidence of muscle atrophy, fasciculation, or weakness.[6]

ALS, PMA, PBP, and PLS are accepted by most, but not all neurologists as interrelated entities. PMA and PLS are clinically defined by the type of motor neuron affected. PBP on the other hand, is defined by site of disease onset, regardless of the type of motor neuron involved. Although survival in PMA and particularly PLS will on average exceed that of ALS, there is considerable overlap.[7-13] Many patients with these initially limited MND (PBP, PMA, and PLS) phenotypes evolve into ALS. Unfortunately, phenotypic classification does not provide a mechanism by which to predict the natural history of disease in an individual patient. Patients with prolonged (>5 years) survival have a similar distribution of phenotypes as do patients with typical natural histories.[14] Individual patients fulfilling ALS criteria may have indolent courses whereas patients with PMA may progress rapidly with approximately a third of PMA patients dying within 3 years of symptom onset.[15,16]

Recognizing the pragmatic limitations imposed by the imprecise MND boundaries, Lord Brain, in his text of 1962, proposed the "lumped" concept of MND, presumably to acknowledge and circumvent uncertainties of the split classification. To this day, MND serves as a synonym for ALS and all other forms of MND in several countries.[6] Arguably, it represents the most intellectually honest means to classify these disorders until a biological basis to justify lumping or splitting becomes available.

There have been four international consensus conferences that have attempted to provide an ALS classification scheme that is both accurate and clinically pragmatic. The first of these met in El Escorial, Spain in 1990. As there were no recognized effective treatments at that time, the primary goal was to define ALS with a high degree of sensitivity and specificity for research purposes. The proceedings of this meeting led to the subsequent publication of the El Escorial criteria (EEC) for ALS diagnosis.[17] Shortly thereafter, Riluzole was reported to alter the natural history of the disease, the first drug treatment shown to do so.[18] In response to this, with promise of other effective treatments, and in recognition that the stringency of the EEC would hamper enrollment into clinical trials, a subsequent meeting was held in Airlie House, Virginia in 1998.[19] The purpose of this convocation was to modify the EEC in order to allow earlier diagnosis without reducing diagnostic specificity thus facilitating for earlier and expedited clinical trial enrollment. These criteria

▶ TABLE 6-1. EL ESCORIAL CRITERIA (EEC)—REVISED

Clinically definite ALS	Defined on clinical evidence alone by the presence of UMN, as well as LMN signs, in three regions.
Clinically probable ALS	Defined on clinical evidence alone by UMN and LMN signs in at least two regions, with some UMN signs necessarily rostral to (above) the LMN signs.
Clinically probable, laboratory-supported ALS	Defined when clinical signs of UMN and LMN dysfunction are in one region, or when clinical UMN signs alone are present in one region—coupled with LMN signs defined by EMG criteria in at least two regions, with proper application of neuroimaging and clinical laboratory protocols to exclude other causes.
Clinically possible ALS	Defined when clinical signs of UMN and LMN dysfunction are found together in only one region or UMN signs are found alone in two or more regions, or LMN signs are found rostral to UMN signs (in absence of EMG evidence of more widespread LMN disease).

ALS, amyotrophic lateral sclerosis; UMN, upper motor neuron; LMN, lower motor neuron; EEC, El Escorial criteria.

became known as the revised EEC (Table 6-1). To this day, these criteria are the most commonly used to assess eligibility for ALS clinical trials. Of note, EEC categories capture the geographic spread of the disease (i.e., whether it affects one or more regions at the time of the exam) and not the degree of diagnostic certainty. Even patients with "possible" ALS are thought to have clear evidence of the disease, though characteristic findings are limited to a specific area.

Despite the virtual universal acceptance of revised EEC as the "gold standard" for eligibility for ALS trials, they may continue to sacrifice sensitivity for specificity.[20] Thus, patients with early ALS may be ineligible to enroll in clinical trials that restrict participation to specific EEC categories. Studies suggest that only 56% of patients clinically thought to have ALS will fulfill definite or probable revised EEC at the time of diagnosis.[12] Furthermore, up to 10% of a clinically defined ALS population will die without achieving either of these levels of diagnostic certainty.[12] In support of this, postmortem examination of patients who would not fulfill definite or probable ALS diagnostic criteria because of phenotypes restricted to upper motor neuron (UMN) or lower motor neuron (LMN) findings will have pathological confirmation of ALS.[21,22] The diagnosis of probable or definite ALS via EEC is dependent upon either clinical or lab demonstration of both UMN and LMN findings in two or three body regions (cranial, cervical, thoracic, lumbosacral), respectively. The reliable demonstration of UMN findings can be difficult and subjective, particularly in the thoracic and cranial regions. In addition, there is no reliable surrogate marker for UMN involvement as there is for lower motor disease (EMG).

In an attempt to improve sensitivity without sacrificing specificity in ALS diagnosis, a third consensus conference of experts convened in Awaji Island, Japan in 2006.[23] The premise of the Awaji criteria is that electrophysiological evidence for chronic neurogenic changes should be taken as equivalent to clinical information in the recognition of involvement of individual muscles in a limb. Conference participants also agreed that fasciculation potentials, particularly when "complex or unstable," represented an adequate surrogate for fibrillation potentials and positive waves as a marker of ongoing denervation. To maintain adequate disease specificity, the authors dictated that these unstable and complex fasciculation potentials had to occur in the context of two additional features: (1) the patient had clinical features suggesting ALS, and (2) fasciculation potentials had to occur in muscles concomitantly with chronic motor unit action potential (MUAP) changes. Subsequent studies supported the Awaji hypothesis by suggesting that diagnostic sensitivity increased by 23% in comparison to EEC while maintaining the same specificity of over 96%.[24,25]

Despite the field's interest in tools to enable early ALS diagnosis, the adoption of the Awaji criteria has been limited by concerns about the ability to distinguish between "complex and unstable," malignant fasciculation potentials and benign fasciculation potentials.[26] In addition, questions remain about whether fasciculation potentials, unstable or otherwise, should be accepted as a surrogate marker of ongoing denervation in the absence of other electrodiagnosis (EDX) abnormalities.[27]

More recently, the Gold Coast criteria were developed to enable earlier diagnosis and to equip the field with diagnostic criteria that are not only rigorous from a research perspective but also practical for clinical use.[28] To support the diagnosis of ALS, three criteria must be met (Table 6-2).[28] UMN dysfunction is assessed clinically (e.g., increased deep tendon reflexes, pathologic reflexes, spasticity). Evidence of LMN dysfunction can be derived from clinical examination and/or

▶ TABLE 6-2. GOLD COAST CRITERIA

1. Progressive motor impairment documented by history or repeated clinical assessment, preceded by normal motor function, AND
2. Presence of UMN and LMN signs in at least one body region (with UMN and LMN dysfunction noted in the same body region if only one body region is involved) or LMN dysfunction in at least two body regions, AND
3. Investigations excluding other disease processes

UMN, upper motor neuron; LMN, lower motor neuron.

EMG. Thus, in a given muscle, LMN dysfunction requires either clinical examination evidence of muscle weakness and wasting or EMG abnormalities (i.e., both evidence of chronic neurogenic changes and ongoing denervation as demonstrated by fibrillation potentials/positive sharp waves or fasciculation potentials). To be classified as an involved region with respect to LMN signs, abnormalities must be present in two limb muscles innervated by different roots and nerves, or one bulbar muscle, or one thoracic muscle either by clinical examination or EMG. These criteria simplify the diagnosis of ALS by collapsing the categories of possible, probable, and definite disease into a single entity, which helps from a clinical management perspective.[29] The performance of these criteria in clinical trials remains to be tested.[30]

Aran first reported the occurrence of ALS in multiple family members in 1848. Nonetheless, the concept of familial ALS (fALS) was dismissed by Charcot and largely ignored until the discovery of the first ALS gene mutation in the SOD1 gene in the early 1990s (Table 6-3). Up to 10%–20% of all ALS cases occur as a result of a single gene (Mendelian) mutation in one of the over 30 genes currently associated with ALS.[31-33] Additional genes have been reported to confer disease susceptibility and/or influence disease course. ALS may be recognized in multiple members of the same family (fALS) in about 10% of cases. In addition, about 5%–10% of apparently sporadic cases (sALS) may be due to a genetic mutation. Chromosome 9 open reading frame 72 (C9ORF72), SOD1, FUS and TARDBP are the most common causative genes. Familial and apparently sALS are clinically indistinguishable.[34]

ALS displays phenotypic heterogeneity. The full spectrum of phenotypic heterogeneity of ALS is evident even within different point mutations of the same gene (Table 6-3). fALS may occur with juvenile or adult onset, slow or fast progression, limb or bulbar onset, UMN or LMN predominance, and in the presence or absence of frontotemporal dysfunction. Not only do all of these different phenotypic variations occur in both fALS and sALS, but they also seem to occur with similar prevalence rates.[35] As in sALS, fALS patients may never fulfill the clinical EEC requirements for probable or definite ALS during the patient's lifetime.

As alluded to previously, the historical conceptualization of ALS, either inherited or sporadic, is that of a degenerative disorder of anterior horn cells and pyramidal tracts. This construct is confounded by the recognition that both the clinical manifestations and pathology of ALS may affect extrapyramidal, cerebellar, and particularly, cognitive systems.[1-3] It has been estimated that about 50% of ALS patients will have subtle or overt abnormalities in executive function, behavior, and/or language if carefully sought for, implicating frontotemporal dysfunction.[5,36] Overt FTD is estimated to affect 15% of the ALS population.[5,36] Conversely, if patients with FTD are carefully examined, it has been suggested that about 15% will have signs of definite ALS and additional 30% signs of possible disease. MND may precede, occur concurrently, or follow the onset of FTD.[5,37] Estimates of FTD prevalence, however, originate in large part from Western cultures where prolonged survival and the use of tracheostomy-assisted mechanical ventilation (TAMV) occur infrequently. Experiences in cultures where long-term ALS survivors are more prevalent, related to increased utilization of TAMV, suggest that the occurrence of dementia increases over time in ALS patients. This further supports the concept of ALS as a multisystem disorder. ALS with dementia or involvement of other neurological systems is designated as ALS plus by the revised EEC.[19] Although the focus of this chapter is ALS, the strong association with FTD and FTLD justifies a few comments relevant to the epidemiology of the latter disorder. In addition to ALS, FTLD may occur in association with cortical basal ganglionic degeneration, progressive supranuclear palsy, or other neurodegenerative conditions. In approximately 30% of cases, it is associated with a known genetic mutation.[38,39] The genes most commonly related to heritable FTD that have been identified to date include C9ORF72, microtubule-associated protein tau (MAPT) and progranulin (PGRN). Mutations of the C9ORF72 gene are the most common cause of genetically based ALS, underscoring that the two diseases exist along a spectrum.[40]

Within the general population, MNDs are relatively uncommon. The incidence of ALS is estimated to be approximately 1.6 per 100,000 people across studies and geographies.[41,42] This incidence appears to be increasing both within and outside the boundaries of an aging population. Disease prevalence is estimated at about 4.5 per 100,000 individuals with a global burden of approximately 300,000 cases worldwide.[43] Most people who develop ALS are between the ages of 40 and 70.[44] The average age of onset is about 56 years for sporadic disease and 46 years for most dominantly inherited forms of the disease. However, the disease can strike at any age: teenagers, young adults, and the elderly may be afflicted as well. Although it is widely believed that environmental factors must play at least some role in ALS pathogenesis, epidemiologic studies have failed to identify any reproducible risks other than age, gender, and potentially cigarette smoking.[45-48] The historical inability to identify environmental risks may be related in part to methodology and relative rarity of the disease. Although ALS has been reproducibly shown to occur 1.5 times more frequently in men, this ratio diminishes with advancing age and may not be true for bulbar-onset disease which seems more prevalent in older women.[49] There have been nests of apparent increased incidence. The ALS–Parkinson–Dementia complex formerly endemic in Guam and other Western Pacific regions is the most notable example.[50] The neuronal inclusions in this disorder contain tau however, not the ubiquitin characteristic of typical (non-SOD1) ALS, suggesting that Guamanian ALS may be a different disorder. Currently, typical ALS is considered to be the product of a complex interplay between time, genes, and environmental factors that may each play different roles in individual patients.[46]

The majority of ALS patients die within 2–5 years from symptom onset without ventilatory and nutritional support.[51-53] The range extends however from less than 1 year

▶ TABLE 6-3. MOST COMMON GENES ASSOCIATED WITH ALS

Gene/Protein	Inheritance	% fALS	% sALS	ALS Phenotype	Overlap With Other Diseases
C9ORF72	AD	20–50%	10%	±FTD	FTD, Parkinsonism
SOD1/superoxide dismutase 1	AD (most mutations) (AR with specific mutation)	10–20%	2%	LMN-D Rate of progression varies greatly by specific mutation (some rapidly and some slowly progressing) FTD rare	
TARDBP/TDP43	AD	5%	<1%	±FTD	PSP
FUS/fused in sarcoma	AD	5%	<1%	±FTD Can be adult onset or juvenile LMN-D	FTD, Parkinsonism
OPTN/optineurin	AD/AR	4%	<1%	Slowly progressive	
VCP/valosin-containing protein	AD	2%	<1%	±FTD	FTD Inclusion body myopathy, Paget disease, dementia
MAT3/matrin 3	AD	<1%	<1%	Slowly progressive ±FTD	Distal myopathy
HNRNPA1/heterogeneous nuclear ribonuclear protein A1	AD	<1%	<1%		Inclusion body myopathy
UBQLN2/ubiquilin 2	X-linked	<1%	<1%	Adult or juvenile ±FTD	FTD
SQSTM1/sequestosome 1	AD	<1%	<1%		Paget disease
TBK1/serine/threonine protein kinase	AD	<1%	<1%	±FTD	FTD
ANG/angiogenin	AD	<1%	<1%	±FTD LMN-D	
PFN1/profilin 1	AD	<1%	<1%		
CHCHD10/coiled-coil-helix-coiled-coil-helix-domain-containing protein 10	AD	<1%	<1%	±FTD	FTD
TUBA4A/tubulin A4A chain	AD	<1%	<1%	±FTD	
ATXN2/ataxin 2	AD, Risk Factor for ALS	<1%	<1%		Spinocerebellar ataxia type 2
FIG4/polyphosphoinositide phosphatase	AD	<1%	<1%		High % bulbar onset CMT4J
SETX/senataxin	AD	<1%	<1%		Juvenile onset, slow progression HSP phenotype with eventual LMN signs—no bulbar involvement Ataxia with oculomotor apraxia 2 Distal SMA

AD, autosomal dominant; ALS, amyotrophic lateral sclerosis; AR, autosomal recessive; fALS, familial ALS; FTD, frontotemporal lobar dysfunction; LMN-D, lower motor neuron dominant; PD, Parkinson disease; PSP, progressive supranuclear palsy; sALS, sporadic ALS; UMN-D, upper motor neuron dominant; HSP, hereditary spastic paraparesis; SMA, spinal muscular atrophy.

to more than 10 years without TAMV. It is estimated that a quarter of individuals will survive more than 5 years.[51] A vital capacity of less than 50% of predicted is associated with the need for hospice, death, or need for mechanical ventilation within 6 months.[54,55] Progression seems to follow a linear course, although the abrupt loss of a critical function may provide the appearance of stepwise deterioration.[56] Patients with bulbar-onset have a shorter average life expectancy, although many lead protracted existences if aspiration risk is minimized and ventilation preserved or supported. Young males seem to live longer on average.[57] Participation in a multidisciplinary clinic, access to disease-modifying treatments, noninvasive positive pressure breathing, and possibly percutaneous gastrostomy are interventions that have modest benefits in prolonging life expectancy.[58]

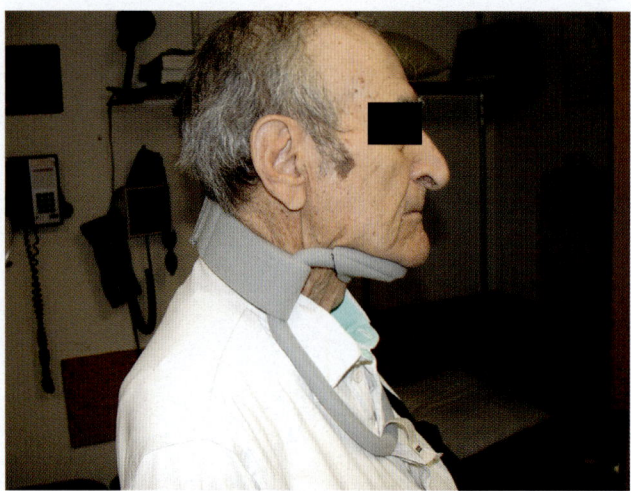

Figure 6-2. Head drop with cervical collar in amyotrophic lateral sclerosis.

▶ CLINICAL FEATURES

ALS is characterized by insidious-onset painless, progressive muscle weakness, and atrophy (Fig. 6-1). The site of onset, the relative predominance of UMN or LMN signs, and the rate of progression are variable. Patients typically present when functional difficulties cause them to acknowledge their deficit. These initial deficits are frequently asymmetric and sometimes monomelic. In instances where the patients do not seek early medical attention, or their physicians do not recognize the significance of the problem, the diagnosis may occur only several months or even a year or more after onset, at a stage when the disease may already be fairly advanced. The initial deficits may be initially limited in distribution but should affect more than one nerve and nerve root distribution in limb-onset cases. A third of cases present with bulbar onset, including dysarthria and/or dysphagia. Less commonly, the initial symptoms may be cramps, unintentional weight loss, or related to impaired ventilation. Occasionally, the initial clinical manifestations may be head drop or bent spine syndromes related to paraspinal muscle weakness (Fig. 6-2). In this latter circumstance, the patient may actually present with back pain due to the disordered posture caused by inadequate spine support.

Fasciculations may be one of the initial manifestations of MND. However, patients presenting with a chief complaint of fasciculations without weakness, atrophy, or abnormal EMGs rarely have or evolve into ALS.[59] In our experience, benign fasciculations are described more than seen, tend to occur most frequently in the calf muscles, and when observed are typically repetitive in the same location in any given muscle at any specific point in time. Conversely, fasciculations that are continuous and multifocal both within and between muscles, even in the absence of weakness, are ominous. This uncommon pattern of visible, frequent, and multifocal fasciculations without weakness is rarely seen in other circumstances other than MND, anticholinesterase overmedication being one notable exception. Lastly, the absence of fasciculations in patients with painless weakness does not preclude the diagnosis of ALS, particularly in those with excessive subcutaneous tissue.[60] An increased frequency of muscle cramping is also common in MND. In our experience, provocation of cramps in muscles (with the exception of the calves) during manual muscle testing is seen with some frequency in ALS patients and is uncommon in other disorders.

As previously alluded to, the clinical diagnosis of ALS is dependent on the demonstration of both LMN and UMN signs, which progress both within and between different body regions. Frequently, ALS may be dominated by LMN or UMN signs. This may occur at onset or, in some patients, may develop during their disease course. Signs of LMN involvement include muscle weakness, atrophy, attenuation or loss of deep tendon reflexes, cramps, and fasciculations.[61] When LMN weakness impairs coordination, it does so to an extent proportionate to the degree of weakness.[61] LMN features in cranial musculature in ALS are most frequently and convincingly manifest in the tongue. Atrophy is noted by

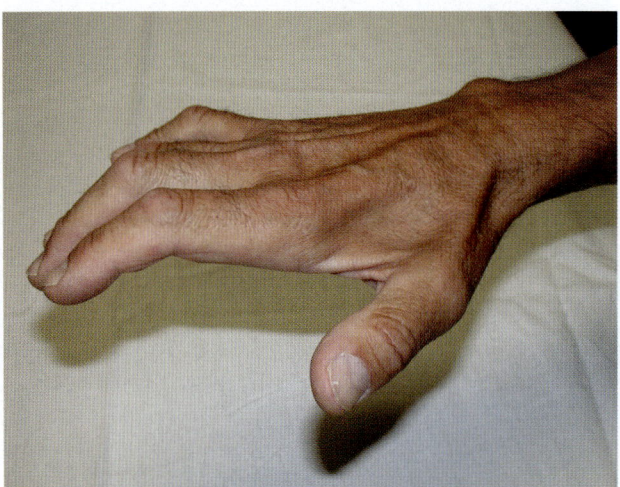

Figure 6-1. Hand atrophy in amyotrophic lateral sclerosis.

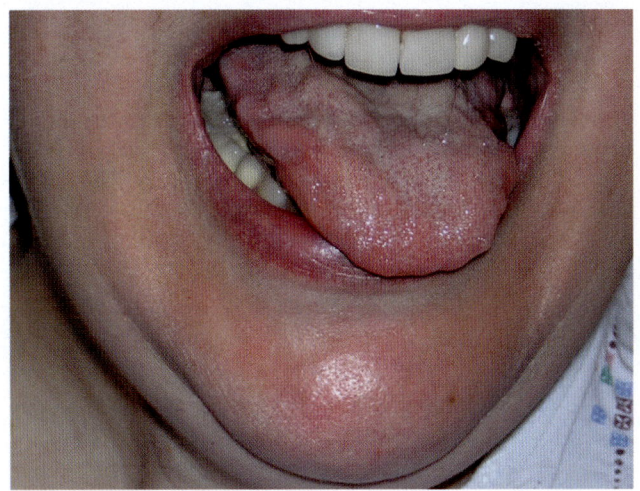

Figure 6-3. Tongue atrophy in amyotrophic lateral sclerosis.

the crenated, as opposed to the normal rounded edges, and fasciculations are best noted with the tongue lying quietly on the floor of the mouth (Fig. 6-3). Tongue strength is best tested by pushing against the bulge in the cheek created by the patient "pocketing" their tongue on either side. Weakness of neck flexion and extension are common in ALS. Weakness of facial (e.g., eye closure) and jaw opening and closing muscles occur but are typically less evident. Ptosis and ophthalmoparesis are notable for their absence.

UMN manifestations are more diverse and, at times, more subjective than their LMN counterparts. The elicitation of Babinski signs, sustained clonus, pathologically hyperactive deep tendon reflexes, and spasticity are objective and universally accepted manifestations of UMN pathology. Unfortunately, they are not overt in a significant percentage of ALS cases, thus confounding and delaying the clinical diagnosis. Other presumptive signs of corticospinal tract pathology include reflex spread (e.g., finger flexion with percussion of the brachioradialis tendon, hip flexion with percussion of the Achilles tendon), synkinesis (coactivation of muscles not required to accomplish a requested movement), Hoffman signs, and preservation of reflexes in a wasted and weak extremity. The latter is arguably the most prevalent of the subjective UMN sign demonstrable in ALS patients. In cranial innervated muscles, unequivocal UMN signs may be difficult to demonstrate. Increased emotional lability (pseudobulbar affect) and spastic dysarthria are perhaps the most frequently occurring UMN signs in this region but are more subjective than objective. Forced yawning is nonspecific. Exaggerated gag or jaw reflexes are more objective but do not occur with particularly great frequency. Arguably, slowness of attempted rapid blinking or tongue movements, in the absence of weakness, implicates central nervous system (CNS) pathology and provides support for UMN involvement in someone whose presentation is otherwise dominated by LMN signs. The same may be said for synkinesis, for example, the concomitant movement of the jaw with requested, rapid side-to-side tongue movements.

Coordination is impaired early with UMN involvement in a manner disproportionate to the degree of weakness.[61] There is frequently a "UMN stickiness" resulting in delayed activation of requested movements associated with the normal or near-normal strength. Often, muscles not required for an attempted motion are inappropriately (synkinetically) activated. For example, contralateral foot tapping may occur with requested unilateral foot-tapping movements. With UMN disease, foot dorsiflexion strength may be normal but delayed in initiation and preceded by great toe dorsiflexion. UMN signs may be transient in ALS, as they may develop and then disappear as LMN-induced weakness evolves and trumps UMN manifestations. For example, a Babinski sign may be lost as the extensor hallucis muscle weakens.

We find it helpful to categorize our patients both by onset site and phenotype. Onset sites include bulbar, upper limb, lower limb, or rarely truncal or ventilatory locations. Phenotypic categories include PMA, lower motor neuron dominant (LMN-D) ALS, ALS, upper motor neuron dominant (UMN-D) ALS, and PLS. We define PMA as muscle weakness and atrophy associated with hypo- or areflexia in involved segments. LMN-D is applied to individuals with dominant LMN features associated with suggestive UMN signs as listed above. Typically, these are individuals mentioned above whose deep tendon reflexes are either preserved or mildly increased in the involved body regions. UMN-D disease is defined by the paucity of LMN signs clinically but with unequivocal signs of denervation on EMG that are not readily explained by an alternative mechanism. PLS is defined as a progressive UMN syndrome occurring without an alternative explanation without either clinical or electrodiagnostic evidence of LMN disease.[7,62]

In most series, ALS is the most common presentation of MND, although even in these patients, the morbidity appears to stem primarily from LMN disease.[61,63] In probability, most classifications consider LMN-D to represent ALS. In approximately two-thirds of cases, the initial site of involvement is in a limb, typically distally and asymmetrically located in a hand or foot.[61] Initial weakness may occur in proximal muscles as well. A definite diagnosis cannot be made until combined UMN and LMN signs spread over a period of months, both within and outside the initially affected body region. The combination of UMN and LMN findings confined to multiple segments in one limb is sinister when unassociated with pain or sensory symptoms.

It is estimated that PMA phenotype represents anywhere between 2% and 10% of MND patients.[10] This variation is undoubtedly based on whether deep tendon reflex preservation in a weak limb is or is not considered to lie within the boundaries of PMA.[10] An LMN-D presentation is estimated to occur in 7%, 26%, 29%, and 18%, respectively in those whose disease begins in the bulbar, cervical, thoracic, and lumbosacral regions.[12] These statistics may be biased however, by the ease or difficulty in identifying UMN or LMN signs in any given region. For example, UMN findings in the thoracic region may be underrepresented due to the insensitive clinical means of detection. Of those who do not manifest UMN signs at onset, 22% will develop them over the course of their disease.[12] Even in the patients who never develop UMN features during life, the pathological features of ALS will be identified on postmortem examination.[64–66]

Other observations, supporting the concept that PMA and ALS exist as a continuum include the documentation that these disorders have overlapping natural histories. Although PMA and LMN-D patients live longer on average than patients classified as having ALS, individual patients in any of these categories may have malignant courses.[10,15] On average, symmetric presentations and individuals who continue to have monomelic involvement after prolonged periods of observation tend to have more indolent courses. As would be expected, those whose measurements of ventilatory or limb strength decline precipitously have life expectancies that parallel ALS despite an absence or paucity of UMN signs.[10,15] Additional arguments in support of PMA and LMN-D as part of the ALS spectrum include the recognition that PMA phenotypes occur in association with at least five different *SOD1* mutations. The A5V (previously known as A4V) *SOD1* mutation, a rapidly progressive PMA phenotype, represents the most common SOD mutation in North America and represents the most dramatic example of this phenomenon.[63,67] FTD prevalence is estimated at 17% in PMA patients, providing further support for a common biology in the two syndromes.[68]

At times, slowly progressive forms of LMN-D ALS may remain confined to both upper extremities over protracted periods, producing a syndrome that has been described as flail arm, brachial amyotrophic diplegia (BAD), or "man-in-the-barrel" syndrome.[69,70] This disorder more commonly affects the shoulder girdles initially in comparison to the more common LMN-D forms of ALS which are more likely to begin distally. A similar more indolent syndrome, referred to a lower extremity amyotrophic diplegia (LAD) may affect both lower extremities, rendering the individual paraparetic for protracted periods before spreading to other regions.[70] In our opinion, both BAD and LAD are best conceptualized as PMA variants.

Between 25% and 40% of individuals with ALS present with "bulbar-onset" disease, that is, dysarthria or less commonly dysphagia as the presenting symptom.[61,71] When the initial presentation is limited to the bulbar region, the term PBP may be used. This PBP presentation more commonly occurs in women than in men. As in limb-onset ALS, PBP may be dominated by UMN characteristics, LMN characteristics, or both. As with limb-onset cases, unequivocal UMN and LMN signs occurring concomitantly in cranial innervated muscles, even in the absence of limb involvement, are ominous. In some individuals with sporadic PBP, signs and symptoms may remain confined to the "bulbar" musculature for considerable time, affecting the physicians' confidence in the accuracy of their diagnosis, particularly with a UMN-D presentation. Most cases do progress to ALS, eventually. As in PMA and PLS, fALS may have a PBP presentation. Life expectancy in bulbar-onset forms of ALS has been repeatedly demonstrated to be on average less than in limb-onset disease particularly if there is an associated FTD.[72,73] This average prognosis does not necessarily apply to individual patients as mortality may be related more to the importance of the functions jeopardized early in the course (breathing and swallowing) than a reflection of the biology of the disease.[73] Some reports suggest both the prevalence and severity of FTD are increased in bulbar as opposed to limb-onset cases whereas others do not. FTD has been reported to occur in as many as 48% of PBP cases if carefully sought for.[74,75] One report suggests that there is an increased incidence of FTD in patients with bulbar-onset disease.[72]

ALS beginning as a UMN exclusive (PLS) or dominant (UMN-D) process is less common than phenotypes dominated by LMN or bulbar dysfunction.[62,76,77] Approximately 2%–5% of ALS cases begin with a PLS phenotype.[7,76,78] The average age of onset in virtually every series is about 50 years, which is younger than typical ALS.[7,76,78] Three-quarters of PLS cases involve the legs, initially creating an inability to effectively run or hop. In most cases, the onset is asymmetric and at times may be hemiparetic, referred to as the Mills variant.[7,76,78] In approximately 15% of cases, PLS affects the bulbar muscles initially. In 10% of cases, the upper extremities are the first region to become symptomatic.[7,76,78] It is commonly held that ALS spares the anterior horn of the sacral segments. As a result, it is commonly held that genitourinary symptoms do not occur in this disease. In our experience, PLS is an exception to this rule as urinary urgency and urgency incontinence may occur. Presumably, these symptoms result from detrusor–sphincter dyssynergia. To further cement the biological relationship between PLS and ALS, PLS patients also appear susceptible to frontotemporal dysfunction and FTLD.[79,80]

The distinction between PLS from UMN-D ALS is based on whether LMN signs are absent (PLS) or present.[8,76] In the aforementioned reports, the authors defined the threshold for LMN involvement by EMG as abnormalities in more than two muscles (minimal number of muscles studied not defined). These abnormalities could include fibrillation potentials/positive waves, fasciculation potentials, or evidence of mild MUAP enlargement consistent with denervation and reinnervation. Presumably, these limits were defined so as to not exclude patients with minor EMG abnormalities secondary to a separate, unrelated, neurogenic injury. It has been suggested that focal weakness, bulbar symptoms at onset, or later development of weight loss and declining ventilatory function predict transition to ALS.

The natural history of PLS is more favorable than PMA or ALS. In several case series, mean disease duration ranged between 7 and 14 years.[8,78,81] The majority (80%) of individuals with PLS who evolve into ALS do so within the first 4 years of their disorder.[7] PLS is extremely rare and only accounts for about 2% of cases of MND. Typically, PLS is considered, and appropriately diagnosed, only after imaging, CSF and other investigations fail to provide an alternative explanation for a patient's worsening spasticity. In an attempt to accelerate research and facilitate therapeutic development in PLS, consensus diagnostic criteria were developed in 2020 by the delegates of the second International PLS Conference.[62] These criteria state that the diagnosis of PLS requires the presence of symptoms of progressive UMN dysfunction for at least 2 years in at least two of three regions (lower extremity, upper extremity, bulbar), as well as the absence of sensory symptoms, active LMN degeneration, and an alternative diagnosis.[62] When these criteria are met, the level of diagnostic certainty depends on the time from symptom onset. Probable PLS is defined by the absence of significant active LMN degeneration 2–4 years from symptom onset while definite PLS is defined by the absence of significant active LMN degeneration 4 or more years from symptom onset.[62] International efforts are ongoing to better define the natural history of both probable and definite PLS and develop biomarkers and outcome measures in preparation for possible future interventional trials.[82,83]

In up to 2.7% of cases, ALS may initially present with symptoms attributable to ventilatory muscle weakness.[84,85] These may escape initial detection due to their sometimes protean clinical manifestations including disordered sleep, early morning headache, fatigue, or altered sensorium. Involvement of ventilatory muscles may not be recognized until the more classic manifestations of dyspnea on exertion or orthopnea occur. It is not rare for patients to notice dyspnea for the first time after meals or while bending over to tie their shoes which restrict movement of weak diaphragms. On occasion, ALS may be first recognized in an individual who cannot be weaned from the ventilator following elective intubation. Paradoxical abdominal movements or a drop in vital capacity of more than 10% in the supine position indicates diaphragmatic weakness in patients with a suspected neuromuscular cause of ventilatory symptoms.

ALS and frontotemporal dysfunction represent overlapping disorders which exist in a continuum.[86] This association is important for a number of reasons including insight into a potential common biology. In addition, a reduced life expectancy in ALS patients with concomitant frontotemporal dysfunction has been suggested.[72,87] Alternative management strategies may be required when ALS and FTD coexist. Both ALS and FTD may occur on either a sporadic or hereditary basis. Certain ALS-causing gene mutations (*C9orf72*, *TARDBP*, *FUS*, *TBK1*, *VCP*, *CHCHD10*, and *SQSTM1*) are more commonly associated with the potential development of FTD than others.[88] Both ALS and FTD may exist as individual disorders or develop collectively, either on a clinically evident or strictly a pathological basis. In the latter circumstance, the second disorder may or may not become clinically manifest during the lifetime of the patient.

ALS and FTD may precede the development of the other, or both may present concomitantly.[89] On occasion, patients with FTD and ALS will be found to have concomitant Parkinsonism as well. The concurrence of ALS, a movement disorder, and dementia should raise the consideration of one of the known genetic causes of this triad (Table 6-3).

Minor cognitive and behavioral changes in MND patients may be overlooked for a number of reasons. They may be subtle and therefore escape detection unless appropriate screening instruments are utilized. The detection of these changes may also be obscured by the patient's writing and speaking difficulties. Behavioral changes, when recognized, may be misattributed to known consequences of ALS such as hypercapnia, depression, or pseudobulbar affect.

Diagnostic criteria to define frontotemporal dysfunction in ALS were first developed in 2009 and then revised in 2017. Key elements of this approach include the recognition that neuropsychological deficits in ALS are extremely heterogeneous, fall along a spectrum (the frontotemporal spectrum disorder of ALS or ALS-FTSD), affect over 50% of patients, and significantly impact survival. ALS patients exist along a spectrum of cognitively normal (ALScn) to ALS with FTD (ALS-FTD) that includes ALS with behavioral impairment (ALSci), ALS with behavioral impairment (ALSbi), and ALS with combined cognitive and behavioral impairment (ALScbi). The most common cognitive impairment observed in ALS is executive dysfunction, which is the loss of the ability to plan and organize tasks by maintenance of attention or the ability to shift sets to accomplish a goal-directed task. Another domain frequently impaired is language. Language deficits may be affecting expressive language with speech that is dysgrammatical, associated with paraphasic errors and word-finding difficulties, or may also manifest as a semantic, predominantly receptive language disorder in which the significance of words and objects loses meaning. Patients may have a behavioral syndrome characterized by apathy, altered social and interpersonal conduct, emotional blunting, and loss of insight.

A battery of neuropsychological tests exists to evaluate different aspects of ALS-FTSD.[90] Tests of verbal fluency provide a sensitive screening method for FTD patients with cognitive impairment.[89] Normal values are 8 and 13 respectively for number of words generated in 1 minute beginning with the letter D and names of animals.[89] Another strategy that may be even more sensitive for detecting set-shifting difficulties is to ask the patient to provide a word beginning with a specific letter alternating with a different category, for example, men's first names. Normative values for this task are seven or more pairs in 1 minute. Perseveration may be readily detected if two consecutive responses belonging to the same category are provided. A potentially useful screening test in individuals with unintelligible speech is "antisaccade" testing (the ability to look in the opposite direction in response to a lateralized visual stimulus). A patient should make no more than 2 errors in 10 attempts to be considered normal. There are numerous standardized tests that can be efficiently administered during a routine clinic visit. It should be pointed out that the minimental state examination is not a particularly sensitive test for detection of early frontotemporal dysfunction. The Montréal cognitive assessment (MOCA) has been used as a screening instrument due to its availability and ease of use but was not specifically designed for ALS. The ALS cognitive behavioral screen (ALS CBS) is often used in ALS clinics as is the Edinburgh Cognitive and Behavioural ALS Screen (ECAS).[91] Behavioral abnormalities are best assessed by specific behavioral inventories.

DIAGNOSIS AND DIFFERENTIAL DIAGNOSIS

sALS remains a clinical diagnosis supported by the exclusion of potentially mimicking disorders for which testing exists. In cases where the clinical diagnosis of ALS is indisputable, it can be argued that the predominant goal of testing is to validate the credibility of the diagnosis in the eyes of the patient and their family. There are a number of suggested algorithms for the evaluation of the ALS suspect based on differential diagnostic considerations.[92] It is our practice to perform limited "routine" testing in ALS suspects, which may be expanded on a case-by-case basis as the differential diagnostic emphasis differs depending on whether it is a UMN-D, LMN-D, or bulbar-onset phenotype (Table 6-4). Disorders that are dominated by LMN features provide the largest number of differential diagnostic considerations.[93,94] The availability of low-cost gene panels, coupled with the advent of targeted treatments for selected genetic mutations, has resulted in broader use of genetic testing for both fALS and sALS cases, though optimal implementation of genetic testing and genetic counseling is still a topic of debate and varies greatly across different geographies.

Multifocal motor neuropathy (MMN) is the most common LMN-D ALS mimic in most series (discussed in detail in Chapter 14).[11,95,96] It is distinguished from ALS by clinical, EDX, and serological means, and in some cases by response to diagnostic trials of IVIG. Potentially distinguishing clinical features include a slower rate of progression, motor deficits occurring in nerve rather than segmental (myotomal) distribution, and absence of cranial nerve and overt UMN signs.[96] Nonetheless, preservation or slight exaggeration of deep tendon reflexes in an affected limb may serve as a confounding variable.[96] The most characteristic laboratory

▶ TABLE 6-4. ANCILLARY TESTING IN SUSPECTED ALS PATIENTS

Tests That Should Be Considered in All Suspected ALS Patients

1. EDX with multipoint motor nerve stimulation for potential conduction block
2. MR imaging of brain, cervical, and/or thoracic spinal cord
3. Pulmonary function tests
4. Routine labs including CBC, complete metabolic panel, CPK, SPEP/IFE, TSH, CRP, or ESR

Additional tests to be considered:
- fALS mutational analysis
- Serum neurofilament light levels

Tests That Could Be Considered in Selected Patients With UMN-Dominant Syndromes

1. B12
2. Serum copper, ceruloplasmin, and zinc
3. Serum HIV and HTLV-1 serology
4. Serum long-chain fatty acid ratios

Additional tests to be considered as clinically indicated:
- Genetic testing for HSP
- CSF examination
- Anti-GAD, antiamphiphysin

Tests That Could Be Considered in Selected Patients With Combined UMN and LMN

1. Genetic testing for selected HSP and dSMA phenotypes that may combine UMN and LMN features

Additional tests to be considered as clinically indicated:
- Nerve biopsy, skin biopsy, fibroblast cultures, or genetic testing for polyglucosan disease
- Hexosaminidase levels

Tests That Could Be Considered in Selected Patients With LMN-Dominant Syndromes

1. GM1 antibodies
2. Acetylcholine receptor and MuSK antibodies

Additional tests to be considered as clinically indicated:
- Lyme serology
- Voltage-gated calcium channel antibodies
- Paraneoplastic antibodies
- Survival motor neuron gene mutational analysis (SMA I–IV)
- Kennedy disease mutational analysis
- CSF examination
- Muscle biopsy
- EDX with repetitive stimulation, single fiber EMG

Tests That Could Be Considered in Selected Patients With Bulbar-Onset Disease

1. EDX with repetitive stimulation, single fiber EMG
2. Acetylcholine receptor antibodies, MuSK antibodies

Additional tests to be considered as clinically indicated:
- Muscle biopsy
- Neck MRI
- Kennedy disease mutational analysis
- Genetic testing for gelsolin or transthyretin amyloidosis

ALS, amyotrophic lateral sclerosis; EDX, electrodiagnosis; CBC, complete blood count; CPK, creatine phosphokinase; SPEP/IFE, serum protein electrophoresis/immunofixation; TSH, thyroid-stimulating hormone; CRP, c-reactive protein; GAD, glutamic acid decarboxylase; ESR, erythrocyte sedimentation rate; MR, magnetic resonance; HIV, human immunodeficiency virus; HTLV-1, human T lymphocytic virus; HSP, hereditary spastic paraplegia; CSF, cerebrospinal fluid; fALS, familial ALS; CK, creatine kinase; MuSK, muscle-specific kinase; EMG, electromyography; dSMA, distal spinal muscular atrophy.

feature is motor nerve conduction block but this can be elusive if located in very proximal or distal nerve segments. Antibodies directed at the GM1 ganglioside have been found in high titer in between 30% and 80% of these patients.[97,98] In adults with sporadic multifocal or diffuse LMN syndromes, we routinely do more extensive motor conductions looking for conduction block and order GM1 antibody screens. In addition, we consider MR imaging of the brachial or lumbosacral plexus in selected cases in an attempt to demonstrate swelling or increased signal of nerve elements which may occur in a third of MMN cases. In selected cases, we have felt compelled to offer a 3-month trial of IVIG when the diagnosis remains uncertain.

Serological tests for disorders of neuromuscular transmission, typically acetylcholine receptor binding, and if negative, muscle-specific kinase antibodies should be considered in any patient with painless weakness. These tests are particularly relevant in bulbar-onset cases without atrophy or fasciculations. In cases presenting with a limb-girdle pattern of weakness, associated with diminished deep tendon reflexes and/or evidence of cholinergic dysautonomia, we would obtain voltage-gated calcium channel antibodies as one means as both a sensitive and specific test for Lambert–Eaton myasthenic syndrome. EDX remains a valuable adjunct in any suspected disorder of neuromuscular transmission evaluation. Edrophonium testing remains useful in selected suspected myasthenia cases.

Kennedy disease should be considered in males with bulbar symptoms and/or proximal weakness.[99–102] Like many MNDs, cramps, fasciculations, and atrophy are common. As with other spinal muscular atrophies, tremor may occur. There is an EDX evidence of sensory involvement which may or may not be evident clinically. Creatine kinase (CK) levels are frequently elevated in the two to five times the upper limits of normal range, similar to ALS, though occasionally can be higher, approaching values up to eight times the upper limit of normal. Features of impaired androgen effect such as gynecomastia occur. Needle EMG is dominated by features of chronic denervation and reinnervation with a relative paucity of ongoing denervation in most cases. The diagnosis is suspected when sensory nerve action potentials (SNAP) amplitudes are reduced on nerve conduction studies in a patient with proximal symmetric weakness and a predominantly chronic MND pattern with EDX. It is confirmed by identifying the characteristic trinucleotide repeats originating from the androgen receptor gene on the X chromosome.

Inclusion body myositis (IBM) and ALS typically affect individuals in the same age range. Both occur with a slightly greater incidence in males. Both are disorders that commonly demonstrate asymmetric limb weakness and atrophy. In addition, both frequently cause dysphagia, have similar levels of CK elevation, and may have fibrillation potentials and large MUAPs on EMG.[103] However, fasciculations and fasciculation potentials are not features of IBM. In addition, the large, polyphasic MUAPs seen on EMG are frequently intermixed with myopathic units in IBM. The course in IBM is typically more indolent than ALS and the pattern of weakness usually distinctive from the segmental pattern and regional spread of ALS. Quadriceps and finger/wrist flexors are typically the most severely affected. Weakness of facial and upper esophageal muscles, neck flexors, and foot dorsiflexors are common. Unlike most myopathies, asymmetric and relatively focal patterns of weakness are common. We have observed distal interphalangeal joint (DIP) flexion weakness in the thumb with relative sparing of DIP flexion of the contiguous digits. The forearm muscles are atrophic in IBM while the hand intrinsic muscles have preserved bulk (see Chapter 33). The diagnosis of IBM is typically confirmed by distinctive muscle biopsy features although most patients with ALS do not need a biopsy to exclude IBM if attentive clinical and EDX examinations are done.

Slowly progressive LMN syndromes are not uncommon in neuromuscular clinics and may be very difficult to distinguish from PMA or LMN-D ALS at onset as it is their protracted course that provides the primary means of discrimination.[11,93,104] In a manner similar to PLS, 4 years has been suggested as the statute of limitations to distinguish the "benign" focal forms of MND from LMN forms of ALS. The benign focal forms of MND have been referred to by a wide variety of names, the most notable of which is Hirayama disease. The classic phenotype is of a sporadic disorder presenting as slowly progressive wasting and weakness of one hand in a teenage or young adult male of Asian heritage.[105,106] The weakness often progresses within the C7–T1 segments for number of years and then arrests. It may or may not affect the opposite upper extremity in a similar distribution. Brachioradialis sparing is a notable clinical feature. Like MMN, deep tendon reflexes may be preserved in an affected extremity, although this may reflect the preferential C8–T1 segmental involvement with anatomic sparing of the C5–C7 segments where the most readily elicitable deep tendon reflexes reside. There is phenotypic heterogeneity in these slowly progressive LMN syndromes. There are cases with simultaneous involvement of the arms.[107] Not all cases occur in those of Asian descent.[108] Lower extremity syndromes exist as well which have a predilection for the posterior compartment of the leg and have been described as benign calf amyotrophy.[109] The younger age of onset, the initial involvement of distal rather than proximal upper extremity muscles, and a frequent signal change within the cervical spinal cord with MR imaging serve to distinguish the symmetrical form of Hirayama disease from the BAD variant of PMA. The differential diagnosis of LMN-dominant forms of ALS also includes benign fasciculation syndrome. This has been previously addressed in the *Clinical Features* section.

The distal forms of spinal muscular atrophy (dSMA) or hereditary motor neuropathy (dHMN) would be uncommonly confused with ALS. They may be inherited in either a dominant or recessive manner. The potential resemblance to ALS originates from the occasional occurrence of UMN features, vocal cord paralysis, facial, and diaphragmatic weakness in some cases in addition to the characteristic LMN features.[110,111] One such genotype, SETX, has been characterized as both a fALS and dSMA because of the potential coexistence of UMN features. To further confuse matters, the authors have had the personal experience of a SETX patient with a hereditary spastic paraparesis (HSP) phenotype. Other dSMA genotypes in which pyramidal signs may occur are mutations of the *Berardinelli–Seip congenital lipodystrophy 2* (*BSCL2*), *heat-shock protein B1* (*HSPB1*), and *dynactin* (*DCTN1*) (in which facial weakness may occur) genes, and an as of yet unidentified gene in a Jordanian cohort. dSMA associated with diaphragmatic palsy occurs in infants associated with mutations of the *immunoglobulin mu–binding protein 2* (*IGHMBP2* gene) or in dSMA4 whose gene has yet to be identified. dSMA associated with vocal cord paralysis results from mutations in either the *DCTN1* or *transient receptor vallanoid 4 gene* (*TRPV4*). dSMA beginning in the upper extremities is associated with the glycyl-tRNA synthetase (GARS) as well as with *BSCL2* gene mutations.[111]

The dSMA phenotype closely resembles and overlaps with Charcot–Marie–Tooth (CMT) disease, both being characterized by slow progression, frequent foot deformities, and a distal symmetric pattern of weakness. The difference is based largely on the presence or absence of clinical and EDX sensory loss.[111] The distinction is semantic in some cases as mutations in certain genes may produce a dSMA or CMT. Mutations in HSPB1 may result in dSMA1 or 2, or CMT2F. Mutations in HSPB8 may result in dSMA1 or 2, or CMT2L. dSMA type 5 is also allelic with CMT2D when caused by the GARS mutation. To further confound the semiology of these diseases, FIG4 mutations may produce both fALS and CMT4J phenotypes.[111] The diagnosis of dSMA is typically based on clinical and EDX criteria, though options for genetic testing are expanding. The reader is referred to the SMA Chapter 8 for further details.

On occasion, patients who have received radiation therapy may develop a delayed disorder that mimics MND.[112] The disorder typically begins within a few years of radiation exposure, progresses for a period of time, and then seemingly stabilizes. In the majority of cases, the syndrome occurs in patients who have received pelvic radiation, particularly for testicular tumors. This syndrome has been presumed to have an anterior horn cell localization as the weakness usually affects both lower extremities, fasciculations are common, with sensory signs and symptoms occurs infrequently. Sphincter involvement may or may not occur. Radiation-induced plexopathy or polyradiculopathy have been suggested as alternative localizations although no single locus need be mutually exclusive. The syndrome does not appear to be solely related to the total amount of radiation delivered, or the radiation per dose, which has led to hypothesis of potential synergistic pathologies such as infectious or genetic influences. Diagnosis in a typical case involves the appropriate timing, deficits that remain confined to the radiation field, potentially supported by the demonstration of myokymic discharges within affected muscles.

We have rarely seen cases of a head and neck cancer presenting as a painless, progressive bulbar syndrome mimicking bulbar ALS. MR imaging of the soft tissues of the head and neck should be considered in an atypical bulbar presentation of ALS, for example, one associated with unilateral involvement of the tongue. Rarely, a bulbar syndrome including tongue atrophy and fasciculations has been seen as one of the presenting symptoms of transthyretin familial amyloid neuropathy (TTR-FAP) though the phenotype is typically associated with other non-ALS symptoms such as severe neuropathy.[113] Another rarely seen mimicker of PBP is hereditary gelsolin amyloidosis, which can present as a slowly progressive bulbar syndrome associated with corneal dystrophy and loss of skin turgor.[114]

The differential diagnosis of PLS or UMN-D ALS phenotypes are predominantly structural and hereditary disorders, less commonly selected infectious and acquired metabolic diseases. HSP and cervical spondylotic myelopathy arguably deserve the greatest consideration.[115] HSP is usually readily recognized by its slow rate of progression and a phenotype which is typically a symmetric spastic paraparesis. The upper extremities may be hyperreflexic but usually display normal strength, tone, and coordination. Bulbar involvement would be distinctly uncommon.[115] Pes cavus and minor proprioceptive deficits in the toes may occur and offer other discriminating features.[115] As with most heritable disorders, the absence of other obviously affected family member does not exclude an HSP diagnosis. The diagnosis of HSP is also rendered more difficult in complicated forms of the disease where other neurological systems, particularly the LMNs, may be involved.[116] LMN involvement has been reported in the SPG9, 10, 14, 15, 17, 20, 22, 26, 30, 38, and 41 genotypes.[115] Recently, commercial availability of genetic testing for many HSP genotypes has increased, though the diagnosis of HSP is still typically made clinically with exclusion of other causes of UMN disease in sporadic cases. The reader is referred to the Chapter 7 on hereditary spastic paraplegia for more detailed information.

Cervical spondylotic myelopathy is usually dominated by UMN features. LMN features including hand atrophy may occur but multisegmental atrophy, weakness, fasciculations, and/or evidence of active denervation should be cautiously attributed to spinal cord compression.[117,118] We have had the unfortunate experience of evaluating many cases of ALS with painless weakness associated with MR imaging evidence of spondylosis that have in retrospect undergone needless surgery.[119] Nonetheless, imaging of the spinal cord should be included in any MND phenotype with prominent UMN signs and no compelling "bulbar" involvement.

There are a number of other disorders that should receive some consideration in the differential diagnosis of UMN-D or PLS presentations of MND. Primary progressive multiple sclerosis (MS) may present as a progressive UMN syndrome that would be addressed by MR imaging of the spinal cord and CSF examination. Dopa-responsive dystonia and stiff person syndrome may resemble progressive UMN disorders. The former diagnosis is supported by response to low-dose dopa and the latter by demonstration of antibodies against glutamic acid decarboxylase (GAD) or amphiphysin. A progressive myelopathy may be the presenting manifestation of adrenoleukodystrophy. While this disorder is X-linked, it has also been reported in females as a slowly progressive myelopathy. In men, the disease has earlier onset and faster progression, and may be accompanied by other symptoms such as impaired adrenal function and concomitant cognitive changes. Diagnosis is made by an elevated C26:C22 long-chain fatty acid ratio or by gene analysis. Retroviral infection, particularly with human T lymphocytic virus 1 (HTLV-1), may present as a progressive myelopathy and serological testing should be considered in symptomatic individuals at risk in residents of endemic areas or in individuals at risk by exposure through transfusion, recreational drug use, or sexual behavior.

A progressive UMN and LMN phenotype unassociated with involvement of other neurological or organ systems is almost always ALS. An ALS phenotype has been reported in association with copper deficiency.[120] The individuals reported had asymmetric foot drop as one of the initial manifestations of a progressive UMN and LMN disorder. Retrospectively, there were clinical clues that could have raised suspicion of copper deficiency in these patients. Patients with suspected ALS who have large fiber sensory loss, malabsorptive risk including prior bariatric surgery, excess zinc absorption, or concomitant anemia or cytopenia should be screened for serum copper, ceruloplasmin, and zinc levels if any of the aforementioned features are present.

Most of the other discretionary tests listed in Table 6-4 are utilized only as clinically indicated in the evaluation of ALS suspects. Although an ALS phenotype rarely if ever occurs in association with Lyme disease, it is a frequent inquiry on the part of patients who live in an endemic area.[121] For this reason, it is a frequent practice to obtain an ELISA screening test on patients from these areas. We would not recommend this in areas where Lyme disease is uncommon. In view of the uncertain associations and rarity of occurrence, we reserve other testing for situations in which clinical context heightens the index of suspicion. This would include testing for HIV, occult neoplasia or lymphoproliferative disorders (with or without) paraneoplastic antibodies, hexosaminidase A deficiency, thyrotoxicosis, heavy metal toxicity, polyglucosan disease, and dural venous malformations.[122-133] Hexosaminidase A deficiency might be considered in a young person with MND and a concomitant spinocerebellar, dystonic, or bipolar syndrome. Polyglucosan disease is a phenotypic variant of glycogen storage disease type IV with phenotypic manifestations that may include distal sensory loss, a neurogenic bladder, cerebellar dysfunction, and cognitive decline.

In the absence of genetic confirmation, ALS remains a clinical diagnosis supported by the absence of evidence of other, potentially mimicking diseases. At the time of initial evaluation, ALS may be suspected but the clinical features may not have developed sufficiently to allow a physician to feel confident in the diagnosis. The physician may feel conflicted as to when to have this conversation. To do so prematurely hazards the possibility of being wrong. In addition, patients may lack confidence in someone who confronts them with a diagnosis of this magnitude without the appearance of due diligence. Balanced against this is the patients' need for answers and early referral to multidisciplinary clinics. Perceived "foot dragging" and uncertainty may have equally deleterious effects on their trust in their physician. Disclosing the suspected diagnosis as early in the course as possible, following exclusion of reasonable differential diagnostic considerations, subsequent to demonstration of progression both within and outside of initially affected regions, would seem to be a reasonable approach. One should not wait for a patient to fulfill EEC for definite or probable ALS before disclosing the diagnosis, and Gold Coast criteria appear more practical than EEC for use in the clinic. In view of the implications of an ALS diagnosis, considering the lack of a confirmatory test, and wishing to facilitate the early initiation of multidisciplinary care and potential research participation, patients are frequently counseled to seek a second opinion from specialized ALS clinics.

▶ LABORATORY FEATURES

With the exception of identification of known pathological mutations in known ALS-causing genes in symptomatic patients, there are no laboratory tests that currently provide disease confirmation. Testing in ALS is done for three general reasons. The first potential goal is to identify either UMN or particularly LMN involvement when it is not obvious clinically, in a patient with either an LMN- or UMN-dominant phenotype. A second diagnostic strategy is to attempt to exclude other disorders that fall within the ALS differential diagnosis. Finally, testing may be performed in an attempt to aid in disease management and prognostication, for example, forced vital capacity (FVC) measurements to identify the appropriate time to discuss positive airway pressure support, percutaneous gastrostomy placement, or end-of-life conversations.

EMG and nerve conduction studies are recommended in virtually all suspected ALS patients, even when the diagnosis is clinically unequivocal. The implications of the ALS diagnosis are such that both patient and clinician wish to be as certain as possible. EMG has the capability of confirming the existence, distribution, and relative duration of LMN degeneration in support of an ALS diagnosis.[134,135] In addition, EDX may identify features more consistent with an alternative diagnosis as described below. The specific goals of the test are to:

1. Identify EDX abnormalities in clinically unaffected muscles to confirm a pattern consistent with ALS, that is, ongoing denervation coupled with changes implying subacute or chronic denervation and reinnervation (a reduced number of large MUAPs, MUAP instability) demonstrable in multiple muscles innervated by multiple segments (≥2 segments in

limb muscles, ≥1 muscle in cranial or thoracic muscles) in more than one body region. As described above, demonstration of ongoing denervation requires the detection of fibrillation potentials and/or positive sharp waves to fulfill EEC criteria, while Gold Coast criteria also accept fasciculation potentials as indicative of LMN dysfunction, as long as other requirements are met.

2. Identify features that might implicate an ALS mimic. Examples of this would include abnormal sensory conductions (Kennedy syndrome), a large decremental response (>20%) to 2–5 Hz repetitive stimulation without evidence of chronic denervation (myasthenia, Lambert–Eaton myasthenic syndrome), motor nerve conduction block or other demyelinating features (MMN), or EMG evidence of both small and large motor units with fibrillation potentials that might suggest IBM in the appropriate clinical context.

3. Offer insight into the rate of progression and prognosis, that is, active denervation without chronic denervation and reinnervation, motor unit variability, and a rapid decline in motor unit estimation being electrodiagnostic indicators of a more rapidly progressive course.

Muscle biopsy can also serve as a surrogate for EMG to confirm LMN involvement by demonstrating a pattern of denervation atrophy characterized by scattered atrophic fibers of both fiber types that are angulated in appearance, and by small groups of atrophic fibers (Fig. 6-4). However, muscle biopsy is not routinely employed in ALS as it is both more invasive and less capable of demonstrating the multifocal or diffuse neurogenic features than EMG.

Unfortunately, there are no widely available and reliable surrogates for the detection of subclinical UMN involvement.

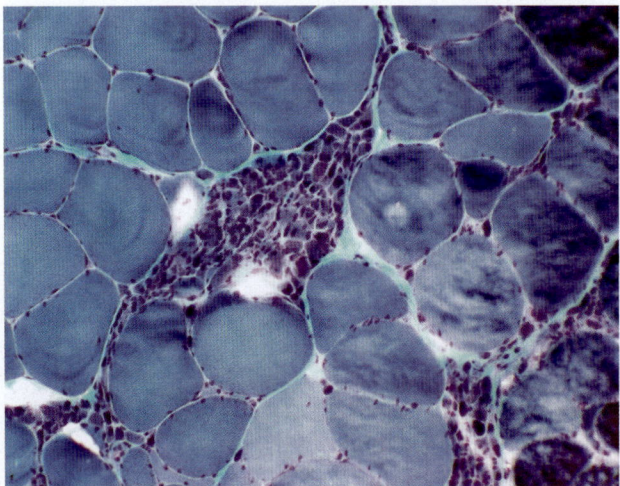

Figure 6-4. Muscle biopsy demonstrating small fiber-type grouped atrophy consistent with neurogenic atrophy and ALS (modified Gomori trichrome).

A test of this nature would be an invaluable tool in patients with PMA or LMN-D presentations. Central motor conduction velocity obtained through transcranial magnetic stimulation, magnetic resonance spectroscopy, and diffusion tensor imaging are some of the methodologies utilized that have been applied with the hope of identifying subclinical cortical spinal, or corticobulbar, tract pathology.[136,137] Single photon emission computerized tomography (SPECT) or positron emission tomography (PET) have also been used to demonstrate extra motor CNS involvement through reduced blood flow or metabolic changes. All of these tests are utilized more for research than for clinical purposes as both their availability and accuracy are currently limited.

The majority of laboratory tests are done in an attempt to exclude other ALS differential diagnostic considerations or to monitor disease progression. CK levels are mildly to moderately elevated in the serum of approximately 23%–75% of ALS patients, though they only rarely rise higher than five times the upper limit of normal.[138,139] It is important to recognize this so as to not confuse an MND with a myopathy in a patient with painless weakness. Serum CK determination may be of value in the appropriate context. For example, an elevated CK value would favor ALS over myasthenia gravis in a patient presenting with bulbar symptoms. Tests of "pulmonary function" are done routinely. Their role is to aid in determination of prognosis and in timing of management decisions. For example, a declining vital capacity may suggest the need for positive airway pressure assistance, percutaneous gastrostomy, or initiation of end-of-life decision-making discussions.

There have been significant additions to our knowledge regarding ALS-causing genes and an increased number of commercially available tests since the previous edition of this book.[35,140,141] There are now over 30 different disease-causing gene mutations. The genotype for approximately 80% of fALS cases can now be identified.

fALS mutations display varying and often incomplete penetrance.[142] As a result, up to 10% of patients with apparent sALS will have heritable disease. Guidelines for genetic testing are rapidly evolving and may continue to be refined as treatments targeting genetic forms of the disease continue to be developed.[140,141]

If testing is performed in asymptomatic individuals, adequate genetic counseling is mandatory with a clear understanding of the implications of both a positive and a negative test result. Ideally, other family members at risk whose genetic status may be revealed by testing of the proband would be involved in the decision making as well. Significant research efforts are ongoing to characterize the first signs of phenoconversion in asymptomatic carriers of ALS-causing mutations with the goal of preventing disease onset and/or intervening at the first sign of disease with targeted treatments in the future in this population.[143]

One focus of current ALS research is the attempt to identify a biomarker or pattern of biomarkers that would provide a gold standard for diagnosis and/or provide prognostic information and data on response to disease-modifying treatments.[144,145] Biomarker identification could provide the opportunity for early therapeutic intervention and disease monitoring, offer insight into disease pathogenesis, and clarify nosology by defining whether MND represents one or more diseases. At present, neurofilament levels are the most promising biomarker for ALS.[146] Neurofilaments are neuronal cytoskeletal proteins that can "leak" from degenerating axons and can be measured in CSF, serum or plasma thus representing a marker of neuronal degeneration. Available assays detect phosphorylated neurofilament heavy chain (pNFH) and neurofilament light chain (NfL). Neurofilament levels rise in presymptomatic individuals about 1 year prior to phenoconversion, higher levels at diagnosis correlate with more aggressive disease course and shorter survival, and, recently, lowering of neurofilament levels in response to treatment with an antisense oligonucleotide targeting the *SOD1* gene supported the accelerated approval of tofersen for *SOD1*-associated ALS.[147,148] Elevated neurofilament levels, however, can also be seen in other neurodegenerative disease and cannot be used alone to diagnose ALS. Additional biomarkers are in development to capture other aspects of ALS pathophysiology including neuroinflammation, oxidative stress, and RNA metabolism.[149]

▶ HISTOPATHOLOGY

Postmortem analysis can reveal atrophy in the motor areas and can also identify extra motor CNS involvement such as atrophy in a frontotemporal lobar pattern (Fig. 6-5).

Light microscopic features in the spinal cord consist of myelinated fiber loss in the corticospinal and corticobulbar pathways as well as loss of motor neurons within the anterior horns of the spinal cord and the motor cranial nerve nuclei at risk (Fig. 6-6). As a result, ventral roots become atrophic while dorsal roots are spared. The anterior horn cell loss occurs within virtually all levels of the spinal cord with cell preservation of the intermediolateral cell columns. There is selective sparing of the third, fourth, and sixth cranial nerves as well as Onuf nucleus within the anterior horn of sacral segments 2–4.

As with the majority of neurodegenerative disease, the immunohistochemical signature of ALS with or without concomitant dementia is the presence of cytoplasmic inclusions representing aggregates of misfolded proteins. In cases of ALS associated with *SOD1* gene mutations, the inclusions consist of misfolded *SOD1* protein. In 97% of ALS cases, that is those not associated with *SOD1* or FUS mutations, and more than half FTLD patients without ALS, these inclusions are labeled with antibodies to ubiquitin but not *SOD1*. These ubiquitinated inclusions (UI) are found within the cytoplasm of relevant neurons and glial cells within the primary motor cortex, brainstem motor nuclei, spinal cord, and associated white matter tracts as well as the cingulate gyrus and dentate nuclei of the cerebellum.[150,151] In patients with FTLD, these inclusions are found in the neocortex and hippocampus as well.[150]

Although UI are not unique to ALS or FTLD, their location and composition may be. In 2006, it was first recognized that these UI stain with TDP-43 in virtually all ALS cases and 80% of FTLD cases associated with UI.[150] UI in ALS also contain the proteins ubiquilin 2 and optineurin whose genes, when mutated, are causative of the disease.[152,153] UI that occur in neurodegenerative disorders other than ALS/FTD stain for other proteins such as tau or α-synuclein rather than TDP-43. TDP-43 is a DNA/RNA binding protein translated from a gene locus on chromosome 1. TDP-43 normally shuttles between the nucleus and cytoplasm of cells although is primarily nuclear in its location.[154] In ALS, TDP-43 incorporated into UI is mislocalized to the cytoplasm of motor neurons (Fig. 6-7). Although TDP-43 is found in UI in the majority of FTLD patients, 20% remain TDP-43 negative.[150] In 2009, the FUS gene/protein, also related to DNA repair and RNA microprocessing, was found to colocalize to UI in non–TDP-43 FTLD cases.[150] Like TDP-43, FUS pathology in FTLD is also concentrated in the frontotemporal neocortex and hippocampus but may affect the striatum, thalamus, and brainstem as well. Like mutations in the TDP-43 gene, mutations in the *FUS* gene may result in either an ALS and/or FTD phenotype. In addition, ubiquilin 2 pathology is prominent in the hippocampus of ALS patients with (but not without) dementia.[152]

As anticipated, the pathology and clinical phenotype do not always perfectly coincide, the latter often underestimating the former. For example, in patients with sporadic FTLD, UI/TDP-43 (+) inclusions may be found in motor neurons in the absence of any premortem evidence of MND. In addition, TDP-43 (+) inclusions are identified postmortem in the distribution characteristic of ALS as described above in patients with restricted PMA, LMN-D, and FTD/PLS phenotypes during life.[155,156] These pathological observations further cement the relationship between ALS and these phenotypically overlapping disorders.

TDP-43 (+) inclusions also occur in heritable as well as sporadic forms of FTD. Specifically, they have been demonstrated in mutations of the *VCP*, *PGRN*, and *TARDBP* genes as well as the *C9ORF72* gene on chromosome 9. Their staining patterns appear to be identical in appearance to the TDP-43 staining pattern seen with sALS and sFTD with UI.[150] These associations add further support for a biological link between ALS and FTD in both their sporadic and familial forms.

One additional histological finding in ALS is the Bunina body. These are dense granular intracytoplasmic inclusions that stain for cystatin C, transferrin, and peripherin that are less commonly identified UI. They may be identified within the cytoplasm of motor neurons, are thought to be specific for ALS, and appear distinctive from but not necessarily independent of TDP-43 aggregates.[157,158]

The vast majority of ALS patients with clinical dementia will be found to have FTLD on gross inspection.

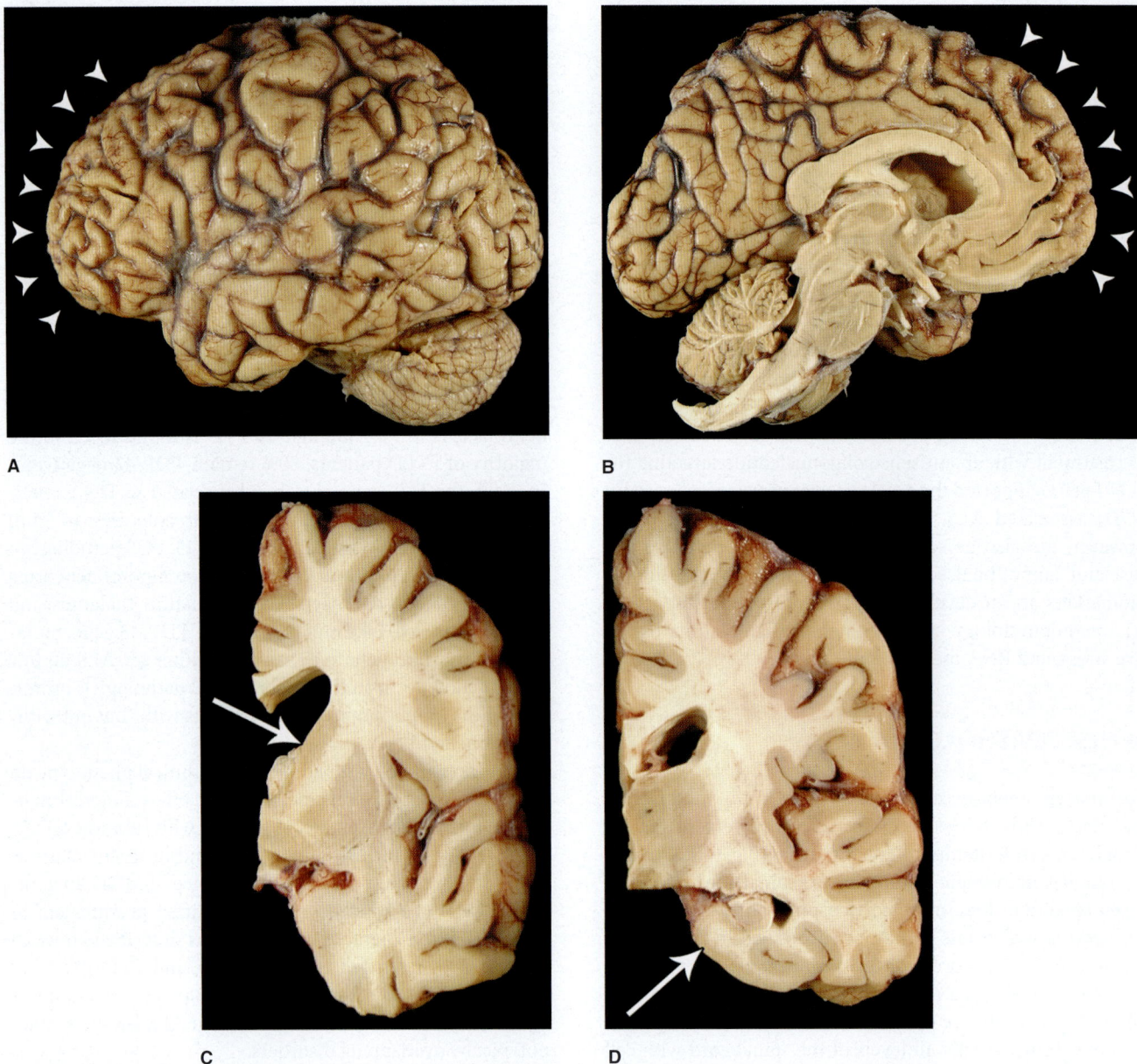

Figure 6-5. Preferential frontal atrophy (*arrowheads*) with lateral (**A**) and parasagittal (**B**) views of the cerebrum with associated enlargement of the frontal horn and caudate flattening (*arrow*) (**C**) and relative hippocampal sparing (*arrow*) (**D**) with coronal views.

Occasionally, either the patient's phenotype, or their pathology will suggest Alzheimer disease. The latter association is currently considered to be coincidental and not related.

The histology of FTLD typically consists of linear spongiosus in the first and second layer of the cortex with prominent neuronal loss in the anterior cingulate and superior frontal gyri regardless of the makeup of the associated cytoplasmic inclusions. These spongiform changes seem to segregate demented from nondemented ALS patients. The immunohistochemical properties of cytoplasmic inclusions in FTLD are varied. In greater than half of all FTLD patients, and virtually all patients with sALS, these inclusions will immunostain with ubiquitin. In approximately 40% of FTLD, the cases, the inclusions will stain for tau. In patients whose inclusions stain for tau, the phenotype will not include MND but may incorporate cortical basal degeneration or progressive supranuclear palsy in addition to their FTD.

▶ PATHOGENESIS

The cause(s) of ALS remains unknown. Current hypotheses regarding disease mechanisms in ALS include defects in RNA metabolism, oxidative damage, accumulation of toxic intracellular protein aggregates, mitochondrial dysfunction, defective axonal transport, growth factor deficiency, neuroinflammation, and/or glutamate excitotoxicity.[159,160] These pathophysiological mechanisms may work in series or in

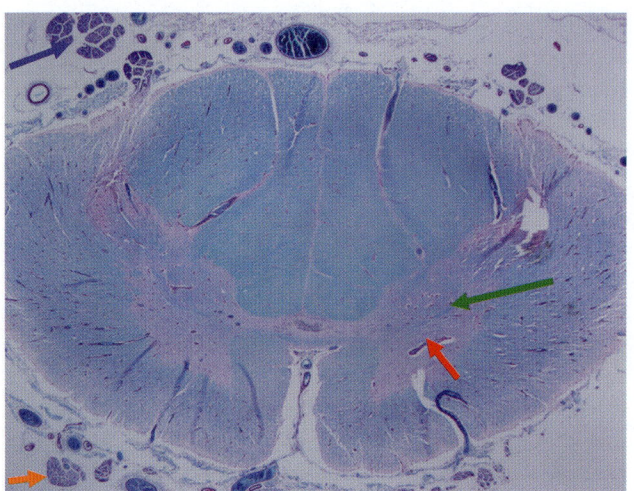

Figure 6-6. Thoracic spinal cord in a patient with amyotrophic lateral sclerosis, demonstrating reduced numbers of anterior horn cells (*red arrow*), normal complement of neurons in intermediolateral cell column (*green arrow*), atrophy of ventral root (*orange arrow*), and normal dorsal root (*blue arrow*). (Luxol fast blue/hematoxylin and eosin.)

parallel with eventual confluence. Although our knowledge of disease pathogenesis has increased, the elements of ALS biology that contribute to disease initiation, disease propagation, or represent consequence of disease remain uncertain.

It is attractive to hypothesize that ALS is a consequence of the complex interplay between environmental exposures, genetic risk, and time.[46] As previously mentioned, there is considerable phenotypic and pathological overlap between sALS and fALS. Consequently, a significant proportion of ALS research in recent years has focused on disease mechanisms in familial disease with the hope that they are relevant to sporadic disease. The recognition that specific gene mutations such as TARDNP and UBQLN may result in both fALS and apparent sALS, and that their protein products (TDP-43 and ubiquilin 2) can be found within neuronal inclusions in sporadic as well as familial forms of the disease lends support for this construct. Epidemiologic studies have failed to reproducibly identify a single environmental culprit or a set of well-defined environmental causes. The gene–environment–time hypothesis suggests a multistep model where a series of environmental exposures over time in combination with genetic predisposition leads to ALS. Ultimately, the biology of ALS will have to account for the identical phenotypic heterogeneity of sporadic and familial disease, the semiselective vulnerability of motor neurons, and the tendency for the disease to spread in a regional fashion.[161] In that regard, one attractive hypothesis holds that misfolded protein aggregates in one cell can proselytize the normal analogous proteins of a neighboring cell to undergo the same pathological process, thus explaining the observed patterns of regional disease spread.[162,163]

Currently, we can only speculate as to whether ALS is a disease of singular cause capable of phenotypic diversity or the final common expression of different insults that prey upon the selected vulnerability of motor neurons. Working from the premise that sALS and fALS must share at least in part a common biology and recognizing that similar phenotypes result from differing gene mutations, the latter paradigm that differing etiologies and disease mechanisms converge to produce a common phenotype would represent the most logical conclusion.

Since the previous edition of this text, knowledge relevant to fALS has expanded at a rapid pace.[32,35,145] As mentioned, it is the hope that insight gained from the pathophysiology of fALS will be relevant to sporadic disease as well. Mutations in several genes are thought to be definitely causative of ALS, and additional genes have strong evidence of a disease-causing link. Within each gene, several mutations have been identified. As an example, about 200 mutations of the superoxide dismutase (*SOD1*) gene have been described, some of which present with characteristic phenotypes. The most common mutations along with a summary of their phenotypes are outlined in Table 6-3. In addition, there are several other ALS-related genes, including genes that have been linked to increased risk of developing ALS and/or genes that may act as modifiers of disease course. Global efforts are underway to continue to update and refine the list of ALS-related genes (details are available on the ALS online genetic database, a resource for information relevant to both disease-causing and disease-related mutations).

Currently, mutations of the *SOD1* gene (ALS1) and *C9ORF72* are the most common causes of fALS and constitute approximately 40%–45% of familial cases.[35,145] Mutations of *C9ORF72* associated with a hexanucleotide repeat mechanism can may cause ALS, FTD, and ALS-FTD.[35,145] Less frequent ALS-causing mutations are located in the FUS and TAR DNA-binding protein (*TARDBP*) genes, each

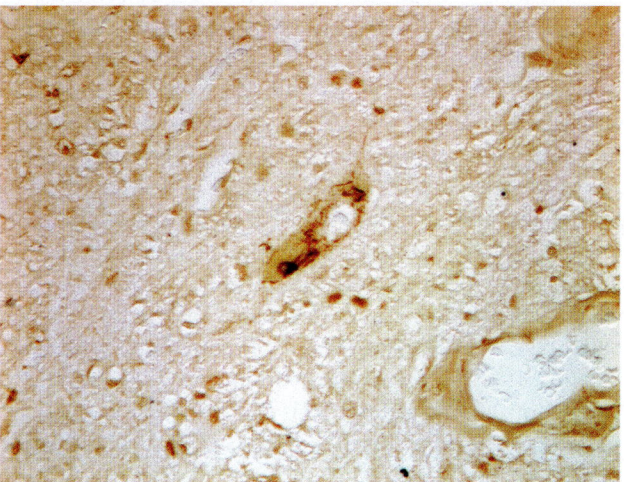

Figure 6-7. TDP-43 (+) skein in a motor neuron (lumbar) in a sporadic patient with amyotrophic lateral sclerosis (40× magnification—rabbit polyclonal antibody to human TDP-43, dilution 1:400). (Reproduced with permission from Michael Strong, MD and Robert Hammond, MD.)

representing approximately 5% of fALS cases, and approximately 1% of all cases.

The majority of ALS-causing gene mutations are transmitted dominantly. ALS2 (alsin) and ALS5 are inherited recessively and are associated with juvenile-onset ALS. Ubiquilin 2 mutations are transmitted in an X-linked fashion. Optineurin seems unique in that both dominant and recessive inheritance patterns have been described. The penetrance of these mutations is variable. *SOD1* mutations were initially thought to be highly penetrant based on a bias originating from the original studies that involved a few large families in which penetrance was understandably high. In reality, less than 50% of identified ALS families have more than two identified family members. Currently, penetrance is estimated to be approximately 80% in *SOD1* mutations by age 85. In the highly penetrant A5V (formerly known as A4V) mutation, the most prevalent *SOD1* mutation in North America, 90% of individuals are clinically affected by age 70. Conversely, the I113T mutation appears to be expressed in only a portion of patients harboring the mutation. This knowledge serves to blur the boundaries between familial and sporadic disease and reinforce that apparent sALS patients can have heritable disease.

Further complicating our understanding of gene expression is the fact that the onset of symptoms in individuals with the same mutation may vary widely and that mutations in the same locus may behave differently in different populations. In individuals harboring two copies of the D90A mutation in the *SOD1* gene, onset may vary from 20 to 94 years of age. This locus behaves as a recessive trait in Scandinavia where heterozygotes are asymptomatic. In North America, except in those of Scandinavian descent, the D90A mutation behaves as a dominant disorder with heterozygotes developing ALS.

The mechanisms by which the aforementioned mutations initiate and/or propagate MND and FTD remain enigmatic. A common theme in ALS is the presence of inclusions within motor neurons consisting of misfolded proteins with the implication that these inclusions confer a toxic gain of function.[164] Alternatively, ALS could represent a loss of function of proteins migrating from their normal nuclear location to a pathological cytoplasmic position. As previously mentioned however, the makeup of the inclusions found in ALS is variable, with *SOD1* inclusions being absent of TDP-43 staining, implicating more than one toxic mechanism. Although potential mechanisms remain unknown, common themes are emerging. Ubiquilin 2 is a constituent of the ubiquitin proteasome system responsible for protein degradation which may confer a toxic gain of function when mutated. Mutations of the *TDP43*, FUS, ANG, SETX, and *C9ORF72* all appear to adversely affect RNA metabolism. For example, RNA generated by pathogenic expansions of the *C9ORF72* gene is hypothesized to sequester normal RNA and proteins resulting in disruption of normal transcription. TDP-43 and FUS are both trapped into stress granules that may further hinder RNA metabolism. The ataxin 2 gene, large expansions of which cause the spinocerebellar ataxia type 2 phenotype, appears to be a potent modifier of TDP-43 toxicity.[165–167] Intermediate expansions in ataxin-2 are now recognized as a risk factor for ALS. The mechanism of action for optineurin mutations in the genesis of ALS is uncertain.[168]

▶ MANAGEMENT

Once the diagnosis has been shared with the patient, we organize their management into three domains: (1) education and psychosocial support to both the patient, the caregivers and the family, (2) disease-specific treatment including consideration of clinical trials, and (3) supportive care, ideally provided in a multidisciplinary setting.[169–172]

In the Internet age, information is readily available to patients and their families. It is the responsibility of any physician caring for an ALS patient to direct them toward reputable educational resources. To that end, the websites provided by the Muscular Dystrophy Association (www.mda.org), the ALS Association (www.alsa.org), and the Motor Neuron Disease Association (www.mndassociation.org) are recommended. The website of the Northeast ALS Consortium (neals.org) provides up-to-date information regarding clinical research and trial opportunities. Unfortunately, there are also websites that provide false hope or false information and patients should be warned about the variable quality of online resources. www.alsuntangled.com is a web-based resource developed by ALS clinician researchers to help patients and their families sort through this potentially confusing terrain.

In part due to the paucity of effective treatments, many patients with ALS seek advice from their physicians regarding alternative, "natural treatments" for their disorder. There is no clear correct response. A dogmatic response on the part of a physician in opposition to this approach runs the risk of losing the patient. Conversely, the physician has a responsibility to dispel what seems to be a generally held perception that "natural" is synonymous with safe. It may be helpful to emphasize to a patient that any substance that is biologically active enough to be beneficial is also biologically active enough to be harmful. "Natural" substances do not benefit from the same underlying science or undergo the same scrutiny and quality control as do pharmaceuticals and pose additional risk for those reasons alone.

There are no known treatments that can reverse or arrest disease progression in ALS. Disease-modifying pharmacotherapy is available to slow down disease progression. At the time of publication of this text, a few disease-modifying drugs have been approved by the FDA for the treatment of ALS and are available in the United States (Table 6-5). Availability of these drugs varies greatly by country and is expected to continue to evolve as clinical trials are completed and new evidence is generated.[173]

Riluzole was approved in the United States in 1995 as the first disease-specific treatment that favorably alters the

▶ TABLE 6-5. FDA-APPROVED MEDICATIONS FOR THE TREATMENT OF ALS

Name	Indication	ROA	Feeding Tube Administration?	Dosage	Safety Laboratory Monitoring	Side Effects	Impact on Disease Progression
Riluzole	ALS	Oral (tablets, suspension, film)	Yes	50 mg bid	Liver function tests monthly for the first 3 months; then every 3 months	Most common: fatigue, dizziness, nausea, GI upset. Rare: hepatotoxicity, pancreatitis, neutropenia	Prolongs survival by about 3 months
Edaravone	ALS	Oral suspension (also available for IV administration)	Yes (suspension)	5 mL/day (oral suspension) or 60 mg/day (IV) First cycle: once daily for 14 consecutive days off. Subsequent cycles: 10 of 14 days followed by 14 consecutive days off of each month	NA	Most common: bruising, gait disturbance, headaches, dermatitis, eczema. Rare: sulfite allergic reactions, hypersensitivity reactions	Slows disease progression by about 30% as measured by the ALSFRS-R (a measure of function); survival effect not known
Tofersen	SOD1-associated ALS	Intrathecal	No	Each dose contains 100 mg (15 mL). Three loading doses administered at 14-day intervals followed by maintenance dose once every 28 days	Not required. Some clinicians monitor plasma neurofilament levels and CSF cell counts and protein	Most common: pain, fatigue, arthralgia, myalgia, and increased white blood cell count in the CSF. Rare: myelitis, radiculitis, papilledema, and elevated intracranial pressure; aseptic meningitis	Reduces neurofilament levels in plasma; it also reduces levels of SOD1 protein in the CSF. In the trial that led to its accelerated approval, trends for reduction in functional decline were seen across multiple outcomes that were not statistically significant.

ALS, amyotrophic lateral sclerosis; IV, Intravenous; ROA, route of administration; SOD1, superoxide dismutase 1.

natural history of the disease.[18] It is thought to exert antiglutamatergic effects and may also modulate sodium channels. In the trials that led to its approval, the drug was associated with modest benefits on survival on the order of about 3 months, though subsequent real-world studies suggested the impact on survival may be longer. It is usually well tolerated although some experience upper gastrointestinal side effects and increased fatigue. Reversible hepatotoxicity may occur with an associated requirement for monitoring of liver function tests.

Edaravone was developed in Japan and approved in the United States for the treatment of ALS in 2017.[174] It was initially available for intravenous administration only, until its oral formulation was approved in 2022.[175] It is thought to protect against oxidative stress thought the exact mechanism is unknown. In the trial that led to its approval, edaravone treatment resulted in slowing of disease progression as measured by the ALS functional rating scale (ALSFRS-R) by about 30% in a cohort who was also taking riluzole. It is contraindicated in those with sulfite allergy and is otherwise well tolerated. The most common side effects include bruising, gait disturbance, and headaches. A trial of edaravone run in Europe and reported in 2024 had negative results, raising questions about the efficacy of the drug.

The combination of sodium phenylbutyrate and taurursodiol (PB-TURSO) was approved in 2022 in the United States and Canada based on the results of the phase 2 CENTAUR trial showing slowing of disease progression by about 25% as measured by the ALSFRS-R and prolongation of survival by about 5 months.[176-178] Unfortunately, results of the phase 3 PHOENIX trial, which became available in March 2024, did not replicate the efficacy results on functional decline. At the time of this writing, the drug is expected to be taken off the market.

Riluzole and edaravone target different disease mechanisms, are approved for all forms of ALS, and are often prescribed as a "cocktail." While their effects might be additive, the real-world effects of this combination requires further research. Given the heterogeneity of ALS, and the effect size of these drugs, it is extremely difficult, if not impossible, for individual clinicians and patients to tell whether a particular patient is benefiting from one or more of these medications. As these drugs become more widely adopted, patient registries and ongoing natural history studies may provide further insights into their real-world impact. Ongoing trials will also help provide more information about their long-term effects.

The first drug for the treatment of *SOD1*-associated ALS, tofersen, was approved in 2023, ushering in the era of gene-targeted treatments for ALS.[148] Tofersen is an antisense oligonucleotide that is delivered intrathecal and received accelerated approval based on reduction in plasma NfL observed in patients treated with the drug compared to placebo. While the primary endpoint of the trial (slowing of functional decline) was not met at 6 months, data from the trial as well as its open-label extension provided encouraging trends across multiple secondary and exploratory endpoints. A study of tofersen in presymptomatic *SOD1* gene mutation carriers is ongoing to test whether administration of the drug can prevent or significantly slow down the disease in this at-risk population.

Recent therapeutic advances in ALS are the fruit of years of investments in basic and translational research. Today, the ALS clinical research community is extremely active, with large and well-organized research consortia in multiple regions and several ongoing clinical trials.[145,173,179] Reasons for hope include the ever-expanding drug pipeline, the launch of innovative clinical trial designs, the development of gene-based approaches, and engagement from multiple stakeholders within the ALS community. Patients and clinicians can be kept abreast of clinical trial availability and enrollment status through several websites. We and others consider clinical research as an integral component of multidisciplinary ALS care.

Optimal management of the patients with ALS and their families requires knowledge and resources that undoubtedly surpass the capabilities of any single health care worker. For this reason, the multidisciplinary clinic provides the recommended care model.[169,172,180-182] Studies have demonstrated that participation in a multidisciplinary clinic improves both quality and duration of life.[58] The goals of the clinic are to anticipate and resolve problems that adversely affect patients' ability to function, their safety, and their comfort. During the clinic, multiple parameters including the patient's psychosocial well-being, the presence or absence of pain, sleep quality, "bulbar" functions, fine motor skills, ventilation, and mobility are assessed. Independence with several functions can be quantified and monitored by capturing the revised ALSFRS-R, a validated 48-point assessment tool that can be acquired both in person and over the phone.[183] Twelve points are assigned to each of four domains assessing ventilation, bulbar function, fine motor skills, and gross motor skills. Predictive models to estimate prognosis have been developed by combining ALSFRS-R scores with other clinical and demographic characteristics.

In addition to the ALSFRS-R, we routinely monitor measurements of ventilatory function. Although at times helpful in reinforcing the initial diagnosis, tests of ventilatory function have the greatest utility in monitoring the disease course. Declining ventilatory muscle strength not only speaks to prognosis and helps to time discussions pertaining to life-sustaining treatments, but it also has management implications regarding the initiation of noninvasive positive airway pressure and percutaneous gastrostomy tube insertion.[55] The most commonly used measurements are FVC, and maximal inspiratory (MIP) and expiratory (MEP) pressures. A drop in FVC in the supine in comparison to the sitting position of more than 10% of the predicted value suggests a disproportionate degree of diaphragmatic weakness.

Clinical guidelines exist to guide ALS care. The ALS practice parameter endorsed by both the American Academy of Neurology and the American Association of Neuromuscular and Electrodiagnostic Medicine was published in 2009.[180–182] Guidelines have also been released in Canada and some European countries and clinical reviews provide experienced, expert opinion.[184] In addition, the American Academy of Neurology published its first ALS quality management set in 2013, which was recently updated in 2023, to address aspects of ALS care for which there is a strong evidence base and that should be offered to all people living with ALS.[182] These key areas include ALS support services, disease-modifying pharmacotherapy, screening for malnutrition and dysphagia and appropriate referral, screening for respiratory impairment and appropriate intervention, multidisciplinary care plan, and patient care preferences. Symptomatic management of poor sleep (due to immobility, depression, urinary frequency, sleep disordered breathing), pain (due to immobility, joint contractures, cramps, and spasticity), sialorrhea, impaired clearance of viscous secretions, laryngospasm, impaired communication, dysphagia, impaired performance of ADLs, and disordered bowel and bladder function are typically addressed with durable medical equipment, physical modalities/therapy, or pharmacologic treatment. These interventions are outlined in (Table 6-6).[169,171]

It also behooves the neurologist to become familiar with the topography and limitations of the patient's residence and if necessary, to arrange for a home safety evaluation to identify areas of home modification that would benefit the patient. Patients and families frequently inquire about the role of genetics. As discussed earlier, knowledge about the genetic causes of ALS, availability of genetic testing, and development of targeted treatments continues to expand. Physicians working in ALS clinics should be familiar with the evolving field of ALS genetics and refer to genetic counseling as clinically indicated. The role of exercise pertaining to its effect on both the disease progression and the preservation of function is a near-universal inquiry by ALS patients. Studies done to date favorably report on the benefits of exercise done in moderation.[185–187] We recommend stretching and consideration of low-level conditioning and nonfatiguing exercise that is safe, for the specific patient. For example, a stationary exercise bicycle would be preferable to a treadmill for a patient with lower extremity weakness or spasticity. The reader is referred to Chapter 5 for a comprehensive review of the role of exercise in Neuromuscular Diseases as well as an outline of additional rehabilitation interventions and equipment considerations.

There are a number of potential interventions that can help enhance quality of life as well as maintenance of independence. It is best to introduce these concepts prior to their actual need to give patients and families a chance to consider and adjust.

Percutaneous gastrostomy, noninvasive ventilation (NIV), and mechanical gait aids are commonly recommended.[180,181] All should be introduced as measures to improve the quality of life rather than duration of life, even though the latter is probably achieved with NIV and may be accomplished with gastrostomy feeding. There are no absolute criteria to determine optimal percutaneous gastrostomy timing.[188] Loss of weight of more than 10% of baseline weight, doubling of eating time, demonstration of laryngeal penetration or aspiration, or recurrent coughing or choking during eating are the most common indicators utilized to prompt gastrostomy tube recommendation. We attempt to place percutaneous gastrostomy before FVC falls below 50% of predicted to limit risk associated with the procedure.

NIV is typically recommended when the patient is symptomatic from shortness of breath, when disturbed sleep is attributed to hypoventilation, when symptoms attributable to hypercapnia such as morning headache or confusion occur, or when FVC decreases to less than 50% of predicted.[189] Initial use usually occurs at night when hypoventilation is most likely to occur. Settings often require titration to patient's comfort and adjustments as disease progresses. NIV appears to have the most dramatic effects on disease survival of any treatment options available. Although it is suspected that early use of NIV is beneficial in prolonging life expectancy, third-party payers typically require an FVC of less than 50% of predicted, an MIP of less than 60 cm H_2O, or evidence of carbon dioxide retention before reimbursement for NIV is authorized.

As the disease progresses, preferentially while the patient remains capable of communicating effectively and before any ventilatory crisis might occur, it is important to discuss with the patient preferences regarding decisions that will inevitably have to be made such as those around the use of life-sustaining treatments, including TAMV. Ideally, this discussion would occur at a time of the patient's choosing but may need to be initiated by the physician in some cases. Family meetings and involvement of palliative care might be helpful. Delicate, but important topics related to TAMV include considerations of cost, location of care, caretaker burden, life expectancy, and potential development of future dementia. The majority of patients with ALS in the United States decline TAMV. The use of TAMV is more prevalent in some Asian and European countries, with considerable geographic variation. Most patients choose to receive their terminal care at home. Hospice services either at home or in hospice facilities provide an invaluable resource. Many, if not all, patients fear that their death will involve physical suffering. Some may be intrepid enough to broach the subject, some may not. Providing patients with the reassurance that adequate palliation will be provided to avert physical discomfort is another important responsibility to fulfill. A frank discussion about the logistics and limits of how this will be accomplished is often appreciated by the patient, family, and caregivers. Typically, ALS clinics and primary care physicians, through hospice nurses, provide for treatment of pain, anxiety, dyspnea, nausea, and any other distressing symptom. This goal is usually achieved often with drugs such as morphine and lorazepam. Fortunately, the vast majority of ALS patients appear to die peacefully and comfortably, as long as adequate palliative care and hospice services are initiated.[171]

▶ TABLE 6-6. SYMPTOMATIC MANAGEMENT OF MND/ALS

Symptom, Management Issue	Potential Treatments	Symptom, Management Issue	Potential Treatments
Sialorrhea	Glycopyrrolate Amitriptyline Hyoscyamine Atropine drops (sublingual) Scopolamine patch Botulinum toxin (salivary glands) Salivary gland radiation	**Mobility issues** Tripping/falls from foot drop and/or quadriceps weakness Bed mobility	Ankle–foot orthoses Canes Crutches Walker Wheelchair, manual, or power Hospital bed with side rails and/or trapeze
Secretion clearance	Cough-assist device Suction Expectorants (e.g., guaifenesin)	Bathroom safety and functionality	Stall shower Shower chair Transfer bench Toilet seat extension Shower and toilet bars
	Nebulized *N*-acetylcysteine and/or albuterol Secretion mobilization vests, chest PT Tracheostomy	House accessibility	Stair lift
Pseudobulbar affect	Dextromethorphan hydrobromide and quinidine sulfate Tricyclic antidepressants Selective serotonin reuptake inhibitors	 ADLs	Hoyer lift Elevators Ramps Velcro for buttons and shoelaces Elastic shoelaces Long-handled grippers Foam collars for pens and utensils
Depression	Tricyclic antidepressants Selective serotonin reuptake inhibitors	Dysphagia	Neck positioning, compensatory strategies during eating Change in food consistency Gastrostomy tubes
Laryngospasm	Antihistamines H$_2$-receptor blockers Antacids Proton pump inhibitors Sublingual lorazepam drops	Constipation Urinary urgency	Hydration Fiber Stool softeners Laxatives Tolterodine, oxybutynin, or other medications for overactive bladder
Neck drop	Cervical collar	Cramps	Magnesium supplements Tonic water Mexiletine Gabapentin Benzodiazepines
	High back wheelchair with supports		
Communication	Augmentative and alternative communication devices		
Hypoventilation	Noninvasive ventilation (NIV)		Quinine sulfate[a]
	Tracheostomy with invasive ventilation	Safety	Lifeline and other medical alert systems Home safety evaluation
Contractures	Range of motion exercises Night splints Botulinum toxin	Spasticity	Tizanidine Baclofen oral (intrathecal in selected cases of PLS) Benzodiazepines Botulinum toxin

ALS, amyotrophic lateral sclerosis; MND, motor neuron disease; ADLs, activities of daily living.
[a]Not FDA approved for this purpose.

In many locations, support groups are available for patients and their families and are integrated with clinic staff to help provide community support beyond the clinic walls. Virtual forums are also available. ALS advocacy has grown exponentially in recent years and has provided substantial contributions to ALS research and care.

▶ SUMMARY

HIV and cancer are disorders that were uniformly fatal within many of our professional lifetimes. Now, in many instances, these are disorders that are controllable and, at times, curable. For patients with ALS, their families, and their physicians, it is important to realize that similar outcomes may be realized for ALS in the foreseeable future. Until that hope is realized, neurologists caring for patients with ALS should provide comprehensive multidisciplinary care including available disease-modifying treatments as well as supportive and palliative care to help patients maintain function and quality of life.

REFERENCES

1. Hardiman O, Al-Chalabi A, Chio A, et al. Amyotrophic lateral sclerosis. *Nat Rev Dis Primers*. 2017;3:17071.
2. Feldman EL, Goutman SA, Petri S, et al. Amyotrophic lateral sclerosis. *Lancet*. 2022;400(10360):1363–1380.
3. Brown RH, Al-Chalabi A. Amyotrophic lateral sclerosis. *N Engl J Med*. 2017;377(2):162–172.
4. Strong MJ, Grace GM, Freedman M, et al. Consensus criteria for the diagnosis of frontotemporal cognitive and behavioural syndromes in amyotrophic lateral sclerosis. *Amyotroph Lateral Scler*. 2009;10(3):131–146.
5. Strong MJ, Abrahams S, Goldstein LH, et al. Amyotrophic lateral sclerosis – frontotemporal spectrum disorder (ALS-FTSD): revised diagnostic criteria. *Amyotroph Lateral Scler Frontotemporal Degener*. 2017;18(3–4):153–174.
6. Swash M, Desai J. Motor neuron disease: classification and nomenclature. *Amyotroph Lateral Scler Other Motor Neuron Disord*. 2000;1(2):105–112.
7. Gordon PH, Cheng B, Katz IB, et al. The natural history of primary lateral sclerosis. *Neurology*. 2006;66(5):647–653.
8. Gordon PH, Cheng B, Katz IB, Mitsumoto H, Rowland LP. Clinical features that distinguish PLS, upper motor neuron-dominant ALS, and typical ALS. *Neurology*. 2009;72(22):1948–1952.
9. Tartaglia MC, Rowe A, Findlater K, Orange JB, Grace G, Strong MJ. Differentiation between primary lateral sclerosis and amyotrophic lateral sclerosis: examination of symptoms and signs at disease onset and during follow-up. *Arch Neurol*. 2007;64(2):232–236.
10. Kim WK, Liu X, Sandner J, et al. Study of 962 patients indicates progressive muscular atrophy is a form of ALS. *Neurology*. 2009;73(20):1686–1692.
11. Visser J, van den Berg-Vos RM, Franssen H, et al. Mimic syndromes in sporadic cases of progressive spinal muscular atrophy. *Neurology*. 2002;58(11):1593–1596.
12. Traynor BJ, Codd MB, Corr B, Forde C, Frost E, Hardiman OM. Clinical features of amyotrophic lateral sclerosis according to the El Escorial and Airlie House diagnostic criteria: a population-based study. *Arch Neurol*. 2000;57(8):1171–1176.
13. Rowland LP. Progressive muscular atrophy and other lower motor neuron syndromes of adults. *Muscle Nerve*. 2010;41(2):161–165.
14. Mateen FJ, Carone M, Sorenson EJ. Patients who survive 5 years or more with ALS in Olmsted County, 1925–2004. *J Neurol Neurosurg Psychiatry*. 2010;81(10):1144–1146.
15. Visser J, van den Berg-Vos RM, Franssen H, et al. Disease course and prognostic factors of progressive muscular atrophy. *Arch Neurol*. 2007;64(4):522–528.
16. Mortara P, Chiò A, Rosso MG, Leone M, Schiffer D. Motor neuron disease in the province of Turin, Italy, 1966–1980. Survival analysis in an unselected population. *J Neurol Sci*. 1984;66(2–3):165–173.
17. Brooks BR. El Escorial World Federation of Neurology criteria for the diagnosis of amyotrophic lateral sclerosis. Subcommittee on motor neuron diseases/amyotrophic lateral sclerosis of the World Federation of Neurology Research Group on Neuromuscular Diseases and the El Escorial "clinical limits of amyotrophic lateral sclerosis" workshop contributors. *J Neurol Sci*. 1994;124:96–107.
18. Bensimon G, Lacomblez L, Meininger V; Group ALRS. A controlled trial of riluzole in amyotrophic lateral sclerosis. *N Engl J Med*. 1994;330(9):585–591.
19. Brooks BR, Miller RG, Swash M, Munsat TL; World Federation of Neurology Research Group on Motor Neuron D. El Escorial revisited: revised criteria for the diagnosis of amyotrophic lateral sclerosis. *Amyotroph Lateral Scler Other Motor Neuron Disord*. 2000;1(5):293–299.
20. Ross MA, Miller RG, Berchert L, et al. Toward earlier diagnosis of amyotrophic lateral sclerosis: revised criteria. rhCNTF ALS Study Group. *Neurology*. 1998;50(3):768–772.
21. Chaudhuri KR, Crump S, al-Sarraj S, Anderson V, Cavanagh J, Leigh PN. The validation of El Escorial criteria for the diagnosis of amyotrophic lateral sclerosis: a clinicopathological study. *J Neurol Sci*. 1995;129:11–12.
22. Ince PG, Evans J, Knopp M, et al. Corticospinal tract degeneration in the progressive muscular atrophy variant of ALS. *Neurology*. 2003;60(8):1252–1258.
23. Carvalho MD, Swash M. Awaji diagnostic algorithm increases sensitivity of El Escorial criteria for ALS diagnosis. *Amyotroph Lateral Scler*. 2009;10(1):53–57.
24. Chen A, Weimer L, Brannagan T, et al. Experience with the Awaji island modifications to the ALS diagnostic criteria. *Muscle Nerve*. 2010;42(5):831–832.
25. Douglass CP, Kandler RH, Shaw PJ, McDermott CJ. An evaluation of neurophysiological criteria used in the diagnosis of motor neuron disease. *J Neurol Neurosurg Psychiatry*. 2010;81(6):646–649.
26. Mills KR. Characteristics of fasciculations in amyotrophic lateral sclerosis and the benign fasciculation syndrome. *Brain*. 2010;133(11):3458–3469.
27. Benatar M, Tandan R. The Awaji criteria for the diagnosis of amyotrophic lateral sclerosis: have we put the cart before the horse? *Muscle Nerve*. 2011;43(4):461–463.
28. Shefner JM, Al-Chalabi A, Baker MR, et al. A proposal for new diagnostic criteria for ALS. *Clin Neurophysiol*. 2020;131(8):1975–1978.

29. Hannaford A, Pavey N, van den Bos M, et al. Diagnostic utility of gold coast criteria in amyotrophic lateral sclerosis. *Ann Neurol.* 2021;89(5):979–986.
30. Shefner JM. Changing amyotrophic lateral sclerosis diagnostic criteria: will it impact clinical trials? *Muscle Nerve.* 2022;66(4):377–379.
31. Andersen PM, Al-Chalabi A. Clinical genetics of amyotrophic lateral sclerosis: what do we really know? *Nat Rev Neurol.* 2011;7(11):603–615.
32. Al-Chalabi A, van den Berg LH, Veldink J. Gene discovery in amyotrophic lateral sclerosis: implications for clinical management. *Nat Rev Neurol.* Feb;13(2):96–104.
33. Shatunov A, Al-Chalabi A. The genetic architecture of ALS. *Neurobiol Dis.* 2021;147:105156.
34. Younger DS, Brown RH Jr. Amyotrophic lateral sclerosis. *Handb Clin Neurol.* 2023;196:203–229.
35. Goutman SA, Hardiman O, Al-Chalabi A, et al. Recent advances in the diagnosis and prognosis of amyotrophic lateral sclerosis. *Lancet Neurol.* 2022;21(5):480–493.
36. Abrahams S. Neuropsychological impairment in amyotrophic lateral sclerosis-frontotemporal spectrum disorder. *Nat Rev Neurol.* 2023;19(11):655–667.
37. McHutchison CA, Wuu J, McMillan CT, et al. Temporal course of cognitive and behavioural changes in motor neuron diseases. *J Neurol Neurosurg Psychiatry.* 2024;;95(4):316–324.
38. Goldman JS, Rademakers R, Huey ED, et al. An algorithm for genetic testing of frontotemporal lobar degeneration. *Neurology.* 2011;76(5):475–483.
39. Greaves CV, Rohrer JD. An update on genetic frontotemporal dementia. *J Neurol.* 2019;266(8):2075–2086.
40. DeJesus-Hernandez M, Mackenzie IR, Boeve BF, et al. Expanded GGGGCC hexanucleotide repeat in noncoding region of C9ORF72 causes chromosome 9p-linked FTD and ALS. *Neuron.* 2011;72(2):245–256.
41. Hardiman O, Al-Chalabi A, Brayne C, et al. The changing picture of amyotrophic lateral sclerosis: lessons from European registers. *J Neurol Neurosurg Psychiatry.* 2017;88(7):557–563.
42. Mehta P, Raymond J, Zhang Y, et al. Prevalence of amyotrophic lateral sclerosis in the United States, 2018. *Amyotroph Lateral Scler Frontotemporal Degener.* 2023:1–7.
43. Wolfson C, Gauvin DE, Ishola F, Oskoui M. Global prevalence and incidence of amyotrophic lateral sclerosis: a systematic review. *Neurology.* 2023;101(6):e613–e623.
44. Raymond J, Punjani R, Larson T, Berry JD, Horton DK, Mehta P. Comparing amyotrophic lateral sclerosis (ALS) patient characteristics from the National ALS Registry and the Massachusetts ALS Registry, data through 2015. *Amyotroph Lateral Scler Frontotemporal Degener.* 2023:1–8.
45. Goutman SA, Savelieff MG, Jang D-G, Hur J, Feldman EL. The amyotrophic lateral sclerosis exposome: recent advances and future directions. *Nat Rev Neurol.* 2023;19(10):617–634.
46. Al-Chalabi A, Hardiman O. The epidemiology of ALS: a conspiracy of genes, environment and time. *Nat Rev Neurol.* 2013;9(11):617–628.
47. Wang H, O'Reilly EJ, Weisskopf MG, et al. Smoking and risk of amyotrophic lateral sclerosis: a pooled analysis of 5 prospective cohorts. *Arch Neurol.* 2011;68(2):207–213.
48. Vasta R, Chia R, Traynor BJ, Chio A. Unraveling the complex interplay between genes, environment, and climate in ALS. *EBioMedicine.* 2022;75:103795.
49. Cashman NR, Cudkowicz ME, Davidson MC, Pioro EP, Rosenfeld J; The ALS patient care database. Gender effects on duration and onset age of amyotrophic lateral sclerosis. Proceedings of the 12th International Symposium on ALS/MND. Oakland, November 18–20, 2001;2(Suppl 2): abstractC60;41.
50. Bradley WG, Mash DC. Beyond Guam: the cyanobacteria/BMAA hypothesis of the cause of ALS and other neurodegenerative diseases. *Amyotroph Lateral Scler.* 2009;10(10):7–20.
51. Chancellor AM, Slattery JM, Fraser H, Swingler RJ, Holloway SM, Warlow CP. The prognosis of adult-onset motor neuron disease: a prospective study based on the Scottish Motor Neuron Disease Register. *J Neurol.* 1993;240(6):339–346.
52. Magnus T, Beck M, Giess R, Puls I, Naumann M, Toyka KV. Disease progression in amyotrophic lateral sclerosis: predictors of survival. *Muscle Nerve.* 2002;25(5):709–714.
53. Larson TC, Goutman SA, Davis B, Bove FJ, Thakur N, Mehta P. Causes of death among United States decedents with ALS: an eye toward delaying mortality. *Ann Clin Transl Neurol.* 2023;10(5):757–764.
54. Lechtzin N, Cudkowicz ME, de Carvalho M, et al. Respiratory measures in amyotrophic lateral sclerosis. *Amyotroph Lateral Scler Frontotemporal Degener.* 2018;19(5-6):321–330.
55. Andrews JA, Meng L, Kulke SF, et al. Association between decline in slow vital capacity and respiratory insufficiency, use of assisted ventilation, tracheostomy, or death in patients with amyotrophic lateral sclerosis. *JAMA Neurol.* 2018;75(1):58–64.
56. Atassi N, Berry J, Shui A, et al. The PRO-ACT database: design, initial analyses, and predictive features. *Neurology.* 2014;83(19):1719–1725.
57. Chio A, Logroscino G, Hardiman O, et al. Prognostic factors in ALS: a critical review. *Amyotroph Lateral Scler.* 2009;10(5-6):310–323.
58. Traynor BJ, Alexander M, Corr B, Frost E, Hardiman O. Effect of a multidisciplinary amyotrophic lateral sclerosis (ALS) clinic on ALS survival: a population based study, 1996–2000. *J Neurol Neurosurg Psychiatry.* 2003;74(9):1258–1261.
59. Blexrud MD, Windebank AJ, Daube JR. Long-term follow-up of 121 patients with benign fasciculations. *Ann Neurol.* 1993;34(4):622–625.
60. Norris F, Shepherd R, Denys E, et al. Onset, natural history and outcome in idiopathic adult motor neuron disease. *J Neurol Sci.* 1993;118(1):48–55.
61. Masrori P, Van Damme P. Amyotrophic lateral sclerosis: a clinical review. *Eur J Neurol.* 2020;27(10):1918–1929.
62. Turner MR, Barohn RJ, Corcia P, et al; Delegates of the 2nd International PLS Conference. Primary lateral sclerosis: consensus diagnostic criteria. *J Neurol Neurosurg Psychiatry.* 2020;91(4):373–377.
63. Andersen PM. Amyotrophic lateral sclerosis associated with mutations in the CuZn superoxide dismutase gene. *Curr Neurol Neurosci Rep.* 2006;6(1):37–46.
64. Brownell B, Oppenheimer DR, Hughes JT. The central nervous system in motor neurone disease. *J Neurol Neurosurg Psychiatry.* 1970;33(3):338–357.
65. Iwanaga K, Hayashi S, Oyake M, et al. Neuropathology of sporadic amyotrophic lateral sclerosis of long duration. *J Neurol Sci.* 1997;146(2):139–143.
66. Lawyer T, Netsky MG. Amyotrophic lateral sclerosis, a clinicoanatomic study of fifty-three cases. *AMA Arch Neurol Psychiatry.* 1953;69:171–192.
67. Cudkowicz ME, McKenna-Yasek D, Chen C, Hedley-Whyte ET, Brown RH. Limited corticospinal tract involvement in

amyotrophic lateral sclerosis subjects with the A4V mutation in the copper/zinc superoxide dismutase gene. *Ann Neurol.* 1998;43(6):703–710.
68. Raaphorst J, de Visser M, van Tol M-J, et al. Cognitive dysfunction in lower motor neuron disease: executive and memory deficits in progressive muscular atrophy. *J Neurol Neurosurg Psychiatry.* 2011;82(2):170–175.
69. Katz JS, Wolfe GI, Andersson PB, et al. Brachial amyotrophic diplegia: a slowly progressive motor neuron disorder. *Neurology.* 1999;53(5):1071–1076.
70. Wijesekera LC, Mathers S, Talman P, et al. Natural history and clinical features of the flail arm and flail leg ALS variants. *Neurology.* 2009;72(12):1087–1094.
71. Robert D, Pouget J, Giovanni A, Azulay JP, Triglia JM. Quantitative voice analysis in the assessment of bulbar involvement in amyotrophic lateral sclerosis. *Acta Otolaryngol.* 1999;119(6):724–731.
72. Coon EA, Sorenson EJ, Whitwell JL, Knopman DS, Josephs KA. Predicting survival in frontotemporal dementia with motor neuron disease. *Neurology.* 2011;76(22):1886–1893.
73. Turner MR, Scaber J, Goodfellow JA, Lord ME, Marsden R, Talbot K. The diagnostic pathway and prognosis in bulbar-onset amyotrophic lateral sclerosis. *J Neurol Sci.* 2010;294(1–2):81–85.
74. Portet F, Cadilhac C, Touchon J, Camu W. Cognitive impairment in motor neuron disease with bulbar onset. *Amyotroph Lateral Scler Other Motor Neuron Disord.* 2001;2(1):23–29.
75. Ringholz GM, Appel SH, Bradshaw M, Cooke NA, Mosnik DM, Schulz PE. Prevalence and patterns of cognitive impairment in sporadic ALS. *Neurology.* 2005;65(4):586–590.
76. Pringle CE, Hudson AJ, Munoz DG, Kiernan JA, Brown WF, Ebers GC. Primary lateral sclerosis. Clinical features, neuropathology and diagnostic criteria. *Brain.* 1992;115(Pt 2):495–520.
77. Strong MJ, Gordon PH. Primary lateral sclerosis, hereditary spastic paraplegia and amyotrophic lateral sclerosis: discrete entities or spectrum? *Amyotroph Lateral Scler Other Motor Neuron Disord.* 2005;6(1):8–16.
78. Singer MA, Statland JM, Wolfe GI, Barohn RJ. Primary lateral sclerosis. *Muscle Nerve.* 2007;35(3):291–302.
79. Caselli RJ, Smith BE, Osborne D. Primary lateral sclerosis: a neuropsychological study. *Neurology.* 1995;45(11):2005–2009.
80. Josephs KA, Dickson DW. Frontotemporal lobar degeneration with upper motor neuron disease/primary lateral sclerosis. *Neurology.* 2007;69(18):1800–1801.
81. Paganoni S, De Marchi F, Chan J, et al. The NEALS primary lateral sclerosis registry. *Amyotroph Lateral Scler Frontotemporal Degener.* 2020;21(sup1):74–81.
82. Mitsumoto H, Jang G, Lee I, et al. Primary lateral sclerosis natural history study – planning, designing, and early enrollment. *Amyotroph Lateral Scler Frontotemporal Degener.* 2023;24(5–6):394–404.
83. Floeter MK, Warden D, Lange D, Wymer J, Paganoni S, Mitsumoto H. Clinical care and therapeutic trials in PLS. *Amyotroph Lateral Scler Frontotemporal Degener.* 2020;21(sup1):67–73.
84. Chen R, Grand'Maison F, Strong MJ, Ramsay DA, Bolton CF. Motor neuron disease presenting as acute respiratory failure: a clinical and pathological study. *J Neurol Neurosurg Psychiatry.* 1996;60(4):455–458.
85. Shoesmith CL, Findlater K, Rowe A, Strong MJ. Prognosis of amyotrophic lateral sclerosis with respiratory onset. *J Neurol Neurosurg Psychiatry.* 2007;78(6):629–631.
86. Strong MJ, Lomen-Hoerth C, Caselli RJ, Bigio EH, Yang W. Cognitive impairment, frontotemporal dementia, and the motor neuron diseases. *Ann Neurol.* 2003;54(5):S20–S23.
87. Elamin M, Phukan J, Bede P, et al. Executive dysfunction is a negative prognostic indicator in patients with ALS without dementia. *Neurology.* 2011;76(14):1263–1269.
88. Wheaton MW, Salamone AR, Mosnik DM, et al. Cognitive impairment in familial ALS. *Neurology.* 2007;69(14):1411–1417.
89. Lomen-Hoerth C, Anderson T, Miller B. The overlap of amyotrophic lateral sclerosis and frontotemporal dementia. *Neurology.* 2002;59(7):1077–1079.
90. Abrahams S, Newton J, Niven E, Foley J, Bak TH. Screening for cognition and behaviour changes in ALS. *Amyotroph Lateral Scler Frontotemporal Degener.* 2014;15(1–2):9–14.
91. Niven E, Newton J, Foley J, et al. Validation of the Edinburgh Cognitive and Behavioural Amyotrophic Lateral Sclerosis Screen (ECAS): a cognitive tool for motor disorders. *Amyotroph Lateral Scler Frontotemporal Degener.* 2015;16(3–4):172–179.
92. Andersen PM, Borasio GD, Dengler R, et al; EFNS Task Force on Diagnosis and Management of Amyotrophic Lateral Sclerosis. EFNS task force on management of amyotrophic lateral sclerosis: guidelines for diagnosing and clinical care of patients and relatives. *Eur J Neurol.* 2005;12(12):921–938.
93. Van Den Berg-Vos RM, Van Den Berg LH, Visser J, de Visser M, Franssen H, Wokke JHJ. The spectrum of lower motor neuron syndromes. *J Neurol.* 2003;250(11):1279–1292.
94. Kwan J, Vullaganti M. Amyotrophic lateral sclerosis mimics. *Muscle Nerve.* 2022;66(3):240–252.
95. Traynor BJ, Codd MB, Corr B, Forde C, Frost E, Hardiman O. Amyotrophic lateral sclerosis mimic syndromes: a population-based study. *Arch Neurol.* 2000;57(1):109–113.
96. Nobile-Orazio E, Cappellari A, Priori A. Multifocal motor neuropathy: current concepts and controversies. *Muscle Nerve.* 2005;31(6):663–680.
97. Cats EA, Jacobs BC, Yuki N, et al. Multifocal motor neuropathy: association of anti-GM1 IgM antibodies with clinical features. *Neurology.* 2010;75(22):1961–1967.
98. Gooch CL, Amato AA. Are anti-ganglioside antibodies of clinical value in multifocal motor neuropathy? *Neurology.* 2010;75(22):1950–1951.
99. Finsterer J. Perspectives of Kennedy's disease. *J Neurol Sci.* 2010;298(1–2):1–10.
100. Rhodes LE, Freeman BK, Auh S, et al. Clinical features of spinal and bulbar muscular atrophy. *Brain.* 2009;132(Pt 12):3242–3251.
101. Kennedy WR, Alter M, Sung JH. Proximal bulbar and spinal muscular atrophy of late onset. A sex-linked recessive trait. *Neurology.* 1968;18(7):671–680.
102. Parboosingh JS, Figlewicz DA, Krizus A, et al. Spinobulbar muscular atrophy can mimic ALS: the importance of genetic testing in male patients with atypical ALS. *Neurology.* 1997;49(2):568–572.
103. Dabby R, Lange DJ, Trojaborg W, et al. Inclusion body myositis mimicking motor neuron disease. *Arch Neurol.* 2001;58(8):1253–1256.
104. Van den Berg-Vos RM, Visser J, Kalmijn S, et al. A long-term prospective study of the natural course of sporadic adult-onset lower motor neuron syndromes. *Arch Neurol.* 2009;66(6):751–757.
105. Sobue I, Saito N, Iida M, Ando K. Juvenile type of distal and segmental muscular atrophy of upper extremities. *Ann Neurol.* 1978;3(5):429–432.
106. Hirayama K, Toyokura Y, Tsubaki T. Juvenile muscular atrophy of unilateral upper extremity: a new clinical entity. *Psychiatr Neurol Jpn.* 1959;61:2190–2197.

107. Pradhan S. Bilaterally symmetric form of Hirayama disease. *Neurology.* 2009;72(24):2083–2089.
108. Patel DR, Knepper L, Jones HR. Late-onset monomelic amyotrophy in a Caucasian woman. *Muscle Nerve.* 2008;37(1):115–119.
109. Felice KJ, Whitaker CH, Grunnet ML. Benign calf amyotrophy: clinicopathologic study of 8 patients. *Arch Neurol.* 2003;60(10):1415–1420.
110. Irobi J, De Jonghe P, Timmerman V. Molecular genetics of distal hereditary motor neuropathies. *Hum Mol Genet.* 2004;13(Spec No 2):R195–R202.
111. Rossor AM, Kalmar B, Greensmith L, Reilly MM. The distal hereditary motor neuropathies. *J Neurol Neurosurg Psychiatry.* 2012;83(1):6–14.
112. Giray E, Karayigit M, Senocak KC, et al. Delayed radiation-induced motor neuron syndrome: a case report. *J Back Musculoskelet Rehabil.* 2023;36(6):1469–1475.
113. Goyal NA, Mozaffar T. Tongue atrophy and fasciculations in transthyretin familial amyloid neuropathy: an ALS mimicker. *Neurol Genet.* 2015;1(2):e18.
114. Park J, Kim YE, Oh KW, et al. Gelsolin variant amyloidosis mimicking progressive bulbar palsy. *Muscle Nerve.* 2022;66(5):E28–E30.
115. Fink JK. The hereditary spastic paraplegias. *Handb Clin Neurol.* 2023;196:59–88.
116. Meyer T, Schwan A, Dullinger JS, et al. Early-onset ALS with long-term survival associated with spastin gene mutation. *Neurology.* 2005;65(1):141–143.
117. Mathews JA. Wasting of the small hand muscles in upper and mid-cervical cord lesions. *QJM.* 1998;91(10):691–700.
118. Stark RJ, Kennard C, Swash M. Hand wasting in spondylotic high cord compression: an electromyographic study. *Ann Neurol.* 1981;9(1):58–62.
119. Srinivasan J, Scala S, Jones HR, Saleh F, Russell JA. Inappropriate surgeries resulting from misdiagnosis of early amyotrophic lateral sclerosis. *Muscle Nerve.* 2006;34(3):359–360.
120. Weihl CC, Lopate G. Motor neuron disease associated with copper deficiency. *Muscle Nerve.* 2006;34(6):789–793.
121. Qureshi M, Bedlack RS, Cudkowicz ME. Lyme disease serology in amyotrophic lateral sclerosis. *Muscle Nerve.* 2009;40(4):626–628.
122. Henning F, Hewlett RH. Brachial amyotrophic diplegia (segmental proximal spinal muscular atrophy) associated with HIV infection. *J Neurol Neurosurg Psychiatry.* 2008;79(12):1392–1394.
123. Verma A, Berger JR. ALS syndrome in patients with HIV-1 infection. *J Neurol Sci.* 2006;240(1–2):59–64.
124. Drory VE, Birnbaum M, Peleg L, Goldman B, Korczyn AD. Hexosaminidase A deficiency is an uncommon cause of a syndrome mimicking amyotrophic lateral sclerosis. *Muscle Nerve.* 2003;28(1):109–112.
125. Jackson CE, Amato AA, Bryan WW, Wolfe GI, Sakhaee K, Barohn RJ. Primary hyperparathyroidism and ALS: is there a relation? *Neurology.* 1998;50(6):1795–1799.
126. Stich O, Kleer B, Rauer S. Absence of paraneoplastic antineuronal antibodies in sera of 145 patients with motor neuron disease. *J Neurol Neurosurg Psychiatry.* 2007;78(8):883–885.
127. Moulignier A, Moulonguet A, Pialoux G, Rozenbaum W. Reversible ALS-like disorder in HIV infection. *Neurology.* 2001;57(6):995–1001.
128. Johnson WG. The clinical spectrum of hexosaminidase deficiency diseases. *Neurology.* 1981;31(11):1453–1456.
129. Younger DS. Motor neuron disease and malignancy. *Muscle Nerve.* 2000;23(5):658–660.
130. Gordon PH, Rowland LP, Younger DS, et al. Lymphoproliferative disorders and motor neuron disease: an update. *Neurology.* 1997;48(6):1671–1678.
131. Verma A, Berger JR. Primary lateral sclerosis with HIV-1 infection. *Neurology.* 2008;70(7):575–577.
132. Atkinson JL, Miller GM, Krauss WE, et al. Clinical and radiographic features of dural arteriovenous fistula, a treatable cause of myelopathy. *Mayo Clin Proc.* 2001;76(11):1120–1130.
133. Armon C, Daube JR. Electrophysiological signs of arteriovenous malformations of the spinal cord. *J Neurol Neurosurg Psychiatry.* 1989;52(10):1176–1181.
134. Makki AA, Benatar M. The electromyographic diagnosis of amyotrophic lateral sclerosis: does the evidence support the El Escorial criteria? *Muscle Nerve.* 2007;35(5):614–619.
135. Daube JR. Electrodiagnostic studies in amyotrophic lateral sclerosis and other motor neuron disorders. *Muscle Nerve.* 2000;23(10):1488–1502.
136. Agosta F, Chiò A, Cosottini M, et al. The present and the future of neuroimaging in amyotrophic lateral sclerosis. *AJNR Am J Neuroradiol.* 2010;31(10):1769–1777.
137. Mitsumoto H, Ulu AM, Pullman SL, et al. Quantitative objective markers for upper and lower motor neuron dysfunction in ALS. *Neurology.* 2007;68(17):1402–1410.
138. Felice KJ, North WA. Creatine kinase values in amyotrophic lateral sclerosis. *J Neurol Sci.* 1998;160:S30–S32.
139. Chahin N, Sorenson EJ. Serum creatine kinase levels in spinobulbar muscular atrophy and amyotrophic lateral sclerosis. *Muscle Nerve.* 2009;40(1):126–129.
140. Roggenbuck J, Eubank BHF, Wright J, Harms MB, Kolb SJ; ALS Genetic Testing and Counseling Guidelines Expert Panel. Evidence-based consensus guidelines for ALS genetic testing and counseling. *Ann Clin Transl Neurol.* 2023;10(11):2074–2091.
141. Dilliott AA, Al Nasser A, Elnagheeb M, et al. Clinical testing panels for ALS: global distribution, consistency, and challenges. *Amyotroph Lateral Scler Frontotemporal Degener.* 2023;24(5–6):420–435.
142. Yamashita S, Ando Y. Genotype-phenotype relationship in hereditary amyotrophic lateral sclerosis. *Transl Neurodegener.* 2015;4:13.
143. Benatar M, Turner MR, Wuu J. Presymptomatic amyotrophic lateral sclerosis: from characterization to prevention. *Curr Opin Neurol.* 2023;36(4):360–364.
144. Benatar M, Boylan K, Jeromin A, et al. ALS biomarkers for therapy development: state of the field and future directions. *Muscle Nerve.* 2016;53(2):169–182.
145. Kiernan MC, Vucic S, Talbot K, et al. Improving clinical trial outcomes in amyotrophic lateral sclerosis. *Nat Rev Neurol.* 2021;17(2):104–118.
146. Benatar M, Wuu J, Turner MR. Neurofilament light chain in drug development for amyotrophic lateral sclerosis: a critical appraisal. *Brain.* 2023;146(7):2711–2716.
147. Benatar M, Wuu J, Andersen PM, Lombardi V, Malaspina A. Neurofilament light: a candidate biomarker of presymptomatic amyotrophic lateral sclerosis and phenoconversion. *Ann Neurol.* 2018;84(1):130–139.
148. Miller TM, Cudkowicz ME, Genge A, et al; VALOR and OLE Working Group. Trial of antisense oligonucleotide tofersen for SOD1 ALS. *N Engl J Med.* 2022;387(12):1099–1110.

149. McMackin R, Bede P, Ingre C, Malaspina A, Hardiman O. Biomarkers in amyotrophic lateral sclerosis: current status and future prospects. *Nat Rev Neurol.* 2023;19(12):754–768.
150. Mackenzie IR, Rademakers R, Neumann M. TDP-43 and FUS in amyotrophic lateral sclerosis and frontotemporal dementia. *Lancet Neurol.* 2010;9(10):995–1007.
151. Hodges JR, Davies RR, Xuereb JH, et al. Clinicopathological correlates in frontotemporal dementia. *Ann Neurol.* 2004;56(3): 399–406.
152. Daoud H, Rouleau GA. A role for ubiquilin 2 mutations in neurodegeneration. *Nat Rev Neurol.* 2011;7(11):599–600.
153. Del Bo R, Tiloca C, Pensato V, et al; SLAGEN Consortium. Novel optineurin mutations in patients with familial and sporadic amyotrophic lateral sclerosis. *J Neurol Neurosurg Psychiatry.* 2011;82(11):1239–1243.
154. Arai T, Hasegawa M, Akiyama H, et al. TDP-43 is a component of ubiquitin-positive tau-negative inclusions in frontotemporal lobar degeneration and amyotrophic lateral sclerosis. *Biochem Biophys Res Commun.* 2006;351(3):602–611.
155. Geser F, Stein B, Partain M, et al. Motor neuron disease clinically limited to the lower motor neuron is a diffuse TDP-43 proteinopathy. *Acta Neuropathol.* 2011;121(4):509–517.
156. Kobayashi Z, Tsuchiya K, Arai T, et al. Clinicopathological characteristics of FTLD-TDP showing corticospinal tract degeneration but lacking lower motor neuron loss. *J Neurol Sci.* 2010;298(1–2):70–77.
157. Mizuno Y, Fujita Y, Takatama M, Okamoto K. Peripherin partially localizes in Bunina bodies in amyotrophic lateral sclerosis. *J Neurol Sci.* 2011;302(1–2):14–18.
158. Mori F, Tanji K, Miki Y, Kakita A, Takahashi H, Wakabayashi K. Relationship between Bunina bodies and TDP-43 inclusions in spinal anterior horn in amyotrophic lateral sclerosis. *Neuropathol Appl Neurobiol.* 2010;36(4):345–352.
159. Rothstein JD. Current hypotheses for the underlying biology of amyotrophic lateral sclerosis. *Ann Neurol.* 2009;65(S1):S3–S9.
160. Pasinelli P, Brown RH. Molecular biology of amyotrophic lateral sclerosis: insights from genetics. *Nat Rev Neurosci.* 2006;7(9):710–723.
161. Ravits JM, La Spada AR. ALS motor phenotype heterogeneity, focality, and spread: deconstructing motor neuron degeneration. *Neurology.* 2009;73(10):805–811.
162. Kuwabara S, Yokota T. Propagation: prion-like mechanisms can explain spreading of motor neuronal death in amyotrophic lateral sclerosis? *J Neurol Neurosurg Psychiatry.* 2011;82(11): 1181–1182.
163. Fujimura-Kiyono C, Kimura F, Ishida S, et al. Onset and spreading patterns of lower motor neuron involvements predict survival in sporadic amyotrophic lateral sclerosis. *J Neurol Neurosurg Psychiatry.* 2011;82(11):1244–1249.
164. Neumann M, Kwong LK, Sampathu DM, Trojanowski JQ, Lee VMY. TDP-43 proteinopathy in frontotemporal lobar degeneration and amyotrophic lateral sclerosis: protein misfolding diseases without amyloidosis. *Arch Neurol.* 2007;64(10):1388–1394.
165. Van Damme P, Veldink JH, van Blitterswijk M, et al. Expanded ATXN2 CAG repeat size in ALS identifies genetic overlap between ALS and SCA2. *Neurology.* 2011;76(24):2066–2072.
166. Fischbeck KH, Pulst SM. Amyotrophic lateral sclerosis and spinocerebellar ataxia 2. *Neurology.* 2011;76(24):2050–2051.
167. Daoud H, Belzil V, Martins S, et al. Association of long ATXN2 CAG repeat sizes with increased risk of amyotrophic lateral sclerosis. *Arch Neurol.* 2011;68(6):739–742.
168. Maruyama H, Morino H, Ito H, et al. Mutations of optineurin in amyotrophic lateral sclerosis. *Nature.* 2010;465(7295):223–226.
169. Paganoni S, Karam C, Joyce N, Bedlack R, Carter GT. Comprehensive rehabilitative care across the spectrum of amyotrophic lateral sclerosis. *NeuroRehabilitation.* 2015;37(1):53–68.
170. Majmudar S, Wu J, Paganoni S. Rehabilitation in amyotrophic lateral sclerosis: why it matters. *Muscle Nerve.* 2014;50(1):4–13.
171. Karam CY, Paganoni S, Joyce N, Carter GT, Bedlack R. Palliative care issues in amyotrophic lateral sclerosis: an evidenced-based review. *Am J Hosp Palliat Care.* 2016;33(1):84–92.
172. Paganoni S, Nicholson K, Leigh F, et al. Developing multidisciplinary clinics for neuromuscular care and research. *Muscle Nerve.* 2017;56(5):848–858.
173. Johnson SA, Fang T, De Marchi F, et al. Pharmacotherapy for amyotrophic lateral sclerosis: a review of approved and upcoming agents. *Drugs.* 2022;82(13):1367–1388.
174. Writing Group, Edaravone (MCI-186) ALS 19 Study Group. Safety and efficacy of edaravone in well defined patients with amyotrophic lateral sclerosis: a randomised, double-blind, placebo-controlled trial. *Lancet Neurol.* 2017;16(7):505–512.
175. Pattee GL, Genge A, Couratier P, et al. Oral edaravone – introducing a flexible treatment option for amyotrophic lateral sclerosis. *Expert Rev Neurother.* 2023;23(10):859–866.
176. Paganoni S, Macklin EA, Hendrix S, et al. Trial of sodium phenylbutyrate-taurursodiol for amyotrophic lateral sclerosis. *N Engl J Med.* 2020;383(10):919–930.
177. Paganoni S, Hendrix S, Dickson SP, et al. Long-term survival of participants in the CENTAUR trial of sodium phenylbutyrate-taurursodiol in amyotrophic lateral sclerosis. *Muscle Nerve.* 2021;63(1):31–39.
178. Paganoni S, Watkins C, Cawson M, et al. Survival analyses from the CENTAUR trial in amyotrophic lateral sclerosis: evaluating the impact of treatment crossover on outcomes. *Muscle Nerve.* 2022;66(2):136–141.
179. Paganoni S, Berry JD, Quintana M, et al; Healey ALS Platform Trial Study Group. Adaptive platform trials to transform amyotrophic lateral sclerosis therapy development. *Ann Neurol.* 2022;91(2):165–175.
180. Miller RG, Jackson CE, Kasarskis EJ, et al; Quality Standards Subcommittee of the American Academy of Neurology. Practice parameter update: the care of the patient with amyotrophic lateral sclerosis: drug, nutritional, and respiratory therapies (an evidence-based review): report of the Quality Standards Subcommittee of the American Academy of Neurology. *Neurology.* 2009;73(15):1218–1226.
181. Miller RG, Jackson CE, Kasarskis EJ, et al; Quality Standards Subcommittee of the American Academy of Neurology. Practice parameter update: the care of the patient with amyotrophic lateral sclerosis: multidisciplinary care, symptom management, and cognitive/behavioral impairment (an evidence-based review): report of the Quality Standards Subcommittee of the American Academy of Neurology. *Neurology.* 2009;73(15):1227–1233.
182. Kvam KA, Benatar M, Brownlee A, et al. Amyotrophic Lateral Sclerosis Quality Measurement Set 2022 Update: quality improvement in neurology. *Neurology.* 2023;101(5):223–232.
183. Cedarbaum JM, Stambler N, Malta E, et al. The ALSFRS-R: a revised ALS functional rating scale that incorporates assessments of respiratory function. BDNF ALS Study Group (Phase III). *J Neurol Sci.* 1999;169(1–2):13–21.

184. Shoesmith C, Abrahao A, Benstead T, et al. Canadian best practice recommendations for the management of amyotrophic lateral sclerosis. *CMAJ*. 2020;192(46):E1453-E1468.
185. Clawson LL, Cudkowicz M, Krivickas L, et al; Neals consortium. A randomized controlled trial of resistance and endurance exercise in amyotrophic lateral sclerosis. *Amyotroph Lateral Scler Frontotemporal Degener*. 2018;19(3-4):250-258.
186. Lunetta C, Lizio A, Sansone VA, et al. Strictly monitored exercise programs reduce motor deterioration in ALS: preliminary results of a randomized controlled trial. *J Neurol*. 2016;263(1):52-60.
187. Dalbello-Haas V, Florence JM, Krivickas LS. Therapeutic exercise for people with amyotrophic lateral sclerosis or motor neuron disease. *Cochrane Database Syst Rev*. 2008;(2):CD005229.
188. Sulistyo A, Abrahao A, Freitas ME, Ritsma B, Zinman L. Enteral tube feeding for amyotrophic lateral sclerosis/motor neuron disease. *Cochrane Database Syst Rev*. 2023;8(8):CD004030.
189. Ackrivo J. Pulmonary care for ALS: progress, gaps, and paths forward. *Muscle Nerve*. 2023;67(5):341-353.

CHAPTER 7

Hereditary Spastic Paraplegia

The diagnosis of hereditary spastic paraplegia (HSP) is based on the identification of a phenotype characterized as a slowly progressive, symmetric, spastic paraparesis in which the morbidity is largely related to impaired leg control rather than weakness, with or without recognition of other family members. The reported prevalence is estimated to range from 0.5 to 12 per 100,000.[1–4] Like many of the disorders discussed in this text, the nosology of HSP is confounded by insights generated by molecular biology. The HSP phenotype is now recognized to result from mutations involving over 80 different genetic loci and over 60 identified genes (Table 7-1).[5–8] Despite the potential precision that a classification system based solely on gene location and gene product would provide, it remains an impractical bedside tool. Due to current limitations of genetic testing, a pragmatic classification system requires at least some consideration of clinical features. This chapter will attempt to provide a classification hybrid that addresses both clinical and genetic considerations (Table 7-1).[5–8]

The concept of a hereditary disorder manifesting as spasticity of the lower extremities was initially championed by Seeligmüller, Strumpell, and Lorrain in the last quarter of the 19th century. It was envisioned as a singular entity with phenotypic variation. The classification system still utilized today was initially promoted by Anita Harding in 1981.[9] She proposed a dominantly inherited HSP dichotomy in which type I was considered to reflect an early-onset phenotype with predominant, if not exclusive, upper motor neuron (UMN) features. In contrast, type II HSP referred to those with late onset in which weakness and presumed lower motor neuron (LMN) involvement overshadowed the UMN signs. In 1983, her classification system was expanded to encompass complicated as well as uncomplicated forms of the syndrome.[10] Uncomplicated HSP still refers to a syndrome of spastic paraparesis in which cavus foot deformities and mild vibratory sense loss may occur as the only other associated features. Complicated HSP is defined by involvement of additional neurological and occasionally nonneurological systems as described below (Table 7-1).[5–8]

In 1996, the nosology of HSP became at the same time both enhanced and complicated with discovery of the first disease-producing mutation.[7] The HSPs are currently genotypically catalogued by a numerical system based on the order of individual gene discovery. Each number is prefaced by the acronym SPG, which stands for spastic paraplegia gene (Table 7-1).[5–8] Unlike other classification systems, subheadings distinguishing dominant from other inheritance patterns are not utilized.

▶ CLINICAL FEATURES

In virtually every case, the presenting symptoms relate to lower extremity spasticity which has a symmetric or near symmetric distribution. Symptom onset is typically recognized in the second or third decade but may become manifest as early as the first or as late as the seventh decade of life. Patients lose the ability to run or hop early in their course due to increased extensor tone in the lower extremities. Consequently, the ability to fully flex the hip and the knee is impaired resulting in reduced stride length and difficulty running. Patients will describe dragging and stiffness of the legs and a tendency to trip on uneven ground. When observed, the legs may be noted to scissor or cross over each other due to increased adductor tone (Fig. 7-1). Circumduction (a rotational rather than linear advancement of the legs) is common in a compensatory attempt to avoid tripping. This risk results from a leg that is tonically extended at the hip and knee and from a tonic foot posture of inversion and plantar flexion (equinovarus posture). High-arched feet and hammer toe deformity are common but not invariable features of the illness. They are more likely to occur with disease onset in childhood at a time when the metatarsals remain malleable and vulnerable to the imbalance of forces produced by disproportionate involvement of specific muscle groups (Fig. 7-2).

HSP morbidity results in large part from the increased lower extremity extensor tone impairing lower extremity coordination. LMN involvement may occur but is typically overshadowed by spasticity. If weakness occurs, it typically does so in a UMN pattern, with hip flexors, knee flexors, and foot dorsiflexors being typically weaker than their respective antagonists. Hyperreflexia of the lower extremities is universal, almost always accompanied by extensor plantar responses. Hyperreflexia of the upper extremities with Hoffman signs and reflex spread is common as well. Significant loss of upper extremity function associated with weakness, increased tone, or impaired coordination occurs infrequently in most genotypes and should lead to consideration of an alternative diagnosis.

Mild posterior column involvement may occur with vibratory sense loss and occasionally position sense loss in the toes. Rarely is it severe enough to produce significant sensory ataxia. A strikingly positive Romberg sign should once again lead to consideration of an alternative diagnosis. Urinary frequency, urgency, and urgency incontinence are common symptoms even in uncomplicated disease.

▶ TABLE 7-1. HEREDITARY SPASTIC PARAPLEGIA

Name	Locus/Gene	Type	Associated Features
Autosomal dominant (AD)			
SPG3A	14q11–q21/atlastin	U	Usually childhood onset, minimal progression mimicking CP +/– distal amyotrophy
SPG4	2p22/Spastin	U/C	Onset any age 40% of AD cases +/– late cognitive, ataxia, seizures, LMN
SPG6	15q11.1/NIPA1	U	Late adolescent—early adult onset
SPG8	8q23–q24/Strumpellin	U	
SPG9	10q23.3–q24.2/ALDH18A1	C	Cataracts, GERD, motor neuronopathy
SPG10	12q13/KIF5A	U/C	+/– distal muscle atrophy
SPG12	19q13/RTN2	U	
SPG13	2q24–q34/HPSD1	U	Late adolescent—early adult
SPG17	11q12–q14 BSCL2/seipin	C	Silver syndrome, amyotrophy of hands
SPG19	9q33–q34	U	
SPG29	1p31.1–p21.1	C	Hearing loss Hiatal hernia Intractable vomiting
SPG31	2p12/REEP1	U/C	+/– peripheral neuropathy
SPG33	10q24.2/ZFYVE2	U	
SPG36	12q23–q24	C	Onset 20–30 years Peripheral neuropathy
SPG37	8p21.1–q13.3/	U	
SPG38	4p16–p15	C	Amyotrophy of hands
SPG40	Unknown	U	Adult onset
SPG41	11p14.1–p11.2	C	Amyotrophy of hands
SPG42	3q24–q26/SLC33A1	U	Onset decade 1–5
SPG73	19q13.33/CPT1C	U	
SPG80	9p13.3/UBAP1	U	
SPG88	13q14/KPNA3	U/C	Peripheral neuropathy, speech delay
Autosomal recessive (AR)			
SPG5A	8p/CYPB1	U/C	Axonal neuropathy Distal amyotrophy White matter changes
SPG7 (AR, AD cases reported)	16q/paraplegin	U/C	Ragged red fibers, dysarthria, dysphagia, optic atrophy, axonal neuropathy, cerebral and cerebellar atrophy
SPG11	15q/spatacsin	U/C	Juvenile onset, thin corpus callosum, intellectual disability, RPD Upper extremity weakness, nystagmus, dysarthria, dementia, distal amyotrophy 50% of AR cases
SPG14	3q27–28	C	Distal amyotrophy, intellectual disability
SPG15	14q/spastizin	C	Pigmentary maculopathy, distal amyotrophy, dysarthria, intellectual disability
SPG18	8p12–p11.21	C	Intellectual disability, thin corpus callosum
SPG20	13q/spartin	C	"Troyer syndrome," distal amyotrophy
SPG21	15q21–q22/maspardin	C	Dementia, cerebellar and extrapyramidal signs, thin corpus callosum, white matter abnormalities, "Mast syndrome"
SPG23	1q24–q32	C	Vitiligo, premature graying, characteristic facies, "Lison syndrome"
SPG24	13q14	C	Spastic dysarthria, pseudobulbar
SPG25	6q23–q21.4	C	Peripheral neuropathy
SPG26	12p11.1–12q14	C	Onset childhood, dysarthria, distal amyotrophy, mild intellectual disability
SPG27	10q22.1–q24.1	U/C	Ataxia, dysarthria, intellectual disability, peripheral neuropathy, facial dysmorphism, short stature

TABLE 7-1. (CONTINUED)

Name	Locus/Gene	Type	Associated Features	
SPG28	14q21.3–q22.3	U	Childhood onset	
SPG29	14q	U	Childhood onset	
SPG30	2q37.3	C	Distal amyotrophy, saccadic pursuit, peripheral neuropathy, cerebellar signs	
SPG32	14q12–q21	C	Mild intellectual disability, cerebellar atrophy, brainstem dysraphia	
SPG35	16q21–q23/fatty acid 2 hydroxylase	C	Childhood onset, extrapyramidal, dysarthria, dementia, seizures, white matter changes, brain iron deposition	
SPG39	19p13	C	Distal amyotrophy	
SPG43	19p13.11–q12	C	Hand wasting, dysarthria	
SPG44	1q41/gap junction protein connexin 47	C	Pelizaeus–Merzbacher, nystagmus, psychomotor delay, ataxia, dysarthria, CNS hypomyelination	No
SPG45 (also referred to as SPG65)	10q24.3–q25.1/NT5C2	C	Intellectual disability, contractures, optic atrophy, pendular nystagmus	No
SPG46	9p21.2–q21.12/GBA2	C	Dementia, cataract, ataxia thin corpus callosum	No
SPG47	1p13.2–1p12/AP4B	C	Intellectual disability, seizures, thin corpus callosum, white matter changes	No
SPG48	7p22.1/AP5Z1	U	Late onset	Research
SPG49	14q32.31/TECPR2	C	Intellectual disability, short stature, microcephaly, seizures	
SPG50	7q22.1/AP4M1	C	Intellectual disability, microcephaly	
SPG51	15q21.2/AP4E1	C	Intellectual disability, microcephaly, limited or absent speech	
SPG52	14q12/AP4S1	C	Intellectual disability, microcephaly, limited or absent speech	
SPG53	8p22/VPS37A	C	Intellectual disability, limited or absent speech, skeletal dysmorphism	
SPG54	8p11.23/DDHD2	C	Delayed psychomotor development, intellectual disability, thin corpus callosum	
SPG55	12q24.31/C12ORF65	C	Optic atrophy, ophthalmoplegia, sensorimotor neuropathy	
SPG56	4q25/CYP2U1	C	Intellectual disability, neuropathy	
SPG57	3q12.2/TFG	C	Optic atrophy, distal wasting of the hands and feet due to an axonal demyelinating sensorimotor neuropathy	
SPG58 (AR or AD)	17p13.2/KIF1C	C	Cerebellar ataxia, dysarthria, nystagmus, distal amyotrophy	
SPG59	15q21.2/USP8	C	Intellectual disability, nystagmus	
SPG60	3p22.2/WDR48	C	Intellectual disability, nystagmus, neuropathy	
SPG61	16p12.3/ARL6IP1	C	Sensorimotor polyneuropathy, loss of terminal digits, and acropathy	
SPG62	10q24.3/ERLIN1	U/C	Cerebellar ataxia, amyotrophy	
SPG63	1p13.3/AMPD2	C	Short stature, periventricular deep white matter changes, normal cognition	
SPG64	10q24.1/ENTPD1	C	Microcephaly, amyotrophy, dysarthria, delayed puberty, intellectual disability	
SPG66	5q32/ARSI	C	Intellectual disability, sensorimotor neuropathy	
SPG67	2q33.1/PGAP1	C	Global developmental delay, intellectual disability, tremor	
SPG68	11q13/KLC2	C	Spastic paraplegia, optic atrophy, and neuropathy (SPOAN syndrome)	
SPG69	1q41/RAB3GAP2	C	Global developmental delay, intellectual disability, dysarthria, cataracts and hearing impairment	
SPG70	12q13/MARS	C	Global developmental delay, intellectual disability, amyotrophy	
SPG71	5p13.3/ZFR	U	Thin corpus callosum	
SPG72 (AR or AD)	5q31/REEP2	U		
SPG74	1q42.1/IBA57	C	SPOAN-like disorder, with spastic paraplegia-optic atrophy-neuropathy	

(continued)

▶ TABLE 7-1. (CONTINUED)

Name	Locus/Gene	Type	Associated Features
SPG75	19q13.1/MAG	C	Cerebellar signs, nystagmus, peripheral neuropathy, intellectual disability
SPG76	11q13.1/CAPN1	C	Dysarthria
SPG77	6p25.1/FARS2	U	
SPG78	1p36.1/ATP13A2	C	Cerebellar signs, oculomotor disturbances, psychiatric symptoms, and cognitive impairment
SPG79	4p13/UCHL1	C	Optic atrophy, cerebellar signs
SPG81	2p23.3/SELENOI	C	Impaired intellectual development, speech delay, seizures
SPG82	17q25.3/PCYT2	C	Global developmental delay
SPG83	1p34.1/HPDL	U	
SPG84	22q11.21/PI4KA	C	Impaired intellectual development, nystagmus
SPG85	8p11.21/RNF170	C	Polyneuropathy, optic atrophy, dysarthria, dysphagia, ataxia, urinary incontinence
SPG86	6p21.33/ABHD16A	C	Impaired intellectual development, speech delay
SPG87	14q24.3/TMEM63C	U/C	Intellectual disability or speech problems
SPG89	16q13/AMFR	U/C	Mildly impaired intellectual development or learning difficulties
None	5p15.31–14.1/chaperonin containing t-complex peptide 1	C	Mutilating sensory neuropathy with spastic paraplegia
X-linked			
SPG1	Xq28 L1CAM	C	Hydrocephalus, intellectual disability, aphasia, adducted thumbs
SPG2	Xq28/PLP1	C	White matter changes, peripheral neuropathy
SPG16	Xq11.2–q23	U/C	Aphasia, visual loss, intellectual disability, nystagmus, urinary dysfunction
SPG22	Xq21/SLC16A2	C	Intellectual disability, ataxia, dysarthria, abnormal facies
SPG34	Xq24-q25/unknown	U	Typical
Mitochondrial			
SPG	Unknown	C	Peripheral neuropathy, cardiomyopathy, dementia

AD, autosomal dominant; AR, autosomal recessive; C, complicated; CP, cerebral palsy; LMN, lower motor neuron; REEP1, receptor expression enhancing protein 1; RPD, retinal pigmentary degeneration; SPG, SPastic parapleGia; U, uncomplicated.

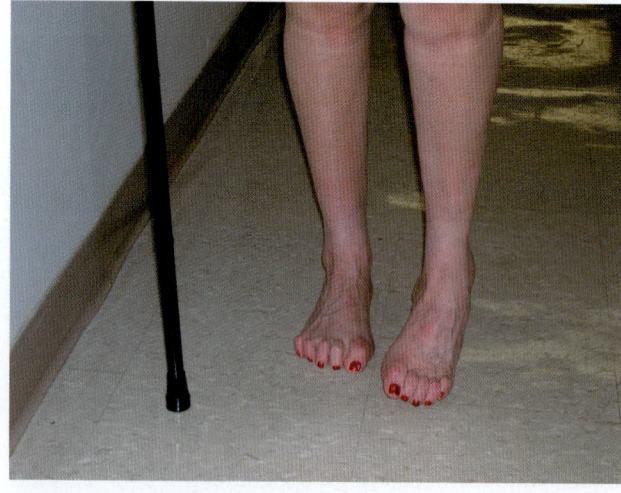

Figure 7-1. Circumducting leg with equinovarus foot posturing in HSP.

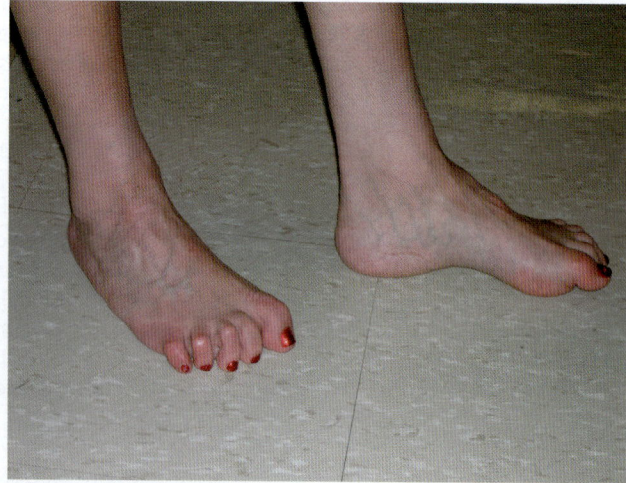

Figure 7-2. Hammer toes and cavus deformity in HSP.

Fecal urgency and incontinence and sexual dysfunction are uncommon.

There is a wide range of associated neurological and non-neurological symptoms that can occur in complicated forms of the disease. Recognition of these additional features may aid in the identification of a specific genotype (Table 7-1).[5–8,11] Some of the more common associated features are amyotrophy of distal limb muscles that may result from either a motor neuronopathy (SPG3A, 4, 5, 9, 10, 11, 14, 15, 17, 20, 26, 30, 38, 39, 41, 43) or peripheral neuropathy (SPG2, 3A, 5, 6, 7, 10, 25, 27, 30, 31, 36, 55, 56, 57, 60, 68, 74, 75, 76, 79, and the one recognized mitochondrial mutation producing an SPG phenotype). Distal amyotrophy may initially affect either the hands or feet, hand wasting and spastic paraparesis being referred to as Silver syndrome.[12,13] Dysarthria can occur in SPG7, 11, 15, 22, 24, 26, 27, 35, 43, 44, 58, 64, 69, 76, 85. Ataxia, nystagmus, dysarthria, and other features of cerebellar dysfunction occur less frequently (SPG21, 22, 58, 64). Extrapyramidal manifestations are relatively uncommon as well (SPG21, 35, 56). Cognitive changes may manifest as either intellectual disability or dementia (SPG4, 11, 14, 15, 16, 18, 20, 21, 22, 26, 27, 32, 35, 44, 45, 46, 47, 49, 50, 51, 52, 53, 54, 56, 75, 78, 81, 82). A thin corpus callosum is a relatively common feature (SPG11, 18, 21, 35, 46, 47, 54, 71, 86). Seizures, deafness, cataracts, ichthyosis, ophthalmoparesis, ocular apraxia, retinal pigmentary degeneration, and optic atrophy with visual loss are some of the other potential associated features.

A uniform age of symptom onset and rate of disease progression are characteristic of uncomplicated HSP genotypes but exceptions to this general rule are not uncommon.[14] The reasons for variations of disease onset and severity of affliction, both within and between families of the same genotype are not understood. This variability does not appear to correlate directly with the mechanism of mutation, at least within the SPG4 genotype. For the most part, individual families will remain segregated into either uncomplicated or complicated phenotypes, but occasional families will have members with both.

▶ DIFFERENTIAL DIAGNOSIS

The differential diagnosis of HSP includes any disorder that results in UMN dysfunction of the lower extremities (Table 7-2).[7,8] In our opinion, the disorder that is most likely to mimic HSP is primary lateral sclerosis (PLS) or UMN-dominant amyotrophic lateral sclerosis (ALS), either on a sporadic or inherited basis.[15,16] Slow progression, symmetry, cavus foot deformity, and loss of vibration perception in the toes favor an HSP diagnosis although these clues are relative and clinical distinction may be difficult in many cases. Rapid progression, notable asymmetry, or impaired upper extremity or bulbar function would favor a PLS/UMN-D ALS diagnosis.[15] The family history needs to be interpreted with caution as ALS like HSP may be hereditary, and absence of other affected family members by no means precludes heritable disease.[17,18] The difficulty in distinguishing between HSP and ALS was

▶ TABLE 7-2. DIFFERENTIAL DIAGNOSIS OF HSP: TESTING CONSIDERATIONS

Disease	Test(s)
ALS/PLS	EMG
	Genetic testing
Compressive myelopathy	Cervical and thoracic spine imaging (MR, myelography)
Dural venous malformation	Cervical and thoracic spine imaging (MR, angiography)
Multiple sclerosis	Brain, cervical, thoracic spine MR imaging, CSF evaluation
Neuromyelitis optica	Aquaporin-4 (AQP4) and myelin oligodendrocyte glycoprotein (MOG) antibodies
Retroviral infection	HIV and HTLV1 serology
Sarcoidosis	CSF evaluation; chest imaging; Gallium scan
Metabolic myelopathy	Vitamin B12
	Copper, zinc, and ceruloplasmin
Adrenoleukodystrophy	Very long-chain fatty acids (VLCFAs)
Spinocerebellar degeneration	Genetic testing
Dopa-responsive dystonia	Response to levodopa

MR, magnetic resonance.

recently emphasized to us in the case of a woman in her mid-30s with 20 years of seemingly sporadic, slowly progressive, spastic paraparesis, and cavus foot deformity suggesting HSP in whom a pathological mutation in a familial ALS gene (senataxin) was identified in both her and her asymptomatic father.

The differential diagnosis of HSP includes another category of heritable neuromuscular disease, distal spinal muscular atrophy/hereditary motor neuropathy.[8] The latter, although dominated by LMN features, may include UMN features as well as providing phenotypic and at times genotypic overlap between these two disease categories (Table 7-1).[8]

Most metabolic or structural myelopathies affect sensory pathways more than HSP typically does. Nonetheless, the differential diagnosis of HSP includes metabolic and structural disorders in which sensory signs or symptoms are limited. In consideration of its chronicity and frequency, cervical spondylotic myelopathy is a common differential diagnostic consideration. We urge caution in attributing spastic paraparesis to cervical canal stenosis in the absence of significant spinal cord compression or abnormal cord signal at the level of compression. Other myelopathic considerations in which imaging may be abnormal include dural venous fistulas, spinal forms of multiple sclerosis, and other inflammatory disorders such as acute disseminated encephalomyelitis, neuromyelitis optica, HIV or HTLV1 inflection, and sarcoidosis. The chronological course in these latter disorders would characteristically progress at a different and usually faster pace than HSP.

Adrenoleukodystrophy and adrenomyeloneuropathy are X-linked disorders that require consideration in young men but also young adult women. Arguably, the latter cohort provides the greatest difficulty as adrenoleukodystrophy frequently presents as a slowly progressive spastic paraparesis in young adult women. Young males typically have a more severe and multisystem phenotype producing varying combinations of adrenal insufficiency, myelopathy, neuropathy, and cognitive decline. Other leukodystrophies may be considered in the differential diagnosis of complicated forms of the disease.

Vitamin B12 and copper deficiency may affect pyramidal tracts although they tend to manifest primarily as posterior column myelopathies with predominant sensory loss. Other inherited disorders with prominent myelopathic features include Friedreich ataxia and spinocerebellar ataxia type III (Machado–Joseph disease). Both are more typically clinically dominated by posterior column and spinocerebellar ataxia, respectively rather than by spasticity.

Cerebral palsy is a differential diagnostic consideration in early-onset cases of HSP. This is particularly true for SPG3A associated with mutations of the atlastin gene.[19,20] Dopa-responsive dystonia may manifest itself as a progressive, spastic gait disorder of childhood. Low-dose therapy with levodopa would serve both a diagnostic and a therapeutic purpose in this disorder.

► LABORATORY FEATURES

Genetic testing has recently become broadly available for suspected HSP patients, though geographic availability and insurance reimbursement are still variable. Extensive gene panels are now available for most of the more than 80 recognized gene loci.[6,8,11] Therefore, testing with a multigene panel targeting known HSP-related genes is often the first approach to determine a genetic diagnosis. Inheritance can be autosomal dominant (AD), autosomal recessive (AR), X-linked recessive (XLR), and mitochondrial. De novo cases can occur. Most HSPs (75%–80%) are due to AD gene mutations, with SPG4 being the most common (40%) of all AD cases.[11] SPG3A is the second-most prevalent AD form, followed by SPG31. The most common AR forms are SPG11, SPG15, and SPG7.[11] Negative genetic testing, however, does not exclude HSP as our knowledge of the genetic causes of HSP is still incomplete and commercial tests do not cover all known genes at present. In addition, commercially utilized methodologies may not detect certain mutational mechanisms, thus providing the opportunity for a false-negative test. For example, partial deletions of the SPAST gene (SPG4 locus) may not be detected by some commercial laboratories.[21]

It is important that the clinician be aware of additional nuances of HSP genetic testing. It is estimated that approximately 10%–20% of apparent sporadic cases will be found to have a gene mutation.[11,14,17,18] Incomplete penetrance does occur in HSP, providing at least one reason for the aforementioned observation. Although anticipation is not a well-described phenomenon in HSP, particularly in uncomplicated forms, it has been reported to occur in SPG4.[22]

If genotypic confirmation of the HSP diagnosis cannot be accomplished, other diagnostic testing such as imaging may be undertaken in an attempt to address other differential diagnostic considerations. Tests that may be considered are summarized in Table 7-2. Imaging in HSP is typically normal in uncomplicated cases, although atrophy of the thoracic spinal cord has been reported.[7] Magnetic resonance imaging (MRI) of the brain may identify some of the features associated with complicated forms of HSP, including atrophy of the corpus callosum, hydrocephalus, or white matter changes. This would be of more value in identifying the type of HSP rather than establishing the initial diagnosis.

► HISTOPATHOLOGY

HSP appears to be a "dying back myelopathy." Affected individuals will have degeneration of both the crossed and uncrossed corticospinal tracts, most notable in the lumbosacral and thoracic segments of the spinal cord. This degeneration becomes less apparent in the cervical regions. Conversely, degeneration of the posterior columns is most evident in the fasciculus gracilis in their most centrifugal locations, that is, at the cervical–medullary junction.[3] Spinocerebellar pathways are involved in some cases to a far lesser extent. Decreased numbers of anterior horn cells and/or cortical motor neurons have been reported.

In a manner similar to the clinical overlap described above, certain HSP genotypes may have TDP-43 positive inclusions, a marker more typically associated with ALS.[23]

► PATHOGENESIS

The multiple HSP genotypes suggest that there is a final common pathway by which mutations of different proteins coalesce into an identical or near-identical phenotype. The proteins implicated in HSP tend to affect a relatively small number of functions such as organelle distribution and morphology, axon pathfinding, axon transport, myelination, mitochondrial function, and lipid metabolism.[11] Although the functions of certain HSP-related proteins are understood, the means by which they induce a fairly uniform phenotype remains unknown.[24] The function of spastin (SPG4) is related to microtubule dynamics. The kinesin 5A gene (SPG10) has a role in axonal transport. Three SPG genes, paraplegin, chaperonin 60, receptor expression enhancing protein 1, and mitochondrial ATPase 6 (SPG7, 13, 31) code for mitochondrial proteins. L1 cell adhesion molecule (SPG1) plays a role in corticospinal tract development. Mutations of the proteolipid protein and the gap junction protein gamma 2 genes (SPG2, 42) result in abnormalities of myelination. The morphology of the endoplasmic reticulum is altered in mutations of the atlastin, spastin, and receptor expression enhancing protein 1 genes (SPG3A, 4, 31). Disturbances of membrane trafficking, protein accumulation, and endoplasmic reticulum stress response are associated with abnormalities of strumpellin and seipin gene function (SPG8, 17).

A recurrent theme throughout this text is the increasing recognition that neuromuscular disorders historically classified as different diseases are allelic. Although this phenomenon is not as prevalent as in spinal muscular atrophy, it is relevant to HSP as well (Table 7-1). SPG3A and hereditary sensory neuropathy type I result from mutations in the atlastin gene.[24] SPG17 is allelic with both hereditary motor neuropathy type V and Charcot–Marie–Tooth disease type II.

▶ MANAGEMENT

HSP management is supportive.[8] The goal is to maintain comfort, function, and, to the extent possible, safe and independent patient mobility. There are a number of different interventions that attempt to reduce spasticity (Table 7-3). Nonpharmacological interventions and oral medications such as baclofen or tizanidine are usually tried first. If sufficient control of spasticity cannot be attained with these first-line interventions, intramuscular injection of botulinum toxin or intrathecal baclofen can be considered. In extreme cases, surgical release of tendons may be considered in nonambulatory patients to facilitate hygiene or improve patient comfort. The treatment of spasticity requires considerable clinical judgment. Improved ambulation, comfort, and range of motion are the desired effects. These need to be balanced with expected common side effects such as sedation and unmasking underlying muscle weakness that may actually add to fall risk and detract from safe mobility. Although spasticity hinders gait, it may also paradoxically reduce fall

▶ **TABLE 7-3. TREATMENT OPTIONS FOR SPASTICITY (LISTED IN APPROXIMATE ORDER OF USE)**

Intervention	Initial Dose	Maximal Dose	Common or Significant Side Effects
First-tier			
Nonpharmacologic interventions described in Chapter 5 such as physical therapy, stretching exercises, bracing, physical modalities (e.g., heat, massage), etc.	Highly individualized	NA	Few side effects reported, may vary by modality
Baclofen	5 mg po qhs-TID	20 mg po QID	Constipation, nausea, emesis, ↓ muscle tone, dizziness, headache, somnolence, coma, seizure, and abrupt withdrawal syndrome
Tizanidine	4 mg po daily	12 mg po TID	Hypotension, xerostomia, asthenia, dizziness, and sedation
Cannabinoids if legally available where patient resides	Different formulations available (po, topical, spray, inhaled). Available by prescription in some regions. Dose varies with product	Varies with product	Products may contain different amounts of tetrahydrocannabinol (THC) and/or cannabidiol (CBD). Side effects depend on the specific active ingredients and formulation
Benzodiazepines (e.g., diazepam)	Diazepam: 2 mg po daily (also available for IM or IV administration)	15 mg po QID	Sedation, ataxia, hypotension, fatigue, respiratory depression, and withdrawal symptoms
Second-tier (if no response to first-tier treatments)			
Botulinum toxin	IM; dose varies with product	Varies with product	Excessive ↓ muscle tone and allergy
Intrathecal baclofen	50 μg test dose adults, 25 μg children, increase dose by 10–30%/day in adults, 5–15 μg in children titrated to response	2,000 μg/day	Pump failure, catheter fracture, CNS infection, CSF leak with intracranial hypotension, and complications of baclofen
Less commonly used			
Dantrolene	25 mg po daily	100 mg po QID	Lightheadedness, constipation, diarrhea, asthenia, headache, sedation, diplopia, visual, CHF and arrhythmia, myelosuppression, and hepatotoxicity
Rhizotomy	NA	NA	CSF leak with intracranial hypotension, excessive weakness

CHF, congestive heart failure; CNS, central nervous system; CSF, cerebrospinal fluid; IM, intramuscular; NA, not applicable.

risk. In an individual who also has considerable underlying weakness, the increased tone of extensor muscles may represent the major source of antigravity resistance. Suppression of this tone may deprive individuals of their ability to stand.

To improve tolerance, oral antispasticity drugs are typically initiated at very low doses and then titrated upward (Table 7-3). Baclofen and tizanidine are preferred as first-line agents by most. Rapid withdrawal of these agents may lead to unwanted central nervous system (CNS) and generalized side effects, including altered mental status, psychosis, fever, worsening of spasticity and weakness, and autonomic instability. Dantrolene is used less frequently because of risks associated with hepatotoxicity. Benzodiazepines have less well-developed antispasticity properties and are frequently used as an adjunct rather than as a primary antispasticity treatment.

Intrathecal baclofen delivered by a programmable pump is an option if oral drugs do not provide the desired effect. The theoretical benefit is to deliver the drug directly to the afflicted end organ in small titratable doses in order to avoid the side effects commonly associated with the larger oral doses required. Intrathecal baclofen may allow certain patients who are spastic to remain ambulatory longer than their natural history would otherwise allow. A more realistic goal is to diminish refractory painful spasms or to diminish lower extremity tone to facilitate hygiene.

Injection of botulinum toxin into spastic muscles provides an alternative means to diminish muscle tone.[25] Although attractive in concept because of the ability to affect only selected muscles, identification of the best dose and obtaining reimbursement for the relatively large volumes often required provide significant obstacles to its use. Many payers limit reimbursement, which may be inadequate to achieve the desired goals. The effect of botulinum toxin is greatest when the toxin is delivered in proximity to the motor point. Identification of the most severely affected muscles and delivery of the lowest effective doses are the two major principles used. Repeat injections are typically required at approximately 3-month intervals.

Urinary urgency from detrusor overactivity is a common source of morbidity in HSP patients. There are a number of pharmacological agents that may ameliorate this problem. The antispasticity agents, baclofen and tizanidine, may provide some relief. Typically, however, the first-line treatments for overactive bladder are either muscarinic anticholinergic agents (e.g., oxybutynin, tolterodine, darifenacin, solifenacin, and trospium) or beta-3 adrenergic agonists (mirabegron, vibegron). If symptoms are refractory to oral treatments, botulinum toxin injections into the detrusor can provide relief. Rarely used interventions include intravesicular delivery of certain drugs including capsaicin and S2–4 ventral root stimulation coupled with analogous dorsal rhizotomies.

Durable medical equipment and home modification can provide substantial benefit to individual patients. The reader is referred to Chapter 5 for more details. Ankle–foot orthoses are of great benefit to individual patients to prevent falls due to tripping. Ideally, they should be custom fitted to improve comfort, particularly in consideration of associated cavus foot deformities. A skilled physical therapist is an invaluable tool to decide whether a cane, Lofstran or Canadian crutches, a walker, or a wheelchair is the best solution for an individual patient. Upright walkers like the Dashaway® walker could be helpful. Power chairs and scooters may benefit some patients. Insurance reimbursement requires coordination and planning. HSP patients are one group of patients where scooters, often preferred by the patient over power chairs, may be recommended. When mobility devices become medically indicated, they should be presented to patients as an opportunity to maintain independence while minimizing the risk of falls and the potential of severe injury. In patients who live in multiple-story dwellings who require access to more than one floor, stair lifts provide a safe and energy-sparing option. Patients should also be encouraged to perform daily stretching exercises to maintain flexibility, help manage spasticity, and prevent contractures.

Like all chronic diseases, HSP patients may benefit from the resources provided by support organizations. Examples include the following:

- National Institute of Neurological Disorders and Stroke
- Spastic Paraplegia Foundation (e-mail: information@sp-foundation.org; www.sp-foundation.org)
- National Ataxia Foundation (e-mail: naf@ataxia.org; www.ataxia.org)

Genetic counseling should be considered for patients with HSP. Although there is phenotypic homogeneity within HSP families, exceptions do exist, complicating conversations about risk and prognosis. Current initiatives within the international scientific community include patient registries to better characterize the natural history of HSP, creation of Centers of Excellent for HSP care and research, and translational efforts toward disease-modifying medications.[26]

▶ SUMMARY

HSP is a heritable disorder in which more than 80 currently recognized gene loci correlate with a fairly homogeneous phenotypic syndrome dominated by spastic paraparesis. It is a disorder that offers the opportunity to understand how semiselective vulnerability of a single component of the nervous system can occur as a result of seemingly disparate pathophysiologies. Like other heritable disorders in which the molecular biology is providing new insights into disease mechanisms, the nosology of the HSP will undoubtedly be revised as the overlapping genetics of different heritable disorders are increasingly clarified.

REFERENCES

1. McMonagle P, Webb S, Hutchinson M. The prevalence of "pure" autosomal dominant hereditary spastic paraparesis in the island of Ireland. *J Neurol Neurosurg Psychiatry*. 2002;72(1):43–46.

2. Stichele GV, Durr A, Yoon G, et al. An integrated modelling methodology for estimating global incidence and prevalence of hereditary spastic paraplegia subtypes SPG4, SPG7, SPG11, and SPG15. *BMC Neurol.* 2022;22(1):115.
3. Racis L, Tessa A, Di Fabio R, et al. The high prevalence of hereditary spastic paraplegia in Sardinia, insular Italy. *J Neurol.* 2014;261(1):52–59.
4. Braschinsky M, Luus SM, Gross-Paju K, Haldre S. The prevalence of hereditary spastic paraplegia and the occurrence of SPG4 mutations in Estonia. *Neuroepidemiology.* 2009;32(2):89–93.
5. Meyyazhagan A, Orlacchio A. Hereditary spastic paraplegia: an update. *Int J Mol Sci.* 2022;23(3):1697.
6. Panza E, Meyyazhagan A, Orlacchio A. Hereditary spastic paraplegia: genetic heterogeneity and common pathways. *Exp Neurol.* 2022;357:114203.
7. Fink JK. Hereditary spastic paraplegia. *Curr Neurol Neurosci Rep.* 2006;6(1):65–76.
8. Fink JK. The hereditary spastic paraplegias. *Handb Clin Neurol.* 2023;196:59–88.
9. Harding AE. Hereditary "pure" spastic paraplegia: a clinical and genetic study of 22 families. *J Neurol Neurosurg Psychiatry.* 1981;44(10):871–883.
10. Harding AE. Classification of the hereditary ataxias and paraplegias. *Lancet.* 1983;1(8334):1151–1155.
11. Blackstone C. Converging cellular themes for the hereditary spastic paraplegias. *Curr Opin Neurobiol.* 2018;51:139–146.
12. Orlacchio A, Patrono C, Gaudiello F, et al. Silver syndrome variant of hereditary spastic paraplegia: a locus to 4p and allelism with SPG4. *Neurology.* 2008;70(21):1959–1966.
13. Rowland LP, Bird TD. Silver syndrome: the complexity of complicated hereditary spastic paraplegia. *Neurology.* 2008;70(21):1948–1949.
14. Mo A, Saffari A, Kellner M, et al. Early-onset and severe complex hereditary spastic paraplegia caused by De Novo variants in SPAST. *Mov Disord.* 2022;37(12):2440–2446.
15. Brugman F, Veldink JH, Franssen H, et al. Differentiation of hereditary spastic paraparesis from primary lateral sclerosis in sporadic adult-onset upper motor neuron syndromes. *Arch Neurol.* 2009;66(4):509–514.
16. Brugman F, Wokke JHJ, Vianney de Jong JMB, Franssen H, Faber CG, Van den Berg LH. Primary lateral sclerosis as a phenotypic manifestation of familial ALS. *Neurology.* 2005;64(10):1778–1779.
17. Brugman F, Wokke JHJ, Scheffer H, Versteeg MHA, Sistermans EA, van den Berg LH. Spastin mutations in sporadic adult-onset upper motor neuron syndromes. *Ann Neurol.* 2005;58(6):865–869.
18. Brugman F, Scheffer H, Wokke JHJ, et al. Paraplegin mutations in sporadic adult-onset upper motor neuron syndromes. *Neurology.* 2008;71(19):1500–1505.
19. Rainier S, Sher C, Reish O, Thomas D, Fink JK. De novo occurrence of novel SPG3A/atlastin mutation presenting as cerebral palsy. *Arch Neurol.* 2006;63(3):445–447.
20. Namekawa M, Ribai P, Nelson I, et al. SPG3A is the most frequent cause of hereditary spastic paraplegia with onset before age 10 years. *Neurology.* 2006;66(1):112–114.
21. Beetz C, Nygren AOH, Schickel J, et al. High frequency of partial SPAST deletions in autosomal dominant hereditary spastic paraplegia. *Neurology.* 2006;67(11):1926–1930.
22. Hashemi SS, Hajati R, Davarzani A, et al. Anticipation can be more common in hereditary spastic paraplegia with spast mutations than it appears. *Can J Neurol Sci.* 2022;49(5):651–661.
23. Martinez-Lage M, Molina-Porcel L, Falcone D, et al. TDP-43 pathology in a case of hereditary spastic paraplegia with a NIPA1/SPG6 mutation. *Acta Neuropathol.* 2012;124(2):285–291.
24. Timmerman V, Clowes VE, Reid E. Overlapping molecular pathological themes link Charcot-Marie-Tooth neuropathies and hereditary spastic paraplegias. *Exp Neurol.* 2013;246:14–25.
25. Comella CL, Pullman SL. Botulinum toxins in neurological disease. *Muscle Nerve.* 2004;29(5):628–644.
26. Trummer B, Haubenberger D, Blackstone C. Clinical trial designs and measures in hereditary spastic paraplegias. *Front Neurol.* 2018;9:1017.

CHAPTER 8

Spinal Muscular Atrophies

The spinal muscular atrophies (SMAs) have been historically conceptualized as hereditary disorders preferentially affecting anterior horn cells and selected motor cranial nerve nuclei.[1] As in all disorders caused or influenced by genetics, molecular biology has served to confound as much as clarify the nosology. We have become very aware that the historical boundaries of hereditary neuromuscular disease are inaccurate. Part of this confusion arises from phenotypic overlap. For example, although lower motor neuron (LMN) morbidity dominates most SMA phenotypes, upper motor neuron (UMN) features may occur in some forms of distal SMA. Conversely, hereditary spastic paraplegia is a predominantly UMN disorder but may have notable LMN features in some genotypes. Even more damaging to the historical nosology of hereditary neuromuscular disease is the discovery that mutations of a single gene may produce variable phenotypes that have been historically represented as two or more diseases (Table 8-1).

In this chapter, we will discuss the SMAs related to mutations of the survival motor neuron (SMN) gene, the non-SMN infantile forms of the disease, the rare childhood bulbar forms of motor neuron disease (MND), Hirayama disease, Kennedy disease, the distal SMAs, the scapuloperoneal forms of SMA, and the uncommon SMA phenotypes that occur in association with multisystem disorders (Tables 8-2 and 8-3).[2-4] We emphasize this predominantly phenotypic classification as this remains, for the most part, the most practical means by which these disorders are recognized if not diagnosed.

► SURVIVAL MOTOR NEURON–RELATED SMAs

The history of SMA dates to the independent descriptions of children with progressive weakness by Werdnig and Hoffman in the last decade of the 19th century. Ironically, their cases would be classified today as SMA II rather than the more severe infantile form (SMA I) that bears their eponym. The molecular genetic era in SMA began in earnest in 1990 when a gene locus 5q13 was linked to the majority of childhood-onset SMA cases.[5] In 1995, deficiency of the SMN protein type 1 (SMN1) was identified in approximately 95% of cases as the primary cause of the disease.[6]

SMA related to mutations of the SMN1 is currently classified into five types, SMA I-IV with SMA III subdivided into SMA IIIa and SMA IIIb.[7] SMA I-III represent the traditional infantile, intermediate, and juvenile forms of the disease. SMA IV is the adult form of the disease which is less frequently associated with SMN mutations than other forms.[8] The childhood SMAs have been historically distinguished from one another, by age of onset and the milestones achieved rather than by significant phenotypic differences. SMN-related SMAs are recessively inherited. They do not differ significantly by phenotype, only by severity which is in turn related to contributions of the SMN2 gene as will be described subsequently. They can be considered as a continuum of a single disorder.[7] Progression and life expectancy correlate with age of onset which in turn correlates with the genetic signature as described below. Age of onset and clinical course tend to be similar in siblings. Of note, the advent of effective disease-modifying medications has revolutionized the natural history of SMA.[9,10] The typical clinical phenotype and disease progression described below are based on the natural history of the disease in the absence of pharmacological interventions.

CLINICAL FEATURES

Werdnig–Hoffman disease or SMA I is the most common form of MND and the prototype of these disorders. Its incidence is estimated to occur in a range of 4-10 per 100,000 live births, depending on the geographic cohort studied.[11] Clinical manifestations are evident within the first 6 months of life. Affected infants are hypotonic with a symmetric, generalized, or proximally predominant pattern of weakness. The legs are usually affected to a greater degree than the arms (Fig. 8-1). As in most MNDs, facial weakness is mild and extraocular muscles are spared. Fasciculations are seen in the tongue but rarely in limb muscles, presumably due to the ample subcutaneous tissue of neonates. Manual tremor, characteristic of SMA II and SMA III, occurs uncommonly. Deep tendon reflexes are typically absent. Abdominal breathing, and bulbar symptoms such as a weak cry, poor suck and feeding, and impaired secretion clearance are commonplace. The characteristic appearance includes pectus excavatum with a diminished anterior–posterior diameter of the chest, a bell-shaped chest, and a protuberant abdomen. These features are due to the relative diaphragmatic sparing in comparison to external intercostals early in the disease course. Mild contractures may occur, but arthrogryposis is not part of the classic phenotype. There is no intellectual impairment. Historically, children with SMA I never developed the capability of independent sitting and without mechanical ventilation,

TABLE 8-1. SMA MUTATIONS ALLELIC WITH OTHER NEUROMUSCULAR PHENOTYPES

Locus (Gene)	SMA	ALS	CMT	HSP	Other
20q13.32 (VAPB)	SMA IV Finkel type	ALS8			
12q24.3 (heat-shock protein 8)	HMN IIA		CMT 2L		Desmin-related myopathy
7q11.23 (heat-shock protein B1)	HMN IIB		CMT 2F		
7p14,3 (GARS)	HMN VA		CMT 2D		
11q12.3 (BSCL2)	HMN VA (Silver syndrome)		CMT 2D	SPG17	
4p16–p15	Silver syndrome			SPG38	
2p22–23 (spastin)	Silver syndrome			SPG4	
6q21 (FIG4)		ALS11	CMT 4J		
12q24.1 (TRPV4)	Scapuloperoneal SMA or dSMA or severe congenital form of SMA		CMT 2C		
17p11.2 (PMP22)	Scapuloperoneal SMA		HNPP		
9q34 (senataxin)	HMN with UMN signs	ALS4		May look phenotypically identical to HSP	
2p13.1 (dynactin)	HMN VII	AR form of ALS1			
1q22 (lamin A/C)	SMA IV		CMT 2B1		Emery–Dreifuss MD, LGMD 1B, congenital MD
14q32.31 (dynein)	HMN I or SMA-lower leg predominant		CMT 2O		This is allelic SMA-LED (lower leg predominant)

VAPB, vesicle-associated membrane protein-associated protein B; HMN, hereditary motor neuropathy; GARS, glycyl-tRNA synthetase; dSMA, distal spinal muscular atrophy; BSCL2, Berardinelli-Seip congenital lipodystrophy; FIG4, polyphosphoinositide phosphatase; PMP22, peripheral myelin protein.

the large majority died in the first 2 years of life usually as a direct or indirect consequence of bulbar and/or ventilatory muscle weakness. Eight percent of individuals would survive to 10 years of age. A 20-year lifespan was unexpected.[12]

SMA II or the intermediate form of childhood SMA typically manifests between 6 and 18 months of age.[13] The disorder is clinically defined by milestone acquisition, that is, a child who sits independently but never walks. Postural hand tremor is the only significant phenotypic variance from Werdnig–Hoffman disease. Tongue fasciculations, areflexia, manual tremor, and a symmetric, proximally predominant pattern of weakness characterize the SMA II phenotype. Symptoms related to impaired bulbar function are less of an issue than in SMA I. Natural history studies preceding the development of disease-modifying medications showed that approximately 98% of these individuals survived to the age of 5 years and two-thirds to the age of 25 years. In view of the more protracted course and the ability to sit, patients with SMA II and SMA III patients commonly acquire kyphoscoliosis and joint contractures.

SMA III is also referred to as the Kugelberg–Welander disease or the juvenile-onset SMA.[13] It differs clinically from the intermediate form by age of onset, life expectancy, and milestones achieved. SMA IIIa is distinguished from SMA IIIb predominantly by age of onset, the former defined by symptom onset between 18 months and 3 years and the latter with symptoms between 3 and 21 years. Afflicted individuals develop the ability to stand and walk which are subsequently lost in childhood, adolescence, or adulthood. Initial symptoms are referable to weakness of proximal leg muscles in the vast majority of cases. For example, the patient depicted in

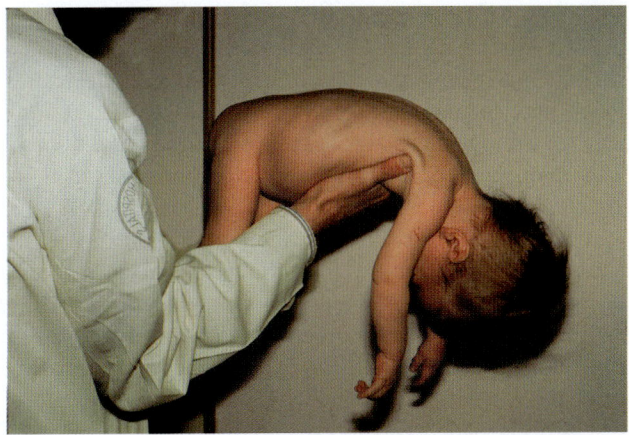

Figure 8-1. Hypotonic SMA I patient. (Used with permission of Dr. Basil Darras, Boston's Children's Hospital.)

TABLE 8-2. SMA CLASSIFICATION—PROXIMAL OR GENERALIZED WEAKNESS

Category	Eponym	Acronym	Gene/Locus	Weakness Pattern	Other Features (Natural History)
Infantile onset	Werdnig–Hoffman	SMA I	SMN	Proximally predominant bulbar	Ventilatory failure
		SMARD 1 HMN VI dSMA I	IGMHBP 2	Generalized severe	Ventilatory failure
		SMA 0	UBE1	Generalized severe	Arthrogryposis facial diplegia
			VRK1	Generalized severe	Pontocerebellar hypoplasia Microcephaly, mental retardation, nystagmus, arthrogryposis
			SCO2	Generalized severe	Cardiomyopathy, lactic acidosis
			GLE1	Generalized severe	Arthrogryposis facial deformities
Childhood onset		SMA II	SMN	Proximally predominant	Hand tremor
Juvenile onset	Kugelberg–Welander	SMA III	SMN	Proximally predominant	Tongue fasciculations hand tremor
Childhood bulbar syndromes	Fazio Londe		C20ORF54	Generalized with multiple cranial neuropathies	Ventilatory weakness, ataxia, UMN signs, optic atrophy, retinal pigmentary degeneration, seizures, dysautonomia
	Brown–Vialetto–Von Laere		C20ORF54	Generalized with multiple cranial neuropathies	Same as Fazio Londe with the addition of *sensorineural hearing loss*
Adult onset	Kennedy disease	SBMA	Androgen receptor	Proximal bulbar	Gynecomastia tremor
		SMA IV	SMN	Proximally predominant	Tongue fasciculations, hand tremor, +/− calf hypertrophy
	Finkel type	fALS8	VAPB	Proximally predominant	
	Finnish type		unknown	Generalized legs > arms proximal > distal	Cramps and fasciculations
	Okinawa type		3q13.1	Proximally predominant	Cramps and fasciculations, sensory loss
	SMA-LED		14q32.31 Dynein	Proximal lower extremities	Allelic to CMT2O (also in Table 8-1)
			LMNA	Proximally predominant	Cardiomyopathy

SMN, survival motor neuron; IGMHBP2, immunoglobulin mu binding protein 2; UBE1, ubiquitin activating enzyme 1; VRK1, vaccinia-related kinase 1; SCO2, cytochrome c oxidase 2; GLE1, S. Cerevisiae homolog like; C20ORF54, chromosome 20 open reading frame 54; VAPB, vesicle-associated membrane protein-associated protein B; LMNA, lamin A/C.

Adapted from Darras BT. Non-5q spinal muscular atrophies: the alphanumeric soup thickens. *Neurology*. 2011;77(4):312–314.

Figure 8-2, was still capable of standing at the age of 30 years and became aware of his problem at age 14 when the crouched position of a hockey goalie became difficult to maintain. In SMA IIIa, 70% of patients are capable of walking 10 years after symptom onset and 20% at 40 years. In SMA IIIb, almost all patients walk at 10 years and 60% of patients remain ambulatory 40 years after symptom onset.[13] Life expectancy in SMA IIIb extends into the sixth decade and may be normal in many individuals. Like SMA II, hand tremor, areflexia, and tongue fasciculations, are commonplace in SMA III. Presumably related to the older age of these patients, and the diminished proportion of subcutaneous tissue, limb fasciculations are more evident in SMA III than in SMA I and SMA II.

Recessively or dominantly inherited adult-onset SMA or SMA IV is uncommon.[14,15] Even though X-linked spinobulbar muscular atrophy is an adult-onset disorder manifesting with the same proximally predominant, symmetric pattern of weakness, it has both distinctive clinical and genetic features and will not be considered as SMA IV in this text.

SMA IV patients do not typically become aware of weakness until age 21 years or older. As with other SMAs, initial symptoms are typically referable to proximal lower extremity

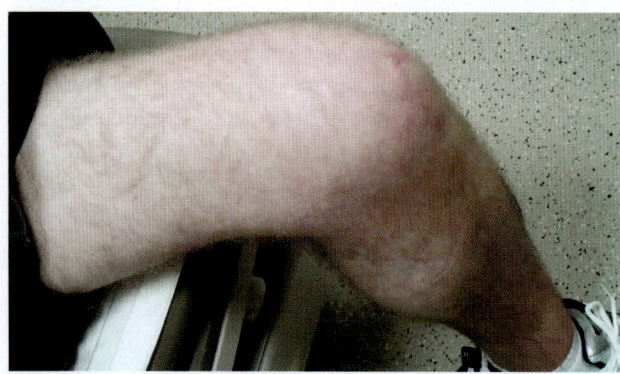

Figure 8-2. A 32-year-old male with SMA IIIb.

▶ **TABLE 8-3. DISTAL HEREDITARY MOTOR NEUROPATHIES/SPINAL MUSCULAR ATROPHIES**

Disease	Inheritance	Gene/Protein Product	Phenotype
dHMN I	AD	7q36 (gene/protein not known)	Juvenile onset; distal LE +/− UMN signs
dHMN II	AD		Adult onset; distal LE +/− UMN signs
dHMN IIA	AD	HSPB8/heat shock protein B8	Adult onset; distal LE +/− UMN signs
dHMN IIB	AD	HSPB1/heat shock protein B1	Adult onset; distal LE +/− UMN signs
dHMN IIC	AD	HSPB3/heat shock protein B3	Adult onset; distal LE +/− UMN signs
dHMN IID	AD	FBX038/F-box only protein 38	Juvenile or adult onset; starts with calf weakness
dHMN III	AR	11q13 (gene/protein not known)	Childhood onset; distal LE +/− UMN signs
dHMN IV	AR	PLEKHG5/Pleckstrin homology domain-containing protein, family G, protein 5	Childhood onset; distal LE, scapular winging, diaphragm weakness
dHMN V	AD		
dHMN VA	AD	GARS1/glycyl-tRNA synthetase 1	Allelic to CMT2D (see CMT chapter)
dHMN VB	AD or AR	REEP1/receptor expression-enhancing protein 1	Allelic to SPG13 (AD); infancy to early adult onset
dHMN VC	AD	BSCL2	Allelic Silver syndrome (SPG13)
dHMN VI	AR	IGHMBP2/immunoglobulin mu-binding protein 2	Allelic to CMT2S (see CMT chapter)
dHMN VII			
dHMN VIIA	AD	SLC5A7/solute carrier family 5 (choline transporter)	Onset in early adult life; vocal cord paralysis; allelic to congenital myasthenic syndrome 20
dHMN VIIB	AD	DCTN1/dynactin 1	Early adult onset; vocal cord paralysis
dHMN VIII	AD	TRPV4/transient receptor protein cation channel, subfamily 5, member 4	Childhood to early adult onset; allelic to CMT2C (see CMT chapter)
dHMN IX	AD	WARS1/tryptophanyl t-RNA synthetase 1	Juvenile onset
dHMN X	AD	EMILIN1/elastin microfibril interfacer 1	Childhood onset; +/− UMN signs
dHMN XI	AD	SPTAN1/spectrin alpha nonerythrocytic 1	Childhood or adult onset; allelic to SPG 91
SCAPULOPERONEAL MOTOR NEUROPATHY			Scapuloperoneal weakness
	AD	PMP22/peripheral myelin protein 22	Allelic to CMT1A
	AD	TRPV4/transient receptor protein cation channel, subfamily 5, member 4	Childhood to early adult onset; allelic to DHMN VIII and CMT2C (see CMT chapter)
Distal HMN Autosomal Recessive 5	AR	DNAJB6/heat shock protein, DNAJ-like 1	Young adult onset
OTHERS			
	AD	SETX/senataxin	Childhood to adult onset; allelic to ALS4
	AR	SIGMAR1/sigma nonopioid intracellular receptor 1	Early childhood to juvenile onset; allelic to ALS16
	XLR	ATP7A/ATPse copper transporting, alpha polypeptide	Childhood onset; males; allelic to Menke's disease

AD, autosomal dominant; AR, autosomal recessive; XLR, X-linked recessive; ALS, amyotrophic lateral sclerosis; CMT, Charcot Marie Tooth; UMN, upper motor neuron.

muscles. Hip flexors and extensors and knee extensors are usually the most severely affected muscles. The shoulder abductors and elbow extensors are the most affected muscles of the arms. Tongue and limb fasciculations, hand tremor, and, in some cases, calf hypertrophy occur. The latter can be confounding, particularly in males, as myopathies are a more common cause of proximal weakness in this age group. Life expectancy is normal.

The first disease-modifying medications became available in 2016.[16] As more patients have access to one or more of these medications early in their disease course, expected motor milestones and prognosis will continue to improve.[17,18]

DIFFERENTIAL DIAGNOSIS

The differential diagnosis of SMA I is the differential diagnosis of the floppy infant.[19] The majority of hypotonic neonates have a central nervous system disorder. Clinical clues implicating a potential but less common neuromuscular cause of a floppy infant include preservation of alertness, depressed or absent deep tendon reflexes, the pattern of weakness, and fasciculations if present. At least two other forms of non-SMN infantile SMA are known to exist. Recessively inherited spinal muscular atrophy with respiratory distress type 1 (SMARD1) and X-linked infantile SMA with arthrogryposis will be described subsequently.[20,21] Neonatal or congenital myasthenia, congenital muscular dystrophy, neonatal myotonic dystrophy, infantile Pompe disease, severe nemaline, myotubular or other congenital myopathies, infantile botulism, and rare hypomyelinating neuropathies are the major neuromuscular considerations in a hypotonic infant. Of note, newborn screening for SMA was introduced in the United States in 2018 and is now implemented in most states, allowing early intervention with disease-modifying treatments which is linked to better outcomes.[22]

SMN-related SMA II–IV need to be distinguished from dominantly inherited SMAs including the Finkel type associated with mutations of the VAPB (fALS8), a disorder linked to the 14q32 locus, mutations of the lamin A/C gene (LMNA) and a disorder described in two Finnish families in which the gene has yet to be identified.[23-26] The differential also includes a wide variety of myopathic disorders, including certain muscular dystrophies (dystrophinopathies, limb girdle, myotonic, congenital, and Emery–Dreifuss), congenital myopathies; mitochondrial disorders; and lipid and glycogen storage disorders. Chronic inflammatory demyelinating polyradiculoneuropathy would be the primary neuropathic consideration. Congenital myasthenic syndromes should also be considered.

LABORATORY FEATURES

In Werdnig–Hoffman disease, creatine kinase (CK) is elevated, typically less than five times the upper limits of normal. In a patient with an SMA I–IV phenotype the most expeditious means to confirm the diagnosis is through SMN1-targeted mutation analysis which identifies the exon 7 deletion, this is the genetic defect in the majority of SMA I–III, and some SMA IV cases. This test will identify a mutation in approximately 95% of childhood and adolescent patients with an SMA phenotype and is felt to be nearly 100% specific.[27-29] In the remaining patients, sequence analysis may be performed to identify other mutations.

Patients with recessively inherited SMA IV are associated with homozygous SMN1 deletions infrequently. Analysis of the vesicle-associated membrane protein-associated protein B (VAPB) gene on chromosome 20, allelic to familial ALS type 8, may provide diagnostic confirmation in some patients with dominantly inherited SMA IV. Asymptomatic adults with SMN 1 genotypes have been described.[30,31] Although SMN mutations are highly specific for SMA, a phenotype suggesting congenital axonal neuropathy with sensory involvement has been described.[32-34]

Genetic testing for SMA I–III is available both for symptomatic patients and to evaluate individuals at risk. Carrier detection and newborn screening are particularly important as the recently developed targeted treatments are more effective when initiated before symptom onset.[35] Although 98% of SMA children have parents who are each heterozygotes for the SMN1 mutation, an SMA child born of only one identified heterozygote parent can occur. This can result from either a spontaneous mutation of the child's second allele, through germline mosaicism in the seemingly normal parent, or from false paternity. Interpretation of carrier testing is also complicated by consideration that both SMN 1 copies may exist on a single chromosome in 4% of individuals.

ELECTRODIAGNOSIS

Historically, electrodiagnosis (EDX) was the major diagnostic tool used to support the clinical diagnosis of childhood SMA. This has been supplanted by genetic testing in the majority of cases. EMG is primarily used in individuals with an SMA phenotype without a detectable SMN mutation or in individuals who have neuromuscular disorders originating from muscle, neuromuscular junction, or nerve that may resemble the SMA phenotype. With SMA or other anterior horn cell diseases, the electromyographer would anticipate a characteristic pattern of abnormal parameters. These would include low-amplitude compound muscle action potentials (CMAPs), normal sensory nerve action potential, and widespread evidence of both ongoing denervation (spontaneous discharge of fibrillation potentials and positive waves) and chronic partial denervation, and reinnervation (reduced numbers of motor unit potentials of increased amplitude and duration with muscle activation). Fasciculation potentials may or may not be identified in part because of the necessary brevity of the needle examination in many children.

EDX has a limited role in the determination of SMA prognosis. The density and geographic distribution of fibrillation potentials in comparison to changes of chronic partial denervation and reinnervation are related to the rapidity with which these disorders progress. Although pragmatically difficult to apply to the pediatric patient, motor unit instability and the rate of decline of motor unit number estimation may also provide prognostic insight.

HISTOPATHOLOGY

The SMN-related SMAs are attributed to anterior horn cell pathology. This observation dates back to the original writings of Werdnig and Hoffman. In SMA, swelling of motor neurons laden with phosphorylated neurofilaments and glial bundles within ventral roots are common. The ubiquitinated inclusions of amyotrophic lateral sclerosis (ALS) are not seen.

As with EDX, the role of muscle biopsy in SMA has greatly diminished. For all intents and purposes, EDX will arrive at the same conclusion provided by the arguably more invasive muscle biopsy. EDX has the additional advantage of more readily demonstrating the geographic distribution of these findings. In SMA I, the biopsy will demonstrate sheets of rounded, atrophic fibers of both types. Hypertrophic fibers are intermixed and are exclusively type I (Fig. 8-3). Type grouping is uncommon. In SMA II, the biopsy may be similar to SMA I or may differ because of the presence of hypertrophic type II fibers and/or the presence of type grouping.

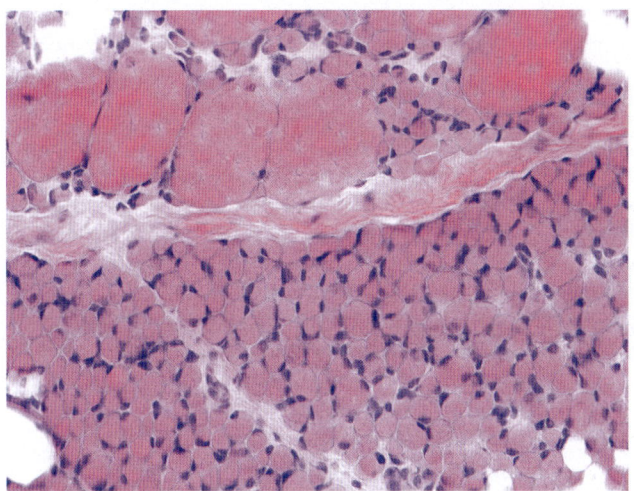

Figure 8-3. Muscle biopsy of SMA patient demonstrating complete fascicles of sheets of round, atrophic muscle fibers and a few preserved normal-sized myofibers (hematoxylin and eosin stain). (Used with permission of Dr. Umberto DeGirolami of Brigham and Women's Hospital, Boston, MA.)

In SMA III, type grouping and group atrophy of both fiber types are common. In addition, as with many chronic neurogenic disorders, "pseudomyopathic" features such as fiber splitting, increased endomysial connective tissue, and an increased number of internal nuclei may be seen.

PATHOGENESIS

SMN-related SMA is caused by a loss of function effect due to deficiency of the SMN1 protein caused in most cases by large deletions of exon 7 or 8 or truncation of the SMN 1 gene.[15] The SMN proteins are found in both the nucleus and cytoplasm of all cells where they have RNA processing functions. The SMN1 protein appears to interact with a number of cytoplasmic proteins to facilitate the formation, nuclear importation, and regeneration of nuclear spliceosomal RNA. The SMN1 protein is also found to traffic in motor axons and may play a role in disordered axonal transport through its influence on β-actin mRNA.[15]

The severity of the SMA phenotype is related in part to the number of copies of the similar, but unstable and significantly less effective than the allelic protein, SMN2.[36] The SMN2 gene is identical to SMN1 with the exception that exon 7 is excluded. SMA 0 is typically associated with one copy of the SMN2 gene, SMA I with two copies, SMA IIIa with three or four copies, and SMA IIIb invariably with four, and recessively inherited SMA IV with anywhere between four and eight gene copies.[7] Individuals homozygous for the SMN1 mutation with five copies of the SMN2 gene have been reported to be asymptomatic. SMN2 gene copy number is not the sole determinant of phenotypic severity. There are other complex genetic influences that are not as yet fully understood. Although 95% of affected individuals have homozygous mutations, 5% have more complex compound heterozygotic mutations with a typical deletion in one allele with a subtle intragenic defect on the other.[37] Prognostication based on SMN2 gene copy number in SMN homozygotes should proceed cautiously. There are no known clinical consequences from mutations of the SMN2 gene alone.

Unlike SMA 0–III, the SMA IV phenotype may be inherited in either dominant or recessive fashion. Autosomal-dominant inheritance, referred to as the Finkel type, is estimated to occur in approximately 30% of these patients. This phenotype is associated with a mutation of the VAPB gene. Autosomal-dominant SMA IV is allelic to ALS 8 as some families with VAPB mutations will have UMN in addition to the more characteristic LMN findings.

MANAGEMENT

The prognosis of SMA improved dramatically in 2016, with the introduction of the first disease-modifying medication.[18] The characteristics of the medications currently on the market in the Unites States and many other countries are summarized in Table 8-4.

With three drugs on the market, selecting the right agent, or combination of agents, depends on the trial efficacy data, the patient's age, safety considerations, and preferred route of administration and treatment frequency.[18,38] Two trials support the dramatic efficacy of nusinersen and onasemnogene abeparvovec-xioi, respectively, in presymptomatic patients (under 2 months of age).[39,40] Several trials were conducted in children between the ages of 2 and 24 months supporting the efficacy of all three drugs currently on the market.[41,42] For both age groups, many clinicians consider onasemnogene abeparvovec-xioi first, which could be followed by treatment with either nusinersen or risdiplam when the child gets older. For children over the age of 24 months (SMA II and SMA III) either nusinersen or risdiplam are typically initiated. Comorbidities, side effects, and family preference may affect the ultimate treatment choice and additional trials are needed to further refine treatment algorithms and drug combinations.[18]

In addition to disease-modifying medications, multidisciplinary care is recommended to support function and quality of life.[38,43] Neuromuscular specialists should provide parents, and when applicable the patient, information related to the natural history of the disease, genetic implications, available treatments, and the role of clinical trials. Like ALS, a multidisciplinary clinic with representation from disciplines that are familiar with the management of the nutritional, psychosocial, mobility/orthopedic, and ventilatory consequences of the disease in this age group is the recommended care model.[44,45] The development of kyphoscoliosis is a common problem in children who become wheelchair bound. Spine stabilization is commonly recommended in individuals whose curves exceed 50 degrees and whose vital capacities exceed 40% of the predicted normal value. The goals of this intervention are patient comfort, ease of patient management, and potential stabilization of restrictive

▶ TABLE 8-4. DISEASE-MODIFYING MEDICATIONS IN 5Q SMA

Medication	Year of US Approval	Indication	MOA	ROA and Dosage	Black-Box Warning	Side Effects	Safety Lab Monitoring
Nusinersen	2016	All ages	Antisense oligonucleotide, improves SMN2 effect	Intrathecal, 4 loading doses followed by dosing every 4 months	NA	Common: upper and lower respiratory infection, constipation. Major: thrombocytopenia and renal toxicity; risks associated with intrathecal access	PLT, PT, PTT, urine protein prior to each dose
Onasemnogene abeparvovec-xioi	2019	Age <24 months, <16 hours a day of mechanical ventilation, not completely paralyzed	SMN1 gene replacement	Intravenous, single infusion, total dose is weight-based	Acute liver injury	Common: fever, vomiting, increased aminotransferases, thrombocytopenia, increased troponin I levels. Major: liver injury, thrombotic microangiopathy	PLT, hemoglobin, PT, liver function tests, creatinine, troponin I weekly for the first month, then every 2 weeks for months 2 and 3 and until values normalize
Risdiplam	2020	Age ≥2 months	RNA splicing modifier, improves SMN2 effect	Oral (liquid), daily dosing, weight-based	NA	Common: fever, diarrhea, rash. Among infantile onset: URI, pneumonia, constipation and vomiting. Major: nausea, vomiting and diarrhea. Adverse effects on male fertility in animal models	No safety labs required

MOA, mechanism of action; PLT, platelet; PT, prothrombin time; PTT, partial thromboplastin time; ROA, route of administration.

pulmonary deficits. Tracheostomy-assisted long-term mechanical ventilation, and percutaneous gastrostomy feeding tube insertion are decisions with enormous emotional and financial consequence to the parents of an affected child. Noninvasive positive pressure ventilation may provide an improved quality and duration of life in a child with symptoms of ventilatory insufficiency until a decision regarding tracheostomy is required.[45] As disease-modifying treatments are implemented more broadly and earlier, new treatments are developed, and prognosis continues to improve, the goals and methods of multidisciplinary care will continue to evolve.

▶ NON–SMN-RELATED SMAS OF INFANCY AND CHILDHOOD

Infantile SMA with arthrogryposis, previously referred to by some as SMA 0 is an X-linked disorder associated with a mutation of the ubiquitin-activating enzyme 1 gene (UBE1) (Xp11.23). Its phenotype is very similar to SMN1 with the exception that contractures are present at birth or early in development.[15]

SMARD1 is also referred to as hereditary motor neuropathy (HMN) type VI or distal SMA type I as the pattern of weakness typically affects distal more than proximal muscles.[15] Its onset is in infancy and as the name implies, is associated with compromise of ventilatory muscles, particularly the diaphragm. Understandably, without mechanical ventilation, life expectancy is limited to months in most cases. It is a recessively inherited disorder resulting from a mutation of the immunoglobulin mu binding protein 2 gene (IGHMPP2) at locus 11q13.2–q13.4.

Recessively inherited SMA may occur in association with pontocerebellar hypoplasia.[15] The phenotype of this congenital or infantile-onset disorder may include microcephaly, mental retardation, nystagmus, upper limb ataxia, or in some cases arthrogryposis. It occurs as a result of mutations of the vaccinia-related kinase 1 gene (VRK1) located at locus 14q32. Recessively inherited SMA may also result from abnormal mitochondrial function due to mutations of the cytochrome oxidase 2 (SCO2) gene on locus 22q13. In addition to clinical features suggestive of SMA I, an associated cardiomyopathy with lactic acidosis may occur. There is also a lethal arthrogryposis with anterior horn cell disorder (LAAHD) associated with severe facial deformities resulting from mutations of the GLE1 gene at locus 9q34.11.

▶ CHILDHOOD BULBAR SMA

The syndromes of Fazio Londe and Brown–Vialetto–Van Laere (BVVLS) historically describe two bulbar syndromes, clinically distinguished from one another by the sensorineural hearing loss that occurs in the latter.[46] Disease onset is typically within the first two decades of life. In BVVLS, the hearing loss typically precedes the development of bulbar and limb weakness. These disorders are complex with the involvement of multiple neurologic systems which typically include LMN weakness of the limbs and ventilatory muscles. Less common UMN signs, as well as ataxia, optic atrophy, retinal pigmentary degeneration, seizures, and dysautonomia occur. The brainstem syndrome is dominated by involvement of cranial nerves VII, IX, and XII which are more commonly affected than III, V, or VI. The disorders are usually inherited in a recessive manner; historically their clinical course was usually progressive and fatal within years of onset. More recently, many cases have been linked to genetic mutations in the SLC52A3 gene which encodes the intestinal (hRFT2) riboflavin transporter. These patients have associated low flavin levels and exhibit strong clinical response to riboflavin supplementation.[47]

▶ X-LINKED BULBOSPINAL MUSCULAR ATROPHY (KENNEDY DISEASE)

In 1968, Kennedy and colleagues described a unique X-linked form of spinal and bulbar muscular atrophy (SBMA) affecting middle-aged men.[48] In 1986, the genetic defect was identified on the proximal aspect of the long arm of the X chromosome by Fishbeck and colleagues.[49] In 2001, LaSpada and colleagues identified a trinucleotide repeat mutation on exon 1 of the androgen receptor (AR) gene.[49]

The prevalence of SBMA is low, estimated at 3.3 per 100,000 although may vary geographically. There appear to be clusters of increased prevalence in Japan and the Vasa region of Western Finland.[50]

CLINICAL FEATURES

SBMA is an X-linked, adult-onset form of SMA.[50–52] Males identify symptoms of bulbar or proximal weakness at a median onset of 41–44 years.[53,54] The average age of diagnosis in one series was 47 years although this may not be reproducible in the general population.[54] The initial symptoms, however, are typically nonspecific and often begin in younger males. These include muscle cramping associated with elevated serum CK levels, tremor, gynecomastia, and/or fatigue.[54] Their significance is commonly overlooked at this age in the absence of disease suspicion prompted by other affected family members.

As the name implies, the clinical manifestations are largely referable to the lower cranial nerve motor nuclei and the anterior horn cells of the spinal cord. Like most disorders, there is some degree of phenotypic heterogeneity. The classic pattern is for proximally predominant and symmetric limb weakness. There are notable exceptions including distal weakness and asymmetric limb weakness that may occur in more than a half of patients.[54] The weakness is insidiously progressive although rapidly progressive weakness has been reported.[54] Hyporeflexia or areflexia is the norm.

Approximately 10% of the time, the initial symptoms pertain to involvement of brainstem motor nuclei with difficulty in swallowing, chewing, or speaking. A dropped jaw may occur as well.[55] The tongue is frequently fasciculating and wasted with scalloped margins and a deep midline furrow in some cases. Facial weakness is common although tends to occur later in the disease. Perioral fasciculations are common. Like all adult-onset MNDs, extraocular movements are clinically unaffected. Breathing difficulty is uncommon but may occur late in the disease. Unlike the majority of MNDs, there is often an associated, but frequently asymptomatic, sensory neuropathy/neuronopathy detected during the performance of the clinical examination or more commonly, nerve conduction studies. Postural tremor of the limbs or perioral tremor are commonplace and on occasion, may be the presenting manifestation.

The median age of wheelchair dependency is 61 years or approximately 15 years after the onset of weakness. Only a third of affected individuals will be wheelchair dependent 20 years following symptom onset.[50] Life expectancy may be minimally compromised with an average life expectancy of 71.[50] Approximately half of the women who are heterozygous for the Kennedy disease mutation will be minimally symptomatic. The phenotype is similar to those experienced by young affected men with cramps, tremor, CK elevation, and perioral fasciculations. The penetrance of SBMA is incomplete as not all males with the mutation will become symptomatic.

The effects of Kennedy disease are not restricted to the neuromuscular system as a mutation of the AR gene would imply. Affected males suffer the consequences of androgen insensitivity, including gynecomastia (Fig. 8-4), impotence, testicular atrophy, and potential infertility. There is an increased incidence of diabetes mellitus and hypertension. Hyperlipidemia and abnormal liver function are thought to occur in this population as well.

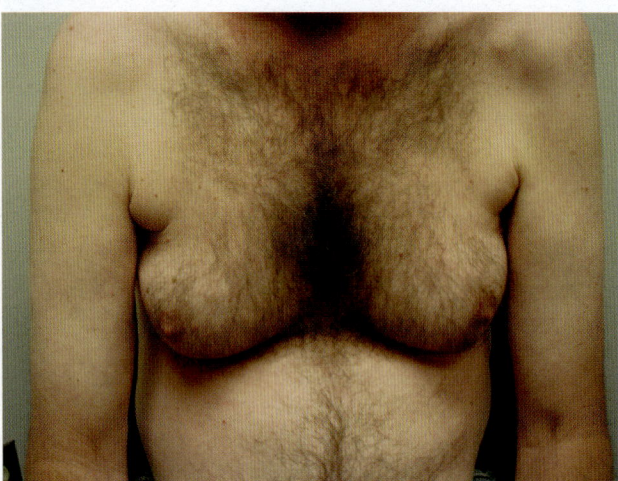

Figure 8-4. Gynecomastia in SBMA disease. (Used with permission of Paul E. Barkhaus, MD.)

DIFFERENTIAL DIAGNOSIS

Kennedy disease may be misdiagnosed as ALS. DNA mutational analysis for X-linked SBMA should be at least considered in any male with suspected LMN-dominant ALS. Rapid progression and UMN signs would favor ALS whereas insidious progression, tremor, sensory neuropathy, and signs of androgen insensitivity would favor SBMA. Less frequently occurring LMN disorders such as progressive muscular atrophy, certain genotypes of fALS, and SMA IV would be more difficult to clinically separate and may require careful pedigree analysis or genetic testing in order to do so. There is a proximal form of hereditary sensory motor neuropathy with locus at 3q13.1 reported in Okinawa, associated with optineurin neuronal inclusions, that may mimic the neurogenic pattern of SBMA limb weakness. It lacks bulbar involvement, however, and progresses in a fashion reminiscent of ALS. In view of its predilection to produce a limb-girdle and bulbar pattern of weakness, disorders of neuromuscular transmission such as the Lambert–Eaton myasthenic syndrome, congenital and acquired myasthenia gravis should be considered.[56] In view of its propensity to affect older individuals and cause symptomatic dysphagia as well as quadriceps weakness, inclusion body myositis, and to a lesser extent oculopharyngeal muscular dystrophy deserve consideration. The differential diagnosis of bulbar-onset SBMA should include syringobulbia, familial amyloidosis associated with gelsolin mutations, Tangier disease, and facial-onset sensory motor neuropathy (FOSMN).[57] The latter typically begins with facial sensory symptoms but may evolve to include limb-girdle weakness thus potentially mimicking SBMA. A single case of an SBMA phenotype has been reported in an individual with elevated estrogen levels.[58]

LABORATORY FEATURES

Serum CK levels may be normal in approximately 10% of patients or as high as 8,000 IU/L. The use of cholesterol-lowering agents may represent a confounding variable in interpreting elevated CK levels in this population.[59] As previously implied, SBMA is consideration in young males with elevated CK even if muscle weakness is not yet evident. Oligo- or azoospermia, elevated levels of testosterone, progesterone, estradiol, follicle stimulating hormone, or luteinizing hormone may occur. The incidence of glucose intolerance is increased. Cerebrospinal fluid is normal. The DNA mutational analysis for Kennedy disease is highly sensitive and specific although is not fully penetrant. MR imaging of muscle has a limited role demonstrating fatty infiltration of affected muscles on T1-weighted images. The pattern is however nonspecific and does not allow distinction from many other neuromuscular diseases.

ELECTRODIAGNOSIS

In Kennedy disease, EDX has a greater role than in childhood SMAs. In the SMN-related SMAs, the clinical diagnosis is commonly suspected prior to electrodiagnostic testing leading directly to genetic testing. In contrast, as neurogenic causes of proximal symmetric weakness in adults are uncommon, SBMA may not be considered until after the EMG is performed and demonstrates a predominantly chronic, neurogenic pattern.

The electrodiagnostic findings in Kennedy disease are similar to any other MND with at least two exceptions. Unlike most MNDs, there is involvement of the sensory system in SBMA manifested by absent or low-amplitude sensory nerve action potentials (SNAPs) and H reflexes.[60] Greater than 95% of individuals will have involvement of at least one sensory nerve. Upper extremity sensory conductions seem just as likely as lower extremity sensory conductions to be abnormal in a manner consistent with a dorsal root ganglionopathy. In addition, the denervation on needle examination in Kennedy disease is typically dominated by chronic features (reduced numbers of enlarged motor unit action potentials [MUAPs]) with a paucity of the markers of ongoing denervation (fibrillation potentials and positive waves) that characterize the more rapidly progressive MNDs.

HISTOPATHOLOGY

In Kennedy disease, the muscle biopsy changes of neurogenic atrophy are typical, including angulated atrophic fibers of both types and pyknotic nuclear clumps. For some reason, fiber-type grouping is unusual. In addition, like many chronic neurogenic disorders, "pseudomyopathic" features including increased numbers of central nuclei, regenerating fibers, and necrotic fibers are seen. Occasionally, inflammatory cells may be seen. Animal modeling would suggest that these findings may be related to a separate myopathic disease component that may precede motor neuron degeneration.[61] Sural nerve biopsy predictably identifies loss of myelinated fibers. On postmortem examination, there is loss of brainstem and spinal motor nuclei as well as dorsal root ganglion cells. Inclusions formed by the accumulation of the mutated

AR are noted. Inclusions are also found through numerous regions of the central nervous system including the basal ganglia. The ubiquitinated inclusions of ALS are not seen.

PATHOGENESIS

Kennedy disease was the first trinucleotide repeat disorder to be described. SBMA results from an expansion of the cytosine–adenine–guanine (CAG) trinucleotide sequence in the first exon of the AR gene on the X chromosome. Normal males will have 21–37 repeats whereas affected males will have 40–62. A normal repeat number will remain stable in subsequent generations whereas progeny of individuals with 38 or 39 repeats may develop disease from gene expansion. The number of repeats correlates inversely with onset age of limb weakness but not necessarily with disease severity, rate of progression, cramps, CK levels, tremor, or endocrine abnormalities.[62] Expansion of the repeat size and anticipation appears to occur in SBMA resulting in earlier disease onset in subsequent generations. The majority of cases appear to be genetically transmitted; spontaneous mutations are thought to occur rarely. Approximately 30% of diagnosed individuals in one series had no other identifiable family members.

The unstable polyglutamine CAG expansion appears to be pathogenic through a toxic gain of function. The expanded AR protein appears to misfold and aggregate in the nuclei of motor neurons and dorsal root ganglia. Although the nuclear presence of this misfolded AR protein is a disease prerequisite, it would not appear to be the sole mechanism of toxicity as the burden of protein accumulation does not appear to correlate with the extent of toxicity. The presence of the normal AR ligands, testosterone and dihydrotestosterone, are necessary for the phenotype to develop. Disease expression is also dependent on AR binding to DNA. This concept is supported by observations of the rare female homozygotes, or in mouse models in which homozygous females and mutant castrated males where little if any disease develops. The actual mechanism(s) by which the misfolded protein and synergistic effects of androgens are toxic to motor neurons and dorsal root ganglia are not fully understood. There is evidence to support attenuation of transcriptional activity of the AR with a resultant decrease in histone acetylation, mitochondrial dysfunction, and caspase-dependent apoptotic contributions. In addition, there is evidence-impaired axonal transport with disordered function of dynactin, a protein whose gene when mutated may produce a distal SMA phenotype.[61]

MANAGEMENT

Treatment for SBMA remains largely symptomatic. Cramps may respond to nightly stretching and medications such as mexiletine gabapentin, tizanidine, baclofen, magnesium, or carbamazepine. Quinine was used in the past as an effective drug for cramps but is currently approved by the FDA solely for the treatment of malaria. Tremor is rarely severe enough to warrant treatment but may respond to propranolol or primidone. Gynecomastia, if problematic, may be treated with hormonal therapy, castration, or surgical reduction. Durable medical equipment to facilitate safe mobility is a mainstay of treatment in the latter stages of the disease. Percutaneous gastrostomy and noninvasive ventilation are important interventions in patients where impaired swallowing and breathing become severe enough to compromise the patient's health or quality of life. The criteria for initiation are similar to that described in Chapter 6.

As the development of SBMA is testosterone dependent, therapeutic strategies have understandably been directed at the androgenic system. Unfortunately, testosterone replacement provides no benefit. Leuprorelin, an luteinizing hormone-releasing hormone agonist that reduces testosterone release, and prevents nuclear relocation of mutated AR, has been shown to have a therapeutic effect on animal models of the disease. A single trial in humans had modest chemical and clinical results.[63] There are other experimental constructs that appear to have beneficial effects on animal disease models but remain to be tested in humans.

▶ BENIGN FOCAL AMYOTROPHIES (HIRAYAMA DISEASE, JUVENILE SEGMENTAL SPINAL MUSCULAR ATROPHY)

In 1959, Hirayama described a slowly progressive, focal motor neuron disorder affecting the upper extremities.[64] It has been referred to by a variety of names including monomelic amyotrophy and juvenile segmental spinal muscular atrophy (JSSMA). JSSMA implies a genetic mechanism, however, and there is no currently known genetic cause. Although there have been occasional reports of more than one first-degree family member involved, the majority of cases appear to be sporadic. The SMN genes 1 and 2 have been excluded from consideration. The construct of monomelic amyotrophy is also flawed. With Hirayama disease and other related phenotypes, bilateral involvement is not rare. For these reasons, we concur with Felice that the classification of these disorders as benign focal amyotrophies (BFAs) represents the most cogent nosology due to their tendency to produce regional patterns of weakness that are indolent and commonly plateau after an initial period of progression.[65]

CLINICAL FEATURES

Hirayama disease typically becomes symptomatic between ages 15 and 25 years, with a range of 2–30 years.[64] Males are affected in 60%–88% of cases.[66] The typical phenotype is atrophy and weakness that develops insidiously in C7–T1 hand and forearm muscles unilaterally, typically in the dominant extremity (Fig. 8-5). Preserved brachioradialis bulk in contrast to the atrophied medial flexor compartment

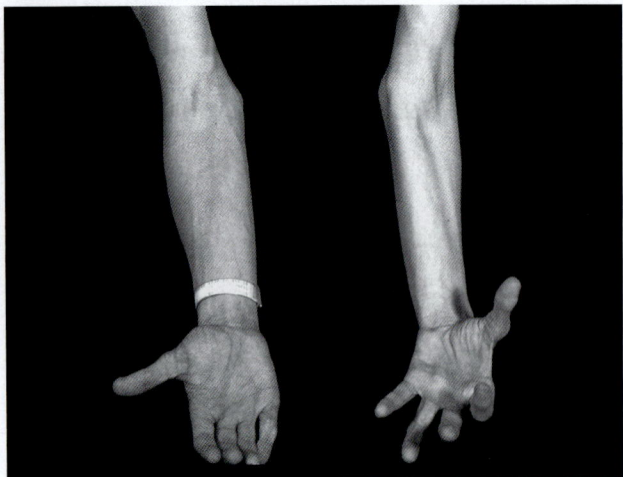

Figure 8-5. Asymmetric forearm and hand atrophy in Hirayama disease.

DIFFERENTIAL DIAGNOSIS

In our experience, focal limb-onset presentations of MND are often attributed to the more commonly occurring compressive mononeuropathies or cervical radiculopathy. If the patient has coincident evidence of cervical spondylosis on imaging or electrodiagnostic evidence of ulnar nerve slowing at the elbow or prolonged median distal latencies, unnecessary surgical intervention may take place. A practical rule of thumb is that painless weakness in the absence of sensory symptoms rarely represents a surgically correctable condition although the Hirayama phenotype provides one possible exception. Another possible exception to this is true thoracic outlet syndrome. In this rare disorder, the inevitable sensory involvement may be masked by the insidiously progressive nature of the disorder so that chronic hand atrophy and weakness becomes the predominant clinical problem. In our experience with this disorder, first rib resection may alleviate associated discomfort and prevent further progression but is unlikely to restore meaningful hand bulk or strength.

In keeping with the purely motor nature of this disorder, the differential diagnosis of Hirayama disease would include other MNDs, particularly progressive muscular atrophy, multifocal motor neuropathy, or perhaps even polio if an accurate onset history cannot be obtained. Pathology of the spinal cord itself, for example, syringomyelia, should be considered. In our experience, surgically amenable spinal cord or nerve root disease is an uncommon cause of painless limb weakness without sensory signs or symptoms. As one potential exception to this general rule, a condition referred to as cervical spondylitic amyotrophy may produce a syndrome of hand amyotrophy presumed to represent central, cervical cord ischemia provoked by spondylitic compression at a more rostral level.[69]

LABORATORY FEATURES

As will be described in the pathophysiology section, many consider Hirayama disease to represent a compressive/ischemic myelopathy. Imaging of the cervical spine in flexion may demonstrate forward movement of the posterior cervical dura mater and ligaments resulting in flattening of the spinal cord against the C5–C6 vertebral bodies in approximately 90% of cases.[70] The posterior cervical subarachnoid space tends to be obliterated and a crescent-shaped posterior epidural space that enhances with contrast is seen. The latter has been attributed to engorgement of the epidural venous plexus.[66,70] These changes seem to be most pronounced in younger individuals in the progressive stages of their disease and dissipate with a course that seems to parallel the natural history of the disease. The patient may be left with an atrophic lower cervical cord with increased T2 signal in the anterior horn.[66]

Like all MNDs, modest elevations of serum CK levels are seen but apparently, only in a minority of cases. Spinal fluid is normal or demonstrates a mild increase in protein content.[71]

muscles is a notable observation in many cases. Over the course of months to years, the weakness may spread gradually to more proximal arm muscles. In 30%–40% of cases, there is clinical weakness of the opposite limb, with an even higher percentage having electrodiagnostic evidence of bilateral involvement.[66] In 75% of cases, disease progression arrests within 5 years.[66] Unlike most non-ALS anterior horn cell diseases, reflexes in the involved limb may be spared although neither overt pyramidal nor bulbar involvement occurs. This may represent a reflection of the C8–T1 segmental involvement which provides no adequate deep tendon reflex for testing. One observation that ties BFA to SMA is the common occurrence of tremor in both. In BFA however, the tremor may occur with or be potentially caused by "contraction fasciculations" of involved muscles. Fasciculations are not commonly observed in muscles at rest. Although a significant decline in affected limb function in the cold is common with all MNDs, "cold paresis" is particularly emphasized in this population. Hyperhidrosis of the involved limb(s) has been described.

BFA has been described less frequently in Western populations. Not all patients with BFA adhere precisely to the phenotype originally described by Hirayama. Precise boundaries are difficult without a reliable biological marker. A bilateral symmetric form of the disease has been described and in one large series represented 10% of cases although even in these cases the disease evolved asymmetrically. There are lower extremity analogs that are similar in every way except topography. The first of these was described in an Indian population in 1981 where most affected individuals had weakness distributed throughout the affected lower limb although preferential quadriceps involvement did occur.[67,68] A syndrome of benign calf amyotrophy represents another phenotype and in our experience, is more common in North Americans than is the Hirayama phenotype. Like Hirayama, it may be either unilateral or bilateral in approximately half of affected individuals and appears to have a similar male predominance.

ELECTRODIAGNOSIS

The electrodiagnostic features of Hirayama disease are no different than any other motor disease, other than for a relative restriction in their distribution. The abnormalities are typically more widespread than would be predicted on a clinical basis.[72] Electromyographic findings in the opposite, asymptomatic hand, for example, occur in approximately 90% of cases. One would expect reduced recruitment of enlarged MUAPs in the majority of patients and abnormal spontaneous activity occurring in a smaller percentage. Unlike thoracic outlet syndrome and ALS, the ulnar CMAP amplitude recording from the abductor digiti minimi is often more severely reduced than the median CMAP recording from the abductor pollicis brevis.[73] This suggests that the C8 segment is more severely affected than the T1 segment. This observation is consistent with the compressive mechanism described below which occurs maximally at C5 to C6. Relevant sensory conductions, in particular the ulnar and medial antebrachial cutaneous SNAPs should be spared. In addition, there should be no suggestion of demyelinating features on motor nerve conductions.

HISTOPATHOLOGY

Muscle biopsies are not routinely performed for Hirayama disease. When performed, they have demonstrated the anticipated findings of a chronic denervating disorder, that is, fiber-type grouping, and small groups of angular, atrophic fibers. The opportunity to study the pathological findings of the cervical spinal cord in Hirayama disease is limited but in a solitary report, reduced numbers of anterior horn cells from C5–T1, most severely seen at the C7–C8 levels, and degeneration of some of the remaining motor neurons was seen. In addition, mild associated central necrosis and gliosis were seen. These changes have been postulated to represent an ischemic mechanism, perhaps secondary to epidural venous congestion.[74]

PATHOPHYSIOLOGY

The proposed ischemic changes in the cervical spinal cord in the single autopsied case of Hirayama disease led to the hypothesis of a compressive mechanism.[74,75] In 2000, Hirayama reported the results of dynamic imaging in 73 patients and 20 controls. Ninety-four percent of patients had significant forward displacement and flattening of the posterior surface of the cervical cord during neck flexion. Presumptively this compromised the cord blood supply, with preferential susceptibility of the anterior horn to ischemia. Other observations from this study that were consistent with clinical observations were the frequent asymmetric flattening of the cord, and the lesser degrees of cord distortion in older patients in whom progression had stopped. It has been hypothesized that the typical onset age of Hirayama disease, the arrest of disease progression, and the resultant reduction of posterior dural compression as affected individuals age, are related to accelerated growth that can occur in young men of this age.[75] In further support of the proposed mechanism, there have been reports of young individuals who engage in repetitive head rocking activities who develop the clinical and imaging features of the disease.[76] Although the compressive/ischemic mechanism of BFA has convincing support and appears to be largely accepted, there has been historical controversy as to the validity of the hypothesis.[71]

MANAGEMENT

The management of BFA is largely symptomatic. Tendon transfer has been utilized in an attempt to improve hand function.[77] Techniques have been utilized to restore hand bulk and appearance if not function.[78] The use of cervical collars has been associated with the observation that the arrest of disease progression occurs earlier than suggested by the normal natural history. Cervical fusion with duraplasty has been utilized with unclear influence on the natural history of the disease.[79]

▶ DISTAL SPINAL MUSCULAR ATROPHY

We, along with other authors, consider distal spinal muscular atrophy (dSMA) and HMN to be synonymous.[80] Presumably, the duplication of terms is based on differing schools of thought about disease pathophysiology. dSMA suggests that the disease begins in the anterior horn, whereas HMN implies initial pathology of the motor axon. To the best of our knowledge, neither motor nerve nor spinal cord pathology has been reported to provide conclusive support for either position. We would speculate that those who support the HMN nomenclature do so because of the length-dependent phenotype in most cases that resembles Charcot–Marie–Tooth (CMT) disease, and sensory nerve biopsy evidence of axon loss in some but not all cases.[81,82] In addition, as described below, molecular biological knowledge of these disorders identifies that at least some cases are related to mutations of genes that code for axon transport proteins. Conversely, we hypothesize that the support for dSMA as a motor neuronopathy is based on normal sensory conductions, normal sensory nerve biopsies in some cases, and an electrodiagnostic and muscle biopsy pattern that is identical to other MNDs.[81] In addition, we suspect that the non–length-dependent pattern of proximal weakness that exists in most SMAs, that would be more consistent with anterior horn cell pathology, has been extrapolated to the nosology of distal forms of the disease as well.

The initial seminal work on the nosology of these disorders was introduced by Harding and Thomas in 1980.[83] It was based on inheritance pattern and phenotype. Currently, the most pragmatic classifications include a hybrid of clinical and genetic considerations.[84,85] Several genetic mutations have been discovered in recent years expanding our understanding of the mechanisms underlying this group of diseases.[84,85]

CLINICAL FEATURES

The dSMAs are conceptualized as slowly progressive disorders that produce symmetric or near symmetric weakness and atrophy of distal muscles.[84,85] Like CMT, dorsiflexion of the toes and feet and foot eversion are usually the initially and the most severely involved functions. It is not rare however for the posterior compartment of the leg to be preferentially affected. In many cases, the hands will eventually become involved. Unlike CMT, there is neither clinical nor electrophysiological evidence of sensory involvement. Fasciculations are uncommonly recognized.

There is, however, considerable phenotypic variability. Although the majority of currently recognized genotypes produce the aforementioned leg-onset disease pattern, other mutations can produce a phenotype that begins in the hands, that involves the vocal cords or diaphragms, or one that produces pyramidal tract findings in addition to LMN features. The combination of an LMN disorder beginning in the hands and UMN features in the legs has been referred to as the eponym, Silver syndrome.[86–88] Like CMT, foot deformities such as pes cavus and hammer toes are common and kyphoscoliosis is estimated to occur in 25% of cases.

There is also heterogeneity in the age of onset and inheritance pattern. Most patients become symptomatic in the second or third decade but distal hereditary motor neuropathy (dHMN) VI can begin at birth or in the first year of life. Inheritance in dSMA is dominant in approximately 30% of cases with recessive, X-linked, or seemingly sporadic representing the remainder.[84,85]

Harding's original classification included seven categories.[89] Types I and II were distinguished only by onset age, type I being juvenile and type II being adult. In both cases, the phenotype was the classic pattern of distal symmetric leg weakness and inheritance was autosomal dominant. Type III disease represents this same classic phenotype inherited in a recessive fashion. Type IV is similar to type III with the addition of diaphragmatic weakness. Type V disease is dominantly inherited and characterized by upper limb predominance. Type VI is a specific recessively inherited disorder associated to date with a single gene mutation that results in a severe form with ventilatory distress, typically beginning within the first year of life. Type VII disease is dominantly inherited and associated with vocal cord paralysis and facial weakness. Individuals with the uncommon mutations that cause dHMN VII may develop frontal temporal dementia as well. X-linked forms of the disease, dSMAs associated with pyramidal tract features, and a congenital form were not considered in the initial Harding classification scheme (Table 8-3).[84,85,89]

Although certain mutations may produce more than one of the aforementioned phenotypic pattern, there is a reasonable phenotype/genotype correlation within the boundaries of dSMA (Table 8-3). Having said that, a number of these genes may produce phenotypes that have been historically designated as other diseases, most notably CMT (Table 8-1).

DIFFERENTIAL DIAGNOSIS

The distal SMAs are frequently diagnosed as CMT. Other than for the presence or absence of sensory involvement, the disorders may be phenotypically identical. That many of the dSMAs are allelic with forms of CMT cast doubt on whether distal SMA and axonal forms of CMT disease will be considered different disorders in the future. The distal SMAs may be readily confused with a number of the distal myopathy genotypes which may present with slowly progressive symmetric weakness of foot plantar or dorsiflexion. The childhood forms of dSMA will need to be distinguished from the more commonly occurring SMN-related disorders. As we alluded, there is both genetic and phenotypic overlap between the distal SMA, ALS, and hereditary spastic paraparesis.

LABORATORY FEATURES

Other than genetic testing, blood work has little relevance in dSMA. CK measurements are rarely reported but appear to be normal or mildly elevated. There are currently over 30 recognized genetic loci for dSMA.[84,85] Genetic testing is now increasingly available and the current rate of genetic diagnosis is about 30%–40%. There is a potential role for MR imaging in dSMA. A pattern of muscle atrophy believed to be unique to the TRPV4 mutation has been described.[90]

ELECTRODIAGNOSIS

Sensory nerve conductions are by definition normal in this disorder, at least in the majority of cases early in the disease course. CMAP amplitudes may be reduced or absent. Conduction velocities and motor latencies are preserved in a manner proportionate to the degree of axon loss. Needle electromyography demonstrates largely findings of chronic denervation and reinnervation in a distribution that extends well beyond the recognized pattern of weakness.

HISTOPATHOLOGY

Muscle biopsy is rarely performed on these patients unless EDX studies do not adequately distinguish between a nerve and muscle disease. If performed, a neurogenic pattern is seen with angulated atrophy, fiber-type grouping, and group atrophy. Sensory nerve biopsy results, as previously mentioned may be either normal or show axon loss. As previously mentioned, we are unaware of any pathological reports of either motor nerve or spinal cord in this disorder.

PATHOGENESIS

A growing list of gene mutations has been reported to produce a dSMA phenotype and many of these genes can now be tested using commercially available gene panels.[84,85] The proteins associated with dSMA loci have diverse functions including protein folding, axonal transport, cation-channel function, and RNA metabolism. The dHMN VII phenotype secondary to the dynactin gene mutation lends strong support to the axonal transport hypothesis as dynactin is a microtubular motor protein responsible for retrograde axonal transport.[91]

MANAGEMENT

The therapy for this disorder remains symptomatic. Patients will frequently benefit from ankle foot orthoses to prevent tripping or night splints to prevent contracture if the hands are involved. Durable equipment is a helpful means by which to preserve safe and independent ambulation. Only a minority of cases will require a wheelchair. Patients with ventilatory weakness may benefit from positive airway pressure devices and patients with vocal cord paralysis may benefit from procedures that may improve vocal cord functionality.

▶ SCAPULOPERONEAL SMA (DAVIDENKOW DISEASE)

Other than the childhood bulbar syndromes, the neurogenic scapuloperoneal syndromes undoubtedly represent the least common SMA phenotype. As will be described below, classifying this syndrome as an SMA may be erroneous. This disorder bears the eponym Davidenkow syndrome after the individual who initially described it in 1939.[92,93]

CLINICAL FEATURES

Recognition typically occurs in late childhood or early adulthood. Asymmetric weakness of the shoulder girdles and foot dorsiflexors are the usual initial manifestations. Weakness may progress to a more generalized pattern over a period of years.

Twelve of Davidenkow's original 13 patients had a familial disorder with apparent-dominant inheritance.[92,93] Sporadic cases have been described as well. Neurogenic scapuloperoneal syndrome has been classified as an SMA even though distal sensory loss was common in Davidenkow's original series. Despite the frequent occurrence of foot deformities and sensory loss, he eschewed any relationship to CMT although others have not shared his conviction.[94]

DIFFERENTIAL DIAGNOSIS

Most scapuloperoneal syndromes are myopathic. Recognized myopathies that may present in this pattern include facioscapulohumeral dystrophy, scapuloperoneal myopathy, Emery–Dreifuss dystrophy, Pompe disease, myofibrillar myopathy, congenital myopathy, and inclusion body myopathy with Paget disease and frontotemporal dementia (IBMPFD).[95,96]

LABORATORY FEATURES

CK is likely to be normal in most if not all cases. Genetic testing for the PMP22 gene mutation may be considered if the patient or other family members have features suggesting CMT or hereditary liability to pressure palsy (HNPP).[97]

ELECTRODIAGNOSIS

EDX in neurogenic scapuloperoneal syndromes may identify features consistent with SMA rather than features suggestive of the more common "myopathic" forms of this phenotype. Although there are limited electrodiagnostic reports of this disorder, abnormal sensory nerve conductions may occur.

HISTOPATHOLOGY

Nerve pathology demonstrates axon loss with secondary demyelinating features. To the best of our knowledge the histological hallmarks of HNPP, tomaculae, have not been demonstrated in any individual with a scapuloperoneal phenotype.

PATHOGENESIS

In our opinion, although the construct of a neurogenic scapuloperoneal is valid and useful, both its classification and causation remain unclear.[93] In keeping with Davidenkow's original (ignored) observations, the disorder appears in many cases to be a nerve disease, not an MND, and allelic to HNPP.[97] The phenotype has also been linked to mutations of the TRPV4 gene which also may cause a dSMA phenotype.[98,99]

MANAGEMENT

Management is supportive and symptomatic. Ankle foot orthoses aid walking and prevent tripping. Scapular fixation braces may be utilized in an attempt at improved scapular stabilization and improved antigravity use of the arms. Although to the best of our knowledge, it has not been used in neurogenic causes of the scapuloperoneal syndrome, scapular arthrodesis represents potential intervention worthy of consideration in selected cases.

► SUMMARY

The SMAs are LMN disorders that are phenotypically and genetically heterogeneous. With the insights provided by molecular biology, it is safe to predict that future nosology of what has been historically considered SMA will be revised considerably. More importantly, molecular biological insights into disease pathogenesis have already resulted in transformative gene-targeted treatments for SMAs associated with the SMN1 gene and provide the hope of future effective treatments for other hereditary motor neuropathies. Supportive care by committed clinicians remains of paramount importance.

REFERENCES

1. Byers RK, Banker BQ. Infantile muscular atrophy. *Arch Neurol.* 1961;5:140–164.
2. Chou SM. Controversy over Werdnig-Hoffmann disease and multiple system atrophy. *Curr Opin Neurol.* 1993;6(6):861–864.
3. Gorgen-Pauly U, Sperner J, Reiss I, Gehl HB, Reusche E. Familial pontocerebellar hypoplasia type I with anterior horn cell disease. *Eur J Paediatr Neurol.* 1999;3(1):33–38.
4. Ryan MM, Cooke-Yarborough CM, Procopis PG, Ouvrier RA. Anterior horn cell disease and olivopontocerebellar hypoplasia. *Pediatr Neurol.* 2000;23(2):180–184.
5. Brzustowicz LM, Lehner T, Castilla LH, et al. Genetic mapping of chronic childhood-onset spinal muscular atrophy to chromosome 5q11.2-13.3. *Nature.* 1990;344(6266):540–541.
6. Lefebvre S, Burglen L, Reboullet S, et al. Identification and characterization of a spinal muscular atrophy-determining gene. *Cell.* 1995;80(1):155–165.
7. Kolb SJ, Kissel JT. Spinal muscular atrophy. *Neurol Clin.* 2015;33(4):831–846.
8. Clermont O, Burlet P, Lefebvre S, Burglen L, Munnich A, Melki J. SMN gene deletions in adult-onset spinal muscular atrophy. *Lancet.* 1995;346(8991-8992):1712–1713.
9. Crisafulli S, Boccanegra B, Vitturi G, Trifiro G, De Luca A. Pharmacological therapies of spinal muscular atrophy: a narrative review of preclinical, clinical-experimental, and real-world evidence. *Brain Sci.* 2023;13(10):1446.
10. Antonaci L, Pera MC, Mercuri E. New therapies for spinal muscular atrophy: where we stand and what is next. *Eur J Pediatr.* 2023;182(7):2935–2942.
11. Verhaart IEC, Robertson A, Wilson IJ, et al. Prevalence, incidence and carrier frequency of 5q-linked spinal muscular atrophy—a literature review. *Orphanet J Rare Dis.* 2017;12(1):124.
12. Bertini E, Burghes A, Bushby K, et al. 134th ENMC International Workshop: Outcome measures and treatment of spinal muscular atrophy, 11–13 February 2005, Naarden, The Netherlands. *Neuromuscul Disord.* 2005;15(11):802–816.
13. Zerres K, Rudnik-Schoneborn S, Forrest E, Lusakowska A, Borkowska J, Hausmanowa-Petrusewicz I. A collaborative study on the natural history of childhood and juvenile onset proximal spinal muscular atrophy (type II and III SMA): 569 patients. *J Neurol Sci.* 1997;146(1):67–72.
14. Brahe C, Servidei S, Zappata S, Ricci E, Tonali P, Neri G. Genetic homogeneity between childhood-onset and adult-onset autosomal recessive spinal muscular atrophy. *Lancet.* 1995;346(8977):741–742.
15. Wee CD, Kong L, Sumner CJ. The genetics of spinal muscular atrophies. *Curr Opin Neurol.* 2010;23(5):450–458.
16. Qiu J, Wu L, Qu R, et al. History of development of the life-saving drug "Nusinersen" in spinal muscular atrophy. *Front Cell Neurosci.* 2022;16:942976.
17. Li Y, Zeng H, Wei Y, Ma X, He Z. An overview of the therapeutic strategies for the treatment of spinal muscular atrophy. *Hum Gene Ther.* 2023;34(5–6):180–191.
18. Cartwright MS, Upadhya S. Selecting disease-modifying medications in 5q spinal muscular atrophy. *Muscle Nerve.* 2021;64(4):404–412.
19. David WS, Jones HR Jr. Electromyography and biopsy correlation with suggested protocol for evaluation of the floppy infant. *Muscle Nerve.* 1994;17(4):424–430.
20. Eckart M, Guenther U-P, Idkowiak J, et al. The natural course of infantile spinal muscular atrophy with respiratory distress type 1 (SMARD1). *Pediatrics.* 2012;129(1):e148–e156.
21. Kobayashi H, Baumbach L, Matise TC, Schiavi A, Greenberg F, Hoffman EP. A gene for a severe lethal form of X-linked arthrogryposis (X-linked infantile spinal muscular atrophy) maps to human chromosome Xp11.3-q11.2. *Hum Mol Genet.* 1995;4(7):1213–1216.
22. De Siqueira Carvalho AA, Tychon C, Servais L. Newborn screening for spinal muscular atrophy—what have we learned? *Expert Rev Neurother.* 2023;23(11):1005–1012.
23. Harms MB, Allred P, Gardner R Jr, et al. Dominant spinal muscular atrophy with lower extremity predominance: linkage to 14q32. *Neurology.* 2010;75(6):539–546.
24. Penttilä S, Jokela M, Huovinen S, et al. Late-onset spinal motor neuronopathy—a common form of dominant SMA. *Neuromuscul Disord.* 2014;24(3):259–268.
25. Nishimura AL, Mitne-Neto M, Silva HCA, et al. A mutation in the vesicle-trafficking protein VAPB causes late-onset spinal muscular atrophy and amyotrophic lateral sclerosis. *Am J Hum Genet.* 2004;75(5):822–831.
26. Rudnik-Schoneborn S, Botzenhart E, Eggermann T, et al. Mutations of the LMNA gene can mimic autosomal dominant proximal spinal muscular atrophy. *Neurogenetics.* 2007;8(2):137–142.
27. Keinath MC, Prior DE, Prior TW. Spinal muscular atrophy: mutations, testing, and clinical relevance. *Appl Clin Genet.* 2021;14:11–25.
28. Brandsema JF, Gross BN, Matesanz SE. Diagnostic testing for patients with spinal muscular atrophy. *Clin Lab Med.* 2020;40(3):357–367.
29. Milligan JN, Blasco-Pérez L, Codina-Solà M, Codina-Sola M, Tizzano EF. Recommendations for interpreting and reporting silent carrier and disease-modifying variants in SMA testing workflows. *Genes (Basel).* 2022;13(9):1657.
30. Hahnen E, Forkert R, Marke C, et al. Molecular analysis of candidate genes on chromosome 5q13 in autosomal recessive spinal muscular atrophy: evidence of homozygous deletions of the SMN gene in unaffected individuals. *Hum Mol Genet.* 1995;4(10):1927–1933.
31. Prior TW, Swoboda KJ, Scott HD, Hejmanowski AQ. Homozygous SMN1 deletions in unaffected family members and modification of the phenotype by SMN2. *Am J Med Genet A.* 2004;130A(3):307–310.
32. Hergersberg M, Glatzel M, Capone A, et al. Deletions in the spinal muscular atrophy gene region in a newborn with neuropathy and extreme generalized muscular weakness. *Eur J Paediatr Neurol.* 2000;4(1):35–38.

33. Korinthenberg R, Sauer M, Ketelsen UP, et al. Congenital axonal neuropathy caused by deletions in the spinal muscular atrophy region. *Ann Neurol.* 1997;42(3):364–368.
34. MacLeod MJ, Taylor JE, Lunt PW, Mathew CG, Robb SA. Prenatal onset spinal muscular atrophy. *Eur J Paediatr Neurol.* 1999;3(2):65–72.
35. Nishio H, Niba ETE, Saito T, Okamoto K, Takeshima Y, Awano H. Spinal muscular atrophy: the past, present, and future of diagnosis and treatment. *Int J Mol Sci.* 2023;24(15):11939.
36. Elsheikh B, Prior T, Zhang X, et al. An analysis of disease severity based on SMN2 copy number in adults with spinal muscular atrophy. *Muscle Nerve.* 2009;40(4):652–656.
37. Fraidakis MJ, Drunat S, Maisonobe T, et al. Genotype-phenotype relationship in 2 SMA III patients with novel mutations in the Tudor domain. *Neurology.* 2012;78(8):551–556.
38. Mercuri E, Sumner CJ, Muntoni F, Darras BT, Finkel RS. Spinal muscular atrophy. *Nat Rev Dis Primers.* 2022;8(1):52.
39. Finkel RS, Mercuri E, Darras BT, et al; ENDEAR Study Group. Nusinersen versus sham control in infantile-onset spinal muscular atrophy. *N Engl J Med.* 2017;377(18):1723–1732.
40. Mendell JR, Al-Zaidy S, Shell R, et al. Single-dose gene-replacement therapy for spinal muscular atrophy. *N Engl J Med.* 2017;377(18):1713–1722.
41. Mercuri E, Darras BT, Chiriboga CA, et al; CHERISH Study Group. Nusinersen versus sham control in later-onset spinal muscular atrophy. *N Engl J Med.* 2018;378(7):625–635.
42. Qiao Y, Chi Y, Gu J, Ma Y. Safety and efficacy of nusinersen and risdiplam for spinal muscular atrophy: a systematic review and meta-analysis of randomized controlled trials. *Brain Sci.* 2023;13(10):1419.
43. Ropars J, Peudenier S, Genot A, Barnerias C, Espil C. Multidisciplinary approach and psychosocial management of spinal muscular atrophy (SMA). *Arch Pediatr.* 2020;27(7S):7S45–7S49.
44. Boulay C, Peltier E, Jouve J-L, Pesenti S. Functional and surgical treatments in patients with spinal muscular atrophy (SMA). *Arch Pediatr.* 2020;27(7S):7S35–7S39.
45. Fauroux B, Griffon L, Amaddeo A, et al. Respiratory management of children with spinal muscular atrophy (SMA). *Arch Pediatr.* 2020;27(7S):7S29–7S34.
46. Bosch AM, Stroek K, Abeling NG, Waterham HR, Ijlst L, Wanders RJA. The Brown-Vialetto-Van Laere and Fazio Londe syndrome revisited: natural history, genetics, treatment and future perspectives. *Orphanet J Rare Dis.* 2012;7:83.
47. Fennessy JR, Cornett KMD, Burns J, Menezes MP. Benefit of high-dose oral riboflavin therapy in riboflavin transporter deficiency. *J Peripher Nerv Syst.* 2023;28(3):308–316.
48. Kennedy WR, Alter M, Sung JH. Progressive proximal spinal and bulbar muscular atrophy of late onset. A sex-linked recessive trait. *Neurology.* 1968;18(7):671–680.
49. Fischbeck KH, Ionasescu V, Ritter AW, et al. Localization of the gene for X-linked spinal muscular atrophy. *Neurology.* 1986;36(12):1595–1598.
50. Finsterer J. Bulbar and spinal muscular atrophy (Kennedy's disease): a review. *Eur J Neurol.* 2009;16(5):556–561.
51. Parboosingh JS, Figlewicz DA, Krizus A, et al. Spinobulbar muscular atrophy can mimic ALS: the importance of genetic testing in male patients with atypical ALS. *Neurology.* 1997;49(2):568–572.
52. Amato AA, Prior TW, Barohn RJ, Snyder P, Papp A, Mendell JR. Kennedy's disease: a clinicopathologic correlation with mutations in the androgen receptor gene. *Neurology.* 1993;43(4):791–794.
53. Atsuta N, Watanabe H, Ito M, et al. Natural history of spinal and bulbar muscular atrophy (SBMA): a study of 223 Japanese patients. *Brain.* 2006;129(Pt 6):1446–1455.
54. Rhodes LE, Freeman BK, Auh S, et al. Clinical features of spinal and bulbar muscular atrophy. *Brain.* 2009;132(Pt 12):3242–3251.
55. Sumner CJ, Fischbeck KH. Jaw drop in Kennedy's disease. *Neurology.* 2002;59(9):1471–1472.
56. Burns TM, Russell JA, LaChance DH, Jones HR. Oculobulbar involvement is typical with Lambert-Eaton myasthenic syndrome. *Ann Neurol.* 2003;53(2):270–273.
57. Hu N, Zhang L, Yang X, Fu H, Cui L, Liu M. Facial onset sensory and motor neuronopathy (FOSMN syndrome): Cases series and systematic review. *Neurol Sci.* 2023;44(6):1969–1978.
58. Luo JJ. Hyperestrogenemia simulating Kennedy disease. *J Clin Neuromuscul Dis.* 2007;9(2):291–296.
59. Chahin N, Sorenson EJ. Serum creatine kinase levels in spinobulbar muscular atrophy and amyotrophic lateral sclerosis. *Muscle Nerve.* 2009;40(1):126–129.
60. Ferrante MA, Wilbourn AJ. The characteristic electrodiagnostic features of Kennedy's disease. *Muscle Nerve.* 1997;20(3):323–329.
61. Katsuno M, Banno H, Suzuki K, Adachi H, Tanaka F, Sobue G. Molecular pathophysiology and disease-modifying therapies for spinal and bulbar muscular atrophy. *Arch Neurol.* 2012;69(4):436–440.
62. Igarashi S, Tanno Y, Onodera O, et al. Strong correlation between the number of CAG repeats in androgen receptor genes and the clinical onset of features of spinal and bulbar muscular atrophy. *Neurology.* 1992;42(12):2300–2302.
63. Banno H, Katsuno M, Suzuki K, et al. Phase 2 trial of leuprorelin in patients with spinal and bulbar muscular atrophy. *Ann Neurol.* 2009;65(2):140–150.
64. Hirayama K, Tsubaki T, Toyokura Y, Okinaka S. Juvenile muscular atrophy of unilateral upper extremity. *Neurology.* 1963;13:373–380.
65. Felice KJ, Whitaker CH, Grunnet ML. Benign calf amyotrophy: clinicopathologic study of 8 patients. *Arch Neurol.* 2003;60(10):1415–1420.
66. Huang Y-C, Ro L-S, Chang H-S, et al. A clinical study of Hirayama disease in Taiwan. *Muscle Nerve.* 2008;37(5):576–582.
67. Gourie-Devi M, Suresh TG, Shankar SK. Monomelic amyotrophy. *Arch Neurol.* 1984;41(4):388–394.
68. Prabhakar S, Chopra JS, Banerjee AK, Rana PV. Wasted leg syndrome: a clinical, electrophysiological and histopathological study. *Clin Neurol Neurosurg.* 1981;83(1):19–28.
69. Mathews JA. Wasting of the small hand muscles in upper and mid-cervical cord lesions. *QJM.* 1998;91(10):691–700.
70. Hirayama K, Tokumaru Y. Cervical dural sac and spinal cord in juvenile muscular atrophy of distal upper extremity. *Neurology.* 2000;54(10):1922–1926.
71. Willeit J, Kiechl S, Kiechl-Kohlendorfer U, Golaszewski S, Peer S, Poewe W. Juvenile asymmetric segmental spinal muscular atrophy (Hirayama's disease): three cases without evidence of "flexion myelopathy." *Acta Neurol Scand.* 2001;104(5):320–322.
72. van den Berg-Vos RM, Visser J, Franssen H, et al. Sporadic lower motor neuron disease with adult onset: classification of subtypes. *Brain.* 2003;126(Pt 5):1036–1047.
73. Lyu R-K, Huang Y-C, Wu Y-R, et al. Electrophysiological features of Hirayama disease. *Muscle Nerve.* 2011;44(2):185–190.
74. Hirayama K, Tomonaga M, Kitano K, Yamada T, Kojima S, Arai K. Focal cervical poliopathy causing juvenile muscular

atrophy of distal upper extremity: a pathological study. *J Neurol Neurosurg Psychiatry*. 1987;50(3):285–290.
75. Hirayama K. Juvenile muscular atrophy of distal upper extremity (Hirayama disease): focal cervical ischemic poliomyelopathy. *Neuropathology*. 2000;20 Suppl:S91–S94.
76. Jeannet P-Y, Kuntzer T, Deonna T, Roulet-Perez E. Hirayama disease associated with a severe rhythmic movement disorder involving neck flexions. *Neurology*. 2005;64(8):1478–1479.
77. Chiba S, Yonekura K, Nonaka M, Imai T, Matumoto H, Wada T. Advanced Hirayama disease with successful improvement of activities of daily living by operative reconstruction. *Intern Med*. 2004;43(1):79–81.
78. Puwanant A, Evangelisti SM, Griggs RC. Treating the chief complaint: hand rejuvenation for Hirayama disease. *Neurology*. 2011;77(2):190–191.
79. Konno S, Goto S, Murakami M, Mochizuki M, Motegi H, Moriya H. Juvenile amyotrophy of the distal upper extremity: pathologic findings of the dura mater and surgical management. *Spine (Phila Pa 1976)*. 1997;22(5):486–492.
80. Rossor AM, Kalmar B, Greensmith L, Reilly MM. The distal hereditary motor neuropathies. *J Neurol Neurosurg Psychiatry*. 2012;83(1):6–14.
81. McLeod JG, Prineas JW. Distal type of chronic spinal muscular atrophy. Clinical, electrophysiological and pathological studies. *Brain*. 1971;94(4):703–714.
82. Frequin ST, Gabreels FJ, Gabreels-Festen AA, Joosten EM. Sensory axonopathy in hereditary distal spinal muscular atrophy. *Clin Neurol Neurosurg*. 1991;93(4):323–326.
83. Irobi J, De Jonghe P, Timmerman V. Molecular genetics of distal hereditary motor neuropathies. *Hum Mol Genet*. 2004; 13 Spec No 2:R195–R202.
84. Frasquet M, Sevilla T. Hereditary motor neuropathies. *Curr Opin Neurol*. 2022;35(5):562–570.
85. Bansagi B, Griffin H, Whittaker RG, et al. Genetic heterogeneity of motor neuropathies. *Neurology*. 2017;88(13): 1226–1234.
86. Rohkamm B, Reilly MM, Lochmuller H, et al. Further evidence for genetic heterogeneity of distal HMN type V, CMT2 with predominant hand involvement and Silver syndrome. *J Neurol Sci*. 2007;263(1–2):100–106.
87. Timmerman V, Clowes VE, Reid E. Overlapping molecular pathological themes link Charcot-Marie-Tooth neuropathies and hereditary spastic paraplegias. *Exp Neurol*. 2013;246:14–25.
88. Orlacchio A, Patrono C, Gaudiello F, et al. Silver syndrome variant of hereditary spastic paraplegia: a locus to 4p and allelism with SPG4. *Neurology*. 2008;70(21):1959–1966.
89. Harding AE, Thomas PK. Genetic aspects of hereditary motor and sensory neuropathy (types I and II). *J Med Genet*. 1980;17(5):329–336.
90. Astrea G, Brisca G, Fiorillo C, et al. Muscle MRI in TRPV4-related congenital distal SMA. *Neurology*. 2012;78(5):364–365.
91. Puls I, Oh SJ, Sumner CJ, et al. Distal spinal and bulbar muscular atrophy caused by dynactin mutation. *Ann Neurol*. 2005; 57(5):687–694.
92. Schwartz MS, Swash M. Scapuloperoneal atrophy with sensory involvement: Davidenkow's syndrome. *J Neurol Neurosurg Psychiatry*. 1975;38(11):1063–1067.
93. Hyser CL, Kissel JT, Warmolts JR, Mendell JR. Scapuloperoneal neuropathy: a distinct clinicopathologic entity. *J Neurol Sci*. 1988;87(1):91–102.
94. Harding AE, Thomas PK. Distal and scapuloperoneal distributions of muscle involvement occurring within a family with type I hereditary motor and sensory neuropathy. *J Neurol*. 1980;224(1):17–23.
95. Barohn RJ, Watts GDJ, Amato AA. A case of late-onset proximal and distal muscle weakness. *Neurology*. 2009;73(19):1592–1597.
96. Selcen D. Myofibrillar myopathies. *Neuromuscul Disord*. 2011; 21(3):161–171.
97. Verma A. Neuropathic scapuloperoneal syndrome (Davidenkow's syndrome) with chromosome 17p11.2 deletion. *Muscle Nerve*. 2005;32(5):668–671.
98. Isozumi K, DeLong R, Kaplan J, et al. Linkage of scapuloperoneal spinal muscular atrophy to chromosome 12q24.1-q24.31. *Hum Mol Genet*. 1996;5(9):1377–1382.
99. Dai J, Cho T-J, Unger S, et al. TRPV4-pathy, a novel channelopathy affecting diverse systems. *J Hum Genet*. 2010;55(7):400–402.

CHAPTER 9

Other Motor Neuron Diseases

The previous three chapters discussed motor neuron diseases (MNDs) that are inherited or degenerative in etiology. This chapter will focus on the less common (of this era), largely acquired motor neuron syndromes including the acute and delayed effects of poliomyelitis and other neurotropic viral infections. In addition, other less common causes of lower motor neuron (LMN) disease such as the potential association with malignancy and radiation exposure will be discussed.

▶ POLIOVIRUS AND OTHER INFECTIOUS CAUSES OF MOTOR NEURON DISEASE

Technically, poliomyelitis implies inflammation of spinal cord grey matter regardless of cause resulting in a phenotype of acute flaccid paralysis (AFP). In this chapter, in order to avoid confusion, we will refer to poliomyelitis as the myelopathy associated with infection with the three strains of the poliovirus, distinguishing it from other infectious myelopathies that may also be dominated by LMN weakness. Other infectious myelopathies or myeloradiculopathies with signs and symptoms of notable sensory or long-tract involvement will not be addressed.

Poliomyelitis dates to antiquity. In 1988, the World Health Organization launched the Global Polio Eradication Initiative. Poliovirus cases decreased by over 99% since then, from an estimated 350,000 cases in more than 125 endemic countries to 6 reported cases in 2021. Of the three strains of wild poliovirus (type 1, type 2, and type 3), poliovirus type 2 was eradicated in 1999 and poliovirus type 3 was eradicated in 2020. As of 2022, endemic poliovirus type 1 remains in very few countries where vaccination programs and public health measures are suboptimal. In these regions, individuals are likely to be exposed early in life. Cases occur more randomly than in epidemic disease and paralytic disease tends to be less severe in this population typically affected at an earlier age. Epidemic polio is a disorder of considerable historical interest. Epidemics tended to occur in the summer and early fall when people were more likely to be in contact with common water sources and each other. Individuals were typically exposed at an older age frequently resulting in more severe disease.

The Salk vaccine, a killed injectable product, became available in 1955. In the early 1960s, the live, attenuated oral vaccine (Sabin) was introduced providing two notable advantages, ease of delivery and long-term immunity. The disadvantage, however, was the potential for infection in vaccinated individuals, or those coming in contact with the vaccinated individuals who were themselves inadequately immunized.

People in the latter category most at risk were those who had emigrated from countries without adequate vaccination programs, those whose religious or cultural beliefs opposed vaccination, or those whose immunity had lapsed from the exclusive use of the Salk vaccine. Since 2000, no cases of AFP from the poliovirus have been reported in the United States coincident with withdrawal of Sabin vaccine usage.[1]

Although poliomyelitis is a disease of largely historical interest in the United States as a public health menace, it continues to have relevance on a number of levels. It is one of the earliest and best models of selective neuronal vulnerability from environmental cause. The development and distribution of effective polio vaccines represents one of the most notable triumphs of translational medicine in the 20th century. The relevance of poliomyelitis persists as well in that survivors of the paralytic polio (PP) epidemics of the late 1940s and early 1950s continue to populate neurology clinics.[1]

CLINICAL FEATURES

Poliomyelitis may occur as a monophasic or biphasic disease. The initial symptoms ("minor illness") are nonspecific, lasting 1–2 days. The symptoms are predominantly constitutional or gastrointestinal in nature consisting of some combination of fever, malaise, pharyngitis, headache, nausea, vomiting, and/or abdominal cramping. In the majority of individuals who are infected, the illness is self-limited and ends at this point. In individuals who fall victim to the "major illness," symptoms may occur immediately or after a delay of up to 10 days. The major illness is defined by any central nervous system (CNS) involvement including aseptic meningitis, encephalitis, or any paralytic component affecting bulbar, trunk, ventilatory, or limb musculature. Stiff neck, back pain, and fever are prominent.

Encephalitis occurs with or without a paralytic component in less than 5% of cases.[2] The manifestations may include tremulousness, obtundation, agitation, autonomic dysfunction (hypertension, hypotension, tachycardia, arrhythmias, excessive sweating), and/or upper motor neuron (UMN) signs.

Although poliomyelitis is best known for its paralytic manifestations, weakness develops in 2% or less of infected individuals. The paresis typically evolves over the course of a few days. In individuals destined to develop paralytic disease, prominent myalgias, cramping, and fasciculations precede paralysis by 48 hours or less. The paresis is typically asymmetric and is confined to the limbs and trunk in half of the cases (Fig. 9-1). There is preferential involvement of the lower

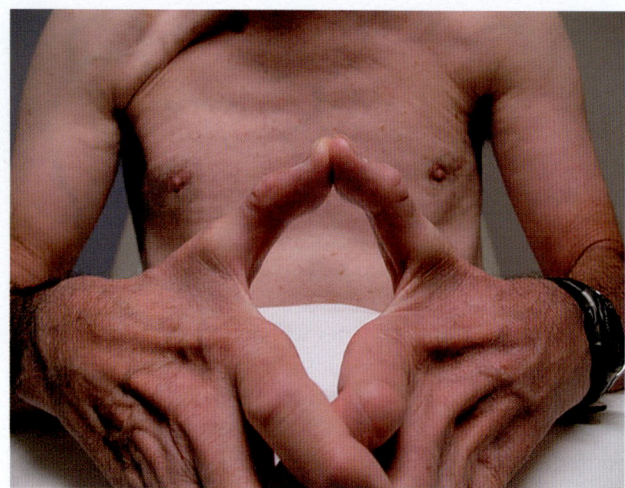

Figure 9-1. Asymmetric pectoralis and severe intrinsic hand muscle wasting in a 67-year-old who contracted polio in 1955 affecting only cervical segments.

extremities and proximal muscles, but these tendencies are relative and of limited value in the evaluation of an individual case. About 10%–15% of cases have weakness limited to bulbar muscles; the majority of these occur in children. A similar percentage is afflicted with both spinal and bulbar weakness. The most frequently affected cranial nerves are the 7th, 9th, and 10th.[2] In adults, bulbar weakness is invariably accompanied by limb weakness. Ventilatory failure is more common in this latter group. Affected limbs are paretic if not plegic with deep tendon reflexes diminished or absent. As in virtually all disorders with a predilection for anterior horn cells, the 3rd, 4th, and 6th cranial nerves are inexplicably spared. Sensory signs and symptoms are atypical although poliomyelitis may rarely result in a transverse myelitis phenotype.[3,4]

The natural history of AFP from the poliovirus is variable, dependent in large part on the severity and extent of the initial illness. Less than 10% of individuals will die from the acute illness, typically due to the complications of ventilatory failure or immobility. Those who survive typically regain strength. Patients with mild weakness typically regain most, if not all, of their strength presumably due to the effectiveness of reinnervation through collateral sprouting of unaffected, neighboring neurons or through recovery of reversibly injured anterior horn cells.[5] The majority of this recovery takes place over the course of the first 3–6 months and plateaus by 2 years. Patients with severe initial weakness typically are left with residual atrophy and weakness. A chronic persistent form of poliomyelitis can occur in children who are immunosuppressed and have received modified live vaccination. It typically begins a few months after vaccination and is invariably lethal.[6,7]

DIAGNOSIS AND DIFFERENTIAL DIAGNOSIS

Differential diagnostic considerations for AFP are listed in Table 9-1. Other nonpolio enterovirus species and neurotropic

▶ TABLE 9-1. DIFFERENTIAL DIAGNOSIS OF ACUTE FLACCID PARALYSIS DUE TO POLIOVIRUS INFECTION

Disorder	Clinical Features	Diagnosis
Other viral causes of acute flaccid paralysis	May be indistinguishable from polio with viral prodrome, followed by aseptic meningitis and acute, asymmetric limb, and bulbar paralysis, ± encephalitic component	Cultures of throat, stool, or CSF PCR and reverse transcriptase PCR for other viruses causing AFP (Table 9-2) Increased T2 signal of anterior horns with spinal MRI
Guillain–Barré syndrome	Acute onset of motor > sensory signs and symptoms affecting limbs and cranial nerves—dysautonomia	Elevated CSF protein without pleocytosis Electrodiagnostic (EDX) pattern of acquired demyelinating neuropathy
Transverse myelitis	Acute-onset paraparesis or quadriparesis with sensory level—back pain	↑ signal, swelling on spinal cord MRI
Botulism	Cranial nerve including extraocular muscle weakness, generalized weakness, and symptoms of cholinergic dysautonomia occurring in appropriate clinical context	EDX findings of a presynaptic disorder of neuromuscular transmission Toxin isolation or organism culture from wound, stool, or ingested food
Rabies	Pain, weakness, and sensory symptoms in the bitten limb in 20% of individuals who are affected	Clinical diagnosis in context of appropriate exposure
Porphyria	Prodrome of abdominal pain, encephalopathy including psychosis, followed by acute, proximally predominant motor > sensory neuropathy	Family history (variable) Increased products of heme synthesis in urine
Spinal epidural abscess	Back pain Rapidly progressive paraparesis/quadriparesis with sensory level	Imaging of spine Blood cultures
Hypokalemia, hypokalemia, and hypophosphatemia	Rapidly progressive, symmetric, and generalized weakness	Potassium <2 mEq/L Potassium >7 mEq/L Phosphorus <1 mg/dL

AFP, acute flaccid paralysis; CSF, cerebrospinal fluid; MRI, magnetic resonance imaging; PCR, polymerase chain reaction.

▶ **TABLE 9-2. OTHER VIRAL AGENTS CAUSING ACUTE FLACCID PARALYSIS**

West Nile virus
Japanese encephalitis virus
Tick-borne encephalitis
Dengue
Enterovirus D68, A71
Coxsackievirus A16
Rabies virus

viral agents are also capable of producing paralytic disease (Table 9-2).[8–10] The most common culprits are the enteroviruses and the flaviviruses, including Japanese encephalitis, dengue, tick-borne encephalitis, and West Nile virus (WNV).[10,11] Since 2014, outbreaks of acute flaccid myelitis affecting mostly young children have occurred in the United States, with approximately 700 cases reported to date. Cases have usually occurred in geographical clusters, most commonly in Western states such as California and Colorado, but have also been recognized in other states and globally, with a distinct seasonal biennial pattern in temperate regions. Though no pathogen was detected in most cases, a few have been linked to nonpolio enteroviruses (most commonly D68, but also A71) and occasionally to coxsackievirus A16. With the decline in poliomyelitis, Japanese encephalitis and WNV appear to be the most common causes of infectious AFP in Southeast Asia and North America, respectively.[11] "Dumb" rabies may present uncommonly as a paralytic illness.[12]

This list is not exhaustive and other viral agents that are more typically associated with encephalitis may occasionally produce an AFP phenotype. Agents such as herpes simplex virus type-2, varicella zoster virus, cytomegalovirus, Epstein–Barr virus, and various strains of Coxsackie A & B viruses may produce weakness but typically affect other aspects of the spinal cord in addition to the anterior horns producing concomitant sensory involvement. Paresis caused by nonpolio agents is typically less severe than that produced by polioviruses, though West Nile infection is a notable exception.[12]

Other notable infectious agents have less certain associations with MND phenotypes. HIV-infected patients have been uncommonly reported with different MND phenotypes resembling amyotrophic lateral sclerosis (ALS); the pathophysiological basis of this rare association is being actively investigated.[13] The pace of progression would be unlikely to be as acute as with poliomyelitis. Importantly, MND is an unlikely phenotypic presentation of Lyme disease.[14]

The differential diagnosis of AFP includes other disorders that present with acute weakness occurring in either a regional or generalized pattern, particularly in the absence of sensory symptoms. Of these, the Guillain–Barré syndrome (GBS) is the most common and notable. Porphyria may produce an acute generalized neuropathy. Disorders of neuromuscular transmission need to be considered, particularly botulism in consideration of its acuity. Severe hypokalemia (<2 mEq/L), hyperkalemia (>7 mEq/L), and hypophosphatemia (<1 mEq/L) are potential causes of acute generalized weakness. In the appropriate context, and in view of their acuity, tick paralysis, intoxication from marine toxins, reptile and insect envenomations, and vasculitic neuropathy need to be considered. In many but not all cases, sensory signs and symptoms will serve as distinguishing features from poliomyelitis and other causes of AFP.

LABORATORY FEATURES

The evaluation of the patient with AFP ideally begins with magnetic resonance (MR) imaging of the relevant aspects of the neuraxis. The findings in poliomyelitis are indistinguishable from other viral myelopathies.[15,16] Hyperintense T2 signal abnormalities which may extend longitudinally over a number of segments are centered in the ventral horns on axial images. Additional findings may include T1 signal abnormalities indicating hemorrhagic necrosis, short-lived enhancement with gadolinium, and cord expansion due to swelling. Routine blood work has a very limited role in the evaluation of a suspected polio patient. Like all anterior horn cell diseases, mild elevations of serum creatine kinase (CK) values are common.

The value of electrodiagnosis in cases of AFP is largely to identify a motor neuron pattern and to distinguish it from an acute neuropathy pattern. As the most common differential diagnostic consideration is GBS, it is particularly important to look for demyelinating features such as prolonged distal and F wave/H reflex latencies [in the setting of normal compound muscle action potential (CMAP) amplitudes], waveform dispersion, and conduction block, none of which would be expected in anterior horn cell diseases. Although interpretation of sensory nerve conduction study results may be difficult in the first week of an illness, reduction in sensory nerve action potential (SNAP) amplitudes is not expected in polio but would be the norm in GBS and other neuropathies. The acute motor axonal neuropathy variant of GBS is a notable exception to this rule.

The electrodiagnostic (EDX) findings in poliomyelitis would include reduced CMAP amplitudes in weak muscles, reduced recruitment of initially normal-appearing motor unit potentials, and within 3 weeks, evidence of ongoing denervation in the form of positive waves and fibrillation potentials occurring in a multifocal, segmental distribution including the paraspinal musculature. The EDX features of postpolio muscular atrophy will be addressed in the postpolio section.

Examination of the cerebrospinal fluid (CSF) is integral to the diagnosis and differential diagnosis of poliomyelitis although may be initially negative in 10% of cases. Within 2 weeks of onset, however, a pleocytosis develops. Initially, there may be a neutrophilic predominance, but 50–200 lymphocytes/mm^3 represent the typical pattern. These cells typically dissipate within 2 weeks. There is a gradual increase in the CSF protein level to a peak of 300 mg/dL or less, which then resolves within 2 months. This pattern is similar to that of the viral agents that may produce a poliomyelitis syndrome. Hypoglycorrhachia would be a rare finding.

CSF viral cultures are rarely positive in poliomyelitis. Currently, the gold standard for viral identification in the CNS is the polymerase chain reaction (PCR) for DNA viruses and reverse transcription PCR for RNA viruses.[10] CSF antibody levels may be helpful, as the presence of IgM antibodies that cannot cross the blood–brain barrier implies production within the CNS. A four-fold rise in serum antibody levels comparing chronic to acute serum provides diagnostic confirmation but are of limited value in acute diagnosis. Viral isolation in culture is the most sensitive method to diagnose poliovirus infection. Poliovirus is most likely to be isolated from stool specimens but may also be isolated from pharyngeal swabs. To increase the probability of isolating the virus, at least two stool specimens should be collected 24 hours apart, ideally as early in the course of disease as possible. The virus will be shed from the saliva for weeks and from the stool for months following infection-aiding diagnosis in cases where the patient is not seen acutely. Unfortunately, identification of a specific viral agent remains elusive in the majority of AFP cases.

HISTOPATHOLOGY

The original pathologic studies of the CNS in acute poliomyelitis were made by Bodian, at times within days of disease onset.[5] The earliest pathologic changes were in motor neurons consisting of dissolution of the cytoplasmic Nissl substance (chromatolysis) occurring in the absence of inflammation. Although neuronal loss appeared independent of inflammation suggesting an apoptotic mechanism of cell death, the presence of inflammation in the anterior horn or neuronophagia was described as a poor prognostic indicator.

The macroscopic spinal cord pathology can include pial inflammation, vascular dilatation, and petechial hemorrhages.[17] In addition to the anterior horn cells, particularly of the cervical and lumbar regions, poliomyelitis may affect neurons of the intermediate, intermediolateral, and posterior horns of the spinal cord; the dorsal root ganglia; the precentral motor cortex; hypothalamus; thalamus; cerebellar roof nuclei and vermis; nucleus ambiguous; nuclei of the facial, hypoglossal, vestibular, and trigeminal nerves; as well as the reticular formation of the brainstem.[5] Other than for hyperplasia of lymphatic tissues, the pathology of poliomyelitis is largely confined to the CNS.[18]

PATHOGENESIS

There are three known serotypes of the poliovirus. Type 1 is most frequently associated with paralytic disease. Poliomyelitis is typically contracted through fecal–oral transmission, infection often initiated within families by infants not adequately toilet trained. The incubation period is typically 6–20 days. The virus replicates in the oropharyngeal and intestinal mucosa, amplifies in lymphatic tissue, and typically goes through two viremic phases, the second of which may result in CNS disease. The exact mechanism of CNS invasion is unclear but either a disrupted blood–brain barrier or entry through neuromuscular junctions with retrograde axonal transport has been suggested. This provides a potential explanation for why AFP is more common and severe in older individuals whose fast axonal transport mechanisms are better established.[19]

Susceptibility to poliomyelitis is conferred by the presence of the poliovirus receptor (PVR) or CV155 that allows viral entry into motor neurons.[20] CV155 is a protein belonging to an immunoglobulin-like class of proteins known as nectins that promote cell surface adhesion. The PVR normally exists only in primates but transgenic mice expressing this gene are disease susceptible and have provided an animal model that has offered valuable insights into disease pathogenesis. For example, the CV155 protein expresses itself embryologically in transgenic mouse neurons destined to become anterior horn cells suggesting a potential mechanism for the selective vulnerability of motor neurons. Genetic susceptibility to PP has been suspected but never proven.

TREATMENT

The best current treatment for poliomyelitis is prevention. The peak incidence of AFP from the poliovirus occurred in the United States in 1952 with more than 20,000 new victims. Subsequent to the introduction of vaccine programs, the annual incidence fell to approximately 10 cases a year, the majority of which were felt to be vaccine related. Since the moratorium on the modified-live virus (Sabin) vaccine in 2000, no new cases in the United States have occurred.

There are no known antiviral agents effective against the poliovirus. Strategies to alter the structure of the PVR to prevent viral access to motor neurons has been theoretically proposed. We are aware of anecdotal reports of intravenous immune globulin (IVIG) being utilized in AFP due to WNV and in postpolio syndrome (PPS) but not in acute poliomyelitis.[21,22]

The treatments for polio and other causes of AFP remain largely symptomatic. Acute care measures include monitoring of, and if needed, support for hypoventilation and dysautonomia. Prevention of pressure injury to skin and nerve is of great importance as is attention to adequate nutrition particularly in patients with bulbar disease. Treatment of the sequelae of polio involves consideration of durable equipment needs and orthopedic procedures and is addressed in Chapter 5.

▶ WEST NILE VIRUS

The WNV has been recognized as a human pathogen since 1937. The first documented cases in humans in the United States were in 1999. WNV has supplanted poliovirus as the most common viral cause of AFP in adults in this country. It is a mosquito-borne pathogen belonging to the *Flavivirus* family, all members of which have been reported to cause an AFP syndrome.

CLINICAL FEATURES

Like poliomyelitis, most individuals who are infected remain asymptomatic or develop minimal symptoms. A minor, flu-like illness develops in approximately 20% of patients. Those who become symptomatic do so suddenly with combination of fever, malaise, anorexia, nausea, emesis, diarrhea, headache, photosensitivity, neck pain and stiffness, myalgia, rash, and/or lymphadenopathy.[23,24]

Meningoencephalitis and/or AFP develops in approximately 1 out of 150 infected individuals. Meningoencephalitis is the more common phenotype. Most, but not all, patients with AFP have concomitant meningeal or encephalitic signs and symptoms. There is at least a suggestion that the elderly and immunocompromised, particularly those with T-cell deficiencies, are most at risk.[24,25]

The clinical spectrum of meningoencephalitis is quite broad and may include high fever, nuchal rigidity, seizures, and cognitive impairment including confusion, memory loss, and aphasia. Movement disorders are a common feature of WNV encephalitis and may have either hyperkinetic manifestations such as tremor or myoclonus or a hypokinetic syndrome with Parkinsonism. Stiff-person syndrome (SPS) has been reported.[26] In addition, patients with WNV infection are more prone to develop systemic manifestations than poliomyelitis. Chorioretinitis is reported to occur in 75% of patients with meningoencephalitis. Hepatitis, pancreatitis, rhabdomyolysis, and myocarditis may occur.[24]

AFP as a consequence of WNV infection is a well-established concept.[23,25,27-32] Like polio, the phenotype is that of an acute onset of asymmetric flaccid weakness which usually develops over a 3–8-day period.[23] Unlike polio, older individuals appear to be at the greatest risk with the mean age of affected individuals being 55 years. The facial nerve is affected frequently, which could prompt confusion with GBS or Lyme polyradiculopathy. Ventilatory muscle involvement with the need for mechanical breathing support occurs. As in AFP secondary to poliomyelitis, the outcome is variable with residual deficits being commonplace. Fatality rates in patients with WNV meningoencephalitis average 9% and are reported to be as high as 14%, invariably affecting those greater than 50 years of age.[24,33] It is estimated that only a third of individuals affected with meningoencephalitis will be fully recovered 1 year after their illness.[24]

DIAGNOSIS AND DIFFERENTIAL DIAGNOSIS

The diagnosis of West Nile should be considered in any case of AFP of acute to subacute onset, particularly if associated with features of meningitis and/or encephalitis. The majority of cases will be seasonal and related to periods of mosquito activity. Nonetheless, the diversity of transmission mechanisms described below, that are not seasonally dependent, allow for potential WNV infection in patients at risk at any time of year. The differential diagnosis of AFP secondary to WNV is identical to that described in the poliomyelitis section.

LABORATORY FEATURES

Imaging has a supportive role in diagnosis. High-resolution MR imaging of the spine may demonstrate increased signal in the ventral horns or ventral roots in West Nile patients with AFP.[25,34,35] Leptomeningeal, ventral root, and cauda equina enhancement, as well as increased signal in the basal ganglia, mesial temporal lobes, brainstem, cerebellum, and thalami have been described with MR imaging in patients with WNV infection.[33,36-37]

The earliest reports of WNV patients with AFP, based on EDX data, suggested polyneuropathy as the likely cause of patient weakness. This is no longer felt to be the case. Subsequent reports of AFP associated with WNV infection describe an EDX pattern identical to poliomyelitis.[25] Sensory nerve conductions are normal. CMAP amplitudes are normal or reduced without demyelinating features. Needle examination reveals evidence of reduced recruitment of normal-appearing motor unit action potentials (MUAPs) if done acutely. Within 1–3 weeks, fibrillation potentials and positive waves develop in a generalized pattern that includes clinically unaffected as well as clinically weak muscles.[25]

Routine laboratory studies have limited utility in suspected WNV infection. Like poliomyelitis, patients with AFP secondary to WNV infection can be anticipated to have modest elevations of serum CK levels. The CSF examination in cases of meningoencephalitis and/or AFP should include enzyme-linked immunosorbent assays for IgM and IgG antibodies for the WNV. WNV reverse transcriptase PCR and viral culture should be utilized as well due to their specificity. Unfortunately, both suffer from inadequate diagnostic sensitivity and cannot be relied upon to exclude the diagnosis. The preliminary CSF results typically include a pleocytosis of between 5 and 500 cells/mm^3 in 96% of cases. Initially, there may be a sizeable proportion of neutrophils, but transition to lymphocytic predominance occurs. CSF protein levels are normal in 7% of cases, elevated to <100 mg/dL in 63% of cases, and elevated to >100 mg/dL in 26% of all meningoencephalitis cases but in 47% of cases with a predominantly encephalitic phenotype.[38]

The Centers for Disease Control and Prevention provide diagnostic criteria for both probable and confirmed meningoencephalitis due to WNV which presumably extrapolate to an AFP syndrome as well. A probable diagnosis requires the appropriate clinical syndrome, occurring at the appropriate time of year associated with a singular serum determination of IgM antibodies to WNV detected by antibody capture enzyme-linked immunosorbent assay.

A definite diagnosis requires the identical clinical context with more complex serologic confirmation provided through one of four potential testing methods. These options include either a four-fold increase in serum antibody concentration (usually over a 4-week interval), isolation of WNV antigen or genomic sequences usually through reverse transcription PCR, detection of virus-specific IgM antibodies in CSF, or serum IgG antibodies in addition to IgM.[24,36,39] These testing paradigms are not mutually exclusive and can be used in a complementary fashion. One unfortunate issue related to WNV serologic testing is the recognition that the latency between infection and seroconversion may be up to 8 days.[40]

HISTOPATHOLOGY

The histopathology of WNV meningoencephalitis is characterized by perivascular and leptomeningeal chronic inflammation, the formation of microglial nodules, neuronal necrosis within gray matter, and neuronophagia with a predilection for the temporal lobes, basal ganglia, and brainstem. In individuals with AFP, similar findings are noted in the spinal cord, particularly in the lumbar region. The predominant inflammatory cells are CD3+ T lymphocytes and CD68+ macrophages.[33,36,41]

PATHOGENESIS

WNV is primarily transmitted to humans by mosquitoes. Most cases occur in August and September in temperate climates when mosquitoes become more likely to feed on humans than birds. Transmission rarely occurs through blood transfusion, organ transplantation, occupational exposure, breast feeding, and via the transplacental route.[24,33,36] Blood collection agencies have been screening all donated blood in the United States for WNV since 2003; very few cases have been reported to occur after blood transfusion.

In addition to humans, other mammals and birds are also susceptible, the latter providing undoubtedly the largest reservoir as well as the probable mechanism for rapid geographic spread. To that point, although the initial United States cases were reported in New York City, the major outbreaks in the United States have occurred in the Midwest. Human epidemics are usually preceded by large kills of infected birds.

In a manner similar to poliomyelitis, viral replication occurs in skin and lymph nodes with two viremic stages. Also similar is the need for blood–brain barrier to be rendered permeable in order to serve as a portal for CNS inoculation. All flaviviruses, including WNV, gain access to targeted cells through receptor-mediated endocytosis and fusion from within acidic endosomes. The cell entry process of flaviviruses is mediated by the viral E glycoprotein.[42] Both the frequency and severity of CNS disease appear to be related to loss of function of the chemokine receptor CCR5 whose normal function is to regulate trafficking of lymphocytes to the infected brain in viral diseases such as HIV and WNV.[24] The WNV infects astrocytes as well as neurons. One theory of motor neuron death in WNV is similar to the one proposed for ALS. Specifically, it has been suggested that anterior horn cells fall victim to excitotoxicity promoted by the impaired reuptake of glutamate resulting from damaged astrocytes.[24]

TREATMENT

There are no antiviral agents proven to be effective against WNV. Vaccines are in development but are not currently available. IVIG, particularly the product obtained in populations where WNV is endemic, has been reported to have anecdotal success in case reports but no support from controlled trials has been provided to date.[22] Similar reports with mixed results in response to interferon α-2b have also been published.[10,43–46] The symptomatic and supportive treatment of WNV patients experiencing AFP is identical to poliomyelitis both in the acute care and rehabilitation settings.

▶ POSTPOLIO SYNDROME/POSTPOLIO PROGRESSIVE MUSCULAR ATROPHY (PPMA)

PPS was first suggested as a specific entity by Cornil and Lépine in 1875 who described the clinical and postmortem features of an individual who developed progressive weakness following a remote episode of poliomyelitis. This concept received no more than cursory attention until 1981 when an international symposium of experts was convened in Chicago in response to the slowly progressive weakness experienced by the large numbers of people affected by the epidemics of the early 1940s and early 1950s with convincing evidence of slowly progressive weakness after a protracted period of disease stability.[47] This has been referred to by the more specific name of postpolio progressive muscular atrophy (PPMA) which will be preferentially used in this chapter.

A number of controversies remain. The clinical boundaries of what is attributable to direct and indirect effects of "old polio" remain incompletely defined. Some symptoms attributed to PPS are not readily explained by the known pathology of the disease. They can be nonspecific and potentially attributable to other disorders prevalent in an aging population. Even with the more readily conceptualized signs and symptoms of PPMA, that is, fatigue and new, progressive muscle atrophy and weakness, no consensus exists to explain the mechanism of new weakness or the latency between the initial illness once thought to be self-limited and the onset of PPMA.

CLINICAL FEATURES

PPMA has been estimated to occur in between 22% and 85% of individuals previously affected with PP with the largest survey suggesting a prevalence of 50%.[48–50] The latency between the acute illness and the onset of PPMA has been reported to range between 8 and 71 years with an average interval of 35 years.[51–53] Risk factors for PPMA appear to be related primarily to the severity of the acute illness which in turn is proportionate to the age of disease onset. An additional risk factor appears to be the degree of recovery from the acute illness. Patients who are more successful in regaining strength after acute illness seem less susceptible to PPMA than those of similar age and whose initial recovery is more successful.[54] Finally, excessive exercise following recovery from the acute illness is a purported risk factor.[54,55]

PPMA tends to affect muscles that were the most severely affected at the time of the acute illness (Fig. 9-2). Less frequently, PPMA may affect muscles, even patients, thought to have been clinically unaffected at the time of initial illness.[5] This theory is supported by the knowledge that 50%–60% loss of motor neurons must occur before weakness is typically detected. Progressive atrophy and weakness in PPMA can affect virtually any limb, trunk, cranial, or ventilatory muscle group. As with all MNDs, clinical involvement of extraocular muscles does not occur in either acute poliomyelitis or PPMA.

As mentioned, the progression in PPMA is insidiously slow. The decline in ventilatory function has been estimated to occur at an annual rate of 2%.[56] Limb muscle strength has been estimated to deteriorate at an annual rate of 1%.[47,57] One study when conducted for only 5 years failed to detect progression which became apparent only after the same cohort was observed for a lengthier period of time.[58,59]

The most common symptoms attributed to PPMA are fatigue, arthralgias, and myalgias; these are estimated to occur in greater than 80%, 70%, and 70% of patients, respectively.[60] The more objective sign of PPMA, progressive weakness, is estimated to occur in 70%–90% of patients in previously afflicted muscles and in 50%–60% of patients in previously unaffected muscles.[60] Dysphagia is the most common bulbar symptom in PPMA patients, developing in approximately 30% of patients.[60] New symptoms attributable to ventilatory insufficiency occur in approximately 40% of patients, typically in those who had ventilatory problems during their acute illness.[60]

Some symptoms that patients with PPMA experience are readily understood. Fatigue has many potential causes directly or indirectly related to the initial illness including declining strength, development of sleep apnea or reactive depression, or declining ventilation. The latter may be the result of PPMA affecting ventilatory muscles or chest wall restriction due to kyphoscoliosis. Both obstructive and central sleep apnea are prevalent in the PPMA cohort.[61] Sleep-disordered breathing occurs most commonly in patients with previous bulbar polio.[62] Hypopharyngeal muscles, normally relaxed during rapid eye movement (REM) sleep, may further weaken as a consequence of the late effects of polio and contribute to airway obstruction. Both aging and reduced exercise capacity related to the acute illness predispose to deconditioning and weight gain which undoubtedly play a role in sleep-disordered breathing as well. Central sleep apnea is likely to represent an adverse late effect on neurons within the breathing center in the brainstem reticular formation.

Other symptoms such as depression, anxiety, and nonspecific pain occur frequently in the postpolio cohort and are less readily attributable to direct effects of prior poliomyelitis.[5] Arthralgias and myalgias are estimated to occur in approximately 40%–80% of PPMA patients.[63] Musculoskeletal complaints are readily understandable. Joint pains are likely related to accelerated degenerative joint disease resulting from years of imbalanced forces brought to bear on joints resulting from weakness of stabilizing muscle groups. Biomechanical alterations may also occur due to polio-related surgeries and osteoporosis and fractures of the limbs affected by polio are common. Adhesive capsulitis secondary to joint immobility is another logical cause of joint discomfort. Myalgias are equally understandable in muscles overworked in their attempts to accomplish the same amount of work with a diminishing number of motor units. Cold intolerance is also readily attributable to declining muscle mass and muscle activity in addition to the effects of advancing age. Acrocyanosis may occur and is presumably due to loss of neurons within the intermediolateral cell column during the acute illness.

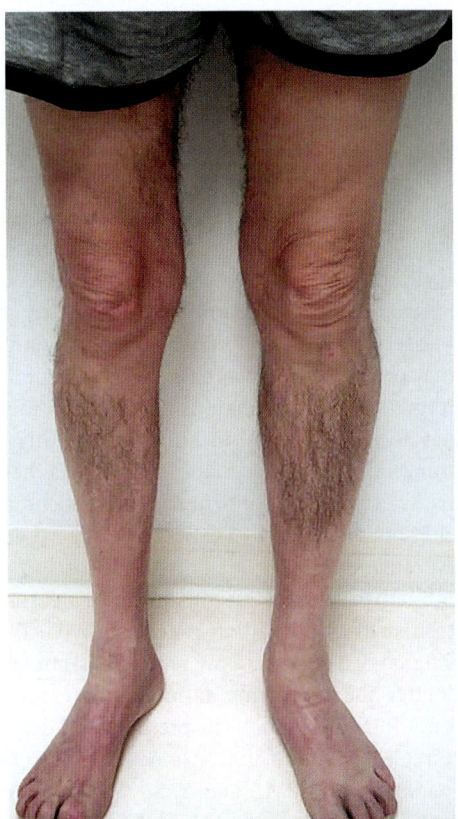

Figure 9-2. Right > left leg atrophy in a patient with childhood poliomyelitis with 2 years of insidiously progressive leg weakness due to PPMA.

Other symptoms are more difficult to attribute to the known pathology of polio.[5,59] Impaired concentration and the ability to process information with the usual speed are complaints sometimes voiced by postpolio patients. This may result as an indirect effect of impaired sleep patterns or CO_2 retention. Alternatively, physicians should be cognizant that adverse psychological effects can result from late polio. Patients' sense of well-being can be seriously undermined by their realization that their muscles are weakening and that they may be losing control of a disease with which they had formerly believed that they had achieved an equilibrium.

DIAGNOSIS AND DIFFERENTIAL DIAGNOSIS

PPMA is a clinical diagnosis of exclusion and the diagnostic criteria are straightforward. They include a history of illness consistent with acute poliomyelitis, chronologically related evidence of motor neuron loss identified either clinically or electrodiagnostically, and a history supportive of at least partial recovery of strength and function in the months following the acute illness. As mentioned, a hiatus between initial illness and subsequent development of fatigue and new, progressive weakness measured in years is required. Electromyographic and muscle biopsy findings cannot reliably identify patients with PPMA. Signs and symptoms of PPMA have been reported to begin as early as 8 years after the initial illness or as late as 71 years, with an average of 35 years. Lastly, other rational differential diagnostic considerations must be excluded.[57]

The most relevant exclusionary considerations in PPMA are other MNDs, particularly ALS. With the increased prevalence of PPMA in the 1970s, it was proposed that new weakness in PP patients might represent ALS, implying that prior polio represented an ALS risk factor.[57] Longitudinal observations in PPMA patients that include slow rates of progression and absence of UMN features have put this hypothesis to rest. Nonetheless, poliomyelitis is not ALS protective and prior PP victims developing ALS have been reported, and have raised the secondary question as to whether ALS in these patients represents reactivation of the poliovirus.[64,65] At least one postmortem study suggests that this is not the case.[64]

Identification of ALS in a prior polio victim may be challenging. Arguably, an accelerated rate of progression atypical of PPMA is the most distinctive clue. UMN findings are understandably unlikely to develop in previously atrophic and weak limbs. Their development in previously unaffected limbs represents the other major clinically distinguishing tool.[65] Fasciculations may occur in both ALS and PPMA although they are less common in the latter.[5] There are differences between the serologic, EDX, and pathologic profiles in ALS and PPMA patients but these are relative and not pathognomonic.[65] These will be discussed in the laboratory section below.

Any disorder that may produce painless weakness must be considered in a prior polio victim who is getting weaker and evaluated for, if the pattern of weakness or rate of progression is atypical for PPMA. These are outlined in detail in the differential diagnosis of ALS in Chapter 7 and include disorders of muscle such as inclusion body myositis (IBM), disorders of neuromuscular transmission such as myasthenia, other MNDs such as benign focal amyotrophy and Kennedy disease, and multifocal motor neuropathy.

In view of the nonspecific nature of many complaints offered by aging PPMA patients such as fatigue, it is prudent to consider and address other common systemic causes of these symptoms by performing a careful general examination and relevant testing before attributing these symptoms to PPMA. In addition, patients with prior PP are likely to be at greater risk of compressive mononeuropathies and monoradiculopathies than an age-matched population, suggesting a need for a greater index of suspicion for these potentially treatable disorders in this population.

LABORATORY FEATURES

There are two potential goals of laboratory testing in patients with prior PP, to identify those who have developed PPMA, and to distinguish PPMA from other disorders that might mimic it. Regarding identification of PPMA, there are no definite serologic, EDX, or pathologic means by which to distinguish patients with prior PP who have transitioned into PPMA from those who have not.[66] There are conflicting opinions as to whether an elevated level of serum CK discriminates between these two groups.[49,67] EDX evidence of ongoing denervation appears to occur with equal prevalence in both symptomatic and asymptomatic patients with PP.[66,68] The same holds true for muscle biopsy where the pathologic hallmark of acute denervation, angulated and atrophic muscle fibers seen either individually or in groups, is evident in both groups.[68] Identification of PPMA is therefore made largely on clinical grounds.

There is an EDX distinction between PPMA and ALS, but it is largely quantitative rather than qualitative. Large MUAPs may occur in both disorders but in view of the rate of disease progression and limitations of reinnervation in ALS, are unlikely to exceed 8 mV in amplitude in this disorder. This information is of limited value; however, as there are no MUAP characteristics that confirm ALS in a patient with prior PP.[65] In addition, the absence of extremely large MUAPs in the 15–25-mV range does not preclude a diagnosis of PPMA.[65] Features of active denervation and unstable neuromuscular transmission such as fibrillation potentials, MUAP variability, decremental responses to slow repetitive stimulation, and increased jitter measurements although more prevalent in ALS, occur in PPMA as well.[65] The presence and degree of elevated serum CK levels also appear to be a poor discriminator between patients with PPMA and ALS.[67] We do not routinely recommend routine muscle biopsy in PPMA patients. When performed, there are characteristics that would aid in distinguishing between PPMA and ALS. Atrophic fibers that are angular in their morphology are seen in both disorders as is

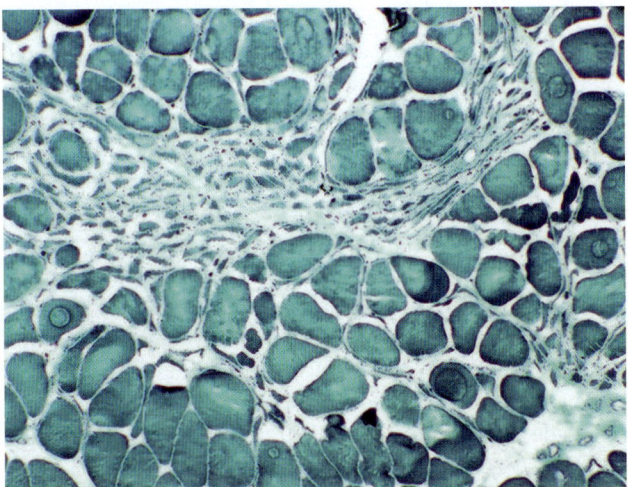

Figure 9-3. Quadriceps muscle biopsy [modified Gömöri trichrome at low (40×) power] demonstrating large group atrophy from patient in Figure 9-2.

type grouping, although large groups are not typical of ALS[65] (Fig. 9-3). CSF biomarkers have been suggested as a potential mechanism to identify PPMA patients.[69]

HISTOPATHOLOGY

Muscle biopsy in PPMA invariably demonstrates evidence of denervation and reinnervation. Type grouping of both type 1 and type 2 fibers occur. Group size may be extremely large with as many as 200 fibers of the same group bunched together.[5,65] Other neurogenic features such as pyknotic nuclear clumping, grouped atrophy, and isolated angular, atrophic fibers may be seen.[47] Like all chronic denervating diseases, "myopathic" features such as rare pockets of endomysial inflammation, increased internal nuclei, and myofiber vacuolization are occasionally evident.[5,70] The spinal cord pathology of patients with PPMA demonstrates the fairly nonspecific findings of perivascular lymphocytic infiltrates, neuronal atrophy, and gliosis proportionate to the degree of neuronal loss.[5]

PATHOGENESIS

Differing opinions persist as to the cause of delayed and slowly progressive weakness in patients with prior AFP from poliomyelitis. The three most popular theories are an increased risk of premature death of enlarged motor units, persistent poliovirus infection, and an immune-mediated mechanism.[60] In our opinion, the enlarged motor unit theory is the most credible. Observations suggest that the largest motor units, those associated with large fiber-type grouping and the most extensive collateral reinnervation, are the motor units most susceptible to premature failure and death.[66] It is logical to believe that the demands placed on these enlarged motor units over time, would predispose them to a premature demise. It is also logical to believe that loss of these larger motor units would lead to a more notable loss in strength than would loss of a normal motor unit during the normal aging process.

There is evidence that poliovirus and other picornaviruses may persist in the CNS of animals.[19] The evidence that this occurs in humans and is the mechanism behind PPMA is limited. Perhaps the most convincing evidence comes from a study that detected the poliovirus genome through PCR technology in over half of the PPMA patients but in none of their controls.[71] The majority of studies, however, have been negative or inconclusive in this regard.[60] To the best of our knowledge, there has been no unequivocal pathologic evidence of the poliovirus genome or evidence of persistent infection in PPMA patients.[5,64] The support for a potential autoimmune mechanism stems in large part from pathologic evidence identifying inflammation in the absence of an infectious agent.[60] Oligoclonal bands and inflammatory cytokines in the CSF have been inconsistently reported.[59]

TREATMENT

The management of PPMA is largely supportive and should be highly individualized. A high index of suspicion is required to identify issues not directly related to the late effects of polio that may have specific and effective treatments. Much of the morbidity of PPMA is related to impaired mobility that may benefit from bracing, durable medical equipment, or the judicious use of orthopedic procedures. The reader is referred to Chapter 6 for more detailed information. Symptomatic treatment of bulbar and ventilatory symptomatology follows the principles outlined in Chapter 7. Secretion clearance issues may be improved upon by hydration, expectorants, suction, oscillating vests, and cough-assist devices. Swallowing issues may be addressed by attention to the consistencies and size of food ingested, head position during swallowing, and eventually by the provision of percutaneous gastrostomy. Ventilatory issues, particularly at night, may benefit from positive airway pressure, usually delivered noninvasively (BiPAP) but occasionally delivered through tracheostomy-assisted mechanical ventilation.

▶ MND AND MALIGNANCY

Malignancy can adversely affect the nervous system through numerous mechanisms. Although relatively uncommon and often controversial, a number of neuromuscular syndromes, usually but not always dominated by LMN features, have been associated with malignancy and its treatments.[72] These include ALS and all of its subtypes including PMA and primary lateral sclerosis (PLS), neurolymphomatosis, paraneoplastic motor neuropathy, multifocal motor neuropathy, subacute motor neuronopathy (SMN), GBS, and SPS.[73–77]

Although LMN syndromes have been described in association with both solid tumors and hematologic malignancies, perusal of existing literature would suggest that the most frequent association and widest phenotypic diversity occur with lymphoma.[72–74,76–80]

The motor neuron disorders described in this chapter, particularly those related to neoplasia, are rare in comparison to the more common degenerative or hereditary disorders. Practical guidelines that would help neurologists to decide when and how to look for underlying malignancy in ALS patients would be helpful. It has been historically suggested that the presence of a monoclonal protein in the serum or urine, a CSF protein value of >75 mg/dL or oligoclonal banding in the spinal fluid should prompt a search for lymphoma in an MND patient.[72] This strategy is no longer frequently employed by most specialists, as its ability to identify a treatable condition is minute.[74] Alternatively, knowledge of the phenotypes and behaviors of these uncommon syndromes and the features that distinguish them from more common MNDs provide another means to identify patients who would be most likely to benefit from a more intense search for an underlying tumor.

RADIATION MYELOPATHY

Radiation therapy was first recognized in 1948 as an uncommon cause of an acquired LMN disorder. There are numerous case reports or reviews describing this syndrome.[51,77,81–91] Radiation-induced motor neuron disease (RIMND) occurs most commonly in association with prophylactic radiation of lower thoracic and lumbar fields for testicular tumors.[77,88] The phenotype may be more representative of the selective vulnerability of motor neurons or ventral roots in the lumbosacral region, rather than the focus of radiation, as RIMND confined to the lower extremities has been described in individuals receiving whole neuraxis radiation.[86] Its incidence appears to increase with radiation dosage, most reported cases having occurred in individuals receiving 40 Gy or more.[88] The authors' perception is that RIMND occurs or is reported less frequently now in comparison to the past which may reflect dose reduction, refinement in radiotherapy technique, or recognition that the concept is no longer novel.[85] The syndrome may also affect other body regions after radiation of the neck, thorax, or abdomen, but is distinctly uncommon, with neurologic injury being more commonly myelopathic in these conditions.[89,90]

Clinical onset is typically delayed for months or more, commonly years following treatment.[77] The disease often progresses for a period of time within the distribution of affected nerve elements, only to plateau and stabilize in many cases.[77,88] Painless weakness is the predominant symptom. It is often monomelic at onset, evolving into an asymmetric, paraparetic distribution affecting multiple nerve and nerve root distributions. It is, commonly associated with amyotrophy, cramps, and fasciculations lending clinical support to an anterior horn localization. The presence of radiation dermatitis probably increases the likelihood that the neurologic syndrome in the appropriate topographic area is causally related. Sensory and genitourinary involvement is notable for its absence in most but not all reports. When present however, sensory symptoms typically represent a delayed and minor component, often with preserved SNAPs in the symptomatic distribution.[88]

The diagnosis of RIMND is based predominantly on a typical phenotype occurring in the appropriate clinical context, coupled with the exclusion of other non–radiation-induced motor neuron syndromes. Localization to motor neurons (or ventral roots/motor nerves) is presumed through combination of clinical and EDX assessment. CSF examination may be normal or demonstrate a mild elevation in protein.[85,86,88]

The EDX features of RIMND are similar to other MNDs. Sensory conductions in involved segments are normal, supporting an anterior horn cell, ventral root, or motor nerve localization.[81] CMAPs are reduced proportionate to the degree of involvement of the analogous spinal cord segment. Needle electromyography demonstrates the usual features of both ongoing denervation (fibrillation potentials and positive waves) and chronic denervation and reinnervation (reduced recruitment of MUAPs that are increased in amplitude and duration). The demonstration of myokymic discharges on EMG has been described in some but not all cases.[83,88]

The implication that RIMND is an anterior horn cell disease is also supported by in vitro studies suggesting disproportionate vulnerability of anterior cells to radiation.[83] Others have argued that RIMND is more properly termed a polyradiculopathy based on imaging and pathologic evidence. Ventral root enhancement on MRI has been reported in some but not all cases.[88] Rare reports of autopsied cases support this conclusion, demonstrating thickening, nodularity, and hemorrhagic discoloration in nerve roots but no abnormalities within the spinal cord.[88] Conversely, others have reported chromatolysis of anterior horn cell.

Regarding the mechanism, it has been hypothesized that radiation may allow for reactivation of a latent virus with predilection for anterior cells, analogous to poliomyelitis. To the best of our knowledge, there is no data to support this theory.[86] The pathologic demonstration of hyalization of blood vessels in response to radiation, particularly in nerve roots, suggests a chronic ischemic mechanism.[88] Selective vulnerability of Schwann cells to radiation as demonstrated in vitro may potentially contribute to disease pathogenesis.[92] Chemotherapy does not appear to play a role.[88]

There is no recognized effective treatment for RIMND. In view of the consideration that vaso-occlusive disease is the basis of nerve injury, attempted treatments have included anticoagulants, and hyperbaric oxygen in addition to immunomodulating agents such as corticosteroids and d-penicillamine.

PARANEOPLASTIC MND

Paraneoplasia is estimated to cause no more than 1% of neurologic syndromes occurring in patients with malignancy.[75]

In general, paraneoplastic syndromes are more common in solid tumors than in hematologic malignancies and are more likely to affect the central rather than the peripheral nervous system. One apparent exception to this generalization is an LMN syndrome. Although rare, and historically controversial, MND appears to be the most common paraneoplastic manifestation of lymphoma affecting the peripheral neuromuscular system.[72,79] Conversely, lymphoma appears to be the tumor most commonly associated with a paraneoplastic LMN syndrome.[79] Although paraneoplastic syndromes associated with lymphoma and CNS disorders may be commonly associated with measurable autoantibodies, LMN syndromes occurring in association with lymphoma have yet to be associated with a reproducible, paraneoplastic antibody.[79]

Paraneoplastic LMN syndromes may occur in isolation as described above or may represent one component of a multisystem paraneoplastic syndrome. This usually occurs within the context of paraneoplastic encephalomyelitis (PEM), often associated with the Hu antibody in CSF and/or serum. In one series, 20% of 71 patients with anti-Hu (+) PEM patients had a recognized LMN component.[93] In further support of the existence of a paraneoplastic LMN syndrome is the knowledge that these Hu antibodies cross react with malignancy and with motor neurons.[80] Although the majority of reported cases of paraneoplastic MNDs preferentially affected LMNs, other motor neuron syndromes (e.g., ALS, PLS, and SPS) have been described as paraneoplastic syndromes as well.[72,75,76] A relationship between ALS and cancer has been long debated.[94] This association has been particularly emphasized in lymphoproliferative disorders. Currently, the association is considered coincidental although a prevalence of cancer of up to 8%–10% in an ALS population has been reported.[95,96] The SPS phenotype frequently overlaps with PLS with the exception of a more typically indolent course in PLS. These paraneoplastic PLS/SPS cases may be associated with breast cancer or lymphoma and amphiphysin antibodies.[76,97]

Paraneoplastic MNDs may respond to successful treatment of the underlying neoplasm in some cases.[77] Insufficient evidence exists to adequately predict treatment responsiveness in these rare syndromes.

SUBACUTE MOTOR NEURONOPATHY

SMN is another presumed MND associated with Hodgkin or non-Hodgkin lymphoma and/or their treatments.[98] Although first described in single case reports, the most comprehensive description was provided by a review of 10 cases in 1979. Eighty percent of these cases had been radiated. Most, but not all, had received differing chemotherapy regimens as well. SMN appears to differ from RIMND in three notable ways, the type of underlying malignancy, the phenotype, and the natural history.

Like RIMND, the pattern of weakness in SMN is notable for its asymmetry. Unlike RIMND, the distribution appears to be more generalized. It may begin in the arms and frequently affects the upper extremities and neck muscles in addition to the legs. At least one of the originally described cases had prominent UMN signs suggesting ALS, although on autopsy, these clinical findings were likely explicable by the demonstration of superimposed progressive multifocal leukoencephalopathy.[98] Differing natural histories also distinguish SMN from RIMND. SMN is characterized by a period of initial progression followed by stabilization. After months or years, significant improvement and even normalization of patient strength may occur.

CSF analysis in SMN may either be normal or demonstrate a modest elevation in protein levels. Reported EDX patterns are typical of MND. Nerve biopsy results, when reported, are normal further supporting an anterior or nerve root localization. Muscle biopsy in reported cases uniformly describe the neurogenic features of angular atrophy in individual fibers and/or in small groups. The pathologic findings in autopsied cases have not been uniform which is understandable in view of the complex nature of the described cases with their associated confounding variables. In both cases in which autopsied findings were described, however, the construct of an MND was supported by significant cell loss in the anterior horns with associated ventral root atrophy. Remaining motor neurons often demonstrated angular atrophy of anterior horn cells, and clumped Nissl substance or eosinophilic staining within them. As SMN patients are immunosuppressed, there is increased theoretical vulnerability of infection from organisms with tropism for anterior horns. For this reason, it is important to note reported absence of microgliosis or any evidence of inflammation or superimposed infection in anterior horns in SMN patients.[98]

OTHER LMN SYNDROMES ASSOCIATED WITH MALIGNANCY

There are a number of neuromuscular syndromes that typically affect the peripheral nerve, root, or plexus rather than the anterior horn cell that are usually readily distinguishable from MND based on clinical or EDX patterns. On certain occasions, these other syndromes may have LMN predominance making the distinction more difficult. For sake of completeness, these disorders will be briefly mentioned here. GBS appears to occur more frequently in certain malignancies, particularly lymphoma.[75] In one of its forms, acute motor axonal neuropathy, there is little or no sensory involvement which could confound the distinction from an MND. Neurolymphomatosis, that is, infiltration of peripheral nerve by lymphoma, is predominantly associated with non-Hodgkin lymphoma. Typically, there is associated pain and sensory loss. The phenotype is variable extending from a progressive mononeuropathy to regional neuropathy syndromes such as a radiculoplexopathy to a more generalized polyneuropathy that undoubtedly represents a confluent, multifocal neuropathy.[73,99–101] Polyradiculopathy may occur from neoplastic meningitis from both solid tumors, lymphoma, and leukemia. It may also occur as a result of certain infections with predilection for nerve roots such as varicella zoster or cytomegalovirus in immunosuppressed individuals. It has also been suggested that the syndrome of multifocal motor neuropathy may occur in patients with lymphoma.[102]

► SUMMARY

This chapter addresses the MNDs that are neither inherited nor degenerative in etiology. Although poliomyelitis, the most notorious of these disorders, is hopefully a disorder of largely historical domestic interest, neurologists and physiatrists remain responsible for the care of many of the disease's victims. In addition, other less prevalent virions have the same apparent affinity for anterior horn cells and the capability of producing an identical or near-identical syndrome of AFP. Consequently, we should remain aware of both the acute and the chronic features of these "other MNDs" of infectious and noninfectious etiology.

REFERENCES

1. Alexander LN, Seward JF, Santibanez TA, et al. Vaccine policy changes and epidemiology of poliomyelitis in the United States. *JAMA*. 2004;292:1696–1701.
2. Jerath A, Reddy C, Jerath N, Johnson RT. Poliomyelitis. 2009. www.medlink.com
3. Plum F. Sensory loss with poliomyelitis. *Neurology*. 1956;6:166–172.
4. Foley KM, Beresford RH. Acute poliomyelitis beginning as transverse myelopathy. *Arch Neurol*. 1974;30:182–183.
5. Dalakas MC. Pathogenetic mechanisms of post-polio syndrome: morphological, electrophysiological, virological, and immunological correlations. *Ann N Y Acad Sci*. 1995;753:167–185.
6. Wyatt HV. Poliomyelitis in hypogammaglobulinemics. *J Infect Dis*. 1973;128:802–806.
7. Wright PF, Hatch MH, Kasselberg AG, Lowry SP, Wadlington WB, Karzon DT. Vaccine-associated poliomyelitis in a child with sex-linked agammaglobulinemia. *J Pediatr*. 1977;91:408–412.
8. Mehrabi Z, Shahmahmoodi S, Eshraghian MR, et al. Molecular detection of different types of non-polio enteroviruses in acute flaccid paralysis cases and healthy children, a pilot study. *J Clin Virol*. 2011;50(2):181–182.
9. Dias APM, Tavares FN, Costa EV, da Silva EE. Evaluation of a protocol for rapid diagnosis of enterovirus associated with acute flaccid paralysis cases. *J Clin Virol*. 2009;46(4):337–340.
10. Kincaid O, Lipton HL. Viral myelitis: an update. *Curr Neurol Neurosci Rep*. 2006;6(6):469–474.
11. Johnson RT, Cornblath DR. Poliomyelitis and flavivirus. *Ann Neurol*. 2003;53(6):691–692.
12. Ghosh JB, Roy M, Lahiri K, Bala AK, Roy M. Acute flaccid paralysis due to rabies. *J Pediatr Neurosci*. 2009;4(1):33–35.
13. Verma A, Berger JR. ALS syndrome in patients with HIV-1 infection. *J Neurol Sci*. 2006;240:59–64.
14. Quereshi M, Bedlack RS, Cudkowicz ME. Lyme disease serology in amyotrophic lateral sclerosis. *Muscle Nerve*. 2009;40:626–628.
15. Kornreich L, Dagan I, Gunebaum M. MRI in acute poliomyelitis. *Neuroradiology*. 1996;38:371–372.
16. Haq A, Wasay M. Magnetic resonance imaging in poliomyelitis. *Arch Neurol*. 2006;63(5):778.
17. Jubelt B, Gallez-Hawkins G, Narayan O, Johnson RT. Pathogenesis of human poliovirus infection in mice. I. Clinical and pathological studies. *J Neuropathol Exp Neurol*. 1980;39:138–148.
18. Erb IH. Pathology of poliomyelitis. *Can Med Assoc J*. 1931;25(5):547–551.
19. Ford DJ, Ropka SL, Collins GH, Jubelt B. The neuropathology observed in wild-type mice inoculated with human poliovirus mirrors human paralytic poliomyelitis. *Microb Pathog*. 2002;33:97–107.
20. Fuchs A, Cella M, Giurisato E, Shaw AS, Colonna M. Cutting edge: CD96 (tactile) promotes NK cell-target cell adhesion by interacting with the poliovirus receptor (CD155). *J Immun*. 2004;172:3994–3998.
21. Koopman FS, Uegaki K, Gilhus NE, Beelen A, de Visser M, Nollet F. Treatment for postpolio syndrome. *Cochrane Database Syst Rev*. 2011;(2):CD007818.
22. Walid MS, Mahmoud FA. Successful treatment with intravenous immunoglobulin of acute flaccid paralysis caused by West Nile virus. *Perm J*. 2009;13(3):43–46.
23. Jeha LE, Sila CA, Lederman RJ, Prayson RA, Isada CM, Gordon SM. West Nile virus infection: a new acute paralytic illness. *Neurology*. 2003;61:55–59.
24. Lanska DJ. West Nile virus. https://www.medlink.com/articles/west-nile-virus.
25. Al-Shekhlee A, Katirji B. Electrodiagnostic features of acute paralytic poliomyelitis associated with West Nile virus infection. *Muscle Nerve*. 2004;29:376–380.
26. Hassin-Baer S, Kirson ED, Shulman L, et al. Stiff-person syndrome following West Nile fever. *Arch Neurol*. 2004;61:938–941.
27. Flaherty ML, Wijdicks EFM, Stevens JC, et al. Clinical and electrophysiologic patterns of flaccid paralysis due to West Nile virus. *Mayo Clin Proc*. 2003;78:1245–1248.
28. Leis AA, Stokic DS, Webb RM, Slavinski SA, Fratkin J. Clinical spectrum of muscle weakness in human West Nile virus infection. *Muscle Nerve*. 2003;28:302–308.
29. Sejvar JJ, Haddad MB, Tierney BC, et al. Neurologic manifestations and outcome of West Nile virus infection. *JAMA*. 2003;290:511–515.
30. Sejvar JJ. West Nile virus and "poliomyelitis." *Neurology*. 2004;63:206–207.
31. Leis AA, Stokic DS, Polk JL, Dostrow V, Winkelmann M. A poliomyelitis-like syndrome from West Nile virus infection. *N Engl J Med*. 2002;347(16):1278–1280.
32. Glass JD, Samuels O, Rich MM. Poliomyelitis due to West Nile virus. *N Engl J Med*. 2002;347(16):1280–1281.
33. Kelley TW, Prayson RA, Isada CM. Spinal cord disease in West Nile virus infection. *N Engl J Med*. 2003;348:564–566.
34. Li J, Loeb JA, Shy ME, et al. Asymmetric flaccid paralysis: a neuromuscular presentation of West Nile virus infection. *Ann Neurol*. 2003;53:703–710.
35. Park M, Hui JS, Bartt RE. Acute anterior radiculitis associated with West Nile virus infection. *J Neurol Neurosurg Psychiatry*. 2003;74:823–825.

36. Roos KL. Fever and asymmetrical weakness in the summer: evidence of a West Nile virus-associated poliomyelitis-like illness. *Mayo Clin Proc.* 2003;78(19):1205-1206.
37. Petropoulou KA, Gordon SM, Prayson RA, Ruggierri PM. West Nile virus meningoencephalitis: MR imaging finding. *AJNR Am J Neuroradiol.* 2005;26(8):1986-1995.
38. Tyler KL, Pape J, Goody RJ, Corkill M, Kleinschmidt-DeMasters BK. CSF findings in 250 patients with serologically confirmed West Nile virus meningitis and encephalitis. *Neurology.* 2006;66(3):361-365.
39. Centers for Disease Control and Prevention. *Epidemic/epizootic West Nile virus in the United States: Guidelines for Surveillance, Prevention, and Control.* U.S. Department of Health and Human Services; 2003.
40. Roos KL. West Nile encephalitis and myelitis. *Curr Opin Neurol.* 2004;17(3):343-346.
41. Doron SI, Dashe JF, Adelman LS, Brown WF, Werner BG, Hadley S. Histopathologically proven poliomyelitis with quadriplegia and loss of brainstem function due to West Nile virus infection. *Clin Infect Dis.* 2003;37:e74-e77.
42. Smit JM, Moesker B, Rodenhuis-Zybert I, Wilschut J. Flavivirus cell entry and membrane fusion. *Viruses.* 2011;3(2):160-171.
43. Chan-Tack KM, Forrest G. Failure of interferon alpha-2b in a patient with West Nile virus meningoencephalitis and acute flaccid paralysis. *Scand J Infect Dis.* 2005;37(11-12):944-946.
44. Anderson JF, Rahal JJ. Efficacy of interferon alpha-2b and ribavirin against West Nile virus in vitro. *Emerg Infect Dis.* 2002;8(1):107-108.
45. Lewis M, Amsden JR. Successful treatment of West Nile virus infection after approximately 3 weeks into the disease course. *Pharmacotherapy.* 2007;27(3):455-458.
46. Hayes EB, Sejvar JJ, Zaki SR, Lanciotti RS, Bode AV, Campbell GL. Virology, pathology, and clinical manifestations of West Nile virus disease. *Emerg Infect Dis.* 2005;11:1174-1179.
47. Dalakas MC, Elder G, Hallett M, et al. A long-term follow-sup study of patients with post-poliomyelitis neuromuscular symptoms. *N Engl J Med.* 1986;314:959-963.
48. Codd MB, Mulder DW, Kurland LT, Berard CM, O'Fallon WM. Poliomyelitis in Rochester, Minnesota, 1935-1955: Epidemiology and long-term sequelae. A preliminary report. In: Halstead LS, Wiechers DO, eds. *Late Effects of Poliomyelitis.* Symposia Foundation; 1985:121-134.
49. Windebank AJ, Litchy WJ, Daube JR, Kurland LT, Codd MB, Iverson R. Late effects of paralytic poliomyelitis in Olmsted County, Minnesota. *Neurology.* 1991;41:501-507.
50. Bruno RL. Post-polio sequelae: research and treatment in the second decade. *Orthopedics.* 1991;14(11): 1169-1170.
51. Mathis S, Dumas P, Neau JP, Gil R. Pure motor neuropathy, an uncommon complication of radiotherapy: report of 3 cases and review of the literature. *Rev Med Interne.* 2007;28(6):377-387.
52. Halstead LS, Diechers DL, Rossi CD. Late effects of poliomyelitis: A national survey. In: Halstead LS, Wiechers DO, eds. *Late Effects of Poliomyelitis.* Symposia Foundation; 1985:11-33.
53. Jubelt B, Cashman NR. Neurological manifestations of the post-polio syndrome. *Crit Rev Neurobiol.* 1987;3:199-220.
54. Klingman J, Chui H, Corgiat M, Perry J. Functional recovery. A major risk factor for the development of postpoliomyelitis muscular atrophy. *Arch Neurol.* 1998;45:645-647.
55. Trojan DA, Cashman NR, Shapiro S, Tansey CM, Esdaile JM. Predictive factors for post-poliomyelitis syndrome. *Arch Phys Med Rehabil.* 1994;75:770-777.
56. Bach JR, Alba AS, Bodofsky E, Curran FJ, Schulteiss M. Glossopharyngeal breathing and noninvasive aids in the management of post-polio respiratory insufficiency. *Birth Defects Orig Artic Ser.* 1987;23(4):99-113.
57. Mulder DW, Rosenbaum RA, Layton DD Jr. Late progression of poliomyelitis or forme fruste amyotrophic lateral sclerosis? *Mayo Clin Proc.* 1972;47:756-761.
58. Sorenson EJ, Daube JR, Windebank AJ. A 15-yr follow up of neuromuscular function in patients with prior poliomyelitis. *Neurology.* 2005;64:1079-1072.
59. Windebank AJ, Litchy WJ, Daube JR, Iverson R. Lack of progression of neurologic deficit in survivors of paralytic polio: a 5-year prospective population-based study. *Neurology.* 1996;46:80-84.
60. Gibson SB. Post-polio Syndrome. https://www.medlink.com/articles/post-polio-syndrome.
61. Guilleminault C, Motta J. Sleep apnea syndrome as a long-term sequela of poliomyelitis. In: Guilleminault C, ed. *Sleep Apnea Syndromes.* Alan R Liss; 1978:309-315.
62. Siegel H, McCutchen C, Dalakas M, et al. Physiologic events initiating REM sleep in patients with the postpolio syndrome. *Neurology.* 1999;52:516-522.
63. Gawne AC, Halstead LS. Post-polio syndrome: pathophysiology and clinical management. *Crit Rev Phys Rehabil Med.* 1995;7:147-188.
64. Roos RP, Viola MV, Wollmann R, Hatch MH, Antel JP. Amyotrophic lateral sclerosis with antecedent poliomyelitis. *Arch Neurol.* 1980;37:312-313.
65. Salajegheh M, Bryan WW, Dalakas MC. The challenge of diagnosing ALS in patients with prior poliomyelitis. *Neurology.* 2006;67:1078-1079.
66. Cashman NR, Maselli R, Wollmann RL, Roos R, Simon R, Antel JP. Late denervation in patients with antecedent paralytic poliomyelitis. *N Engl J Medi.* 1987;317(1):7-12.
67. Nelson KR. Creatine kinase and fibrillation potentials in patients with late sequelae of polio. *Muscle Nerve.* 1990;13(8):722-725.
68. Ravits J, Hallett M, Baker M, Nilsson J, Dalakas MC. Clinical and electromyographic studies of postpoliomyelitis muscular atrophy. *Muscle Nerve.* 1990;13:667-674.
69. Gonzalez H, Ottervald J, Nilsson KC, et al. Identification of novel candidate protein biomarkers for the post-polio syndrome: implications for diagnosis, neurodegeneration and neuroinflammation. *J Proteomics.* 2009;71(6):670-681.
70. Semino-Mora C, Dalakas MC. Rimmed vacuoles with beta-amyloid and ubiquitinated filamentous deposits in the muscles of patients with long-standing denervation (postpoliomyelitis muscular atrophy): similarities with inclusion body myositis. *Hum Pathol.* 1998;29(10):1128-1133.
71. Julien J, Leparc-Goffart I, Lina B, et al. Postpolio syndrome: poliovirus persistence is involved in the pathogenesis. *J Neurol.* 1999;246(6):472-476.
72. Younger DS, Rowland LP, Latov N, et al. Lymphoma, motor neuron diseases, and amyotrophic lateral sclerosis. *Ann Neurol.* 1991;29:78-86.
73. Kelly JJ, Karcher DS. Lymphoma and peripheral neuropathy: a clinical review. *Muscle Nerve.* 2005;31:301-313.
74. Gordon PH, Rowland LP, Younger DS, et al. Lymphoproliferative disorders and motor neuron disease: an update. *Neurology.* 1997;48:1671-1678.

75. Rudnicki SA, Dalmau J. Paraneoplastic syndromes of the spinal cord, nerve, and muscle. *Muscle Nerve*. 2000;23:1800–1818.
76. Forsyth PA, Dalmau J, Graus F, Cwik V, Rosenblum MK, Posner JB. Motor neuron syndromes in cancer patients. *Ann Neurol*. 1997;41:722–730.
77. Rowland LP. Diagnosis of amyotrophic lateral sclerosis. *J Neurol Sci*. 1998;160(Suppl 1):S6–S24.
78. Stern BV, Baehring JM, Kleopa KA, Hochberg FH. Multifocal motor neuropathy with conduction block associated with metastatic lymphoma of the nervous system. *J Neurooncol*. 2006;78(1):81–84.
79. Briani C, Vitaliani R, Grisold W, et al. Spectrum of paraneoplastic disease associated with lymphoma. *Neurology*. 2011;76:705–710.
80. Younger DS. Motor neuron disease and malignancy. *Muscle Nerve*. 2000;23:658–660.
81. Van den Berg-Vos RM, Van den Berg LH, Visser J, de Visser M, Franssen H, Wokke JH. The spectrum of lower motor neuron syndromes. *J Neurol*. 2003;250:1279–1292.
82. Greenfield MM, Stark FM. Post-irradiation neuropathy. *AJR Am Roentgenol*. 1948;60:617–622.
83. Lamy C, Mas JL, Varet B, Ziegler M, de Recondo J. Postradiation lower motor neuron syndrome presenting as monomelic amyotrophy. *J Neurol Neurosurg Psychiatry*. 1991;347:648–649.
84. Walton JN, Tomlinson BE, Pearce GW. Subacute "poliomyelitis" and Hodgkin's disease. *J Neurol Sci*. 1068;6:435–445.
85. Tallaksen CM, Jetne V, Fosså S. Postradiation lower motor neuron syndrome–a case report and brief literature review. *Acta Oncol*. 1997;36(3):345–347.
86. Sadowsky CH, Sachs E, Ochoa J. Post-radiation motor neuron syndrome. *Arch Neurol*. 1976;33:786–786.
87. Horowitz SL, Stewart JD. Lower motor neuron syndrome following radiotherapy. *Can J Neurol Sci*. 1983;10:56–58.
88. Bowen J, Gregory R, Squier M, Donaghy M. The post-irradiation lower motor neuron syndrome neuronopathy or radiculopathy? *Brain*. 1996;119:1429–1439.
89. Malapert D, Brugieres P, Degos JD. Motor neuron syndrome in arms after radiation treatment. *J Neurol Neurosurg Psychiatry*. 1991;54:1123–1124.
90. Shapiro BE, Bordorf G, Schwann L, Preston DC. Delayed radiation-induced bulbar palsy. *Neurology*. 1996;46:1604–1606.
91. DeCarolis P, Montagna P, Cipulli M, Baldrati A, d'Alessandro R, Sacquegna T. Isolated lower motorneuron involvement following radiotherapy. *J Neurol Neurosurg Psychiatry*. 1986;49:718–719.
92. Cavanagh JB. Effects of x-radiation on the proliferation of cells in peripheral nerve during wallerian degeration in the rat. *Br J Radiol*. 1968;41:275–281.
93. Dalmau J, Graus F, Rosenblum MK, Posner JB. Anti-Hu associated paraneoplastic encephalomyelitis/sensory neuronopathy. A clinical study of 71 patients. *Medicine*. 1992;71:59–72.
94. Rowland LP. Paraneoplastic primary lateral sclerosis and amyotrophic lateral sclerosis. *Ann Neurol*. 1997;41(6):703–705.
95. Norris FR Jr, Engel WK. Carcinomatous amyotrophic lateral sclerosis. In: Brain WR, Norris FH Jr, eds. *The Remote Effects of Cancer on the Nervous System*. Grune and Statton; 1965:24–34.
96. Gubbay SS, Kahana E, Zilber N, Cooper G, Pintov S, Leibowitz Y. Amyotrophic lateral sclerosis. A study of its presentation and prognosis. *J Neurol*. 1985;232:295–300.
97. McKeon A, Robinson MT, McEvoy KM, et al. Stiff-man syndrome and variants: clinical course, treatments, and outcomes. *Arch Neurol*. 2012;69(2):230–238.
98. Schold SC, Cho ES, Somasundaram M, Posner JV. Subacute motor neuronopathy: a remote effect of lymphoma. *Ann Neurol*. 1979;5:271–287.
99. Viala K, Béhin A, Maisonobe T, et al. Neuropathy in lymphoma: a relationship between the pattern of neuropathy, type of lymphoma and prognosis. *J Neurol Neurosurg Psychiatry*. 2008;79:778–782.
100. Walk D, Handelsman A, Beckmann E, Kozloff M, Shapiro C. Mononeuropathy multiplex due to infiltration of lymphoma in hematologic remission. *Muscle Nerve* 1998;21:823–826.
101. Diaz-Arrastia R, Younger DS, Hair L, et al. Neurolymphomatosis: a clinicopathologic syndrome re-emerges. *Neurology*. 1992;42:1136–1141.
102. Noguchi M, Mori K, Yamazaki S, Suda K, Sato N, Oshimi K. Multifocal motor neuropathy caused by a B-cell lymphoma producing a monoclonal IgM autoantibody against peripheral nerve myelin glycolipids GM1 and GD1B. *Br J Haemotol*. 2003;123:600–605.

CHAPTER 10

Disorders of Motor Nerve Hyperactivity

Complaints referable to muscle such as pain, spasm, stiffness, fatigue, and/or abnormal movements within a muscle are commonplace in the practice of medicine. As the cause is often elusive, both patients and physicians may become frustrated as many with these complaints will remain undiagnosed despite thorough investigation. There are many sources for this diagnostic elusiveness. With the exception of cramps and fasciculations, the disorders described in this chapter are uncommon. In addition, most of the disorders that will be described have nonspecific and overlapping clinical features. Successful diagnosis requires a heightened index of clinical suspicion, detailed knowledge concerning each disorder's phenotypic characteristics, and awareness of the serologic and electrodiagnostic (EDX) features of each syndrome.

Motor nerve hyperactivity disorders frequently result in reduced exercise intolerance and impaired mobility. They originate from numerous central and neuromuscular system localizations. This chapter will restrict itself to disorders thought to originate from motor nerves and the upper motor neurons that control them. Cramps, fasciculations, tetany, tetanus, the cramp–fasciculation syndrome (CFS), Isaacs syndrome, Satoyoshi syndrome, stiff person syndrome (SPS), and hyperekplexia will all be discussed.[1,2] As the differential diagnosis of many of these disorders overlaps, the majority of the differential diagnostic considerations will be primarily emphasized in the first section devoted to muscle cramping.

Historical writings on motor nerve hyperactivity disorders have been potentially confusing. Different names have been used for the same syndrome. Nomenclature to describe clinical observations has overlapped with that used to describe frequently associated electromyographic waveforms. In an attempt to avoid this, and as neurologists deeply appreciative of history and those who created it, we will be preferentially referring to these syndromes by their eponyms whenever appropriate.

▶ CRAMPS, FASCICULATIONS, AND CRAMP–FASCICULATION SYNDROME

CLINICAL FEATURES

Cramps refer to a sudden, involuntary, and painful shortening of an entire muscle belly accompanied by a squeezing sensation and visible, palpable muscle induration.[3,4] As cramps tend to incorporate multiple if not all the motor units in one or more muscles, they typically generate sufficient force to induce abnormal posturing of relevant joints. Cramps are characteristically relieved by massage or stretching. They tend to recur if the muscle is prematurely returned to its unstretched position. They will spontaneously remit within minutes in most cases.

Cramps occur commonly. Their prevalence in a "normal" population is estimated at 35% in one study and in 95% of young, healthy people who recently initiated exercise in another.[3,4] Their prevalence is increased in the elderly, in pregnant females, and subsequent to exercise in those who have recently begun unaccustomed activity. Cramps are a considerable source of morbidity for afflicted individuals, particularly if nocturnal. In the majority of cases however, they are not associated with serious disease and considered benign. Benign cramps are most prevalent in the calf. Familial cramp syndromes have been reported.

Pathologic cramps as a symptom of an underlying neuromuscular disease are less common.[5,6] Although potentially representative of nerve or nerve root diseases, their most notorious association is with the motor neuron diseases (MNDs). In MND, they are frequently mentioned in passing and represent a minor component of the illness in most but may represent a significant source of morbidity in some. Like fasciculations, they tend to dissipate as the disease progresses.

In general, benign cramps occur at rest or following exercise. In our experience, cramping provoked by manual muscle testing occurs with some regularity in MND patients. Exertional cramping during protracted or intense exercise is more typically associated with metabolic muscle disease.

Fasciculations, unlike cramps, represent the discreet, random contraction of the muscle fibers in an individual motor unit. Unlike cramps, the patient may not be aware of them. As fasciculations represent activation of a single motor unit, movement at a relevant joint is uncommon. In our experience, if movement at a joint occurs, it tends to be seen in situations where reinnervated and enlarged motor units act on a small joint (i.e., the first dorsal interosseous on the metacarpophalangeal joint of the index finger). Fasciculations, when occurring in isolation, are typically benign. Characteristics of benign fasciculations are their tendency to occur repetitively for seconds at a single site, in a single muscle. Randomly occurring fasciculations throughout face and body are also suggestive of a benign process. Disconcerting signs are when fasciculations are evident in an atrophic and weakness muscle as well as when accompanied by pathogenic hyperreflexia.

Cramps and fasciculations occurring in together are also a cause for concern and increase the likelihood of an underlying neuromuscular disease, particularly when not localized to a singular muscle like the calf. This association may suggest CFS in which patients experience myalgias, cramps, stiffness, myokymia, and fasciculations in some combination.[7] The symptoms of CFS are frequently provoked by exercise and promote exercise intolerance. Patients can find these disabling. CFS may be conceptualized as a limited expression of Isaacs syndrome with which it may share not only clinical but serologic and/or electrophysiologic features.[8,9]

DIAGNOSIS AND DIFFERENTIAL DIAGNOSIS

Muscle cramps remain a largely clinical diagnosis dependent for the most part on patient description. Differential diagnostic strategies are twofold: (1) to distinguish cramps from other causes of unwanted muscle contraction and pain and (2) to identify an underlying cause for the cramping. Cramps represent one of many potential causes of myalgia or muscle pain.

The differential diagnosis of cramps includes disorders originating from the central nervous system (CNS) and other neuromuscular locations. Although the mechanism of unwanted muscle activation is not fully understood in many of the following disorders, it may be accurate to conceptualize neural disorders of involuntary muscle contraction as positive events resulting from a lower threshold for nerve activation or prolonged depolarization. In contrast, myopathies producing unwanted muscle contraction may be considered as a negative phenomenon, that is, a failure of muscle relaxation after voluntary activation. Myopathies capable of producing involuntary muscle contraction, myalgia, or/and stiffness will be covered more extensively in later chapters of this textbook but will be briefly mentioned here for completeness.

Myotonia may be considered as the prototypic disorder of failed muscle relaxation. Myotonia differs from benign cramps in that it is typically painless and provoked by muscle activation. Myotonia is characterized by a completely different EDX signature, that is, myotonic as opposed to cramp discharges demonstrable with needle electromyography.

As described above, metabolic myopathies may produce unwanted muscle contraction, induration and myalgia by physiologic contracture. These inherited defects result in most cases from impaired glycogen metabolism, leading to muscle energy failure, and resulting in painful muscle shortening. Intense or protracted exercise is typically required to deplete readily available muscle fuel sources and provoke contractures. Physiologic contractures are also distinguished from cramps by their EDX signature of electrical silence which is also a feature of rippling muscle disease (RMD) and Brody disease.

RMD is clinically defined by observation of wave-like rippling of muscles, typically provoked by muscle stretch or percussion. Patients may complain of muscle stiffness and muscle hypertrophy may be observed on examination.[10] RMD can be inherited in an autosomal dominant fashion caused by mutations of the caveolin-3 gene, *CAV3* (see Chapter 27 for further discussion regarding the evaluation of the numerous phenotypes associated with mutations of in *CAV3*). RMD may also occur as an acquired disorder in association with myasthenia gravis (MG), thymoma, and AChR antibodies.[10–12] Recently, antibodies have been found to be directed against autoantibody specific to caveolae-associated protein 4 (cavin-4) that localizes to T-tubules where it interacts with cavelin-3.[12] Unlike disorders of motor nerve hyperactivity, the EDX signature of rippling muscles is electrical silence. The EDX examination, however, may identify features of an underlying myopathy. Patients with RMD typically have a 3–25-fold increase in their serum CK levels.

Brody disease is another rare, inherited myopathy producing physiologic contractures through disruption of calcium reuptake within the sarcoplasmic reticulum of muscle (see Chapter 32).[13–15] It results from a mutation in the fast-twitch skeletal muscle sarcoplasmic reticulum Ca–ATPase gene (*SERCA1*).[15] Its morbidity stems from impaired muscle relaxation that is exercise induced, associated with stiffness affecting muscle of the limbs and face. A more detailed description may be found in Chapter 32 regarding nondystrophic myotonias and periodic paralysis. Cold may aggravate the symptoms of Brody disease as it may aggravate the stiffness associated with myotonic disorders.

Malignant hyperthermia and neuroleptic malignant syndrome are other disorders resulting in unwanted muscle rigidity, typically recognized by associated signs and symptoms and the context in which they occur. Malignant hyperthermia is an inherited disorder and, like Brody disease, represents disordered sarcoplasmic reticulum function. The neuroleptic malignant syndrome appears to be related to dopaminergic receptor dysfunction, presumably within the CNS.

The palmaris brevis syndrome is characterized by a spontaneous, irregular, non-painful contraction of the palmaris brevis muscle resulting in "wrinkling" motions of the palm.[16] It has been associated with C8–T1 radiculopathy, pathology of the deep branch of the ulnar nerve in Guyon canal, and occupational risk. The EDX features of the palmaris brevis syndrome have been reported as spontaneous rapid discharges of single motor unit action potentials (MUAPs) of normal morphology and myokymic discharges associated with normal motor and sensory conduction studies.

Focal dystonias such as writer's cramp produce unwanted muscle contraction and are uncomfortable, although are typically not as painful as cramps. They are most readily identified by the characteristic activities that provoke them.

The characteristic features of all of these disorders are involuntary muscle contraction and the stiffness that may accompany it. Many of these disorders are accompanied by discomfort or pain. The differential diagnosis of disorders that are dominated by generalized or focal myalgias, unassociated with unwanted muscle contraction, stiffness, and movement is far more extensive and exceeds the scope of this book.

The differential diagnosis of cramps also has to take into consideration whether the cramps are primary or secondary in their etiology. The latter is defined by their association with another underlying illness. Primary cramping occurs with the greatest frequency in calf and intrinsic foot muscles and as previously mentioned in older individuals, often at rest (particularly at night) or following unaccustomed exercise. Volume depletion is generally considered a benign cause of cramping that may be related in turn to exercise, hemodialysis, emesis, diarrhea, and diuretic use.

Secondary cramping (Table 10-1) associates with a variety of toxic or metabolic disturbances and the MNDs. These associated conditions are identified through careful history taking, and by clinical, EDX, and judicious laboratory assessment. Metabolic conditions associated with cramping include hypoadrenalism, hypothyroidism, pregnancy, uremia, and cirrhosis. Cramps may also be hereditary in nature, either related or unrelated to a definable disease. Cramps may be provoked by a number of medications (Table 10-1). Finally, cramps and fasciculations are most commonly associated with disorders of anterior horn cells and, to a lesser extent, neuropathy and radiculopathy.

LABORATORY FEATURES

The EDX evaluation of patients with suspected cramps is done primarily to exclude secondary causes of cramping such as MND or to identify other forms of spontaneous discharges that might suggest an alternative cause of motor nerve hyperactivity. The EDX signature of cramping is the cramp discharge, an involuntary, often irregular and "sputtering" discharge of multiple, normal appearing MUAPs. Cramp discharges begin abruptly and fire at a collective frequency of up to 150 Hz. Cramp discharges are most commonly encountered in normal individuals during activation of the gastrocnemius muscle. They are usually readily identifiable by both their morphologic characteristics and firing pattern. The discharges are made up of multiple, normal MUAPs. Like the cramp itself, the number of MUAPs contributing to the cramp discharge builds up and then dissipates. Fasciculation potentials may be recognizable both at the initial and terminal portions of cramp potentials.

In SPS and tetanus, there are many more MUAP discharges that are continuous without the aforementioned crescendo–decrescendo pattern. A more commonly occurring potential EDX mimic of cramp potentials is normal, voluntarily activated MUAPs in patients who have an underlying tremor or are experiencing respiratory alkalosis related to anxiety or hyperventilation. MUAPs in this situation are also normal but differ as they are voluntarily activated and discharge in clusters. Once again, the similarities are based on waveform morphology, not firing pattern. End-plate potentials are the waveform most likely to be confused with cramp

▶ **TABLE 10-1. CAUSES OF MUSCLE CRAMPING, FASCICULATION, STIFFNESS**

By localization
  CNS
  • Dystonia
  Brain/Spinal cord
  • Stiff-person syndrome
  • Tetanus
  • Demyelination (e.g., multiple sclerosis)
  Anterior horn cell diseases
  • ALS
  • Spinal muscular atrophy
  • Postpolio syndrome
  Radiculopathy
  • Compressive—discogenic/spondylotic, tumor
  • Tumor infiltration
  • Nonstructural (e.g., diabetes mellitus, sarcoidosis, infection, radiation induced)
  Peripheral Nerve
  • Cramp-fasciculation syndrome
  • Isaacs syndrome
  • Polyneuropathy
  • Tetany
  • Palmaris brevis syndrome
  Muscle (not fasciculations but cramping and stiffness)
  • Rippling muscle disease
  • Dystrophic and nondystrophic myotonias
  • Metabolic muscle diseases (glycogen storage, lipid storage, mitochondrial)
  • Brody disease
  Uncertain
  • Satoyoshi syndrome

By etiology
  Benign
  • Advanced age
  • Postexercise
  • Pregnancy
  Metabolic
  • Hypocalcemia
  • Hypomagnesemia
  • Hypothyroidism
  • Hypoadrenalism
  • Uremia
  • Cirrhosis
  • Dialysis
  • Dehydration with electrolyte loss
  Medication (common)
  • Diuretics
  • Cholesterol-lowering agents
  • β-adrenergic agonists
  • H_2 receptor blockers
  • Nifedipine
  • Ethanol

discharges based upon firing pattern. They discharge with the same sputtering pattern as cramp discharges, but their waveform morphology is readily distinguishable.

The EDX signatures of other disorders of muscle induration and stiffness when symptomatic are typically distinctive. They include the electrical silence of the muscle diseases as described above, the myotonic discharges seen in the myotonic disorders, and the myokymic, grouped, and neuromyotonic discharges characteristic of Isaacs syndrome.

In a patient with true cramps, it would be reasonable to obtain blood for thyroid stimulating hormone (TSH), creatinine, magnesium, and calcium as well as to assess for orthostatic hypotension and serum potassium as screening tests for adrenal insufficiency. Genetic testing for familial forms of MND (ALS, spinal muscular atrophy) may be considered if warranted by clinical and EDX context. An elevation in serum CK in a patient with cramping may be more confounding than helpful. If cramps are persistent, an elevation of serum CK may occur and may take 3–8 days to normalize.[17] This is important to recognize so as to not assume CK elevations in this setting implicate an underlying myopathy.

Fasciculation potentials are readily recognized electromyographically by their morphology and firing pattern. They are MUAPs that fire individually in a random fashion unlike those that are voluntarily activated (Fig. 10-1). Consecutive fasciculation potentials usually represent different motor units. Like fasciculations, the distinction between benign and pathologic fasciculation potentials is in large part determined by the clinical and electrophysiologic company that they keep. Attempts to assign pathologic significance to fasciculation potentials based on their morphology has been described,[18–20] but in our opinion is of more academic than pragmatic clinical interest.

The EDX findings in CFS include fasciculation potentials, cramp discharges, multiplets, and even neuromyotonic discharges.[7,8] In addition, repetitive stimulation of peripheral nerves may produce after-discharges in some cases in a manner similar to Isaacs syndrome (Fig. 10-2).[8,21] Other EDX abnormalities including myokymic and complex repetitive discharges; fibrillation potentials and positive waves; and morphologic changes of MUAPs suggesting chronic partial denervation and reinnervation are typically notable for their absence.[7]

In patients with complaints of cramps and/or fasciculations, it is our tendency to be conservative in our testing unless there are historical or examination features of concern. A family history suggestive of neuromuscular disease, visible fasciculations, or other adventitious movements of muscle such as myokymia or muscle weakness/atrophy would be indications for EDX testing. We would reserve autoantibody testing for patients with clinical myokymia or EMG demonstrating neuromyotonic or myokymic discharges, thus raising the suspicion for Isaacs syndrome (see below).

HISTOPATHOLOGY

Patients with CFS may have features of neurogenic atrophy with muscle biopsy.[7] As neurogenic atrophy can be accurately and less invasively be predicted by electromyographic examination, and as muscle biopsy rarely identifies the etiology of the neurogenic condition, muscle biopsy is uncommonly performed in these patients.

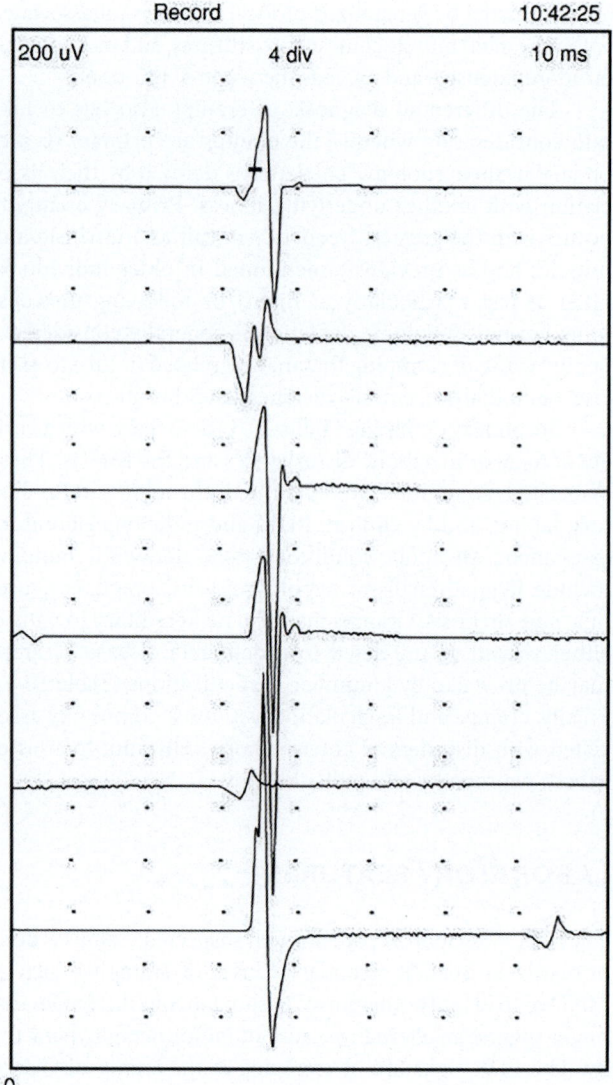

Figure 10-1. Fasciculation potential—single, random, and spontaneous discharges of normal appearing but differing motor unit action potentials.

PATHOGENESIS

The weight of experimental evidence supports a neurogenic origin for both cramps and fasciculations. Specifically, the generator appears to be located within distal nerve terminals. There are a number of lines of evidence to support this. Cramps can be provoked in normal humans by repetitive stimulation of motor nerves distal to a complete, pharmacologically induced nerve block. Cramps are often preceded and followed by fasciculation potentials, implicating a shared generator. The waveform morphology of cramp potentials is that of MUAP. This does not preclude a CNS generator but diminishes the likelihood of a muscle or neuromuscular generator. Cramps may seemingly occur in a single muscle at any given time, sparing other muscles in the same myotome, making a CNS generator unlikely.

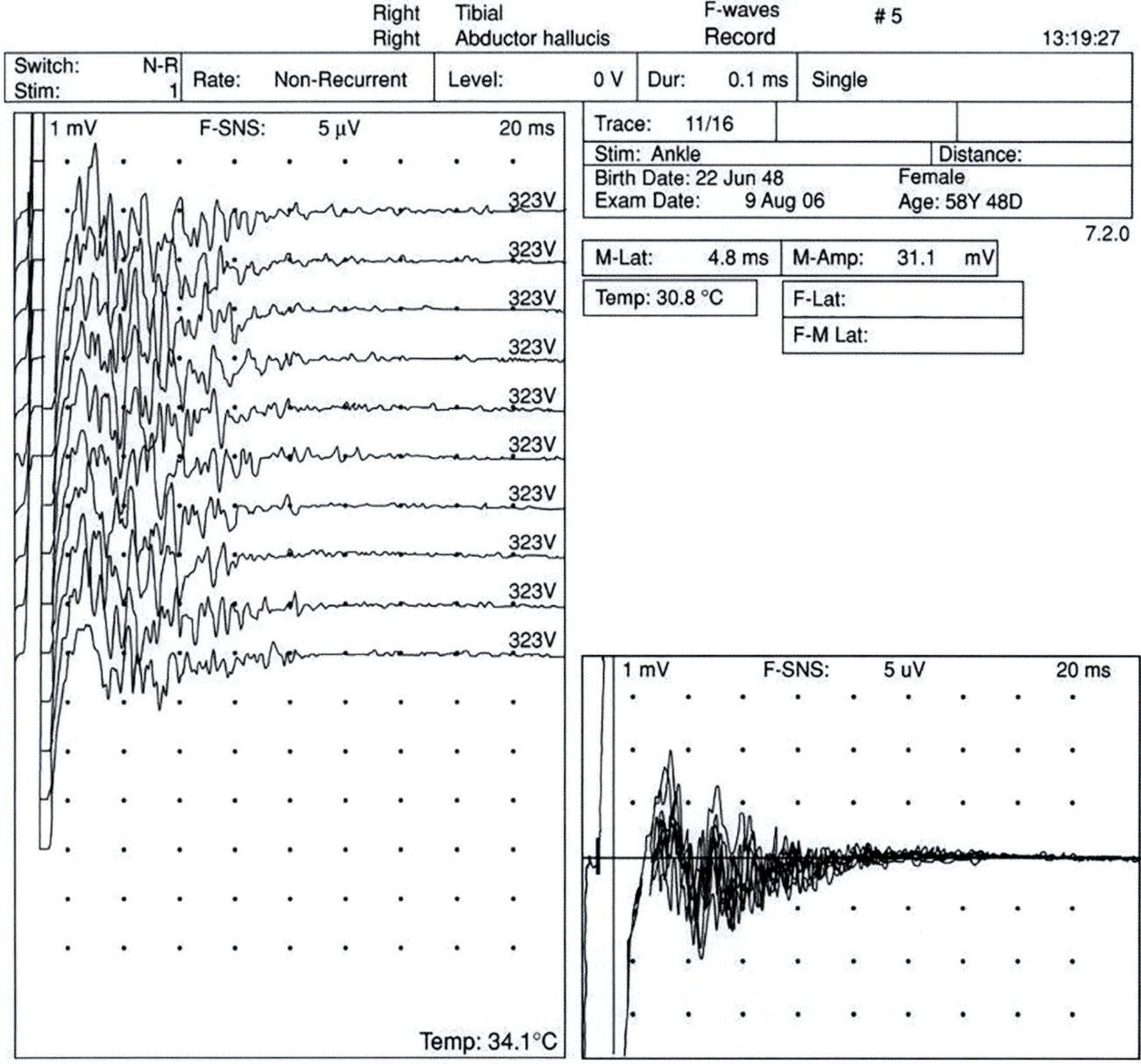

Figure 10-2. Rastered CMAPs from the tibial nerve in response to single stimuli resulting in repetitive after-discharges. (Used with permission of Dr. Steven Vernino, University of Texas Southwestern.)

Even though cramps occur more commonly in patients who are pregnant or who exercise, no measurable metabolic differences have been identified in either group compared to those who do not experience cramping.[3] Cramping has been precipitated by infusion of hypotonic fluids implicating fluid or solute movement between extracellular and intracellular compartments as the causative mechanism.[3]

TREATMENT

Evidence to guide clinicians in the prevention and treatment of cramps is limited and may be reviewed in an American Academy of Neurology (AAN) evidence-based publication.[17] Prevention of cramping related to exertion and fluid loss can be attempted with the prophylactic use of salt tablets, hydration, and routine or pre- or post-exercise stretching. Successful prevention of cramps occurring under other circumstances may be achieved with the avoidance of offending drugs or, when necessary, by using prophylactic medication.[3,17] Typically, these agents are dispensed preferentially at night, as sleep interruption is usually the most bothersome source of morbidity. Medications that have been used for this purpose are reviewed in Table 10-2. Of these, only quinine sulfate has achieved level A support as an efficacious treatment.[17] Unfortunately, the FDA considers the use of quinine to be associated with unacceptable risk for any condition except malaria.[22] The incidence of serious side effects with

► TABLE 10-2. DRUGS UTILIZED IN THE TREATMENT OF CRAMPS

Drug	Dosage Range	Comments	Common or Serious Adverse Effects/Monitoring
Drugs where adequate trials have been performed suggesting efficacy			
Mexiletine	150 mg bid	Level A support for efficacy with cramps related to ALS	Dizziness/lightheadedness
Quinine sulfate	324 mg qhs	Level A support for efficacy FDA warning against off-label use of quinine products (cramps) "Should be avoided for routine use in the management of muscle cramps because of the potential of toxicity, but in select patients they can be considered for an individual therapeutic trial once potential side effects are taken into account."	Nausea/vomiting Tremulousness Cinchonism (visual, auditory and GI symptoms, headache, fever) Prolonged QT interval Thrombotic thrombocytopenic purpura
Vitamin B complex	Including 30-mg pyridoxine	Level C support for efficacy	Lightheadedness Nausea Dyspepsia
Naftidrofuryl	300 mg bid	Level C support for efficacy	Not available in the United States
Diltiazem	30 mg qhs	Level C support for efficacy in frequency but not severity	No side effects reported at this dose
Drugs where trials have been performed suggesting inefficacy			
Gabapentin	3,600 mg/day	Class 1 study	Lightheadedness Drowsiness Limb swelling
Vitamin E	800 U qhs	No benefit suggested	
Magnesium citrate	900 mg	Class 2 study—no benefit suggested	Diarrhea Lightheadedness Nausea Dyspepsia
Magnesium sulfate	300 mg	Class 2 study—no benefit suggested	Diarrhea Lightheadedness Nausea Dyspepsia
Drugs utilized without benefit of adequate trials			
Baclofen	20–80 mg day	No adequate trials	Drowsiness
Levetiracetam	500–1,500 mg bid	Benefit in cramp frequency and severity in open-label trial of ALS patients	Drowsiness
Verapamil	120 mg qhs	Benefit in cramp frequency in unblended elderly population	
Carbamazepine	200 mg bid–tid	Anecdotal benefit	Leukopenia Transaminitis Hyponatremia Vestibular symptoms
Phenytoin	300 qhs	Anecdotal benefit	Vestibular symptoms
Tocainide	200–400 mg bid	Anecdotal benefit	
Calcium	0.5–1 g qd	Anecdotal benefit	
Amitriptyline	25–100 mg qhs	Anecdotal benefit	Sedation Sicca symptoms Urinary retention
Benadryl	50 mg qhs	Anecdotal benefit	Sedation Sicca symptoms Urinary retention
Botulinum toxin	Varies	Reported benefit when injected locally	Local or distant weakness
Creatinine	12 mg prior to dialysis	Reported benefit in dialysis patients	No adverse effects reported

De Wel B, Claeys KG. Neuromuscular hyperexcitability syndromes. *Curr Opin Neurol.* 2021;34(5):714–720; Katzberg HD, Khan AH, So YT. Assessment: symptomatic treatment for muscle cramps (an evidence based review). *Neurology.* 2010;74:691–696; Garrison SR, Kor quinine is estimated at 2%–4%.[17] The official position of the AAN regarding quinidine, which can still be prescribed as Qualaquin®, is that "select patients can be considered for an individual therapeutic trial once potential side effects are taken into account."[17] The AAN suggests that quinine be utilized in the setting of significant cramp morbidity and failure of other agents. Unfortunately, other agents possess only anecdotal or equivocal efficacy (Table 10-2). Since the AAN paper, a recent Cochrane review found no benefit for magnesium, though it is frequently prescribed.[23] However, a randomized trial of mexiletine in patients with amyotrophic lateral sclerosis reported Class I evidence that mexiletine is safe, well tolerated, and efficacious in reducing cramps at a total dosage of 300 mg daily (150 mg twice daily).[24]

The traditional approach to the treatment of symptomatic cramps if related to dehydration or exercise includes intravenous saline (not dextrose) solutions with electrolyte replacement.[3,17] An acute cramp can usually be aborted by stretching the involved muscle(s) although this will not necessarily prevent recurrence.

In our experience, patients who are psychologically troubled by an apparent benign fasciculation syndrome are reassured by providing them with a copy of the notable Mayo Clinic manuscript describing what is almost always a benign natural history.[25] Patients with CFS typically respond to treatment with anticonvulsants such as carbamazepine or phenytoin, again demonstrating similarities to Isaacs syndrome.

▶ ISAACS/MORVAN SYNDROME (ACQUIRED NEUROMYOTONIA)

CLINICAL FEATURES

Isaacs syndrome was first described by Denny-Brown in 1948.[26] Its eponym originates from the description of two patients by Isaacs in 1961 manifesting as progressive muscle stiffness associated with continuous muscle fiber activity.[27] Isaacs syndrome has also been referred to as acquired neuromyotonia, and when it affects the CNS and autonomic nervous system, Morvan syndrome or Morvan fibrillary chorea.[28,29] The encephalopathy of Morvan syndrome manifests as confusion, agitation, insomnia, amnesia, hallucinations, and seizures.[9,26,29] Dysautonomia has been reported in as many as 93% of patients with concomitant CNS involvement (see below).[9,28,29] Features of dysautonomia include cardiovascular instability, excessive sweating and lacrimation, and constipation.

Neoplasms, particularly thymoma, may be found in as many as 40% of patients with Isaacs and Morvan syndrome; some with concurrent myasthenia gravis.[30,31] Small cell carcinoma of the lung, Hodgkin lymphoma, and rarely plasmacytoma, ovarian, renal, bladder, and thyroid cancers are other associated tumors.[9,28,32–38] Like other paraneoplastic disorders, Isaacs may precede the recognition of lung cancer by years.

Isaacs syndrome may affect individuals of any age including neonates but is most commonly a disorder of adolescents and young adults.[9,39] The cardinal clinical feature is muscle stiffness, typically provoked by use, resulting from motor nerve hyperactivity and the associated involuntary and undesired muscle contraction. A very characteristic feature is the adventitious movements that are observed in muscles, notably continuous muscle undulation or rippling (myokymia) and intermittent, focal muscle twitching (fasciculations).[40–43] "Pseudomyotonia" often results in abnormal posturing mimicking the joint positioning of tetany such as carpopedal spasm, plantar flexion of the foot at the ankle, enhanced spinal curvature, facial grimacing, and flexion of the elbows, wrists, hips, and knee. In addition to the continuous muscle fiber activity, muscle hypertrophy, and weight loss are frequent concomitants, all of which may result from excessive muscular activity. Some patients complain of numbness, paresthesia, or neuropathic pain probably from spontaneous discharges of sensory nerves.

The signs and symptoms of Isaacs syndrome may be generalized or focal in distribution. In addition to the limbs and trunk, the tongue, face, and pharynx may be involved, resulting in difficulty in speaking (hoarseness or dysarthria) and swallowing. Dyspnea, believed to result from stiffness of chest wall muscles, was a prominent symptom in Isaacs' initial cases.[27] Ocular neuromyotonia has been implicated as a cause of intermittent, spasmodic diplopia, occurring either spontaneously or in response to sustained eccentric gaze.[44–46] Ocular neuromyotonia may occur either as a component of the Isaacs syndrome or as an isolated event following parasellar radiation.

The physical examination may include observations of stiff posture with slight trunk flexion, shoulder elevation and abduction, and elbow flexion.[40] Involuntary finger flexion has also been described as an isolated manifestation of this syndrome.[47] Widespread fasciculations and myokymia are seen and appear as continuous undulating or quivering of the underlying muscles.[48] These adventitious movements may be particularly prominent in the facial, pectoral, and calf muscles and may be provoked by muscle contraction. Delayed relaxation of eye or hand opening following forceful eye closure or a strong grip resembling myotonia may be appreciated. Length-dependent sensory loss, weakness, and reflex loss are indicative of axonal polyneuropathy which occurs in approximately a third of cases. Diminished or lost deep tendon reflexes provide another distinguishing feature from SPS. Muscle hypertrophy may be focal or generalized. The trapezius muscles may appear particularly prominent when the patient is viewed from the front. Chvostek and Trousseau signs may be appreciated despite normal calcium levels.

DIAGNOSIS AND DIFFERENTIAL DIAGNOSIS

The diagnosis of Isaacs or Morvan syndrome is established by the clinical features, supported by the characteristic EDX findings, and in many cases, the presence of autoantibodies. The differential diagnosis of Isaacs syndrome needs

▶ TABLE 10-3. NEUROMYOTONIA/NEUROMYOTONIC/ MYOKYMIC DISCHARGES—SECONDARY CAUSES

By localization
   Motor neuron
- ALS

   Neuropathies
- Charcot–Marie–Tooth disease (e.g., HINT-1 mutations)
- Guillain–Barré syndrome
- Chronic inflammatory demyelinating polyneuropathy
- Isaacs syndrome

By etiology
   Radiation
- Brain/Spinal cord
- Plexus

   Neoplasia
- Small-cell carcinoma of the lung
- Thymoma
- Hodgkin disease

   Drugs
- Penicillamine

   Immune mediated
- Primary systemic sclerosis
- Bone marrow transplantation

   Familial
- Autosomal dominant neuromyotonia
- Familial amyloid polyneuropathy

to be considered in three domains: disorders that mimic the clinical phenotype, disorders that appear to occur at increased frequency in patients with either Isaacs or Morvan syndrome, and disorders that share the EDX features of the disorder (Table 10-3).

The differential diagnosis of Isaacs syndrome consists largely of the other disorders discussed in this chapter, as well as those previously summarized in the cramps and fasciculations section. Causes of muscle stiffness that originate from the extrapyramidal system are beyond the scope of this book. The differential diagnosis of each of the EDX features that may be seen in Isaacs syndrome patients (fasciculation potentials, cramp, myokymic and neuromyotonic discharges, multiplets) can be found in appropriate tables in Chapter 2.

Neuromyotonic discharges do not occur as a universal feature of Isaacs syndrome nor are they unique to this disorder. They can occur as a consequence of radiation injury to affected nerves.[45,46,49] Neuromyotonic discharges have been reported as an association with certain neuropathies, particularly those as autosomal recessive, axonal Charcot–Marie–Tooth type 2 caused by mutations HINT1 gene that encodes for histidine triad nucleotide-binding protein 1,[50–52] Guillain–Barré syndrome, and chronic inflammatory demyelinating polyradiculoneuropathy.[53] They have been rarely described in association with ALS, amyloidosis, and rattlesnake envenomation as well as disorders also felt to have autoimmune mechanisms such as primary systemic sclerosis, systemic lupus, celiac disease, bone marrow transplantation, graft versus host disease, and penicillamine therapy.[9,40,54–61]

LABORATORY FEATURES

Isaacs and Morvan syndromes are associated with antibodies to leucine-rich glioma-inactivated 1 (LGI1) and contactin-associated protein like-2 (CASPR2) in both the serum and cerebrospinal fluid (CSF) in up to 80% patients.[9,31,62–65] Importantly, voltage-gated potassium channel (VGKC) antibodies that lack LGI1 or CASPR2 reactivities ("double-negative") are common in healthy controls and are not associated with any distinct pathogenic syndrome.[64,65] Although these antibodies appear to be most closely associated with Isaacs and Morvan syndromes, they may occur with other forms of autoimmune encephalitis and polyneuropathy. Furthermore, other neuronal and often paraneoplastic antibodies, notably, antinicotinic AChR, CRMP-5, amphiphysin, and antinuclear neuronal type 4 have been identified in a small portion of patients with Isaacs or Morvan syndrome. Patients may have other markers of autoimmunity including increased protein, immunoglobulins, and oligoclonal bands within the CSF.[9] Serum abnormalities including elevated CK levels from continuous muscle fiber activity and hyponatremia related to SIADH.

Motor and sensory nerve conduction studies (NCS) are often normal although may indicate a concomitant polyneuropathy in some patients.[9,40,42,66,67] If one looks closely, however, repetitive after-discharges are often evident following standard motor conduction and F-wave studies similar to what may be identified in organophosphate poisoning (Fig. 10-2).[68] Microneurographic recordings demonstrate after-discharges in sensory as well as motor nerve fibers.

Multiple potential types of abnormal spontaneous activity are apparent on needle EMG in patients with Isaacs syndrome.[9,43,61,66] Neuromyotonic, myokymic or cramps discharges, fasciculation or fibrillation potentials, and positive sharp waves may occur individually or in combination.[9,43] One of the most characteristic EDX signatures are spontaneous bursts of grouped MUAPs known as multiplets.[43] These are similar in appearance to myokymic discharges but are distinguished by their random rather than semirhythmic discharge pattern and by their faster intraburst frequency. Myokymic discharges typically have slower intrabursts discharge frequencies. The discharge frequency is always less than 150 Hz and is more typically in the 40–80 Hz range. Although there is some overlap, the intraburst discharge frequency of multiplets is typically higher and overlaps with the neuromyotonic discharge range, reaching 350 Hz in some cases.[43] Neuromyotonic discharges are high-frequency discharges of single MUAPs that occur at random intervals with intradischarge frequencies of greater than 150 Hz and up to 500 Hz or intraspike intervals in the 2–5 ms range. They cannot sustain themselves at these frequencies and rapidly dissipate in a decrescendo pattern. It is this decrescendo pattern that distinguishes them from multiplets. They begin and end abruptly with a duration measured in seconds (Fig. 10-3). The resultant sound has been described as "pinging" or likened to the scream of a Formula 1 engine.

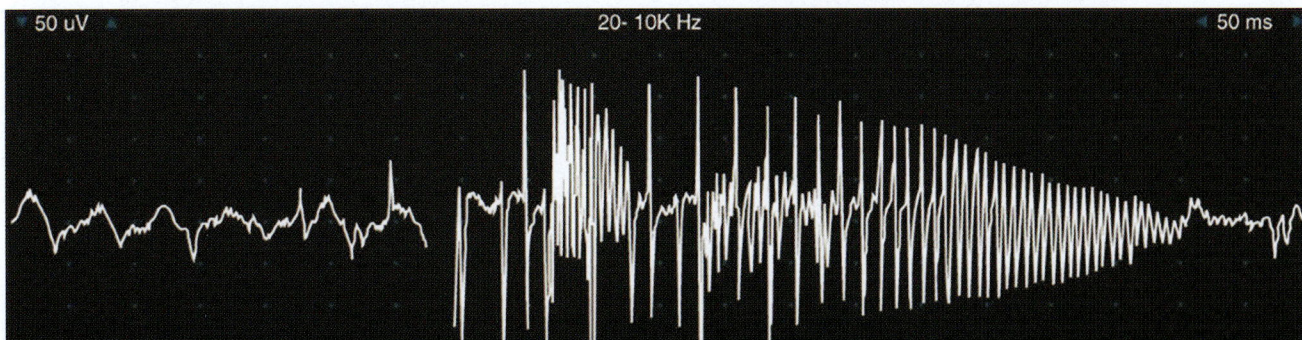

Figure 10-3. Neuromyotonic discharge—abrupt onset, high frequency and high pitched, and rapidly dissipating. (Used with permission of Devon Rubin, MD, Mayo Clinic, Jacksonville, FL.)

Myokymic discharges are seen at a greater frequency in Isaacs syndrome than neuromyotonic discharges.[40] Their distinction from neuromyotonic discharges may be artificial in that each individual burst of discharges are felt to originate from motor nerve and are constituted from individual MUAPs. Myokymic discharges are considered different from neuromyotonic discharges by their intraburst frequency as described above, by their firing pattern, and by the diseases they associate with. They are defined and recognized as spontaneously firing grouped discharges that occur in a repetitive, semirhythmic pattern with intervening periods of electrical silence (Fig. 10-4), thus differing from the singular decrescendo burst of a neuromyotonic discharge. Their intradischarge frequency is considerably slower than neuromyotonic discharges. The associated sound has been likened to troops marching in unison.

MRI of the brain in Morvan syndrome is typically normal, although positron emission tomography (PET) scanning can demonstrate focal or generalized hypometabolism. Lumbar puncture may reveal elevated CSF protein levels, lymphocytic pleocytosis, oligoclonal banding, and antibodies LGI1 or CASPR2 are found in approximately half of Morvan syndrome patients. Imaging of the chest is recommended to address the potential for thymoma, lung cancer, or lymphoma.

HISTOPATHOLOGY

Neither nerve nor muscle biopsy are routinely performed in suspected Isaacs syndrome cases. If performed, sural nerve biopsies may be normal or reveal evidence of a concomitant neuropathy with a reduction in myelinated fibers numbers or evidence of demyelination. Grouped atrophy and fiber-type grouping that may be demonstrable on muscle biopsy is also consistent with a peripheral neuropathy. Histopathologic evidence of an inflammatory myopathy has been reported.[32]

PATHOGENESIS

Isaacs syndrome is a disorder that appears to originate from terminal nerve twigs or the neuromuscular junction. Neuromyotonic discharges are abolished by curare or botulinum toxin and persist following general or spinal anesthesia, and

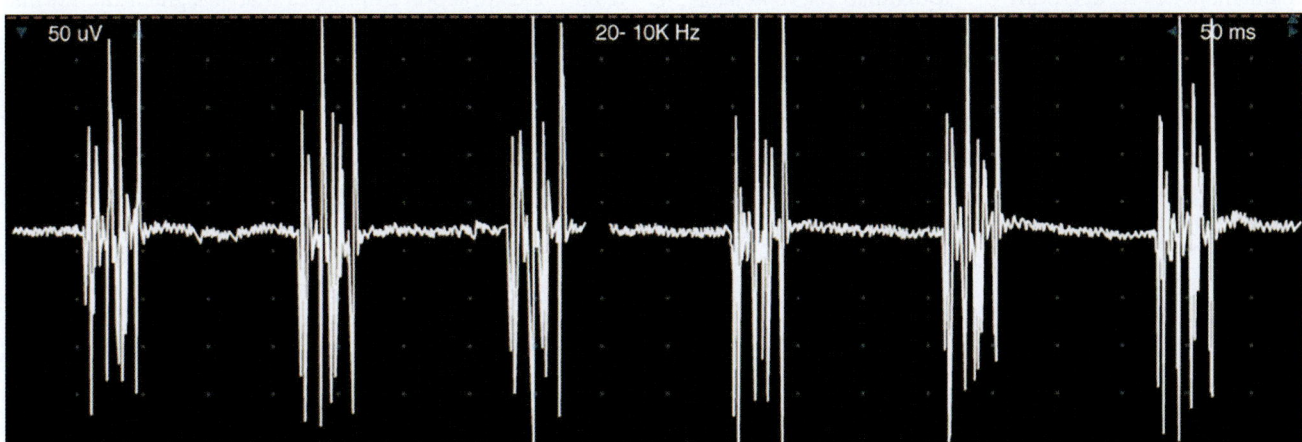

Figure 10-4. Myokymic discharges—semirhythmic-grouped discharges. (Used with permission of Devon Rubin, MD, Mayo Clinic, Jacksonville, FL.)

in most cases, proximal nerve block.[69] In some cases however, discharges appear to originate from more proximal aspects of nerve.[67,70-75]

The demonstration of CASPR2 and LGI1 antibodies in the serum and CSF provide both incontrovertible evidence of autoimmunity and a potential pathophysiological explanation for peripheral nerve hyperexcitability.[9,31,62-65,73] There is a high prevalence of antigen-specific antibodies of the IgG4 subclass in both CASPR and LGI1 subgroups, however, IgG1 antibodies are also evidently the second most commonly detected subclass.[65] The importance of this observation is that IgG4 antibodies do not bind complement and therefore associated diseases are less responsive to intravenous immunoglobulin (IVIG), but may respond to rituximab. CASPR2 appears to concentrate VGKC in the juxtaparanodal regions of both peripheral and CNS axons. CASPR2 autoantibodies may lead to potassium channel dysfunction through impaired clustering and appears to be the principal antigenic target in neuromyotonia.[76] LGl1 appears to be the principal antigenic target in limbic encephalitis. That it localizes to specific brain regions in experimental animals may well explain the selected vulnerability of certain neuronal populations and the nature of the characteristic clinical manifestations of Morvan syndrome. Disruption of the VGKC reduces the hyperpolarizing effect of channel activation, preventing the nerve action potential from dissipating and leading to retrograde depolarization of certain terminal twigs and reactivation of other terminal twigs belonging to the same motor unit.[55,74]

TREATMENT

Various forms of immunotherapy have partial efficacy in patients with Isaacs and Morvan syndromes.[1,2,31,64,65] Plasma exchange (PLEX) and IVIG are generally considered to have a faster onset of action than oral immunomodulating drugs. Corticosteroid and second-line immunosuppressive agents (e.g., azathioprine) are usually utilized in addition in an attempt to avoid the inconvenience and cost associated with maintenance IVIG or PLEX.[9,77-81] Rituximab is a reasonable option and some feel is the preferred treatment of choice in patients with IgG4 antibody syndromes.[82]

Symptomatic treatment with antiepileptic medications that block sodium channels such as phenytoin or carbamazepine or decrease neuronal excitability through other mechanisms (e.g., baclofen, mexiletine, valproic acid, and gabapentinoids) may provide some measure of symptomatic relief.[66,68]

▶ TETANUS

CLINICAL FEATURES

Despite their entirely different causes and mechanisms, both tetanus and tetany are derived from the Greek word for spasm, "tetanus." Tetanus is a disorder of sustained muscle rigidity with superimposed painful spasms. The natural history of tetanus consists of an incubation period varying from a few days to weeks with a mean of 8 days.[83] A shorter duration between exposure and symptom onset portends the development of severe disease with intense spasms and bulbar symptoms. Once begun, the clinical manifestations tend to progress for 10–14 days. If the patient avoids secondary complications of the illness and survives, recovery typically begins approximately a month after symptom onset and is often complete. However, the mortality rate may be as high as 30%, particularly in neonates, in older patients with comorbidities, and in locations where supportive medical care may be limited.

The clinical manifestations of tetanus are dependent upon the inoculation site, the extent of toxin spread, and the patient's premorbid immunization status.[83] Tetanus may begin and remain local in proximity to the wound site producing "local" or "cephalic" tetanus. This is a somewhat artificial distinction as the majority of these patients will progress to a generalized form of the disease. If the disease remains localized, for example, as monomelic rigidity, the diagnosis may be difficult. Cephalic tetanus may mimic one or more cranial nerve palsies, the effects of which may include laryngospasm with associated breathing and phonation difficulties, dysphagia, as well as impaired extraocular movement and pupillary function. Evidence of muscle overactivity provides a helpful clue as to the cause of these symptoms which more commonly occurs with diseases that produce muscle weakness.

In generalized tetanus, the initial symptoms that typically precede the development of the more recognizable spasms are nonspecific, including irritability, akathisia, diaphoresis, and tachycardia.[84] The most distinctive symptom of tetanus is painful muscle spasms that more often than not begin either near the wound or in the masseter or facial muscles. The former, trismus or lockjaw, is the disease's most notorious manifestation. Trismus may be provoked by tactile stimulation of the posterior pharyngeal wall, a reflex thought to represent both a sensitive and a specific bedside test. Involvement of muscles innervated by the facial nerve may produce a characteristic facial posture known as risus sardonicus, resulting from the contraction of muscles that straighten the normal bowed appearance of the upper lip (Fig. 10-5).

Paraspinal and abdominal muscles are the next groups that are most commonly affected and may contribute to ventilatory insufficiency or mimic an abdominal emergency. In severe cases, violent stimulus-induced spasms may produce opisthotonus, a dramatic overarching of the back along with a fisted posture of the hands (Fig. 10-6). If the limbs are involved, proximal more than distal muscles are typically affected. However, there are exceptions with severe generalized cases in which proximal and distal muscles may be equally affected or local involvement in proximity to the wound site representing potential exceptions. Spasms are often triggered by an emotional or sensory stimuli, or by attempted patient movement.[83]

Dysautonomia, primarily expressing itself through excessive adrenergic influence, manifests as hypertensive

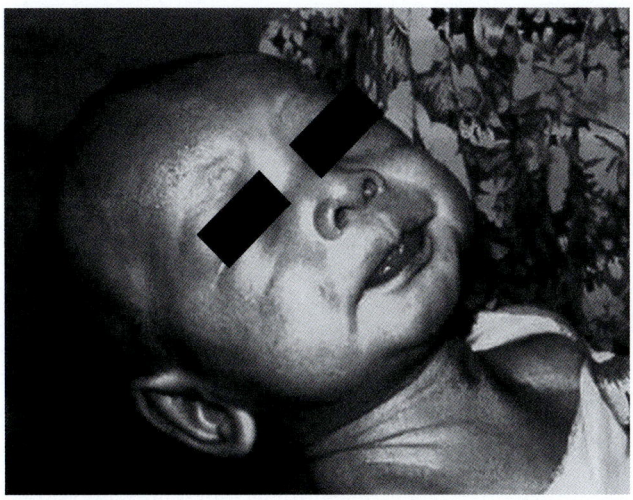

Figure 10-5. Risus sardonicus in infantile tetanus. (Used with permission of the Immunization Action Coalition, St. Paul, MN.)

crises, arrhythmia, and hyperhidrosis.[83] Prominent sialorrhea may contribute to airway compromise. Fever occurs commonly. Alteration of consciousness represents an effect of hypoxia. The offending tetanus toxin (tetanospasmin) does not cause permanent neurologic injury. Complete recovery may occur if the patient can be spared from hypoxic and other secondary consequences of the disease.

Uncommonly, tetanus may result from anaerobic infection of the middle ear or paranasal sinuses.[83] This may result in "local" tetanus, producing trismus as well as motor cranial nerve dysfunction as described, potentially including ophthalmoparesis. Tetanus may also proliferate in the uterus and represents a feared complication of parturition or abortion in nonhygienic facilities.

Neonatal tetanus is predominantly a disease of underdeveloped countries.[83] It typically originates from an umbilical stump infection in a child born of an unimmunized mother. Local customs that include the application of substances to the umbilical stump that unknowingly harbor spores may contribute to the risk of the disease. Symptom onset is typically within the first 2 weeks of life, manifesting as a poorly feeding infant with prominent muscle twitching. Changes

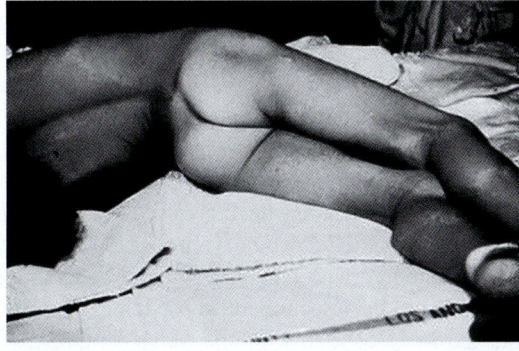

Figure 10-6. Opisthotonus. (Used with permission of the Immunization Action Coalition, St. Paul, MN.)

in cranial musculature provide valuable clues. The jaw may clamp tight on a finger placed in the mouth. The upper lip stiffens, the eyelids are closed tightly, and the forehead is continuously wrinkled. Mortality in neonatal tetanus is high. Neonatal tetanus accounted for two-thirds of the 300,000 deaths attributed to tetanus worldwide in the year 2000.[84]

The differential diagnosis of trismus includes dental infection and paraneoplastic brainstem encephalitis. Trismus and painful spasms are not typical of most dystonias. Drug-induced dystonias have to be considered in cephalic tetanus as they may affect ocular movements. A chronologic relationship to drug exposure and a prompt and dramatic response to anticholinergic drugs provide diagnostic clues. Rabies needs to be considered in the differential diagnosis of cephalic tetanus when dysphagia is part of the symptom complex. Patients with rabies are frequently encephalopathic, have dysautonomic symptoms that are more likely to be cholinergic in nature (sialorrhea), do not tend to have continuous muscular rigidity, and have a CSF pleocytosis if tested.

Other extrapyramidal disorders in which dystonia is a prominent feature may resemble generalized tetanus but are typically chronic and result in distorted postures that are recognizably different from those of the disorders described above, for example, torticollis. Meningoencephalitis may be associated with fever, nuchal, and paraspinal rigidity. Associated seizures may further contribute to tonic and phasic increases in the trunk and limb tone. SPS is characterized by the same axial rigidity and superimposed spasm as tetanus but is typically more insidious in onset and typically lacks the prominent cephalic involvement of tetanus. Neuroleptic malignant syndrome produces profound muscular rigidity and significant dysautonomia. Exposure to an offending drug, fever, altered mental status, and absence of spasms are potential distinguishing features from tetanus. Peritonitis and localized tetanus affecting the abdominal wall may be confused with each other. Spasticity is never acute, although spasms and involuntary jerking of the extremities may occur. The pattern of increased muscle tone is usually distinctive, affecting flexors in the upper extremities and extensors in the lower extremities preferentially. The limbs are affected more so than the trunk and head in contrast to tetanus. Strychnine is a CNS glycine antagonist, which is used primarily as rat poison. It impedes postsynaptic inhibition of motor neurons in the spinal cord. The phenotype is almost identical to tetanus other than the absence of trismus and the onset that occurs within minutes to hours of exposure. The diagnosis is dependent on a history of exposure in addition to the expected clinical manifestations. Reflex spasms are superimposed upon tonic rigidity affecting upper extremity flexors, lower extremity extensors, and facial muscles resulting in risus sardonicus.

LABORATORY FEATURES

Clostridium tetani can be cultured in approximately a third of infected wounds. No other organism-specific diagnostic test available as toxin assays are not available in either serum or CSF. Regarding differential diagnostic considerations, strychnine assays can be performed by specialized laboratories. CSF examination should be obtained, if possible, if meningoencephalitis is considered. Elevated levels of CSF protein and immunoglobulins may occur in some cases of tetanus but are nonspecific and of little clinical value. Testing for glutamic acid decarboxylase (GAD) autoantibodies is reasonable if there is any suspicion for SPS. Electromyographic evaluation may reveal MUAP activation occurring involuntarily and simultaneously in agonist and antagonist muscles. Secondary complications such as inappropriate secretion of antidiuretic hormone and rhabdomyolysis require monitoring of serum sodium, CK, and creatinine.

PATHOGENESIS

Tetanus results from wounds, often penetrating, that are contaminated by spores of the organism *C. tetani*, a gram-positive anaerobic rod. In underdeveloped countries, septic abortion, infected umbilical stumps, burns, intramuscular injections, and compound fractures provide common portals of entry. In developed countries, the organism is commonly introduced by contaminated puncture wounds sustained through recreational drug use or in areas where fecal debris from animals is prevalent, such as farms.

Outside of the human body, the organism is resilient, surviving exposure to certain disinfectants and boiling for short periods of time. The spores may remain viable for decades. They thrive particularly in warm, moist soil contaminated by animal fecal material. Germination and proliferation occurs under optimal conditions, including those provided by wounds with tissue necrosis, foreign bodies, tissue ischemia, or coinfection with other organisms.

Under anaerobic conditions, the spores will germinate and release two exotoxins: tetanospasmin and tetanolysin. The role of the latter in disease expression is unknown. There are three known mechanisms by which tetanospasmin may adversely affect the nervous system. Localized tetanus is thought to occur as a consequence of direct binding to peripheral nerve terminals proximate to the wound site. Generalized disease results from retrograde transport of toxin into the CNS via motor nerves. Within the CNS, the toxin migrates transynaptically into GABAergic (brainstem) and glycinergic (spinal cord) inhibitory interneurons. Tetanospasmin blocks neurotransmitter release by cleaving synaptobrevin [vesicle-associated membrane protein (VAMP)], a protein essential for vesicle docking at synaptic membrane release sites.[85,86] Hematogenous dissemination of toxin may contribute to generalized disease by adversely affecting neuromuscular transmission through a presynaptic effect, similar but of far lesser magnitude to botulism.[87,88] It is hypothesized that this lower motor neuron effect, typically overshadowed by CNS hyperactivity, may be particularly relevant to cranial nerve dysfunction. Glycine inhibition is also believed to have an adverse effect on preganglionic sympathetic neurons translating to increased plasma catecholamine levels and heightened sympathetic activity.

The early involvement of cranial muscles is presumptively due to their shorter length and early arrival of neurotoxin to brainstem via this retrograde transport mechanism. Cranial, trunk, and limb muscles are usually affected in that order presumably due to the relationship of nerve length and retrograde neurotoxin transport. Recovery from tetanus is dependent on the genesis of new presynaptic nerve terminals of inhibitory interneurons.[83,89]

TREATMENT

The primary treatment strategy for tetanus is prevention. Tetanus is an uncommon illness due to the existence of effective vaccination programs. During a 2-year period in the United States in the 1990s, only 124 cases were reported. To further amplify the efficacy of prevention, a vaccination program for pregnant women with tetanus toxoid in India reduced the annual number of cases of neonatal tetanus from 9,313 to 653 over a 21-year period of time.[90] Although vaccination is extremely effective, rare individuals may develop tetanus even with a complete and up-to-date tetanus vaccination program and demonstration of preexisting tetanus antibodies.[91] In countries where vaccination programs and medical access are limited, neonatal tetanus is more prevalent. In developed countries, the incidence of tetanus is higher in older individuals. Waning immunity from remote immunization may play a significant role in this observation.[83]

Vaccination against tetanus can be delivered either passively (tetanus toxoid) or actively (tetanus-specific immunoglobulin). The former, developed in the 1940s, is the preferred vaccination method. Primary vaccination for infants consists of five doses of tetanus toxoid delivered at 2, 4, and 6 months of age, as well as at 15–18 months and 4–6 years. The fifth dose is not required if the fourth was received after age 4. Typically, tetanus toxoid is combined with pertussis and diphtheria vaccines for the first five doses. Following these initial five doses, pertussis is deleted, and tetanus toxoid/diphtheria boosters are recommended at 10-year intervals.

Primary vaccination is indicated in adults when their childhood vaccination history is uncertain or if a bone marrow transplant is planned. It consists of three injections, the first two of which are separated by a minimum of 4 weeks, and the last dose done 6–12 months subsequent to the second. In individuals who have received a "clean" wound, vaccination is considered adequate if previously vaccinated and if a tetanus booster has been received within 10 years. In the setting of a "dirty" wound, a booster within 5 years would be considered with adequate primary vaccination. In a patient who has been wounded, whose tetanus immunization has "expired," or their immune status compromised by HIV infection, dialysis, chronic chloroquine exposure (and potentially other immunosuppressant agents), both primary vaccination with tetanus toxoid and human tetanus immunoglobulin (250 units intramuscularly) should be administered at different sites.

With the development of symptomatic tetanus, the goals are to: (1) limit further production of tetanospasmin by wound debridement and antimicrobial therapy; (2) neutralize if possible, the effects of existing, unbound toxin by active immunization; (3) provide symptomatic treatment of painful spasms, impaired ventilation, and swallowing; and (4) treat symptoms referable to dysautonomia. Patients with tetanus without obvious wounds should have orifices examined, such as the external ear or rectum, with removal of foreign bodies if relevant. Patients with tetanus should be considered for early lumbar puncture if indicated, and particularly prophylactic intubation and enteral feeding tube placement as both are frequently required and become technically difficult once rigidity and spasms begin in earnest.

Elimination of the toxin source involves removal of any foreign body, debridement of any necrotic tissue, and delivery of antibiotics with anaerobic efficacy. The latter is recommended despite absence of proven efficacy. Metronidazole, penicillin, third-generation cephalosporins, clindamycin, or erythromycin are typically administered and may reduce the need for muscle relaxants and sedatives. Penicillin G is given in doses ranging from 10 to 12 million units per day. Metronidazole appears to be equally effective and may be preferential in view of penicillin's stimulatory effect on the cortex. The customary dose is 500 mg IV q6h for 7–10 days.

Conversely, neutralization of unbound circulating toxin has documented efficacy in shortening disease duration and improving recovery rates. Human tetanus immune globulin should be administered at a dose of 500 units intramuscularly as soon as possible, ideally before the wound is manipulated. The addition of intrathecal (1,000 units) to intramuscular administration appears to result in even better outcomes.[92] Equine-derived tetanus immune globulin may be used if human-derived immune globulin is not available. Infection with C. tetani does not stimulate active immunity by the host.

Treatment of symptomatic spasms is important for patient comfort, to improve ventilation, and to prevent thermal and mechanical injury from excessive and sustained muscular contraction. Treatment should be titrated to patient response. Benzodiazepines (lorazepam—up to 80 mg a day, diazepam—up to 500 mg a day, or midazolam) with preservation of consciousness. Neuromuscular blocking agents, and/or baclofen are commonly used. Vecuronium at a dose of 6–8 mg/h is preferred over pancuronium, as the latter has catecholamine reuptake-blocking properties that may contribute to autonomic instability. Baclofen may be administered orally or intrathecally. The initial intrathecal dose is 40–200 μg followed by a continuous infusion of 20 μg/h.[93,94] Meticulous catheter care is required to minimize the risk of meningitis from prolonged intrathecal catheter placement. Labetalol (0.25–1.0 mg/min), morphine (0.5–1.0 mg/kg/h), magnesium sulfate, atropine, clonidine, and epidural bupivacaine have all been used with some degree of reported benefit for hyperadrenergic and other autonomic manifestations.[89] As with all illnesses associated with protracted recovery periods, vigorous supportive care including tracheostomy is frequently required to minimize the risk of secondary complications to which these patients are susceptible.

▶ TETANY

CLINICAL FEATURES

Tetany is a disorder of nerve hyperexcitability provoked by hypocalcemia with or without vitamin D deficiency, hypomagnesemia or alkalosis. The syndrome has both motor and sensory features and is characterized by the development of paresthesias which initially occur in the digits and in a circumoral distribution. The paresthesias may in some cases have a lateralized preponderance and may spread to the proximal extremities. Paresthesias are followed by manifestations of motor nerve hyperactivity manifesting as spasmodic muscle contraction resulting in characteristic patterns of extremity posturing. The most characteristic of these is "carpal spasm" consisting of a "fisted" posture with the thumb adducted against the palm covered by fingers that are flexed at the metacarpophalangeal joints, extended at the proximal interphalangeal joints, and adducted against each other. In more severe cases, the wrists and elbows may assume a flexed posture as well. In the lower extremities, the pedal portion of carpal pedal spasm, the tendency is for the toes to flex and the ankle to assume the equinovarus posture, that is, plantar flexed and inverted. Unlike tetanus, the effects of tetany are more pronounced in limb as opposed to cranial and axial muscles and influence sensory as well as motor function due to their peripheral nerve effects. In severe cases however, laryngospasm may occur, and trunk muscles may be affected, potentially resulting in opisthotonus.

Carpal spasm may be elicited in patients at risk by inflating a blood pressure cuff to greater than systolic blood pressure for ≤3 minutes (Trousseau sign). Spasm of facial muscles may be provoked in these patients by digital percussion of the facial nerve at the angle of the jaw (Chvostek sign).

Tetany is diagnosed by recognition of the characteristic pattern of paresthesias, typical hand-and-foot postures, and a positive response to the provocative maneuvers described above. The diagnosis is further supported by identification of reduced serum levels of ionized calcium or magnesium. Cases of normocalcemic, normomagnesemic tetany do however occur.[95] Cases in which reduced ionized calcium has been detected in arterial but not venous blood have been described as well.

The differential diagnosis of tetany once again includes any disorder that produces cramps or cramp-like painful muscle contractions. Diagnostic considerations should include consideration of drug-induced tetany, typically resulting from alterations in magnesium homeostasis. Potential offenders include proton pump inhibitors, diuretics, epidermal growth factor receptor modulators, some antimicrobials and chemotherapeutic agents, and of particular interest to neuromuscular clinicians, calcineurin inhibitors such as tacrolimus and certain monoclonal antibodies including bevacizumab.[96–98]

LABORATORY FEATURES

All patients with unwanted muscle contractions should have ionized calcium, 25 hydroxy-vitamin D, and magnesium levels assessed in their serum. Tetany induced by hyperventilation will be associated with an arterial blood gas pattern consistent with acute respiratory alkalosis (i.e., a reduced PCO_2 and elevated pH). The EDX signature of tetany is grouped discharges that may occur spontaneously (myokymic discharges) or in response to voluntary activation (multiplets).

PATHOGENESIS

The effects of tetany are believed to result from a neural generator.[99] Concomitant sensory and motor symptoms support this. The neural hyperexcitability of tetany is thought to result from the effects of hypocalcemia or hypomagnesemia on sodium channels.[98,99] Reduction in serum calcium or magnesium levels are thought to result in preferential and enhanced sodium channel opening resulting in prolonged nerve depolarization and hyperexcitability. Calcineurin inhibitors are thought to promote hypomagnesemia by inhibition of the transient receptor ion channel 6 (TRPM6) channel that is responsible for the renal tubular reabsorption of magnesium. In addition, there is a potential direct effect of calcineurin inhibitors on the muscle. These drugs inhibit calmodulin-mediated calcium uptake in muscle, potentially augmenting unwanted muscle contraction through prolonged sodium channel activation at this level as well.[97]

TREATMENT

The treatment of tetany involves recognition and correction of hypocalcemia and/or hypomagnesemia if detectable. With symptomatic hypocalcemia, the goal is to elevate the corrected serum calcium to greater than 7.0 mg/dL. This can be accomplished by infusions of calcium gluconate at doses of 15–20 mEq/kg delivered over 4–6 hours. Conditions causing chronic hypocalcemia can be managed with 1–3 g of elemental calcium replacement a day. In the case of acute symptomatic hypomagnesemia, magnesium sulfate can be delivered either intramuscularly or intravenously. The intravenous dose is typically a bolus of 4–6 g followed by 2–3 g per hour as required. Vitamin D deficiency is treated with oral replacement. Vitamin D2 is the most economical way to accomplish this at daily doses of 25,000–150,000 IU.

If hyperventilation is the cause, breathing into a paper bag will address this problem acutely. Addressing the underlying cause of hyperventilation is important if a patient is repeatedly symptomatic. Drugs that potentially cause symptomatic hypomagnesemia should be removed if possible with consideration of patient comorbidities.

▶ SATOYOSHI SYNDROME

CLINICAL FEATURES

Satoyoshi syndrome is a rare, presumed autoimmune disorder, predominantly affecting individuals in the first two decades of life.[100–106] Females are affected twice as frequently as males. Satoyoshi syndrome occurs worldwide but appears to have the greatest prevalence in Japan.[101] It is characterized by painful muscle spasms of the extremities, typically beginning in the legs, but progressing to involve the entire body including the trunk, neck, and masticatory muscles. In Japan, it has been also referred to as "komura-gaeri" (calf-spasm) disease.[104] The spasms, like those of Isaacs syndrome, are commonly provoked by movement, persist during sleep, and interfere with gait.[101,104] Unlike Isaacs syndrome, adventitious muscle movements such as myokymia and fasciculations are not described.[102,103] The spasms commonly distort posture, typically last for a few minutes, and recur after short intervals. Although these paroxysms may be the sole manifestation of Satoyoshi syndrome, the syndrome is best conceptualized as a multisystem disorder associated with alopecia, diarrhea, and short stature. Short stature may occur as a result of impaired nutrition and/or endocrine abnormalities that may include amenorrhea as well as growth retardation.[102,106] The amenorrhea, at least in some cases, is a consequence of hypergonadotropic hypogonadism and primary ovarian failure. Bony deformities may occur in Satoyoshi syndrome. They have been hypothesized to result from the influence of repeated forceful muscle spasm on developing bone.[101] Life expectancy is reduced, attributed predominantly to nutritional deficiency.[101,104]

DIAGNOSIS AND DIFFERENTIAL DIAGNOSIS

Satoyoshi syndrome remains a clinical diagnosis, suspected when movement-related painful muscle spasms develop in children and adolescents, accompanied by alopecia, diarrhea, short stature, and in postpubescent females, amenorrhea. The laboratory abnormalities and responsiveness to immunomodulating treatment described below provide diagnostic support.

LABORATORY FEATURES

Lab testing results may reflect malnutrition or malabsorption. Consistent with this conclusion are duodenal imaging abnormalities felt to be consistent with chronic inflammatory change. Endoscopy may demonstrate atrophic gastric mucosa and multiple ulcerations.[104,105] X-rays may reveal osteolytic lesions of the epiphysis and metaphysis of bone.[101] Serum CK levels may be elevated.[104,105,107] The serum IgE level has been elevated in at least two cases.[106,107] In post-pubescent females, levels of sex hormones may be reduced and gonadotropin levels elevated.[101] Although a number of circulating autoantibodies including those directed at the acetylcholine receptor and GAD enzyme have been anecdotally reported, there has been no consistent pattern identified to date.[105,107] Despite the presence of acetylcholine receptor antibodies in some cases, we are unaware of any reports of Satoyoshi syndrome associated with thymic abnormality. As titers of anti-GAD autoantibodies are frequently elevated in high titers in the SPS, the significance of low-level titers of these antibodies in Satoyoshi syndrome awaits further clarification. Routine EDX studies done in Satoyoshi syndrome patients when muscles are quiescent are normal. Surface EMG recordings during involuntary muscle contraction reveals high amplitude, synchronous motor unit discharges that are pervasive throughout the entire muscle belly.[107]

PATHOGENESIS

Satoyoshi syndrome is suspected to have an autoimmune mechanism. Other autoimmune diseases such as myasthenia, idiopathic thrombocytopenia, and immune-mediated nephropathies appear to occur with increased frequency in Satoyoshi syndrome.[104] As previously mentioned, a nonspecific pattern of autoantibodies may be identified in the serum of Satoyoshi syndrome patients. A single report has described a circulating antibody reacting to a 90-kDa protein found in the brain, stomach, and duodenum but not the uterus.[104]

The pathophysiology of muscle contraction in Satoyoshi syndrome is unknown. It appears to differ from cramps in that surface EMG recordings of motor unit discharges are synchronous, not random, and occur in uniform rather than a migrating pattern throughout the muscle belly.

TREATMENT

In view of its rarity, there is no standardized approach to the treatment of Satoyoshi syndrome. A variety of agents have been used unsuccessfully for the treatment of spasms. Botulinum toxin may be locally effective (e.g., masticatory spasm) but is impractical for widespread application. Carbamazepine was effective in at least one case whereas baclofen provided no benefit.[101] Case reports suggest that immunomodulation may favorably alter the natural history of the disease in some but not all cases. Significantly beneficial responses to muscle spasms, alopecia, and gastrointestinal symptoms have been reported with tacrolimus, methotrexate, corticosteroids, and IVIG.[101,104,105] Conversely, both corticosteroids and IVIG have been reported to be ineffective.[101,105,107–109] Appropriate hormonal replacement may be considered.

▶ STIFF-PERSON SYNDROME AND THE ANTI-GAD SPECTRUM DISORDERS

CLINICAL FEATURES

Moersch and Woltman described "stiff-man syndrome" in 1956 based on their experience with 14 patients afflicted with a syndrome of fluctuating but progressive muscle rigidity and spasm that preferentially affected the axial muscles.[110] For multiple reasons including its greater prevalence in women, this disorder is now commonly referred to as the SPS.[111–114] As will be discussed in Laboratory section, SPS was later found to be associated with antibodies targeting GAD. Subsequently, other clinical syndromes were associated with anti-GAD antibodies and are now referred to as "GAD antibody-spectrum disorders (GAD-SD)."[115–124] In addition to SPS, these include autoimmune cerebellar ataxia, parkinsonism, limbic encephalitis, seizures, progressive encephalomyelitis with rigidity and myoclonus variant of this disease (PERM), and a vestibular–ocular disorder. Furthermore, in addition to GAD, other autoantibodies targeting, amphiphysin, glycine receptors, γ-aminobutyric acid-A (GABA-A) receptor, and gephyrin, have been less frequently associated with SPS-SD.[116,125–129]

Like other autoimmune disorders, the onset is often acute to subacute although it may go undiagnosed for years. SPS affects women twice as frequently as men with a median onset of 35–40 years of age. In view of its rarity and the often protean nature of its onset symptoms (i.e., low back pain), the diagnosis is often delayed by an average of 6 years following symptom onset.[111,112]

In the classic form of the disease, the initial symptom is typically painful muscle stiffness in the lumbosacral and abdominal regions.[113,114,130] One of the key features of SPS is the co-contraction of agonist and antagonist muscles leading to muscle rigidity in the axial muscles and extremities, particularly the legs. Eventually, any muscle under voluntary control may be affected. Limb involvement may be symmetric or asymmetric. Falls constitute a significant risk and source of morbidity. Fear of falling is a significant source of anxiety for these patients.

At onset, paroxysmal muscle spasms are the norm. They usually become more persistent as the disease worsens. These spasms, superimposed upon baseline muscle stiffness, may begin abruptly, last for seconds to minutes as individual events, and may recur in clusters that may persist for hours.[112,130–132] They are often provoked or intensified by movement, by tactile, emotional, or auditory stimuli, or by cold weather or intercurrent infection. The spasms may be powerful enough to break bones, dislocate joints, or incite rhabdomyolysis. The spasms may be so dramatic as to mimic the opisthotonic posturing of tetanus.[112,131] Unlike Isaacs syndrome, spasms are typically diminished, if not alleviated, by general anesthesia, benzodiazepines, and sleep.[113] The paroxysms of SPS may be associated with adrenergic symptoms of dysautonomia including diaphoresis, hypertension, tachycardia, tachypnea, and pupillary dilatation.[130] Rarely, the dysautonomia may result in sudden death.[112,133]

Like many clinical syndromes, the clinical manifestations of SPS may be heterogeneous.[134] Focal presentations have been referred to as "stiff-limb" syndrome.[115,134–138] Focal-onset SPS may or may not progress to more generalized disorder. If the phenotype remains focal, SPS may not be readily suspected. Cervical involvement may result in restricted head movement. Thoracoabdominal rigidity may result in symptoms whose mechanism may not be initially recognized as being related to restricted muscle movement including ventilatory insufficiency (dyspnea on exertion, orthopnea, exercise intolerance, inability to swim underwater) and impaired gastric distention (early satiety). Facial involvement resulting in facial masking has been described in some cases, leading to the diagnosis of Parkinson disease.[111]

The PERM variant, also known as "jerking stiff-man syndrome," is associated with progressive rigidity, myoclonus, nystagmus, opsoclonus, impaired ocular motility, dysarthria, dysphagia, and cognitive impairment.[112,113,134–137] Seizures may occur in up to 10% of cases. Peripheral neuropathy and motor neuronopathy have also been reported to occur as part of the PERM complex.[115] The course of PERM is relentless, and death may occur within weeks to months of onset. Other manifestations of GAD-SD include a subacute cerebellar syndrome with prominent ataxia, dysarthria, and eye movement abnormalities superimposed on muscle stiffness and spasms.[113,114] Another variant involves vestibular–ocular motor (VOM) dysfunction.[118,119] One series of 22 patients with GAD-SD reported 8 patients with early dominant VOM dysfunction.[118] Seven had features of cerebellar ataxia, and four had additional features of classic SPS. The common symptoms were dizziness and diplopia. On examination, the most common VOM abnormalities were downbeating and gaze-evoked nystagmus and saccadic pursuit.[118]

The clinical examination of "classic" SPS patient often reveals accentuation of the normal lumbar lordosis with resultant restriction of spine mobility. As a result, a patient's lower back may fail to flatten and contact the bed when lying supine. Their ability to touch their toes may be severely restricted similar to a spondyloarthropathy patient. The lumbar lordotic curve is increased rather than decreased both in the upright and attempted flexed positions. Although nonspecific, the paraspinal muscles in SPS are typically indurated to palpation. As a result, the patient's flexibility, mobility, and ambulation are hampered. The patient's gait may be described as stiff, robotic, and spastic in nature. In addition to abnormal axial postures, other abnormal postures during spasms may include extension and slight abduction of the leg, inversion and plantar flexion of the foot that may be mistaken as foot drop, or pronation and extension of the upper extremity.[112,133] Deep tendon reflexes may be increased, but pathologic reflexes (e.g., clonus and Babinski signs) should not be seen. The head retraction reflex is a bedside test that can be utilized in an SPS suspect. A positive response is contraction of neck muscles, with or without head movement, in response to a gentle tap to the glabella, bridge of the nose, lip or cheek in a patient whose eyes are closed.

SPS is thought to be paraneoplastic in approximately 5% of individuals.[111,112] Patients with paraneoplastic SPS may have a preferential involvement of the upper extremities and cranial nerves.[111,112] Malignancies reported in SPS include breast cancer and small-cell carcinoma of the lung, and less commonly Hodgkin disease, thymoma, colon, and ovarian cancer. The majority of these occur in GAD-65 seronegative patients.[56,112,113]

Other nonparaneoplastic autoimmune disorders both within and outside of the nervous system associate with SPS. This is particularly true in those who possess GAD antibodies. These comorbidities may include encephalomyelitis with seizures, cerebellitis, myasthenia gravis, hypo- and hyperthyroidism, pernicious anemia, celiac disease, adrenal insufficiency, systemic lupus erythematosus, rheumatoid arthritis, ovarian failure, and vitiligo.[111,112,139,140] Diabetes mellitus is particularly prevalent and may exist in up to 70% of patients with SPS.

The decision regarding potential evaluation for underlying malignancy should probably depend on the context of the individual patient. The presence of amphiphysin antibodies, a strong family history of breast or ovarian cancer or smoking, and predominant upper extremity or cranial nerve involvement are features that will increase the diagnostic yield of identifying an underlying malignancy.[59,131,141] In an environment where neither cost nor availability are considerations, ^{18}F fluorodeoxyglucose PET (FDG PET) scanning would represent the presumed screening method of choice to search for an occult malignancy.

LABORATORY FEATURES

The association of glutamic acid decarboxylase autoantibodies (anti-GAD) and SPS was first reported in 1988.[142] Antibodies directed against the 65KD isoform of GAD (GAD-65) may be found in high titer in 85% of SPS patients as well as individuals with the other described syndromes associated with GAD-SD.[113,114,142,143,144–146] Importantly, low titers of anti–GAD-65 antibodies occur in up to 8% of the population, particularly in people with diabetes mellitus.[124] Only high antibody titers (>10,000 IU) by enzyme-linked immunosorbent assay or greater than 20 nmol/L using radioimmunoassay are considered clinically relevant.[120–122] A major source of diagnostic error is basing a diagnosis of SPS because of subjective symptoms only and a slightly elevated anti-GAD level.[123,124] If only patients with the classic phenotype are considered, the prevalence of anti-GAD antibodies in SPS may exceed 90%.[134] GAD-65 autoantibodies are also demonstrable in the CSF in 75% of cases.[113,147] They are present in the CSF in lower titer than in serum but with a 10-fold increase when indexed against serum implicating intrathecal synthesis.[113] GAD-65 autoantibody titers do not correlate with disease severity, duration, or treatment responsiveness. GAD-65 autoantibodies may occur rarely in individuals with SPS who have an underlying malignancy.[113,138,147–149]

In addition to GAD-65, autoantibodies directed against the amphiphysin, glycine receptor alpha-1 subunit (GLRA1), GABA-A receptor, gephyrin, and the NMDA receptor have been reported in SPS.[113,114,125–129,150–153] Amphiphysin antibodies are found in approximately 5% of SPS cases, almost always in women. As with anti-GAD antibodies, the clinical phenotype of patients with antiamphiphysin antibodies can be variable. Amphiphysin autoantibodies may occur in other non-SPS paraneoplastic syndromes including limbic encephalitis, cerebellar degeneration, polyradiculopathy, and sensory neuronopathy.[114,125] Paraneoplastic SPS appears to be more commonly associated with autoantibodies directed against amphiphysin than GAD-65.[113,114,150,152,153] In a large series from 53 amphiphysin-IgG–positive cases identified at the Mayo Clinic, 33 patients (60%) manifested with a peripheral neuropathy, including sensory ganglionopathy and polyradiculopathy.[125] Stiff-person spectrum disorder was seen in 45% and among these cases, 12 had cancer (small cell cancer of lung in 9, 1 had breast cancer, and 2 had "limited cancer"). There are also reports linking paraneoplastic SPS with antigephyrin antibodies.[114,154,155] In addition to SPS, antiglycine receptor antibodies have been associate with PERM and isolated exaggerated startle (hyperekplexia).[127,128]

Oligoclonal bands in the CSF are common in SPS. Their presence may provide valuable support for the diagnosis of SPS in an individual who does not possess identifiable antibodies in either serum or their CSF. Other organ-specific autoantibodies may be found in SPS including antithyroid, anti-intrinsic factor, antinuclear, anti-RNP, and antigliadin.[113] Routine testing for these less specific autoantibodies is not generally recommended as they are more likely representative of an underlying autoimmune diathesis than indicative of SPS.

Regarding EDX evaluation, routine NCS are normal. Needle electromyography of symptomatic muscles will reveal MUAPs with normal morphology and firing rates. The only difference between SPS and normal patients is that these MUAPs fire involuntarily and simultaneously in both agonist and antagonist muscle groups. This pattern must be interpreted with caution, however, as spontaneously firing MUAPs in a single muscle is common in a normal, tense individual. In addition, it is possible for a normal individual to consciously activate agonist and antagonist and feign this pattern of abnormality should they be incentivised to do so. In our opinion, the greatest value of EDX in a suspected SPS patient is to exclude the waveforms that characterize other disorders that should be considered in the SPS differential diagnosis.

Other electrophysiologic techniques, not routinely applied in clinical settings, may demonstrate abnormalities consistent with known SPS pathophysiology.[112,113] In keeping with the lack of CNS inhibition that occurs in this disease, hyperexcitability of the reflex arc in SPS can be demonstrated. Vibration-induced inhibition of H reflexes is a GABAergic phenomenon that may be suppressed in SPS. Enhancement of exteroceptive reflexes appears to be specific for SPS. This phenomenon involves the demonstration of prolonged, tonic activity in multiple muscles not typically activated by a brief train of suprathreshold electrical stimuli to peripheral sensory nerve. With the blink reflex, it may be possible to demonstrate a contralateral R1 response. Excessive muscle activation in response to auditory stimuli (startle response), both in degree and in distribution, can be recorded in SPS.[112] The electrical analogue of the head retraction reflex described in the clinical section is one example of this where discharges from the trapezius muscles can be obtained by electrical stimulation of a trigeminal nerve branch.

MR imaging of the brain and spinal cord in SPS patients is usually normal.[114,156] Specifically, SPS patients with cerebellar syndromes do not demonstrate cerebellar atrophy.[114] MR spectroscopy, however, may demonstrate a significant regional decrease in GABA levels in the motor cortices in these patients.[114,139,156]

HISTOPATHOLOGY

Histologic findings in SPS are limited and inconsistent, thus suggesting a predominantly physiologic rather than histologic pathogenesis.[110,112] Postmortem examination may reveal loss of anterior horn cells, interneurons, and small alpha and gamma motor neurons within the spinal cord or cerebellum, but these findings are inconsistent. More overt pathology is seen in PERM in which perivascular inflammation in the cord, brain, and brainstem may be identified.[112,155,157]

PATHOGENESIS

SPS is an autoimmune disease, related to circulating autoantibodies to proteins involved in GABA neurotransmission, resulting in impaired GABAergic inhibition of α-motor neurons within the brain and spinal cord. The exact pathogenic mechanisms, specifically whether these autoantibodies are causal, remains unknown.

GAD is an enzyme that catalyzes the decarboxylation of glutamate to GABA. GAD is widely prevalent in the cytosol, specifically the inner surface of synaptic vesicles of GABA-secreting neurons within the CNS. GABA is the major inhibitory neurotransmitter within the forebrain, whereas both GABA and glycine serve in this capacity within the spinal cord. There are other proteins relevant to SPS and CNS, which causes neuromuscular hyperexcitability. Amphiphysin is another cytosolic presynaptic protein that is responsible for the retrieval of the vesicular protein following GABA exocytosis.[113]

GABA-receptor–associated protein (GABARAP) is a postsynaptic protein that stabilizes and surface expression of GABA-A receptors as well as modulating their conductance.[114] Approximately 65%–70% of GAD-65 seropositive SPS patients will have antibodies that react with this protein.[113,114] These antibodies inhibit the surface expression and impair the stability of GABA-A receptors.[114] Gephyrin (GHPN) is a postsynaptic protein responsible for the clustering of glycine receptors in the spinal cord and GABA-A receptors within the brain, essential for their proper functioning.[114] Accordingly, knockout of the *GHPN* gene in mice results in an SPS phenotype.

The exact roles of the autoantibodies remain, however, uncertain. GAD-65–specific autoantibodies harvested from SPS patients inhibit GAD activity and GABA synthesis in vitro. They are presumed to adversely affect inhibitory GABA interneurons in the spinal gray matter and cortex, leading to continuous tonic firing of α-motor neurons.[112,141,158] Given the logic of this hypothesis, the high prevalence of GAD-65 autoantibodies in high-titer in SPS patients, and their apparent intrathecal synthesis, it is tempting to suggest that GAD-65 have a direct pathogenic role. Inhibition of GABA synthesis and interference with GABA vesicle exocytosis are proposed mechanisms.[113]

TREATMENT

The treatment of SPS involves the use of both symptomatic agents to enhance GABAergic influences and immunomodulating treatments aimed at the presumed autoimmune basis of the disease.[1,2,113,114] In the case of paraneoplastic SPS, treatment and, if possible, eradication of the underlying tumor represent the initial therapeutic goal. Patients are typically treatment responsive, although complete eradication of symptoms is the exception rather than the rule. A significant portion of affected individuals remain dependent on others for at least some activities of daily living.

Benzodiazepines have been the historical mainstay of symptomatic treatment.[114] Patients require and are tolerant of large doses, with a median daily diazepam dose of 40 mg required to provide efficacy without excessive side effects. Although many SPS patients tolerate doses of benzodiazepines that normal patients would not, unwanted CNS side effects still represent a limitation of this therapy. Antispasticity drugs provide a second line of symptomatic treatment. Baclofen, tizanidine, and dantrolene have been used with some success.[114] Baclofen can also be used intrathecally and has been shown to have some benefit in controlled trials but is associated with the potential risk of significant complication.[141] A number of anticonvulsants with mechanisms of action that augment GABA effect have been tried with anecdotal reports of benefit including gabapentin, valproic acid, levetiracetam, vigabatrin, and tiagabine. Botulinum toxin may benefit individual patients as well but is limited by its cost, and the need for large doses to adequately address large axial muscle groups.

We reported a small series of six patients with SPS who appeared to have objective improvement with IVIG.[159] Subsequently a randomized, placebo-controlled trial of IVIG in 16 patients with PSP and reported clinical improvement associated with a reduction in GAD autoantibody titers with IVIG.[160] There have been several case reports of rituximab leading to beneficial and protracted responses,[161,162] however, a randomized, double-blind, placebo-controlled trial found no benefit.[163] It is conceivable though that rituximab works in a subset of patients and that the clinical scales utilized in the study were not responsible to change, particularly in less severely affected patients.

There have been many reports describing anecdotal responses to other immunomodulating therapies but a limited evidence basis by which to judge efficacy. In general, efforts to assess treatment efficacy in SPS are hampered not only by the rarity of the condition but by the lack of adequate parameters by which to measure it. PLEX has benefited some patients. Corticosteroids are less attractive than in other diseases, in view of the high concordance of diabetes. Azathioprine, methotrexate, and mycophenolate have been tried. As in other paraneoplastic syndromes, successful treatment of the underlying malignancy may lessen the morbidity of the associated SPS.

▶ HYPEREKPLEXIA

CLINICAL FEATURES

Hyperekplexia originates from the Greek "ekplexis" meaning surprise, an apt description for the exaggerated startle response that characterizes the syndrome. It is characterized by nonepileptic, paroxysmal rigidity, and hyperreflexia in response to external, often auditory stimuli. The startle response frequently includes eye blinking and trunk flexion similar to a salaam attack in West syndrome. Voluntary movement is typically precluded during the spasm.

Hyperekplexia can be hereditary or autoimmune in nature.[164,165] As previously discussed, hyperekplexia can been seen patients with anti-GAD spectrum disorder as well as SPS with other autoantibodies (i.e., α1-subunit of the glycine receptor or GlyR).[126–128] Hereditary hyperekplexia is more common and typically a newborn disorder, but it often persists to some degree during adult life. Affected adults often experience drop attacks as their major manifestation. In neonates, it may be provoked by handling. Childcare, such as changing a diaper, may be impaired due to the inability to passively abduct the legs. The spasms tend to disappear during sleep but may occur at night during arousals. The clinical examination may reveal an exaggerated head retraction response as is described above in the SPS. Gentle tapping of the tip of the nose will elicit a startle response in affected babies. The severity of hyperekplexia varies and in extreme cases, it can result in neonatal cardiac arrest and death.

LABORATORY FEATURES

The most common cause of hereditary hyperekplexia (hyperekplexia-1 or HKPX1) is mutations (both autosomal dominant and recessive) in the human glycine receptor α1-subunit gene, *GLRA1*.[164,165] HKPX2 is caused by AR mutations in *GLRB* encoding the glycine receptor β subunit.[166,167] HKPX3 is caused by AD or AR mutations in the *SLC6A5* that encodes for glycine transporter, GlyT2.[168] HKPX4 is caused by AR mutations in the *ATAD1* which encodes for ATPase family, AAA+ domain containing 1-protein.[169] Additionally, rare mutations in the rho guanine nuclear exchange factor 9 gene, *ARHGEF9*,[170] and the gephyrin gene, *GPHN*, can result in hyperekplexia.[171]

PATHOGENESIS

The hereditary forms predominantly involve the glycine receptors or those organizational proteins that are important in clusters and localizes the inhibitory glycine (GlyR) and GABA-A receptors to the microtubular matrix of the neuronal postsynaptic membrane. The mutations in relevant genes as well as antibodies in the rare autoimmune etiologies lead to a lack of inhibition within the pontomedullary reticular formation and the exaggerated response to startle and other stimuli.

TREATMENT

There have been no studies addressing therapeutic intervention in hyperekplexia. Clonazepam has been reported to have a beneficial effect. Phenytoin, carbamazepine, piracetam, clobazam, vigabatrin, phenobarbital, 5-hydroxytryptophan, and diazepam have been used anecdotally with uncertain benefit. Positioning a child in a flexed, fetal position may abort a spasm. Autoimmune forms may be responsive to immunotherapies as discussed in the section regarding SPS.

▶ SUMMARY

With the exception of cramps and fasciculations, the disorders described in this chapter are uncommon. Most of these disorders have, to some extent, overlapping clinical features. Successful diagnosis requires a heightened index of clinical suspicion, detailed knowledge concerning each disorder's phenotypic characteristics, and awareness of the serologic and EDX features of each syndrome. Many of these disorders appear to have an autoimmune pathogenesis, some of which are in turn related to underlying malignancies. No singular treatment paradigm exists for any of these disorders. In many cases, both immunomodulating therapies and symptomatic measures will provide relief from disease morbidity.

REFERENCES

1. Sawlani K, Katirji B. Peripheral nerve hyperexcitability syndromes. *Continuum (Minneap Minn)*. 2017;23(5, Peripheral Nerve and Motor Neuron Disorders):1437–1450.
2. De Wel B, Claeys KG. Neuromuscular hyperexcitability syndromes. *Curr Opin Neurol*. 2021;34(5):714–720.
3. Miller TM, Layzer RB. Muscle cramps. *Muscle Nerve*. 2005;32:431–442.
4. Norris FH Jr, Gasteiger EL, Chatfield PO. An electromyographic study of induced and spontaneous muscle cramps. *Electroencephalogr Clin Neurophysiol*. 1957;9(1):139–147.
5. Dijkstra JN, Boon E, Kruijt N, et al. Muscle cramps and contractures: causes and treatment. *Pract Neurol*. 2023;23(1):23–34.
6. Bordoni B, Sugumar K, Varacallo M. Muscle cramps. In: *StatPearls [Internet]*. StatPearls Publishing; 2022.
7. Tahmoush AJ, Alonso RJ, Tahmoush GP, Heiman-Patterson TD. Cramp–fasciculation syndrome: a treatable hyperexcitable peripheral nerve disorder. *Neurology*. 1991;41:1021–1024.
8. Masland RL. Cramp-fasciculation syndrome. *Neurology*. 1992;42(2):466.
9. Newsom-Davis J, Mills KR. Immunological associations of acquired neuromyotonia (Isaacs' syndrome). Report of five cases and literature review. *Brain*. 1993;116:453–469.
10. Lo HP, Bertini E, Mirabella M, et al. Mosaic caveolin-3 expression in acquired rippling muscle disease without evidence of myasthenia gravis or acetylcholine receptor autoantibodies. *Neuromuscul Disord*. 2011;21(3):194–203.
11. George JS, Harikrishnan S, Ali I, Baresi R, Hanemann CO. Acquired rippling muscle disease in association with myasthenia gravis. *J Neurol Neurosurg Psychiatry*. 2010;81(1):125–126.
12. Dubey D, Beecher G, Hammami MB, et al. Identification of caveolae-associated protein 4 autoantibodies as a biomarker of immune-mediated rippling muscle disease in adults. *JAMA Neurol*. 2022;79(8):808–816.
13. Brody IA. Muscle contracture induced by exercise. A syndrome attributable to decreased relaxing factor. *N Engl J Med*. 1969;281:187–192.
14. Karpati G, Charuk J, Carpenter S, Jablecki C, Holland P. Myopathy caused by a deficiency of Ca^{2+}-adenosine triphosphatase in sarcoplasmic reticulum (Brody's disease). *Ann Neurol*. 1986;20:38–49.
15. Odermatt A, Taschner PE, Khanna VK, et al. Mutations in the gene-encoding SERCA1, the fast-twitch skeletal muscle sarcoplasmic reticulum Ca2-ATPase, are associated with Brody disease. *Nat Genet*. 1996;14:191–194.
16. Liguori R, Donadio V, DiStasi V, Cianchi C, Montagna P. Palmaris brevis spasm: an occupational syndrome. *Neurology*. 2003;60:1705–1707.
17. Katzberg HD, Khan AH, So YT. Assessment: symptomatic treatment for muscle cramps (an evidence based review): report of the therapeutics and technology assessment subcommittee of the American academy of neurology. *Neurology*. 2010;74:691–696.
18. de Carvalho M, Swash M. Fasciculation potentials: a study of amyotrophic lateral sclerosis and other neurogenic disorders. *Muscle Nerve*. 1998;21:336–344.
19. Daube JR, Rubin DI. Needle electromyography. *Muscle Nerve*. 2009;39:244–270.
20. Mills KR. Characteristics of fasciculations in amyotrophic lateral sclerosis and the benign fasciculation syndrome. *Brain*. 2010;133:3458–3469.

21. Verdru P, Leenders J, Van Hees J. Cramp–fasciculation syndrome. *Neurology.* 1992;42:1846–1847.
22. Food and Drug Administration, Department of Health and Human Services. Drug products containing quinine; enforcement action dates. *Federal Register.* 2006;71:75557–75560.
23. Garrison SR, Korownyk CS, Kolber MR, et al. Magnesium for skeletal muscle cramps. *Cochrane Database Syst Rev.* 2020; 9(9):CD009402.
24. Weiss MD, Macklin EA, Simmons Z, et al; Mexiletine ALS Study Group. A randomized trial of mexiletine in ALS: safety and effects on muscle cramps and progression. *Neurology.* 2016;86(16):1474–1481.
25. Blexrud MD, Windebank AJ, Daube JR. Long-term follow-up of 121 patients with benign fasciculations. *Ann Neurol.* 1993; 34:622–625.
26. Denny-Brown D, Foley JM. Myokymia and the benign fasciculation of muscle cramps. *Trans Assoc Am Physicians.* 1948;61:88–96.
27. Isaacs H. A syndrome of continuous muscle fiber activity. *J Neurol Neurosurg Psychiatry.* 1961;24:319–325.
28. Irani SR, Pettingill P, Kleopa KA, et al. Morvan syndrome: clinical and serological observations in 29 cases. *Ann Neurol.* 2012;72:241–255.
29. Masood W, Sitammagari KK. Morvan syndrome. In: *StatPearls [Internet].* StatPearls Publishing; 2022.
30. Gastaldi M, De Rosa A, Maestri M, et al. Acquired neuromyotonia in thymoma-associated myasthenia gravis: a clinical and serological study. *Eur J Neurol.* 2019;26(7):992–999.
31. Comperat L, Pegat A, Honnorat J, Joubert B. Autoimmune neuromyotonia. *Curr Opin Neurol.* 2022;35(5):597–603.
32. Rubio-Agusti I, Perez-Miralles F, Sevilla T, et al. Peripheral nerve hyperexcitability; a clinical and immunologic study of 38 patients. *Neurology.* 2011;76:172–178.
33. Waerness E. Neuromyotonia and bronchial carcinoma. *Electromyogr Clin Neurophysiol.* 1974;14:527–535.
34. Rosin L, De Camilli P, Butler M, et al. Stiff-man syndrome in a woman with breast cancer: an uncommon central nervous system paraneoplastic syndrome. *Neurology.* 1998;50(1):94–98.
35. Caress JB, Abend WK, Preston DC, Logigian EL. A case of Hodgkin's lymphoma producing neuromyotonia. *Neurology.* 1997;49:258–259.
36. García-Merino A, Cabello A, Mora JS, Liaño H. Continuous muscle fiber activity, peripheral neuropathy, and thymoma. *Ann Neurol.* 1991;29:215–218.
37. Partanen VS, Soininen H, Saksa M, Riekkinen P. Electromyographic and nerve conduction findings in a patient with neuromyotonia, normocalcemic tetany, and small-cell lung cancer. *Acta Neurol Scand.* 1980;61(4):216–226.
38. Issa SS, Herskovitz S, Lipton RB. Acquired neuromyotonia as a paraneoplastic manifestation of ovarian cancer. *Neurology.* 2011;76:100–101.
39. Balck JT, Garcia-Mullin R, Good E, Brown S. Muscle rigidity in a newborn due to continuous peripheral nerve excitability. *Arch Neurol.* 1972;27(5):413–425.
40. Jamieson PW, Katirji MG. Idiopathic generalized myokymia. *Muscle Nerve.* 1994;17:42–51.
41. Isaacs H, Frere G. Syndrome of continuous muscle fiber activity. Histochemical, nerve terminal and end-plate study of two cases. *S Afr Med J.* 1974;48:1601–1607.
42. Isaacs H. Continuous muscle fiber activity in an Indian male with additional evidence of terminal motor fiber activity. *J Neurol Neurosurg Psychiatry.* 1967;30:126–133.
43. Maddison P, Mills KR, Newsom-Davis J. Clinical electrophysiological characterization of the acquired neuromyotonia phenotype of autoimmune peripheral nerve hyperexcitability. *Muscle Nerve.* 2006;33(6):801–808.
44. Barroso L, Hoyt W. Episodic exotropia from lateral rectus neuromyotonia-appearance and remission after radiation therapy for a thalamic glioma. *J Pediatr Ophthalmol Strabismus.* 1993;30:56–57.
45. Lessell S, Lessell IM, Rizzo JF III. Ocular neuromyotonia after radiation therapy. *Am J Ophthalmol.* 1986;102:766–770.
46. Yuruten B, Ilhan S. Ocular neuromyotonia: a case report. *Clin Neurol Neurosurg.* 2003;105(2):140–142.
47. Modarres H, Samuel M, Schon F. Isolated finger flexion: a novel form of focal neuromyotonia. *J Neurol Neurosurg Psychiatry.* 2000;69:110–113.
48. Lublin FD, Tsairis P, Streletz LJ, et al. Myokymia and impaired muscular relaxation with continuous motor unit activity. *J Neurol Neurosurg Psychiatry.* 1979;42:557–562.
49. Weiss N, Behin A, Psimaras D, Delattre J-Y. Post-irradiation neuromyotonia of spinal accessory nerves. *Neurology.* 2011;76: 1188–1189.
50. Hahn AF, Parkes AW, Bolton CW, Stewart SA. Neuromyotonia in hereditary motor neuropathy. *J Neurol Neurosurg Psychiatry.* 1991;54(3):230–235.
51. Zimoń M, Baets J, Almeida-Souza L, et al. Loss-of-function mutations in HINT1 cause axonal neuropathy with neuromyotonia. *Nat Genet.* 2012;44(10):1080–1083.
52. Peeters K, Chamova T, Tournev I, Jordanova A. Axonal neuropathy with neuromyotonia: there is a HINT. *Brain.* 2017;140(4):868–877.
53. Odabasi Z, Joy JL, Claussen GC, Herrera GA, Oh SJ. Issacs' syndrome associated with chronic inflammatory demyelinating polyneuropathy. *Muscle Nerve.* 1996;19:210–215.
54. Lee EK, Maselli RA, Ellis WG, Agius MA. Morvan's fibrillary chorea: a paraneoplastic manifestation of thymoma. *J Neurol Neurosurg Psychiatry.* 1998;65:857–862.
55. Kleopa KA, Elman LB, Lang B, Vincent A, Scherer SS. Neuromyotonia and limbic encephalitis sera target mature Shaker-type K^+ channels: subunit specificity correlates with clinical manifestations. *Brain.* 2006;129:1570–1584.
56. Evoli A, Monaco ML, Marra R, Lino MM, Batocchi AP, Tonali PA. Multiple paraneoplastic diseases associated with thymoma. *Neuromuscul Disord.* 1999;9(8):601–603.
57. Heidenreich F, Vincent A. Antibodies to ion-channel proteins in thymoma with myasthenia, neuromyotonia, and peripheral neuropathy. *Neurology.* 1998;50:1483–1485.
58. Martinelli P, Patuelli A, Minardi C, Cau A, Riviera AM, Dal Posso F. Neuromyotonia, peripheral neuropathy and myasthenia gravis. *Muscle Nerve.* 1996;19:505–510.
59. Reeback J, Benton S, Swash M, Schwartz MS. Penicillamine-induced neuromyotonia. *Br Med J.* 1979;1(6176):1464–1465.
60. Welch LK, Appenzeller O, Bicknell JM. Peripheral neuropathy with myokymia, sustained muscular contraction, and continuous motor unit activity. *Neurology.* 1972;22:161–169.
61. Gutmann L, Gutmann L. Myokymia and neuromyotonia 2004. *J Neurol.* 2004;251(2):138–142.
62. Hart IK, Waters C, Vincent A, et al. Autoantibodies detected to expressed K^+ channels are implicated in neuromyotonia. *Ann Neurol.* 1997;41(2):238–256.
63. Tan KM, Lennon VA, Klein CJ, Boeve EF, Pittock SJ. Clinical spectrum of voltage-gated potassium channel autoimmunity. *Neurology.* 2008;70:1883–1890.

64. Michael S, Waters P, Irani SR. Stop testing for autoantibodies to the VGKC-complex: only request LGI1 and CASPR2. *Pract Neurol.* 2020;20(5):377–384.
65. Binks SNM, Klein CJ, Waters P, Pittock SJ, Irani SR. LGI1, CASPR2 and related antibodies: a molecular evolution of the phenotypes. *J Neurol Neurosurg Psychiatry.* 2018;89(5):526–534.
66. Brown TJ. Isaacs' syndrome. *Arch Phys Med Rehabil.* 1984;65:27–29.
67. Lütschg J, Jerusalem F, Ludin H, Vassella F, Mumenthaler M. The syndrome of 'continuous muscle fiber activity.' *Arch Neurol.* 1978;35:198–205.
68. Dhand UK. Issacs's syndrome: clinical and electro-physiological response to gabapentin. *Muscle Nerve.* 2006;34:646–650.
69. Deymeer F, Emre Öge A, Serdaroglu P, Yazici JK, Özdemir C, Baslo A. The use of botulinum toxin in localizing neuromyotonia to the terminal branches of the peripheral nerve. *Muscle Nerve.* 1998;21:643–646.
70. Jackson DL, Satya-Murti S, Davis L, Drachman DB. Isaacs syndrome with laryngeal involvement: an unusual presentation of myokymia. *Neurology.* 1979;29:1612–1615.
71. Irani PF, Purohit AV, Wadia NH. The syndrome of continuous muscle fiber activity. Evidence to suggest proximal neurogenic causation. *Acta Neurol Scand.* 1977;55:273–288.
72. Sakai T, Hosokawa S, Shibasaki H, et al. Syndrome of continuous muscle-fiber activity: increased CSF GABA and effect of dantrolene. *Neurology.* 1983;33(4):495–498.
73. Hart IK. Acquired neuromyotonia: a new autoantibody-mediated neuronal potassium channelopathy. *Am J Med Sci.* 2000;319:209–216.
74. Ruff RL. Upsetting the balance among membrane channels can produce hyperexcitablity or inexcitability. *Neurology.* 2007;69:2036–2037.
75. Wallis WE, Van Poznak A, Plum F. Generalized muscular stiffness, fasciculations, and myokymia of peripheral nerve origin. *Arch Neurol.* 1970;22:430–439.
76. Lancaster E, Huijbers MG, Bar C, et al. Investigations of caspr2, an autoantigen of encephalitis and neuromyotonia. *Ann Neurol.* 2011;69(2):303–311.
77. Sinha S, Newsom-Davis J, Mills K, Byrne N, Lang B, Vincent A. Autoimmune aetiology for acquired neuromyotonia (Isaacs' syndrome). *Lancet.* 1991;338:75–77.
78. Alessi G, De Reuck J, De Bleecker J, Vancayzeele S. Successful immunoglobulin treatment in a patient with neuromyotonia. *Clin Neurol Neurosurg.* 2000;102:173–175.
79. Ho WK, Wilson JD. Hypothermia, hyperhidrosis, myokymia and increased urinary excretion of catecholamines associated with a thymoma. *Med J Aust.* 1993;158:787–788.
80. Ishii A, Hayashi A, Ohkoshi N, et al. Clinical evaluation of plasma exchange and high dose intravenous immunoglobulin in a patient with Isaacs' syndrome. *J Neurol Neurosurg Psychiatry.* 1994;57(7):840–842.
81. van den Berg JS, van Engelen BG, Boerman RH, de Baets MH. Acquired neuromyotonia: superiority of plasma exchange over high-dose intravenous immunoglobulin. *J Neurol.* 1999;246:623–625.
82. Dalakas MC. IgG4-mediated neurologic autoimmunities: Understanding the pathogenicity of IgG4, ineffectiveness of IVIg, and long-lasting benefits of Anti-B cell therapies. *Neurol Neuroimmunol Neuroinflamm.* 2021;9(1):e1116.
83. Roos KL. Tetanus. *Semin Neurol.* 1991;11(3):205–214.
84. Vandelaer J, Birmingham M, Gasse F, Kurian M, Shaw C, Garnier S. Tetanus in developing countries: an update on the Maternal and Neonatal Tetanus Elimination Initiative. *Vaccine.* 2003;21(24):3442.
85. Schiavo G, Benfata F, Poulain B, et al. Tetanus and botulinum toxin-B neurotoxins block neurotransmitter release by proteolytic cleavage of synaptobrevin. *Nature.* 1992;359(6398):832–835.
86. Link E, Edelman L, Chou JH, et al. Tetanus toxin action: inhibition of neurotransmitter release linked to synaptobrevin proteolysis. *Biochem Biophys Res Commun.* 1992;189(2):1017–1023.
87. Price DL, Griffin JW. Tetanus toxin: retrograde axonal transport of systemically administered toxin. *Neurosci Lett.* 1977;4:61–65.
88. Montecucco C, Schiavo G. Structure and function of tetanus and botulinum neurotoxins. *Q Rev Biophys.* 1995;28:423–472.
89. Sexton DJ, Westerman EL. Tetanus. *UpToDate.* 2006;14:3.
90. Verma R, Khanna P. Tetanus toxoid vaccine: elimination of neonatal tetanus in selected states of India. *Hum Vaccin Immunother.* 2012;8(10):1439–1442.
91. Berger SA, Cherubin CE, Nelson S, Levine L. Tetanus despite preexisting antitetanus antibody. *JAMA.* 1978;240:769–770.
92. Kabura L, Ilibagiza D, Menten J, Van den Ende J. Intrathecal versus intramuscular administration of human anti-tetanus immunoglobulin or equine tetanus antitoxin in the treatment of tetanus: a meta-analysis. *Trop Med Int Health.* 2006;11:1075–1081.
93. Engrand N, Guerot E, Rouamba A, Vilain GA. The efficacy of intrathecal baclofen in severe tetanus. *Anesthesiology.* 1999;90:1773–1776.
94. Santos ML, Mota-Miranda A, Alves-Pereira A, Gomes A, Correia J, Marçal N. Intrathecal baclofen for the treatment of tetanus. *Clin Infect Dis.* 2004;38:321–328.
95. Sehgal V, Vijayan S, Yasmin S, Srirangalingam U, Pati J, Drake WM. Normocalcaemic tetany. *Clin Med (Lond).* 2011;11(6):594–595.
96. Anwikar SR, Bandekar MS, Patel TK, Patel PB, Kshirsagar NA. Tetany: possible adverse effect of bevacizumab. *Indian J Cancer.* 2011;48(1):31–33.
97. Lameris AL, Monnens LA, Bindels RJ, Hoenderop JG. Drug-induced alterations in Mg2+ homoeostasis. *Clin Sci (Lond).* 2012;123(1):1–14.
98. Aiyangar A, Chowdhary P, Rao K, Kiran K. Normocalcaemic, normomagnesaemic tetany with tacrolimus. *Nephrology (Carlton).* 2011;16(8):784–785.
99. Brick JF, Gutmann L, McComas CF. Calcium effect on generation and amplification of myokymic discharges. *Neurology.* 1982;32:618–622.
100. Satoyoshi E, Yamada K. Recurrent muscle spasms of central origin. A report of two cases. *Arch Neurol.* 1967;16:254–264.
101. Heger S, Kuester RM, Volk R, Stephani U, Sippell WG. Satoyoshi syndrome: a rare multisystemic disorder requiring systemic and symptomatic treatment. *Brain Dev.* 2006;28(5):300–304.
102. Satoyoshi E. A syndrome of progressive muscle spasm, alopecia, and diarrhea. *Neurology.* 1978;28:458–471.
103. Ikeda K, Satoyoshi E, Kinoshita M, Wakata N, Iwasaki Y. Satoyoshi's syndrome in an adult: a review of the literature of adult onset cases. *Intern Med.* 1998;37:784–787.
104. Matsuura E, Matsuyama W, Sameshima T, Arimura K. Satoyoshi syndrome has antibody against brain and gastrointestinal tissue. *Muscle Nerve.* 2007;36:400–403.
105. Endo K, Yamamoto T, Nakamura K, et al. Improvement of Satoyoshi syndrome with tacrolimus and corticosteroids. *Neurology.* 2003;600(12):2014–2015.

106. Uddin AB, Walters AS, Ali A, Brannan T. A unilateral presentation of 'Satoyoshi syndrome.' *Parkinsonism Relat Disord.* 2002;8(3):211–213.
107. Drost G, Verrips A, Hooijkass H, Zwarts M. Glutamic acid decarboxylase antibodies in Satoyoshi syndrome. *Ann Neurol.* 2004;55(3):450–451.
108. Cecchin CR, Felix TM, Magalhaes RB, Furlanetto TW. Satoyoshi syndrome in a Caucasian girl improved with glucocorticoids—a clinical report. *Am J Med Genet A.* 2003;118A:52–54.
109. Arita J, Hamano S, Nara T, Maekawa K. Intravenous gammaglobulin therapy of Satoyoshi syndrome. *Brain Dev.* 1996;18:409–411.
110. Moersch FP, Woltman HW. Progressive fluctuating rigidity and spasm (stiff-man syndrome): report of a case and some observations in 13 other cases. *Proc Staff Meet Mayo Clin.* 1956;31:421–427.
111. Dalakas M, Fujii M, Li M, McElroy B. The clinical spectrum of anti-GAD antibody-positive patients with stiff-person syndrome. *Neurology.* 2000;55:1531–1535.
112. Espay AJ, Chen R. Rigidity and spasms from autoimmune encephalomyelopathies: stiff-person syndrome. *Muscle Nerve.* 2006;34:677–690.
113. Rakocevic G, Floeter MK. Autoimmune stiff person syndrome and related myelopathies: understanding of electrophysiological and immunological processes. *Muscle Nerve.* 2012;45:623–634.
114. Dalakas MC. Advances in the pathogenesis and treatment of patients with stiff person syndrome. *Curr Neurol Neurosci Rep.* 2008;8:48–55.
115. McKeon A, Robinson MT, McEvoy KM, et al. Stiff-man syndrome and variants: clinical course, treatments, and outcomes. *Arch Neurol.* 2012;69(2):230–238.
116. Dalakas MC. Stiff-person syndrome and GAD antibody-spectrum disorders: GABAergic neuronal excitability, immunopathogenesis and update on antibody therapies. *Neurotherapeutics.* 2022;19(3):832–847.
117. Madlener M, Strippel C, Thaler FS, et al; German Network for Research on Autoimmune Encephalitis (GENERATE). Glutamic acid decarboxylase antibody-associated neurological syndromes: clinical and antibody characteristics and therapy response. *J Neurol Sci.* 2022;445:120540.
118. Wang Y, Tourkevich R, Bosley J, Gold DR, Newsome SD. Ocular motor and vestibular characteristics of antiglutamic acid decarboxylase-associated neurologic disorders. *J Neuroophthalmol.* 2021;41(4):e665–e671.
119. Newsome SD, Johnson T. Stiff person syndrome spectrum disorders; more than meets the eye. *J Neuroimmunol.* 2022;369:577915.
120. Budhram A, Sechi E, Flanagan EP, et al. Clinical spectrum of high-titre GAD65 antibodies. *J Neurol Neurosurg Psychiatry.* 2021;92(6):645–654.
121. Muñoz-Lopetegi A, de Bruijn MAAM, Boukhrissi S, et al. Neurologic syndromes related to anti-GAD65: clinical and serologic response to treatment. *Neurol Neuroimmunol Neuroinflamm.* 2020;7(3):e696.
122. Graus F, Saiz A, Dalmau J. GAD antibodies in neurological disorders—insights and challenges. *Nat Rev Neurol.* 2020;16:353–365.
123. Dalmau J, Graus F. Autoimmune encephalitis—misdiagnosis, misconceptions, and how to avoid them. *JAMA Neurol.* 2023;80(1):12–14.
124. Flanagan EP, Geschwind MD, Lopez-Chiriboga AS, et al. Autoimmune encephalitis misdiagnosis in adults. *JAMA Neurol.* 2023;80(1):30–39.
125. Dubey D, Jitprapaikulsan J, Bi H, et al. Amphiphysin-IgG autoimmune neuropathy: a recognizable clinicopathologic syndrome. *Neurology.* 2019;93(20):e1873–e1880.
126. Piquet AL, Khan M, Warner JEA, et al. Novel clinical features of glycine receptor antibody syndrome: a series of 17 cases. *Neurol Neuroimmunol Neuroinflamm.* 2019;6(5):e592.
127. Hinson SR, Lopez-Chiriboga AS, Bower JH, et al. Glycine receptor modulating antibody predicting treatable stiff-person spectrum disorders. *Neurol Neuroimmunol Neuroinflamm.* 2018;5(2):e438.
128. Martinez-Hernandez E, Ariño H, McKeon A, et al. Clinical and immunologic investigations in patients with stiff-person spectrum disorder. *JAMA Neurol.* 2016;73(6):714–720.
129. Butler MH, Hayashi A, Ohkoshi N, et al. Autoimmunity to gephyrin in stiff-man syndrome. *Neuron.* 2000;26(2):307–312.
130. McEvoy KM. Stiff-man syndrome. *Mayo Clin Proc.* 1991;66:300–304.
131. Miller F, Korsvik H. Baclofen in the treatment of stiff-man syndrome. *Ann Neurol.* 1981;9(5):511–512.
132. Folli F. Stiff-man syndrome, 40 years later. *J Neurol Neurosurg Psychiatry.* 1998;65:618.
133. Mitosumoto H, Schwartzman MJ, Estes ML, et al. Sudden death and paroxysmal autonomic dysfunction in stiff-man syndrome. *J Neurol.* 1991;238(2):91–96.
134. Barker RA, Revesz T, Thom M, Marsden CD, Brown P. Review of 23 patients affected by the stiff man syndrome: clinical subdivision into stiff trunk(man) syndrome, stiff limb syndrome, and progressive encephalomyelitis with rigidity. *J Neurol Neurosurg Psychiatry.* 1998;65:633–640.
135. Brown P, Marsden CD. The stiff man and stiff man plus syndromes. *J Neurol.* 1999;246:648–652.
136. Saiz A, Graus F, Valldeoriola F, Valls-Solé J, Tolosa E. Stiff-leg syndrome: a focal form of stiff-man syndrome. *Ann Neurol.* 1998;43:400–403.
137. Souza-Lima CF, Ferraz HB, Braz CA, Araüjo AM, Manzano GM. Marked improvement in a stiff-limb patient treated with intravenous immunoglobulin. *Mov Disord.* 2000;15:358–359.
138. Silverman IE. Paraneoplastic stiff limb syndrome. *J Neurol Neurosurg Psychiatry.* 1999;67(1):126–127.
139. Levy LM, Dalakas MC, Floeter MK. The stiff-person syndrome: an autoimmune disorder affecting neurotransmission of gamma-aminobutyric acid. *Ann Intern Med.* 1999;131:522–530.
140. Amato AA, Cornmann EW, Kissel JT. Treatment of stiff-man syndrome with intravenous immunoglobulin. *Neurology.* 1994;44:1652–1654.
141. Silbert PL, Masumoto JY, McManis PG, Stolp-Smith KA, Elliott BA, McEvoy KM. Intrathecal baclofen therapy in stiff-man syndrome: a double-blind, placebo-controlled trial. *Neurology.* 1995;45:1893–1897.
142. Solimena M, Folli F, Denis-Donini S, et al. Autoantibodies to glutamic acid decarboxylase in a patient with stiff-man syndrome, epilepsy, and type I diabetes mellitus. *N Engl J Med.* 1988;318(16):1012–1020.
143. Solimena M, Folli F, Aparisi R, Pozza G, De Camilli P. Autoantibodies to GABA-ergic and pancreatic beta cells in stiff-man syndrome. *N Engl J Med.* 1990;322:1555–1560.

144. Whiteley AM, Swash M, Urich H. Progressive encephalomyelitis with rigidity. *Brain*. 1976;99:27–42.
145. Howell DA, Lees AJ, Toghill PJ. Spinal internuncial neurones in progressive encephalomyelitis with rigidity. *J Neurol Neurosurg Psychiatry*. 1979;42:773–785.
146. Leigh PN, Rothwell JC, Traub M, Marsden CD. A patients with reflex myoclonus and muscle rigidity: "jerking stiff-man syndrome." *J Neurol Neurosurg Psychiatry*. 1980;43:1125–1131.
147. Rakocevic G, Faju R, Dalakas MC. Anti-glutamic acid decarboxylase antibodies in the serum and cerebrospinal fluid of patients with stiff-person syndrome: correlation with clinical severity. *Arch Neurol*. 2004;61:902–904.
148. Thomas S, Critchley P, Lawden M, et al. Stiff person syndrome with eye movement abnormality, myasthenia gravis, and thymoma. *J Neurol Neurosurg Psychiatry*. 2005;76:141–142.
149. McHugh JC, Murray B, Renganathan R, Connolly S, Lynch T. GAD antibody positive paraneoplastic stiff person syndrome in a patient with renal cell carcinoma. *Mov Disord*. 2007;22:1343–1346.
150. Petzold GC, Marcucci M, Butler MH, et al. Rhabdomyolysis and paraneoplastic stiff-man syndrome with amphiphysin autoimmunity. *Ann Neurol*. 2004;55:286–290.
151. Turner MR, Irani SR, Leite MI, Nithi K, Vincent A, Ansorge O. Progressive encephalomyelitis with rigidity and myoclonus: glycine and NMDA receptor antibodies. *Neurology*. 2011;77:439–443.
152. De Camilli P, Thomas A, Cofiell R, et al. The synaptic vesicle-associated protein amphiphysin is the 128 kD autoantigen of stiff-man syndrome with breast cancer. *J Exp Med*. 1993;178(6):2219–2223.
153. Folli F, Solimena M, Cofiell R, et al. Autoantibodies to a 128-kd synaptic protein in three women with the stiff-man syndrome and breast cancer. *N Engl J Med*. 1993;328(8):546–551.
154. Feng G, Tintrup H, Kirsch J, et al. Dual requirement for gephyrin in glycine receptor clustering and molybdoenzyme activity. *Science*. 1998;282:1321–1324.
155. McCabe DJ, Turner NC, CChao D, et al. Paraneoplastic "stiff-person syndrome" with metastatic adenocarcinoma and anti-Ri antibodies. *Neurology*. 2004;62(8):1402–1404.
156. Levy LM, Levy-Reis I, Fujii M, Dalakas MC. Brain gamma-aminobutyric acid changes in stiff-person syndrome. *Arch Neurol*. 2005;62:970–974.
157. Warren JD, Scott G, Blumbergs PC, Thompson PD. Pathological evidence of encephalomyelitis in the stiff man syndrome with anti-GAD antibodies. *J Clin Neurosci*. 2002;9:328–329.
158. Ishida K, Mitoma H, Song SY, et al. Selective suppression of cerebellar GABAergic transmission by an autoantibody to glutamic acid decarboxylase. *Ann Neurol*. 1999;46(2):263–267.
159. Amato AA, Cornman EW, Kissel JT. Treatment of stiff-man syndrome with intravenous immunoglobulin. *Neurology*. 1994;44(9):1652–1654.
160. Dalakas MC, Fujii M, Li M, Lufti B, Kyhos J, McElroy B. High-dose intravenous immune globulin for stiff-person syndrome. *N Engl J Med*. 2001;345:1870–1876.
161. Baker MR, Das M, Isaacs J, Fawcett PRW, Bates D. Treatment of stiff person syndrome with rituximab. *J Neurol Neurosurg Psychiatry*. 2005;76:999–1001.
162. Dupond JL, Essalmi L, Gil H, Meaux-Ruault N, Hafsaoui C. Rituximab treatment of stiff-person syndrome in a patient with thymoma, diabetes mellitus and autoimmune thyroiditis. *J Clin Neurosci*. 2010;17(3):389–391.
163. Dalakas MC, Rakocevic G, Dambrosia JM, Alexopoulos H, McElroy B. A double-blind, placebo-controlled study of rituximab in patients with stiff person syndrome. *Ann Neurol*. 2017;82(2):271–277.
164. Saini AG, Pandey S. Hyperekplexia and other startle syndromes. *J Neurol Sci*. 2020;416:117051.
165. Zhan F-X, Wang S-G, Cao L. Advances in hyperekplexia and other startle syndromes. *Neurol Sci*. 2021;42(10):4095–4107.
166. López-Corcuera B, Arribas-González E, Aragón C. Hyperekplexia-associated mutations in the neuronal glycine transporter 2. *Neurochem Int*. 2019;123:95–100.
167. Rees MI, Lewis TM, Kwok JBJ, et al. Hyperekplexia associated with compound heterozygote mutations in the beta-subunit of the human inhibitory glycine receptor (GLRB). *Hum Molec Genet*. 2002;11(7):853–860.
168. Rees MI. Harvey K, Pearce BR, et al. Mutations in the gene encoding GlyT2 (SLC6A5) define a presynaptic component of human startle disease. *Nat Genet*. 2006;38(7):801–806.
169. Ahrens-Nicklas RC, Umanah GKE, Sondheimer N, et al. Precision therapy for a new disorder of AMPA receptor recycling due to mutations in ATAD1. *Neurol Genet*. 2017;3(1):e130.
170. Harvey K, Duguid IC, Alldred MJ, et al. The GDP-GTP exchange factor collybistin: an essential determinant of neuronal gephyrin clustering. *J Neurosci*. 2004;24:5816–5826.
171. Rees MI, Harvey K, Ward H, et al. Isoform heterogeneity of the human gephyrin gene (GPHN), binding domains to the glycine receptor, and mutation analysis in hyperekplexia. *J Biol Chem*. 2003;278(27):24688–24696.

CHAPTER 11

Charcot–Marie–Tooth Disease and Related Disorders

Hereditary neuropathies may account for as many as 50% of previously undiagnosed peripheral neuropathies referred to large neuromuscular centers. Charcot–Marie–Tooth (CMT) disease is the most common type of hereditary neuropathy. Rather than one disease, CMT is a syndrome of several genetically distinct disorders (Table 11-1). The prevalence of CMT ranges from 9.7 to 82 per 100,000.[1,2] In this chapter, we discuss CMT and related neuropathies. In the other chapters, we will review other less common hereditary neuropathies (Chapter 8 for hereditary distal motor neuropathies, Chapter 17 for familial amyloid polyneuropathy, Chapter 31 for mitochondrial neuropathies, and Chapter 13 for other hereditary neuropathies).

The various subtypes of CMT are classified according to the nerve conduction velocities (NCVs), presumed pathology (e.g., demyelinating or axonal), mode of inheritance (autosomal dominant, autosomal recessive, or X-linked), age of onset (e.g., infancy or childhood/adulthood), and the specific mutated gene (Table 11-1).[1–8] Traditionally, CMT type 1 or CMT1 has referred to inherited demyelinating motor and sensory neuropathies, whereas the axonal motor and sensory neuropathies are classified as CMT2. By definition, CMT1 is associated with ulnar motor NCV less than 38 m/s while CMT2 is associated with NCV of 38 m/s or greater. However, most CMT1 have NCVs in the 20 m/s range. So, the "Intermediate" category includes patients with NCS in between 35 and 45 m/s. Both CMT1 and CMT2 usually begin in childhood or early adult life; however, onset later in life can occur, particularly in CMT2. CMT1 is associated with autosomal dominant inheritance, while forms of CMT2 can be inherited in an autosomal dominant or recessive fashion. Dejérine–Sottas neuropathy appears in infancy and is associated with severe demyelination or hypomyelination and was initially classified as CMT3. However, it was subsequently found be caused by autosomal dominant mutations in various genes that are more typically associated with CMT1. Therefore, the term "CMT3" is no longer recommended by many authorities, and this neuropathy has been classified as CMT1, if autosomal dominant, and as CMT4, in cases of autosomal recessive inheritance.

In this era of widely available next-generation sequencing (NGS), the traditional classification of these neuropathies has not been straightforward. Mutations of the same gene can lead to neuropathies associated with nerve conduction studies (NCSs) and histopathology that may reflect either a primary demyelinating or an axonal process, an autosomal dominant or recessive or X-linked inheritance, and a clinical phenotype with overlap between CMT and hereditary motor neuropathy [distal spinal muscular atrophy (SMA)], hereditary sensory and autonomic neuropathy (HSAN), and hereditary spastic paraplegia (HSP) (Fig. 11-1). Therefore, a new classification system was proposed that utilizes four modules for each disease category.[7,8] The first is generic term (e.g., CMT, dHMN, HSAN). The second module is the neuro/pathophysiological phenotype (e.g., "De" for demyelination, "Ax" for axonal, or "In" for intermediate), the third is the inheritance pattern (AD, AR, or X-linked), and finally the specific associated abnormal gene.[1,7,8] Whether or not this new proposed classification systems catches on is unclear, but for the purpose of this chapter, we will refer to both the traditional classification and the newly proposed classification systems.

The many genes associated with the various forms of CMT and related neuropathies have many different functions (Table 11-2, Fig. 11-2). More research needs to be done to better understand how mutations in these genes lead to neuropathy. Currently, there are no specific medical therapies for any of the CMTs, but there is active research in specific gene therapies. Importantly, physical and occupational therapy can be beneficial as can bracing (e.g., ankle–foot orthotics for foot drop) and other orthotic devices.

▶ CMT TYPE 1 (CMT1)/ CMT-DEMYELINATING

CLINICAL FEATURES

CMT1 is the most common form of hereditary neuropathy, with the ratio of CMT1:CMT2 being approximately 2:1. Individuals with CMT1 usually present in the first to third decades with distal leg weakness, although patients may remain asymptomatic even late in life.[1–8] There is an early predilection for the anterior compartment (peroneal muscle group), resulting in progressive foot drop. This leads to poor clearance of the toes when walking particularly on uneven surfaces. People with CMT1 often present with frequent tripping, falling, and recurrent ankle sprains. Affected individuals generally do not complain numbness or tingling, which can be helpful in distinguishing CMT from acquired forms of neuropathy.

▶ TABLE 11-1. CLASSIFICATION OF CHARCOT–MARIE–TOOTH DISEASE AND RELATED NEUROPATHIES

Traditional Nomenclature	Proposed New Nomenclature	Inheritance	Gene
CMT1			
CMT1A	CMT-De-AD-PMP22	AD	PMP-22 (duplication of gene)
CMT1B	CMT-De-AD-MPZ	AD	MPZ
CMT1C	CMT-De-AD-LITAF	AD	LITAF
CMT1D	CMT-De-AD-ERG2	AD	ERG2
CMT1E	CMT-De-AD-PMP22	AD	PMP-22 (point mutation in gene)
CMT1F	CMT-De-AD-NEFL	AD	NEFL
CMT1G	CMT-De-AD-PMP22	AD	PMP-22 (point mutation in gene)
HNPP	HNPP	AD	PMP-22 (deletion of gene)
CMT2	CMT-Ax		
CMT2A1	CMT-Ax-AD-KIF1B	AD	KIF1B
CMT2A2	CMT-Ax-AD-MFN2	AD	MFN2
CMT2B	CMT-Ax-AD-RAB7A1	AD	RAB7A1
CMT2B1	CMT-Ax-AD-LMNA	AD	LMNA
CMT2B2	CMT-Ax-AR- PNKP	AR	PNKP
CMT2C	CMT-Ax-AD-TRPV4	AD	TRPV4
CMT2D	CMT-Ax-AD-GARS1	AD	GARS1
CMT2DD	CMT-Ax-AD-ATP1A1	AD	ATP1A1
CMT2E	CMT-Ax-AD-NEFL	AD	NEFL
CMTEE	CMT-Ax-AD-MPV17	AD	MPV17
CMT2F	CMT-Ax-AD-HSPB1	AD	HSPB1
CMT2I	CMT-Ax-In-AD-MPZ	AD	MPZ
CMT2J	CMT-Ax-AD-MPZ	AD	MPZ
CMT2K	CMT-Ax-AD-GDAP1	AD	GDAP1
CMT2L	CMT-Ax-AD-HSPB8	AD	HSPB8
CMT2M	CMT-Ax-In-AD-DNM2	AD	DNM2
CMT2N	CMT-Ax-AD-AARS1	AD	AARS1
CMT2O	CMT-Ax-AD-DYNC1H1	AD	DYNC1H1
CMT2P	CMT-Ax-AD-LRSAM1	AD	LRSAM1
	CMT-Ax-AR-LRSAM1	AR	LRSAM1
CMT2Q	CMT-Ax-AD-DHTKD1	AD	DHTKD1
CMT2R	CMT-Ax-AD-TRIM2	AD	TRIM2
CMT2S	CMT-Ax-AD-IGHMBP2	AD	IGHMBP2
CMT2T	CMT-Ax-AD-MME	AD	MME
CMT2U	CMT-Ax-AD-MARS1	AD	MARS1
CMT2V	CMT-Ax-AD-NAGLU	AD	NAGLU
CMT2W	CMT-Ax-AD-HARS1	AD	HARS1
CMT2X	CMT-Ax-AR-SPG11	AR	SPG11
CMT2Y	CMT-Ax-AD-VCP	AD	VCP
CMT2Z	CMT-Ax-MORC2	AD	MORC2
CMT-Dominant Intermediate			
CMTDIB	CMT-In-AD-DNM2	AD	DMN2
CMTDIC	CMT-In-AD-YARS	AD	YARS1
CMTDID	CMT-In-AD-MPZ	AD	MPZ
CMTDIE	CMT-In-AD-IFN2	AD	IFN2
CMTDIF	CMT-In-AD-GNB4	AD	GNB4
CMTDIG	CMT-In-AD-NEFL	AD	NEFL
CMT-Recessive Intermediate			
CMTRIA	CMT-In-AR-GDAP1	AR	GDAP1
CMTRIB	CMT-In-AR-KARS1	AR	KARS1
CMTRC	CMT-In-AR-PLEKHG5	AR	PLEKHG5
CMTRID	CMT-In-AR-COX6A1	AR	COX6A1

(continued)

▶ TABLE 11-1. (CONTINUED)

Traditional Nomenclature	Proposed New Nomenclature	Inheritance	Gene
CMT4			
CMT4A	CMT-De-AR-GDAP1	AR	*GDAP1*
CMT4B1	CMT-De-AR-MTMR2	AR	*MTMR2*
CMT4B2	CMT-De-AR-SBF2	AR	*SBF2*
CMT4B3	CMT-De-AR-SBF1	AR	*SBF1*
CMT4C	CMT-De-AR-SH3TC2	AR	SH3TC2
CMT4D (HMSN-Lom)	CMT-De-AR-NDRG1	AR	*NDRG1*
CMT4E	CMT-De-AR-ERG2	AR	*ERG2*
CMT4F	CMT-De-AR-PRX	AR	*PRX*
CMT4G	CMT-De-AR-HK1	AR	*HK1*
CMT4H	CMT-De-AR-FGD4	AR	*FGD4*
CMT4J	CMT-De-AR-FIG4	AR	*FIG4*
CMT4K	CMT-De-AR-SURF1	AR	*SURF1*
CMTX			
CMTX1	CMT-In-XLD-GJB1	XLD	*GJB1*
CMTX4	CMT-Ax-XLR-AIFM1	XLR	*AIFM1*
CMTX5	CMT-Ax-XLR-PRPS1	XLR	*PRPS1*
CMTX6	CMT-Ax-XLD-PDK3	XLD	*PDK3*
Others			
SORD		AR	*SORD*
Hereditary Neuropathy with Neuromyotonia		AR	*HINT*
HNA		AD	*SEPT9*
HMSN-P		AD	*TFG*
Scapuloperoneal Neuropathy		AD	*TRPV4*

AD, autosomal dominant; AR, autosomal recessive; CMT, Charcot–Marie–Tooth; HMSN-P, hereditary motor and sensory neuropathy proximal; HNA, hereditary neuralgic amyotrophy; HNPP, hereditary neuropathy with liability to pressure palsies; HSAN, hereditary sensory and autonomic neuropathy; SORD, sorbitol dehydrogenase deficiency with peripheral neuropathy.

▶ TABLE 11-2. PATHOGENIC TARGETS INVOLVED IN INHERITED NEUROPATHIES

Myelin structure and function (PMP22, MPZ, GJB1, ERG2, LITAF, FGD4, PRX, MMTR2, SBF1, SBF2, IFN2)
Axonal structure (DYN2, DYS, NGF, NEFL, FGD4, SPG11, SEPT9, PRX)
Axonal transport (ATL1, ATL3, DYN2, DYNC1H, DYS, NEFL, KIF1A, RAB7, WNK1, KIF1B, NDRG1, SH3TC2, TFG, DMN2)
Golgi body formation (RETREG1/FAM134B)
Endoplasmic reticulum formation (ATL1, ATL3)
Sphingolipid metabolism (SPTLC1, SPTLC2)
Nuclear structure (LMNA)
DNA transcription regulation (ERG2, LRSAM1, MORC1)
DNA repair (PNKP)
RNA splicing and translation (LRSAM1, IGHMBP2, GARS1, YARS1, AARS1, KARS1, MARS1, HARS1, BCL2, VCP)
DNA methylation (DNMT1)
Protein degradation chaperones and stress regulation (LITAF, BAG3, HSPB1, HSPB8, HSP27, HSJ1)
Mitochondrial DNA maintenance (see Chapter 30)
Mitochondrial fission or fusion (MFN2, GDAP1)
Ion channels (TRPV4, TRPA, SCN9A, SCN10A, SCN11A, HINT1)

Although people with CMT1 usually do not complain of sensory loss, reduced sensation to all modalities is apparent on examination. Muscle stretch reflexes are unobtainable or reduced throughout. There is often atrophy of the muscles below the knee (particularly the anterior compartment), leading to the appearance of the so-called inverted champagne bottle legs. However, rare individuals have asymmetric pseudohypertrophy of the calves.[9] Most will have pes cavus, equinovarus, or hammertoe deformities (Fig. 11-3), which lead to aching in the feet. Rather than having a heel strike while ambulating, affected people land flat-footed or on their toes and thus use a steppage gait to help prevent tripping. Approximately two-thirds of individuals with CMT1 also have distal weakness and atrophy of the arms. Claw–hand deformities of the hands may develop in the most severely affected. Mild-to-moderate proximal weakness can develop over time as well, which can lead to diagnostic confusion with chronic inflammatory demyelinating polyneuropathy (CIDP). In addition, some individuals manifest with phrenic nerve involvement leading to respiratory weakness.[10] Rarely, patients with hypertrophy of nerve roots can be severe enough such that it leads to compression of the spinal cord or cauda equina. Hypertrophy of the nerves, especially posterior to

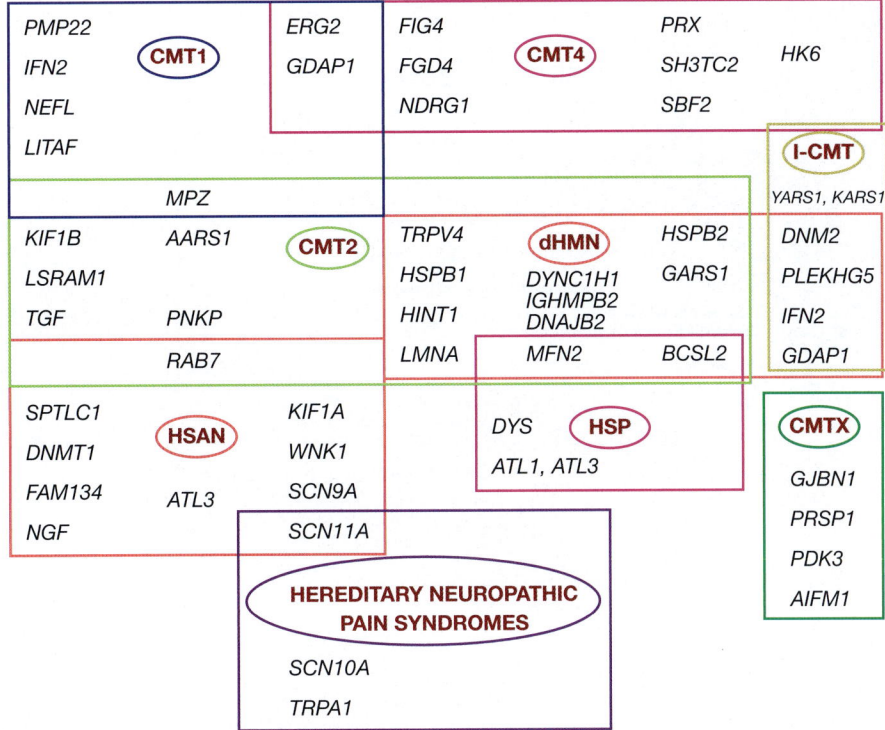

Figure 11-1. The overlap of CMT, HSAN, dHMN, HSP, episodic pain syndrome, and related disorders. Diseases: CMT, Charcot–Marie–Tooth disease (CMT1, demyelinating, autosomal dominant; CMT2, axonal, autosomal dominant or recessive; CMT4, demyelinating, autosomal recessive; CMTX, X-linked; I-CMT, intermediate CMT); dHMN, distal hereditary motor neuropathies; HSN, hereditary sensory neuropathies; HSP, hereditary spastic paraplegia. Genes: AARS, alanyl-tRNA synthetase; ATL, atlastin; BSCL2, Berardinelli–Seip congenital lipodystrophy type 2; DNM2, dynamin 2; DNMT1, DNA methyltransferase 1; DYNCH1H1, cytoplasmic dynein 1 heavy chain 1; DYS, dystonin; EGR2, early-growth response 2; FAM134B, family with sequence similarity 134, member B; GARS, glycyl-tRNA synthetase; GDAP1, ganglioside-induced differentiation-associated protein 1; GJB1, gap junction B1/connexin-32; HSJ1 (or DNAJB2), heat-shock protein J1 (or DNAJ Hsp40); HSPB1 (or HSP27), heat-shock 27-kDa protein 1; HSPB8 (or HSP22), heat-shock 22-kDa protein 8; HK6, hexokinase 6; HINT1, histidine triad nucleotide-binding protein 1; IFN2, inverted formin 2; LITAF, lipopolysaccharide-induced tumor necrosis factor-alpha factor; LMNA, lamin A/C nuclear envelope protein; LSRAM1, leucine-rich repeat and sterile alpha motif containing 1; MED25, mediator complex subunit; MFN2, mitofusin 2; MTMR2, myotubularin-related protein 2; SBF2, SET-binding factor 2; SH3TC2, SH3 domain and tetratricopeptide repeat domain 2; NDRG1, N-myc downstream-regulated gene 1; NEFL, neurofilament light chain; NGF, nerve growth factor; MPZ, myelin protein zero; PLEKHG5, pleckstrin homology domain-containing protein; PMP22, peripheral myelin protein 22; PDK3, pyruvate dehydrogenase kinase isoenzyme 3; PRSP1, phosphoribosyl pyrophosphate synthetase 1; PRX, periaxin; RAB7, small GTPase late endosomal protein RAB7; SPTLC1, serine palmitoyltransferase long chain base 1; TRPA1, transient receptor potential A 1; TRPV4, transient receptor potential cation channel subfamily V, member 4; YARS, tyrosyl-tRNA synthetase; WNK1, protein kinase, lysine-deficient 1.

the ear and arm regions, may be visualized and palpated. Approximately one-third of patients with CMT1 have an essential tremor (Roussy–Levy syndrome). Some individuals who are affected also develop deafness or Adie's pupils. It is important to examine family members of patients with possible CMT. Although there may be no family history of CMT, careful examination of the family may demonstrate other members with features of the neuropathy. This can be important in clarifying a diagnosis and in providing genetic counseling.

LABORATORY FEATURES

Cerebrospinal fluid (CSF) protein levels may be elevated. Besides genetic testing, NCSs are the most important

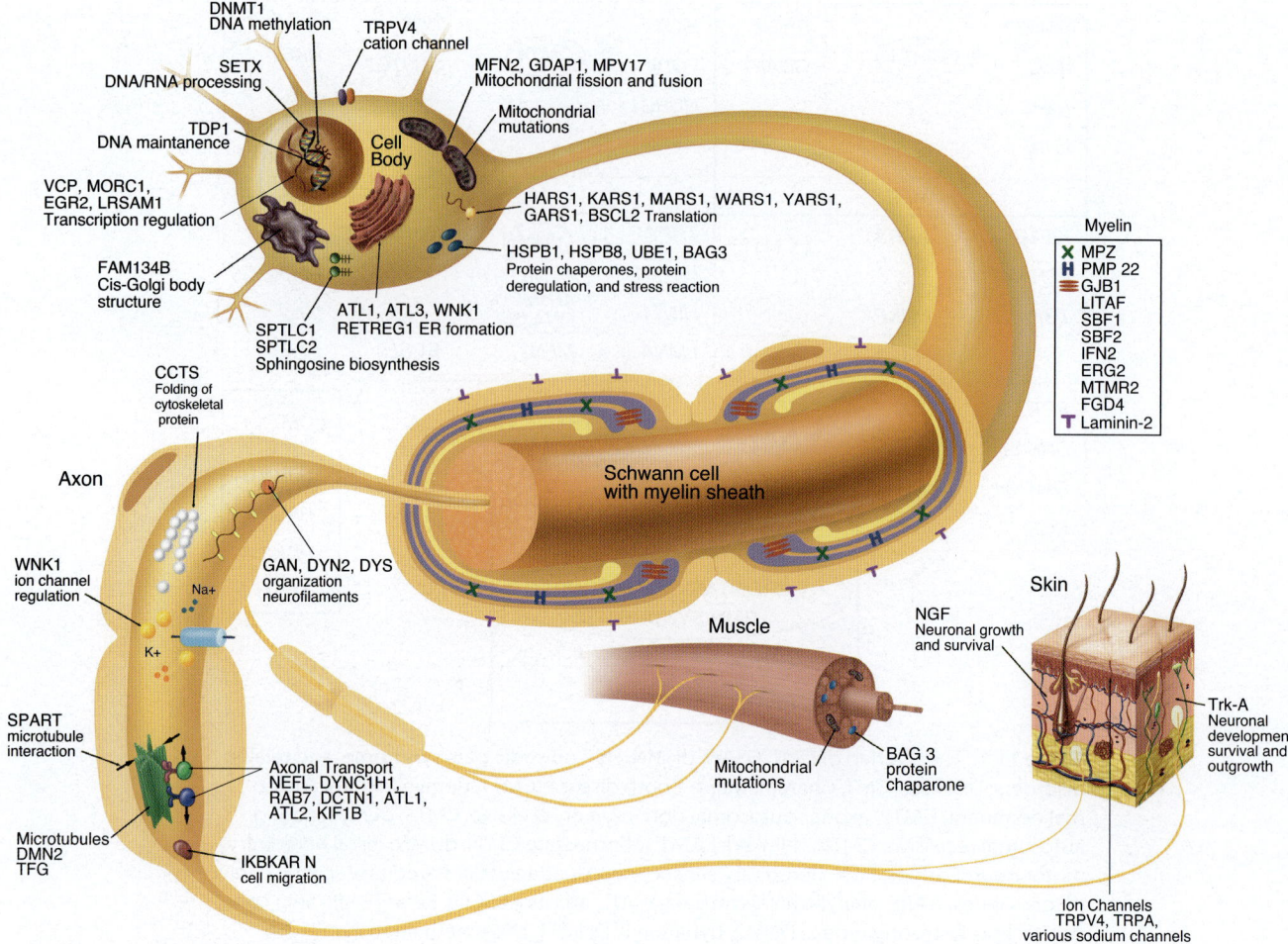

Figure 11-2. Molecular targets of inherited neuropathies demonstrate the diverse pathogenesis of these different neuropathies.

laboratory tests in the evaluation of people suspected of having CMT. The NCSs are invaluable in determining if patients have a demyelinating or axonal neuropathy and, if demyelinating, if it is uniform or multifocal, which is useful in distinguishing CMT from CIDP.[11,12] Uniform slowing of NCVs is suggestive of a hereditary demyelinating neuropathy, while multifocal slowing is more typical of CIDP. At birth and in infancy, NCVs may be normal or only minimally slowed in children with CMT1. However, the NCVs rapidly decline, and, by 3–5 years of age, the nadir in NCV slowing is achieved and remains stable throughout the rest of the person's life. However, the compound muscle action potential (CMAP) amplitudes continue to diminish over time, reflecting ongoing loss of axons. Distal motor latencies at birth are commonly borderline abnormal. These latencies continue to increase until approximately the age of 10 years, at which time there is little further prolongation of the distal latencies. A detailed discussion of specific nerve conduction abnormalities in CMT1 follows.

Motor NCSs

Motor NCVs by definition are slowed to less than 38 m/s in the upper extremities, but in most cases the NCVs are in the 20–25 m/s range.[7,11–13] Patients with point mutations in peripheral myelin protein 22 (*PMP22*) and myelin protein zero (*MPZ*) genes can have even slower conduction velocities (CVs) approaching that seen in CMT3 (10 m/s or less).[14,15] As will be discussed in the subsequent section, some people with *MPZ* mutations have only slightly slow or normal NCVs and thus by NCV criteria can be classified as having CMT2.[13,16] Demyelination is generally uniform; therefore, patients with CMT1 do not usually demonstrate conduction block or temporal dispersion on NCSs.[12,17] However, there are well-documented cases of genetically proven CMT1A with nonuniform slowing and CVs over 42 m/s and thus might mimic an acquired neuropathy.[9]

Distal motor latencies are usually markedly prolonged. The CMAPs may be absent when recordings are attempted from severely atrophic muscles. It is useful in people with wasted foot intrinsics to perform motor NCSs in the lower limb by recording from the tibialis anterior muscle. F-waves are usually absent but, when obtainable, the latencies are extremely prolonged.

There is no correlation between the NCVs and the clinical severity of the neuropathy. The NCVs are quite slow in childhood, even when there are minimal clinical deficits. Further,

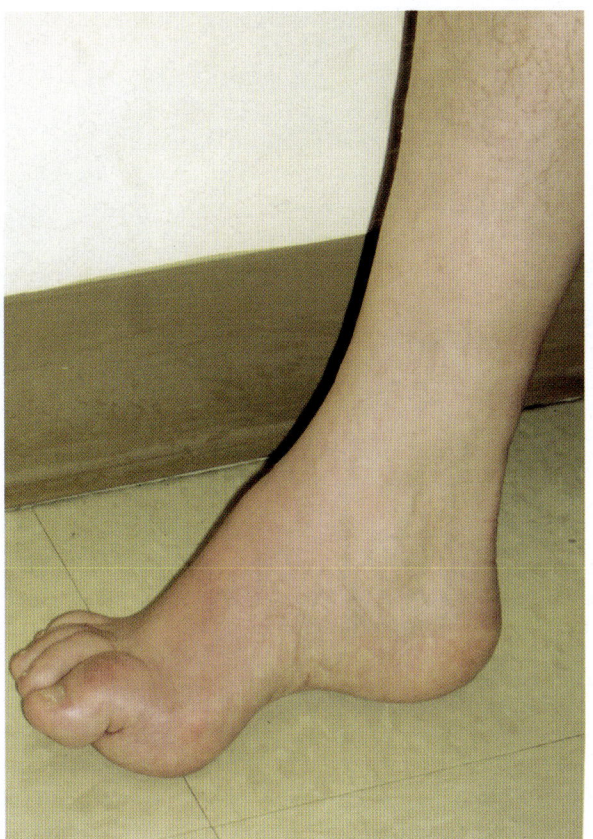

Figure 11-3. CMT1. Note the high arch (pes cavus) of the foot and hammertoes of a patient with CMT1.

asymptomatic adults can have prolonged distal motor latencies and slow NCV. It is apparent that weakness and loss of function are more related to the degree of axon loss, rather than the extent of demyelination and slowing of nerve conduction.

Sensory NCSs

The sensory nerve action potentials (SNAPs) are usually unobtainable or very low in amplitude.[18–26] When recordable, the distal latencies are very prolonged and NCVs are markedly slow.

Evoked Potentials

Somatosensory-evoked potentials have demonstrated slowing of central conduction in CMT1. Visual-evoked potentials also reveal similar slowing in the optic pathways.

Needle Electromyography

Electromyography (EMG) reveals positive sharp waves and fibrillation potentials along with reduced recruitment of long-duration, high-amplitude, and polyphasic motor unit action potentials (MUAPs) in the distal legs and lesser in the arms.[21] Evidence of active denervation and reinnervation may also be found in some of the proximal muscles.

HISTOPATHOLOGY

We do not perform nerve biopsies on people suspected of having CMT1, as the diagnosis can usually be made by less invasive testing (e.g., NCSs and genetic studies). Nevertheless, nerve biopsies, when done, are strikingly abnormal.[1,7,13,22] The enlarged gross appearance of the peripheral nerves led to the early designation of CMT1 as a hypertrophic neuropathy. Light microscopy reveals reduction of myelinated nerve fibers with a predilection for the loss of the large-diameter fibers.[21,22] The diameters of the axons are also decreased; on the whole there is an increase in the density of neurofilaments within these atrophic axons. Early in life, the peripheral nerves may appear normally myelinated, but over time axons become thinly myelinated. Recurrent demyelination and remyelination lead to reduced internodal length, while Schwann cell proliferation results in the formation of the so-called onion bulbs (Fig. 11-4). In patients with CMT1B, occasionally biopsies reveal tomacula, uncompacted myelin, and focally folded or widened myelin sheaths (Fig. 11-5).[4,14,24] Demyelination, neuronal loss, and axonal atrophy are slightly more prominent distally. Autopsy studies demonstrate the loss of myelinated fibers in the posterior columns in the spinal cord.

MOLECULAR GENETICS AND PATHOGENESIS

CMT1 is a genetically heterogeneous disorder (Tables 11-1 and 11-2 and Figs. 11-1 and 11-2).[1–8] In addition, there is phenotypic heterogeneity associated with mutations in specific genes. CMT1A (*PMP22* duplication) is by far the most common form of CMT1, representing 70% of cases, while 20% have CMT1B, and 10% have one of the other subtypes.

CMT1A (CMT-DE-AD-PMP22)

Approximately 85% of people with CMT1A have a 1.5-megabase (MB) duplication within chromosome 17p11.2–12 where the *PMP22* gene lies.[25,26] Thus, these individuals carry three copies of the *PMP22* rather than two. In contrast, inheritance of the chromosome with the deleted segment results in affected individuals having only one copy of the *PMP22* gene and leads to hereditary neuropathy with liability to pressure palsies (HNPP). Although these disorders are inherited in an autosomal dominant fashion, de novo mutations do occur. Most de novo duplications are paternally inherited and are believed to arise due to unequal crossover during meiosis. De novo mutations of maternal origin are probably caused by intrachromosomal rearrangement.[27] In keeping with this abnormal dosage effect of *PMP22*, people affected with trisomy 17p (thus, containing three copies of the *PMP22*) also have a demyelinating sensorimotor polyneuropathy.[28]

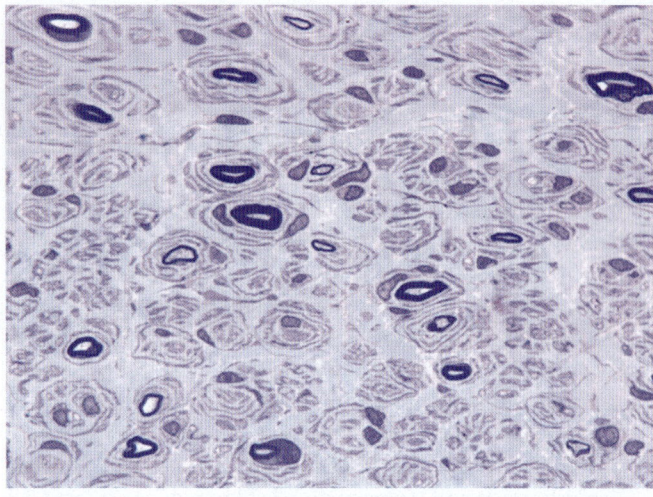
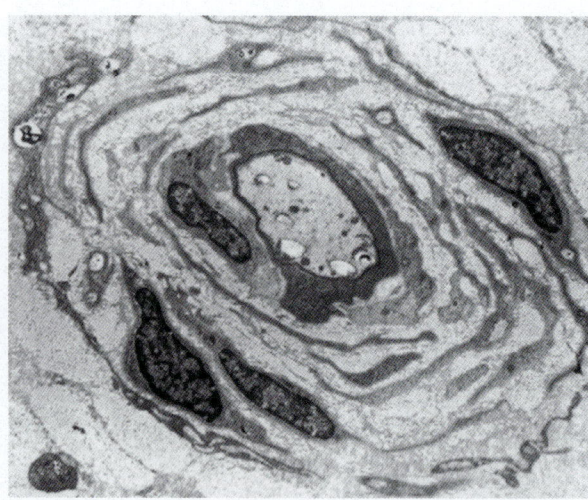

Figure 11-4. CMT1. Nerve biopsy demonstrates a reduction of myelinated nerve fibers, thinly myelinated fibers, and onion-bulb formations (**A**, semithin section). (Reproduced with permission from www.neuropathologyweb.org/chapter12.) Electron microscopy reveals proliferation of Schwann cell processes surrounding demyelinated fiber forming a so-called onion bulb (**B**). (Reproduced with permission from www.neuropathologyweb.org/chapter12.)

Some individuals with CMT1A have point mutations in *PMP22*.[29] These individuals can more closely resemble Dejérine–Sottas (previous also called CMT3) phenotypically, in which they are more severely affected at an earlier age, demonstrate slower NCVs (<10 m/s), and have more prominent histopathology than those with the classic duplication.[15] Other individuals present with a milder phenotype with pressure-induced palsies (e.g., HNPP as discussed in a subsequent section).

The pathogenic basis for CMT1A is likely due to a toxic gain of function of the PMP22 protein. This protein accounts for 2%–5% of myelin protein and is expressed in compact portions of the peripheral myelin sheath. An increased expression of PMP22 mRNA and the protein itself in the myelin sheaths has been demonstrated on nerve biopsies in CMT1A; however, late in the course PMP22 expression actually decreases.[30-33] The exact function of PMP22 in the peripheral nerves is not known, but it may be important in maintaining the structural integrity of myelin, acting as an adhesion molecule, or regulating the cell cycle. Regeneration-associated remyelination is delayed in nerve xenografts implanted from individuals with CMT1A into mice.[34] Further, PMP22 must also be essential for

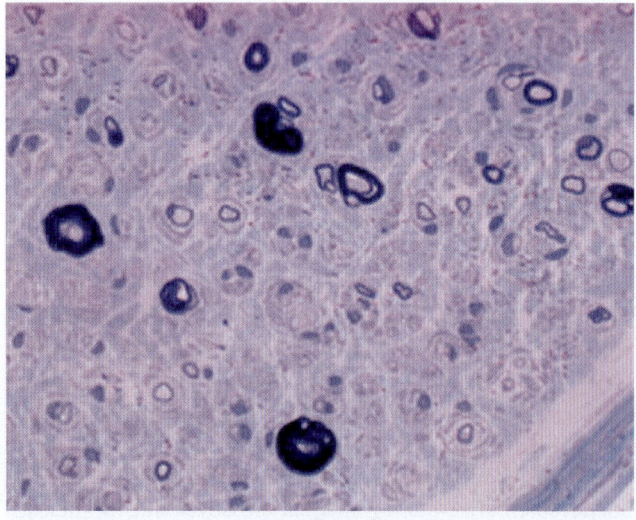
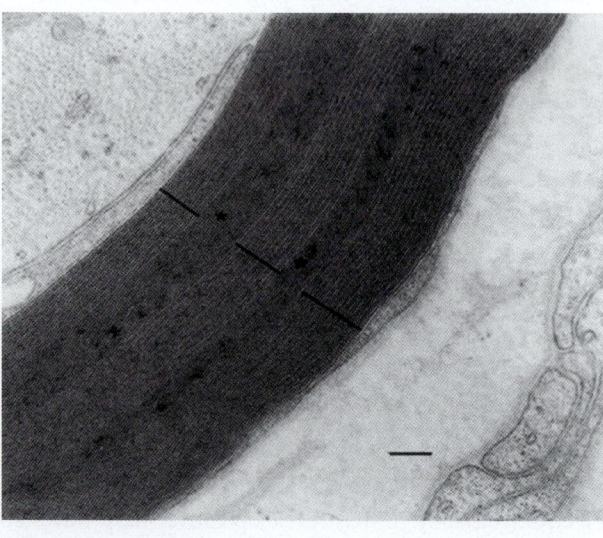

Figure 11-5. CMT1B. Semithin section reveals rarefaction of myelinated fibers, foldings of myelin, and onion-bulb proliferations of Schwann cells (**A**). Note the alternate disposition of normal (*stars*) and uncompacted myelin lamellae (*lines*), Scale bar = 0.2 μm (**B**). (Reproduced with permission from Vallat JM, Magy L, Lagrange E, et al. Diagnostic value of ultrastructural nerve examination in Charcot Marie Tooth disease: Two CMT1B cases with pseudo-recessive inheritance. *Acta Neuropathol*. 2007;113(4):443–449.)

maintaining the integrity of the axon itself, as there is evidence of axonal atrophy on nerve biopsies in people with CMT1A.

CMT1B (CMT-De-AD-MPZ)

Approximately 20% of people with CMT1 have CMT1B, which is caused by mutations in the *MPZ* gene that encodes for myelin protein zero.[35-37] CMT1B is for the most part clinically, electrophysiologically, and histologically indistinguishable from CMT1A. However, some patients with *MPZ* mutations are more likely to have more "axonal" physiology on NCSs than those patients with *PMP22* mutations (CMT2A or CMT-Ax-AD-MPZ). Also, CMT associated with Adie's pupils is more common in patients with *MPZ* mutations. MPZ is an integral myelin protein and accounts for more than half of the myelin protein in peripheral nerves. It is a member of the immunoglobulin superfamily and consists of an extracellular immunoglobulin-like domain, a transmembrane domain, and a cytoplasmic domain. MPZ localizes to the tight compact regions of myelin, where it may play a role in maintaining tight compaction by forming links between adjacent myelin layers. Nerve biopsies in people with CMT1B reveal abnormalities similar to that noted in CMT1A. However, occasionally tomaculae and uncompacted myelin are apparent, which are not typically seen on nerve biopsy in CMT1A.[4,14,38] Immunohistochemistry and ultrastructural studies on nerve biopsy specimens may demonstrate decreased expression of MPZ protein.[39] Some mutations in the *MPZ* gene have been associated with a severe demyelinating CMT3 phenotype, while others are associated with NCSs suggestive of an axonopathy or CMT2. The specific location of the mutations in the *MPZ* gene and how these affect the function of the myelin protein probably account for the phenotypic heterogeneity.

CMT1C (CMT-De-AD-LITAF)

This rare neuropathy is caused by mutations in the *LITAF* gene (lipopolysaccharide-induced tumor necrosis factor-alpha).[40,41] In a large study of 968 unrelated cases of CMT1, the percentage of patients with LITAF mutations was only 0.6%.[41] *LITAF*, also known as *SIMPLE* (small integral membrane protein of the lysosome/late endosome), encodes a protein that is expressed on Schwann cells and may play a role in protein degradation pathways.[42]

CMT1D (CMT-De-AD-ERG2)

Autosomal dominant mutations in the early growth response 2 gene, *ERG2* are responsible for CMT1D.[43] Autosomal recessive mutations in ERG2 cause the more severe CMT4D (CMT-De-AR-ERG2). ERG2 is believed to be a transcription factor that binds DNA through three zinc finger domains and likely has an important action in regulating myelin genes in Schwann cells. CMT1D accounts for <1% of molecular-defined cases of CMT1.

CMT1E (CMT-De-AD-PMP22)

This refers to kinships with CMT1 associated with deafness. It has been demonstrated to be allelic to CMT1A and caused by point mutations in *PMP22*.[5]

CMT1F (CMT-De-AD-NEFL)

CMT1F is caused by mutations in the neurofilament light chain (*NEFL* or *NFL*) gene.[44,45] It is usually associated with low-amplitude CMAPs and normal or only slightly slow NCVs and thus has also been categorized as an axonal form of CMT (CMT2E) or dominant intermediate CMT (CMTDIF or CMT-In-AD-NEFL). However, some cases have been reported with motor NCVs in the mid-20s and thus have been classified as a CMT1F.

CMT1G (CMT-De-AD-PMP22)

CMT1G, like CMT1E, is caused by point mutations in *PMP22*.[46,47]

▶ HEREDITARY NEUROPATHY WITH LIABILITY TO PRESSURE PALSIES

Because HNPP is associated with mutations affecting *PMP22* and less commonly *MPZ*, we discuss it here before moving on to CMT2.

CLINICAL FEATURES

HNPP or tomaculous neuropathy is inherited in an autosomal dominant manner.[18,48-54] The neuropathy usually manifests within the second or third decade, although some affected individuals present earlier and others remain asymptomatic their entire life. People usually describe painless numbness and weakness in the distribution of a single peripheral nerve, although multiple mononeuropathies and cranial neuropathies can occur. Symptomatic mononeuropathy or multiple mononeuropathies are often precipitated by trivial compression of nerve(s), as it can occur with wearing a backpack, leaning on the elbows, or crossing one's legs for even a short period of time. These pressure-related mononeuropathies usually resolve, although it may take several weeks or months. The most commonly affected sites are the median nerve at the wrist (carpal tunnel syndrome), ulnar nerve at the elbow (cubital tunnel syndrome), radial nerve in the arm (spiral groove insult), and peroneal nerve at the fibular head. In addition, the brachial plexus can be involved after carrying a heavy shoulder bag or backpack. Further, some individuals who are affected manifest with a progressive or relapsing, generalized, and symmetric sensorimotor peripheral neuropathy that resembles CMT or even CIDP.[18,48] On examination, there is decreased sensation to all modalities, particularly large fiber functions. Muscle stretch reflexes are usually reduced throughout, but these can be normal. Pes cavus deformities and hammertoes are often evident, as seen in CMT.

LABORATORY FEATURES

Although the clinical symptoms and signs are typically focal, NCSs often reveal diffuse abnormalities.[18,48-56] Sensory and motor NCSs usually demonstrate moderately prolonged distal latencies and slightly slow NCVs with normal or reduced amplitudes. Slowing of NCVs, conduction block, and temporal dispersion are accentuated across typical sites of entrapment or compression (i.e., the carpal and cubital tunnel, Guyon's canal, and across the fibular head). In addition, there also appears to be a distal accentuation of nerve conduction slowing, irrespective of possible compression.[48] However, this length-dependent slowing has not been appreciated by all.[53,55] NCSs may also be abnormal in asymptomatic family members who carry the mutation. Findings of widespread conduction slowing superimposed on the focal demyelinating lesions that correlate with the mononeuropathies, whether clinically evident or not, are a clue to this disorder.

HISTOPATHOLOGY

Nerve biopsies demonstrate focal globular thickening of the myelin sheath, which is best appreciated on teased fiber preparations.[48,50,55,57] The thickened myelin resembles as a sausage, hence the name tomaculous neuropathy (Latin: sausage) (Fig. 11-6). These tomaculae represent redundant loops of myelin. In addition, nerve biopsies reveal a reduction in large, myelinated fibers, segmental demyelination and remyelination, and axonal atrophy and degeneration similar to but not as severe as that seen in CMT1.

MOLECULAR GENETICS AND PATHOGENESIS

Approximately 85% of cases of HNPP are caused by an inverse of the mutation that is responsible for most cases of CMT1A.[18,48,58] While CMT1A is usually associated with a 1.5-MB duplication in chromosome 17p11.2, an extra copy of the *PMP22* gene, HNPP is caused by inheritance of the chromosome with the corresponding 1.5-MB deletion of this segment and thus have only one copy of the *PMP22* gene. De novo deletions are usually paternally inherited and arise due to unequal crossing-over during meiosis, while rare de novo mutations are of female origin and the result of intrachromosomal rearrangements.[27] In addition, rare point mutations within the *PMP22* gene itself can cause HNPP.[59] Why some point mutations in the *PMP22* gene result in a CMT1 clinical phenotype and others are associated with an HNPP phenotype is not known. It is speculated that mutations causing CMT1A produce a gain of function of the PMP22 protein, while mutations causing HNPP cause a loss of function of the PMP22 protein. Nerve biopsies demonstrate an underexpression of PMP22 mRNA and the protein[30,32] that inversely correlate with the mean diameter of the axons and clinical severity.[60] Normal expression of PMP22 protein appears important for proper axonal development.

▶ CMT TYPE 2 (CMT2)/CMT-AXONAL

CLINICAL FEATURES

CMT2 refers to the "axonal" hereditary motor and sensory neuropathies (HMSNs).[1] Most of these are associated with autosomal dominant inheritance (CMT-Ax-AD), but they can be inherited in an autosomal recessive manner (CMT-Ax-AR). The prevalence of CMT2 is about half that of CMT1. There are many well-defined subtypes based on the clinical features and genetic localization (Table 11-1).[1,7,20-22,61-156] CMT2A2 (CMT-Ax-AD-MFN2) caused by mutations in the mitofusin 2 gene, *MFN2*, is the most common subtype accounting for approximately one-third of CMT2 cases overall.[66-68] The different subtypes can be difficult to distinguish from one another and even from CMT1; however, there are clinical features that may be helpful. CMT2 tends to present later in life compared to CMT1. Individuals who are affected usually become symptomatic by the second decade, but some remain asymptomatic into late adult life while others present in the first decade of life.[65,70] People with CMT2 tend to have less severe involvement of the intrinsic hand muscles than that appreciated in CMT1. In contrast, CMT2 is more likely to have profound atrophy and weakness of the posterior compartments (gastrocnemius and soleus) of the distal legs in addition to the anterior compartment involvement (peroneal and anterior tibial) compared to CMT1. Generalized areflexia is rare in CMT2, while it is rather common in CMT1. Ankle reflexes are usually absent in both types. Individuals with CMT2 are less likely to have a tremor (Roussy–Levy syndrome) than people with CMT1. Although patients generally do not complain of sensory loss or paresthesia, 50%–70% of those with CMT2 have significant reductions in light touch, pain, joint position, and vibration sense on examination. While pes cavus and hammertoe deformities may be seen in CMT2, these are less frequent than in CMT1.

There are some features that also help distinguish the different subtypes of CMT2. For example, optic atrophy, hearing loss, pyramidal tract, and subcortical white matter abnormalities on brain magnetic resonance imaging findings

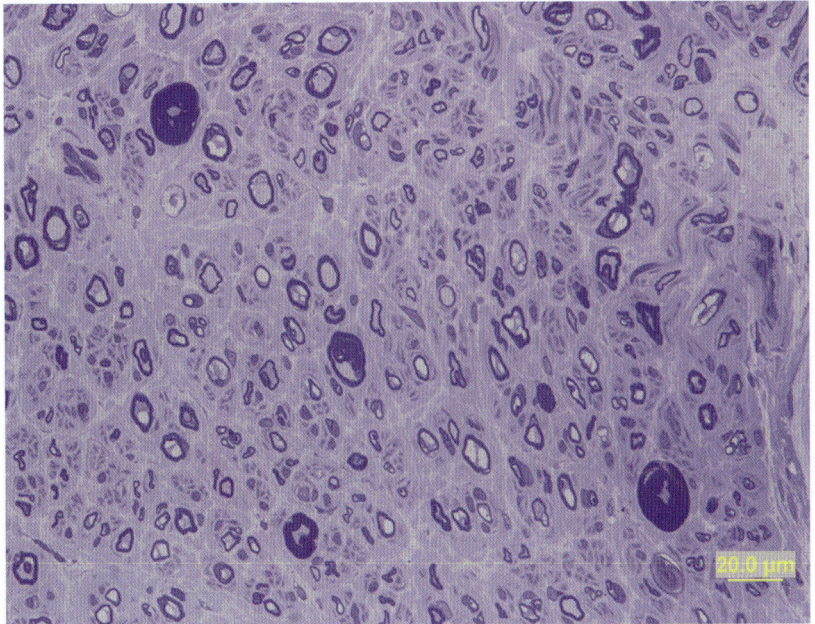

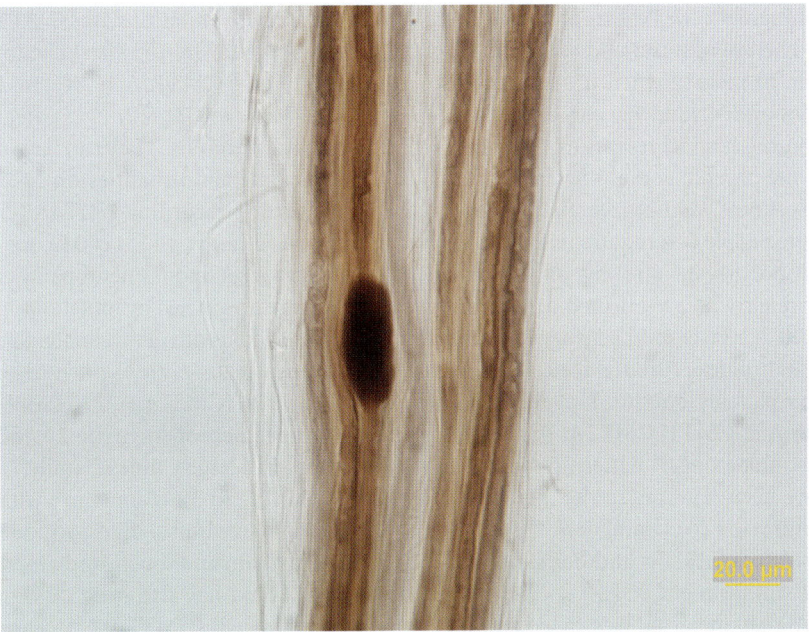

Figure 11-6. HNPP nerve biopsy. Transverse section of toluidine blue-stained epon-embedded sural nerve from a patient with HNPP reveals scattered thinly myelinated nerve fibers and fibers with redundant myelin swellings (**A**). Teased fiber preparation demonstrates a sausage-shaped myelin swelling or tomacula (**B**).

are sometimes seen in CMT2A2 (CMT-Ax-AD-MFN2), which was previously reported as hereditary motor and sensory neuropathy type 6 (HMSN VI) and overlaps with the HSPs.[71,72] Severe mutilating neuropathic ulcerations similar to those typically seen in HSAN type 1 (HSAN1) sometimes complicate CMT2B (CMT-Ax-AD-RAB7).[73-76]

CMT2B1 (CMT-Ax-AR-LMN) is usually inherited in an autosomal recessive fashion and early cases were initially reported in North Africa and the Middle East, where consanguineous marriages are not uncommon.[77-80] The age of onset has ranged from 6 to 27 years in these small series, and the course of the neuropathy is variable. The neuropathy can progress rapidly with severe distal and proximal weakness of the arms and legs evolving in a few years, while other affected individuals have only mild weakness two decades after the onset of symptoms.

CMT2B2 (CMT-Ax-AR-PNKP) has a variable age of onset and severity is variable, but most affected individuals have onset in the third decade. Other clinical features can include oculomotor apraxia, ataxia, dysarthria, cerebellar atrophy, and eye movement abnormalities. It has also been given the designation oculomotor apraxia type 4 (AOA4).[81]

CMT2C (CMT-Ax-AD-TRPV) is associated with vocal cord paralysis and diaphragmatic weakness, in addition to limb involvement.[3,82-85] The age of onset and symptoms are variable, and it can begin in infancy when it may manifest with breathing difficulties and stridor. Laryngeal weakness is more often insidious in onset and presents as progressive hoarseness. In addition, the phrenic nerves may be affected, leading to diaphragm weakness, reduced ventilatory function, and orthopnea. Some people will require tracheostomy and mechanical ventilation. Severe atrophy of the distal limbs is common. Individuals who are affected can develop proximal weakness as well. There is mild sensory loss to all modalities and deep tendon reflexes are reduced. Pes cavus can be appreciated in some patients, but such foot deformities are not as common as seen in CMT1, CMT2A, or CMT2B. Patients may have a "scapuloperoneal" pattern of weakness as well. Similar cases have been reported in the literature as hereditary distal SMA with vocal cord paralysis.[83,86]

CMT2D (CMT-Ax-AD-GARS1) is another genetically distinct autosomal dominant form of CMT2.[87-90] The hands are more severely affected than the distal legs. Selected wasting of the first interosseous muscles is often appreciated. Onset of weakness is usually appreciated in the late teens (range between the ages of 12 and 36 years), and the neuropathy has a slowly progressive course. Distal hypesthesia to all sensory modalities and areflexia are appreciated. Pes cavus, hammertoes, and scoliosis are variably present. Enlarged palpable nerves are not appreciated. This disorder is allelic to distal SMA type 5.[87-89]

CMT2E (CMT-Ax-AD-NEFL) is allelic with CMT1F (CMT-De-AD-NEFL) and CMTDIG (CMT-In-AD-NEFL) a rare neuropathy usually manifested in early childhood or adult life with progressive distal leg weakness.[44,45,91,92] Some patients develop deafness. Distal weakness, sensory loss, pes cavus, and areflexia are also often appreciated on examination. Additional features including ataxia, dysphagia, dysarthria, dementia, ptosis, waddling gait, tremor, hearing loss, and reduced vision.[92]

CMT2EE (CMT-Ax-AD-MPV17) is an autosomal recessive disorder that more typically cause mitochondrial DNA depletion syndrome-6 (MTDPS6), also known as Navajo neurohepatopathy (see Chapter 30).[93,94] Affected individuals usually manifest with cerebral leukoencephalopathy, severe sensory and motor neuropathy, liver disease, recurrent metabolic acidosis, and failure to thrive. However, some patients resent with a nonsyndromic axonal sensorimotor neuropathy.[94]

CMT2F (CMT-Ax-AD-AR-HSPB1) is allelic to distal hereditary motor neuropathy 2B (dHMN2B). It was initially reported in a Russian family with symmetric weakness and atrophy of the distal legs greater than the arms, with onset age 15–25 years but subsequently has been reported elsewhere and with later adult onset.[95-101] Some have preferential involvement of plantar flexors.[99] CMT2G and CMT2H are terms no longer used. The family reported as CMT2G was later found to have been linked incorrectly and was subsequently found to have CMT2P. CMT2H is found to be linked to autosomal mutations in GDAP1 and CMT2K. CMT2K (CMT-Ax-AD-GDAP1) is allelic to CMT4A (CMT-Ax-AR-GDAP1) and CMTRIA (CMT-In-AR-GDAP1) and caused by mutations in *GDAP1*.[102,103] Affected individuals may have vocal cord paralysis. They can have axonal, demyelinating, or intermediate abnormalities on NCSs. We discuss this more in the section regarding CMT4A (CMT-Ax-AR-GDAP1).

CMT2I and CMT2J (CMT-Ax-AD-MPZ) are associated with late-onset axonal neuropathy, Adie's pupil, and hearing loss. These are caused by mutations in *MPZ* that are more typically associated with demyelinating neurophysiology (CMT1B) and clinical features are as previously discussed.

CMT2L (CMT-Ax-AD-HSPB8) is allelic to distal hereditary motor neuropathy type 2A (dHMN2A). It was initially reported in a large Chinese family.[105] Onset of the disease was between 15 and 33 years of age with symmetric weakness of the distal lower limbs, mild-to-moderate sensory impairment including pain and touch, and absent muscle stretch reflexes.

CMT2M has also been classified dominant intermediate CMT type B (CMTDIB) because NCVs are usually in the intermediate range. The newer proposed classification system lists this as CMT-Ax-In-AD-DNM2. It is also allelic to a form of centronuclear myopathy.[106-108]

CMT2N (CMT-Ax-AD-AARS1) is associated with an age of onset ranging from early childhood to sixth decade of variable severity.[111-113] Sensorineural hearing loss may be seen in some individuals. NCVs are in the intermediate range.

CMT2O (CMT-Ax-AD-DYNC1H1) is allelic to SMA with lower extremity predominance 1 (SMALED1).[114,115] Most patients present with SMALED1 phenotype which is associated with early childhood onset of lower extremity weakness and atrophy without sensory loss.[115] However, some have motor and sensory loss involving upper and lower extremities.

CMT2P (CMT-Ax-AD-LRSAM1 and CMT-Ax-AD-AR-LRSAM1) is associated with a relatively mild, very slowly progressive axonal neuropathy with age of onset in the second or third decade of life.[116–119] The original family was erroneously reported as CMT2G.

CMT2Q (CMT-Ax-AD-DHTKD1) is a rare autosomal dominant form of axonal CMT reported in a 5 generation Chinese family.[120] Age of symptom onset ranged between ages 13 and 25 years.

CMT2R (CMT-Ax-AR-TRIM2) is a rare autosomal recessive neuropathy associated with infantile or childhood axial hypotonia, muscle weakness, hammertoes, pes equinus, and pes cavus.[121–123] Additional features may include involvement of several other cranial nerves leading to vocal cord paralysis, facial weakness, dysphagia, dyspnea, and hearing loss.

CMT2S (CMT-Ax-AR-IGHMBP2) is an autosomal recessive axonal neuropathy characterized by onset in the first two decades of life (most in early childhood) of slowly progressive distal muscle weakness of the arms and legs.[124–127] Some individuals also exhibit signs of autonomic neuropathies (bladder and gastrointestinal dysfunction, achalasia). It is allelic to spinal muscular atrophy with respiratory distress type 1 (SMARD1) which as the name implies is associated with severe ventilatory muscle weakness.

CMT2T (CMT-Ax-AD-MME) is a slowly progressive, autosomal dominant, sensorimotor peripheral neuropathy with mid- to late-adult onset.[128,129]

CMT2U (CMT-Ax-AD-MARS1) is another rare autosomal dominant form of axonal CMT, although there are very rare reports of NCSs in the demyelinating range. Onset of symptoms is typically mid- to late-adulthood.[130–133]

CMT2V (CMT-Ax-AD-NAGLU) is a rare autosomal dominant disorder initially described in a large French Canadian family in which 21 individuals had a late-onset, painful, sensory neuropathy.[134] Although weakness was not detected, CMAPs on NCSs gradually decreased over time suggesting some degree of axon motor involvement as well. Subsequently, a patient with early onset of motor neuropathy was reported.[135]

CMT2W (CMT-Ax-AD-HARS1) is an autosomal dominant, axonal CMT with a variable age at onset ranging from childhood to late adulthood (age 62 years) in the reported series of patients.[136,137]

CMT2X (CMT-Ax-AR-SPG11) is an autosomal recessive, slowly progressive, axonal peripheral sensorimotor neuropathy with an onset that usually occurs in the first two decades of life (range 4–35).[138] Notably, it is allelic to autosomal recessive hereditary spastic paraplegia type 11 (SPG11) and autosomal recessive juvenile-onset amyotrophic lateral sclerosis type 5 (fALS5) for which there can be overlapping features. For example, some patients had thin corpus callosum on brain imaging and mild cognitive impairment.

CMT2Y (CMT-Ax-AD-VCP) is an autosomal disorder that is allelic to multisystem proteinopathy type 1 that includes the spectrum of hereditary inclusion body myopathy, familial amyotrophic lateral sclerosis, frontotemporal dementia, and Paget disease of bone.[139] Rare patients manifest with only a length-dependent motor and sensory polyneuropathy in middle or late adulthood.[140,141]

CMT2Z (CMT-Ax-AD-MORC2) is associated with a wide clinical spectrum. Onset can be in infancy to late adulthood.[142–144] In early-onset cases affected patients have an SMA type phenotype with proximal greater than distal weakness. Rarely, there is cognitive impairment with global developmental delay. Adult-onset cases may have more distal motor weakness and sensory loss, though onset with proximal weakness can occur. Electrophysiological studies can show features of asymmetric axonal motor and sensory neuropathies. Notably, myokymic discharges and fasciculations have been frequently appreciated in needle EMG.

LABORATORY FEATURES

The similarities between the CMT1 and CMT2 make it difficult to definitely distinguish between these neuropathies on clinical grounds alone; thus, NCSs are invaluable. It is usually not difficult to differentiate CMT2 from the more common chronic idiopathic axonal neuropathy. Although there is electrophysiological evidence of motor involvement in chronic idiopathic axonal neuropathy, sensory symptoms predominate the clinical picture in this neuropathy, while motor signs and symptoms are the major clinical features in CMT2.

NCSs can help distinguish CMT1 from CMT2[7,11,21,62,63]; however, these do not help ascertain the various subtypes of CMT2. Sensory NCSs reveal reduced or absent SNAP amplitudes in both the upper and lower limbs. CVs are normal or only slightly reduced. Likewise, the distal sensory latencies are either normal or only mildly prolonged. The motor NCSs demonstrate reduced CMAP amplitudes, particularly in the legs. One notable exception is (CMT-AD-Ax-GARS1) in which the distal arms are affected more than the legs. Distal motor latencies are normal or only mildly prolonged. NCVs are normal or only slightly slow, usually greater than 37 m/s in the upper extremities. However, rare cases of CMT2E (CMT-Ax-AD-NEFL) have been reported with motor NCVs in the mid-20s.[45] Some have had slowing of NCVs in an intermediate range and are designated as having dominant intermediate CMT. Needle EMG reveals fasciculation and fibrillation potentials, particularly in distal extremity muscles. A few patients with CMT2 have been reported to have continuous MUAP firing resembling neuromyotonia; these discharges are abolished with peripheral neuromuscular blockade. The MUAPs can be increased in amplitude and duration with a higher-than-normal number of polyphasic potentials. Recruitment is reduced in weak muscles as well.

HISTOPATHOLOGY

Nerve biopsies in CMT2 demonstrate a generalized reduction in myelinated fibers, particularly the large, myelinated fibers.[148] Axonal atrophy, Wallerian degeneration, and small clusters of thinly myelinated fibers representing regenerating axons can be appreciated. As opposed to CMT1, onion bulbs are not a prominent feature in CMT2. Abnormal accumulations of mitochondria may be appreciated on electron microscopy (EM) in CMT2A2. Some forms such as CMT2E are associated with giant axons and accumulation of disorganized neurofilaments.[44]

MOLECULAR GENETICS AND PATHOGENESIS

CMT2 is a genetically heterogeneous group of disorders (Table 11-1).[1,3-8]

CMT2A1 is caused by mutations in a microtubule motor kinesin-like protein gene, *KIF1B*.[149,150] The kinesin superfamily is involved in axonal transport and likely impairment of this function leads to axon degeneration.

The majority of patients with CMT2A have *MFN2* mutations (CMT2A2), which account for one-third of CMT2 cases overall.[67,69,151] Mitofusin 2 localizes to the outer mitochondrial membrane, where it regulates the mitochondrial network architecture by fusion of mitochondria. Mitochondria undergo a dynamically regulated balance between fusion and fission reactions of their tubular and branched membrane network in order to maximize cell functions, such as equilibrating mitochondrial gene products to overcome acquired somatic mutations of mitochondrial DNA and establishing a uniform membrane potential at the mitochondrial double membrane and regulation of apoptosis.[151] Mutations in *MFN2* lead to abnormal mitochondrial trafficking, which may explain the length-dependent severity of the associated neuropathy.[69,152]

CMT2B is caused by mutations in a small GTPase late endosomal protein encoded by the *RAB7* gene.[75,153] Mutations in this gene also cause a form of HSAN1 (see below). The encoded protein serves as a guanine-nucleotide exchange factor for the Rho family of GTPase enzymes (RhoGTPases). Rho guanine-nucleotide exchange factors regulate the activity of small RhoGTP-ase by catalyzing the exchange of bound GDP by GTP. In turn, RhoGTPases play a pivotal role in regulating the actin cytoskeleton by their ability to influence cell polarity, microtubule dynamics, membrane-transport pathways, and transcription-factor activity, as well as RhoGTPases in neuronal morphogenesis, including cell migration, axonal growth and guidance, dendrite elaboration and plasticity, and synapse formation.[75]

CMT2B1 is usually caused by homozygous mutations in the *LMNA* gene.[77-80] This gene encodes for the nuclear envelop protein, lamin A/C. This gene is also mutated in patients with LGMD (limb girdle muscular dystrophy) 1B and EDMD2 (Emery Dreifuss 2) (see Chapter 27).

CMT2B2 (CMT-Ax-AR-PNKP) is an autosomal recessive disorder that was previously thought to be caused by mutations in the MED25 gene, but subsequently was found to be actually caused by mutations in polynucleotide kinase 3′-phosphatase (*PNKP*) gene.[81] The age at onset and severity is variable, but most have onset in the third decade. Other clinical features can include oculomotor apraxia, ataxia, dysarthria, cerebellar atrophy, and eye movement abnormalities. It has also been given the designation oculomotor apraxia type 4 (AOA4). Polynucleotide kinase 3′-phosphatase is an important enzyme repair of DNA damage.

CMT2C (CMT-Ax-AD-TRPV4) is caused by mutations in the transient receptor potential cation channel, subfamily V, member 4 gene (*TRPV4*).[85,86] CMT2C is allelic to some forms of distal HMN and scapuloperoneal neuropathy/SMA.[87] How mutations involving this cation channel that mediates calcium influx causes neuropathy is not exactly known.

CMT2D (CMT-Ax-AD-GARS1) and distal SMA type 5 are allelic disorders caused by mutations in the glycyl-tRNA synthetase 1 (*GARS1*) gene on chromosome 7p14.[88-90] Glycyl-tRNA synthetase 1 is a member of the family of aminoacyl-tRNA synthetases (ARSs), responsible for charging tRNAs with their cognate amino acids. The pathogenic mechanism by which mutations in this gene lead to CMT2D/distal SMA type 5 is not completely understood.

CMT2E (CMT-Ax-AD-NEFL) is allelic with CMT1F (CMT-De-AD-NEFL) and CMTDIG (CMT-In-AD-NEFL) and is caused by autosomal dominant mutations in the *NEFL* gene.[44,45,91,92] Neurofilaments are important for proper organization, function, and regeneration of axons as well as for axonal transport. Furthermore, neurofilament light chain encoded by *NEFL* plays a major role in regulating the expression and function of other neurofilament proteins.

CMT2EE (CMT-Ax-AR-MPV17) is an autosomal recessive disorder caused by mutations in *MPV17* gene that encodes a mitochondrial inner membrane protein involved in mitochondrial deoxynucleotide homeostasis and maintenance of mtDNA.[93,94] As previously mentioned, this is allelic to mitochondrial DNA depletion syndrome-6, also known as Navajo neurohepatopathy (see Chapter 30).

CMT2F (CMT-Ax-AD-AR-HSPB1) is caused by mutations in the *HSPB1* gene that encodes for 27-kDa small heat-shock or HSP27.[95-101] Mutations in this gene are also responsible for some patients categorized as having distal spinal muscular atrophy (dHMN2).[96] Most cases are inherited in an autosomal dominant fashion but there are rare reports of autosomal recessive inheritance.[100,101] The pathogenic basis is unclear but may be related to disturbances in chaperone function, cellular neurofilament and microtubule structure and function, or mitochondrial and metabolic dysfunction.[97]

CMT2I and CMT2J (CMT-Ax-AD-MPZ) refer to late-onset cases with mutations in *MPZ* gene (CMT1B) but in which the neurophysiology and nerve biopsies look more axonal and thus can be classified as a form of CMT2.[16,154] Affected patients may have hearing loss and Adie's pupil.

CMT2K refers to early-onset neuropathy (usually before the age of 2 years), which is caused by autosomal dominant or recessive mutations in *GDAP1* and is allelic to CMT4A (CMT-Ax-AD-GDAP1 and CMT-Ax-AR-GDAP1).[80,102-104] Some individuals who are affected have vocal cord paralysis. GDAP1 is an outer mitochondrial membrane protein and helps regulate the mitochondrial network.

CMT2L (CMT-Ax-AD-HSPB8) is caused by mutations in the *HSPB8* gene that encodes for small heat-shock protein 22-kDa protein 8.[105,155] Mutations in this gene are also responsible for dHMN2B.HSPB8 forms homodimers and larger oligomers with other HSPs. The mutation may lead to an increased tendency to form cytoplasmic protein aggregates by weakening chaperone-assisted selective autophagy.[155,156]

CMT2M is allelic to CMTDIB (and thus termed CMT-Ax-In-AD-DNM2) and is caused by mutations in the *DNM2* gene. This gene encodes for dynamin 2 that belongs to a subfamily of GTP-binding proteins.[106-108] Dynamins are associated with microtubules and bind proteins that bind actin and other cytoskeletal proteins.

CMT2N (CMT-Ax-AD-AARS) is caused by mutations in alanyl-tRNA synthetase (*AARS*) 1.[111-113] AARS catalyzes the attachment of alanyl to the appropriate tRNA. ARSs are essential enzymes in the first step of protein synthesis by attaching specific amino acids to their specific, cognate tRNA molecules. As will become apparent in discussion of other CMT disorders there is an increasing number of other CMT neuropathies caused by mutations in ARS genes (e.g., *HARS1*, *GARS1*, *MARS1*, and *YARS1*).

CMT2O (CMT-Ax-AD-DYNC1H1) is caused by heterozygous mutation in the dynein, cytoplasmic 1, heavy chain 1 (*DYNC1H1*) gene.[114,115] Dyneins are a group of microtubule-activated ATPases that have a role in retrograde axonal transport and organelle movement.

CMT2P (CMT-Ax-AD-LRSAM and CMT-Ax-AR-LRSAM1) is caused by homozygous or heterozygous mutations in the leucine-rich repeat and sterile alpha motif containing 1 gene, *LRSAM1* and thus inheritance can be autosomal recessive or autosomal dominant.[116,117] The encoded protein regulates cell adhesion molecules, has ubiquitin ligase activity, and plays a role in receptor endocytosis.[118] Some studies suggest that mutations may affect the formation of RNA-binding protein complex and normal splicing of mRNA.[119]

CMT2Q (CMT-Ax-AD-DHTKD1) is caused by pathogenic alterations in DHTKD1 that encodes for dehydrogenase E1 and transketolase domain-containing 1.[120] The mechanism by which this causes CMT is unclear.

CMT2R (CMT-Ax-AR-TRIM2) is a rare autosomal recessive neuropathy caused by mutations in the tripartite motif containing 2 gene, *TRIM2*.[121-123] The gene encodes a ligase that ubiquitinates the neurofilament light chain, which as previously discussed leads to neuropathy.

CMT2S (CMT-Ax-AR-IGHMBP2) is an autosomal recessive disorder associated with pathogenic alterations in *IGHMBP2* that encodes for immunoglobulin heavy-chain μ-DNA-binding protein 2.[124-127] This is an ATP-dependent 5′→3′ helicase for both DNA and RNA and appears to be important for normal translation of proteins.

CMT2T (CMT-Ax-AD-MME) is an autosomal recessive neuropathy caused by pathogenic mutations in *MME* that encodes for membrane metalloendopeptidase, also known as neprilysin.[128,129] The mechanism by which mutations cause neuropathy is not known.

CMT2U (CMT-Ax-AD-MARS1) is an autosomal dominant disorder caused by mutations in the methionyl-tRNA synthetase gene, *MARS*.[130-133] The pathogenic mechanism is not known.

CMT2V (CMT-Ax-AD-NAGLU) is caused by autosomal dominant mutations in *NAGLU*, which encodes α–N-acetylglucosaminidase.[134,135] Notably, autosomal recessive mutations in *NAGLU*, cause the severe childhood lysosomal disease mucopolysaccharidosis IIIB (Sanfilippo syndrome). α-N-acetyl-glucosaminidase is involved in the degradation of the glycosaminoglycan compound heparan sulfate. It has been speculated that the neuropathy could be caused by neurotoxicity due to the accumulation of mucopolysaccharides with secondary accumulation of tau, GM2, and GM3 in lysosomes, as in MPS IIIB.[134]

CMT2W (CMT-Ax-AD-HARS1) is the result of autosomal dominant mutations in the gene that encodes for histidyl-tRNA synthetase, *HARS*.[136,137] The ARSs are essential enzymes that catalyze the first step of protein translation.

CMT2X (CMT-Ax-AR-SPG11), hereditary spastic paraplegia type 11 (SPG11), and juvenile-onset amyotrophic lateral sclerosis type 5 (fALS5) are allelic disorders caused by autosomal recessive mutations in *SPG11* that encodes for spatacsin.[138] This protein is located in axons and dendrites in central and peripheral nerves, where co-localizes with cytoskeletal and synaptic vesicles and in synaptosomes.

CMT2Y (CMT-Ax-AD-VCP) is an autosomal dominant disorder that is part of the multisystem proteinopathy clinical spectrum that includes hereditary inclusion body myopathy, amyotrophic lateral sclerosis, dementia, and Paget disease of bone. These disorders are caused by mutations in the valosin-containing protein gene, *VCP*, which is widely expressed in central and peripheral nerves.[139-141] Pathogenic mutations are believed to lead to impaired autophagic function of VCP, accumulation of immature autophagosomes, and impairment in membrane fusion, nuclear envelope reconstruction, Golgi reassembly, DNA damage response, suppressor of apoptosis, RNA binding, and ubiquitin-dependent protein degradation.[139]

CMT2X (CMT-Ax-AD-MORC2) is caused by mutations in *MORC2* that encodes for microrchidia family CW-type zinc finger 2.[142-144] This ubiquitously expressed nuclear protein has a role involved in chromatin remodeling, DNA repair, and transcriptional regulation.

▶ DOMINANT AND RECESSIVE INTERMEDIATE CMT (CMTDI AND CMTRI)

Intermediate CMT refers to forms of CMT in which the CVs show only mild slowing (>38 m/s) in the upper extremities and in which there are both demyelinating and axonal features on nerve biopsies. They are inherited in an autosomal dominant fashion (CMTDI) or recession fashion (CMTRI), and by the recently proposed nomenclature are classified as CMT-In-AD-Gene or CMT-In-AR-Gene (Table 11-1).[1,7,8] The clinical features are for the most part similar to what was described previously in CMT1 and CMT2 sections.

An Italian family reported as CMTDIA was linked to chromosome 10q24.1–q25.1, but the causal gene has not been found.

CMTDIB (CMT-In-AD-DNM2) is caused by mutations in dynamin 2 gene, *DYN2*.[106–108] Of note, mutations in the same gene have been found in adult-onset centronuclear myopathy (see Chapter 28). *DYN2* mutations should be considered in those with a classical mild to moderately severe CMT phenotype, particularly when seen in combination with neutropenia or cataracts.[107] Dynamin 2 belongs to the family of large GTPases and is important in endocytosis, membrane trafficking, actin assembly, and centrosome cohesion.[108]

CMTDIC (CMT-In-AD-YARS1) is caused by mutations in *YARS1* that encodes for tyrosyl-tRNA synthetase.[157–159] As discussed in with other forms CMT caused by mutations in different ARSs, these are essential enzymes that catalyzes the first step of protein translation. Onset of length-dependent weakness and sensory loss ranged from first to sixth decades of life. NCVs ranged from 29 m/s to normal velocities.

CMTDIE (CMT-In-AD-IFN2) is caused by mutations in the gene that codes for inverted formin 2, *INF2*.[109,110] This neuropathy is associated with focal segmental glomerulosclerosis (FSGS) and notably mutations in *IFN2* are also a major cause of isolated FSGS. Approximately one-third of patients has sensorineural hearing loss. Some affected individuals have intellectual disabilities and abnormalities in the white matter and ventricular dilatation on brain MRI. Formin 2 interacts with Rho-GTPase CDC42 and myelin and lymphocyte protein (MAL) and is felt to be important in the essential steps of myelination and myelin maintenance.

CMTDIF (CMT-In-AD-GNB4) is caused by mutations in *GNB4*, encoding guanine-nucleotide-binding protein subunit beta-4.[160,161] This protein is abundantly expressed in the axons and Schwann cells of peripheral nerves and may be important in transmitting extracellular signals into cells. Age of onset ranged from 5 to 45 years, and individuals ranged in clinical severity from being asymptomatic to being wheelchair-bound. The median motor NCVs ranged from 3.9 to 45.7 m/s. Sural nerve biopsies have showed severe loss of myelinated fibers and many onion bulb formations.

CMTDIG (CMT-In-AD-NEFL) is allelic with CMT1F (CMT-De-AD-NEFL) and CMT2E (CMT-Ax-AD-NEFL) and is caused by autosomal dominant mutations in *NEFL* that encodes for neurofilament light chain.[45,92] This neuropathy is discussed in greater detail in the sections on CMT1F and CMT2E and the phenotypes overlap. CMTR1A (CMT-In-AR-GDAP1) is allelic to CMT2K (CMT-Ax-AD-GDAP1) and CMT4A (CMT-De-AR-GDAP1) and is caused by mutations in *GDAP1*.[102–104] Affected individuals may have axonal, demyelinating, or intermediate abnormalities on NCSs. We discuss this more detail in the section regarding CMT4A (CMT-Ax-AR-GDAP1).

CMTRIB (CMT-In-AR-KARS1) has been reported in one patient with a mutation in lysyl-tRNA synthetase gene, *KARS1*.[162] The patient had developmental delay, self-abusive behavior, dysmorphic features, and vestibular Schwannoma with intermediate slowing of motor NCVs in the 30s. As discussed with CMTs associated with mutations in other ARS genes, these are essential enzymes that catalyze the first step of protein translation.

CMTRIC (CMT-In-AR-PLEKHG5) is caused by mutations in *PLEKHG5* that encodes for the pleckstrin homology domain-containing protein, family G, member 5.[163–165] Mutations in this gene also cause autosomal recessive distal SMA type 4. The encoded protein activates the nuclear factor kappa B signaling pathway. Affected individuals developed distal weakness and atrophy that were worse in the legs and associated with foot deformities, areflexia, and moderately slow NCVs. The age at onset was variable. Nerve biopsies demonstrated a loss of large, myelinated fibers and thinly myelinated fibers.

CMTRID (CMT-In-AR-COX6A1) has been reported in only a few individuals. Clinical features were not well described in one report outside of motor NCSs showing mild slowing of NCVs and sural nerve biopsy showing onion bulbs.[166] Another case report described a patient with a severe neuropathy starting at the age of 5 years.[167] Autosomal recessive mutations were identified in the *COX6A1* gene that encodes for cytochrome *c* oxidase subunit VIa polypeptide 1. This is a component of mitochondrial respiratory complex IV (cytochrome *c* oxidase).

▶ CMT TYPE 3 (DEJÉRINE–SOTTAS DISEASE, CONGENITAL HYPOMYELINATING NEUROPATHY)

CLINICAL FEATURES

CMT3 was originally described by Dejérine and Sottas as a hereditary demyelinating or hypomyelinating sensorimotor polyneuropathy presenting in infancy or early childhood.[1,168–179] Although initially CMT3 was believed to be an autosomal recessive disorder because of a lack of family history, some cases are due to spontaneous mutations in the *PMP22*, *ERG2*, or *MPZ* genes and are now currently classified as forms of CMT1 (AD), CMT4 (AR), or CMTX.[1,11,169]

The neuropathy usually manifests as generalized weakness at birth or in early childhood. Affected infants can be hypotonic and often have distal contractures (arthrogryposis multiplex). Ventilatory distress and swallowing difficulties can develop in severe cases, leading to death in several months. In less severe cases, infants may appear normal at birth, but motor milestones are delayed. Some children achieve independent ambulation, although it may take several years. Distal muscles are affected more than proximal muscles. Weakness can progress and render some ambulatory patients to a wheelchair.

The peripheral nerves may be visible or palpably enlarged. There is a reduction in all sensory modalities, particularly those conveyed by large, myelinated fibers (i.e., vibration and proprioception) and generalized areflexia. Sensory ataxia of the limbs and trunk can be profound. Sensorineural hearing and abnormal pupillary reaction to light can be detected in some children. Skeletal deformities (e.g., pes cavus and kyphoscoliosis) are common.

LABORATORY FEATURES

CSF protein levels are usually elevated. Motor NCVs are markedly slow, typically 5–10 m/s or less; the distal motor latencies are markedly increased; and the amplitudes are reduced.[20,173,176,177] Sensory responses are usually unobtainable. Needle EMG demonstrates increased insertional activity with variable degrees of positive sharp waves and fibrillation potentials, and reduced recruitment of MUAPs.[179] In milder cases of CMT3 in which reinnervation can occur, large-amplitude, long-duration, polyphasic MUAPs are apparent. However, in severe cases, the MUAPs can appear small and almost "myopathic" in appearance.

HISTOPATHOLOGY

Nerve biopsies in CMT3 are markedly abnormal.[175,180–182] One can see hypomyelination with redundant basal lamina or classical onion bulbs as well as amyelination. There is an increase in the size of nerve fasciculi with a reduction in the numbers of myelinated fibers, while unmyelinated nerve fibers are less affected.

The most common histopathological abnormality is hypomyelination with basal lamina onion bulbs. There is marked loss of myelinated nerve fibers with the remaining axons surrounded by onion bulbs composed of multiple layers of basement membranes, with only one or two thin Schwann cell lamella in the outer ring. These abnormalities are typically found in cases of infantile or early-onset neuropathy. Although some of the infants have respiratory and swallowing problems, nearly all survive. However, affected children rarely achieve independent ambulation and most are wheelchair dependent.

Occasionally, nerve biopsies reveal hypomyelination, with classical onion bulbs composed of concentrically arranged thin Schwann cell lamellae, enclosing nearly all the fibers. This histopathological appearance is associated with a more benign neuropathy. Affected children can appear normal at birth but subsequently fail to meet normal motor milestones. They usually are eventually able to ambulate but may require assistance over time.

Other cases are associated with a marked reduction of nerve fibers with the remaining fibers having minimal myelin. Onion bulbs are not apparent. These so-called congenital amyelinating neuropathies are the most severe form of CMT3 and are usually lethal.

MOLECULAR GENETICS AND PATHOGENESIS

This is a genetically heterogeneous disorder. As previously discussed, the neuropathy was initially felt to be an autosomal recessive disorder and classified as "CMT3." However, autosomal dominant, de novo heterozygous point mutations also have been discovered in the genes for *PMP22*, *MPZ*, and *ERG2*, which are also genes responsible for CMT1.[1,43,171,183] Thus, there exists a wide spectrum of clinical, electrophysiological, and histological phenotypes associated with mutations in *PMP22*, *MPZ*, and the *ERG2* genes. Some individuals who are affected have a mild phenotype with only asymptomatic slowing of NCV, while others manifest with severe congenital amyelinating neuropathy, resulting in severe generalized weakness and death in infancy. The severity of CMT is probably related to the exact locations of the mutations in the *PMP22*, *MPZ*, and the *ERG2* genes and how these mutations specifically affect the function of the myelin proteins or how these interact with one another and the axons.

▶ CMT TYPE 4 (CMT4)

CLINICAL FEATURES

This subgroup of CMT is characterized by a severe, childhood-onset, sensorimotor polyneuropathy that is usually inherited in an autosomal recessive fashion. The electrophysiological and histological features are usually demyelinating but are rarely axonal.[1,184] Using the newly proposed nomenclature, subtypes CMT4 are called CMT-De-AR-GENE or CMT-Ax-AR-GENE.[7,8]

CMT4A (CMT-De-AR-GDAP1) was initially reported in Tunisian families but has subsequently been reported elsewhere.[80,102–104,185–192] As previously mentioned, it is allelic to CMT2H and CMT2K as well as CMTRIA (CMT-In-AR-GDAP1). Distal weakness is usually noted within the first 2 years of life. Motor development is generally delayed, and progressive weakness involving the proximal muscles is apparent by the end of the first decade. Some individuals who are affected become wheelchair dependent by the third decade of life. Vocal cord paresis and diaphragm paralysis can occur.[186,193] Mild sensory loss and areflexia are evident on clinical examination, as are scoliosis, pes cavus, and other skeletal deformities.

CMT4B1 (CMT-De-AR-MTMR2) is characterized clinically by distal greater than proximal weakness affecting the legs more than the arms and histologically by the abundance of focally folded myelin sheaths on nerve biopsy.[194,195] Weakness is usually apparent at birth or within the first year of life but may not be apparent until the third decade. Motor milestones are often delayed but children do generally become ambulatory. Weakness is progressive and the ability to ambulate without a wheelchair may be lost over time. Sensation is reduced, particularly large fiber function, and muscle stretch reflexes are generally unobtainable. Some people develop scoliosis. It appears to be more severe than CMT4B2 that is closely related.

CMT4B2 (CMT-De-AR-SBF2) is a demyelinating HMSN that is also characterized by abnormal folding of myelin sheaths.[196–198] Onset is typically in first decade of life. Some affected individuals have early-onset glaucoma.

CMT4B3 (CMT-De-AR-SBF1) is similar to CMT4B1 and CMT4B2 clinically, electrophysiologically, and histologically with abnormal folding of myelin sheaths on sural nerve biopsy may be seen.[199,200] One series reported that children had normal development but later in adolescence developed progressive neuropathy. They also had significant microcephaly, severe strabismus, and syndactyly.[200]

CMT4C (CMT-De-AR-SG3TC2) was initially described in two Algerian kinships[201] but has since been reported elsewhere.[202–205] The main clinical features are delay in walking until 18–24 months, deformities in the feet and spine by 5 years of age, and distal greater than proximal leg and arm weakness. Reduced sensation primarily affects large fiber modalities and is evident prominently in patients with severe motor weakness. Some patients develop sensorineural hearing loss. Muscle stretch reflexes are reduced or absent. Hypertrophy of the nerves may be appreciated. However, there is phenotypic variability even within affected families. Some have late-onset of symptoms, asymmetric involvement, and lack of scoliosis. NCSs are demyelinating.[204] Sural nerve biopsy has revealed severe hypomyelination, basal lamina onion bulbs, and in some the abundant presence of focal myelin foldings.

CMT4D (CMT-De-AR-NDRG1) is allelic to HMSN with deafness—Lom (HMSN-Lom). It is a rare autosomal recessive demyelinating neuropathy that was initially recognized in Bulgarian gypsies from the town of Lom.[206–209] However, not all affected people are of gypsy ancestry.[208,209] Individuals who are affected develop distal leg weakness in the first decade of life, which progresses to involve the hands by the second decade of life. Subsequently, hearing loss is generally noted in the third decade. Reduced sensation to all modalities and hyporeflexia are appreciated on examination. Pes cavus, hammer toes, clawing of the hands, and scoliosis are also common. NCSs reveal a demyelinating sensorimotor polyneuropathy.[206,207] Sural nerve biopsies reveal a loss of large and small myelinated nerve fibers with relative preservation of unmyelinated axons. Remaining axons are thinly myelinated, and onion-bulb formations may also be evident.

CMT4E is allelic to CMT1D (CMT-Di-AD-ERG2) and some cases of autosomal recessive Dejérine–Sottas disease (CMT-AR-De-ERG2).[43,210] Clinical features were discussed in these sections.

CMT4F (CMT-De-AR-PRX) is an autosomal recessive neuropathy that usually manifests with weakness leading to developmental motor delay, sensory loss, and areflexia in early childhood, although adult-onset cases have also been described.[211–215] Pes cavus and kyphoscoliosis are common.

CMT4G (CMT-De-AR-HK1), also known as CMT-Russe type, has been reported in several gypsy kinships. Distal lower extremity weakness develops in the first two decades of life followed by distal upper extremity weakness.[216,217] Motor NCSs have shown slowing to low 30 m/s range in the arms to being absent in the legs.

CMT4H (CMT-De-AR-FGD4) typically presents in the first 2 years of life with severe weakness.[218–220] Nerve biopsies have shown excessive redundant myelin outfoldings.[220]

CMT4J (CMT-De-AR-FIG4) manifests at birth to early adulthood with severe and often rapidly progressive motor weakness.[221–224] Weakness can be quite asymmetric and resemble motor neuron disease. NCSs can show nonuniform slowing of CVs, conduction block, and temporal dispersion on NCSs, which resemble those found in acquired demyelinating polyneuropathies.[221–224] Some patients also have CNS abnormalities and brain MRI can show features suggestive of a leukoencephalopathy.[222,224]

CMT4K (CMT-De-AR-SURF1) is a rare autosomal recessive demyelinating peripheral neuropathy that was reported in two Algerian siblings.[225] Onset of distal weakness and sensory loss was in the first decade of life. Over time they developed nystagmus and ataxia. Brain MRI revealed putaminal and periaqueductal lesions. Serum lactate levels were elevated. Skeletal muscle biopsies revealed cytochrome oxidate negative fibers and reduced enzyme activity.

LABORATORY FEATURES

As noted above NCSs are markedly abnormal in the different subtypes of CMT4. SNAPs are generally unobtainable, while CMAPs are usually reduced in amplitude. CMT4J (CMT-De-AR-FIG4) may show nonuniform slowing of CVs, conduction block, and temporal dispersion on NCSs.[221–224]

HISTOPATHOLOGY

In CMT4A, nerve biopsies reveal a marked reduction of myelinated nerve fibers, severe hypomyelination, and basal lamina onion bulbs.[185,187–192] Hypomyelination, loss of myelinated nerve fibers, basal lamina onion bulbs, and numerous fibers with excessively folded myelin sheaths are features of different forms of CMT4B, CMT4C, CMT4F, and CMT4H (Fig. 11-7).[24,202,203,211–213,220,226]

MOLECULAR GENETICS AND PATHOGENESIS

CMT4A is caused by mutations in the ganglioside-induced differentiation-associated protein 1 gene (*GDAP1*).[80,102–104,185–193,227]

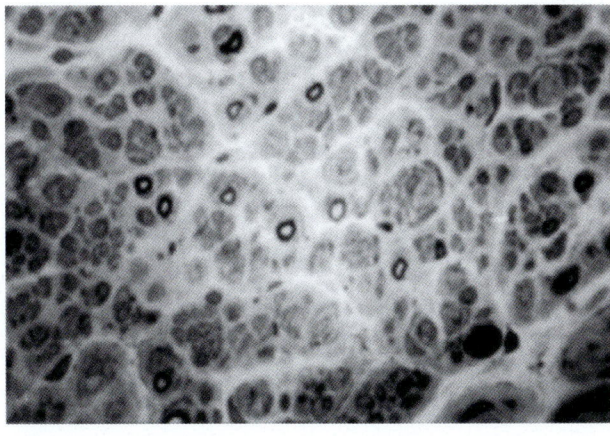
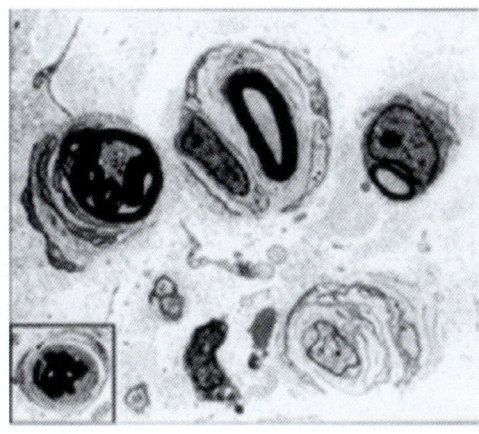

Figure 11-7. CMT4F. (**A**) Light microscopy. Cross semithin–epon section of the sural nerve. Loss of myelinated fibers of all diameters, small onion-bulb structures, and tomacula. (**B**) Electron microscopy. Onion-bulb formations, fiber with focally folded myelin. *Inset*: A naked axon with myelin infoldings surrounded by an onion bulb of mixed type. (Reproduced with permission from Kabzinska D, Drac H, Sherman DL, et al. Charcot–Marie–Tooth type 4 F disease caused by S399fsx410 mutation in the PRX gene. *Neurology*. 2006;66(5):745–747.)

Both neurons and Schwann cells express GDAP1, which may explain why mutations may be associated with electrophysiological and histopathological features of either an axonal or a demyelinating neuropathy. The GDAP1 protein is located in the mitochondrial outer membrane and helps regulate the mitochondrial network, which when abnormal leads to CMT.

CMT4B1 with focally folded myelin sheaths appears to be genetically heterogeneic.[194,195] Focally folded myelin sheaths are not specific for CMT4B, as these have also been described in patients with point mutations in the *MPZ* gene, which is the causative gene in CMT1B.[228] CMT4B1 is caused by mutations in the myotubularin-related protein 2 (*MTMR2*) gene.[195,229–231] The MTMR2 protein is a dual specificity phosphatase, and its deficiency may lead to the phosphorylation of an as-yet-unknown substrate that results in Schwann cell proliferation and abnormal myelinogenesis. Of note, a related member of this same protein family, MTM1, is responsible for X-linked myotubular myopathy (see Chapter 28). Mutations in *MTMR2* may lead to malfunction of neural membrane recycling, membrane trafficking, and/or endocytic or exocytotic processes, combined with altered axon–Schwann cell interactions. Studies suggest that the loss of MTMR2 protein decreases Schwann cells proliferation and survival and may impair the first stages of myelination of the peripheral nervous system.

CMT4B2 (CMT-De-AR-SBF2) is caused by mutation in the myotubularin-related 13 gene (*MTMR13*), better known as SET-binding factor 2 (SBF2).[197] This protein is a member of the pseudophosphatase branch of myotubularins and bears striking homology to MTMR2. Myotubularin-related proteins have been suggested to work in phosphoinositide-mediated signaling events, which may also convey control of myelination.

CMT4B3 (CMT-De-AR-SBF1) is caused by mutations in myotubularin-related protein 5 gene better known as SET-binding factor 1 (*SBF1*).[199,200] Pathogenic basis is similar to the related CMT4B1 and CMT4B2.

CMT4C is caused by mutations in *SH3TC2* that encodes a protein called SH3 domain and tetratricopeptide repeats 2.[203–205] SH3TC2 localizes to the intracellular recycling endosome on Schwann cells and abnormalities may lead to abnormalities in endocytic pathways.

CMT4D, also known as HSMN-Lom, is caused by mutations in the N-myc downstream-regulated gene 1, *NDRG1*.[206–209] NDRG1 is expressed on Schwann cells may function as a signaling protein shuttling between the cytoplasm and nucleus.

CMT4E is caused by mutations in the early growth response 2 gene, *ERG2* is responsible for CMT1D.[43,210] Autosomal recessive mutations in ERG2 cause the more severe CMT4D (CMT-De-AR-ERG2). CMT4F is caused by mutations in the gene that encodes for periaxin, *PRX*.[211,213–215,226] Periaxin normally localizes to the Schmidt–Lanterman incisures and paranodal membranes and is thought to be important in myelin–axon interactions and maintenance of normal myelin structure.

CMT4G (CMT-De-AR-HK1) has been linked to mutations in the hexokinase 1 gene, *HK1*.[217] Hexokinase 1 catalyzes the first step in glucose metabolism, using ATP for the phosphorylation of glucose to glucose-6-phosphate. Mutations in *HK1* can also cause hemolytic anemia. The mechanisms by which mutations in this gene cause neuropathy are not known.

CMT4H (CMT-De-AR-FGD4) is caused by mutations in the *FGD4* gene that encodes for FYVE, RhoGEF, and PH domain-containing protein 4 also known as frabin.[219,220] Frabin is a GDP/GTP nucleotide exchange factor and may have a role in mediating actin cytoskeleton changes during cell migration, morphogenesis-polarization, and division. Mutations in *FGD4* may lead to impaired Rho GTPase signaling. Recent evidence suggests that frabin regulates the NRG1 type III/ERBB2/3 pathway and dysfunction leads to demyelination and myelin outfolding on peripheral nerves.[220]

CMT4J (CMT-De-AR-FIG4) is caused by mutations in the *FIG4* gene that encodes for FIG4 homolog, CAC1 phosphatase domain containing *Saccharomyces cerevisiae*.[221–224] This enzyme is a phosphoinositide phosphatase and is felt to regulate intracellular membrane trafficking by recruiting effector proteins to the surface of specific organelles. However, the mechanism by which neuropathy is caused is not understood.

CMT4K (CMT-De-AR-SURF1) is caused by mutations in *SURF1* that encodes for surfeit locus protein 1 cytochrome c oxidase (COX) assembly factor.[208] This leads to a reduction in COX activity.

▶ X-LINKED CMT

CMTX1 (CMT-In-XLD-GJB1)

Clinical Features

CMTX1 (CMT-In-XLD-GJB1) is an X-linked dominant disorder with clinical features similar to CMT1, except that the neuropathy is much more severe in men than in women.[1,13,232–238] It accounts for approximately 12% of the overall CMT cases. Men usually present in the first two decades of life with atrophy and weakness of the distal arms and legs, areflexia, pes cavus, hammertoes, and claw–hand deformities. Some patients have disproportionate involve of hand intrinsic muscles with the abductor policis brevis being more involved than the first dorsal interossei, the so-called "split hand syndrome." Most do not complain of a sensory disturbance, although reduced sensation to all modalities can be demonstrated on examination. As opposed to men, obligate women carriers are frequently asymptomatic, and if they manifest with symptoms the onset is usually after the second decade of life. The neuropathy is also typically less severe in affected women. Rarely, patients with CMTX1 can present with transient CNS symptoms and marked white matter lesions on magnetic resonance imaging scans.[239–241]

Laboratory Features

NCSs reveal features of both demyelination and axonal degeneration, which are more severe in men compared to women.[1,13,232–245] SNAPs are reduced in amplitude or absent in the majority of patients but, when obtainable, the distal latencies are prolonged and CVs are slow. Peroneal CMAPs are absent in as many as two-thirds of patients, while median and ulnar CMAPs are often reduced in amplitude.[233,235] Distal motor latencies are prolonged in men more than in women with CMTX1.[233]

In men, motor NCVs in the arms and legs are moderately slow (median nerve 31 +/− 6 m/s; peroneal nerve 31.0 +/− 3.9 m/s).[235] NCVs in men with CMTX1 are approximately 10 m/s faster than that usually seen in autosomal dominant forms of CMT1. By comparison, motor NCVs in women with CMTX1 are usually only slightly slow (median nerve 44.6 +/− 8.8 m/s; peroneal nerve 33.8 +/− 8.1 m/s).[235] As previously discussed, uniform slowing of motor NCVs is the rule in CMT1 and helps distinguish hereditary from acquired forms of demyelinating polyneuropathy.[17] However, nonuniform slowing of CVs between different nerves and along different segments of individual nerves resulting in temporal dispersion has been described in some cases of CMTX1, particularly in women.[244,245] Motor unit nerve estimates demonstrate a reduction in units, which correlates with clinical severity.[236]

Histopathology

Sensory nerve biopsies reveal a loss of myelinated nerve fibers, especially of large-diameter fibers, along with axonal degeneration and atrophy, and clusters of thinly myelinated regenerating fibers.[13,233,242,244] A mild degree of Schwann cell proliferation (onion bulbs) can also be seen surrounding some of the thinly myelinated fibers. A mixture of demyelination and remyelination is evident on teased fiber preparations.

Molecular Genetics and Pathogenesis

CMTX1 is caused by mutations in the *GJB1* gene that encodes for Gap junction beta 1 protein, also known as connexin 32.[1,2,234,238,246–248] Connexins are gap junction structural proteins, which are important in cell-to-cell communication. Connexin 32 oligomerizes into a hexameric structure on the Schwann cell lamella in the paranodal region and Schmidt–Lanterman incisures, where it forms intercellular channels. These channels allow diffusion of ions, nutrients, and other small molecules through the compact myelin to the inner most layers of the myelin sheath and the axon itself. The mutations in *GJB1* lead to demyelination and axonal degeneration.[244]

OTHER FORMS OF CMTX

CMT4X (CMT-Ax-XLR-AIFM1) is an X-linked recessive disorder also known as Cowchock syndrome.[249–253] Affected males can manifest with an axonal sensorimotor neuropathy, delayed motor milestones, hearing loss, cognitive impairment, spasticity, dysarthria, nystagmus, and cerebellar ataxia from infancy to young adulthood. MRI scans can show a leukoencephalopathy and cerebellar atrophy. It is caused by mutations in *AIDM1* that encodes for the apoptosis inducing factor mitochondria-associated 1 protein. How this leads to the associated central and peripheral nervous system abnormalities is unclear.

CMTX5 (CMT-Ax-XLR-PRPS1) is associated with distal weakness, atrophy, and sensory loss in early childhood and is caused by mutations in *PRPSI* that encodes for phosphoribosyl pyrophosphate synthetase 1.[254–257] This enzyme is necessary for the de novo and salvage pathways of purine and pyrimidine biosynthesis. Mutations in this *PRPSI* also cause Arts syndrome, an X-linked disorder characterized by mental retardation, early-onset hypotonia, ataxia, delayed motor development, hearing impairment, and optic atrophy. In addition, some patients with *PRPS1* mutations manifest with isolated X-linked sensorineural deafness. The typical trial of CMTX comprises the triad of optic atrophy, deafness, and polyneuropathy.

CMTX6 (CMT-In-XLD-PDK3) was reported in a large family affecting five males and eight carrier females over two generations.[258,259] Males had symptom onset before the age of 13 years and were more severely affected then manifesting women carriers who were asymptomatic or had only minor symptoms and signs (foot deformity or tremor). Electrophysiological studies revealed findings suggestive of an axonal sensorimotor polyneuropathy. The neuropathy is caused by mutations in the pyruvate dehydrogenase kinase isoenzyme 3 gene, *PDK3*.[258,259] PDK3 is an enzyme located in the mitochondrial matrix that assists in regulating the pyruvate dehydrogenase complex, by reversible phosphorylation.

▶ MISCELLANEOUS HEREDITARY MOTOR AND SENSORY NEUROPATHIES

PROXIMAL HEREDITARY MOTOR AND SENSORY NEUROPATHY/ NEURONOPATHY (HMSN-P)

Clinical Features

Proximal hereditary motor and sensory neuropathy/neuronopathy resembles Kennedy disease (see Chapter 8), except that it is inherited in an autosomal dominant fashion rather than being an X-linked disorder.[260–264] Muscle cramps are often the earliest symptoms. Affected individuals usually develop progressive proximal muscle atrophy, weakness, and fasciculations in the legs worse than in the arms after the age of 30 years (mean 45 +/− 6 years) and typically become nonambulatory 5–20 years after the onset of symptoms. Facial muscles are also slightly weak, but neck flexors and extensors remain relatively strong. The tongue may be slightly weak, but dysphagia and dysarthria are not common. Nevertheless, bulbar and respiratory muscle weakness can develop late in the course of the disease. Some patients complain of mild dysesthesias in the distal legs and hands. Decreased sensation to all modalities, particularly vibratory perception and proprioception, is evident on examination. As in Kennedy disease, muscle stretch reflexes are diminished or absent, neurogenic tremor is common, and there is an association with type 2 diabetes mellitus.

Laboratory Features

Serum creatine kinase (CK) levels are often mildly elevated. SNAPs are reduced in amplitude or unobtainable as in Kennedy disease. CMAP amplitudes can be moderately decreased, while the distal latencies and NCVs are relatively preserved. Needle EMG reveals diffuse fasciculation and fibrillation potentials and decreased recruitment of long-duration, large-amplitude, polyphasic MUAPs.

Histopathology

Nerve biopsies show a loss of large and small myelinated nerve fibers with preservation of unmyelinated nerve fibers.[260] An autopsy demonstrated only a few remaining atrophic anterior horn cells along with significant loss off neurons in the spinal roots, cauda equina, and dorsal root ganglia.[260]

Molecular Genetics and Pathogenesis

This disorder is caused by heterozygous mutations in *TFG* that encodes the trafficking from ER to Golgi regulator protein *TFG* (Table 11-1).[262–264] This protein plays a role in the normal dynamic function of the endoplasmic reticulum (ER) and its associated microtubules. Mutations in *TFG* are also responsible for autosomal recessive familial spastic paraplegia type 57.

HEREDITARY NEURALGIC AMYOTROPHY

Clinical Features

Hereditary neuralgic amyotrophy (HNA) is an autosomal dominant disorder, characterized by recurrent attacks of pain, weakness, and sensory loss in the distribution of the brachial plexus often beginning in childhood.[265–267] These attacks are similar to those seen with idiopathic brachial plexitis (Parsonage–Turner syndrome), and most patients fully or at least partially recover over several weeks or months. Varying degrees of hypotelorism, epicanthal folds, cleft palate, syndactyly, micrognathia, and facial asymmetry are seen in some patients. HNA can be distinguished from brachial plexopathy that can occur in HNPP because of the lack of severe pain in HNPP. Rarely, HNA can affect the lumbosacral plexus, lower cranial nerves, and phrenic nerves.[1]

Laboratory Features

The electrodiagnostic findings are typically of classic brachial plexitis.[265–267] Amplitudes of SNAPs and CMAPs of the affected trunks, cords, divisions, and individual nerves are reduced, while the distal latencies and CVs relatively preserved. Needle EMG reveals fibrillation and positive sharp waves in affected muscle groups along with decreased recruitment of MUAPs. Following reinnervation, especially after recurrent attacks of paresis, large polyphasic MUAPs become evident. NCSs and EMG of the unaffected arm and the lower limbs are normal. The electrophysiological studies in HNA reflect an axonal process localized to the brachial plexus, while HNPP is a generalized or multifocal process, which is demyelinating in nature.

Histopathology

Sural nerve biopsies should be normal in patients with HNA. Although tomaculae have been reported in some patients,[56] these were most likely cases of HNPP rather than HNA.

Molecular Genetics and Pathogenesis

HNA is caused by mutations in the gene encoding for septin 9 (*SEPT9*).[265–267] Septins may be important in formation of the neuronal cytoskeleton and have a role in cell division.

SCAPULOPERONEAL NEUROPATHY

Clinical Features

A scapuloperoneal distribution of weakness can be seen in several different myopathic and neurogenic disorders, including scapuloperoneal muscular dystrophy (some cases of which have also been termed myofibrillar myopathy—see Chapter 27), a scapuloperoneal neuropathy (Davidenkow syndrome), and a pure motor neuropathy/SMA form.[85,86,268–275] In regard to scapuloperoneal neuropathy or motor neuropathy, symptoms usually develop insidiously in the second or third decade of life. The early symptoms are related to progressive foot drop, with individuals complaining of tripping easily and recurrent ankle sprains similar to CMT. Gradually, proximal weakness of the legs and shoulder girdle arises. Examination reveals muscle wasting about the shoulder girdle (pectoralis, serratus anterior, rhomboids, supraspinatus, infraspinatus, trapezius, deltoid, and brachioradialis) muscles as well as the anterior compartment (peroneal innervated) muscles of the legs. Distal musculature of the arms is relatively spared. The unusual muscle distribution of proximal upper limb and distal lower limb muscles is the clinical distinguishing characteristic of the scapuloperoneal syndromes. Sensation may be normal or reduced. Muscle stretch reflexes may be normal or reduced and the plantar responses are flexor. Pes cavus and hammertoes are commonly appreciated.

Laboratory Features

Median and ulnar CMAPs and NCSs are typically normal in the arms; however, peroneal CMAPs are usually reduced in amplitude with the preservation of distal latency and CV. The SNAPs may be reduced in amplitude in the legs and arms, but individuals with scapuloperoneal motor neuropathy or SMA have normal sensory studies. The needle EMG examination reveals reduced recruitment of large-amplitude, long-duration, polyphasic MUAPs in weak muscle groups.

Histopathology

Sural and superficial peroneal nerve biopsies demonstrate axonal degeneration. Autopsies have demonstrated degeneration of the anterior horn cells. Muscle biopsy demonstrates small, angulated fibers, grouped atrophy, and fiber-type grouping, which can help distinguish the neuropathy from cases of scapuloperoneal myopathy.

Molecular Genetics and Pathogenesis

Autosomal dominant scapuloperoneal neuropathy or SMA and congenital distal SMA are caused by autosomal dominant mutations in the *TRPV4* gene. They are allelic disorders to CMT2C (CMT-Ax-AD-TRPV4) that is discussed in greater detail in the section on CMT2.[85,86]

SORBITOL DEHYDROGENASE DEFICIENCY WITH PERIPHERAL NEUROPATHY (SORD)

Sorbitol dehydrogenase deficiency with peripheral neuropathy (SORD) is a recently reported hereditary neuropathy that is very important as it appears to be the most common autosomal recessive inherited form of neuropathy to date.[276] The authors identified 45 cases from 38 families from multiple ethnicity that presented as slowly progressive, length-dependent, axonal motor greater than sensory polyneuropathy. The clinical and electrophysiological diagnosis was CMT2 51% ($N = 23$), distal HMN in 40% ($N = 18$), and intermediate CMT in 9% ($N = 4$). As of onset was 17+/− 8 years. Other large series likewise reported similar findings.[277,278] Abnormal sequence alterations were found in *SORD* gene. SORD is second enzyme of the two-step polyol pathway. First aldose reductase catalyzes the conversion of glucose into sorbitol, a relatively nonmetabolizable sugar. Next SORD oxidizes sorbitol into fructose. Serum sorbitol levels are markedly increased. How mutations affecting this enzyme cause the neuropathy is unclear.

HEREDITARY NEUROPATHY WITH NEUROMYOTONIA

There are reports of patients with a hereditary motor or sensorimotor polyneuropathy with neuromyotonia.[146,279–282] Most affected individuals have been of European heritage and presented with distal weakness and impaired relaxation (action myotonia). Most have few sensory symptoms and signs; however sural nerve biopsy has revealed a loss of myelinated nerve fibers in some. Some have neurodevelopmental or psychiatric features as generalized anxiety disorder, obsessive-compulsive disorder, mood disorder, and attention-deficit hyperactivity disorder.[282] NCSs usually reveal low-amplitude CMAPs while EMG demonstrates neuromyotonic discharges. Autosomal recessive mutations in the histidine triad nucleotide-binding protein 1 gene, *HINT1*, are the cause. This is a tumor suppressor that participates in several apoptotic pathways, but the pathogenic mechanism by which these mutations cause neuropathy are unknown.

HEREDITARY SENSORY AND AUTONOMIC NEUROPATHIES

HSANs constitute a rare group of hereditary neuropathies in which sensory and autonomic dysfunction predominate over motor function loss, unlike CMT in which motor findings are most prominent (Table 11-3).[1,283–289] Nevertheless, affected individuals can develop motor weakness and thus can overlap with CMT (Fig. 11-1). Patients with autosomal dominant HSAN (HSAN1) usually present in adulthood, whereas autosomal recessive HSANs (HSAN2 to HSAN8) typically express at birth. HSAN1 is caused by pathogenic variants in *SPTLC1*, *SPTLC2*, *ATL1*, *DNMT1*, and *ATL3*. HSAN2 by mutations in *WNK1*, *KIF1A*, *FAM134B*, *SCN9A*, while mutations in *IKBKAP* cause HSAN3, *NTRK1* causes HSAN4, *NGF* causes HSAN5, *DST* causes HSAN6, *SCN11A* causes HSAN7, and *PRDM12* results in HSAN8. Furthermore, mutations in RAB7 that cause CMT2B can cause a mutilating neuropathy that resembles HSAN.[288] Likewise, repeat expansions in *RFC1* that have been more commonly associated with cerebellar ataxia, neuropathy, and vestibular areflexia syndrome (CANVAS) can also manifest with an HSAN phenotype (see Chapter 12).[285,286] Although recently proposed nomenclature advocates for renaming these as HSAN-Ax-AD-GENE or HSAN-Ax-AR-GENE the traditional nomenclature is still most commonly used.[7,8] There are no specific medical therapies available to treat these neuropathies, other than prevention and treatment of mutilating skin and bone lesions. Affected individuals are advised to utilize a night light to limit risk of nocturnal falls, to avoid walking in their bare feet, and to inspect their feet frequently for foreign bodies in order to minimize risk of infection and the subsequent morbidity that delayed detection of an infection may cause.

HSAN TYPE 1

Clinical Features

The HSAN1 is the most common of the HSANs and is inherited in an autosomal dominant fashion. HSAN1 usually presents in the second to fourth decades and this later age of onset is helpful in distinguishing it from other subtypes of HSANs, which typically manifest in infancy or childhood.[1,287–290] HSAN1 is slowly progressive and predominantly affects the small myelinated and unmyelinated nerve fibers, resulting in the loss of pain and temperature sensation in the feet and hands. This can lead to the development of deep dermal ulcerations, recurrent osteomyelitis, Charcot joints, bone loss, gross foot and hand deformities, and amputated digits. Although most people with HSAN1 do not complain of numbness, they often describe burning, aching, or lancinating pains. Autonomic neuropathy is not a prominent feature, but bladder dysfunction and reduced sweating in the feet may occur.

On examination, there is reduced sensation to all modalities, particularly to pin prick and temperature. Mild-to-moderate distal arm and leg weakness develop over time. However, some individuals develop severe distal extremity weakness early in the course.[290] Muscle stretch reflexes are usually absent at the ankles but may be normal or reduced elsewhere. As with CMT, pes cavus and hammertoe deformities can be seen.

Laboratory Features

CSF examination is usually normal. Increased levels of IgA in the serum may be seen. Sensory NCSs reveal normal or only mildly reduced amplitudes with normal distal latencies and NCVs.[290,291] Reduced amplitudes of Aδ and C potentials reflecting the loss of small myelinated and unmyelinated nerve fibers can be appreciated on near-nerve recordings. Motor NCSs are relatively spared; however, reduced amplitudes and slowing of conduction can develop over time. Needle EMG can demonstrate positive sharp waves and fibrillation potentials, with large MUAPs suggesting chronic reinnervation. Sympathetic skin responses are often unobtainable.[291]

Histopathology

Peripheral nerve biopsies demonstrate reduced density of all fiber sizes with a preferential loss of small myelinated and unmyelinated fibers.[290] Muscle biopsies demonstrate features of neurogenic atrophy due to motor nerve involvement. Autopsy studies have revealed degeneration of dorsal root ganglia neurons and of the posterior columns, suggesting a primary sensory neuronopathy or ganglionopathy.

Molecular Genetics and Pathogenesis

HSAN1-like neuropathy is genetically heterogeneous as mentioned earlier.[292–301]

HSAN1A is the most common subtype and is caused by mutations in the serine palmitoyltransferase long chain base 1 gene, *SPTLC1*.[292–294] Serine palmitoyltransferase catalyzes the rate-limiting, regulatory step in the biosynthesis of sphingolipids, and the autosomal dominant inheritance suggests that the mutations either cause a gain of function of the enzyme or result in dominant-negative inhibition.[293] Mutations in *SPTLC1* in lymphoblast cell lines cause an increase in the de novo synthesis of ceramide (a sphingolipid) that appears to trigger apoptotic cell death.[294]

HSAN1B associated with cough and gastroesophageal reflux in a large Australian family was linked to chromosome 3p22–p24, but the gene has not been identified.[297]

▶ TABLE 11-3. HEREDITARY SENSORY AND AUTONOMIC NEUROPATHIES

Traditional Nomenclature	Proposed Nomenclature	Inheritance	Gene	Onset	Clinical Features	Neurophysiology	Pathology
HSAN1A	HSAN-Ax-AD-SPTLC1	AD	SPTLC1	2nd–4th decade	Loss of pain and temperature sensation; autonomic functions relatively spared (except for reduced sweating); arthropathies and foot ulcers are common; distal weakness may develop	Normal or only mildly reduced CMAP and SNAP amplitudes; near nerve recordings: reduced amplitudes of Aδ and C-fibers; abnormal QST (particularly temperature perception); SSR: absent	Distal greater than proximal loss of small myelinated and unmyelinated fibers more than large, myelinated fibers
HSAN1C	HSAN-Ax-AD-SPTLC2	AD	SPTLC2	2nd decade+	As above	As above	As above
HSAN1D (allelic to SPG3A)	HSAN-Ax-AD-ATL1	AD	ATL1	2nd decade+	As above.	As above	As above
HSAN1E	HSAN-Ax-AD-DNMT1	AD	DNMT1	2nd decade+	As above. Hearing loss and dementia.	As above	As above
HSAN1F	HSAN-Ax-AD-ATL3	AD	ATL3	2nd decade+	Loss of pain and temperature sensation; autonomic functions relatively spared (except for reduced sweating); arthropathies and foot ulcers are common; distal weakness may develop		
HSAN2A	HSAN-Ax-AR-WNK1	AR	WNK1	Infancy–early childhood	Severe loss of sensation to all modalities (particularly touch-pressure/vibration); mutilation of hands and feet; impaired sweating, impotence, and bladder function	Absent SNAPs; normal or only mildly reduced CMAPs amplitudes; abnormal QST (particularly vibratory perception)	Virtual absence of large, myelinated fibers; mild loss of small myelinated and unmyelinated fibers
HSAN2B	HSAN-Ax-AR-RETREG1	AR	RETREG1 (FAM134B)	Infancy–early childhood	Severe loss of sensation to all modalities	Absent SNAPs; normal or only mildly reduced CMAPs amplitudes	Loss of large, myelinated fibers
HSAN2C (allelic to SPG30)	HSAN-Ax-AR-KIF1A	AR	KIF1A	First decade	Severe loss of sensation to all modalities; spastic paraplegia	Absent SNAP and reduced CMAP amplitudes	As above
HSAN2D	HSAN-Ax-AR-SCN9A	AR	SCN9A	Infancy–early childhood	Congenital insensitivity to pain; hyposmia, hearing loss, bone dysplasia, and hypogeusia; erythromelalgia, and paroxysmal extreme pain disorder	NCSs and autonomic studies are usually normal	Decreased IENFD

Disease	Inheritance	Gene	Onset	Clinical Features	Electrophysiology	Pathology
HSAN3 (familial dysautonomia; Riley–Day syndrome)	AR	ELP1 (IKBKAP)	Infancy	Severe autonomic dysfunction (labile BP, sweating, and temperature); decreased pain-temperature sensation more than touch/vibration; absence of fungiform papillae and taste; increased mortality	Decreased SNAP amplitudes; mild slowing of CMAP NCVs; abnormal QST; normal SSR	Marked reduction of small myelinated and unmyelinated fibers and to a lesser extent large, myelinated fibers; loss of neurons in sympathetic ganglia
HSAN4	AR	NTRK1	Infancy	Absence of pain and temperature sensation; episodic fevers, postural hypotension, anhidrosis; self-mutilation; mental retardation	Mildly reduced amplitudes and slow NCVs of SNAPs and to a lesser extent of CMAPs; abnormal QST (particularly temperature perception); SSR: intact	Virtual absence of small myelinated and unmyelinated fibers and a moderate loss of large, myelinated fibers
HSAN5	AR	NGF	Infancy	Congenital indifference to painful stimuli despite intact sensation to all modalities and normal deep tendon reflexes	Normal SNAPs, CMAPs, QST, and SSR	May show loss of unmyelinated fibers and selected loss of small myelinated fibers
HSAN6	AR	DST	Infancy–early adult life	Neonatal hypotonia, feeding and respiratory difficulties, pain insensitivity, autonomic abnormalities, mutilation, lack of psychomotor development that is lethal in infants to milder involvement in early adulthood; epidermolysis bullosa simplex	Absent SNAPs; distal CMAPs may have reduced amplitudes. QST abnormal for all modalities. Sudomotor testing is abnormal.	Decreased IENFD
HSAN7	AD	SCN11A	Infancy–early adult life	Congenital insensitivity to pain; severe pruritus; familial episodic pain syndrome 3	Normal NCS	Normal sural nerve biopsy in one patient
HSAN8	AR	PRDM12	Infancy	Congenital insensitivity to pain; mutilation of lips, tongue and extremities	Normal NCS	Reduced small, myelinated fibers and IENFD

AD, autosomal dominant; AR, autosomal recessive; HSAN, hereditary sensory and autonomic neuropathy; IENFD, intraepidermal nerve fiber density; NCV, nerve conduction velocity; NCS, nerve conduction study; SNAP, sensory nerve action potential; CMAP, compound muscle action potential; QST, quantitative sensory testing; SSR, sympathetic skin response.

HSAN1C is caused by mutations in the serine palmitoyltransferase long chain base 2 gene, SPTLC2.[295,296] Pathogenic mechanism is not clear but likely similar to HSAN1A.

HSAN1D is caused by mutations in the gene that encodes for atlastin 1, ATL1.[298] In addition to features of HSAN1, affected individuals may have spasticity of their lower extremities. In this regard, mutations in ATL1 are also responsible for early-onset HSP (SPG3A). Atlastin-1 interacts with spastin and has a role in both in intracellular membrane trafficking as well as in expansion at the axonal growth cone.

HSAN1E is caused by mutations in the DNA methyltransferase 1 gene, DNMT1, that is associated with an autosomal dominant inheritance of sensory neuropathy with sensorineural hearing loss and early-onset dementia.[299–301] The neurological deficits began between the second and fourth decades and were progressive, with death occurring in the fifth and sixth decades. It is also autosomal dominant cerebellar ataxia, deafness, and narcolepsy (ADCA-DN).[302] DNA methyltransferase adds methyl groups to DNA which effects gene expression, but how this causes neuropathy is unclear.

HSAN1F is caused by mutations in the gene that encodes for atlastin 3, ATL3.[303–305] Pathogenic mutations appear to cause a disruption in the ER with reduced lysosomal transport down neuronal axons.[305]

HSAN TYPE 2

Clinical Features

HSAN2 is an autosomal recessive disorder that manifests at birth or early childhood, with severe sensory loss to all modalities and areflexia.[23,305–309] Unlike HSAN1, patients with HSAN2 do not complain of lancinating pains. Autonomic dysfunction manifests with impaired sweating, bladder dysfunction, and impotence. However, postural hypotension is not common. Muscle strength is relatively normal. Scoliosis may be present. The severe sensory loss leads to pressure ulcers, Charcot joints, osteomyelitis, and bone resorption, and amputation of digits in the hands and feet can occur (Fig. 11-8).

Laboratory Features

Sensory NCSs usually absent, while the CMAPs are normal or have slightly reduced amplitudes.[24,306,309] Needle EMG can reveal positive sharp waves, fibrillation potentials, and a reduced recruitment of large, polyphasic MUAPs, particularly in the distal legs.

Histopathology

Nerve biopsies demonstrate a virtual absence of all myelinated fibers with less severe diminution of unmyelinated fibers (Fig. 11-9).

Molecular Genetics and Pathogenesis

HSAN2A is caused by mutations in the protein kinase, lysine-deficient 1 gene, PRKWNK1, now better known as just WNK1 (With No Lysine 1).[310] This protein may play a role functions as an assembly factor for the ER membrane protein complex that is important in the development and/or maintenance of peripheral sensory neurons and their supporting Schwann cells.[311]

HSAN2B is caused by mutations in the FAM134B (family with sequence similarity 134, member B; KIF1 A, kinesin family 1 A) gene that was remained RETREG1 (reticulophagy regulator 1).[312–315] This protein is expressed on the Golgi complex, but how it causes HSAN is unclear. The FAM134 protein families are ER-resident receptors that bind to autophagy modifiers and facilitate ER degradation by autophagy. Mutations appear to inhibit ER turnover, sensitize cells to stress-induced apoptotic cell death, and degeneration of sensory neurons.

HSAN2C is caused by homozygous or compound heterozygous mutation in the kinesin, heavy chain member 1A gene, KIF1A.[316,317] Mutations in the KIF1A can also cause HSP type 30. The encoded protein interacts with WNK1 and is involved in the anterograde transport of synaptic-vesicle precursors along axons.[316]

HSAN2D is caused by mutations in SCN9A that encodes Na(v)1.7 sodium channels.[318] Additional symptoms in affected patients included hyposmia, hearing loss, bone dysplasia, and hypogeusia. Interestingly, mutations in SCN9A have also been associated with a congenital indifference to pain, hereditary small fiber polyneuropathy, erythromelalgia, and paroxysmal extreme pain disorder (discussed at the end of this chapter).[319] NCSs and autonomic studies are usually normal.

HSAN3 (RILEY–DAY SYNDROME; FAMILIAL DYSAUTONOMIA)

Clinical Features

HSAN3 is a rare autosomal recessive disorder that manifests in infancy with feeding difficulties due to poor suck, crying without tears (alacrima), blotchy skin, unexplained fluctuations in body temperature and blood pressure, and repeated vomiting.[170,320–322] Other autonomic features include esophageal and gastrointestinal dysmotility, excessive sweating, tonic pupils, and postural hypotension. Recurrent pulmonary infections are common. Developmental delay and seizures may also occur, although intelligence is normal. Most patients are of Ashkenazi Jewish heritage in whom the incidence of the disease is 1:3,700 live births and carrier frequency is 1:32.[323] HSAN3 is associated with an increased mortality, with a 30-year survival of approximately 50%.[253] However, there have been a few cases with clinical features of HSAN3 and contractures (clubbed feet and clenched hands) and a more severe lethal course.[324] These affected infants were found to have a different gene than more common form of HSAN3.

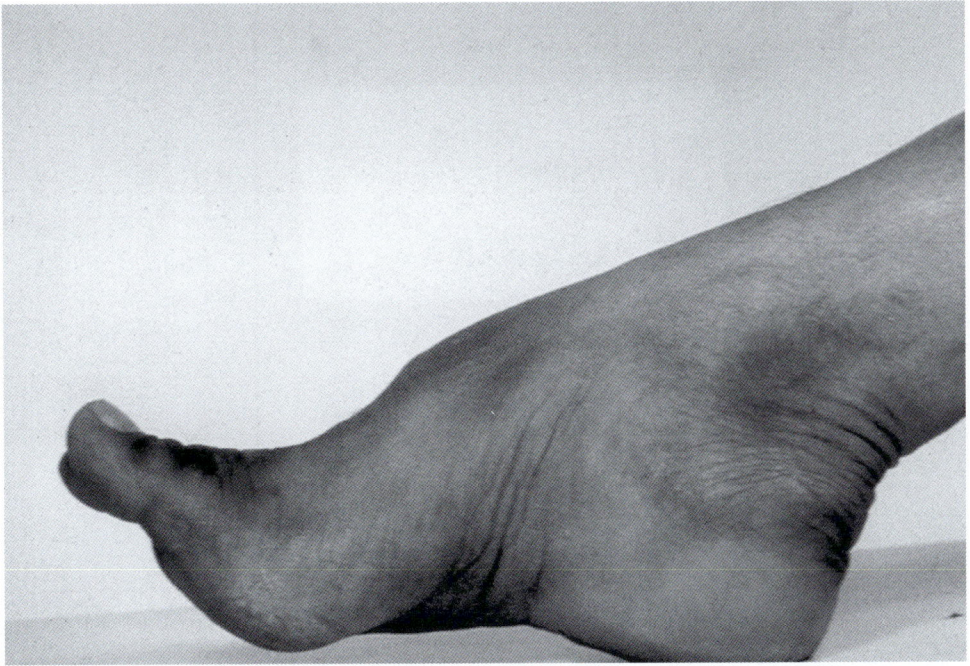

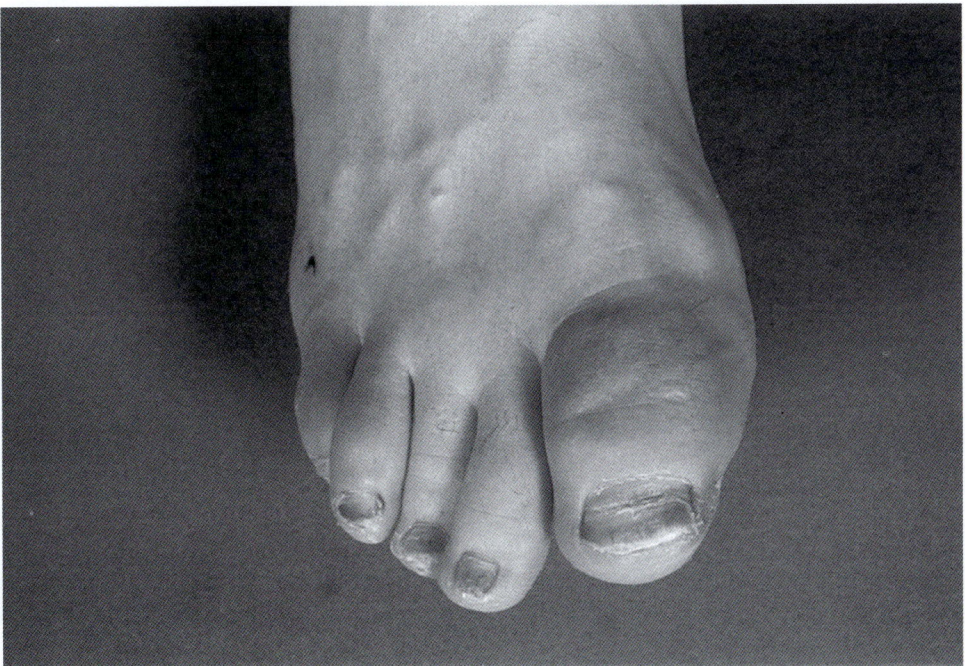

Figure 11-8. Hereditary sensory and autonomic neuropathy type 2. Foot deformities such as pes cavus are common (**A**). Because of the severe lack of sensation, these patients are prone to developing neurogenic arthropathies (**B**). (Reproduced with permission from Amato AA, Dumitru D. Hereditary neuropathies. In: Dumitru D, Amato AA, Swartz MJ, eds. *Electrodiagnostic Medicine*. 2nd ed. Hanley & Belfus; 2002:889–936.)

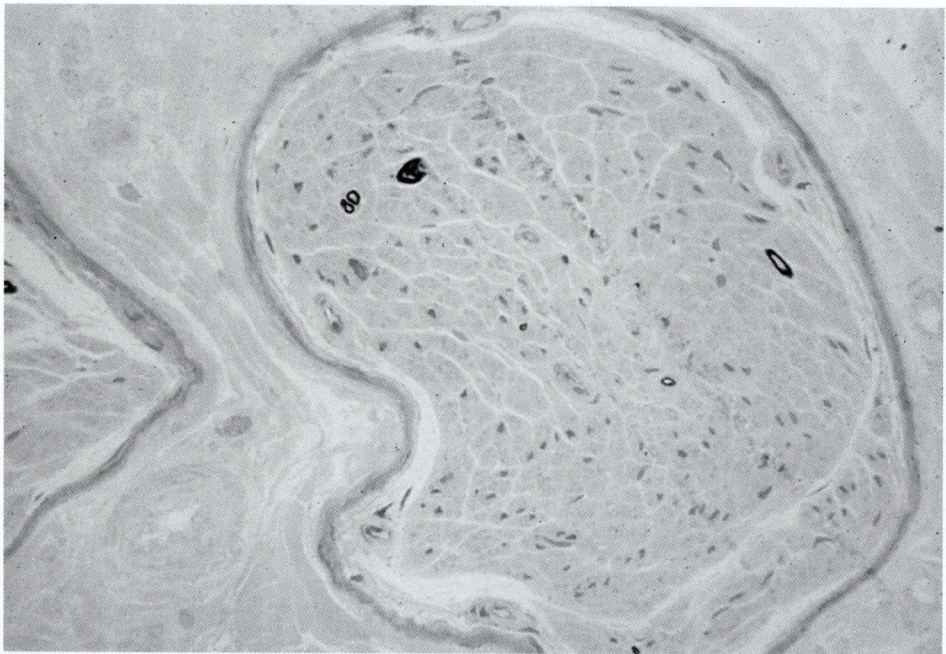

Figure 11-9. Hereditary sensory and autonomic neuropathy type 2. Sural nerve biopsy reveals a severe loss of myelinated and unmyelinated nerve fibers. Semithin, epoxy resin. (Reproduced with permission from Amato AA, Dumitru D. Hereditary neuropathies. In: Dumitru D, Amato AA, Swartz MJ, eds. *Electrodiagnostic Medicine*. 2nd ed. Philadelphia, PA: Hanley & Belfus; 2002:889–936.)

Examination reveals reduced pain and temperature perception and, to a lesser extent, a reduction in proprioception and vibration. Of note, there is an absence of fungiform papillae of the tongue and impaired taste sensation. Muscle strength is usually normal. Muscle stretch reflexes are reduced or absent. Corneal reflexes are also often absent. Mutilation and amputations of the distal extremities are not usually seen in HSAN3, but occasional Charcot joints occur. Short stature and scoliosis are common.

Laboratory Features

SNAPs have only slightly reduced amplitudes and slow CVs, while CMAPs are normal. Sympathetic skin responses are preserved, but quantitative sensory testing reveals impaired heat, cold, and vibratory perception.[170]

Histopathology

Autopsy studies have demonstrated a loss of neurons within the cervical and thoracic sympathetic ganglia as well as in the dorsal root ganglia and trigeminal sensory nucleus. Sural nerve biopsies reveal a marked reduction of unmyelinated fibers (5%–15% of normal) and a less severe reduction in the number of large, myelinated fibers (15%–50% of normal).

Molecular Genetics and Pathogenesis

HSAN3A is caused by mutations in the $I_\kappa B$ kinase complex-associated protein gene, *IKAP*.[323–327] The IKAP protein may activate genes important in the development of sensory and autonomic neurons. Importantly, carrier detection and prenatal diagnosis can be made.

HSAN4 (CONGENITAL INSENSITIVITY TO PAIN WITH ANHIDROSIS)

Clinical Features

HSAN4 is an extremely rare autosomal recessive disorder that manifests in infancy or childhood with an insensitivity to pain, self-mutilation, anhidrosis, and reduced mentation.[170,328] Individuals who are affected become extremely poikilothermic and are at risk of hyperthermia due to their inability to sweat in hot temperatures. In addition, they can develop severe postural hypotension. Sensory examination demonstrates a prominent loss of pain and temperature perception, while vibratory sensation and proprioception are less severely affected. Motor strength and reflexes are preserved.

Laboratory Features

NCSs reveal normal or only slightly reduced SNAP and CMAP amplitudes and CVs. Quantitative sensory testing reveals markedly abnormal heat and cold perception and to a lesser extent vibratory perception.[170] Unlike HSAN3, sympathetic skin responses are unobtainable in HSAN4.[170,329]

Histopathology

As expected on the basis of the clinical examination, sural nerve biopsies reveal a virtual absence of unmyelinated and small myelinated fibers and to a lesser extent a reduction of large fibers to 45%–65% of normal.[170,330]

Molecular Genetics and Pathogenesis

HSAN4 is caused by mutations in *NTRK1* that encodes for neurotrophic receptor tyrosine kinase 1.[331-333] However, no mutations in this gene have been identified in some individuals with a similar phenotype, suggesting genetic heterogeneity of HSAN4. Tyrosine kinase receptors are ligands for neurotrophins. In this regard, NGF, a neurotrophin, binds to trkA receptors, which are highly expressed on dorsal root ganglia and sympathetic neurons. Once bound to the receptor, the trkA–NGF complex is internalized into the nucleus of the neuron, where it regulates the expression of genes important for neuronal maturation, growth, and survival. Mutations affecting the trkA/NGF receptor results in a loss of function of this receptor–ligand complex, which in turn leads to degeneration of sympathetic ganglion neurons and nociceptive sensory neurons derived from the neural crest.[331,333]

HSAN5 (CONGENITAL INDIFFERENCE TO PAIN)

Clinical Features

HSAN5 is similar to HSAN4 is that affected individuals have a congenital insensitivity or indifference to pain. Those with HSAN5 do not appear to recognize or react to painful stimuli (i.e., withdrawal) from birth despite having normal sensitivity to other sensory modalities, normal strength, and muscle stretch reflexes.[334-338] There is no obvious dysautonomia.

Laboratory Features

Motor and sensory NCSs, quantitative sensory testing, and autonomic testing are all usually normal.

Histopathology

Reports of sural nerve biopsies have yielded mixed results. Some have reported normal densities of myelinated and unmyelinated nerve fibers,[334] while other studies have described a loss of small myelinated and unmyelinated fibers.[335-338] Skin biopsy may show reduced intraepidermal nerve fiber density (IENF).

Molecular Genetics and Pathogenesis

Mutations in the *NGF* gene were identified in one family classified as having HSAN5.[337,338] Some could argue that this family actually represents a more benign subtype of HSAN4 because the nerve biopsies were abnormal although neurophysiological testing was normal. In this regard, it is interesting that NGFB binds to trkA, which is mutated in HSAN4 (see "HSAN Type 4" section).

Mutations in *SCN9A*, aside from causing HSAN2D, also can cause HSAN with congenital indifference to pain.[268-270]

▶ HSAN6

CLINICAL FEATURES

HSAN6 was initially reported as a severe sensory neuropathy that was lethal in infancy, the spectrum has increased to include result in milder forms of the disease with onset in early adult life.[324,339-343] The severe form is associated with neonatal hypotonia, feeding and respiratory difficulties, insensitivity to pain leading to corneal scaring, ulceration and mutilation of distal extremities, severe autonomic abnormalities, lack of psychomotor development, and early death. Mutations in the gene have also been associated with epidermolysis bullosa simplex.

LABORATORY FEATURES

NCSs show evidence of a severe sensory axonal neuropathy. Distal motor amplitudes may be reduced. Autonomic testing reveals reduced sudomotor testing.[340]

HISTOPATHOLOGICAL FEATURES

Skin biopsies show a decrease of IENF density.[340]

MOLECULAR GENETICS AND PATHOGENESIS

HSAN6 is by mutations in the gene that encodes dystonin, *DYS*.[324,339-343] Dystonin belongs to the spectraplakin family of proteins and serve as cytoskeletal linker that is essential in maintaining structural integrity and intracellular trafficking.[343]

▶ HSAN7

CLINICAL FEATURES

HSAN7 is associated with congenital insensitivity to pain with mutilation injuries, severe pruritus, intestinal dysmotility, and familial episodic pain syndrome.[344-346] It is also allelic to adult-onset familial episodic pain syndrome type 3.[347]

LABORATORY FEATURES

NCSs are unremarkable.

HISTOPATHOLOGICAL FEATURES

Sural nerve biopsy in one patient was normal.[344]

MOLECULAR GENETICS AND PATHOGENESIS

HSAN7 is caused by mutations in *SCN11A*, which encodes the voltage-gated sodium channel Nav1.9 that is highly expressed in nociceptive neurons of dorsal root ganglia and trigeminal ganglia.[344–347]

▶ HSAN8

CLINICAL FEATURES

HSAN8 was reported in 11 families with congenital insensitivity to pain.[348] Affected children suffered from painless mutilating lesions of the tongue, perioral tissues, and fingers. Sweating and tearing occurred but were reduced compared to normal. Examination revealed normal large fiber sensory functions (light touch, vibration, proprioception).

LABORATORY FEATURES

NCSs are normal.

HISTOPATHOLOGICAL FEATURES

Sural nerve biopsy in two patients revealed a severe loss of small-diameter, myelinated fibers.[348] Skin biopsies demonstrated reduced IENF densities.

MOLECULAR GENETICS AND PATHOGENESIS

HSAN8 is caused by homozygous mutations in *PRDM12* that encodes for positive regulator domain-containing protein 12.[348] PRDM12 is expressed in nociceptors and appears to be required for initiation of neurogenesis of pain-initiating neurons.[349]

▶ ERYTHROMELALGIA (ERYTHERMALGIA)

CLINICAL FEATURES

Erythromelalgia, also known as erythermalgia, is a rare disorder characterized by episodic erythema, intense burning pain and warmth of the hands or feet.[319,350–353] It can occur in an inherited condition (autosomal dominant) or may be acquired. The acquired or secondary form can occur in association with myeloproliferative diseases, neuropathies, and autoimmune diseases. Onset of symptoms can begin or may begin spontaneously at any age in the hereditary form.

LABORATORY FEATURES

NCSs, quantitative sensory testing, and sudomotor testing may be normal or abnormal.[351]

HISTOPATHOLOGICAL FEATURES

Skin biopsies may reveal reduced epidermal nerve fiber density. In addition, perivascular inflammation and edema, fibrosis or arterioles, thickening of arteriolar basement membranes, and smooth muscle hyperplasia may be observed.[351]

MOLECULAR GENETICS AND PATHOGENESIS

Autosomal dominant hereditary erythromelalgia is caused by mutations in the *SCN9A* gene that encodes the Nav1.7 channel.[319,352–354] As previously discussed, mutations in this gene also cause HSAN2D and a form of congenital insensitivity to pain. The Nav1.7 sodium channel is preferentially expressed in most nociceptive dorsal root ganglion neurons and in sympathetic neurons and plays an important role in nociception and vasomotor regulation. Some mutations produced a hyperpolarized voltage-dependence of activation, slower kinetics of deactivation, and impaired steady-state slow inactivation while others do not.

▶ TREATMENT

This is a very difficult to treat disorder. Some patients respond to lidocaine-like medications (e.g., lidoderm patches, mexiletine) and antiepileptic medication (e.g., gabapentin) but many are refractory and require opiates.[353,355]

▶ OTHER SODIUM CHANNELOPATHIES

Paroxysmal extreme pain disorder (formerly known as familial rectal pain) is an autosomal dominant disorder characterized by severe episodes of perineal and rectal, ocular, and mandibular pain that is often associated with dysautonomia including flushing, lacrimation, rhinorrhea, bradycardia, and apnea.[319,356,357] Interestingly, it is also caused by mutations in *SCN9A* which again encodes the Nav1.7 channel.

Familial episodic pain syndrome type 1 is an autosomal dominant disorder associated with severe episodes of pain, predominantly in the chest and arms, but occasionally involving the abdomen and legs.[319,358] The onset is usually in infancy. The episodes of pain typically lasts about 60–90 minutes, can be triggered by hunger and cold, and are typically refractory to standard pain medications. The neurological examination, NCS, and IENF densities are usually normal. This disorder is caused by mutations in *TRPA*, which encodes the transient receptor potential A1 channel.

Familial episodic pain syndrome type 2 is an autosomal dominant disorder characterized by adult-onset of paroxysmal pain mainly affecting the distal lower extremities. It is caused by mutations in *SCNA10A* encoding the Nav1.8 channel.[359]

Familial episodic pain syndrome type 3 is yet another autosomal dominant disorder associated with paroxysmal pain affecting distal hands and feet that has been reported in two Chinese kindreds and was found to be caused by a mutation in *SCN11A* that encodes the Nav1.9 channel.[360]

Interestingly, approximately 30% of patients in one series with otherwise idiopathic painful, small fiber neuropathy had missense substitutions in *SCN9A*.[361,362] This is an overestimate as some of the sequence changes reported have subsequently been found to be benign sequence changes.[319] Nonetheless, mutations in *SCN9A* are a cause of small fiber neuropathy and have been reported in other series of patients.[363,364] Symptoms and signs are similar to idiopathic small fiber polyneuropathy discussed in detail in Chapter 22. Affected individuals however tended to be younger than the older patients who more typically develop small fiber polyneuropathy. Nav1.7 is expressed in the sensory dorsal root ganglion and sympathetic ganglion neurons and their small-diameter peripheral axons. Some mutations impair slow inactivation can produce DRG neuron hyperexcitability that contributes to pain.[362–368]

Rare patients with otherwise idiopathic small fiber neuropathy also have been found to have mutations in *SCN10A* that encodes for a different sodium channel, Nav1.8.[319,369,370] This sodium channel is preferentially expressed in small-diameter dorsal root neurons. Mutations have been demonstrated to shift activation in a hyperpolarizing direction, thus rendering neurons hyperexcitability.

▶ OTHER HEREDITARY SENSORY NEUROPATHIES

Pathogenic sequence variants in the replication factor complex subunit 1 gene, *RFC1*, are most commonly associated with autosomal recessive cerebellar ataxia, neuropathy, vestibular areflexia (CANVAS) syndrome (see Chapter 12). However, patients can present with only sensory symptoms and signs.[285,286,371,372] In regard to small fiber neuropathies, at least 80 pathogenic mutations have been reported in a variety of different sodium channel genes, the most common of which include *SCN7A*, *SCN9A*, *SCN10A*, and *SCN11A* as mentioned above.[373–375]

▶ APPROACH TO GENETIC TESTING

Genetic testing is invaluable in diagnosing, aiding in prognosis, genetic counseling, and helping to avoid of unnecessary and invasive tests (e.g., nerve biopsies), and perhaps unnecessary trials of potentially harmful treatments and (e.g., immunosuppressive agents, intravenous immunoglobulin) when there is diagnostic doubt (e.g., possible CIDP). One good argument for genetic testing and following up carefully phenotyped patients is to learn more about the natural history of all types of hereditary neuropathy, including the rare types so that we can provide a more accurate prediction of the natural history of disease in individual patients in the future.[376–378]

The diagnostic approach to patients with a possible hereditary neuropathy can be daunting given the large number a causal genes and phenotypic variability even within a genotype. Fortunately, useful guidelines are available to help direct which genetic tests should be ordered on the basis of inheritance pattern, age of onset, severity, and motor NCVs.[376,377] A large study and proposed diagnostic algorithms from Dr. Shy's group based on the results of genetic testing on their very large cohort of presumed CMT patients (787 patients of which 527 were genotyped) is particularly helpful.[377] Importantly, approximately 92% of the 527 genetically defined CMT patients in their cohort had mutations in one of only four genes (*PMP22*, *MPZ*, *GJB1*, and *MFN2*).[377]

They proposed that patients with a classical CMT phenotype with slow NCVs (between 16 and 35 m/s), initially should be screened for *PMP22* duplications as this is the most common mutation.[377] If this is negative, they suggested that patients should next be screened for *GJB1* mutations (CMT1X), or if there is clear male-to-male transmission, *MPZ* (CMT1B). Only if these targets are negative would they suggest screening for point mutations in *PMP22*, *LITAF/SIMPLE*, and *EGR2*.

Those with severely slow NCV (≤15 m/s) and who begin to walk after 15 months of age should have testing for both the *PMP22* duplication and *MPZ* mutations.[377] Affected individuals with such severely slow NCVs who walk before 15 months of age should be tested only for the *PMP22* duplication. If no *PMP22* duplication or *MPZ* mutations are found, they suggested sequencing *PMP22*.

Individuals with intermediate MNCVs (between 35 and 45 m/s) usually have CMT1X or CMT1B. For patients with no male-to-male transmission, intermediate conductions, and a classical phenotype, the authors recommend first screening for *GJB1* mutations.[377] If this testing is negative, testing should proceed to *MPZ* mutations. Alternatively, if there is male-to-male transmission, patients should be first screened for *DNM2* mutations as seen in CMT1B. As no patients with CMT1A had intermediate CVs, testing for a *PMP22* duplication would not be warranted. If testing for *MPZ* and *GJB1* is negative, patients could be screened for mutations in the less common dominant intermediate forms of CMT including *DNM2* (DI-CMTB) and *YARS* (DI-CMTC). *DYN2* mutations should also be considered those with cataracts and neutropenia.

In severe childhood onset CMT2 screening should begin with testing of *MFN2* gene as this is the most common cause of CMT2.[377] If this is negative, testing for *MPZ* and *GJB1* would be reasonable. Sequencing *MPZ* and *GJB1* also would be the initial genes to screen for late-onset CMT2; if there was male-to-male transmission in the pedigree only *MPZ* screening is necessary.

Genetic testing for the much rarer forms of hereditary neuropathy (e.g., HSAN) is likewise based on age of onset, inheritance pattern, and the clinical phenotype as discussed in this chapter.

Given the overlap in clinical and electrophysiological phenotypes of the various hereditary neuropathies and the increasing availability and reduced cost of NGS panels most authorities now order these panels instead of sequencing of individual genes. Approximately 90% of demyelinating forms of CMT can be picked up on commercially available NGS panels, however still only 40% of axonal CMT and distal motor neuropathies are successfully genotyped at this time.

▶ SUMMARY

As one can see, there is marked variability in clinical phenotype associated with mutations in individual genes and the same clinical phenotype can be caused by mutation in various genes associated with CMT. Further, there is much overlap of CMT with distal motor neuropathies and HSAN. A practical approach to diagnosis is based on clinical and electrodiagnostic features. Clear autosomal dominant, autosomal recessive, or X-linked pattern of inheritance combined with data from NCSs (e.g., demyelinating, axonal, or intermediate physiology) can be helpful in directing which genes that could be preferentially check for mutations, but more and more NGS panels are utilized to aid in efficient diagnosis. Unfortunately, there are no specific medical treatments available at this time but genetic counseling and supportive therapies (e.g., physical and occupational therapy, bracing) are important and certainly can improve function and quality of life (see Chapter 5).

REFERENCES

1. Klein CJ. Charcot-Marie-Tooth disease and other hereditary neuropathies. *Continuum (Minneap Minn)*. 2020;26(5):1224–1256.
2. Barreto LC, Oliveira FS, Nunes PS, et al. Epidemiologic study of Charcot-Marie-Tooth disease: a systematic review. *Neuroepidemiology*. 2016;46(3):157–165.
3. Lewis RA, Sumner AJ, Shy ME. Electrophysiological features of inherited demyelinating neuropathies: a reappraisal in the era of molecular diagnosis. *Muscle Nerve*. 2000;23:1472–1487.
4. Carroll AS, Burns J, Nicholson G, Kiernan MC, Vucic S. Inherited neuropathies. *Semin Neurol*. 2019;39(5):620–639.
5. Ouvrier RA. Correlation between the histopathologic, genotypic, and phenotypic features of hereditary peripheral neuropathies in children. *J Child Neurol*. 1996;11:133–146.
6. Klein CJ, Duan X, Shy ME. Inherited neuropathies: clinical overview and update. *Muscle Nerve*. 2013;48(4):604–622.
7. Mathis S, Goizet C, Tazir M, Magdelaine C, Lia AS, Magy L, Vallat JM. Charcot-Marie-Tooth diseases: an update and some new proposals for the classification. *J Med Genet*. 2015;52(10):681–690.
8. Magy L, Mathis S, Le Masson G, Goizet C, Tazir M, Vallat JM. Updating the classification of inherited neuropathies: results of an international survey. *Neurology*. 2018 6;90(10):e870–e876.
9. Krampitz DE, Wolfe GI, Fleckenstein JL, Barohn RJ. Charcot–Marie–Tooth type 1 A presenting as calf hypertrophy and muscle cramps. *Neurology*. 1998;51:1508–1509.
10. Carger GT, Kilmer DD, Bonekat WH, Lieberman JS, Fowler WM Jr. Evaluation of phrenic nerve and pulmonary function in hereditary motor and sensory neuropathy, type I. *Muscle Nerve*. 1992;15:459–462.
11. Harding AE, Thomas PK. The clinical features of hereditary motor and sensory neuropathy type I and II. *Brain*. 1980;103:259–280.
12. Kaku DA, Parry GJ, Malamut R, Lupski JR, Garcia CA. Uniform slowing of conduction velocities in Charcot–Marie–Tooth polyneuropathy type 1. *Neurology*. 1993;43:2664–2667.
13. Hattori N, Yamamoto M, Yoshihara T, et al.; Study Group for Hereditary Neuropathy in Japan. Demyelinating and axonal features of Charcot–Marie–Tooth disease with mutations of myelin-related proteins (PMP22, MPZ and Cx32): a clinicopathological study of 205 Japanese patients. *Brain*. 2003;126(Pt 1):134–151.
14. Bird TD, Kraft GH, Lipe GH, Kenney KL, Sumi SM. Clinical and pathological phenotype of the original family with Charcot–Marie–Tooth type 1B: a 20-year study. *Ann Neurol*. 1997;41:463–469.
15. Gabreëls-Festen AA, Bolhuis PA, Hoogendijk JE, Vaentijn LJ, Eshuis EJ, Gabreëls FJ. Charcot–Marie–Tooth disease type 1 A: morphological phenotype of the 17p duplication versus PMP22 point mutations. *Acta Neuropathol (Berl)*. 1995;90:645–649.
16. Santoro L, Manganelli F, Di Maria E, et al. A novel mutation of myelin protein zero associated with an axonal form of Charcot–Marie–Tooth disease. *J Neurol Neurosurg Psychiatry*. 2004;75(2):262–265.
17. Lewis RA, Sumner AJ. The electrodiagnostic distinctions between chronic familial and acquired demyelinating neuropathies. *Neurology*. 1982;32:592–596.
18. Amato AA, Barohn RJ. Hereditary liability to pressure palsies: association with central nervous system demyelination. *Muscle Nerve*. 1996;19:770–773.
19. Combarros O, Calleja J, Figols J, Cabello A, Berciano J. Dominantly inherited motor and sensory neuropathy type I: genetic, clinical, electrophysiological and pathological features in four families. *J Neurol Sci*. 1983;61:181–191.
20. Dyck PJ, Lambert EH. Lower motor and primary sensory neuron diseases with peroneal muscular atrophy. *Arch Neurol*. 1968;18:603–618.
21. Buchthal F, Behse F. Peroneal muscular atrophy (PMA) and related disorders: I. Clinical manifestations as related to biopsy findings, nerve conduction and electromyography. *Brain*. 1977;100:41–66.
22. Behse F, Buchthal F. Peroneal muscular atrophy (PMA) and related disorders: II. Histological findings in sural nerves. *Brain*. 1977;100:67–85.

23. Dyck PJ. Histologic measurements and fine structure of biopsied sural nerve: normal and in peroneal muscular atrophy, hypertrophic neuropathy, and congenital sensory neuropathy. *Mayo Clin Proc.* 1966;41:742–774.
24. Kochanski A, Drac H, Kabzinska D, Hausmanowa-Petrusewicz I. A novel mutation, Thr65Ala, in the MPZ gene in a patient with Charcot–Marie–Tooth type 1B disease with focally folded myelin. *Neuromuscul Disord.* 2004;14(3):229–232.
25. Lupski JR, deOca-Luna RM, Slaugenhaupt S, et al. DNA duplication associated with Charcot–Marie–Tooth disease type 1 A. *Cell.* 1991;66:219–232.
26. Raemakears P, Timmerman V, Nellis E, et al. Duplication in chromosome 17p11.2 in Charcot–Marie–Tooth disease type 1 a (CMT1 a). The HMSN Collaborative Group. *Neuromuscul Disord.* 1991;1:93–97.
27. Lopes J, Ravise N, Vandenberghe A, et al. Fine mapping of de novo CMT1 A and HNPP rearrangements within CMT1 A-REPS evidences two distinct sex-dependent mechanisms and candidate sequences involved in recombination. *Hum Mol Genet.* 1998;7:141–148.
28. Chance PF, Bird TD, Matsunami N, Lensch MW, Brothman AR, Feldman GM. Trisomy 17p associated with Charcot–Marie–Tooth neuropathy type 1 A phenotype: evidence for gene dosage as a mechanism in CMT1 A. *Neurology.* 1992;42:2295–2299.
29. Roa BB, Garcia CA, Suter U, et al. Evidence for Charcot–Marie–Tooth disease type 1 A association with point mutation in the PMP22 gene. *N Engl J Med.* 1993;5:189–194.
30. Gabriel JM, Erne B, Pareyson D, Sghirlanzoni A, Taroni F, Steck AJ. Gene dosage effects in hereditary peripheral neuropathy. Expression of peripheral myelin protein 22 in Charcot–Marie–Tooth disease type 1 A and hereditary neuropathy with liability to pressure palsies nerve biopsies. *Neurology.* 1997;49:1635–1640.
31. Hanemann CO, Stoll G, D'Urso D, et al. Peripheral myelin protein-22 expression in Charcot–Marie–Tooth disease type 1 A sural nerve biopsies. *J Neurosci Res.* 1994;37:654–659.
32. Vallat JM, Sindou P, Preux PM, et al. Ultrastructural PMP22 expression in inherited demyelinating neuropathies. *Ann Neurol.* 1996;39:813–817.
33. Yoshikawa H, Nishimura T, Nakatsuji Y, et al. Elevated expression of messenger RNA for peripheral myelin protein 22 in biopsied peripheral nerves of patients with Charcot–Marie–Tooth disease type 1 A. *Ann Neurol.* 1994;35:445–450.
34. Sahenk Z, Chen L, Mendell JR. Effects of PMP22 duplication and deletion on the axonal cytoskeleton. *Ann Neurol.* 1999;45:16–24.
35. Hayasaka K, Himoro M, Sato W, et al. Charcot–Marie–Tooth neuropathy type 1B is associated with mutations of the myelin P0 gene. *Nat Genet.* 1993;5:31–34.
36. Kulkens T, Bulhuis PA, Wolterman RA, et al. Deletion of serine 34 codon from the major peripheral myelin protein P0 gene in Charcot–Marie–Tooth disease type 1B. *Nat Genet.* 1993;5:35–39.
37. Su Y, Brooks DG, Li L, et al. Myelin protein zero gene mutated in Charcot–Marie–Tooth type 1B. *Proc Natl Acad Sci USA.* 1993;90:10856–10860.
38. Vallat JM, Magy L, Lagrange E, et al. Diagnostic value of ultrastructural nerve examination in Charcot–Marie–Tooth disease: two CMT 1B cases with pseudo-recessive inheritance. *Acta Neuropathol (Berl).* 2007;113(4):443–449.
39. Sindou P, Vallat JM, Chapon F, et al. Ultrastructural protein zero expression in Charcot–Marie–Tooth type 1B disease. *Muscle Nerve.* 1999;22:99–104.
40. Street VA, Bennett CL, Goldy JD, et al. Mutation of a putative protein degradation gene LITAF/SIMPLE in Charcot–Marie–Tooth disease 1 C. *Neurology.* 2003;60(1):22–26.
41. Latour P, Gonnaud PM, Ollagnon E, et al. SIMPLE mutation analysis in dominant demyelinating Charcot–Marie–Tooth disease: three novel mutations. *J Peripher Nerv Syst.* 2006;11(2):148–155.
42. Shirk AJ, Anderson SK, Hashemi SH, Chance PF, Bennett CL. SIMPLE interacts with NEDD4 and TSG101: evidence for a role in lysosomal sorting and implications for Charcot–Marie–Tooth disease. *J Neurosci Res.* 2005;82(1):43–50.
43. Warner LE, Mancias P, Butler IJ, et al. Mutations in the early growth response 2 (ERG2) gene are associated with hereditary myelinopathies. *Nat Genet.* 1998;18:382–384.
44. Fabrizi GM, Cavallaro T, Angiari C, et al. Giant axon and neurofilament accumulation in Charcot–Marie–Tooth disease type 2E. *Neurology.* 2004;62(8):1429–1431.
45. Zuchner S, Vorgerd M, Sindern E, Schroder JM. The novel neurofilament light (NEFL) mutation Glu397Lys is associated with a clinically and morphologically heterogeneous type of Charcot–Marie–Tooth neuropathy. *Neuromuscul Disord.* 2004;14(2):147–157.
46. Motley WW, Palaima P, Yum SW, et al. De novo PMP2 mutations in families with type I Charcot-Marie-Tooth disease. *Brain.* 2016;139:1649–1656.
47. Punetha J, Mackay-Loder L, Harel T, et al. Identification of a pathogenic PMP2 variant in a multi-generational family with CMT type 1: clinical gene panels versus genome-wide approaches to molecular diagnosis. *Molec Gene Metab.* 2018; 125: 302–304, 2018.
48. Amato AA, Gronseth G, Callerame K, Kagan-Hallet KS, Bryan W, Barohn RJ. Tomaculous neuropathy: a clinical and electrophysiological study in patients with and without 1.5 Mb deletions in chromosome 17p11.2. *Muscle Nerve.* 1996;19:16–22.
49. Lenssen PPA, Gabreels-Festen AAWM, Valentijn LJ, et al. Hereditary neuropathy with liability to pressure palsies. Phenotypic differences between patients with the common deletion and a PMP22 frame shift mutation. *Brain.* 1998; 121:1451–1458.
50. Madrid R, Bradley WG. The pathology of neuropathies with focal thickening of the myelin sheath (Tomaculous neuropathy). *J Neurol Sci.* 1975;25:415–448.
51. Mouton P, Tardieu S, Goudier R, et al. Spectrum of clinical and electrophysiologic features in HNPP patients with the 17p11.2 deletion. *Neurology.* 1999;52:1440–1446.
52. Verhagen WIM, Gabreels-Festen AAWM, van Wensen PJM, et al. Hereditary neuropathy with liability to pressure palsies: a clinical, electrophysiological, and morphological study. *J Neurol Sci.* 1993;116:176–184.
53. Li J, Krajewski K, Shy ME, Lewis RA. Hereditary neuropathy with liability to pressure palsy: the electrophysiology fits the name. *Neurology.* 2002;58(12):1769–1773.
54. Li J, Krajewski K, Lewis RA, Shy ME. Loss-of-function phenotype of hereditary neuropathy with liability to pressure palsies. *Muscle Nerve.* 2004;29(2):205–210.
55. Behse F, Buchthal F, Carlsen F, et al. Hereditary neuropathy with liability to pressure palsies. *Brain.* 1972;95:777–794.
56. Stögbauer F, Young P, Kerschensteiner M, Ringelsein EB, Assman G, Funke H. Recurrent brachial plexus palsies as the only

clinical expression of neuropathy with liability to pressure palsies associated with a de novo deletion of peripheral myelin protein-22 gene. *Muscle Nerve*. 1998;21:1199–1201.
57. Bosch EP, Chui HC, Martin MA, Cancilla PA. Brachial plexus involvement in familial pressure-sensitive neuropathy: electrophysiological and morphological findings. *Ann Neurol*. 1980;8:620–624.
58. Chance PF, Alderson MK, Leppig KA, et al. DNA deletion associated with hereditary neuropathy with liability to pressure palsies. *Cell*. 1993;72:143–151.
59. Sahenk Z, Chen L, Freimer M. A novel PMP22 point mutation causing HNPP phenotype. Studies on nerve xenografts. *Neurology*. 1998;51:702–707.
60. Schenone A, Nobbio L, Caponnetto C, et al. Correlation between PMP-22 messenger RNA expression and phenotype in hereditary neuropathy with liability to pressure palsies. *Ann Neurol*. 1997;42:866–872.
61. Berciano J, Combarros O, Figols J, et al. Hereditary motor and sensory neuropathy type II. *Brain*. 1986;109:897–914.
62. Bouche' P, Gherardi R, Cathala HP, Lhermitte F, Castaigne P. Peroneal muscular atrophy: Part 1. Clinical and electrophysiological study. *J Neurol Sci*. 1983;61:389–399.
63. Dyck PJ, Lambert EH. Lower motor and primary sensory neuron disease with peroneal muscular atrophy. *Arch Neurol*. 1968;18:619–625.
64. Teunissen LL, Notermans NC, Franssen H, Van Engelen BG, Baas F, Wokke JH. Disease course of Charcot–Marie–Tooth disease type 2: a 5-year follow-up study. *Arch Neurol*. 2003;60(6):823–828.
65. Bienfait HM, Verhamme C, van Schaik IN, et al. Comparison of CMT1 A and CMT2: similarities and differences. *J Neurol*. 2006;253(12):1572–1580.
66. Bienfait HME, Baas F, Koelman JHTM, et al. Phenotype of Charcot–Marie–Tooth disease Type 2. *Neurology*. 2007;68:1658–1667.
67. Lawson VH, Graham BV, Flanigan KM. Clinical and electrophysiologic features of CMT2 A with mutations in the mitofusin 2 gene. *Neurology*. 2005;65(2):197–204.
68. Verhoeven K, Claeys KG, Zuchner S, et al. MFN2 mutation distribution and genotype/phenotype correlation in Charcot–Marie–Tooth type 2. *Brain*. 2006;129(Pt 8):2093–2102.
69. Loiseau D, Chevrollier A, Verny C, et al. Mitochondrial coupling in Charcot–Marie–Tooth Type 2 A disease. *Ann Neurol*. 2007;61:315–323.
70. Gabreëls-Festen AAWM, Joosten EMG, Gabreëls FJM, Jennekens FG, Gooskens RH, Stegeman DF. Hereditary motor and sensory neuropathy of neuronal type with onset in early childhood. *Brain*. 1991;114:1855–1870.
71. Chung KW, Kim SB, Park KD, et al. Early onset severe and late-onset mild Charcot–Marie–Tooth disease with mitofusin 2 (MFN2) mutations. *Brain*. 2006;129:2103–2118.
72. Zuchner S, De Jonghe P, Jordanova A, et al. Axonal neuropathy with optic atrophy is caused by mutations in mitofusin 2. *Ann Neurol*. 2006;59(2):276–281.
73. De Jonghe P, Timmerman V, Fitzpatrick D, Spoelders P, Martin J-J, Van Broeckhoven C. Mutilating neuropathic ulcerations in a chromosome 3q13–q22 linked Charcot–Marie–Tooth disease type 2B family. *J Neurol Neurosurg Psychiatry*. 1997;62:570–573.
74. Auer-Grumbach M, De Jonghe P, Verhoeven K, et al. Autosomal dominant inherited neuropathies with prominent sensory loss and mutilations: a review. *Arch Neurol*. 2003;60(3):329–334.
75. Verhoeven K, De Jonghe P, Coen K, et al. Mutations in the small GTP-ase late endosomal protein RAB7 cause Charcot–Marie–Tooth type 2B neuropathy. *Am J Hum Genet*. 2003;72:722–727.
76. Meggouh F, Bienfait HM, Weterman MA, de Visser M, Baas F. Charcot–Marie–Tooth disease due to a de novo mutation of the RAB7 gene. *Neurology*. 2006;67(8):1476–1478.
77. De Sandre-Giovannoli A, Chaouch M, Kozlov S, et al. Homozygous defects in LMNA, encoding lamin A/C nuclear-envelope proteins, cause autosomal recessive axonal neuropathy in human (Charcot–Marie–Tooth disorder type 2) and mouse. *Am J Hum Genet*. 2002;70(3):726–736. Erratum in *Am J Hum Genet*. 2002;70(4):1075.
78. Chaouch M, Allal Y, De Sandre-Giovannoli A, et al. The phenotypic manifestations of autosomal recessive axonal Charcot–Marie–Tooth due to a mutation in Lamin A/C gene. *Neuromuscul Dis*. 2003;13(1):60–67.
79. Tazir M, Azzedine H, Assami S, et al. Phenotypic variability in autosomal recessive axonal Charcot–Marie–Tooth disease due to the R298 C mutation in lamin A/C. *Brain*. 2004;127(Pt 1):154–163.
80. Bouhouche A, Birouk N, Azzedine H, et al. Autosomal recessive axonal Charcot–Marie–Tooth disease (ARCMT2): phenotype–genotype correlations in 13 Moroccan families. *Brain*. 2007;130(Pt 4):1062–1075.
81. Leal A, Bogantes-Ledezma S, Ekici AB, et al. The polynucleotide kinase 3-prime-phosphatase (PNKP) is involved in Charcot-Marie-Tooth disease (CMT2B2) previously related to MED25. *Neurogenetics*. 2018;19:215–225.
82. Dyck PJ, Litchey WJ, Minnerath S, et al. Hereditary motor and sensory neuropathy with diaphragm and vocal cord paresis. *Ann Neurol*. 1994;35:608–615.
83. Pridmore C, Baraister M, Brett EM, Harding AE. Distal spinal muscular atrophy with vocal cord paralysis. *J Med Genet*. 1992;29:197–199.
84. Klein CJ, Cunningham JM, Atkinson EJ, et al. The gene for HMSN2 C maps to 12q23–24: a region of neuromuscular disorders. *Neurology*. 2003;60:1151–1156.
85. Echaniz-Laguna A, Dubourg O, et al. Phenotypic spectrum and incidence of TRPV4 mutations in patients with inherited axonal neuropathy. *Neurology*. 2014;82(21):1919–1926.
86. Deng H-X, Klein CJ, Yan J, et al. Scapuloperoneal spinal muscular atrophy and CMT2 C are allelic disorders caused by alterations in TRPV4. *Nat Genet*. 2010;42:165–169.
87. Sambuughin N, Sivakumar K, Selenge B, et al. Autosomal dominant distal spinal muscular atrophy type V (dsSMA-V) and Charcot–Marie–Tooth disease type 2D (CMT2D) segregate within a large kindred and map to a refined region on chromosome 7p15. *J Neurol Sci*. 1998;161:23–28.
88. Antonellis A, Ellsworth RE, Sambuughin N, et al. Glycyl tRNA synthetase mutations in Charcot–Marie–Tooth disease type 2D and distal spinal muscular atrophy type V. *Am J Hum Genet*. 2003;72:1293–1299.
89. Sivakumar K, Kyriakides T, Puls I, et al. Phenotypic spectrum of disorders associated with glycyl-tRNA synthetase mutations. *Brain*. 2005;128(Pt 10):2304–2314.
90. James PA, Cader MZ, Muntoni F, Childs AM, Crow YJ, Talbot K. Severe childhood SMA and axonal CMT due to anticodon binding domain mutations in the GARS gene. *Neurology*. 2006;67(9):1710–1712. Erratum in *Neurology*. 2007;68(9):711.
91. Jordanova A, De Jonghe P, Boerkoel CF, et al. Mutations in the neurofilament light chain gene (NEFL) cause early onset severe Charcot–Marie–Tooth disease. *Brain*. 2003;126:590–597.

92. Kim HJ, Kim SB, Kim HS, et al. Phenotypic heterogeneity in patients with NEFL-related Charcot-Marie-Tooth disease. *Mol Genet Genomic Med.* 2022;10(2):e1870.
93. Zaman Q, Khan MA, Sahar K, et al. Novel variants in *MPV17, PRX, GJB1,* and *SACS* cause Charcot-Marie-Tooth and spastic ataxia of Charlevoix-Saguenay type diseases. *Genes (Basel).* 2023;14(2):328.
94. Baumann M, Schreiber H, Schlotter-Weigel B. MPV17 mutations in juvenile- and adult-onset axonal sensorimotor polyneuropathy. *Clin Genet.* 2019;95(1):182–186.
95. Ismailov SM, Fedotov VP, Dadali EL, et al. A new locus for autosomal dominant Charcot–Marie–Tooth disease type 2 (CMT2F) maps to chromosome 7q11–q21. *Eur J Hum Genet.* 2001;9:646–650.
96. Evgrafov OV, Mersiyanova I, Irobi J, et al. Mutant small heat-shock protein 27 causes axonal Charcot–Marie–Tooth disease and distal hereditary motor neuropathy. *Nat Genet.* 2004;36(6):602–606.
97. Schwartz NU. Charcot-Marie-Tooth 2F (Hsp27 mutations): a review. *Neurobiol Dis.* 2019;130:104505
98. Greenbaum L, Ben-David M, Nikitin V, et al. Early and late manifestations of neuropathy due to HSPB1 mutation in the Jewish Iranian population. *Ann Clin Transl Neurol.* 2021;8(6):1260–1268.
99. Taga A, Cornblath DR. A novel HSPB1 mutation associated with a late onset CMT2 phenotype: Case presentation and systematic review of the literature. *J Peripher Nerv Syst.* 2020;25(3):223–229.
100. Abati E, Magri S, Meneri M, et al. Charcot-Marie-Tooth disease type 2F associated with biallelic HSPB1 mutations. *Ann Clin Transl Neurol.* 2021;8(5):1158–1164.
101. Houlden H, Laura M, Wavrant-De Vrièze F, Blake J, Wood N, Reilly MM. Mutations in the HSP27 (HSPB1) gene cause dominant, recessive, and sporadic distal HMN/CMT type 2. *Neurology.* 2008;71(21):1660–1668.
102. Crimella C, Tonelli A, Airoldi G, et al. The GST domain of GDAP1 is a frequent target of mutations in the dominant form of axonal Charcot Marie Tooth type 2K. *J Med Genet.* 2010;47(10):712–716.
103. Cassereau J, Chevrollier A, Gueguen N, et al. Mitochondrial complex I deficiency in GDAP1-related autosomal dominant Charcot-Marie-Tooth disease (CMT2K). *Neurogenetics.* 2009;10(2):145–150.
104. Wu R, Lv H, Wang H, Wang Z, Yuan Y. The pathological features of common hereditary mitochondrial dynamics neuropathy. *Front Neurosci.* 2021;15:705277.
105. Tang BS, Zhao GH, Luo W, et al. Small heat-shock protein 22 mutated in autosomal dominant Charcot–Marie–Tooth disease type 2 L. *Hum Genet.* 2005;116(3):222–224.
106. Zuchner S, Noureddine M, Kennerson M, et al. Mutations in the pleckstrin homology domain of dynamin 2 cause dominant intermediate Charcot-Marie-Tooth disease. *Nat Genet.* 2005;37(3):289–294.
107. Claeys KG, Züchner S, Kennerson M. Phenotypic spectrum of dynamin 2 mutations in Charcot-Marie-Tooth neuropathy. *Brain.* 2009;132(Pt 7):1741–1752.
108. Fischer D, Herasse M, Bitoun M, et al. Characterization of the muscle involvement in dynamin 2-related centronuclear myopathy. *Brain.* 2006;129(Pt 6):1463–1469.
109. Mademan I, Deconinck T, Dinopoulos A, et al. De novo INF2 mutations expand the genetic spectrum of hereditary neuropathy with glomerulopathy. *Neurology.* 2013;81(22):1953–1958.
110. Boyer O, Nevo F, Plaisier E, et al. INF2 mutations in Charcot-Marie-Tooth disease with glomerulopathy. *N Engl J Med.* 2011;365:2377–2388.
111. Latour P, Thauvin-Robinet C, Baudelet-Mery C, et al. A major determinant for binding and aminoacylation of tRNA-Ala in cytoplasmic alanyl-tRNA synthetase is mutated in dominant axonal Charcot-Marie-Tooth disease. *Am J Hum Genet.* 2010;86:77–82.
112. Lin K-P, Soong B-W, Yang C-C, et al. The mutational spectrum in a cohort of Charcot-Marie-Tooth disease type 2 among the Han Chinese in Taiwan. *PLoS One.* 2011;6:e29393.
113. McLaughlin HM, Sakaguchi R, Giblin W, et al. A recurrent loss-of-function alanyl-tRNA synthetase (AARS) mutation in patients with Charcot-Marie-Tooth disease type 2 N (CMT2 N). *Hum Mutat.* 2012;33:244–253.
114. Weedon MN, Hastings R, Caswell R, et al. Exome sequencing identifies a DYNC1H1 mutation in a large pedigree with dominant axonal Charcot-Marie-Tooth disease. *Am J Hum Genet.* 2011;89:308–312.
115. Li JT, Dong SQ, Zhu DQ, et al. Expanding the phenotypic and genetic spectrum of neuromuscular diseases caused by *DYNC1H1* mutations. *Front Neurol.* 2022;13:943324.
116. Guernsey DL, Jiang H, Bedard K, et al. Mutation in the gene encoding ubiquitin ligase LRSAM1 in patients with Charcot-Marie-Tooth disease. *PLoS Genet.* 2010;6:1–7.
117. Weterman MA, Sorrentino V, Kasher PR, et al. A frameshift mutation in LRSAM1 is responsible for a dominant hereditary polyneuropathy. *Hum Mol Genet.* 2011;21:358–370.
118. Palaima P, Berciano J, Peeters K, Jordanova A. LRSAM1 and the RING domain: Charcot-Marie-Tooth disease and beyond. *Orphanet J Rare Dis.* 2021;16(1):74.
119. Hu B, Arpag S, Zuchner S, Li J. A novel missense mutation of CMT2P alters transcription machinery. *Ann Neurol.* 2016;80(6):834–845.
120. Xu WY, Gu MM, Sun LH, et al. A nonsense mutation in DHTKD1 causes Charcot-Marie-Tooth disease type 2 in a large Chinese pedigree. *Am J Hum Genet.* 2012;91(6):1088–1094.
121. Ylikallio E, Poyhonen R, Zimon M, et al. Deficiency of the E3 ubiquitin ligase TRIM2 in early-onset axonal neuropathy. *Hum Mol Genet.* 2013;22:2975–2983.
122. Pehlivan D, Coban Akdemir Z, Karaca E, et al. Exome sequencing reveals homozygous TRIM2 mutation in a patient with early onset CMT and bilateral vocal cord paralysis. *Hum Genet.* 2015;134:671–673.
123. Magri S, Danti FR, Balistreri F, et al. Expanding the phenotypic spectrum of TRIM2-associated Charcot-Marie-Tooth disease. *J Peripher Nerv Syst.* 2020;25(4):429–432.
124. Cottenie E, Kochanski A, Jordanova A, et al. Truncating and missense mutations in IGHMBP2 cause Charcot-Marie-Tooth disease type 2. *Am J Hum Genet.* 2014;95(5):590–601.
125. Schottmann G, Jungbluth H, Schara U, et al. Recessive truncating IGHMBP2 mutations presenting as axonal sensorimotor neuropathy. *Neurology.* 2015;84:523–531.
126. Rzepnikowska W, Kochański A. Models for IGHMBP2-associated diseases: an overview and a roadmap for the future. *Neuromuscul Disord.* 2021;31(12):1266–1278.
127. Lei L, Zhiqiang L, Xiaobo L, et al. Clinical and genetic features of Charcot-Marie-Tooth disease patients with IGHMBP2 mutations. *Neuromuscul Disord.* 2022;32(7):564–571.
128. Higuchi Y, Hashiguchi A, Yuan J, et al. Mutations in MME cause an autosomal-recessive Charcot-Marie-Tooth disease type 2. *Ann Neurol.* 2016;79(4):659–672.

129. Auer-Grumbach M, Toegel S, Schabhüttl M, et al. Rare variants in MME, encoding metalloprotease neprilysin, are linked to late-onset autosomal-dominant axonal polyneuropathies. *Am J Hum Genet.* 2016;99(3):607–623.
130. Hyun YS, Park HJ, Heo SH, et al. Rare variants in methionyl- and tyrosyl-tRNA synthetase genes in late-onset autosomal dominant Charcot-Marie-Tooth neuropathy. *Clin Genet.* 2014;86(6):592–594.
131. Gonzalez M, McLaughlin H, Houlden H, et al. Exome sequencing identifies a significant variant in methionyl-tRNA synthetase (MARS) in a family with late-onset CMT2. *J Neurol Neurosurg Psychiatry.* 2013;84(11):1247–1249.
132. Hirano M, Oka N, Hashiguchi A, et al. Histopathological features of a patient with Charcot-Marie-Tooth disease type 2U/AD-CMTax-MARS. *J Peripher Nerv Syst.* 2016;21(4):370–374.
133. Ma Z, Lv H, Zhang H, et al. Clinicopathological features in two families with MARS-related Charcot-Marie-Tooth disease. *Neuropathology.* 2022;42(6):505–511.
134. Tétreault M, Gonzalez M, Dicaire MJ, et al. Adult-onset painful axonal polyneuropathy caused by a dominant NAGLU mutation. *Brain.* 2015;138(Pt 6):1477–1483.
135. Lopergolo D, Salvatore S, Sorrentino V, Malandrini A, Santorelli FM, Battisti C. Early-onset motor polyneuropathy associated with a novel dominant NAGLU mutation. *Neurol Sci.* 2023;44(4):1415–1418.
136. Safka Brozkova D, Deconinck T, Griffin LB, et al. Loss of function mutations in HARS cause a spectrum of inherited peripheral neuropathies. *Brain.* 2015;138(Pt 8):2161–2172.
137. Vester A, Velez-Ruiz G, McLaughlin HM, et al. A loss-of-function variant in the human histidyl-tRNA synthetase (HARS) gene is neurotoxic in vivo. *Hum Mutat.* 2013;34:191–199.
138. Montecchiani C, Pedace L, Lo Giudice T, et al. ALS5/SPG11/KIAA1840 mutations cause autosomal recessive axonal Charcot-Marie-Tooth disease. *Brain.* 2016;139(Pt 1):73–85.
139. Schiava M, Ikenaga C, Villar-Quiles RN. Genotype-phenotype correlations in valosin-containing protein disease: a retrospective multicentre study. *J Neurol Neurosurg Psychiatry.* 2022;jnnp-2022-328921.
140. Gonzalez MA, Feely SM, Speziani F, et al. A novel mutation in VCP causes Charcot-Marie-Tooth type 2 disease. *Brain.* 2014;137(Pt 11):2897–2902.
141. Gite J, Milko E, Brady L, Baker SK. Phenotypic convergence in Charcot-Marie-Tooth 2Y with novel VCP mutation. *Neuromuscul Disord.* 2020;30(3):232–235.
142. Sevilla T, Lupo V, Martínez-Rubio D, et al. Mutations in the MORC2 gene cause axonal Charcot-Marie-Tooth disease. *Brain.* 2016;139(Pt 1):62–72.
143. Ando M, Okamoto Y, Yoshimura A, et al. Clinical and mutational spectrum of Charcot-Marie-Tooth disease type 2Z caused by MORC2 variants in Japan. *Eur J Neurol.* 2017;24(10):1274–1282.
144. Jacquier A, Ribault S, Mendes M, et al. Expanding the phenotypic variability of MORC2 gene mutations: from Charcot-Marie-Tooth disease to late-onset pure motor neuropathy. *Hum Mutat.* 2022;43(12):1898–1908.
145. Teunissen LL, Notermans NC, Fransen H, et al. Difference between hereditary motor and sensory neuropathy type 2 and chronic idiopathic axonal neuropathy. A clinical and electrophysiological study. *Brain.* 1997;120:955–962.
146. Hahn AF, Parkes AW, Bolton CF, Stewart SA. Neuromyotonia in hereditary motor neuropathy. *J Neurol Neurosurg Psychiatry.* 1991;54:230–235.
147. Vasilescu C, Marilena A, Dan A. Neuronal type of Charcot-Marie-Tooth disease with a syndrome of continuous motor unit activity. *J Neurol Sci.* 1984;63:11–25.
148. Schroder JM. Neuropathology of Charcot-Marie-Tooth and related disorders. *Neuromol Med.* 2006;8(1–2):23–42.
149. Zhao C, Takita J, Tanaka Y, et al. Charcot-Marie-Tooth disease type 2 A caused by mutation in a microtubule motor KIF1Bbeta. *Cell.* 2001;105(5):587–597. Erratum in *Cell.* 2001;106(1):127.
150. Ben Othame K, Middleton LT, Loprest LJ. Localization of a gene (CMT2 A) for autosomal dominant Charcot-Marie-Tooth type 2 to chromosome 1p and evidence for genetic heterogeneity. *Genomics.* 1993;17:370–375.
151. Zuchner S, Mersiyanova IV, Muglia M, et al. Mutations in the mitochondrial GTPase mitofusin 2 cause Charcot-Marie-Tooth neuropathy type 2 A. *Nat Genet.* 2004;36(5):449–451.
152. Baloh RH, Schmidt RE, Pestronk A, Milbrandt J. Altered axonal mitochondrial transport in the pathogenesis of Charcot-Marie-Tooth disease from mitofusin 2 mutations. *J Neurosci.* 2007;27(2):422–430.
153. Kwon JM, Eliott JL, Yee W, et al. Assignment of a second Charcot-Marie-Tooth type II locus to chromosome 3q. *Am J Hum Genet.* 1995;57:853–858.
154. Auer-Grumbach M, Strasser-Fuchs S, Robl T, Windpassinger C, Wagner K. Late onset Charcot-Marie-Tooth 2 syndrome caused by two novel mutations in the MPZ gene. *Neurology.* 2003;61(10):1435–1437.
155. Fontaine JM, Sun X, Hoppe AD, et al. Abnormal small heat shock protein interactions involving neuropathy-associated HSP22 (HSPB8) mutants. *FASEB J.* 2006;20(12):2168–2170.
156. Tedesco B, Vendredy L, Adriaenssens E, et al. HSPB8 frameshift mutant aggregates weaken chaperone-assisted selective autophagy in neuromyopathies. *Autophagy.* 2023;19(8):2217–2239.
157. Jordanova A, Thomas FP, Guergueltcheva V, et al. Dominant intermediate Charcot-Marie-Tooth type C maps to chromosome 1p34-p35. *Am J Hum Genet.* 2003;73(6):1423–1430.
158. Jordanova A, Irobi J, Thomas FP, et al. Disrupted function and axonal distribution of mutant tyrosyl-tRNA synthetase in dominant intermediate Charcot-Marie-Tooth neuropathy. *Nat Genet.* 2006;38:197–202.
159. Hyun YS, Park H, Heo S-H. Rare variants in methionyl- and tyrosyl-tRNA synthetase genes in late-onset autosomal dominant Charcot-Marie-Tooth neuropathy. *Clin Genet.* 2014;86: 592–594.
160. Soong BW, Huang YH, Tsai PC, et al. Exome sequencing identifies GNB4 mutations as a cause of dominant intermediate Charcot-Marie-Tooth disease. *Am J Hum Genet.* 2013;92(3):422–430.
161. Kwon HM, Kim HS, Kim SB, et al. Clinical and neuroimaging features in Charcot-Marie-Tooth patients with *GNB4* mutations. *Life (Basel).* 2021;11(6):494.
162. McLaughlin HM, Sakaguchi R, Liu C, et al. Compound heterozygosity for loss-of-function lysyl-tRNA synthetase mutations in a patient with peripheral neuropathy. *Am J Hum Genet.* 2010;87(4):560–566.
163. Azzedine H, Zavadakova P, Plante-Bordeneuve V, et al. PLEKHG5 deficiency leads to an intermediate form of autosomal-recessive Charcot-Marie-Tooth disease. *Hum Molec Genet.* 2013;22:4224–4232.
164. Kim HJ, Hong YB, Park JM, et al. Mutations in the PLEKHG5 gene is relevant with autosomal recessive intermediate Charcot-Marie-Tooth disease. *Orphanet J Rare Dis.* 2013;8:104.

165. Maystadt I, Rezsohazy R, Barkats M, et al. The nuclear factor kappa-beta-activator gene PLEKHG5 is mutated in a form of autosomal recessive lower motor neuron disease with childhood onset. *Am J Hum Genet.* 2007;81:67–76.
166. Tamiya G, Makino S, Hayashi M, et al. A mutation of COX6A1 causes a recessive axonal or mixed form of Charcot-Marie-Tooth disease. *Am J Hum Genet.* 2014;95(3):294–300.
167. Laššuthová P, Beharka R, Krůtová M, Neupauerová J, Seeman P. COX6A1 mutation causes axonal hereditary motor and sensory neuropathy - the confirmation of the primary report. *Clin Genet.* 2016;89(4):512–514.
168. Déjérine J, Sottas J. Sur la névrite: Interstitielle, hypertrophique et progressive de l'enfance. *CR Soc Biol (France).* 1893;45:63–96.
169. Harding AE, Thomas PK. Autosomal recessive forms of hereditary motor and sensory neuropathy. *J Neurol Neurosurg Psychiatry.* 1980;43:669–678.
170. Hilz MJ, Stemper B, Axelrod FB. Sympathetic skin response differentiates hereditary sensory autonomic neuropathies III and IV. *Neurology.* 1999;52:1652–1657.
171. Roa BB, Dyck PJ, Marks HG, Chance PF, Lupski JR. Dejerine-Sottas syndrome associated with point mutation in the peripheral myelin protein 22 (PMP22) gene. *Nat Genet.* 1993;5:269–273.
172. Timmerman V, De Jonghe P, Ceuterick C, et al. Novel missense mutation in the early growth response 2 gene associated with Dejerine–Sottas syndrome phenotype. *Neurology.* 1999;52:1827–1832.
173. Dyck PJ, Lambert EH, Sanders K, O'Brien PC. Severe hypomyelination and marked abnormality of conduction in Dejerine-Sottas hypertrophic neuropathy: myelin thickness and compound action potential of sural nerve in vitro. *Mayo Clin Proc.* 1971;46:432–436.
174. Guzzetta F, Ferriere G, Lyon G. Congenital hypomyelination polyneuropathy: pathological findings compared with polyneuropathies starting later in life. *Brain.* 1982;105:395–416.
175. Gabreëls-Festen AAWM, Gabreëls FJM, Jennekens FGI, Janssen-van Kempen TW. The status of HMSN type III. *Neuromuscul Disord.* 1994;4:63–69.
176. Andermann F, Lloyd-Smith DL, Mavor H, Mathieson G. Observations on hypertrophic neuropathy of Dejerine and Sottas. *Neurology.* 1962;12:712–724.
177. Joostens E, Gabreëls F, Gabreëls-Festen A, Vrensen G, Korten J, Notermans S. Electron microscopic heterogeneity of onionbulb neuropathies of the Dejerine–Sottas type. *Acta Neuropathol.* 1974;27:105–118.
178. Kennedy WR, Shung JH, Berry JF. A case of congenital hypomyelination neuropathy. *Arch Neurol.* 1977;34:337–345.
179. Harati Y, Butler IJ. Congenital hypomyelinating neuropathy. *J Neurol Neurosurg Psychiatry.* 1985;48:1269–1276.
180. Dyck PJ, Gomez MR. Segmental demyelination in Dejerine–Sottas disease: light, phase-contrast, and electron microscopic studies. *Mayo Clin Proc.* 1968;43:280–296.
181. Dyck PJ, Ellefson RD, Lais AC, Smith RC, Taylor WF, Van Dyke RA. Histologic and lipid studies of sural nerves in inherited hypertrophic neuropathy: preliminary report of a lipid abnormality in nerve and liver in Dejerine–Sottas disease. *Mayo Clin Proc.* 1970;45:286–327.
182. Towfighi J. Congenital hypomyelination neuropathy: glial bundles in cranial and spinal nerve roots. *Ann Neurol.* 1981;10:570–573.
183. Ionasescu V, Searby C, Ionasescu R, Chatkupt S, Patel N, Koenigsberger R. Dejerine–Sottas neuropathy in mother and son with the same point mutation of PMP22 gene. *Muscle Nerve.* 1997;20:97–99.
184. Nicholson G, Ouvrier R. GDAP1 mutations in CMT4: axonal and demyelinating phenotypes? The exception "proves the rule". *Neurology.* 2002;59(12):1835–1836.
185. Ben Othame K, Hentani F, Lennon F, et al. Linkage of a locus (CMT4 A) for autosomal recessive Charcot–Marie–Tooth disease to chromosome 8q. *Hum Mol Genet.* 1993;2:1625–1628.
186. Stojkovic T, Latour P, Viet G, et al. Vocal cord and diaphragm paralysis, as clinical features of a French family with autosomal recessive Charcot-Marie-Tooth disease, associated with a new mutation in the GDAP1 gene. *Neuromuscul Disord.* 2004;14(4):261–264.
187. Ammar N, Nelis E, Merlini L, et al. Identification of novel GDAP1 mutations causing autosomal recessive Charcot–Marie–Tooth disease. *Neuromuscul Disord.* 2003;13(9):720–728.
188. Sevilla T, Cuesta A, Chumillas MJ, et al. Clinical, electrophysiological and morphological findings of Charcot–Marie–Tooth neuropathy with vocal cord palsy and mutations in the GDAP1 gene. *Brain.* 2003;126(Pt 9):2023–2033.
189. Birouk N, Azzedine H, Dubourg O, et al. Phenotypical features of a Moroccan family with autosomal recessive Charcot-Marie-Tooth disease associated with the S194X mutation in the GDAP1 gene. *Arch Neurol.* 2003;60(4):598–604.
190. Boerkoel CF, Takashima H, Nakagawa M, et al. CMT4 A: identification of a Hispanic GDAP1 founder mutation. *Ann Neurol.* 2003;53(3):400–405.
191. Senderek J, Bergmann C, Ramaekers VT, et al. Mutations in the ganglioside-induced differentiation-associated protein-1 (GDAP1) gene in intermediate type autosomal recessive Charcot–Marie–Tooth neuropathy. *Brain.* 2003;126(Pt 3):642–649.
192. Nelis E, Erdem S, Van Den Bergh PY, et al. Mutations in GDAP1: autosomal recessive CMT with demyelination and axonopathy. *Neurology.* 2002;59(12):1865–1872.
193. Cuesta A, Pedrola L, Sevilla T, et al. The gene encoding ganglioside-induced differentiation-associated protein-1 is mutated in Charcot–Marie–Tooth type 4 A disease. *Nat Genet.* 2002;1:22–25.
194. Sander SA, Ouvrier RA, McLeod JG, Nicholson GA, Pollard JS. Clinical syndromes associated with tomacula or myelin swellings in sural nerve biopsies. *J Neurol Neurosurg Psychiatry.* 2000;68:483–488.
195. Nelis E, Erdem S, Tan E, et al. A novel homozygous missense mutation in the myotubularin-related protein 2 gene associated with recessive Charcot–Marie–Tooth disease with irregularly folded myelin sheaths. *Neuromuscul Disord.* 2002;12(9):869–873.
196. Pareyson D, Stojkovic T, Reilly MM, et al. A multicenter retrospective study of Charcot-Marie-Tooth disease type 4B (CMT4B) associated with mutations in myotubularin-related proteins (MTMRs). *Ann Neurol.* 2019;86(1):55–67.
197. Azzedine H, Bolino A, Taïeb T, et al. Mutations in MTMR13, a new pseudophosphatase homologue of MTMR2 and Sbf1, in two families with an autosomal recessive demyelinating form of Charcot-Marie-Tooth disease associated with early-onset glaucoma. *Am J Hum Genet.* 2003;72(5):1141–1153.
198. Senderek J, Bergmann C, Weber S, et al. Mutation of the SBF2 gene, encoding a novel member of the myotubularin family, in Charcot–Marie–Tooth neuropathy type 4 B2/11p15. *Hum Mol Genet.* 2003;12(3):349–356.
199. Nakhro K, Park JM, Hong YB, et al. SET binding factor 1 (SBF1) mutation causes Charcot-Marie-Tooth disease type 4B3. *Neurology.* 2013;81(2):165–173.

200. Alazami AM, Alzahrani F, Bohlega S, Alkuraya FS. SET binding factor 1 (SBF1) mutation causes Charcot-Marie-tooth disease type 4B3. *Neurology*. 2014;82:1665–1666.
201. Kessali M, Zemmouri R, Guilbot A, et al. A clinical, electrophysiologic, neuropathologic, and genetic study of two large Algerian families with an autosomal recessive demyelinating form of Charcot-Marie-Tooth disease. *Neurology*. 1997;48(4):867–873.
202. Gabreëls-Festen A, van Beersum S, Eshuis L, et al. Study on the gene and phenotypic characterisation of autosomal recessive demyelinating motor and sensory neuropathy (Charcot-Marie-Tooth disease) with a gene locus on chromosome 5q23-q33. *J Neurol Neurosurg Psychiatry*. 1999;66:569–574.
203. Senderek J, Bergmann C, Stendel C, et al. Mutations in a gene encoding a novel SH3/TPR domain protein cause autosomal recessive Charcot-Marie-Tooth type 4 C neuropathy. *Am J Hum Genet*. 2003;73:1106–1119.
204. Varley TL, Bourque PR, Baker SK. Phenotypic variability of CMT4C in a French-Canadian kindred. *Muscle Nerve*. 2015;52(3):444–449.
205. Jerath NU, Mankodi A, Crawford TO, et al. Charcot-Marie-Tooth disease type 4C: novel mutations, clinical presentations, and diagnostic challenges. *Muscle Nerve*. 2018;57(5):749–755.
206. Kalaydjieva L, Gresham D, Gooding R, et al. N-myc downstream-regulated gene 1 is mutated in hereditary motor and sensory neuropathy—Lom. *Am J Hum Genet*. 2000;67:47–58.
207. Ishpekova BA, Christova LG, Alexandrov AS, Thomas PK. The electrophysiological profile of hereditary motor and sensory neuropathy—Lom. *J Neurol Neurosurg Psychiatry*. 2005;76(6):875–878.
208. Echaniz-Laguna A, Degos B, Bonnet C, et al. NDRG1-linked Charcot–Marie–Tooth disease (CMT4D) with central nervous system involvement. *Neuromuscul Disord*. 2007;17(2):163–168.
209. Pravinbabu P, Holla VV, Phulpagar P, et al. A splice altering variant in NDRG1 gene causes Charcot-Marie-Tooth disease, type 4D. *Neurol Sci*. 2022;43(7):4463–4472.
210. Timmerman V, De Jonghe P, Ceuterick C, et al. Novel missense mutation in the early growth response 2 gene associated with Dejerine-Sottas syndrome phenotype. *Neurology*. 1999;52(9):1827–1832.
211. Boerkoel CF, Takashima H, Stankiewicz P, et al. Periaxin mutations cause recessive Dejerine–Sottas neuropathy. *Am J Hum Genet*. 2001;68:325–333.
212. Delague V, Bariel C, Tuffery S, et al. Mapping of a new locus for autosomal recessive demyelinating Charcot–Marie–Tooth disease to 19q13.1–13.3 in a large consanguineous Lebanese family: exclusion of MAG as a candidate gene. *Am J Hum Genet*. 2000;67:236–243.
213. Kabzinska D, Drac H, Sherman DL, et al. Charcot–Marie–Tooth type 4 F disease caused by S399fsx410 mutation in the PRX gene. *Neurology*. 2006;66(5):745–747.
214. Takashima H, Boerkoel CF, De Jonghe P, et al. Periaxin mutations cause a broad spectrum of demyelinating neuropathies. *Ann Neurol*. 2002;51(6):709–715.
215. Tokunaga S, Hashiguchi A, Yoshimura A, et al. Late-onset Charcot-Marie-Tooth disease 4F caused by periaxin gene mutation. *Neurogenetics*. 2012;13(4):359–365.
216. Thomas PK, Kalaydjieva L, Youl B, et al. Hereditary motor and sensory neuropathy-Russe: new autosomal recessive neuropathy in Balkan Gypsies. *Ann Neurol*. 2001;50:452–457.
217. Sevilla T, Martinez-Rubio D, Marquez C, et al. Genetics of the Charcot-Marie-Tooth disease in the Spanish Gypsy population: the hereditary motor and sensory neuropathy-Russe in depth. *Clin Genet*. 2013;83:565–570.
218. Delague V, Jacquier A, Hamadouche T, et al. Mutations in FGD4 encoding the Rho GDP/GTP exchange factor FRABIN cause autosomal recessive Charcot-Marie-Tooth type 4 H. *Am J Hum Genet*. 2007;81(1):1–16.
219. Stendel C, Roos A, Deconinck T, et al. Peripheral nerve demyelination caused by a mutant Rho GTPase guanine nucleotide exchange factor, frabin/FGD4. *Am J Hum Genet*. 2007;81(1):158–164.
220. El-Bazzal L, Ghata A, Estève C, et al. Imbalance of NRG1-ERBB2/3 signalling underlies altered myelination in Charcot-Marie-Tooth disease 4H. *Brain*. 2023;146(5):1844–1858.
221. Chow CY, Zhang Y, Dowling JJ, et al. Mutation of FIG4 causes neurodegeneration in the pale tremor mouse and patients with CMT4 J. *Nature*. 2007;448:68–72.
222. Zhang X, Chow CY, Sahenk Z, Shy ME, Meisler MH, Li J. Mutation of FIG4 causes a rapidly progressive, asymmetric neuronal degeneration. *Brain*. 2008;131:1990–2001.
223. Lenk GM, Ferguson CJ, Chow CY, et al. Pathogenic mechanism of the FIG4 mutation responsible for Charcot-Marie-Tooth disease CMT4 J. *PLoS Genet*. 2011;7:e1002104.
224. Hu B, McCollum M, Ravi V, et al. Myelin abnormality in Charcot-Marie-Tooth type 4J recapitulates features of acquired demyelination. *Ann Neurol*. 2018;83(4):756–770.
225. Echaniz-Laguna A, Ghezzi D, Chassagne M, et al. SURF1 deficiency causes demyelinating Charcot-Marie-Tooth disease. *Neurology*. 2013;81(17):1523–1530.
226. Shintaku M, Maeda K, Shiohara M, Namura T, Kushima R. Neuropathology of the spinal nerve roots, spinal cord, and brain in the first autopsied case of Charcot-Marie-Tooth disease 4F with a D651N mutation in the periaxin gene. *Neuropathology*. 2021;41(4):281–287.
227. Baxter RV, Ben Othmane K, Rochelle JM, et al. Ganglioside-induced differentiation-associated protein-1 is mutant in Charcot–Marie–Tooth disease type 4 A/8q21. *Nat Genet*. 2002;1:21–22.
228. Nakagawa M, Suehara M, Saito A, et al. A novel MPZ gene mutation in dominantly inherited neuropathy with focally folded myelin sheaths. *Neurology*. 1999;52:1271–1275.
229. Berger P, Bonneick S, Willi S, Wymann M, Suter U. Loss of phosphatase activity in myotubularin-related protein 2 is associated with Charcot–Marie–Tooth disease type 4B1. *Hum Mol Genet*. 2002;11(13):1569–1579.
230. Chojnowski A, Ravise N, Bachelin C, et al. Silencing of the Charcot–Marie–Tooth associated MTMR2 gene decreases proliferation and enhances cell death in primary cultures of Schwann cells. *Neurobiol Dis*. 2007;26:323–331.
231. Bolino A, Muglia M, Conforti FL, et al. Charcot-Marie-Tooth type 4B is caused by mutations in the gene encoding myotubularin-related protein-2. *Nat Genet*. 2000;25:17–19.
232. Gutierrez A, England JD, Sumner AJ, et al. Unusual electrophysiological findings in X-linked dominant Charcot–Marie–Tooth disease. *Muscle Nerve*. 2000;23:182–188.
233. Hahn AF, Brown WF, Koopman WJ, Feasby TE. X-linked dominant hereditary motor and sensory neuropathy. *Brain*. 1990;113:1511–1525.
234. Lewis RA. The challenge of CMTX and connexin 32 mutations. *Muscle Nerve*. 2000;23:147–149.
235. Nicholson G, Nash J. Intermediate nerve conduction velocities define X-linked Charcot–Marie–Tooth neuropathy families. *Neurology*. 1993;43:2555–2564.

236. Shy ME, Siskind C, Swan ER, et al. CMT1X phenotypes represent loss of GJB1 gene function. *Neurology*. 2007;68(11):849–855.
237. Panosyan FB, Laura M, Rossor AM, et al. Cross-sectional analysis of a large cohort with X-linked Charcot-Marie-Tooth disease (CMTX1). *Neurology*. 2017;89(9):927–935.
238. Record CJ, Skorupinska M, Laura M, et al. Genetic analysis and natural history of Charcot-Marie-Tooth disease CMTX1 due to GJB1 variants. *Brain*. 2023:awad187.
239. Hanemann CO, Bergmann C, Senderek J, Zerres K, Sperfeld AD. Transient, recurrent, white matter lesions in X-linked Charcot–Marie–Tooth disease with novel connexin 32 mutation. *Arch Neurol*. 2003;60(4):605–609.
240. Schelhaas HJ, Van Engelen BG, Gabreels-Festen AA, et al. Transient cerebral white matter lesions in a patient with connexin 32 missense mutation. *Neurology*. 2002;59(12):2007–2008.
241. Paulson HL, Garbern JY, Hoban TF, et al. Transient central nervous system white matter abnormality in X-linked Charcot–Marie–Tooth disease. *Ann Neurol*. 2002;52(4):429–434.
242. Birouk N, LeGuern E, Maisonobe T, et al. X-linked mutations Charcot–Marie–Tooth disease with connexin-32 mutations: Clinical and electrophysiological study. *Neurology*. 1998;50:1074–1082.
243. Nicholson G, Yeung L, Corbett A. Efficient neurophysiologic selection of X-linked Charcot–Marie–Tooth families. Ten novel mutations. *Neurology*. 1998;51:1412–1416.
244. Tabaraud F, LaGrange E, Sindou P, Vandenberghe A, Levy N, Vallat JM. Demyelinating X-linked Charcot–Marie–Tooth disease: unusual electrophysiological findings. *Muscle Nerve*. 1999;22:1442–1447.
245. Dubourg O, Tardieu S, Birouk N, et al. Clinical, electrophysiological and molecular genetic characteristics of 93 patients with X-linked Charcot–Marie–Tooth disease. *Brain*. 2001;124:1958–1967.
246. Bergoffen J, Scherer SS, Wang S, et al. Connexin mutations in X-linked Charcot–Marie–Tooth disease. *Am J Hum Genet*. 1993;262:2039–2042.
247. Fairweather N, Bell C, Cochrane S, et al. Mutation in the connexin 32 gene in X-linked dominant Charcot–Marie–Tooth neuropathy. *Hum Mol Genet*. 1994;3:355–358.
248. Ionasescu V, Searby C, Ionasescu R. Point mutations of connexin 32 (GJB1) gene in X-linked dominant Charcot–Marie–Tooth neuropathy. *Hum Mol Genet*. 1994;3:355–358.
249. Cowchock FS, Duckett SW, Streletz LJ, Graziani LJ, Jackson LG. X-linked motor-sensory neuropathy type-II with deafness and mental retardation: a new disorder. *Am J Med Genet*. 1985;20:307–315.
250. Priest JM, Fischbeck KH, Nouri N, Keats BJ. A locus for axonal motor-sensory neuropathy with deafness and mental retardation maps to Xq24-q26. *Genomics*. 1995;29:409–412.
251. Ardissone A, Piscosquito G, Legati A, et al. A slowly progressive mitochondrial encephalomyopathy widens the spectrum of AIFM1 disorders. *Neurology*. 2015;84: 2193–2195.
252. Bogdanova-Mihaylova P, Alexander MD, Murphy RP, et al. Clinical spectrum of AIFM1-associated disease in an Irish family, from mild neuropathy to severe cerebellar ataxia with colour blindness. *J Peripher Nerv Syst*. 2019;24: 348–353.
253. Rinaldi C, Grunseich C, Sevrioukova IF, et al. Cowchock syndrome is associated with a mutation in apoptosis-inducing factor. *Am J Hum Genet*. 2012;91:1095–1102, 2012.
254. Kim H-J, Sohn K-M, Shy ME, et al. Mutations in PRPS1, which encodes the phosphoribosyl pyrophosphate synthetase enzyme critical for nucleotide biosynthesis, cause hereditary peripheral neuropathy with hearing loss and optic neuropathy (CMT5X). *Am J Hum Genet*. 2007;81:552–558.
255. Synofzik M, Muller vom Hagen J, Haack TB, et al. X-linked Charcot-Marie-Tooth disease, Arts syndrome, and prelingual non-syndromic deafness form a disease continuum: evidence from a family with a novel PRPS1 mutation. *Orphanet J Rare Dis*. 2014;9:24.
256. Almoguera B, He S, Corton M, et al. Expanding the phenotype of PRPS1 syndromes in females: neuropathy, hearing loss and retinopathy. *Orphanet J Rare Dis*. 2014;9:190.
257. Robusto M, Fang M, Asselta R, et al. The expanding spectrum of PRPS1-associated phenotypes: three novel mutations segregating with X-linked hearing loss and mild peripheral neuropathy. *Europ J Hum Genet*. 2015;23:766–773.
258. Kennerson ML, Yiu EM, Chuang DT, et al. A new locus for X-linked dominant Charcot-Marie-Tooth disease (CMTX6) is caused by mutations in the pyruvate dehydrogenase kinase isoenzyme 3 (PDK3) gene. *Hum Mol Genet*. 2013;22(7):1404–1416.
259. Kennerson ML, Kim EJ, Siddell A, et al. X-linked Charcot-Marie-Tooth disease type 6 (CMTX6) patients with a p.R158H mutation in the pyruvate dehydrogenase kinase isoenzyme 3 gene. *J Peripher Nerv Syst*. 2016;21(1):45–51.
260. Takashima H, Nakagawa M, Nakahara K, et al. A new type of hereditary motor and sensory neuropathy linked to chromosome 3. *Ann Neurol*. 1997;41:771–780.
261. Ishiura H, Sako W, Yoshida M, et al. The TRK-fused gene is mutated in hereditary motor and sensory neuropathy with proximal dominant involvement. *Am J Hum Genet*. 2012; 91:320–329.
262. Lee SS, Lee HJ, Park JM, Hong YB. Proximal dominant hereditary motor and sensory neuropathy with proximal dominance association with mutation in the TRK-fused gene. *JAMA Neurol*. 2013;70(5):607–615.
263. Khani M, Shamshiri H, Alavi A, Nafissi S, Elahi E. Identification of novel TFG mutation in HMSN-P pedigree: emphasis on variable clinical presentations. *J Neurol Sci*. 2016; 369:318–323.
264. Fujisaki N, Suwazono S, Suehara M, et al. The natural history of hereditary motor and sensory neuropathy with proximal dominant involvement (HMSN-P) in 97 Japanese patients. *Intractable Rare Dis Res*. 2018;7(1):7–12.
265. Chance PF, Lensch MW, Lipe H, Brown RH Sr, Brown RH Jr, Bird TD. Hereditary neuralgic amyotrophy and hereditary neuropathy with liability to pressure palsies: two distinct genetic disorders. *Neurology*. 1994;44:2253–2257.
266. van Alfen N, van Engelen BG. The clinical spectrum of neuralgic amyotrophy in 246 cases. *Brain*. 2006;129(Pt 2):438–450.
267. Ueda M, Kawamura N, Tateishi T, et al. Phenotypic spectrum of hereditary neuralgic amyotrophy caused by the SEPT9 R88W mutation. *J Neurol Neurosurg Psychiatry*. 2010;81(1):94–96.
268. Kuhlenbaumer G, Hannibal MC, Nelis E, et al. Mutations in SEPT9 cause hereditary neuralgic amyotrophy. *Nat Genet*. 2005;37:1044–1046.
269. Davidenkow S. Scapuloperoneal amyotrophy. *Arch Neurol*. 1939;41:694.
270. Emery ES, Fenichel GM, Eng G. A spinal muscular atrophy with scapuloperoneal distribution. *Arch Neurol*. 1968;18:129–133.
271. Ricker K, Mertens HG, Schimrig K. The neurogenic scapuloperoneal syndrome. *Eur Neurol*. 1968;1:257–274.
272. Mercelis R, Demeester J, Martin JJ. Neurogenic scapuloperoneal syndrome in childhood. *J Neurol Neurosurg Psychiatry*. 1980;43:888–896.

273. Harding AE, Thomas PK. Distal and scapuloperoneal distribution of muscle involvement occurring within a family with type 1 hereditary motor and sensory neuropathy. *J Neurol.* 1980;224:17-23.
274. Hyser CL, Kissel JT, Warmolts JR, Mendell JR. Scapuloperoneal neuropathy: a distinct clinicopathologic entity. *J Neurol Sci.* 1988;87:91-102.
275. Tandan R, Verma A, Mohire M. Adult onset autosomal recessive neurogenic scapuloperoneal syndrome. *J Neurol Sci.* 1989;94:201-209.
276. Cortese A, Zhu Y, Rebelo AP, et al. Biallelic mutations in SORD cause a common and potentially treatable hereditary neuropathy with implications for diabetes [published correction appears in *Nat Genet.* 2020;52(6):640] *Nat Genet.* 2020;52:473-481.
277. Liu X, He J, Yilihamu M, Duan X, Fan D. Clinical and genetic features of biallelic mutations in *SORD* in a series of Chinese patients with Charcot-Marie-Tooth and distal hereditary motor neuropathy. *Front Neurol.* 2021;12:733926.
278. Pons N, Fernández-Eulate G, Pegat A, et al. SORD-related peripheral neuropathy in a French and Swiss cohort: clinical features, genetic analyses, and sorbitol dosages. *Eur J Neurol.* 2023;30(7):2001-2011.
279. Zhao H, Race V, Matthijs G, et al. Exome sequencing reveals HINT1 mutations as a cause of distal hereditary motor neuropathy. *Eur J Hum Genet.* 2014;22(6):847-850.
280. Zimoń M, Baets J, Almeida-Souza L, et al. Loss-of-function mutations in HINT1 cause axonal neuropathy with neuromyotonia. *Nat Genet.* 2012;44(10):1080-1083.
281. Peeters K, Chamova T, Tournev I, Jordanova A. Axonal neuropathy with neuromyotonia: there is a HINT. *Brain.* 2017;140(4):868-877.
282. Morel V, Campana-Salort E, Boyer A. HINT1 neuropathy: expanding the genotype and phenotype spectrum. *Clin Genet.* 2022;102(5):379-390.
283. Palma JA, Yadav R, Gao D, Norcliffe-Kaufmann L, Slaugenhaupt S, Kaufmann H. Expanding the genotypic spectrum of congenital sensory and autonomic neuropathies using whole-exome sequencing. *Neurol Genet.* 2021;7(2):e568.
284. Houlden H, King RH, Muddle JR, et al. A novel RAB7 mutation associated with ulcero-mutilating neuropathy. *Ann Neurol.* 2004;56(4):586-590.
285. Yuan JH, Higuchi Y, Ando M, et al. Multi-type RFC1 repeat expansions as the most common cause of hereditary sensory and autonomic neuropathy. *Front Neurol.* 2022;13:986504.
286. Beijer D, Dohrn MF, De Winter J, et al. RFC1 repeat expansions: a recurrent cause of sensory and autonomic neuropathy with cough and ataxia. *Eur J Neurol.* 2022;29(7):2156-2161.
287. Davidson G, Murphy S, Polke J, et al. Frequency of mutations in the genes associated with hereditary sensory and autonomic neuropathy in a UK cohort. *J Neurol.* 2012;259(8):1673-1685.
288. Rotthier A, Baets J, De Vriendt E, et al. Genes for hereditary sensory and autonomic neuropathies: a genotype-phenotype correlation. *Brain.* 2009;132(Pt 10):2699-2711.
289. Denny-Brown D. Hereditary sensory radicular neuropathy. *J Neurol Neurosurg Psychiatry.* 1951;14:237-252.
290. Houlden H, King R, Blake J, et al. Clinical, pathological and genetic characterization of hereditary sensory and autonomic neuropathy type 1 (HSAN I). *Brain.* 2006;129(Pt 2):411-425.
291. Shivji ZM, Ashby P. Sympathetic skin responses in hereditary sensory and autonomic neuropathy and familial amyloid neuropathy are different. *Muscle Nerve.* 1999;22:1283-1286.
292. Bejaoui K, McKenna-Yasek D, Hosler BA, et al. Confirmation of linkage of type 1 hereditary sensory neuropathy to human chromosome 9q22. *Neurology.* 1999;52:510-515.
293. Bejaoui K, Wu C, Scheffler MD, et al. SPTLC1 is mutated in hereditary sensory neuropathy, type 1. *Nat Genet.* 2001;27:261-262.
294. Dawkins JL, Hulme DJ, Brambhatt SB, Auer-Grumbach M, Nicholson GA. Mutations in SPTLC1, encoding serine palmitoyl transferase long chain base subunit-1, cause hereditary sensory neuropathy type 1. *Nat Genet.* 2001;27:309-312.
295. Rotthier A, Auer-Grumbach M, Janssens K, et al. Mutations in the SPTLC2 subunit of serine palmitoyltransferase cause hereditary sensory and autonomic neuropathy type I. *Am J Hum Genet.* 2010;87:513-522.
296. Murphy SM, Ernst D, Wei Y, et al. Hereditary sensory and autonomic neuropathy type 1 (HSANI) caused by a novel mutation in SPTLC2. *Neurology.* 2013;80(23):2106-2011.
297. Kok C, Kennerson ML, Spring PJ, Ing AJ, Pollard JD, Nicholson GA. A locus for hereditary sensory neuropathy with cough and gastroesophageal reflux on chromosome 3p22-p24. *Am J Hum Genet.* 2003;73(3):632-637.
298. Guelly C, Zhu P-P, Leonardis L, et al. Targeted high throughput sequencing identifies mutations in atlastin-1 as a cause of hereditary sensory neuropathy type I. *Am J Hum Genet.* 2011;88:99-105.
299. Wright A, Dyck PJ. Hereditary sensory neuropathy with sensorineural deafness and early-onset dementia. *Neurology.* 1995;45:560-562.
300. Klein CJ, Botuyan MV, Wu Y, et al. Mutations in DNMT1 cause hereditary sensory neuropathy with dementia and hearing loss. *Nat Genet.* 2011;43:595-600.
301. Klein CJ, Bird T, Ertekin-Taner N, et al. DNMT1 mutation hot spot causes varied phenotypes of HSAN1 with dementia and hearing loss. *Neurology.* 2013;80(9):824-828.
302. Catania A, Peverelli L, Tabano S, Ghezzi D, Lamperti C. DNMT1-complex disorder caused by a novel mutation associated with an overlapping phenotype of autosomal-dominant cerebellar ataxia, deafness, and narcolepsy (ADCA-DN) and hereditary sensory neuropathy with dementia and hearing loss (HSN1E). *Neurol Sci.* 2019;40(9):1963-1966.
303. Kornak U, Mademan I, Schinke M, et al. Sensory neuropathy with bone destruction due to a mutation in the membrane-shaping atlastin GTPase 3. *Brain.* 2014;137(Pt 3):683-692.
304. Behrendt L, Hoischen C, Kaether C. Disease-causing mutated ATLASTIN 3 is excluded from distal axons and reduces axonal autophagy. *Neurobiol Dis.* 2021;155:105400.
305. Nukada H, Pollock M, Haas LF. The clinical spectrum and morphology of type II hereditary sensory neuropathy. *Brain.* 1982;105:647-665.
306. Schoene WC, Asbury AK, Astrom KE, et al. Hereditary sensory neuropathy. *J Neurol Sci.* 1970;11:463-487.
307. Winkelmann RK, Lambert EH, Hayles AB. Congenital absence of pain. *Arch Dermatol.* 1962;85:325-338.
308. Loggia ML, Bushnell MC, Tétreault M, et al. Carriers of recessive WNK1/HSN2 mutations for hereditary sensory and autonomic neuropathy type 2 (HSAN2) are more sensitive to thermal stimuli. *J Neurosci.* 2009;29:2162-2166.
309. Ohta M, Ellefson RD, Lambert EH, et al. Hereditary sensory neuropathy, Type II. *Arch Neurol.* 1973;29:23-37.
310. Lafreniere RG, MacDonald ML, Dube MP, et al. Study of Canadian Genetic Isolates. Identification of a novel gene (HSN2) causing hereditary sensory and autonomic neuropathy type II through the Study of Canadian genetic isolates. *Am J Hum Genet.* 2004;74(5):1064-1073.

311. Pleiner T, Hazu M, Tomaleri GP, et al. WNK1 is an assembly factor for the human ER membrane protein complex. *Mol Cell.* 2021;81(13):2693–2704.
312. Kurth I, Pamminger T, Hennings JC, et al. Mutations in FAM134B, encoding a newly identified Golgi protein, cause severe sensory and autonomic neuropathy. *Nat Genet.* 2009; 41:1179–1181.
313. Ilgaz Aydinlar E, Rolfs A, Serteser M, Parman Y. Mutation in FAM134B causing hereditary sensory neuropathy with spasticity in a Turkish family. *Muscle Nerve.* 2014;49(5):774–775.
314. Rivière JB, Verlaan DJ, Shekarabi M, et al. A mutation in the HSN2 gene causes sensory neuropathy type II in a Lebanese family. *Ann Neurol.* 2004;56:572–575.
315. Kanamori A, Hinaga S, Hirata Y, Amaya F, Oh-Hashi K. Molecular characterization of wild-type and HSAN2B-linked FAM134B. *Mol Biol Rep.* 2023;50(7):6005–6017.
316. Riviere J-B, Ramalingam S, Lavastre V, et al. KIF1 A, an axonal transporter of synaptic vesicles, is mutated in hereditary sensory and autonomic neuropathy type 2. *Am J Hum Genet.* 2011;89:219–230.
317. Shekarabi M, Girard N, Rivière JB, et al. Mutations in the nervous system—Specific HSN2 exon of WNK1 cause hereditary sensory neuropathy type II. *J Clin Invest.* 2008;118:2496–2505.
318. Yuan J, Matsuura E, Higuchi Y, et al. Hereditary sensory and autonomic neuropathy type IID caused by an SCN9 A mutation. *Neurology.* 2013;80:1641–1649.
319. Bennett DL, Woods CG. Painful and painless channelopathies. *Lancet Neurol.* 2014;13(6):587–599.
320. Aguayo AJ, Nair CPV, Bray GM. Peripheral nerve abnormalities in the Riley–Day syndrome. *Arch Neurol.* 1971;24:106–116.
321. Brown JC. Nerve conduction in familial dysautonomia (Riley–Day syndrome). *J Am Med Assoc.* 1967;201:200–202.
322. Brown WJ, Beauchemin JA, Linde LM. A neuropathological study of familial dysautonomia (Riley–Day syndrome) in siblings. *J Neurol Neurosurg Psychiatry.* 1964;27:131–139.
323. Blumenfeld A, Slaugenhaupt SA, Liebert CB, et al. Precise genetic mapping and haplotype analysis of familial dysautonomia gene on human chromosome 9q31. *Am J Hum Genet.* 1999;64:1110–1118.
324. Edvardson S, Cinnamon Y, Jalas C, et al. Hereditary sensory autonomic neuropathy caused by a mutation in dystonin. *Ann Neurol.* 2012;71(4):569–572.
325. Anderson SL, Coli R, Daly IW, et al. Familial dysautonomia is caused by mutations of the IKAP gene. *Am J Hum Genet.* 2001;68:753–758.
326. Eng CM, Slaugenhaupt SA, Blumenfeld A, Axelrod FB, Gusella JF, Desnick RJ. Prenatal diagnosis of familial dysautonomia by analysis of linked CA-repeat polymorphisms on chromosome 9q31-33. *Am J Med Genet.* 1995;59:349–355.
327. Slaugenhaupt SA, Blumenfeld A, Gil SP, et al. Tissue-specific expression of a splicing mutation in the IKBKAP gene causes familial dysautonomia. *Am J Hum Genet.* 2001;68:598–605.
328. Swanson AG, Buchan GC, Alvord EC. Anatomic changes in congenital insensitivity to pain: absence of small primary sensory neurons in ganglia, roots, and Lissauer's tract. *Arch Neurol.* 1965;12:12–19.
329. Shorer Z, Moses SW, Hershkovitz E, Pinsk V, Levy J. Neurophysiologic studies in congenital insensitivity to pain with anhidrosis. *Pediatr Neurol.* 2001;25(5):397–400.
330. Goebel HH, Veit S, Dyck PJ. Confirmation of virtual unmyelinated fiber absence in hereditary sensory neuropathy type IV. *J Neuropathol Exp Neurol.* 1980;39:670–675.
331. Greco A, Villa R, Tubino B, Romano L, Penso D, Pierotti MA. A novel NTRK1 mutation associated with congenital insensitivity to pain with anhidrosis. *Am J Hum Genet.* 1999;64: 1207–1210.
332. Indo Y, Tsuruta M, Hayashida Y, et al. Mutations in the trkA/NGF receptor gene in patients with congenital insensitivity to pain with anhidrosis. *Nat Genet.* 1996;13:485–488.
333. Indo Y. Molecular basis of congenital insensitivity to pain with anhidrosis (CIPA): mutations and polymorphisms in TRKA (NTRK1) gene encoding the receptor tyrosine kinase for nerve growth factor. *Hum Mutat.* 2001;18(6):462–471.
334. Landrieu P, Said G, Alaire C. Dominantly transmitted congenital indifference to pain. *Ann Neurol.* 1990;27:574–578.
335. Dyck PJ, Mellinger JF, Reagan TJ, et al. Not "indifference to pain" but varieties of hereditary sensory and autonomic neuropathy. *Brain.* 1983;106:373–390.
336. Low PA, Burke WJ, McLeod JG. Congenital sensory neuropathy with selective loss of small myelinated nerve fibers. *Ann Neurol.* 1978;3:179–182.
337. Einarsdottir E, Carlsson A, Minde J, et al. A mutation in the nerve growth factor beta gene (NGFB) causes loss of pain perception. *Hum Mol Genet.* 2004;13(8):799–805.
338. Houlden H, King RH, Hashemi-Nejad A, et al. A novel TRK A (NTRK1) mutation associated with hereditary sensory and autonomic neuropathy type V. *Ann Neurol.* 2001;49(4):521–525.
339. Edvardson S, Cinnamon Y, Jalas C, et al. Hereditary sensory autonomic neuropathy caused by a mutation in dystonin. *Ann Neurol.* 2012;71:569–572.
340. Manganelli F, Parisi S, Nolano M, et al. Novel mutations in dystonin provide clues to the pathomechanisms of HSAN-VI. *Neurology.* 2017;88:2132–2140.
341. Cappuccio G, Pinelli M, Torella A, et al. Expanding the phenotype of DST-related disorder: a case report suggesting a genotype/phenotype correlation. *Am J Med Genet A.* 2017;173:2743–2746.
342. Fortugno P, Angelucci F, Cestra G, et al. Recessive mutations in the neuronal isoforms of DST, encoding dystonin, lead to abnormal actin cytoskeleton organization and HSAN type VI. *Hum Mutat.* 2019;40:106–114.
343. Lynch-Godrei A, Kothary R. HSAN-VI: a spectrum disorder based on dystonin isoform expression. *Neurol Genet.* 2020;6(1):e389.
344. Leipold E, Liebmann L, Korenke GC, et al. A de novo gain-of-function mutation in SCN11A causes loss of pain perception. *Nature Genet.* 2013;45:1399–1404.
345. Woods CG, Babiker MOE, Horrocks I, Tolmie J, Kurth I. The phenotype of congenital insensitivity to pain due to the Nav1.9 variant pL811P. *Europ J Hum Genet.* 2015;23:561–563.
346. Salvatierra J, Diaz-Bustamante M, Meixiong J, Tierney E, Dong X, Bosmans F. A disease mutation reveals a role for Na(v)1.9 in acute itch. *J Clin Invest.* 2018;128: 5434–5447.
347. Zhang XY, Wen J, Yang W, et al. Gain-of-function mutations in SCN11A cause familial episodic pain. *Am J Hum Genet.* 2013;93:957–966.
348. Chen YC, Auer-Grumbach M, Matsukawa S, et al. Transcriptional regulator PRDM12 is essential for human pain perception. *Nat Genet.* 2015;47(7):803–808.
349. Bartesaghi L, Wang Y, Fontanet P, et al. PRDM12 is required for initiation of the nociceptive neuron lineage during neurogenesis. *Cell Rep.* 2019;26(13):3484–3492.
350. Kalgaard OM, Seem E, Kvernebo K. Erythromelalgia: a clinical study of 87 cases. *J Intern Med.* 1997;242(3):191–197.

351. Davis MD, Weenig RH, Genebriera J, Wendelschafer-Crabb G, Kennedy WR, Sandroni P. Histopathologic findings in primary erythromelalgia are nonspecific: special studies show a decrease in small nerve fiber density. *J Am Acad Dermatol.* 2006;55(3):519–522.
352. Yang Y, Wang Y, Li S, et al. Mutations in SCN9 A, encoding a sodium channel alpha subunit, in patients with primary erythermalgia. *J Med Genet.* 2004;41(3):171–174.
353. Lampert A, Dib-Hajj SD, Tyrrell L, Waxman SG. Size matters: Erythromelalgia mutation S241 T in Nav1.7 alters channel gating. *J Biol Chem.* 2006;281(47):36029–36035.
354. Michiels JJ, te Morsche RH, Jansen JB, Drenth JP. Autosomal dominant erythermalgia associated with a novel mutation in the voltage-gated sodium channel alpha subunit Nav1.7. *Arch Neurol.* 2005;62(10):1587–1590.
355. McGraw T, Kosek P. Erythromelalgia pain managed with gabapentin. *J Anesthesiol.* 1997;86(4):988–990.
356. Fertleman CR, Ferrie CD, Aicardi J, et al. Paroxysmal extreme pain disorder (previously familial rectal pain syndrome). *Neurology.* 2007;69:586–595.
357. Choi JS, Boralevi F, Brissaud O, et al. Paroxysmal extreme pain disorder: a molecular lesion of peripheral neurons. *Nat Rev Neurol.* 2011;7:51–55.
358. Kremeyer B, Lopera F, Cox JJ, et al. A gain-of-function mutation in TRPA1 causes familial episodic pain syndrome. *Neuron.* 2010;66:671–680.
359. Faber CG, Lauria G, Merkies ISJ, et al. Gain-of-function Nav1.8 mutations in painful neuropathy. *Proc Nat Acad Sci.* 2012;109:19444–19449.
360. Zhang XY, Wen J, Yang W, et al. Gain-of-function mutations in SCN11 A cause familial episodic pain. *Am J Hum Genet.* 2013;93:957–966.
361. Faber CG, Hoeijmakers JG, Ahn HS, et al. Gain of function Nav1.7 mutations in idiopathic small fiber neuropathy. *Ann Neurol.* 2012;71:26–39.
362. Persson AK, Liu S, Faber CG, Merkies IS, Black JA, Waxman SG. Neuropathy-associated Nav1.7 variant I228M impairs integrity of dorsal root ganglion neuron axons. *Ann Neurol.* 2013;73:140–145.
363. Han C, Hoeijmakers JG, Liu S, et al. Functional profiles of SCN9 A variants in dorsal root ganglion neurons and superior cervical ganglion neurons correlate with autonomic symptoms in small fibre neuropathy. *Brain.* 2012;135:2613–2628.
364. Han C, Hoeijmakers JG, Ahn HS, et al. Nav1.7-related small fiber neuropathy: impaired slow-inactivation and DRG neuron hyperexcitability. *Neurology.* 2012;78:1635–1643.
365. Ahn HS, Vasylyev DV, Estacion M, et al. Differential effect of D623 N variant and wild-type Na(v)1.7 sodium channels on resting potential and interspike membrane potential of dorsal root ganglion neurons. *Brain Res.* 2013;1529:165–177.
366. Fertleman CR, Baker MD, Parker KA, et al. SCN9 A mutations in paroxysmal extreme pain disorder: allelic variants underlie distinct channel defects and phenotypes. *Neuron.* 2006;52:767–774.
367. Estacion M, Dib-Hajj SD, Benke PJ, et al. NaV1.7 gain-of-function mutations as a continuum: A1632E displays physiological changes associated with erythromelalgia and paroxysmal extreme pain disorder mutations and produces symptoms of both disorders. *J Neurosci.* 2008;28:11079–11088.
368. Dib-Hajj SD, Estacion M, Jarecki BW, et al. Paroxysmal extreme pain disorder M1627K mutation in human Nav1.7 renders DRG neurons hyperexcitable. *Mol Pain.* 2008;4:37.
369. Huang J, Yang Y, Zhao P, et al. Small-fiber neuropathy Nav1.8 mutation shifts activation to hyperpolarized potentials and increases excitability of dorsal root ganglion neurons. *J Neurosci.* 2013;33:14087–14097.
370. Han C, Vasylyev D, Macala LJ, et al. The G1662 S NaV1.8 mutation in small fibre neuropathy: impaired inactivation underlying DRG neuron hyperexcitability. *J Neurol Neurosurg Psychiatry.* 2014;85(5):499–505.
371. Currò R, Salvalaggio A, Tozza S, et al. RFC1 expansions are a common cause of idiopathic sensory neuropathy. *Brain.* 2021;144(5):1542–1550.
372. Tagliapietra M, Cardellini D, Ferrarini M, et al. RFC1 AAGGG repeat expansion masquerading as chronic idiopathic axonal polyneuropathy. *J Neurol.* 2021;268(11):4280–4290.
373. Chan ACY, Kumar S, Tan G, et al. Expanding the genetic causes of small-fiber neuropathy: SCN genes and beyond. *Muscle Nerve.* 2023;67(4):259–271.
374. Eijkenboom I, Sopacua M, Hoeijmakers JGJ, et al. Yield of peripheral sodium channels gene screening in pure small fibre neuropathy. *J Neurol Neurosurg Psychiatry.* 2019;90(3):342–352.
375. Almomani R, Sopacua M, Marchi M, et al. Genetic profiling of sodium channels in diabetic painful and painless and idiopathic painful and painless neuropathies. *Int J Mol Sci.* 2023;24(9):8278.
376. England JD, Gronseth GS, Franklin G, et al. Evaluation of distal symmetric polyneuropathy: the role of laboratory and genetic testing (an evidence-based review). *Muscle Nerve.* 2009;39:116–125.
377. Saporta AS, Sottile SL, Miller LJ, Feely SM, Siskind CE, Shy ME. Charcot-Marie-Tooth disease subtypes and genetic testing strategies. *Ann Neurol.* 2011;69:22–33.
378. Klein CJ, Middha S, Duan X, et al. Application of whole exome sequencing in undiagnosed inherited polyneuropathies. *J Neurol Neurosurg Psychiatry.* 2014;85(11):1265–1272.

CHAPTER 12

Other Hereditary Neuropathies

In Chapter 11, we reviewed Charcot–Marie–Tooth syndrome and related hereditary neuropathies. Here we discuss some of the other types of hereditary neuropathies (Table 12-1).[1]

▶ NEUROPATHIES ASSOCIATED WITH LYSOSOMAL STORAGE DISORDERS

The lysosomal storage disorders are associated with abnormal accumulation of lysosomal products (e.g., sphingolipids, mucolipids, etc.) within neurons, leading to dysmyelination and axonal degeneration of both central and peripheral nerves (Table 12-1). Usually, the central nervous system (CNS) manifestations overshadow the peripheral neuropathy in most of these disorders. However, some patients present with peripheral neuropathy, which can be associated with significant disability.

METACHROMATIC LEUKODYSTROPHY

Clinical Features

There are three characteristic forms of metachromatic leukodystrophy (MLD) defined by age of onset: (1) late infantile, (2) juvenile, and (3) adult onset.[1-17] Most patients have the late infantile-onset MLD variant and develop progressive generalized weakness, decline in mental functions, dysarthria, and worsening gait between 1 and 2 years of age. Children become quadriparetic, spastic, and cortically blind and often develop seizures. On examination, generalized muscle weakness, hypotonia, hyporeflexia, and extensor plantar responses are appreciated. Most children die within 5–6 years after onset of symptoms.

The juvenile form of MLD typically presents later in childhood or adolescence but is associated with clinical features similar to the late infantile form of the disease. Patients with adult-onset MLD usually develop slowly progressive dementia, psychosis, spasticity, ataxia, extrapyramidal signs, visual impairment, and incontinence in the third or fourth decade of life.[15]

Laboratory Features

Magnetic resonance imaging (MRI) of the brain often demonstrates increased signal on T2-weighted images in the subcortical white matter.

The diagnosis is suggested by demonstrating decreased arylsulfatase A (ARSA) activity in urine, from leukocytes, or from cultured fibroblasts and can be confirmed with genetic testing. Levels of ARSA activity inversely correlates with clinical severity.[15] Prenatal diagnosis can be made by amniocentesis. Cerebral spinal fluid (CSF) protein is usually markedly elevated in the 100–300 mg/dL range. In late infantile patients, nerve conduction studies (NCS) and brainstem auditory evoked responses are usually quite abnormal, but these are variably affected in juvenile and adult-onset cases.[17] Motor NCS reveal mild to moderately reduced amplitudes, prolonged distal latencies, and marked slowing of nerve conduction velocities (NCVs) that range from 10 to 20 m/s in the legs and 20 to 40 m/s in the arms.[2,4,5,7-12,15-21] Rarely, conduction block or temporal dispersion is appreciated.[11,21] Sensory NCS are often unobtainable, but when recordable the sensory nerve action potentials (SNAPs) are reduced in amplitude with slightly to moderately prolonged latencies and slow NCVs. Visual, brainstem, and somatosensory-evoked potentials are delayed. Ultrasound may reveal homogenous enlargement of the peripheral nerves.[22]

Histopathology

Autopsy studies reveal degeneration of myelin in the CNS and peripheral nerves (Fig. 12-1).[3,6,10,12,15] Nerve biopsies are not routinely performed but can also demonstrate a decrease in myelinated fibers with evidence of demyelination and remyelination. The characteristic abnormality is the accumulation of metachromatically staining inclusions in cytoplasm of Schwann cells (Fig. 12-2). On electron microscopy (EM), these inclusions appear as lamellated bodies within Schwann cells.

Molecular Genetics and Pathogenesis

MLD is an autosomal-recessive disorder caused by mutations in the *ARSA* or the prosaposin (*PSAP*) genes.[23] ARSA and PSAP are both enzymes required for metabolizing galactosylsulfatide (cerebroside sulfatase), a glycolipid, present in myelin membranes. Deficiency of ARSA or the proteolytic product of PSAP results in the accumulation of sulfatides (inclusions) in Schwann cells and oligodendrocytes resulting in dysmyelination.

Treatment

No specific medications are helpful, but bone marrow and hematopoietic stem cell transplantation have been tried, but their therapeutic effectiveness is not proven.[24,25]

▶ **TABLE 12-1. RARE HEREDITARY NEUROPATHIES**

Hereditary Disorders of Lipid Metabolism
    Metachromatic leukodystrophy
    Krabbe disease (globoid cell leukodystrophy)
    Fabry disease
    Adrenoleukodystrophy/adrenomyeloneuropathy
    Refsum disease
    Tangier disease
    Cerebrotendinous xanthomatosis
Hereditary Ataxias With Neuropathy
    Friedreich ataxia
    Vitamin E deficiency
    Spinocerebellar ataxia
    Abetalipoproteinemia (Bassen–Kornzweig disease)
    Ataxia–telangiectasia
    Oculomotor apraxia type 1
    Oculomotor apraxia type 2
DNA-Repair Disorders
    Cerebellar Ataxia Neuropathy Vestibular Areflexia Syndrome (CANVAS)
    Ataxia telangiectasia
    Cockayne syndrome
    Xeroderma pigmentosa
Porphyria
    Acute intermittent porphyria (AIP)
    Hereditary coproporphyria (HCP)
    Variegate porphyria (VP)
Others
    Giant axonal neuropathy
    Infantile neuroaxonal dystrophy
    Polyglucosan body neuropathy
    Familial amyloid polyneuropathy

KRABBE DISEASE (GLOBOID CELL LEUKODYSTROPHY)

Clinical Features

Krabbe disease is another autosomal-recessive myelinopathy, affecting both the CNS and the peripheral nervous system (PNS). As with MLD, Krabbe typically presents early in infancy or less frequently, in adulthood.[1,26–38] Krabbe disease usually manifests between 3 and 8 months of age. Infants who are affected often appear normal at birth but later become extremely irritable and appear hypersensitive to various stimuli which may provoke opisthotonos.[38] They develop feeding difficulties, recurrent vomiting, and often generalized tonic–clonic seizures. Progressive weakness and spasticity, blindness, and deafness ensue. Muscle stretch reflexes initially may be pathologically brisk but become hypoactive as concurrent polyneuropathy worsens. Plantar responses are extensor. Death generally occurs by the age of 2 years.

Less commonly, Krabbe disease presents later in childhood or adult life with progressive dementia, spastic paraparesis or hemiparesis, cerebellar ataxia, cortical blindness, and optic atrophy.[33,37–42] Although peripheral neuropathy is common, it is overshadowed by the CNS abnormalities. Pes cavus and scoliosis may be seen. Rarely, it may manifest as an isolated polyneuropathy.[43]

Laboratory Features

Diagnosis is made by demonstrating decreased β-galactosidase activity in leukocytes or cultured fibroblasts and can be confirmed by genetic testing. Chorionic villi can be biopsied for

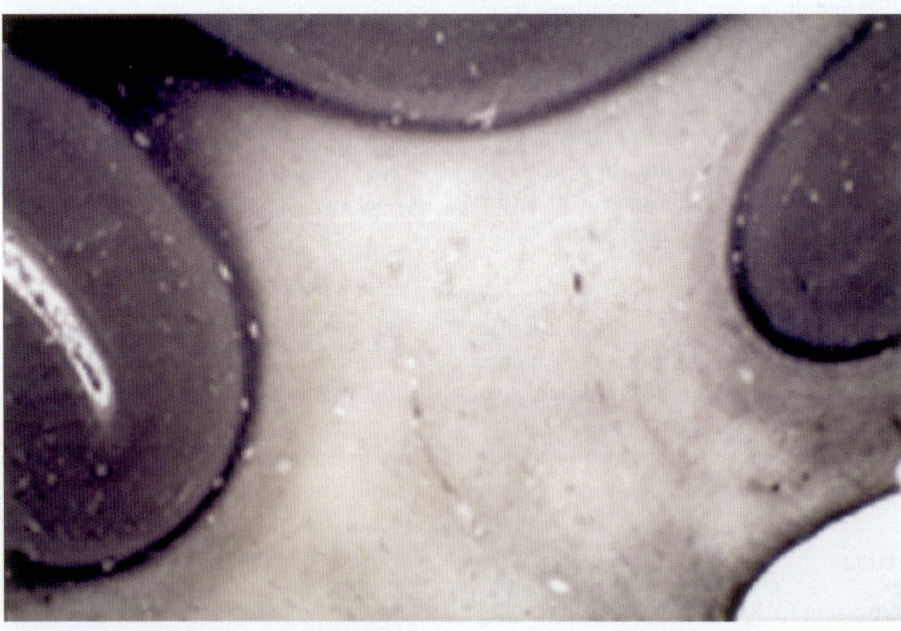

Figure 12-1. MLD pathology. Lysosomal storage of sulfatides kills oligodendrocytes and Schwann cells. Sulfatides discharged from dying cells are picked up by histiocytes. The white matter shows diffuse loss of myelin, which spares the subcortical fibers. (Reproduced with permission from http://neuropathology-web.org/. Chapter 10.)

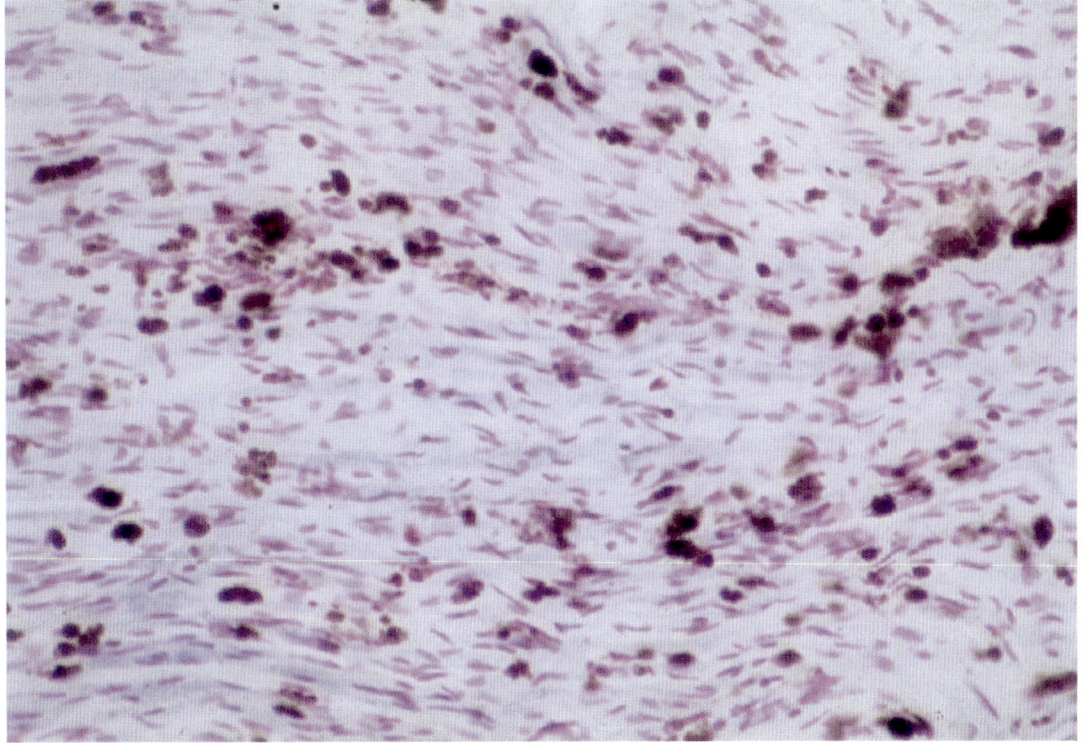

Figure 12-2. Nerve biopsy stained with cresyl violet demonstrating dense metachromatic deposits within Schwann cells obscuring the nerve fibers in the endoneurium. With acid cresyl violet, these take on a brown color (brown metachromasia), hence the term metachromatic leukodystrophy. (Reproduced with permission from www.neuropathologyweb.org/chapter10/chapter 10.)

prenatal diagnosis. Approximately 50% of the individuals affected have increased CSF protein concentrations.[33,37] MRI of the brain reveals evidence of demyelination involving the corticospinal tracts and optic radiations as well as demyelination or atrophy of the posterior part of the corpus callosum.[37,39,40] Motor NCS demonstrate mild to moderately reduced compound muscle action potential (CMAP) amplitudes, moderately prolonged distal latencies, moderately slow NCV, and delayed or absent F-waves.[26–31,33,34,36–40,42,43] Sensory NCS reveal absent responses or SNAPs with markedly reduced amplitudes and mildly prolonged distal latencies and slow CV.

Histopathology

Moderate cortical atrophy, loss of CNS white matter, gliosis, and globoid cells (macrophages filled with galactocerebroside) are appreciated on autopsy. Nerve biopsies also demonstrate a loss of myelinated fibers and segmental demyelination or hypomyelination, and macrophages filled with galactocerebroside.[27,33,37–40,42–44] The abnormal inclusions within macrophages stain with periodic acid Schiff (indicating glycogen), faintly with Sudan black (indicating lipid), and with acid phosphate (suggesting that these are within lysosomes). Unlike MLD, the inclusions in Krabbe disease are not metachromatic. On EM, electron-dense granules and tubular crystalloid inclusions are evident in the cytoplasm of these histiocytes.

Molecular Genetics and Pathogenesis

Krabbe disease is autosomal recessive caused by mutations in the β-galactosidase gene (*GALC*) located on chromosome 14q24.3-q32.1.[37,39,40] β-Galactosidase metabolizes galactocerebroside to ceramide and galactose as well as catalyzes the hydrolysis of psychosine. The abnormal accumulation of galactocerebroside and psychosine leads to the degeneration of Schwann cells and oligodendrocytes.

Treatment

There is no proven effective therapy for Krabbe disease, although bone marrow and hematopoietic stem cell transplantation may prove to be useful treatments.[24,45,46]

FABRY DISEASE

Clinical Features

Fabry disease (angiokeratoma corporis diffusum) is an X-linked disorder that usually affects males in childhood or adolescence.[1,13,47–62] Individuals who are affected typically present with burning or lancinating dysesthesia in the hands and feet. Angiokeratomas, which appear as reddish–purple maculopapular lesions, are characteristically found around the umbilicus, scrotum, inguinal region, and perineum. In addition, tiny red angiectasia may be visualized in the nailbeds, oral mucosa, and conjunctiva. The major cause of morbidity and mortality is related to accumulation of ceramide trihexoside or globotriaosylceramide (Gb3) in walls of blood vessels leading to hypertension, renal failure, coronary artery disease, strokes, and death by the fifth decade of life. Occasionally, women develop a mild painful sensory neuropathy, but only rarely do they have significant atherosclerotic disease.

Laboratory Features

A decrease in α-galactosidase activity can be demonstrated in leukocytes or cultured fibroblasts. Diagnosis can be confirmed by genetic testing. Prenatal diagnosis can be made by amniocentesis. NCS are usually normal but mildly decreased amplitudes of motor, and sensory NCS may be seen.[47–54] Quantitative sensory testing may reveal impaired temperature perception indicative of small fiber dysfunction.[51,52,54,56,59] MRI scans may demonstrate symmetric enlargement of dorsal root ganglia and sciatic nerves in affected males as well as in manifesting females, but less so.[57,58]

Histopathology

Nerve biopsies are not routinely done, but they can reveal a marked reduction of small myelinated and unmyelinated nerve fibers (Fig. 12-3). Glycolipid granules may be appreciated in ganglion cells of the peripheral and sympathetic nervous systems and in perineurial cells.[49,50] Reduced epidermal nerve fiber density may also be seen on skin biopsies.[53,55,56,59]

Molecular Genetics and Pathogenesis

Fabry disease is caused by mutations in the α-galactosidase gene (*GLA*) located on chromosome Xq21–22.[1,62] Decreased α-galactosidase enzyme activity leads to the accumulation of globotriaosylceramide (Gb3) in nerves and blood vessels.

Treatment

Studies have suggested that enzyme replacement therapy (ERT) with agalsidase alfa or beta may reduce microvascular endothelial deposits of globotriaosylceramide and improve pain-related quality of life in patients with Fabry disease and very low or undetectable levels of alpha-galactosidase.[1,59,60,63–67] FDA-approved recombinant ERTs include agalsidase-α or Replagal (0.2 mg/kg body weight), agalsidase-β or Fabrazyme (1 mg/kg body weight), and pegunigalsidase or Elfabrio (1 mg/kg), which are each given intravenously every 2 weeks. There is no evidence to support the alfa or beta form being superior or what the optimal dose or frequency might be. In addition, migalastat is an oral pharmacological chaperone that increases the enzyme activity of "amenable" mutations (amenable being defined as a mutation affecting the catalytic domain of the enzyme that leads to misfolding of the enzyme, but otherwise would not significantly impair its function).[68,69] Such mutations occur in about 50% of patients. Migalastat is another FDA-approved therapy that has been shown to reduce in left ventricular mass and stabilize kidney function, but there are no studies that have assessed efficacy of treating the neuropathy.

▶ PEROXISOMAL DISORDERS

Peroxisomes are organelles within the cytoplasm that contain enzymes essential in fatty acid oxidation (distinct from mitochondrial enzymes associated with β-oxidation), bile acid and cholesterol synthesis, and amino acid metabolism. These disorders are the result of mutations in genes encoding for structural proteins or specific peroxisomal enzymes.

ADRENOLEUKODYSTROPHY/ ADRENOMYELONEUROPATHY

Clinical Features

Adrenoleukodystrophy (ALD) and adrenomyeloneuropathy (AMN) are allelic X-linked dominant disorders. ALD is more common and manifests in young males as progressive dementia, optic atrophy, cortical blindness, hearing loss, seizures, and spasticity.[1,13,70–78] At least 90% of patients with ALD also have adrenal insufficiency. The onset of symptoms in ALD is usually between the ages of 4 and 8 years, and death usually occurs within 2 years of onset of symptoms. Less commonly, ALD develops in adolescence or young adult life and progresses at a slower rate. Affected individuals may be misdiagnosed as having multiple sclerosis. Later-onset cases may also present with psychiatric symptoms leading to misdiagnosis as schizophrenia.

Approximately 30% of cases present with the AMN phenotype and usually manifests in the third to fifth decade of life.[73,76,79] Individuals affected develop progressive spastic paraplegia along with a mild to moderate peripheral neuropathy. Muscle stretch reflexes may be normal or reduced. Progressive dementia indicative of cerebral involvement can develop in some patients later in the course of the disease. Adrenal insufficiency is evident in approximately two-thirds of patients. Rare patients present with an adult-onset spinocerebellar ataxia or only with adrenal insufficiency.

Although these are X-linked disorders, women occasionally develop symptoms.[77] A large study of ALD/AMD, 46 women carriers in a prospective cross-sectional cohort study reported symptoms of myelopathy (29/46, 63%) and/or peripheral neuropathy (26/46, 57%).[77] The frequency of symptomatic women carriers increases with age from 18% in women less than 40 years of age to 88% in women over the age of 60 years. Manifesting women carriers are often misdiagnosed with multiple sclerosis or familial spastic paraparesis.[73]

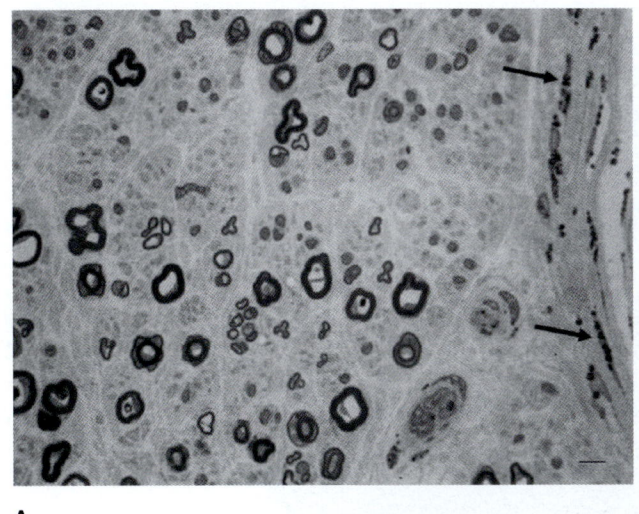
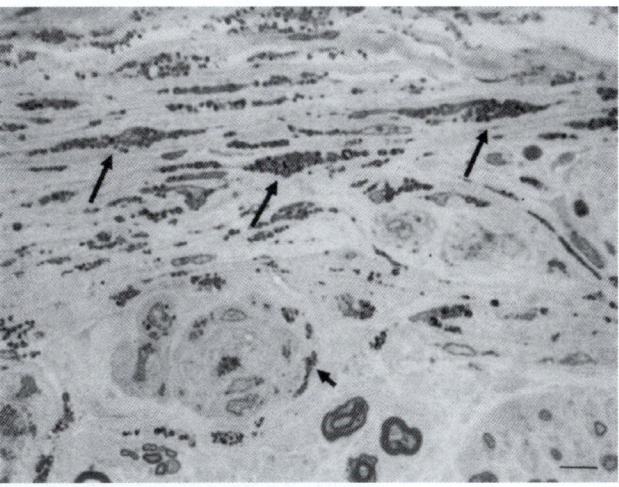

Figure 12-3. Fabry disease. Nerve biopsy. A toluidine blue-stained, semithin, plastic-embedded section reveals mild, patchy loss of large, myelinated fibers, a few thinly myelinated axons, and several regenerative axon clusters (**A**). The perineurium (right edge) contains osmiophilic inclusions (*arrows*). Higher power reveals dark osmiophilic deposits in the perineurium (*long arrows*) and in association with blood vessels (*short arrow*) (**B**). An electron photomicrograph of the muscle biopsy specimen reveals electron-dense amorphous and lamellated inclusions in the perinuclear, subsarcolemmal region (**C**). (Reproduced with permission from Lacomis D, Roeske-Anderson L, Mathie L. Neuropathy and Fabry disease. *Muscle Nerve*. 2005;31:102–107. Figure 1 & Figure 2AB.)

Laboratory Features

Diagnosis is made on finding that very long–chain fatty acid (VLCFA) levels (C24, C25, and C26) are increased in the serum.[76,80] The ratio of hexacosanoic acid to docosanoic or erucic acid (C26:C22) and tetracosanoic acid to docosanoic acid (C24:C22) are increased in both ALD and AMN. VLCFA levels can be assessed in neonates and can be used to screen for the disease shortly after birth. Because VLCFA levels are similar in ALD and AMN, these are not helpful in predicting the clinical phenotype. As many as 85% of obligate female carriers also have elevated VLCFA levels. Some, but not all, individuals have laboratory evidence of adrenal insufficiency. Diagnosis is confirmed by genetic testing.

MRI scans reveal confluent subcortical white matter demyelination in ALD, preferentially in the posterior parietal–occipital regions.[75] MRI abnormalities of the cerebral white matter also develop later in the course in nearly half of patients with AMD but are not uniformly present in late-onset cases.

NCS are usually normal in ALD. However, AMN is usually associated with a sensorimotor polyneuropathy. Typically, sensory and motor NCS reveal slightly reduced amplitudes, prolonged distal latencies, and slight slow CVs, suggesting a primary axonopathy with secondary demyelination.[70,71,74,78,79,81-84] Occasionally, patients fulfill electrophysiological criteria for a primary demyelination.[83] Somatosensory and visual-evoked potentials demonstrate evidence of central slowing.[72,74]

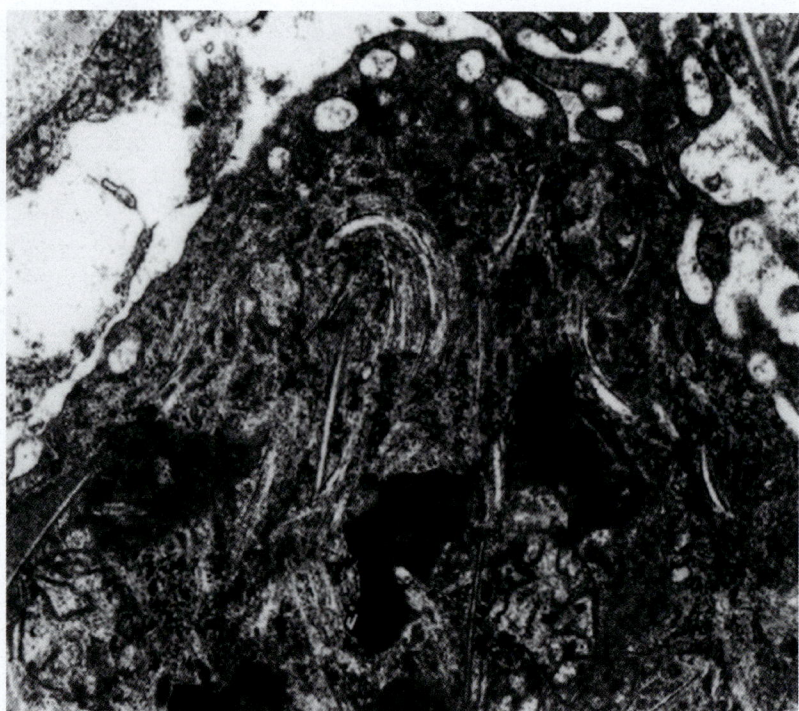

Figure 12-4. Adrenoleukodystrophy. Characteristic cellular inclusions (trilamellar membranes containing VLCFA cholesterol esters) are seen with the electron microscope in adrenal cortical cells, white matter histiocytes, Leydig cells, and Schwann cells. (Reproduced with permission from www.neuropathologyweb.org/chapter10/chapter 10.)

Histopathology

We do not perform nerve biopsies routinely, but they can demonstrate a loss of myelinated and unmyelinated nerve fibers. On EM, lamellar inclusions are evident in the cytoplasm of Schwann cells (Fig. 12-4). Autopsies in ALD demonstrate demyelination and perivascular inflammation, particularly in the parietal and occipital regions.[73] The spinal cord displays bilateral, usually symmetrical, long tract degeneration, particularly of the gracile tract in a dying-back pattern.[83]

Molecular Genetics and Pathogenesis

ALD and AMN are caused by mutations in the peroxisomal transmembrane adenosine triphosphate-binding cassette transporter gene (ABCD1), located on chromosome Xq28.[73,76] The ABC transporter protein is part of peroxins family of proteins, which are involved in the transport, biogenesis, and proliferation of peroxisomes. There is no clear genotype–phenotype correlation associated with any specific mutation, and phenotypic heterogeneity can be found even within the family members who carry the same genetic mutation. Mutations in the gene cause impaired transport of VLCFA or VLCFA CoA synthetase into peroxisomes, thus decreasing β-oxidization of VLCFA. How this leads to dysmyelination and axonal degeneration is not known.

Treatment

Allogeneic stem-cell transplantation and elivaldogene autotemcel (Skysona™, eli-cel; Lenti-D™ gene therapy) may be beneficial in early-stage cerebral ALD but is not likely effective in AMN.[85,86] Diets low in VLCFAs and supplemented with Lorenzo oil (erucic and oleic acids) reduce the levels of VLCFAs and increase the levels of C22 in serum, fibroblasts, and liver; however, such changes have not been consistently noted in the brain.[87] Rare reports suggest clinical and MRI improvement in individual patients treated with Lorenzo oil, but several large open-label trials of Lorenzo oil failed to demonstrate significant efficacy.[78,88,89]

REFSUM DISEASE (HMSN IV)

Clinical Features

Refsum disease is a peroxisomal disorder associated with impaired α-oxidation of phytanic acid. The disease can manifest in infancy to early adulthood with the classic tetrad of (1) peripheral neuropathy, (2) retinitis pigmentosa (often the earliest symptom which manifests as night blindness), (3) cerebellar ataxia, and (4) elevated CSF protein concentration.[90–95] Patients with Refsum disease may also develop sensorineural hearing loss, cardiac conduction abnormalities, ichthyosis, and anosmia. Some or all of these clinical findings are usually manifest in the majority of patients by the end of the second decade. Infantile Refsum disease falls within the clinical spectrum of Zellweger syndrome and neonatal ALD, albeit much milder in severity.

Although not typically a presenting manifestation, most individuals who are affected develop distal numbness and paresthesia in the legs by their 20s. The distal legs become atrophic and weak, and patients develop progressive foot drop. Subsequently, the proximal leg and arm muscles may become weak. Interestingly, the neuropathy can have a fluctuating course. On examination, a length-dependent loss of vibration, proprioception, and light touch is appreciated. Hypertrophic nerves may be palpated. Muscle stretch reflexes are reduced or absent throughout.

Laboratory Features

Serum phytanic acid levels are elevated, usually greater than 200 μmol/L, as may the CSF protein concentration. Other abnormalities include an increased phytanic acid/pristanic acid ratio, elevated pipecolic acid concentration, and reduced phytanoyl-CoA hydroxylase enzyme activity. Genetic testing can be done to confirm the disorder. Sensory NCS reveal reduced amplitudes and prolonged latencies/slow CVs.[94] Motor NCS demonstrate normal or moderately reduced amplitudes, mildly or moderately prolonged distal latencies, and mild to marked slowing of CV to the 10–30 m/s range.[90,92,93]

Histopathology

Nerve biopsies demonstrate a loss of myelinated nerve fibers with remaining axons often thinly myelinated and associated with onion-bulb formation.

Molecular Genetics and Pathogenesis

Refsum disease is autosomal recessive and can be caused by mutations in two different genes.[96] Classical Refsum disease with childhood or early adult onset is caused by mutations in the gene that encodes for phytanoyl-CoA α-hydroxylase (*PHYX*) located on chromosome 10p13 in 90% of affected individuals.[97,98] This peroxisomal enzyme helps catalyze α-oxidation of phytanic acid. The defect leads to the accumulation of phytanic acid in various organs including the CNS and PNS, leading to neuronal degeneration. Less common, mutations in the gene that encodes for peroxin 7 receptor protein (*PRX7*) located on chromosome 6q22–24 are responsible for Refsum disease.[96,99,100] Mutations in the *PEX7* gene that encodes for the peroxisome-targeting signal type 2 receptor are seen in less than 10% of individuals. Mutations in PEX7 also cause rhizomelic chondrodysplasia punctata type 1, a severe peroxisomal disorder.

Treatment

Refsum disease is treated by removing phytanic precursors (phytols: fish oils, dairy products, and ruminant fats) from the diet. In addition to the noticed clinical improvement, the NCS also improves with appropriate dietary restrictions as well as with plasma exchange.[90–93]

TANGIER DISEASE

Clinical Features

Tangier disease is a rare autosomal-recessive disorder associated with a deficiency of high-density lipoprotein. The first reported patients came from Tangier Island located in Chesapeake Bay—thus the name. Tangier disease may present as (1) an asymmetric mononeuropathy multiplex, (2) a slowly progressive symmetric polyneuropathy predominantly in the legs, or (3) a pseudo syringomyelia appearance in which there is dissociation between loss of pain/temperature and position/vibration in the arms.[101–112] Deposition of cholesterol esters within the tonsils leads to their swollen, yellowish–orange appearance. In addition, splenomegaly and lymphadenopathy may be apparent.

Laboratory Features

Serum high-density lipoprotein cholesterol levels are markedly reduced while triacylglycerol levels are increased. Genetic testing is available to confirm the diagnosis. Motor and sensory NCS can be normal or associated with moderately reduced amplitudes, prolonged distal latencies, partial conduction block, and slow CVs.[102–106,108,109,111] The asymmetric nature of the polyneuropathy and demyelinating features including conduction block may mimic Lewis–Sumner syndrome (e.g., multifocal acquired demyelinating sensory and motor neuropathy or MADSAM neuropathy—see Chapter 13).[108,109]

Histopathology

Nerve biopsies are not required for the diagnosis, but studies have reported they reveal axonal degeneration with demyelination, remyelination, and redundant myelin folds (i.e., tomacula).[101,110–114] EM demonstrates abnormal accumulation of lipids in Schwann cells, particularly those encompassing unmyelinated and small myelinated nerves (Fig. 12-5).[101,110] There appears to be preferential involvement of noncompacted myelin region of the paranode for lipid storage in the myelinated Schwann cells.

Molecular Genetics and Pathogenesis

Tangier disease is caused by mutations in the ATP-binding cassette-1 gene (*ABCA1*) located in chromosome 9q22–31.[115,116] The pathogenic basis of the peripheral neuropathy

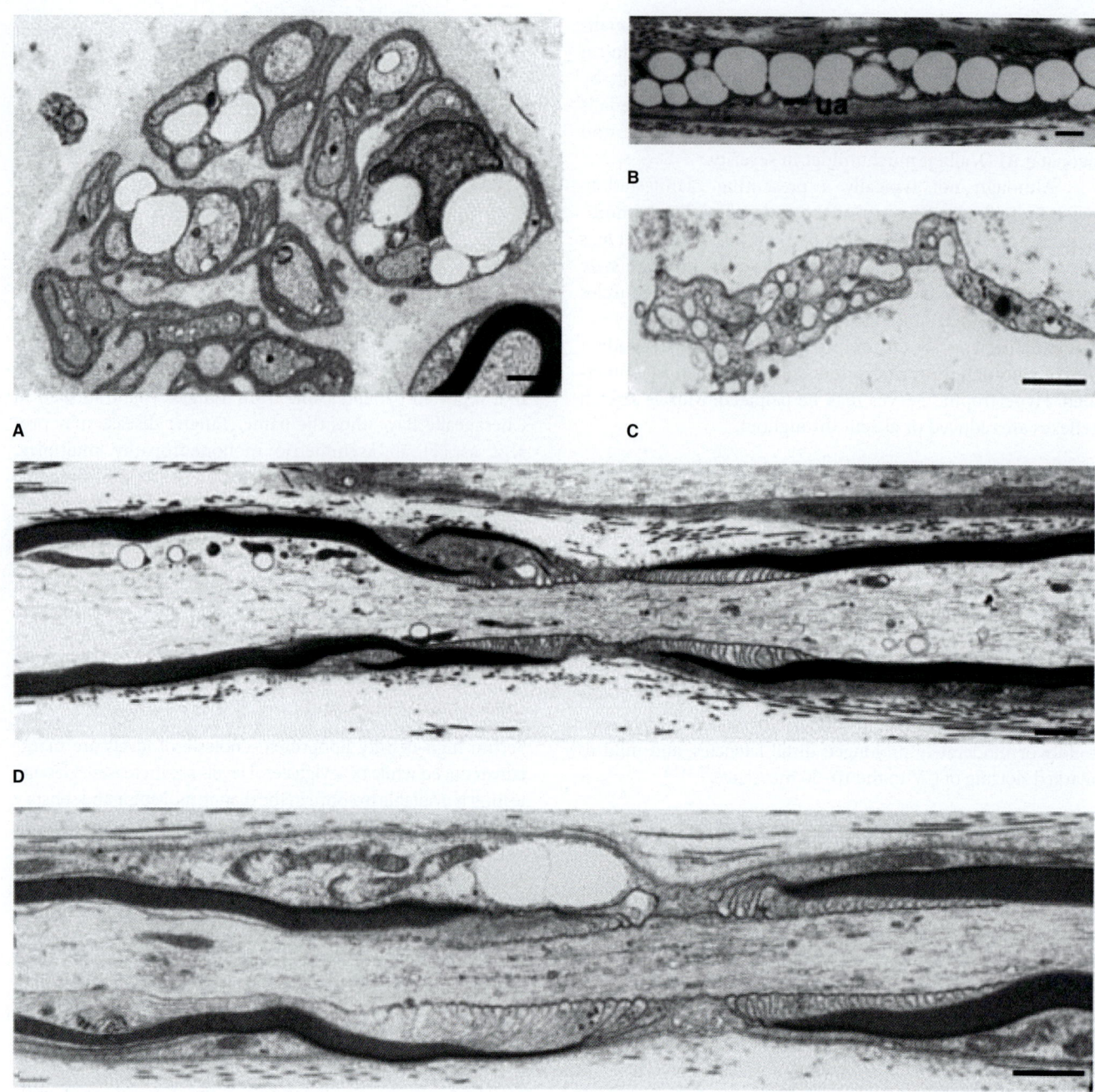

Figure 12-5. Tangier disease. Electron micrographs. (**A**) Transverse section showing multiple electron-lucent vacuoles in the cytoplasm of unmyelinated Schwann cells. (**B**) Longitudinal section showing linearly arranged vacuoles in Schwann cell cytoplasm of an unmyelinated axon (ua). (**C**) Multiple vacuoles in a fibroblast. (**D**) Small vacuoles in the disrupted paranodal myelin terminal loops. (**E**) Large vacuoles in the paranodal abaxonal Schwann cell cytoplasm. Bar = 1 μm. (Reproduced with permission from Cai Z, Blumbergs PC, Cash K, et al. Paranodal pathology in Tangier disease with remitting-relapsing multifocal neuropathy. *J Clin Neurosci.* 2006;13(4):492–497. Figure 1, p. 494.)

is unknown but may be similar to ALD/AMN, which are also caused by mutations involving the ABC transporter superfamily.

Treatment

There is no specific treatment.

CEREBROTENDINOUS XANTHOMATOSIS (CHOLESTANOLOSIS)

Clinical Features

Cerebrotendinous xanthomatosis is a rare autosomal-recessive disorder that usually presents after the second decade with progressive dementia, spasticity, ataxia, and mild sensory neuropathy.[117–125] The name of the disorder arises because of the common occurrence of xanthomas on tendons and the skin. Cataracts are another frequent complication. Most individuals who are affected die in the fourth decade of life because of complications from premature atherosclerosis.

Laboratory Features

Serum level of cholestanol is increased. Genetic testing can be performed to confirm the diagnosis. NCS are variable, depending on the presence and the degree of severity of peripheral neuropathy.[117–121,124] Motor and sensory may be normal or reveal absent amplitudes, with slightly prolonged distal latencies, and mildly slow CVs suggestive of an axonal sensorimotor polyneuropathy.

Histopathology

Nerve biopsies reveal a loss of myelinated nerve fibers with variable degrees of demyelination and onion-bulb formation. Lipid inclusions are evident in Schwann cells.

Molecular Genetics and Pathogenesis

This disorder is caused by mutations in the sterol 27 hydroxylase gene located on chromosome 2, which results in impaired metabolism of cholestanol, the 5α-dihydro derivative of cholesterol.[126] Cholestanol accumulates in body tissues, including peripheral nerves, thereby resulting in the associated clinical features.

Treatment

Early treatment with chenodeoxycholic acid may lead to a decrease in serum cholestanol and diminished excretion of bile alcohols in urine accompanied by clinical improvement.[119] Motor and sensory NCS improved in one patient following plasma exchange and treatment with chenodeoxycholic acid.[120]

▶ HEREDITARY ATAXIAS

The hereditary ataxias are a group of progressive neurodegenerative disorders characterized by varying degrees of degeneration of the cerebral cortex, basal ganglia, cerebellum, brainstem, corticospinal tracts, spinocerebellar tracts, motor neurons, and peripheral nerves (Table 12-1). The associated peripheral neuropathy with some of these disorders is usually overshadowed by the CNS abnormalities. However, the neuropathy can be quite prominent in Friedreich ataxia (FA) and an inherited form of vitamin E deficiency.

FRIEDREICH ATAXIA

Clinical Features

FA usually presents between 2 and 16 years of age with gait ataxia (63%), generalized clumsiness (25%), difficulty ambulating (4%), scoliosis (5%), tremor (1%), and cardiomyopathy (2%).[127–134] However, several genetically confirmed late-onset cases have been described.[129,135,136] FA is the most common form of autosomal-recessive ataxia. Dysarthria, optic atrophy, pigmentary retinopathy, nystagmus, reduced hearing, ataxia, pyramidal and lower motor neuron weakness, distal limb atrophy, scoliosis, and pes cavus are evident on examination. In addition, reduced vibratory sensation and proprioception associated with diminished muscle stretch reflexes are seen often associated with extensor plantar responses.[129,135,136] Rarely, affected individuals have retained reflexes.[137] Some patients develop dementia. FA is a progressive disorder, and most patients are wheelchair dependent with 15 years of onset of symptoms. There is increased mortality with the mean age of death in the mid to late thirties.

Laboratory Features

Genetic testing is available for diagnosis. MRI of the brain is usually normal, but the cervical spinal cord is often atrophic.[135–137] Electrocardiogram reveals nonspecific abnormalities (e.g., nonspecific ST and T-wave changes, low-voltage QRS complexes, deep Q-waves, and conduction defects) in at least 30% of patients. Echocardiogram reveals increased thickness of the interventricular septum in approximately two-thirds of affected individuals; later in the course, a dilated cardiomyopathy may develop. Sensory NCS are associated with absent or reduced amplitudes.[122,127–129,132,135,138] H-reflexes are absent. Motor NCS are less affected[128,129,139]; however, central motor conduction may be slow on magnetic stimulation studies.[140,141] Somatosensory-evoked potentials demonstrate reduced or absent cortical potentials and slowing of central conduction.[139,142,143]

Histopathology

Sural nerve biopsies reveal a loss of large, myelinated fibers.[143] On autopsy, the posterior columns are markedly atrophied, and the dorsal roots are considerably decreased in size compared to the ventral roots.

Molecular Genetics and Pathogenesis

FA is an autosomal recessive disorder that is usually caused by an expanding GAA trinucleotide repeat mutation within the first intron of the frataxin gene (*FXN*) located on chromosome 9q13.[144,145] The normal gene contains 40 or fewer copies of the GAA triplet repeats, while patients with FA usually have 100 to more than 1,700 repeats. Approximately 2% of cases are caused by point mutations within the frataxin gene.[146] The mutations result in low or absent levels of frataxin, a mitochondrial protein of unclear function. Frataxin is speculated to have a role in iron metabolism, protection against free radical toxicity, or mitochondrial DNA replication.[146]

Treatment

There is no medical treatment for FA. However, patients may benefit from speech, occupational, and physical therapy. Cardiac function needs to be monitored and treated appropriately.

VITAMIN E DEFICIENCY

Clinical Features

Vitamin E or α-tocopherol is a lipid-soluble vitamin present in the lipid bilayer of cell membranes.[143,147–153] Vitamin E deficiency can arise due to (1) deficient fat absorption (e.g., cystic fibrosis, chronic cholestasis, short-bowel syndrome, and intestinal lymphangiectasia), (2) deficient fat transport (abetalipoproteinemia, hypobetalipoproteinemia, normotriglyceridemic abetalipoproteinemia, and chylomicron retention disease), or (3) secondary to mutations in α-tocopherol transfer protein.

The clinical manifestations of hereditary and secondary vitamin E deficiency resemble those seen in FA. Onset in the hereditary cases is usually between the ages of 5 and 10 years. Affected individuals manifest with slowly progressive ataxia, dysarthria, reduced vibratory perception and proprioception, diminished or absent muscle stretch reflexes with extensor plantar responses, and generalized weakness. Pes cavus deformities and scoliosis are common. Ophthalmoplegia, optic neuropathy, and retinitis pigmentosa are seen in acquired cases of vitamin E deficiency but are not typically present in the hereditary form.

Laboratory Features

Serum vitamin E levels are reduced. Patients deficient in vitamin E secondary to malabsorption of fat also have low serum levels of cholesterol, triglycerides, very low-density lipoproteins (VLDLs), vitamin A, and vitamin C. These levels are normal in patients with hereditary vitamin E deficiency in which there is isolated vitamin E deficiency. Hereditary cases can be confirmed with genetic testing. Sensory NCS reveal absent potentials or low amplitudes.[143,148,149,151,152] Motor conduction studies are usually normal, although slightly prolonged distal latencies and slow NCVs may be found.[143,149] Somatosensory-evoked potentials may be unobtainable but, when recordable, demonstrate slowing of central conduction and reduced amplitudes.

Histopathology

Autopsies and nerve biopsies demonstrate a marked loss of dorsal root ganglion cells, large-diameter myelinated fibers, and degeneration of the dorsal columns, and reductions in the cells of the gracile and cuneate nuclei. Vacuoles may be evident in the myelin sheath and the Schmidt–Lanterman incisures may appear disrupted.

Molecular Genetics and Pathogenesis

Isolated vitamin E deficiency is inherited in an autosomal-recessive manner and is caused by mutations in the α-tocopherol transfer protein gene (*TTPA*) located on chromosome 8q13.[147,150] As a result, there is reduced incorporation of vitamin E into serum VLDLs.[153] Although absorption of vitamin E in the intestines and incorporation into chylomicrons are normal, recycling of vitamin E is dependent on α-tocopherol transfer protein into VLDL. Thus, vitamin E is rapidly eliminated, and levels are diminished in the CNS and PNS.

Vitamin E may have antioxidant properties and may assist in modulating against glutamate excitotoxicity. The dorsal root ganglia and the posterior column nuclei have the lowest concentrations of vitamin E in the nervous system and might therefore be particularly sensitive to diminishing concentrations of vitamin E and its possible neuroprotective effects.

Treatment

Early treatment may stabilize or improve neurological function. Patients are started on vitamin E 400 mg twice a day, and the dosage is gradually increased up to 100 mg/kg per day until vitamin E levels normalize.[149]

ABETALIPOPROTEINEMIA (BASSEN–KORNZWEIG DISEASE)

Clinical Features

Abetalipoproteinemia or Bassen–Kornzweig disease is characterized by the combination of ataxia, retinitis pigmentosa, steatorrhea, and loss of sensation in the distal arms and legs.[154–157] Affected individuals usually present with ataxia and vision loss at night within the first two decades of life. The ataxia is progressive and leads to the loss of independent ambulation by the fourth or fifth decades of life. On physical examination, patients are often short in stature and have pes cavus and hammer toes. Reduction in vibration sensation and proprioception is apparent along with sensory ataxia. Muscle stretch reflexes are reduced or absent. Mild distal muscle atrophy and weakness may be appreciated. Ophthalmoparesis may be observed in some patients.

Laboratory Features

Acanthocytes are seen on blood smear. Total serum cholesterol, low-density lipoproteins and VLDLs, and chylomicrons are reduced, as are serum concentrations of the fat-soluble vitamins A, E, and K. The electrophysiological abnormalities are very similar to those found in FA and vitamin E deficiency.[158–160] The sensory SNAPs are absent or reveal reduced amplitudes with minimal slowing of conduction and normal or borderline distal sensory latencies. The CMAP amplitudes are normal or only slightly reduced, while distal latencies and CVs are preserved or only mildly slow. Central conduction slowing may be appreciated on somatosensory and visual-evoked potential studies.[159,161] Brainstem auditory-evoked responses are characteristically normal, which is the only distinguishing electrophysiological feature between this disorder and FA.

Histopathology

Nerve biopsies demonstrate axonal degeneration with a loss of large-diameter myelinated fibers as well as demyelination and remyelination on teased nerve fiber analysis. Degeneration of the posterior columns and the ventral spinocerebellar tracts has been appreciated on autopsies.

Molecular Genetics and Pathogenesis

This is an autosomal-recessive disorder caused by mutations in the *MTTP* gene that encodes for microsomal triglyceride transfer protein large subunit. This protein is important in lipoprotein assembly and absorption of fat-soluble vitamins from the intestinal tract. This most likely leads to decreased vitamin E, leading to the neurological deficits in this disorder.

Treatment

Patients should be treated by replacing fat-soluble vitamins, in particular vitamin E.

ATAXIA WITH OCULOMOTOR APRAXIA TYPE 1

Clinical Features

Ataxia with oculomotor apraxia type 1 (AOA1) was initially described in Japanese patients and characterized by early-onset, slowly progressive cerebellar ataxia, mental retardation (though some have normal intellect), choreoathetosis, followed by oculomotor apraxia and an axonal motor peripheral neuropathy.[162–166] Typically, patients present with gait imbalance between the ages of 2 and 10 years, followed by slurred, then poor coordination of the arms with mild intention tremor. Oculomotor apraxia develops a few years after the onset of ataxia and progresses to external ophthalmoplegia. Progressive generalized weakness and areflexia evolve with loss of ambulation usually occurring about 7–10 years after onset.

Laboratory Features

MRI scans demonstrated cerebellar atrophy.[162–165] Electrodiagnostic studies reveal evidence of an axonal sensorimotor polyneuropathy.[165,166] Serum concentration of AFP is usually elevated. In addition, hypoalbuminemia and hypercholesterolemia become evident, particularly during the later stages of the disease. Diagnosis is confirmed by genetic testing.

Histopathology

Sural nerve biopsy is not routinely done but has revealed severe loss of small and large myelinated fibers with preservation of the unmyelinated nerve fibers.[162]

Molecular Genetics and Pathogenesis

AOA1 is caused by mutations in the *APTX* gene that encodes for aprataxin, which is involved in DNA single-strand break repair.[163,166] The mechanism by which defects in aprataxin result in central and peripheral nerve damage is not at all clear.

Treatment

There is no specific treatment.

ATAXIA WITH OCULOMOTOR APRAXIA TYPE 2

Clinical Features

Ataxia with oculomotor apraxia type 2 (AOA2) is characterized by progressive cerebellar atrophy, choreoathetosis, axonal sensorimotor polyneuropathy, and oculomotor apraxia (the latter in approximately 60% of affected individuals) with an onset between the ages of 3 and 30 years.[167–174]

Laboratory Features

There is usually elevated serum concentration of AFP. Electrodiagnostic studies reveal features of a mixed demyelinating, and axonal sensorimotor neuropathy. Diagnosis is made by genetic testing.

Histopathology

Sural nerve biopsy has reportedly showed severe depletion of large and small myelinated fibers.[170] Autopsy studies have demonstrated a marked loss of Purkinje cells in the cerebellar cortex, loss of neurons in the dentate nucleus, chromatolysis of the oculomotor and raphe nuclei in the brainstem, severe demyelination of the gracilis and cuneatus funiculi, and degeneration of the Clarke columns with gliosis in the spinal cord.[170]

Molecular Genetics and Pathogenesis

AOA2 is caused by mutations in *SETX*, the gene that encodes the protein senataxin. Mutations in this gene are also responsible for the dominant juvenile form of familial amyotrophic lateral sclerosis type 4. Senataxin may modulate neurite growth through fibroblast growth factor 8 signaling.[174] However, the exact mechanism by which defects in senataxin result in central and peripheral nerve damage is not known.

Treatment

There is no specific treatment.

▶ DISORDERS OF DNA REPAIR

There are several disorders of DNA repair that are associated with axonal polyneuropathies, including Cerebellar ataxia, neuropathy, and vestibular areflexia syndrome (CANVAS), ataxia–telangiectasia, Cockayne syndrome, and xeroderma pigmentosum—the latter two are closely related and some forms are allelic. These disorders are also associated with ataxia.

CEREBELLAR ATAXIA, NEUROPATHY, AND VESTIBULAR AREFLEXIA SYNDROME (CANVAS)

Clinical Features

CANVAS usually manifests in middle adult life with a sensory neuropathy/neuropathy that progresses over the course of 10–15 years to cerebellar and vestibular dysfunction, as well as a dry cough.[175–182] Examination reveals loss of large fiber sensory modalities with a sensory ataxia as well as cerebellar ataxia. The vestibulopathy leads to a diminished vestibulo-ocular reflex (VOR) an oscillopsia may be apparent. Upper and lower motor neuron involvement may also be appreciated in some patients (spasticity, brisk reflexes, muscle atrophy, and fasciculations) as well as dysautonomia and features of parkinsonism.[182] So, the clinical spectrum is quite broad.

Laboratory Features

NCS reveal low amplitude or absent sensory responses that are in a non–length-dependent pattern suggestive of a sensory neuropathy/ganglionopathy.[175–181] Patients with lower motor neuron involvement may have evidence of active denervation and chronic reinnervation changes on electromyography (EMG).[182] Cerebellar atrophy may be appreciated on MRI scans.[177,179]

Histopathology

Sural nerve biopsies have shown the loss of large myelinated axons.[178] Autopsy studies have demonstrated degeneration of the dorsal root ganglia and posterior columns.[179,180] There is degeneration of the vestibulospinal and spinocerebellar tracts depletion of cerebellum Purkinje cells and gliosis in the cerebellum, the pars compacta of the substantia nigra was depleted, with widespread Lewy bodies in the locus coeruleus, substantia nigra, hippocampus, entorhinal cortex, and amygdala, as well as and loss of motor neurons.[182]

Molecular Genetics and Pathogenesis

In most cases, CANVAS is associated with biallelic $(AAGGG)_n$ repeat expansions in the second intron of the replication factor complex subunit 1 (*RFC1*).[175–184] Notably, this is probably the most common cause of autosomal recessive ataxia.[177] A few cases with typical CANVAS have a heterozygous expansion in one allele and together with a second truncating variant *in trans* in *RFC1*.[183] There is a DNA polymerase accessory protein required for the coordinated synthesis of both DNA strands during replication and after DNA damage.[178]

Treatment

There is no specific medical therapy at this time, but patients may benefit from physical and occupational therapy.

ATAXIA–TELANGIECTASIA

Clinical Features

Ataxia–telangiectasia is characterized by childhood onset (usually in first 5 years of life) of cerebellar ataxia, oculocutaneous telangiectasia, oculomotor dyspraxia, and frequent sinopulmonary infections.[184–187] Motor milestones are delayed, but mental functioning is well preserved. Affected children develop choreoathetotic movements and dysarthric speech within the first decade. Sensory examination reveals a marked loss of proprioception and vibration sense, and muscle stretch reflexes are reduced or absent. Distal motor weakness may become apparent over time.

Laboratory Features

Variable immune deficiency with reduced levels of IgA and IgG can be seen along with an increase in serum α-fetoprotein (AFP) levels. The electrophysiological abnormalities are similar to those found in FA with absent or reduced amplitudes of the SNAPs, with only a mild reduction in the NCVs or prolongation in the distal sensory latencies.[109,141] Similar but less striking abnormalities can be seen on motor NCS. Genetic testing is done to confirm the diagnosis.

Histopathology

Sural nerve biopsies reveal a loss of large, myelinated nerve fibers.

Molecular Genetics and Pathogenesis

The disorder is inherited in an autosomal-recessive manner and is caused by mutations in the ataxia telangiectasia mutated (*ATM*) gene located on chromosome 11q23, which encodes for phosphatidylinositol-3 kinase.[184,187] This enzyme is important in signal transduction, meiotic recombination, and cell-cycle regulation, and the mutations in the ATM gene result in impaired DNA repair. Cytogenetic testing reveals a 6- to 10-fold increase in chromosome breakage following ionizing irradiation. Further, there is increased spontaneous breakage and specific translocations involving the T-cell receptor genes on chromosome 7 and 14.

Treatment

There is no specific treatment.

COCKAYNE SYNDROME

Clinical Features

Cockayne syndrome is a rare disorder caused by defects in DNA repair and is associated with various systemic abnormalities, including central and PNS dysmyelination.[184,188–193] Most children appear normal at birth, but by the end of the first year of their life, they are noted to have reduced growth rates and signs of aging. Between 4 and 10 years of age, they develop progeric facial appearance, cognitive decline, ataxia, areflexia, hearing loss, photosensitivity, pigmentary retinopathy, and dwarfism.

Laboratory Features

Motor and sensory NCS may demonstrate moderate to marked reduction in NCVs and prolonged distal latencies, though abnormalities may not be apparent before the age of 2 years.[184,191–193,195,196]

Histopathology

Nerve biopsies reveal segmental demyelination and inclusions within Schwann cells.[194–197]

Molecular Genetics and Pathogenesis

Cockayne syndrome is an autosomal-recessive disorder that can be caused by mutations in two different genes that encode for DNA excision repair proteins: group 6 excision repair cross-complementing protein (*ERCC6*); in group 8 excision repair cross-complementing protein (*ERCC8*), group 5 excision repair cross-complementing protein (*ERCC5*), and group 4 excision repair cross-complementing protein (*ERCC4*).[184] Defects in these transcription factors interact with RNA polymerase II and result in impaired transcription initiation, nucleotide excision, and DNA repair.[198] The inability to properly excise and repair spontaneous DNA mutations results in accelerated signs of aging and increased risk of malignancy.

Treatment

There is no specific treatment.

XERODERMA PIGMENTOSUM

Clinical Features

Xeroderma pigmentosum (XP) is another rare disorder caused by defects in DNA repair and is associated with various systemic abnormalities, including central and PNS dysmyelination.[184,199–204] Approximately 20%–30% manifest with sensory and sensorimotor peripheral neuropathies as well as ataxia and hearing loss.

Laboratory Features

NCS demonstrate features of an axonal sensory or sensorimotor polyneuropathy.[184,199,204]

Histopathology

Autopsies and nerve biopsies reveal motor and sensory axon loss of myelinated and unmyelinated nerve fibers.[203,204] Zebra–body-like structures have been detected in Schwann cell cytoplasm.[204]

Molecular Genetics and Pathogenesis

XP is an autosomal-recessive disorder caused by pathogenic mutations various complementation groups—XP-A to XP-G (involved in nucleotide excision repair) and one variant form, XPV, caused by mutations affecting translesional DNA polymerase eta.[205]

XP complementation group A (XPA) is caused by homozygous or compound heterozygous mutation in the *XPA* gene. XPB is caused by mutation in the DNA excision repair gene, *ERCC3*. XPC is caused by mutation in the *XPC* gene. XPD is caused by homozygous or compound heterozygous mutation in the excision repair gene *ERCC2*. XPE is caused by a homozygous mutation in the *DDB2* gene that encodes DNA damage-binding protein 2. XPF/Cockayne syndrome is caused by homozygous or compound heterozygous mutation in the *ERCC4* gene. XPG/Cockayne syndromes are caused by homozygous or compound heterozygous mutation in the ERCC5 gene. Xeroderma pigmentosum variant (XPV) is caused by mutations in the DNA polymerase eta gene.

Treatment

There is no specific treatment. However, protective measures such as systematic sun protection (e.g., sunscreen, long-sleeved clothing, and broad-brimmed hats) and frequent cancer screenings. Skin cancers are treated according to standard of care.

▶ MISCELLANEOUS HEREDITARY NEUROPATHIES

GIANT AXONAL NEUROPATHY

Clinical Features

Giant axonal neuropathy presents in the first decade of life with progressive gait difficulty.[206–218] Children who are affected appear to have a normal birth and meet early motor milestones. However, around the age of 2 years, they begin to exhibit signs of imbalance. By about 4 years of age, signs of a sensorimotor polyneuropathy and cerebellar ataxia are evident. Cognitive impair ensues. Sensory examination reveals a decrease in all sensory modalities in a length-dependent distribution along with mild distal muscle atrophy and weakness. Muscle stretch reflexes are usually absent in the legs and reduced in the arms, while extensor plantar responses are appreciated. Truncal and limb ataxias are evident. Pes cavus is evident in most affected individuals and all have characteristic curly or kinky hair.[217]

Laboratory Features

NCS reveal absent or reduced amplitudes of SNAPs and CMAPs with normal or slightly prolonged distal latencies and mildly slow CVs.[212,214–218] Diagnosis is confirmed by genetic testing (see below). Brain MRI shows cerebral and cerebellar white matter abnormalities.[217]

Histopathology

Nerve biopsies demonstrate loss of myelinated axons with segmental demyelination and, notably, giant axonal swellings.[206–212] On EM, these axonal swellings consist of abnormal accumulations of densely packed intermediate-sized neurofilaments that are most prominent distally and in the paranodal regions. Similar giant axons occur in toxic neuropathies caused by exposure to *n*-hexane, methyl *n*-butyl ketone, acrylamide, carbon disulfide, 2,5-hexanedione, and triorthocresyl (tri-*o*-cresyl) phosphate.

Molecular Genetics and Pathogenesis

Giant axonal neuropathy is caused by mutations in the gigaxonin gene (*GAN*) located on chromosome 16q24.[217–219] Gigaxonin is a cytoskeletal protein, which may be important in actin–cytoskeletal interactions.

Treatment

There is no specific treatment.

INFANTILE NEUROAXONAL DYSTROPHY

Clinical Features

Infantile neuroaxonal dystrophy presents in the first or second year of life, with progressive psychomotor regression, visual loss, generalized hypotonia, and weakness.[220–224] Those children who eventually ambulate usually lose the ability to walk independently over time due to progressive weakness, spasticity, and ataxia. Some affected children develop complex partial or generalized tonic–clonic seizures. Muscle stretch reflexes are usually reduced. Optic atrophy is apparent on funduscopic examination.

Laboratory Features

MRI scans reveal cerebellar and cerebral atrophy, hyperintensity on T2-weighted images in the periventricular white matter and dentate nuclei, and hypointense T2 images in the globus pallidus and substantia nigra.[221] The optic chiasm is often thin. Motor and sensory NCS may reveal decreased amplitudes and mild to moderate slowing of CV.[220–223] EMG demonstrates active denervation and features of a motor neuron disease. Visual-evoked potentials are unobtainable or have prolonged latencies.

Histopathology

Axonal swellings with spheroid bodies can be found on biopsies of peripheral nerves, muscle, skin, and conjunctiva.[220–223]

Molecular Genetics and Pathogenesis

Infantile neuroaxonal dystrophy is usually caused by mutations in *PLA2G6*, which encodes for encoding phospholipase A2.[224] This enzyme catalyzes the hydrolysis of the sn-2 acyl-ester bonds in phospholipids, leading to the release of arachidonic acid and other fatty acids. In addition, mutations in the gene, *NAGA*, which encodes for the lysosomal enzyme, α-*N*-acetyl-galactosaminidase, has been identified in some cases that is also known as Schindler disease.[221,223]

Treatment

There is no specific medical treatment.

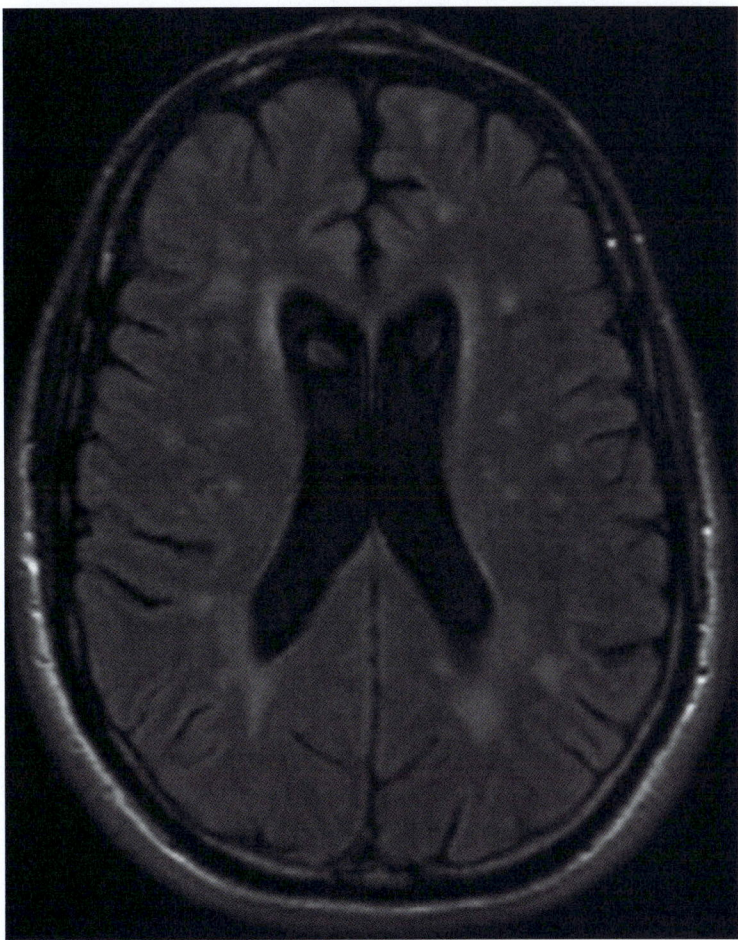

Figure 12-6. MRI of brain in a patient with adult polyglucosan body disease reveals scattered hyperintense white matter abnormalities fluid-attenuated inversion recovery sequences.

ADULT POLYGLUCOSAN BODY DISEASE

Clinical Features

Adult polyglucosan body disease (APBD) is allelic to glycogen storage disease type IV [glycogen branching enzyme (GBE) deficiency] that typically manifests as a myopathy and is discussed in Chapter 29. In contrast, APBD usually presents in adults as progressive upper and lower motor neuron loss, sensory nerve involvement, cerebellar ataxia, neurogenic bladder, and dementia.[225–236] Occasionally, polyglucosan body neuropathy manifests in children. There is a predilection for APBD in the Ashkenazi population.

Laboratory Features

The serum creatine kinase level (CK) may be normal or slightly elevated. An axonal sensorimotor neuropathy is apparent on NCS while the EMG abnormalities reflect a superimposed polyradiculopathy.[225,228,230] APBD may be diagnosed by demonstrating a reduction of GBE activity in leukocytes or cultured skin fibroblasts. MRI of the brain reveals hyperintense white matter abnormalities on T2- and fluid-attenuated inversion recovery sequences predominantly in the periventricular regions, the posterior limb of the internal capsule, the external capsule, the pyramidal tracts, and medial lemniscus of the pons and medulla (Fig. 12-6).[225]

Histopathology

Routine light and EM reveals deposition of varying amounts of finely granular and filamentous polysaccharide (polyglucosan bodies) in the CNS, peripheral nerves (axons and Schwann cells), and skin (Figs. 12-7 and 12-8).[225,226,228,229,234] These polyglucosan bodies are PAS positive and diastase resistant, suggesting the accumulation of polysaccharides other than glycogen. They are not specific for this disorder and can be seen occasionally in nerve biopsies from patients with other diseases. This polysaccharide resembles amylopectin in that it has longer than normal peripheral chains and few branch points. Autopsy studies have demonstrated

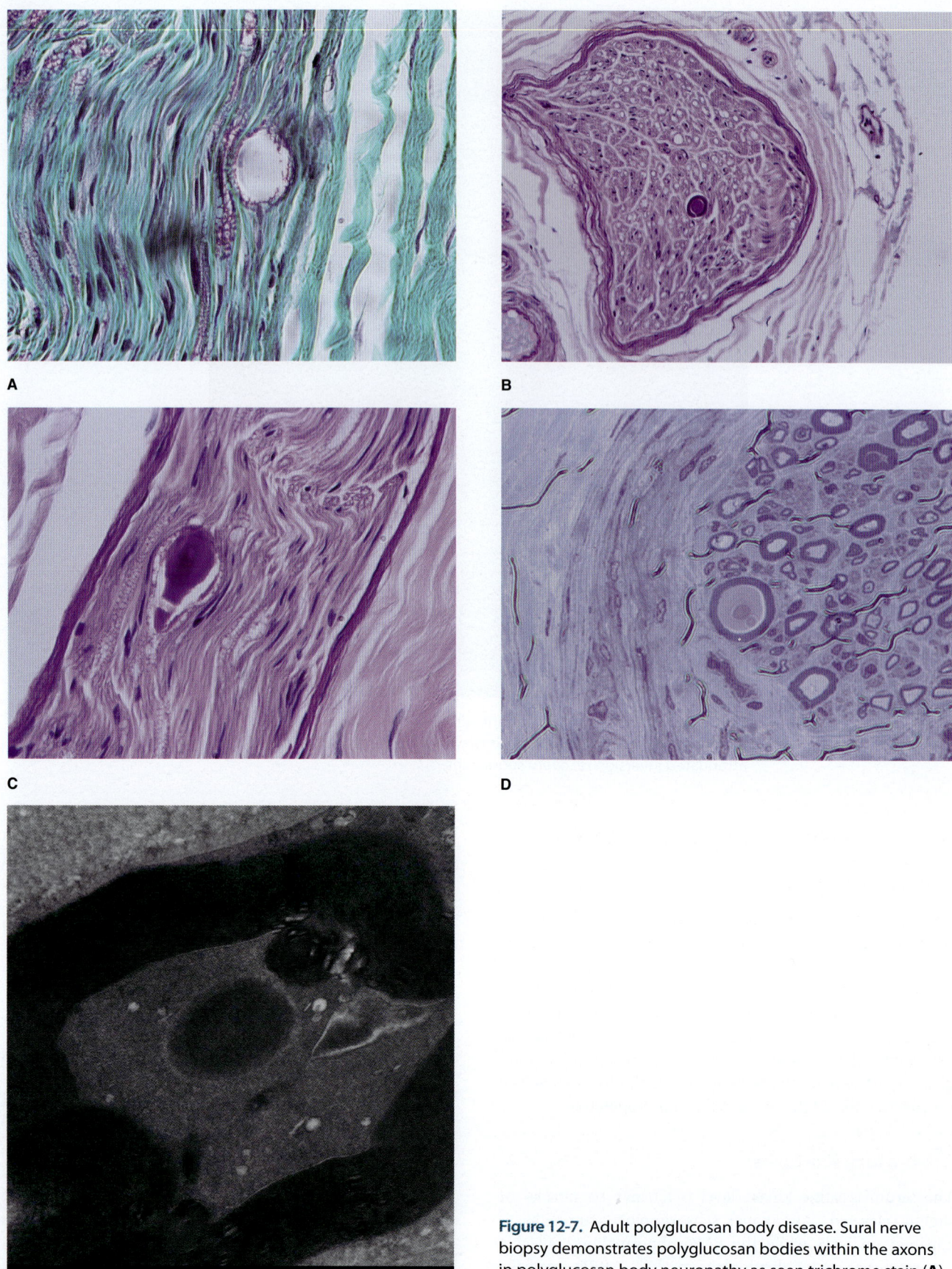

Figure 12-7. Adult polyglucosan body disease. Sural nerve biopsy demonstrates polyglucosan bodies within the axons in polyglucosan body neuropathy as seen trichrome stain (**A**), PAS in cross-section (**B**), PAS in longitudinal section (**C**), on semithin section (**D**), and electron microscopy (**E**).

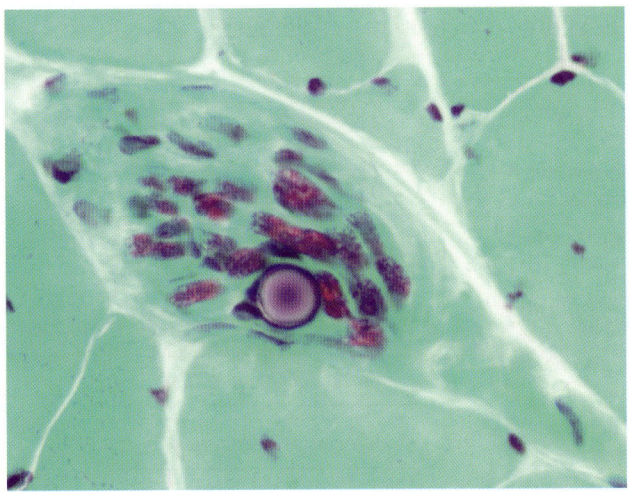
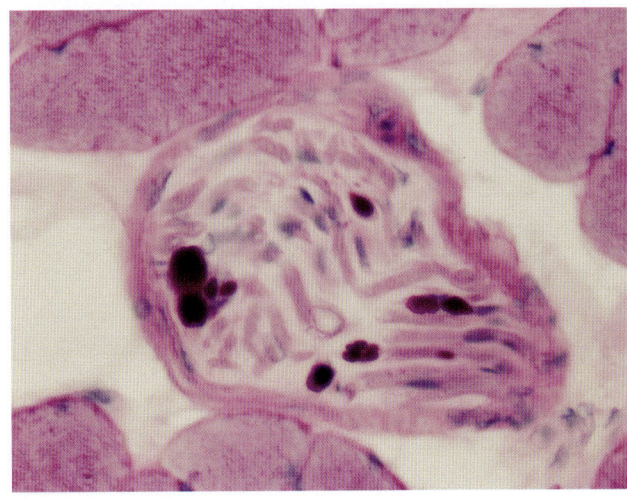

Figure 12-8. Polyglucosan bodies can also be appreciated in nerve twigs on muscle biopsy, modified Gomori trichrome (**A**) and PAS (**B**).

abnormal polysaccharide material in the motor neurons in the brainstem and spinal cord.[226,229]

Molecular Genetics and Pathogenesis

Polyglucosan body neuropathy is inherited in an autosomal-recessive manner and is caused by mutations in the glycogen branching enzyme gene (*GBE1*).[225,231,233,235] The mechanism by which the abnormal accumulation of polysaccharide results in nerve damage is not known.

Treatment

There is no specific medical treatment.

PORPHYRIA

Clinical Features

Porphyria is a group of inherited disorders caused by defects in heme biosynthesis. There are three forms of porphyria that are associated with peripheral neuropathy as well as CNS abnormalities: acute intermittent porphyria (AIP), hereditary coproporphyria (HCP), and variegate porphyria (VP) (Fig. 12-9).[1,237–247] The acute neurological manifestations are quite similar; however, a photosensitive rash is seen with HCP and VP but not in AIP. Attacks of porphyria can be precipitated by certain drugs (usually those metabolized by the P450 system), hormonal changes (e.g., pregnancy and luteal phase of the menstrual cycle), and dietary restrictions.

An acute attack of porphyria is often heralded by acute abdominal pain. Subsequently, patients may develop agitation, hallucinations, or seizures. Several days later, back and leg pain followed by weakness can occur and may mimic Guillain–Barré syndrome. Motor involvement can be asymmetric and can preferentially involve either proximal or distal muscles, or either the arms or legs. Cranial nerves can also be affected, leading to facial weakness and dysphagia. Sensory impairment may be difficult to determine if the patient is encephalopathic. Muscle stretch reflexes are often reduced. Autonomic dysfunction manifested by signs of sympathetic overactivity (e.g., pupillary dilatation, tachycardia, and hypertension) is common. Constipation, urinary retention, and incontinence can also be seen. Recovery is usually good, provided treatment is instituted rapidly to prevent excessive amounts of axonal damage.

Laboratory Features

The CSF protein can be normal or mildly elevated. Liver function tests and blood counts are usually normal. Some patients are hyponatremic due to inappropriate secretion of antidiuretic hormone. The urine may appear brownish in color secondary to the high concentration of porphyrin metabolites. The diagnosis is made by evaluating the urine or stool for the accumulating intermediary precursors of heme (i.e., δ-aminolevulinic acid, porphobilinogen, uroporphobilinogen, coproporphyrinogen, and protoporphyrinogen).[196] The reduced activity of specific enzymes can also be measured in erythrocytes and leukocytes. Genetic testing is available to confirm the specific defect.

Sensory NCS usually demonstrate normal NCVs and distal sensory latencies, but the amplitudes may be slightly reduced, although not to the same degree as the CMAPs are reduced.[237,240,241,243,244,246–251] Motor NCVs are only mildly reduced or normal, and distal motor latencies are normal or only slightly prolonged. The primary abnormality on NCS is the marked reduction in CMAP amplitudes.[237,240,241,243,244,246–251] Needle EMG demonstrates primarily a reduced recruitment, fibrillation potentials, and positive sharp waves.

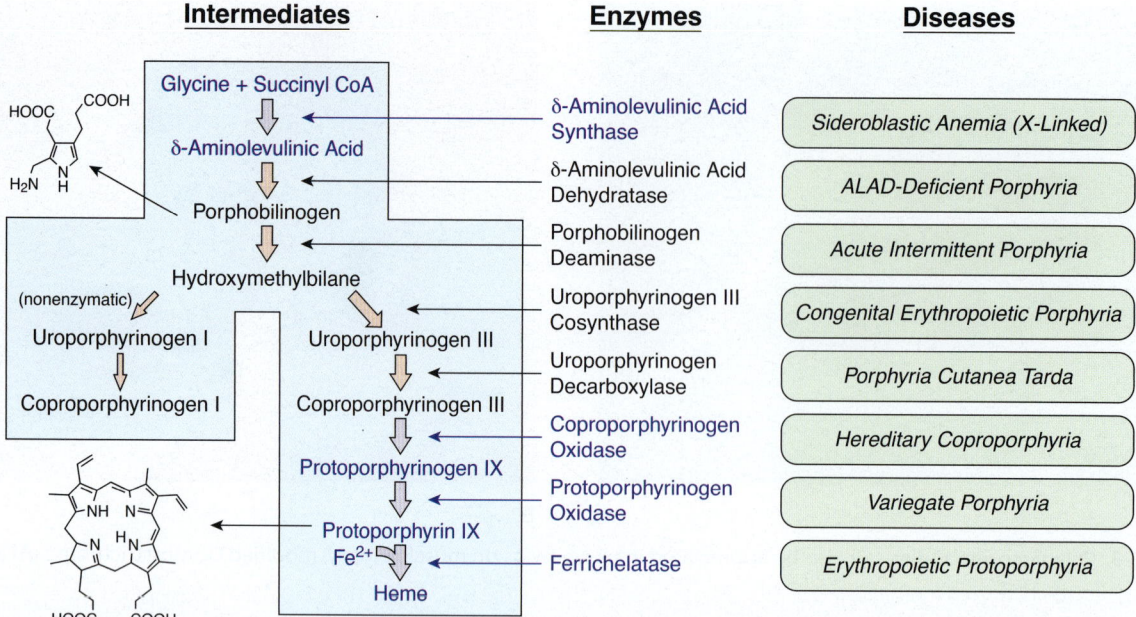

Figure 12-9. Porphyria pathway. Schematic representation of hepatic heme synthesis pathway. Defects in specific enzymes at various intermediate steps (boxes) controlling the synthesis of heme can lead to different clinical forms of porphyria. All of the noted diseases (boxes) have the potential to result in a neuropathy except porphyria cutanea tarda.

Histopathology

Axonal degeneration is apparent on nerve biopsies.

Molecular Genetics and Pathogenesis

The porphyrias are inherited in an autosomal-dominant fashion.[237] AIP is associated with porphobilinogen deaminase deficiency, HCP is caused by defects in coproporphyrin oxidase, and VP is associated with protoporphyrinogen oxidase (Fig. 12-9). The pathogenesis of the neuropathy is not completely understood. The biochemical alterations in heme production may affect the production of energy via effects on oxidative phosphorylation in the mitochondria. The inability to detoxify various drugs in the liver may have secondary toxic effects on the nervous system. Finally, some studies suggest that porphyrin precursor neurotoxicity may arise due to the activation of transcription factors pivotal in regulating cell survival.[252,253]

Treatment

Patients should be treated with hematin and glucose to reduce the accumulation of heme precursors.[237] Intravenous glucose is started at a rate of 10–20 g/h. If there is no improvement within 24 hours, intravenous hematin 2–5 mg/kg per day for 3–14 days should be given. This hematin dose can be infused over a 30–60-minute period. Drugs that can precipitate the acute porphyric attack should be avoided.

Both the FDA and EMA have approved givosiran, a small interfering RNA (siRNA) that neutralizes excess aminolevulinic acid mRNA in hepatocytes, for treatment of patients with recurrent attacks of AIP. Randomized, placebo-controlled trials and open-label extension trials demonstrated that givosiran 2.5 mg/kg subcutaneously per month led to reduced attack frequency, better daily pain scores for pain, improved quality of life lower levels of urinary ALA and porphobilinogen, and fewer days of hemin than placebo.[254,255]

▶ FAMILIAL AMYLOID POLYNEUROPATHIES

Although frequently clinically indistinguishable from primary amyloidosis, familial amyloid polyneuropathy (FAP) is phenotypically and genetically heterogeneous. It is caused by mutations in the genes for transthyretin (TTR), apolipoprotein A1, or gelsolin.[1,256–280] Diagnosis of familial amyloidosis is made by detection of amyloid deposition in abdominal fat pad, rectal, or nerve biopsies or with genetic testing (Fig. 12-10). The amyloid deposits may stain for TTR, apolipoprotein A1, or gelsolin, but not light chains as seen in AL amyloidosis.

Nerve biopsies in the different forms of FAP reveal findings similar to that seen in AL amyloidosis. Amyloid deposition can be multifocal or diffuse within the endoneurium, epineurium, or perineurium, as well as around blood vessels in autonomic ganglia and in peripheral nerves.[275] Importantly, in approximately 50% of FAP, nerve biopsies do not demonstrate amyloid deposits perhaps secondary to sampling error.[281] Immunohistochemistry and even laser microdissection and mass spectrometric-based proteomic analysis can be used to distinguish specific types of amyloid.

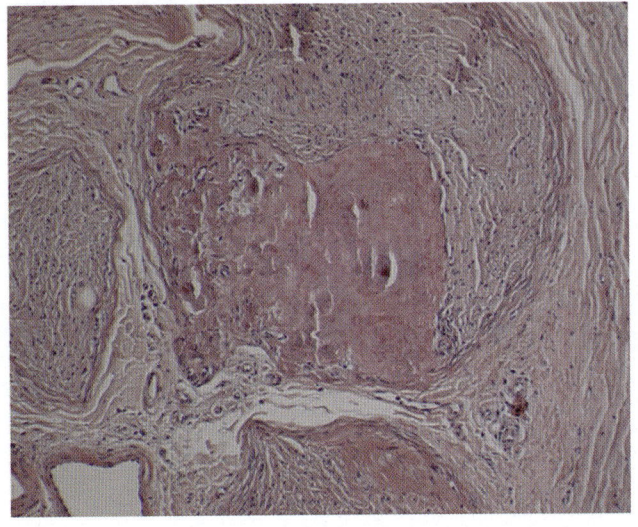
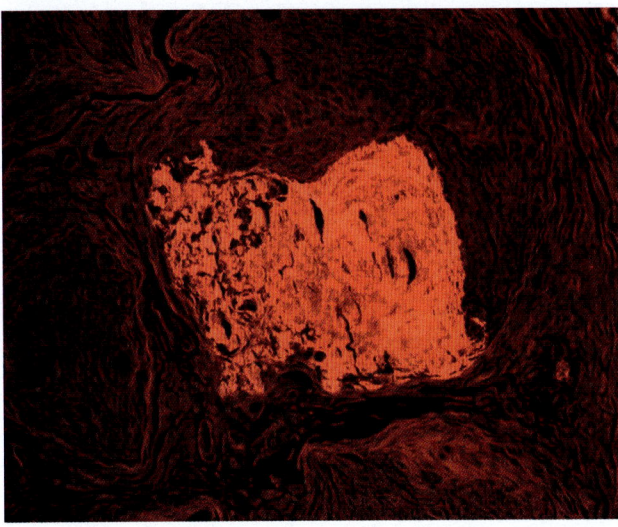
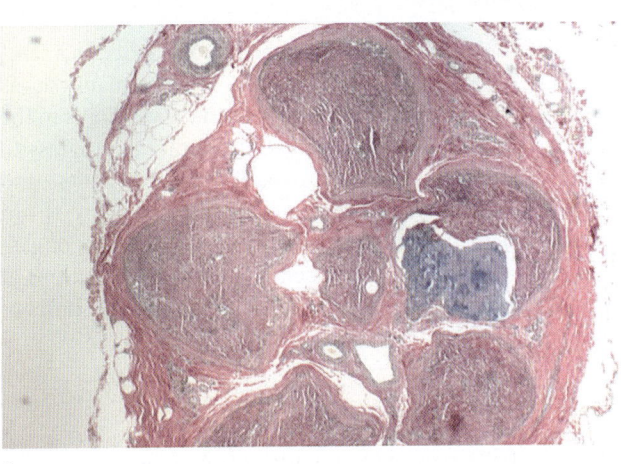

Figure 12-10. Familial amyloid polyneuropathy (ATTRv). Sural nerve biopsy in a patient with mutations in the transthyretin gene (*TTR*) reveals large globular deposition of amyloid in the endoneurium that is appreciated using Congo red stain. (**A**) The amyloid stains pinkish-red under routine light microscope without polarization, and under rhodamine fluorescence (**B**) the amyloid deposition appears bright red. The amyloid deposit stains blue with Alcian blue (**C**).

There is a loss of myelinated nerve fibers, particularly small myelinated and unmyelinated nerve fibers. These deposits encroach upon the nerve fibers, resulting in axonal degeneration and segmental demyelination. The clinical features, histopathology, and electrophysiological studies reveal abnormalities consistent with a generalized or multifocal, predominantly axonal but occasionally demyelinating, sensorimotor polyneuropathy.[265,271–283] Cerebrospinal fluid can reveal elevated protein levels with normal cell count again mimicking chronic inflammatory demyelinating polyneuropathy (CIDP). The pathogenic bases for the FAP neuropathies are likely similar to that noted with AL neuropathy.

TTR-RELATED AMYLOIDOSIS (FAP TYPES I AND II)

Clinical Features

The majority of patients with FAP have mutations in the *TTR* gene. There appear to be two somewhat different clinical phenotypes associated with TTR-related amyloidosis: FAP I and a less severe FAP II. These are now classified as "ATTRv" to distinguish from sporadic senile or wild-type ATTRwt. FAP I was originally reported in the Portuguese,[172] but it affects multiple ethnic groups with particularly large foci in Sweden and Japan.[1,273,276–278,284–288] Patients usually develop insidious onset of numbness and painful paresthesia in the distal lower limbs in the third to fourth decade of life, although some patients develop the disorder later in life.[254] Pain and thermal sensation are the most common modalities affected. Carpal tunnel syndrome is uncommon. Autonomic involvement can be severe, leading to postural hypotension, constipation or persistent diarrhea, erectile dysfunction, and impaired sweating. Distal and later proximal muscle atrophy and weakness develop over time such that the patients may be mistaken for having CIDP.[265,283] Occasional cranial neuropathies, leading to pupillary changes, decreased saliva secretion, diminished facial (including corneal) sensation, dysphonia, dysphagia, and facial weakness occurs. Amyloid deposition also occurs in the heart, kidneys, liver, and the corneas. Patients usually die by 10–15 years after the onset of symptoms from cardiac failure or complications from malnutrition.

A milder form of TTR-associated FAP (type II FAP) was initially described in families in Indiana and Switzerland and is characterized by the development of carpal tunnel syndrome and later by a mild generalized sensorimotor polyneuropathy.[1,276] Although erectile dysfunction can be seen, severe autonomic dysfunction is unusual. As with FAP I, vitreous opacities may be appreciated. Although there can be systemic involvement, severe nephropathy or cardiomyopathy usually does not develop. Thus, most patients with FAP II have a relatively long survival, with little morbidity related to the amyloidosis. The symptoms of carpal tunnel syndrome can be relieved with surgical decompression.

Molecular Genetics and Pathogenesis

More than 100 different mutations within the *TTR* gene located on chromosome 18q11.2–12.1 have been associated with FAP types I and II.[1,276,282,286,289] A mutation involving a methionine to valine substitution at position 30 (Val30Met) in the *TTR* gene is the most common mutation associated with type I FAP, while serine substitutions at position 84 and histidine at position 58 are the most common mutations associated with FAP type II. There can be variability in the age of onset and severity even within families with the Val30Met mutations. TTR functions as a transport protein for vitamin A and thyroxin. Over 90% of the body's TTR is synthesized in the liver. The amino acid substitutions lead to the formation of the β-pleated sheet structure of the protein and its resistance to degradation by proteases, thus its amyloidogenic properties.

Treatment

Because the liver produces much of the body's TTR, liver transplantation has been used to treat FAP related to TTR mutations. Serum TTR levels decrease after transplantation and improvement in clinical and neurophysiological features has been reported.[283,286,289,290] However, abnormal TTR can continue to be synthesized in the CNS (by the choroid plexus) and within the eyes, potentially resulting in progressive deficits from local accumulation in these areas.

Randomized, placebo-controlled trials of both tafamidis 20 mg orally daily and diflunisal 250 mg orally twice daily have been demonstrated to slightly reduce progression of TTR-associated polyneuropathy compared to placebo.[291–293] Both work by binding to mutant misfolded TTR and preventing their aggregation in amyloid fibrils.

Gene silencers including several small interfering RNAs and antisense oligonucleotides have been should to be beneficial in clinical trials and are now FDA approved. These include patisiran 0.3 mg per kilogram intravenous every 3 weeks,[294,295] vutrisiran 25 mg subcutaneous every 3 months,[296] eplontersen 45 mg subcutaneous every 4 weeks, and inotersen 300 mg subcutaneous weekly.[297] These drugs block expression of both mutant and wild type TTR reducing amyloid precursor protein synthesis and have been found to be useful in reducing progression of the associated neuropathy in the familial form TTR FAP.[291] Mild to moderate infusion-related reactions occur in approximately 20% of patients receiving patisiran. Vitamin A deficiency has been reported with vutrisiran, so supplementation at the recommended daily allowance (RDA) of vitamin A is advised for patients taking this medication. Rare patients treated with inotersen develop severe glomerulonephritis or thrombocytopenia as adverse complications, so frequent monitoring of platelets and renal function are required.

APOLIPOPROTEIN A1-RELATED AMYLOIDOSIS (TYPE III FAP OR VAN ALLEN TYPE)

Clinical Features

FAP type III was originally described by Van Allen in a family from Iowa.[298,299] The neuropathy usually manifests as numbness and painful dysesthesias in the lower limbs in the fourth decade of life. Gradually, the symptoms progress to the distal upper limbs and proximal muscle weakness and atrophy develops. Although autonomic neuropathy is not severe, some patients develop diarrhea, constipation, or gastroparesis. Most patients die from systemic complications of amyloidosis (e.g., renal failure) 12–15 years after the onset of the neuropathy.

Molecular Genetics and Pathogenesis

FAP type III is caused by mutations leading to arginine for glycine substitution at position 26 (Arg26Gly) in the apolipoprotein A1 gene on chromosome 11q23–qter.[300] Apolipoprotein A1 is a major component of high-density lipoproteins. As with TTR mutations, the amino acid substitution probably impairs its degradation by proteases.

Treatment

There are no specific medical therapies.

GELSOLIN-RELATED AMYLOIDOSIS (FAP TYPE IV, FINNISH)

Clinical Features

FAP IV was initially described in Finland and is characterized by the combination of lattice corneal dystrophy, multiple cranial neuropathies (e.g., facial palsies and bulbar weakness), and cutis laxa.[301–305] Onset of symptoms is usually in the third decade of life. Over time, a mild generalized sensorimotor polyneuropathy develops. Autonomic dysfunction does not occur. Cutis laxa manifests as loose or hanging skin affecting the scalp and face.

Histopathology

Autopsy studies have demonstrated a different distribution of amyloid deposition in FAP type IV than the other types of amyloidosis.[306] Histological, immunohistochemical, and electron microscopic studies reveal deposition of gelsolin amyloid, particularly in the vascular walls and perineurial sheaths. Nerve roots are more severely affected than distal nerves. The marked proximal nerve involvement with gelsolin-related angiopathy is a characteristic feature of FAP type IV. There was also preferential large fiber loss, not generally seen in other forms of amyloid neuropathy.

Molecular Genetics and Pathogenesis

Type IV amyloidosis is caused by mutations in the gelsolin gene.[307-309] Gelsolin is an actin-binding protein found in plasma, leukocytes, and other cells. The resultant mutations and amino acid substitutions lead to a charge change on the protein, which may render the molecule resistant to proteases.

Treatment

There are no specific medical therapies. However, facial plastic surgical procedures can help fix the cosmetic problems associated with cutis laxa.[301]

▶ SUMMARY

These hereditary neuropathies are uncommon but need to be considered in the right clinical context. Because of the hereditary nature of these neuropathies, some of which are quite devastating, diagnosis is important, particularly for genetic counseling. With the exception of Fabry disease in which ERT is available and perhaps ALD/AMN in which patients may be treated with Lorenzo oil, most of these disorders can only be treated symptomatically.

REFERENCES

1. Klein CJ. Charcot-Marie-Tooth disease and other hereditary neuropathies. *Continuum (Minneap Minn)*. 2020;26(5):1224–1256.
2. Cruz Martinez A, Ferrer MT, Fueyo E, Galdos L. Peripheral neuropathy detected on electrophysiological study as first manifestation of metachromatic leukodystrophy in infancy. *J Neurol Neurosurg Psychiatry*. 1975;38:169–174.
3. Dayan AD. Peripheral neuropathy of metachromatic leukodystrophy: observations on segmental demyelination and remyelination and the intracellular distribution of sulphatide. *J Neurol Neurosurg Psychiatry*. 1967;30:311–318.
4. Fullerton PM. Peripheral nerve conduction in metachromatic leukodystrophy (Sulphatide lipidosis). *J Neurol Neurosurg Psychiatry*. 1964;27:100–105.
5. Hahn AF, Gordon BA, Hinton GG, Gilbert JJ. A variant form of metachromatic leukodystrophy without arylsulfatase deficiency. *Ann Neurol*. 1982;12:33–36.
6. Martin JJ, Ceuterick C, Mercelis R, Joris C. Pathology of peripheral nerves in metachromatic leukodystrophy: a comparative study of ten cases. *J Neurol Sci*. 1982;53:95–112.
7. Shapiro LJ, Aleck KA, Kaback MM, et al. Metachromatic leukodystrophy without arylsulfatase deficiency. *Pediatr Res*. 1979;13:1179–1181.
8. Yudell A, Gomez MR, Lambert EH, Dockerty MB. The neuropathy of sulfatide lipidosis (metachromatic leukodystrophy). *Neurology*. 1967;17:103–111.
9. Cameron CL, Kang PB, Burns TM, Darras BT, Jones HR Jr. Multifocal slowing of nerve conduction in metachromatic leukodystrophy. *Muscle Nerve*. 2004;29(4):531–536.
10. Coulter-Mackie MB, Applegarth DA, Toone JR, Gagnier L, Anzarut AR, Hendson G. Isolated peripheral neuropathy in atypical metachromatic leukodystrophy: a recurrent mutation. *Can J Neurol Sci*. 2002;29:159–163.
11. Comabella M, Waye JS, Raguer N, et al. Late-onset metachromatic leukodystrophy clinically presenting as isolated peripheral neuropathy: compound heterozygosity for the IVS2+1G->A mutation and a newly identified missense mutation (Thr408Ile) in a Spanish family. *Ann Neurol*. 2001;50:108–112.
12. Bindu PS, Mahadevan A, Taly AB, Christopher R, Gayathri N, Shankar SK. Peripheral neuropathy in metachromatic leucodystrophy. A study of 40 cases from south India. *J Neurol Neurosurg Psychiatry*. 2005;76:1698–1701.
13. Kararizou E, Karandreas N, Davaki P, Davou R, Vassilopoulos D. Polyneuropathies in teenagers: a clinicopathological study of 45 cases. *Neuromuscul Disord*. 2006;16:304–307.
14. MacFaul R, Cavanagh N, Lake BD, Stephens R, Whitfield AE. Metachromatic leucodystrophy: review of 38 cases. *Arch Dis Child*. 1982;57:168–175.
15. Beerepoot S, Nierkens S, Boelens JJ, Lindemans C, Bugiani M, Wolf NI. Peripheral neuropathy in metachromatic leukodystrophy: current status and future perspective. *Orphanet J Rare Dis*. 2019;14(1):240.
16. De Silva KL, Pearce J. Neuropathy of metachromatic leucodystrophy. *J Neurol Neurosurg Psychiatry*. 1973;36(1):30–33.
17. Fumagalli F, Zambon AA, Rancoita PMV, et al. Metachromatic leukodystrophy: a single-center longitudinal study of 45 patients. *J Inherit Metab Dis*. 2021;44(5):1151–1164.
18. Wulff CH, Trojaborg W. Adult metachromatic leukodystrophy: neurophysiologic findings. *Neurology*. 1985;35:1776–1778.
19. Pilz H, Hopf HC. A preclinical case of late adult metachromatic leukodystrophy? Manifestation only with lipid abnormalities in urine, enzyme deficiency and decrease of nerve conduction velocity. *J Neurol Neurosurg Psychiatry*. 1972;35:360–364.
20. Thomas PK, King RH, Kocen RS, Brett EM. Comparative ultrastructural observations on peripheral nerve abnormalities in the late infantile, juvenile and late onset forms of metachromatic leukodystrophy. *Acta Neuropathol (Berl)*. 1977;39:237–245.
21. Raina A, Nair SS, Nagesh C, Thomas B, Nair M, Sundaram S. Electroneurography and advanced neuroimaging profile in pediatric-onset metachromatic leukodystrophy. *J Pediatr Neurosci*. 2019;14(2):70–75.
22. Grimm A, Schaffer E, Just J, et al. Thickening of the peripheral nerves in metachromatic leukodystrophy. *J Neurol Sci*. 2016;368:399–401.
23. Gieselmann V, Zlotogora J, Harris A, Wenger DA, Morris CP. Molecular genetics of metachromatic leukodystrophy. *Hum Mutat*. 1994;4:233–242.

24. Krivit W, Peters C, Shapiro EG. Bone marrow transplantation as effective therapy of central nervous system disease in globoid cell leukodystrophy, metachromatic leukodystrophy, adrenoleukodystrophy, mannosidosis, fucosidosis, aspartylglucosaminuria, Hurler, Maroteaux–Lamy, Sly syndromes, and Gaucher disease type III. *Curr Opin Neurol.* 1999;12:167–176.
25. Shaimardanova AA, Chulpanova DS, Solovyeva VV, et al. Metachromatic leukodystrophy: diagnosis, modeling, and treatment approaches. *Front Med (Lausanne).* 2020;7:576221.
26. Darras BT, Kwan ES, Gilmore HE, Ehrenberg BL, Rabe EF. Globoid cell leukodystrophy: cranial computed tomography and evoked potentials. *J Child Neurol.* 1986;1:126–130.
27. Dunn HG, Lake BD, Dolman CL, Wilson J. The neuropathy of Krabbe's infantile cerebral sclerosis (globoid cell leucodystrophy). *Brain.* 1969;92:329–344.
28. Dunn HG, Dolman CL, Farrell DF, Tischler B, Hasinoff C, Woolf LI. Krabbe's leukodystrophy without globoid cells. *Neurology.* 1976;26:1035–1041.
29. Gutmann L, Hogan G, Chou SM. The peripheral neuropathy of Krabbe's (globoid) leukodystrophy. *Electroencephalogr Clin Neurophysiol.* 1969;27:715–716.
30. Adachi H, Ishihara K, Tachibana H, et al. Adult-onset Krabbe disease presenting with an isolated form of peripheral neuropathy. *Muscle Nerve.* 2016;54:152–7.
31. Hogan GR, Gutmann L, Chou SM. The peripheral neuropathy of Krabbe's (globoid) leukodystrophy. *Neurology.* 1969;19:1094–1100.
32. Lieberman JS, Oshtory M, Taylor RG, Dreyfus PM. Perinatal neuropathy as an early manifestation of Krabbe's leukodystrophy. *Arch Neurol.* 1980;37:446–447.
33. Loonen MC, Van Diggelsen OP, Janse HC, Kleijer WJ, Arts WF. Late-onset globoid cell leukodystrophy (Krabbe's disease). Clinical and genetic delineation of two forms and their relation to the early infantile form. *Neuropediatrics.* 1985;16:137–142.
34. Thomas PK, Halpern JP, King RH, Patrick D. Galactosylceramide lipidosis: novel presentation as a slowly progressive spinocerebellar degeneration. *Ann Neurol.* 1984;16:618–620.
35. Korn-Lubetzki I, Dor-Wollman T, Soffer D, Raas-Rothschild A, Hurvitz H, Nevo Y. Early peripheral nervous system manifestations of infantile Krabbe disease. *Pediatr Neurol.* 2003;28:115–118.
36. Siddiqi ZA, Sanders DB, Massey JM. Peripheral neuropathy in Krabbe disease: electrodiagnostic findings. *Neurology.* 2006;67:263–267.
37. Debs R, Froissart R, Aubourg P, et al. Krabbe disease in adults: phenotypic and genotypic update from a series of 11 cases and a review. *J Inherit Metab Dis.* 2013;36:859–868.
38. Malandrini A, D'Eramo C, Palmeri S, et al. Peripheral neuropathy in late-onset Krabbe disease: Report of three cases. *Neurol Sci.* 2013;34:79–83.
39. Marks HG, Scavina MT, Kolodny EH, Palmieri M, Childs J. Krabbe's disease presenting as a peripheral neuropathy. *Muscle Nerve.* 1997;20:1024–1028.
40. Sato JI, Tokumoto H, Kurohara K, et al. Adult-onset Krabbe disease with homozygous T1853 C mutation in the galactocerebroside gene. Unusual MRI findings of corticospinal tract demyelination. *Neurology.* 1997;49:1392–1399.
41. Jardim LB, Giugliani R, Pires RF, et al. Protracted course of Krabbe disease in an adult patient bearing a novel mutation. *Hum Mol Genet.* 1999;56:1014–1017.
42. Sabatelli M, Quaranta L, Madia F, et al. Peripheral neuropathy with hypomyelinating features in adult-onset Krabbe's disease. *Neuromuscul Disord.* 2002;12:386–391.
43. Adachi H, Ishihara K, Tachibana H, et al. Adult-onset Krabbe disease presenting with an isolated form of peripheral neuropathy. *Muscle Nerve.* 2016;54(1):152–157.
44. Matsumoto R, Oka N, Nagahama Y, Akiguchi I, Kimura J. Peripheral neuropathy in late-onset Krabbe's disease: histochemical and ultrastructural findings. *Acta Neuropathol (Berl).* 1996;92:635–639.
45. Krivit W, Shapiro EG, Peters C, et al. Hematopoietic stem cell transplantation in globoid-cell leukodystrophy. *N Engl J Med.* 1998;338:1119–1126.
46. Siddiqi ZA, Sanders DB, Massey JM. Peripheral neuropathy in Krabbe disease: effect of hematopoietic stem cell transplantation. *Neurology.* 2006;67:268–272.
47. Fukuhara N, Suzuki M, Fujita N, Tsubaki T. Fabry's disease on the mechanism of the peripheral nerve involvement. *Acta Neuropathol (Berl).* 1975;33:9–21.
48. Kocen RS, Thomas PK. Peripheral nerve involvement in Fabry's disease. *Arch Neurol.* 1970;22:81–88.
49. Ohnishi A, Dyck PJ. Loss of small peripheral sensory neurons in Fabry's disease. Histologic and morphometric evaluation of cutaneous nerves, spinal ganglia, and posterior columns. *Arch Neurol.* 1974;31:120–127.
50. Sheth KJ, Swick HM. Peripheral nerve conduction in Fabry's disease. *Ann Neurol.* 1980;7:319–323.
51. Lacomis D, Roeske-Anderson L, Mathie L. Neuropathy and Fabry's disease. *Muscle Nerve.* 2005;31:102–107.
52. Dutsch M, Marthol H, Stemper B, Brys M, Haendl T, Hilz MJ. Small fiber dysfunction predominates in Fabry neuropathy. *J Clin Neurophysiol.* 2002;19(6):575–586.
53. Scott LJ, Griffin JW, Luciano C, et al. Quantitative analysis of epidermal innervation in Fabry disease. *Neurology.* 1999;52:1249–1254.
54. Luciano CA, Russell JW, Banerjee TK, et al. Physiological characterization of neuropathy in Fabry's disease. *Muscle Nerve.* 2002;26:622–629.
55. Toyooka K. Fabry disease. *Handb Clin Neurol.* 2013;115:629–642.
56. Üçeyler N, Kahn AK, Kramer D, et al. Impaired small fiber conduction in patients with Fabry disease: a neurophysiological case-control study. *BMC Neurol.* 2013;13:47.
57. Godel T, Bäumer P, Pham M, et al. Human dorsal root ganglion in vivo morphometry and perfusion in Fabry painful neuropathy. *Neurology.* 2017 Sep 19;89(12):1274–1282.
58. Godel T, Köhn A, Muschol N, et al. Dorsal root ganglia in vivo morphometry and perfusion in female patients with Fabry disease. *J Neurol.* 2018;265(11):2723–2729.
59. Üçeyler N, He L, Schönfeld D, et al. Small fibers in Fabry disease: baseline and follow-up data under enzyme replacement therapy. *J Peripher Nerv Syst.* 2011;16:304–314.
60. Bersano A, Lanfranconi S, Valcarenghi C, Bresolin N, Micieli G, Baron P. Neurological features of Fabry disease: clinical, pathophysiological aspects and therapy. *Acta Neurol Scand.* 2012;126:77–97.
61. Liguori R, Di Stasi V, Bugiardini E, et al. Small fiber neuropathy in female patients with Fabry disease. *Muscle Nerve.* 2010;41:409–412.
62. Schiffmann R. Fabry disease. *Handb Clin Neurol.* 2015;132:231–248.

63. Hilz MJ, Brys M, Marthol H, Stemper B, Dutsch M. Enzyme replacement therapy improves function of C-, Adelta-, and Abeta-nerve fibers in Fabry neuropathy. *Neurology*. 2004;62:1066–1072.
64. Schiffmann R, Floeter MK, Dambrosia JM, et al. Enzyme replacement therapy improves peripheral nerve and sweat function in Fabry disease. *Muscle Nerve*. 2003;28:703–710.
65. El Dib R, Gomaa H, Carvalho RP, et al. Enzyme replacement therapy for Anderson-Fabry disease. *Cochrane Database Syst Rev*. 2016;7(7):CD006663.
66. Keating GM. Agalsidase alfa: a review of its use in the management of Fabry disease. *BioDrugs*. 2012;26(5):335–354.
67. Arends M, Biegstraaten M, Wanner C, et al. Agalsidase alfa versus agalsidase beta for the treatment of Fabry disease: an international cohort study. *J Med Genet*. 2018;55(5):351–358.
68. Perretta F, Jaurretche S. Fabry Disease: switch from enzyme replacement therapy to oral chaperone migalastat: what do we know today? *Healthcare (Basel)*. 2023;11(4):449.
69. Hughes DA, Nicholls K, Shankar SP, et al. Oral pharmacological chaperone migalastat compared with enzyme replacement therapy in Fabry disease: 18-month results from the randomised phase III ATTRACT study. *J Med Genet*. 2017;54(4):288–296.
70. Aubourg P, Scotto J, Rocchiccioli F, Feldmann-Pautrat D, Robain O. Neonatal adrenoleukodystrophy. *J Neurol Neurosurg Psychiatry*. 1986;49:77–86.
71. Griffin JW, Goren E, Schaumburg H, Engel WK, Loriaux L. Adrenomyeloneuropathy: a probable variant of adrenoleukodystrophy. *Neurology*. 1977;27:1107–1113.
72. Martin JJ, Lowenthal A, Ceuterick C, Gacoms H. Adrenomyeloneuropathy: a report on two families. *J Neurol*. 1982;226:221–232.
73. Moser HW. Adrenoleukodystrophy: phenotype, genetics, pathophysiology, and therapy. *Brain*. 1997;120:1485–1508.
74. Vercruyssen A, Martin JJ, Mercelis R. Neurophysiologic studies in adrenomyeloneuropathy: a report of five cases. *J Neurol Sci*. 1982;56:327–336.
75. van Geel BM, Assies J, Wanders RJ, Barth PG. X linked adrenoleukodystrophy: clinical presentation, diagnosis, and therapy. *J Neurol Neurosurg Psychiatry*. 1997;63:4–14.
76. Moser H, Dubey P, Fatemi A. Progress in X-linked adrenoleukodystrophy. *Curr Opin Neurol*. 2004;17:263–269.
77. Engelen M, Barbier M, Dijkstra IME, et al. X-linked adrenoleukodystrophy in women: a cross-sectional cohort study. *Brain*. 2014;137(Pt 3):693–706.
78. Engelen M, van der Kooi AJ, Kemp S, et al. X-linked adrenomyeloneuropathy due to a novel missense mutation in the ABCD1 start codon presenting as demyelinating neuropathy. *J Peripher Nerv Syst*. 2011;16:353–355.
79. Chaudhry V, Moser HW, Cornblath DR. Nerve conduction studies in adrenomyeloneuropathy. *J Neurol Neurosurg Psychiatry*. 1996;61(2):181–185.
80. Moser AB, Kreiter N, Bezman L, et al. Plasma very long chain fatty acids in 3,000 peroxisomal disease patients and 29,000 controls. *Ann Neurol*. 1999;45:100–110.
81. Toifl K, Mamoli B, Waldhauser F. A combination of spastic paraparesis, polyneuropathy and adrenocortical insufficiency—a childhood form of adrenomyeloneuropathy? *J Neurol*. 1981;225:47–55.
82. van Geel BM, Koelman JH, Barth PG, Ongerboer de Visser BW. Peripheral nerve abnormalities in adrenomyeloneuropathy: a clinical and electrodiagnostic study. *Neurology*. 1996;46:112–118.
83. Powers JM, DeCiero DP, Cox C, et al. The dorsal root ganglia in adrenomyeloneuropathy: neuronal atrophy and abnormal mitochondria. *J Neuropathol Exp Neurol*. 2001;60:493–501.
84. Baumgartner MR, Poll-The BT, Verhoeven NM, et al. Clinical approach to inherited peroxisomal disorders. *Ann Neurol*. 1998;44:720–730.
85. Eichler F, Duncan C, Musolino PL, et al. Hematopoietic stem-cell gene therapy for cerebral adrenoleukodystrophy. *N Engl J Med*. 2017;377(17):1630–1638.
86. Engelen M, van Ballegoij WJC, Mallack EJ, et al. International recommendations for the diagnosis and management of patients with adrenoleukodystrophy: a consensus-based approach. *Neurology*. 2022;99(21):940–951.
87. Poulos A, Gibson R, Sharp P, Beckman K, Grattan-Smith P. Very long chain fatty acids in X-linked adrenoleukodystrophy brain after treatment with Lorenzo's oil. *Ann Neurol*. 1994;36:741–746.
88. Aubourg P, Adamsbaum C, Lavallard-Rousseau MC, et al. A two year trial of oleic acid and erucic acids ("Lorenzo's oil") as treatment for adrenomyeloneuropathy. *N Engl J Med*. 1993;329:745–752.
89. Van Geel B, Assies J, Haverkort EB, et al. Progression of abnormalities in adrenomyeloneuropathy and neurologically asymptomatic X-linked adrenoleukodystrophy despite treatment with "Lorenzo's oil." *J Neurol Neurosurg Psychiatry*. 1999;67:290–299.
90. Eldjarn L, Try K, Stokke O, et al. Dietary effects on serum-phytanic acid levels and on clinical manifestations in heredopathia atactica polyneuritiformis. *Lancet*. 1966;1:691–693.
91. Gibberd FB, Billimoria JD, Page NG, Retsas S. Heredopathia atactica polyneuritiformis (Refsum's disease) treated by diet and plasma exchange. *Lancet*. 1979;1:575–578.
92. Refsum S. Heredopathia atactica polyneuritiformis phytanic-acid storage disease, Refsum's disease: a biochemically well-defined disease with specific dietary treatment. *Arch Neurol*. 1981;38:605–606.
93. Steinberg D, Mize CE, Herndon JH, Fales HM, Engel WK, Vroom FQ. Phytanic acid in patients with Refsum's syndrome and response to dietary treatment. *Arch Intern Med*. 1970;125:75–87.
94. Tuck RR, McLeod JG. Retinitis pigmentosa, ataxia, and peripheral neuropathy. *J Neurol Neurosurg Psychiatry*. 1983;46:206–213.
95. Verny C, Prundean A, Nicolas G, et al. Refsum's disease may mimic familial Guillain Barre syndrome. *Neuromuscul Disord*. 2006;16:805–808.
96. Jansen GA, Waterham HR, Wanders RJA. Molecular basis of Refsum disease: sequence variations in phytanoyl-CoA hydroxylase (PHYH) and the PTS2 receptor (PEX7). *Hum Mutat*. 2004;23:209–218.
97. Jansen GA, Ofman R, Ferndinandusse S, et al. Refsum's disease is caused by mutations in the phytanoyl-CoA hydroxylase gene. *Nat Genet*. 1997;17:190–193.
98. Wierzbicki AS, Lloyd MD, Schofield CJ, Feher MD, Gibberd FB. Refsum's disease: a peroxisomal disorder affecting phytanic acid alpha-oxidation. *J Neurochem*. 2002;80:727–735.
99. Jansen GA, Hogenhout EM, Ferdinandusse S, et al. Human phytanoyl-CoA hydroxylase: resolution of the gene structure

and the molecular basis of Refsum's disease. *Hum Mol Genet.* 2000;9:1195–1200.
100. van den Brink DM, Brites P, Haasjes J, et al. Identification of PEX7 as the second gene involved in Refsum disease. *Am J Hum Genet.* 2003;72:471–477.
101. Dyck PJ, Ellefson RD, Yao JK, Herbert PN. Adult-onset of Tangier disease: 1. Morphometric and pathologic studies suggesting delayed degradation of neutral lipids after fiber degeneration. *J Neuropathol Exp Neurol.* 1978;37:119–137.
102. Engel WK, Dorman JD, Levy RI, Fredrickson DS. Neuropathy in Tangier disease. Alpha-Lipoprotein deficiency manifesting as familial recurrent neuropathy and intestinal lipid storage. *Arch Neurol.* 1967;17:1–9.
103. Gibbels E, Schaefer HE, Runne U, Schröder JM, Haupt WF, Assmann G. Severe polyneuropathy in Tangier's disease mimicking syringomyelia or leprosy. Clinical, biochemical, electrophysiological, and morphological evaluation, including electron microscopy of nerve, muscle, and skin biopsies. *J Neurol.* 1985;232:283–294.
104. Haas LF, Austad WI, Bergin JD. Tangier disease. *Brain.* 1974;97:351–354.
105. Kocen RS, LLoyd JK, Lascelles PT, Fosbrooke AS, Willims D. Familial alpha-lipoprotein deficiency (Tangier disease) with neurological abnormalities. *Lancet.* 1967;1:1341–1345.
106. Kocen RS, King RH, Thomas PK, Haas LF. Nerve biopsy findings in two cases of Tangier disease. *Acta Neuropathol (Berl).* 1973;26:317–326.
107. Pollock M, Nukada H, Frith RW, Simcock JP, Allpress S. Peripheral neuropathy in Tangier disease. *Brain.* 1983;106:911–928.
108. Zyss J, Béhin A, Couvert P, et al. Clinical and electrophysiological characteristics of neuropathy associated with Tangier disease. *J Neurol.* 2012;259:1222–1226.
109. Théaudin M, Couvert P, Fournier E, et al. Lewis-Sumner syndrome and Tangier disease. *Arch Neurol.* 2008;65:968–970.
110. Cai Z, Blumbergs PC, Cash K, et al. Paranodal pathology in Tangier disease with remitting-relapsing multifocal neuropathy. *J Clin Neurosci.* 2006;13:492–497.
111. Mercan M, Yayla V, Altinay S, Seyhan S. Peripheral neuropathy in Tangier disease: a literature review and assessment. *J Peripher Nerv Syst.* 2018;23(2):88–98.
112. Sabatelli E, Luigetti M, Costantini U, Lucioli G, Conte A. Sensory-motor not length-dependent multineuropathy followed by the syringomyelia-like phenotype: a novel presentation of Tangier disease. *Neurol Sci.* 2022;43(12):6975–6978.
113. Hager H, Zimmermann P. Licht- und electronenmikroskopische sowie cytometrische untersuchungern an peripheren nerven bei morbus Tangier. *Acta Neuropathol (Berl).* 1979;45:53–59.
114. Zuchner S, Sperfeld AD, Senderek J, Sellhaus B, Hanemann CO, Schroder JM. A novel nonsense mutation in the ABC1 gene causes a severe syringomyelia-like phenotype of Tangier disease. *Brain.* 2003;126(Pt 4):920–927.
115. Bodzioch M, Orso E, Klucken J, et al. The gene encoding ATP-binding cassette transporter 1 is mutated in Tangier disease. *Nat Genet.* 1999;22:347–351.
116. Rust S, Rosier M, Funke H, et al. Tangier disease is caused by mutations in the gene encoding ATP-binding cassette transporter 1. *Nat Genet.* 1999;22:352–355.
117. Argov Z, Soffer D, Eisenberg S, Zimmerman Y. Chronic demyelinating peripheral neuropathy in cerebrotendinous xanthomatosis. *Ann Neurol.* 1986;20:89–91.
118. Zhang S, Li W, Zheng R, et al. Cerebrotendinous xanthomatosis with peripheral neuropathy: a clinical and neurophysiological study in Chinese population. *Ann Transl Med.* 2020;8(21):1372.
119. Berginer VM, Salen G, Shefer S. Long-term treatment of cerebrotendinous xanthomatosis with chenodeoxycholic acid. *N Engl J Med.* 1984;311:1649–1653.
120. Donaghy M, King RH, McKeran RO, Schwartz MS, Thomas PK. Cerebrotendinous xanthomatosis: clinical, electrophysiological and nerve biopsy findings, and response to treatment with chenodeoxycholic acid. *J Neurol.* 1990;237:216–219.
121. Katz DA, Scheinberg L, Horoupian DS, Salen G. Peripheral neuropathy in cerebrotendinous xanthomatosis. *Arch Neurol.* 1985;42:1008–1010.
122. Ohnishi A, Yamashita Y, Goto I, Kuroiwa Y, Murakami S, Ikeda M. De- and remyelination and onion bulb in cerebrotendinous xanthomatosis. *Acta Neuropathol (Berl).* 1979;45:43–45.
123. Philippart M, van Bogaert L. Cholestanolosis (cerebrotendinous xanthomatosis). *Arch Neurol.* 1969;21:603–610.
124. Salen G, Berginer B, Shore V, et al. Increased concentrations of cholestanol and apolipoprotein B in the cerebrospinal fluid of patients with cerebrotendinous xanthomatosis. Effect of chenodeoxycholic acid. *N Engl J Med.* 1987;316:1233–1238.
125. Kuritzky A, Berginer VM, Korczyn AD. Peripheral neuropathy in cerebrotendinous xanthomatosis. *Neurology.* 1979;29:880–881.
126. Leitersdorf E, Safadi R, Meiner V, et al. Cerebrotendinous xanthomatosis in the Israeli Druze: molecular genetics and phenotype characteristics. *Am J Hum Genet.* 1994;55:907–915.
127. Ackroyd RS, Finnegan JA, Green SH. Friedreich's ataxia. A clinical review with neurophysiological and echocardiographic findings. *Arch Dis Child.* 1984;59:217–221.
128. Caruso G, Santoro L, Perretti A, et al. Friedreich's ataxia: electrophysiological and histologic findings in patients and relatives. *Muscle Nerve.* 1987;10:503–515.
129. Cruz-Martinez A, Anciones B, Palau F. GAA trinucleotide repeat expansion in variant Friedreich's ataxia families. *Muscle Nerve.* 1997;20:1121–1126.
130. Dunn H. Nerve conduction studies in children with Friedreich's ataxia and ataxia telangiectasia. *Dev Med Child Neurol.* 1973;15:324–337.
131. Harding AE. Friedreich's ataxia: a clinical and genetic study of 90 families with an analysis of early diagnostic criteria and intrafamilial clustering of clinical features. *Brain.* 1981;104:589–620.
132. McLeod JG. An electrophysiological and pathological study of peripheral nerves in Friedreich's ataxia. *J Neurol Sci.* 1971;12:333–349.
133. Santoro L, Perretti A, Crisci C, et al. Electrophysiological and histological follow-up study in 15 Friedreich's ataxia patients. *Muscle Nerve.* 1990;13:536–540.
134. Salih MA, Ahlesten G, Stalberg E, et al. Friedreich's ataxia in 13 children: presentation and evolution with neurophysiologic, electrocardiographic, and echocardiographic features. *J Child Neurol.* 1990;5:321–326.
135. Klockgether T, Chamberlain S, Wüller U, et al. Late-onset Friedreich's ataxia. Molecular genetics, clinical neurophysiology, and magnetic resonance imaging. *Arch Neurol.* 1993;50:803–806.
136. Ragno M, De Michele G, Cavalcanti F, et al. Broadened Friedreich's ataxia phenotype after gene cloning. Minimal GAA expansion causes late-onset spastic ataxia. *Neurology.* 1997;49:1617–1620.

137. Klockgether T, Zühlke C, Schulz JB, et al. Friedreich's ataxia with retained tendon reflexes: molecular genetics, clinical neurophysiology, and magnetic resonance imaging. *Neurology.* 1996;46:118–121.
138. Caruso G, Santoro L, Perretti A, et al. Friedreich's ataxia: electrophysiological and histological findings. *Acta Neurol Scand.* 1983;67:26–40.
139. Pedersen L, Trojaborg W. Visual, auditory and somatosensory pathway involvement in hereditary cerebellar ataxia, Friedreich's ataxia and familial spastic paraplegia. *Electroencephalogr Clin Neurophysiol.* 1981;52:283–297.
140. Claus D, Harding AE, Hess CW, Mills KR, Murray NM, Thomas PK. Central conduction in degenerative ataxic disorders: a magnetic stimulation study. *J Neurol Neurosurg Psychiatry.* 1988;51:790–795.
141. Cruz Martinez A, Anciones B. Central motor conduction to upper and lower limbs after magnetic stimulation of the brain and peripheral nerve abnormalities in 20 patients with Friedreich's ataxia. *Acta Neurol Scand.* 1992;85:323–326.
142. Jones SJ, Baraister M, Halliday AM. Peripheral and central somatosensory nerve conduction studies in Friedreich's ataxia. *J Neurol Neurosurg Psychiatry.* 1980;43:495–503.
143. Zouri M, Feki M, Ben Hamida C, et al. Electrophysiology and nerve biopsy: comparative study in Friedreich's ataxia and Friedreich's ataxia phenotype with vitamin E deficiency. *Neuromuscul Disord.* 1998;8:416–425.
144. Campuzano V, Montermini L, Molto MD, et al. Friedreich's ataxia: autosomal recessive disease caused by intronic GAA triplet repeat expansion. *Science.* 1996;27:1423–1427.
145. Gray JV, Johnson KJ. Waiting for frataxin. *Nat Genet.* 1997;16:323–325.
146. Pandolfo M. Molecular pathogenesis of Friedreich's ataxia. *Arch Neurol.* 1999;56:1201–1208.
147. Gotoda T, Arita M, Arai H, et al. Adult-onset spinocerebellar dysfunction caused by a mutation in the gene for the alpha-tocopherol transfer protein. *N Engl J Med.* 1995;333:1313–1318.
148. Guggenheim MA, Ringel SP, Silverman A, Grabert BE. Progressive neuromuscular disease in children with chronic cholestasis and vitamin E deficiency: diagnosis and treatment with alpha tocopherol. *J Pediatr.* 1982;100:51–58.
149. Jackson CE, Amato AA, Barohn RJ. Isolated vitamin E deficiency. *Muscle Nerve.* 1996;19:1161–1165.
150. Ouachi K, Arita M, Kayden H, et al. Ataxia with isolated vitamin E deficiency is caused by mutations in the alpha-tocopherol transfer protein. *Nat Genet.* 1995;9:141–145.
151. Krendel DA, Gilchrist JM, Johnson AO, Bossen EH. Isolated deficiency of vitamin E with progressive neurologic deterioration. *Neurology.* 1987;37:538–540.
152. Werlin SL, Harb JM, Swick H, Blank E. Neuromuscular dysfunction and ultrastructural pathology in children with chronic cholestasis and vitamin E deficiency. *Ann Neurol.* 1983;13:291–296.
153. Traber MG, Sokol RJ, Burton GW, et al. Impaired ability of patients with familial isolated vitamin E deficiency to incorporate alpha-tocopherol into lipoproteins secreted by the liver. *J Clin Invest.* 1990;85:397–407.
154. Kott E, Delpre G, Kadish U, Dziatelovsky M, Sandbank U. Abetalipoproteinemia (Bassen-Kornzweig syndrome). *Acta Neuropathol (Berl).* 1977;37:255–258.
155. Muller DP, Lloyd JK. Effect of large oral doses of vitamin E on the neurological sequelae of patients with abetalipoproteinemia. *Ann N Y Acad Sci.* 1982;393:133–144.
156. Scwhartz JF, Rowland LP, Eder HA, et al. Bassen-Kornweig syndrome. Neuromuscular disorder resembling Friedreich's ataxia associated with retinitis pigmentosa, acanthocytosis, steatorrhea, and an abnormality of lipid metabolism. *Trans Am Neurol Assoc.* 1961;86:49–53.
157. Sobrevilla LA, Goodman JL, Kane CA. Demyelinating central nervous system disease, macular atrophy and acanthocytosis (Bassen–Kornzweig syndrome). *Am J Med.* 1964;37:821–828.
158. Brin MF, Pedley TA, Lovelace RE, et al. Electrophysiologic features of abetalipoproteinemia: functional consequences of vitamin E deficiency. *Neurology.* 1986;36:669–673.
159. Lowry NJ, Taylor MJ, Belknapp W, Logan WJ. Electrophysiological studies in five cases of abetalipoproteinemia. *Can J Neurol Sci.* 1984;11:60–63.
160. Miller RG, Davis CJ, Illingworth DR, Bradley W. The neuropathy of abetalipoproteinemia. *Neurology.* 1980;30:1286–1291.
161. Fagan ER, Taylor MJ. Longitudinal multimodal evoked potentials studies in abetalipoproteinemia. *Can J Neurol Sci.* 1987;14:617–621.
162. Le Ber I, Moreira MC, Rivaud-Péchoux S, et al. Cerebellar ataxia with oculomotor apraxia type 1: clinical and genetic studies. *Brain.* 2003;126:2761–2772.
163. Castellotti B, Mariotti C, Rimoldi M, et al. Ataxia with oculomotor apraxia type1 (AOA1): novel and recurrent aprataxin mutations, coenzyme Q10 analyses, and clinical findings in Italian patients. *Neurogenetics.* 2011;12:193–201.
164. Amouri R, Moreira M, Zouari M, et al. Aprataxin gene mutations in Tunisian families. *Neurology.* 2004;63:928–929.
165. Barbot C, Coutinho P, Chorão R, et al. Recessive ataxia with ocular apraxia: review of 22 Portuguese patients. *Arch Neurol.* 2001;58:201–205.
166. Renaud M, Moreira MC, Ben Monga B, et al. Clinical, biomarker, and molecular delineations and genotype-phenotype correlations of ataxia with oculomotor apraxia type 1. *JAMA Neurol.* 2018;75(4):495–502.
167. Vantaggiato C, Cantoni O, Guidarelli A, et al. Novel SETX variants in a patient with ataxia, neuropathy, and oculomotor apraxia are associated with normal sensitivity to oxidative DNA damaging agents. *Brain Dev.* 2014;36(8):682–689.
168. Fogel BL, Perlman S. Clinical features and molecular genetics of autosomal recessive cerebellar ataxias. *Lancet Neurol.* 2007;6:245–257.
169. Le Ber I, Brice A, Dürr A. New autosomal recessive cerebellar ataxias with oculomotor apraxia. *Curr Neurol Neurosci Rep.* 2005;5:411–417.
170. Criscuolo C, Chessa L, Di Giandomenico S, et al. Ataxia with oculomotor apraxia type 2: a clinical, pathologic, and genetic study. *Neurology.* 2006;66:1207–1210.
171. Gazulla J, Benavente I, López-Fraile IP, et al. Sensory neuronopathy in ataxia with oculomotor apraxia type 2. *J Neurol Sci.* 2010;298:118–120.
172. Nanetti L, Cavalieri S, Pensato V, et al. SETX mutations are a frequent genetic cause of juvenile and adult onset cerebellar ataxia with neuropathy and elevated serum alpha-fetoprotein. *Orphanet J Rare Dis.* 2013;8:123.
173. Moreira MC, Klur A, Watanabe M, et al. Senataxin, the ortholog of a yeast RNA helicase, is mutant in ataxia–ocular apraxia 2. *Nat Genet.* 2004;36:225–227.

174. Vantaggiato C, Bondioni S, Airoldi G, et al. Senataxin modulates neurite growth through fibroblast growth factor 8 signalling. *Brain*. 2011;134:1808–1828.
175. Migliaccio AA, Halmagyi GM, McGarvie LA, Cremer PD. Cerebellar ataxia with bilateral vestibulopathy: description of a syndrome and its characteristic clinical sign. *Brain*. 2004;127:280–293.
176. Cortese A, Tozza S, Yau WY, et al. Cerebellar ataxia, neuropathy, vestibular areflexia syndrome due to RFC1 repeat expansion. *Brain*. 2020;143(2):480–490.
177. Cortese A, Curro' R, Vegezzi E, Yau WY, Houlden H, Reilly MM. Cerebellar ataxia, neuropathy and vestibular areflexia syndrome (CANVAS): genetic and clinical aspects. *Pract Neurol*. 2022;22(1):14–18.
178. Cortese A, Simone R, Sullivan R, et al. Biallelic expansion of an intronic repeat in RFC1 392 is a common cause of late-onset ataxia. *Nat Genet*. 2019;51(4):649–658.
179. Szmulewicz DJ, Roberts L, McLean CA, MacDougall HG, Halmagyi GM, Storey E. Proposed diagnostic criteria for cerebellar ataxia with neuropathy and vestibular areflexia syndrome (CANVAS). *Neurol Clin Pract*. 2016;6(1):61–68.
180. Szmulewicz DJ, McLean CA, Rodriguez ML, et al. Dorsal root ganglionopathy is responsible for the sensory impairment in CANVAS. *Neurology*. 2014;22:1410–1415.
181. Sánchez-Tejerina D, Alvarez PF, Laínez E, et al. RFC1 repeat expansions and cerebellar ataxia, neuropathy and vestibular areflexia syndrome: experience and perspectives from a neuromuscular disorders unit. *J Neurol Sci*. 2023;446:120565.
182. Huin V, Coarelli G, Guemy C, et al. Motor neuron pathology in CANVAS due to RFC1 expansions. *Brain*. 2022;145(6):2121–2132.
183. Ronco R, Perini C, Currò R, et al. Truncating variants in *RFC1* in cerebellar ataxia, neuropathy, and vestibular areflexia syndrome. *Neurology*. 2023;100(5):e543–e554.
184. Maguina M, Kang PB, Tsai AC, Pacak CA. Peripheral neuropathies associated with DNA repair disorders. *Muscle Nerve*. 2023;67(2):101–110.
185. Martinez AC, Barrio M, Gutierrez AM, López. Abnormalities in sensory and mixed evoked potentials in ataxia telangiectasia. *J Neurol Neurosurg Psychiatry*. 1977;40:44–49.
186. Woods GG. DNA repair disorders. *Arch Dis Child*. 1998;78:78–184.
187. Savitsky L, Bar-Shira A, Gilad S, et al. A single ataxia telangiectasia gene product similar to PI-3 kinase. *Science*. 1995;268:1749–1753.
188. Sugarman GI, Landing BH, Reed WB. Cockayne syndrome: clinical study of two patients and neuropathologic findings in one. *Clin Pediatr*. 1977;16:225–232.
189. Rapin I, Lindenbaum Y, Dickson DW, Kraemer KH, Robbins JH. Cockayne syndrome and xeroderma pigmentosum. *Neurology*. 2000;55:1442–1449.
190. Moosa A, Dubowitz V. Peripheral neuropathy in Cockayne's syndrome. *Arch Dis Child*. 1970;45:674–677.
191. Weidenheim KM, Dickson DW, Rapin I. Neuropathology of Cockayne syndrome: Evidence for impaired development, premature aging, and neurodegeneration. *Mech Ageing Dev*. 2009;130:619–36.
192. Vos A, Gabreels-Festen A, Joosten E, Gabreëls F, Renier W, Mullaart R. The neuropathy of Cockayne syndrome. *Acta Neuropathol (Berl)*. 1983;61:153–156.
193. Gitiaux C, Blin-Rochemaure N, Hully M, et al. Progressive demyelinating neuropathy correlates with clinical severity in Cockayne syndrome. *Clin Neurophysiol*. 2015;126:1435–1439.
194. Roy S, Srivastava RN, Gupta PC, Mayekar G. Ultrastructure of peripheral nerve in Cockayne's syndrome. *Acta Neuropathol (Berl)*. 1973;24:345–349.
195. Grunnet ML, Zimmerman AW, Lewis RA. Ultrastructure and electrodiagnosis of peripheral neuropathy in Cockayne's syndrome. *Neurology*. 1983;33:1606–1609.
196. Ohnishi A, Mitsudome A, Murai Y. Primary segmental demyelination in the sural nerve in Cockayne's syndrome. *Muscle Nerve*. 1987;10:163–167.
197. Lehky TJ, Sackstein P, Tamura D, et al. Differences in peripheral neuropathy in xeroderma pigmentosum complementation groups A and D as evaluated by nerve conduction studies. *BMC Neurol*. 2021;21:393.
198. Lindenbaum Y, Dickson D, Rosenbaum P, Kraemer K, Robbins I, Rapin I. Xeroderma pigmentosum/cockayne syndrome complex: first neuropathological study and review of eight other cases. *Eur J Paediatr Neurol*. 2001;5:225–242.
199. Anttinen A, Koulu L, Nikoskelainen E, et al. Neurological symptoms and natural course of xeroderma pigmentosum. *Brain*. 2008;131:1979–1989.
200. Tsuji Y, Ueda T, Sekiguchi K, et al. Progressive length-dependent polyneuropathy in xeroderma pigmentosum group a. *Muscle Nerve*. 2020;62:534–540.
201. Kanda T, Oda M, Yonezawa M, et al. Peripheral neuropathy in xeroderma pigmentosum. *Brain*. 1990;113(Pt 4):1025–1044.
202. Tachi N, Sasaki K, Kusano T, et al. Peripheral neuropathy in four cases of group a xeroderma pigmentosum. *J Child Neurol*. 1988;3:114–119.
203. Martens MC, Emmert S, Boeckmann L. Xeroderma pigmentosum: gene variants and splice variants. *Genes (Basel)*. 2021;12(8):1173.
204. Smits MG, Gabreels FJ, Renier WO, et al. Peripheral and central myelinopathy in Cockayne's syndrome. Report of 3 siblings. *Neuropediatrics*. 1982;13:161–167.
205. Tatin D. RNA polymerase II elongation complexes containing the Cockayne syndrome group b protein interact with a molecular complex containing transcription factor IIH components xeroderma pigmentosum B and p62. *J Biol Chem*. 1998;273:27794–27799.
206. Asbury AK, Gale MK, Cox SC, Baringer JR, Berg BO. Giant axonal neuropathy—a unique case with segmental neurofilamentous masses. *Acta Neuropathol (Berl)*. 1972;20:237–247.
207. Igisu H, Ohta M, Tabira T, Hosokawa S, Goto I. Giant axonal neuropathy. A clinical entity affecting the central as well as the peripheral nervous system. *Neurology*. 1975;25:717–721.
208. Koch T, Schultz P, Williams R, Lampert P. Giant axonal neuropathy: a childhood disorder of microfilaments. *Ann Neurol*. 1977;1:438–451.
209. Kumar K, Barre P, Nigro M, Jones MZ. Giant axonal neuropathy: clinical, electrophysiologic, and neuropathologic features in two siblings. *J Child Neurol*. 1990;5:229–234.
210. Mohri I, Taniike M, Yoshikawa H, Higashiyama M, Itami S, Okada S. A case of giant axonal neuropathy showing focal aggregation and hypophosphorylation of intermediate filaments. *Brain Dev*. 1998;20:594–597.

211. Prineas JW, Ouvrier RA, Wright RG, Walsh JC, McLeod JG. Giant axonal neuropathy—a generalized disorder of cytoplasmic microfilament formation. *J Neuropathol Exp Neurol*. 1976;35:458–470.
212. Demir E, Bomont P, Erdem S, et al. Giant axonal neuropathy: clinical and genetic study in six cases. *J Neurol Neurosurg Psychiatry*. 2005;76(6):825–832.
213. Ouvrier RA, Prineas J, Walsh JC, Reye RD, McLeod JG. Giant axonal neuropathy—a third case. *Proc Aust Assoc Neurol*. 1974;11:137–144.
214. Berg BO, Rosenberg SH, Asbury AK. Giant axonal neuropathy. *Pediatrics*. 1972;49:894–899.
215. Carpenter S, Karpati G, Andermann F, Gold R. Giant axonal neuropathy. A clinically and morphologically distinct neurological disease. *Arch Neurol*. 1974;31:312–316.
216. Mizuno Y, Otsuka S, Takano Y, et al. Giant axonal neuropathy. *Arch Neurol*. 1979;36:107–108.
217. Echaniz-Laguna A, Cuisset JM, Guyant-Marechal L, et al. Giant axonal neuropathy: a multicenter retrospective study with genotypic spectrum expansion. *Neurogenetics*. 2020;21(1):29–37.
218. Bharucha-Goebel DX, Norato G, Saade D, et al. Giant axonal neuropathy: cross-sectional analysis of a large natural history cohort. *Brain*. 2021;144(10):3239–3250.
219. Bomont P, Cavalier P, Bondeau F, et al. The gene encoding gigaxonin, a member of the cytoskeletal BTB/Kelch repeat family is mutated in giant axonal neuropathy. *Nat Genet*. 2000;26:370–374.
220. Aicardi J, Castelein P. Infantile neuroaxonal dystrophy. *Brain*. 1979;102:727–748.
221. Nardocci N, Zorzi G, Farina L, et al. Infantile neuroaxonal dystrophy. Clinical spectrum and diagnostic criteria. *Neurology*. 1999;52:1472–1478.
222. Raemakers VT, Lake BD, Harding B, et al. Diagnostic difficulties in infantile neuroaxonal dystrophy. A clinicopathological study of eight cases. *Neuropediatrics*. 1987;18:170–175.
223. Schindler D, Bishop DF, Wolfe DE, et al. Neuroaxonal dystrophy due to lysosomal α-N-acetyl-galactosaminase deficiency. *N Engl J Med*. 1989;320:1735–1740.
224. Khateeb S, Flusser H, Ofir R, et al. PLA2G6 mutation underlies infantile neuroaxonal dystrophy. *Am J Hum Genet*. 2006;79(5):942–948.
225. Mochel F, Schiffmann R, Steenweg ME, et al. Adult polyglucosan body disease: natural history and key magnetic resonance imaging findings. *Ann Neurol*. 2012;72:433–441.
226. Robitaille Y, Carpenter S, Karpati G, DiMauro SD. A distinct form of adult polyglucosan body disease with massive involvement of central and peripheral neuronal processes and astrocytes: a report of four cases and a review of the occurrence of polyglucosan bodies in other conditions such as Lafora's disease and normal ageing. *Brain*. 1980;103:315–336.
227. Klein CJ, Boes CJ, Chapin JE, et al. Adult polyglucosan body disease: case description of an expanding genetic and clinical syndrome. *Muscle Nerve*. 2004;29:323–328.
228. Cafferty MS, Lovelace RE, Hays AP, Servidei S, Dimauro S, Rowland LP. Polyglucosan body disease. *Muscle Nerve*. 1991;14:102–107.
229. Sindern E, Ziemssen F, Ziemssen T, et al. Adult polyglucosan body disease: a postmortem correlation study. *Neurology*. 2003;61:263–265.
230. Vucic S, Pamphlett R, Wills EJ, Yiannikas C. Polyglucosan body disease myopathy: an unusual presentation. *Muscle Nerve*. 2007;35:536–539.
231. Massa R, Bruno C, Martorana A, de Stefano N, van Diggelen OP, Federico A. Adult polyglucosan body disease: proton magnetic resonance spectroscopy of the brain and novel mutation in the GBE1 gene. *Muscle Nerve*. 2008;37:530–536.
232. Bruno C, Servidei S, Shanske S, et al. Glycogen branching enzyme deficiency in adult polyglucosan body disease. *Ann Neurol*. 1993;33:88–93.
233. Bruno C, van Diggelen OP, Cassandrini D, et al. Clinical and genetic heterogeneity of branching enzyme deficiency (glycogenosis type IV). *Neurology*. 2004;63:1053–1058.
234. McMaster KR, Powers JM, Hennigar GR, Wohltmann HJ, Farr GH Jr. Nervous system involvement in type IV glycogenosis. *Arch Neurol*. 1979;103:105–111.
235. Lossos A, Meiner Z, Barash V, et al. Adult polyglucosan body disease in Ashkenazi Jewish patients carrying the Tyr329 Ser mutation in the glycogen-branching enzyme gene. *Ann Neurol*. 1998;44:867–872.
236. Koch RL, Soler-Alfonso C, Kiely BT, et al. Diagnosis and management of glycogen storage disease type IV, including adult polyglucosan body disease: a clinical practice resource. *Mol Genet Metab*. 2023;138(3):107525.
237. Gandhi Mehta RK, Caress JB, Rudnick SR, Bonkovsky HL. Porphyric neuropathy. *Muscle Nerve*. 2021;64(2):140–152.
238. Bonkowsky HL, Schady W. Neurologic manifestations of acute porphyria. *Semin Liver Dis*. 1982;2:108–124.
239. Ridley A. The neuropathy of acute intermittent porphyria. *Q J Med*. 1969;38:307–333.
240. Wenger S, Meisinger V, Brucke T, Deecke L. Acute porphyric neuropathy during pregnancy—effect of hematin therapy. *Eur Neurol*. 1998;39:187–188.
241. Albers JW, Fink JK. Porphyric neuropathy. *Muscle Nerve*. 2004;30(4):410–422.
242. King PH, Petersen NE, Rakhra R, Schreiber WE. Porphyria presenting with bilateral radial motor neuropathy: evidence of a novel gene mutation. *Neurology*. 2002;58:1118–1121.
243. Kochar DK, Poonia A, Kumawat BL, Shubhakaran, Gupta BK. Study of motor and sensory nerve conduction velocities, late responses (F-wave and H-reflex) and somatosensory evoked potential in latent phase of intermittent acute porphyria. *Electromyogr Clin Neurophysiol*. 2000;40(2):73–79.
244. Muley SA, Midani HA, Rank JM, Carithers R, Parry GJ. Neuropathy in erythropoietic protoporphyrias. *Neurology*. 1998;51(1):262–265.
245. Marcelis R, Hassoun A, Verstraeten L, De Bock R, Martin JJ. Porphyric neuropathy and hereditary delta-aminolevulinic acid dehydratase deficiency in adults. *J Neurosci*. 1990;95:39–47.
246. Hengstman GJ, de Laat KF, Jacobs B, van Engelen BG. Sensorimotor axonal polyneuropathy without hepatic failure in erythropoietic protoporphyria. *J Clin Neuromuscul Dis*. 2009;11:72–76.
247. Lin CS, Park SB, Krishnan AV. Porphyric neuropathy. *Handb Clin Neurol*. 2013;115:613–627.
248. Albers JW, Robertson WC, Daube JR. Electrodiagnostic findings in acute porphyric neuropathy. *Muscle Nerve*. 1978;1:292–296.
249. Anzil AP, Dozic S. Peripheral nerve changes in porphyric neuropathy: findings in a sural nerve biopsy. *Acta Neuropathol (Berl)*. 1978;42:121–126.

250. Bosch EP, Pierach CA, Bossenmaier I, Cardinal R, Thorson M. Effect of hematin in porphyric neuropathy. *Neurology*. 1977;27:1053–1056.
251. Flugel KA, Druschky KF. Electromyogram and nerve conduction in patients with acute intermittent porphyria. *J Neurol*. 1977;214:267–279.
252. Wilson GN. Tales from the neural genome: the lessons of homozygous porphyria. *Arch Neurol*. 2004;61:1650–1651.
253. Solis C, Martinez-Bermejo A, Naidich TP, et al. Acute intermittent porphyria: studies of the severe homozygous dominant disease provides insights into the neurologic attacks in acute porphyrias. *Arch Neurol*. 2004;61:1764–1770.
254. Balwani M, Sardh E, Ventura P, et al. Phase 3 trial of RNAi therapeutic givosiran for acute intermittent porphyria. *N Engl J Med*. 2020;382:2289–2301.
255. Ventura P, Bonkovsky HL, Gouya L, et al. Efficacy and safety of givosiran for acute hepatic porphyria: 24-month interim analysis of the randomized phase 3 ENVISION study. *Liver Int*. 2022;42(1):161–172.
256. Adams D. Hereditary and acquired amyloid polyneuropathy. *J Neurol*. 2001;248:647–657.
257. Lachmann HJ, Chir B, Booth DR, et al. Misdiagnosis of hereditary amyloidosis as AL (primary) amyloidosis. *N Engl J Med*. 2002;346:1786–1791.
258. Rajani B, Rajani V, Prayson RA. Peripheral nerve amyloidosis in sural nerve biopsies: a clinicopathologic analysis of 13 cases. *Arch Pathol Lab Med*. 2000;124(1):114–118.
259. Klein CJ, Vrana JA, Theis JD, et al. Mass spectrometric-based proteomic analysis of amyloid neuropathy type in nerve tissue. *Arch Neurol*. 2011;68:195–199.
260. Duston MA, Skinner M, Anderson J, Cohen AS. Peripheral neuropathy as an early marker of AL amyloidosis. *Arch Intern Med*. 1989;149:358–360.
261. Kelly JJ Jr, Kyle RA, O'Brien PC, Dyck PJ. The natural history of peripheral neuropathy in primary systemic amyloidosis. *Ann Neurol*. 1979;6:1–7.
262. Kyle RA, Greipp PR. Amyloidosis (AL). Clinical and laboratory features in 229 cases. *Mayo Clin Proc*. 1983;58:665–683.
263. Vucic S, Chon PS, Cros D. Atypical presentations of amyloid neuropathy. *Muscle Nerve*. 2003;28(6):696–702.
264. Tracy JA, Dyck PJ, Dyck PJ. Primary amyloidosis presenting as upper limb multiple mononeuropathies. *Muscle Nerve*. 2010;41:710–715.
265. Mathis S, Magy L, Diallo L, Boukhris S, Vallat JM. Amyloid neuropathy mimicking chronic inflammatory demyelinating polyneuropathy. *Muscle Nerve*. 2012;45:26–31.
266. Andersson R, Blom S. Neurophysiological studies in primary hereditary amyloidosis with polyneuropathy. *Acta Med Scand*. 1972;191:233–239.
267. Dyck PJ, Lambert EH. Dissociated sensation in amyloidosis. *Arch Neurol*. 1969;20:490–507.
268. Thomas PK, King RH. Peripheral nerve changes in amyloid neuropathy. *Brain*. 1974;97:395–406.
269. Berghoff M, Kathpal M, Khan F, Skinner M, Falk R, Freeman R. Endothelial dysfunction precedes C-fiber abnormalities in primary (AL) amyloidosis. *Ann Neurol*. 2003;53(6):725–730.
270. Skinner M, Sanchorowala V, Seldin DC, et al. High dose melphalan and autologous stem-cell transplantation in patients with AL amyloidosis. An 8-year study. *Ann Intern Med*. 2004;140:85–93.
271. Dispenzieri A, Kyle RA, Lancy MG, et al. Superior survival in primary systemic amyloidosis patients undergoing peripheral blood stem cell transplantation: a case control study. *Blood*. 2004;101:3960–3963.
272. Dingli D, Tan TS, Kumar SK, et al. Stem cell transplantation in patients with autonomic neuropathy due to primary (AL) amyloidosis. *Neurology*. 2010;74:913–918.
273. Blom S, Steen L, Zetterlund B. Familial amyloidosis with polyneuropathy type I. *Acta Neurol Scand*. 1981;63:99–110.
274. Boysen G, Galassi G, Kamieniecka Z, Schlaeger J, Trojaborg W. Familial amyloidosis with cranial neuropathy and corneal lattice dystrophy. *J Neurol Neurosurg Psychiatry*. 1979;42:1020–1030.
275. Hanyu N, Ikeda S, Nakadai A, Yanagisawa N, Powell HC. Peripheral nerve pathological findings in familial amyloid polyneuropathy: a correlative study of proximal sciatic nerve and sural nerve lesions. *Ann Neurol*. 1989;25:340–350.
276. Hund E, Linke RP, Willig F, Graus A. Transthyretin-associated neuropathic amyloidosis. Pathogenesis and treatment. *Neurology*. 2001;56:431–435.
277. Luis ML. Electroneurophysiological studies in familial amyloid polyneuropathy—Portuguese type. *J Neurol Neurosurg Psychiatry*. 1978;41:847–850.
278. Sobue G, Nakao N, Murakami K, et al. Type I familial amyloid polyneuropathy. *Brain*. 1990;113:903–919.
279. Tozza S, Severi D, Spina E, et al. The neuropathy in hereditary transthyretin amyloidosis: a narrative review. *J Peripher Nerv Syst*. 2021;26(2):155–159.
280. Zampino S, Sheikh FH, Vaishnav J, et al. Phenotypes associated with the Val122Ile, Leu58His, and late-onset Val30Met variants in patients with hereditary transthyretin amyloidosis. *Neurology*. 2023;100(19):e2036–e2044.
281. Luigetti M, Conte A, Del Grande A, et al. TTR-related amyloid neuropathy: clinical, electrophysiological and pathological findings in 15 unrelated patients. *Neurol Sci*. 2013;34(7):1057–1063.
282. Blanco-Jerez CR, Jimenez-Escrig A, Gobernado JM, et al. Transthyretin Tyr77 familial amyloid polyneuropathy: a clinicopathological study of a large kindred. *Muscle Nerve*. 1998;21:1478–1485.
283. Briemberg HR, Amato AA. Transthyretin amyloidosis presenting with multifocal demyelinating mononeuropathies. *Muscle Nerve*. 2004;29(2):318–322.
284. Anrade C. A peculiar form of peripheral neuropathy. *Brain*. 1952;75:408–426.
285. Plante-Bordeneuve V, Lalu T, Misrahi M, et al. Genotypic-phenotypic variations in a series of 65 patients with familial amyloid polyneuropathy. *Neurology*. 1998;51:708–714.
286. Planté-Bordeneuve V, Said G. Familial amyloid polyneuropathy. *Lancet Neurol*. 2011;10:1086–1097.
287. Benson MD, Kincaid JC. The molecular biology and clinical features of amyloid neuropathy. *Muscle Nerve*. 2007;36:411–423.
288. Cappellari M, Cavallaro T, Ferrarini M, et al. Variable presentations of TTR-related familial amyloid polyneuropathy in seventeen patients. *J Peripher Nerv Syst*. 2011;16:119–129.
289. Bergethon PR, Sabin TD, Lewis D, Simms RW, Cohen AS, Skinner M. Improvement in the polyneuropathy associated with familial amyloid polyneuropathy after liver transplantation. *Neurology*. 1996;47:944–951.
290. Adams D, Samule D, Goulin-Goeau C, et al. The course and prognostic factors of familial amyloid polyneuropathy after liver transplantation. *Brain*. 2000;123:1495–1504.
291. Magrinelli F, Fabrizi GM, Santoro L, et al. Pharmacological treatment for familial amyloid polyneuropathy. *Cochrane Database Syst Rev*. 2020 ;4(4):CD012395.

292. Coelho T, Maia LF, Martins da Silva A, et al. Tafamidis for transthyretin familial amyloid polyneuropathy: a randomized, controlled trial. *Neurology*. 2012;79(8):785–792.
293. Berk JL, Suhr OB, Obici L, et al. Repurposing diflunisal for familial amyloid polyneuropathy: a randomized clinical trial. *JAMA*. 2013;310(24):2658–2667.
294. Adams D, Gonzalez-Duarte A, O'Riordan WD, et al. Patisiran, an RNAi therapeutic, for hereditary transthyretin amyloidosis. *New England Journal of Medicine*. 2018;379(1):11–21.
295. Adams D, Polydefkis M, González-Duarte A, et al. Long-term safety and efficacy of patisiran for hereditary transthyretin-mediated amyloidosis with polyneuropathy: 12-month results of an open-label extension study. *Lancet Neurol*. 2021;20(1):49–59.
296. Adams D, Tournev IL, Taylor MS, et al. Efficacy and safety of vutrisiran for patients with hereditary transthyretin-mediated amyloidosis with polyneuropathy: a randomized clinical trial. *Amyloid*. 2023;30(1):1–9.
297. Benson MD, Waddington-Cruz M, Berk JL, et al. Inotersen treatment for patients with hereditary transthyretin amyloidosis. *New England Journal of Medicine*. 2018;379(1):22–31.
298. Van Allen MW, Frolich JA, Davis JR. Inherited predisposition to generalized amyloidosis. *Neurology*. 1969;19:10–25.
299. Joy T, Wang J, Hahn A, Hegele RA. APOA1 related amyloidosis: a case report and literature review. *Clin Biochem*. 2003;36:641–645.
300. Nichols WC, Gregg RE, Brewer BH, Benson MD. A mutation in apolipoprotein A1 Iowa type of familial amyloidotic polyneuropathy. *Genomics*. 1990;8:318–323.
301. Pihlamaa T, Suominen S, Kiuru-Enari S. Familial amyloidotic polyneuropathy type IV–gelsolin amyloidosis. *Amyloid*. 2012;19:30–33.
302. Asahina A, Yokoyama T, Ueda M, et al. Hereditary gelsolin amyloidosis: a new Japanese case with cutis laxa as a diagnostic clue. *Acta Derm Venereol*. 2011;91:201–203.
303. Kiuru-Enari S, Keski-Oja J, Haltia M. Cutis laxa in hereditary gelsolin amyloidosis. *Br J Dermatol*. 2005;152:250–257.
304. Meretoja J. Familial systemic paramyloidosis with lattice dystrophy of the cornea, progressive cranial neuropathy, skin changes and various internal symptoms. *Ann Clin Res*. 1969;1:314–324.
305. Haltia M, Levy E, Meretohi J, Fernandez-Madrid I, Koivunene O, Frangione B. Gelsolin gene mutation at codon 187 in familial amyloidosis, Finnish: DNA-diagnostic assay. *Am J Med*. 1992;42:357–359.
306. Kiuru-Enari S, Somer H, Seppalainen AM, Notkola IL, Haltia M. Neuromuscular pathology in hereditary gelsolin amyloidosis. *J Neuropathol Exp Neurol*. 2002;61(6):565–571.
307. Gorevic PD, Munoz PC, Gorgone G, et al. Amyloidosis due to a mutation in the gelsolin gene in an American family with lattice corneal dystrophy type II. *N Engl J Med*. 1991;325:1780–1785.
308. Kiuru S. Gelsolin-related familial amyloidosis, Finnish type (FAF), and its variants found worldwide. *Amyloid*. 1998;5:55–66.
309. Maury CP, Liljestrom M, Boysen G, Tornroth T, de la Chapelle A, Nurmiaho-310. Lassila EL. Danish type gelsolin related amyloidosis: 654G-T mutation is associated with a disease pathogenetically and clinically similar to that caused by the 654G-A mutation (familial amyloidosis of the Finnish type). *J Clin Pathol*. 2000;53:95–99.

CHAPTER 13

Guillain–Barré Syndrome and Related Disorders

Landry described a condition characterized by acute ascending paralysis in 1859. Later, Guillain, Barré, and Strohl noted the areflexia and the albuminocytologic dissociation in the cerebral spinal fluid (CSF) associated with this neuropathy.[1] This neuropathy has most commonly been referred to as Guillain–Barré syndrome (GBS), neglecting the contributions of Landry and Strohl. In 1949, Haymaker and Kernohan detailed the histopathologic features seen in 50 fatal cases of GBS. The earliest features noted were edema of the proximal nerves and the subsequent degeneration of the myelin sheaths within the first week of the illness. They did not appreciate inflammatory cell infiltrate until later in the course of the illness.[2] However, another group reported on 19 autopsy cases of GBS, showing prominent perivascular inflammation in the spinal roots, dorsal root ganglia, cranial nerves, and randomly along the whole length of peripheral nerves, along with segmental demyelination adjacent to the areas of inflammation.[3] Thus, the term acute inflammatory demyelinating polyradiculoneuropathy (AIDP), which is quite descriptive of the disease process, has historically been used synonymously with GBS.[4–7]

It is now appreciated that GBS is not a single disorder, but rather an umbrella syndrome including several acute immune-mediated polyneuropathies (Table 13-1).[8–10] In addition to AIDP, acute motor–sensory axonal neuropathy (AMSAN) and acute motor axonal neuropathy (AMAN) have been described. Further, some disorders that appear clinically different from AIDP [e.g., the Miller Fisher syndrome (MFS), acute small fiber neuropathy, and acute autonomic neuropathy] may share similar pathogenesis and can be considered variants of GBS. Of these, MFS has been best described and understood. Multiple other rare phenotypes have been described in the literature, including idiopathic cranial polyneuropathy, pharyngeal–cervical–brachial weakness with or without ophthalmoparesis, facial diplegia with limb paresthesias, and paraparetic weakness.[11–15] These disorders may represent oligosymptomatic or forme frustes of GBS.

▶ EPIDEMIOLOGY OF GBS AND ANTECEDENT ILLNESS

GBS has an estimated annual incidence ranging from 0.9 to 4 per 100,000 population.[9,10,16–19] There may be a slight male predominance. AIDP is the most common subtype of GBS, especially in the United States and Europe. There is notable regional variation.[20] McKhann and colleagues initially described the acute motor axonal variant (AMAN) in patients with seasonal outbreaks of acute flaccid paralysis in northern China.[21,22] AMAN is now recognized as the most common subtype of GBS in northern China and elsewhere in Asia. While less frequent elsewhere, AMAN is not rare; 27 of the 147 (18%) patients enrolled in the Dutch GBS trial comparing intravenous immune globulin (IVIg) to plasma exchange (PLEX) were later classified as having AMAN.[23,24] Miller Fisher syndrome may also be more common in Asia.[20]

Approximately 60%–75% of patients with GBS have a history of a recent infection within the 8 weeks prior to the onset of the neuropathy.[10,20,25] *Campylobacter jejuni* is most commonly identified, with roughly 30% of patients having serologic evidence of recent infection.[25–28] *C. jejuni* is particularly associated with axonal variants of GBS. Sixty-seven percent to 92% of patients have specific serologic evidence of a recent *C. jejuni* infection, which may explain the seasonal variation of this syndrome in China.[22,24,29]

Cytomegalovirus (CMV) infection, which can be identified in 4%–13% of patients with GBS, is by contrast associated with a demyelinating phenotype.[25,26] Patients with GBS following CMV infection may also have a longer time to nadir compared to others. Serologic evidence of recent Epstein–Barr virus or *Mycoplasma pneumoniae* infection may be found in 5%–10% of patients. A possible infrequent link with SARS-CoV-2/Covid-19 infection has emerged.[30–32] Other infectious agents associated with GBS include influenza, hepatitis A, B, C, and E, Zika virus, and human immunodeficiency virus (HIV).[7,9,33–37] In HIV infection, AIDP usually occurs at the time of seroconversion or early in the course of the disease.

Vaccinations have at times been associated with GBS, most notably the swine flu vaccine in the 1970s.[38] Some but not all contemporary studies examining the seasonal influenza vaccine have demonstrated a slight increased risk of GBS.[39–49] When this has been demonstrated, however, the estimated risk is fewer than one case per 1 million vaccines administered. By contrast, the risk of GBS following influenza infection is estimated to be 17 cases per 1 million infections. An increased risk of GBS has been associated with the adenovirus-vector SARS-CoV-2 vaccines developed early in

▶ **TABLE 13-1. GUILLAIN–BARRÉ SYNDROME AND RELATED DISORDERS**

Acute inflammatory demyelinating polyradiculoneuropathy (AIDP)
Acute motor and sensory axonal neuropathy (AMSAN)
Acute motor axonal neuropathy (AMAN)
Other GBS variants
    Miller Fisher syndrome
    Idiopathic cranial polyneuropathy
    Pharyngeal–cervical–brachial
    Paraparetic GBS
    Acute sensory neuronopathy/ganglionopathy
    Acute small fiber neuropathy
    Acute autonomic neuropathy
Acute-onset CIDP (can mimic GBS)
Nodopathy/Paranodopathy (can mimic GBS, especially pan-neurofascin antibodies)

GBS, Guillain–Barré syndrome; CIDP, chronic inflammatory demyelinating polyneuropathy.

▶ **TABLE 13-2. DIAGNOSTIC FEATURES OF ACUTE INFLAMMATORY DEMYELINATING POLYRADICULONEUROPATHY**

I. Required for diagnosis
  1. Progressive weakness of variable degree from mild paresis to complete paralysis
  2. Generalized hypo- or areflexia
II. Supportive of diagnosis
  1. Clinical features
    a. Symptom progression: Motor weakness rapidly progresses initially but ceases by 4 weeks. Nadir attained by 2 weeks in 50%, 3 weeks in 80%, and 4 weeks in 90%.
    b. Demonstration of relative limb symmetry regarding paresis.
    c. Mild to moderate sensory signs.
    d. Frequent cranial nerve involvement: Facial (cranial nerve VII) 50% and typically bilateral but asymmetric; occasional involvement of cranial nerves XII, X, and occasionally III, IV, and VI as well as XI.
    e. Recovery typically begins 2–4 weeks following plateau phase.
    f. Autonomic dysfunction can include tachycardia, other arrhythmias, postural hypotension, hypertension, and other vasomotor symptoms.
    g. A preceding gastrointestinal illness (e.g., diarrhea) or upper respiratory tract infection is common.
  2. Cerebrospinal fluid features supporting diagnosis
    a. Elevated or serial elevation of CSF protein.
    b. CSF cell counts are <10 mononuclear cell/mm^3.
  3. Electrodiagnostic medicine findings supportive of diagnosis
    a. 80% of patients have evidence of NCV slowing/conduction block at some time during disease process.
    b. Patchy reduction in NCV attaining values <60% of normal.
    c. Distal motor latency increase may reach three times the normal values.
    d. F-waves indicate proximal NCV slowing.
    e. About 15–20% of patients have normal NCV findings.
    f. No abnormalities on nerve conduction studies may be seen for several weeks.
III. Findings reducing possibility of diagnosis
  1. Asymmetric weakness
  2. Failure of bowel/bladder symptoms to resolve
  3. Severe bowel/bladder dysfunction at initiation of disease
  4. Greater than 50 mononuclear cells/mm^3 in CSF
  5. Well-demarcated sensory level
IV. Exclusionary criteria
  1. Diagnosis of other causes of acute neuromuscular weakness (e.g., myasthenia gravis, botulism, poliomyelitis, and toxic neuropathy)
  2. Abnormal CSF cytology suggesting carcinomatous invasion of the nerve roots

CSF, cerebral spinal fluid; NCS, nerve conduction velocity.
Reproduced with permission from Amato AA, Dumitru D. Acquired neuropathies. In: Dumitru D, Amato AA, Swartz MJ, eds. *Electrodiagnostic Medicine*. 2nd ed. Hanley & Belfus, 2002.

the Covid-19 pandemic.[50–53] At the time of this publication, no increased risk has been found with the mRNA SARS-CoV-2 vaccines.

Other disorders have been associated with a possible increased risk of GBS, including other autoimmune disorders (i.e., systemic lupus erythematosus), lymphoma and other malignancies, organ rejection or graft versus host disease following solid organ and bone marrow transplantation, and perhaps recent surgery.[9,54–56] Certain immunomodulating agents, such as tumor-necrosis alpha blockers or immune checkpoint inhibitors, may increase the risk of developing acute neuropathy akin to GBS.[57,58]

GBS can occur at any age. Though it is most common in older adults (the incidence increases with each decade of life), children can also be affected.[18] Peak incidence in childhood is 2 years of age.[59] Childhood GBS has clinical, laboratory, and electrophysiologic findings similar to adult cases.[60–67] AIDP is also the most common subtype in children. An antecedent infection is appreciated in approximately 66%–75% of cases.

▶ ACUTE INFLAMMATORY DEMYELINATING POLYRADICULONEUROPATHY (AIDP)

CLINICAL FEATURES

AIDP usually presents with numbness and tingling in the feet that gradually progresses up the legs and then into the arms[7,9,10,68] (Table 13-2). Numbness and paresthesia can also involve the face and trunk. Severe, aching, prickly, or burning neuritic pain sensations in the back and limbs are present in at least half the patients and may be particularly common in children. Large fiber modalities (touch, vibration, and position sense) are more severely affected than small fiber functions (pain and temperature perception).

Although initial symptoms are often sensory in nature, progressive muscle weakness quickly becomes the dominant feature in most cases. The severity can range from mild distal weakness to complete quadriplegia and the need for mechanical ventilation. The "ascending paralysis" that has been at times associated with AIDP is somewhat misleading, in that the pattern of weakness is usually not length dependent. Rather, weakness is usually first noted somewhere in the legs and ascends to involve the arms, trunk, head, and neck. Ropper reported that 56% had onset of weakness in the legs, 12% in the arms, and 32% simultaneously in the arms and legs.[7,9] Occasionally, there is a descending presentation with onset in the cranial nerves, with subsequent progression to the arms and legs. At nadir, however, the vast majority of patients will have some weakness in all four limbs.[69] Weakness in AIDP is symmetric—so much so that asymmetry should prompt careful consideration of mimicking conditions. Facial weakness and/or bulbar weakness is apparent in at least half of patients, though mild in most.[69] Preceding CMV, Zika, and Covid-19 infection have all been suggested to confer a higher frequency of facial weakness.[32,36,70] Ophthalmoparesis and ptosis develop in 5%–15% of patients.

Muscle stretch reflexes progressively diminish and frequently become unobtainable, due to desynchronization of action potential transmission caused by the multifocal demyelination characteristic of AIDP. If reflexes remain normal at first presentation, ongoing observation will typically find eventual diminishment or absence.[69] Bowel and bladder function are usually spared, although these may become involved in particularly severe disease states.

Approximately 25%–30% of patients with AIDP develop ventilatory failure due to respiratory muscle weakness. It is important to follow the strength of neck flexors and extensors and shoulder abductors closely. These muscle groups are innervated by cervical roots close to the phrenic nerve (C3/C4) and thus correlate well with diaphragmatic strength and impending ventilatory failure.[71] Autonomic instability is also common in AIDP. Both hypotension and hypertension can occur, with labile extremes between the two. Progressive reversible leukoencephalopathy syndrome (PRES) has also been reported in this setting and may rarely be the initial disease manifestation.[72–78] Cardiac arrhythmias can occur in severe cases and can be one cause of mortality in this disorder.

Symptoms usually progress over the course of 2–4 weeks. Approximately 80% of patients reach their nadir by 2 weeks, and 90% by 4 weeks.[7,9,69] Progression of symptoms and signs for over 8 weeks excludes GBS and suggests the diagnosis of chronic inflammatory demyelinating polyneuropathy (CIDP). Subacute onset with progression of the disease over 4 to 8 weeks occurs in a small subset and has been termed subacute inflammatory demyelinating polyneuropathy.[79–81] Patients with subacute inflammatory demyelinating polyneuropathy may have a monophasic illness like AIDP or may behave like CIDP and continue to progress unless treated with immunosuppressive or immunomodulating agents. Once the disease nadir is reached, there is an expected plateau phase of several days to weeks followed by gradual recovery over several months.

LABORATORY FEATURES

Albuminocytologic dissociation—elevated CSF protein levels accompanied by no or only a few mononuclear cells—is present in over 80% of AIDP patients 2 weeks after symptom onset.[20,69] However, within the first week of symptoms, CSF protein levels are normal in one-third to one-half of patients.[69,82] When CSF pleocytosis of more than 10 WBCs/mm^3 (particularly with cell counts >50/mm^3) is found, acute neuropathies related to Lyme disease, recent HIV infection, or sarcoidosis need to be considered.

Elevated liver function tests are common and may be attributed to viral hepatitis (A, B, C, and E), Epstein–Barr virus, or CMV infection. Some patients develop hyponatremia due to inappropriate antidiuretic hormone (SIADH) secretion.[83,84] Unlike the axonal forms of GBS, antiganglioside antibodies appear to be uncommon in AIDP (Fig. 13-1). Thickening or enhancement of the nerve roots may be appreciated on magnetic resonance imaging of the spine.[85]

ELECTRODIAGNOSTIC FEATURES

When GBS is suspected clinically, electrodiagnostic studies (EDX) are typically obtained to confirm localization to the peripheral nerves and, in the case of AIDP, specifically identify features of demyelination. It is critical to be aware that electrodiagnostic findings evolve throughout the course of illness. Within the first week of symptom onset, motor conduction studies can be normal or show only minor abnormalities. Because of the early predilection for the proximal nerve segments and spinal roots in AIDP, the absence of the H reflexes and/or abnormalities of the F-waves are among the most frequent findings early in the course.[86–89] In one cohort, 97% of patients had absent H reflexes and 84% had abnormal F waves on nerve conduction studies (NCS) performed within 1 week of symptom onset.[89] Prolonged or absent F-waves and prolonged distal motor latencies were the earliest abnormal features appreciated by the North American Guillain–Barré Syndrome Study Group.[86,87] Prolonged distal latencies and diminished compound muscle action potential (CMAP) amplitude were the earliest NCS abnormalities in another cohort described by Albers and colleagues.[88] Characteristic findings of demyelination including slowing of motor nerve conduction velocities (NCVs), temporal dispersion of the CMAP waveforms, and conduction block typically do not become apparent until later in the course. The maximum degree of motor conduction abnormality occurs within 3–8 weeks, with 80%–90% of patients with AIDP having abnormalities in at least one of the motor nerve parameters (distal CMAP latency, F-wave latency, conduction velocity, and/or conduction block) within 5 weeks of onset.[86–92]

Subtypes and variants	IgG autoantibodies to
Guillain-Barré syndrome	
Acute inflammatory demyelinating polyneuropathy	None
Facial variant: Facial diplegia and paresthesia	None
Acute motor axonal neuropathy	GM1, GD1a
More and less extensive forms	
Acute motor–sensory axonal neuropathy	GM1, GD1a
Acute motor-conduction-block neuropathy	GM1, GD1a
Pharyngeal–cervical–brachial weakness	GT1a > GQ1b >> GD1a
Miller Fisher syndrome	GQ1b, GT1a
Incomplete forms	
Acute ophthalmoparesis (without ataxia)	GQ1b, GT1a
Acute ataxic neuropathy (without ophthalmoplegia)	GQ1b, GT1a
CNS variant: Bickerstaff's brain-stem encephalitis	GQ1b, GT1a

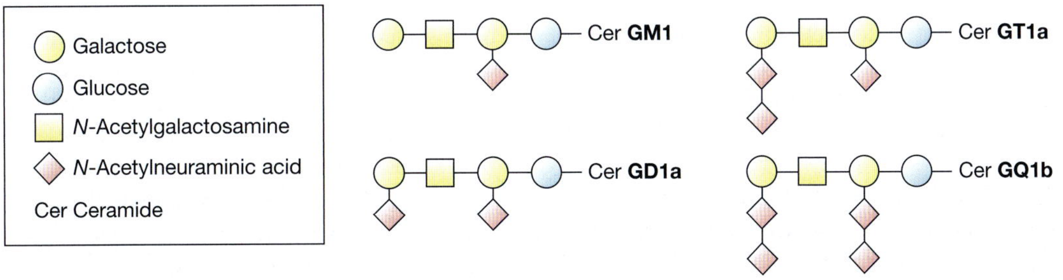

Figure 13-1. Spectrum of disorders in the Guillain–Barré syndrome and associated antiganglioside antibodies. IgG autoantibodies against GM1 or GD1a are strongly associated with acute motor axonal neuropathy, as well as the more extensive acute motor–sensory axonal neuropathy. IgG anti-GQ1b antibodies, which cross-react with GT1a, are strongly associated with the Miller Fisher syndrome, its incomplete forms [acute ophthalmoparesis (without ataxia) and acute ataxic neuropathy (without ophthalmoplegia)], and its more extensive form, Bickerstaff brain-stem encephalitis. Pharyngeal–cervical–brachial weakness is categorized as a localized form of acute motor axonal neuropathy or an extensive form of the Miller Fisher syndrome. Half the patients with pharyngeal–cervical–brachial weakness have IgG anti-GT1a antibodies, which often cross-react with GQ1b. IgG anti-GD1a antibodies have also been detected in a small percentage of patients. The anti-GQ1b antibody syndrome includes the Miller Fisher syndrome, acute ophthalmoparesis, acute ataxic neuropathy, Bickerstaff brain-stem encephalitis, and pharyngeal–cervical–brachial weakness. The presence of clinical overlap also indicates that the Miller Fisher syndrome is part of a continuous spectrum with these conditions. Patients who have had the Guillain–Barré syndrome overlapped with the Miller Fisher syndrome or with its related conditions have IgG antibodies against GM1 or GD1a as well as against GQ1b or GT1a, supporting a link between AMAN and the anti-GQ1b syndrome. CNS, central nervous system. (Reproduced with permission from Hughes RA, Cornblath DR. Guillain-Barre syndrome. *Lancet.* 2005; 366(9497):1653–1666.)

Therefore, while various EDX criteria for demyelination have been developed to aid in the diagnosis of AIDP,[88,93–95] their usefulness may vary depending on when studies are performed in the course of illness. Early on, many patients with apparent GBS will have an ambiguous pattern on EDX studies that does not allow for clear distinction between a demyelinating or axonal physiology.[29,69,96,97] Some patients will simply have unexcitable nerves. Absence of the F waves, as another example, are nonspecific; prolongation of F-wave minimum latency is more specific for demyelination. Complicating matters further, patients with AMAN may be noted to have conduction block, without motor NCV slowing or temporal dispersion of the CMAP waveform. This has been referred to as reversible conduction failure and likely reflects direct alterations at the nodes of Ranvier rather than demyelination. Recent proposed diagnostic criteria have specifically recognized the features that may overlap between AIDP and AMAN and their application generally results in more cases being classified as axonal in nature.[98,99] Since repeat studies at a later timepoint have been shown to change the electrodiagnostic classification in some patients, some authors specifically advocate the importance of serial testing for accurate diagnosis of GBS subtype.[100]

Sensory NCS can also be helpful diagnostically. By definition, the AMAN variant of GBS is associated with normal sensory conduction studies. Sensory studies in the arms can be affected more severely and earlier than the sural sensory nerve action potentials (SNAPs) in AIDP, resulting in a pattern known as "sural sparing."[88] This may be present in up to 50% of patients within the first two weeks of symptom onset. By some accounts, this is the most specific electrodiagnostic finding for AIDP when considering other mimicking causes of polyneuropathy or polyradiculopathy.[89,101] Sural sparing is not unique to GBS, however, and can be seen in other non–length-dependent neuropathy syndromes such as sensory neuronopathies.

About 40%–60% of patients eventually demonstrate either amplitude reduction or slow conduction velocities, with maximal abnormalities seen after 4–6 weeks.[88,102] Reduced SNAP amplitudes can be the result of secondary axonal degeneration, conduction block, or phase cancellation related to differential demyelination of various sensory nerve fibers. Rarely, patients may present with what appears to be pure sensory symptoms and signs, but careful evaluation usually reveals some motor nerve conduction abnormalities.[103,104]

The earliest abnormality on electromyography (EMG) is reduced recruitment of motor unit action potentials.[88] Positive sharp waves and fibrillation potentials may be appreciated 2–4 weeks after onset of weakness, as some degree of axon loss is common even in AIDP.[105] Myokymic discharges may be seen, especially in facial muscles.

DIFFERENTIAL DIAGNOSIS

Arguably, the most important alternative to consider is CIDP. Up to 18% of cases of CIDP begin acutely, mimicking GBS; 2%–5% of patients diagnosed as AIDP will go on to have CIDP instead.[106] Related, as many as 5%–10% of patients with GBS who initially improve with treatment will have a relapse within a few days or up to 3 weeks later. These have been deemed "treatment-related fluctuations (TRF)."[20,106,107] At the time of relapse, it can be very difficult to ascertain whether a patient is having a TRF or instead they are evolving into CIDP and require long-term immunotherapy. Cranial nerve involvement and respiratory failure would generally favor GBS with TRF, since these are uncommon in acute-onset CIDP, but this is not a perfect distinction. Time is the most important factor—when a patient thought to have GBS deteriorates again after 8 weeks from onset or when there are three or more relapses, acute-onset CIDP must be considered instead.[106,108] A few cases of acute neuropathy mimicking GBS have also been reported in association with either IgG2 and IgG3 antibodies targeting Caspr-1 or the "pan-neurofascin" antibodies (see Chapter 14).[109,110]

When identified, certain features should always prompt reconsideration of a potential GBS diagnosis (see Table 13-2): (1) marked asymmetry of sensory loss or weakness, (2) the presence of a sensory level on the trunk, (3) preserved reflexes, (4) early or severe bladder and bowel dysfunction, or (5) severe sensory signs with little to no weakness.[94] Asymmetry, for example, might prompt consideration of a vasculitic neuropathy, an infectious cause of polyradiculitis such as Lyme disease, or carcinomatous meningitis. The presence of a sensory level or preservation of the reflexes requires heightened scrutiny for a myelopathy and spinal imaging should be obtained. Bowel and bladder dysfunction can also be suggestive of a myelopathy, or alternative causes of cauda equina syndrome. Finally, severe sensory signs without weakness suggests sensory ganglionopathy. Because severe proprioceptive loss can interfere with the ability to perceive the amount of force one is generating with voluntary muscle activation, it can be very easy to mistakenly identify "weakness" on examination in such patients. Ensuring the patient is visually attending to the desired movement can help avoid this pitfall.

Occasionally, alternative causes of polyneuropathy might be mistaken for GBS. Neuropathy related to malnutrition can occasionally present acutely and be quite severe.[111] This can be seen after bariatric surgery, for example, in the setting of rapid weight loss. CSF protein is normal in these cases, and electrodiagnostic studies should reveal an axonal pattern. Urgent caloric supplementation is required, alongside correction of any specific micronutrient deficiencies that are identified. Although rare, neuropathy associated with acute intermittent porphyria, diphtheria, or heavy metal poisoning can present acutely. It is also wise to look for ticks, particularly in children, as tick paralysis can mimic GBS.[8,112] Removal of the tick leads to improvement of strength and function.

Some patients with a chronic polyneuropathy may report a pseudoacute onset when they first notice positive symptoms, perhaps failing to recognize more insidious negative symptoms that would have been accompanied by deficits on neurologic examination. In one case series, 13% of patients in whom an initial suspected GBS diagnosis was later refuted indeed had a chronic axonal polyneuropathy.[101] Notably, another 13% were eventually diagnosed with a somatoform disorder instead of GBS.

HISTOPATHOLOGY

Nerve biopsies are not routinely performed in patients suspected of having GBS. Nonetheless, biopsies have demonstrated endoneurial and perivascular mononuclear cell infiltrate consisting of macrophages and lymphocytes.[7,60,113,114] There may be an initial predilection for the nerve root region, areas where peripheral nerves are commonly entrapped (e.g., carpal and cubital tunnels), and the motor nerve terminals. The earliest pathophysiologic features are often appreciated at the nodes of Ranvier, where there is loosened paranodal myelin and subsequent demyelination of the internodal segments. Monocellular infiltrates may be appreciated in areas of segmental demyelination (Fig. 13-2). Polymorphonuclear cells, in addition to monocytes, may be associated with axonal

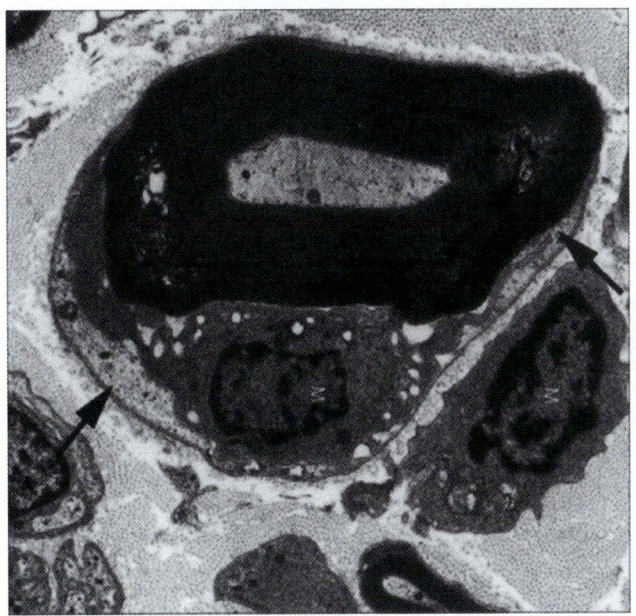

Figure 13-2. Nerve fiber from patient with AIDP. Electron micrograph shows that a macrophage (M) has invaded a Schwann cell basement membrane and stripped the abaxonal Schwann cell cytoplasm (*arrows*). (Reproduced with permission from Hughes RAC. Pathology of Guillain-Barré syndrome. In: *Guillain-Barré Syndrome. Clinical Medicine and the Nervous System.* Springer, London; 1990: 83–100. Figure 4.7: p. 94. https://doi.org/10.1007/978-1-4471-3175-5_4.)

degeneration in severe cases. During the recovery phase, remyelination is appreciated. Myelin thickness is reduced and the number of internodes is increased compared to normal peripheral nerve.

Autopsy studies of patients in China who died early in the course of their illness have shed light on the pathology of GBS, including AIDP, AMSAN, and AMAN.[22,115–117] In two patients who died at 7 and 9 days after onset of the neuropathy, autopsies revealed completely demyelinated peripheral nerves accompanied by extensive lymphocytic infiltrate.[116] However, in a patient who died only 3 days after symptom onset, the peripheral nerves had only scant inflammatory infiltrate and just a few of the nerves were completely demyelinated. Markers of complement activation were demonstrated on the outermost surface of the Schwann cells, and early vesicular changes in the myelin sheaths, beginning in the outer lamellae, were appreciated on electron microscopy.

PATHOGENESIS

Cellular immunity likely plays a role in the pathogenesis of AIDP, given the T-cells and macrophages apparent in the nerves, markers of T-cell activation (e.g., soluble interleukin-2 receptor and interferon-γ) in the serum, and the resemblance to experimental allergic neuritis.[8,118–121] In animal models, depleting the animal of these effector cells prevents the disease.[18] The humoral arm of the immune system has also been implicated, both by the demonstration of complement system products on Schwann cells in affected patients and frequent clinical improvement following plasmapheresis.[116,119] Further, injection of serum from patients with AIDP into nerves of animal models induces complement-dependent demyelination and conduction block.[122]

The nature of the responsible epitope is not known but probably is a glycolipid. Unlike AMAN, which has been more clearly linked with autoantibodies targeting the GM1 ganglioside, autoantibodies against gangliosides, neurofascins, or otherwise are very rarely detected in humans with AIDP. Molecular similarity between myelin epitope(s) and glycolipids expressed on *Campylobacter*, *Mycoplasma*, CMV, and other infectious agents, which precede attacks of AIDP, may be the underlying trigger for the immune attack.[10,116] Antibodies directed against these infectious agents may cross-react with specific antigens on the Schwann cell because of this molecular mimicry. These autoantibodies may bind to the Schwann cells and then activate the complement cascade, leading to lysis of myelin sheaths (Fig. 13-3).[10,116] Inflammatory cells are subsequently recruited to complete the demyelinating process.

TREATMENT

Plasma exchange (PLEX)[123–127] and intravenous immune globulin (IVIg)[23,124] are proven effective treatments for AIDP (Table 13-3).[61,128,129] Six randomized, placebo-controlled trials demonstrate the benefit of PLEX. Treated patients have a higher likelihood of improving one or more clinical disability grades and regaining the ability to walk with assistance after 4 weeks. PLEX treatment is also associated with a shorter time to walking without assistance and a shorter time on a ventilator.[128] A standard course of PLEX requires 5 alternate-day exchanges.

IVIg has generally replaced PLEX as the treatment of choice for AIDP. Several randomized trials treating adults within 2 weeks of symptom onset have demonstrated no difference in the improvement in clinical disability grade at 4 weeks between IVIg and PLEX treatment.[129] Patients enrolled in trials have generally been less likely to discontinue IVIg treatment than PLEX treatment. A retrospective database review study also suggests that PLEX treatment is associated with longer hospitalization by 7.5 days, increased hospitalization costs, and increased risk of in-hospital death (OR 2.78) when compared to IVIg treatment. These trends persisted even when controlling for the severity of illness.[130] The dose of IVIg is 2.0 g/kg body weight infused over 2–5 days.

Treatment with IVIg or PLEX should ideally begin within the first 14 days of symptoms, as this was the cutoff used in most clinical trials. Likewise, most patients treated in clinical trials have some disability related to their symptoms (e.g., inability to walk); mildly affected patients are understudied. The French cooperative trial for PLEX did include some patients

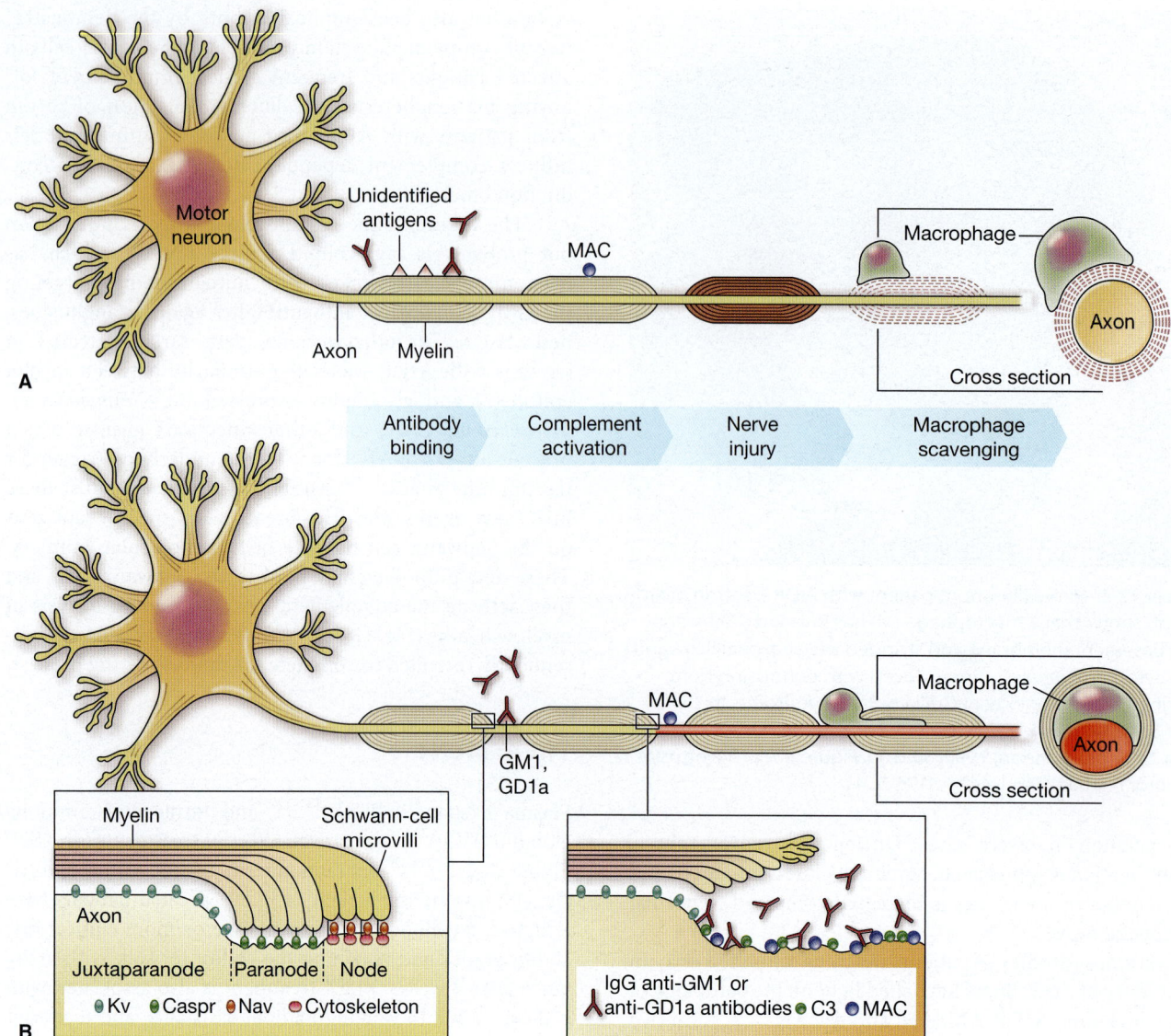

Figure 13-3. Possible immune mechanisms in GBS. Panel A shows the immunopathogenesis of AIDP. Although autoantigens have yet to be unequivocally identified, autoantibodies may bind to myelin antigens and activate complement. This is followed by the formation of membrane-attack complex (MAC) on the outer surface of Schwann cells and the initiation of vesicular degeneration. Macrophages subsequently invade myelin and act as scavengers to remove myelin debris. Panel B shows the immunopathogenesis of acute axonal forms of GBS (AMAN and AMSAN). Myelinated axons are divided into four functional regions: the nodes of Ranvier, paranodes, juxtaparanodes, and internodes. Gangliosides GM1 and GD1a are strongly expressed at the nodes of Ranvier, where the voltage-gated sodium (Nav) channels are localized. Contactin-associated protein (Caspr) and voltage-gated potassium (Kv) channels are respectively present at the paranodes and juxtaparanodes. IgG anti-GM1 or anti-GD1a autoantibodies bind to the nodal axolemma, leading to MAC formation. This results in the disappearance of Nav clusters and the detachment of paranodal myelin, which can lead to nerve-conduction failure and muscle weakness. Axonal degeneration may follow at a later stage. Macrophages subsequently invade from the nodes into the periaxonal space, scavenging the injured axons. (From Yuki N, Hartung HP. Guillain-Barré syndrome. *N Engl J Med*. 2012;366(24):2294–2304. Copyright © 2012 Massachusetts Medical Society. Reprinted with permission from Massachusetts Medical Society.)

who could still walk and stand unaided; the onset of motor recovery occurred in 4 days in those treated with an abbreviated course of PLEX compared to 8 days in those receiving placebo.[131] The improvement with PLEX and IVIg is often not immediate and it is impossible to know in an individual whether the time to nadir has been shortened, so it is often tempting to augment the initial treatment attempt. There is, however, no evidence that PLEX beyond 250 mL/kg[125,132–134] or IVIg greater than 2 g/kg is of any added benefit. In fact, one randomized trial included patients with poor prognosis for recovery and gave a second course of IVIg 7–9 days after the initial course. This showed no benefit compared to placebo and was associated with a higher risk of serious adverse events including thromboembolism.[135] Likewise, there is no evidence that giving IVIg after treating with PLEX confers additional benefit; it makes no mechanistic sense to administer PLEX

▶ TABLE 13-3. **GUILLAIN–BARRÉ SYNDROME: PLASMAPHERESIS AND IVIG TRIALS**[54,90,91,93]

	Plasmapheresis Group	Control Group	IVIg Group
North American Trial			
Number of patients	122	123	
Time to improve one clinical grade (days)	19	40	
Time to walk unaided (all patients) (days)	53	85	
Time to walk unaided (ventilator patients) (days)	97	169	
Time on ventilator (days)	9	23	
Percentage improved at 1 month	59	39	
Percentage improved at 6 months	97	87s	
French Trial			
Number of patients	109	111	
Percentage of patients on ventilator after study (days)	18	31	
Time to wean from ventilator (days)	70	111	
Time to walk unaided (days)	28	45	
Time in hospital	21	42	
Dutch IVIg Trial			
Number of patients	73		74
% of patients improving one clinical grade after 4 weeks	34		53
Time to improve one clinical grade (days)	41		27
Time to clinical grade 2 (days)	69		55
Ventilator dependent by week 2 (%)	42		27
Number of multiple complications	16		5
PE/Sandoglobulin Trial Group			
Number of patients	121		130
Mean change in clinical grade after 4 weeks	0.9		0.8
Time to wean from ventilator (days)	29		26
Time to walk unaided (days)	49		51
Number of patients unable to walk after 48 weeks	19 (16.7%)		21 (16.5%)

Reproduced with permission from Amato AA, Dumitru D. Acquired neuropathies. In: Dumitru D, Amato AA, Swartz MJ, eds. *Electrodiagnostic Medicine*. 2nd ed. Hanley & Belfus; 2002.

after treating with IVIg. When patients develop a TRF, we generally re-treat with the initial modality.[107,125,132–134]

Unlike CIDP, corticosteroids do not appear to be beneficial in the treatment of GBS, and some patients have done worse with steroids. A small study of 25 patients treated with IVIg and intravenous methylprednisolone[136] did better than a historical control group treated with IVIg alone.[23] However, a much larger British study of 142 patients treated with methylprednisolone or placebo (approximately half the patients in each group were also treated with PLEX) failed to demonstrate the efficacy of corticosteroids.[137] A double-blind, placebo-controlled randomized study of IVIg plus intravenous methylprednisolone compared to IVIg plus placebo in 233 patients with GBS revealed no significant difference between treatment with methylprednisolone and IVIg versus IVIg alone.[138] Thus, there is no strong support in the medical literature for supplemental corticosteroid use in patients with GBS.

PROGNOSIS AND LONG-TERM MANAGEMENT

The estimated mortality rate in GBS ranges from 2% to 5%, related to respiratory failure, aspiration pneumonia, pulmonary embolism, cardiac arrhythmias, and sepsis related to secondarily acquired infections.[7,9,139] Most patients die during the recovery period and not while they are actually getting weaker.[139] Older age and preexisting medical comorbidities are associated with a higher risk of mortality.

Improvement in strength and disability can be slow. About 60% of patients are still unable to walk unaided after 4 weeks and 20% at 6 months.[140] There may be some regional variation in this, perhaps related to the predominant subtype of GBS—one study estimated that 91% of patients in Asia walked unaided at 1 year compared to 83% in Europe and the Americas and 69% in Bangladesh.[20] Risk factors for a slower and incomplete recovery include: age greater than 50–60 years, abrupt onset of profound weakness, the need for mechanical ventilation, delay from onset of weakness to treatment, preceding diarrheal illness, and cumulative distal CMAP amplitudes less than 10%–20% of normal.[86,87,123,124,139,141] The modified Erasmus score, for example, uses age, diarrhea, and severity of weakness to stratify likelihood of regaining ambulation at 4 weeks and 6 months.[140,142] Even though most patients regain strength, 50%–85% of patients have some degree of residual deficits as many as 7 years after disease onset.[7,9,10,68,143–146] Pain, fatigue, and depression are common long-term sequelae.

Motor nerve conduction abnormalities reach their nadir somewhere between 1 and 3 months—later than clinical nadir.[88,147] There is no correlation between the NCVs or distal motor latencies and clinical severity of the neuropathy, although distal CMAP amplitudes less than 10%–20% of normal are associated with a poorer prognosis.[86,87,123,124,148–150] Findings gradually improve over the next several weeks to months. Importantly, NCS findings suggestive of demyelination can persist well over 1 year in a minority of patients. Occasionally, these can even meet electrodiagnostic criteria for CIDP; relying on clinical symptom evolution is therefore critical.[147]

An estimated 2%–5% of patients with GBS will have a recurrent episode later in life.[151–154] The same syndrome (e.g., AIDP) tends to repeat itself. Infectious triggers for a recurrence are most common, noted in 78% of recurrent bouts in one series. Perhaps in light of this risk, patients and clinicians alike can be hesitant about pursuing vaccination after GBS. If a specific vaccine was given within 6 weeks of the onset of GBS, then that vaccine should indeed never be given again. Expert consensus guidance also advises against giving routine vaccines within the first year after GBS though this has never been studied in a prospective manner.[155] Otherwise, GBS is not an absolute contraindication to future vaccination, as vaccination has not generally been associated with recurrent GBS. The Covid-19 pandemic provided some further reassurance in this regard. A registry study from Israel included 579 patients with a prior history of GBS who received at least one dose of an mRNA Covid-19 vaccine. Only one of these patients presented with concern for GBS recurrence; their symptoms improved with PLEX treatment.[156] In another survey study, zero of 160 patients with a history of GBS had recurrence after receiving a Covid vaccine.[157]

▶ ACUTE MOTOR AXONAL NEUROPATHY

CLINICAL FEATURES

Feasby and colleagues were the first to detail an axonal variant of GBS in 1986.[158] AMAN occurs in children and adults and begins with the abrupt onset of generalized weakness without sensory symptoms.[10,21,22,60,65,159,160] There is a very strong association between AMAN and preceding diarrheal illness, specifically with *C. jejuni*.[29,93] The distal muscles are often more severely affected than proximal limb muscles. Cranial nerve deficits and ventilatory failure requiring mechanical ventilation can be seen, but are likely less common than with AIDP.[21,22,24,96] Unlike AIDP and AMSAN, there are no sensory signs or symptoms. However, autonomic dysfunction (e.g., cardiac arrhythmias, blood pressure fluctuations, and hyperhidrosis) may still occur. Muscle stretch reflexes are typically absent, but normal reflexes at presentation are seen more frequently than with AIDP; some patients develop hyperactive reflexes during the recovery period.[22,69,91,159,161,162]

The median time of recovery is similar to that seen in typical AIDP, and most affected individuals have a good recovery within 1 year. Residual distal limb weakness is common.[160] Second attacks of the illness have been described in northern Chinese patients, but the actual recurrence rate is not known.[22]

LABORATORY FEATURES

As with AIDP, albuminocytologic dissociation in the CSF is expected. The absence of prominent CSF pleocytosis helps distinguish AMAN from poliomyelitis, which it would otherwise mimic.[21,22,24,159] Both serologic evidence of recent *C. jejuni* infection and IgG autoantibodies against either GM1, GM1b, GalNAc-GD1a, or GD1b are demonstrated in the majority of patients with AMAN (Fig. 13-1).[10,22,24,93,96,163] Gangliosides, which are proteins located on peripheral nerves, are composed of a ceramide attached to one or more sugar residues and contain sialic acid. The major gangliosides in regard to GBS differ with regard to the number and position of their sialic acids (Fig. 13-3).[10]

A purely motor clinical presentation clearly raises strong suspicion for AMAN, but the typical distinction between this disorder and AIDP rests in the EDX findings. The electrodiagnostic distinction between demyelinating and axonal cases is less straightforward than one might expect, however. The findings on EDX in patients with AMAN occur on a spectrum, can be dynamic over time, and reflect the complex underlying pathophysiology of this disorder.

In the acute phase of illness, NCS typically reveals low-amplitude or unobtainable CMAPs with normal SNAPs.[22,96,100,164,165] F-waves are frequently also unobtainable. While distal motor latencies, proximal segment conduction velocities, and the obtainable F-waves latencies are typically normal, conduction block—traditionally considered a feature of demyelination—is frequently encountered in AMAN. If NCS are repeated, conduction block(s) can be shown to resolve very quickly in some patients, within even 2–5 weeks, without any residual evidence of demyelination (e.g., temporal dispersion). In other patients, however, repeat studies will no longer show conduction block but instead a progressive decline in the distal CMAP amplitudes. Both patterns can even be seen in the same patient.

This suggests a spectrum of pathophysiologic possibilities. In some, conduction block is due to reversible conduction failure at the node of Ranvier. This may reflect the pathophysiologic effects of ganglioside antibodies at the nodal region (discussed further below). In others, the responsible immunologic attack may persist or be especially severe, leading to eventual underlying axonal damage and degeneration.

Thus, in some patients the evolution of EDX findings over time will help solidify a demyelinating or axonal phenotype.[29,96] Caution is required early, since low CMAP amplitudes and absent F waves are among the most frequent early NCS findings in AIDP and conduction block may be seen in both.[98] As an important corollary to this point, distal CMAP amplitudes should not be taken as a surrogate for axonal degeneration early in the course of GBS, as this could simply reflect distal reversible conduction failure past the distal-most stimulation site. Findings of fibrillation potentials/positive sharp waves on needle EMG would be a more reliable indicator of underlying axonal degeneration.

HISTOPATHOLOGY

The earliest histologic abnormality is the lengthening of the nodal gaps. Immunocytochemistry reveals deposition of IgG and complement activation products (i.e., C3 and C5b-9) on the nodal and internodal axolemma of motor fibers.[116] This is in contrast to AIDP, where there is early deposition of immunoglobulin and complement on Schwann cells rather than the axons.[116] Macrophages are recruited into the affected nodes of Ranvier and periaxonal space via complement-derived chemotropic factors.[116] T-cells are usually absent. The macrophages migrate through the Schwann cell basal lamina into the nodal gap, where these inflammatory cells dissect beneath the myelin sheath into the periaxonal space (Fig. 13-4).

As macrophages enter the periaxonal space, paranodal detachment occurs and the axon retracts away from the adaxonal Schwann cell. This disruption of the usual nodal/paranodal architecture is likely responsible for the conduction block seen on NCS in some patients. If the immune attack abates quickly, the node can quickly reassemble and the conduction block may be quickly reversible, in turn. In severe cases, however, the underlying axons begin to degenerate while the innermost myelin sheath (adaxonal lamella) appears intact.[96] Active degeneration and severe loss of large myelinated intramuscular nerve fibers can be demonstrated on biopsy in these cases.[160]

PATHOGENESIS

AMAN is most likely caused by an immune-mediated attack against the nodal axolemma (Figs. 13-1 and 13-3).[10,164,166–168] As discussed above, many patients harbor autoantibodies against gangliosides which may be due to cross-reactivity with similar molecules on the lipopolysaccharide membrane of *Campylobacter*.[27,116,169,170] Immunizing rabbits against GM1 gangliosides can produce a similar neuropathy phenotype.[171] Experimental studies demonstrate that GBS sera containing ganglioside antibodies cause neuronal cell lysis by targeting specific cell-surface gangliosides and, secondly, that this cell lysis is complement dependent. Of note, IVIg significantly decreased this complement-dependent cytotoxicity. Binding of GM1 antibodies and the subsequent activation of complement has also been shown to lead to paranodal detachment and destruction of Na_V channels.

When comparing the recovery of patients with AMAN to that of patients with AIDP, the median time required to regain the ability to walk with assistance is similar.[160] This would not be possible if significant motor axonal degeneration occurs, since axonal regeneration is a slow process. As discussed above, in such cases, reversible conduction failure is likely the predominant pathophysiologic mechanism. If complement-mediated cytotoxicity is significant, axonal damage can occur and lead to a more protracted recovery period.[93,96,167,168]

TREATMENT

There have not been any treatment trials devoted to AMAN, although 27 of the 147 (18%) patients enrolled in the Dutch GBS trial comparing IVIg to PLEX were later classified as having AMAN.[23,24] There was no significant difference in outcome, regardless of treatment (IVIg, PLEX, or PLEX followed by IVIg) between AIDP and AMAN, in a subgroup analysis of 369 patients.[93] Treating patients in a similar fashion to AIDP is therefore appropriate.

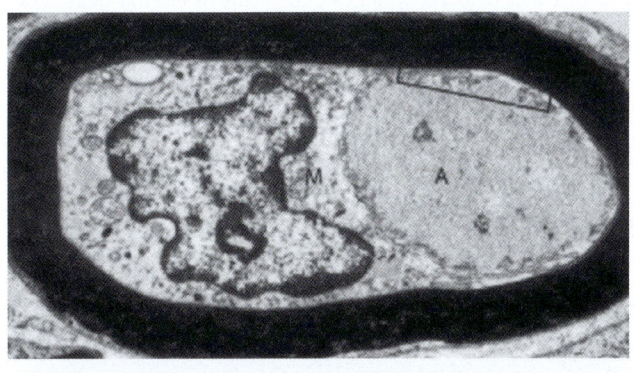
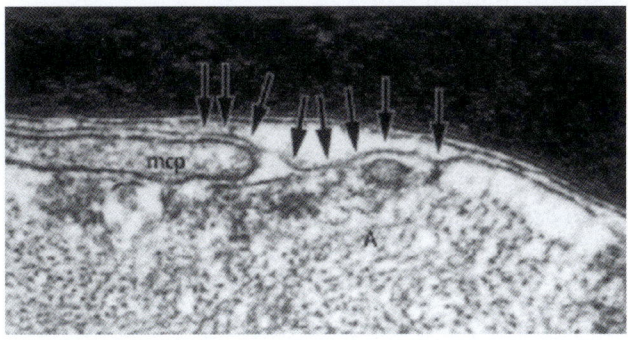

Figure 13-4. Nerve fiber from patient with AMAN. Lower panel is enlargement of box in upper panel. Electron micrograph shows macrophage (M) that has invaded the periaxonal space and axolemma (*arrows*) surrounding the axon (A); mcp, macrophage process. (Reproduced with permission from Griffin JW, Li CY, Macko C, et al. Early nodal changes in the acute motor axonal neuropathy pattern of the Guillain Barré syndrome. *J Neurocytol.* 1996;25(1):33–51. Figure 8. Pg. 44.)

▶ ACUTE MOTOR AND SENSORY AXONAL NEUROPATHY (AMSAN)

CLINICAL FEATURES

Clinically, patients with acute motor and sensory axonal neuropathy (AMSAN) may initially be indistinguishable from those with AIDP.[10,22,60,115,148,151,158,172–177] Usually, sensory symptoms begin in the hands or feet and later progress. Sensation to all modalities is reduced and areflexia is usually evident. Patients with AMSAN rapidly develop progressive and severe generalized weakness over only a few days, as opposed to progression over a couple of weeks in most patients with AIDP. Ophthalmoplegia, dysphagia, and ventilatory muscle weakness can occur. Dysautonomia including labile blood pressure and cardiac arrhythmias may complicate AMSAN as well. Only a few children have been reported with AMSAN, and there is some suggestion that the prognosis is better than in adults.[158,172]

LABORATORY FEATURES

Albuminocytologic dissociation of the CSF protein is usually seen. As in AMAN, antiganglioside antibodies, particularly GM1 and GD1a IgG antibodies, are found in some patients with AMSAN and correlate with recent *C. jejuni* infection (Fig. 13-1).[10,93,170,178,179]

NCS reveal markedly diminished amplitudes or absent CMAPs and SNAPs within 7–10 days of onset.[87,149,158,173,174,176,180,181] As discussed earlier, low-amplitude CMAPs are one of the earliest electrophysiologic abnormalities noted in AIDP; thus, low-amplitude CMAPs do not necessarily imply axonal degeneration. Distal conduction block with or without demyelination can also lead to low-amplitude distal CMAPs.[148,177] It is therefore often impossible to distinguish AIDP from AMSAN by NCSs early in the course of illness. Serial NCSs are helpful.[177] Patients with AIDP will eventually develop other features of demyelination (e.g., significantly prolonged distal latencies and F-wave latencies, slow CVs, more proximal conduction block, or temporal dispersion). The distal latencies of the CMAPs and the NCVs, when obtainable, should be normal or only mildly affected in AMSAN.

Needle EMG demonstrates a markedly abnormal reduction in recruitment. Several weeks after the presentation of major motor weakness, abundant fibrillation potentials, and positive sharp waves can be detected in most muscles, especially those located in the distal regions of the limbs.[169,182,183]

HISTOPATHOLOGY

Nerve biopsies are not typically indicated in clinical practice. Nerves biopsied late in the disease course of AIDP or AMSAN may show axonal degeneration, so it can be difficult to distinguish a primary axonopathy from secondary axonal degeneration. Sensory and motor nerve biopsies in several patients with in-excitable motor and sensory conduction studies revealed severe demyelination rather than primary axonal degeneration.[180,183–186] Nevertheless, some patients with inexcitable CMAPs and SNAPs have features that suggest a primary axonal insult.[22,115,158,175] Unlike AIDP, demyelination and lymphocytic infiltrates are absent or only minimally present on nerve biopsy or at autopsy in patients with AMSAN[115]; rather, prominent axonal degeneration affecting the ventral and dorsal roots and the peripheral nerves is appreciated. As many as 80% of teased fibers reveal axonal degeneration, while demyelinating features are rare.[158,175]

PATHOGENESIS

The pathogenic basis of AMSAN is unknown but is most likely due to an immune-mediated attack directed against epitopes on the axon.[8,10,115,121] AMSAN often follows *C. jejuni* infection and may be associated with the production of the antibodies directed against various nerve gangliosides (e.g., GM1 or GM1a) (Figs. 13-1 and 13-3).[10] These gangliosides are present on the nodal axolemma and may be the target of the immune attack due to molecular mimicry.[10,169,182] It follows then that AMSAN may represent the severe end of the spectrum of disease that is defined by an immune insult on the axon and that also includes AMAN.[22,115,160,187,188] As discussed previously, early in the course or with mild disease, binding of the antibodies to neural epitopes may result in only reversible conduction block. However, complement activation on nodal and later internodal axolemma and recruitment of macrophages can result in axonal degeneration. Due to the axonal loss, recovery of strength and function is slow and often incomplete compared to AIDP.[174]

TREATMENT

There have been no prospective treatment studies specifically for AMSAN; however, we treat patients with IVIg or PLEX.

▶ MILLER FISHER SYNDROME

CLINICAL FEATURES

MFS, first described in 1956,[11] is characterized by ataxia, areflexia, and ophthalmoplegia.[7,10,15,61,189–193] There is a spectrum between MFS and the syndrome of Bickerstaff encephalitis, which is associated with altered consciousness in addition to ataxia and ophthalmoplegia.[189,190,194] There may also be an overlap with the pharyngeal–cervical–brachial subtype of GBS.[195] The mean age of onset of MFS is in the early forties, but it can occur in children. There is a 2:1 male predominance. As with other forms of GBS, an antecedent infection is common, occurring in over two-thirds of the cases. Double vision is usually the earliest symptom (39%), followed by unsteadiness and incoordination due to a sensory ataxia (21%). Asymmetric oculomotor weakness may be seen, but this often progresses to complete ophthalmoplegia. Ptosis also occurs but pupillary involvement is uncommon. Other cranial nerves are also affected with facial weakness evident in 57%, dysphagia in 40%, and dysarthria in 13% patients. Approximately 50%

of the patients complain of paresthesias of the face and distal limbs during the course, and areflexia is evident on examination in over 80%. Mild proximal limb weakness may develop in approximately one-third of cases, and some patients progress to develop severe generalized weakness similar to typical AIDP.[15,191–193] Recovery usually begins within about 2 weeks following the onset of symptoms, and a full return of function is usually seen within 3–5 months.

LABORATORY FEATURES

CSF protein is usually elevated without significant pleocytosis.[7,15] Serologic evidence of recent infection by *C. jejuni* and ganglioside antibodies, in particular anti-GQ1b, is evident in many patients.[194,196,197] A large study of 123 patients with MFS demonstrated CSF albuminocytologic dissociation in 59% of patients during the first 3 weeks of illness, while serum GQ1b IgG antibodies were positive in 85%. While the incidence of CSF albuminocytologic dissociation increased from the first to second weeks, GQ1b IgG antibodies peaked in the first week. GQ1b IgG antibodies are also seen in Bickerstaff encephalitis.

NCS reveals reduced amplitudes of SNAPs out of proportion to any prolongation of the distal latencies or slowing of sensory conduction velocities.[198–202] CMAPs in the arms and legs are usually normal. However, mild-to-moderate reduction of facial CMAP amplitudes is evident in over 50% of patients with MFS.[199] A loss or mild delay of R1 and R2 responses may be appreciated on blink reflex testing.[192,199,203]

HISTOPATHOLOGY

Nerve biopsy and autopsy data are limited and need to be viewed cautiously, as some of the cases began with ophthalmoplegia, ataxia, and areflexia but later evolved to severe quadriparesis characteristic of more typical AIDP.[204] The brainstem appeared normal or revealed only secondary chromatolysis of the oculomotor, trochlear, or abducens nuclei. Demyelination and mild inflammatory infiltrates were noted along the course of these cranial nerves and in the sensory ganglia of peripheral nerves.

PATHOGENESIS

The pathogenic basis for the disorder is not known, although it is likely autoimmune, with preferential early attack directed against the sensory ganglia and oculomotor nerve fibers.[7,15] Antecedent infections (e.g., *C. jejuni*) suggest that autoantibodies directed against these infectious agents cross-react with neuronal epitopes (e.g., GQ1b) (Figs. 13-1 and 13-3).[10] In this regard, oculomotor fibers and the sensory ganglion are enriched in GQ1b, and antibodies directed against this protein are detected in most patients with MFS. Immunohistochemistry studies reveal that GQ1b antibodies stain sensory neurons in the dorsal root as well as cerebellar nuclei. In mice infused with serum from patients with MFS, the GQ1b antibodies bound to neuromuscular junctions and, in a complement-dependent process, this resulted in massive quantal release of acetylcholine from nerve terminals; this lead to blockage of neuromuscular transmission.[205] The similarities between MFS and Bickerstaff encephalitis suggests that these disorders fall along a spectrum and there may be central nervous system (CNS) as well as peripheral nervous system (PNS) involvement in MFS.[189]

TREATMENT

There are no controlled treatment trials of patients with MFS. A large retrospective study of 92 patients with MFS (28 treated with IVIg, 23 treated with PLEX, and 41 who did not receive treatment) suggested that IVIg might have slightly hastened the improvement of the ophthalmoplegia and ataxia, while PLEX was of no benefit.[190,206] This may be explained by the natural history of untreated MFS—most patients have a good recovery anyways. Nonetheless, in the absence of any controlled trials, we treat patients with IVIg.[190] IVIg inhibits the binding of GQ1b antibodies to GQ1b, thereby preventing complement activation and subsequent pathophysiologic effects in ex vivo mouse models, suggesting that it might be beneficial.[207]

▶ ACUTE SMALL FIBER SENSORY NEUROPATHY

CLINICAL FEATURES

Small fiber neuropathies typically present insidiously, with slowly progressive burning pain and paresthesia in the distal lower extremities (see Chapter 22). Rarely, patients present acutely, akin to a variant of GBS.[208–211] An antecedent infection is common; cases have been reported after Covid-19 infection, for example.[212] Neurologic examination discloses normal muscle strength, length-dependent or non–length-dependent sensory loss for pain and temperature, normal proprioception, and vibration senses with normal or brisk muscle stretch reflexes. However, non–length-dependent sensory loss and burning sensation can also be seen.[209] In untreated patients, the burning dysesthesia usually disappears within several months; however, the numbness and objective sensory loss tend to persist longer.

LABORATORY FEATURES

CSF examination may reveal albuminocytologic dissociation. Motor and sensory conduction studies that primarily assess large fiber function are normal. Autonomic testing may be abnormal.

HISTOPATHOLOGY

Nerve biopsies have not been reported. However, skin biopsies in some patients have shown reduced nerve fiber density, which in most cases was worse in the thigh compared to calf.[213]

PATHOGENESIS

The acute clinical presentation often follows an infection and CSF findings suggest that this may be a rare GBS variant.

TREATMENT

No randomized trials have been performed, but in case series steroids and IVIg have been used with variable success.

▶ AUTOIMMUNE AUTONOMIC NEUROPATHY

CLINICAL FEATURES

Young et al. were the first to report a detailed clinical, laboratory, and histologic description of a patient with acute pandysautonomia.[214,215] Subsequently, there have been a number of small reports of idiopathic autonomic neuropathy.[216–232] Many of these cases are presumed to have an autoimmune basis. This is a heterogeneous neuropathy in terms of onset, the type of autonomic deficits, the presence or absence of somatic involvement, and the degree of recovery. A series of 27 cases of idiopathic autonomic neuropathy followed for a mean of 32 months found that approximately 20% of patients had selective cholinergic dysfunction, while 80% had various degrees of widespread sympathetic and parasympathetic dysfunction.[228] The most common symptom is orthostatic dizziness or lightheadedness, occurring in about 80% of patients. Gastrointestinal involvement is present in over 70%, with patients complaining of nausea, vomiting, diarrhea, constipation, ileus, or postprandial bloating. Heat intolerance and poor sweating are also present in the majority of patients. Blurred vision, dry eyes and mouth, urinary retention or incontinence, and impotence are common. Numbness, tingling, and dysesthesia of the distal extremities are evident in about 30% of patients, but muscle strength is normal. An acute autonomic and sensory neuropathy (AASN) has been described in one case series in which severe autonomic failure was the predominant symptom, but varying degrees of diffuse small- and large-fiber sensory dysfunction were also present.[233] Most patients have a monophasic course similar to GBS with progression, followed by a plateau and slow recovery or a stable deficit.[228] Although some patients exhibit a complete recovery,[214,230] it tends to be incomplete in most.[228]

LABORATORY FEATURES

The CSF often reveals slightly elevated protein without pleocytosis.[228] Supine plasma norepinephrine levels are not different, but standing levels are significantly reduced, when compared to normal controls.[228] In a large study of patients with idiopathic autonomic neuropathy, 18/106 (18%) had high levels of ganglionic acetylcholine receptor (AchR) autoantibodies.[232,234] The seropositive group had a significant overrepresentation of abnormal pupillary responses, sicca complex, and lower gastrointestinal tract dysautonomia. A subacute mode of onset was more common in the seropositive group. In this regard, rabbits immunized with a neuronal AchR alpha3 subunit fusion protein produce ganglionic AchR antibodies and develop autonomic failure.[235] Immunohistochemical staining of superior cervical ganglia and myenteric plexus neurons reveals intact presynaptic nerve terminals and postsynaptic neurons containing cytoplasmic AchR, but lacking surface AchR.

Routine motor and sensory NCS and EMG are usually unremarkable.[228] Quantitative sensory testing may reveal abnormalities in thermal thresholds.[222] Autonomic testing can show abnormalities.[236,237] Orthostatic hypotension and reduced variability of the heart rate on deep breathing are evident in over 60% of affected individuals.[228] An abnormal response to Valsalva maneuver (i.e., exaggerated fall in blood pressure during early phase II of the response, absent recovery of systolic and diastolic blood pressure during late phase II, or reduced or absent overshoot of systolic and diastolic pressures during phase IV) has been demonstrated in over 40% of patients. Sympathetic skin response may be absent.[218,238] Abnormal quantitative sudomotor axon reflex test scores are seen in 85% of patients.[228] Most patients have abnormal thermoregulatory sweat tests, with areas of anhidrosis in 12%–97% of the body. Gastrointestinal studies may reveal hypomotility anywhere from the esophagus to the rectum.

HISTOPATHOLOGY

Nerve biopsies reveal reduced density of mainly small-diameter myelinated nerve fibers, along with stacks of empty Schwann cell profiles and collagen pockets.[214,219,221,225,228,238] Scant epineurial perivascular inflammation may be seen.

PATHOGENESIS

The disorder is suspected to be the result of an autoimmune attack directed against peripheral autonomic fibers or the ganglia.[221] A subset of patients may have antibodies directed against calcium channels, which are present on presynaptic autonomic nerve terminals.

TREATMENT

PLEX, prednisone, IVIg, and other immunosuppressive agents have been tried with variable success.[220,221,227,228] The most important aspect of management is supportive therapy for orthostatic hypotension and bowel and bladder symptoms.[205,206] Fludrocortisone is effective at increasing plasma volume but should be administered only in the morning or in the morning and at lunch to avoid nocturnal/supine hypertension. We begin treatment at 0.1 mg/day and increase by 0.1 mg every 3–4 days until their standing time and blood pressure are controlled. Midodrine, a peripheral alpha1 adrenergic agonist, may also be effective and can be used in combination with fludrocortisone.[239,240] Midodrine is started at 2.5 mg/day and can gradually be increased to 40 mg/day in divided doses (every 2–4 hours) as necessary. Gastrointestinal hypomotility can be treated with metoclopramide, cisapride, or erythromycin. Bulking agents, laxatives, and enemas may be needed in patients with constipation. Urology should be consulted in patients with neurogenic bladder. Patient may require cholinergic agonists (e.g., bethanechol), intermittent self-catheterization, or other modes of therapy.

▶ SUMMARY

GBS is an acquired immune-mediated neuropathy. It most commonly presents in the Western hemisphere as AIDP in which the immune attack is directed against myelin in peripheral nerves. Occasionally, the immune attack is directed against the axons of motor (AMAN) or motor and sensory nerves (AMSAN). These axonal variants of GBS are more common in Asia but do occur worldwide and are more common following *C. jejuni* infection. Other immune-mediated neuropathies such as MFS, acute autonomic neuropathy, acute sensory neuronopathies, and acute small fiber neuropathies may also fall into the spectrum of GBS. The natural history of most of these neuropathies is for gradual spontaneous improvement that may be facilitated with IVIg or PLEX.

REFERENCES

1. Guillain G, Barré J, Strohl A. Sur un syndrome de radiculo-nevrite avec hyper albiminose du loquide cephalo-rachiden sas raection cellulaire. Remarques sur les catarcteres cliniques et graphiques des reflexes tendeneux. *Bulletins et Memories de la Societe Medicale des Hospitaux de Paris, Masson et Cie*. 1916;40:1462–1470.
2. Haymaker WE, Kernohan JW. The Landry–Guillain–Barré syndrome; a clinicopathologic report of 50 fatal cases and a critique of the literature. *Medicine (Baltimore)*. 1949;28(1):59–141.
3. Asbury AK, Arnason BG, Adams RD. The inflammatory lesion in idiopathic polyneuritis. Its role in pathogenesis. *Medicine (Baltimore)*. 1969;48(3):173–215.
4. Brown WF, Feasby TE. Sensory evoked potentials in Guillain-Barre polyneuropathy. *J Neurol Neurosurg Psychiatry*. 1984;47(3):288–291.
5. Kennedy RH, Danielson MA, Mulder DW, Kurland LT. Guillain-Barré syndrome: a 42-year epidemiologic and clinical study. *Mayo Clin Proc*. 1978;53(2):93–99.
6. Ropper AH. Severe acute Guillain-Barre syndrome. *Neurology*. 1986;36(3):429–429.
7. Ropper A, Wijdicks E, Traux B. Guillain–Barré syndrome. Philadelphia, PA: *FA Davis*; 1991.
8. Hughes RA, Cornblath DR. Guillain-Barré syndrome. The *Lancet*. 2005;366(9497):1653–1666.
9. Ropper AH. The Guillain–Barré syndrome. *N Engl J Med*. 1992;326(17):1130–1136.
10. Yuki N, Hartung HP. Guillain–Barré syndrome. *N Engl J Med*. 2012;366(24):2294–2304.
11. Fisher M. An unusual variant of acute idiopathic polyneuritis (syndrome of ophthalmoplegia, ataxia and areflexia). *N Engl J Med*. 1956;255(2):57–65.
12. Ropper AH. Unusual clinical variants and signs in Guillain-Barre syndrome. *Arch Neurol*. 1986;43(11):1150–1152.
13. Ropper AH. Further regional variants of acute immune polyneuropathy. Bifacial weakness or sixth nerve paresis with paresthesias, lumbar polyradiculopathy, and ataxia with pharyngeal-cervical-brachial weakness. *Arch Neurol*. 1994;51(7):671–675.
14. Wakerley BR, Yuki N. Pharyngeal-cervical-brachial variant of Guillain-Barre syndrome. *J Neurol Neurosurg Psychiatry*. 2014;85(3):339–344.
15. Berlit P, Rakicky J. The Miller Fisher syndrome. Review of the literature. *J Clin Neuroophthalmol*. 1992;12(1):57–63.
16. Alter M. The epidemiology of Guillain-Barré syndrome. *Ann Neurol*. 1990;27(S1):S7–S12.
17. Shui IM, Rett MD, Weintraub E, et al; Vaccine Safety Datalink Research Team. Guillain-Barré syndrome incidence in a large United States cohort (2000–2009). *Neuroepidemiology*. 2012;39(2):109–115.
18. Shahrizaila N, Lehmann HC, Kuwabara S. Guillain-Barré syndrome. *Lancet*. 2021;397(10280):1214–1228.
19. McGrogan A, Madle GC, Seaman HE, de Vries CS. The epidemiology of Guillain-Barré syndrome worldwide. A systematic literature review. *Neuroepidemiology*. 2009;32(2):150–163.
20. Doets AY, Verboon C, van den Berg B, et al; IGOS Consortium. Regional variation of Guillain-Barré syndrome. *Brain*. 2018;141(10):2866–2877.
21. McKhann GM, Cornblath DR, Ho T, et al. Clinical and electrophysiological aspects of acute paralytic disease of children and young adults in northern China. *Lancet*. 1991;338(8767):593–597.
22. Griffin JW, Li CY, Ho TW, et al. Guillain-Barré syndrome in northern China: the spectrum of neuropathological changes in clinically defined cases. *Brain*. 1995;118(3):577–595.
23. van der Meché FGA, Schmitz PI. A randomized trial comparing intravenous immune globulin and plasma exchange in Guillain–Barré syndrome. *N Engl J Med*. 1992;326(17):1123–1129.
24. Visser LH, Van Der Meché FGA, Van Doorn PA, et al. Guillain-Barré syndrome without sensory loss (acute motor neuropathy). A subgroup with specific clinical, electrodiagnostic and laboratory features. Dutch Guillain-Barré Study Group. *Brain*. 1995;118(4):841–847.
25. Leonhard SE, Van Der Eijk AA, Andersen H, et al; IGOS Consortium. An international perspective on preceding infections in Guillain-Barré syndrome: The IGOS-1000 cohort. *Neurology*. 2022;99(12):E1299–E1313.
26. Jacobs BC, Rothbarth PH, van der Meché FGA, et al. The spectrum of antecedent infections in Guillain-Barré syndrome. *Neurology*. 1998;51(4):1110–1115.

27. Feasby TE, Hughes RA. Campylobacter jejuni, antigangliosides antibodies, and Guillain–Barré syndrome. *Neurology*. 1998;51(2):340–342.
28. Griffin JW, Ho TW. The Guillain-Barré syndrome at 75: the *Campylobacter* connection. *Ann Neurol*. 1993;34(2):125–127.
29. Uncini A, Manzoli C, Notturno F, Capasso M. Pitfalls in electrodiagnosis of Guillain-Barré syndrome subtypes. *J Neurol Neurosurg Psychiatry*. 2010;81(10):1157–1163.
30. Palaiodimou L, Stefanou MI, Katsanos AH, et al. Prevalence, clinical characteristics and outcomes of Guillain–Barré syndrome spectrum associated with COVID-19: a systematic review and meta-analysis. *Eur J Neurol*. 2021;28(10):3517–3529.
31. Keddie S, Pakpoor J, Mousele C, et al. Epidemiological and cohort study finds no association between COVID-19 and Guillain-Barré syndrome. *Brain*. 2021;144(2):682–693.
32. Luijten LWG, Leonhard SE, van der Eijk AA, et al; IGOS consortium. Guillain-Barré syndrome after SARS-CoV-2 infection in an international prospective cohort study. *Brain*. 2021;144(11):3392–3404.
33. Van Koningsveld R, Van Doorn PA, Schmitz PI, Ang CW, Van der Meche FG. Mild forms of Guillain-Barre syndrome in an epidemiologic survey in the Netherlands. *Neurology*. 2000;54(3):620–620.
34. Geurtsvankessel CH, Islam Z, Mohammad QD, Jacobs BC, Endtz HP, Osterhaus ADME. Hepatitis E and Guillain-Barré syndrome. *Clin Infect Dis*. 2013;57(9):1369–1370.
35. van den Berg B, van der Eijk AA, Pas SD, et al. Guillain-Barre syndrome associated with preceding hepatitis E virus infection. *Neurology*. 2014;82(6):491–497.
36. Dirlikov E, Major CG, Medina NA, et al. Clinical features of Guillain-Barré syndrome with vs without zika virus infection, Puerto Rico, 2016. *JAMA Neurol*. 2018;75(9):1089–1097.
37. Cao-Lormeau VM, Blake A, Mons S, et al. Guillain-Barré syndrome outbreak caused by Zika virus infection in French Polynesia. *Lancet*. 2016;387:1531–1539.
38. Schonberger LB, Bregman DJ, Sullivan-Bolyai JZ, et al. Guillain-Barre syndrome following vaccination in the National Influenza Immunization Program, United States, 1976–1977. *Am J Epidemiol*. 1979;110(2):105–123.
39. Dodd CN, Romio SA, Black S, et al. International collaboration to assess the risk of Guillain Barré syndrome following Influenza A (H1N1) 2009 monovalent vaccines. *Vaccine*. 2013;31(40):4448–4458.
40. De Wals P, Deceuninck G, Toth E, et al. Risk of Guillain-Barré syndrome following H1N1 influenza vaccination in Quebec. *JAMA*. 2012;308(2):175–181.
41. Crawford NW, Cheng A, Andrews N, et al. Guillain-Barré syndrome following pandemic (H1N1) 2009 influenza A immunisation in Victoria: a self-controlled case series. *Med J Aust*. 2012;197(10):574–578.
42. Salmon DA, Proschan M, Forshee R, et al. Association between Guillain-Barré syndrome and influenza A (H1N1) 2009 monovalent inactivated vaccines in the USA: a meta-analysis. *Lancet*. 2013;381(9876):1461–1468.
43. Polakowski LL, Sandhu SK, Martin DB, et al. Chart-confirmed Guillain-Barre syndrome after 2009 H1N1 influenza vaccination among the medicare population, 2009–2010. *Am J Epidemiol*. 2013;178(6):962–973.
44. Hughes RA, Charlton J, Latinovic R, Gulliford MC. No association between immunization and Guillain-Barré syndrome in the United Kingdom, 1992 to 2000. *Arch Intern Med*. 2006;166(12):1301–1304.
45. Juurlink DN, Stukel TA, Kwong J, et al. Guillain–Barré syndrome after influenza vaccination in adults: a population-based study. *Arch Intern Med*. 2006;166(20):2217–2221.
46. Grave C, Boucheron P, Rudant J, et al. Seasonal influenza vaccine and Guillain-Barré syndrome: a self-controlled case series study. *Neurology*. 2020;94(20):E2168–E2179.
47. Levison LS, Thomsen RW, Andersen H. Guillain–Barré syndrome following influenza vaccination: a 15-year nationwide population-based case–control study. *Eur J Neurol*. 2022;29(11):3389–3394.
48. Kwong JC, Vasa PP, Campitelli MA, et al. Risk of Guillain-Barré syndrome after seasonal influenza vaccination and influenza health-care encounters: a self-controlled study. *Lancet Infect Dis*. 2013;13(9):769–776.
49. Galeotti F, Massari M, D'Alessandro R, et al. Risk of Guillain-Barré syndrome after 2010–2011 influenza vaccination. *Eur J Epidemiol*. 2013;28(5):433–444.
50. Hanson KE, Goddard K, Lewis N, et al. Incidence of Guillain-Barré syndrome after COVID-19 vaccination in the vaccine safety datalink. *JAMA Netw Open*. 2022;5(4):e228879.
51. Maramattom BV, Krishnan P, Paul R, et al. Guillain-Barré syndrome following ChAdOx1-S/nCoV-19 vaccine. *Ann Neurol*. 2021;90(2):312–314.
52. Keh RYS, Scanlon S, Datta-Nemdharry P, et al; BPNS/ABN COVID-19 Vaccine GBS Study Group. COVID-19 vaccination and Guillain-Barré syndrome: analyses using the National Immunoglobulin Database. *Brain*. 2023;146(2):739–748.
53. Pegat A, Vogrig A, Khouri C, Masmoudi K, Vial T, Bernard E. Adenovirus COVID-19 vaccines and Guillain-Barré syndrome with facial paralysis. *Ann Neurol*. 2022;91(1):162–163.
54. Levison LS, Thomsen RW, Sindrup SH, Andersen H. Association of hospital-diagnosed infections and antibiotic use with risk of developing Guillain-Barré syndrome. *Neurology*. 2021;96(6):E831–E839.
55. Levison LS, Thomsen RW, Sindrup SH, Andersen H. Association between incident cancer and Guillain-Barré syndrome development. A nationwide case-control study. *Neurology*. 2022;98(15):E1555–E1561.
56. Rudant J, Dupont A, Mikaeloff Y, Bolgert F, Coste J, Weill A. Surgery and risk of Guillain-Barré syndrome: a French nationwide epidemiologic study. *Neurology*. 2018;91(13):e1220–e1227.
57. Alvarez-Lario B, Prieto-Tejedo R, Colazo-Burlato M, Macarrón-Vicente J. Severe Guillain–Barré syndrome in a patient receiving anti-TNF therapy. Consequence or coincidence. A case-based review. *Clin Rheumatol*. 2013;32(9):1407–1412.
58. Kao JC, Brickshawana A, Liewluck T. Neuromuscular complications of programmed cell death-1 (PD-1) inhibitors. *Curr Neurol Neurosci Rep*. 2018;18(10):63.
59. Levison LS, Thomsen RW, Markvardsen LK, Christensen DH, Sindrup SH, Andersen H. Pediatric Guillain-Barré syndrome in a 30-year nationwide cohort. *Pediatr Neurol*. 2020;107:57–63.
60. Lu JL, Sheikh KA, Wu HS, et al. Physiologic-pathologic correlation in Guillain-Barre syndrome in children. *Neurology*. 2000;54(1):33–39.
61. Hung PL, Chang WN, Huang LT, et al. A clinical and electrophysiologic survey of childhood Guillain-Barré syndrome. *Pediatr Neurol*. 2004;30(2):86–91.
62. Delanoe C, Sebire G, Landrieu P, Huault G, Metral S. Acute inflammatory demyelinating polyradiculopathy in children:

63. Bradshaw DY, Jones HR Jr. Guillain-Barré syndrome in children: clinical course, electrodiagnosis, and prognosis. *Muscle Nerve*. 1992;15(4):500–506.
64. Rantala H, Uhari M, Niemela M. Occurrence, clinical manifestations, and prognosis of Guillain-Barre syndrome. *Arch Dis Child*. 1991;66(6):706–709.
65. Tekgul H, Serdaroglu G, Tutuncuoglu S. Outcome of axonal and demyelinating forms of Guillain-Barré syndrome in children. *Pediatr Neurol*. 2003;28(4):295–299.
66. Devos D, Magot A, Perrier-Boeswillwald J, et al. Guillain-Barré syndrome during childhood: particular clinical and electrophysiological features. *Muscle Nerve*. 2013;48(2):247–251.
67. Kalita J, Kumar M, Misra UK. Prospective comparison of acute motor axonal neuropathy and acute inflammatory demyelinating polyradiculoneuropathy in 140 children with Guillain-Barré syndrome in India. *Muscle Nerve*. 2018;57(5):761–765.
68. González-Suárez I, Sanz-Gallego I, Rodríguez de Rivera FJ, Arpa J. Guillain-Barré syndrome: natural history and prognostic factors: a retrospective review of 106 cases. *BMC Neurol*. 2013;13(1):95.
69. Fokke C, Van Den Berg B, Drenthen J, Walgaard C, Van Doorn PA, Jacobs BC. Diagnosis of Guillain-Barré syndrome and validation of Brighton criteria. *Brain*. 2014;137(1):33–43.
70. Susuki K, Koga M, Hirata K, Isogai E, Yuki N. A Guillain-Barré syndrome variant with prominent facial diplegia. *J Neurol*. 2009;256(11):1899–1905.
71. Luijten LWG, Doets AY, Arends S, et al. Modified Erasmus GBS respiratory insufficiency score: a simplified clinical tool to predict the risk of mechanical ventilation in Guillain-Barré syndrome. *J Neurol Neurosurg Psychiatry*. 2023;94(4):300–308.
72. Rigamonti A, Basso F, Scaccabarozzi C, Lauria G. Posterior reversible encephalopathy syndrome as the initial manifestation of Guillain-Barré syndrome: case report and review of the literature. *J Peripher Nerv Syst*. 2012;17(3):356–360.
73. Abraham A, Ziv S, Drory VE. Posterior reversible encephalopathy syndrome resulting from Guillain-Barré-like syndrome secondary to West Nile virus infection. *J Clin Neuromuscul Dis*. 2011;12(3):113–117.
74. Bavikatte G, Gaber T, Eshiett MUA. Posterior reversible encephalopathy syndrome as a complication of Guillain-Barré syndrome. *J Clin Neurosci*. 2010;17(7):924–926.
75. Delalande S, de Sèze J, Hurtevent JP, Stojkovic T, Hurtevent JF, Vermersch P. Cécité corticale associée à un syndrome de Guillain-Barré. Une complication de la dysautonomie? *Rev Neurol (Paris)*. 2005;161(4):465–467.
76. Elahi A, Kelkar P, St. Louis EK. Posterior reversible encephalopathy syndrome as the initial manifestation of Guillain-Barré syndrome. *Neurocrit Care*. 2004;1(4):465–468.
77. Sutter R, Mengiardi B, Lyrer P, Czaplinski A. Posterior reversible encephalopathy as the initial manifestation of a Guillain-Barré syndrome. *Neuromuscul Disord*. 2009;19(10):709–710.
78. Etxeberria A, Lonneville S, Rutgers MP, Gille M. Posterior reversible encephalopathy syndrome as a revealing manifestation of Guillain-Barré syndrome. *Rev Neurol (Paris)*. 2012;168(3):283–286.
79. Hughes R, Sanders E, Hall S, Atkinson P, Colchester A, Payan P. Subacute idiopathic demyelinating polyradiculoneuropathy. *Arch Neurol*. 1992;49(6):612–616.
80. Oh SJ, Kurokawa K, de Almeida DF, Ryan HF, Claussen GC. Subacute inflammatory demyelinating polyneuropathy. *Neurology*. 2003;61(11):1507–1512.
81. Rodriguez-Casero MV, Shield LK, Kornberg AJ. Subacute inflammatory demyelinating polyneuropathy in children. *Neurology*. 2005;64(10):1786–1788.
82. Bourque PR, Brooks J, McCudden CR, Warman-Chardon J, Breiner A. Age matters: impact of data-driven CSF protein upper reference limits in Guillain-Barré syndrome. *Neurol Neuroimmunol Neuroinflamm*. 2019;6(4):e576.
83. Ramanathan S, McMeniman J, Cabela R, Holmes-Walker DJ, Fung VSC. SIADH and dysautonomia as the initial presentation of Guillain–Barré syndrome: Table 1. *J Neurol Neurosurg Psychiatry*. 2012;83(3):344–345.
84. Hoffmann O, Reuter U, Schielke E, Weber JR. SIADH as the first symptom of Guillain-Barre syndrome. *Neurology*. 1999;53(6):1365–1365.
85. Gorson KC, Ropper AH, Muriello MA, Blair R. Prospective evaluation of MRI lumbosacral nerve root enhancement in acute Guillain-Barre syndrome. *Neurology*. 1996;47(3):813–817.
86. Cornblath DR. Electrophysiology in Guillain-Barre syndrome. *Ann Neurol*. 1990;27(S1):S17–S20.
87. Cornblath DR, Mellits ED, Griffin JW, et al. Motor conduction studies in Guillain-Barré syndrome: description and prognostic value. *Ann Neurol*. 1988;23(4):354–359.
88. Albers JW, Donofrio PD, McGonagle TK. Sequential electrodiagnostic abnormalities in acute inflammatory demyelinating polyradiculoneuropathy. *Muscle Nerve*. 1985;8(6):528–539.
89. Gordon PH, Wilbourn AJ. Early electrodiagnostic findings in Guillain-Barré syndrome. *Arch Neurol*. 2001;58(6):913–917.
90. Brown WF, Feasby TE. Conduction block and denervation in Guillain–Barré polyneuropathy. *Brain*. 1984;107(1):219–239.
91. Capasso M, Caporale CM, Pomilio F, Gandolfi P, Lugaresi A, Uncini A. Acute motor conduction block neuropathy Another Guillain–Barré syndrome variant. *Neurology*. 2003;61(5):617–622.
92. Ropper AH, Wijdicks EF, Shahani BT. Electrodiagnostic abnormalities in 113 consecutive patients with Guillain-Barre syndrome. *Arch Neurol*. 1990;47(8):881–887.
93. Hadden RD, Cornblath DR, Hughes RAC, et al. Electrophysiological classification of Guillain-Barré syndrome: clinical associations and outcome. *Ann Neurol*. 1998;44(5):780–788.
94. Sejvar JJ, Kohl KS, Gidudu J, et al. Guillain-Barré syndrome and Fisher syndrome: case definitions and guidelines for collection, analysis, and presentation of immunization safety data. *Vaccine*. 2011;29(3):599–612.
95. Asbury AK, Cornblath DR. Assessment of current diagnostic criteria for Guillain-Barre syndrome. *Ann Neurol*. 1990;27(S1):S21–S24.
96. Kokubun N, Nishibayashi M, Uncini A, Odaka M, Hirata K, Yuki N. Conduction block in acute motor axonal neuropathy. *Brain*. 2010;133(10):2897–2908.
97. Meulstee J, van der Meche FG. Electrodiagnostic criteria for polyneuropathy and demyelination: application in 135 patients with Guillain-Barre syndrome. Dutch Guillain-Barre Study Group. *J Neurol Neurosurg Psychiatry*. 1995;59(5):482–486.
98. Rajabally YA, Durand MC, Mitchell J, Orlikowski D, Nicolas G. Electrophysiological diagnosis of Guillain-Barré syndrome subtype: could a single study suffice? *J Neurol Neurosurg Psychiatry*. 2015;86(1):115–119.
99. Van den Bergh PYK, Piéret F, Woodard JL, et al; University of Louvain GBS Electrodiagnosis Study Group. Guillain-Barré

syndrome subtype diagnosis: a prospective multicentric European study. *Muscle Nerve*. 2018;58(1):23–28.
100. Uncini A, Kuwabara S. The electrodiagnosis of Guillain-Barré syndrome subtypes: where do we stand? *Clin Neurophysiol*. 2018;129(12):2586–2593.
101. Derksen A, Ritter C, Athar P, et al. Sural sparing pattern discriminates Guillain-Barré syndrome from its mimics. *Muscle Nerve*. 2014;50(5):780–784.
102. Olney RK, Aminoff MJ. Electrodiagnostic features of the Guillain-Barré syndrome: the relative sensitivity of different techniques. *Neurology*. 1990;40(3 Part 1):471–471.
103. Dawson DM, Samuels MA, Morris J. Sensory form of acute polyneuritis. *Neurology*. 1988;38(11):1728–1728.
104. van der Meche' FG, Meulstee J, Vermeulen M, Kievit A. Patterns of conduction failure in the Guillain–Barré syndrome. *Brain*. 1988;111(2):405–416.
105. Eisen A, Humphreys P. The Guillain-Barré syndrome. *Arch Neurol*. 1974;30(6):438–443.
106. Ruts L, Drenthen J, Jacobs BC, van Doorn PA. Distinguishing acute-onset CIDP from fluctuating Guillain-Barré syndrome: a prospective study. *Neurology*. 2010;74(21):1680–1686.
107. Verboon C, Doets AY, Galassi G, et al; IGOS Consortium. Current treatment practice of Guillain-Barré syndrome. *Neurology*. 2019;93(1):E59–E76.
108. Alessandro L, Pastor Rueda JM, Wilken M, et al. Differences between acute-onset chronic inflammatory demyelinating polyneuropathy and acute inflammatory demyelinating polyneuropathy in adult patients. *J Peripher Nerv Syst*. 2018;23(3):154–158.
109. Appeltshauser L, Brunder AM, Heinius A, et al. Antiparanodal antibodies and IgG subclasses in acute autoimmune neuropathy. *Neurol Neuroimmunol Neuroinflamm*. 2020;7(5):e817.
110. Stengel H, Vural A, Brunder AM, et al. Anti-pan-neurofascin IgG3 as a marker of fulminant autoimmune neuropathy. *Neurol Neuroimmunol Neuroinflamm*. 2019;6(5):e603.
111. Thaisetthawatkul P, Collazo-Clavell ML, Sarr MG, Norell JE, Dyck PJB. A controlled study of peripheral neuropathy after bariatric surgery. *Neurology*. 2004;63(8):1462–1470.
112. Vedanarayanan VV, Evans OB, Subramony SH. Tick paralysis in children: electrophysiology and possibility of misdiagnosis. *Neurology*. 2002;59(7):1088–1090.
113. Honavar M, Tharakan JKJ, Hughes RA, Leibowitz S, Winer JB. A clinico-pathological study of the Guillain–Barré syndrome: nine cases and literature review. *Brain*. 1991;114(3):1245–1269.
114. Kanda T, Hayashi H, Tanabe H, Tsubaki T, Oda M. A fulminant case of Guillain-Barré syndrome: topographic and fibre size related analysis of demyelinating changes. *J Neurol Neurosurg Psychiatry*. 1989;52(7):857–864.
115. Griffin JW, Li CY, Ho TW, et al. Pathology of the motor-sensory axonal Guillain-Barré syndrome. *Ann Neurol*. 1996;39(1):17–28.
116. Hafer-Macko C, Hsieh ST, Ho TW, et al. Acute motor axonal neuropathy: an antibody-mediated attack on axolemma. *Ann Neurol*. 1996;40(4):635–644.
117. Hafer-Macko CE, Sheikh KA, Li CY, et al. Immune attack on the Schwann cell surface in acute inflammatory demyelinating polyneuropathy. *Ann Neurol*. 1996;39(5):625–635.
118. Hartung HP, Hughes RA, Taylor WA, Heininger K, Reiners K, Toyka KV. T cell activation in Guillain-Barre syndrome and in MS: elevated serum levels of soluble IL-2 receptors. *Neurology*. 1990;40(2):215–215.
119. Hartung HP, Toyka KV, Pollard JD, Harvey GK. Immunopathogenesis and treatment of the Guillain-Barre syndrome part I. *Muscle Nerve*. 1995;18(2):137–153.
120. Hartung HP, Toyka KV, Pollard JD, Harvey GK. Immunopathogenesis and treatment of the Guillain-Barre syndrome part II. *Muscle Nerve*. 1995;18(2):154–164.
121. Willison HJ. The immunobiology of Guillain-Barre syndromes. *J Peripher Nerv Syst*. 2005;10(2):94–112.
122. Feasby TE, Hahn AF, Gilbert JJ. Passive transfer studies in Guillain-Barre polyneuropathy. *Neurology*. 1982;32(10):1151–1151.
123. McKhann GM, Griffin JW, Cornblath DR, Mellits ED, Fisher RS, Quaskey SA. Plasmapheresis and Guillain-Barré syndrome: analysis of prognostic factors and the effect of plasmapheresis. *Ann Neurol*. 1988;23(4):347–353.
124. Randomised trial of plasma exchange, intravenous immunoglobulin, and combined treatments in Guillain-Barré syndrome. Plasma Exchange/Sandoglobulin Guillain-Barré Syndrome Trial Group. *Lancet*. 1997;349:225–230.
125. French Cooperative Group on Plasma Exchange in Guillain-Barré syndrome. Efficiency of plasma exchange in Guillain-Barré syndrome: role of replacement fluids. *Ann Neurol*. 1987;22(6):753–761.
126. Plasmapheresis and acute Guillain-Barré syndrome. The Guillain-Barré syndrome Study Group. *Neurology*. 1985;35(8):1096–1104.
127. Appropriate number of plasma exchanges in Guillain-Barré syndrome. *Ann Neurol*. 1997;41(3):298–306.
128. Chevret S, Hughes RAC, Annane D. Plasma exchange for Guillain-Barré syndrome. *Cochrane Database of Syst Rev*. 2017;2017(2):CD001798.
129. Hughes RAC, Swan AV, van Doorn PA. Intravenous immunoglobulin for Guillain-Barré syndrome. *Cochrane Database of Syst Rev*. 2014;2014(9):CD002063.
130. Beydoun HA, Beydoun MA, Hossain S, Zonderman AB, Eid SM. Nationwide study of therapeutic plasma exchange vs intravenous immunoglobulin in Guillain-Barré syndrome. *Muscle Nerve*. 2020;61(5):608–615.
131. Appropriate number of plasma exchanges in Guillain-Barré syndrome: the French Cooperative Group on plasma exchange in Guillain-Barre syndrome. *Ann Neurol*. 1997;41(3):298–306.
132. Castro LH, Ropper AH. Human immune globulin infusion in Guillain-Barre syndrome: worsening during and after treatment. *Neurology*. 1993;43(5):1034–1034.
133. Irani DN, Cornblath DR, Chaudhry V, Borel C, Hanley DF. Relapse in Guillain-Barre syndrome after treatment with human immune globulin. *Neurology*. 1993;43(5):872–875.
134. Ropper AH, Albers JW, Addison R. Limited relapse in Guillain-Barre syndrome after plasma exchange. *Arch Neurol*. 1988;45(3):314–315.
135. Walgaard C, Jacobs BC, Lingsma F B, et al; Dutch GBS Study Group. Second intravenous immunoglobulin dose in patients with Guillain-Barré syndrome with poor prognosis (SID-GBS): a double-blind, randomised, placebo-controlled trial. *Lancet Neurol*. 2021;20(4):275–283.
136. Treatment of Guillain-Barré syndrome with high-dose immune globulins combined with methylprednisolone: a pilot study group. *Ann Neurol*. 1994;35(6):749–752.
137. Double-blind trial of intravenous methylprednisolone in Guillain-Barré syndrome. Guillain-Barré Syndrome Steroid Trial Group. *Lancet*. 1993;341(8845):586–590.

138. van Koningsveld R, Schmitz PIM, van der Meché FG, Visser L, Meulstee J, van Doorn PA: Dutch GBS study group. Effect of methylprednisolone when added to standard treatment with intravenous immunoglobulin for Guillain-Barré syndrome: randomised trial. *Lancet*. 2004;363(9404):192–196.
139. van den Berg B, Bunschoten C, van Doorn PA, Jacobs BC. Mortality in Guillain-Barre syndrome. *Neurology*. 2013;80(18):1650–1654.
140. Walgaard C, Lingsma HF, Ruts L, Van Doorn PA, Steyerberg EW, Jacobs BC. Early recognition of poor prognosis in Guillain-Barré syndrome. *Neurology*. 2011;76(11):968–975.
141. Visser LH, Schmitz PI, Meulstee J, van Doorn PA, van der Meche FG. Prognostic factors of Guillain-Barre syndrome after intravenous immunoglobulin or plasma exchange. *Neurology*. 1999;53(3):598–604.
142. Doets AY, Lingsma HF, Walgaard C, et al; IGOS Consortium. Predicting outcome in Guillain-Barré syndrome: international validation of the modified Erasmus GBS outcome score. *Neurology*. 2022;98(5):E518–E532.
143. de la Cour CD, Jakobsen J. Residual neuropathy in long-term population-based follow-up of Guillain-Barre syndrome. *Neurology*. 2005;64(2):246–253.
144. Garssen MPJ, Bussmann JBJ, Schmitz PIM, et al. Physical training and fatigue, fitness, and quality of life in Guillain-Barré syndrome and CIDP. *Neurology*. 2004;63(12):2393–2395.
145. Merkies ISJ, Kieseier BC. Fatigue, pain, anxiety and depression in Guillain-Barré syndrome and chronic inflammatory demyelinating polyradiculoneuropathy. *Eur Neurol*. 2016;75(3–4):199–206.
146. Levison LS, Thomsen RW, Andersen H. Increased risk of depression after Guillain-Barré syndrome. *Muscle Nerve*. 2023;67(6):497–505.
147. Guémy C, Durand MC, Brisset M, Nicolas G. Changes in electrophysiological findings suggestive of demyelination following Guillain-Barré syndrome: a retrospective study. *Muscle Nerve*. 2023;67(5):394–400.
148. Triggs WJ, Cros D, Gominak SC, et al. Motor nerve excitability in Guillain-Barré syndrome: the spectrum of conduction block and axonal degeneration. *Brain*. 1992;115(5):1291–1302.
149. van der Meché FG, Meulstee J, Kleyweg RP. Axonal damage in Guillain-Barré syndrome. *Muscle Nerve*. 1991;14(10):997–1002.
150. Winer JB, Hughes RA, Osmond C. A prospective study of acute idiopathic neuropathy. I. Clinical features and their prognostic value. *J Neurol Neurosurg Psychiatry*. 1988;51(5):605–612.
151. Kuitwaard K, Van Koningsveld R, Ruts L, Jacobs BC, van Doorn PA. Recurrent Guillain-Barré syndrome. *J Neurol Neurosurg Psychiatry*. 2009;80(1):56–59.
152. Kuitwaard K, Bos-Eyssen ME, Blomkwist-Markens PH, Van Doorn PA. Recurrences, vaccinations and long-term symptoms in GBS and CIDP. *J Peripher Nerv Syst*. 2009;14(4):310–315.
153. Mossberg N, Nordin M, Movitz C, et al. The recurrent Guillain-Barré syndrome: a long-term population-based study. *Acta Neurol Scand*. 2012;126(3):154–161.
154. Grand-Maison F, Feasby TE, Hahn AF, Koopman WJ. Recurrent Guillain-Barre' syndrome. *Brain*. 1992;115(4):1093–1106.
155. Hughes RAC, Wijdicks EFM, Benson E, et al. Supportive care for patients with Guillain-Barré syndrome. *Arch Neurol*. 2005;62(8):1194–1198.
156. Shapiro Ben David S, Potasman I, Rahamim-Cohen D. Rate of recurrent Guillain-Barré syndrome after mRNA COVID-19 vaccine BNT162b2. *JAMA Neurol*. 2021;78(11):1409–1411.
157. Baars AE, Kuitwaard K, De Koning LC, et al. SARS-CoV-2 vaccination safety in Guillain-Barré syndrome, chronic inflammatory demyelinating polyneuropathy, and multifocal motor neuropathy. *Neurology*. 2023;100(2):E182–E191.
158. Feasby TE, Gilbert JJ, Brown WF, et al. An acute axonal form of Guillain-Barré polyneuropathy. *Brain*. 1986;109(6):1115–1126.
159. Jackson CE, Barohn RJ, Mendell JR. Acute paralytic syndrome in three American men. *Arch Neurol*. 1993;50(7):732–735.
160. Ho TW, Hsieh ST, Nachamkin I, et al. Motor nerve terminal degeneration provides a potential mechanism for rapid recovery in acute motor axonal neuropathy after Campylobacter infection. *Neurology*. 1997;48(3):717–724.
161. Kuwabara S, Nakata M, Sung JY, et al. Hyperreflexia in axonal Guillain-Barré syndrome subsequent to Campylobacter jejuni enteritis. *J Neurol Sci*. 2002;199(1-2):89–92.
162. Yuki N, Kokubun N, Kuwabara S, et al. Guillain-Barré syndrome associated with normal or exaggerated tendon reflexes. *J Neurol*. 2012;259(6):1181–1190.
163. Ho TW, Willison HJ, Nachamkin I, et al. Anti-GD1a antibody is associated with axonal but not demyelinating forms of Guillain-Barré syndrome. *Ann Neurol*. 1999;45(2):168–173.
164. Tamura N, Kuwabara S, Misawa S, et al. Time course of axonal regeneration in acute motor axonal neuropathy. *Muscle Nerve*. 2007;35(6):793–795.
165. Kuwabara S, Yuki N, Koga M, et al. IgG anti-GM1 antibody is associated with reversible conduction failure and axonal degeneration in Guillain-Barre syndrome. *Ann Neurol*. 1998;44(2):202–208.
166. Takigawa T, Yasuda H, Kikkawa R, Shigeta Y, Saida T, Kitasato H. Antibodies against GM1 ganglioside affect K+ and NA+ currents in isolated rat myelinated nerve fibers. *Ann Neurol*. 1995;37(4):436–442.
167. Susuki K, Yuki N, Schafer DP, et al. Dysfunction of nodes of Ranvier: a mechanism for anti-ganglioside antibody-mediated neuropathies. *Exp Neurol*. 2012;233(1):534–542.
168. Susuki K, Rasband MN, Tohyama K, et al. Anti-GM1 antibodies cause complement-mediated disruption of sodium channel clusters in peripheral motor nerve fibers. *J Neurosci*. 2007;27(15):3956–3967.
169. Yuki N, Yoshino H, Sato S, Miyatake T. Acute axonal polyneuropathy associated with anti-GM1 antibodies following Campylobacter enteritis. *Neurology*. 1990;40(12):1900–1902.
170. Rees JH, Gregson NA, Hughes RA. Anti-ganglioside GM1 antibodies in Guillain-Barré syndrome and their relationship to Campylobacter jejuni infection. *Ann Neurol*. 1995;38(5):809–816.
171. Yuki N, Yamada M, Koga M, et al. Animal model of axonal Guillain-Barré syndrome induced by sensitization with GM1 ganglioside. *Ann Neurol*. 2001;49(6):712–720.
172. Reisin RC, Cersósimo R, Alvarez MG, Massaro M, Fejerman N. Acute "axonal" Guillain-Barré syndrome in childhood. *Muscle Nerve*. 1993;16(12):1310–1316.
173. Wexler I. Sequence of demyelination-remyelination in Guillain-Barre disease. *J Neurol Neurosurg Psychiatry*. 1983;46(2):168–174.
174. Miller RG, Peterson GW, Daube JR, Albers JW. Prognostic value of electrodiagnosis in Guillain-Barré syndrome. *Muscle Nerve*. 1988;11(7):769–774.
175. Feasby TE, Hahn AF, Brown WF, Bolton CF, Gilbert JJ, Koopman WJ. Severe axonal degeneration in acute Guillain-Barré

176. Brown WF, Feasby TE, Hahn AF. Electrophysiological changes in the acute "axonal" form of Guillain-Barre syndrome. *Muscle Nerve*. 1993;16(2):200–205.
177. Triggs WJ, Cros D, Gominak SC, et al. Inexcitable motor nerves and low amplitude motor responses in the Guillain–Barré syndrome: distal conduction block or severe axonal degeneration. *Brain*. 1992;115(5):1291–1302.
178. Rees JH, Soudain SE, Gregson NA, Hughes RAC. Campylobacter jejuni infection and Guillain–Barré syndrome. *N Engl J Med*. 1995;333(21):1374–1379.
179. Vriesendorp FJ, Mishu B, Blaser MJ, Koski CL. Serum antibodies to GM1, GD1b, peripheral nerve myelin, and Campylobacter jejuni in patients with Guillain-Barré syndrome and controls: correlation and prognosis. *Ann Neurol*. 1993;34(2):130–135.
180. Hall SM, Hughes RAC, Atkinson PF, McColl I, Gale A. Motor nerve biopsy in severe Guillain-Barré syndrome. *Ann Neurol*. 1992;31(4):441–444.
181. Yokota T, Kanda T, Hirashima F, Hirose K, Tanabe H. Is acute axonal form of Guillain-Barré syndrome a primary axonopathy? *Muscle Nerve*. 1992;15(10):1211–1213.
182. Yuki N, Yamada M, Sato S, et al. Association of IgG anti-GD_{1a} antibody with severe Guillain-Barré syndrome. *Muscle Nerve*. 1993;16(6):642–647.
183. Berciano J, Coria F, Montón F, Calleja J, Figols J, Lafarga M. Axonal form of Guillain-Barré syndrome: evidence for macrophage-associated demyelination. *Muscle Nerve*. 1993;16(7):744–751.
184. Bohlega SA, Stigsby B, Haider A, McLean D. Guillain-Barre syndrome with severe demyelination mimicking axonopathy. *Muscle Nerve*. 1997;20(4):514–516.
185. Fuller GN, Jacobs JM, Lewis PD, Lane RJ. Pseudoaxonal Guillain-Barre syndrome: severe demyelination mimicking axonopathy. A case with pupillary involvement. *J Neurol Neurosurg Psychiatry*. 1992;55(11):1079–1083.
186. Massaro ME, Rodriguez EC, Pociecha J, et al. Nerve biopsy in children with severe Guillain-Barré syndrome and inexcitable motor nerves. *Neurology*. 1998;51(2):394–398.
187. Yuki N, Kuwabara S, Koga M, Hirata K. Acute motor axonal neuropathy and acute motor-sensory axonal neuropathy share a common immunological profile. *J Neurol Sci*. 1999;168(2):121–126.
188. Kuwabara S, Asahina M, Koga M, Mori M, Yuki N, Hattori T. Two patterns of clinical recovery in Guillain-Barre syndrome with IgG anti-GM1 antibody. *Neurology*. 1998;51(6):1656–1660.
189. Odaka M, Yuki N, Yamada M, et al. Bickerstaff's brainstem encephalitis: clinical features of 62 cases and a subgroup associated with Guillain–Barré syndrome. *Brain*. 2003;126(10):2279–2290.
190. Overell JR, Hseih ST, Odaka M, Yuki N, Willison HJ. Treatment for Fisher syndrome, Bickerstaff's brainstem encephalitis and related disorders. *Cochrane Database of Syst Rev*. 2007;2010(1):CD004761.
191. Blau I, Casson I, Liberman A, Weiss E. The not-so-benign Miller Fisher syndrome. *Arch Neurol*. 1980;37(6):384.
192. Hatanaka T, Higashino H, Yasuhara A, Kobayashi Y. Miller Fisher syndrome: etiological significance of serial blink reflexes and MRI study. *Electromyogr Clin Neurophysiol*. 1992;32(6):317–319.
193. Shuaib A, Becker WJ. Variants of Guillain-Barré syndrome: Miller Fisher syndrome, facial diplegia and multiple cranial nerve palsies. *Can J Neurol Sci*. 1987;14(4):611–616.
194. Umapathi T, Tan EY, Kokubun N, Verma K, Yuki N. Non-demyelinating, reversible conduction failure in Fisher syndrome and related disorders. *J Neurol Neurosurg Psychiatry*. 2012;83(9):941–948.
195. Nagashima T, Koga M, Odaka M, Hirata K, Yuki N. Continuous spectrum of pharyngeal-cervical-brachial variant of Guillain-Barré syndrome. *Arch Neurol*. 2007;64(10):1519–1523.
196. Chiba A, Kusunoki S, Shimizu T, Kanazawa I. Serum IgG antibody to ganglioside GQ1b is a possible marker of Miller Fisher syndrome. *Ann Neurol*. 1992;31(6):677–679.
197. Yuki N, Sato S, Tsuji S, Ohsawa T, Miyatake T. Frequent presence of anti-GQ1b antibody in Fisher's syndrome. *Neurology*. 1993;43(2):414–414.
198. de Pablos C, Calleja J, Fernández F, Berciano J. Miller Fisher syndrome: an electrophysiologic case study. *Electromyogr Clin Neurophysiol*. 1988;28(1):21–25.
199. Fross RD, Daube JR. Neuropathy in the Miller Fisher syndrome: clinical and electrophysiologic findings. *Neurology*. 1987;37(9):1493–1493.
200. Jamal GA, MacLeod WN. Electrophysiologic studies in Miller Fisher syndrome. *Neurology*. 1984;34(5):685–685.
201. Sauron B, Bouche P, Cathala HP, Chain F, Castaigne P. Miller Fisher syndrome: clinical and electrophysiologic evidence of peripheral origin in 10 cases. *Neurology*. 1984;34(7):953–953.
202. Weiss JA, White JC. Correlation of 1A afferent conduction with the ataxia of Fisher syndrome. *Muscle Nerve*. 1986;9(4):327–332.
203. Dehaene I, Martin JJ, Geens K, Cras P. Guillain-Barre syndrome with ophthalmoplegia: clinicopathologic study of the central and peripheral nervous systems, including the oculomotor nerves. *Neurology*. 1986;36(6):851–851.
204. Phillips MS, Stewart S, Anderson JR. Neuropathological findings in Miller Fisher syndrome. *J Neurol Neurosurg Psychiatry*. 1984;47(5):492–495.
205. Plomp JJ, Molenaar PC, O'Hanlon GM, et al. Miller Fisher anti-GQ1b antibodies: alpha-latrotoxin-like effects on motor end plates. *Ann Neurol*. 1999;45(2):189–199.
206. Mori M, Kuwabara S, Fukutake T, Hattori T. Intravenous immunoglobulin therapy for Miller Fisher syndrome. *Neurology*. 2007;68(14):1144–1146.
207. Jacobs BC, O'Hanlon G, Bullens R, Veitch J, Plomp J, Willison H. Immunoglobulins inhibit pathophysiological effects of anti-GQ1b-positive sera at motor nerve terminals through inhibition of antibody binding. *Brain*. 2003;126(10):2220–2234.
208. Seneviratne U, Gunasekera S. Acute small fibre sensory neuropathy: another variant of Guillain–Barre syndrome?. *J Neurol Neurosurg Psychiatry*. 2002;72:540–542.
209. Gorson KC, Herrmann DN, Thiagarajan R, et al. Non-length dependent small fibre neuropathy/ganglionopathy. *J Neurol Neurosurg Psychiatry*. 2008;79(2):163–169.
210. Dabby R, Gilad R, Sadeh M, Lampl Y, Watemberg N. Acute steroid responsive small-fiber sensory neuropathy: a new entity? *J Peripher Nerv Syst*. 2006;11(1):47–52.
211. Yuki N, Chan AC, Wong AHY, et al. Acute painful autoimmune neuropathy: a variant of Guillain-Barré syndrome. *Muscle Nerve*. 2018;57(2):320–324.
212. Abrams RMC, Simpson DM, Navis A, Jette N, Zhou L, Shin SC. Small fiber neuropathy associated with SARS-CoV-2 infection. *Muscle Nerve*. 2022;65(4):440–443.

213. Velentgas P, Amato AA, Bohn RL, et al. Risk of Guillain-Barré syndrome after meningococcal conjugate vaccination. *Pharmacoepidemiol Drug Saf*. 2012;21(12):1350–1358.
214. Young R, Asbury A, Corbet JL, Adams R. Pure pandysautonomia with recovery. Description and discussion of diagnostic criteria. *Brain*. 1975;98(4):613–636.
215. Young RR, Asbury AK, Adams RD, Corbett JL. Pure pandysautonomia with recovery. *Trans Am Neurol Assoc*. 1969;94:355–357.
216. Bennett JL, Mahalingam R, Wellish MC, Gilden DH. Epstein-Barr virus-associated acute autonomic neuropathy. *Ann Neurol*. 1996;40(3):453–455.
217. Colan RV, Snead OC, Oh SJ, Benton JW. Steroid-responsive polyneuropathy with subacute onset in childhood. *J Pediatr*. 1980;97(3):374–377.
218. Fagius J, Westerberg CE, Olsson Y. Acute pandysautonomia and severe sensory deficit with poor recovery. A clinical, neurophysiological and pathological case study. *J Neurol Neurosurg Psychiatry*. 1983;46(8):725–733.
219. Feldman EL, Bromberg MB, Blaivas M, Junck L. Acute pandysautonomic neuropathy. *Neurology*. 1991;41(5):746–748.
220. Heafield MTE, Wiliams AC, Nightingale S, Gammage MD. Idiopathic dysautonomia treated with intravenous gammaglobulin. *Lancet*. 1996;347(8993):28–29.
221. Koike H, Watanabe H, Sobue G. The spectrum of immune-mediated autonomic neuropathies: insights from the clinicopathological features: Table 1. *J Neurol Neurosurg Psychiatry*. 2013;84(1):98–106.
222. Low PA, Dyck PJ, Lambert EH, et al. Acute panautonomic neuropathy. *Ann Neurol*. 1983;13(4):412–417.
223. Mericle RA, Triggs WJ. Treatment of acute pandysautonomia with intravenous immunoglobulin. *J Neurol Neurosurg Psychiatry*. 1997;62(5):529–531.
224. McLeod JG, Tuck RR. Disorders of the autonomic nervous system: Part 1. Pathophysiology and clinical features. *Ann Neurol*. 1987;21(5):419–430.
225. Neville BG, Sladen GE. Acute autonomic neuropathy following primary herpes simplex infection. *J Neurol Neurosurg Psychiatry*. 1984;47(6):648–650.
226. Pavesi G, Gemignani F, Macaluso GM, et al. Acute sensory and autonomic neuropathy: possible association with coxsackie B virus infection. *J Neurol Neurosurg Psychiatry*. 1992;55(7):613–615.
227. Smit AAJ, Vermeulen M, Koelman JHTM, Wieling W. Unusual recovery from acute panautonomic neuropathy after immunoglobulin therapy. *Mayo Clin Proc*. 1997;72(4):333–335.
228. Suarez GA, Fealey RD, Camilleri M, Low PA. Idiopathic autonomic neuropathy: clinical, neurophysiologic, and follow-up studies on 27 patients. *Neurology*. 1994;44(9):1675–1682.
229. Taubner RW, Salanova V. Acute dysautonomia and polyneuropathy. *Arch Neurol*. 1984;41(10):1100–1101.
230. Venkataraman S, Alexander M, Gnanamuthu C. Postinfectious pandysautonomia with complete recovery after intravenous immunoglobulin therapy. *Neurology*. 1998;51(6):1764–1765.
231. Yahr MD, Frontera AT. Acute autonomic neuropathy. *Arch Neurol*. 1975;32(2):132.
232. Klein CM, Vernino S, Lennon VA, et al. The spectrum of autoimmune autonomic neuropathies. *Ann Neurol*. 2003;53(6):752–758.
233. Koike H, Atsuta N, Adachi H, et al. Clinicopathological features of acute autonomic and sensory neuropathy. *Brain*. 2010;133(10):2881–2896.
234. Sandroni P, Vernino S, Klein CM, et al. Idiopathic autonomic neuropathy. *Arch Neurol*. 2004;61(1):44.
235. Vernino S, Low PA, Lennon VA. Experimental autoimmune autonomic neuropathy. *J Neurophysiol*. 2003;90(3):2053–2059.
236. McDougall AJ, McLeod JG. Autonomic neuropathy, I. Clinical features, investigation, pathophysiology, and treatment. *J Neurol Sci*. 1996;137(2):79–88.
237. McLeod JG, Tuck RR. Disorders of the autonomic nervous system: part 2. Investigation and treatment. *Ann Neurol*. 1987;21(6):519–529.
238. Yokota T. Dysautonomia with acute sensory motor neuropathy. *Arch Neurol*. 1994;51(10):1022.
239. Jankovic J, Gilden JL, Hiner BC, et al. Neurogenic orthostatic hypotension: a double-blind, placebo-controlled study with midodrine. *Am J Med*. 1993;95(1):38–48.
240. Low PA, Gilden JL, Freeman R, Sheng KN, McElligott MA. Efficacy of midodrine vs placebo in neurogenic orthostatic hypotension. A randomized, double-blind multicenter study. Midodrine Study Group. *JAMA*. 1997;277(13):1046–1051.

CHAPTER 14

Chronic Inflammatory Demyelinating Polyradiculoneuropathy and Related Neuropathies

Like Guillain–Barré syndrome (GBS), chronic inflammatory demyelinating polyradiculoneuropathy (CIDP) is a syndrome with both classic and variant phenotypes. In the case of GBS, the classic phenotype is referred to as acute inflammatory demyelinating polyradiculoneuropathy (AIDP), a disorder characterized by areflexia, generalized and usually symmetric weakness, and sensory involvement. Likewise, the classic phenotype of CIDP, sometimes called "typical CIDP," shares many of the characteristic clinical and electrodiagnostic (EDX) features of GBS.

There are multiple well-described variant syndromes that share some critical features with typical CIDP—for example, features indicative of focal demyelination demonstrable on EDX studies, evidence suggestive of inflammation on other ancillary tests, and frequent therapeutic response to immunomodulatory therapies. These syndromes have their own well-described clinical features to set them apart from typical CIDP, such as asymmetry and focality of weakness and sensory change in the case of multifocal acquired demyelinating sensory and motor neuropathy (MADSAM) or distal predominance in the case of distal acquired demyelinating sensorimotor neuropathy (DADS). The appropriate classification of this spectrum of illness has been a matter of debate over time, with over 17 diagnostic criteria put forth to date.[1–3] The 2021 European Academy of Neurology/Peripheral Nerve Society (EAN/PNS) guideline takes a step toward consensus and clarity by providing separate diagnostic criteria for "typical CIDP" and five variants. (1) Multifocal CIDP (also referred to as MADSAM or Lewis Sumner syndrome), (2) focal CIDP, (3) distal CIDP (also referred to as DADS), (4) motor CIDP, and (5) sensory CIDP (Table 14-1). The relative reported frequencies of these syndromes are quite variable in the literature, owing in part to the varying diagnostic schema used over time. That said, typical CIDP is most common, encompassing more than 50% of patients in representative patient series.[4]

Many related conditions with significant clinical overlap are now explicitly excluded from the CIDP umbrella. While the syndrome of polyneuropathy, organomegaly, endocrinopathy, monoclonal gammopathy, and skin changes (POEMS) shares both clinical and EDX features with typical CIDP and variants, it is set apart by its association with osteosclerotic myeloma and unique treatment paradigm; we discuss POEMS in Chapter 19. Neuropathy seen with myelin-associated glycoprotein antibodies and an IgM paraprotein (anti-MAG neuropathy) is a less straightforward exception. The CIDP diagnostic criteria suggest that this is a separate disorder, outside the spectrum of CIDP. Distal CIDP as defined, however, has a near identical clinical phenotype and can share very similar EDX features to anti-MAG neuropathy. We cover distal CIDP here, and then IgM-associated neuropathies including anti-MAG neuropathy again in Chapter 19. The recent discovery that patients with CIDP-like neuropathies can harbor one or multiple autoantibodies directed against proteins found at the node of Ranvier or the paranodal region have allowed for the most recent distinct disease carve out: the nodopathies and paranodopathies. A distinct pathophysiology and important differences in treatment responses to various therapies have led to this distinction.

Two chronic, presumably inflammatory conditions bear special mention and are covered in this chapter, as well. Multifocal motor neuropathy (MMN) is now considered as a separate entity by virtually all neuromuscular experts owing to its distinct natural history, pathophysiology, and treatment approach. Chronic immune sensory polyradiculopathy (CISP) is similar to CIDP in many respects, but due the localization to the dorsal nerve roots, diagnosis is more challenging.

As we cover these various chronic, immune-mediated neuropathies in this chapter, we will attempt to offer practical clinical pearls on how to distinguish between these distinct phenotypes. We will also outline key differences in both the diagnostic approach and the treatment paradigm for these distinct phenotypes (Fig. 14-1).

▶ CHRONIC INFLAMMATORY DEMYELINATING POLYRADICULONEUROPATHY

The first report of apparent CIDP, referred to as recurrent polyneuritis, is credited to Eichorst in 1890.[5] In the mid-1950s, animal models of both acute and chronic experimental allergic neuritis provided scientific support for an autoimmune pathophysiology. This concept was further cemented by a seminal report by Austin in 1958 describing steroid responsiveness in patients with relapsing polyneuritis.[6] Nonetheless, "chronic relapsing polyneuritis" was often considered to be a form of

TABLE 14-1. COMPARISON OF CHRONIC ACQUIRED IMMUNE-MEDIATED POLYNEUROPATHIES

	CIDP	DADS	MADSAM	MMN	Nodopathies	CISP/CISP-Plus
Clinical Features						
Weakness	Symmetric proximal and distal	None or only mild symmetric distal	Asymmetric, distal > proximal, arms > legs	Asymmetric, distal > proximal, arms > legs	Severe, symmetric; proximal vs. distal varies	None in CISP; mild toe weakness in CISP-Plus
Sensory loss	Yes; symmetric	Yes; distal and symmetric; sensory ataxia may be prominent	Yes; asymmetric	No	Yes; symmetric; sensory ataxia may be prominent; tremor and cerebellar dysfunction occur	Yes, non-length-dependent and often asymmetric; sensory ataxia is prominent
Reflexes	Symmetrically reduced or absent	Symmetrically reduced or absent	Asymmetrically reduced or absent	Asymmetrically reduced or absent	Symmetrically reduced or absent	Symmetrically or asymmetrically reduced or absent
Electrophysiology						
CMAPs	Demyelinating features including CB	Demyelinating features excluding CB but including prominent DML prolongation	Demyelinating features including CB	Demyelinating features including CB	Demyelinating features including CB	Normal in CISP; mild F-wave or CMAP abnormalities in CISP-Plus
SNAPs	Abnormal	Abnormal	Abnormal	Normal	Abnormal	SSEPs usually required to identify abnormalities; SNAPs may be mildly abnormal in CISP-Plus
Laboratory Findings						
CSF protein	Usually elevated	Usually elevated	Usually elevated	Usually normal	Usually very elevated	Usually elevated
Monoclonal protein	Occasionally present, usually IgG or IgA	IgM usually present	Rarely present	Rarely present	Rarely present	No reported association
Serum autoantibodies	N/A	Anti-MAG frequently present	N/A	IgM-GM1 frequently present	IgG4-NF155, IgG4-CNTN1, IgG-pan-neurofascin, or IgG4-Caspr-1	N/A
Sensory nerve biopsies	Demyelinating/remyelinating features are common	Demyelinating/remyelinating features are common, with IgM deposition evident in paranodal regions and widened myelin lamellae	Demyelinating/remyelinating features are common	Demyelinating/remyelinating features are scant, if present	Separation of axon and myelin at the paranode; inflammatory cell infiltrate and onion bulbs not seen	Decreased density of myelinated fibers with demyelinated axons, onion-bulb formation
Treatment Response						
Prednisone	Yes	Poor	Yes	No	Occasional	Yes
Plasma exchange	Yes	Poor	Not adequately studied	No	Occasional	Not adequately studied
IVIg	Yes	Poor	Yes	Yes	Poor or fleeting benefit	Yes
Rituximab	Case series suggest benefit in refractory cases	Occasional benefit	Not adequately studied	Not adequately studied	Case series demonstrate overwhelming benefit	Not adequately studied

CIDP, chronic inflammatory demyelinating polyneuropathy; DADS, distal acquired demyelinating symmetrical; MADSAM, multifocal acquired demyelinating sensory and motor; MMN, multifocal motor neuropathy; CISP, chronic immune sensory polyradiculopathy; CMAPs, compound motor action potentials; SNAPs, sensory nerve action potentials; CB, conduction block; DML, distal motor latency; CSF, cerebrospinal fluid; MAG, myelin-associated glycoprotein; NF, neurofascin; CNTN1, contactin-1; IVIg, intravenous immunoglobulin; SSEP, somatosensory-evoked potential.

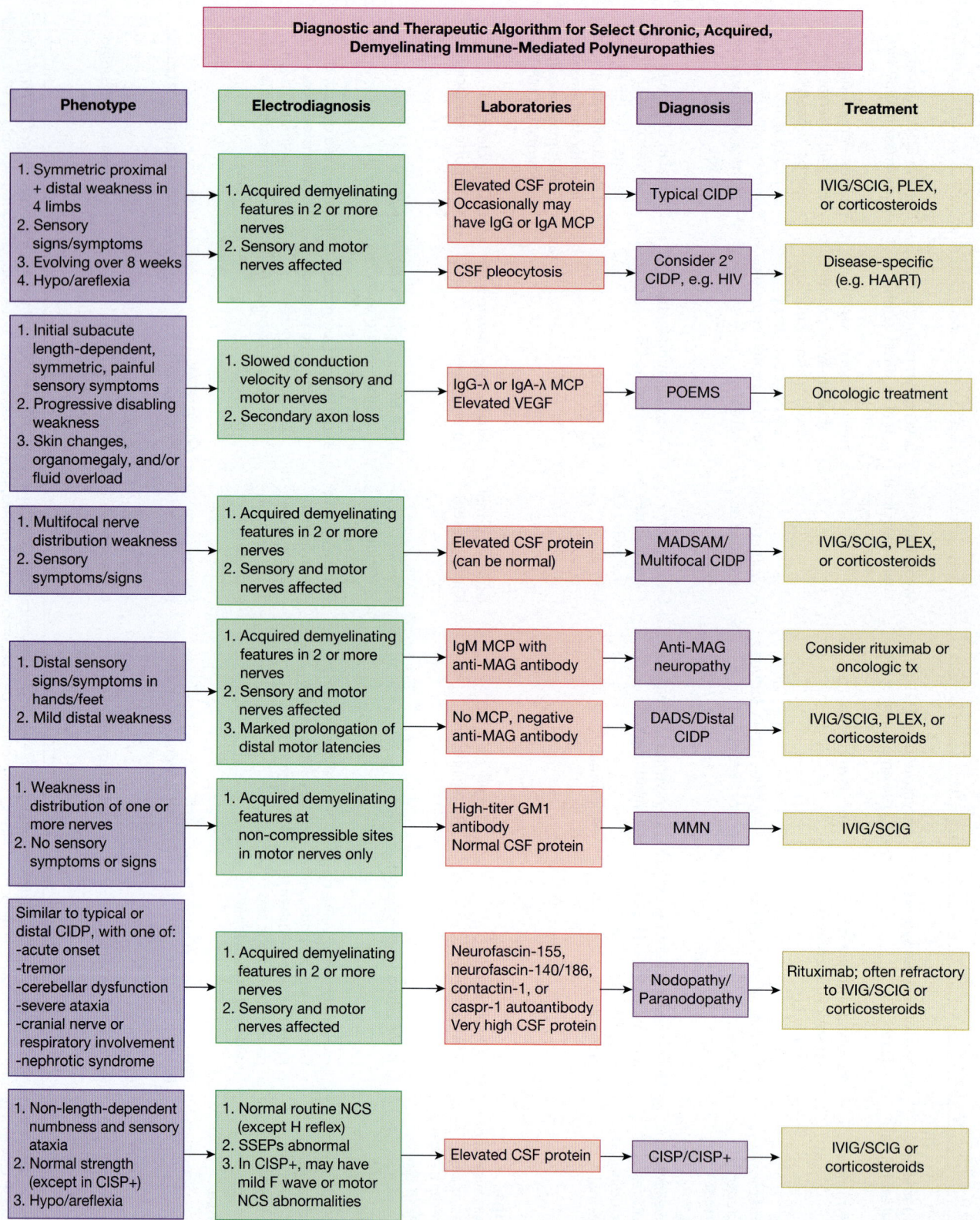

Figure 14-1. Chronic acquired demyelinating polyneuropathies. Diagnostic flow diagram: Diagnosis of CIDP and related neuropathy syndromes derives from clinical phenotype coupled with electrodiagnostic assessment. Other supportive testing is applied when necessary to clarify the diagnosis. CSF, cerebrospinal fluid; MCP, monoclonal protein; NCS, nerve conduction study; CIDP, chronic inflammatory demyelinating polyradiculoneuropathy; HIV, human immunodeficiency virus; SSEP, somatosensory-evoked potential; IVIg, intravenous immunoglobulin; SCIG, subcutaneous immunoglobulin; PLEX, plasma exchange; HAART, highly active antiretroviral therapy; VEGF, vascular endothelial growth factor; POEMS, polyneuropathy, organomegaly, endocrinopathy, monoclonal protein, skin changes; MADSAM, multifocal acquired demyelinating sensory and motor neuropathy; MAG, myelin-associated glycoprotein; DADS, distal acquired demyelinating sensory neuropathy; tx, treatment; MMN, multifocal motor neuropathy; CISP, chronic immune sensory polyradiculopathy.

GBS in early publications until the mid-1970s.[7,8] Arguably, two developments promoted widespread neurological awareness of CIDP. The first was the availability and widespread utilization of nerve conduction studies (NCSs), techniques that allowed for the noninvasive recognition of the demyelinating features that characterize this syndrome. The second seminal moment in the history of CIDP occurred with the 1975 publication by Peter Dyck and colleagues.[9]

CLINICAL FEATURES

The prevalence of CIDP has been reported to range from 0.8 to 8.9/10[10] patients depending on the population studied. Although this may suggest different susceptibility between different geographical locations or ethnicities, this data may be heavily biased based on the diagnostic criteria utilized in different studies.[11] CIDP usually presents in adults (peak incidence at about 30–60 years of age) but it can manifest at any age including infants and children.[9,12–19] The relapsing form tends to present earlier, usually in the 20s.[9,12] There is a slightly increased male prevalence, up to two-thirds of cases in some series.[4,9,20,21] Like GBS, CIDP may begin or relapse in association with an antecedent event that may include infection (10%–30%), vaccination, surgery, trauma, or pregnancy.[9,11,13,22–24] CIDP may account for 10%–33% of initially undiagnosed peripheral neuropathies in some series.[12,25,26] It is possible however, that these statistics represent a biased perspective considering that CIDP patients with their attendant morbidity are more likely to be referred to academic neuropathy clinics than are the far more abundant, indolent, length-dependent, sensory predominant, and frequently idiopathic axonopathies common among the elderly.

The natural history of CIDP needs to be considered both with and without the influence of treatment. Up to 18% of CIDP patients will evolve acutely in such a manner to be initially confused with GBS.[21,27–29] Approximately 12% will evolve subacutely over a 4–8-week period, also confounding the distinction of CIDP from GBS in some cases.[30–33] These subacute cases may have a monophasic course with recovery reminiscent of GBS or have a progressive or relapsing course clearly justifying a CIDP diagnosis. In our minds, subacute inflammatory demyelinating polyradiculoneuropathy represents a "holding" diagnosis until such time as categorization of GBS or CIDP can be made.

Regarding the natural history of treatment naïve CIDP patients, the seminal paper by Peter Dyck and colleagues in 1975 describes four disease trajectories: (1) chronic monophasic (15%), (2) chronic relapsing (fluctuations of weakness or improvement over weeks or months) (34%), (3) stepwise progressive (34%), and (4) steady progressive (15%).[9] With treatment, the majority of patients improve but many will require ongoing treatment to sustain this improvement. Case series have suggested that ~25%–30% of patients will achieve a complete remission off therapy with perhaps 10% achieving "cure" (defined as stable examination off treatment for more than 5 years).[4,20,34] Half of the patients deemed to be cured had normal examinations and the remainder had apparent mild and presumably minor clinical findings. Subacute onset and response to corticosteroids as first-line therapy may be correlated with a higher likelihood of achieving remission off therapy.[34]

Typical CIDP is a subacute to chronic, motor-predominant disorder that presents with a non–length-dependent and symmetric pattern of weakness affecting the arms and the legs.[2,9,11,12,21,25,35–37] Approximately 50%–60% of CIDP patients present in this manner.[4,38] In one series, 53% of patients who initially presented with symptoms and signs compatible with a variant form later evolved into a typical CIDP phenotype.[38] Although distal limb muscles may be more severely affected early, significant and at times dominant involvement of proximal limb muscles is characteristic of the syndrome. This is estimated to occur in approximately 75%–90% of patients, 90% of which will have a symmetric pattern.[6,8,11–13,20,39,40] In addition, approximately 80%–94% of CIDP patients, like GBS, will have sensory symptoms.[11,20,40] While these may be the presenting or relapsing manifestation, they are usually rapidly overshadowed by the morbidity of their weakness. Although the sensory symptoms are usually most pronounced in the distal extremities, they can be frequently identified as being nonlength dependent by affecting the hands before, at the same time, or soon after involvement of the feet. This is notably different from most length-dependent axonal neuropathies. Loss of large fiber sensory modalities is typically more pronounced than the small fiber modalities, but loss of all sensory modalities is not rare. Dysesthesias occur in 15%–50% of affected individuals.[9,13,41] When back pain occurs early in the syndrome in a manner similar to GBS, it is presumed to represent nerve root inflammation.[42] CIDP patients have generalized areflexia (70%) or hyporeflexia in 97% of cases. Pathophysiologically, this is a presumptive effect of desynchronous impulse transmission associated with the temporal dispersion so frequently identified electrodiagnostically.[11,20]

Involvement of cranial nerves, phrenic nerves, and the nerves innervating intercostal and other ventilatory muscles may occur in CIDP but are far less prevalent than in GBS.[20] Bifacial weakness, typically mild, occurs in 15% estimated in the literature.[9,12,13,20,40] Ophthalmoplegia, vestibulocochlear symptoms, and bulbar weakness are less common manifestations.[9,12,13,39,43–45] Neck extensor weakness leading to the dropped head syndrome is even more rare.[46] Papilledema may be seen in rare patients with CIDP, but its presence should heighten consideration toward POEMS syndrome or a nodopathy.[9,47] Symptoms of dysautonomia are uncommon and typically mild when present, affecting distal postganglionic axons and producing mild, cholinergic, predominantly sudomotor dysfunction.[9,13,48–50] Ventilatory failure in CIDP also occurs much less frequently than in GBS, but can occur perhaps more commonly in POEMS patients and is one source of mortality in this disease.[4,50–52] While postural tremor can occur in CIDP, its presence should prompt evaluation for a nodopathy. Likewise, sensory ataxia out of proportion to other sensory changes should also prompt consideration of a nodopathy.[3]

Pure motor forms of CIDP are estimated to occur in 5%–15% of CIDP patients and pure sensory forms in 15%–35%.[4,21] These statistics have to be interpreted with caution, however, as older series may include patients that may represent DADS, MMN, or MADSAM neuropathies. The 2021 EAN/PNS Guidelines require symmetric weakness involving all four limbs in pure motor CIDP, to specifically distinguish this disorder from MMN. Pure motor forms are fairly easy to diagnose, as the EDX features of acquired demyelination characteristic of typical CIDP are the norm. Some patients with purely motor symptoms and examination findings will have sensory abnormalities identified on NCSs; such cases may be referred to as "motor-predominant CIDP."[3]

Sensory CIDP is often a transient state, as up to 70% of patients initially classified this way will later develop weakness in a pattern consistent with either typical CIDP or distal CIDP.[13,21,38,53–55] Keeping this in mind, in one case series half of the patients classified as sensory CIDP actually had EDX features of demyelination on motor NCSs despite the absence of any clinical evidence of motor involvement[4]; these patients may be better referred to as "sensory-predominant CIDP."[3] True sensory CIDP should have sensory symptoms and signs only, abnormalities in at least two nerves on sensory NCSs, but normal motor NCSs. The historical evidence allowing for these patients to be classified as having a variant of CIDP is the demonstration of characteristic nerve histopathology in select patients.[4,13] Given the relatively nonspecific EDX abnormalities used to define this syndrome, it is critical to keep in mind that patients could instead have an alternative diagnosis, such as a sensory ganglionopathy or other causes of axonal sensory polyneuropathy. Patients with CISP also have a pure sensory clinical presentation, usually with sensory ataxia. These patients by definition have normal routine motor and sensory NCSs, distinguishing them from sensory CIDP.

As many as 3% of patients with CIDP develop evidence of central nervous system (CNS) demyelination clinically, electrophysiologically (evoked potential studies), or by magnetic resonance imaging (MRI).[56–62] Attacks of CNS demyelination can precede or follow the onset of CIDP. Like multiple sclerosis (MS), asymptomatic lesions may be detected by MRI and may represent a CIDP variant or coexisting MS. The presence of CNS demyelination should raise suspicion for a nodopathy/paranodopathy, in particular related to neurofascin-155 antibodies.[63–66]

DIAGNOSIS AND DIFFERENTIAL DIAGNOSIS

Making an accurate diagnosis of CIDP requires starting from the recognition of an appropriate clinical phenotype. An overreliance on or an overinterpretation of certain EDX findings or other ancillary testing such as cerebrospinal fluid (CSF) protein levels can lead to diagnostic errors. The appropriate role of NCS/electromyography (EMG) is to support the diagnosis in a patient with a compatible phenotype, not to establish it in the absence of a compatible clinical picture. This is supported by the knowledge that an EDX pattern compatible with an acquired demyelinating neuropathy can be seen with a number of disparate phenotypes whose natural history and response to treatment may vary considerably from CIDP, for example, POEMS syndrome and even forms of hereditary neuropathy.[48,67–69] We do not adhere to the concept that a diagnosis of CIDP can be established by EDX features alone.

Formal published diagnostic criteria have over time increasingly emphasized this point. Historically, proposed criteria have placed variable emphasis on clinical features, EDX findings, CSF, nerve root imaging, nerve biopsy features, and response to treatment. The 2006 criteria (and later 2010 revision) proposed by the European Federation of Neurological Societies (EFNS) in conjunction with the PNS give primacy to the clinical presentation and EDX features.[10,36] This approach results in an overall improved diagnostic accuracy compared to prior criteria, with an estimated sensitivity of 73%–95% and specificity of 91%–96%.[2,21,36] The application of these criteria demonstrated that misdiagnosis remained more common for "atypical CIDP" as defined. An update was therefore made in 2021 [now referred to as the European Academy of Neurology (EAN)/PNS guideline][3] which eliminated the distinction of "atypical CIDP." Instead, specific clinical criteria were defined for each of the specific "variant" forms of CIDP. Sensory NCS abnormalities were also considered to be mandatory EDX features in the 2021 update.

A diagnosis of typical CIDP using the 2021 guidelines first requires that patients have (1) progressive or relapsing, symmetric, proximal and distal muscle weakness of upper and lower limbs, (2) sensory involvement of at least two limbs, (3) development over at least 8 weeks, and (4) absent or reduced tendon reflexes in all limbs. To then confirm this diagnosis, relevant EDX abnormalities in two motor nerves and two sensory nerves are required (discussed further in the "Electrodiagnostic Features" section below). Patients with less robust EDX abnormalities but the proper clinical presentation can be considered to have "possible CIDP." The guidelines consider the results of CSF analysis, MRI, nerve biopsy, and response to treatment to be supportive. These supportive criteria can be used to upgrade diagnostic certainty in those patients lacking sufficient EDX findings. When compared to the 2010 guidelines, the 2021 update leads to a somewhat lower sensitivity but higher specificity.[70,71]

We believe the most important value of accurate diagnosis is to decide who to treat and what to treat them with. Avoiding expensive and potentially harmful treatment without likely benefit while at the same time ensuring that potentially treatment responsive individuals are identified are two self-evident benefits of accurate diagnosis. Accurate diagnosis is also important for research purposes, both in consideration of clinical trial inclusion and in order to be able to eventually illuminate the cause(s) of this syndrome. We follow the lead of the EAN/PNS in considering a characteristic CSF pattern, found in approximately 90% of patients, to be helpful but not diagnostically mandatory. For a number of reasons, we do not routinely recommend nerve biopsy as a means to diagnose CIDP, particularly when the diagnosis is well established by clinical and EDX means. We are more apt to perform nerve biopsies in atypical cases with the primary goal of excluding alternative diagnosis.

The differential diagnosis of CIDP begins in its distinction from GBS. As previously mentioned, up to 18% of individuals who will eventually develop a relapsing or progressing course justifying a CIDP diagnosis will have an initial evolution rapid enough to suspect GBS.[24–26,72] In these individuals, it would be pragmatic to initiate treatment with either intravenous immunoglobulin (IVIg) or plasma exchange (PLEX) and reserve any consideration of corticosteroids until the trajectory of the illness justifies a CIDP diagnosis.

CIDP is typically considered a primary diagnosis. In approximately one-quarter of individuals, however, a concomitant systemic disease may be identifiable, with monoclonal gammopathy of uncertain significance (MGUS), lymphoma, and diabetes being the most prevalent (Table 14-2).[2,12,22,36,73–79] Other autoimmune diseases are also frequently encountered in patients with CIDP. Associations between CIDP and other disorders may represent two different diseases sharing a common pathophysiological mechanism or in the case of diabetes, a common disorder with a similar phenotype occurring coincidentally.[80–85] Alternatively, and probably less commonly, CIDP might be caused by consequences of the primary systemic disease. The last consideration is the coexistence of two unrelated conditions, the second disorder being identified as a by-product of the diagnostic scrutiny provided by the evaluation of the first. In patients with diabetes, it is wise to exercise additional caution when making a diagnosis of CIDP, since patients with diabetes tend to have higher CSF protein levels and patients with diabetic polyneuropathy routinely have slowed conduction velocities (CVs) on EDX.[86–90] Again, a careful focus on the clinical phenotype of patients should help avoid diagnostic errors.[91,92]

IgA/IgG-associated neuropathies frequently have an axonal EDX profile, but occasionally they may manifest with both the clinical and EDX features of CIDP.[93] Cases of CIDP associated with IgG or IgA paraproteinemia tend to resemble idiopathic CIDP with notable motor involvement, faster progression, and similar treatment responsiveness.[94] For these reasons, we do not consider the presence of an IgG or IgA monoclonal gammopathy to preclude a CIDP diagnosis and cases can often be managed similar to idiopathic CIDP (aside from the required hematologic work-up of the monoclonal gammopathy). Patients with IgM monoclonal gammopathy may also occasionally have a clinical phenotype consistent with typical CIDP. These patients can also be managed similar to idiopathic CIDP. However, patients with IgM monoclonal gammopathy and neuropathy more frequently have a phenotype consistent with distal CIDP. These patients, especially when anti-MAG antibodies are identified, should be managed differently as they have a distinct natural history, distinct histopathology, and different responses to typical CIDP treatments.[12,94–96] These issues are discussed further in Chapter 19.

The most relevant mimics to consider in the differential diagnosis of CIDP will vary based on the specific variant phenotype (see Table 14-2). Failure to respond to multiple lines of effective therapy for CIDP should always prompt reconsideration of alternative diagnoses.[97,98] Notably, neurolymphomatosis and hereditary transthyretin amyloidosis neuropathy can occasionally mimic CIDP clinically and electrodiagnostically.[99,100] In those patients with "CIDP-like" clinical phenotypes but with axonal EDX signatures, amyloidosis warrants special

▶ **TABLE 14-2. DISEASE ASSOCIATIONS, DISEASE MIMICS, AND DIAGNOSTIC CONSIDERATIONS IN CIDP**

Conditions That May Be Concomitant With CIDP
Diabetes mellitus
Lymphoma
MGUS
HIV infection (CSF pleocytosis is more common in these patients)
Bone marrow or solid organ transplantation
Systemic autoimmune disorders (autoimmune thyroiditis is most common)
Pregnancy (patients with CIDP may be more likely to relapse during pregnancy or postpartum)
Membranous glomerulonephritis (should prompt antibody testing for nodopathy/paranodopathy, especially CNTN-1)

Important Disease Mimics for CIDP and Variants
Typical CIDP
Guillain–Barré syndrome
AL Amyloidosis
Hereditary TTR Amyloidosis
Immune checkpoint inhibitor–associated neuropathy
Neurolymphomatosis
POEMS syndrome

Distal-predominant symptoms
AL or hereditary TTR amyloidosis
Anti-MAG neuropathy
Charcot–Marie–Tooth (CMT) or other forms of hereditary neuropathy including TTR
Diabetes or other causes of distal symmetric axonal polyneuropathy
Nodopathies/Paranodopathies (e.g., neurofascin-155)

Prominent sensory ataxia
Anti-MAG neuropathy
CANOMAD
CANVAS
CISP
Myelopathy
Nodopathies/Paranodopathies (e.g., neurofascin-155)
Sensory ganglionopathy

Multifocal/Asymmetric symptoms
Brachial plexitis/Parsonage Turner syndrome
Radiculoplexus neuropathy (diabetic or idiopathic)
Hereditary neuropathy with liability to pressure palsies (HNPP)
Multifocal motor neuropathy
Neurolymphomatosis or other nerve tumors
Radiation plexopathy
Vasculitic neuropathy
AL and TTR amyloidosis
Lepromatous neuropathy

Prominent tremor
Anti-MAG neuropathy
Multifocal motor neuropathy
Nodopathies/Paranodopathies (e.g., neurofascin-155)
CMT (Roussy–Lévy syndrome)
Friedreich ataxia

MGUS, monoclonal gammopathy of uncertain significance; CNTN-1, contactin-1; TTR, transthyretin; POEMS, polyneuropathy, organomegaly, endocrinopathy, monoclonal plasma cell disorder, skin changes; MAG, myelin-associated glycoprotein; CANOMAD, chronic ataxic neuropathy with ophthalmoplegia, M-protein- agglutination, and disialosyl antibodies; CANVAS, cerebellar ataxia with neuropathy and vestibular areflexia syndrome; CISP, chronic immune sensory polyradiculopathy.

consideration—especially if there are symptoms of multisystemic or autonomic involvement.[101] Inflammatory polyradiculoneuropathies akin to CIDP have been described in association with immune checkpoint inhibitors, as well (see Chapter 19).

ELECTRODIAGNOSTIC FEATURES

EDX assessment is an integral component of making a CIDP diagnosis, but it cannot determine the diagnosis independent of clinical assessment. When CIDP or a variant is suspected on clinical grounds, multiple nerves should be evaluated on NCSs because of the multifocal nature of the disease process. Some nerves can have normal conduction studies, while other nerves are abnormal. The expected distribution and nature of EDX abnormalities will vary based on the specific CIDP variant.

Motor NCSs include assessment of compound muscle action potential (CMAP) amplitudes, distal latencies, CVs, F-wave latencies, and waveform morphological changes such as temporal dispersion or conduction block. These are the most useful EDX tools in the evaluation of a patient with suspected CIDP.[1–3,12] As previously mentioned, there are at minimum 16 EDX criteria for CIDP that have been proposed. For purposes of simplicity, we will summarize those EDX criteria proposed by the EAN/PNS. For typical CIDP, these require demonstration of one or more of the following characteristic demyelinating abnormalities in at least two motor nerves (Table 14-3)[3]:

1. Prolongation of motor distal latencies by >50% of the upper limits of normal (ULN).
2. Reduction in CV below the lower limits of normal (LLN) by ≥30%.
3. ≥20% prolongation in F-wave latency, increasing to ≥50% prolongation in F-wave latency if CMAP amplitude is <80% LLN. The absence of F waves in two motor nerves with CMAP amplitudes ≥20% LLN is also considered to meet criteria if at least one other demyelinating feature is seen in at least one other nerve.
4. Conduction block as defined by CMAP reduction of ≥30%, if the CMAP amplitude is ≥20% the LLN.
5. Temporal dispersion as defined by >30% increase in CMAP duration in proximal compared to distal CMAP. Absolute prolongation of the CMAP duration is also considered, with specific criteria for each nerve.

Importantly, slowed CV or conduction block at common sites of compression or for the tibial nerve stimulating at the popliteal fossa are excluded from these considerations. We are also cautious about using the absence of the F waves of the peroneal nerve toward fulfilling the diagnostic criteria for CIDP. It is worth emphasizing that an amplitude-dependent reduction in CV can occur with axon loss alone; failure to account for this can lead to overdiagnosis of CIDP.[102] Patients with diabetic polyneuropathy, for example, frequently have slowed CVs, without conduction block.[103]

The EAN/PNS 2021 guidelines also require sensory conduction abnormalities [prolonged latency, reduced sensory nerve action potentials (SNAP) amplitude, or slowed CV outside of normal limits] in two or more nerves. Most patients with CIDP have SNAPs that are reduced in amplitude or absent in both the upper and the lower extremities.[7,12,13,39,53,104–106] When present, SNAPs may demonstrate conduction slowing, but usually not as severe as that demonstrated in motor nerves.[91] A helpful feature when present is the identification of median, ulnar, or radial SNAPs abnormalities when the sural or superficial peroneal SNAPs are normal. This pattern of "sural" sparing suggests a non–length-dependent process (most axonal neuropathies are length dependent). When sensory EDX abnormalities are worse in the arms than in the legs, one needs to consider either a predominantly demyelinating neuropathy or sensory ganglionopathy. Patients with a clinical phenotype compelling for CIDP frequently may have EDX abnormalities demonstrated in only one motor and/or sensory nerve; these patients may be considered to have "possible CIDP" based on the 2021 guidelines.[107]

As patients' strength and function improve, repeat NCSs may demonstrate evidence of improvement with increases in CMAP amplitudes and CVs along with a reduction in the magnitude of conduction block.[39,92,93,105,108–111] Clinical improvement is primarily the result of resolving conduction block, although some may be attributed to improved ion channel function without remyelination, collateral sprouting, or regeneration of axons.

Insertional[13,17–19,65,109,112–114] and spontaneous activities are often normal on needle EMG. However, fibrillation potentials are not rare as there is often some element of secondary axonal loss. Occasionally, myokymic discharges may be seen related to ephaptic transmission between demyelinated nerve fibers. The earliest and perhaps only abnormality one might see on EMG is reduced recruitment (fast-firing) motor unit action potentials (MUAPs) that otherwise appear morphologically normal.

LABORATORY AND NEUROIMAGING FEATURES

Blood testing in CIDP is done largely in consideration of alternative diagnoses, associated diseases, or secondary causes. As previously discussed, a monoclonal gammopathy (IgA, IgG, or IgM) is present in up to 30% of patients with CIDP.[12,40,41,84,104,115,116] In cases in which a monoclonal gammopathy is detected, evaluation for POEMS syndrome, lymphoma, myeloma, and amyloid are undertaken as warranted. A complete blood count, glycosylated hemoglobin, renal function, and liver function should generally be tested. Otherwise, the specific clinical phenotype should determine the highest yield testing to pursue.[3]

CSF analysis is generally not required if patients meet clinical and EDX criteria. As mentioned, an over-reliance on CSF findings in patients with inconsistent clinical phenotypes may lead to misdiagnosis.[86,90,117] Diabetes, spinal stenosis, or even simply older age may be associated with

▶ **TABLE 14-3. EUROPEAN ACADEMY OF NEUROLOGY/PERIPHERAL NERVE SOCIETY DIAGNOSTIC CRITERIA FOR CIDP–2021 REVISION**

First Step: To consider a diagnosis of CIDP, clinical criteria for typical CIDP or a variant syndrome must first be met:
Clinical Criteria:
For all syndromes, symptoms must develop over at least 8 weeks
Typical CIDP: Progressive or relapsing, symmetric, proximal + distal weakness of arms and legs; sensory involvement of at least two limbs; absent or reduced tendon reflexes in all limbs
Distal CIDP: Distal sensory loss and muscle weakness, predominantly in the lower limbs[a]
Multifocal CIDP: Sensory loss and muscle weakness in a multifocal pattern, usually asymmetric, typically upper limb predominant; must involve more than one limb[a]
Focal CIDP: Sensory loss and muscle weakness in only one limb[a]
Motor CIDP: Motor symptoms and signs without sensory involvement; otherwise as in typical CIDP
Sensory CIDP: Sensory symptoms and signs without motor involvement; otherwise as in typical CIDP

Second Step: To support a suspected diagnosis of CIDP, electrodiagnostic (EDX) criteria are used:
EDX Criteria:
(1) At least one of the following on motor NCS:
   (a) Motor distal latency prolongation ≥50% above ULN in two nerves (excluding median neuropathy at the wrist from carpal tunnel syndrome)
   (b) Reduction of motor conduction velocity ≥30% below LLN in two nerves, excluding compressible sites
   (c) Prolongation of F-wave latency ≥20% above ULN in two nerves (≥50% if amplitude of distal negative peak CMAP<80% of LLN)
   (d) Absence of F-waves in two nerves (if these nerves have distal negative peak CMAP amplitudes ≥20% of LLN) + ≥1 other demyelinating parameter in ≥1 other nerve
   (e) Motor conduction block: ≥30% reduction of the proximal relative to distal negative peak CMAP amplitude, excluding the tibial nerve or compressible sites, and distal negative peak CMAP amplitude ≥20% of LLN in two nerves; or in one nerve + ≥1 other demyelinating parameter except absence of F-waves in ≥1 other nerve
   (f) Abnormal temporal dispersion: >30% duration increase between the proximal and distal negative peak CMAP (at least 100% in the tibial nerve) in ≥2 nerves
   (g) Distal CMAP duration (interval between onset of the first negative peak and return to baseline of the last negative peak) prolongation in ≥1 nerve + ≥1 other demyelinating parameter in ≥1 other nerve

–>Relevant findings in only one nerve are considered weakly supportive
AND, (2) sensory conduction abnormalities in at least two nerves (prolonged distal latency, reduced SNAP amplitude, or slowed conduction velocity)
–>relevant findings in only one nerve are considered weakly supportive

Third Step: Determine diagnostic "certainty"
An example is provided for Typical CIDP:
Typical CIDP =
- Clinical criteria + motor conduction criteria in two nerves + sensory conduction abnormalities in two nerves; or
- "Possible typical CIDP" based on EDX criteria as outlined below + at least two supportive criteria (see next section)

Possible typical CIDP =
- Clinical criteria + motor conduction criteria in one nerve + sensory conduction abnormalities in two nerves; or
- Clinical criteria + motor conduction abnormalities (but not fulfilling CIDP motor conduction criteria) in one nerve + sensory conduction abnormalities in two nerves + objective response to treatment + one other supportive criterion

Supportive criteria (only necessary if clinical + EDX is insufficient):
Albuminocytologic dissociation on CSF testing
MR imaging evidence of nerve root or plexus enhancement or hypertrophy; or nerve ultrasound evidence of nerve enlargement at least two noncompressible sites
Biopsy features of demyelination/remyelination
Objective improvement following immunomodulatory treatment

CIDP, chronic inflammatory demyelinating polyneuropathy; CMAP, compound motor action potential; SNAP, sensory nerve action potential; LLN, lower limits of normal; ULN, upper limits of normal.

[a]Tendon reflexes may be normal in unaffected limbs.

Adapted with permission from Van den Bergh PYK, van Doorn PA, Hadden RDM, et al. European Academy of Neurology/Peripheral Nerve Society guideline on diagnosis and treatment of chronic inflammatory demyelinating polyradiculoneuropathy: Report of a joint Task Force-Second revision. *Eur J Neurol*. 2021;28(11):3556–3583.

mild elevations in CSF protein. Most patients with CIDP (80%–95%) do have an elevated CSF protein (>45 mg/dL), with a mean of 135 mg/dL.[7-9,12,39,41] Occasionally CSF protein levels may exceed 1,200 mg/dL, but very high CSF protein levels should prompt consideration of POEMS syndrome or blockade of the spinal canal from hypertrophic nerve roots. Similar to GBS, the CSF cell count is usually normal, although up to 10% of patients have greater than 5 lymphocytes/mm.[67] Elevated CSF cell counts should lead to the consideration of HIV infection, sarcoidosis, Lyme disease, and lymphomatous or leukemic infiltration of nerve roots. Oligoclonal bands may be demonstrated in the CSF in approximately 65% of patients.[118,119]

Testing for specific autoantibodies can help distinguish typical CIDP from variants or from alternative diagnoses when there is clinical uncertainty. Identification of anti-MAG antibodies, for example, might help solidify a case of distal CIDP/DADS. Patients with nodopathy/paranodopathy generally have distinct phenotypes from those with typical CIDP and other defined variants. It is therefore not necessary to send these antibodies in every patient suspected to have CIDP. The 2021 EAN/PNS guidelines suggest that testing is of highest yield in patients with acute onset suggestive of GBS or acute-onset CIDP, tremor, ataxia disproportionate to other sensory involvement, cerebellar dysfunction, respiratory failure, cranial nerve involvement, distal-predominant weakness, concurrent nephrotic syndrome and/or resistance to standard CIDP treatment (IVIg and/or corticosteroids).

In those patients in which CIDP is suspected but the requisite EDX features are lacking, neuroimaging can serve as a helpful adjunct. Hypertrophy and/or contrast enhancement of the cervical or lumbar nerve roots, or the brachial or lumbar plexus can be seen in 44%–82% of patients with CIDP.[120-122] Neuromuscular ultrasound has similar diagnostic performance to MRI,[123,124] and the EAN/PNS guidelines now favor its use in patients with possible CIDP to try to help secure the diagnosis.[3] Enlargement of nerves at noncompressible sites, specifically the proximal median nerve and portions of the brachial plexus, has been shown to accurately discriminate CIDP from axonal neuropathies or ALS and to increase diagnostic sensitivity for CIDP above and beyond EDX alone.[123,125] The specificity of nerve enlargement, however, is modest and the existing case series addressing this matter do not include many patients with relevant disease mimics (e.g., POEMS).

HISTOPATHOLOGY

Nerve biopsies in CIDP should be interpreted with the realization that a sensory nerve is being examined in a disorder that typically has a motor predominant phenotype. As a result, neither the extent nor type of abnormality identified may be fully representative of the entire disease process. Nerve biopsy is a useful, but not requisite diagnostic tool, for CIDP, arguably of greater utility in excluding other disorders than in proving the existence of CIDP.[126,127] Biopsies are particularly useful when vasculitis, lymphomatous infiltration, amyloidosis, or sarcoidosis are considered.

Nerve biopsies may reveal segmental demyelination and remyelination which may not be evident due to the multifocal nature of the process (Fig. 14-2).[9,12,57,126,128,129] Chronic demyelination and remyelination result in proliferation of surrounding Schwann cell processes known as "onion bulbs." These are the basis of hypertrophic nerves and are seen CIDP although they are not as prominent as in demyelinating forms of Charcot–Marie–Tooth disease (see Fig. 3-31). Myelinated fibers are usually reduced in number. Fibers examined in semithin sections demonstrate myelin thickness that is disproportionately thin in relationship to axon diameter indicate remyelination (Fig. 14-2C). Teased nerve fiber analysis demonstrates segmental demyelination and/or remyelination in 23%–46%, axonal degeneration in 21%–42%, mixed demyelinating and axonal features in 12.5%, and normal findings in 18%–43.5% of nerve biopsies from studied CIDP patients[9,12] (see Fig. 3-30).

Endoneurial and perineurial edema may also be appreciated on biopsy. Inflammatory cell infiltrate may be evident in the epineurium, perineurium, or endoneurium. It is often perivascular when detectable but often quite subtle or absent in nerve biopsy specimens (Fig. 14-2A).[9,12] Inflammatory cells are better appreciated with immunostaining for lymphocytes (Fig. 14-2B).[130,131] This inflammatory component comprises of macrophages, CD3+-activated T cells (mainly CD8+ but also CD4+ cells lymphocytes), and dendritic cells.[131,132] Of note, a similar frequency of inflammatory cell infiltrate within nerves is seen in a variety of neuropathies, raising questions concerning the pathogenic role of these cells.[130] The matrix metalloproteinases MMP-2 and MMP-9 (gelatinase A and B) are overexpressed in the peripheral nerves in patients with CIDP.[133] These enzymes are secreted by T cells and are capable of digesting basement membrane proteins, thereby facilitating the infiltration of inflammatory cells into peripheral nerves.

On electron microscopy (EM), macrophages may be noted to penetrate the basement membrane with displacement of the Schwann cell cytoplasm, lyse superficial myelin lamellae, penetrate along intraperiod lines, and engulf the disrupted myelin by endocytosis. By doing so, they disrupt the nodes of Ranvier, and by doing so, presumptively saltatory conduction.[112] Subsequently, Schwann cells are recruited to remyelinate the demyelinated internodes. The demyelinated axons diminish in diameter as much as 50% but later regain some of their diameter following remyelination.

PATHOGENESIS

Physiologically, conduction block is most frequently attributed to paranodal and internodal demyelination which impairs action potential propagation.[107,113,114] Demyelination of a nerve segment produces an increased transverse capacitance, causing a leakage of current. This increases the time required for the

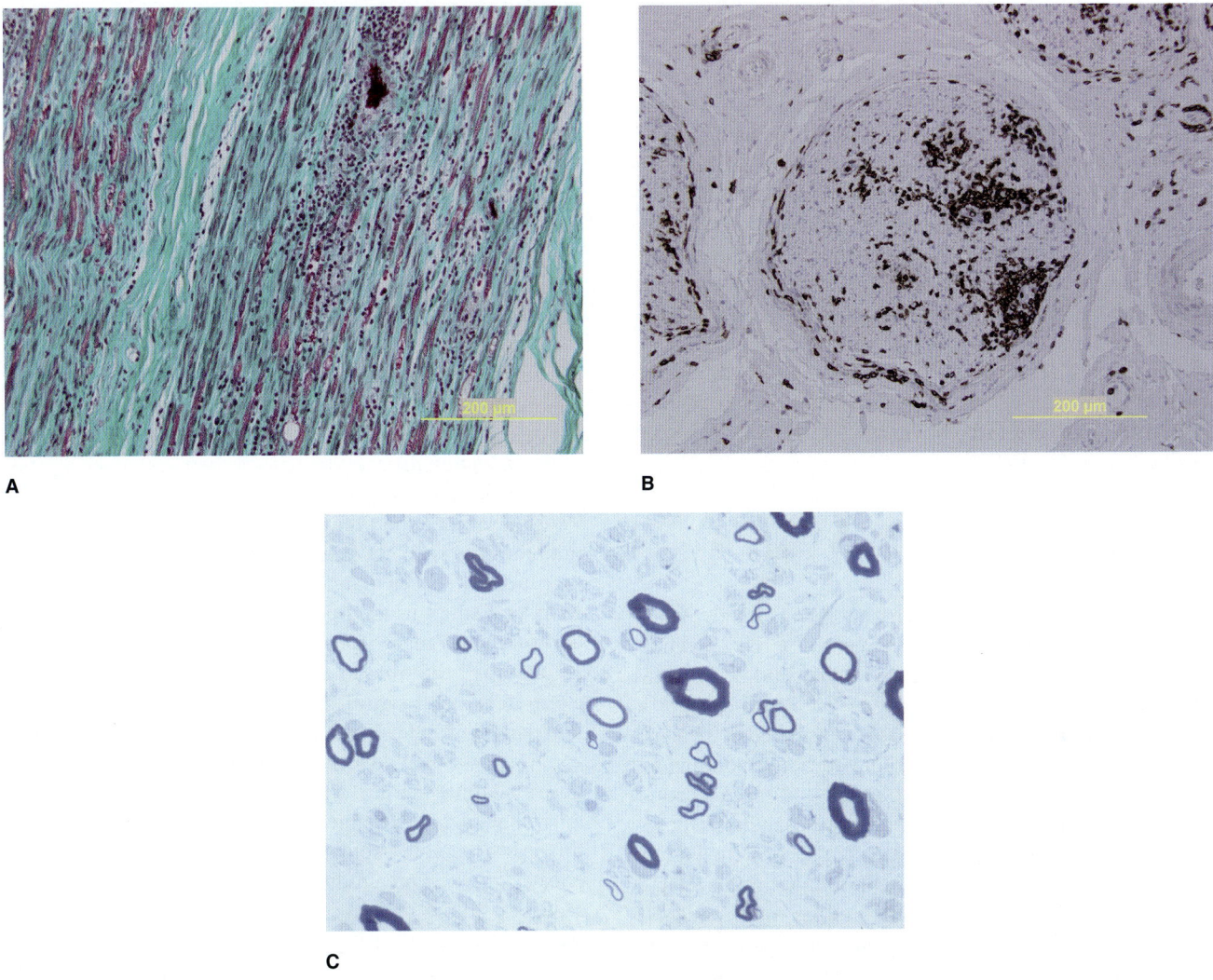

Figure 14-2. Chronic inflammatory demyelinating polyradiculoneuropathy. Nerve biopsy reveals endoneurial inflammatory cell infiltration (paraffin section, modified Gomori trichrome) (**A**). Immunostaining demonstrates that many of these cells are CD3-positive T cells (**B**). Semithin sections reveal scattered thinly myelinated nerve fibers (**C**).

longitudinal current to reach the next node of Ranvier. If current leakage is too excessive, it may be insufficient to depolarize the next node of Ranvier. It is this conduction block, rather than slowed conduction, which is responsible for motor weakness.[107,113,114] Weakness may also occur as a result of axon loss, the mechanism of which in CIDP is poorly understood.

Many lines of evidence solidify CIDP as an autoimmune disorder, although disease mechanisms remain poorly understood.[113] Anatomically, the pathological changes associated with CIDP are demonstrable at the root, plexus, and nerve level.[113] However, the antigen(s) to which the immune attack is targeted and the specific roles of the humoral and cellular immune system remain unknown for most patients. The efficacy of plasma exchange as well as IVIg implies an important role of the humoral immune system in the pathogenesis of CIDP. Indeed, CIDP patients have been shown to have upregulated activating FcγR1-receptors on monocytes and downregulated inhibitory Fc receptors on B cells.[134] The identification of autoantibodies targeted against nodal and paranodal antigens have allowed for the subclassification of another category of autoimmune neuropathies, which will be discussed later in the chapter.

Autoantibodies against other glycolipids such as GM1 and GD1a would be logical suspects as responsible pathogenic agents in CIDP, as these antigenic targets are located on the nodal axolemma of motor nerves. These gangliosides are found on the cell surface of *Campylobacter jejuni*, the precipitating agent in many cases of the acute motor axonal neuropathy (AMAN) variant of GBS with which these autoantibodies have been so closely associated. GM1 and GD1a autoantibodies are capable of interfering with ion channel function, although perhaps not at an order of magnitude sufficient to disrupt impulse transmission. In addition, GM1 and GD1 knockout mice demonstrate that these gangliosides are essential for the integrity of nodal architecture. Myelin loops at the paranodal region do not attach to the axolemma, sodium channels are disrupted, and potassium channels are mislocated to the paranode.[114] Nonetheless, ganglioside autoantibodies have not been routinely identifiable in most CIDP patients.[135]

The failure of regulatory T-cell mechanisms is also thought to underlie persistent or recurrent disease, differentiating CIDP from the acute inflammatory demyelinating polyneuropathy form of GBS.[36,136] CD8+ T-cell–mediated autoimmunity has been demonstrated.[132] The rapid improvement that occasionally follows PLEX or IVIg and the demonstration of immunoglobulin and complement on peripheral nerve tissues suggest a role of the humoral arm of the immune system as well.[39,137] Theoretically, autoantibodies may impair ion channel function and by doing so produce an EDX pattern suggesting rapidly reversible axon loss similar to the AMAN variant of GBS. Ion channel dysfunction may also theoretically result in EDX evidence of conduction block as well.[113]

TREATMENT

Corticosteroids, PLEX, and IVIg have consistently been found to be beneficial for the treatment of CIDP in randomized controlled trials and observational studies, both in adults and children (Table 14-4).[4,109,138–144] Based on short-term efficacy, all three are reasonably considered equivalent first-line options, with ~60%–75% of patients responding to the first therapy (of these three) chosen.[4,145,146] Practical considerations often dictate which therapy is chosen first. Due to the logistical burden of PLEX, corticosteroids or IVIg tend to be favored for most patients. Due to the long-term side effects of corticosteroids, IVIg is used first line for many patients. IVIg is quite costly and can be inconvenient, however, and some studies have suggested that pulse-dose regimens of corticosteroids are associated with a higher frequency and longer duration of remission off therapy compared with IVIg (see below).[4,147] Regardless, treatment response is often very favorable; in one study, 40% of patients treated with IVIg and/or corticosteroids became independent in activities of daily living, achieving a modified Rankin scale of two or less.[4]

Failure[4,124,148] to respond to one of these three treatments does not predict failure with the other two.[11] In one study, half of the patients who failed corticosteroids responded to IVIg.[149] In another retrospective analysis of 281 patients treated with IVIg as first-line therapy, 76% responded to IVIg. Of those that failed IVIg, 67% responded to PLEX as a second choice and 59% responded to corticosteroids as a second choice. Of the 12 patients who failed the second-line choice, 75% responded to the third option.[146] Given these high response rates, when patients fail to respond to a first-line therapy it is always reasonable to reconfirm that CIDP is the correct diagnosis.[17,44]

Corticosteroids

Anecdotal cases and small series,[4,12,13,17,19,150] a randomized control trial of oral prednisone,[151] and a Cochrane systematic review all support the benefit of corticosteroids for the treatment of CIDP.[152] The one exception is for pure motor CIDP, as some patients have been reported to deteriorate after corticosteroid treatment. IVIg is accordingly considered first-line therapy for these patients.[3,153,154]

When we treat CIDP with corticosteroids, we usually use oral prednisone, initiated at a dose of 1–1.5 mg/kg (up to 100 mg) per day for 2–4 weeks, with transition to alternate day treatment as outlined in Chapter 4 (e.g., either 100 mg QOD or 60 mg alternating with 50 mg every other day).[12,25] Patients remain on relatively high doses of prednisone until their strength is normalized or there is a clear plateau in clinical improvement. When weaning begins, the trajectory it takes is dependent on the contextual features of the individual case. Typically, we begin the taper after a month or two of the induction dose, particularly if there are either signs of improvement or the development of unwanted side effects. We slowly taper the prednisone by 5 mg every 2–3 weeks until the dose is 20 mg every other day. At that point, dosing is reduced no faster than 2.5 mg every week or 5 mg every 2 weeks. Using this method of treatment, the time of initial improvement ranges from several days to 5 months (mean 1.9 months), the time to maximum improvement averages 6.6 months, with significant improvement in strength and function appreciated in 95% of treated patients after 1 year.[12]

Others have advocated for regimens using pulse-dosed steroids—either with intravenous methylprednisolone or with oral dexamethasone—with the rationale that this leads to more rapid therapeutic onset and fewer side effects.[149,155–157] One study using pulsed dexamethasone at a dose of 40 mg daily for 4 consecutive days for a total of 6 cycles (if required) demonstrated faster improvement, longer remissions, fewer relapses, and fewer side effects in comparison to a more conventional oral prednisolone regimen.[149] Two other studies, however, were unable to demonstrate any difference in efficacy or safety for pulsed regimens compared to standard daily oral dosing.[157,158] Further information regarding the use of corticosteroids including mechanism(s) of action and adverse effects can be found in Chapter 4.

Plasma Exchange

PLEX is less likely to be used as a CIDP treatment in comparison to corticosteroids or IVIg[159,160] based on considerations of availability and convenience as well as safety concerns.[144,161] It remains an effective option in patients who are refractory or have contraindications to IVIg and/or corticosteroids. A therapeutic/diagnostic trial of PLEX may also be useful in patients in whom the CIDP diagnosis is uncertain, as the relatively rapid response to treatment can allow for an earlier determination of whether the patient has a treatment-responsive inflammatory neuropathy.

Efficacy of PLEX was demonstrated in prospective, randomized, double-blinded, placebo-controlled trials using sham PLEX.[109,111] The characteristic regimen is to exchange approximately 200–250 mL/kg body weight five to six times

▶ TABLE 14-4. IMMUNOMODULATING THERAPY FOR CHRONIC ACQUIRED IMMUNE-MEDIATED POLYNEUROPATHIES

Therapy	Neuropathy Used for	Route	Dose	Side Effects	Monitor
Prednisone	CIDP, MADSAM, CISP	p.o.	1–1.5 mg/kg/day for 2–4 weeks, then switch to QOD	Hypertension, fluid and weight gain, hyperglycemia, hypokalemia, cataracts, glaucoma, gastric irritation, and osteoporosis	Weight, blood pressure, glucose, potassium, ophthalmologic examination
Intravenous immunoglobulin (IVIg)	CIDP, MMN, MADSAM, CISP	i.v.	0.4 g/kg/day over 5 days, or 1 g/kg/day over 2 days; 1 g/kg every three weeks often used for maintenance	Hypotension, arrhythmia, diaphoresis, flushing, nephrotoxicity, headache, aseptic meningitis, thromboembolic complications, hemolytic anemia, and anaphylaxis	Heart rate Blood pressure Renal function
Subcutaneous immunoglobulin (SCIg)	CIDP, MMN, MADSAM, CISP	s.c.	200–400 mg/kg/week administered in 1 or 2 sessions over 1 or 2 consecutive days	Infusion site pain, swelling, or reaction; headache, diarrhea, fever, fatigue, back pain, nausea; risk of systemic reactions including aseptic meningitis likely reduced compared to IVIg	Renal function Injection site(s)
Plasmapheresis	CIDP, MADSAM	i.v.	Remove total of 200–250 cc/kg plasma over 7–14 days; may require periodic exchanges	Hypotension, arrhythmia, electrolyte imbalance, anemia, and coagulation disorders	Heart rate, blood pressure, blood count, electrolytes, PT/PTT, volume removed, and replaced
Azathioprine	CIDP, MADSAM	p.o.	2–3 mg/kg/day; single AM dose	Flu-like illness, hepatotoxicity, leukopenia, macrocytosis, and neoplasia	Monthly blood count and liver enzymes × 3 months then yearly
Cyclophosphamide	CIDP, MMN, MADSAM	p.o.	1.5–2 mg/kg/day; single AM dose	Leukopenia, hemorrhagic cystitis, alopecia, infections, and neoplasia	Monthly blood count and urinalysis for duration of treatment Urine cytology
		i.v.	0.5–3 g/m^2 (max 85 mg/kg)	Same as p.o. (although more severe) and nausea/vomiting	Same
Cyclosporine	CIDP, MADSAM	p.o.	3–6 mg/kg/day; BID.	Nephrotoxicity, hypertension, hepatotoxicity, hirsutism, tremor, and gum hyperplasia	Blood pressure Trough cyclosporine level Creatinine Liver enzymes
Rituximab	MMN, DADS, Nodopathies	i.v.	375 mg/m^2 weekly × 4 weeks or 1 g × 2 weeks; usually the course will need to be repeated in 6–12 months	Infusion-related symptom complex (e.g., hypotension, rash, chills, urticaria, angioedema, and bronchospasm), asthenia, headaches, nausea vomiting, dizziness, and infection	CBC

p.o., oral; i.v., intravenous; CIDP, chronic inflammatory demyelinating polyneuropathy; MMN, multifocal motor neuropathy; MADSAM, multifocal acquired demyelinating sensory and motor neuropathy; PT, prothrombin time; PTT, partial thromboplastin time; BUN, blood urea nitrogen; Red type, strong evidence of efficacy; Blue type, possible efficacy.

over a 2-week period. The response to PLEX is transient, usually lasting only a few weeks. Intermittent maintenance treatment would therefore be required, but protracted PLEX is often inconvenient, impractical, and not endorsed by the evidence-based guideline from the American Academy of Neurology.[161] PLEX can be used in combination with prednisone in patients with severe generalized weakness, as the combination may provide a more rapid response than prednisone alone.[94,160] Further detail regarding PLEX and potential adverse effects may be found in Chapter 4.

Intravenous and Subcutaneous Immunoglobulin

IVIg has been demonstrated to be effective for CIDP in controlled clinical trials and supported by a Cochrane meta-analysis.[111,141,148,149,162-165] Three of four trials comparing IVIg against placebo and another three comparing IVIg against either steroids or PLEX demonstrated benefit.[166] Efficacy is estimated to be as high as 82% in one study.[4] It is generally accepted that the long-term side effect profiles favor IVIg over corticosteroids. Time to response is also often faster for IVIg than with corticosteroids. IVIg should certainly be favored when there is diagnostic uncertainty between acute-onset CIDP and GBS.

Typically, treatment induction consists of 2 g/kg body weight given over 2-5 days. As the effects of IVIg are often transient, repeated courses of IVIg are typically necessary. 1 g/kg given every 3 weeks is often used as a maintenance regimen since it was shown to be effective in a trial.[167] Another recent study found no compelling reason to systematically favor a lower (0.5 g/kg every 3 weeks) or higher (2 g/kg every 3 weeks) dose. Ideally, the regimen should be individualized to the needs of the specific patient, utilizing the minimally effective dose at the longest effective duration. The optimal dosing scheme can range between 1 and 2 g/kg every 3-8 weeks.[167] One study that titrated dose to response at the individual patient level found that the mean required dose was 1.4 g/kg every 4.3 weeks.[168]

Retrospective studies have demonstrated that approximately 65% of patients achieve clinical stability with long-term IVIg treatment.[159] In patients who become refractory to IVIg, courses of PLEX may restore IVIg responsiveness.[169] When IVIg is stopped, approximately 25% of patients remain in a durable remission.[169,170] Periodic trials of an IVIg taper or even cessation are therefore reasonable, especially considering that >90% of patients quickly restabilize when IVIg is resumed after a relapse.[170,171] Compared with IVIg, initial treatment with corticosteroids may be associated with higher frequency of remission off therapy. In one randomized trial, patients stopped therapy after 6 months of treatment with either IVIg or corticosteroids. In the 6 months thereafter, 8 of 21 (38%) IVIg-responsive patients required retreatment compared to 0 of 10 corticosteroid-responsive patients ($P = .03$).[172] Additional observation of this cohort demonstrated that after a median follow-up of 43 months, overall relapse rates were similar but the median time to relapse was longer for corticosteroid-treated patients (14 months) compared to IVIg-treated patients (4.5 months).[147] In a separate retrospective analysis including 72 treated patients with CIDP, 55% of IVIg-treated patients remained dependent on maintenance therapy (>18 months) compared to 18% of prednisone-treated patients.[4]

IVIg is generally well tolerated. Although it has been suggested that individuals with IgA deficiency may be at risk for anaphylaxis from IVIg,[150] we agree with others that this reaction is rare and that the risk may be overstated.[166,173,174] Other adverse effects are addressed in Chapter 4. For those patients who are intolerant of IVIg, subcutaneous administration of Ig (SCIg) has emerged as an effective option for maintenance therapy.[175-179] Two different dosing regimens—0.2 g/kg or 0.4 g/kg body weight given weekly—have been shown to be effective. The higher dose may be associated with a lower risk of relapse in the long term. When switching a patient from maintenance IVIg, their weekly dose of SCIg can simply be calculated as a 1:1 conversion (e.g., a patient receiving 80 g of IVIg every 4 weeks could start 20 g of SCIg weekly).[3] Systemic side effects such as headache are generally less common with SCIg compared with IVIg. Local infusion site reactions are common, however. To improve tolerability in patients requiring higher doses, twice-weekly administration or splitting the dose between multiple anatomic injection sites can be helpful.

Other Treatment Options

Numerous agents have been identified as possible second-line therapies for CIDP.[140] None have demonstrated benefit according to a Cochrane review with the caveat that the studies may have been too small to identify a modest benefit.[180] The 2021 guidelines actively recommend against using interferons, methotrexate, TNF-blockers, fingolimod, alemtuzumab, bortezomib, fludarabine, immunoadsorption, abatacept, natalizumab, and tacrolimus due to insufficient evidence of efficacy or safety concerns.[3] This leaves azathioprine, mycophenolate, cyclosporine, rituximab, and cyclophosphamide as possible options.

In essentially all cases, treatments other than IVIg, PLEX, and corticosteroids are used only as secondary agents, only when an acceptable response cannot be obtained by the three primary treatments. Small anecdotal reports suggest a beneficial effect of azathioprine at doses of 100-300 mg/day.[13,39,160,181-183] A prospective, randomized, but nonblinded 9-month study of 27 patients with CIDP failed to demonstrate a benefit of azathioprine (2 mg/kg/day) when added to prednisone.[184] The dose of azathioprine may have been too small however (we go up to 3 mg/kg/day) and the duration of this study may have been too short for a beneficial effect to become evident. A beneficial response from azathioprine may require a longer-than 9-month exposure to adequate doses.

Cyclosporine also appears effective in some patients with CIDP, even in those refractory to other modes of therapy, including prednisone, PLEX, IVIg, and cyclophosphamide.[58,185-192] A few small studies have suggested that mycophenolate mofetil may benefit patients with CIDP.[193] Other reports have been less favorable.[194] There appears to be a modest benefit in approximately 20% of CIDP patients with stabilization and successful reduction in steroid or IVIg therapy.[195] The response in general appears to be infrequent and modest.[185,196-199]

In several case series, rituximab has been suggested as an effective option for patients refractory to the first-line therapies.[145,200-210] This remains to be proven in a randomized trial, however. A number of small series also suggest that both oral and monthly pulses of intravenous cyclophosphamide can be beneficial in patients with CIDP.[7,13,39,185,211-216] We prefer a monthly pulsed intravenous cyclophosphamide regimen as it is associated with less risks of hemorrhagic cystitis. We use cyclophosphamide as a last resort because of its side effect profile. Nonetheless, we have seen patients rendered essentially quadriplegic by their disease and refractory to multiple other therapies regain complete independence in activities of daily living after a 6-month course of 1 g/m^2/month treatment.[217]

Due to the lack of proven secondary treatment options, FcRn inhibitors and complement inhibitors are under active investigation in clinical trials for the treatment of CIDP. Multiple drugs in these classes have already been approved for use in generalized myasthenia gravis (See Chapter 25). At the time of the publication of this edition, however, none of these have yet been approved for the indication of CIDP in the United States.

▶ MULTIFOCAL AND FOCAL CIDP [MULTIFOCAL ACQUIRED AND DEMYELINATING SENSORY AND MOTOR NEUROPATHY (MADSAM), OR LEWIS SUMNER SYNDROME]

CLINICAL FEATURES

Lewis and colleagues described the first cases of patients with multifocal demyelinating neuropathy with persistent conduction block.[218] As the name implies, the pattern of signs and symptoms in MADSAM neuropathy patients are those of a multifocal sensorimotor neuropathy (Table 14-1).[21,219-226] This is in contrast with MMN, the other notably multifocal chronic, acquired, immune-mediated demyelinating neuropathy, which is a motor disorder.[219] That said, around 50% of patients with MADSAM may have a pure motor onset, so distinguishing this from MMN can be less straightforward than expected.[227] In those with pure motor onset, sensory symptoms emerged on average 18 months later. As with MMN, there is a male predominance with an average age of onset in the early 50s typically in the upper extremities.[228]

Asymmetry is the hallmark that distinguishes MADSAM from typical CIDP. Very focal forms affecting a single limb or even a single nerve have been reported; accordingly, these presentations may mimic a brachial plexus neuritis.[229-232] Onset in the lower extremities may occur however, and commonly develops over time without treatment in the more typical upper extremity-onset cases.

Motor and sensory symptoms occur in the distribution of discrete peripheral nerves if the patient is evaluated before the disease progresses to a more confluent pattern. Other causes of mononeuropathy multiplex such as vasculitic neuropathy or hereditary neuropathy with liability to pressure palsies (HNPP) are therefore important to consider in these patients. Some patients describe pain and paresthesias, but this is typically less prominent than what is seen in brachial neuritis. Cranial neuropathies occur in 30%–48% of patients, more frequent than with typical CIDP.[233,234] Involvement of the optic, oculomotor, trigeminal, and facial nerves have been reported, and many of these are unilateral.[235] Dysautonomia is apparently rare but has been reported. Muscle stretch reflexes can be normal or reduced depending on the nerves affected.[236,237]

LABORATORY FEATURES

Laboratory and EDX testing can be helpful in distinguishing MADSAM from MMN. CSF protein levels are often mildly elevated (mean level of around 70 mg/dL), in contrast to MMN in which CSF protein levels are typically normal.[219,233,238] CSF protein levels can be normal, however. Antiglycolipid autoantibodies such as GM1 are rarely encountered but may be more common among those with an associated paraprotein.[219-225,227] In one series, 25% of patients had an associated monoclonal gammopathy identified.

The EDX pattern in MADSAM is that of an acquired, predominantly demyelinating neuropathy. Conduction block and/or temporal dispersion has been reported in 82% of patients, prolonged distal latencies in 23%, abnormal (typically prolonged) F responses in two-thirds, and slow CVs in 44% of patients in one or more motor nerves.[219-225,233] These demyelinating features are identical to CIDP with the understandable exception that they may be less widespread in their distribution. Abnormalities in the SNAPs are critical for distinguishing this disorder from MMN. As with typical CIDP, the EAN/PNS 2021 guidelines require abnormalities in two motor nerves and two sensory nerves to diagnose multifocal (more than one limb) or focal (single limb) CIDP. As mentioned above, MADSAM may frequently have a pure motor onset. Repeating EDX studies is important, as they may later identify clear sensory involvement. Ultrasound and MRI may also be useful in improving the identification of MADSAM,[239-241] as they frequently identify nerve enlargement especially within the brachial plexus.

HISTOPATHOLOGY

Sensory nerve biopsies, not routinely recommended, demonstrate many thinly myelinated nerve fibers, subperineurial and endoneurial edema, mild onion-bulb formations, and occasional inflammatory cell infiltrates.[219,221–225] Inflammatory cells are often perivascular.[224] Asymmetric loss of large myelinated nerve fibers between and within fascicles may be appreciated.[219,221,223] Findings suggestive of demyelination are reported to occur in 77% of individuals.[233]

TREATMENT

Most patients with MADSAM improve with IVIg treatment (Table 14-4).[220–225,233,236,242,243] Also, in contrast to MMN but similar to CIDP, most patients with MADSAM respond to treatment with corticosteroids.[219,220,223–244] In one retrospective study, response rates were higher for IVIg (94%) than for dexamethasone (30%).[245] Protocols are identical to those utilized for CIDP.

▶ DADS NEUROPATHY OR DISTAL CIDP

CLINICAL FEATURES

DADS neuropathy was first described as a distinct syndrome in 2000 (Table 14-1).[116] The mean age of onset is 59–67 years and the disorder appears to be more common in males.[38,246,247] The DADS phenotype is clinically and electrodiagnostically distinct from typical CIDP. Clinically, it is dominated by distal, symmetric sensory signs and symptoms, frequently associated with sensory ataxia.[35,246] Sensory symptoms typically begin in the feet symmetrically and eventually involve the hands.[246] Wavering or loss of balance accentuated by eye closure is the norm even early in the course. Conversely, compatible with the seemingly large fiber predominance of this disorder, pain is rarely a significant clinical feature. Postural tremor is common, whereas involvement of cranial nerves is very rare and should suggest an alternative diagnosis.[246–250]

Despite the notable demyelinating EDX features affecting motor nerves, there is little if any motor involvement at first.[38] Weakness eventually develops in a majority, usually after years, and typically found initially in toe and foot dorsiflexors. Hand weakness occurs in some, and weakness may become more widespread in those affected for many years. It is important to recognize that weakness on examination may be overestimated in some patients due to the degree of proprioceptive loss. Making sure that the patient sees the tested body part during manual muscle testing is important in this regard. In keeping with its acquired, demyelinating pathophysiology, generalized hyporeflexia or areflexia is also typical.

The natural history is variable. DADS is typically an insidious disorder that progresses very slowly, at a pace notably distinctive from typical CIDP.[12,246] A chronic progressive course is the norm, with few patients having a relapsing/remitting course. It may become incapacitating for some, largely due to loss of balance from the sensory ataxia.[247] A considerable number of patients, however, will retain the ability to walk independently without gait aids, years or even a decade or more after symptom onset. It has been reported that DADS patients with anti-MAG antibodies are more likely to have a more indolent course with less disability.[247]

There is ongoing debate as to whether some or all patients with the DADS phenotype are rightfully considered to have a CIDP-spectrum disorder, or something else entirely. Depending on the case series, up to 85% of patients with DADS also have monoclonal gammopathy, usually IgM Kappa.[116,251] In turn, about two-thirds of those patients with an IgM monoclonal gammopathy also have autoantibodies directed against MAG or a related epitope. It is now generally accepted that patients with the DADS clinical and EDX phenotype, IgM monoclonal gammopathy, and detectable anti-MAG antibodies should be considered to have a distinct disorder, not a form of CIDP. This is owing to the differences in natural history outlined above, as well as key differences in EDX findings, observed pathologic features, and expected treatment response to various therapies. This disorder is now sometimes simply defined as anti-MAG neuropathy and can be seen in association with either Waldenstrom macroglobulinemia or IgM MGUS. This is therefore covered in additional detail in Chapter 19, but we will highlight some key principles below.

Conversely, it has been argued that those patients with DADS but *without* anti-MAG antibodies should be best considered to have a form of CIDP. This is referred to as distal CIDP in the latest EAN/PNS guidelines. A major justification for this schema is that patients with so-called distal CIDP respond to traditional CIDP treatments at a higher frequency than anti-MAG neuropathy patients. This remains an imperfect distinction, however, with some key caveats worth noting. Anti-MAG antibodies can be occasionally found in patients with contrasting phenotypes. Some patients, for example, have EDX findings more reminiscent of typical CIDP and lack the expected pathologic findings of anti-MAG neuropathy on biopsy.[252] Higher titers, above 7,000 BTU, may be more specific for the DADS phenotype.[253,254] This suggests that the clinical phenotype, not a serologic test, may be more important for defining this syndrome and making management decisions.[236]

ELECTRODIAGNOSTIC FEATURES

Like with CIDP, EDX in patients with DADS demonstrates unequivocal demyelinating features. In contrast to CIDP, however, slowed nerve conduction is more prominent in distal as opposed to proximal segments of nerve. Marked prolongation of distal motor latencies are a hallmark of this disorder. It has been reported by some, not all, that the terminal latency index (TLI), a parameter that directly contrasts conduction speed in the distal as opposed to more proximal segments of nerve, is affected to a greater extent in DADS than in other chronic, acquired, demyelinating neuropathy syndromes.[35] In addition, conduction block in motor nerves occurs uncommonly with this disorder.[94,246] This is consistent with the initial absence of weakness in most cases. Most patients with DADS will have widespread absence of SNAPs or reduction in their amplitudes.

To diagnose distal CIDP, the 2021 EAN/PNS guidelines require abnormalities in two motor nerves and two sensory nerves, in the same manner as typical CIDP. Again, it is the clinical syndrome that drives the diagnostic distinction between typical and distal CIDP in these guidelines. Notably, it is specifically required that two upper limb motor nerves demonstrate demyelinating abnormalities despite the distal nature of the initial symptoms in DADS. Patients with abnormalities in only two lower limbs are deemed to have "possible" distal CIDP. This in part provides an implicit reminder that axonopathies can lead to length-dependent, amplitude-dependent reduction in CVs.

LABORATORY FEATURES

As alluded to above, it is essential to test patients with DADS for the presence of a monoclonal gammopathy. Anti-MAG antibodies should also be checked routinely; rarely, these will be found in patients without monoclonal gammopathy. In the rare patient in whom an IgA lambda or IgG lambda paraprotein is found, testing of vascular endothelial growth factor (VEGF) levels in the serum is also recommended as part of an assessment for early POEMS (see Chapter 19). In patients with weakness and without anti-MAG antibodies, nodal/paranodal antibodies can be considered. Patients with neurofascin-155–related neuropathy may have distal-predominant weakness and sensory ataxia. In contrast to DADS, the motor deficits tend to overshadow the sensory deficits in these patients. Finally, in patients with an especially indolent disease course, genetic testing to exclude hereditary demyelinating neuropathies could also be considered.

An elevation of CSF protein levels without a cellular response is characteristic of DADS patients. There appears to be no significant difference in comparison to CIDP, either the number of patients with elevated CSF protein levels, or magnitude of protein elevation.[12,38]

HISTOPATHOLOGY

Nerve biopsies, which should be infrequently performed, characteristically identify features suggestive of demyelination and remyelination in DADS patients.[35,246] Not unexpectedly, concomitant axon loss may occur as well.[237] A characteristic feature however is that patients with MAG autoantibodies may be shown to have binding of these autoantibodies to peripheral nerve myelin with immunohistochemical staining of nerve biopsy specimens. In addition, a characteristic separation of myelin lamella demonstrable with EM, consistent with the known function of MAG, suggests a pathogenic rather than simply a reactionary role for these autoantibodies in this disease. This finding is described in 95% of individuals with neuropathy, IgM monoclonal gammopathy, and anti-MAG autoantibodies.[246]

PATHOGENESIS

Myelin-associated glycoprotein is a transmembrane, structural glycoprotein found in noncompact myelin on its abaxonal surface, on paranodal loops, and in Schmidt–Lanterman incisures.[113,114] As mentioned, the binding of MAG autoantibodies to myelin, the characteristic widening of myelin lamellae found in DADS patients consistent with disruption of normal MAG function, and the ability to reproduce the pathology in passive-transfer experiments utilizing human MAG autoantibodies and chickens suggests a pathogenic role for MAG autoantibodies and perhaps for the almost invariably associated IgM monoclonal gammopathy.[113,246]

TREATMENT

Patients with DADS are generally less responsive to the immunomodulatory treatments typically used for typical and multifocal CIDP (IVIg, corticosteroids, and plasma exchange).[21,35,255] The presence of an IgM monoclonal gammopathy and/or anti-MAG antibodies may influence the treatment responsiveness. As alluded to above, it has been well established that the majority of patients with IgM monoclonal gammopathy and anti-MAG antibodies are refractory to traditional CIDP treatments; only 16%–25% of these patients respond to IVIg, for example.[246,256,257] Some patients with anti-MAG neuropathy may respond to rituximab; this is discussed in further detail in Chapter 19.

Treatment responsiveness has been most clearly established in those patients without monoclonal gammopathy (described also as DADS-I). Even still, their treatment response remains less frequent than for typical CIDP.[35,38,258] Considering the indolent nature of the disorder in many, this alters the risk/benefit analysis of treatment decision-making considerably compared to typical CIDP. It has not been clearly established whether patients with DADS and IgM monoclonal gammopathy (DADS-M) without anti-MAG antibodies have significantly different responses to treatment than those with anti-MAG antibodies,[259,260] so decision making may be even more nuanced for this patient population.

▶ NODOPATHIES AND PARANODOPATHIES

Recently, a small number of patients that previously would have been considered to have GBS or CIDP have been shown to harbor autoantibodies targeting novel antigens residing in nodal and paranodal regions. These antigens are found on cell adhesion molecules responsible for the positioning and anchoring of ion channels and myelin folds in strategic locations along the axolemma.[114] Disruption of these molecules leads to the breakdown of the typical nodal and paranodal architecture and conduction failure of the affected axons.

To date, autoantibodies targeting neurofascin-155, neurofascin-140, neurofascin-186, contactin-1 (CNTN-1), and contactin-associated protein-1 (Caspr-1) have been implicated in cases of autoimmune neuropathy. The frequency of these antibodies among patients diagnosed with CIDP identified through database studies has varied widely, ranging from 1% to 18%.[66,112,228,235,261-264] The largest of these series to date has included 1,500 patients diagnosed with CIDP from Europe; 1% of patients were found to have IgG4 antibodies against neurofascin-155, 0.7% had IgG4 antibodies against CNTN1, and 0.2% had IgG4 antibodies against Caspr-1.[263] Neurofascin-155 has consistently been the most frequently identified antibody across published studies. The frequency of both neurofascin-155 and these antibodies overall has thus far been higher in published East Asian cohorts.[66,262,265] Neurofascin-155 paranodopathy has been associated with the HLA-DRB1*15 haplotype, with 91% of all affected patients in one series having this haplotype.[266] HLA-DRB1*15 is enriched in East Asian populations, which could explain the discrepancy in reported frequencies.[261]

Patients harboring these autoantibodies can have unique clinical features not typically seen with CIDP or other variants thereof. More importantly, patients are frequently refractory to standard treatments for CIDP (corticosteroids and IVIg) but instead appear to respond uniquely well to rituximab. Because the impairments resulting from these disorders can be quite severe, identification of the correct syndrome through autoantibody testing is therefore essential to guide appropriate treatment. For this reason, the 2021 EAN/PNS Guidelines explicitly excluded the nodopathies and paranodopathies from the CIDP umbrella, creating a new disease carve-out.[3]

CLINICAL FEATURES

The specific clinical features vary depending on the specific autoantibody identified. Patients with IgG4 antibodies against neurofascin-155 commonly present with the subacute to chronic onset of symmetric, distally predominant weakness and sensory loss.[66,112,262-264,266-270] Notably, neurofascin-155 patients are often younger than patients with typical CIDP. The mean age of onset was 42 in the largest published series to date, with some patients affected in their 20s.[266] Sensory ataxia is especially prominent, affecting 75% of patients. Cerebellar ataxia may also be apparent, and some patients have additional signs of cerebellar dysfunction including nystagmus or dysarthria. Tremor, often severe and disabling, is seen in 50%–75%. Postural tremor and intention tremor can both occur. The arms are most affected by the tremor, but the head, tongue, and voice can also be involved. About 30% of patients have cranial nerve abnormalities. A small subset of neurofascin-155 patients have been reported to have combined central and peripheral demyelination (CCPD).[64-66] The CNS demyelinating lesions seen in these patients can clinically and radiologically resemble those seen in MS, and some patients will meet the McDonald criteria for MS. The central and peripheral demyelinating syndromes in these patients can occur either simultaneously or separated in time.

Patients with IgG4 antibodies against CNTN-1 frequently present with subacute weakness and sensory loss.[235,263,264,271-276] Both motor-predominant and sensory-predominant presentations have been reported; weakness and sensory loss are distally predominant in some patients. Neuropathic pain is notable in ~50% of patients. Similar to neurofascin-155, CNTN-1 patients almost always have sensory ataxia and frequently have tremors. Reported patients have had greater levels of disability than those with neurofascin-155, suggesting a more severe disease overall. Facial paralysis is also more common than with typical CIDP or with neurofascin-155. Three of ten patients in one case series were possibly paraneoplastic (thymoma, breast cancer, and plasmacytoma).[271]

Uniquely, renal failure and nephrotic syndrome from membranous glomerulonephritis frequently co-occur in patients with CNTN-1 neuropathy.[263,272,274,276,277] A handful of patients have even been identified who have only glomerulonephritis without neuropathy. The contactin-1 protein is also present on podocytes within the kidney; granular deposits of IgG4 can be seen along the glomerular basement membrane on renal biopsy. The renal involvement is also treatment responsive.

Fewer cases of Caspr-1 neuropathy have been reported thus far.[235,263,264,268,278-281] In cell-based assays, these autoantibodies seem to react most strongly to the Caspr-1/CNTN1 complex,[282] but since some published reports refer only to Caspr-1 antibodies we will refer to them as such. The published cases to date suggest that the clinical syndrome may vary depending on the type of antibodies involved in the immune response. Acute cases resembling monophasic GBS have been reported in association with IgG2 and IgG3 antibodies targeting Caspr-1.[278,279] By contrast, those patients with IgG4 antibodies can still have acute to subacute onset of symptoms but tend to develop a more chronic neuropathy. One patient with a syndrome resembling acute-onset CIDP was demonstrated to have IgG3 antibodies during the acute onset of symptoms with a later switch to IgG4 antibodies in the chronic phase.[279] As with other paranodopathies, patients with chronic neuropathy have very commonly had sensory ataxia. Cranial nerve involvement is more frequent than with typical CIDP and neuropathic pain has also frequently been reported.

Antibodies reactive against neurofascin-140 and neurofascin-186, the nodal isoforms of neurofascin, have been the least common. A range of IgG1, IgG3, and IgG4 antibodies have been described. Five patients with antibodies against these paired antigens have been reported to have the subacute onset of weakness and sensory ataxia; two also had nephrotic syndrome.[283] Other patients have been identified with the so-called "pan-neurofascin" antibodies, reactive to a shared epitope on neurofascin-140, -155, and -186.[267,284–287] The clinical syndrome reported in these patients is best thought of as a severe GBS mimic. Affected patients present with severe and fulminant weakness that can lead to severe tetraplegia. As with GBS, severe cranial nerve involvement, respiratory failure, and autonomic dysfunction can all occur. Some cases have progressed to a nearly locked-in state. Three patients with concurrent nephrotic syndrome have been reported.[284]

While these cases can be very severe and frequently fatal, those patients that survive have consistently had a monophasic course without requirement for ongoing maintenance treatment. Patients can regain functional independence despite their severe initial weakness. In follow-up, the autoantibodies often become undetectable.

LABORATORY FEATURES

Due to the overall low prevalence of these disorders, it is not practical nor cost-effective to screen all patients suspected to have CIDP for nodal/paranodal autoantibodies. The 2021 EAN/PNS Guidelines helpfully suggested circumstances under which testing is of higher yield and therefore recommended: (1) acute or subacute aggressive onset, leading to a suspected diagnosis of acute onset CIDP; (2) presence of a low-frequency tremor, and/or ataxia disproportionate to the sensory involvement or other cerebellar features; (3) predominantly distal weakness; (4) respiratory failure and cranial nerve involvement in a patient otherwise suspected to have typical CIDP; (5) associated renal dysfunction due to nephrotic syndrome; (6) very high CSF protein levels; and/or (7) resistance to standard CIDP therapy with IVIg and corticosteroids.[3] Identification of these autoantibodies in the serum typically relies on cell-based assays which maximize reliability.[261]

As described above, most of the cases described to date have been associated with IgG4 autoantibodies. While neurofascin-155 antibodies of other IgG subclasses have been identified in some publications, no consistent associated clinical phenotype distinct from seronegative CIDP has emerged for these yet.[235,267] By contrast, IgG1, IgG2, and IgG3 Caspr-1 or pan-neurofascin antibodies may be identified in patients with acute cases resembling fulminant GBS.

CSF protein levels are elevated in nearly all patients with chronic nodopathies/paranodopathies, often to a greater degree than patients with seronegative CIDP.[235,263,264,266,269,271,275,281] CSF pleocytosis is not expected. Some of the GBS-like cases associated with pan-neurofascin antibodies have had normal CSF protein within the first 2 weeks of illness.[284] While unnecessary to perform in most patients, MRI of the spine will frequently reveal nerve root hypertrophy in affected patients.[269–271,284] In one series of patients with neurofascin-155 antibodies, diffuse or multifocal nerve enlargement was also demonstrable on ultrasound.[288]

A wide spectrum of demyelinating features can be seen in motor NCSs in patients with nodopathy/paranodopathy: prolonged distal motor latencies, slowed CVs for proximal nerve segments, prolonged F-wave minimum latencies, prolonged CMAP duration, conduction block, and temporal dispersion.[263,266,268,269,271,281,289] SNAPs may have low amplitude, and a "sural sparing" pattern has been seen in many patients. Needle EMG can show features suggestive of denervation. The vast majority of affected patients would accordingly meet EDX criteria for CIDP based on the latest guidelines.[266,289] This again underscores the importance of recognizing the unique clinical features of these disorders that should prompt confirmatory antibody testing. That said, one series suggested that CVs may be especially low and that this can help distinguish cases from seronegative CIDP. In this study of 40 patients with seronegative CIDP and 22 patients with neurofascin-155 or CNTN-1 paranodopathy, motor CV for the median nerve <24 m/s, motor CV for the ulnar nerve <26 m/s, or distal motor latency for the ulnar nerve >7.4 ms carried a sensitivity of 59% and a specificity of 93% for paranodopathy.[289]

PATHOGENESIS AND HISTOPATHOLOGY

Understanding the typical nodal architecture is critical for understanding the pathologic processes underlying the nodopathies/paranodopathies. To facilitate the propagation of the action potential down axons, the nodes of Ranvier and nearby regions are enriched with ion channels. Cell adhesion molecules, including the neurofascins, help cluster ion channels in this space and help situate myelin loops at the paranode (Fig. 14-3). Neurofascin-140 and -186 help cluster voltage-gated sodium channels within the nodes of Ranvier via anchors to the axonal cytoskeleton and gliomedin on Schwann cell microvilli. The paranodal region is defined by loops of myelin that are tightly affixed to the underlying axon. These septate junctions behave like a fence, sequestering ion channel clusters from one another on opposite sides of the paranodes. Potassium channels are clustered in the juxtaparanodal portion of the axons. Neurofascin-155 is expressed by Schwann cells at the paranodes. It affixes these myelin loops to the axon via binding to CNTN-1 and Caspr-1, which form a complex together on the axonal cell membrane.[290]

In vitro studies and animal models have demonstrated the pathogenic potential of autoantibodies targeting these nodal and paranodal proteins.[235,291,292] Studies utilizing sciatic nerve preparations incubated with purified patient sera have demonstrated that IgG4 CNTN-1 antibodies and IgG4 Caspr-1 antibodies can physically penetrate the paranodal barrier and slowly diffuse throughout the paranodal space. These antibodies exert a blocking function on the CNTN-1/Caspr-1 complex, preventing its interaction with

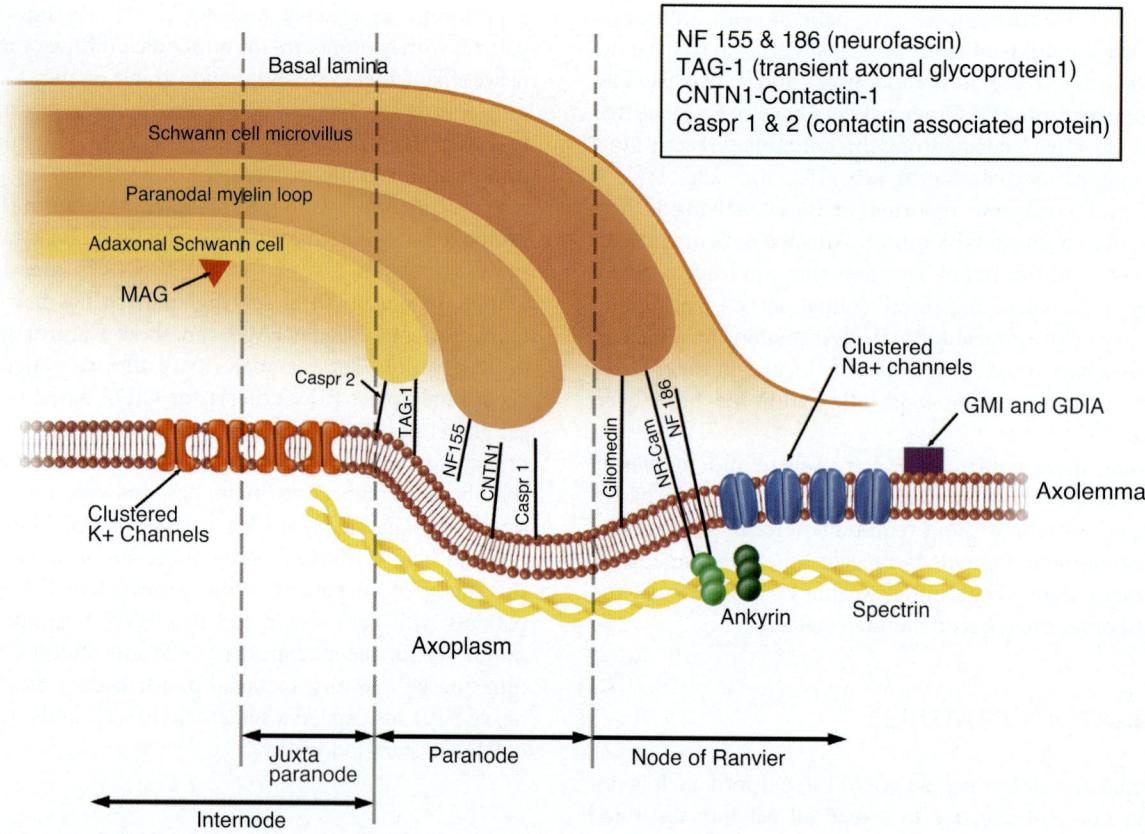

Figure 14-3. Simplified schematic of a peripheral nerve fiber (motor) node/internode junction with locations of proteins and ion channels potentially relevant to the pathogenesis of chronic, acquired, demyelinating polyneuropathies.

neurofascin-155. Over time, this leads to a progressive separation of the myelin loops from the axon and paranodal dismantling. Passive transfer of CNTN-1 patient sera into rats led to similar paranodal disruption, as well as progressive proximal weakness and ataxia in the animals. Antibodies targeting neurofascin-155, by contrast, appear to deplete the protein from the myelin surface entirely. This ultimately leads to the same consequence—dismantling of the paranode. In both cases, disruption of the paranodal architecture impairs the ordered separation of these ion channels, interfering with saltatory conduction and potentially leading to conduction failure.

Utilizing EM, nerve biopsies from affected patients have also shown this characteristic detachment of myelin loops at the paranodes.[293] Overall, the histopathologic findings from patients with IgG4 paranodal antibodies have been quite distinct from what is typically seen in CIDP.[269,271,276,293,294] The density of myelinated nerve fibers is reduced, primarily due to axonal degeneration. Widening of the nodes can be seen and myelin ovoids may be evident. Typical features of demyelination, however, are conspicuously absent—onion bulbs are not present, macrophage-mediated demyelination is not seen, and inflammation is overall scant.

These findings likely relate to the immunologic nature of the IgG4 antibodies which are seen in these conditions. IgG4 antibodies have reduced ability to bind and activate Fc receptors on immune effector cells and are unable to activate the complement cascade. Their effects are therefore primarily exerted through a blocking function on the targeted protein rather than internalization or destruction by immune effector cells. IgG4 antibodies typically result from a class-switching response after prolonged immune response to a specific target.[295] This point is nicely highlighted by the contrasting pathologic features reported to result from pan-neurofascin antibodies, which are primarily of the IgG1 and IgG3 subclasses. The destructive effects on paranodal architecture are overall more severe and the complement system is involved.[286]

TREATMENT

The majority of patients reported in the literature with paranodopathies/nodopathies have been poorly responsive to IVIg.[66,112,235,267,269–271,275,281] This relates to the fact that most patients harbor IgG4 antibodies. IVIg exerts its therapeutic effect in part by inhibiting the activation of the complement system and the Fcγ receptor (FcγRIIb); these are irrelevant to the pathogenesis of IgG4 antibodies as described above. IVIg also saturates the neonatal Fc receptors responsible for extending the half-life of IgG in the serum, thereby increase clearance of pathogenic IgG; IVIg consists largely of IgG1 antibodies, however, so the clearance of IgG4 is minimally affected. Those nodopathies/paranodopathies mediated by IgG1 or IgG3 antibodies—to date, largely the pan-neurofascin cases—can accordingly still be responsive to IVIg.[283,286] Some reported patients have had an initial response to IVIg, but then later become refractory to it; this may be due to the "class-switching" from IgG1/IgG3 → IgG4 described above.[235,269,271,279] Corticosteroids and plasma exchange, by contrast, remain effective options for some patients but most patients have required additional therapy even if they respond.

Similar to what has been described with other IgG4-mediated neurologic diseases, rituximab has been highly effective for many patients with IgG4 nodopathy/paranodopathy. Response rates reported from observational studies have ranged from 75% to 100%.[112,210,235,263,264,266,268,269,281,296,297] Those patients with a very long delay to treatment and significant axonal degeneration may be more refractory. However, some very severely affected patients and some patients with disease duration over 2 years have still had meaningful improvements in disability after treatment.

▶ MULTIFOCAL MOTOR NEUROPATHY

CLINICAL FEATURES

MMN is a presumed immune-mediated demyelinating neuropathy characterized as a potentially reversible form of motor neuropathy, frequently with demonstrable conduction block.[298–301] Like MADSAM, MMN typically presents with a multifocal neuropathy pattern affecting individual peripheral nerves. Unlike MADSAM, it is typically a pure motor syndrome characterized by asymmetrical weakness, cramps, fasciculations, and in many cases eventual atrophy (Table 14-1).[298,302–319] There is a male-to-female ratio of approximately 3:1. The age of symptom onset ranges from the early 20s to late 60s with a mean of approximately 40 years of age.[319,320] Rarely, childhood onsets are encountered.[321] The onset is usually insidious, and the weakness typically progresses, often stepwise, over the course of several years to involve other nerve distributions and other limbs.

Like MADSAM, MMN typically commences in distal muscles of the upper extremities. Most patients present with intrinsic hand weakness, wrist drop, or in some cases foot drop. Unlike MADSAM, sensory signs and abnormal SNAPs are not typically encountered early in the course of MMN. Case series suggest that several years after disease onset, some patients will develop sensory symptoms accompanied by a reduction in SNAP amplitudes.[322]

The differential diagnosis of MMN is largely those disorders that are either predominantly motor or that have a multifocal pattern of weakness. As a disorder of motor nerves with frequent monomelic onset, amyotrophic lateral sclerosis (ALS) is arguably the major consideration. In one series, MMN was the most common ALS mimic[323] although MMN occurs far less commonly than its more malignant counterpart.[304,319,324] The cramps and fasciculations that can occur in MMN contribute to the potential confusion between the two disorders. Demonstrating a nerve rather than myotomal/segmental pattern of weakness is a helpful, discriminating clinical feature in favor of MMN. Other features of MMN include weakness in the absence of atrophy and absence of overt upper motor neuron signs although neither of these features exclude ALS with certainty. Unequivocal corticospinal tract signs (i.e., clonus, spasticity, and extensor plantar responses) are not seen in MMN. Assessment of deep tendon reflexes should be interpreted with caution, as suppressed reflexes can occur in lower motor neuron dominant ALS and preserved or even enhanced reflexes can occur in MMN if no nerve associated with a deep tendon reflex is affected. Other differential diagnostic considerations that may be relatively focal and purely motor include occasional cases of acquired or congenital myasthenia which may have a predilection for wrist and finger extensors in some cases and certain myopathies such as inclusion body myositis. In consideration of multifocality, MADSAM, MAMA (see below), acute brachial plexus neuropathy, and vasculitic neuropathy should be considered as well.

Although MMN is predominantly a disorder of limb weakness, a number of atypical features may occur. Abnormal vibration sense has been reported in a fifth of patients by at least one author.[320] Muscle hypertrophy, believed to be secondary to the underlying myokymic discharges has been reported although eventual axon loss and atrophy are common. Cranial nerve involvement including ophthalmoparesis as a presenting manifestation has been reported.[325,326] Phrenic nerve involvement and ventilatory failure appear to be uncommon but potential features of the syndrome.[327,328]

As implied by its name, MMN affects two or more motor nerves. The astute neuromuscular clinician will consider MMN in cases of monofocal motor neuropathy and will search diligently for conduction block or MR evidence of focal, inflammatory nerve lesions.[329] Intuitively, however, MMN often starts as a mononeuropathy.[317,318,320,321,323–332] The concern in these cases is that the mononeuropathy will be misattributed to an entrapment syndrome, leading to unnecessary surgical intervention. Clinicians should be wary of this potential trap, particularly if the mononeuropathy is pure motor, or has clinical or EDX features suggesting localization to an uncommon compression or entrapment site.

In summary, the current consensus diagnostic criteria for MMN include weakness in two or more nerves, with the demonstration of conduction block in two or more nerves, in the absence of upper motor neuron signs, and clinical and EDX sensory deficits.[315] A minimum of 50% reduction in CMAP amplitude in a proximal location is required for the designation of conduction block. This standard may sacrifice sensitivity for specificity, potentially disqualifying a patient from effective treatment. This criterion for conduction block does not account for the length of the segment tested. Many would consider a sudden drop in CMAP amplitude and associated reduced area under the curve to represent definitive conduction block even if it does meet the 50% criteria. In addition, conduction blocks often occur in inaccessible nerve segments, thus limiting the ability to identify them and increasing the probability of a false-negative study. Accordingly, we agree with those who recommend treatment in those with a typical phenotype, in the absence of demonstrable conduction block or antiglycolipid antibodies, where the response to treatment may be equally effective in comparison to those who fulfill all diagnostic criteria.[318,333–336]

LABORATORY FEATURES

Autoantibodies directed against gangliosides or glycolipids concentrated on the axonal membranes of motor axons and Schwann cell membranes have been purported to be diagnostic biomarkers and potentially pathogenic agents in MMN.[313,316,320,337–339] The GM1 autoantibody is the most notable of these. Asialo-GM1, GM2, and GD1b autoantibodies are less prevalent, and are therefore presumably less significant. The prevalence of GM1 autoantibodies in this disorder is variable. Anywhere from 22% to 84% of patients with MMN will have IgM GM1 autoantibodies; the difference is often attributed to methodological differences.[320,340] In one series of 88 patients, IgM, IgG, and IgA GM1 autoantibodies were found in 43%, 1%, and 5% of cases, respectively with IgM GM2 autoantibodies in 6% of cases and IgM GD1b in 9%.[320,340] In this same series, the presence and higher titer of GM1 autoantibodies correlated with more severe weakness and disability, correlating as well with more severe axon loss as might be anticipated. Despite these observations suggesting a "dose-effect" relationship, the significance of these antibodies regarding their role in disease pathogenesis is still not clear.[340,341] In addition, both the limited sensitivity and specificity of GM1 autoantibodies even in high titers make them a supportive but neither diagnostic nor exclusionary biomarker for MMN.

The other and undoubtedly more important diagnostic tool in suspected MMN, is the ability to identify persistent conduction block in motor nerve segments not usually associated with compression or entrapment.[306,307,309–315] There are no universally accepted criteria for defining definitive conduction block.[342] Consensus criteria for conduction block have been published and are site and nerve specific.[315] A reduction in the distal CMAP amplitude can be seen in chronic lesions due to secondary axonal loss, or at least theoretically as a consequence of distal conduction block.

Although motor conduction block has been considered the EDX hallmark of MMN, other features of demyelination (i.e., prolonged distal latencies, temporal dispersion, slow CVs, and prolonged or absent F waves) are frequently identified on motor NCS.[306,308,333,343] Among those patients with a clinical history compelling for MMN but no conduction block identified on motor NCS, one study suggested that the presence of abnormal A waves when testing late responses may predict patients who will respond to IVIg.[344] As previously mentioned, early in the course of illness there should be no sensory conduction abnormalities including across the region where conduction block can be demonstrated in motor fibers.[309,315] Later in the course, a minority of patients may have some reduction in SNAP amplitudes.[322] Predictably, EDX evidence of demyelination is found more often in the nerves of the arms and is distributed randomly over the lower arm, upper arm, and shoulder segments.[308,345] Approximately one-third of electrophysiological abnormalities are found in nerves innervating muscles considered clinically normal.[345]

Needle EMG demonstrates decreased recruitment in weak muscles.[298,308,325,346] Fibrillation potentials and positive sharp waves can be seen due to secondary axonal loss, more commonly in long-standing cases. Fasciculation potentials, complex repetitive discharges, and myokymic discharges are observed occasionally, not routinely recommended.

CSF protein is usually normal in patients with MMN, which can help differentiate the neuropathy from CIDP and MADSAM. Both MR imaging, particularly MR neurography, and ultrasound may be useful tools for demonstrating enlargement or enhancement of peripheral nerve, particularly within the brachial plexus.[120,125,347,348] Ultrasound has been reported to detect enlargement of nerves at noncompressible sites in the majority of MMN cases.[341]

HISTOPATHOLOGY

Sensory nerve biopsies in MMN are usually normal, although slight reduction of myelinated fibers or axonal degeneration has been appreciated.[309,310,313,349,350] Motor axons studied from forearm nerves, the brachial plexus and the obturator nerve may reveal thinly myelinated axons and small onion bulbs indicative of demyelination as well as evidence of axonal degeneration in the form of regenerating clusters and loss of myelinated axons.[133] Mild perivascular inflammation has been reported.[165]

PATHOGENESIS

Although initially considered to be a variant of CIDP, most authorities now regard MMN as a distinct entity.[3,11,21,317] It is tempting to hypothesize that antibodies targeting specific gangliosides are pathogenic because of the location of their target antigens which are largely sequestered on motor axons in paranodal regions.[114] In addition, it has been demonstrated that GM1 autoantibodies not only bind to GM1 but activate complement in vivo making it conceivable that IgM mediates motor nerve injury at the nodes of Ranvier. Further support for complement-mediated motor nerve dysfunction triggered by IgM GM1 autoantibodies comes from the demonstration that IVIg in vitro can inhibit complement activation.[351] Nonetheless, a pathogenic role for asialo-GM1, GM2, and GD1b autoantibodies has yet to be conclusively demonstrated. Further undermining a potential pathogenic role for GM1 autoantibodies is the observation that the reduction of antibody titers correlates with clinical improvement following immunotherapy in some[312,313] but not all patients.[305,352] Further, there has been no association between the presence or absence of ganglioside antibodies and response to immunotherapy in some series.[308,349,353,354] MMN patient's sera injected into rat nerve in vivo and in vitro has been demonstrated to induce conduction block in some[345,355–357] but not all studies.[358] Not all patients with MMN have detectable ganglioside antibodies. Currently, GM1 autoantibodies are considered to be a biomarker without a defined causative role.[132]

The mechanism of conduction block and the muscle weakness that follows is conceivably a consequence of ion channel dysfunction rather than demyelination. This hypothesis is extrapolated from one report of AMAN associated with GM1 autoantibodies where conduction block and slowing occurred rapidly in the absence of remyelinating electrophysiological features.[359] In that vein, GM1 autoantibodies have been demonstrated to adversely affect sodium and potassium currents in different in vitro models.[360,361] It is possible that demyelination in MMN may not be the initial pathophysiological mechanism but the consequence of a prolonged autoimmune attack.

There have been a number of potential associations with other conditions that could potentially provide insight into the cause or mechanisms of the disease. Given the known existence of the GM1 antigen on the cell surface of C. jejuni and the association between this organism and another motor neuropathy, the AMAN variant of GBS, it is understandable that an association between MMN and C. jejuni might exist. A 1996 report identified such an association in one case but a subsequent study of MMN patients found serological evidence of C. jejuni infection in only 1 in 20 patients.[362,363] MMN has been reported to complicate treatment with tumor necrosis factor alpha blockers, probably through modulation of the immune system.[364,365] MMN has also been reported to worsen during pregnancy.[366]

TREATMENT

Unlike CIDP and MADSAM, patients with MMN generally do not respond to corticosteroids or PLEX.[154,307,309,310,313,325,352,367,368] In the short term, most patients with MMN will respond to IVIg by contrast.[320,368,369–372] Induction treatment is typically a dose of 2 g/kg over 2–5 days. Patients with long-standing disease before starting treatment, those with a later age of onset, and patients who have significant muscle atrophy and presumptive axon loss are less likely to respond.[198,354] We advocate three monthly courses of IVIg before concluding that a patient has failed treatment. We recognize however that the failure of IVIg to reverse well-established axon loss does not mean treatment failure and that maintenance IVIg treatment may prevent further attacks in someone who seems unresponsive, attacks that often occur unpredictably.

Most patients deteriorate after IVIg is withdrawn, suggesting that patients typically require maintenance therapy.[373] Doses ranging from 0.4 g/kg weekly to 1–2 g/kg monthly split over 2–5 days have been used. Subcutaneous Ig, with or without hyaluronidase used to facilitate absorption of Ig, has been shown to be similarly effective as a maintenance therapy in small trials and case series.[178,237,305,370,374–376] Subcutaneous administration can be associated with local infusion reactions, but the rate of systemic side effects such as headache is lower so this may be an appealing option in patients who are intolerant of IVIg.

Even with ongoing maintenance Ig therapy, it seems that most patients with MMN will slowly continue to deteriorate over time.[303,319,320,377] In case series following patients on maintenance IVIg over 4–8 years, there is a general trend of decreased strength and increased disability. Most patients will still remain stronger than the pretreatment baseline despite this. Some authors suggest that increasing the dose or frequency of IVIg can help delay or limit this deterioration, but likely not completely avoid it.

Unfortunately, the evidence base for second-line treatments utilized in MMN after Ig therapy is scant. There have been case reports of MMN patients treated with interferon-β1 A, azathioprine, cyclosporine, methotrexate, and mycophenolate mofetil with at best equivocal results.[378–380] Intravenous cyclophosphamide was the first therapy noted to be useful in MMN, although no double-blinded, placebo-controlled trials have been performed.[307,309,310,313,346,353] When given in combination with IVIg it may prolong the interval between IVIg infusions.[381] Rituximab has also been used to treat a number of immune-mediated neuropathies including MMN.[207,346,382] Those who respond require periodic maintenance dosing.[250,339] Randomized control trials are necessary to confirm the efficacy of these therapies, but they remain the best studied options to date. We reserve cyclophosphamide or rituximab for patients who fail IVIg or lose benefit over time.

MULTIFOCAL ACQUIRED MOTOR AXONOPATHY

Rare patients have the clinical phenotype of MMN but have only axonal features on EDX studies.[383,384] The "MAMA" acronym has been used to describe these patients.[383] Unlike patients with MMN, most patients with MAMA lack GM1 antibodies and by definition lack demyelinating EDX features. As the causes of axon loss multifocal neuropathy is far more extensive than demyelinating etiologies, a diagnosis of MAMA should be made cautiously so as to not miss a vasculitic illness or another disorder capable of infarcting or infiltrating nerves in a multifocal pattern. Some individuals with MAMA improve with prednisone or IVIg. It is felt that this rare subgroup of patients is distinct from typical MMN and other established motor neuron disorders (e.g., ALS). The implication is that if a patient has the clinical appearance of MMN with weakness in the distribution of individual nerves rather than myotomes and no upper motor neuron abnormalities, then a therapeutic trial of immunomodulating treatment may be warranted.

► CHRONIC IMMUNE SENSORY POLYRADICULOPATHY (CISP)

CLINICAL FEATURES

CISP is an apparent inflammatory neuropathy in which the autoimmune attack on nerves is directed exclusively at the level of the sensory nerve roots.[385–388] Patients present with an insidious onset of progressive, non-length dependent numbness and paresthesia of the extremities, and frequently, sensory ataxia. Symptoms and signs may be asymmetric. On examination, large fiber sensory functions are profoundly affected. Muscle stretch reflexes are reduced or absent. In contrast, muscle strength is preserved. The differential diagnosis includes a paraneoplastic sensory neuronopathy/ganglionopathy (e.g., anti-Hu syndrome), sensory ganglionopathy associated with Sjogren syndrome, or pure sensory CIDP.

More recently, the concept of CISP-plus was introduced.[389] Like CISP, patients with CISP-plus have sensory-predominant symptoms, dominated by distal large fiber sensory loss and gait ataxia. Unlike CISP, however, these patients also have mild distal weakness evident on examination (usually toe extension or flexion). Additional recent reports highlight overlapping phenotypes with motor nerve root involvement, referring to these cases as chronic immune sensory motor polyradiculopathy (CISMP).[390,391] CISP was notably excluded from the CIDP umbrella in the EAN/PNS 2021 CIDP Diagnostic Guidelines. We and others feel that the pathophysiology and treatment paradigm for CISP and its expanding spectrum of disease are similar enough to CIDP that it should best be considered a variant of CIDP.

LABORATORY FEATURES

CSF protein should be elevated; this is one important manner of inferring the inflammatory nature of this disorder. CSF cell counts should be normal. Serology is negative for GM1, GD1b, GQ1b, antinuclear, anti-Ro, and anti-La antibodies. MRI may reveal thickening and enhancement of nerve roots (Fig. 14-4).[385,387]

The typical EDX signature of CISP is normal routine sensory and motor NCSs but abnormal somatosensory-evoked potentials (SSEPs), reflective of the localization to the dorsal roots.[385–389] SSEPs classically demonstrate prolonged N13 (cervical spine) latencies or N9–N13 interpeak latencies in the arms, and/or prolonged N22 (lumbar spine) latencies in the legs. H reflexes may also be abnormal since they rely on transmission through the dorsal root.

Routine EDX studies in patients with CISP-Plus may be mildly abnormal by contrast.[389–391] Mildly prolonged F-wave latencies are the most common finding. Some patients will have mild reduction in CMAP or SNAP amplitudes. Mild slowing of CVs in either motor or sensory nerves is also possible, but not sufficient to meet EDX criteria for CIDP based on the EAN/PNS Guidelines. This is a key factor differentiating this syndrome from distal CIDP/DADS.

HISTOPATHOLOGY

Biopsies of lumbar sensory rootlets have been reported to demonstrate a decreased density of large myelinating fibers, demyelinated axons, endoneurial edema, and onion-bulb formation (Fig. 14-5).[385,389]

TREATMENT

Patients may respond to corticosteroids or IVIg in a manner similar to CIDP.

► IDIOPATHIC PERINEURITIS

CLINICAL FEATURES

Perineuritis is a nonspecific histological abnormality characterized by inflammation and thickening of the perineurium, found in neuropathies associated with diabetes mellitus, connective tissue diseases, ulcerative colitis, vasculitis (including cryoglobulinemia), lymphoma, and other malignancies.[392–397] However, perineuritis can occur as an isolated disorder without an apparent underlying systemic disorder.[384,392–398] The clinical presentation associated is variable.[396,398,399] Some patients develop sensory loss, dysesthesias, hyperpathia, and weakness in the distribution of multiple individual nerves, while others manifest with generalized symmetric motor and sensory loss indistinguishable from AIDP or CIDP. Migrating areas of sensory loss have also been described. The course of the neuropathy can be remitting and relapsing. Hyperesthesia is often appreciated on examination and a positive Tinel sign may be present over involved nerves. Large fiber sensory functions are typically less affected than small fiber modalities. Muscle strength is usually preserved, but cases with generalized weakness, suggestive of GBS or CIDP, have been reported.[396] Muscle stretch reflexes are often normal in patients with pure sensory symptoms.

LABORATORY FEATURES

CSF, ANA, ESR, liver function tests, serum protein electrophoresis, and vasculitic profile are usually normal.[392,398] The

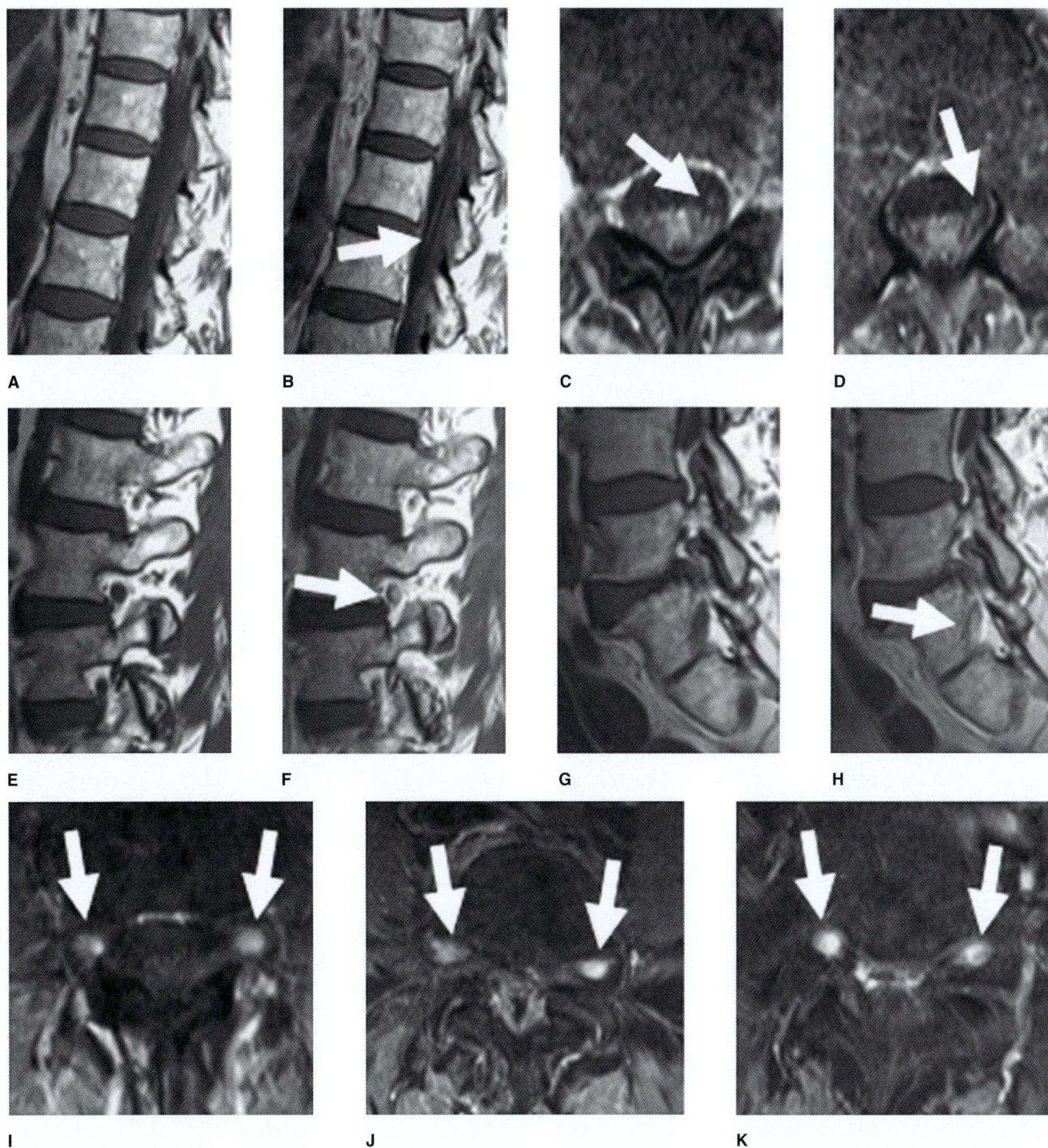

Figure 14-4. MRI of lumbosacral spine in a patient with CISP. Sagittal T1-weighted MRI with fat saturation before (**A**) and after (**B**) IV administration of gadolinium contrast shows abnormal enhancement of a left-sided nerve root at the T12–L1 vertebral level (**B**, *arrow*), also seen on axial postcontrast images (**C, D**, *arrows*). Multiple other nerve roots of the cauda equina demonstrated abnormal contrast enhancement though none were enlarged or clumped. Sagittal precontrast (**E, G**) and postcontrast (**F, H**) images of the intervertebral foramina show abnormal enhancement of right-sided dorsal root ganglia at L2–L3 (**F**, *arrow*) and L4–L5 (**H**, *arrow*). Axial postcontrast images show abnormal enhancement of the bilateral dorsal root ganglia at L2–L3 (**I**, *arrows*), L4–L5 (**J**, *arrows*), and L5–S1 (**K**, *arrows*). (Reproduced with permission from Berkowitz AL, Jha RM, Klein JP. Clinical reasoning: An 85-year-old man with paresthesias and an unsteady gait. *Neurology*. 2013;80(12):e120–e126. Figure 1A-K.)

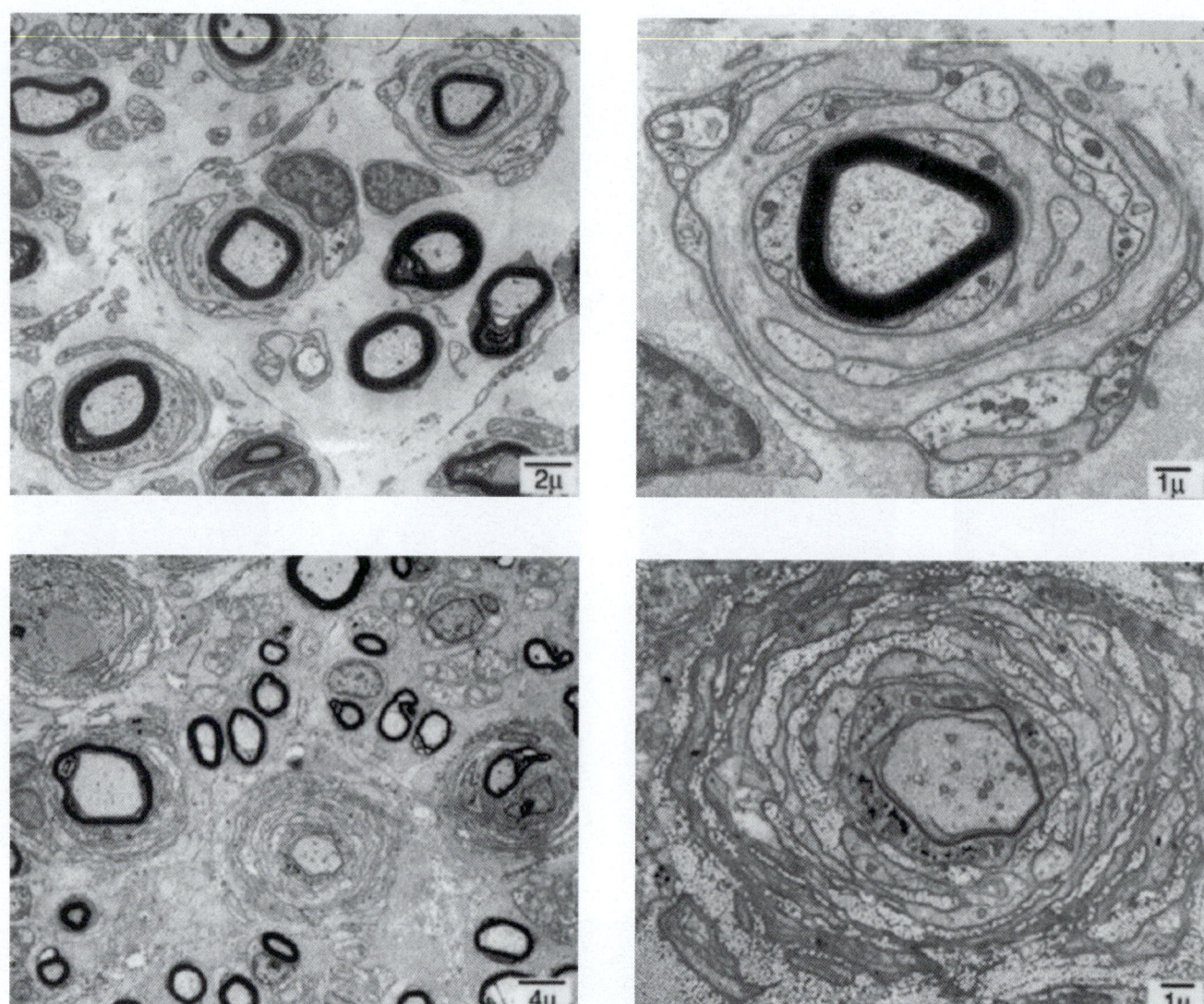

Figure 14-5. Electron micrographs from lumbar dorsal rootlet biopsies of patients with CISP reveal evidence of chronic demyelination and abortive repair. The left column (taken at low power) shows frequent onion-bulb formations associated with thinly myelinated and demyelinated profiles. The right column demonstrates two of these onion bulbs at higher power; the one on the bottom right shows an axon with only a few layers of myelin lamellae. Onion bulbs like these were very common in these two biopsies. (Reproduced with permission from Sinnreich M, Klein CJ, Daube JR, Engelstad J, Spinner RJ, Dyck PJB. Chronic immune sensory polyneuropathy. A possibly treatable sensory ataxia. *Neurology*. 2004;63(9):1662–1669. Figure 6. Pg. 1667.)

presence of an abnormal laboratory workup should lead to the consideration of an underlying systemic disorder such as vasculitis. NCSs demonstrate SNAPs that are either reduced in amplitude or absent, occurring in a multifocal or generalized pattern. Motor NCSs and EMG are normal unless patients have a multifocal neuropathy or radiculoplexopathy with both motor and sensory involvement.[395,396]

HISTOPATHOLOGY

Nerve biopsies reveal the prominent thickening and fibrosis of the perineurium along with perineural infiltration with lymphocytes and macrophages.[392,396,398] Mild perivascular inflammation may be evident as well. Myelinated nerve fiber loss due to axonal degeneration is expected.

PATHOGENESIS

The pathogenic basis for the disorder is unknown but likely to be autoimmune in nature. Perineuritis may inflict damage via ischemia, impairment of nutrient or toxin flow to and from nerve fibers in the endoneurium, or by direct humoral or cellular autoimmune attack against the nerve fibers.

TREATMENT

Response to immunotherapy is variable and difficult to ascertain because the natural history of the neuropathy may be one of remissions and relapses. We have tried prednisone and IVIg in such idiopathic cases with variable success in patients with mainly sensory disturbances.

▶ SUMMARY

The acquired chronic inflammatory polyneuropathies include CIDP, MADSAM, DADS, nodopathies and paranodopathies, MMN, and CISP. These neuropathies are distinguished from one another based on their clinical phenotypes, natural history, and treatment responsiveness. They are distinguished from their far more prevalent axonal counterparts predominantly by their phenotype coupled with their EDX features. Their importance is underscored as they represent collectively, the largest group of treatable neuropathy syndromes. Accordingly, early and accurate diagnosis and prompt treatment are of paramount importance.

REFERENCES

1. Bromberg MB. Review of the evolution of electrodiagnostic criteria for chronic inflammatory demyelinating polyradicoloneuropathy. *Muscle Nerve.* 2011;43(6):780–794.
2. Breiner A, Brannagan TH. Comparison of sensitivity and specificity among 15 criteria for chronic inflammatory demyelinating polyneuropathy. *Muscle Nerve.* 2014;50(1):40–46.
3. Van den Bergh PYK, van Doorn PA, Hadden RDM, et al. European Academy of Neurology/Peripheral Nerve Society guideline on diagnosis and treatment of chronic inflammatory demyelinating polyradiculoneuropathy: Report of a joint Task Force—Second revision. *Eur J Neurol.* 2021;28(11):3556–3583.
4. Viala K, Maisonobe T, Stojkovic T, et al. A current view of the diagnosis, clinical variants, response to treatment and prognosis of chronic inflammatory demyelinating polyradiculoneuropathy. *J Peripher Nerv Syst.* 2010;15(1):50–56.
5. Burns TM. Chronic inflammatory demyelinating polyradiculoneuropathy; with five-year observations of a placebo-controlled case treated with corticotrophin, cortisone, and prednisone. *Arch Neurol.* 2004;61(6):973–975.
6. Austin JH. Recurrent polyneuropathies and their corticosteroid treatment; with five-year observations of a placebo-controlled case treated with corticotrophin, cortisone, and prednisone. *Brain.* 1958;81(2):157–192.
7. Prineas JW, McLeod JG. Chronic relapsing polyneuritis. *J Neurol Sci.* 1976;27(4):427–458.
8. Thomas PK, Lascelles RG, Hallpike JF, Hewer RL. Recurrent and chronic relapsing Guillain–Barre polyneuritis. *Brain.* 1969;92(3):589–606.
9. Dyck PJ, Lais AC, Ohta M, Bastron JA, Okazaki H, Groover RV. Chronic inflammatory polyradiculoneuropathy. *Mayo Clin Proc.* 1975;50(11):621–637.
10. van Schaik I, Léger J, Nobile-Orazio E. European Federation of Neurological Societies/Peripheral Nerve Society Guideline on management of chronic inflammatory demyelinating polyradiculoneuropathy: report of a joint task force of the European Federation of Neurological Societies and the Peripheral Nerve Society—First Revision. *J Peripher Nerv Syst.* 2010;15(1):1–9.
11. Nobile-Orazio E. Chronic inflammatory demyelinating polyradiculoneuropathy and variants: where we are and where we should go. *J Peripher Nerv Syst.* 2014;19(1):2–13.
12. Barohn RJ, Kissel J, Warmolts J, Mendell J. Chronic inflammatory demyelinating polyradiculoneuropathy. Clinical characteristics, course, and recommendations for diagnostic criteria. *Arch Neurol.* 1989;46(8):878–884.
13. Mcombre PA, Pollard JD, McLeod JG. Chronic inflammatory demyelinating polyradiculoneuropathy: a clinical and electrophysiological study of 92 cases. *Brain.* 1987;110(6):1617–1630.
14. Simmons Z, Wald JJ, Albers JW. Chronic inflammatory demyelinating polyradiculoneuropathy in children: II. Long-term follow-up, with comparison to adults. *Muscle Nerve.* 1997;20(12):1569–1575.
15. Simmons Z, Wald JJ, Albers JW. Chronic inflammatory demyelinating polyradiculoneuropathy in children: I. Presentation, electrodiagnostic studies, and initial clinical course, with comparison to adults. *Muscle Nerve.* 1997;20(8):1008–1015.
16. Markowitz JA, Jeste SS, Kang PB. Child neurology: chronic inflammatory demyelinating polyradiculoneuropathy in children. *Neurology.* 2008;71(23):e74–e78.
17. DeVivo DC, Engel WK. Remarkable recovery of a steroid-responsive recurrent polyneuropathy. *J Neurol Neurosurg Psychiatry.* 1970;33(1):62–69.
18. Vedanarayanan VV, Kandt RS, Lewis DV, DeLong GR. Chronic inflammatory demyelinating polyradiculoneuropathy of childhood: treatment with high-dose intravenous immunoglobulin. *Neurology.* 1991;41(6):828–830.
19. Nevo Y, Topaloğlu H. 88th ENMC International Workshop: childhood chronic inflammatory demyelinating polyneuropathy (including revised diagnostic criteria), Naarden, The Netherlands, December 8–10, 2000. *Neuromuscular Disorders.* 2002;12(2):195–200.
20. Gorson KC, van Schaik IN, Merkies ISJ, et al. Chronic inflammatory demyelinating polyneuropathy disease activity status: recommendations for clinical research standards and use in clinical practice. *J Peripher Nerv Syst.* 2010;15(4):326–333.
21. Tackenberg B, Lunemann JD, Steinbrecher A, et al. Classifications and treatment responses in chronic immune-mediated demyelinating polyneuropathy. *Neurology.* 2007;68(19):1622–1629.
22. McCombe PA, McManis PG, Frith JA, Pollard JD, McLeod JG. Chronic inflammatory demyelinating polyradiculopathy associated with pregnancy. *Ann Neurol.* 1987;21(1):102–104.
23. Rajabally YA, Peric S, Bozovic I, et al. Antecedent infections and vaccinations in chronic inflammatory demyelinating polyneuropathy: a European collaborative study. *Muscle Nerve.* 2021;64(6):657–661.
24. Doneddu PE, Bianchi E, Cocito D, et al. Risk factors for chronic inflammatory demyelinating polyradiculoneuropathy (CIDP): antecedent events, lifestyle and dietary habits. Data from the Italian CIDP Database. *Eur J Neurol.* 2020;27(1):136–143.
25. Mendell JR. Chronic inflammatory demyelinating polyradiculoneuropathy. *Annu Rev Med.* 1993;44(1):211–219.
26. Dyck PJ, Oviatt KF, Lambert EH. Intensive evaluation of referred unclassified neuropathies yields improved diagnosis. *Ann Neurol.* 1981;10(3):222–226.

27. Mori K, Hattori N, Sugiura M, et al. Chronic inflammatory demyelinating polyneuropathy presenting with features of GBS. *Neurology*. 2002;58(6):979–982.
28. Ruts L, Drenthen J, Jacobs BC, van Doorn PA; Dutch GBS Study Group. Distinguishing acute-onset CIDP from fluctuating Guillain-Barre syndrome: a prospective study. *Neurology*. 2010;74(21):1680–1686.
29. Mygland A, Monstad P, Vedeler C. Onset and course of chronic inflammatory demyelinating polyneuropathy. *Muscle Nerve*. 2005;31(5):589–593.
30. Hughes R, Sanders E, Hall S, Atkinson P, Colchester A, Payan P. Subacute idiopathic demyelinating polyradiculoneuropathy. *Arch Neurol*. 1992;49(6):612–616.
31. Oh SJ, Kurokawa K, de Almeida DF, Ryan HF, Claussen GC. Subacute inflammatory demyelinating polyneuropathy. *Neurology*. 2003;61(11):1507–1512.
32. Ruts L, van Koningsveld R, van Doorn PA. Distinguishing acute-onset CIDP from Guillain-Barre syndrome with treatment related fluctuations. *Neurology*. 2005;65(1):138–140.
33. Rodriguez-Casero MV, Shield LK, Kornberg AJ. Subacute inflammatory demyelinating polyneuropathy in children. *Neurology*. 2005;64(10):1786–1788.
34. Kuwabara S, Misawa S, Mori M, Tamura N, Kubota M, Hattori T. Long term prognosis of chronic inflammatory demyelinating polyneuropathy: a five year follow up of 38 cases. *J Neurol Neurosurg Psychiatry*. 2006;77(1):66–70.
35. Saperstein DS, Katz JS, Amato AA, Barohn RJ. Clinical spectrum of chronic acquired demyelinating polyneuropathies. *Muscle Nerve*. 2001;24(3):311–324.
36. Hughes RAC, Bouche P, Cornblath DR, et al. European Federation of Neurological Societies/Peripheral Nerve Society guideline on management of chronic inflammatory demyelinating polyradiculoneuropathy: report of a joint task force of the European Federation of Neurological Societies and the Peripheral Nerve Society. *Eur J Neurol*. 2006;13(4):326–332.
37. Köller H, Kieseier BC, Jander S, Hartung HP. Chronic inflammatory demyelinating polyneuropathy. *New England Journal of Medicine*. 2005;352(13):1343–1356.
38. Doneddu PE, Cocito D, Manganelli F, et al. Atypical CIDP: diagnostic criteria, progression and treatment response. Data from the Italian CIDP Database. *J Neurol Neurosurg Psychiatry*. 2019;90(2):125–132.
39. Dalakas MC, Engel WK. Chronic relapsing (dysimmune) polyneuropathy: pathogenesis and treatment. *Ann Neurol*. 1981;9(S1):134–145.
40. Simmons Z, Albers JW, Bromberg MB, Feldman EL. Presentation and initial clinical course in patients with chronic inflammatory demyelinating polyradiculoneuropathy. *Neurology*. 1993;43(11):2202–2209.
41. Gorson KC, Allam G, Ropper AH. Chronic inflammatory demyelinating polyneuropathy: clinical features and response to treatment in 67 consecutive patients with and without a monoclonal gammopathy. *Neurology*. 1997;48(2):321–328.
42. Boukhris S, Magy L, Khalil M, Sindou P, Vallat JM. Pain as the presenting symptom of chronic inflammatory demyelinating polyradiculoneuropathy (CIDP). *J Neurol Sci*. 2007;254(1–2):33–38.
43. Costello F, Lee AG, Afifi AK, Kelkar P, Kardon RH, White M. Childhood-onset chronic inflammatory demyelinating polyradiculoneuropathy with cranial nerve involvement. *J Child Neurol*. 2002;17(11):819–823.
44. Frohman EM, Tusa R, Mark AS, Cornblath DR. Vestibular dysfunction in chronic inflammatory demyelinating polyneuropathy. *Ann Neurol*. 1996;39(4):529–535.
45. Chalmers AC, Miller RG. Chronic inflammatory polyradiculoneuropathy with ophthalmoplegia. *J Clin Neuroophthalmol*. 1986;6(3):166–168.
46. Hoffman D, Gutmann L, Griggs RC, Mendell JR, Miller RG. The dropped head syndrome with chronic inflammatory demyelinating polyneuropathy. *Muscle Nerve*. 1994;17(7):808–810.
47. Nakanishi T, Sobue I, Toyokura Y, et al. The Crow-Fukase syndrome: a study of 102 cases in Japan. *Neurology*. 1984;34(6):712–712.
48. Stamboulis E, Katsaros N, Koutsis G, Iakovidou H, Giannakopoulou A, Simintzi I. Clinical and subclinical autonomic dysfunction in chronic inflammatory demyelinating polyradiculoneuropathy. *Muscle Nerve*. 2006;33(1):78–84.
49. Yamamoto K, Watarai M, Hashimoto T, Ikeda SI. Chronic inflammatory demyelinating polyradiculoneuropathy with autonomic involvement. *Muscle Nerve*. 2005;31(1):108–112.
50. Figueroa JJ, Dyck PJB, Laughlin RS, et al. Autonomic dysfunction in chronic inflammatory demyelinating polyradiculoneuropathy. *Neurology*. 2012;78(10):702–708.
51. Henderson RD, Sandroni P, Wijdicks EFM. Chronic inflammatory demyelinating polyneuropathy and respiratory failure. *J Neurol*. 2005;252(10):1235–1237.
52. Živković SA, Peltier AC, Iacob T, Lacomis D. Chronic inflammatory demyelinating polyneuropathy and ventilatory failure: report of seven new cases and review of the literature. *Acta Neurol Scand*. 2011;124(1):59–63.
53. Oh SJ, Joy JL, Kuruoglu R. "Chronic sensory demyelinating neuropathy": chronic inflammatory demyelinating polyneuropathy presenting as a pure sensory neuropathy. *J Neurol Neurosurg Psychiatry*. 1992;55(8):677–680.
54. Oh SJ, Joy JL, Sunwoo I, Kuruoglu R. A case of chronic sensory demyelinating neuropathy responding to immunotherapies. *Muscle Nerve*. 1992;15(2):255–258.
55. van Dijk GW, Wokke JHJ, Notermans NC, van den Berg LH, Bär PR. Indications for an immune-mediated etiology of idiopathic sensory neuronopathy. *J Neuroimmunol*. 1997;74(1–2):165–172.
56. Feasby TE, Hahn AF, Koopman WJ, Lee DH. Central lesions in chronic inflammatory demyelinating polyneuropathy. *Neurology*. 1990;40(3 Part 1):476–476.
57. Mendell JR, Kolkin S, Kissel JT, Weiss KL, Chakeres DW, Rammohan KW. Evidence for central nervous system demyelination in chronic inflammatory demyelinating polyradiculoneuropathy. *Neurology*. 1987;37(8):1291–1291.
58. Ormerod IE, Waddy HM, Kermode AG, Murray NM, Thomas PK. Involvement of the central nervous system in chronic inflammatory demyelinating polyneuropathy: a clinical, electrophysiological and magnetic resonance imaging study. *J Neurol Neurosurg Psychiatry*. 1990;53(9):789–793.
59. Pakalnis A, Drake ME, Barohn RJ, Chakeres DW, Mendell JR. Evoked potentials in chronic inflammatory demyelinating polyneuropathy. *Arch Neurol*. 1988;45(9):1014–1016.
60. Rubin M, Karpati G, Carpenter S. Combined central and peripheral myelinopathy. *Neurology*. 1987;37(8):1287–1290.
61. Thomas PK, Walker RWH, Rudge P, et al. Chronic demyelinating peripheral neuropathy associated with multifocal central nervous system demyelination. *Brain*. 1987;110(1):53–76.

62. Uncini A, Gallucci M, Lugaresi A, Porrini AM, Onofrj M, Gambi D. CNS involvement in chronic inflammatory demyelinating polyneuropathy: an electrophysiological and MRI study. *Electromyogr Clin Neurophysiol.* 1991;31(6):365–371.
63. Kira JI. Anti-Neurofascin 155 antibody-positive chronic inflammatory demyelinating polyneuropathy/combined central and peripheral demyelination: strategies for diagnosis and treatment based on the disease mechanism. *Front Neurol.* 2021;12:665136.
64. Ogata H, Matsuse D, Yamasaki R, et al. A nationwide survey of combined central and peripheral demyelination in Japan. *J Neurol Neurosurg Psychiatry.* 2016;87(1):29–36.
65. Kawamura N, Yamasaki R, Yonekawa T, et al. Anti-neurofascin antibody in patients with combined central and peripheral demyelination. *Neurology.* 2013;81(8):714–722.
66. Devaux JJ, Miura Y, Fukami Y, et al. Neurofascin-155 IgG4 in chronic inflammatory demyelinating polyneuropathy. *Neurology.* 2016;86(9):800–807. Epub 2016 Feb 3.
67. Mauermann ML, Sorenson EJ, Dispenzieri A, et al. Uniform demyelination and more severe axonal loss distinguish POEMS syndrome from CIDP. *J Neurol Neurosurg Psychiatry.* 2012;83(5):480–486.
68. Nasu S, Misawa S, Sekiguchi Y, et al. Different neurological and physiological profiles in POEMS syndrome and chronic inflammatory demyelinating polyneuropathy. *J Neurol Neurosurg Psychiatry.* 2012;83(5):476–479.
69. Ryan MM, Jones HR. CMTX mimicking childhood chronic inflammatory demyelinating neuropathy with tremor. *Muscle Nerve.* 2005;31(4):528–530.
70. Doneddu PE, De Lorenzo A, Manganelli F, et al. Comparison of the diagnostic accuracy of the 2021 EAN/PNS and 2010 EFNS/PNS diagnostic criteria for chronic inflammatory demyelinating polyradiculoneuropathy. *J Neurol Neurosurg Psychiatry.* 2022;93(12):1239–1246.
71. Rajabally YA, Afzal S, Loo LK, Goedee HS. Application of the 2021 EAN/PNS criteria for chronic inflammatory demyelinating polyneuropathy. *J Neurol Neurosurg Psychiatry.* 2022;93(12):1247–1252.
72. Byers RK, Taft LT. Chronic multiple peripheral neuropathy in childhood. *Pediatrics.* 1957;20(3):517–537.
73. Cornblath D, Asbury A, Albers J, Feasby T. Research criteria for diagnosis of chronic inflammatory demyelinating polyneuropathy (CIDP). Report from an Ad Hoc Subcommittee of the American Academy of Neurology AIDS Task Force. *Neurology.* 1991;41(5):617–618.
74. Amato AA, Collins MP. Neuropathies associated with malignancy. *Semin Neurol.* 1998;18(01):125–144.
75. Amato AA, Barohn RJ, Sahenk Z, Tutschka PJ, Mendell JR. Polyneuropathy complicating bone marrow and solid organ transplantation. *Neurology.* 1993;43(8):1513–1518.
76. Antoine JC, Mosnier JF, Lapras J, et al. Chronic inflammatory demyelinating polyneuropathy associated with carcinoma. *J Neurol Neurosurg Psychiatry.* 1996;60(2):188–190.
77. Doneddu PE, Cocito D, Manganelli F, et al. Frequency of diabetes and other comorbidities in chronic inflammatory demyelinating polyradiculoneuropathy and their impact on clinical presentation and response to therapy. *J Neurol Neurosurg Psychiatry.* 2020;91(10):1092–1099.
78. Rajabally YA, Attarian S. Chronic inflammatory demyelinating polyneuropathy and malignancy: a systematic review. *Muscle Nerve.* 2018;57(6):875–883.
79. Viala K, Béhin A, Maisonobe T, et al. Neuropathy in lymphoma: a relationship between the pattern of neuropathy, type of lymphoma and prognosis? *J Neurol Neurosurg Psychiatry.* 2008;79(7):778–782.
80. Gorson KC, Ropper AH, Adelman LS, Weinberg DH. Influence of diabetes mellitus on chronic inflammatory demyelinating polyneuropathy. *Muscle Nerve.* 2000;23(1):37–43.
81. Haq RU, Pendlebury WW, Fries TJ, Tandan R. Chronic inflammatory demyelinating polyradiculoneuropathy in diabetic patients. *Muscle Nerve.* 2003;27(4):465–470.
82. Sharma KR, Cross J, Ayyar DR, Sherbert R, Bradley W. Diabetic demyelinating polyneuropathy responsive to intravenous immunoglobulin therapy. *Arch Neurol.* 2002;59(5):751.
83. Sharma KR. Demyelinating Neuropathy in Diabetes Mellitus. *Arch Neurol.* 2002;59(5):758–765.
84. Jann S, Beretta S, Bramerio MA. Different types of chronic inflammatory demyelinating polyneuropathy have a different clinical course and response to treatment. *Muscle Nerve.* 2005;32(3):351–356.
85. Ayyar DR, Sharma KR. Chronic inflammatory demyelinating polyradiculoneuropathy in diabetes mellitus. *Curr Diab Rep.* 2004;4(6):409–412.
86. Allen JA, Lewis RA. CIDP diagnostic pitfalls and perception of treatment benefit. *Neurology.* 2015;85(6):498–504.
87. Bril V, Blanchette CM, Noone JM, Runken MC, Gelinas D, Russell JW. The dilemma of diabetes in chronic inflammatory demyelinating polyneuropathy. *J Diabetes Complications.* 2016;30(7):1401–1407.
88. Rajabally YA, Stettner M, Kieseier BC, Hartung HP, Malik RA. CIDP and other inflammatory neuropathies in diabetes—diagnosis and management. *Nat Rev Neurol.* 2017;13(10):599–611.
89. Kobessho H, Oishi K, Hamaguchi H, Kanda F. Elevation of cerebrospinal fluid protein in patients with diabetes mellitus is associated with duration of diabetes. *Eur Neurol.* 2008;60(3):132–136.
90. Broers MC, Bunschoten C, Drenthen J, et al. Misdiagnosis and diagnostic pitfalls of chronic inflammatory demyelinating polyradiculoneuropathy. *Eur J Neurol.* 2021;28(6):2065–2073.
91. Krarup C, Trojaborg W. Sensory pathophysiology in chronic acquired demyelinating neuropathy. *Brain.* 1996;119(1):257–270.
92. Cruz Martínez A, Rabano J, Villoslada C, Cabello A. Chronic inflammatory demyelinating polyneuropathy as first manifestation of human immunodeficiency virus infection. *Electromyogr Clin Neurophysiol.* 1990;30(6):379–383.
93. Grand-Maison F, Feasby TE, Hahn AF, Koopman WJ. Recurrent Guillain–Barré syndrome. *Brain.* 1992;115(4):1093–1106.
94. Joint Task Force of the EFNS and the PNS. European Federation of Neurological Societies/Peripheral Nerve Society Guideline on management of paraproteinemic demyelinating neuropathies. Report of a Joint Task Force of the European Federation of Neurological Societies and the Peripheral Nerve Society—first revision. *J Peripher Nerv Syst.* 2010;(3):185–195.
95. Simmons Z. Paraproteinemia and neuropathy. *Curr Opin Neurol.* 1999;12(5):589–595.
96. Dyck PJ, Low PA, Windebank AJ, et al. Plasma exchange in polyneuropathy associated with monoclonal gammopathy of undetermined significance. *N Engl J Med.* 1991;325(21):1482–1486.
97. Kaplan A, Brannagan TH. Evaluation of patients with refractory chronic inflammatory demyelinating polyneuropathy. *Muscle Nerve.* 2017;55(4):476–482.

98. Levine TD, Katz JS, Barohn R, et al. Review process for IVIg treatment: lessons learned from INSIGHTS neuropathy study. *Neurol Clin Pract.* 2018;8(5):429–436.
99. Tomita M, Koike H, Kawagashira Y, et al. Clinicopathological features of neuropathy associated with lymphoma. *Brain.* 2013;136(Pt 8):2563–2578.
100. Lozeron P, Mariani LL, Dodet P, et al. Transthyretin amyloid polyneuropathies mimicking a demyelinating polyneuropathy. *Neurology.* 2018;91(2):e143–e152. Epub 2018 Jun 15.
101. Mathis S, Magy L, Diallo L, Boukhris S, Vallat JM. Amyloid neuropathy mimicking chronic inflammatory demyelinating polyneuropathy. *Muscle Nerve.* 2012;45(1):26–31.
102. Allen JA, Ney J, Lewis RA. Electrodiagnostic errors contribute to chronic inflammatory demyelinating polyneuropathy misdiagnosis. *Muscle Nerve.* 2018;57(4):542–549.
103. Davies JL, Lodermeier KA, Klein DM, et al. Composite nerve conduction scores and signs for diagnosis and somatic staging of diabetic polyneuropathy: Mid North American ethnic cohort survey. *Muscle Nerve.* 2023;68(1):29–38.
104. Bromberg MB, Feldman EL, Albers JW. Chronic inflammatory demyelinating polyradiculoneuropathy: comparison of patients with and without an associated monoclonal gammopathy. *Neurology.* 1992;42(6):1157–1157.
105. Van der Merche FGA, Vermeulen M, Busch HF. Chronic inflammatory demyelinating polyneuropathy: conduction failure before and during immunoglobulin or plasma therapy. *Brain.* 1989;112(6):1563–1571.
106. Bragg JA, Benatar MG. Sensory nerve conduction slowing is a specific marker for CIDP. *Muscle Nerve.* 2008;38(6):1599–1603.
107. Kaji R. Physiology of conduction block in multifocal motor neuropathy and other demyelinating neuropathies. *Muscle Nerve.* 2003;27(3):285–296.
108. Dyck PJ, Litchy WJ, Kratz KM, et al. A plasma exchange versus immune globulin infusion trial in chronic inflammatory demyelinating polyradiculoneuropathy. *Ann Neurol.* 1994;36(6):838–845.
109. Dyck PJ, Daube J, O'Brien P, et al. Plasma Exchange in Chronic Inflammatory Demyelinating Polyradiculoneuropathy. *N Engl J Med.* 1986;314(8):461–465.
110. Hahn AF, Bolton CF, Zochodne D, Feasby TE. Intravenous immunoglobulin treatment in chronic inflammatory demyelinating polyneuropathy: a double-blind, placebo-controlled, cross-over study. *Brain.* 1996;119(4):1067–1077.
111. Hahn AF, Bolton CF, Pillay N, et al. Plasma-exchange therapy in chronic inflammatory demyelinating polyneuropathy: a double-blind, sham-controlled, cross-over study. *Brain.* 1996;119(4):1055–1066.
112. Querol L, Nogales-Gadea G, Rojas-Garcia R, et al. Neurofascin IgG4 antibodies in CIDP associate with disabling tremor and poor response to IVIg. *Neurology.* 2014;82(10):879–886.
113. Franssen H, Straver DCG. Pathophysiology of immune-mediated demyelinating neuropathies-Part II: Neurology. *Muscle Nerve.* 2014;49(1):4–20.
114. Franssen H, Straver DCG. Pathophysiology of immune-mediated demyelinating neuropathies-part I: Neuroscience. *Muscle Nerve.* 2013;48(6):851–864.
115. Simmons Z, Albers JW, Bromberg MB, Feldman EL. Long-term follow-up of patients with chronic inflammatory demyelinating polyradiculoneuropathy, without and with monoclonal gammopathy. *Brain.* 1995;118(2):359–368.
116. Berger AR, Herskovitz S, Kaplan J. Late motor involvement in cases presenting as "chronic sensory demyelinating polyneuropathy." *Muscle Nerve.* 1995;18(4):440–444.
117. Breiner A, Bourque PR, Allen JA. Updated cerebrospinal fluid total protein reference values improve chronic inflammatory demyelinating polyneuropathy diagnosis. *Muscle Nerve.* 2019;60(2):180–183.
118. Dalakas MC, Houff SA, Engel WK, Madden DL, Sever JL. CSF "monoclonal" bands in chronic relapsing polyneuropathy. *Neurology.* 1980;30(8):864–864.
119. Segurado OG, Kruger H, Mertens HG. Clinical significance of serum and CSF findings in the Guillain-Barre syndrome and related disorders. *J Neurol.* 1986;233(4):202–208.
120. Jongbloed BA, Bos JW, Rutgers D, van der Pol WL, van den Berg LH. Brachial plexus magnetic resonance imaging differentiates between inflammatory neuropathies and does not predict disease course. *Brain Behav.* 2017;7(5):e00632.
121. Shibuya K, Sugiyama A, Ito SI, et al. Reconstruction magnetic resonance neurography in chronic inflammatory demyelinating polyneuropathy. *Ann Neurol.* 2015;77(2):333–337.
122. Ishikawa T, Asakura K, Mizutani Y, et al. MR neurography for the evaluation of CIDP. *Muscle Nerve.* 2017;55(4):483–489.
123. Goedee HS, Jongbloed BA, van Asseldonk JTH, et al. A comparative study of brachial plexus sonography and magnetic resonance imaging in chronic inflammatory demyelinating neuropathy and multifocal motor neuropathy. *Eur J Neurol.* 2017;24(10):1307–1313.
124. Oudeman J, Eftimov F, Strijkers GJ, et al. Diagnostic accuracy of MRI and ultrasound in chronic immune-mediated neuropathies. *Neurology.* 2020;94(1):e62–e74.
125. Herraets IJT, Goedee HS, Telleman JA, et al. Nerve ultrasound for diagnosing chronic inflammatory neuropathy: a multicenter validation study. *Neurology.* 2020;95(12):E1745–E1753.
126. Vallat JM, Tabaraud F, Magy L, et al. Diagnostic value of nerve biopsy for atypical chronic inflammatory demyelinating polyneuropathy: evaluation of eight cases. *Muscle Nerve.* 2003;27(4):478–485.
127. Molenaar DS, Vermeulen M, de Haan R. Diagnostic value of sural nerve biopsy in chronic inflammatory demyelinating polyneuropathy. *J Neurol Neurosurg Psychiatry.* 1998;64(1):84–89.
128. Krendel DA, Parks HP, Anthony DC, St. Clair MB, Graham DG. Sural nerve biopsy in chronic inflammatory demyelinating polyradiculoneuropathy. *Muscle Nerve.* 1989;12(4):257–264.
129. Bosboom WMJ, van den Berg LH, Franssen H, et al. Diagnostic value of sural nerve demyelination in chronic inflammatory demyelinating polyneuropathy. *Brain.* 2001;124(12):2427–2438.
130. Cornblath DR, Griffin DE, Welch D, Griffin JW, McArthur JC. Quantitative analysis of endoneurial T-cells in human sural nerve biopsies. *J Neuroimmunol.* 1990;26(2):113–118.
131. Matsumuro K, Izumo S, Umehara F, Osame M. Chronic inflammatory demyelinating polyneuropathy: histological and immunopathological studies on biopsied sural nerves. *J Neurol Sci.* 1994;127(2):170–178.
132. Schneider-Hohendorf T, Schwab N, Uceyler N, Gobel K, Sommer C, Wiendl H. CD8+ T-cell immunity in chronic inflammatory demyelinating polyradiculoneuropathy. *Neurology.* 2012;78(6):402–408.
133. Leppert D, Hughes P, Huber S, et al. Matrix metalloproteinase upregulation in chronic inflammatory demyelinating polyneuropathy and nonsystemic vasculitic neuropathy. *Neurology.* 1999;53(1):62–70.

134. Quast I, Cueni F, Nimmerjahn F, Tackenberg B, Lünemann JD. Deregulated Fcγ receptor expression in patients with CIDP. *Neurol Neuroimmunol Neuroinflamm.* 2015;2(5):e148.
135. Mizuno K, Nagamatsu M, Hattori N, et al. Chronic inflammatory demyelinating polyradiculoneuropathy with diffuse and massive peripheral nerve hypertrophy: distinctive clinical and magnetic resonance imaging features. *Muscle Nerve.* 1998;21(6):805–808.
136. Hughes RAC, Allen D, Makowska A, Gregson NA. Pathogenesis of chronic inflammatory demyelinating polyradiculoneuropathy. *J Peripher Nerv Syst.* 2006;11(1):30–46.
137. Kwa MSG, van Schaik IN, De Jonge RR, et al. Autoimmunoreactivity to Schwann cells in patients with inflammatory neuropathies. *Brain.* 2003;126(2):361–375.
138. Van den Bergh P, Hadden R, Pouche P. European Federation of Neurological Societies/Peripheral Nerve Society Guideline on management of multifocal motor neuropathy. Report of a Joint Task Force of the European Federation of Neurological Societies and the Peripheral Nerve Society—first revision. *J Peripher Nerv Syst.* 2010;15(4):295–301.
139. Hughes R, Bensa S, Willison H, et al. Randomized controlled trial of intravenous immunoglobulin versus oral prednisolone in chronic inflammatory demyelinating polyradiculoneuropathy. *Ann Neurol.* 2001;50(2):195–201.
140. Brannagan TH. Current treatments of chronic immune-mediated demyelinating polyneuropathies. *Muscle Nerve.* 2009;39(5):563–578.
141. Eftimov F, Winer JB, Vermeulen M, de Haan R, van Schaik IN. Intravenous immunoglobulin for chronic inflammatory demyelinating polyradiculoneuropathy. *Cochrane Database Syst Rev.* 2013:(12):CD001797.
142. Lunn MPT, Willison HJ. Diagnosis and treatment in inflammatory neuropathies. *Postgrad Med J.* 2009;85(1006):437–446.
143. Mehndiratta MM, Hughes RA. Corticosteroids for chronic inflammatory demyelinating polyradiculoneuropathy. In: Mehndiratta MM, ed. *Cochrane Database of Systematic Reviews.* John Wiley & Sons, Ltd; 2002.
144. Mehndiratta MM, Hughes RA, Agarwal P. Plasma exchange for chronic inflammatory demyelinating polyradiculoneuropathy. In: Mehndiratta MM, ed. *Cochrane Database of Systematic Reviews.* John Wiley & Sons, Ltd; 2004.
145. Godil J, Barrett MJ, Ensrud E, Chahin N, Karam C. Refractory CIDP: clinical characteristics, antibodies and response to alternative treatment. *J Neurol Sci.* 2020;418:117098.
146. Kuitwaard K, Hahn AF, Vermeulen M, Venance SL, Van Doorn PA. Intravenous immunoglobulin response in treatment-naïve chronic inflammatory demyelinating polyradiculoneuropathy. *J Neurol Neurosurg Psychiatry.* 2015;86(12):1331–1336.
147. Nobile-Orazio E, Cocito D, Jann S, et al. Frequency and time to relapse after discontinuing 6-month therapy with IVIg or pulsed methylprednisolone in CIDP. *J Neurol Neurosurg Psychiatry.* 2015;86(7):729–734.
148. Nobile-Orazio E, Pujol S, Kasiborski F, et al. An international multicenter efficacy and safety study of IqYmune in initial and maintenance treatment of patients with chronic inflammatory demyelinating polyradiculoneuropathy: PRISM study. *J Peripher Nerv Syst.* 2020;25(4):356–365.
149. Eftimov F, Vermeulen M, van Doorn PA, Brusse E, van Schaik IN. Long-term remission of CIDP after pulsed dexamethasone or short-term prednisolone treatment. *Neurology.* 2012;78(14):1079–1084.
150. Duhem C, Dicato M, Ries F. Side-effects of intravenous immune globulins. *Clin Exp Immunol.* 1994;97 Suppl 1(Suppl 1):79–83.
151. Dyck PJ, O'Brien PC, Oviatt KF, et al. Prednisone improves chronic inflammatory demyelinating polyradiculoneuropathy more than no treatment. *Ann Neurol.* 1982;11(2):136–141.
152. Hughes RA, Mehndiratta MM, Rajabally YA. Corticosteroids for chronic inflammatory demyelinating polyradiculoneuropathy. *Cochrane Database Syst Rev.* 2017;2017(11):CD002062.
153. Pegat A, Boisseau W, Maisonobe T, et al. Motor chronic inflammatory demyelinating polyneuropathy (CIDP) in 17 patients: clinical characteristics, electrophysiological study, and response to treatment. *J Peripher Nerv Syst.* 2020;25(2):162–170.
154. Donaghy M, Mills KR, Boniface SJ, et al. Pure motor demyelinating neuropathy: deterioration after steroid treatment and improvement with intravenous immunoglobulin. *J Neurol Neurosurg Psychiatry.* 1994;57(7):778–783.
155. Molenaar DS, van Doorn PA, Vermeulen M. Pulsed high dose dexamethasone treatment in chronic inflammatory demyelinating polyneuropathy: a pilot study. *J Neurol Neurosurg Psychiatry.* 1997;62(4):388–390.
156. Lopate G, Pestronk A, Al-Lozi M. Treatment of chronic inflammatory demyelinating polyneuropathy with high-dose intermittent intravenous methylprednisolone. *Arch Neurol.* 2005;62(2):249–254.
157. van Schaik IN, Eftimov F, van Doorn PA, et al. Pulsed high-dose dexamethasone versus standard prednisolone treatment for chronic inflammatory demyelinating polyradiculoneuropathy (PREDICT study): a double-blind, randomised, controlled trial. *Lancet Neurol.* 2010;9(3):245–253.
158. van Lieverloo GGA, Peric S, Doneddu PE, et al. Corticosteroids in chronic inflammatory demyelinating polyneuropathy: a retrospective, multicentre study, comparing efficacy and safety of daily prednisolone, pulsed dexamethasone, and pulsed intravenous methylprednisolone. *J Neurol.* 2018;265(9):2052–2059.
159. Querol L, Rojas-Garcia R, Casasnovas C, et al. Long-term outcome in chronic inflammatory demyelinating polyneuropathy patients treated with intravenous immunoglobulin: a retrospective study. *Muscle Nerve.* 2013;48(6):870–876.
160. Cendrowski W. Treatment of polyneuropathy with azathioprine and adrenal steroids. *Acta Med Pol.* 1977;18(2):147–156.
161. Cortese I, Chaudhry V, So YT, Cantor F, Cornblath DR, Rae-Grant A. Evidence-based guideline update: plasmapheresis in neurologic disorders: report of the Therapeutics and Technology Assessment Subcommittee of the American Academy of Neurology. *Neurology.* 2011;76(3):294–300.
162. Doorn PA, Brand A, Strengers PF, Meulstee J, Vermeulen M. High-dose intravenous immunoglobulin treatment in chronic inflammatory demyelinating polyneuropathy: a double-blind, placebo-controlled, crossover study. *Neurology.* 1990;40(2):209–209.
163. Mendell JR, Barohn RJ, Freimer ML, et al. Randomized controlled trial of IVIg in untreated chronic inflammatory demyelinating polyradiculoneuropathy. *Neurology.* 2001;56(4):445–449.
164. Vermeulen M, van Doorn PA, Brand A, Strengers PF, Jennekens FG, Busch HF. Intravenous immunoglobulin treatment in patients with chronic inflammatory demyelinating polyneuropathy: a double blind, placebo controlled study. *J Neurol Neurosurg Psychiatry.* 1993;56(1):36–39.

165. Leger JM, Viala K, Nicolas G, et al. Placebo-controlled trial of rituximab in IgM anti-myelin-associated glycoprotein neuropathy. *Neurology*. 2013;80(24):2217–2225.
166. Donofrio PD, Berger A, Brannagan TH, et al. Consensus statement: the use of intravenous immunoglobulin in the treatment of neuromuscular conditions report of the AANEM ad hoc committee. *Muscle Nerve*. 2009;40(5):890–900.
167. Hughes RA, Donofrio P, Bril V, et al. Intravenous immune globulin (10% caprylate-chromatography purified) for the treatment of chronic inflammatory demyelinating polyradiculoneuropathy (ICE study): a randomised placebo-controlled trial. *Lancet Neurol*. 2008;7(2):136–144.
168. Lunn MP, Ellis L, Hadden RD, Rajabally YA, Winer JB, Reilly MM. *A Proposed Dosing Algorithm for the Individualized Dosing of Human Immunoglobulin in Chronic Inflammatory Neuropathies.* 2016;21.
169. Berger AR, Herskovitz S, Scelsa S. The restoration of IVIg efficacy by plasma exchange in CIDP. *Neurology*. 1995;45(8):1628–1629.
170. Adrichem ME, Lucke IM, Vrancken AFJE, et al. Withdrawal of intravenous immunoglobulin in chronic inflammatory demyelinating polyradiculoneuropathy. *Brain*. 2022;145(5):1641–1652.
171. Kapoor M, Compton L, Rossor A, et al. An approach to assessing immunoglobulin dependence in chronic inflammatory demyelinating inflammatory polyneuropathy. *J Peripher Nerv Syst*. 2021;26(4):461–468.
172. Nobile-Orazio E, Cocito D, Jann S, et al. Intravenous immunoglobulin versus intravenous methylprednisolone for chronic inflammatory demyelinating polyradiculoneuropathy: a randomised controlled trial. *Lancet Neurol*. 2012;11(6):493–502.
173. Ropper AH. Current treatments for CIDP. *Neurology*. 2003;60(Issue 8, Supplement 3):S16–S22.
174. Ruzhansky K, Brannagan TH. Intravenous immunoglobulin for treatment of neuromuscular disease. *Neurol Clin Pract*. 2013;3(5):440–445.
175. van Schaik IN, Bril V, van Geloven N, et al. Subcutaneous immunoglobulin for maintenance treatment in chronic inflammatory demyelinating polyneuropathy (PATH): a randomised, double-blind, placebo-controlled, phase 3 trial. *Lancet Neurol*. 2018;17(1):35–46.
176. van Schaik IN, Mielke O, Bril V, et al. Long-term safety and efficacy of subcutaneous immunoglobulin IgPro20 in CIDP: PATH extension study. *Neurol Neuroimmunol Neuroinflamm*. 2019;6(5):e590.
177. Goyal NA, Karam C, Sheikh KA, Dimachkie MM. Subcutaneous immunoglobulin treatment for chronic inflammatory demyelinating polyneuropathy. *Muscle Nerve*. 2021;64(3):243–254.
178. Racosta JM, Sposato LA, Kimpinski K. Subcutaneous versus intravenous immunoglobulin for chronic autoimmune neuropathies: a meta-analysis. *Muscle Nerve*. 2017;55(6):802–809.
179. Markvardsen LH, Debost JC, Harbo T, et al. Subcutaneous immunoglobulin in responders to intravenous therapy with chronic inflammatory demyelinating polyradiculoneuropathy. *Eur J Neurol*. 2013;20(5):836–842.
180. Mahdi-Rogers M, van Doorn PA, Hughes RA. Immunomodulatory treatment other than corticosteroids, immunoglobulin and plasma exchange for chronic inflammatory demyelinating polyradiculoneuropathy. In: Mahdi-Rogers M, ed. *Cochrane Database of Systematic Reviews.* John Wiley & Sons, Ltd; 2013.
181. Palmer K. Polyradiculoneuropathy treated with cytotoxic drugs. *Lancet*. 1966;1(265).
182. Pentland B, Adams GG, Mawdsley C. Chronic idiopathic polyneuropathy treated with azathioprine. *J Neurol Neurosurg Psychiatry*. 1982;45(10):866–869.
183. Walker GL. Progressive polyradiculoneuropathy: treatment with azathioprine. *Aust N Z J Med*. 1979;9(2):184–187.
184. Dyck PJ, O'Brien P, Swanson C, Low P, Daube J. Combined azathioprine and prednisone in chronic inflammatory-demyelinating polyneuropathy. *Neurology*. 1985;35(8):1173–1176.
185. Cocito D, Grimaldi S, Paolasso I, et al. Immunosuppressive treatment in refractory chronic inflammatory demyelinating polyradiculoneuropathy. A nationwide retrospective analysis. *Eur J Neurol*. 2011;18(12):1417–1421.
186. Barnett MH, Pollard JD, Davies L, McLeod JG. Cyclosporin A in resistant chronic inflammatory demyelinating polyradiculoneuropathy. *Muscle Nerve*. 1998;21(4):454–460.
187. Hodgkinson SJ, Pollard JD, McLeod JG. Cyclosporin A in the treatment of chronic demyelinating polyradiculoneuropathy. *J Neurol Neurosurg Psychiatry*. 1990;53(4):327–330.
188. Mahattanakul W, Crawford TO, Griffin JW, Goldstein JM, Cornblath DR. Treatment of chronic inflammatory demyelinating polyneuropathy with cyclosporin-A. *J Neurol Neurosurg Psychiatry*. 1996;60(2):185–187.
189. Hefter H, Sprenger KBG, Arendt G, Hafner D. Treatment of chronic relapsing inflammatory demyelinating polyneuropathy by cyclosporin A and plasma exchange. *J Neurol*. 1990;237(5):320–323.
190. Kolkin S, Nahman NS, Mendell JR. Chronic nephrotoxicity complicating cyclosporine treatment of chronic inflammatory demyelinating polyradiculoneuropathy. *Neurology*. 1987;37(1):147–147.
191. Matsuda M, Hoshi K, Gono T, Morita H, Ikeda SI. Cyclosporin A in treatment of refractory patients with chronic inflammatory demyelinating polyradiculoneuropathy. *J Neurol Sci*. 2004;224(1-2):29–35.
192. Odaka M. Intractable chronic inflammatory demyelinating polyneuropathy treated successfully with ciclosporin. *J Neurol Neurosurg Psychiatry*. 2005;76(8):1115–1120.
193. Chaudhry V, Cornblath DR, Griffin JW, O'Brien R, Drachman DB. Mycophenolate mofetil: a safe and promising immunosuppressant in neuromuscular diseases. *Neurology*. 2001;56(1):94–96.
194. Umapathi T, Hughes R. Mycophenolate in treatment-resistant inflammatory neuropathies. *Eur J Neurol*. 2002;9(6):683–685.
195. Gorson KC, Amato AA, Ropper AH. Efficacy of mycophenolate mofetil in patients with chronic immune demyelinating polyneuropathy. *Neurology*. 2004;63(4):715–717.
196. Radziwill AJ, Schweikert K, Kuntzer T, Fuhr P, Steck AJ. Mycophenolate mofetil for chronic inflammatory demyelinating polyradiculoneuropathy. *Eur Neurol*. 2006;56(1):37–38.
197. Mowzoon N, Sussman A, Bradley WG. Mycophenolate (CellCept) treatment of myasthenia gravis, chronic inflammatory polyneuropathy and inclusion body myositis. *J Neurol Sci*. 2001;185(2):119–122.
198. Benedetti L, Grandis M, Nobbio L, et al. Mycophenolate mofetil in dysimmune neuropathies: a preliminary study. *Muscle Nerve*. 2004;29(5):748–749.
199. Bedi G, Brown A, Tong T, Sharma KR. Chronic inflammatory demyelinating polyneuropathy responsive to mycophe-

nolate mofetil therapy. *J Neurol Neurosurg Psychiatry*. 2010; 81(6):634–636.
200. Briani C, Zara G, Zambello R, Trentin L, Rana M, Zaja F. Rituximab-responsive CIDP. *Eur J Neurol*. 2004;11(11):788.
201. Benedetti L, Franciotta D, Beronio A, et al. Rituximab efficacy in CIDP associated with idiopathic thrombocytopenic purpura. *Muscle Nerve*. 2008;38(2):1076–1077.
202. Benedetti L, Briani C, Franciotta D, et al. Rituximab in patients with chronic inflammatory demyelinating polyradiculoneuropathy: a report of 13 cases and review of the literature. *J Neurol Neurosurg Psychiatry*. 2011;82(3):306–308.
203. D'Amico A, Catteruccia M, De Benedetti F, et al. Rituximab in a childhood-onset idiopathic refractory chronic inflammatory demyelinating polyneuropathy. *Eur J Paediatr Neurol*. 2012;16(3):301–303.
204. Knecht H, Baumberger M, Tobon A, Steck A. Sustained remission of CIDP associated with Evans syndrome. *Neurology*. 2004;63(4):730–732.
205. Münch C, Anagnostou P, Meyer R, Haas J. Rituximab in chronic inflammatory demyelinating polyneuropathy associated with diabetes mellitus. *J Neurol Sci*. 2007;256(1-2):100–102.
206. Sadnicka A, Reilly MM, Mummery C, Brandner S, Hirsch N, Lunn MPT. Rituximab in the treatment of three coexistent neurological autoimmune diseases: chronic inflammatory demyelinating polyradiculoneuropathy, Morvan syndrome and myasthenia gravis. *J Neurol Neurosurg Psychiatry*. 2011;82(2):230–232.
207. Gorson KC, Natarajan N, Ropper AH, Weinstein R. Rituximab treatment in patients with IVIg-dependent immune polyneuropathy: a prospective pilot trial. *Muscle Nerve*. 2007;35(1):66–69.
208. Rosenberg NL, Lacy JR, Kennaugh RC, Holers VM, Neville HE, Kotzin BL. Treatment of refractory chronic demyelinating polyneuropathy with lymphoid irradiation. *Muscle Nerve*. 1985;8(3):223–232.
209. Muley SA, Jacobsen B, Parry G, et al. Rituximab in refractory chronic inflammatory demyelinating polyneuropathy. *Muscle Nerve*. 2020;61(5):575–579.
210. Chaganti S, Hannaford A, Vucic S. Rituximab in chronic immune mediated neuropathies: a systematic review. *Neuromuscular Disorders*. 2022;32(8):621–627.
211. Bouchard C, Lacroix C, Plante V, et al. Clinicopathologic findings and prognosis of chronic inflammatory demyelinating polyneuropathy. *Neurology*. 1999;52(3):498–498.
212. Good JL, Chehrenama M, Mayer RF, Koski CL. Pulse cyclophosphamide therapy in chronic inflammatory demyelinating polyneuropathy. *Neurology*. 1998;51(6):1735–1738.
213. Koski C. Guillain-Barré syndrome and chronic inflammatory demyelinating polyneuropathy: pathogenesis and treatment. *Semin Neurol*. 1994;14(02):123–130.
214. Brannagan TH, Alaedini A, Gladstone DE. High-dose cyclophosphamide without stem cell rescue for refractory multifocal motor neuropathy. *Muscle Nerve*. 2006;34(2):246–250.
215. Fowler H, Vulpe M, Marks G, Egolf C, Dau PC. Recovery from chronic progressive polyneuropathy after treatment with plasma exchange and cyclophosphamide. *Lancet*. 1979;2(8153):1193.
216. Brannagan TH, Pradhan A, Heiman-Patterson T, et al. High-dose cyclophosphamide without stem-cell rescue for refractory CIDP. *Neurology*. 2002;58(12):1856–1858.
217. Gladstone DE, Prestrud AA, Brannagan TH. High-dose cyclophosphamide results in long-term disease remission with restoration of a normal quality of life in patients with severe refractory chronic inflammatory demyelinating polyneuropathy. *J Peripher Nerv Syst*. 2005;10(1):11–16.
218. Lewis RA, Sumner AJ, Brown MJ, Asbury AK. Multifocal demyelinating neuropathy with persistent conduction block. *Neurology*. 1982;32(9):958–958.
219. Saperstein DS, Amato AA, Wolfe GI, et al. Multifocal acquired demyelinating sensory and motor neuropathy: The Lewis-Sumner syndrome. *Muscle Nerve*. 1999;22(5):560–566.
220. Amato AA, Jackson CE, Kim JY, Worley KL. Chronic relapsing brachial plexus neuropathy with persistent conduction block. *Muscle Nerve*. 1997;20(10):1303–1307.
221. Gibbels E, Behse F, Kentenich M, Haupt WF. Chronic multifocal neuropathy with persistent conduction block (Lewis-Sumner syndrome). A clinico-morphologic study of two further cases with review of the literature. *Clin Neuropathol*. 1993;12(6):343–352.
222. Gorson KC, Ropper AH, Weinberg DH. Upper limb predominant, multifocal chronic inflammatory demyelinating polyneuropathy. *Muscle Nerve*. 1999;22(6):758–765.
223. Nukada H, Pollock M, Haas LF. Is ischemia implicated in chronic multifocal demyelinating neuropathy? *Neurology*. 1989;39(1):106–110.
224. Oh SJ, Claussen GC, Kim DS. Motor and sensory demyelinating mononeuropathy multiplex (multifocal motor and sensory demyelinating neuropathy): a separate entity or a variant of chronic inflammatory demyelinating polyneuropathy? *J Peripher Nerv Syst*. 1997;2(4):362–369.
225. Viala K, Renié L, Maisonobe T, et al. Follow-up study and response to treatment in 23 patients with Lewis-Sumner syndrome. *Brain*. 2004;127(9):2010–2017.
226. Oh SJ, LaGanke C, Powers R, Wolfe GI, Quinton RA, Burns DK. Multifocal motor sensory demyelinating neuropathy: inflammatory demyelinating polyradiculoneuropathy. *Neurology*. 2005;65(10):1639–1642.
227. Beecher G, Shelly S, Dyck PJB, et al. Pure motor onset and IgM-gammopathy occurrence in multifocal acquired demyelinating sensory and motor neuropathy. *Neurology*. 2021;97(14):e1392–e1403.
228. Bunschoten C, Jacobs BC, Van den Bergh PYK, Cornblath DR, van Doorn PA. Progress in diagnosis and treatment of chronic inflammatory demyelinating polyradiculoneuropathy. *Lancet Neurol*. 2019;18(8):784–794.
229. Puwanant A, Herrmann DN. Multifocal acquired demyelinating sensory and motor neuropathy. *Neurology*. 2012;79(16):1742.
230. Simo M, Casasnovas C, Martinez-Yelamos S, Martinez-Matos JA. Multifocal acquired demyelinating sensory and motor neuropathy presenting as idiopathic hypertrophic brachial neuropathy. *J Neurol Neurosurg Psychiatry*. 2009;80(6):674–675.
231. Thomas PK, Claus D, Jaspert A, et al. Focal upper limb demyelinating neuropathy. *Brain*. 1996;119(3):765–774.
232. van den Bergh PY, Thonnard JL, Duprez T, Laterre EC. Chronic demyelinating hypertrophic brachial plexus neuropathy. *Muscle Nerve*. 2000;23(2):283–288.
233. Rajabally YA, Chavada G. Lewis-Sumner syndrome of pure upper-limb onset: diagnostic, prognostic, and therapeutic features. *Muscle Nerve*. 2009;39(2):206–220.
234. Shibuya K, Tsuneyama A, Misawa S, et al. Cranial nerve involvement in typical and atypical chronic inflammatory

demyelinating polyneuropathies. *Eur J Neurol.* 2020;27(12): 2658–2661.
235. Cortese A, Lombardi R, Briani C, et al. Antibodies to neurofascin, contactin-1, and contactin-associated protein 1 in CIDP: clinical relevance of IgG isotype. *Neurol Neuroimmunol Neuroinflamm.* 2020;7(1):E639.
236. Kawagashira Y, Kondo N, Atsuta N, et al. IgM MGUS anti-MAG neuropathy with predominant muscle weakness and extensive muscle atrophy. *Muscle Nerve.* 2010;42(3):433–435.
237. Harbo T, Andersen H, Jakobsen J. Long-term therapy with high doses of subcutaneous immunoglobulin in multifocal motor neuropathy. *Neurology.* 2010;75(15):1377–1380.
238. Ikeda S, Koike H, Nishi R, et al. Clinicopathological characteristics of subtypes of chronic inflammatory demyelinating polyradiculoneuropathy. *J Neurol Neurosurg Psychiatry.* 2019;90(9):988–996.
239. Rajabally YA, Knopp MJ, Martin-Lamb D, Morlese J. Diagnostic value of MR imaging in the Lewis–Sumner syndrome: a case series. *J Neurol Sci.* 2014;342(1–2):182–185.
240. Scheidl E, Böhm J, Simó M, et al. Ultrasonography of MADSAM neuropathy: focal nerve enlargements at sites of existing and resolved conduction blocks. *Neuromuscular Disorders.* 2012;22(7):627–631.
241. Beecher G, Howe BM, Shelly S, et al. Plexus MRI helps distinguish the immune-mediated neuropathies MADSAM and MMN. *J Neuroimmunol.* 2022;371:577953.
242. Bayas A, Gold R, Naumann M. Long-term treatment of Lewis–Sumner syndrome with subcutaneous immunoglobulin infusions. *J Neurol Sci.* 2013;324(1–2):53–56.
243. Attarian S, Verschueren A, Franques J, Salort-Campana E, Jouve E, Pouget J. Response to treatment in patients with Lewis-Sumner syndrome. *Muscle Nerve.* 2011;44(2):179–184.
244. Kerasnoudis A. Ultrasonography of MADSAM neuropathy: focal nerve enlargements at sites of existing and resolved conduction blocks. *Neuromuscular Disorders.* 2012;22(11):1032.
245. Lucke IM, Wieske L, van der Kooi AJ, van Schaik IN, Eftimov F, Verhamme C. Diagnosis and treatment response in the asymmetric variant of chronic inflammatory demyelinating polyneuropathy. *J Peripher Nerv Syst.* 2019;24(2):174–179.
246. Ellie E, Vital A, Steck A, Boiron JM, Vital C, Julien J. Neuropathy associated with "benign" anti-myelin-associated glycoprotein IgM gammapathy: clinical, immunological, neurophysiological pathological findings and response to treatment in 33 cases. *J Neurol.* 1995;243(1):34–43.
247. Niermeijer JMF, Fischer K, Eurelings M, Franssen H, Wokke JHJ, Notermans NC. Prognosis of polyneuropathy due to IgM monoclonal gammapathy: a prospective cohort study. *Neurology.* 2010;74(5):406–412.
248. Dalakas MC, Teräväinen H, Engel W. Tremor as a feature of chronic relapsing and dysgammaglobulinemic polyneuropathies. *Arch Neurol.* 1984;41(7):711.
249. Smith IS. The natural history of chronic demyelinating neuropathy associated with benign IgM paraproteinaemia. *Brain.* 1994;117(5):949–957.
250. Yeung KB, Thomas PK, King RH, et al. The clinical spectrum of peripheral neuropathies associated with benign monoclonal IgM, IgG and IgA paraproteinaemia: comparative clinical, immunological and nerve biopsy findings. *J Neurol.* 1991;238(7):383–391.
251. Donofrio PD. Immunotherapy of idiopathic inflammatory neuropathies. *Muscle Nerve.* 2003;28(3):273–292.
252. Bardel B, Molinier-Frenkel V, Le Bras F, et al. Revisiting the spectrum of IgM-related neuropathies in a large cohort of IgM monoclonal gammapathy. *J Neurol.* 2022;269(9): 4955–4960.
253. Magy L, Kaboré R, Mathis S, et al. Heterogeneity of polyneuropathy associated with anti-MAG antibodies. *J Immunol Res.* 2015;2015:450391.
254. Liberatore G, Giannotta C, Sajeev BP, et al. Sensitivity and specificity of a commercial ELISA test for anti-MAG antibodies in patients with neuropathy. *J Neuroimmunol.* 2020;345: 577288.
255. Mygland Å, Monstad P. Chronic acquired demyelinating symmetric polyneuropathy classified by pattern of weakness. *Arch Neurol.* 2003;60(2):260.
256. Cook D, Dalakas M, Galdi A, Biondi D, Porter H. High-dose intravenous immunoglobulins in the treatment of demyelinating neuropathy associated with monoclonal gammapathy. *Neurology.* 1990;40(2):212–214.
257. Gorson KC, Ropper AH, Weinberg DH, Weinstein R. Treatment experience in patients with anti-myelin-associated glycoprotein neuropathy. *Muscle Nerve.* 2001;24(6):778–786.
258. Kuwabara S, Isose S, Mori M, et al. Different electrophysiological profiles and treatment response in 'typical' and 'atypical' chronic inflammatory demyelinating polyneuropathy. *J Neurol Neurosurg Psychiatry.* 2015;86(10):1054–1059.
259. Gosselin S, Kyle RA, Dyck PJ. Neuropathy associated with monoclonal gammapathies of undetermined significance. *Ann Neurol.* 1991;30(1):54–61.
260. Niermeijer JMF, Eurelings M, Lokhorst HL, et al. Rituximab for polyneuropathy with IgM monoclonal gammapathy. *J Neurol Neurosurg Psychiatry.* 2009;80(9):1036–1039.
261. Gupta P, Mirman I, Shahar S, Dubey D. Growing Spectrum of Autoimmune Nodopathies. *Curr Neurol Neurosci Rep.* 2023;23(5):201–212.
262. Ogata H, Yamasaki R, Hiwatashi A, et al. Characterization of IgG4 anti-neurofascin 155 antibody-positive polyneuropathy. *Ann Clin Transl Neurol.* 2015;2(10):960–971.
263. Delmont E, Brodovitch A, Kouton L, et al. Antibodies against the node of Ranvier: a real-life evaluation of incidence, clinical features and response to treatment based on a prospective analysis of 1500 sera. *J Neurol.* 2020;267(12):3664–3672.
264. Liberatore G, De Lorenzo A, Giannotta C, et al. Frequency and clinical correlates of anti-nerve antibodies in a large population of CIDP patients included in the Italian database. *Neurol Sci.* 2022;43(6):3939–3947.
265. Zhang X, Zheng P, Devaux JJ, et al. Chronic inflammatory demyelinating polyneuropathy with anti-NF155 IgG4 in China. *J Neuroimmunol.* 2019;337:577074.
266. Martín-Aguilar L, Lleixà C, Pascual-Goñi E, et al. Clinical and laboratory features in anti-NF155 autoimmune nodopathy. *Neurol Neuroimmunol Neuroinflamm.* 2022;9(1):e1098.
267. Burnor E, Yang L, Zhou H, et al. Neurofascin antibodies in autoimmune, genetic, and idiopathic neuropathies. *Neurology.* 2018;90(1):E31–E38.
268. Dong M, Tai H, Yang S, Gao X, Pan H, Zhang Z. Characterization of the patients with antibodies against nodal-paranodal junction proteins in chronic inflammatory demyelinating polyneuropathy. *Clin Neurol Neurosurg.* 2022;223:107521.
269. Shelly S, Klein CJ, Dyck JPB, et al. Neurofascin-155 immunoglobulin subtypes clinicopathologic associations and neurologic outcomes. *Neurology.* 2021;97(24):E2392–E2403.

270. Wang W, Liu C, Li W, et al. Clinical and diagnostic features of anti-neurofascin-155 antibody-positive neuropathy in Han Chinese. *Ann Clin Transl Neurol*. 2022;9(5):695–706.
271. Dubey D, Honorat JA, Shelly S, et al. Contactin-1 autoimmunity: serologic, neurologic, and pathologic correlates. *Neurol Neuroimmunol Neuroinflamm*. 2020;7(4):e771.
272. Hashimoto Y, Ogata H, Yamasaki R, et al. Chronic inflammatory demyelinating polyneuropathy with concurrent membranous nephropathy: an anti-paranode and podocyte protein antibody study and literature survey. *Front Neurol*. 2018;9:997.
273. Tang Y, Liu J, Gao F, et al. CIDP/autoimmune nodopathies with nephropathy: a case series study. *Ann Clin Transl Neurol*. 2023;10(5):706–718.
274. Taieb G, Le Quintrec M, Pialot A, et al. "Neuro-renal syndrome" related to anti-contactin-1 antibodies. *Muscle Nerve*. 2019;59(3):E19–E21.
275. Miura Y, Devaux JJ, Fukami Y, et al. Contactin 1 IgG4 associates to chronic inflammatory demyelinating polyneuropathy with sensory ataxia. *Brain*. 2015;138(6):1484–1491.
276. Doppler K, Appeltshauser L, Wilhelmi K, et al. Destruction of paranodal architecture in inflammatory neuropathy with anti-contactin-1 autoantibodies. *J Neurol Neurosurg Psychiatry*. 2015;86(7):720–728.
277. Fehmi J, Davies AJ, Antonelou M, et al. Contactin-1 links autoimmune neuropathy and membranous glomerulonephritis. *PLoS One*. 2023;18:e0281156.
278. Doppler K, Appeltshauser L, Villmann C, et al. Auto-antibodies to contactin-associated protein 1 (Caspr) in two patients with painful inflammatory neuropathy. *Brain*. 2016;139(10):2617–2630.
279. Appeltshauser L, Brunder AM, Heinius A, et al. Antiparanodal antibodies and IgG subclasses in acute autoimmune neuropathy. *Neurol Neuroimmunol Neuroinflamm*. 2020;7(5):e817.
280. Lorenzo B, Alessandro S, Elisa V, et al. Caspr1 antibodies autoimmune paranodopathy with severe tetraparesis: potential relevance of antibody titers in monitoring treatment response. *J Peripher Nerv Syst*. 2023;28(3):522–527.
281. Pascual-Goñi E, Fehmi J, Lleixà C, et al. Antibodies to the Caspr1/contactin-1 complex in chronic inflammatory demyelinating polyradiculoneuropathy. *Brain*. 2021;144(4):1183–1196.
282. Pascual-Goñi E, Martín-Aguilar L, Querol L. Autoantibodies in chronic inflammatory demyelinating polyradiculoneuropathy. *Curr Opin Neurol*. 2019;32(5):651–657.
283. Delmont E, Manso C, Querol L, et al. Autoantibodies to nodal isoforms of neurofascin in chronic inflammatory demyelinating polyneuropathy. *Brain*. 2017;140(7):1851–1858.
284. Fehmi J, Davies AJ, Walters J, et al. IgG1 pan-neurofascin antibodies identify a severe yet treatable neuropathy with a high mortality. *J Neurol Neurosurg Psychiatry*. 2021;92(10):1089–1095.
285. Stengel H, Vural A, Brunder AM, et al. Anti-pan-neurofascin IgG3 as a marker of fulminant autoimmune neuropathy. *Neurol Neuroimmunol Neuroinflamm*. 2019;6(5):e603.
286. Appeltshauser L, Junghof H, Messinger J, et al. Anti-pan-neurofascin antibodies induce subclass-related complement activation and nodo-paranodal damage. *Brain*. 2023;146(5):1932–1949.
287. Fels M, Fisse AL, Schwake C, et al. Report of a fulminant anti-pan-neurofascin-associated neuropathy responsive to rituximab and bortezomib. *J Peripher Nerv Syst*. 2021;26(4):475–480.
288. Garg N, Park SB, Yiannikas C, et al. Neurofascin-155 IGG4 neuropathy: pathophysiological insights, spectrum of clinical severity and response to treatment. *Muscle Nerve*. 2018;57(5):848–851.
289. Kouton L, Boucraut J, Devaux J, et al. Electrophysiological features of chronic inflammatory demyelinating polyradiculoneuropathy associated with IgG4 antibodies targeting neurofascin 155 or contactin 1 glycoproteins. *Clinical Neurophysiology*. 2020;131(4):921–927.
290. Stathopoulos P, Alexopoulos H, Dalakas MC. Autoimmune antigenic targets at the node of Ranvier in demyelinating disorders. *Nat Rev Neurol*. 2015;11(3):143–156.
291. Manso C, Querol L, Mekaouche M, Illa I, Devaux JJ. Contactin-1 IgG4 antibodies cause paranode dismantling and conduction defects. *Brain*. 2016;139(6):1700–1712.
292. Manso C, Querol L, Lleixà C, et al. Anti–neurofascin-155 IgG4 antibodies prevent paranodal complex formation in vivo. *J Clin Invest*. 2019;129(6):2222–2236.
293. Koike H, Kadoya M, Kaida KI, et al. Paranodal dissection in chronic inflammatory demyelinating polyneuropathy with anti-neurofascin-155 and anti-contactin-1 antibodies. *J Neurol Neurosurg Psychiatry*. 2017;88(6):465–473.
294. Vallat JM, Yuki N, Sekiguchi K, et al. Paranodal lesions in chronic inflammatory demyelinating polyneuropathy associated with anti-Neurofascin 155 antibodies. *Neuromuscul Disord*. 2017;27(3):290–293.
295. Rispens T, Huijbers MG. The unique properties of IgG4 and its roles in health and disease. *Nat Rev Immunol*. 2023;23(11):763–778.
296. Hu J, Sun C, Lu J, Zhao C, Lin J. Efficacy of rituximab treatment in chronic inflammatory demyelinating polyradiculoneuropathy: a systematic review and meta-analysis. *J Neurol*. 2022;269(3):1250–1263.
297. Liu B, Hu J, Sun C, et al. Effectiveness and safety of rituximab in autoimmune nodopathy: a single-center cohort study. *J Neurol*. 2023;270(9):4288–4295.
298. Chad DA, Hammer K, Sargent J. Slow resolution of multifocal weakness and fasciculation: a reversible motor neuron syndrome. *Neurology*. 1986;36(9):1260–1260.
299. Parry GJ, Holtz SJ, Ben-Zeev D, Drori JB. Gammopathy with proximal motor axonopathy simulating motor neuron disease. *Neurology*. 1986;36(2):273–273.
300. Rowland LP, Defendini R, Sherman W, et al. Macroglobulinemia with peripheral neuropathy simulating motor neuron disease. *Ann Neurol*. 1982;11(5):532–536.
301. Tucker T, Layzer RB, Miller RG, Chad D. Subacute, reversible motor neuron disease. *Neurology*. 1991;41(10):1541–1544.
302. Auer RN, Bell RB, Lee MA. Neuropathy with onion bulb formations and pure motor manifestations. *Can J Neurol Sci*. 1989;16(2):194–197.
303. Van den Berg-Vos RM, Franssen H, Wokke JHJ, Van den Berg LH. Multifocal motor neuropathy: long-term clinical and electrophysiological assessment of intravenous immunoglobulin maintenance treatment. *Brain*. 2002;125(8):1875–1886.
304. Chaudhry V. Multifocal motor neuropathy. *Semin Neurol*. 1998;18(01):73–81.
305. Chaudhry V, Corse AM, Cornblath DR, et al. Multifocal motor neuropathy: response to human immune globulin. *Ann Neurol*. 2004;33(3):237–242.
306. Chaudhry V, Corse AM, Cornblath DR, Kuncl RW, Freimer ML, Griffin JW. Multifocal motor neuropathy: electrodiagnostic features. *Muscle Nerve*. 1994;17(2):198–205.

307. Feldman EL, Bromberg MB, Albers JW, Pestronk A. Immunosuppressive treatment in multifocal motor neuropathy. *Ann Neurol.* 1991;30(3):397–401.
308. Katz JS, Wolfe GI, Bryan WW, Jackson CE, Amato AA, Barohn RJ. Electrophysiologic findings in multifocal motor neuropathy. *Neurology.* 1997;48(3):700–707.
309. Krarup C, Stewart JD, Sumner AJ, Pestronk A, Lipton SA. A syndrome of asymmetric limb weakness with motor conduction block. *Neurology.* 1990;40(1):118–118.
310. Parry GJ, Clarke S. Multifocal acquired demyelinating neuropathy masqurading as motor neuron disease. *Muscle Nerve.* 1988;11(2):103–107.
311. Parry GJ, Sumner AJ. Multifocal motor neuropathy. *Neurol Clin.* 1992;10(3):671–684.
312. Pestronk A, Chaudhry V, Feldman EL, et al. Lower motor neuron syndromes defined by patterns of weakness, nerve conduction abnormalities, and high titers of antiglycolipid antibodies. *Ann Neurol.* 1990;27(3):316–326.
313. Pestronk A, Cornblath DR, Ilyas AA, et al. A treatable multifocal motor neuropathy with antibodies to GM1 ganglioside. *Ann Neurol.* 1988;24(1):73–78.
314. Roth G, Rohr J, Magistris MR, Ochsner F. Motor Neuropathy with proximal multifocal persistent conduction block, fasciculations and myokymia. *Eur Neurol.* 1986;25(6):416–423.
315. Olney RK, Lewis RA, Putnam TD, Campellone JV. Consensus criteria for the diagnosis of multifocal motor neuropathy. *Muscle Nerve.* 2003;27(1):117–121.
316. Parry G. Motor neuropathy with multifocal conduction block. *Semin Neurol.* 1993;13(03):269–275.
317. Vlam L, van der Pol WL, Cats EA, et al. Multifocal motor neuropathy: diagnosis, pathogenesis and treatment strategies. *Nat Rev Neurol.* 2012;8(1):48–58.
318. Slee M, Selvan A, Donaghy M. Multifocal motor neuropathy: the diagnostic spectrum and response to treatment. *Neurology.* 2007;69(17):1680–1687.
319. Löscher WN, Oberreiter EM, Erdler M, et al. Multifocal motor neuropathy in Austria: a nationwide survey of clinical features and response to treatment. *J Neurol.* 2018;265(12):2834–2840.
320. Cats EA, van der Pol WL, Piepers S, et al. Correlates of outcome and response to IVIg in 88 patients with multifocal motor neuropathy. *Neurology.* 2010;75(9):818–825.
321. Moroni I, Bugiani M, Ciano C, Bono R, Pareyson D. Childhood-onset multifocal motor neuropathy with conduction blocks. *Neurology.* 2006;66(6):922–924.
322. Lambrecq V, Krim E, Rouanet-Larrivière M, Lagueny A. Sensory loss in multifocal motor neuropathy: a clinical and electrophysiological study. *Muscle Nerve.* 2009;39(2):131–136.
323. Traynor BJ, Codd MB, Corr B, Forde C, Frost E, Hardiman O. Amyotrophic lateral sclerosis mimic syndromes. *Arch Neurol.* 2000;57(1):109.
324. Miyashiro A, Matsui N, Shimatani Y, et al. Are multifocal motor neuropathy patients underdiagnosed? An epidemiological survey in Japan. *Muscle Nerve.* 2014;49(3):357–361.
325. Kaji R, Shibasaki H, Kimura J. Multifocal demyelinating motor neuropathy. *Neurology.* 1992;42(3):506–509.
326. Pringle CE, Belden J, Veitch JE, Brown WF. Multifocal motor neuropathy presenting as ophthalmoplegia. *Muscle Nerve.* 1997;20(3):347–351.
327. Boonyapisit K, Katirji B. Multifocal motor neuropathy presenting with respiratory failure. *Muscle Nerve.* 2000;23(12):1887–1890.
328. Beydoun SR, Copeland D. Bilateral phrenic neuropathy as a presenting feature of multifocal motor neuropathy with conduction block. *Muscle Nerve.* 2000;23(4):556–559.
329. Felice KJ, Goldstein JM. Monofocal motor neuropathy: improvement with intravenous immunoglobulin. *Muscle Nerve.* 2002;25(5):674–678.
330. Manganelli F, Pisciotta C, Iodice R, Calandro S, Santoro L. Nine-year case history of monofocal motor neuropathy. *Muscle Nerve.* 2008;38(1):927–929.
331. Jafari H, Carlander B, Camu W. Letter to the editor. *Muscle Nerve.* 2000;23(10):1610–1611.
332. Alentorn A, Albertí MA, Montero J, Casasnovas C. Monofocal motor neuropathy with conduction block associated with adalimumab in rheumatoid arthritis. *Joint Bone Spine.* 2011;78(5):536–537.
333. Pakiam ASI, Parry GJ. Multifocal motor neuropathy without overt conduction block. *Muscle Nerve.* 1998;21(2):243–245.
334. Nobile-Orazio E, Cappellari A, Meucci N, et al. Multifocal motor neuropathy: clinical and immunological features and response to IVIg in relation to the presence and degree of motor conduction block. *J Neurol Neurosurg Psychiatry.* 2002;72(6):761–766.
335. Delmont E, Azulay JP, Giorgi R, et al. Multifocal motor neuropathy with and without conduction block: a single entity? *Neurology.* 2006;67(4):592–596.
336. Chaudhry V, Swash M. Multifocal motor neuropathy: Is conduction block essential? *Neurology.* 2006;67(4):558–559.
337. Kaji R, Hirota N, Oka N, et al. Anti-GM1 antibodies and impaired blood-nerve barrier may interfere with remyelination in multifocal motor neuropathy. *Muscle Nerve.* 1994;17(1):108–110.
338. Kornberg AJ, Pestronk A. The clinical and diagnostic role of anti-GM1 antibody testing. *Muscle Nerve.* 1994;17(1):100–104.
339. Pestronk A, Florence J, Miller T, Choksi R, Al-Lozi M, Levine T. Treatment of IgM antibody associated polyneuropathies using rituximab. *J Neurol Neurosurg Psychiatry.* 2003;74(4):485–489.
340. Gooch CL, Amato AA. Are anti-ganglioside antibodies of clinical value in multifocal motor neuropathy? *Neurology.* 2010;75(22):1950–1951.
341. Parry GJG. Antiganglioside antibodies do not necessarily play a role in multifocal motor neuropathy. *Muscle Nerve.* 1994;17(1):97–99.
342. Cornblath DR, Sumner AJ, Daube J, et al. Conduction block in clinical practice. *Muscle Nerve.* 1991;14(9):869–871.
343. Comi G, Amadio S, Galardi G, Fazio R, Nemni R. Clinical and neurophysiological assessment of immunoglobulin therapy in five patients with multifocal motor neuropathy. *J Neurol Neurosurg Psychiatry.* 1994;57(Suppl):35–37.
344. Lange DJ, Nijjar R, Voustianiouk A, Seidel G, Panchal J, Wang AK. Do a-waves help predict intravenous immunoglobulin response in multifocal motor neuropathy without block? *Muscle Nerve.* 2011;43(4):537–542.
345. Van Asseldonk JTH, Van den Berg LH, Van den Berg-Vos RM, Wieneke GH, Wokke JHJ, Franssen H. Demyelination and axonal loss in multifocal motor neuropathy: distribution and relation to weakness. *Brain.* 2003;126(1):186–198.
346. Levine TD, Pestronk A. IgM antibody-related polyneuropathies: B-cell depletion chemotherapy using Rituximab. *Neurology.* 1999;52(8):1701–1701.

347. Beekman R, van den Berg LH, Franssen H, Visser LH, van Asseldonk JTH, Wokke JHJ. Ultrasonography shows extensive nerve enlargements in multifocal motor neuropathy. *Neurology*. 2005;65(2):305–307.
348. Kronlage M, Knop KC, Schwarz D, et al. Amyotrophic lateral sclerosis versus multifocal motor neuropathy: utility of MR neurography. *Radiology*. 2019;292(1):149–156.
349. Bouche P, Moulonguet A, Younes-Chennoufi AB, et al. Multifocal motor neuropathy with conduction block: a study of 24 patients. *J Neurol Neurosurg Psychiatry*. 1995;59(1):38–44.
350. Corse AM, Chaudhry V, Crawford TO, Cornblath DR, Kuncl RW, Griffin JW. Sensory nerve pathology in multifocal motor neuropathy. *Ann Neurol*. 1996;39(3):319–325.
351. Yuki N, Watanabe H, Nakajima T, Spath PJ. IVIG blocks complement deposition mediated by anti-GM1 antibodies in multifocal motor neuropathy. *J Neurol Neurosurg Psychiatry*. 2011;82(1):87–91.
352. Nobile-Orazio E, Meucci N, Barbieri S, Carpo M, Scarlato G. High-dose intravenous immunoglobulin therapy in multifocal motor neuropathy. *Neurology*. 1993;43(3, Part 1):537–537.
353. Tan E. Immunosuppressive treatment of motor neuron syndromes. *Arch Neurol*. 1994;51(2):194.
354. Markson L, Janzen D, Bril V. Response to therapy in demyelinating motor neuropathy. *Muscle Nerve*. 1998;21(12):1769–1771.
355. Arasaki K, Kusunoki S, Kudo N, Kanazawa I. Acute conduction block in vitro following exposure to antiganglioside sera. *Muscle Nerve*. 1993;16(6):587–593.
356. Roberts M, Willison HJ, Vincent A, Newsom-Davis J. Multifocal motor neuropathy human sera block distal motor nerve conduction in mice. *Ann Neurol*. 1995;38(1):111–118.
357. Santoro M, Uncini A, Corbo M, et al. Experimental conduction block induced by serum from a patient with anti-GM1 antibodies. *Ann Neurol*. 1992;31(4):385–390.
358. Harvey GK, Toyka KV, Zielasek J, Kiefer R, Simonis C, Hartung HP. Failure of anti-GM1 IgG OR IgM to induce conduction block following intraneural transfer. *Muscle Nerve*. 1995;18(4):388–394.
359. Kuwabara S, Yuki N, Koga M, et al. IgG Anti-GM1 antibody is associated with reversible conduction failure and axonal degeneration in Guillain-Barré syndrome. *Ann Neurol*. 1998;44(2):202–208.
360. Takigawa T, Yasuda H, Kikkawa R, Shigeta Y, Saida T, Kitasato H. Antibodies against GM1 ganglioside affect K+ and NA+ currents in isolated rat myelinated nerve fibers. *Ann Neurol*. 1995;37(4):436–442.
361. Weber F, Rudel R, Aulkemeyer P, Brinkmeier H. Anti-GM1 antibodies can block neuronal voltage-gated sodium channels. *Muscle Nerve*. 2000;23(9):1414–1420.
362. White JR, Sachs GM, Gilchrist JM. Multifocal motor neuropathy with conduction block and Campylobacter jejuni. *Neurology*. 1996;46(2):562–563.
363. Terenghi F, Allaria S, Scarlato G, Nobile-Orazio E. Multifocal motor neuropathy and *Campylobacter jejuni* reactivity. *Neurology*. 2002;59(2):282–284.
364. Rodriguez-Escalera C, Belzunegui J, Lopez-Dominguez L, Gonzalez C, Figueroa M. Multifocal motor neuropathy with conduction block in a patient with rheumatoid arthritis on infliximab therapy. *Rheumatology*. 2005;44(1):132–133.
365. Tektonidou MG, Serelis J, Skopouli FN. Peripheral neuropathy in two patients with rheumatoid arthritis receiving infliximab treatment. *Clin Rheumatol*. 2006;26(2):258–260.
366. Chaudhry V, Escolar DM, Cornblath DR. Worsening of multifocal motor neuropathy during pregnancy. *Neurology*. 2002;59(1):139–141.
367. Charles N, Vial C, Moreau T, Benoit P, Bierme T, Bady B. Intravenous immunoglobulin treatment in multifocal motor neuropathy. *Lancet*. 1992;340(8812):182.
368. Léger JM, Chassande B, Musset L, Meininger V, Bouche P, Baumann N. Intravenous immunoglobulin therapy in multifocal motor neuropathy: a double-blind, placebo-controlled study. *Brain*. 2001;124(Pt 1):145–153.
369. Azulay JP, Blin O, Pouget J, Boucraut J, Billé-Turc F, Carles G, Serratrice G. Intravenous immunoglobulin treatment in patients with motor neuron syndromes associated with anti-GM1 antibodies: a double-blind, placebo-controlled study. *Neurology*. 1994;44(3 Pt 1):429–432.
370. Keddie S, Eftimov F, van den Berg LH, Brassington R, de Haan RJ, van Schaik IN. Immunoglobulin for multifocal motor neuropathy. *Cochrane Database Syst Rev*. 2022;1(1):CD004429.
371. Chaudhry V, Corse AM, Cornblath DR, Kuncl RW, Drachman DB, Freimer ML, Miller RG, Griffin JW. Multifocal motor neuropathy: response to human immune globulin. *Ann Neurol*. 1993;33(3):237–242.
372. Van den Berg LH, Kerkhoff H, Oey PL, Franssen H, Mollee I, Vermeulen M, Jennekens FG, Wokke JH. Treatment of multifocal motor neuropathy with high dose intravenous immunoglobulins: a double blind, placebo controlled study. *J Neurol Neurosurg Psychiatry*. 1995;59(3):248–252.
373. Hahn AF, Beydoun SR, Lawson V, et al. A controlled trial of intravenous immunoglobulin in multifocal motor neuropathy. *J Peripher Nerv Syst*. 2013;18(4):321–330.
374. Eftimov F, Vermeulen M, de Haan RJ, van den Berg LH, van Schaik IN. Subcutaneous immunoglobulin therapy for multifocal motor neuropathy. *J Peripher Nerv Syst*. 2009;14(2):93–100.
375. Harbo T, Andersen H, Hess A, Hansen K, Sindrup SH, Jakobsen J. Subcutaneous versus intravenous immunoglobulin in multifocal motor neuropathy: a randomized, single-blinded cross-over trial. *Eur J Neurol*. 2009;16(5):631–638.
376. Herraets IJT, Bakers JNE, van Eijk RPA, Goedee HS, van der Pol WL, van den Berg LH. Human immune globulin 10% with recombinant human hyaluronidase in multifocal motor neuropathy. *J Neurol*. 2019;266(11):2734–2742.
377. Herraets I, Van Rosmalen M, Bos J, et al. Clinical outcomes in multifocal motor neuropathy: a combined cross-sectional and follow-up study. *Neurology*. 2020;95(14):E1979–E1987.
378. van Schaik IN, Bouche P, Illa I, et al. European Federation of Neurological Societies/Peripheral Nerve Society guideline on management of multifocal motor neuropathy. *Eur J Neurol*. 2006;13(8):802–808.
379. Jinka M, Chaudhry V. Treatment of multifocal motor neuropathy. *Curr Treat Options Neurol*. 2014;16(2):269.
380. Van den Berg-Vos RM, Van den Berg LH, Franssen H, Van Doorn PA, Merkies ISJ, Wokke JHJ. Treatment of multifocal motor neuropathy with interferon-1A. *Neurology*. 2000;54(7):1518–1521.
381. Meucci N, Cappellari A, Barbieri S, Scarlato G, Nobile-Orazio E. Long term effect of intravenous immunoglobulins and oral cyclophosphamide in multifocal motor neuropathy. *J Neurol Neurosurg Psychiatry*. 1997;63(6):765–769.
382. Ruegg SJ, Fuhr P, Steck AJ. Rituximab stabilizes multifocal motor neuropathy increasingly less responsive to IVIg. *Neurology*. 2004;63(11):2178–2179.

383. Katz JS, Barohn RJ, Kojan S, et al. Axonal multifocal motor neuropathy without conduction block or other features of demyelination. *Neurology*. 2002;58(4):615–620.
384. Sansa-Fayos G, Viguera-Martínez ML, Ribera-Perpiñá G, Martínez-Pérez JM. Axonal multifocal motor neuropathy. A case report. *Rev Neurol*. 2005;41(7):444–446.
385. Sinnreich M, Klein CJ, Daube JR, Engelstad J, Spinner RJ, Dyck PJB. Chronic immune sensory polyradiculopathy: a possibly treatable sensory ataxia. *Neurology*. 2004;63(9):1662–1669.
386. Citak KA, Dickoff DJ, Simpson DM. Progressive sensory radiculopathy responsive to corticosteroid therapy. *Muscle Nerve*. 1993;16(6):679–680.
387. Burton M, Anslow P, Gray W, Donaghy M. Selective hypertrophy of the cauda equina nerve roots. *J Neurol*. 2002;249(3):337–340.
388. Caporale CM, Staedler C, Gobbi C, Bassetti CL, Uncini A. Chronic inflammatory lumbosacral polyradiculopathy: a regional variant of CIDP. *Muscle Nerve*. 2011;44(5):833–837.
389. Shelly S, Shouman K, Paul P, et al. Expanding the spectrum of chronic immune sensory polyradiculopathy: CISP-Plus. *Neurology*. 2021;96(16):E2078–E2089.
390. Khadilkar SV, Patel R, Shah N, Deshmukh ND, Patel BA, Mansukhani KA. Chronic immune polyradiculopathies: three clinical variants of one disease? *Muscle Nerve*. 2021;63(1):99–103.
391. Thammongkolchai T, Suhaib O, Termsarasab P, Li Y, Katirji B. Chronic immune sensorimotor polyradiculopathy: report of a case series. *Muscle Nerve*. 2019;59(6):658–664.
392. Asbury AK, Picard EH, Baringer JR. Sensory Perineuritis. *Arch Neurol*. 1972;26(4):302–312.
393. Chad DA, Smith TW, DeGirolami U, Hammer K. Perineuritis and ulcerative colitis. *Neurology*. 1986;36(10):1377–1377.
394. Konishi T, Saida K, Ohnishi A, Nishitani H. Perineuritis in mononeuritis multiplex with cryoglobulinemia. *Muscle Nerve*. 1982;5(2):173–177.
395. Simmons Z, Albers JW, Sima AAF. Case-of-the-month: perineuritis presenting as mononeuritis multiplex. *Muscle Nerve*. 1992;15(5):630–635.
396. Sorenson EJ, Sima AAF, Blaivas M, Sawchuk K, Wald JJ. Clinical features of perineuritis. *Muscle Nerve*. 1997;20(9):1153–1157.
397. Yamada M, Owada K, Eishi Y, Kato A, Yokota T, Furukawa T. Sensory perineuritis and non-Hodgkin's T-Cell lymphoma. *Eur Neurol*. 1994;34(5):298–299.
398. Matthews WB, Squier MV. Sensory perineuritis. *J Neurol Neurosurg Psychiatry*. 1988;51(4):473–475.
399. Colan RV, Snead OC, Oh SJ, Benton JW. Steroid-responsive polyneuropathy with subacute onset in childhood. *J Pediatr*. 1980;97(3):374–377.

CHAPTER 15

Vasculitic Neuropathies

Vasculitis is an immune-mediated disorder directed against blood vessels, which results in ischemia to end organs supplied by the affected blood vessels.[1-5] The vasculitides can be distinguished and classified based on at least three nosologic categories. They can be differentiated based on the caliber of vessel involved (i.e., small, medium, or large vessel). They can be distinguished on whether the disorder is primary [e.g., polyarteritis nodosa (PAN), microscopic polyangiitis (MPA), granulomatosis with polyangiitis (GAN, formerly known as Wegener granulomatosis), and eosinophilic granulomatosis with polyangiitis (EGPA, previously referred to as Churg–Strauss syndrome)] or secondary to other systemic disorders (e.g., connective tissue disease, malignancy, infection, or drug reaction). Furthermore, the vasculitides can be separated based on whether they are systemic or isolated to the peripheral nervous system (PNS), and if associated with antineutrophil cytoplasmic antibodies (ANCAs) (Table 15-1). Vasculitis is much more common in adults but can develop in children.[6]

▶ CLINICAL FEATURES

PNS vasculitis can present as (1) a mononeuropathy or multiple mononeuropathies, (2) overlapping mononeuropathies, or (3) distal symmetric polyneuropathies (Fig. 15-1).[1-8] In the first pattern, patients may present with just a mononeuropathy, but usually multiple nerves eventually become affected over time, giving a distinct asymmetric pattern of involvement in the distribution of individual nerves. With the second pattern, different nerves on both sides of the body are affected but to varying degrees, leading to a generalized, yet asymmetric, pattern of involvement. Finally, with gradual progression, somewhat uniform and generalized involvement of peripheral nerves results in what looks like a distal symmetric polyneuropathy. Approximately 60%–70% of patients present with mononeuropathy or multiple mononeuropathies (multifocal neuropathy or mononeuropathy multiplex pattern), while 30%–40% of patients present as a distal symmetric polyneuropathy.[7] There is a large differential diagnosis of patients with a multiple mononeuropathy (Table 15-2). For this reason, multifocal neuropathy, multiple mononeuropathies, or mononeuropathy multiplex are preferable terminologies to mononeuritis multiplex because the latter term implies a histologically defined disorder rather than a clinically defined syndrome.

Patients usually complain of burning or tingling pain in the distribution of the affected nerve(s). On examination, weakness and sensory loss are evident as well. Rare patients have purely sensory symptoms and signs.[9] Muscle stretch reflexes may be normal or diminished, depending on whether or not the involved nerve innervating is in a reflex arc. For example, involvement of the sciatic nerve could lead to a diminished ankle jerk, but a median nerve infarct would not result in a loss of a biceps or triceps reflex.

▶ LABORATORY FINDINGS

Most patients have elevated erythrocyte sedimentation rate (ESR) or C-reactive protein (CRP).[1-5,10] Some vasculitides are associated with ANCAs, antinuclear antibodies (ANAs), cryoglobulins, rheumatoid factor, leukocytosis, and anemia. ANCAs are of particular importance as they are 85% sensitive and 99% specific for vasculitis.[11] The ANCAs are subclassified as cytoplasmic (cANCA) or perinuclear (pANCA) based on their immunofluorescence staining pattern and antigenic target; cANCAs are directed against proteinase 3 (PR3), while pANCAs target myeloperoxidase (MPO). PR3/cANCA is associated with GAN, while MPO/pANCA is typically associated with MPA and to a lesser extent with EGPA and PAN. MPO/pANCA has also been seen in minocycline-induced vasculitis.

Affected nerves may appear enlarged and hypoechoic with ultrasound.[12-14] MR imaging may also be useful to identify nerve lesions.[15,16] Motor and sensory nerve conduction studies (NCSs) demonstrate unobtainable potentials or reduced amplitudes.[4,7,8,17-21] In particular, it is important to look for side-to-side asymmetries in amplitudes that reflect the multifocal nature of the pathology. Distal latencies are normal or slightly prolonged, while conduction velocities are normal or only mildly reduced. Conduction block or pseudoconduction block may be demonstrated in some affected nerves.[22-25] The presence of persistent conduction block or temporal dispersion in a patient with a multifocal neuropathy pattern should suggest a disorder such as the multifocal acquired demyelinating sensory and motor (MADSAM) neuropathy variant of chronic inflammatory demyelinating polyneuropathy (CIDP). The needle electromyography (EMG) reveals denervation changes in affected muscle groups. Again, the needle EMG abnormalities are often also asymmetric.

▶ HISTOPATHOLOGY

The sural, superficial peroneal (sensory branch), and superficial radial sensory nerves are the most common nerves

TABLE 15-1. VASCULITIDES ASSOCIATED WITH PERIPHERAL NEUROPATHY

Primary Vasculitis
    Large vessel vasculitis
        Giant cell (temporal) arteritis
    Medium and small vessel vasculitis
        Polyarteritis nodosa
        Eosinophilic granulomatosis with polyangiitis (Churg–Strauss syndrome)
        Granulomatosis with angiitis
        Microscopic polyangiitis
        Nonsystemic vasculitic neuropathy
Secondary Vasculitis
    Vasculitis associated with connective tissue diseases
    Vasculitis associated with diabetes mellitus
    Vasculitis associated with Behçet disease
    Vasculitis associated with sarcoidosis
    Vasculitis associated with malignancies
    Vasculitis associated with infections
    Vasculitis associated with cryoglobulinemia
    Vasculitis associated with hypersensitivity reaction (leukocytoclastic angiitis)—uncommonly associated with a peripheral neuropathy

TABLE 15-2. MULTIFOCAL NEUROPATHIES/MULTIPLE MONONEUROPATHIES: DIFFERENTIAL DIAGNOSIS

Peripheral Nerve Vasculitis
    Polyarteritis nodosa
    Granulomatosis with angiitis
    Eosinophilic granulomatosis with polyangiitis (Churg–Strauss syndrome)
    Microscopic polyangiitis
    Connective tissue disorders associated with vasculitic neuropathies (e.g., SLE, RA, mixed connective tissue disease)
    Remote effect of cancer
    Nonsystemic vasculitic neuropathy
Other Immune-Medicated Neuropathies
    Multifocal acquired demyelinating sensory and motor neuropathy [MADSAM, asymmetric chronic inflammatory demyelinating polyradiculoneuropathy (CIDP)]
    Multifocal motor neuropathy
    Sensory perineuritis
    Lumbosacral/brachial plexus neuritis (diabetic and nondiabetic)
    Postsurgical inflammatory neuropathy
Granulomatous Infiltration
    Sarcoid
    Lymphomatoid granulomatosis
Infectious Neuropathies
    Leprosy
    Herpes zoster
    Lyme disease
    HIV
    CMV
    Hepatitis B and C
Compression Neuropathy
    Primary compression neuropathies (e.g., traumatically induced)
    Secondary compression neuropathies (e.g., superimposed on generalized peripheral nerve disease; e.g., diabetes mellitus and carpal/cubital tunnel syndrome)
    Hereditary liability to pressure palsy
Other Disorders
    Diabetes mellitus (some cases may be due to a microvasculitis)
    Amyloidosis (hereditary and acquired)
    Neoplastic infiltration (particularly lymphoma and leukemia)
    Peripheral nerve tumors (e.g., neurofibromatosis, perineurioma)
    Atherosclerotic vascular disease (monomelic neuropathy secondary to acute large artery occlusion of AV shunts/fistulas)
    Drug induced (e.g., interferon-α, leukotriene receptor antagonist, tumor necrosis factor-α inhibitors, leflunomide, amphetamine, sulfonamides, minocycline)

CMV, cytomegalovirus; HIV, human immunodeficiency virus; RA, rheumatoid arthritis; SLE, systemic lupus erythematosus.

that are biopsied.[1–5,26] Suspected vasculitis is one of the few clinical situations in which we routinely perform nerve biopsy. We usually biopsy the superficial peroneal nerve if it is involved clinically and by NCSs. This is because the peroneus brevis muscle can also be biopsied from the same incision site, and the diagnostic yield is increased when the nerve and muscle both are biopsied (Fig. 15-2).[5,26–28] Diagnostic criteria for pathologically definite vasculitis include transmural inflammatory cell infiltration and fibrinoid necrosis

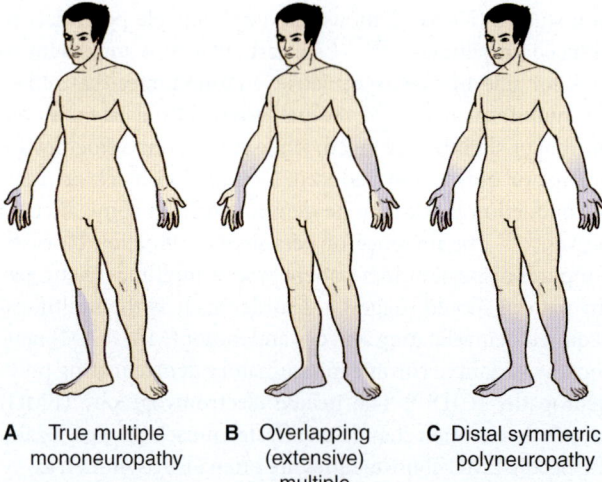

A True multiple mononeuropathy
B Overlapping (extensive) multiple mononeuropathy
C Distal symmetric polyneuropathy

Figure 15-1. Patterns of involvement in vasculitic neuropathy. Vasculitis can present as (**A**) a mononeuropathy or multiple mononeuropathies, (**B**) overlapping mononeuropathies, or (**C**) distal symmetric polyneuropathies.

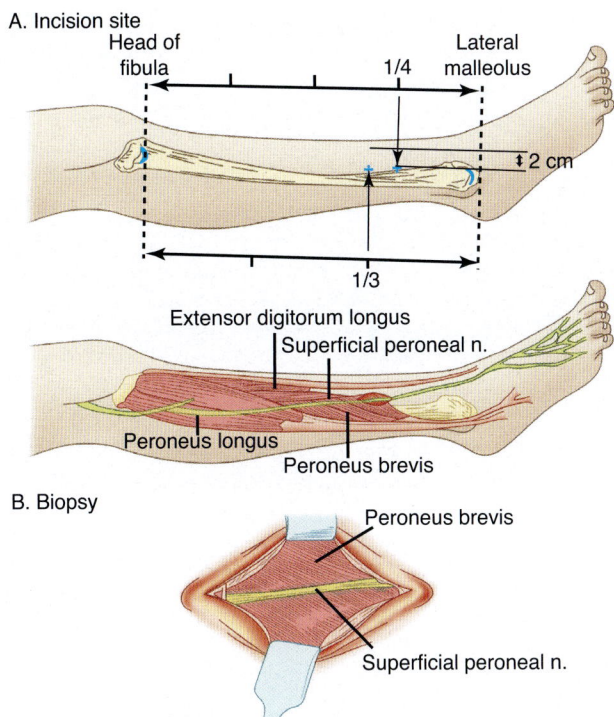

Figure 15-2. Superficial peroneal nerve and peroneus brevis muscle biopsy. The superficial peroneal nerve can usually be biopsied at a site between one-third and one-fourth the distance between the lateral aspect of the ankle and the fibular head and about 1.5–2 cm anterior to the fibula. After the nerve is biopsied, the underlying peroneus brevis muscle can be biopsied. This combination increases the yield of finding vasculitis and can be made through one incision. (Modified from Mendell JR, Erdem S, Agamonolis DR. Peripheral nerve and skin biopsies. In: Mendell JR, Kissel JT, Cornblath DR, eds. *Diagnosis and Management of Peripheral Nerve Disorders*. Oxford University Press; 2001.)

of the vessel wall (Fig. 15-3).[1–3,7,19,29–31] Supportive features of acute vasculitis also include loss or fragmentation of internal elastic lamina and loss/fragmentation/separation of smooth muscles in the media (can be highlighted by elastin and antismooth muscle actin staining), vascular or perivascular hemorrhage, acute thrombosis, and leukocytoclasia.

Immunocytochemistry may reveal immunoglobulin (IgM and/or IgG), complement, and membrane attack complex deposition on blood vessels.[32] Signs of repair may be seen in chronic vasculitis and include intimal hyperplasia, fibrosis of media, adventitial/periadventitial fibrosis, and recanalization of the lumen. Common findings are asymmetrical nerve fiber loss between and within individual nerve fascicles and active axonal degeneration. Nerve biopsies can also demonstrate immunostaining for the receptor for advanced glycosylation end products, nuclear factor-kappa B, and interleukin-6 that are expressed by CD4(+), CD8(+), and CD68(+) cells invading nerves. Such immunostaining can be identified in mononuclear cells, epineurial and endoneurial vessels, and in the perineurium.[33] This data suggests that the receptor for advanced glycosylation end products pathway plays a critical proinflammatory role in vasculitic neuropathy. Matrix metalloproteinases (e.g., MMP-9) are upregulated as well and may play an important role as means for inflammatory cell invasion.[34]

There are different histopathological features associated with the different types of vasculitic neuropathy.[35–38] ANCA-associated vasculitis is often associated with neutrophils adjacent to endothelial cells in the epineurium. Additionally, MPA with or without MPO-ANCA antibodies is characterized by the attachment of neutrophils to the endothelial cells of epineurial small vessels, necrotizing vasculitis, but no complement deposition. Granulomatous inflammation is seen in EGPA with PR3-ANCA. EGPA with MPO-ANCA is associated with necrotizing vasculitis, while EPGA without MPO-ANCA antibodies are more likely to have of eosinophil infiltration in the endoneurium, eosinophils in the lumen of epineurial vessels walls, epineurial vessels occluded by intraluminal eosinophils, are less likely to have disruption of vascular walls and fibrinoid necrosis.

In addition to vasculitis, muscle biopsies may show evidence of muscle infarction (Fig. 15-4). Skin biopsies have also demonstrated reduced epidermal nerve fiber density in some cases of vasculitic neuropathy.[27,39,40]

▶ PRIMARY SYSTEMIC VASCULITIC DISORDERS AFFECTING LARGE- AND MEDIUM-SIZED VESSELS

GIANT CELL VASCULITIS

Temporal arteritis and Takayasu arteritis are the two forms of giant cell arteritis, but peripheral neuropathy only occurs in the setting of temporal arteritis.[10,41–43] Giant cell arteritis affects medium- and large-sized vessels, particularly the aortic arch and the internal and external carotid arteries, and the vertebral arteries. Patients may present with headaches, jaw and tongue claudication, generalized myalgias, vision loss secondary to ischemic optic neuropathy, or stroke. Approximately 14% of patients develop multifocal neuropathy/multiple mononeuropathies, radiculopathies, plexopathies, or a generalized sensorimotor peripheral neuropathy.[10] The temporal artery is often tender, and a palpable cord can be felt. Ultrasound of the temporal artery may reveal a hypoechoic "halo sign" that is strongly suggestive of temporal arteritis.[44–46] Other imaging modalities such as MRA and PET/CT are also highly sensitive in picking up inflamed large vessels throughout the body (see Chapter 33 on Inflammatory Myopathies, Fig. 33-21).[44–46] Temporal artery biopsies reveal inflammatory infiltrate with giant cells in only two-thirds of suspected cases. There is limited information available in regard to peripheral nerve biopsies in GCA patients with polyneuropathy. Patients generally respond quite well to treatment with corticosteroids.

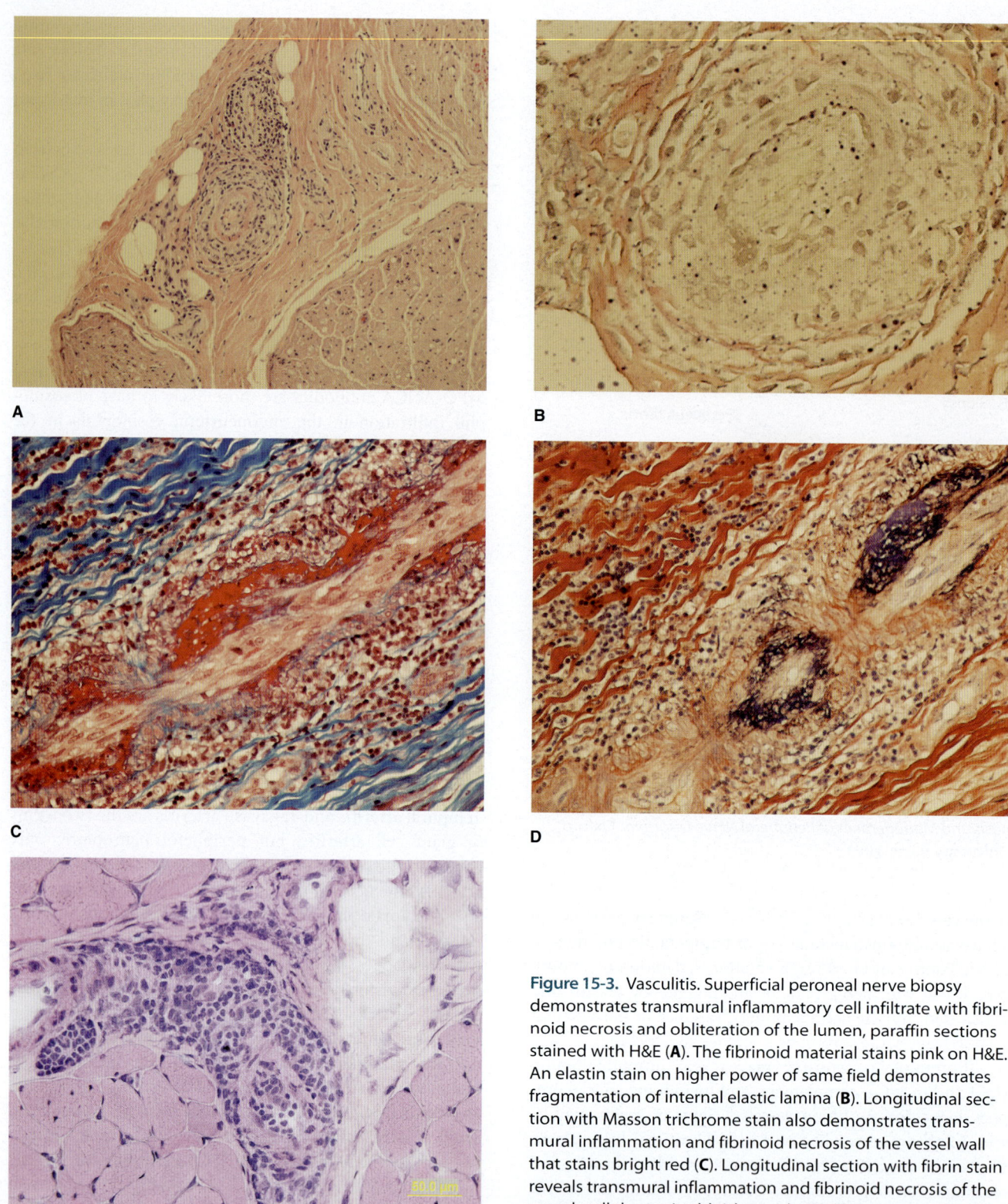

Figure 15-3. Vasculitis. Superficial peroneal nerve biopsy demonstrates transmural inflammatory cell infiltrate with fibrinoid necrosis and obliteration of the lumen, paraffin sections stained with H&E (**A**). The fibrinoid material stains pink on H&E. An elastin stain on higher power of same field demonstrates fragmentation of internal elastic lamina (**B**). Longitudinal section with Masson trichrome stain also demonstrates transmural inflammation and fibrinoid necrosis of the vessel wall that stains bright red (**C**). Longitudinal section with fibrin stain reveals transmural inflammation and fibrinoid necrosis of the vessel wall that stains bluish-purple (**D**). The peroneus brevis muscle biopsy also demonstrates vasculitis on frozen section stained with hematoxylin and eosin (**E**).

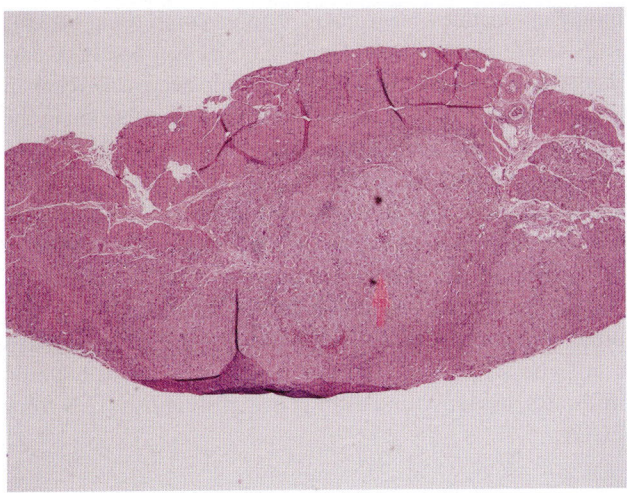
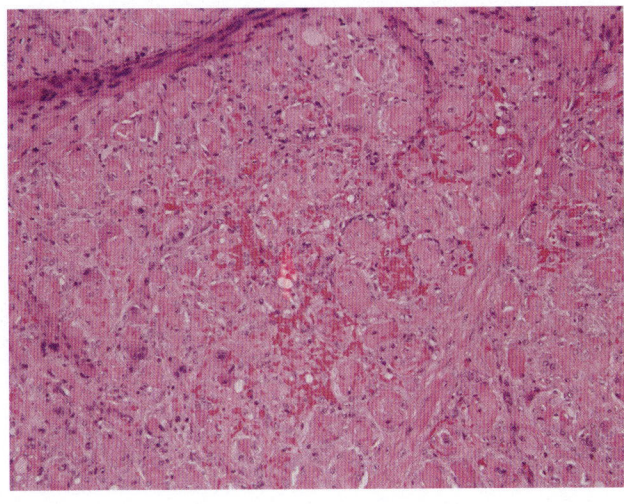

Figure 15-4. Muscle biopsy demonstrates an area of muscle infarct and some hemorrhagic conversion at low- (**A**) and high-power (**B**) paraffin sections stained with H&E.

▶ PRIMARY SYSTEMIC VASCULITIC DISORDERS AFFECTING MEDIUM- AND SMALL-SIZED VESSELS

POLYARTERITIS NODOSA

PAN, the most common of the necrotizing vasculitides, is a systemic disorder involving small- and medium-caliber arteries in multiple organs.[1–5,11,47] PAN has an incidence ranging from 2 to 9 per million and usually presents between 40 and 60 years of age. The most common pattern of nerve involvement is multifocal neuropathy/multiple mononeuropathies. The sciatic nerve or its peroneal or tibial branches are the most frequently involved nerves. Cranial neuropathies and central nervous system (CNS) involvement are rare but can occur. Other organ systems affected include the heart, liver, kidneys, gastrointestinal that may lead to liver or renal failure, abdominal pain, and gastrointestinal bleeding. Notably, the lungs are generally spared. Myalgias and arthralgias occur in 30%–70% of patients. Vasculitis involving the skin can result in petechiae, livedo reticularis, subcutaneous nodules, and distal gangrene.[47] Orchitis is also a common complication. Constitutional symptoms include weight loss, fever, and loss of appetite.

Although not as commonly found as in MPA and EGPA, approximately 10%–20% of PAN patients have MPO/pANCA. Elevated ESR and CRP are evident in the majority of patients.[1–3] One-third of cases are associated with hepatitis B antigenemia,[47] but PAN can also complicate hepatitis C virus (HCV) and human immunodeficiency virus (HIV) infections.[48] Abdominal angiograms can reveal a vasculitic aneurysm, a useful finding in patients with nondiagnostic biopsies.

Medium-sized arteries are usually affected; however, smaller-sized vessels can be involved in PAN.[1–5,11] Nerve biopsies may demonstrate transmural infiltration of CD8+ T cells, macrophages, and polymorphonuclear cells along with fibrinoid necrosis of the vessel wall. IgM, IgG, complement, and membrane attack complex deposition may be appreciated on blood vessels. Unlike EGPA, granulomas and eosinophilic infiltration are not seen on nerve biopsies in PAN. The pathogenic mechanism of PAN is unknown but is believed to be a T cell–dependent process with secondary complement-mediated vascular damage.

EOSINOPHILIC GRANULOMATOSIS WITH POLYANGIITIS (CHURG–STRAUSS SYNDROME)

EGPA was previously referred to as Churg–Strauss syndrome (CSS) or allergic granulomatosis and angiitis. EGPA manifests with signs and symptoms similar to PAN except that respiratory involvement is common in EGPA.[1–5,49–53] The incidence of EGPA is about one-third that of PAN, but the frequency of neurological complications is about the same. In this regard, multifocal neuropathy/multiple mononeuropathies develop in as many as 75% of individuals who are affected.[2] Patients with EGPA typically present with allergic rhinitis, nasal polyposis, sinusitis, and late-onset asthma (after the age of 35 years). Symptoms and signs of systemic vasculitis occur an average of 3 years after the onset of asthma and even longer after the onset of nasal symptoms. Anywhere from 16% to 49% of patients with EGPA develop a necrotizing glomerulonephritis as opposed to an ischemic nephropathy that can complicate PAN. Several cases of EGPA have been reported in patients treated with leukotriene antagonists after weaning corticosteroids.[54]

Routine laboratory workup reveals eosinophilia, leukocytosis, elevated ESR, CRP, rheumatoid factor, and serum IgG and IgE levels. One should consider EGPA in any patient

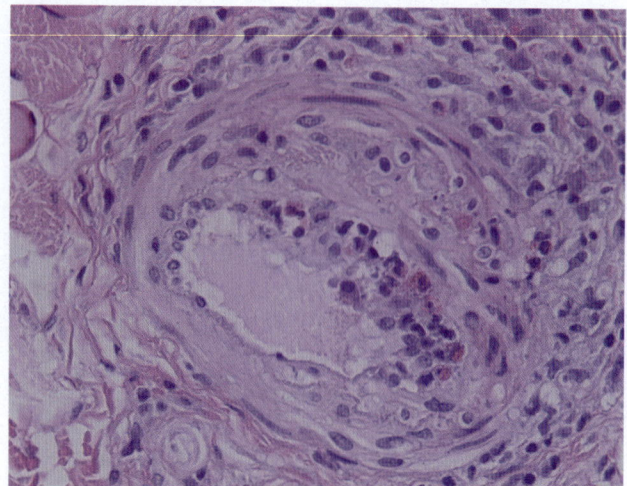

Figure 15-5. Eosinophilic granulomatosis with polyangiitis. Nerve biopsy demonstrates transmural infiltration of a vessel wall that includes eosinophils and obliteration of the lumen. Paraffin section stained with H&E.

with a neuropathy and peripheral eosinophilia. Approximately two-thirds of individuals who are affected have MPO/pANCA.[1,2,11] Chest x-rays reveal that pulmonary infiltrates are present in nearly half of patients.

Nerve biopsies may demonstrate necrotizing vasculitis with CD8+ cytotoxic T lymphocytes, CD4+ cells and, to a lesser extent, eosinophilic infiltrates (Fig. 15-5).[1,2,51,55] In addition, intravascular and extravascular granulomas are occasionally found in and around affected blood vessels in EGPA with PR3-ANCA. EGPA with MPO-ANCA is associated with necrotizing vasculitis. In contrast, EPGA without MPO-ANCA antibodies are more likely to have of eosinophil infiltration in the endoneurium, eosinophils in the lumen of epineurial vessels walls, and epineurial vessels occluded by intraluminal eosinophils, but are less likely to have disruption of vascular walls and fibrinoid necrosis.[35,36]

GRANULOMATOSIS WITH POLYANGIITIS

Granulomatosis with polyangiitis (GAN) was formerly referred to as Wegener granulomatosis. The latter term is no longer recommended as Dr. Wegener was a high-ranking Nazi physician, and the facility he was assigned to in Poland was associated with unethical humane experimentation. GAN is characterized by necrotizing vasculitis and granulomas involving the upper and lower respiratory tract and kidneys (glomerulonephritis).[1,2,56-63] Early respiratory symptoms (e.g., nasal discharge, cough, hemoptysis, and dyspnea) can help distinguish this from other vasculitides. In a large prospective study of 128 patients with granulomatosis with polyangiitis, 64 patients (50%) developed CNS or PNS involvement.[56] Peripheral neuropathy occurred in 56 patients and in 9 cases the CNS was involved. Thirty-one patients had a distal symmetric polyneuropathy, while 25 had multifocal neuropathy/multiple mononeuropathies. Neuropathy is more common in patients with severe renal involvement.[60] Cranial neuropathies, particularly the second, sixth, and seventh nerves, develop in approximately 5%–10% of cases as a result of extension of the nasal or paranasal granulomas rather than vasculitis.[56,62]

The majority of affected individuals have PR3-cANCA, and this test has a specificity of 98% and sensitivity of 95%.[60] The histological appearance of the vasculitis is similar to PAN, with involvement of medium- and small-sized blood vessels. In addition, granulomatous infiltration of the respiratory tract and necrotizing glomerulonephritis are also seen. The absence of peripheral eosinophilia, eosinophilic infiltrates on biopsy, and asthma help distinguish GAN from EGPA.

MICROSCOPIC POLYANGIITIS

MPA clinically resembles PAN and EGPA, except that diffuse alveolar damage and interstitial fibrosis develop due to involvement of pulmonary capillaries.[1,2,11,52,64] The incidence of MPA is about one-third that of PAN. The average age of onset is 50 years and polyneuropathy develops 14%–36% of MPA cases.[1,2,11,64]

Laboratory evaluation is remarkable for renal insufficiency, hematuria, and MPO/pANCA in most patients. PR3/cANCA can also occasionally be detected. As suggested by the name, MPA affects small arterioles, veins, and capillaries.[1,2,11] Nerve biopsies usually reveal neutrophils attached to endothelial cells of epineurial small vessels along with fibrinoid necrosis but without complement deposition.[35-38] Kidney biopsies reveal focal segmental thrombosis and necrotizing glomerulonephritis.

BEHÇET SYNDROME

This disorder is characterized by recurrent oral and genital ulcerations, inflammation of the eye, arthritis, thrombophlebitis, skin lesions, and vasculitic lesions of these organs involving the small- to medium-sized arteries.[65-68] The CNS complications (brainstem strokes, meningoencephalitis, and psychosis) are more common than peripheral neuropathy.

▶ SECONDARY SYSTEMIC VASCULITIDES

VASCULITIS ASSOCIATED WITH CONNECTIVE TISSUE DISEASE

Neuropathies are not uncommon in people with connective tissue diseases, although necrotizing are not uncommon in people with connective tissue diseases, although necrotizing vasculitis as the cause is infrequent (see Chapter 16). That said, secondary vasculitis can complicate rheumatoid arthritis, systemic lupus erythematosus, mixed connective tissue disease, Sjögren syndrome, and, less frequently, systemic sclerosis.[18,69,70] The clinical, histological, and electrophysiological features are similar to PAN. In addition, vasculitis may be seen in sarcoidosis (see Chapter 16).

MICROVASCULITIS ASSOCIATED WITH DIABETES MELLITUS

Some forms of neuropathy associated with diabetes are suspected be due to a microvasculitis and are discussed in Chapter 21 regarding neuropathies associated with endocrine disorders.

INFECTION-RELATED VASCULITIS

Vasculitic neuropathy can arise as a complication of a variety of infections.[48,71–73] The most common infectious agents associated with vasculitic neuropathy are HIV, hepatitis B and C, cytomegalovirus, Epstein–Barr viruses, and herpes varicella zoster (discussed in Chapter 17). Multifocal neuropathy/multiple mononeuropathies related to HIV or cytomegalovirus infection occur in up to 3% of patients with acquired immune deficiency syndrome (AIDS).[73] As previously discussed, hepatitis B and C infections are associated with PAN, a medium-sized systemic vasculitis, as well as a small vessel vasculitis associated with cryoglobulinemia. Vasculitic neuropathy may also complicate Lyme disease.

MALIGNANCY-RELATED VASCULITIS

Rarely, cancers have been associated with vasculitic neuropathy. Small cell lung cancer and lymphoma are the most common implicated malignancies, but leukemia, other myelodysplastic syndromes, and carcinomas of the kidneys, bile duct, prostate, and stomach have also been described.[74–83] However, most of the reported cases were not associated with a necrotizing vasculitis, rather only nonspecific transmural or perivascular inflammation of small blood vessels without fibrinoid necrosis was seen on biopsy. In this regard, several of the cases with "vasculitic" neuropathy associated with lung cancer and anti-Hu antibodies were reported as having vasculitis, although this disorder is not a true necrotizing vasculitis (see Chapter 19).[74] Multiple mononeuropathies or generalized neuropathies associated with lymphomas are often paraneoplastic in etiology or due to lymphomatous infiltration of the nerves. However, rare cases of vasculitic neuropathy have been reported in the setting of lymphoma.[81]

DRUG-INDUCED HYPERSENSITIVITY VASCULITIS

Hypersensitivity vasculitis is often secondary to drug reactions and is a self-limited process as opposed to the systemic

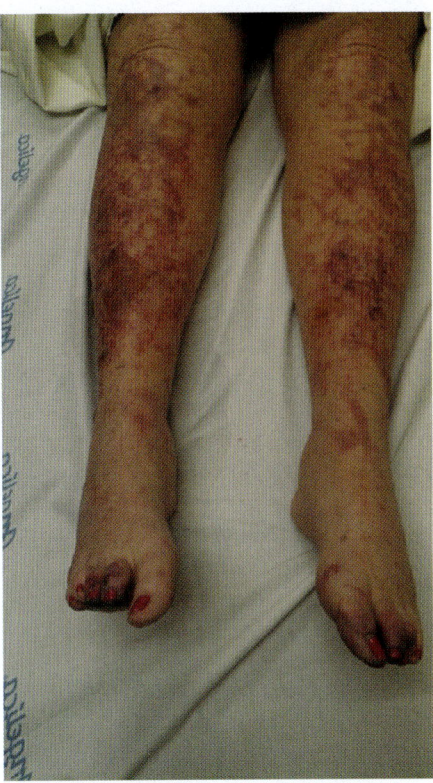

Figure 15-6. Hypersensitivity vasculitis. Severe petechial lesions are evident on bilateral lower extremities.

necrotizing vasculitides. Skin manifestations (e.g., petechiae) predominate the clinical picture of hypersensitivity vasculitis and neuropathy is uncommon (Fig. 15-6). Minocycline may be an exception as we and others have seen typical vasculitic neuropathy as a complication.[16,84,85] Drugs of abuse (e.g., amphetamine, cocaine, and opioids) also can cause vasculitis of the CNS or PNS.[86,87] The pathogenesis most likely relates to a complement-mediated leukocytoclastic reaction.

VASCULITIS SECONDARY TO ESSENTIAL MIXED CRYOGLOBULINEMIA

Cryoglobulins are circulating immune complexes consisting of immunoglobulins directed against polyclonal immunoglobulins. These complexes precipitate out of solution when exposed to a cool temperature but dissolve back into solution when rewarmed—thus the name cryoglobulin. There are actually three types of cryoglobulins. Type I cryoglobulins are monoclonal immunoglobulins, usually IgM, directed against polyclonal IgG. These are most commonly seen in individuals with plasma cell dyscrasias. Type II cryoglobulins are composed of a combination of monoclonal IgM and polyclonal immunoglobulins directed against polyclonal IgG. Type III cryoglobulins are a mixture of polyclonal IgM, IgG, and IgA directed against polyclonal IgG. Type II and III cryoglobulins are seen in patients with the so-called mixed cryoglobulinemia and typically occur in the setting of lymphoproliferative disorders, connective tissue diseases, HIV, and hepatitis B and hepatitis C infection. Most patients with mixed cryoglobulinemia are associated with hepatitis C antigenemia. *Essential* mixed cryoglobulinemia is the term used when mixed cryoglobulinemia is found in the absence of an underlying disease. Peripheral neuropathy develops in 25%–90% of patients with cryoglobulinemia of any type.[22,88–98] The neuropathy may manifest as a painful, distal, symmetric sensory or sensorimotor polyneuropathy; as multifocal/multiple mononeuropathies; or rarely as a pure small fiber neuropathy.[22]

The lack of local HCV replication in nerve biopsies suggests that that HCV-mixed cryoglobulinemia-associated neuropathy results from virus-triggered immune-mediated mechanisms rather than direct nerve infection and in situ replication.[93,95] The neuropathy may arise due to ischemia from hyperviscosity or due to vasculitis related to immune complex deposition in small epineurial blood vessels. NCSs are similar to PAN. Conduction block was appreciated on motor NCSs in one report.[22]

NONSYSTEMIC OR ISOLATED PNS VASCULITIS

Nearly 60% of vasculitis is restricted to peripheral nerves.[1,2,6,7,11,26,30,38,99–104] This so-called nonsystemic vasculitis or isolated PNS vasculitis is usually seen in adults, but children can also be affected.[6] The clinical, electrophysiological, and histopathological features of isolated PNS vasculitis are quite similar to PAN, except that there is no significant involvement of other organ systems. Affected individuals may present with multiple mononeuropathies or a generalized symmetric sensorimotor polyneuropathy. Laboratory testing may demonstrate elevated ESR or positive ANA titers. Vasculitis may be apparent on muscle biopsies,[5] but the peripheral nerves are predominantly involved. The diagnostic yield of finding vasculitis is increased by biopsying both muscle and nerve.

The vasculitis typically involves small- and medium-sized arteries of the epineurium and perineurium, and immune complex deposition on these blood vessels may be appreciated on biopsy.[38] MMPs, in particular MMP-2 and MMP-9 (gelatinase A and B), are upregulated in the peripheral nerves in patients with nonsystemic vasculitis.[103] T-cells are the predominant source of MMP-2 and MMP-9, although stromal cells of the perineurium and endoneurium may also secrete MMP. These enzymes digest the subendothelial basement membrane and thus facilitate inflammatory cells to penetrate the blood–nerve barrier.

The prognosis for isolated PNS vasculitis is much better than that for systemic vasculitic disorders. In one large series, corticosteroids were effective in over 70% of patients, but one-third of these patients experienced relapses.[104] Approximately 50% of patients required second-line immunosuppressive agents. Those started quickly on prednisone at a dose of 1 mg/kg/day had better neurological outcomes, while those with longer diagnostic delay and treated with low-dose prednisone were associated need to also treat with a second-line therapy.

POSTSURGICAL INFLAMMATORY NEUROPATHY

Most neuropathies that occur following surgery are felt to be due to stretching or compression of nerves. Recent studies suggest that some of these neuropathies may be secondary to inflammation.[105–109] The initial report from the Mayo Clinic described 23 patients who developed neuropathies following a surgical procedure, 12 had no history of direct trauma to a nearby nerve and were suspected of having an autoimmune neuritis.[105] A total of 21 patients had abnormal nerve biopsies that showed increased epineurial perivascular lymphocytic inflammation (9 small, 5 moderate, and 7 large), with 15 having findings suggestive of microvasculitis. Subsequent reports supported these initial findings.[106–109] Some affected patients apparently improved upon treatment with immunotherapy, but we do not know if the natural history might be gradual improvement. This entity seems similar to idiopathic brachial plexus and lumbosacral radiculoplexus neuropathy—some of which may occur after surgeries. Fibrinoid necrosis of vessel walls is not typical, but there is transmural or perivascular inflammation.

TREATMENT OF VASCULITIC NEUROPATHY

There is a lack of randomized therapeutic trials of corticosteroids and other immunosuppressive agent therapies in vasculitic neuropathy.[1–5,11,30,36,52,110–114] Nonetheless, the mainstay of initial treatment of systemic vasculitis in the past has been the combination of corticosteroids and cyclophosphamide. Since the use of corticosteroids to treat systemic vasculitis began in the 1950s, the 5-year survival rate increased from 10% to 55% by the mid-to-late 1970s. The addition of cyclophosphamide to corticosteroids further increased the 5-year survival rate to more than 80%.[113,114] We tend to be aggressive in our treatment approach because treatment failure in a disease such as PAN may be lead to a catastrophic event, such as a bowel or myocardial infarction. Hypersensitivity vasculitis and sometimes isolated PNS vasculitis may be treated with only prednisone. However, a large retrospective series suggested that the combination of corticosteroids and cyclophosphamide was more effective than corticosteroids alone as mentioned previously.[26] There is less experience with other immunotherapies in the treatment of vasculitis. Methotrexate (0.15–0.3 mg/kg/week) in combination with corticosteroids can be effective in GAN.[63,114] Azathioprine, cyclosporine, tacrolimus, chlorambucil, and intravenous immunoglobulin have been tried in refractory cases with variable success.[111,112,115,116] Rituximab has gained popularity as it appears effective in ANCA-associated vasculitis and cryoglobulinemia. The current recommended treatment strategy is dependent on the type of vasculitis.

Treatment of ANCA-Associated Vasculitis (MPA, EGPA, and GAN)

As mentioned, treatment of ANCA-associated vasculitis has been induction with corticosteroids and cyclophosphamide and then replacing cyclophosphamide with another second-line agent after 3–6 months as outlined in the previous section. However, there have been several reports suggesting rituximab may be beneficial[117–124] and two randomized clinical trials[125,126] showing that the combination of rituximab and corticosteroids is not inferior to cyclophosphamide and corticosteroids. Thus, the combination of corticosteroids (e.g., prednisone 1.0–1.5 mg/kg daily) and rituximab is increasingly recommended as the standard initial treatment of choice. In adults, rituximab is often given at a dosage of 375 mg/m^2 IV weekly for 4 weeks or 1 g IV followed by another 1 g IV 2 weeks later. Subsequent maintenance therapy is 1 g IV every 6 months thereafter based on clinical evaluation. In pediatric patients, the induction dose is typically 375 mg/m^2 once weekly for 4 weeks followed by 250 mg/m^2 intravenous infusion every 6 months as needed.

Avacopan is small molecule that selectively blocks the effects of C5a through the C5a receptor and also inhibits chemoattraction and activation of neutrophils.[127] A phase 3 randomized trial (ADVOCATE) avacopan (30 mg orally twice daily) with a tapering schedule of prednisone in patients with ANCA-associated vasculitis that included patients with vasculitic neuropathy.[127] All the patients also concurrently received cyclophosphamide or rituximab. Avacopan was found to be noninferior but not superior to prednisone taper with respect to remission at week 26 and was superior to prednisone taper with respect to sustained remission at week 52.

Treatment of Vasculitis Associated with HCV-Mixed Cryoglobulinemia

Treatment of mixed cryoglobulinemia requires removal of the antigen. In patients with mixed cryoglobulinemia due to hepatitis C infection, treatment with α-interferon appears to be effective.[11,75,92,128–135] Combination of α-interferon and ribavirin also has yield positive results though no randomized, controlled trials have been performed.[136–138] Use of high-dose corticosteroids and cyclophosphamide may allow the virus to persist and replicate, thus increasing the risk of liver failure. Methotrexate is avoided due to the risk of direct hepatotoxicity. Plasma exchange in combination with immunosuppressive therapy is often considered as first line treatment in patients with severe complications from the vasculitis.[97,98] There have been several reports suggesting rituximab may be beneficial in cryoglobulinemic vasculitis.[97,98,139–152] Two randomized, open-label studies comparing rituximab to standard treatment with immunosuppressive agents (glucocorticoids, azathioprine, cyclophosphamide, or plasmapheresis) demonstrated a greater response rate with rituximab.[149,150] Two studies compared treatment with rituximab and antivirals (Peg-interferon-alpha/riboflavin) to antiviral alone and, again, the rituximab-treated patients seemed to do better.[151,152] We usually initiate treatment with plasma exchange followed by the combination of rituximab and antiviral therapy. It is important though to first assess for hepatitis B infection as there is an increased risk of hepatitis reactivation in both HBsAg-positive as well as in HBsAg-negative and anti–HBc-positive patients with resulting liver failure.

Treatment of Non-ANCA Vasculitis (PAN and Isolated PNS Vasculitis)

We typically treat with oral prednisone 1.0 to 1.5 mg/kg/day (up to 100 mg/day) as a single dose in the morning in addition to cyclophosphamide. After 2–4 weeks, we switch from daily to alternate-day prednisone (i.e., 100 mg every other day). However, if a patient is diabetic, we treat with daily corticosteroids (e.g., prednisone 50 mg daily) so as not to have wide fluctuations in blood glucose. In patients with severe vasculitis, we may initiate treatment with a pulse of intravenous methylprednisolone (1 g intravenously every day for 3 days), then switch to oral corticosteroids. Patients are concurrently started on calcium and vitamin D supplementation and sometimes on a bisphosphonate to prevent and treat steroid-induced osteoporosis.

In addition, oral or intravenous cyclophosphamide is started. Oral cyclophosphamide at a dose of 1.0–2.0 mg/kg is a more potent suppressor of the immune system but is associated with more adverse side effects (e.g., hemorrhagic cystitis) than intravenous doses. Thus, we usually treat patients with monthly intravenous pulses of cyclophosphamide at a dose of 500–1,000 mg/m^2 of body surface area. Hydration is essential to minimize bladder toxicity. We also often premedicate patients with sodium 2-mercaptoethane sulfonate to reduce the incidence of bladder toxicity and with antiemetics to diminish nausea. Following intravenous pulses of cyclophosphamide, the leukocyte count drops. The nadir of the leukopenia occurs between 7 and 18 days, during which time the risk of infection is greatest. We check complete blood counts and urinalysis prior to each treatment. Urinalysis is obtained every 3–6 months after treatment because of the risk of future bladder cancer.

If patients do not respond to pulsed cyclophosphamide, oral dosing should be tried before concluding that the patient failed cyclophosphamide treatment. High-dose corticosteroids and cyclophosphamide are continued until the patient begins to improve or at least the deficit stabilizes. This usually occurs within 3–6 months. Subsequently, we discontinue cyclophosphamide and start methotrexate (7.5 mg/week). The methotrexate dose is gradually increased as necessary. At the same time, we begin to taper the prednisone by 5 mg every 2–3 weeks. In our experience, the disease may "burn itself out" and immunomodulating drugs may be successfully weaned after a year or more resulting in a prolonged drug-free remission in some cases.

Extrapolating to ANCA-associated vasculitis, rituximab might be beneficial in isolated PNS vasculitis, but we just do not have literature to support its use at this time. However, we certainly would use it in patients refractory to prednisone and cyclophosphamide and perhaps prior to cyclophosphamide use. In patients with hepatitis B–associated vasculitis, we usually treat with antiviral medications, plasma exchange, and a short course of corticosteroids. IVIG and rituximab have been used but the literature is scant; we also worry about increasing viral load with immunosuppressive agents and rituximab use.

▶ SUMMARY

There are a number of causes of systemic vasculitis that can affect peripheral nerves, and many times the vasculitis may be isolated to the peripheral nerves. Individuals who are affected may manifest with mononeuropathy, multifocal neuropathy/multiple mononeuropathies, and overlapping mononeuropathies, or even as a generalized symmetric sensorimotor polyneuropathy. It is important to take a detailed medical history for disorders that may be associated with vasculitis (e.g., connective tissue diseases, viral hepatitis, and late-onset asthma). Useful laboratory tests include assessment for eosinophilia, ANAs, MPO/pANCA, PR3/cANCA, ESR, CRP, rheumatoid factor, cryoglobulins, hepatitis serology, Lyme disease, and urinalysis. We like to have histological confirmation of vasculitis before initiating what can turn out to be long-term immunosuppressive therapy. The diagnostic yield of a combined superficial peroneal nerve and peroneus brevis muscle biopsy, when clinically affected, is high. Most patients improve with immunotherapy.

REFERENCES

1. Gwathmey KG, Tracy JA, Dyck PJB. Peripheral nerve vasculitis: classification and disease associations. *Neurol Clin.* 2019;37(2):303–333.
2. Beachy N, Satkowiak K, Gwathmey KG. Vasculitic neuropathies. *Semin Neurol.* 2019;39(5):608–619.
3. Collins MP, Hadden RD. The nonsystemic vasculitic neuropathies. *Nat Rev Neurol.* 2017;13(5):302–316.
4. Hawke SH, Davies L, Pamphlet R, Guo YP, Pollard JD, McLeod JG. Vasculitic neuropathy. A clinical and pathological study. *Brain.* 1991;114:2175–2190.
5. Said G, Lacroix-Ciaudo C, Fujimura H, Blas C, Faux N. The peripheral neuropathy of necrotizing arteritis: a clinicopathological study. *Ann Neurol.* 1988;23:461–465.
6. Ryan MM, Tilton A, De Girolami U, Darras BT, Jones HR Jr. Paediatric mononeuritis multiplex: a report of three cases and review of the literature. *Neuromuscul Disord.* 2003;13(9):751–756.
7. Kissel JT, Slivka AP, Warmolts JR, Mendell JR. The clinical spectrum of necrotizing angiopathy of the peripheral nervous system. *Ann Neurol.* 1985;18:251–257.
8. Amato AA, Dumitru D. Acquired neuropathies. In: Dumitru D, Amato AA, Swartz MJ, eds. *Electrodiagnostic Medicine.* 2nd ed. Hanley & Belfus; 2002:937–1041.
9. Seo JH, Ryan HF, Claussen GC, Thomas TD, Oh SJ. Sensory neuropathy in vasculitis. A clinical, pathologic, and electrophysiologic study. *Neurology.* 2004;63:874–878.
10. Caselli RJ, Daube JR, Hunder GG, Whisnant JP. Peripheral neuropathic syndromes in giant cell (temporal) arteritis. *Neurology.* 1988;38:685–689.
11. Collins MP. The vasculitic neuropathies: an update. *Curr Opin Neurol.* 2012;25:573–585.
12. Ito T, Kijima M, Watanabe T, Sakuta M, Nishiyama K. Ultrasonography of the tibial nerve in vasculitic neuropathy. *Muscle Nerve.* 2007;35:379–382.
13. Schmidt WA, Seifert A, Gromnica-Ihle E, Krause A, Natusch A. Ultrasound of proximal upper extremity arteries to increase the diagnostic yield in large-vessel giant cell arteritis. *Rheumatology (Oxford).* 2008;47:96–101.
14. Nodera H, Sato K, Terasawa Y, Takamatsu N, Kaji R. High-resolution sonography detects inflammatory changes in vasculitic neuropathy. *Muscle Nerve.* 2006;34:380–381.
15. Sanada M, Terada M, Suzuki E, Kashiwagi A, Yasuda H. MR angiography for the evaluation of non-systemic vasculitic neuropathy. *Acta Radiol.* 2003;44:316–318.
16. Thaisetthawatkul P, Sundell R, Robertson CE, Dyck PJ. Vasculitic neuropathy associated with minocycline use. *J Clin Neuromuscul Dis.* 2011;12:231–234.
17. Bouche P, Léger JM, Travers MA, Cathala HP, Castaigne P. Peripheral neuropathy in systemic vasculitis: clinical and electrophysiologic study of 22 patients. *Neurology.* 1986;36:1598–1602.
18. Hietaharju A, Jääskeläinen S, Kalimo H, Hietarinta M. Peripheral neuromuscular manifestations in systemic sclerosis (scleroderma). *Muscle Nerve.* 1993;16:1204–1212.
19. Wees SJ, Sunwoo IN, Oh SJ. Sural nerve biopsy in systemic vasculitis. *Am J Med.* 1981;71:525–532.
20. Zivkovic SA, Ascherman D, Lacomis D. Vasculitic neuropathy: electrodiagnostic findings and association with malignancies. *Acta Neurol Scand.* 2007;115(6):432–436.
21. Davalos L, Watanabe M, Gallagher GW, et al. Diagnostic characteristics of nerve conduction study parameters for vasculitic neuropathy. *Muscle Nerve.* 2023;67(1):45–51.
22. Lippa CF, Chad DA, Smith TW, Kaplan MH, Hammer K. Neuropathy associated with cryoglobulinemia. *Muscle Nerve.* 1986;9:626–631.
23. McCluskey L, Feinberg D, Cantor C, Bird S. "Pseudo-conduction block" in vasculitic neuropathy. *Muscle Nerve.* 1999;22:1361–1366.
24. Mohamed A, Davies L, Pollard JD. Conduction block in vasculitic neuropathy. *Muscle Nerve.* 1988;21:1084–1088.
25. Ropert A, Metral S. Conduction block in neuropathies with necrotizing vasculitis. *Muscle Nerve.* 1990;13:102–105.
26. Collins MP, Periquet MI, Mendell JR, Sahenk Z, Nagaraja HN, Kissel JT. Nonsystemic vasculitic neuropathy: insights from a clinical cohort. *Neurology.* 2003;61(5):623–630.
27. Agadi JB, Raghav G, Mahadevan A, Shankar SK. Usefulness of superficial peroneal nerve/peroneus brevis muscle biopsy in the diagnosis of vasculitic neuropathy. *J Clin Neurosci.* 2012;19:1392–1396.
28. Vrancken AF, Gathier CS, Cats EA, Notermans NC, Collins MP. The additional yield of combined nerve/muscle biopsy in vasculitic neuropathy. *Eur J Neurol.* 2011;18:49–58.

29. Kissel JT, Riethman JL, Omerza J, Rammohan KW, Mendell JR. Peripheral nerve vasculitis: immune characterization of the vascular lesions. *Ann Neurol.* 1989;25:291–297.
30. Panegyres PK, Blumbergs PC, Leong AS, Bourne AJ. Vasculitis of peripheral nerve and skeletal muscle: clinicopathological correlation and immunopathic mechanism. *J Neurol Sci.* 1990;100:193–202.
31. Collins MP, Dyck PJ, Gronseth GS, et al; Peripheral Nerve Society. Peripheral Nerve Society Guideline on the classification, diagnosis, investigation, and immunosuppressive therapy of non-systemic vasculitic neuropathy: executive summary. *J Peripher Nerv Syst.* 2010;15:176–184.
32. Collins MP, Periquet-Collins I, Sahenk Z, Kissel JT. Direct immunofluoresence in vasculitic neuropathy: specificity of vascular immune deposits. *Muscle Nerve.* 2010;42:62–69.
33. Haslbeck KM, Bierhaus A, Erwin S, et al. Receptor for advanced glycation end product (RAGE)-mediated nuclear factor-kappaB activation in vasculitic neuropathy. *Muscle Nerve.* 2004;29(6):853–860.
34. Renaud S, Erne B, Fuhr P, et al. Matrix metalloproteinases-9 and -2 in secondary vasculitic neuropathies. *Acta Neuropathol.* 2003;105(1):37–42.
35. Nishi R, Koike H, Ohyama K, et al. Differential clinicopathologic features of EGPA-associated neuropathy with and without ANCA. *Neurology.* 2020;94(16):e1726–e1737.
36. Koike H, Nishi R, Ohyama K, et al. ANCA-associated vasculitic neuropathies: a review. *Neurol Ther.* 2022;11(1):21–38.
37. Koike H, Furukawa S, Mouri N, Fukami Y, Iijima M, Katsuno M. Early ultrastructural lesions of anti-neutrophil cytoplasmic antibody- versus complement-associated vasculitis. *Neuropathology.* 2022;42(5):420–429.
38. Takahashi M, Koike H, Ikeda S, et al. Distinct pathogenesis in nonsystemic vasculitic neuropathy and microscopic polyangiitis. *Neurol Neuroimmunol Neuroinflamm.* 2017;4(6):e407.
39. Chao CC, Hsieh ST, Shun CT, Hsieh SC. Skin denervation and cutaneous vasculitis in eosinophilia-associated neuropathy. *Arch Neurol.* 2007;64(7):959–965.
40. Uçeyler N, Devigili G, Toyka KV, Sommer C. Skin biopsy as an additional diagnostic tool in non-systemic vasculitic neuropathy. *Acta Neuropathol.* 2010;120:109–116.
41. Koorey DJ. Cranial arteritis: a twenty-year review of cases. *Aust N Z J Med.* 1984;14:143–147.
42. Pfadenhauer K, Roesler A, Golling A. The involvement of the peripheral nervous system in biopsy proven active giant cell arteritis. *J Neurol.* 2007;254(6):751–755.
43. Nesher G, Rosenberg P, Shorer Z, Gilai A, Solomonovich A, Sonnenblick M. Involvement of the peripheral nervous system in temporal arteritis-polymyalgia rheumatica. Report of 3 cases and review of the literature. *J Rheumatol.* 1987;14(2):358–360.
44. Younger DS. Giant cell arteritis. *Neurol Clin.* 2019;37(2):335–344.
45. Buttgereit F, Matteson EL, Dejaco C. Polymyalgia rheumatica and giant cell arteritis. *JAMA.* 2020;324(10):993–994.
46. Serling-Boyd N, Stone JH. Recent advances in the diagnosis and management of giant cell arteritis. *Curr Opin Rheumatol.* 2020;32(3):201–207.
47. Guillevin L, Lhote F, Jarrousse B, Fain O. Treatment of polyarteritis nodosa and Churg–Strauss syndrome. A meta-analysis of 3 prospective controlled trials including 182 patients over 12 years. *Ann Med Interne (Paris).* 1992;143:405–416.
48. Cacoub P, Maisonobe T, Thibault V, et al. Systemic vasculitis in patients with hepatitis C. *J Rheumatol.* 2001;28(1):109–118.
49. Chumbley LC, Harrison EG Jr, DeRemee RA. Allergic granulomatosis and angiitis (Churg–Strauss syndrome). Report and analysis of 30 cases. *Mayo Clin Proc.* 1977;52:477–484.
50. Cooper BJ, Bacal E, Patterson R. Allergic angiitis and granulomatosis. Prolonged remission induced by combined prednisone-azathioprine therapy. *Arch Intern Med.* 1978;138:367–371.
51. Hattori N, Ichimura M, Nagamatsu M, et al. Clinicopathological features of Churg–Strauss syndrome-associated neuropathy. *Brain.* 1999;122:427–439.
52. Hattori N, Mori K, Misu K, Koike H, Ichimura M, Sobue G. Mortality and morbidity in peripheral neuropathy associated Churg–Strauss syndrome and microscopic polyangiitis. *J Rheumatol.* 2002;29(7):1408–1414.
53. Oh SJ, Herrera GA, Spalding DM. Eosinophilic vasculitis neuropathy in the Churg–Strauss syndrome. *Arthritis Rheum.* 1986;29:1173–1175.
54. Boccagni C, Tesser F, Mittino D, et al. Churg–Strauss syndrome associated with the leukotriene antagonist Montelukast. *Neurol Sci.* 2004;25(1):21–22.
55. Nagashima T, Cao B, Takeuchi N, et al. Clinicopathological studies of peripheral neuropathy in Churg–Strauss syndrome. *Neuropathology.* 2002;22(4):299–307.
56. de Groot K, Schmidt DK, Arlt AC, Gross WL, Reinhold-Keller E. Standardized neurologic evaluations of 128 patients with Wegener granulomatosis. *Arch Neurol.* 2001;58(8):1215–1221.
57. Drachman DA. Neurological complications of Wegener's granulomatosis. *Arch Neurol.* 1963;8:145–155.
58. Fauci AS, Haynes BF, Katz P, Wolff SM. Wegener's granulomatosis: prospective clinical and therapeutic experience with 85 patients for 21 years. *Ann Intern Med.* 1983;98:76–85.
59. Hoffman GS, Kerr GS, Leavitt RY, et al. Wegener granulomatosis: an analysis of 158 patients. *Ann Intern Med.* 1992;116:488–498.
60. Jaffe IA. Wegener's granulomatosis and ANCA syndromes. *Neurol Clin.* 1997;15:887–891.
61. Jimenez-Mendez HJ, Yablon SA. Electrodiagnostic characteristics of Wegener's granulomatosis-associated peripheral neuropathy. *Am J Phys Med Rehabil.* 1992;71:6–11.
62. Nishino H, Rubino FA, DeRemmee RA, Swanson JW, Parisi JE. Neurological involvement in Wegener's granulomatosis: an analysis of 324 consecutive patients at the Mayo Clinic. *Ann Neurol.* 1993;33:4–9.
63. Stern GM, Hoffbrand AV, Urich H. The peripheral nerves and skeletal muscle in Wegener's granulomatosis: a clinicopathological study of four cases. *Brain.* 1965;88:151–164.
64. Savage CO, Winearls CG, Evans DJ, Rees AJ, Lockwood CM. Microscopic polyarteritis: presentation, pathology and prognosis. *Q J Med.* 1985;56:467–483.
65. Frayha RA, Afifi AK, Bergman RA, Nader S, Bahuth NB. Neurogenic muscular atrophy in Behçet's disease. *Clin Rheumatol.* 1985;4:202–211.
66. Namer IJ, Karabudak R, Zileh T, Ruacan S, Küçükali T, Kansu E. Peripheral nervous system involvement in Behçet's disease. *Eur Neurol.* 1987;26:235–240.
67. Takeuchi A, Kodama M, Takatsu M, Hashimoto T, Miyashita H. Mononeuritis multiplex in incomplete Behçet's disease: a case report and the review of the literature. *Clin Rheumatol.* 1989;8:375–380.

68. Wakayama T, Takayaniagi T, Iida M, et al. A nerve biopsy study in two cases of neuro-Behçet's syndrome. *Clin Neurol (Tokyo)*. 1975;14:519–525.
69. Mawrin C, Brunn A, Röcken C, Schröder JM. Peripheral neuropathy in systemic lupus erythematosus: pathomorphological features and distribution pattern of matrix metalloproteinases. *Acta Neuropathol*. 2003;105(4):365–372.
70. Rosenbaum R. Neuromuscular complications of connective tissue diseases. *Muscle Nerve*. 2001;24(2):154–169.
71. Gerber O, Roque C, Colye PK. Vasculitis owing to infection. *Neurol Clin*. 1997;15:903–925.
72. Kanai K, Kuwabara S, Mori M, Arai K, Yamamoto T, Hattori T. Leukocytoclastic-vasculitic neuropathy associated with chronic Epstein–Barr virus infection. *Muscle Nerve*. 2003;27(1):113–116.
73. Brannagan TH III. Retroviral-associated vasculitis of the nervous system. *Neurology*. 1997;15:927–944.
74. Amato AA, Collins MP. Neuropathies associated with malignancy. *Semin Neurol*. 1998;18:125–144.
75. Naarendorp M, Kallemuchikkal U, Nuovo GJ, Gorevic PD. Longterm efficacy of interferon-alpha for extrahepatic disease associated with hepatitis C virus infection. *J Rheumatol*. 2001;28(11):2466–2473.
76. Oh SJ, Slaughter R, Harrell L. Paraneoplastic vasculitic neuropathy: a treatable neuropathy. *Muscle Nerve*. 1991;14:152–156.
77. Saif MW, Hopkins JL, Gore SD. Autoimmune phenomena in patients with myelodysplastic syndromes and chronic myelomonocytic leukemia. *Leuk Lymphoma*. 2002;43(11):2083–2092.
78. Sánchez-Guerrero J, Gutiérrez-Ureña S, Vidaller A, Reyes E, Iglesias A, Alarcón-Segovia D. Vasculitis as a paraneoplastic syndrome. Report of 11 cases and review of the literature. *J Rheumatol*. 1990;17:1458–1462.
79. Torvik A, Berntzen AE. Necrotizing vasculitis without visceral involvement. Postmortem examination of three cases with affection of skeletal muscles and peripheral nerves. *Acta Med Scand*. 1968;184:69–77.
80. Turner MR, Warren JD, Jacobs JM, et al. Microvasculitic paraproteinaemic polyneuropathy and B-cell lymphoma. *J Peripher Nerv Syst*. 2003;8(2):100–107.
81. Vincent D, Dubas F, Haue JJ, et al. Nerve and muscle microvasculitis in peripheral neuropathy: a remote effect of cancer. *J Neurol Neurosurg Psychiatry*. 1986;49:1007–1010.
82. Younger DS, Dalmau J, Inghirami G, Sherman WH, Hays AP. Anti-Hu-associated peripheral nerve and muscle vasculitis. *Neurology*. 1994;44:181–183.
83. Fain O, Hamidou M, Cacoub P, et al. Vasculitides associated with malignancies: analysis of sixty patients. *Arthritis Rheum*. 2007;57:1473–1480.
84. Ogawa N, Kawai H, Yamakawa I, Sanada M, Sugimoto T, Maeda K. Case of minocycline-induced vasculitic neuropathy. *Rinsho Shinkeigaku*. 2010;50:301–305.
85. Kermani TA, Ham EK, Camilleri MJ, Warrington KJ. Polyarteritis nodosa-like vasculitis in association with minocycline use: a single-center case series. *Semin Arthritis Rheum*. 2012;42:213–221.
86. Brust JCM. Vasculitis owing to substance abuse. *Neurol Clin*. 1997;15:945–957.
87. Stafford CR, Bogdanoff BM, Green L, Spector HB. Mononeuropathy multiplex as a complication of amphetamine angiitis. *Neurology*. 1975;25:570–572.
88. Cavaletti G, Petruccioli MG, Crespi V, Pioltelli P, Marmiroli P, Tredici G. A clinico-pathological and follow-up study of 10 cases of essential type II cryoglobulinemic neuropathy. *J Neurol Neurosurg Psychiatry*. 1990;53:886–889.
89. David WS, Peine C, Schlesinger P, Smith SA. Nonsystemic vasculitic mononeuropathy multiplex, cryoglobulinemia, and hepatitis C. *Muscle Nerve*. 1996;19:1596–1602.
90. Ferri C, La Civita L, Cirafisi C, et al. Peripheral neuropathy in mixed cryoglobulinemia: clinical and electrophysiologic investigations. *J Rheumatol*. 1992;19:889–895.
91. Gemignani F, Pavesi G, Fiocchi A, Manganelli P, Ferraccioli G, Marbini A. Peripheral neuropathy in essential mixed cryoglobulinemia. *J Neurol Neurosurg Psychiatry*. 1992;55:116–120.
92. Khella SL, Frost S, Hermann GA, et al. Hepatitis C infection, cryoglobulinemia, and vasculitis neuropathy. Treatment with interferon alpha: case report and literature review. *Neurology*. 1995;45:407–411.
93. Nemni R, Corbo M, Fazio R, Quattrini A, Comi G, Canal N. Cryoglobulinemic neuropathy. *Brain*. 1988;111:541–552.
94. Valli G, De Vecchi A, Gaddi L, Nobile-Orazio E, Tarantino A, Barbieri S. Peripheral nervous system involvement in essential cryoglobulinemia and nephropathy. *Clin Exp Rheumatol*. 1989;7:479–483.
95. Authier FJ, Bassez G, Payan C, et al. Detection of genomic viral RNA in nerve and muscle of patients with HCV neuropathy. *Neurology*. 2003;60(5):808–812.
96. Kolopp-Sarda MN, Miossec P. Cryoglobulinemic vasculitis: pathophysiological mechanisms and diagnosis. *Curr Opin Rheumatol*. 2021;33(1):1–7.
97. Quartuccio L, Bortoluzzi A, Scirè CA, et al. Management of mixed cryoglobulinemia with rituximab: evidence and consensus-based recommendations from the Italian Study Group of Cryoglobulinemia (GISC). *Clin Rheumatol*. 2023;42(2):359–370.
98. Galli M, Monti G, Marson P, et al. Recommendations for managing the manifestations of severe and life-threatening mixed cryoglobulinemia syndrome. *Autoimmun Rev*. 2019;18(8):778–785.
99. Davies L, Spies JM, Pollard JD, McLeod JG. Vasculitis confined to peripheral nerves. *Brain*. 1996;119:1441–1448.
100. Dyck PJ, Benstead TJ, Conn DL, Stevens JC, Windebank AJ, Low PA. Nonsystemic vasculitic neuropathy. *Brain*. 1987;110:843–854.
101. Nicholai A, Bonetti B, Lazzarino LG, Ferrari S, Monaco S, Rizzuto N. Peripheral nerve vasculitis: a clinic-pathological study. *Clin Neuropathol*. 1995;14:137–141.
102. Said G. Necrotizing peripheral nerve vasculitis. *Neurol Clin*. 1997;15:835–848.
103. Leppert D, Hughes P, Hiber S, et al. Matrix metalloproteinase upregulation in chronic inflammatory demyelinating polyneuropathy and nonsystemic vasculitic neuropathy. *Neurology*. 1999;53:62–70.
104. Quirins M, Théaudin M, Cohen-Aubart F, et al; French Vasculitis Study Group (FVSG). Nonsystemic vasculitic neuropathy: Presentation and long-term outcome from a French cohort of 50 patients. *Autoimmun Rev*. 2021;20(8):102874.
105. Staff NP, Engelstad J, Klein CJ, et al. Post-surgical inflammatory neuropathy. *Brain*. 2010;133:2866–2880.
106. Rattananan W, Thaisetthawatkul P, Dyck PJ. Postsurgical inflammatory neuropathy: a report of five cases. *J Neurol Sci*. 2014;337(1-2):137–140.

107. Laughlin RS, Dyck JB, Watson JC, et al. Ipsilateral inflammatory neuropathy after hip surgery. *Mayo Clin Proc.* 2014; 89:454–461.
108. Laughlin RS, Johnson RL, Burkle CM, Staff NP. Postsurgical neuropathy: a descriptive review. *Mayo Clin Proc.* 2020;95(2): 355–369.
109. Godlewski CA, Kalagara H, Vazquez Do Campo R, Northern T, Kukreja P. Post-surgical inflammatory neuropathy: an underappreciated but critical and treatable cause of postoperative neuropathy. *Cureus.* 2020;12(12):e11927.
110. Vrancken AF, Hughes RA, Said G, Wokke JH, Notermans NC. Immunosuppressive treatment for non-systemic vasculitic neuropathy. *Cochrane Database Syst Rev.* 2007;(1):CD006050.
111. Callabrese LH. Therapy of systemic vasculitis. *Neurol Clin.* 1997;15:973–991.
112. Donofrio PD. Immunotherapy of idiopathic inflammatory neuropathies. *Muscle Nerve.* 2003;28:273–292.
113. Mathew L, Talbot K, Love S, Puvanarajah S, Donaghy M. Treatment of vasculitic peripheral neuropathy: a retrospective analysis of outcome. *QJM.* 2007;100(1):41–51.
114. Langford CA, Talar-Williams C, Barron KS, Sneller MC. Use of a cyclophosphamide-induction methotrexate-maintenance regimen for the treatment of Wegener's granulomatosis: extended follow-up and rate of relapse. *Am J Med.* 2003;114(6): 463–469.
115. Levy Y, Uziel Y, Zandman GG, et al. Intravenous immunoglobulins in peripheral neuropathy associated with vasculitis. *Ann Rheum Dis.* 2003;62(12):1221–1223.
116. Richter C, Schanbel E, Csernok E, et al. Treatment of ANCA-associated vasculitis with high-dose intravenous immunoglobulin. *Arthritis Rheum.* 1994;37:S353.
117. Jones RB, Ferraro AJ, Chaudhry AN, et al. A multicenter survey of rituximab therapy for refractory antineutrophil cytoplasmic antibody-associated vasculitis. *Arthritis Rheum.* 2009;60:2156–2168.
118. Holle JU, Dubrau C, Herlyn K, et al. Rituximab for refractory granulomatosis with polyangiitis (Wegener's granulomatosis): comparison of efficacy in granulomatous versus vasculitic manifestations. *Ann Rheum Dis.* 2012;71:327–333.
119. Eriksson P. Nine patients with anti-neutrophil cytoplasmic antibody-positive vasculitis successfully treated with rituximab. *J Intern Med.* 2005;257:540–548.
120. Brihaye B, Aouba A, Pagnoux C, Cohen P, Lacassin F, Guillevin L. Adjunction of rituximab to steroids and immunosuppressants for refractory/relapsing Wegener's granulomatosis: a study on 8 patients. *Clin Exp Rheumatol.* 2007;25(1 suppl 44): S23–S27.
121. Ramos-Casals M, Garcia-Hernandez FJ, de Ramon E, et al; BIOGEAS Study Group. Off-label use of rituximab in 196 patients with severe, refractory systemic autoimmune diseases. *Clin Exp Rheumatol.* 2010;28:468–476.
122. de Menthon M, Cohen P, Pagnoux C, et al. Infliximab or rituximab for refractory Wegener's granulomatosis: long-term follow up. A prospective randomised multicentre study on 17 patients. *Clin Exp Rheumatol.* 2011;29(1 suppl 64):S63–S71.
123. Rees F, Yazdani R, Lanyon P. Long-term follow-up of different refractory systemic vasculitides treated with rituximab. *Clin Rheumatol.* 2011;30:1241–1245.
124. Roccatello D, Sciascia S, Rossi D, et al. Long-term effects of rituximab added to cyclophosphamide in refractory patients with vasculitis. *Am J Nephrol.* 2011;34:175–180.
125. Jones RB, Tervaert JW, Hauser T, et al; European Vasculitis Study Group. Rituximab versus cyclophosphamide in ANCA-associated renal vasculitis. *N Engl J Med.* 2010;363:211–220.
126. Stone JH, Merkel PA, Spiera R, et al; RAVE-ITN Research Group. Rituximab versus cyclophosphamide for ANCA-associated vasculitis. *N Engl J Med.* 2010;363:221–232.
127. Jayne DRW, Merkel PA, Schall TJ, Bekker P; ADVOCATE Study Group. Avacopan for the treatment of ANCA-associated vasculitis. *N Engl J Med.* 2021;384(7):599–609.
128. Guillevin L, Lhote F, Cohen P, et al. Polyarteritis nodosa related to hepatitis B virus. A prospective study with long-term observation of 41 patients. *Medicine (Baltimore).* 1995;74:238–253.
129. Casato M, Lagana B, Antonelli G, Dianzani F, Bonomo L. Long-term results of therapy with interferon-alpha for type II essential mixed cryoglobulinemia. *Blood.* 1991;78:3142–3147.
130. Davis GL, Balart LA, Schiff ER, et al; Hepatitis Interventional Therapy Group. Treatment of chronic hepatitis C with recombinant interferon alpha. A multicenter randomized controlled trial. *N Engl J Med.* 1989;321:1501–1506.
131. DiBisceglie AM, Martin P, Kassianides CK, et al. Recombinant interferon alpha therapy for chronic hepatitis C. A randomized, double-blind, placebo controlled trial. *N Engl J Med.* 1989;321:1501–1506.
132. Ferri C, Marzo E, Longombardo G, et al. Interferon-alpha in mixed cryoglobulinemia patients: a randomized, crossover-controlled trial. *Blood.* 1993;81:1132–1136.
133. Dammacco F, Sansonno D, Han JH, et al. Natural interferon-alpha versus its combination with 6-methyl-prednisolone in the therapy of type II mixed cryoglobulinemia: a long-term, randomized, controlled study. *Blood.* 1994;84:3336–3343.
134. Misiani R, Bellavita P, Fenili D, et al. Interferon alfa-2 a therapy in cryoglobulinemia associated with hepatitis C virus. *N Engl J Med.* 1994;330:751–756.
135. Lauta VM, De Sangro MA. Long-term results regarding the use of recombinant interferon alpha-2b in the treatment of II type mixed essential cryoglobulinemia. *Med Oncol.* 1995; 12:223–230.
136. Saadoun D, Resche-Rigon M, Thibault V, Piette JC, Cacoub P. Antiviral therapy for hepatitis C virus–associated mixed cryoglobulinemia vasculitis: a long-term followup study. *Arthritis Rheum.* 2006;54:3696–3706.
137. Mazzaro C, Monti G, Saccardo F, et al. Efficacy and safety of peginterferon alfa-2b plus ribavirin for HCV-positive mixed cryoglobulinemia: a multicentre open-label study. *Clin Exp Rheumatol.* 2011;29:933–941.
138. El Khayat HR, Fouad YM, El Amin H, Rizk A. A randomized trial of 24 versus 48 weeks of peginterferon alpha-2a plus ribavirin in Egyptian patients with hepatitis C virus genotype 4 and rapid viral response. *Trop Gastroenterol.* 2012;33: 112–117.
139. Lamprecht P, Lerin-Lozano C, Merz H, et al. Rituximab induces remission in refractory HCV associated cryoglobulinaemic vasculitis. *Ann Rheum Dis.* 2003;62(12):1230–1233.
140. Zaja F, De Vita S, Mazzaro C, et al. Efficacy and safety of rituximab in type II mixed cryoglobulinemia. *Blood.* 2003; 101(10):3827–3834.
141. Ramos-Casals M, Stone JH, Cid MC, Bosch X. The cryoglobulinaemias. *Lancet.* 2012;379:348–360.
142. Saadoun D, Delluc A, Piette JC, Cacoub P. Treatment of hepatitis C-associated mixed cryoglobulinemia vasculitis. *Curr Opin Rheumatol.* 2008;20:23–28.

143. Pietrogrande M, De Vita S, Zignego AL, et al. Recommendations for the management of mixed cryoglobulinemia syndrome in hepatitis C virus-infected patients. *Autoimmun Rev.* 2011;10:444–454.
144. Ferri C, Cacoub P, Mazzaro C, et al. Treatment with rituximab in patients with mixed cryoglobulinemia syndrome: results of multicenter cohort study and review of the literature. *Autoimmun Rev.* 2011;11:48–55.
145. Sansonno D, De Re V, Lauletta G, Tucci FA, Boiocchi M, Dammacco F. Monoclonal antibody treatment of mixed cryoglobulinemia resistant to interferon alpha with an anti-CD20. *Blood.* 2003;101:3818–3826.
146. Saadoun D, Resche-Rigon M, Sene D, Perard L, Karras A, Cacoub P. Rituximab combined with Peg-interferon-ribavirin in refractory hepatitis C virus-associated cryoglobulinaemia vasculitis. *Ann Rheum Dis.* 2008;67:1431–1436.
147. Petrarca A, Rigacci L, Caini P, et al. Safety and efficacy of rituximab in patients with hepatitis C virus-related mixed cryoglobulinemia and severe liver disease. *Blood.* 2010;116:335–342.
148. Visentini M, Ludovisi S, Petrarca A, et al. A phase II, single-arm multicenter study of low-dose rituximab for refractory mixed cryoglobulinemia secondary to hepatitis C virus infection. *Autoimmun Rev.* 2011;10:714–719.
149. De Vita S, Quartuccio L, Isola M, et al. A randomized controlled trial of rituximab for the treatment of severe cryoglobulinemic vasculitis. *Arthritis Rheum.* 2012;64:843–853.
150. Sneller MC, Hu Z, Langford CA. A randomized controlled trial of rituximab following failure of antiviral therapy for hepatitis C virus-associated cryoglobulinemic vasculitis. *Arthritis Rheum.* 2012;64:835–842.
151. Dammacco F, Tucci FA, Lauletta G, et al. Pegylated interferon-alpha, ribavirin, and rituximab combined therapy of hepatitis C virus-related mixed cryoglobulinemia: a long-term study. *Blood.* 2010;116:343–353.
152. Saadoun D, Resche Rigon M, Sene D, et al. Rituximab plus Peg-interferon-alpha/ribavirin compared with Peg-interferon-alpha/ribavirin in hepatitis C-related mixed cryoglobulinemia. *Blood.* 2010;116:326–334.

CHAPTER 16

Neuropathies Associated with Systemic Disease

Neuropathies are associated with a number of systemic disorders (Table 16-1).[1] Neuropathies related to vasculitis, infection, endocrinopathies, amyloidosis (hereditary and acquired), cancer, and medications are discussed in other chapters. The neuropathies discussed in this chapter may be directly or indirectly related to the systemic disorder (e.g., connective tissue diseases, nutritional deficiency due to malabsorption in gastrointestinal disease).

▶ NEUROPATHIES ASSOCIATED WITH CONNECTIVE TISSUE DISEASES

SJÖGREN SYNDROME

Clinical Features

Sjögren syndrome is characterized by the sicca complex: xerophthalmia (dry eyes), xerostomia (dry mouth), and dryness of other mucous membranes. It is more common in women and typically presents in middle adult life. Sjögren syndrome can be complicated by central nervous system (CNS) and peripheral nervous system (PNS) involvement. The CNS manifestations can mimic transverse myelitis or multiple sclerosis. Peripheral neuropathy occurs in 2%–22% of patients with Sjögren syndrome.[1–21]

Furthermore, peripheral neuropathy can be the presenting feature of Sjögren syndrome and develop in patients without the typical sicca symptoms. The most common form of peripheral neuropathy is a length-dependent axonal sensorimotor neuropathy characterized by numbness and tingling in the distal portions of the limbs.[1–3,7,8,10–13,17,19] Mild distal muscle weakness may also be seen. Occasionally, patients with SS can manifest with GBS (AIDP, AMAN, AMSAN) or CIDP.[22] A pure small fiber neuropathy characterized by burning discomfort and tingling is also common.[20–24] Signs of autonomic nervous system dysfunction involving the cardiovascular system are often evident.[25–29] Necrotizing vasculitis may be responsible for as many as one-third of the cases of neuropathy associated with Sjögren syndrome. Vasculitis should be suspected in patients with an asymmetric, multiple mononeuropathy pattern of involvement. Cranial neuropathies, particularly involving the trigeminal nerve, can also be seen.[30]

Sjögren syndrome is also associated with sensory neuronopathy/ganglionopathy that can be large or small fiber in nature.[1–4,8,11,16–18,20,31–36] Patients with sensory ganglionopathies develop progressive numbness and tingling of the limbs, trunk, and face. Symptoms and signs may be length-dependent or non–length-dependent, the later suggesting a small fiber ganglionopathy. Symptoms can involve the arms more than the legs, and involvement can be quite asymmetric or even unilateral. Patches of numbness may occur in unusual locations like the perioral regions, the back of the head, or the trunk. The onset can be acute or insidious. Sensory examination demonstrates severe vibratory and proprioceptive loss leading to sensory ataxia. Romberg sign is noted in patients with lower limb involvement. The lack of proprioception may lead to pseudoathetotic posturing of affected arms and legs. There can also be diminished sensation in the face. Signs of autonomic neuropathy also may be appreciated: Adie pupil, anhidrosis, fixed tachycardia, and orthostatic hypotension. Muscle stretch reflexes are often reduced or absent with large fiber involvement. Muscle strength is usually normal.

Laboratory Features

Patients with neuropathy due to Sjögren syndrome may have antinuclear antibodies (ANA), SS-A/Ro, and SS-B/La antibodies in the serum, but many do not.[8,34,35] Cerebrospinal fluid is usually normal. Schirmer test and Rose-Bengal stain are useful for diagnosing keratoconjunctivitis. The diagnosis can be confirmed by parotid gland or lip biopsies demonstrating a lymphocytic invasion of salivary glands. Salivary gland biopsies can demonstrate histopathological features of Sjögren syndrome even in patients without complaints of dry mouth.[8,34,35]

Nerve conduction studies (NCSs) in patients with distal sensorimotor polyneuropathy demonstrate absent or reduced amplitudes of sensory nerve action potentials (SNAPs) with normal or only mildly slow conduction velocities.[1–3,7,13] Motor conduction studies are less affected but may show slightly reduced amplitudes. Abnormal blink reflexes and cutaneous masseter inhibitory reflexes may be appreciated in patients with trigeminal neuropathy.[30] Patients with GBS or CIDP can have demyelinating features on NCS.[22]

NCSs in patients with sensory neuronopathy/ganglionopathy demonstrate absent or reduced amplitudes of the SNAPs in a non–length-dependent manner such that these may be abnormal in the arms while normal in the legs.[1–4,6,13,31–36] In addition, there may be asymmetric involvement. Motor

▶ **TABLE 16-1. NEUROPATHIES ASSOCIATED WITH SYSTEMIC DISORDERS**

Connective tissue disease
    Sjögren syndrome or sicca complex
    Rheumatoid arthritis
    Systemic lupus erythematosus
    Scleroderma
    Mixed connective tissue disease
    Drug-induced (e.g., TNF-alpha blockers)
Sarcoidosis
Celiac disease
Inflammatory bowel disease
    Ulcerative colitis
    Crohn disease
    Drug-induced (e.g., TNF-alpha blockers)
Hypereosinophilic syndrome
Uremia
Primary biliary sclerosis
Liver disease
Whipple disease
Gout
Critical illness polyneuropathy
Amyloidosis
    Acquired
    Familial
Vasculitis
    Giant cell arteritis
    Isolated peripheral nerve vasculitis
    Vasculitis associated with other systemic disease
        Granulomatosis with angiitis
        Polyarteritis nodosa
        Churg–Strauss syndrome
        Microscopic polyangiitis
Infection
    HIV
    HTLV1
    CMV
    EBV
    SARS-CoV-2
    Lyme
    Syphilis
Cancer
    Direct tumor infiltration of nerves
    Paraneoplastic
    Chemotherapy-induced (including checkpoint inhibitors)

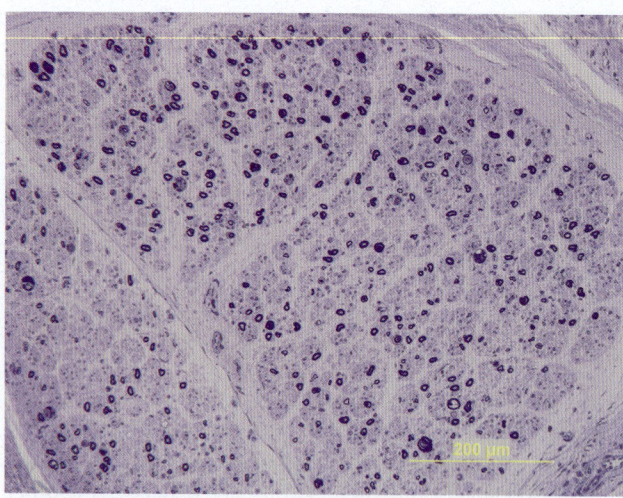

Figure 16-1. Sjögren syndrome. Sural nerve biopsy demonstrates a moderate reduction of large and small myelinated nerve fibers and evidence of axonal degeneration. Plastic section stained with toluidine blue.

conduction studies and electromyography (EMG) are usually normal. If the trigeminal nerve is affected, blink reflexes may also be abnormal.[37] An important clinical and electrophysiological feature that can help distinguish length-dependent sensory neuropathy from a sensory neuronopathy/ganglionopathy is the preservation of the masseter reflex or jaw jerk in the latter.[38] The masseter reflex is unique among the stretch reflexes in that the cell bodies of the afferent limb lie in the mesencephalic nucleus within the CNS as opposed to the dorsal root ganglia where the sensory cell bodies innervating the extremities lie. Thus, the mesencephalic nucleus is often spared in ganglionopathies and so the associated masseter reflex is preserved. In contrast, the Gasserian ganglion, which is responsible for conveying sensory nerves responsible for facial sensation and the blink reflex, reside outside the CNS, and thus the blink reflex may be abnormal.

Histopathology

Peripheral nerve biopsies in patients with the more common sensorimotor polyneuropathy demonstrate axonal degeneration and some degree of secondary segmental demyelination (Fig. 16-1).[1–3,7] Nonspecific perivascular inflammation involving perineurial or endoneurial blood vessels is occasionally seen. Rarely, necrotizing vasculitis is appreciated.

Biopsy of sensory nerves in patients with sensory neuronopathy/ganglionopathy may reveal a loss of large, myelinated fibers and perivascular lymphocytic (CD8 T cells) inflammation involving endoneurial or perineurial vessels.[2–4] Biopsy of the dorsal root ganglion have shown lymphocytic (mainly CD8 T cells) infiltration and degeneration of cell bodies.[4]

Reduced epidermal nerve fiber density or abnormal morphology may be demonstrated on skin biopsies and when seen in a non–length-dependent pattern suggests small fiber sensory neuronopathy/ganglionopathy rather than a "dying-back" axonopathy.[20–23]

Pathogenesis

The pathogenic basis of the distal sensory or sensorimotor polyneuropathy is unknown but is presumably autoimmune in nature. Some cases may be caused by vasculitis. The sensory neuronopathy/ganglionopathy appears to be the result of cell-mediated autoimmune attack directed against the sensory ganglia. The specific antigen(s) and trigger of the autoimmune attack are not known.

Treatment

There are no proven therapies for the neuropathies related to Sjögren syndrome. When vasculitis is suspected, immunosuppressive agents may be beneficial. IVIG may be useful in nonvasculitic sensory and sensorimotor neuropathies, however the benefit of such therapy in sensory neuronopathy/ganglionopathy is much less clear.[1,4,12,15–17,19,31,34–36,39–41]

RHEUMATOID ARTHRITIS

Clinical Features

Peripheral neuropathy occurs in at least 50% of patients with rheumatoid arthritis (RA).[1,14–16,42–49] Vasculitic neuropathy has been reported in develops in 35%–50% of patients with RA. Neuropathic symptoms usually manifest 10–15 years after manifestations of other symptoms of RA, although rarely the neuropathy can be the presenting feature. Rheumatoid vasculitis can present with multiple neuropathies or generalized symmetric pattern of involvement. In addition, the neuropathy associated with RA may be secondary to amyloid deposition.[42] Carpal tunnel syndrome is not uncommon, occurring in 10% of patients in one series.[42]

Demyelinating neuropathies [sensorimotor or pure sensory chronic inflammatory demyelinating polyneuropathy (CIDP), multifocal motor neuropathy] may develop as a complication of drugs used to treat the RA [e.g., antitumor necrosis factor-alpha (TNF-α) therapy and leflunomide].[50,51] These neuropathies may or may not improve after discontinuation of the TNF-α blocker. In cases in which the neuropathy does not get better, treatment with other immunotherapies (e.g., corticosteroids or IVIG) may be warranted.

Laboratory Features

ANA, elevated ESR, CRP, and rheumatoid factor are often detected in the serum.[49] NCSs in patients with vasculitic neuropathy demonstrate absent or reduced amplitudes of SNAPs and compound muscle action potentials (CMAPs), often in an asymmetric, non–length-dependent pattern with normal or only mildly slow conduction velocities. Those with neuropathy related to medications typically have features of demyelination.

Histopathology

Nerve biopsies often reveal thickening of the epineurial and endoneurial blood vessels as well as perivascular inflammation, perhaps related to the so-called microvasculitis (Fig. 16-2). Occasionally, there is necrotizing vasculitis with transmural inflammatory cell infiltration and fibrinoid necrosis of vessel walls. In a retrospective series of 108 patients with RA, 23 underwent sural nerve biopsies.[42] Abnormalities included perineurial thickening ($n = 5$), amyloid deposits ($n = 4$), perivascular infiltrate ($n = 4$), loss of myelin fibers ($n = 2$), and necrotizing vasculitis ($n = 1$).

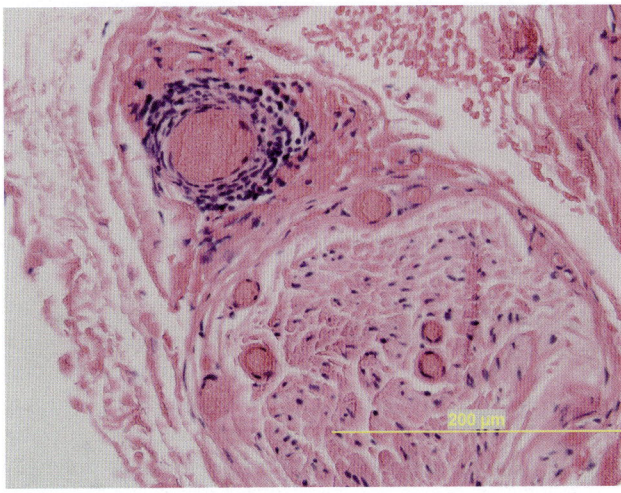

Figure 16-2. Rheumatoid arthritis. Sural nerve biopsy reveals an epineurial vessel with perivascular inflammation and scattered perineurial and endoneurial dilated capillaries with thickened walls. Paraffin section stained with hematoxylin and eosin (H&E).

Treatment

In most cases, the neuropathy is presumably autoimmune in nature and may respond to immunomodulating therapies used to treat RA. Of course, those with demyelinating polyneuropathy secondary to TNF-α blockage should first go off the medication. If the neuropathy does not improve, they may need to be treated as well with IVIG or corticosteroids; they should also avoid treatment with other TNF-α blockers in the future.

SYSTEMIC LUPUS ERYTHEMATOSUS

Clinical Features

Systemic lupus erythematosus (SLE) is a common connective tissue disease with prevalence in adults of approximately 1 in 2,000. SLE can be associated with multiple organ system involvement and associated laboratory abnormalities. CNS complications are more common than peripheral neuropathies, although 2%–41% of individuals with SLE clinically develop a peripheral neuropathy.[1,15,52–65] Most of the time the neuropathy manifests as slowly progressive sensory loss beginning in the feet. Some patients develop burning pain and paresthesia with normal reflexes and NCSs suggestive of a pure small fiber neuropathy.[57,58] Less common are mononeuropathies, cranial neuropathies, and multiple mononeuropathies. The longer the disease progresses, the more likely the multiple mononeuropathies are to fuse and overlap, creating an increasingly symmetric pattern that mimics a length-dependent axonal sensorimotor polyneuropathy. Of 1,533 patients in a large SLE database, 207 (14%) had a peripheral neuropathy.[52] Of these, 40% were non–SLE-related. Polyneuropathy was diagnosed in 56%, multiple mononeuropathies in

9%, cranial neuropathy in 13%, and mononeuropathy in 11% of patients. Most presentations were asymmetric (59%) and distal weakness occurred in 34%. Some patients present with a large or small fiber sensory ganglionopathy.[34,35,61] Additionally, patients may manifest with generalized sensorimotor polyneuropathy meeting clinical, laboratory, electrophysiological, and histological criteria for either acute or chronic inflammatory demyelinating polyneuropathy (AIDP or CIDP).[66-68]

Laboratory Features

ANA, anti–double-stranded DNA, and anti-Ro antibodies may be demonstrated in the serum. Abnormal NCSs occur in 24%–56% of patients with SLE.[55,56] Most commonly, the NCSs reveal a length-dependent, axonal sensory polyneuropathy.[69] However, as many as 20% of patients may have features of demyelination on NCSs.[52,66-68]

Histopathology

Nerve biopsies may demonstrate endoneurial mononuclear inflammatory infiltrates and increased expression of class II antigens within nerve fascicles and on endothelial cells, suggesting an autoimmune pathogenesis.[55] Upregulation of matrix metalloproteinase-3 and matrix metalloproteinase-9 within the vessel walls has also been observed.[70] Skin biopsies may reveal decreased density of epidermal nerve fibers suggestive of a small fiber neuropathy.[57,58]

Pathogenesis

The pathogenic basis of the associated neuropathy is likely multifactorial. Neuropathy may be related to the underlying vasculopathy characteristic of SLE, which however is rare associated with histological evidence of necrotizing vasculitis. Some patients may develop neuropathy due to other systemic complications of SLE (i.e., renal failure and uremic neuropathy).

Treatment

Immunosuppressive therapy is beneficial in patients with vasculitic neuropathy. Immunosuppressive agents are less likely to be effective in patients with a generalized sensory or sensorimotor polyneuropathy without evidence of vasculitis. Patients with an AIDP- or CIDP-like neuropathy should be treated accordingly (see Chapters 13 and 14).

SYSTEMIC SCLEROSIS (SCLERODERMA)

Scleroderma is associated with progressive fibrosis of the skin, gastrointestinal tract, kidney, and lung. A distal symmetric, mainly sensory, polyneuropathy complicates 5%–67% of cases.[14,16,71-79] Cranial mononeuropathies can also develop, most commonly affecting the trigeminal nerve, leading to numbness and dysesthesias in the face. Occasionally, seventh and ninth cranial neuropathies develop.

The CREST syndrome (calcinosis, Raynaud phenomenon, esophageal dysmotility, sclerodactyly, and telangiectasia) is considered a limited form of scleroderma. Multiple mononeuropathies have been described in a small percentage (1%–2%) of patients with CREST syndrome.[80] The electrophysiological and histological features of nerve biopsies are those of an axonal sensory greater than motor polyneuropathy.

MIXED CONNECTIVE TISSUE DISEASE

Mixed connective tissue disease represents an overlap syndrome of SLE, scleroderma, and myositis. A mild distal axonal sensorimotor polyneuropathy reportedly occurs in approximately 10% of patients.[14,81] Trigeminal neuropathy is also a recognized complication of this syndrome.

▶ OTHER PRESUMABLY IMMUNE-MEDIATED NEUROPATHIES

SARCOIDOSIS

Clinical Features

Sarcoidosis, a systemic granulomatous disorder, can affect the CNS, peripheral nerves, and muscle.[82-85] The etiology is unknown. Women are more commonly affected than men. Nonspecific constitutional symptoms of fever, weight loss, arthralgias, and fatigue are usually the presenting complaints of most patients. Erythematous subcutaneous nodules about the anterior shin and enlarged peripheral lymph nodes may be noted. Granulomatous uveitis can lead to significant visual impairment and even blindness. Pulmonary involvement as well as mucosal lesions of the nose and sinuses are common.

The PNS or CNS is involved in about 5% of patients with sarcoidosis and may be the presenting manifestation.[1,16,82-102] In the CNS, granulomas most typically involve the meninges, hypothalamus, and pituitary gland. Cranial nerves are also frequently involved. The most common cranial nerve to be involved is the seventh nerve, which can be affected bilaterally. Any cranial nerve may be affected however, particularly the second and eighth. Often the neuropathy is relapsing and remitting in nature. Some patients develop a radiculopathy or a polyradiculopathy. With a generalized root involvement, the clinical presentation can mimic AIDP or CIDP.[86-89] Rarely, patients may present with an acute sensory ataxia with sphincter dysfunction.[90] Patients can also present with mononeuropathies, multiple mononeuropathies, or a generalized, slowly progressive, primarily sensory greater than motor polyneuropathy.[91,92] Some have features of a pure small fiber neuropathy or a non–length-dependent neuronopathy/ganglionopathy pattern that is characterized by burning pain, paresthesia, allodynia, and occasional dysautonomia.[91-96,101,102]

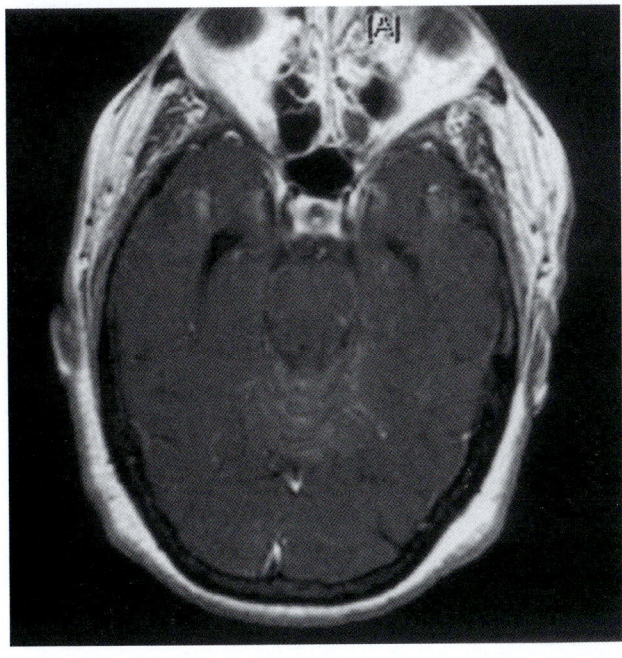 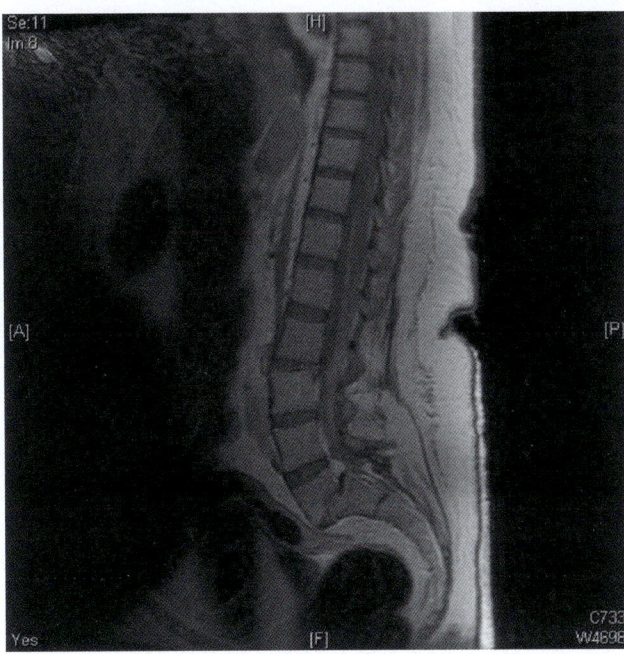

Figure 16-3. Sarcoidosis. MRI scan of the brain with contrast demonstrates enhancement of the meninges around the cerebellum (**A**) and of the cauda equina (**B**) in a patient who presented with multiple cranial neuropathies and a polyradiculopathy.

Laboratory Features

Hilar adenopathy is often but not always appreciated on chest radiographs. MRI scans may demonstrate enhancement of the meninges in the brain, particularly in the posterior fossa, and of affected spinal roots in patients with radiculopathy (Fig. 16-3).[91] PET and gallium scans can also demonstrate abnormalities. CSF may reveal pleocytosis and an elevated white blood cell count.[91] Angiotensin-converting enzyme (ACE) levels may be elevated in those with lung disease, but it is neither a very sensitive test nor a specific test. In patients with subclinical neuropathy, the most common finding is an absence or reduction in SNAP amplitudes in a mononeuropathy multiplex pattern.[85,97] In patients with the symmetric sensorimotor peripheral neuropathy, the SNAPs may be absent or reduced in amplitude.[85,98] Motor NCSs may also reveal reduced or absent CMAP amplitudes in the lower limbs, with decreased or borderline normal CMAPs in the upper limbs. Needle EMG can show features suggestive of a radiculopathy or polyradiculopathy.[83] Quantitative sensory testing often reveals abnormal thermal thresholds, and autonomic testing may be abnormal indicative of small fiber involvement.[94,96]

Histopathology

Nerve biopsies can reveal noncaseating granulomas infiltrating the endoneurium, perineurium, and epineurium along with lymphocytic necrotizing angiitis (Fig. 16-4).[85,92,99] There is a combination of axonal loss as well as demyelination. Muscle biopsies likewise can demonstrate noncaseating granulomas in the endomysium even in patients without an underlying myopathy.[85] Skin biopsies may reveal reduced intraepidermal nerve fiber density suggestive of a small fiber neuropathy in some patients.[93,95]

Pathogenesis

Sarcoidosis is an autoimmune disorder, although the etiology and pathogenic mechanism of the disorder is unclear. Neuropathies may result from invasion or direct compression

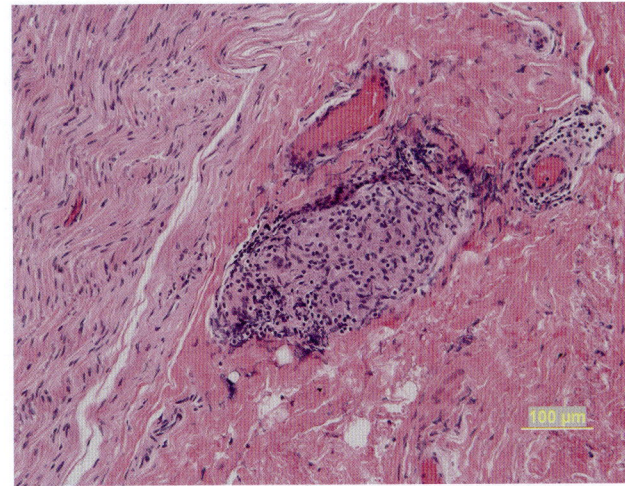

Figure 16-4. Sarcoidosis. Superficial peroneal nerve biopsy reveals a noncaseating granuloma and perivascular inflammation in the epineurium. Paraffin section stained with H&E.

by granulomas or as a result of ill-defined factors associated with inflammation such as cytokine toxicity or ischemic damage.[92] One also needs to consider a neuropathy associated with TNF-α blockade (in cases of demyelinating polyneuropathy).[50,51]

Treatment

There is a lack of randomized, controlled trials, but there is expert consensus that neurosarcoidosis, particularly of the cranial nerves, may respond well to corticosteroid treatment.[1,16,83,91,101,102] If patients are resistant to corticosteroids, other immunosuppressive/immunomodulating therapies can be tried (e.g., cyclosporine, methotrexate, IVIG, and TNF-α blockers).[1,16,100–102] Uncontrolled small series suggest that some patients with small fiber neuropathy may also respond to IVIG or TNF-α blockers (e.g., infliximab) as well.[101–103]

CELIAC DISEASE (GLUTEN-INDUCED ENTEROPATHY OR NONTROPICAL SPRUE)

Clinical Features

Intolerance to gluten, which is a protein found in wheat and wheat products, results in a malabsorption syndrome (weight loss, abdominal distention, and steatorrhea). Diagnosis of celiac disease is based on the documentation of (1) malabsorption, (2) demonstration of blunting and flattening of jejunal villi, and (3) clinical and histological improvement following the institution of a gluten-free diet.[104] A causal relationship between celiac disease and potential neurological complications remains somewhat controversial. The prevalence of neurological complications is variable and is estimated to occur in 2%–40% of patients with celiac disease, with ataxia and peripheral neuropathy being the most common problems.[1,104–107] The neuropathy associated with celiac disease usually manifests as distal sensory loss, paresthesias, and imbalance. Generalized sensorimotor polyneuropathy, motor neuropathy, multiple mononeuropathies, autonomic neuropathy, and neuromyotonia have also been reported in association with celiac disease or antigliadin/antiendomysial transglutaminase 6 (TG6) antibodies.[1,104–119] Neurological examination often demonstrates loss of large fiber sensory modalities, mild distal muscle weakness, reduced or absent muscle stretch reflexes, and an ataxic gait. Signs of a small fiber neuropathy or autonomic neuropathy may be evident.[113,114]

Laboratory Features

Antigliadin and anti-TG6 antibodies may be detected in the serum of patients with celiac disease but are neither sensitive nor specific.[120] NCSs usually demonstrate reduced SNAP amplitudes with only mildly reduced nerve conduction velocities (NCVs) or prolonged distal latencies.[105,106,111,112,115,116] Motor conduction studies demonstrate a mild reduction in the NCVs with preservation of distal motor latencies and CMAP amplitudes. Autonomic studies may be abnormal in patients with autonomic neuropathy.[114] Rare cases with neuromyotonic discharges have been appreciated.[111]

Histopathology

Nerve biopsy may reveal a loss of large myelinated fibers.[105] Skin biopsies can demonstrate loss of epidermal nerve fibers suggestive of a small fiber neuropathy in some patients.[113] In one small series, autopsy of three patients revealed inflammation in the dorsal root ganglia with degeneration of the posterior columns of the spinal cord.[117] In another report, a loss of Purkinje cells in the cerebellum was described along with degeneration of the posterior columns and corticospinal tracts, cortical atrophy and loss of neurons in the thalamus, basal ganglia, and brainstem.[110]

Pathogenesis

The neuropathy may be secondary to malabsorption of vitamins B12 and E. However, some patients have no appreciable vitamin deficiencies. The pathogenic basis for the neuropathy in these patients is unclear but may be autoimmune in etiology.[105,115]

Treatment

Some patients may improve with gluten-free diet,[108] many others do not.[104,117] In patients with vitamin B12 or E deficiency, replacement therapy may improve or stabilize the neuropathy.

Response to IVIG has been variable with some reporting no benefit,[105] while others noting improvement.[121]

INFLAMMATORY BOWEL DISEASE

Ulcerative colitis and Crohn disease are inflammatory disorders of the bowel and are associated with various neurological abnormalities including peripheral neuropathy.[1,122–132] Most patients present with a distal numbness, paresthesias, and pain and electrophysiological features of axonal distal, length-dependent sensory greater than motor polyneuropathy.[125,127,128,130,131] Demyelinating neuropathies occur in approximately one-third of patients.[122–125,127,132] In addition, small fiber neuropathy,[127,131] brachial plexopathy,[125,133] multiple mononeuropathies,[125] and cranial neuropathies[125] can complicate ulcerative colitis and Crohn disease. The neuropathies associated with inflammatory bowel disease may be autoimmune in nature, nutritional (e.g., vitamin B12 deficiency), secondary to toxicity of treatment (e.g., metronidazole, TNF-α blockers), or idiopathic. Toxic neuropathies associated with metronidazole and TNF-α blockers (discussed in greater detail in Chapter 19 regarding Toxic

Neuropathies).[134] Patients should be treated with immunotherapy when an autoimmune etiology is suspected (e.g., proximal and distal weakness and demyelination on NCSs; see Chapters 13 and 14). In addition, patients can develop weakness secondary to myasthenia gravis or myositis (including polymyositis, dermatomyositis, and granulomatous myositis), which likewise are treated with immunotherapy.

PRIMARY BILIARY CIRRHOSIS

Clinical Features

Primary biliary cirrhosis (PBC) is an autoimmune disorder directed against the biliary ducts in the liver. Peripheral neuropathy is the most common neurological complication of PBC. The neuropathy usually manifests with distal numbness and tingling.[135–137] Large fiber sensory modalities are predominantly affected, leading to reduced or absent muscle stretch reflexes. Muscle strength is typically normal but may be reduced in patients with a CIDP-like neuropathy.

Laboratory Features

Liver function tests are elevated, and antimitochondrial antibodies can be detected in the sera of some patients with PBC. NCS demonstrates reduced or absent SNAPs. The motor conduction and needle EMG portions of the evaluation are typically normal.

Histopathology

Nerve biopsies may reveal a loss of large, myelinated fibers without evidence of segmental demyelination.

Pathogenesis

The neuropathy could have an immunological basis or may be related to unknown toxins that might be accumulating secondary to the liver failure. In addition, the neuropathy may be associated with treatments (e.g., TNF-α blockade or metronidazole).

Treatment

PBC is treated with immunosuppressive therapy and ultimately liver transplantation. Whether or not transplantation affects the peripheral neuropathy has not been adequately addressed.

HYPEREOSINOPHILIC SYNDROME

The hypereosinophilic syndrome is characterized by eosinophilia associated with various skin, cardiac, hematologic, and neurological abnormalities.[138–140] Multiple mononeuropathies or a generalized, symmetric polyneuropathy occurs in 6%–14% of patients. In addition, some develop an inflammatory myopathy (see Chapter 33). NCSs reveal features suggestive of axonal sensorimotor peripheral neuropathy. The pathogenic basis for the neuropathy is not known but may be autoimmune in nature. The multiple organ dysfunction, including the PNS, is believed to occur as a result of the eosinophilia or some byproducts of the eosinophils.

▶ OTHER NEUROPATHIES ASSOCIATED WITH SYSTEMIC DISEASE

UREMIC NEUROPATHY

Clinical Features

Renal failure is associated with both CNS and PNS complications.[1,141–145] At least 60% of patients with renal failure (usually with glomerular filtration rates below 12 mL/min) develop neuropathy characterized by length-dependent numbness, tingling, and allodynia. Muscle cramps in the distal legs and restless legs syndrome are also common. Reduced sensation, particularly large fiber modalities, and diminished muscle stretch reflexes are appreciated on neurological examination. Mild distal greater than proximal muscle weakness may be noted. Rarely, patients develop rapidly progressive weakness and sensory loss very similar to AIDP, which improves with an increase in renal dialysis or transplantation.[141,142,145]

Mononeuropathies can also occur, the most common of which is carpal tunnel syndrome. These neuropathies are often related to hemodialysis equipment that uses a cuprophane membrane. This is because this membrane fails to completely remove a small β2-microglobulin, that is normally catabolized by the healthy kidney. β2-Microglobulin can deposit throughout the body, including the transverse carpal ligament. Individuals who are affected are also prone to developing ulnar neuropathy at the elbow and peroneal nerve injury about the fibular head. Damage to the brachial plexus or the peripheral nerves may also occur secondary to improper limb positioning or traction during renal transplant surgery. Ischemic monomelic neuropathy affecting the median, ulnar, and radial nerves can complicate arteriovenous shunts created in the arm for dialysis.[146]

NCSs in patients with uremia reveal features of a length-dependent, primarily axonal, sensorimotor polyneuropathy.[143,144,147–151] Sensory studies are reduced in amplitude, if obtainable, distal latencies are prolonged, and conduction velocities are slow. Most patients have either prolonged or absent H-reflexes, and somatosensory-evoked potential studies reveal both peripheral and central slowing of conduction. Motor conduction studies reveal normal or mildly reduced amplitudes. Distal latencies and conduction velocities can be normal or reflect moderate slowing of conduction. F-waves are usually absent or demonstrate delayed latencies. The posterior tibial and peroneal motor studies are affected earlier than the median and ulnar studies.

Patients with mononeuropathies often have NCSs compatible with superimposed focal demyelination or axonal loss.

With ischemic monomelic neuropathy, the EMG and NCS abnormalities reveal severe axonopathy in the territory of the ischemic insult.[146] The median, radial, and ulnar SNAPs may be absent or reduced in amplitude, depending on the degree and duration of ischemia. If CMAPs are elicited, the distal motor latencies are relatively normal as are the conduction velocities. Pseudoconduction block or actual conduction block may be seen across the ischemic segments, particularly within the first week of injury before complete Wallerian degeneration of the affected nerve distal to the nerve infarct can occur. Needle EMG demonstrates a marked reduction in motor unit action potentials (MUAPs) with abundant positive sharp waves and fibrillation potentials along with decreased recruitment. The pattern of EMG abnormalities is typically length dependent, affecting distal more than proximal muscles innervated by the same peripheral nerve.

Histopathology

In uremic neuropathy, sural nerve biopsies demonstrate a loss of nerve fibers, particularly the large, myelinated nerve fibers; active axonal degeneration; and segmental and paranodal demyelination.[152] At autopsy, chromatolysis of anterior horn cells and degeneration of the fasciculus gracilis have been noted in the spinal cord.

Pathogenesis

It is unclear what the primary pathophysiological mechanism of uremic neuropathy is and equally unclear whether the Schwann cell or the axon is the primary target of the essential metabolic or toxic abnormality.

Treatment

The sensorimotor polyneuropathy may be stabilized by hemodialysis and improved upon successful renal transplant, if performed prior to the loss of large numbers of axons.[144,145,153–157] Patients with carpal tunnel syndrome can be treated with surgical release. Median neuropathy at the wrist related to amyloid deposition in the form of β2-microglobulin is much less common nowadays with newer dialysis techniques currently in use. Patients with ischemic monomelic neuropathy should undergo revision of their shunt so as to allow more blood flow to the nerves. If treated early enough, the motor and sensory symptoms can resolve quickly, indicating an ischemic-induced conduction block rather than peripheral nerve infarction. Severe ischemia resulting in infarction is associated with a delayed and incomplete recovery.

CHRONIC LIVER DISEASE

Generalized sensorimotor peripheral neuropathy, characterized by numbness, tingling, and minor weakness in the distal aspects of primarily the lower limbs, commonly occurs in patients with chronic liver failure.[158–162] In addition, autonomic dysfunction is present in approximately 50% of patients with severe liver disease.[162] The cause of the neuropathy is quite variable. Neuropathy may be directly related to the underlying cause of the liver disease (e.g., alcoholism, viral infection, porphyria, amyloidosis, mitochondrial cytopathy), associated nutritional deficiencies, and complications of treatment such as transplantation (e.g., toxic effect of drugs or altered immunity related to immunosuppression). It is not known if hepatic failure in and of itself can cause peripheral neuropathy. Perhaps, toxins may accumulate secondary to the liver disease that could damage peripheral nerves. Electrophysiological abnormalities are thus variable and dependent on the cause of the liver failure. Most often, NCSs demonstrate reduced SNAP amplitudes, while motor NCSs are usually normal or show only slightly diminished amplitudes. Quantitative sensory and autonomic tests are abnormal in most patients.[162] Sural nerve biopsies reveal both segmental demyelination and axonal loss.

WHIPPLE DISEASE

Clinical Features

Whipple disease is characterized by abdominal pain, diarrhea, malabsorption, weight loss, arthralgias, fever, and peripheral lymphadenopathy, accompanied by enlargement of the celiac, mesenteric, and periaortic lymph nodes.[163–166] CNS involvement can lead to dementia, supranuclear ophthalmoparesis, convergence nystagmus, myoclonus, oromandibular myorhythmia, insomnia, hyperphagia, and polydipsia. Rarely, patients develop a sensorimotor polyneuropathy.[163–166]

Laboratory Features

The cerebrospinal fluid examination in patients with CNS involvement typically demonstrates polymorphonuclear cells and macrophages. MRI scans reveal gadolinium enhancement suggestive of ependymitis/meningitis. Sensory and motor NCSs may demonstrate reduced amplitudes with mild impairment of conduction velocities.[163]

Histopathology

Small bowel biopsies demonstrate PAS-positive macrophages containing the gram-positive rod-shaped bacterium, *Tropheryma whippeli*, in the mucosa. The organism can also be identified in the CNS, but there have been no reports of peripheral nerve or muscle histopathology in patients with suspected neuropathy or myopathy.

Pathogenesis

Whipple disease is caused by the actinomycete—*T. whippeli*. The pathogenic basis of the neuropathy is not known, but some symptoms of the polyneuropathy may be the result of malabsorption of necessary vitamins. Another possibility is that the neuropathy may be caused by bacterial infiltration and subsequent inflammatory involvement of the peripheral nerves.

Treatment

Whipple disease can be treated with chloramphenicol and trimethoprim-sulfamethoxazole.[73]

▶ GOUT

Gout is the most common cause of inflammatory arthritis in the world, and one large cross-sectional study of 442 patients with gout from China reported a prevalence of neuropathy in this population to be approximately 11%.[167] Some patients with gout develop a length-dependent sensory loss or mononeuropathies at the usual sites of compression at the wrist and elbow.[167,168] Sensory and motor NCSs may reveal reduced amplitudes with normal or only mild alterations of conduction velocities or distal latencies.

CRITICAL ILLNESS POLYNEUROPATHY

Background

The most common causes of acute generalized weakness leading to admission to a medical intensive care unit (ICU) are Guillain–Barré syndrome (GBS) and myasthenia gravis. However, weakness developing in patients who are critically ill while in the ICU is usually caused by critical illness polyneuropathy (CIP),[169–172] critical illness myopathy (CIM) (also known as acute quadriplegic myopathy),[173–179] or, much less commonly, prolonged neuromuscular blockade.[180] From a clinical and electrophysiological standpoint, it can be quite difficult to distinguish these disorders. Although a few authorities believe that CIP is more frequent than CIM, most specialists and the authors' own anecdotal experiences suggest that CIM is much more common than CIP.[176,178,181] In a series of 88 patients who developed weakness while in an ICU, CIM was three times as common as CIP (42% vs. 13%); prolonged neuromuscular blockade occurred in only one patient who also had CIM.[176] In patients who survive the underlying sepsis and multiorgan failure, muscle strength recovers slowly over several months.

Clinical Features

CIP can develop as a complication of sepsis and multiple organ failure.[169–172] Neuropathies are common in the subset of critically ill patients due to extensive burn surfaces.[182,183] Often, CIP presents as an inability to wean a patient from a ventilator. Concomitant encephalopathy may limit the neurological examination, in particular the sensory examination; however, generalized weakness can still be appreciated. Cranial nerves are relatively spared, although mild facial weakness can occur. Muscle stretch reflexes are absent or reduced.

Laboratory Features

Serum creatine kinase (CK) is usually normal. An elevated serum CK would point to CIM as opposed to CIP. Ultrasound may demonstrate abnormal swelling and hypoechogenicity of nerves in CIP.[184,185]

The electrophysiological hallmark is markedly reduced amplitudes or absent CMAPs with preserved motor conduction velocities and distal motor latencies.[172–179,186] Repetitive stimulation studies should be normal. The SNAPs are significantly diminished in amplitude or absent. Importantly, it is important to recognize that low-amplitude SNAPs do not necessarily implicate CIP as the cause of weakness. Patients may have an age-related decrease in SNAP amplitudes or the SNAPs may be abnormal secondary to an underlying coincidental condition (e.g., diabetes mellitus and uremia). In addition, lower extremity edema is common in these patients potentially obscuring SNAPs on a technical basis. Thus, the patients could still have CIM rather than CIP even if the SNAPs are abnormal. Lastly, CIP and CIM are not mutually exclusive and may occur concurrently.[187]

Needle EMG in CIP usually reveals profuse positive sharp waves and fibrillation potentials. It is not unusual for patients with severe weakness to be unable to recruit MUAPs. When MUAPs are recruited, these are often small and polyphasic in morphology. These small units have been attributed to early reinnervation but may occur because there is degeneration of distal motor nerve terminals without reinnervation early in the course. Thus, MUAP morphology may resemble what is commonly seen in myopathies. Most published studies fail to discuss the recruitment pattern of MUAPs. One would expect to see decreased recruitment of these small MUAPs in a neurogenic process. However, decreased recruitment can also be seen in severe myopathies when all the muscle fibers of a motor unit have degenerated. Nevertheless, if one sees early recruitment of small duration, polyphasic MUAPs, CIM is most likely.

Direct muscle stimulation may help distinguish CIP from CIM, as it bypasses the distal motor nerve and neuromuscular junction.[177,178] In a neuropathic process or prolonged neuromuscular blockade, the muscle membranes should retain its excitability and the direct muscle stimulation CMAP amplitude should be near normal compared to the low or absent nerve stimulation–evoked CMAP. In contrast, in CIM in which there is reduced muscle membrane excitability, both the nerve stimulation–evoked and the direct muscle stimulation CMAPs are reduced. The ratio of nerve stimulation–evoked CMAP to direct muscle stimulation CMAP should be close to 1:1 (>0.9) in CIM and should approach zero (0.1 or less) in a CIP or neuromuscular junction disorder.

Histopathology

Nerve biopsies demonstrate axonal degeneration.[172] On autopsies, chromatolysis of anterior horn cells, loss of dorsal root ganglion cells, and axonal degeneration of motor and sensory nerves have been observed.[172] Muscle biopsies may reveal atrophic and targetoid or core-like lesion fibers suggestive of acute neurogenic process.[172] However, these light microscopic features can be seen in myopathies. Other studies have found loss of myosin thick filaments on muscle biopsy and morphology of intramuscular nerves and those of multiple nerve roots and proximal nerves to be normal on autopsy, suggesting that these cases may all be CIM.[181]

Pathogenesis

The pathogenic basis of CIP is not known. Perhaps, circulating toxins and metabolic abnormalities associated with sepsis and multiorgan failure impair axonal transport or mitochondrial function, leading to axonal degeneration.[172] As mentioned, some have questioned the existence of CIP and suggested that most, if not all, such cases are CIM.

Treatment

There is no specific therapy for critical illness neuropathy other than supportive care and treatment of the underlying sepsis and organ failure.

► SUMMARY

As discussed, neuropathies may complicate many different systemic disorders. It is important to distinguish neuropathies that may be directly related to the underlying disorder, caused by treatment (toxic neuropathy), or just be coincidental occurrence as management may differ according to the etiology. Thus, as discussed in Chapter 1, it is always important to take a detailed medical history and examination to assess for an underlying systemic disorder that may be associated with the neuropathy.

REFERENCES

1. Bowley MP, Ropper AH. Neuropathies in systemic disease. *Semin Neurol.* 2015;35(4):431–447.
2. Gemignani F, Marbini A, Pavesi G, et al. Peripheral neuropathy associated with primary Sjögren's syndrome. *J Neurol Neurosurg Psychiatry.* 1994;57(8):983–986.
3. Grant IA, Hunder GG, Homburger HA, Dyck PJ. Peripheral neuropathy associated with sicca complex. *Neurology.* 1997;48:855–862.
4. Griffin JW, Cornblath DR, Alexander E, et al. Ataxic sensory neuropathy and dorsal root ganglionitis associated with Sjögren's syndrome. *Ann Neurol.* 1990;27(3):304–315.
5. Kennett RP, Harding AE. Peripheral neuropathy associated with sicca syndrome. *J Neurol Neurosurg Psychiatry.* 1986;49:90–92.
6. Malinow K, Yannakakis GD, Glusman SM, et al. Subacute sensory neuronopathy secondary to dorsal root ganglionitis in primary Sjögren's syndrome. *Ann Neurol.* 1986;20(4):535–537.
7. Mellgren S, Conn DL, Steven JC, Dyck PJ. Peripheral neuropathy in primary Sjögren's syndrome. *Neurology.* 1989;39(3):390–394.
8. Gorson KC, Ropper AH. Positive salivary gland biopsy, Sjögren syndrome, and neuropathy: clinical implications. *Muscle Nerve.* 2003;28(5):553–560.
9. Ramos-Casals M, Anaya J-M, García-Carrasco M, et al. Cutaneous vasculitis in primary Sjögren syndrome: classification and clinical significance of 52 patients. *Medicine (Baltimore).* 2004;83(2):96–106.
10. Mori K, Iijima M, Sugiura M, et al. Sjögren's syndrome associated painful sensory neuropathy without sensory ataxia. *J Neurol Neurosurg Psychiatry.* 2003;74(9):1320–1322.
11. Mori K, Iijima M, Koike H, et al. The wide spectrum of clinical manifestations in Sjögren's syndrome-associated neuropathy. *Brain.* 2005;128(Pt 11):2518–2534.
12. Font J, Ramos-Casals M, de la Red G, et al. Pure sensory neuropathy in primary Sjögren's syndrome. Longterm prospective followup and review of the literature. *J Rheumatol.* 2003;30(7):1552–1557.
13. Pavlakis PP, Alexopoulos H, Kosmidis ML, et al. Peripheral neuropathies in Sjögren syndrome: a new reappraisal. *J Neurol Neurosurg Psychiatry.* 2011;82(7):798–802.
14. Rosenbaum R. Neuromuscular complications of connective tissue diseases. *Muscle Nerve.* 2001;24(2):154–169.
15. Pavlakis PP. Rheumatologic disorders and the nervous system. *Continuum (Minneap Minn).* 2020;26(3):591–610.
16. Gwathmey KG, Satkowiak K. Peripheral nervous system manifestations of rheumatological diseases. *J Neurol Sci.* 2021;424:117421.
17. Liampas A, Parperis K, Erotocritou MF, et al. Primary Sjögren syndrome-related peripheral neuropathy: a systematic review and meta-analysis. *Eur J Neurol.* 2023;30(1):255–265.
18. Pereira PR, Viala K, Maisonobe T, et al. Sjögren sensory neuronopathy (Sjögren ganglionopathy): long-term outcome and treatment response in a series of 13 cases. *Medicine (Baltimore).* 2016;95(19):e3632.
19. Cafaro G, Perricone C, Carubbi F, et al. Peripheral nervous system involvement in Sjögren's syndrome: analysis of a cohort from the Italian Research Group on Sjögren's syndrome. *Front Immunol.* 2021;12:615656.
20. Descamps E, Henry J, Labeyrie C, et al. Small fiber neuropathy in Sjögren syndrome: comparison with other small fiber neuropathies. *Muscle Nerve.* 2020;61(4):515–520.
21. Seeliger T, Dreyer HN, Siemer JM, et al. Clinical and paraclinical features of small fiber neuropathy in Sjögren's syndrome. *J Neurol.* 2023;270(2):1004–1010.
22. Cao X, Guo J, Yang Y, Yu Z, Pan H, Zhou W. Clinical characteristics of Guillain-Barré syndrome in patients with primary Sjögren's syndrome. *Sci Rep.* 2024;14(1):5783.
23. Chai J, Herrmann DN, Stanton M, Barbano RL, Logigian EL. Painful small-fiber neuropathy in Sjögren syndrome. *Neurology.* 2005;65:925–927.
24. Lopate G, Pestronk A, Al-Lozi M, et al. Peripheral neuropathy in an outpatient cohort of patients with Sjögren's syndrome. *Muscle Nerve.* 2006;33(5):672–676.
25. Kovács L, Paprika D, Tákacs R, et al. Cardiovascular autonomic dysfunction in primary Sjögren's syndrome. *Rheumatology (Oxford).* 2004;43(1):95–99.
26. Goto H, Matsuo H, Fukudome T, Shibuya N, Ohnishi A, Nakamura H. Chronic autonomic neuropathy in a patient with primary Sjögren's syndrome. *J Neurol Neurosurg Psychiatry.* 2000;69(1):135.
27. Kaur D, Tiwana H, Stino A, Sandroni P. Autonomic neuropathies. *Muscle Nerve.* 2021;63(1):10–21.

28. Brunetta E, Shiffer D, Mandelli P, et al. Autonomic abnormalities in patients with primary Sjogren's syndrome - preliminary results. *Front Physiol*. 2019;10:1104.
29. Koh JH, Kwok SK, Lee J, Park SH. Autonomic dysfunction in primary Sjogren's syndrome: a prospective cohort analysis of 154 Korean patients. *Korean J Intern Med*. 2017;32(1):165–173.
30. Urban PP, Keilmann A, Teichmann EM, Hopf HC. Sensory neuropathy of the trigeminal, glossopharyngeal, and vagal nerves in Sjögren's syndrome. *J Neurol Sci*. 2001;186(1–2):59–63.
31. Asahina M, Kuwabuara S, Asahina M, Nakajima M, Hattori T. D-penicillamine treatment for chronic sensory ataxia neuropathy associated with Sjögren's syndrome. *Neurology*. 1998; 51:1451–1453.
32. Hankey GJ, Gubbay SS. Peripheral neuropathy associated with sicca syndrome. *J Neurol Neurosurg Psychiatry*. 1987;50:1085–1086.
33. Laloux P, Brucher JM, Guerit JM, Sindic CJ, Laterre EC. Subacute sensory neuronopathy associated with Sjögren's sicca syndrome. *J Neurol*. 1988;235:352–354.
34. Amato AA, Ropper AH. Sensory ganglionopathy. *N Engl J Med*. 2020;383(17):1657–1662.
35. Gwathmey KG. Sensory neuronopathies. *Muscle Nerve*. 2016; 53(1):8–19.
36. Sheikh SI, Amato AA. The dorsal root ganglion under attack: the acquired sensory ganglionopathies. *Pract Neurol*. 2010;10(6):326–334.
37. Auger RG, Windebank AJ, Lucchinetti CF, Chalk CH. Role of the blink reflex in the evaluation of sensory neuronopathy. *Neurology*. 1999;53:407–408.
38. Auger RG. The role of the masseter reflex in the assessment of subacute sensory neuropathy. *Muscle Nerve*. 1998;21:800–801.
39. Kizawa M, Mori K, Iijima M, Koike H, Hattori N, Sobue G. Intravenous immunoglobulin treatment in painful sensory neuropathy without sensory ataxia associated with Sjögren's syndrome. *J Neurol Neurosurg Psychiatry*. 2006;77(8):967–969.
40. Chen WH, Yeh JH, Chiu HC. Plasmapheresis in the treatment of ataxic sensory neuropathy associated with Sjögren's syndrome. *Eur Neurol*. 2001;45(4):270–274.
41. Rist S, Sellam J, Hachulla E, et al; Club Rhumatismes et Inflammation. Experience of intravenous immunoglobulin therapy in neuropathy associated with primary Sjögren's syndrome: a national multicentric retrospective study. *Arthritis Care Res*. 2011;63(9):1339–1344.
42. Agarwal V, Singh R, Wiclaf, et al. A clinical, electrophysiological, and pathological study of neuropathy in rheumatoid arthritis. *Clin Rheumatol*. 2008;27(7):841–844.
43. Bayrak AO, Durmus D, Durmaz Y, Demir I, Canturk F, Onar MK. Electrophysiological assessment of polyneuropathic involvement in rheumatoid arthritis: relationships among demographic, clinical and laboratory findings. *Neurol Res*. 2010;32:711–714.
44. Chamberlain MA, Bruckner FE. Rheumatoid neuropathy: clinical and electrophysiologic features. *Ann Rheum Dis*. 1970; 29:609–616.
45. Peyronnard J-M, Charron L, Beaudet F, Couture F. Vasculitic neuropathy in rheumatoid disease and Sjögren's syndrome. *Neurology*. 1982;32:839–845.
46. Scott DG, Bacon PA, Elliott PJ, Tribe CR, Wallington TB. Systemic vasculitis in a district general hospital 1972-1980: clinical and laboratory features, classification and prognosis of 80 cases. *Q J Med*. 1982;51(203):292–311.
47. Weller RO, Bruckner FE, Chamberlain MA. Rheumatoid neuropathy: a histological and electrophysiological study. *J Neurol Neurosurg Psychiatry*. 1970;33:592–604.
48. Conn DL, McDuffie FC, Dyck PJ. Immunopathologic study of sural nerves in rheumatoid arthritis. *Arthritis Rheum*. 1972;15(2):135–143.
49. Makol A, Crowson CS, Wetter DA, Sokumbi O, Matteson EL, Warrington KJ. Vasculitis associated with rheumatoid arthritis: a case-control study. *Rheumatology (Oxford)*. 2014; 53(5):890–899.
50. Lozeron P, Denier C, Lacroix C, Adams D. Long-term course of demyelinating neuropathies occurring during tumor necrosis factor-alpha-blocker therapy. *Arch Neurol*. 2009;66:490–497.
51. Alshekhlee A, Basiri K, Miles JD, Ahmad SA, Katirji B. Chronic inflammatory demyelinating polyneuropathy associated with tumor necrosis factor-alpha antagonists. *Muscle Nerve*. 2010;41:723–727.
52. Florica B, Aghdassi E, Su J, Gladman DD, Urowitz MB, Fortin PR. Peripheral neuropathy in patients with systemic lupus erythematosus. *Semin Arthritis Rheum*. 2011;41:203–211.
53. Hughes RA, Cameron JS, Hass SM, Heaton J, Payan J, Teoh R. Multiple mononeuropathy as an initial presentation of systemic lupus erythematosus—nerve biopsy and response to plasma exchange. *J Neurol*. 1982;228:239–247.
54. McCombe PA, McLeod JG, Pollard JD, Guo YP, Ingall TJ. Peripheral sensorimotor and autonomic neuropathy associated with systemic lupus erythematosus. Clinical, pathological and immunological features. *Brain*. 1987;110:533–549.
55. McNicholl JM, Glynn D, Mongey A-B, Hutchinson M, Bresihan B. A prospective study of neurophysiologic, neurologic, and immunologic abnormalities in systemic lupus erythematosus. *J Rheumatol*. 1994;21:1061–1066.
56. Sivri A, Hasçelik Z, Celiker R, Başgöze O. Early detection of neurological involvement in systemic lupus erythematosus patients. *Electromyogr Clin Neurophysiol*. 1995;35:195–199.
57. Omdal R, Mellgren SI, Gøransson L, et al. Small nerve fiber involvement in systemic lupus erythematosus: a controlled study. *Arthritis Rheum*. 2002;46(5):1228–1232.
58. Goransson LG, Tjensvoll AB, Herigstad A, Mellgren SI, Omdal R. Small-diameter nerve fiber neuropathy in systemic lupus erythematosus. *Arch Neurol*. 2006;63(3):401–404.
59. Enevoldson TP, Wiles CM. Severe vasculitic neuropathy in systemic lupus erythematosus and response to cyclophosphamide. *J Neurol Neurosurg Psychiatry*. 1991;54:468–469.
60. Jasmin R, Sockalingam S, Ramanaidu LP, Goh KJ. Clinical and electrophysiological characteristics of symmetric polyneuropathy in a cohort of systemic lupus erythematosus patients. *Lupus*. 2015;24(3):248–255.
61. Oomatia A, Fang H, Petri M, Birnbaum J. Peripheral neuropathies in systemic lupus erythematosus: clinical features, disease associations, and immunologic characteristics evaluated over a twenty-five-year study period. *Arthritis Rheum*. 2014;66(4):1000–1009.
62. Hanly JG, Li Q, Su L, et al. Peripheral nervous system disease in systemic lupus erythematosus: results from an international inception cohort study. *Arthritis Rheumatol*. 2020;72(1):67–77.
63. Bortoluzzi A, Silvagni E, Furini F, Piga M, Govoni M. Peripheral nervous system involvement in systemic lupus erythematosus: a review of the evidence. *Clin Exp Rheumatol*. 2019;37(1):146–155.

64. Toledano P, Orueta R, Rodríguez-Pintó I, Valls-Solé J, Cervera R, Espinosa G. Peripheral nervous system involvement in systemic lupus erythematosus: prevalence, clinical and immunological characteristics, treatment and outcome of a large cohort from a single centre. *Autoimmun Rev.* 2017;16(7):750–755.
65. Kissel JT, Slivka AP, Warmolts JR, Mendell JR. The clinical spectrum of necrotizing angiopathy of the peripheral nervous system. *Ann Neurol.* 1985;18:251–257.
66. Rechtland E, Cornblath DR, Stern BJ, Meyerhoff JO. Chronic demyelinating polyneuropathy in systemic lupus erythematosus. *Neurology.* 1984;34:1375–1377.
67. Lewis M, Gibson T. Systemic lupus erythematosus with recurrent Guillain–Barré-like syndrome treated with intravenous immunoglobulins. *Lupus.* 2003;12:857–859.
68. Ait Benhaddou E, Birouk N, El Alaoui-Faris M, et al. Acute Guillain–Barré-like polyradiculoneuritis revealing acute systemic lupus erythematosus: two case studies and review of the literature. *Rev Neurol.* 2003;159(3):300–306.
69. Omdal R, Løseth S, Torbergsen T, Koldingsnes W, Husby G, Mellgren SI. Peripheral neuropathy in systemic lupus erythematosus—a longitudinal study. *Acta Neurol Scand.* 2001;103(6):386–391.
70. Mawrin C, Brunn A, Röcken C, Schröder JM. Peripheral neuropathy in systemic lupus erythematosus: pathomorphological features and distribution pattern of matrix metalloproteinases. *Acta Neuropathol (Berl).* 2003;105(4):365–372.
71. Dierckx RA, Aichner F, Gerstenbrand F, Fritsch P. Progressive systemic sclerosis and nervous system involvement. *Eur Neurol.* 1987;26:134–140.
72. Hietaharju A, Jääskeläinen S, Kalimo H, Hietarinta M. Peripheral neuromuscular manifestations in systemic sclerosis (scleroderma). *Muscle Nerve.* 1993;16:1204–1212.
73. Lecky BR, Hughes RA, Murray NM. Trigeminal sensory neuropathy: a study of 22 cases. *Brain.* 1987;110:1463–1485.
74. Lee P, Bruni J, Sukenik S. Neurological manifestations in systemic sclerosis (scleroderma). *J Rheumatol.* 1984;11:480–483.
75. Poncelet AN, Connolly MK. Peripheral neuropathy in scleroderma. *Muscle Nerve.* 2003;28:330–335.
76. AlMehmadi BA, To FZ, Anderson MA, Johnson SR. Epidemiology and treatment of peripheral neuropathy in systemic sclerosis. *J Rheumatol.* 2021;48(12):1839–1849.
77. Raja J, Balaikerisnan T, Ramanaidu LP, Goh KJ. Large fiber peripheral neuropathy in systemic sclerosis: a prospective study using clinical and electrophysiological definition. *Int J Rheum Dis.* 2021;24(3):347–354.
78. Amaral TN, Peres FA, Lapa AT, Marques-Neto JF, Appenzeller S. Neurologic involvement in scleroderma: a systematic review. *Semin Arthritis Rheum.* 2013;43(3):335–347.
79. Paik JJ, Mammen AL, Wigley FM, Shah AA, Hummers LK, Polydefkis M. Symptomatic and electrodiagnostic features of peripheral neuropathy in scleroderma. *Arthritis Care Res (Hoboken).* 2016;68(8):1150–1157.
80. Dyck PJ, Hunder GG, Dyck PJ. A case-control and nerve biopsy study of CREST multiple mononeuropathy. *Neurology.* 1997;49:1641–1645.
81. Bennet RM, Bong DM, Spargo BH. Neuropsychiatric problems in mixed connective tissue disease. *Am J Med.* 1978;65:955–962.
82. Delaney P. Neurologic manifestations of sarcoidosis. *Ann Intern Med.* 1977;87:336–345.
83. Koffman B, Junck L, Elias SB, Feit HW, Levine SR. Polyradiculopathy in sarcoidosis. *Muscle Nerve.* 1999;22:608–613.
84. Zuniga G, Ropper AH, Frank J. Sarcoid peripheral neuropathy. *Neurology.* 1991;41:1558–1561.
85. Said G, Lacroix C, Planté-Bordeneuve V, et al. Nerve granulomas and vasculitis in sarcoid peripheral neuropathy: a clinicopathological study of 11 patients. *Brain.* 2002;125(Pt 2):264–275.
86. Pawate S. Sarcoidosis and the nervous system. *Continuum (Minneap Minn).* 2020;26(3):695–715.
87. Singhal NS, Irodenko VS, Margeta M, Layzer RB. Sarcoid polyneuropathy masquerading as chronic inflammatory demyelinating polyneuropathy. *Muscle Nerve.* 2015;52(4):664–668.
88. Saifee TA, Reilly MM, Ako E, et al. Sarcoidosis presenting as acute inflammatory demyelinating polyradiculoneuropathy. *Muscle Nerve.* 2011;43(2):296–298.
89. Fahoum F, Drory VE, Issakov J, Neufeld MY. Neurosarcoidosis presenting as Guillain-Barré-like syndrome. A case report and review of the literature. *J Clin Neuromuscul Dis.* 2009;11(1):35–43.
90. De Marco O, Riffaud L, Pinel JF, Edan G. Systemic sarcoidosis revealed by acute ataxic sensory polyradiculoneuropathy. *Rev Neurol.* 2003;159(11):1060–1062.
91. Burns TM, Dyck PJ, Aksamit AJ, Dyck PJ. The natural history and long-term outcome of 57 limb sarcoidosis neuropathy cases. *J Neurol Sci.* 2006;244(1–2):77–87.
92. Vital A, Lagueny A, Ferrer X, Louiset P, Canron MH, Vital C. Sarcoid neuropathy: clinico-pathological study of 4 new cases and review of the literature. *Clin Neuropathol.* 2008;27:96–105.
93. Bakkers M, Merkies IS, Lauria G, et al. Intraepidermal nerve fiber density and its application in sarcoidosis. *Neurology.* 2009;73(14):1142–1148.
94. Khan S, Zhou L. Characterization of non-length-dependent small-fiber sensory neuropathy. *Muscle Nerve.* 2012;45:86–91.
95. Hoitsma E, Marziniak M, Faber CG, et al. Small fibre neuropathy in sarcoidosis. *Lancet.* 2002;359(9323):2085–2086.
96. Hoitsma E, Drent M, Verstraete E, et al. Abnormal warm and cold sensation thresholds suggestive of small-fibre neuropathy in sarcoidosis. *Clin Neurophysiol.* 2003;114(12):2326–2333.
97. Challenor YB, Felton CP, Brust JC. Peripheral nerve involvement in sarcoidosis: an electrodiagnostic study. *J Neurol Neurosurg Psychiatry.* 1984;47:1219–1222.
98. Nemni R, Galassi G, Cohen M, et al. Symmetric sarcoid polyneuropathy: analysis of a sural nerve biopsy. *Neurology.* 1981;31:1217–1223.
99. Souayah N, Chodos A, Krivitskaya N, Efthimiou P, Lambert WC, Sharer LR. Isolated severe vasculitic neuropathy revealing sarcoidosis. *Lancet Neurol.* 2008;7:756–760.
100. Heaney D, Geddes JF, Nagendren K, Swash M. Sarcoid polyneuropathy responsive to intravenous immunoglobulin. *Muscle Nerve.* 2004;29(3):447–450.
101. Tavee J. Peripheral neuropathy in sarcoidosis. *J Neuroimmunol.* 2022;368:577864.
102. Tavee JO, Karwa K, Ahmed Z, Thompson N, Parambil J, Culver DA. Sarcoidosis-associated small fiber neuropathy in a large cohort: clinical aspects and response to IVIG and anti-TNF alpha treatment. *Respir Med.* 2017;126:135–138.
103. Parambil JG, Tavee JO, Zhou L, Pearson KS, Culver DA. Efficacy of intravenous immunoglobulin for small fiber neuropathy associated with sarcoidosis. *Respir Med.* 2011;105:101–105.
104. Perkin GD, Murray-Lyon I. Neurology and the gastrointestinal system. *J Neurol Neurosurg Psychiatry.* 1998;65:291–300.
105. Chin RL, Sander HW, Brannagan TH, et al. Celiac neuropathy. *Neurology.* 2003;60:1581–1585.

106. Hadjivassiliou M, Grünewald R, Sharrack B, et al. Gluten ataxia in perspective: epidemiology, genetic susceptibility and clinical characteristics. *Brain*. 2003;126(Pt 3):685–691.
107. Shen DT, Lebwohl B, Verma H, et al. Peripheral neuropathic symptoms in celiac disease and inflammatory bowel disease. *Clin Neuromuscul Dis*. 2012;13:137–145.
108. Hadjivassiliou M, Rao DG, Wharton SB, Sanders DS, Grünewald RA, Davies-Jones AG. Sensory ganglionopathy due to gluten sensitivity. *Neurology*. 2010;75:1003–1008.
109. Collin P, Maki M. Associated disorders in coeliac disease: clinical adult coeliac disease. *Scand J Gastroenterol*. 1994;29:769–775.
110. Cooke WT, Smith WT. Neurological disorders associated with coeliac disease. *Brain*. 1966;86:686–718.
111. Hadjivassiliou M, Chattopadhyay AK, Davies-Jones GA, Gibsin A, Grunewald RA, Lobo AJ. Neuromuscular disorder as a presenting feature of coeliac disease. *J Neurol Neurosurg Psychiatry*. 1997;63:770–775.
112. Kaplan JG, Horoupian D, DeSouza T, Brin M, Schaumburg H, Pack D. Distal axonopathy associated with chronic gluten enteropathy: a treatable disorder. *Neurology*. 1988;38:642–645.
113. Brannagan TH III, Hays AP, Chin SS, et al. Small-fiber neuropathy/neuronopathy associated with celiac disease: skin biopsy findings. *Arch Neurol*. 2005;62(10):1574–1578.
114. Gibbons CH, Freeman R. Autonomic neuropathy and coeliac disease. *J Neurol Neurosurg Psychiatry*. 2005;76(4):579–581.
115. Chin RL, Tseng VG, Green PH, Sander HW, Brannagan TH III, Latov N. Multifocal axonal polyneuropathy in celiac disease. *Neurology*. 2006;66(12):1923–1925.
116. Luostarinen L, Himanen SL, Luostarinen M, Collin P, Pirttila T. Neuromuscular and sensory disturbances in patients with well treated coeliac disease. *J Neurol Neurosurg Psychiatry*. 2003;74(4):490–494.
117. Cicarelli G, Della Rocca G, Amboni M, et al. Clinical and neurological abnormalities in adult celiac disease. *Neurol Sci*. 2003;24(5):311–317.
118. Thawani SP, Brannagan TH III, Lebwohl B, Green PH, Ludvigsson JF. Risk of neuropathy among 28,232 patients with biopsy-verified celiac disease. *JAMA Neurol*. 2015;72(7):806–811.
119. Zis P, Sarrigiannis P, Artemiadis A, Sanders DS, Hadjivassiliou M. Gluten neuropathy: electrophysiological progression and HLA associations. *J Neurol*. 2021;268(1):199–205.
120. McKeon A, Lennon VA, Pittock SJ, Kryzer TJ, Murray J. The neurologic significance of celiac disease biomarkers. *Neurology*. 2014;83(20):1789–1796.
121. Souayah N, Chin RL, Brannagan TH, et al. Effect of intravenous immunoglobulin on cerebellar ataxia and neuropathic pain associated with celiac disease. *Eur J Neurol*. 2008;15(12):1300–1303.
122. Chad DA, Smith TW, DeGirolami U, Hammer K. Perineuritis and ulcerative colitis. *Neurology*. 1986;36:1377–1379.
123. Humbert P, Monnier G, Billerey C, Birgen C, Dupond JL. Polyneuropathy: an unusual extraintestinal manifestation if Crohn's disease. *Acta Neurol Scand*. 1989;80:301–306.
124. Konagaya Y, Konagaya M, Takayanagi T. Chronic polyneuropathy and ulcerative colitis. *Jpn J Med*. 1989;28:72–74.
125. Lossos A, River Y, Eliakim A, Steiner I. Neurologic aspects of inflammatory bowel disease. *Neurology*. 1995;45(3 Pt 1):416–421.
126. Zimmerman J, Steiner I, Gavish D, Argov Z. Guillain–Barré syndrome: a possible extraintestinal manifestation of ulcerative colitis? *J Clin Gastroenterol*. 1985;7:301–303.
127. Gondim FA, Brannagan TH III, Sander HW, Chin RL, Latov N. Peripheral neuropathy in patients with inflammatory bowel disease. *Brain*. 2005;128(Pt 4):867–879.
128. Nemni R, Fazio R, Corbo M, Sessa M, Comi G, Canal N. Peripheral neuropathy associated with Crohn's disease. *Neurology*. 1987;37:1414–1417.
129. Singh S, Kumar N, Loftus EV Jr, Kane SV. Neurologic complications in patients with inflammatory bowel disease: increasing relevance in the era of biologics. *Inflamm Bowel Dis*. 2013;19(4):864–872.
130. Sassi SB, Kallel L, Ben Romdhane S, Boubaker J, Filali A, Hentati F. Peripheral neuropathy in inflammatory bowel disease patients: a prospective cohort study. *Scand J Gastroenterol*. 2009;44:1268–1269.
131. Oliveira GR, Teles BCV, Brasil EF, et al. Peripheral neuropathy and neurological disorders in an unselected Brazilian population based cohort of IBD patients. *Inflamm Bowel Dis*. 2008;14(3):389–395.
132. Benavente L, Morís G. Neurologic disorders associated with inflammatory bowel disease. *Eur J Neurol*. 2011;18(1):138–143.
133. Cohen MG, Webb J. Brachial neuritis with colitic arthritis [letter]. *Ann Intern Med*. 1987;106:780–781.
134. Singer OS, Otto B, Steinmetz H, Zieman U. Acute neuropathy with multiple conduction blocks after TNFα monoclonal antibody therapy. *Neurology*. 2004;63:1754.
135. Charron L, Peyronnard J-M, Marchand L. Sensory neuropathy associated with primary biliary cirrhosis. Histologic and morphometric studies. *Arch Neurol*. 1980;37:84–87.
136. Murata K-Y, Ishiguchi H, Ando R, Miwa H, Kondo T. Chronic inflammatory demyelinating polyneuropathy associated with primary biliary cirrhosis. *J Clin Neurosci*. 2013;20(12):1799–1801.
137. Brites L, Ribeiro J, Luis M, Santiago M, Negrão L, Duarte C. Neuromuscular manifestations of primary biliary cholangitis: two case reports and literature review. *Acta Reumatol Port*. 2018;43(4):304–308.
138. Chusid MJ, Dale DC, West BC, Wolff SM. The hypereosinophilic syndrome: analysis of fourteen cases with review of the literature. *Medicine*. 1975;54:1–27.
139. Dorfman LJ, Ransom BR, Forno LS, Kelts A. Neuropathy in the hypereosinophilic syndrome. *Muscle Nerve*. 1983;6:291–298.
140. Monaco S, Lucci B, Laperchia N, et al. Polyneuropathy in hypereosinophilic syndrome. *Neurology*. 1988;38:494–496.
141. Bolton CF, McKneown MJ, Chen R, Toth B, Remtulla H. Subacute uremic and diabetic polyneuropathy. *Muscle Nerve*. 1997;20:59–64.
142. Ropper AH. Accelerated neuropathy of renal failure. *Arch Neurol*. 1993;50:536–539.
143. Amato AA, Dumitru D. Acquired neuropathies. In: Dumitru D, Amato AA, Zwarts M, eds. *Electrodiagnostic Medicine*. 2nd ed. Hanley & Belfus, Inc; 2002:937–1041.
144. Krishnan AV, Kiernan MC. Uremic neuropathy: clinical features and new pathophysiological insights. *Muscle Nerve*. 2007;35:273–290.
145. Ho DT, Rodig NM, Kim HB, et al. Rapid reversal of uremic neuropathy following renal transplantation in an adolescent. *Pediatr Transplant*. 2012;16(7):E296–E300.
146. Bolton CF, Driedger AA, Lindsay RM. Ischaemic neuropathy in uraemic patients caused by bovine arteriovenous shunt. *J Neurol Neurosurg Psychiatry*. 1979;42:810–814.

147. Ogura T, Makinodan A, Kubo T, Hayashida T, Hirasawa Y. Electrophysiological course of uraemic neuropathy in haemodialysis patients. *Postgrad Med J*. 2001;77(909):451–454.
148. Thomas PK, Hillinrake K, Lascelles RG, et al. The polyneuropathy of chronic renal failure. *Brain*. 1971;94:761–780.
149. Van den Neucker K, Vanderstraeten G, Vanholder R. Peripheral motor and sensory nerve conduction studies in haemodialysis patients. A study of 54 patients. *Electromyogr Clin Neurophysiol*. 1998;38(8):467–474.
150. Laaksonen S, Metsärinne K, Voipio-Pulkki L-M, Falck B. Neurophysiologic parameters and symptoms in chronic renal failure. *Muscle Nerve*. 2002;25(6):884–890.
151. Krishnan AV, Phoon RKS, Pussell BA, Charlesworth JA, Bostock H, Kiernan MC. Altered motor nerve excitability in end-stage kidney disease. *Brain*. 2005;128(Pt 9):2164–2174.
152. Dyck PJ, Johnson WJ, Lambert EH, O'Brien PC. Segmental demyelination secondary to axonal degeneration in uremic neuropathy. *Mayo Clin Proc*. 1971;46:400–431.
153. Bolton CF, Baltzan MA, Baltzan RF. Effects of renal transplantation in uremic neuropathy. A clinical and electrophysiologic study. *N Engl J Med*. 1971;284:1170–1175.
154. Bolton CF, Lindasy RM, Linton AL. The course of uremic neuropathy during chronic hemodialysis. *Can J Neurol Sci*. 1975;2:332–333.
155. Bolton CF. Electrophysiologic changes in uremic neuropathy after successful renal transplantation. *Neurology*. 1976;26:152–161.
156. Bolton CF. Peripheral neuropathies associated with chronic renal failure. *Can J Neurol Sci*. 1980;7:89–96.
157. Oh SJ, Clements RS, Lee YW, Diethelm AG. Rapid improvement in nerve conduction velocity following renal transplantation. *Ann Neurol*. 1978;4:369–373.
158. Kardel T, Nielsen VK. Hepatic neuropathy. A clinical and electrophysiological study. *Acta Neurol Scand*. 1974;50:513–526.
159. Knill-Jones RP, Goodwill CJ, Dayan AD, Williams R. Peripheral neuropathy in chronic liver disease: clinical, electrodiagnostic, and nerve biopsy findings. *J Neurol Neurosurg Psychiatry*. 1972;35:22–30.
160. Seneviratne KN, Peiris OA. Peripheral nerve function in chronic liver disease. *J Neurol Neurosurg Psychiatry*. 1970;33:609–614.
161. Lee JH, Jung WJ, Choi KH, Chun MH, Ha SB, Lee SK. Nerve conduction study on patients with severe liver syndrome and its change after transplantation. *Clin Transplant*. 2002;16(6):430–432.
162. McDougall AJ, Davies L, McCaughan GW. Autonomic and peripheral neuropathy in endstage liver disease and following liver transplantation. *Muscle Nerve*. 2003;28(5):595–600.
163. Cruz Martinez A, González P, Garza E, Bescansa E, Anciones B. Electro-physiologic follow-up in Whipple's disease. *Muscle Nerve*. 1987;10:616–620.
164. Halperin JJ, Landis DM, Kleinman GM. Whipple disease of the nervous system. *Neurology*. 1982;32:612–617.
165. Gerard A, Sarrot-Reynauld F, Liozon E, et al. Neurologic presentation of Whipple disease: report of 12 cases and review of the literature. *Medicine*. 2002;81(6):443–457.
166. Pauletti C, Pujia F, Accorinti M, et al. An atypical case of neuro-Whipple: clinical presentation, magnetic resonance spectroscopy and follow-up. *J Neurol Sci*. 2010;297:97–100.
167. Guo K, Liang N, Wu M, Chen L, Chen H. Prevalence and risk factors for peripheral neuropathy in Chinese patients with gout. *Front Neurol*. 2022;13:789631.
168. Delaney P. Gouty neuropathy. *Arch Neurol*. 1983;40:823–824.
169. Bolton CF, Gilbert JJ, Hahn AF, Sibbald WJ. Polyneuropathy in critically ill patients. *J Neurol Neurosurg Psychiatry*. 1984;47:1223–1231.
170. Bolton CF, Laverty DA, Brown JD, Witt NJ, Hahn AF, Sibbald WJ. Critically ill polyneuropathy: electrophysiological studies and differentiation from Guillain–Barré syndrome. *J Neurol Neurosurg Psychiatry*. 1986;49:563–573.
171. Leijten FS, Harink-de Weerd JE, Poortvleit DC, de Weerd AW. The role of polyneuropathy in motor convalescence after prolonged mechanical ventilation. *JAMA*. 1995;274:1221–1225.
172. Zochodne DW, Bolton CF, Wells GA, et al. Critical illness polyneuropathy. A complication of sepsis and multiple organ failure. *Brain*. 1987;110:819–842.
173. Deconinck N, Van Parijs V, Beckers-Bleukx G, Van den Bergh P. Critical illness myopathy unrelated to corticosteroids or neuromuscular blocking agents. *Neuromuscul Disord*. 1998;8:186–192.
174. Lacomis D, Smith TW, Chad DA. Acute myopathy and neuropathy in status asthmaticus: case report and literature review. *Muscle Nerve*. 1993;16:84–90.
175. Lacomis D, Giuliani MJ, Van Cott A, Kramer DJ. Acute myopathy of the intensive care: clinical, electromyographic, and pathological aspects. *Ann Neurol*. 1996;40:645–654.
176. Lacomis D, Petrella JT, Giuliani MJ. Causes of neuromuscular weakness in the intensive care unit: a study of ninety-two patients. *Muscle Nerve*. 1998;21:610–617.
177. Rich MM, Teener JW, Raps EC, Schotland DL, Bird SJ. Muscle is electrically inexcitable in acute quadriplegic myopathy. *Neurology*. 1996;46:731–736.
178. Rich MM, Bird SJ, Raps EC, McClaskey LF, Teener JW. Direct muscle stimulation in acute quadriplegic myopathy. *Muscle Nerve*. 1997;20:665–673.
179. Zochodne DW, Ramsey DA, Saly V, Shelley S, Moffatt S. Acute necrotizing myopathy of the intensive care: electrophysiological studies. *Muscle Nerve*. 1994;17:285–292.
180. Barohn RJ, Jackson CE, Rogers SJ, Ridings LW, McVey AL. Prolonged paralysis due to nondepolarizing neuromuscular blocking agents and corticosteroids. *Muscle Nerve*. 1994;17:647–654.
181. Sander HW, Golden M, Danon MJ. Quadriplegic areflexic ICU illness: selective thick filament loss and normal nerve histology. *Muscle Nerve*. 2002;26(4):499–505.
182. Carver N, Logan A. Critical illness polyneuropathy associated with burns: a case report. *Burns*. 1989;15:179–180.
183. Marquez S, Turley JJ, Peters WJ. Neuropathy in burn patients. *Brain*. 1993;116:471–483.
184. Gruber L, Loizides A, Gruber H, et al. Differentiation of critical illness myopathy and critical illness neuropathy using nerve ultrasonography. *J Clin Neurophysiol*. 2023;40(7):600–607.
185. Fisse AL, May C, Motte J, et al. New approaches to critical Illness polyneuromyopathy: high-resolution neuromuscular ultrasound characteristics and cytokine profiling. *Neurocrit Care*. 2021;35(1):139–152.
186. Z'Graggen WJ, Lin CS, Howard RS, Beale RJ, Bostock H. Nerve excitability changes in critical illness polyneuropathy. *Brain*. 2006;129(Pt 9):2461–2470.
187. Ojha A, Zivkovic SA, Lacomis D. Electrodiagnostic studies in the intensive care unit: a comparison study 2 decades later. *Muscle Nerve*. 2018;57(5):772–776.

CHAPTER 17

Neuropathies Associated with Infections

Neuropathies can result directly from various bacterial and viral infections, as well as from an indirect or parainfectious autoimmune response to the infection (Table 17-1). Parainfectious neuropathies [e.g., Guillain–Barré syndrome (GBS) associated with various infections and vasculitis associated with hepatitis] are discussed in detail in other chapters.

▶ LEPROSY (HANSEN DISEASE)

CLINICAL FEATURES

Leprosy is caused by the acid-fast bacteria *Mycobacterium leprae*. Leprosy is the most common cause of peripheral neuropathy in Southeast Asia, Africa, and South America. The main route of transmission is felt to be from person-to-person spread via nasal droplets. The bacteria are very slow growing with an incubation period that can vary between 2 and 40 years, customarily between 5 and 7 years.[1]

There is a spectrum of clinical manifestations ranging from tuberculoid leprosy at one end to lepromatous leprosy on the other end of the spectrum, with borderline leprosy in between based upon the Ridley–Joplin classification (Table 17-2).[1–6] The World Health Organization (WHO) introduced a simpler classification based on the number of skin lesions to help guide treatment: multibacillary (six more skin lesions) and paucibacillary (fewer than six skin lesions) leprosy.[1] In general, lepromatous leprosy is always multibacillary, and tuberculoid leprosy is usually paucibacillary; borderline leprosy can be either multibacillary or paucibacillary. The clinical manifestations of the disease are determined by the immunological response of the host to the infection. In tuberculoid leprosy, the cell-mediated immune response is intact.[1–5] Thus, there are focal, circumscribed inflammatory responses to the bacteria within the affected areas of skin and nerves. The resulting skin lesions appear as well-defined, scattered hypopigmented patches and plaques with raised, erythematous borders (Figs. 17-1 and 17-2). Cutaneous nerves are often affected, resulting in a loss of sensation in the center of these skin lesions. Cooler regions of the body (e.g., face and limbs) are more susceptible than warmer regions such as the groin or axilla. In addition, the ulnar nerve at the medial epicondyle, the median nerve at the distal forearm, the peroneal nerve at the fibular head, the sural nerve, the greater auricular nerve, and the superficial radial nerve at the wrist are common sites of involvement and become encased with granulomas, leading to mononeuropathy or mononeuropathy multiplex. These nerves are thickened and often palpable.

In lepromatous leprosy, cell-mediated immunity is severely impaired, leading to extensive infiltration of the bacilli and hematogenous dissemination, producing confluent and symmetrical areas of rash, anesthesia, and anhidrosis.[1–6] Neuropathies tend to be more severe in the lepromatous subtype. As in the tuberculoid form, there is a predilection for the involvement of cooler regions of the body. Infiltration of the organism in the face leads to the loss of eyebrows and eyelashes and exaggeration of the natural skin folds, leading to the so-called "leonine facies." Superficial cutaneous nerves of the ears and distal limbs are also commonly affected. A slowly progressive symmetric sensorimotor polyneuropathy gradually develops due to widespread invasion of the bacilli into the epi-, peri-, and endoneurium. Distal extremity weakness may be seen, but large fiber sensory modalities and muscle stretch reflexes are relatively spared. Involvement of nerve trunks leads to superimposed mononeuropathies, including facial neuropathy.

Neuropathies are most common in patients with borderline leprosy.[2,3,5] Patients can develop generalized symmetric sensorimotor polyneuropathies, mononeuropathies, and mononeuropathy multiplex, including multiple mononeuropathies in atypical locations, such as the brachial plexus. Borderline leprosy is associated with clinical and histological features of both the lepromatous and the tuberculoid forms of leprosy (Table 17-2 and Fig. 17-3). There is partial impairment in cellular immunity in patients with borderline leprosy, such that there is some degree of mycobacterial spread as well as an inflammatory response. The immunological state is considered unstable in patients with borderline leprosy in that the immune response and clinical manifestations can shift up and down the spectrum.

Patients with leprosy may present with isolated peripheral neuropathy without skin lesions, particularly in endemic areas.[7,8] Most cases of the so-called pure neuritic leprosy have the tuberculoid or borderline tuberculoid subtypes of the disease.

LABORATORY FEATURES

Sensory nerve conduction studies (NCSs) are usually absent in the lower limb and are reduced in amplitude in the arms.[1,7,8] Motor NCSs may demonstrate reduced amplitudes

TABLE 17-1. INFECTIOUS AGENTS ASSOCIATED WITH NEUROPATHIES

Bacterial:
Mycobacterium leprae (Leprosy)
Borrelia burdorferi (Lyme disease)
Corynebacterium diphtheriae (Diphtheria)
Treponema pallidum (Syphilis)
Viral:
Human immunodeficiency virus (HIV)
    Distal symmetric polyneuropathy
    Acute inflammatory demyelinating polyradiculoneuropathy
    Chronic inflammatory demyelinating polyradiculoneuropathy
    Other polyradiculoneuropathy
    Mononeuropathy multiplex
    Autonomic neuropathy
    Sensory ganglionopathy
Human T-lymphocytic type 1 (HTLV-1)
Cytomegalovirus (CMV)
Ebstein-Barr virus (EBV)
Hepatitis B and C
Herpes varicella-zoster (HVZ)
Severe acute respiratory syndrome coronavirus 2 (SARS-CoV-2)

in affected nerves.[9,10] Motor conduction velocities are normal or slightly reduced; however, a few patients may demonstrate values less than 20 m/s in both the upper and the lower limb. Electromyography (EMG) reveals mild-to-moderate degrees of active denervation. The pattern of involvement on the EMG and NCSs can be generalized as symmetric or reflective of a mononeuropathy or multiple mononeuropathies, as apparent from the clinical features. Ultrasound can demonstrate enlarged axons, particularly of the median nerve in distal forearm near the carpal tunnel and of the ulnar nerve just proximal to the medial epicondyle (Fig. 17-4).[11]

HISTOPATHOLOGY

Leprosy is usually diagnosed with skin lesion biopsy and using the Fite method to stain the acid-fast bacilli red (Fig. 17-3).[3] The morphological index (MI) is the ratio of viable to nonviable organisms on skin smears. The bacteriological index (BI) is a logarithmically scaled measure of the density of bacilli in the dermis. Both the MI and BI have been used to measure treatment response. The host's immune response to the bacilli

TABLE 17-2. CLINICAL, LABORATORY, IMMUNOLOGICAL, AND HISTOPATHOLOGICAL FEATURES OF LEPROSY

	Tuberculous Leprosy (TT)	Mid-Borderline Leprosy (BB)	Lepromatous Leprosy (LL)
Lepromin test	Positive (>5 mm induration)	+/− (2–5 mm induration)	Negative (0–2 mm induration)
Bacterial index	0	2–4	5–6
Morphological index (MI)	Low (down to zero)	Moderate	High (up to 10)
Immunology	Cell-mediated immunity: intact; CD4 > CD8 lymphocytes; Th1 cytokines expressed: IL-2 and γ-IF	Cell-mediated immunity: unstable (can range and switch from intact to absent)	Cell-mediated immunity: absent; CD8 > CD4 lymphocytes; Th2 cytokines expressed: IL-4, IL-5, and IL-10
Skin lesions	Few localized and well-demarcated large skin lesions; erythematous macules and plaques with raised borders; centers of lesions may be hypopigmented	Size, number, and appearance of the skin lesions are intermediate between that seen in the TT and LL poles	Multiple, symmetrical small macules and papules; older lesions form plaques and nodules
Histopathology	Localized granulomas and giant cells encompassed by dense lymphocytic infiltrate extending to epidermis; Fite stain: negative for bacteria	Granulomas with epithelioid cells but no giant cells. Not localized by zones of lymphocytes. Lymphocytes, if present, are diffusely infiltrating. Fite stain: slightly positive	Scant lymphocytes, but if present diffuse along with organism-laden foamy macrophages. Fite stain: marked positive
Neuropathies	Mononeuropathy of the superficial cutaneous nerves or large nerve trunks (i.e., ulnar, median, and peroneal nerves), multiple mononeuropathies; pure neuritic leprosy may be seen	The neuropathies can range in the spectrum of that seen in TT to LL	Distal symmetric sensory and sensorimotor polyneuropathies are more common than mononeuropathy; pure neuritic leprosy is not seen
Treatment[a]	Paucibacillary. Dapsone 100 mg daily. Rifampin 600 mg per month. Clofazimine 300 mg per month and 50 mg twice a week. Duration: 6 months		Multibacillary. Dapsone 100 mg daily. Rifampin 600 mg per month. Clofazimine 300 mg per month and 50 mg twice a week. Duration: 12 months or until skin smears is zero

The features of the borderline tuberculoid (BT) form ranges between the TT and BB forms. The features of the borderline lepromatous (BL) form ranges between that seen in BB and LL forms of leprosy.
[a]Treatment based on World Health Organization recommendations.

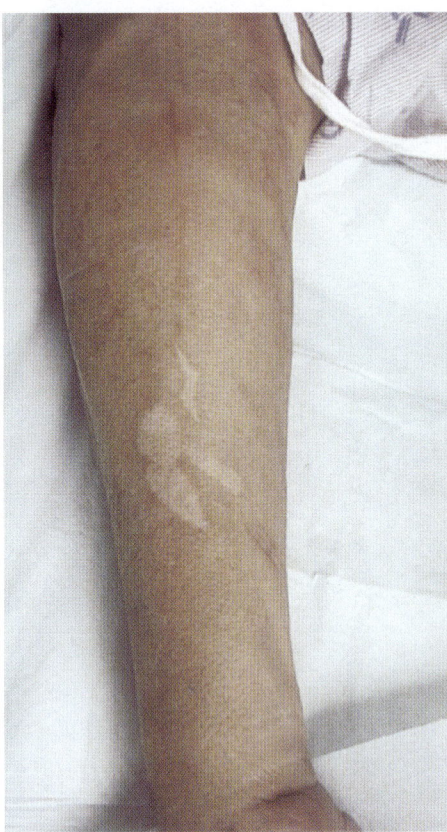

Figure 17-1. Tuberculoid leprosy. Hypopigmented skin lesions are evident on lateral aspect of forearm in a patient with tuberculoid leprosy.

determines the histopathology (Table 17-2).[1–5,12,13] Nerve biopsies can also be diagnostic, particularly when there are no apparent skin lesions. The tuberculoid form is characterized by granulomas formed by macrophages and T lymphocytes (CD4 T lymphocytes greater than CD8). Caseating granulomas may or may not be present. Importantly, bacilli are not seen. In contrast, with lepromatous leprosy, large number of infiltrating bacilli, CD8 greater than CD4 lymphocytes, and organism-laden, foamy macrophages with minimal granulomatous infiltration are evident (Fig. 17-5A). The bacilli are best appreciated using the Fite stain, in which they can be seen as red staining rods in clusters within the endoneurium, within macrophages, or within Schwann cells (Fig. 17-5B). Nonmyelinated Remak Schwann cells are particularly vulnerable.[12] On electron microscopy, the bacilli appear as dense osmiophilic rods surrounded by a clear halo (Fig. 17-5C and D). Borderline leprosy can have histological features of both tuberculoid and lepromatous leprosy. Morphometric analysis of nerve biopsy reveals axonal atrophy, Wallerian degeneration, and demyelination, with axonal degeneration predominating over demyelination in chronic stages.[13]

PATHOGENESIS

The clinical and pathological spectrum of the disease is dependent on the host's immune response to *M. leprae* and reflects the relative balance between the Th1 and Th2 response (Table 17-2).[1–5] The tuberculoid form defines one end of the spectrum, in which the CD4 T cells predominate. These CD4 T cells produce interleukin-2 and gamma-interferon which in turn lead to activation of macrophages. On the other extreme, the lepromatous form is dominated by CD8 cells, which produce interleukin-4, interleukin-5, and interleukin-10, thereby downregulating cell-mediated immunity and inhibiting macrophages. The borderline subtypes exhibit immune responses spanning the spectrum between the tuberculoid and lepromatous forms. *M. leprae* laminin-binding protein (LBP21) is a major protein expressed on the surface of the bacteria binds to the G domain of the laminin alpha-2 chain that is expressed on the basal lamina of Schwann cells.[12,14] The binding triggers the Schwann cells to engulf the bacteria.

TREATMENT

Patients are treated with multiple drugs: dapsone, rifampicin, and clofazimine depending on the form of leprosy they have (Table 17-2).[1–4,6,12,15,16] The current WHO recommendations for adults with multibacillary leprosy are as follows: rifampicin (600 mg once a month), dapsone (100 mg daily), and clofazimine (300 mg once a month and 50 mg twice a week) for 12 months.[11] For adults with paucibacillary leprosy, the WHO recommends the same three drug regimen for 6 months.[16] For adults with single skin lesion paucibacillary leprosy the recommended WHO regimen is a single dose of rifampicin 600 mg, ofloxacin 400 mg, and minocycline 100 mg. Proven relapses are re-treated with multidrug regimen.

The WHO recommendations have been controversial as the relapse rate of multibacillary leprosy can be high. Thus, some advocate for more aggressive treatment based in part on Ridley–Joplin classification: tuberculoid leprosy to be treated with dapsone 100 mg daily for 5 years and lepromatous leprosy to be treated with rifampin 600 mg daily for 3 years and dapsone 100 mg daily for life.[1] However, a recent meta-analysis on 25 studies conducted to evaluate the effectiveness on diverse treatment regimens, found that the WHO antibiotic regimen for leprosy was the most effective treatment.[15]

Patients should be instructed on the side effects of these medications before starting treatment. Rifampicin may make the urine turn a slightly reddish color for a few hours after its intake. Clofazimine causes brownish-black discoloration and dryness of skin. However, this disappears within few months after stopping treatment. The main side effect of dapsone is allergic reaction, causing itchy skin rashes and exfoliative dermatitis. Patients known to be allergic to drugs containing sulfa should not be given dapsone.

Treatment is sometimes complicated by the so-called reversal reaction, particularly in borderline leprosy.[1–3,12] The reversal reaction can occur at any time during treatment and develops because of a shift to the tuberculoid end of the

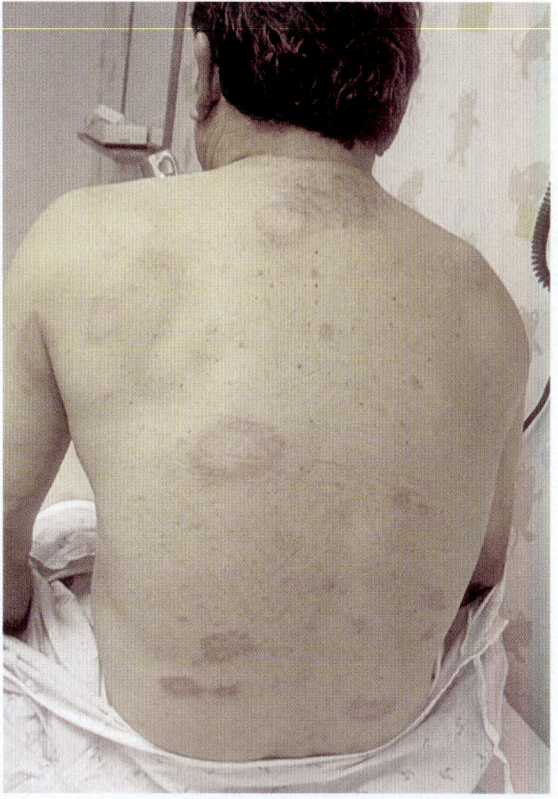 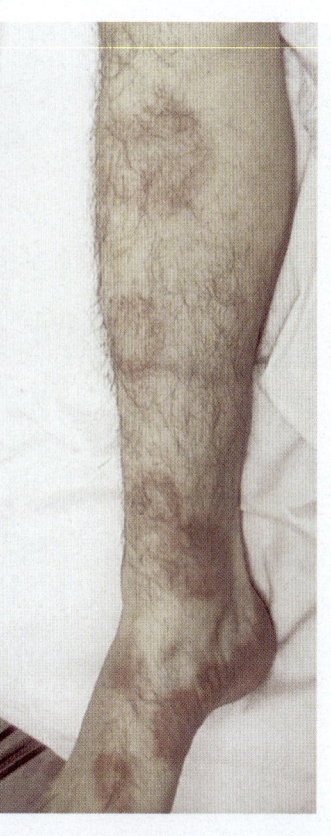

Figure 17-2. Borderline leprosy. A patient with borderline leprosy has multiple skin lesions with hypopigmented center with raised erythematous borders on the back (**A**) (Reproduced with permission from Amato AA, Dumitru D. Acquired neuropathies. In: Dumitru D, Amato AA, Swartz MJ, eds. *Electrodiagnostic Medicine*. 2nd ed. Hanley & Belfus; 2002.) and on the leg (**B**). (Reproduced with permission from Amato AA, Dumitru D. Acquired neuropathies. In: Dumitru D, Amato AA, Swartz MJ, eds. *Electrodiagnostic Medicine*, 2nd ed. Philadelphia, PA: Hanley & Belfus; 2002.)

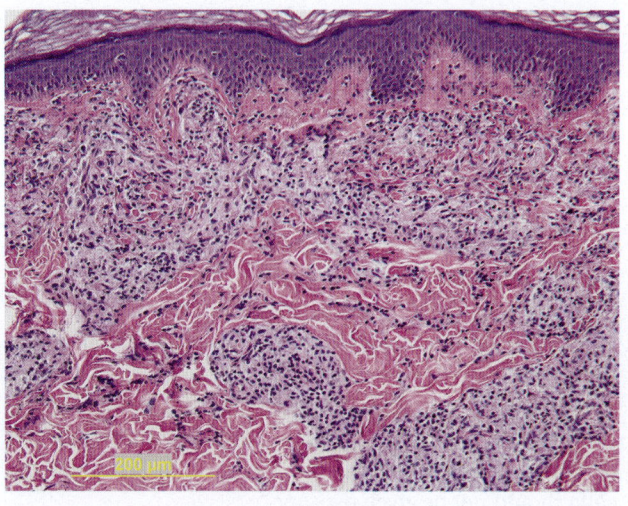 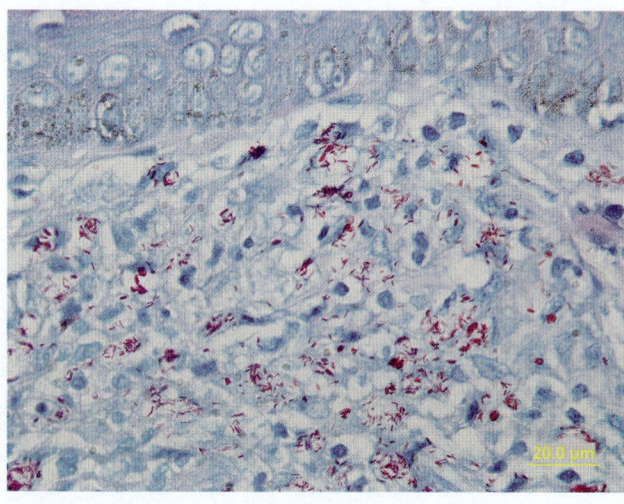

Figure 17-3. Borderline leprosy. Skin biopsy demonstrates marked inflammatory cell infiltrate, H&E (**A**). Red staining bacilli are evident on higher power with a Fite stain (**B**).

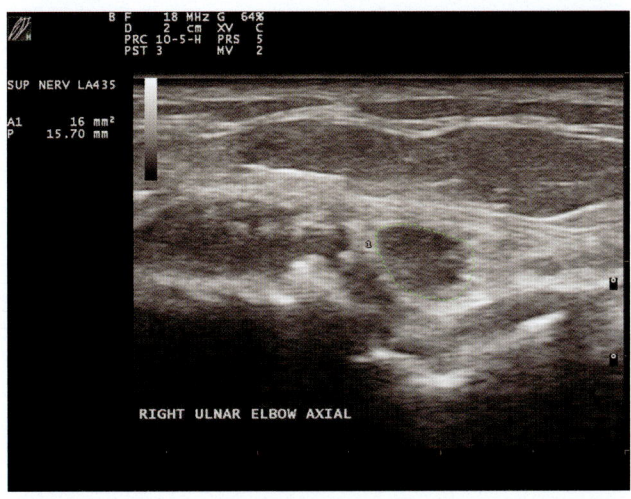
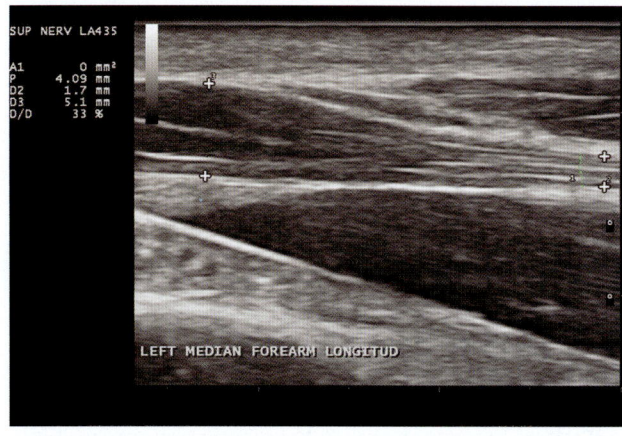

Figure 17-4. Ultrasound in patient with lepromatous leprosy demonstrates swelling of the ulnar nerve at the elbow just proximal to the medial epicondyle with an area of 16 mm² (normal <10 mm²) (**A**). There was also swelling of the median nerve in the distal forearm as it approached the carpel tunnel as the diameter 1.4 mm at D2 to 5.1 mm (**B**).

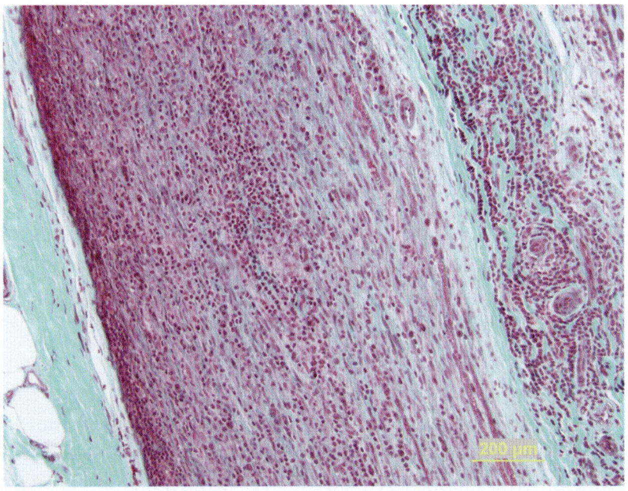

Figure 17-5. Borderline leprosy. Sural nerve biopsy perivascular and diffuse endoneurial inflammation consisting of lymphocytes and macrophages, paraffin section stained with trichrome (**A**). Fite stain reveals red staining bacilli (the so-called "red snappers") sometimes in clusters in the endoneurium and within Schwann cells (**B**). Electron microscopy reveals electron-dense bacilli with surrounding clear halos within the cytoplasm of a Schwann cell surrounding a myelinated axon (**C**) and on higher power within a Remak Schwann cell surrounding unmyelinated axons (**D**).

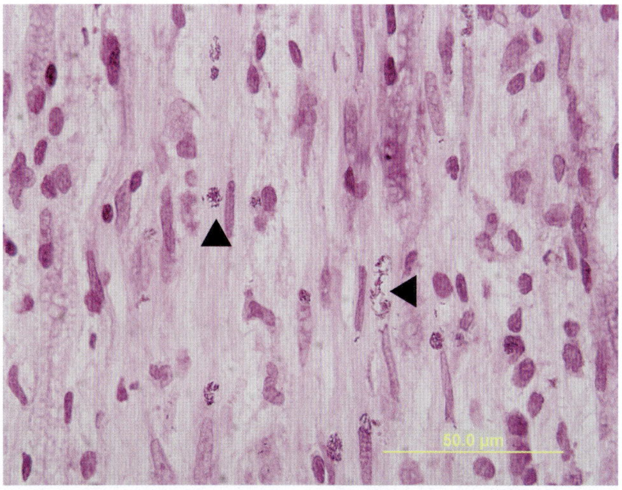

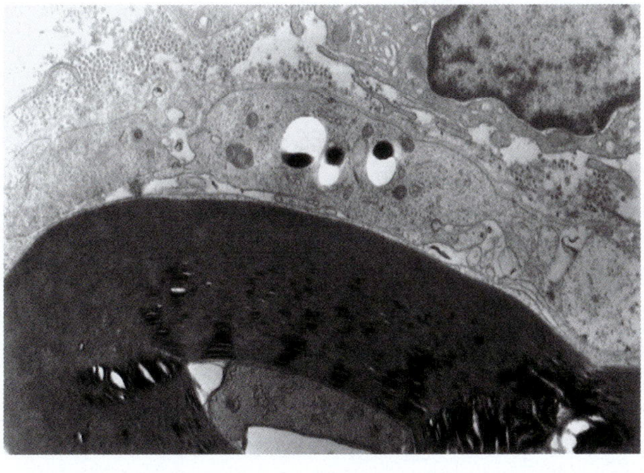

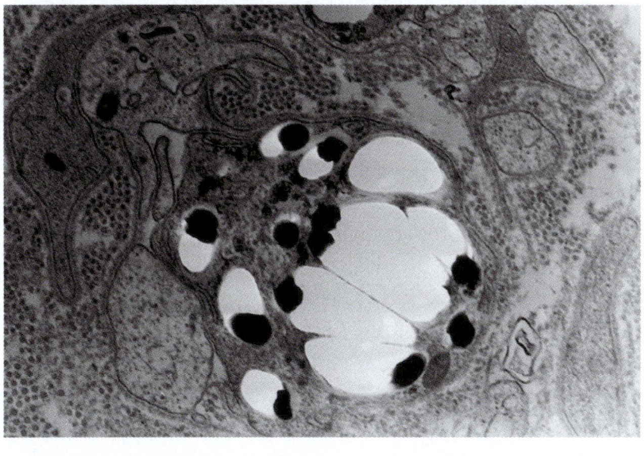

spectrum, as the result of an increase in cellular immunity during treatment. The cellular response is upregulated as evidenced by an increased release of tumor necrosis factor-alpha, gamma-interferon, and interleukin-2 with new granuloma formation. This can result in an exacerbation of the skin lesions and the neuropathy. High-dose corticosteroids blunt this adverse reaction and are often used prophylactically in high-risk patients (i.e., those with borderline leprosy) at treatment onset.

Erythema nodosum leprosum is another adverse reaction that usually occurs during treatment of patients with lepromatous leprosy.[1–3,12,17] Multiple erythematous, sometimes painful, subcutaneous nodules appear, and may be associated with worsening of the neuropathy. Erythema nodosum leprosum probably results from slow degradation of bacilli and release of new antigens. Subsequently, antigen–antibody complexes form and complement is activated in affected tissue. Erythema nodosum leprosum is commonly treated with corticosteroids, clofazimine, or thalidomide.

A review looked at 13 studies involving 445 participants treated for erythema nodosum leprosum with corticosteroids, clofazimine, thalidomide, and other agents (i.e., pentoxifylline, indomethacin, and levamisole).[18] The quality of the trials was generally poor and results could not be pooled due to the treatments being so heterogeneous. That said, clofazimine treatment was felt to be superior to prednisolone and thalidomide.[17]

Prevention of leprosy is of primary importance. It is recommended that children exposed to leprosy in the household be prophylactically treated with rifampin daily for 6 months.[2,3] Various vaccinations are available, including BCG, killed leprae, and chemically modified organisms.

▶ LYME DISEASE

CLINICAL FEATURES

Lyme disease is caused by infection with *Borrelia burgdorferi*, a spirochete, transmitted by ticks. The deer tick, *Ixodes dammini*, is responsible for the disease in most cases. Ticks acquire the spirochetes by feeding on an infected host (e.g., deer) and then transmit the spirochetes to the next host (e.g., humans) at a later feed. It takes approximately 12–24 hours of tick attachment to transfer the spirochetes.

There are three recognized stages of Lyme disease: (1) early infection with localized erythema migrans, (2) disseminated infection, and (3) late-stage infection. The localized response occurs within 1 month of a tick bite. It consists of an erythematous circular region centered around the area of the original tick bite. The erythematous area gradually expands and the center of the lesion becoming clear creating a bull's eye appearance. The rash resolves spontaneously after approximately a month. Importantly, not all patients with Lyme disease develop erythema migrans. The second stage of the illness is marked by dissemination of the spiro-

▶ **TABLE 17-3. NEUROLOGICAL DISORDERS ASSOCIATED WITH LYME DISEASE**

Encephalitis/meningitis
Myelitis
Cranial neuropathies (e.g., facial nerve palsy)
Peripheral neuropathy
Mononeuropathies
Multiple mononeuropathies
Radiculopathy
Plexopathy
Inflammatory myopathy

chetes throughout the body. Patients develop systemic symptoms including fever, chills, localized adenopathy, fatigue, myalgias, headache, neck and back pain, and additional skin lesions about the body. Cardiac involvement may lead to pericarditis and heart block. Inflammatory arthritis of large and small joints may also occur.

Neurological complications may develop during the second and third stages of infection (Table 17-3).[19–29] Facial nerve palsy is the most common neurological manifestation of Lyme disease and is bilateral in about half of cases, which is rare for idiopathic Bell palsy. Involvement of nerves is frequently asymmetric. Patients with Lyme disease may also manifest with multiple mononeuropathies or, more commonly in our experience, with radiculopathy or polyradiculopathy. Although often considered in the differential diagnosis of GBS, it usually does not resemble cases of GBS given the asymmetric nature and electrophysiological features (see below). Rarely, affected patients develop an inflammatory myopathy as opposed to neuropathy.[29]

The late stage of infection is characterized by further destructive inflammatory changes in the joints. The distal extremities develop a bluish discoloration of the skin (acrodermatitis chronica atrophicans). Spirochetes may be readily cultured from biopsies of these sites. Approximately 50% of patients have numbness, paresthesia, weakness, and cramps in the distal extremities, and proprioception and vibration are reduced as are muscle stretch reflexes.

LABORATORY FEATURES

Examination of the cerebrospinal fluid (CSF) should demonstrate lymphocytic pleocytosis and increased protein in patients with polyradiculitis, cranial neuropathies, and central nervous system involvement. Immunofluorescent or enzyme-linked immunosorbent assay may detect antibodies directed against the spirochete in the serum and CSF. False-positive reactions are not uncommon and, therefore, Western blot analysis should be performed to confirm a positive enzyme-linked immunosorbent assay.

Electrodiagnostic studies are suggestive of a primary axonopathy. In a patient with a mononeuropathy or multiple mononeuropathies, NCSs typically reveal reduced compound muscle action potential (CMAP) and sensory nerve action potential (SNAP) amplitudes.[20,24–29] Those with facial nerve palsies can have reduced facial nerve CMAPs and abnormal blink reflexes.[22] The electrophysiological abnormalities are often asymmetric.[30,31] Needle EMG reveals increased insertional and spontaneous activity in the form of fibrillation potentials and positive sharp waves and decreased recruitment of neurogenic-appearing motor unit action potentials (MUAPs). Patients presenting with a radiculopathy may have normal motor and sensory NCSs, but the EMG is abnormal as above.

HISTOPATHOLOGY

Nerve biopsies are not typically performed in patients with Lyme disease complicated by neuropathy, but when done have shown perivascular infiltration of plasma cells and lymphocytes around small endoneurial, perineurial, and epineurial blood vessels without clear necrotizing vasculitis. Axonal degeneration and secondary demyelination can be seen.

PATHOGENESIS

Peripheral nerve involvement may be the result of an indirect immunological response and/or some form of vasculopathy.

TREATMENT

Recommended treatment of facial nerve palsies in adults is the combination of amoxicillin 500 mg p.o. q.i.d. plus probenecid 500 mg q.i.d. for 2–4 weeks. Patients who are allergic to penicillin can be treated with doxycycline 100 mg p.o. b.i.d. for 2–4 weeks. Children less than 4 years of age can be treated with amoxicillin 20–40 mg/kg/day in four divided doses for 2–4 weeks. If allergic to penicillin, children can be treated with erythromycin 30 mg/kg/day in four divided doses for 2–4 weeks.

Adult patients with other types of peripheral neuropathy are treated with intravenous (IV) penicillin 20–24 million units/day for 10–14 days or ceftriaxone 2 g IV daily for 2–4 weeks. Those allergic to penicillin should receive doxycycline 100 mg p.o. b.i.d. for 30 days. Children with Lyme neuropathy can receive IV penicillin G 250,000 U/kg/day in divided doses for 10–14 days or ceftriaxone 50–80 mg/kg/day IV for 2–4 weeks.

▶ SYPHILIS

CLINICAL FEATURES

Syphilis is caused by the spirochete bacterium *Treponema pallidum* that invades the nervous system within days after primary infection. Neurosyphilis can be categorized as asymptomatic or symptomatic and develop as early 1–2 years after primary infection or many years later. Early neurosyphilis is often asymptomatic but be associated with headache, meningismus, cranial nerve palsies, and blindness or deafness. Late neurosyphilis is associated dementia and tabes dorsalis that is characterized by severe stabbing pain an ataxic gait.[32–35] Patients report lancinating pains in their extremities and trunk. Visceral crises may result in recurrent attacks of severe epigastric pain due to gastric crises, along with nausea and vomiting. Urinary retention and overflow incontinence may occur in the early stages due to bladder dysfunction.

On examination most patients exhibit a loss of light touch, vibratory perceptions, and proprioception.[32–34] Gait is often wide based and associated with foot slapping and a sensory ataxia. Deep tendon reflexes are reduced. Charcot joints (neuropathic arthropathy) may be evident. Tabes dorsalis is often associated with Argyll Robertson pupils (constriction of the pupils when the eyes are focused on a nearby object but not when the bright light is shined into the pupils)—pupils accommodate but do not respond.

LABORATORY FEATURES

Diagnosis of syphilis requires two-stage testing with positive nontreponemal [e.g., rapid plasma reagin or RPR, venereal disease research laboratory (VDRL) test], as well as a treponemal test (e.g., treponema pallidum particle agglutination or TPPA).[32–34] Serum nontreponemal tests are reactive in almost all cases of neurosyphilis during and after the secondary stage of syphilis but can become negative in late neurosyphilis because of waning titers over time, especially after treatment. In CSF, nontreponemal tests such as VDRL have a higher specificity than treponemal tests but are only 30%–70% sensitive. If the CSF VDRL test is negative in a patient with a syndrome that is consistent with neurosyphilis, CSF treponemal tests are advised. CSF is also usually associated with a mild, chronic pleocytosis, and increased protein. NCSs would be expected to show absent or reduced amplitudes of SNAPs. Affected patients should be tested for human immunodeficiency virus (HIV).

HISTOPATHOLOGY AND PATHOGENESIS

Nerve biopsies are not typically performed in patients with syphilis. Autopsy studies have demonstrated degeneration of the dorsal root ganglia and the dorsal columns in the spinal cord. Perivascular infiltration composed of CD4+ and CD8+ T lymphocytes, macrophages, and plasma cells with a reductio in the number of small blood vessel is evident.[33,34] Gummas (central caseous necrosis surrounded by granulomatous inflammation) may be found throughout the brain and spinal cord. Spirochetes, however, are not typically identified.[33,34]

TREATMENT

Patients with neurosyphilis should be treated with aqueous crystalline penicillin G, 3–4 million units IV every 4 hours or 18–24 million units every 24 hours as a continuous infusion, for 10–14 days. If compliance can be ensured, an alternative is penicillin G procaine, 2.4 million units IM daily, plus probenecid, 500 mg orally four times a day, for 10–14 days.[32–34] If signs and symptoms persist in conjunction with clinical assessment of interval serologies and CSF testing, additional courses of penicillin are required in patients with persistent symptoms and signs along with abnormal serology and CSF.

▶ DIPHTHERITIC NEUROPATHY

CLINICAL FEATURES

Diphtheria is caused by the bacteria *Corynebacterium diphtheriae*. Individuals who are infected present with "flu-like" symptoms of generalized myalgias, headache, fatigue, low-grade fever, and irritability within a week to 10 days of the exposure. A whitish membranous exudate may be appreciated in the pharynx with or without swollen or tender cervical lymph nodes. Cardiovascular involvement can manifest as cardiac arrhythmias and hypotension. About 20%–70% of patients develop a peripheral neuropathy caused by a toxin released by the bacteria.[36–39] Three to four weeks after infection, patients may note decreased sensation in their throat and begin to develop dysphagia, dysarthria, or hoarseness. Around the same time, patients develop blurred vision, particularly when looking at near objects. Pupils react to light but fail to accommodate. Additional cranial nerves may also become involved. Ventilatory muscle weakness can develop due to phrenic nerve involvement. A generalized polyneuropathy may manifest 2 or 3 months following the initial infection characterized by numbness, paresthesia, and weakness of the arms and legs. Neurological examination reveals a reduction in perception of all sensory modalities. Distal greater than proximal weakness is seen. Weakness may progress over a period of weeks, such that patients are unable to ambulate. Muscle stretch reflexes are diminished or absent throughout in keeping with the demyelinating nature of the neuropathy. Rarely, bowel and bladder function are affected.

LABORATORY FEATURES

CSF protein can be elevated with or without a lymphocytic pleocytosis.[40] Sensory NCSs often reveal absent SNAPs.[38] Motor NCSs demonstrate markedly reduced conduction velocities (<50% of mean values) in the arms and legs.[37,38,40,41] The distal motor latencies are only mildly to moderately prolonged. The NCSs become abnormal by 2 weeks following onset of neuropathic symptoms and reach their nadir by 5–8 weeks. Subsequently, there is slow and steady improvement in the NCSs that lag behind clinical recovery.

HISTOPATHOLOGY

Segmental demyelination and axonal degeneration have been appreciated in the nerve roots and the more distal segments of the peripheral nerve.[36] Degeneration of dorsal root ganglia may be observed as well.

PATHOGENESIS

The bacteria release diphtheria exotoxin which binds to Schwann cells and inhibits synthesis of myelin proteins.[42]

TREATMENT

Antitoxin and antibiotics should be given within 48 hours of symptom onset. Although early treatment reduces the incidence and severity of some complications (i.e., cardiomyopathy), it does not appear to alter the natural history of the associated peripheral neuropathy. The neuropathy usually resolves after several months. Patients need to be managed with supportive care (e.g., mechanical ventilation, PE prophylaxis, physical therapy) as discussed in the chapter on GBS (Chapter 13).

▶ HUMAN IMMUNODEFICIENCY VIRUS

HIV infection can result in a variety of neuromuscular complications (Table 17-4), including peripheral neuropathies.

▶ **TABLE 17-4. NEUROLOGICAL COMPLICATIONS ASSOCIATED WITH HIV INFECTION**

Central nervous system
    Opportunistic infections
    Progressive multifocal leukoencephalopathy
    HIV-associated encephalopathy (AIDS dementia)
    Lymphomas and other malignancies
    Subacute combined degeneration (B12 deficiency)
    Vacuolar myelopathy
Peripheral nervous system disorders
    Distal symmetric polyneuropathy
    Motor neuronopathy
    Acute and chronic inflammatory demyelinating polyradiculoneuropathy
    Polyradiculoneuropathy/multiple mononeuropathies caused by other infections (e.g., cytomegalovirus, hepatitis B or C, and herpes zoster)
    Autonomic neuropathy
    Sensory ganglionopathy
    Toxic neuropathy (antiretroviral medications)
Myopathy
    Toxic myopathy (antiretroviral medications)
    Inflammatory (polymyositis or inclusion body myositis)
    Infectious (opportunistic infections)
    Myopathy secondary to wasting/cachexia

Approximately 20% of individuals infected with HIV develop a neuropathy which may be as a direct result of the virus itself, other associated viral infections [e.g., cytomegalovirus (CMV) infection], or neurotoxicity secondary to antiviral medications.[43–56] The neuropathy associated with antiviral medications are discussed in Chapter 20. The major presentations of peripheral neuropathy associated with HIV infection include: (1) distal symmetric polyneuropathy (DSP), (2) inflammatory demyelinating polyneuropathy (including both AIDP and CIDP), (3) multiple mononeuropathies (e.g., vasculitis, CMV related), (4) polyradiculopathy (usually CMV related), (5) autonomic neuropathy, and (6) sensory ganglionitis.[43–56]

▶ HIV-RELATED DISTAL SYMMETRIC POLYNEUROPATHY

CLINICAL FEATURES

DSP is the most common form of peripheral neuropathy associated with HIV infection and usually is seen in patients with AIDS.[43,44,46–48,57,58] It is characterized by numbness and painful paresthesia involving the distal legs and arms. Some patients are asymptomatic but have reduced sensation to all modalities on examination. Mild distal muscle weakness may be appreciated. Proximal leg and distal arm weakness may develop late in the course of the disease. Muscle stretch reflexes are reduced at the ankles but are relatively preserved at the knees and in the arms.

LABORATORY FEATURES

CSF examination may demonstrate an increased protein and mild lymphocytic pleocytosis in patients with HIV infection regardless of the stage of the infection and the presence or absence of peripheral neuropathy.[59,60] Vitamin B12 deficiency is noted in some[61,62] but not all patients.[63–65] NCSs and EMG reveal abnormalities suggestive of a symmetric, axonal sensory greater than motor polyneuropathy.[43,45,66–69]

HISTOPATHOLOGY

Nerve biopsies are not routinely performed in HIV patients with DSP but typically reveal axonal degeneration and a loss in the total number of both myelinated and demyelinated axons (Fig. 17-6).[54,66,69–72] A reduction of cell bodies in the dorsal root ganglia may be appreciated, as well as secondary degeneration of the dorsal columns. Mild perivascular inflammation consisting of macrophages and T lymphocytes is seen along with the evidence of increased cytokine expression. Reduced density of small myelinated epidermal nerve fibers is appreciated in the epidermis with skin biopsy along with an increase in large mitochondrial DNA deletions.[73,74]

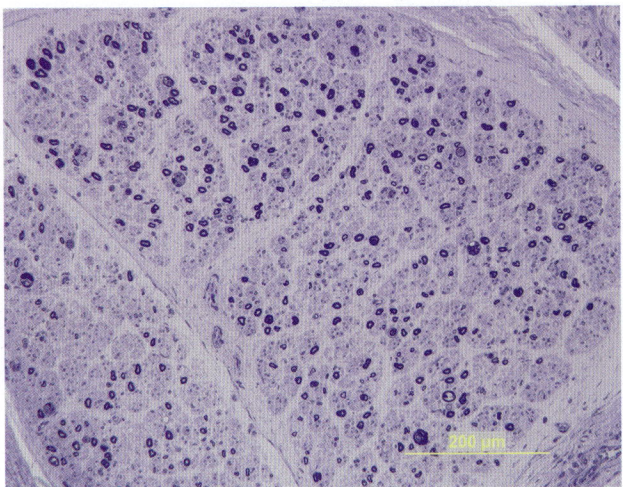

Figure 17-6. HIV neuropathy. Sural nerve biopsy in a patient with distal symmetric sensory neuropathy demonstrates a mild reduction in myelinated nerve fibers. Epoxy embedded, toluidine blue stain.

PATHOGENESIS

The pathogenic basis for DSP is unknown but is not due to actual infection of the peripheral nerves. Viral coat proteins, in particular gp120, may mediate nerve fiber damage and hyperalgesia through direct and indirect mechanisms.[58] In addition, the glial and macrophage response activated by virus may indirectly damage neurons by the release of cytokines from surrounding inflammatory cells. Vitamin B12 deficiency may contribute to some cases but is not a major cause of most cases of DSP. Various antiretroviral agents (e.g., dideoxycytidine, dideoxyinosine, and stavudine) are also neurotoxic and may cause a painful sensory neuropathy.[68,75–77] The HIV itself, secondary inflammatory response, and antiviral treatments appear to cause abnormal mitochondrial function, in part related to impaired mitochondrial DNA replication.[74,78]

TREATMENT

The neuropathy is not responsive to treatment with antiretroviral medications and therapy is largely symptomatic. We usually initiate treatment with neuropathic pain medications (see Chapter 22, Table 23-2).

▶ HIV-RELATED INFLAMMATORY DEMYELINATING POLYRADICULONEUROPATHY

CLINICAL FEATURES

Both AIDP and CIDP can occur as a complication of HIV infection.[48,58,79] AIDP usually develops at the time of seroconversion, whereas CIDP can occur anytime in the course of the infection. Clinical features are indistinguishable from idiopathic AIDP or CIDP.

LABORATORY FEATURES

In addition to elevated protein levels, lymphocytic pleocytosis is evident in the CSF—a finding that helps distinguish HIV-associated polyradiculoneuropathy from idiopathic AIDP/CIDP. Motor and sensory NCSs are similar to that seen in idiopathic AIDP and CIDP (Chapters 13 and 14).[41,79–81] Motor and sensory NCSs may demonstrate slow conduction velocities, prolonged distal latencies and F waves, conduction block, and/or temporal dispersion.

HISTOPATHOLOGY

Nerve biopsies are not routinely performed for this indication, but can show features identical to those found in idiopathic AIDP and CIDP.[41,70]

TREATMENT

We usually treat patients with HIV-associated AIDP or CIDP with intravenous immunoglobulin (IVIg) though plasmapheresis (PE) can also be used.[41,80] Prednisone can be used in HIV-associated CIDP, but we try to avoid steroids and other second-line immunosuppressive agents because of the long-term implications of immunosuppression in patients with HIV.

▶ HIV-RELATED PROGRESSIVE POLYRADICULOPATHY (SECONDARY CMV INFECTION)

CLINICAL FEATURES

An acute, progressive lumbosacral polyradiculoneuropathy secondary to CMV infection can develop in patients with AIDS.[48,58] Patients usually present with severe radicular pain, numbness, and weakness in the legs, which is usually asymmetric. Loss of perineal sensation with bowel and bladder incontinence is common. The arms and cranial nerves may also be affected. Reduced or absent muscle stretch reflexes are appreciated on examination. Plantar responses are usually flexor but can be extensor if a superimposed CMV myelitis is also present. Patients usually have evidence of CMV infection in other parts of the body (i.e., CMV retinitis).

LABORATORY FEATURES

CSF is abnormal, demonstrating an increased protein level along with a reduced glucose concentration and, notably, a neutrophilic pleocytosis. CMV can be cultured from the CSF, blood, and urine. NCSs often demonstrate an asymmetric reduction of amplitudes of the SNAPs and CMAPs with active denervation changes on EMG in muscles innervated by affected nerve roots and nerves including the paraspinals.[82,83] The axonal nature and distribution of these abnormalities are quite distinct from those found in both CIDP and DSP, respectively, helping to differentiate these various disorders.

HISTOPATHOLOGY

With postmortem examination, inflammatory infiltrates associated with varying degrees of axonal loss are evident in the ventral and dorsal roots, particularly in the lumbar regions. Occasionally, the cranial nerves exiting from the brainstem may be involved in association with the myelitis. CMV inclusions may be found in endothelial cells and macrophages on nerve biopsy specimens when obtained.[84]

PATHOGENESIS

The polyradiculoneuropathy may be caused by the direct infection of neurons by CMV or ischemia secondary to associated vasculitis.

TREATMENT

The polyradiculoneuropathy may improve with ganciclovir or foscarnet, if treatment is started early.[83,85] However, the prognosis is poor, and most patients die within several weeks or months.

▶ HIV-RELATED MULTIPLE MONONEUROPATHIES

CLINICAL FEATURES

Multiple mononeuropathies can also develop in patients with HIV infection usually in the context of AIDS.[48,58] Weakness, numbness, paresthesia, and pain are evident in the distribution of affected nerves.

LABORATORY FEATURES

Elevated CSF protein and mononuclear pleocytosis may be seen. EMG and NCSs demonstrate features of axon loss as seen with other forms of multiple mononeuropathies caused by vasculitis (see Chapter 15).[86]

HISTOPATHOLOGY

Nerve biopsies can reveal axonal degeneration with necrotizing vasculitis or perivascular inflammation.[87] CMV inclusions may be seen in endothelial cells and macrophages on electron microscopy.[84]

PATHOGENESIS

The pathogenic basis for this disorder is likely multifactorial. The neuropathy may be caused by vasculitis related to deposition of HIV antigen–antibody complexes in the walls of blood vessel, concomitant hepatitis B or C infection, or CMV infection.

TREATMENT

Corticosteroid treatment is indicated in vasculitis directly due to HIV infection. Multiple mononeuropathies secondary to concurrent hepatitis B or C infection can be treated with plasma exchange, antiviral agents (e.g., vidarabine), or α-interferon. Short courses of prednisone and cyclophosphamide may be necessary. If CMV is suspected, treatment with ganciclovir or foscarnet should be initiated.

▶ HIV-RELATED AUTONOMIC NEUROPATHY

CLINICAL FEATURES

An autonomic neuropathy characterized by orthostatic hypotension, impaired sweating, diarrhea, impotence, and bladder dysfunction can develop acutely or insidiously in patients with HIV infection.[88–90] Clinical features are similar to those seen with idiopathic autonomic neuropathy.

LABORATORY FEATURES

CSF can reveal pleocytosis and increased protein. Most patients have electrodiagnostic features similar to that noted in DSP. In addition, autonomic function testing is usually abnormal.[89]

PATHOGENESIS

An immune-mediated mechanism similar to that suspected in idiopathic autonomic neuropathy is likely.

TREATMENT

A trial of corticosteroids, IVIg, or PE may be tried. Symptoms of autonomic neuropathy are treated symptomatically.

▶ HIV-RELATED SENSORY NEURONOPATHY/ GANGLIONOPATHY

Dorsal root ganglionitis is a very rare complication of HIV infection, but neuronopathy can be the presenting manifestation.[91] Patients develop sensory ataxia similar to idiopathic sensory neuronopathy/ganglionopathy. Autopsies have demonstrated inflammatory cell infiltrate in the dorsal root ganglia along with the loss of cell bodies and degeneration of myelinated nerve fibers in the peripheral nerves. NCSs reveal amplitudes or absence of SNAPs. Again, a trial of corticosteroids, IVIg, or PE may be considered.

▶ HUMAN T-LYMPHOCYTE TYPE 1 INFECTION

Besides the more common myelopathy (tropical spastic paraparesis), human T-lymphocyte type 1 (HTLV-1) infection is also associated with an axonal sensorimotor polyneuropathy.[92–94] The neuropathy can be seen even in patients without a myelopathy. HTLV-1 infection has also been associated with myositis. NCSs demonstrate abnormalities suggestive of an axonal, sensory greater than motor, length-dependent neuropathy.[94] Sural nerve biopsy when performed can reveal axonal degeneration with secondary demyelination and inflammatory cell infiltrates. There is one report of CIDP occurring in the setting of HTLV-1 infection.[95]

▶ CYTOMEGALOVIRUS

CMV can cause an acute lumbosacral polyradiculopathy and multiple mononeuropathies in patients with HIV infection or other causes of severe immunosuppression as previously noted.

▶ EPSTEIN–BARR VIRUS

Epstein–Barr virus infection has been associated with AIDP, cranial neuropathies, mononeuropathy multiplex, brachial plexopathy, lumbosacral radiculoplexopathy, and sensory neuronopathies.[96]

▶ HEPATITIS VIRUSES

Hepatitis B and C can cause multiple mononeuropathies related to vasculitis, AIDP, or CIDP, as previously discussed (Chapters 13, 14, and 15).

▶ HERPES VARICELLA-ZOSTER VIRUS

CLINICAL FEATURES

Peripheral neuropathy from herpes varicella-zoster (HVZ) infection is the result of reactivation of latent virus or a primary infection. Primary infection is the cause of "chicken pox." Reactivation of the virus later in life leads to dermal zoster. In patients who are immunocompromised, HVZ infection can be associated with severe disseminated zoster. Two-thirds of infections in adults are characterized by dermal zoster, in which severe pain and paresthesias develop in a dermatomal region, followed within a week or two by a vesicular rash in the same distribution. The vesicular skin lesions clear by 2 weeks. Approximately 25% of patients who are affected have continued pain (postherpetic neuralgia). In a large series of patients, zoster developed in thoracic dermatomes in nearly 50%, lumbosacral region in 18%, trigeminal distribution in the head in an additional 18%, and the cervical dermatomes in the remainder.

Weakness in muscles innervated by roots corresponding to the dermatomal distribution of skin lesions occurs in 5%–30% of patients.[97-99] The weakness usually develops within the first 2 weeks of the skin eruption but can vary between several hours and a month. Unilateral phrenic nerve involvement can lead to hemidiaphragmatic paralysis.[100] When the thoracic myotomes are involved, hernias can occur through weakened abdominal wall musculature.[101,102] Muscle strength usually improves over time. Rarely, patients develop AIDP following HVZ infection.[103,104] Additional neurological manifestations of herpes zoster infection include encephalitis and angiitis leading to vascular events.

LABORATORY FEATURES

CSF protein may be elevated with or without pleocytosis. The virus is difficult to culture from the CSF, but polymerase chain reaction can be used to confirm the presence of the virus in the CSF. Sensory NCSs reveal reduced or absent SNAPs amplitudes in affected nerves.[105-107] Motor NCSs may also demonstrate normal or reduced CMAP amplitudes.[98,99,105,107] Positive sharp waves and fibrillation potentials and neurogenic-appearing MUAPs and recruitment can be observed on needle EMG in muscles of affected myotomes.[98,99,105,107]

HISTOPATHOLOGY

The basic pathological neural reaction is that of axonal degeneration with some degree of secondary segmental demyelination. With respect to the sensory system, severe infections can result in the destruction of dorsal root ganglion cells with the secondary loss of posterior column fibers.

PATHOGENESIS

Following initial infection, the HVZ migrates up the sensory nerves and takes residence in the sensory ganglia, where the virus appears to be insulated from the host's immune defense mechanisms. When the host becomes immunosuppressed, the virus can reactivate and replicate. HVZ travels down the sensory nerves including cutaneous nerves and result in the typical cutaneous zoster lesions. The inflammatory response in the spinal nerve may involve motor axons resulting in muscle weakness.

TREATMENT

Acyclovir helps improve the rate of healing of the skin lesions, but acyclovir neither alone nor in combination with corticosteroids reduces the frequency or severity of postherpetic neuralgia. IV acyclovir should be administered in immunocompromised patients with severe infections. The treatment of postherpetic neuralgia is symptomatic. Our first-line treatment of choice is lidoderm patches applied over the regions with neuralgic pain. Gabapentin,[108] carbamazepine, topical capsaicin ointment, and tricyclic antidepressants[109] may also reduce the pain in some patients. Opioids are warranted as well in patients with refractory pain.[110]

▶ SEVERE ACUTE RESPIRATORY SYNDROME CORONAVIRUS 2 (SARS-COV-2)

Coronavirus disease 2019 (COVID-19) is caused by severe acute respiratory syndrome coronavirus 2 (SARS-CoV-2). Even in the early days of the pandemic, we postulated on the possible neuromuscular complications that may arise, including the possibility of GBS occurring in patients with COVID-19 or possibly the result of vaccinations that might develop.[111] Not surprising, since the start of the pandemic there have been hundreds of reports of various neuropathies, in particular GBS, complicating the acute infection, as well as vaccinations.[112-114] There also arose many cases of patients with persistent symptoms long after acute infection cleared, the so-called "long-haulers" or postacute COVID-19 syndrome (PACS).[115] The problem with many of these case reports and series is that association does not imply causation,[116] so much more research needs to be done in this regard.

There have been many observational studies looking at the potential relationship between GBS and COVID-19.[18,112-114,117-126] Several studies noted that GBS was more common in COVID-19-positive than COVID-19-negative.[120-122] However, other studies found that the incidence of GBS during the pandemic decreased compared with prior years.[118,119,126] This was likely due to increased hygiene measures during the pandemic leading to a reduction in the number of GBS cases associated with other infections. In our opinion, the best epidemiological study to date from the United Kingdom showed no significant increase in the incidence of GBS during the second wave of COVID-19.[118,119] Importantly, there was no correlation between the number of COVID cases and GBS in different regions of the United Kingdom which argues against a causal association. Aside from GBS, other forms of neuropathy have been reported in the setting of COVID-19, including Miller Fisher syndrome, cranial neuropathies, other focal mononeuropathies, and radiculoplexopathies.[18,127–129,130–135] Some cases were felt to arise from compression of various nerves from prone positioning of critically ill patients. Additionally, there have been a number of case reports, small series, and observational studies that report an association with small fiber neuropathy, including dysautonomia, with COVID-19, particularly in long-haulers.[136–144] Again the problem is the small sample size, confounding or bias, which prevent firm establishment of a causative link.[113] Further epidemiological studies are warranted.

There have also been many studies looking at the risk of GBS with the various COVID-19 vaccines. We reported two cases of GBS in the Jannsen/Johnson & Johnson trial using a viral vector—one participant received the vaccine, while the other received placebo. Thus, again we urged caution that temporal associations due not imply causation.[116] However, subsequent accumulating evidence indeed do support an association between viral vector vaccines (Janssen and AstraZeneca) and GBS, but not with mRNA vaccines

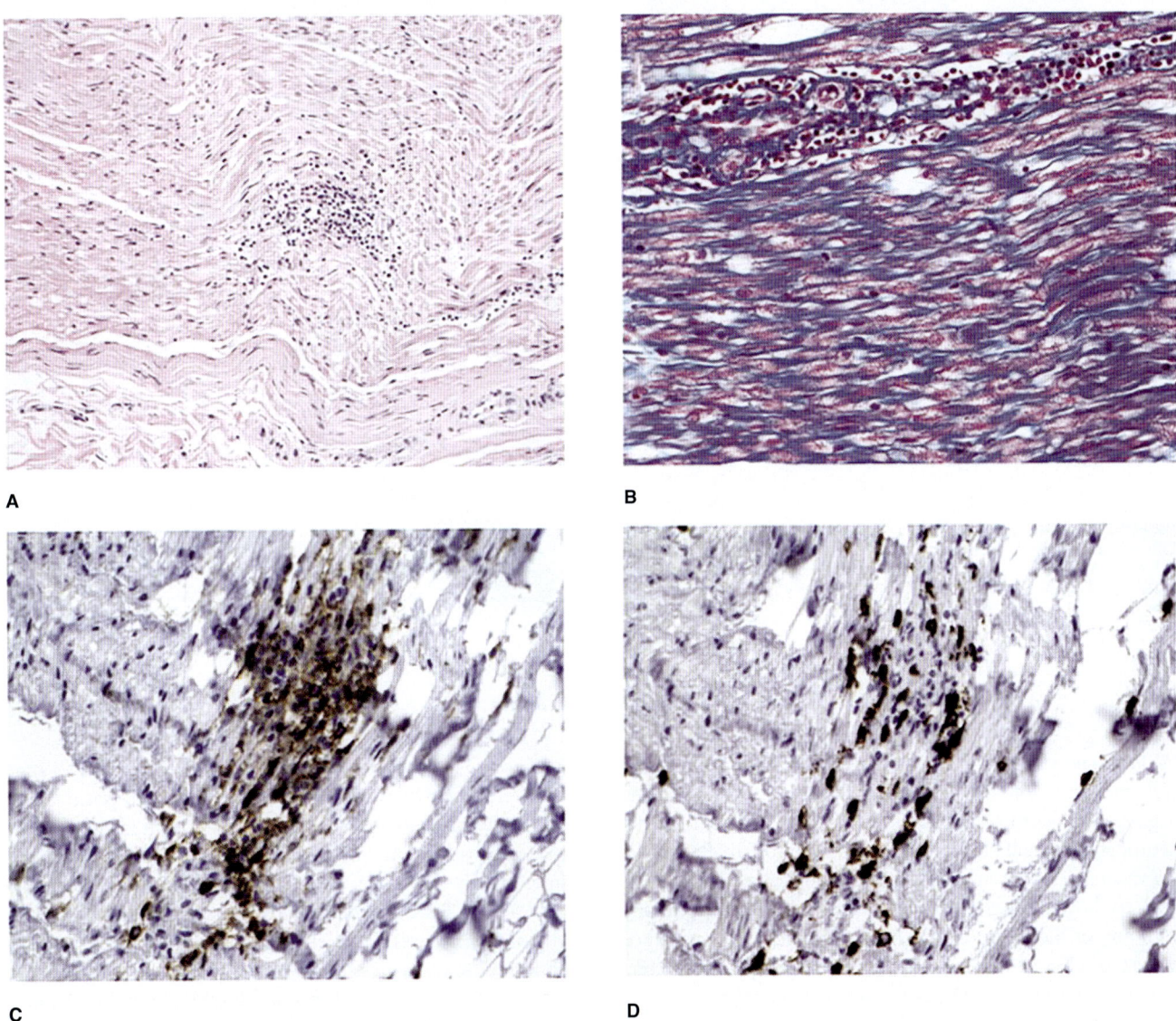

Figure 17-7. Femoral nerve histopathology on an autopsy study of 35 consecutive patients who died from COVID-19 early in the pandemic. Histologic findings include (**A**) perivascular and endoneurial inflammation, in the absence of (**B**) demyelination, comprising mixed (**C**) CD4, (**D**) CD8, (**E**) CD20, and (**F**) CD68 immune cell infiltrates. (**G**) Severe acute respiratory syndrome coronavirus 2 (SARS-CoV-2) immunohistochemistry (IHC) was negative in all cases. (**H**) Human myxovirus resistance protein A (MxA) IHC highlights scattered capillary cell walls (*arrows*). Panel H is from patient 19; panels B and G are from patient 20; panel A is from patient 25; and panels C–F are from patient 26. Section from panel A stained with hematoxylin and eosin, panel B with Masson trichrome, panel C with CD4 IHC, panel D with CD8 IHC, panel E with CD20 IHC, panel F with CD68 IHC, panel G with SARS-CoV-2 nucleocapsid IHC, and panel H with MxA IHC. Image in panel A taken with ×20 objective; images in panels B–G with ×40 objective; and images in panel H with ×60 objective. (With permission from Suh J, Mukerji SS, Collens SI, et al. Muscle and Peripheral Nerve Histopathology in COVID-19. *Neurology*. 2021 ;97(8):e849–e858.) *(continued)*

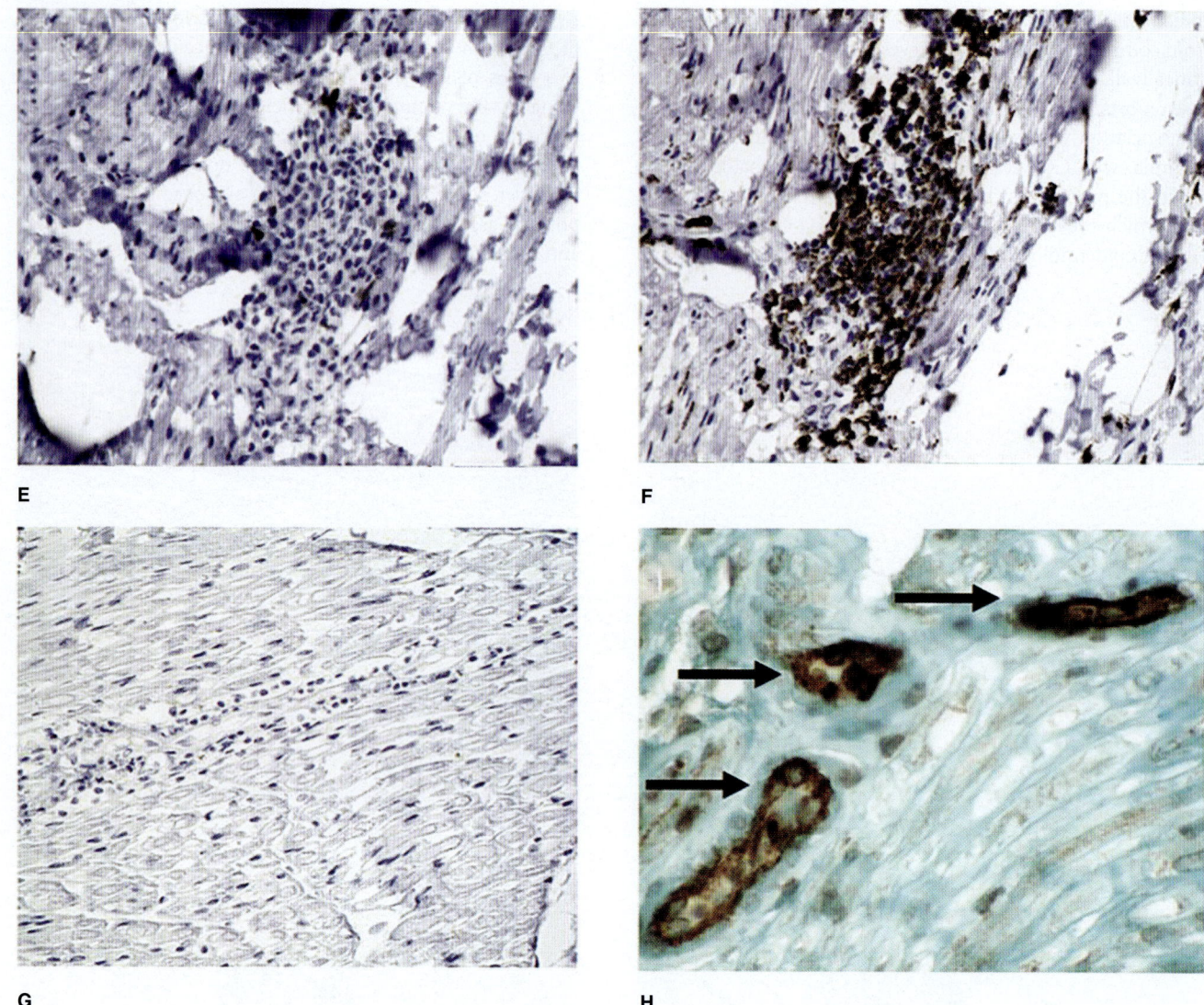

Figure 17-7. (continued)

(Moderna and Pfizer).[113,145–152] There are also many case reports and small series of other potential inflammatory neuropathies (e.g., cranial neuropathies, mononeuropathies, radiculoplexus neuropathies, small fiber and autonomic neuropathies) following vaccinations but no strong epidemiological study has been done to show a causal relationship with of these complications with any of the types of COVID-19 vaccines. Importantly, a history of GBS or any autoimmune neuropathy are not contraindications for receiving a COVID-10 vaccination.[153,154]

There is limited nerve histopathology on patient with COVID-19. We did an autopsy study looking at muscle (iliopsoas) and peripheral nerve (femoral) from 5 consecutive autopsies of patients who died after SARS-CoV-2 infection and 10 SARS-CoV-2-negative controls were examined under light microscopy.[155] Microscopic examination of nerve showed neuritis in nine patients (Fig. 17-7), consisting of perivascular inflammatory cells in six, endoneurial infiltrates in one, and both perivascular and endoneurial inflammatory cells in two patients. The most abundant inflammatory cells were CD68-positive histiocytes were evident in all nine but were sometimes co-predominant with CD8-positive and less frequently with CD4-positive T cells. MxA immunostaining was observed in 7 of 35 (20%) cases in the capillaries, but interestingly only one of whom had neuritis. Importantly SARS-CoV-2 was not detected by immunohistochemistry in any of the 35 cases. Neither inflammatory cell infiltrates nor abnormal MxA expression was observed in the control cases. None had signs or symptoms of GBS. MxA is a type 1 interferon–inducible protein that is normally expressed in response to viral infections and prevents viral replication in the host. However, overexpression of type 1 interferons may be toxic to nerves and muscle (e.g., dermatomyositis and systemic lupus erythematosus). Peripheral nerve was felt to be bystander victim of the host response and cytokine dysregulation. Given the findings it is possible thought that some reported cases of polyneuropathy around the time of infection or in long haulers may be related to such inflammation or a possible exaggerated type 1 interferon response at the time of acute infection.

SUMMARY

Neuropathies associated with infection are not uncommon. In fact, lepromatous neuropathy may be the most common form of neuropathy, particularly in nonindustrialized nations. Further, neuropathies related to HIV infection have increased, owing to the spread of this infection and longer life span of treated individuals rendering them susceptible to the neurotoxic effects of the infection and antiretroviral infections. Lyme disease likewise needs to be considered in endemic regions. Notably, many of these neuropathies are treatable; thus, diagnosis is essential.

REFERENCES

1. Rodrigues LC, Lockwood DN. Leprosy now: epidemiology, progress, challenges, and research gaps. *Lancet Infect Dis.* 2011;11(6):464–470.
2. Altman D, Amato A. Lepromatous neuropathy. *J Clin Neuromuscul Dis.* 1999;1(2):68–73.
3. Nations SP, Katz JS, Lyde CB, Barohn RJ. Leprous neuropathy: an American perspective. *Semin Neurol.* 1998;18(1):113–124.
4. Ooi WW, Srinivasan J. Leprosy and the peripheral nervous system: basic and clinical aspects. *Muscle Nerve.* 2004;30(4):393–409.
5. Ridley DS, Jopling WH. Classification of leprosy according to immunity. A five-group system. *Int J Lepr Other Mycobact Dis.* 1966;34(3):255–273.
6. Khadilkar SV, Patil SB, Shetty VP. Neuropathies of leprosy. *J Neurol Sci.* 2021;420:117288.
7. Rodriguez G, Sanchez W, Chaleta JG, Soto J. Primary neuritic leprosy. *J Am Acad Dermatol.* 1993;29(6):1050–1052.
8. Jardim MR, Chimelli L, Faria SC, et al. Clinical, electroneuromyographic and morphological studies of pure neural leprosy in a Brazilian referral centre. *Lepr Rev.* 2004;75(3):242–253.
9. McLeod JG, Hargrave JC, Walsh JC, Booth GC, Gye RS, Barron A. Nerve conduction studies in leprosy. *Int J Lepr Other Mycobact Dis.* 1975;43(1):21–31.
10. Amato AA, Dumitru D. Acquired neuropathies. In: Dumitru D, Amato AA, Swartz MJ, eds. *Electrodiagnostic Medicine.* 2nd ed. Hanley & Belfus; 2002:937–1041.
11. Bathala L, Kumar K, Pathapati R, Jain S, Visser LH. Ulnar neuropathy in hansen disease: clinical, high-resolution ultrasound and electrophysiologic correlations. *J Clin Neurophysiol.* 2012;29(2):190–193.
12. Ebenezer GJ, Scollard DM. Treatment and evaluation advances in leprosy neuropathy. *Neurotherapeutics.* 2021;18(4):2337–2350.
13. Antunes SLG, Fazan VPS, Jardim MR, et al. Morphometric analysis of nerve fibers in neural leprosy. *Muscle Nerve.* 2021;63(4):593–599.
14. Shimoji Y, Ng V, Matsumura K, Fischetti VA, Rambukkana A. A 21-kDa surface protein of Mycobacterium leprae binds peripheral nerve laminin-2 and mediates Schwann cell invasion. *Proc Natl Acad Sci USA.* 1999;96(17):9857–9862.
15. Lazo-Porras M, Prutsky GJ, Barrionuevo P, et al. World Health Organization (WHO) antibiotic regimen against other regimens for the treatment of leprosy: a systematic review and meta-analysis. *BMC Infect Dis.* 2020;20(1):62.
16. World Health Organization (WHO) recommended MDT regimens. https://iris.who.int/bitstream/handle/10665/274127/9789290226383-eng.pdf?ua=1
17. Van Veen NH, Lockwood DN, Van Brakel WH, Ramirez J Jr, Richardus JH. Interventions for erythema nodosum leprosum. A Cochrane review. *Lepr Rev.* 2009;80(4):355–372.
18. Gutiérrez-Ortiz C, Méndez-Guerrero A, Rodrigo-Rey S, et al. Miller Fisher syndrome and polyneuritis cranialis in COVID-19. *Neurology.* 2020;95(05):e601–e605.
19. Halperin JJ, Eikeland R, Branda JA, Dersch R. Lyme neuroborreliosis: known knowns, known unknowns. *Brain.* 2022;145(8):2635–2647.
20. Halperin JJ, Little BW, Coyle PK, Dattwyler RJ. Lyme disease: cause of a treatable peripheral neuropathy. *Neurology.* 1987;37(11):1700–1706.
21. Halperin J, Luft BJ, Volkman DJ, Dattwyler RJ. Lyme neuroborreliosis. Peripheral nervous system manifestations. *Brain.* 1990;113(Pt 4):1207–1221.
22. Krishnamurthy KB, Liu GT, Logigian EL. Acute Lyme neuropathy presenting with polyradicular pain, abdominal protrusion, and cranial neuropathy. *Muscle Nerve.* 1993;16(11):1261–1264.
23. Logigian EL, Steere AC. Clinical and electrophysiologic findings in chronic neuropathy of Lyme disease. *Neurology.* 1992;42(2):303–311.
24. Oey PL, Franssen H, Bersen RA, Wokke JH. Multifocal conduction block in a patient with *Borrelia burgdorferi* infection. *Muscle Nerve.* 1991;14(4):375–377.
25. Scelsa SN, Hershkovitz S, Berger AR. A predominantly motor polyradiculopathy of Lyme disease. *Muscle Nerve.* 1996;19(6):780–783.
26. Pachner AR, Steere AC. The triad of neurologic manifestations of Lyme disease: meningitis, cranial neuritis, and radiculoneuritis. *Neurology.* 1985;35(1):47–53.
27. Vallat JM, Hugon J, Lubeau M, Leboutet MJ, Dumas M, Desproges-Gotteron R. Tick-bite meningoradiculoneuritis: clinical, electrophysiologic, and histologic findings in 10 cases. *Neurology.* 1987;37(5):749–753.
28. Wulff CH, Hansen K, Strange P, Trojaborg W. Multiple mononeuritis and radiculitis with erythema, pain, elevated CSF protein and pleocytosis (Bannwarth's syndrome). *J Neurol Neurosurg Psychiatry.* 1983;46(6):485–490.
29. Schoenen J, Sianard-Gainko J, Carpentier M, Reznik M. Myositis during *Borrelia burgdorferi* infection (Lyme disease). *J Neurol Neurosurg Psychiatry.* 1989;52(8):1002–1005.
30. Halperin JJ, Volkman DJ, Luft BJ, Dattwyler RJ. Carpal tunnel syndrome in Lyme borrelliosis. *Muscle Nerve.* 1989;12(5):397–400.
31. Halperin JJ, Pass HL, Anand AK, Luft BJ, Volkman DJ, Dattwyler RJ. Nervous system abnormalities in Lyme disease. *Ann N Y Acad Sci.* 1988;539:24–34.
32. Gonzalez H, Koralnik IJ, Marra CM. Neurosyphilis. *Semin Neurol.* 2019;39(4):448–455.
33. Ropper AH. Neurosyphilis. *N Engl J Med.* 2019;381(14):1358–1363.
34. Bhandari J, Thada PK, Ratzan RM. Tabes dorsalis. 2022. In: *StatPearls [Internet].* StatPearls Publishing; 2023.
35. Chu M, Kumar S, Sturm J. Syphilitic meningitis presenting with multiple cranial neuropathies. *BMJ Case Rep.* 2021;14(6):e241765.
36. Fisher CM, Adams RD. Diphtheritic polyneuritis; a pathological study. *J Neuropathol Exp Neurol.* 1956;15(3):243–268.

37. Kazemi B, Tahernia AC, Zandian K. Motor nerve conduction in diphtheria and diphtheritic myocarditis. *Arch Neurol.* 1973;29(2):104–106.
38. Kurdi A, Abdul-Kader M. Clinical and electrophysiological studies of diphtheritic neuritis in Jordan. *J Neurol Sci.* 1979;42(2):243–250.
39. Solders G, Nennesmo I, Persson A. Diphtheritic neuropathy, an analysis based on muscle and nerve biopsy and repeated neurophysiological and autonomic function tests. *J Neurol Neurosurg Psychiatry.* 1989;52(7):876–880.
40. Créange A, Meyrignac C, Roualdes B, Degos JD, Gherardi RK. Diphtheritic neuropathy. *Muscle Nerve.* 1995;18(12):1460–1463.
41. Cornblath DR, McArthur JC, Kennedy PG, Witte AS, Griffin JW. Inflammatory demyelinating peripheral neuropathies associated with human T-cell lymphotropic virus type III infection. *Ann Neurol.* 1987;21(1):32–40.
42. Pleasure DE, Feldmann B, Prockop DJ. Diphtheria toxin inhibits the synthesis of myelin proteolipid and basic proteins by peripheral nerve in vitro. *J Neurochem.* 1973;20(1):81–90.
43. Floeter MK, Civetello LA, Everett CR, Dambrosia J, Luciano CA. Peripheral neuropathy in children with HIV infection. *Neurology.* 1997;49(1):207–212.
44. Marra CM, Boutin P, Collier AC. Screening for distal sensory peripheral neuropathy in HIV-infected persons in research and clinical settings. *Neurology.* 1998;51(6):1678–1681.
45. Tagliati M, Grinnell J, Godbold J, Simpson DM. Peripheral nerve function in HIV infection: clinical, electrophysiologic, and laboratory findings. *Arch Neurol.* 1999;56(1):84–89.
46. Julian T, Rekatsina M, Shafique F, Zis P. Human immunodeficiency virus-related peripheral neuropathy: a systematic review and meta-analysis. *Eur J Neurol.* 2021;28(4):1420–1431.
47. Jazebi N, Evans C, Kadaru HS, et al. HIV-related neuropathy: pathophysiology, treatment and challenges. *J Neurol Exp Neurosci.* 2021;7(1):15–24.
48. Robinson-Papp J, Simpson DM. Neuromuscular diseases associated with HIV-1 infection. *Muscle Nerve.* 2009;40(6):1043–1053.
49. Barohn RJ, Gronseth GS, LeForce BR, et al. Peripheral nervous system involvement in a large cohort of human immunodeficiency virus-infected individuals. *Arch Neurol.* 1993;50(2):167–171.
50. Cornblath DR, McArthur JC. Predominantly sensory neuropathy in patients with AIDS and AIDS-related complex. *Neurology.* 1988;38(5):794–796.
51. Dalakas MC, Pezeshkpour GH. Neuromuscular diseases associated with human immunodeficiency virus infection. *Ann Neurol.* 1988;23:S38–S48.
52. de la Monte SM, Gabuzda DH, Ho DD, et al. Peripheral neuropathy in the acquired immunodeficiency syndrome. *Ann Neurol.* 1988;23(5):485–492.
53. Fuller GN, Jacobs JM, Guiloff RJ. Nature and incidence of peripheral nerve syndromes in HIV infection. *J Neurol Neurosurg Psychiatry.* 1993;56(4):372–381.
54. Hall CD, Snyder CR, Messenheimer JA, et al. Peripheral neuropathy in a cohort of human immunodeficiency virus-infected patients. Incidence and relationship to other nervous system dysfunction. *Arch Neurol.* 1991;48(12):1273–1274.
55. Lange DJ. AAEM minimonograph #41: neuromuscular diseases associated with HIV-1 infection. *Muscle Nerve.* 1994;17(1):16–30.
56. McArthur JC, Cohen BA, Selnes OA, et al. Low prevalence of neurological and neuropsychological abnormalities in otherwise healthy HIV-1-infected individuals: results from the multicenter AIDS Cohort Study. *Ann Neurol.* 1989;26(5):601–611.
57. Kamerman PR, Moss PJ, Weber J, Wallace VC, Rice AS, Huang W. Pathogenesis of HIV-associated sensory neuropathy: evidence from in vivo and in vitro experimental models. *J Peripher Nerv Syst.* 2012;17(1):19–31.
58. Simpson DM, Olney RK. Peripheral neuropathies associated with human immunodeficiency virus infection. *Neurol Clin.* 1992;10(3):685–711.
59. Barohn RJ, Gronseth GS, Amato AA, et al. Cerebrospinal fluid and nerve conduction abnormalities in HIV positive individuals. *J Neurol Sci.* 1996;136(1-2):81–85.
60. Marshall DW, Brey RL, Butzin CA, Lucey DR, Abbadessa, Boswell RN. CSF changes in a longitudinal study of 124 neurologically normal HIV-1-infected U.S. Air Force personnel. *J Acquir Immune Defic Syndr.* 1991;4(8):777–781.
61. Beach RS, Morgan R, Wilkie F, et al. Plasma vitamin B12 level as a potential cofactor in studies of human immunodeficiency virus type 1-related cognitive changes. *Arch Neurol.* 1992;49(5):501–506.
62. Kieburtz KD, Giang DW, Schiffer RB, Vakil N. Abnormal vitamin B12 metabolism in human immunodeficiency virus infection. Association with neurological dysfunction. *Arch Neurol.* 1991;48(3):312–314.
63. Dal Pan GJ, Allen RH, Glass JD, et al. Cobalamin (vitamin B12)-dependent metabolism is not altered in HIV-1-associated vacuolar myelopathy. *Ann Neurol.* 1993;34:281–282.
64. Robertson KR, Stern RA, Hall CD, et al. Vitamin B12 deficiency and nervous system disease in HIV infection. *Arch Neurol.* 1993;50(8):807–811.
65. Veilleux M, Paltiel O, Falutz J. Sensorimotor neuropathy and abnormal vitamin B12 metabolism in early HIV infection. *Can J Neurol Sci.* 1995;22(1):43–46.
66. Bailey RO, Baltch AL, Venkatesh R, Singh JK, Bishop MB. Sensory motor neuropathy associated with AIDS. *Neurology.* 1988;38(6):886–891.
67. Chavanet P, Solary E, Giroud M, et al. Infraclinical neuropathies related to immunodeficiency virus infection associated with higher T-helper cell count. *J Acquir Immune Defic Syndr.* 1989;2(6):564–569.
68. Dubinsky RM, Yarchoan R, Dalakas M, Broder S. Reversible axonal neuropathy from treatment of AIDS and related disorders with 2′,3′-dideoxycytidine (ddC). *Muscle Nerve.* 1989;12(10):856–860.
69. Fuller GN, Jacobs JM, Guiloff RJ. Subclinical peripheral nerve involvement in AIDS: an electrophysiological and pathological study. *J Neurol Neurosurg Psychiatry.* 1991;54(4):318–324.
70. Chaunu MP, Ratinahirana H, Raphael M, et al. The spectrum of the changes on 20 nerve biopsies in patients with HIV infection. *Muscle Nerve.* 1989;12(6):452–459.
71. Fuller GN, Jacobs JM, Guiloff RJ. Axonal atrophy in the painful peripheral neuropathy in AIDS. *Acta Neuropathol.* 1990;81(2):198–203.
72. Rance NE, McArthur JC, Cornblath DR, Landstrom DL, Griffin JW, Price DL. Gracile tract degeneration in patients with sensory neuropathy and AIDS. *Neurology.* 1998;38(2):265–271.
73. Herrman DN, Griffin JW, Hauer P. Cornblath DR, McArthur JC. Epidermal nerve fiber density and sural nerve

morphometry in peripheral neuropathies. *Neurology.* 1999; 53(8):1634–1640.
74. Roda RH, Bargiela D, Chen W, et al. Large mitochondrial DNA deletions in HIV sensory neuropathy. *Neurology.* 2021; 97(2):e156–e165.
75. Berger AR, Arezzo JC, Schaumburg HH, et al. 2′,3′-dideoxycytidine (ddC) toxic neuropathy: a study of 52 patients. *Neurology.* 1993;43(2):358–362.
76. Kieburtz KD, Seidlin M, Lambert JS, Dolin R, Reichman R, Valentine F. Extended follow-up of peripheral neuropathy in patients with AIDS and AIDS-related complex treated with dideoxyinosine. *J Acquir Immune Defic Syndr.* 1992;5(1):60–64.
77. Leung GP. Iatrogenic mitochondriopathies: a recent lesson from nucleoside/nucleotide reverse transcriptase inhibitors. *Adv Exp Med Biol.* 2012;942:347–369.
78. Roda RH, Hoke A. Mitochondrial dysfunction in HIV-induced peripheral neuropathy. *Int Rev Neurobiol.* 2019;145:67–82.
79. Brannagan TH III, Zhou Y. HIV-associated Guillain–Barre syndrome. *J Neurol Sci.* 2003;208(1–2):39–42.
80. Leger JM, Bouche P, Bolgert F, et al. The spectrum of polyneuropathies in patients infected with HIV. *J Neurol Neurosurg Psychiatry.* 1989;52(12):1369–1374.
81. Przedbroski S, Liesnard C, Voordecker P, et al. Inflammatory demyelinating polyradiculoneuropathy associated with human immunodeficiency virus infection. *J Neurol.* 1988; 235(6):359–361.
82. Dalakas MC, Yarchoan R, Spitzer R, Elder G, Sever JL. Treatment of human immunodeficiency virus-related polyneuropathy with 3′-azido-2′,3′-dideoxythymidine. *Ann Neurol.* 1988;23:S92–S94.
83. Miller RG, Storey JR, Greco CM. Ganciclovir in the treatment of progressive AIDS-related polyradiculopathy. *Neurology.* 1990;40(4):569–574.
84. Roullet E, Assueurs V, Gozlan J, et al. Cytomegalovirus multifocal neuropathy in AIDS: analysis of 15 consecutive cases. *Neurology.* 1994:44(11):2174–2182.
85. Kim YS, Hollander H. Polyradiculopathy due to cytomegalovirus: report of two cases in which improvement occurred after prolonged therapy and review of the literature. *Clin Infect Dis.* 1993;17(1):32–37.
86. Lipkin WI, Parry G, Kiprov D, Abrams D. Inflammatory neuropathy in homosexual men with lymphadenopathy. *Neurology.* 1985;35(10):1479–1483.
87. Said G, Lacroix-Ciaudo C, Fujimura H, Blas C, Faux N. The peripheral neuropathy of necrotizing arteritis: a clinicopathological study. *Ann Neurol.* 1988;23(5):461–465.
88. Cohen JA, Laudenslager M. Autonomic nervous system involvement in patients with human immunodeficiency virus infection. *Neurology.* 1989;39(8):1111–1112.
89. Craddock C, Pasvol G, Bull R, Protheroe A, Hopkin J. Cardiorespiratory arrest and autonomic neuropathy in AIDS. *Lancet.* 1987;2(8549):16–18.
90. Lin-Greenberger A, Taneja-Uppal N. Dysautonomia and infection with the human immunodeficiency virus. *Ann Intern Med.* 1987;106(1):167.
91. Elder G, Dalakas M, Pezeshkpour G, Sever J. Ataxic neuropathy due to ganglioneuronitis after probable acute human immunodeficiency virus infection. *Lancet.* 1986;2(8518):1275–1276.
92. Kiwaki T, Umehara F, Arimura Y, et al. The clinical and pathological features of peripheral neuropathy accompanied with HTLV-I associated myelopathy. *J Neurol Sci.* 2003;206(1):17–21.
93. Leite AC, Silva MT, Alamy AH, et al. Peripheral neuropathy in HTLV-I infected individuals without tropical spastic paraparesis/HTLV-I-associated myelopathy. *J Neurol.* 2004; 251(7):877–881.
94. Saeidi M, Sasannejad P, Foroughipour M, Shahami S, Shoeibi A. Prevalence of peripheral neuropathy in patients with HTLV-1 associated myelopathy/tropical spastic paraparesis (HAM/TSP). *Acta Neurol Belg.* 2011;111(1):41–44.
95. Ali A, Char G, Hanchard B. Chronic inflammatory demyelinating polyneuropathy in a patient infected with human T lymphotropic virus type I. *BMJ Case Rep.* 2009;2009: bcr03.2009.1680.
96. Rubin DI, Daube JR. Subacute sensory neuropathy associated with Epstein–Barr virus. *Muscle Nerve.* 1999;22(11):1607–1610.
97. Greenberg MK, McVey AL, Hayes T. Segmental motor involvement in herpes zoster: an EMG study. *Neurology.* 1992;42(5):1122–1123.
98. Haanpää M, Häkkinen V, Nurmikko T. Motor involvement in acute herpes zoster. *Muscle Nerve.* 1997;20(11):1433–1438.
99. Modelli M, Scarpini C, Malandrini A, Romano C. Painful neuropathy after diffuse herpes zoster. *Muscle Nerve.* 1997; 20(2):229–231.
100. Dutt AK. Diaphragmatic paralysis caused by herpes zoster. *Am Rev Respir Dis.* 1970;101(5):755–758.
101. Glantz RH, Ristanovic RK. Abdominal muscle paralysis from herpes zoster. *J Neurol Neurosurg Psychiatry.* 1988;51(6): 885–886.
102. Gottschau P, Trojaborg W. Abdominal muscle paralysis associated with herpes zoster. *Acta Neurol Scand.* 1991;84(4): 344–347.
103. Dayan AD, Ogul E, Graveson GS. Polyneuritis and herpes zoster. *J Neurol Neurosurg Psychiatry.* 1972;35(2):170–175.
104. Sanders EA, Peters AC, Gratana JW, Hughes RA. Guillain–Barré syndrome after varicella-zoster infection. *J Neurol.* 1987;234(6):437–439.
105. Gardner-Thorpe C, Foster JB, Barwick DD. Unusual manifestations of herpes zoster. A clinical and electrophysiological study. *J Neurol Sci.* 1976;28(4):427–447.
106. Rosenfeld T, Price MA. Paralysis in herpes zoster. *Aust N Z J Med.* 1985;15(6):712–716.
107. Sachs GM. Segmental zoster paresis: an electrophysiological study. *Muscle Nerve.* 1996;19(6):784–786.
108. Segal AZ, Rordorf G. Gabapentin as a novel treatment for postherpetic neuralgia. *Neurology.* 1996;46(4):1175–1176.
109. Max MB. Treatment of post-herpetic neuralgia: antidepressants. *Ann Neurol.* 1994;35:S50–S53.
110. Rowbotham MC. Managing post-herpetic neuralgia with opioids and local anesthetics. *Ann Neurol.* 1994;35:S46–S49.
111. Guidon AC, Amato AA. COVID-19 and neuromuscular disorders. *Neurology.* 2020;94(22):959–969.
112. Suh J, Amato AA. Neuromuscular complications of coronavirus disease-19. *Curr Opin Neurol.* 2021;34(5):669–674.
113. Suh J, Amato AA. Neuromuscular complications of COVID-19: evidence from the third year of the global pandemic. *Seminars Neurol*; 2023;43(2):251–259.
114. Ellul MA, Benjamin L, Singh B, et al. Neurological associations of COVID-19. *Lancet Neurol.* 2020;19(9):767–783.
115. Nalbandian A, Sehgal K, Gupta A, et al. Post-acute COVID-19 syndrome. *Nat Med.* 2021;27(4):601–615.
116. Márquez Loza AM, Holroyd KB, Johnson SA, Pilgrim DM, Amato AA. Guillain-Barré syndrome in the placebo and

117. Petrelli C, Scendoni R, Pagliorti M, Logullo FO. Acute motor axonal neuropathy related to COVID-19 infection: a new diagnostic overview. *J Clin Neuromuscul Dis.* 2020;22(02): 120–121.
118. Keddie S, Pakpoor J, Mousele C, et al. Epidemiological and cohort study finds no association between COVID-19 and Guillain-Barré syndrome. *Brain.* 2021;144(02):682–693.
119. Lunn MP, Carr AC, Keddie S, Pakpoor J, Pipis M, Willison HJ. Reply: Guillain-Barré syndrome, SARS-CoV-2 and molecular mimicry and ongoing challenges in unravelling the association between COVID-19 and Guillain-Barré syndrome and unclear association between COVID-19 and Guillain-Barré syndrome and currently available data regarding the potential association between COVID-19 and Guillain-Barré syndrome. *Brain.* 2021;144(05):e47.
120. Miró Ò, Llorens P, Jiménez S, et al; Spanish Investigators in Emergency Situations TeAm (SIESTA) network. Frequency of five unusual presentations in patients with COVID-19: results of the UMC-19-S1. *Epidemiol Infect.* 2020;148:e189.
121. Patone M, Handunnetthi L, Saatci D, et al. Neurological complications after first dose of COVID-19 vaccines and SARS-CoV-2 infection. *Nat Med.* 2021;27(12):2144–2153.
122. Luijten LWG, Leonhard SE, van der Eijk AA, et al; IGOS Consortium. Guillain-Barré syndrome after SARS-CoV-2 infection in an international prospective cohort study. *Brain.* 2021;144(11):3392–3404.
123. Garnero M, Del Sette M, Assini A, et al. COVID-19-related and not related Guillain-Barré syndromes share the same management pitfalls during lock down: the experience of Liguria region in Italy. *J Neurol Sci.* 2020;418:117114.
124. Gigli GL, Bax F, Marini A, et al. Guillain-Barré syndrome in the COVID-19 era: just an occasional cluster? *J Neurol.* 2021;268(04):1195–1197.
125. Filosto M, Cotti Piccinelli S, Gazzina S, et al. Guillain-Barré syndrome and COVID-19: an observational multicentre study from two Italian hotspot regions. *J Neurol Neurosurg Psychiatry.* 2021;92(07):751–756.
126. Umapathi T, Er B, Koh JS, Goh YH, Chua L. Guillain-Barré syndrome decreases in Singapore during the COVID-19 pandemic. *J Peripher Nerv Syst.* 2021;26(02):235–236.
127. Taga A, Lauria G. COVID-19 and the peripheral nervous system. A 2-year review from the pandemic to the vaccine era. *J Peripher Nerv Syst.* 2022;27(1):4–30.
128. Michaelson NM, Malhotra A, Wang Z, Heier L, Tanji K, Wolfe S, Gupta A, MacGowan D. Peripheral neurological complications during COVID-19: a single center experience. *J Neurol Sci.* 2022;434:120118.
129. Meixedo S, Correia M, Machado Lima A, Carneiro I. Parsonage-Turner syndrome post-COVID-19 Oxford/AstraZeneca vaccine inoculation: a case report and brief literature review. *Cureus.* 2023;15(2):e34710.
130. Wan EYF, Chui CSL, Lai FTT, et al. Bell's palsy following vaccination with mRNA (BNT162b2) and inactivated (CoronaVac) SARS-CoV-2 vaccines: a case series and nested case-control study. *Lancet Infect Dis.* 2022;22(01):64–72.
131. Ozonoff A, Nanishi E, Levy O. Bell's palsy and SARS-CoV-2 vaccines—an unfolding story—authors' reply. *Lancet Infect Dis.* 2021;21(09):1211–1212.
132. Sato K, Mano T, Niimi Y, Toda T, Iwata A, Iwatsubo T. Facial nerve palsy following the administration of COVID-19 mRNA vaccines: analysis of a self-reporting database. *Int J Infect Dis.* 2021;111:310–312.
133. Shemer A, Pras E, Einan-Lifshitz A, Dubinsky-Pertzov B, Hecht I. Association of COVID-19 vaccination and facial nerve palsy: a case-control study. *JAMA Otolaryngol Head Neck Surg.* 2021;147(08):739–743.
134. Shasha D, Bareket R, Sikron FH, et al. Real-world safety data for the Pfizer BNT162b2 SARS-CoV-2 vaccine: historical cohort study. *Clin Microbiol Infect.* 2022;28(01):130–134.
135. Renoud L, Khouri C, Revol B, et al. Association of facial paralysis with mRNA COVID-19 vaccines: a disproportionality analysis using the World Health Organization Pharmacovigilance Database. *JAMA Intern Med.* 2021;181(09): 1243–1245.
136. Gemignani F, Bellanova MF, Saccani E. Long-COVID phenotypes and small fiber neuropathy. *J Neurol Sci.* 2023;444: 120490.
137. Shouman K, Vanichkachorn G, Cheshire WP, et al. Autonomic dysfunction following COVID-19 infection: an early experience. *Clin Auton Res.* 2021;31(3):385–394.
138. Abrams RMC, Simpson DM, Navis A, Jette N, Zhou L, Shin SC. Small fiber neuropathy associated with SARS-CoV-2 infection. *Muscle Nerve.* 2022;65(4):440–443.
139. Oaklander AL, Mills AJ, Kelley M, et al. Peripheral neuropathy evaluations of patients with prolonged long COVID. *Neurol Neuroimmunol Neuroinflamm.* 2022;9(03):e1146.
140. Scala I, Bellavia S, Luigetti M, et al. Autonomic dysfunction in noncritically ill COVID-19 patients during the acute phase of disease: an observational, cross-sectional study. *Neurol Sci.* 2022;43(08):4635–4643.
141. Odozor CU, Kannampallil T, Ben Abdallah A, et al. Post-acute sensory neurological sequelae in patients with severe acute respiratory syndrome coronavirus 2 infection: the COVID-PN observational cohort study. *Pain.* 2022;163(12):2398–2410.
142. Abrams RMC, Simpson DM, Navis A, Jette N, Zhou L, Shin SC. Small fiber neuropathy associated with SARS-CoV-2 infection. *Muscle Nerve.* 2022;65(04):440–443.
143. Novak P, Mukerji SS, Alabsi HS, et al. Multisystem involvement in post-acute sequelae of coronavirus disease 19. *Ann Neurol.* 2022; 91(03):367–379.
144. Barizien N, Le Guen M, Russel S, Touche P, Huang F, Vallée A. Clinical characterization of dysautonomia in long COVID-19 patients. *Sci Rep.* 2021;11(01):14042.
145. Woo EJ, Mba-Jonas A, Dimova RB, Alimchandani M, Zinderman CE, Nair N. Association of receipt of the Ad26.COV2.S COVID-19 vaccine with presumptive Guillain-Barré syndrome, February-July 2021. *JAMA.* 2021;326(16):1606–1613.
146. Hanson KE, Goddard K, Lewis N, et al. Incidence of Guillain-Barré syndrome after COVID-19 vaccination in the Vaccine Safety Datalink. *JAMA Netw Open.* 2022;5(04):e228879.
147. Atzenhoffer M, Auffret M, Pegat A, et al. Guillain-Barré syndrome associated with COVID-19 vaccines: a perspective from spontaneous report data. *Clin Drug Investig.* 2022;42(07): 581–592.
148. Keh RYS, Scanlon S, Datta-Nemdharry P, et al. BPNS/ABN COVID-19 Vaccine GBS Study Group. COVID-19 vaccination and Guillain-Barré syndrome: analyses using the National Immunoglobulin Database. *Brain.* 2023;146(02):739–748.

149. Maramattom BV, Krishnan P, Paul R, et al. Guillain-Barré syndrome following ChAdOx1-S/nCoV-19 vaccine. *Ann Neurol*. 2021;90(02):312–314.
150. Osowicki J, Morgan H, Harris A, Crawford NW, Buttery JP, Kiers L. Guillain-Barré syndrome in an Australian state using both mRNA and adenovirus-vector SARS-CoV-2 vaccines. *Ann Neurol*. 2021;90(05):856–858.
151. COVID-19 Vaccine Safety Update. COVID-19 vaccine Janssen. European Medicines Agency. Updated August 11, 2021. Accessed August 30, 2022. https://www.ema.europa.eu/en/documents/covid-19-vaccine-safety-update/covid-19-vaccine-safety-update-covid-19-vaccine-janssen-11-august-2021_en.pdf.
152. Shapiro Ben David S, Potasman I, Rahamim-Cohen D. Rate of recurrent Guillain-Barré syndrome after mRNA-COVID-19 vaccine BNT162b2. *JAMA Neurol*. 2021;78(11):1409–1411.
153. Baars AE, Kuitwaard K, de Koning LC, et al. SARS-CoV-2 vaccination safety in Guillain-Barré syndrome, chronic inflammatory demyelinating polyneuropathy, and multifocal motor neuropathy. *Neurology*. 2023;100(2):e182–e191.
154. Allen JA. SARS-CoV-2 vaccination and autoimmune neuropathies: rebalancing the risk. *Neurology*. 2023;100(2):55–56.
155. Suh J, Mukerji SS, Collens SI, et al. Skeletal muscle and peripheral nerve histopathology in COVID-19. *Neurology*. 2021;97(08):e849–e858.

CHAPTER 18

Neuropathies Related to Nutritional Deficiencies

Patients can develop neuropathies due to inadequate nutrition and subsequent vitamin deficiency (Table 18-1).[1-6] Nutritional deficiency-related polyneuropathies are currently uncommon, especially in developed countries. However, these neuropathies do occur and are important because they are potentially treatable. Malnutrition may occur in chronic alcoholics and in patients with chronic illness, unusual diets, and obesity surgery. Some vitamin deficiencies (e.g., vitamins B12 and E) often occur because of impaired gastrointestinal absorption rather than poor dietary intake. In other cases, neuropathy may develop secondary to the effects of medications (e.g., isoniazid causing vitamin B6 deficiency). The clinical and laboratory features of most nutritional polyneuropathies are similar to those of the more common polyneuropathies. Most are insidious but some present acutely.[5,6] Timely and accurate diagnosis is important because patients can improve with replacement therapy.

▶ THIAMINE (VITAMIN B1) DEFICIENCY

CLINICAL FEATURES

Thiamine deficiency or beriberi is uncommon nowadays and primarily occurs as a consequence of chronic alcohol abuse, recurrent vomiting, total parenteral nutrition, inappropriately restrictive diets, and bariatric surgery.[1-7] Wernicke encephalopathy, Korsakoff syndrome, and beriberi can arise from insufficient dietary intake of thiamine Wernicke encephalopathy is characterized by delerium, ataxia, and eye movement abnormalities (e.g., ophthalmoparesis, nystagmus), while Korsakoff syndrome is associated with severe short term memory loss and confabulation. Beriberi may present in two forms: dry beriberi and wet beriberi. The difference between these two types of beriberi is simply the presence (wet beriberi) or absence (dry beriberi) of congestive heart failure and lower limb edema. Beriberi usually presents with numbness, tingling, and burning in the distal lower extremities, which subsequently spread to involve the proximal legs and upper extremities.[8] On examination, a mild-to-moderate reduction in all sensory modalities is noted in a stocking distribution along with diminished muscle stretch reflexes. Mild, predominantly distal weakness may be appreciated.

Rarely, there is motor involvement without sensory changes.[6] Onset can be acute with only a minority of patients with beriberi also having Wernicke encephalopathy.[6] Congestive heart failure with edema of the lower legs is seen in the so-called wet beriberi.

LABORATORY FEATURES

Measuring thiamine concentration in serum and urine is not very reliable.[9] Assay of erythrocyte transketolase activity and the increase in activity after adding thiamine pyrophosphate (TPP) appears to be more accurate and reliable.[10-13] Sensory nerve conduction studies (NCSs) usually reveal reduced or absent sensory nerve action potentials (SNAPs) amplitudes with relative preservation of distal sensory latencies and conduction velocities.[1-6,8] The motor NCSs may be normal or demonstrate slightly reduced amplitudes.

HISTOPATHOLOGY

Sural nerve biopsies reveal loss of primarily large, myelinated axons.[7,14] Necropsy studies have demonstrated chromatolysis of the anterior horn cells and dorsal root ganglia cells along with axonal degeneration and secondary demyelination of the posterior columns.

PATHOGENESIS

Most meats and vegetables contain adequate amounts of thiamine, in particular unrefined cereal grains, wheat germ, yeast, soybean flour, and pork.[9] It is absorbed in the small intestine by both passive diffusion and active transport. Here, thiamine is converted to TPP.[9] Because stores of thiamine in the body are limited and its half-life is only 10–14 days, 1–1.5 mg daily of thiamine should be part of any routine diet else deficiency can arise.[9]

Thiamine and TPP catalyze the decarboxylation of alpha-ketoacids to coenzyme A moieties, an important process in ATP synthesis in mitochondria.[9] TPP plays a role in the formation of myelin.[15] Thiamine may also affect neuronal conduction by altering membrane sodium channel function.[16,17]

▶ TABLE 18-1. NUTRITIONAL DEFICIENCY ASSOCIATED WITH PERIPHERAL NEUROPATHY

Thiamine (vitamin B1) deficiency
Riboflavin (vitamin B2)
Pyridoxine (vitamin B6) deficiency
Folate (vitamin B9) deficiency
Cobalamin (vitamin B12) deficiency
Vitamin E deficiency
Copper deficiency
Hypophosphatemia

TREATMENT

Thiamine 100 mg/day should be given intravenously or intramuscularly in deficient patients. In patients with thiamine deficiency secondary to alcohol use, discontinuation of alcohol is imperative. In addition to the likely direct toxic influences on Schwann cells and peripheral nerves, ethanol is likely to impair thiamine utilization even when blood levels are normal.[18] Cardiomyopathy usually is quite responsive to thiamine replacement, although improvement in neurologic function is more variable and less dramatic.[19] Some improvement is expected in most patients, motor more so than sensory, but this typically occurs slowly over 6–12 months.[4,20] In patients with severe acute nutritional neuropathy permanent deficits are typical.[5,6,8]

▶ RIBOFLAVIN (VITAMIN B2 DEFICIENCY)

Riboflavin deficiency is a rare autosomal recessive disorder that usually presents in children as sensory ataxia, axonal sensorimotor polyneuropathy, ventilatory muscle weakness, and cranial neuropathies (optic atrophy, hearing loss).[2,21] It is caused by pathogenic mutations in either *SLC52A2* or *SLC52A3* genes that encode transporter proteins for riboflavin required for absorption from the small intestines. The result is deficiency of riboflavin (vitamin B2) and consequent impairment of flavoprotein-dependent metabolic pathways. High-dose oral supplementation of riboflavin between 10 mg and 50 mg/kg/day may improve symptoms and signs and normalize acylcarnitine levels.

▶ PYRIDOXINE (VITAMIN B6 DEFICIENCY)

Pyridoxine not only is neurotoxic when taken in large dosages (see Chapter 20),[1-6,22-25] but can also be associated with a sensorimotor polyneuropathy when deficient. Pyridoxine deficiency is often associated with isoniazid and hydralazine treatment.[26-28] Pyridoxine deficiency may also result from malnutrition (e.g., chronic alcoholism) or in patients receiving chronic peritoneal dialysis.[29] The symptoms of vitamin B6 deficiency are nonspecific. Affected individuals manifest with a sensory greater than motor polyneuropathy similar to most idiopathic neuropathies, however onset can be acute.[5,6] The electrophysiology studies reflect an axonal sensorimotor polyneuropathy but can be pure sensory or pure motor.[5,6,26,27] Vitamin B6 levels can be measured in blood. Deficient patients should be treated with 50–100 mg/day of vitamin B6.[30] This should also be given prophylactically in patients being treated with isoniazid or hydralazine.[31]

▶ COBALAMIN (VITAMIN B12) DEFICIENCY

CLINICAL FEATURES

Patients with vitamin B12 deficiency can present with central nervous system (CNS) or peripheral nervous system (PNS) abnormalities with or without hematologic findings (megaloblastic anemia).[1,2,4,32-40] Those affected may manifest with numbness and sensory ataxia due to posterior column dysfunction and spastic weakness due to pyramidal tract insult (subacute combined degeneration). In addition, they may have altered mental status. Most patients have signs and symptoms of both CNS and PNS involvement, with reduction of vibratory perception and proprioception, positive Romberg sign, sensory ataxia, decreased or absent reflexes at the ankles, and brisk reflexes elsewhere. Plantar responses can be either extensor or flexor. Because of the myelopathy, patients may present with numbness restricted to the hands potentially mimicking carpal tunnel syndrome. A subacute onset and constant, rather than intermittent numbness would favor vitamin B12 deficiency. A positive Lhermitte sign may be present owing to swelling in the cervical spinal cord.

Several studies have demonstrated an association between treatment with metformin in patients with type 2 diabetes and vitamin B12 deficiency. In turn, metformin is associated with an increased prevalence of distal symmetrical polyneuropathy and autonomic neuropathy.[41,42] Thus, periodic monitoring of vitamin B12 is recommended in all patients taking metformin, particularly if used for over 5 years.[41] The mechanism by which metformin blocks B12 absorption is not known.

LABORATORY FEATURES

Serum vitamin B12 assays are not sensitive, as many symptomatic patients may have serum vitamin B12 levels that are within the normal range.[43,44] Serum levels of the vitamin B12 metabolites, methylmalonic acid (MMA) and homocysteine (Hcy), are much more sensitive in detecting deficiency of B12.[44,45] MMA and Hcy levels are increased (i.e., evidence of B12 deficiency) in 5%–10% of patients with serum vitamin B12 levels less than 300 pg/mL and in 0.1%–1% of those with levels greater than 300 pg/mL.[45] We measure MMA and Hcy levels in patients with polyneuropathy who are suspected of having vitamin B12 deficiency (e.g., those with a sudden onset of symptoms, symptoms beginning in the hands, findings suggestive of myelopathy, or risk factors for vitamin B12 malabsorption). In addition, we routinely measure copper, ceruloplasmin, and zinc levels in the same group of patients as copper deficiency manifests in a virtually identical manner.

In the absence of symptomatic gastrointestinal disease, it probably is not necessary to seek a diagnosis of pernicious anemia in a patient with vitamin B12 deficiency because this information will not alter management.[46] A Schilling test can be done to diagnose pernicious anemia.[47] It is a multistep and therefore inconvenient test which is now uncommonly utilized. Anti-intrinsic factor antibodies are specific for pernicious anemia but are found in only 50% of patients.[48] The combination of elevated gastrin and antiparietal cell antibodies is more sensitive and specific for pernicious anemia.[49]

NCSs reveal absent or reduced SNAP amplitudes with CMAPs amplitudes that are normal or slightly reduced.[32–36,40,50] Motor and sensory distal latencies and conduction velocities are essentially normal or only mildly abnormal. Somatosensory-evoked potentials and magnetic stimulation studies may reveal prolongation of central conduction time.[35,38] Magnetic resonance imaging (MRI) scans of the cervical cord can reveal increased signal on T2 images in the posterior columns (Fig. 18-1).[51]

HISTOPATHOLOGY

Degeneration of the posterior columns and corticospinal tracts has been found at autopsies. Nerve biopsies reveal loss of large, myelinated fibers, axonal degeneration, and secondary segmental demyelination.[37,40,52]

PATHOGENESIS

Cobalamin is found in meat, fish, and dairy products but is not present in fruits, vegetables, and grains. Vitamin B12 requires a transport molecule, intrinsic factor, which is synthesized and secreted by gastric parietal cells. Vitamin B12 deficiency can result from lack of dietary intake (strict vegetarian diet), lack of intrinsic factor (pernicious anemia with autoimmune destruction of parietal cells or gastrectomy), malabsorption syndromes (sprue or lower ileum resection), genetic defects in methionine synthetase, and bacteria (blind-loop syndrome) or bacterial or parasitic consumption prior to its absorption. Cobalamin functions as an enzyme necessary for demethylation of methyltetrahydrofolate.[53] Tetrahydrofolate, in turn, is required for the production of folate coenzymes that are necessary for DNA synthesis.

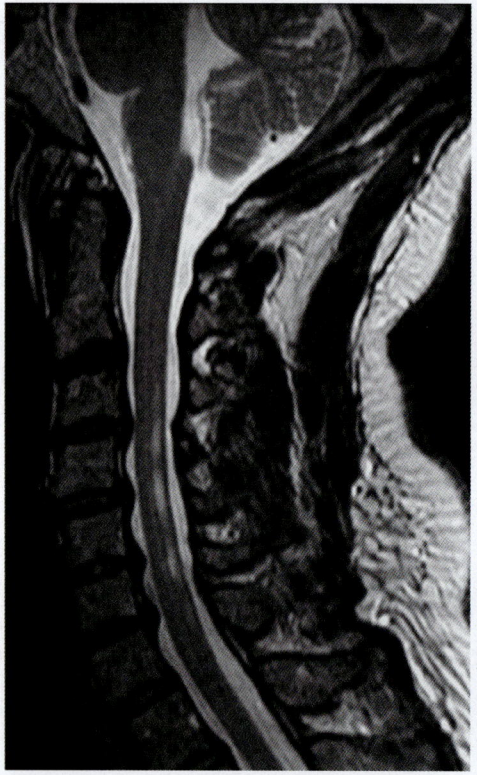 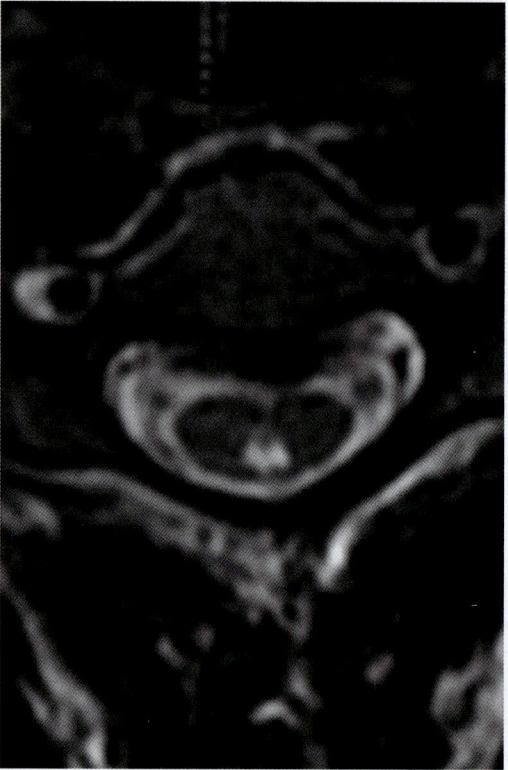

Figure 18-1. Vitamin B12 deficiency. Sagittal (*left image*) and axial (*right image*) T2 MRI in subacute combined degeneration (SCD) showing abnormal hyperintensity in the posterior columns. The patient had markedly reduced vibration and position sense and a Romberg sign; the tendon reflexes were preserved and there were no corticospinal tract or peripheral nerve signs. (Reproduced with permission from Ropper AH, Samuels MA, Klein JP, eds. *Adams and Victor's Principles of Neurology*, 10th ed. New York, NY: McGraw-Hill; 2014. FIGURE 41-3.)

The pathogenic mechanism for the neuropathy/myelopathy associated with cobalamin deficiency is not known but may be related to impairment in DNA synthesis, decreased methylation of myelin phospholipids, or buildup of methylmalonic and propionic acids that serve as abnormal substrates for fatty acid synthesis, leading to aberrant myelination.[53]

TREATMENT

We generally treat deficient patients with B12 1,000 μg IM week/year for 1 month, followed by 1,000 μg IM monthly thereafter. It may be possible to treat vitamin B12 deficiency with oral replacement. A randomized trial comparing treatment with 2,000-mg oral vitamin B12/day to 1,000-mg intramuscular vitamin B12/month showed similar improvements in hematologic indices, serum MMA and Hcy, and neurologic symptoms.[54] However, a minority of subjects had neurologic symptoms, and the methods by which clinical efficacy was assessed were lacking.

Approximately 2% of patients experience worsening sensory symptoms for unclear reasons during the first month of treatment.[55] The response to treatment of vitamin B12 deficiency polyneuropathy, separate from other neurologic complications of vitamin B12, has not been well studied. Patients with vitamin B12 deficiency polyneuropathy/myelopathy probably do not show an immediate response to treatment and may not respond at all.[40,56] The duration of symptoms is an important determinant of treatment response.[55,57,58]

▶ VITAMIN B12 DEFICIENCY SECONDARY TO NITROUS OXIDE INHALATION

Nitrous oxide can inactivate methylcobalamin, leading to neuropathy and subacute combine degeneration in individuals with low or borderline vitamin B12 levels, euphemistically referred to as "anesthetica paresthetica."[59-63] Physical examination, electrodiagnostic findings, and nerve biopsies are similar to those seen in B12 deficiency, as described in the previous section.

▶ FOLATE DEFICIENCY

CLINICAL FEATURES

Folate (vitamin B9) deficiency is associated with neurologic abnormalities similar to those complicating B12 deficiency.[5,6,64,65] Subacute combined degeneration of the posterior columns and corticospinal tracts, sensorimotor peripheral neuropathy, and altered mental status can develop.

LABORATORY FEATURES

Serum folate levels should be reduced. It is necessary to measure both serum folate and vitamin B12 levels to define a pure folic acid deficiency. Megaloblastic anemia may be evident on a complete blood count and smear. Sensory and motor NCSs are similar to those seen with B12 deficiency.[6]

PATHOGENESIS

Folate is found in fruit and vegetables and in liver. It is primarily absorbed in the proximal jejunum. Isolated folic acid deficiencies are extremely rare but can occur in the elderly on poor diets, those with alcohol abuse, young persons' consuming only snack foods, partial gastrectomies, duodenojejunal resections, celiac disease, and disorders of the jejunal mucosa.[64,65] Several drugs (e.g., phenytoin, phenobarbital, sulfasalazine, and colchicine) can also interfere with the optimal utilization of folic acid. The mechanism by which folic acid deficiency results in a polyneuropathy is not known; however, folic acid is required in DNA synthesis.

TREATMENT

Administration of folic acid usually results in good clinical recovery.

▶ VITAMIN E DEFICIENCY

CLINICAL FEATURES

Vitamin E or alpha-tocopherol is a lipid-soluble antioxidant vitamin that is present in the lipid bilayer constituting the cell membrane.[66,67] There is a close relationship between the metabolism of lipids and that of vitamin E. There are three major mechanisms associated with vitamin E deficiency: (1) deficient fat absorption (e.g., cystic fibrosis, chronic cholestasis, short-bowel syndrome, and intestinal lymphangiectasia), (2) deficient fat transport (abetalipoproteinemia, hypobetalipoproteinemia, normotriglyceridemic abetalipoproteinemia, and chylomicron retention disease), and (3) a genetically based abnormality of vitamin E metabolism. Patients with vitamin E deficiency usually present with progressive difficulty ambulating and impaired coordination of the hands.[68-71] Some individuals complain of weakness and sensory loss. Dysarthria can also occur.

Physical examination is remarkable for ataxia of the trunk and upper and lower extremities.[68-71] There is prominent loss of proprioception and vibratory perception. Muscle stretch reflexes are reduced or absent. Manual muscle testing can be difficult secondary to the ataxia, but there can be proximal muscle weakness, suggesting a superimposed myopathic process. Ocular examination may reveal ophthalmoplegia and retinopathy.

LABORATORY FEATURES

Vitamin E (alpha-tocopherol) levels in the serum are low. With hyperlipidemia, the vitamin E level may be normal.

In such cases, the ratio of total serum vitamin E to the total serum lipid concentration is a more sensitive indicator of vitamin E deficiency.[72]

NCSs reveal reduced amplitudes or absent SNAPs.[63–73] The sensory nerve conduction velocities are normal or only slightly reduced. Somatosensory-evoked potentials demonstrate normal peripheral nerve potentials with marked slowing and attenuation of central responses consistent with slowing of central conduction with loss of posterior column fibers.[74] Motor NCSs are normal.

HISTOPATHOLOGY

Autopsy studies demonstrate swelling and degeneration of axons in the posterior columns and spinocerebellar tracts along with neuronal loss and lipofuscin accumulation in the gracile and cuneate nuclei.[69,75,76] Changes within the basal ganglia may be seen. Sural nerve biopsies show nonspecific abnormalities including the loss of large, myelinated fibers, axonal degeneration, regenerating sprouts, occasional vacuoles in the myelin sheath, and breakup of the Schmidt–Lanterman incisures, but little in the way of primary demyelination.[77,78]

PATHOGENESIS

There are four main types of vitamin E, the most active of which is alpha-tocopherol. Vitamin E is lipid soluble and absorbed in the small intestine. Vitamin E is incorporated into chylomicrons and is transported to the liver. Here, vitamin E is incorporated into very low-density lipoproteins in a step requiring alpha-tocopherol transfer protein. Deficiency of this transfer protein is associated with hereditary vitamin E deficiency (discussed in Chapter 11). Vitamin E may serve to eliminate free radicals and stabilize cell membrane structure.[79]

Vitamin E deficiency is usually due to factors other than insufficient intake.[80] As mentioned, deficiency can result secondary to disorders of lipid malabsorption or transport. Abetalipoproteinemia is a rare autosomal-dominant disorder characterized by steatorrhea, pigmentary retinopathy, acanthocytosis, and progressive ataxia that is associated with vitamin E deficiency.[81] Cystic fibrosis can also be complicated by vitamin E deficiency secondary to malabsorption. There are also genetic forms of isolated vitamin E.[82,83] Mutations in the alpha-tocopherol transfer protein gene, *TTPA*, located on chromosome 8q13 result in loss of vitamin E.[84,85] Vitamin E deficiency may also complicate various liver and biliary disorders as well as surgical removal of parts of the intestines leading to short bowel or dumping syndrome.[73,86,87]

TREATMENT

Therapy is aimed at preventing progression, but improvement in neurologic function may occur. The specific dose of vitamin E is dependent upon the cause of deficiency.[80] In cases of isolated vitamin E deficiency, patients are treated with 1,500–6,000 international units (IU)/day in divided doses. Patients with chronic cholestasis are initially treated with 50 IU/kg/day and the dose is increased in 50 IU/kg increments up to a 200 IU/kg/day as required to obtain a normal serum tocopherol to lipid ratio. Patients with cystic fibrosis, who are receiving oral pancreatic enzyme therapy, require doses of 5–10 IU/kg/day. Those with short bowel syndrome are given 300–5,400 IU/day. Abetalipoproteinemia is treated with vitamin E 150–300 IU/kg/day and vitamin A 15,000–20,000 IU/day.

▶ POSTGASTRECTOMY/BARIATRIC SURGERY DEFICIENCIES

Polyneuropathy may complicate gastric/bariatric surgery for gastric ulcers, cancer, or morbid obesity.[5,6,20,88–91] The clinical picture is variable and may include acute or subacute sensory loss, burning feet, generalized weakness that can resemble Guillain–Barré syndrome, mononeuropathies, and radiculoplexus neuropathy.[5,6,91–95] Some cases are complicated by CNS dysfunction resembling Wernicke–Korsakoff syndrome. In the largest retrospective series, 71 out of 435 (16%) of patients who underwent bariatric surgery developed some type of peripheral neuropathy. The neuropathy is associated with malnutrition and the rapidity of weight loss and usually develops within the first 1½ years following weight loss surgery.[88,91,95] The latency between surgery and symptoms ranges from a few months to years in patients following total or partial gastrectomy for ulcer or cancer.[20,96]

Weight reduction surgical procedures include gastrojejunostomy, gastric stapling, vertical banded gastroplasty, and gastrectomy with Roux-en-Y anastomosis. Although thiamine deficiency seems to be a factor (given the frequent cooccurrence of the Wernicke–Korsakoff syndrome), there is no good documentation of thiamine deficiency in the reported cases. In some cases, one or more vitamin deficiencies are identified.[97] In many cases, no specific deficiency is identified. Electrodiagnostic studies most commonly reveal evidence of a length-dependent, axonal, sensory greater than motor polyneuropathy.

HISTOPATHOLOGY

Sural nerve biopsies when obtained may reveal active axonal degeneration and mild perivascular, endoneurial, and epineurial infiltrate.

PATHOGENESIS

The basis of the neuropathies is unclear but likely to result from multiple nutritional deficiencies.

TREATMENT

Patients should be treated with parenteral vitamin supplementation and, on occasion, reversal of the surgical bypass.[91,97,98] Patients with protracted vomiting after weight reduction surgery should receive total parenteral nutrition and vitamins. Patients can recover if started on treatment early, though some will have persistent sensory loss and weakness. The duration and severity of deficits before identification and treatment of neuropathy are important predictors of the final outcome.

▶ COPPER DEFICIENCY

CLINICAL FEATURES

Copper deficiency is associated with an unusual myeloneuropathy, neutropenia, and sometimes pancytopenia.[99–109] The clinical phenotype is similar to vitamin B12 deficiency. Most patients manifest with numbness and tingling in the legs, weakness, spasticity, and gait difficulties. Large fiber sensory function is impaired, reflexes are brisk, and plantar responses are extensor. In some cases, light touch and pinprick sensation are affected and NCSs indicate sensorimotor axonal polyneuropathy in addition to myelopathy.[100,102] A severe motor axonopathy can also be seen.[103] The weakness and sensory loss in some cases is primarily due to a myelopathy.[104] Demyelinating lesions may be appreciated on brain MRI, and some patients have ocular dysmetria indicating brain involvement.[104]

LABORATORY FEATURES

Besides low serum copper levels, some cases are associated with high levels of zinc. Microcytic anemia and neutropenia,[99,102–107,110,111] and occasionally pancytopenia[100] are also seen. Bone marrow biopsy may reveal abnormalities of a myelodysplastic syndrome. Cerebrospinal fluid may be normal or show mildly elevated protein or immunoglobulin synthesis rate.[100,103,104,106] MRI may demonstrate abnormal T2-weighted signal in the dorsal columns.[99,103,104,106,107] NCSs may reveal features of an axonal, sensorimotor polyneuropathy.[100,102,106,107] Somatosensory-evoked potentials demonstrate impaired conduction in the central pathway in those with myelopathy.[106,107]

HISTOPATHOLOGY

Sural nerve biopsies may show evidence of axonal degeneration.[106,107]

PATHOGENESIS

Copper is absorbed in the stomach and proximal jejunum accounting for why deficiency may complicate gastric surgery.[99,102,112] The reason that zinc can lead to copper deficiency is that it upregulates the production of metallothionein in the gut, which in turn reduces copper absorption.[113,114] Interestingly, some denture creams used to contain a large amount of zinc and can lead to hypocupremia and neurologic disease.[105] Copper deficiency may also result from malnutrition, prematurity, total parenteral nutrition, and copper chelating agents.[110,112]

TREATMENT

The myeloneuropathy may improve with oral or intravenous copper replacement quickly,[99,101,102] but benefits may not be seen for months or years,[100,104,106] and some patients do not improve at all.[103] In contrast to the variable clinical improvement, the pancytopenia usually normalizes with copper replacement therapy.[106]

HYPOPHOSPHATEMIA

Hyperalimentation with inadequate phosphate supplementation can lead to hypophosphatemia and the development of a subacute and severe sensorimotor peripheral neuropathy, which can clinically resemble Guillain–Barré syndrome.[115,116] Typically, serum phosphate levels need to be below 1 mg/dL for this to occur. Paresthesias are initially noted in the feet and ascend to involve the upper limbs and remainder of the body. Impaired ambulation secondary to both weakness and sensory ataxia occurs over the course of hours to days. Generalized weakness, ataxia, depressed muscle stretch reflexes, and reduced perception of all sensory modalities are appreciated on examination. Weakness may also involve the ventilatory muscles requiring mechanical assistance. NCSs reveal an absence of SNAPs, reduced CMAP amplitudes, and slow conduction velocities. Correction of the hypophosphatemia results in clinical and electrophysiologic improvement.

▶ ALCOHOL-RELATED NEUROPATHY

CLINICAL FEATURES

Patients with a history of alcohol abuse can develop a generalized axonal sensorimotor polyneuropathy.[18,117–124] Usually the neuropathy is slowly progressive, although some cases with acute or subacute presentation resembling Guillain–Barré syndrome have been reported.[122,123] Unlike Guillain–Barré syndrome, CSF protein in alcohol-related acute axonal polyneuropathy is usually normal or only slightly elevated. Most cases are preceded by prominent weight loss for 2–3 months. Most patients manifest with an insidious onset of numbness, paresthesia, and burning pain suggestive of a small fiber polyneuropathy. It is estimated that the equivalent of 10 oz of 86 proof-distilled spirits were 3 L of beer a day for 3 or more years, which is the threshold for alcoholic neuropathy. It has also been hypothesized that the lead content of wine may also contribute to the pathogenesis of alcoholic neuropathy.[18]

Examination demonstrates a reduction of all sensory modalities in a glove and stocking distribution, worse in the lower compared to upper limbs. Muscle stretches are reduced or absent. Mild distal leg weakness may be appreciated, but proximal leg and arm strength is usually normal. An occasional patient presents with symptoms and signs suggestive of a myopathy as opposed to neuropathy. NCSs reveal features suggestive of a generalized axonal sensory or sensorimotor polyneuropathy.[18,117–119,121]

HISTOPATHOLOGY

Nerve biopsies may reveal loss of large- and small-caliber myelinated fibers along with Wallerian degeneration and secondary segmental demyelination.[121,123]

PATHOGENESIS

The exact etiology of peripheral nerve associated with alcohol abuse is unknown but may in part be related to both a nutritional deficiency (e.g., vitamin B group and folate) and a direct toxic effect of alcohol on peripheral nerves.[18]

TREATMENT

Abstaining from alcohol and consuming an optimal diet can result in an improvement of the peripheral neuropathy.[123]

▶ SUMMARY

Nutritional neuropathies are not particularly common. However, because they can be treatable with correction of the deficit, it is important to be vigilant for signs and symptoms that would suggest a nutritional deficiency. In particular, those patients with gastrointestinal disease, history of gastric bypass, and alcohol abuse may be particularly vulnerable.

REFERENCES

1. Gwathmey KG, Grogan J. Nutritional neuropathies. *Muscle Nerve*. 2020;62(1):13–29.
2. Kramarz C, Murphy E, Reilly MM, Rossor AM. Nutritional peripheral neuropathies. *J Neurol Neurosurg Psychiatry*. 2023; 95(1):61–72.
3. Mathis S, Soulages A, Vallat JM, Le Masson G. Epidemics and outbreaks of peripheral nervous system disorders: II. Toxic and nutritional causes. *J Neurol*. 2021;268(3):892–902.
4. Stein J, Geisel J, Obeid R. Association between neuropathy and B-vitamins: a systematic review and meta-analysis. *Eur J Neurol*. 2021;28(6):2054–2064.
5. Hamel J, Logigian EL. Acute nutritional axonal neuropathy. *Muscle Nerve*. 2018;57(1):33–39.
6. Hamel JI, Logigian EL. Clinical spectrum and prognosis in patients with acute nutritional axonal neuropathy. *Neurology*. 2023;100(20):e2134–e2140.
7. Ohnishi A, Tsuji S, Igisu H, et al. Beriberi neuropathy. Morphometric study of sural nerve. *J Neurol Sci*. 1980;45:177–190.
8. Hong CZ. Electrodiagnostic findings of persisting polyneuropathies due to previous nutritional deficiency in former prisoners of war. *Electromyogr Clin Neurophysiol*. 1986;26:351–363.
9. McCormick DB, Greene HL. Vitamins. In: Burtis CA, Ashwood ER, eds. *Tierz Textbook of Clinical Chemistry*. Saunders; 1999:999–1028.
10. Brin M, Tai M, Ostashever AS, Kalinsky H. The effect of thiamine deficiency on the activity of erythrocyte hemolysate transketolase. *J Nutr*. 1960;71:273–281.
11. Brin M. Erythrocyte transketolase in early thiamine deficiency. *Ann N Y Acad Sci*. 1962;98:528–541.
12. Jeyasingham MD, Pratt OE, Burns A, Shaw GK, Thomson AD, Marsh A. The activation of red blood cell transketolase in groups of patients especially at risk from thiamin deficiency. *Psychol Med*. 1987;17:311–318.
13. Jeyasingham MD, Pratt OE, Shaw GK, Thomson AD. Changes in the activation of red blood cell transketolase of alcoholic patients during treatment. *Alcohol*. 1987;22:259–365.
14. Takahashi K, Nakamura H. Axonal degeneration in beriberi neuropathy. *Arch Neurol*. 1976;33:836–841.
15. Collins RC, Lonergan ET. Transketolase and myelin. *N Engl J Med*. 1971;285:751–752.
16. Cooper JR, Pincus JH. The role of thiamine in nervous tissue. *Neurochem Res*. 1979;4:223–229.
17. Schoffeniels E. Thiamine phosphorylated derivatives and bioelectrogenesis. *Arch Int Physiol Biochim*. 1983;91:233–242.
18. Mellion M, Gilchrist JM, de la Monte S. Alcohol—related peripheral neuropathy: nutritional, toxic, or both? *Muscle Nerve*. 2011;43:309–316.
19. Jolliffe N. The diagnosis, treatment and prevention of vitamin B1 deficiency. *Bull N Y Acad Med*. 1939;15:469–478.
20. Koike H, Misu K, Hattori N, et al. Postgastrectomy polyneuropathy with thiamine deficiency. *J Neurol Neurosurg Psychiatry*. 2001;71:357–362.
21. Jaeger B, Bosch AM. Clinical presentation and outcome of riboflavin transporter deficiency: mini review after five years of experience. *J Inherit Metab Dis*. 2016;39:(4)559–64.
22. Albin RL, Albers JW, Greenberg HS, et al. Acute sensory neuropathy-neuronopathy from pyridoxine overdose. *Neurology*. 1987;37:1729–1732.
23. Dalton K, Dalton MJ. Characteristics of pyridoxine overdose neuropathy syndrome. *Acta Neurol Scand*. 1987;76:8–11.
24. Parry GJ, Bredesen DE. Sensory neuropathy with low dose pyridoxine. *Neurology*. 1985;35:1466–1468.
25. Schaumburg H, Kaplan J, Windsbank A, et al. Sensory neuropathy from pyridoxine abuse. A new megavitamin syndrome. *N Engl J Med*. 1983;309:445–448.
26. Gammon GD, Burge FW, King G. Neural toxicity in tuberculous patients treated with isoniazid (isonicotinic acid hydrazide). *AMA Arch Neurol Psychiatry*. 1953;70:64–69.

27. Lubing HN. Peripheral neuropathy in tuberculosis patients treated with isoniazid. *Am Rev Tuberc.* 1953;68:458–461.
28. Selikoff IJ, Robitzek EH, Ornstein CG. Treatment of pulmonary tuberculosis with hydrazide derivatives of nicotinic acid. *J Am Med Assoc.* 1952;150(10):973–980.
29. Moriwaki K, Kanno Y, Nakamoto H, Okada H, Suzuki H. Vitamin B6 deficiency in elderly patients on chronic peritoneal dialysis. *Adv Perit Dial.* 2000;16:308–312.
30. Ruffin JM, Smith DT. Treatment of pellagra with special reference to the use of nicotinic acid. *South Med J.* 1939;32:40–47.
31. Marcus R, Coulston AN. Water-soluble vitamins. In: Gilman AG, Goodman LS, Rall TW, Murad F, eds. *Goodman and Gilman's the Pharmacological Basis of Therapeutics.* 7th ed. Macmillan Publishing Company; 1985:1551–1572.
32. Fine EJ, Hallett M. Neurophysiological study of subacute combined degeneration. *J Neurol Sci.* 1980;45:331–336.
33. Fine EJ, Soria E, Paroski MW, Petryk D, Thomasula L. The neurophysiological profile of vitamin B_{12} deficiency. *Muscle Nerve.* 1990;13:158–164.
34. Hahn AF, Gilbert JJ, Brown WF. A study of the sural nerve in pernicious anemia. *Can J Neurol Sci.* 1976;3:217.
35. Hemmer B, Glocker FX, Schumacher M, Deuschl G, Lucking CH. Subacute combined degeneration: clinical, electrophysiological, and magnetic resonance imaging findings. *J Neurol Neurosurg Psychiatry.* 1998;65:822–827.
36. Kayser-Gatchalian MC, Neundorfer B. Peripheral neuropathy with vitamin B_{12} deficiency. *J Neurol.* 1977;214:183–193.
37. Kosik KS, Mullins TF, Bradley WG, Tempelis LD, Cretella AJ. Coma and axonal degeneration in vitamin B12 deficiency. *Arch Neurol.* 1980;37:590–592.
38. Krumholz A, Weiss HD, Goldstein PJ, Harris KC. Evoked responses in vitamin B12 deficiency. *Ann Neurol.* 1981;9:407–409.
39. Lockner D, Reizenstein P, Wennberg A, Widén L. Peripheral nerve function in pernicious anemia before and after treatment. *Acta Haematol.* 1969;41:257–263.
40. McCombe PA, McLeod JG. The peripheral neuropathy of vitamin B12 deficiency. *J Neurol Sci.* 1984;66:117–126.
41. Bell DSH. Metformin-induced vitamin B12 deficiency can cause or worsen distal symmetrical, autonomic and cardiac neuropathy in the patient with diabetes. *Diabetes Obes Metab.* 2022;24(8):1423–1428.
42. Gupta K, Jain A, Rohatgi A. An observational study of vitamin b12 levels and peripheral neuropathy profile in patients of diabetes mellitus on metformin therapy. *Diabetes Metab Syndr.* 2018;12(1):51–58.
43. Carmel R. Current concepts in cobalamin deficiency. *Annu Rev Med.* 2000;51:357–375.
44. Savage DG, Lindenbaum J, Stabler SP, Allen RH. Sensitivity of serum methylmalonic acid and total homocysteine determinations for diagnosing cobalamin and folate deficiencies. *Am J Med.* 1994;96:239–246.
45. Lindenbaum J, Savage DG, Stabler SP, Allen RH. Diagnosis of cobalamin deficiency: II. Relative sensitivities of serum cobalamin, methylmalonic acid, and total homocysteine concentrations. *Am J Hematol.* 1990;34:99–107.
46. Stabler SP. Screening the older population for cobalamin (vitamin B12) deficiency. *J Am Geriatr Soc.* 1995;43:1290–1297.
47. Swain R. An update of vitamin B12 metabolism and deficiency states. *J Fam Pract.* 1995;41:595–600.
48. Chanarin I. *The Megaloblastic Anemias.* 2nd ed. Blackwell Scientific Publications; 1979.
49. Metz J, Bell AH, Flicker L, et al. The significance of subnormal serum vitamin B12 concentration in older people: a case control study. *J Am Geriatr Soc.* 1996;44:1355–1361.
50. Saperstein DS, Wolfe GI, Gronseth GS, Nations SP, Herbelin LL, Bryan WW, Barohn RJ. Challenges in the identification of cobalamin-deficiency polyneuropathy. *Arch Neurol.* 2003;60(9):1296–301.
51. Bou-Haidar P, Peduto AJ, Karunaratne N. Differential diagnosis of T2 hyperintense spinal cord lesions: part B. *J Med Imaging Radiat Oncol.* 2009;53:152–159.
52. Abarbanel JM, Frishers S, Osimani A. Vitamin B12 deficiency neuropathy: sural nerve biopsy study. *Isr J Med Sci.* 1986;22:909–911.
53. Green R, Kinsella LJ. Current concepts in the diagnosis of cobalamin deficiency. *Neurology.* 1995;45:1435–1440.
54. Kuzminski AM, Del Giacco EJ, Allen RH, Stabler SP, Lindenbaum J. Effective treatment of cobalamin deficiency with oral cobalamin. *Blood.* 1998;92:1191–1198.
55. Healton EB, Savage DG, Brust JC, Garrett TJ, Lindenbaum J. Neurologic aspects of cobalamin deficiency. *Medicine (Baltimore).* 1991;70:229–245.
56. Saperstein DS, Wolfe GI, Gronseth GS, et al. Challenges in the identification of cobalamin-deficiency polyneuropathy. *Arch Neurol.* 2003;60:1296–1301.
57. Hyland HH, Watts GO, Farquharson RF. The course of subacute combined degeneration of the spinal cord. *Can Med Assoc J.* 1951;65(4):295–302.
58. Ungley CC. Subacute combined degeneration of the cord: I. Response to liver extracts. II. Trials with vitamin B12; quantitative method of assessing neurological status. *Brain.* 1949;72:382–427.
59. Heyer EJ, Simpson DM, Bodis-Wollner I, Diamond SP. Nitrous oxide: clinical and electrophysiologic investigation of neurologic complications. *Neurology.* 1986;36:1618–1622.
60. Layzer RB, Fishman RA, Schafer JA. Neuropathy following abuse of nitrous oxide. *Neurology.* 1978;28:504–506.
61. Sahenk Z, Mendell JR, Couri D, Nachtman J. Polyneuropathy from inhalation of N_2O cartridges through a whipped-cream dispenser. *Neurology.* 1978;28:485–487.
62. Vishnubhakat SM, Beresford HR. Reversible myeloneuropathy of nitrous oxide abuse: serial electrophysiological studies. *Muscle Nerve.* 1991;14:22–26.
63. Fang X, Yu M, Zheng D, Gao H, Li W, Ma Y. Electrophysiologic characteristics of nitrous-oxide-associated peripheral neuropathy: a retrospective study of 76 patients. *J Clin Neurol.* 2023;19(1):44–51.
64. Enk C, Hougaard K, Hippe E. Reversible dementia and neuropathy associated with folate deficiency 16 years after partial gastrectomy. *Scand J Haematol.* 1980;25:63–66.
65. Fehling C, Jagerstad M, Linstrand K, Elmqvist D. Folate deficiency and neurological disease. *Arch Neurol.* 1974;30:263–265.
66. Guggenheim MA, Ringel SP, Silverman A, Grabert BE. Progressive neuromuscular disease in children with chronic cholestasis and vitamin E deficiency: diagnosis and treatment with alpha tocopherol. *J Pediatr.* 1982;100:51–58.
67. Harding AE. Vitamin E and the nervous system. *Crit Rev Neurobiol.* 1987;3(1):89–103.

68. Bertoni JM, Abraham FA, Falls HF, Itabashi HH. Small bowel resection with vitamin E deficiency and progressive spinocerebellar syndrome. *Neurology*. 1984;34:1046–1052.
69. Rosenblum JL, Keating JP, Prensky AL, Nelson JS. A progressive neurologic syndrome in children with chronic liver disease. *N Engl J Med*. 1981;304:503–508.
70. Ko HY, Park-Ko I. Electrophysiologic recovery after vitamin E-deficient neuropathy. *Arch Phys Med Rehab*. 1999;80:964–967.
71. Brin MF, Pedley TA, Lovelace RE, et al. Electrophysiologic features of abetalipoproteinemia: functional consequences of vitamin E deficiency. *Neurology*. 1986;36:669–673.
72. Sokol RJ, Heubi JE, Iannaccone ST, Bove KE, Balistreri WF. Vitamin E deficiency with normal serum vitamin E concentrations in children with chronic cholestasis. *N Engl J Med*. 1984;310:1209–1212.
73. Satya-Murti S, Howard L, Krohel G, Wolf B. The spectrum of neurologic disorder from vitamin E deficiency. *Neurology*. 1986; 36:917–921.
74. Kaplan PW, Rawal K, Erwin CW, D'Souza BJ, Spock A. Visual and somatosensory evoked potentials in vitamin E deficiency with cystic fibrosis. *Electroencephalogr Clin Neurophysiol*. 1988; 71:266–272.
75. Jeffrey GP, Muller DPR, Burroughs AK, et al. Vitamin E deficiency and its clinical significance in adults with primary biliary cirrhosis and other forms of chronic liver disease. *J Hepatol*. 1987;4:307–317.
76. Sung JH, Stadlan EM. Neuroaxonal dystrophy in congenital biliary atresia. *J Neuropathol Exp Neurol*. 1966;25:341–361.
77. Traber MG, Sokol RJ, Ringel SP, Neville HE, Thellman CA, Kayden HJ. Lack of tocopherol in peripheral nerves of vitamin E-deficient patients with peripheral neuropathy. *N Engl J Med*. 1987;317:262–265.
78. Yokota T, Wada Y, Furukawa T, Tsukagoshi H, Uchihara T, Watabiki S. Adult-onset spinocerebellar syndrome with idiopathic vitamin E deficiency. *Ann Neurol*. 1987;22:84–87.
79. Tappel AL. Vitamin E and free radical peroxiadation of lipids. *Ann NY Acad Sci*. 1972;203:12–28.
80. Sokol RJ. Vitamin E and neurologic deficits. *Adv Pediatr*. 1990;37:119–148.
81. Muller DP, Harries JT, Lloyd JK. The relative importance of the factors involved in the absorption of vitamin E in children. *Gut*. 1974;15:966–971.
82. Harding AE, Matthews S, Jones S, Ellis CJ, Booth IW, Muller DP. Spinocerebellar degeneration associated with a selective defect of vitamin E absorption. *N Engl J Med*. 1985;313: 32–35.
83. Sokol RJ, Kayden HJ, Bettis DB, et al. Isolated vitamin E deficiency in the absence of fat malabsorption–familial and sporadic cases: characterization and investigation of causes. *J Lab Clin Med*. 1988;111:548–559.
84. Ouahchi K, Arita M, Kayden H, et al. Ataxia with isolated vitamin E deficiency is caused by mutations in the α-tocopherol transfer protein. *Nat Genet*. 1995;9:141–145.
85. Gotoda T, Arita M, Arai H, et al. Adult-onset spinocerebellar dysfunction caused by a mutation in the gene for α-tocopherol transfer protein. *N Engl J Med*. 1995;333:1313–1318.
86. Harding AE, Muller DP, Thomas PK, Willison HJ. Spinocerebellar degeneration secondary to chronic intestinal malabsorption: a vitamin E deficiency syndrome. *Ann Neurol*. 1982; 12:419–424.
87. Howard L, Ovensen L, Satya-Murti S, Chu R. Reversible neurological symptoms caused by vitamin E deficiency in a patient with short bowel syndrome. *Am J Clin Nutr*. 1982;36:1243–1249.
88. Cirignotta F, Manconi M, Mondini S, Buzzi G, Ambrosetto P. Wernicke–Korsakoff encephalopathy and polyneuropathy after gastroplasty for morbid obesity. *Arch Neurol*. 2000;57:1356–1359.
89. Harwood SC, Chodoroff G, Ellenberg MR. Gastric partitioning complicated by peripheral neuropathy with lumbosacral plexopathy. *Arch Phys Med Rehab*. 1987;68:310–312.
90. Somer H, Bergstrom L, Mustajoki P, Rovamo L. Morbid obesity, gastric application and a severe neurological deficit. *Acta Med Scand*. 1985;217:575–576.
91. Koffman BM, Greenfield LJ, Ali II, Pirzada NA. Neurologic complications after surgery for obesity. *Muscle Nerve*. 2006; 33(2):166–176.
92. Feit H, Glasberg M, Ireton C, Rosenberg RN, Thal E. Peripheral neuropathy and starvation after gastric partitioning for morbid obesity. *Ann Intern Med*. 1982;96:453–455.
93. Williams JA, Hall GS, Thompson AG, Cooke WT. Neurological disease after partial gastrectomy. *Br Med J*. 1969;3: 210–212.
94. Abarbanel JM, Berginer VM, Osimani A, Solomon H, Charuzi I. Neurologic complications after gastric restriction surgery for morbid obesity. *Neurology*. 1987;37:196–200.
95. Thaisetthawatkul P, Collazo-Clavell ML, Sarr MG, Noreel JE, Dyck PJ. A controlled study of peripheral neuropathy after bariatric surgery. *Neurology*. 2004;63:1462–1470.
96. Hoffman PM, Brody JA. Neurological disorders in patients following surgery for peptic ulcer. *Neurology*. 1972;22:450.
97. Rudnicki SA. Prevention and treatment of peripheral neuropathy after bariatric surgery. *Curr Treat Options Neurol*. 2010;12:29–36.
98. Thaisetthawatkul P, Collazo-Clavell ML, Sarr MG, Norell JE, Dyck PJ. Good nutritional control may prevent polyneuropathy after bariatric surgery. *Muscle Nerve*. 2010;42:709–714.
99. Schleper B, Stuerenburg HJ. Copper deficiency-associated myelopathy in a 46-year-old woman. *J Neurol*. 2001;248: 705–706.
100. Hedera P, Fink JK, Bockenstedt PL, Brewer GJ. Myelopolyneuropathy and pancytopenia due to copper deficiency and high zinc levels of unknown origin: further support for existence of a new zinc overload syndrome. *Arch Neurol*. 2003;60: 1303–1306.
101. Kumar N, Gross JB Jr, Ahlskog JE. Myelopathy due to copper deficiency. *Neurology*. 2003;61:273–274.
102. Kumar N, McEvoy KM, Ahlskog JE. Myelopathy due to copper deficiency following gastrointestinal surgery. *Arch Neurol*. 2003;60:1782–1785.
103. Greenberg SA, Briemberg HR. A neurological and hematological syndrome associated with zinc and excess and copper deficiency. *J Neurol*. 2004;251:111–114.
104. Prodan CI, Holland NR, Wisdom PJ, Burstein SA, Bottomley SS. CNS demyelination associated with copper deficiency and hyperzincemia. *Neurology*. 2002;59:1453–1456.
105. Nations SP, Boyer PJ, Love LA, et al. Denture cream: an unusual source of excess zinc, leading to hypocupremia and neurologic disease. *Neurology*. 2008;71:639–643.
106. Kumar N, Gross JB Jr, Ahlskog JE. Copper deficiency myelopathy produces a clinical picture like subacute combined degeneration. *Neurology*. 2004;63:33–39.

107. Kumar N. Copper deficiency myelopathy (human sway-back). *Mayo Clin Proc.* 2006;81(10):1371–1384.
108. Rowin J, Lewis SL. Copper deficiency myeloneuropathy and pancytopenia secondary to overuse of zinc supplementation. *J Neurol Neurosurg Psychiatry.* 2005;76(5):750–751.
109. Prodan CI, Bottomley SS, Holland NR, Lind SE. Relapsing hypocupraemic myelopathy requiring high-dose oral copper replacement. *J Neurol Neurosurg Psychiatry.* 2006;77(9):1092–1093.
110. Bottomley SS. Sideroblastic anemias. In: Lee GR, Foerster J, Lukens J, et al., eds. *Wintrobe's Clinical Hematology.* 10th ed. Lippincott Williams & Wilkins; 1999:1022–1045.
111. Gregg XT, Reddy V, Prchal JT. Copper deficiency masquerading as myelodysplastic syndrome. *Blood.* 2002;100:1493–1495.
112. Solomons NW. Biochemical, metabolic, and clinical role of copper in human nutrition. *J Am Coll Clin Nutr.* 1985;4:83–105.
113. Irving JA, Mattman A, Lockitch G, Farrell K, Wadsworth LD. Element of caution: a case of reversible cytopenias associated with excessive zinc supplementation. *CMAJ.* 2003;169:129–131.
114. Fiske DN, McCoy HE III, Kitchens CS. Zinc-induced sideroblastic anemia: report of a case, review of the literature, and description of the hematologic syndrome. *Am J Hematol.* 1994;46:147–150.
115. Weintraub MI. Hypophosphatemia mimicking acute Guillain–Barré–Strohl syndrome: a complication of hyperalimentation. *JAMA.* 1976;235:1040–1041.
116. Yagnik P, Singh N, Burns R. Peripheral neuropathy with hypophosphatemia in patient receiving intravenous hyperalimentation. *Muscle Nerve.* 1982;5:562.
117. Casey EB, Le Quesne PM. Electrophysiological evidence for a distal lesion in alcoholic neuropathy. *J Neurol Neurosurg Psychiatry.* 1972;35:624–630.
118. Mawdsley C, Mayer RF. Nerve conduction in alcoholic polyneuropathy. *Brain.* 1985;88:335–356.
119. Shankar K, Maloney FP, Thompson C. An electrodiagnostic study in chronic alcoholic subjects. *Arch Phys Med Rehab.* 1987;68:803–805.
120. Shields RW Jr. Alcoholic polyneuropathy. *Muscle Nerve.* 1985;8:183–187.
121. Walsh JC, McLeod JG. Alcoholic neuropathy: an electrophysiological and histological study. *J Neurol Sci.* 1970;10:457–469.
122. Julian T, Glascow N, Syeed R, Zis P. Alcohol-related peripheral neuropathy: a systematic review and meta-analysis. *J Neurol.* 2019;266(12):2907–2919.
123. Tabaraud F, Vallat JM, Hugon J, Ramiandrisoa H, Dumas M, Signoret JL. Acute or subacute alcoholic neuropathy mimicking Guillain–Barré syndrome. *J Neurol Sci.* 1990;97:195–205.
124. Wöhrle JC, Spengos K, Steinke W, Goebel HH, Hennerici M. Alcohol-related acute axonal polyneuropathy. A differential diagnosis of Guillain–Barré syndrome. *Arch Neurol.* 1998;55:1329–1334.

CHAPTER 19

Neuropathies Associated with Malignancy

Patients with malignancy can develop peripheral neuropathies as the result of (1) a direct effect of the cancer by invasion or compression of the nerves, (2) a remote or paraneoplastic effect including vasculitis, (3) a direct toxic effect of treatment, or (4) an alteration of immune status caused by immunosuppression (Table 19-1).[1] It is difficult to estimate the frequency of polyneuropathy in patients with cancer because it is dependent on a number of factors including the type, stage, and location of the malignancy, as well as confounding variables such as malnutrition, the toxic effects of therapy, and the background incidence of neuropathy in this frequently older population. Nevertheless, some series indicate that 1.7%–5.5% of patients with cancer have clinical symptoms or signs of a peripheral neuropathy, while neurophysiologic testing [quantitative sensory testing and nerve conduction studies (NCSs)] demonstrates evidence of peripheral neuropathy in as many as 30%–40% of patients with cancer.[2]

▶ PARANEOPLASTIC NEUROPATHIES

Neuropathies related to remote effects of carcinoma or the so-called paraneoplastic syndromes are quite interesting but quite rare.[1,3]

PARANEOPLASTIC SENSORY NEURONOPATHY/GANGLIONOPATHY

In 1948, Denny-Brown reported two patients with small-cell lung cancer (SCLC) and sensory neuronopathy (SN).[4] Autopsies revealed dorsal root ganglionitis with degeneration of the posterior columns as well as peripheral sensory axons. Subsequently, there have been many reports of patients presenting with SN, sometimes associated with a concurrent paraneoplastic encephalomyelitis (PEM).[2,4–17] SCLC is the most common malignancy associated with PEM/SN, but cases of carcinoma of the esophagus, breast, ovaries, kidney, and lymphoma have also been reported.[2,4,5] Approximately 13% of patients with SCLC have another type of concomitant malignancy.[2] Therefore, finding a malignancy other than SCLC in a patient with PEM/SN does not obviate the need to look for concurrent lung cancer.

Clinical Features

PEM/SN most commonly develops in the sixth or seventh decade.[2,4,5,18] The disease is more common in women than in men (up to a 2:1 ratio). The neurologic symptoms usually precede the diagnosis of cancer. Most malignancies are detected within 4–12 months, although there are reports of cancer being diagnosed 8 years or more following the onset of the neurologic symptoms.[2,4] Patients usually present with numbness, dysesthesia, and paresthesia, usually in the distal extremities. These symptoms begin in the hands in up to 60% and may be asymmetric in 27%–40% of cases, a pattern that provides a helpful clue in distinguishing an SN from the more typical length-dependent axonal sensory polyneuropathy.[2,4,17] The onset can be quite acute or insidiously progressive. Diminished touch, pain, and temperature sensation and prominent loss of vibratory and position sense occur, resulting in sensory ataxia and pseudoathetosis. The causes of sensory ataxia are limited and should lead to a malignancy workup in any patient who exhibits such signs (Table 19-2). Muscle stretch reflexes are diminished or absent. While sensory symptoms predominate, mild weakness is evident in at least 20% of patients.[2] Weakness can be secondary to an associated myelitis, motor neuronopathy, or concurrent Lambert–Eaton myasthenic syndrome (LEMS).[2,4,17,18] Autonomic neuropathy may occur as an isolated disturbance or as part of the spectrum of a paraneoplastic syndrome in up to 28% of patients and can be the presenting feature in as many as 12%.[2,4,18]

Another clue suggesting a paraneoplastic etiology is the concomitant involvement of other anatomically unrelated neurologic systems. As many as 21% of affected individuals also present with limbic encephalitis manifesting as confusion, memory loss, depression, hallucinations, or seizures.[2,4,18] Approximately 32% of patients develop brainstem dysfunction (e.g., diplopia, vertigo, nausea, and vomiting). Cranial neuropathies, especially of the eighth cranial nerve, occur in up to 15% of patients. Cerebellar ataxia, scanning dysarthria, tremor, and peduncular reflexes attributed to cerebellar dysfunction are evident in 25% of patients. Abnormal ocular movements such as nystagmus, opsoclonus, and internal and external ophthalmoplegia are seen in up to 32% of patients. Myoclonus develops in approximately 1% of patients. Myelitis with secondary degeneration of the anterior horn is the presenting feature in as many as 14% of those affected.

▶ **TABLE 19-1. NEUROPATHIES ASSOCIATED WITH CANCER**

Direct effect of the cancer by invasion or compression of the nerves
Paraneoplastic
    Sensory ganglionopathy (anti-Hu syndrome)
    Sensorimotor neuropathy
    Autonomic neuropathy
Direct toxic effect of treatment
    Neurotoxicity secondary to chemotherapy
    Radiation toxicity
Alteration of immune status caused by immunosuppressive medications
    Often occur in setting of bone marrow transplantation or treatment of GVHD

GVHD, graft-versus-host disease.

Laboratory Features

Polyclonal antineuronal antibodies (IgG) directed against a 35–40 kDa protein or complex of proteins, the so-called Hu antigen or antineuronal nuclear antigen 1 (ANNA1), are found in the sera or cerebrospinal fluid (CSF) in the majority of patients with paraneoplastic PEM/SN.[2,4–8,18–22] The presence of anti-Hu antibodies in the serum correlates with SN,[8] while antibodies in the CSF are associated with the development of PEM.[21] In a study of 49 patients with paraneoplastic sensory neuropathy, anti-Hu antibodies were present in the serum of 40 out of 49 patients.[5] In 77 patients with idiopathic sensory neuropathy, anti-Hu antibodies were found in only one patient.[5] Thus, the sensitivity and specificity of the anti-Hu antibodies are high. More than 10% of patients with paraneoplastic SN do not have anti-Hu antibodies, so all patients suspected of having PEM/SN should undergo periodic screening for an underlying malignancy, regardless of their anti-Hu antibody status. Among those patients without anti-Hu antibodies, antibodies in the sera or CSF may instead be found against anticollapsin response mediator protein 5 (CRMP5) or ampiphysin.[17,23–25] These antibodies can also be identified in addition to anti-Hu antibodies in some patients. As with anti-Hu, concurrent neurologic syndromes may be seen in patients with these antibodies (see **paraneoplastic sensorimotor polyneuropathy** below).

CSF may be normal or may demonstrate mild lymphocytic pleocytosis and elevated protein.[2,4,18,21] Oligoclonal bands and increased CSF IgG synthesis and index are evident in the majority of patients suggestive of intrathecal synthesis of the autoantibody. Magnetic resonance imaging (MRI) of the brain is usually unremarkable. However, some patients with encephalomyelitis have signal abnormalities on T2-weighted and FLAIR images in the temporal or frontal lobes.[17,26] Periventricular white matter hypodensities, and atrophy of the frontal and temporal lobes and cerebellum also have been reported.

NCSs in pure SN reveal low-amplitude or absent sensory nerve action potentials (SNAPs).[27] Compound muscle action potentials (CMAPs) and needle electromyography (EMG) are normal unless the patient has a concurrent motor neuropathy or LEMS. The blink reflex study is usually abnormal, while the masseter reflex study can be normal.[28,29]

Histopathology

Sural nerve biopsies may demonstrate perivascular inflammation comprised of plasma cells, macrophages, B cells, and T cells.[17,27] Autopsy studies reveal inflammation and degeneration of the dorsal root ganglia with secondary degeneration of sensory neurons and the posterior columns (Fig. 19-1).[2,16,22,30] In addition, inflammation and degeneration of neurons in the autonomic ganglia, including the myenteric plexus, may be evident.[30–32] Lennon et al. reported autoantibodies (presumably anti-Hu) directed against a nuclear antigen of myenteric neurons in patients with intestinal pseudo-obstruction due to autonomic involvement.[32] In patients with PEM, autopsies have revealed perivascular and perineuronal inflammation and degeneration of neurons in the brainstem and limbic system (medial temporal lobe, cingulate gyrus, piriform cortex, orbital surface of the frontal lobes, and the insular cortex) (Fig. 19-2).[2,7,18,22] The thalamus, hypothalamus, subthalamic nucleus, deep cerebellar nuclei, and Purkinje cells may also be involved. Inflammation and degeneration of the anterior horn cells and the ventral spinal roots are evident in patients with myelitis. In addition to deposition on tumor cells, deposits of

▶ **TABLE 19-2. CAUSES OF SENSORY NEUROPATHY/GANGLIONOPATHY**

Type of Ganglionopathy	Causes
Genetic	CANVAS, certain spinocerebellar ataxias, certain mitochondrial disorders, and Friedreich's ataxia
Paraneoplastic	Small-cell lung cancer, bronchial carcinoma, breast cancer, ovarian cancer, prostate cancer, lymphoma, neuroendocrine tumors, or sarcoma
Systemic autoimmune	Sjögren syndrome, systemic lupus erythematosus, MCTD, or rheumatoid arthritis
Infection related	HIV, HTLV-1, EBV, Zika virus, enterovirus, or VZV infection or leprosy
Drug or toxicity related	Platinum-based chemotherapy (cisplatin, oxaliplatin, or carboplatin) Vitamin B6 (pyridoxine) toxicity Checkpoint inhibitors
Idiopathic	Large fiber sensory ganglionopathy Small fiber sensory ganglionopathy

MCTD, mixed connective tissue disease; HIV, human immunodeficiency virus; HTLV-1, human T-lymphotrophic virus-1; EBV, Epstein-Barr virus; VZV, Varicella zoster virus; CANVAS, Cerebellar ataxia with neuropathy and vestibular areflexia syndrome.

From Amato AA, Ropper AH. Sensory ganglionopathy. *N Eng J Med*. 2020;383:1657–1662. Copyright © 2020 Massachusetts Medical Society. Reprinted with permission from Massachusetts Medical Society.

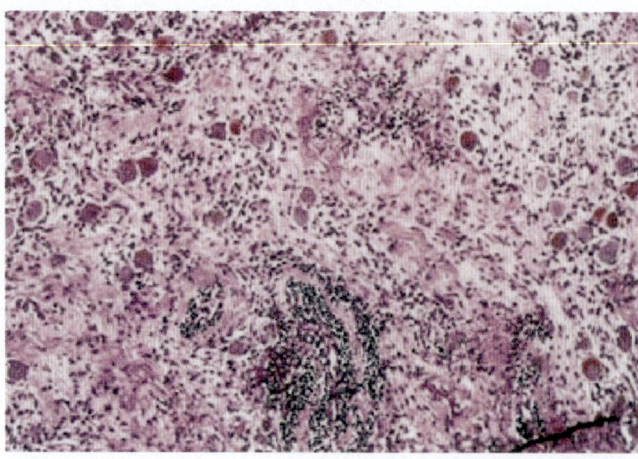
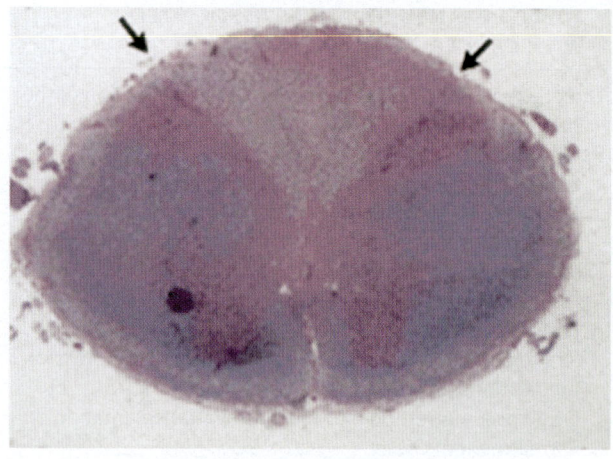

Figure 19-1. (**A**) Dorsal-root ganglia of the cervical cord, showing marked parenchymal and perivascular inflammation, loss of ganglion cells, and fibrosis (H&E, ×100). (**B**) Section of cervical spinal cord showing marked pallor of the dorsal columns (*arrows*) (Luxol Fast Blue—H&E, ×5). (Reproduced with permission from Amato AA, Anderson MP. A 51 year old woman with lung cancer and neuropsychiatric abnormalities (Case 38 2001). *N Engl J Med*. 2001;345(24):1758–1765. Figure 5 & Figure 7, pp. 1763–1764.)

anti-Hu antibody have been demonstrated in areas of the nervous system that correlate with the clinical symptoms.[9,22,30–32]

Pathogenesis

PEM/SN is probably the result of antigenic similarity between proteins expressed in the tumor cells and the neuron cells (e.g., Hu antigens), leading to an immune response directed against both tumor and neuronal cells.[2,4,10,18,33] The Hu antigen is a family of four similar RNA-binding proteins (HuD, HuC/ple21, Hel-N1, and Hel-N2). The Hu antigen is expressed in the nuclei and to a lesser extent in the cytoplasm of neurons and SCLC cells.[20] The function of this group of proteins is not known, but these are thought to be crucial in the development and maintenance of the nervous system.[10] The role of the anti-Hu antibodies in the development of PEM/NS is also unclear. The antibodies appear to bind to CNS and PNS neurons affected in the syndrome.[9,22,30–32] There is a correlation of high anti-Hu titers in the CSF and the development of PEM,[21] and the serum titer with the occurrence of SN.[8] However, the anti-Hu antibodies have not been proved to be pathogenic. Passive transfer of autoantibodies from patients with PEM/SN and immunization with purified HuD protein have failed to reproduce the disease in animal studies.[34] Further, the anti-Hu antibodies exhibit only weak complement activation.[32,35]

The cellular immune response also appears to be involved in the pathogenesis of PEM/SN.[12] The perivascular infiltrate in tumors and the nervous system consists mainly of CD4+ cells, B cells, and macrophages, while CD8+ cells, cytotoxic T cells, and microglia-like cells predominate in the tissue immediately surrounding neurons.[12,32] T-cell receptor studies on the inflammatory infiltrates in the nervous system and within the tumors of anti-Hu-positive PEM/SN patients reveal a limited Vβ repertoire and clonal expansion suggestive of an antigen-driven cytotoxic T-cell response.[13] Studies have demonstrated an increase of CD45RO+CD4+ memory helper T cells in the peripheral blood of patients with anti-PEM/SN.[12] Antigen-specific proliferations of these T cells occur following in vitro stimulation of cultured lymphocytes with purified HuD antigen. In addition, the cells secreted interferon-γ, suggesting that these lymphocytes were primarily of the Th1 helper subtype. The authors speculated that neoplastic cells express the Hu antigen previously produced by fetal cells but lie sequestered in adult neurons. Autoreactive CD4+ T cells that escaped thymic deletion may become activated by the tumor expressing the Hu

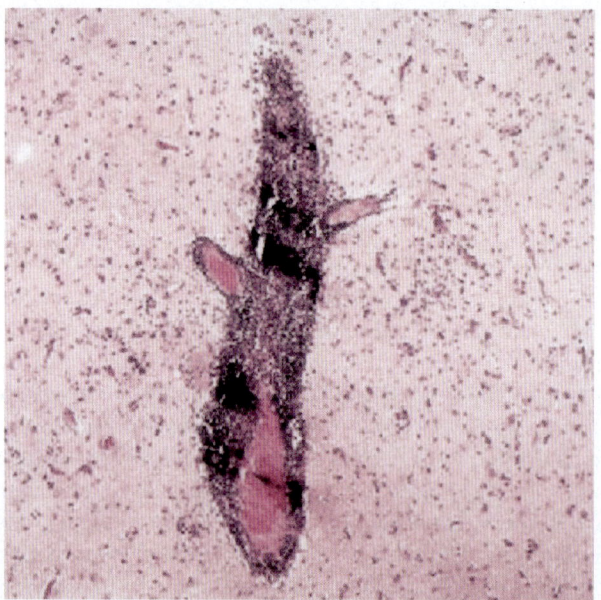

Figure 19-2. Amygdalar complex with a perivascular lymphocytic infiltrate and microglial nodules (H&E, ×100). (Reproduced with permission from Amato AA, Anderson MP. A 51 year old woman with lung cancer and neuropsychiatric abnormalities (Case 38 2001). *N Engl J Med*. 2001;345(24):1758–1765. Figure 6, p. 1764.)

antigen. These cells, in turn, activate CD4+ Th1 T cells that migrate to the tumor and into the nervous system as well, inducing a direct cytotoxic effect on tumor cells and on neurons.

Treatment

Treatment of the underlying cancer generally does not affect the course of PEM/SN.[2,27] However, some patients may improve with treatment of the tumor. Unfortunately, plasmapheresis (PE), intravenous immunoglobulin (IVIg), rituximab, and immunosuppressive agents have been disappointing.[2,4,15,36] To maximize the changes of improvement, diagnosis and initiation of treatment must come before permanent neuronal loss has occurred.[37]

PARANEOPLASTIC SENSORIMOTOR POLYNEUROPATHY

Clinical Features

Sensorimotor polyneuropathies occasionally can be paraneoplastic in nature.[5] Distal symmetric polyneuropathy patterns are not an expected paraneoplastic phenotype; instead an asymmetric sensorimotor polyradiculoneuropathy is most common.[23–25,38,39] Pain is very common and can be quite severe and disabling. While CRMP-5 and/or amphiphysin antibodies can be seen in association with sensory ganglionopathy, both are more commonly associated with this phenotype instead. SCLC is the most common cancer associated with CRMP-5 antibodies, while breast cancer is most common with amphiphysin antibodies.[24,38] Polyradiculoneuropathy in association with either of these antibodies can also occur as an autoimmune process in patients *without* malignancy. Patients with CRMP-5 antibodies frequently have overlap syndromes of either myeloneuropathy or cerebellar ataxia with neuropathy.[25,40] Concurrent retinitis or optic neuritis can also occur. Patients with amphiphysin may also have stiff person syndrome spectrum disorders. Separately, multiple mononeuropathies attributed to paraneoplastic vasculitis have rarely been reported in patients with lymphoma, SCLC, adenocarcinoma of the lungs, endometrium, prostate, and kidneys.[41–46]

Laboratory Features

The majority of patients with detectable CRMP-5 and/or amphiphysin antibodies have either an elevated CSF protein or pleocytosis.[23,24] Sensory NCSs show absent or low-amplitude SNAPs with normal or only borderline slowing of conduction velocities and slightly prolonged distal latencies, while motor studies demonstrated normal or only mild abnormalities reflective of axon loss.[3] A primarily demyelinating neuropathy may be seen as a complication of melanoma, lymphoma, and myeloma/plasmacytoma.[47,48]

Histopathology

Nerve biopsies may reveal a generalized reduction in numbers of myelinated fibers, often with perivascular or microvascular inflammation.[3,23,24] Necrotizing vasculitis is extremely rare.

Treatment

Outcomes are more favorable than anti-Hu-associated sensory ganglionopathy and case series suggest that some patients improve with immunotherapy.[23,24]

PARANEOPLASTIC AUTONOMIC NEUROPATHY

Autonomic dysfunction can occur as an isolated disturbance or as part of the spectrum of the anti-Hu–associated PEM/SN.[5,27] Autonomic neuropathy is most commonly described as a paraneoplastic effect of SCLC but has also occurred with adenocarcinoma and carcinoid tumor of the lungs, breast, testicular and ovarian cancer, pancreatic malignancy, and lymphoma.[5,49] Symptoms and signs of autonomic neuropathy include orthostatic hypotension, gastroparesis, intestinal pseudo-obstruction, urinary retention, dry eyes and mouth, and pupillary dysfunction. In a study of 71 patients with anti-Hu–associated PEM/SN, 10% presented with severe orthostatic hypotension and 28% had varying degrees of dysautonomia during the course of their illness.[5] Autopsies have demonstrated loss of neurons and inflammatory infiltrate in the dorsal root and autonomic ganglia (e.g., myenteric plexus). Autoantibodies directed against a nuclear antigen in myenteric neurons have been shown.[49]

COINCIDENTAL IDIOPATHIC SENSORY OR SENSORIMOTOR POLYNEUROPATHY ASSOCIATED WITH MALIGNANCY

Clinical Features

Idiopathic sensory or sensorimotor polyneuropathy complicating cancer is much more common than paraneoplastic neuropathies. The polyneuropathy is more frequent in individuals with SCLC but can be seen in most cancers. In the majority of cases, etiology of sensory or sensorimotor polyneuropathy complicating cancer remains unknown.

Most patients develop slowly progressive, distal, symmetric numbness beginning in the feet and later progressing to involve the hands. All sensory modalities can be affected, but the prominent sensory ataxia associated with PEM/SN does not occur. If weakness is appreciated it is usually mild and distal. Muscle stretch reflexes are diminished or absent distally.

Laboratory Features

There are no specific laboratory abnormalities. NCSs demonstrate features of a length-dependent, axonal, sensory, or sensorimotor polyneuropathy with reduced or absent amplitudes and relatively preserved distal latencies and conduction velocities.[2] EMG may reveal mild denervation changes distally.

Histopathology

Nerve biopsies and autopsies reveal axonal degeneration and regeneration with secondary segmental demyelination and remyelination.

Pathogenesis

The pathogenic basis for this neuropathy is not known. Neuropathies can develop in untreated patients, so neurotoxicity from chemotherapies is not the cause in all. Patients with cancer may lose weight and appear cachectic; however, the neuropathy can manifest before they appear malnourished, and vitamin supplementation does not help. Perhaps, toxic or cytokine factors released by an inflammatory response to the tumor lead to neuronal damage. Alterations in protein and fat metabolism that are associated with cancers conceivably might cause neuropathy.

Treatment

There is no specific treatment for neuropathy other than treating the underlying malignancy and maintaining adequate nutrition.

▶ NEUROPATHY SECONDARY TO TUMOR INFILTRATION

Malignant cells, in particularly leukemic and lymphomatous cells, can occasionally infiltrate peripheral nerves. Manifestations are diverse and include mononeuropathy, multifocal neuropathy/multiple mononeuropathies, cranial neuropathies, polyradiculopathy, plexopathy, or even rarely a generalized symmetric distal or proximal and distal polyneuropathy.[50–57] The sixth and fifth cranial nerves are most commonly affected in nasopharyngiomas, while the sixth cranial nerve followed by the third, fifth, and seventh are more commonly affected in metastatic processes. The so-called "numb chin syndrome," characterized by numbness of the lower lip and chin, is particularly worrisome for malignant invasion of the mental or alveolar branches of the mandibular nerve. Direct invasion of the peripheral nerves or nerve roots is typically a poor prognostic indicator.

NEUROLYMPHOMATOSIS

Clinical Features

Neuropathy related to tumor infiltration can be the presenting clinical manifestation of leukemia or lymphoma or the heralding of a relapse. Peripheral neuropathy occurs in up to 5.5% of patients with leukemia, for example.[53,57–61] Neurolymphomatosis refers to the direct invasion of peripheral nerves and/or nerve roots by lymphoma cells. Lymphoma can also cause neuropathy by compression of nearby nerves or via a paraneoplastic process. While both Hodgkin disease and non-Hodgkin lymphoma (NHL) have been associated with polyneuropathies, the vast majority of cases of neurolymphomatosis occur in patients with high-grade B-cell NHL.[52,60,62–65] Secondary cases sometimes evolve from a low-grade lymphoma.

Patients may initially present with a single painful mononeuropathy.[66–69] This may explain why diagnosis is frequently delayed—a mean of 20 months after symptom onset in one series, for example.[68] The sciatic nerve is the most commonly reported mononeuropathy.[65] Other patients develop a clear mononeuropathy multiplex picture. When the affected nerve territories are confluent, a painful asymmetric sensory disturbance or even a pattern reminiscent of distal symmetric polyneuropathy can result. In addition to the peripheral nerves, the leptomeninges, cranial nerves, and nerve roots can be invaded by tumor cells; this explains the diverse clinical presentations. Polyradiculopathies manifest as radicular pain and sensory loss, weakness, and hypo- or areflexia. If the spinal cord is involved, superimposed upper motor neuron signs are seen. Multiple cranial neuropathies can also occur.

Vasculitic neuropathy may also rarely complicate hairy cell leukemia.[42,43] Two additional rare types of lymphoma have a unique association with neuropathy. Angiotrophic large-cell lymphoma is characterized by intravascular proliferation of large, atypical, lymphoid B cells.[51,52,70–72] The CNS and skin are the most common sites of involvement. Nearly a quarter of patients develop a radiculopathy or polyradiculopathy, while 5% develop mononeuropathies. Biopsy of affected nerves demonstrates intravascular and endoneurial lymphocytic infiltration (primarily B cells). Lymphomatoid granulomatosis is an angiocentric immunoproliferative disorder associated with a pleomorphic lymphoid infiltrate of blood vessels. Infection of T cells by Epstein–Barr virus drives this inflammatory response of reactive T cells.[73] There is a predisposition for evolution into NHL. Distal symmetric polyneuropathy, multifocal neuropathy/multiple mononeuropathies, polyradiculoneuropathies, and cranial neuropathies develop in 10%–15% of patients.[74–77] These neuropathies can begin acutely or have a more slow, insidious onset.

Laboratory Features

Imaging studies (e.g., MRI, CT, neuromuscular ultrasound, or PET) may demonstrate infiltration or compression of the nerve roots (Figs. 19-3 to 19-5).[65,66,68,69,78,79] If the neurologic examination or electrodiagnostic studies clearly localize to a specific peripheral nerve, MRI is quite sensitive. Nerve ultrasound may be a timely, useful adjunct to electrodiagnostic studies as neurolymphomatosis will lead to both enlargement and increased vascularity of the affected nerve segment.

CSF protein is elevated in about two-thirds of affected patients and an increased CSF cell count occurs in 40%–60%. Signs of lymphoma are seen on cytology and/or flow

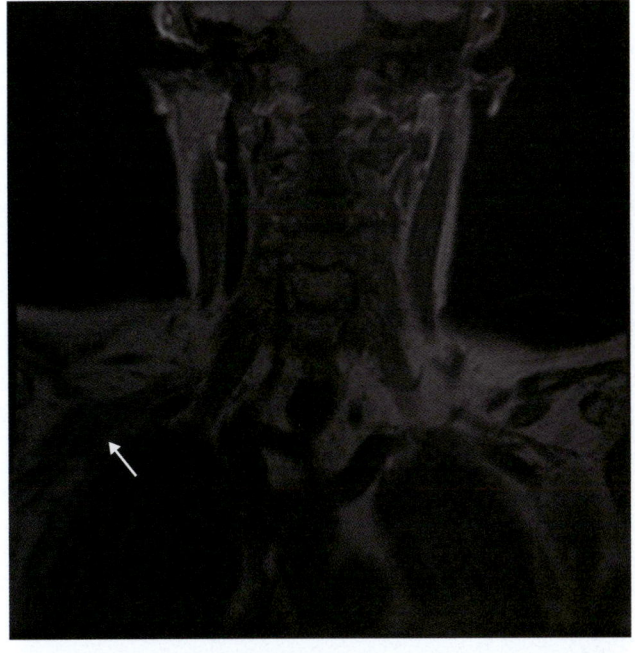
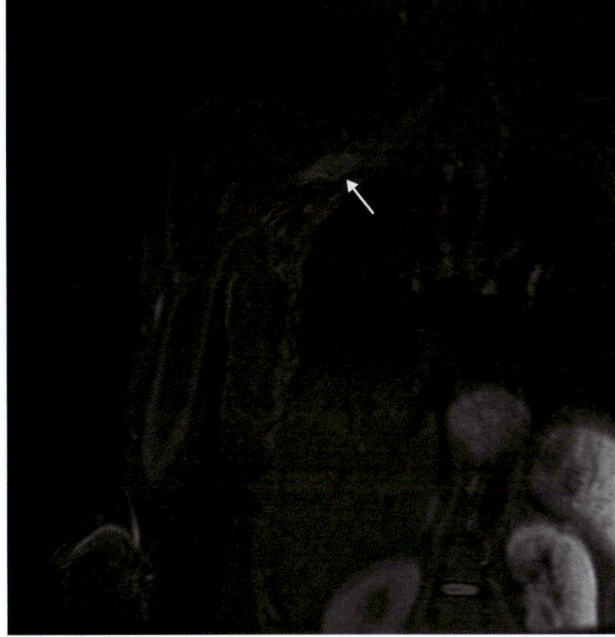
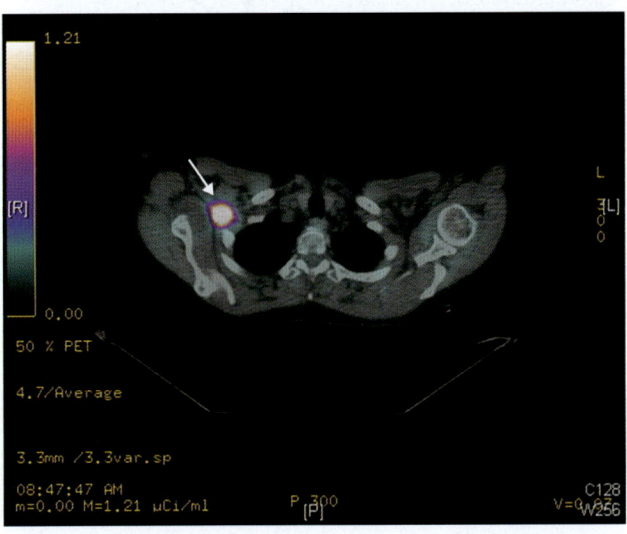

Figure 19-3. MRI T1 without contrast (**A**) and with contrast (**B**) demonstrates lymphoma compressing the right brachial plexus. PET/CT scan shows increased signal highlighting the tumor in the plexus (**C**).

cytometry in less than 50% of patients, likely because the site of malignant infiltration is peripheral to the CSF space in many of these patients.

Electrodiagnostic studies can be useful to localize the site of the lesion(s) and aid eventual biopsy. A frequent pattern is that of multiple axonal mononeuropathies or polyradiculopathy. Demyelinating features, however, can be seen in a sizeable minority of patients with neurolymphomatosis. Since patients frequently also have elevated CSF protein and may initially respond to steroids (see below), CIDP is a frequent misdiagnosis.[69] Conduction block may be seen without other signs of demyelination and may reflect Wallerian degeneration in action—"pseudo-conduction block." Repeat studies in such cases reflect eventual axon loss.[68]

Histopathology

Nerve biopsy may be essential for making this diagnosis, since CSF cytology is often negative. Given the patchy nature of infiltration, imaging studies should be used to guide the biopsy site. Endoneurial inflammatory cells can be seen in both infiltrative and presumed paraneoplastic neuropathies complicating lymphoma (Fig. 19-5). A monoclonal population of cells would favor lymphomatous invasion.[62,80]

Treatment

Patients may temporarily improve when given corticosteroids.[69] This may be done out of initial concern for an inflammatory neuropathy such as CIDP and lead to further diagnostic

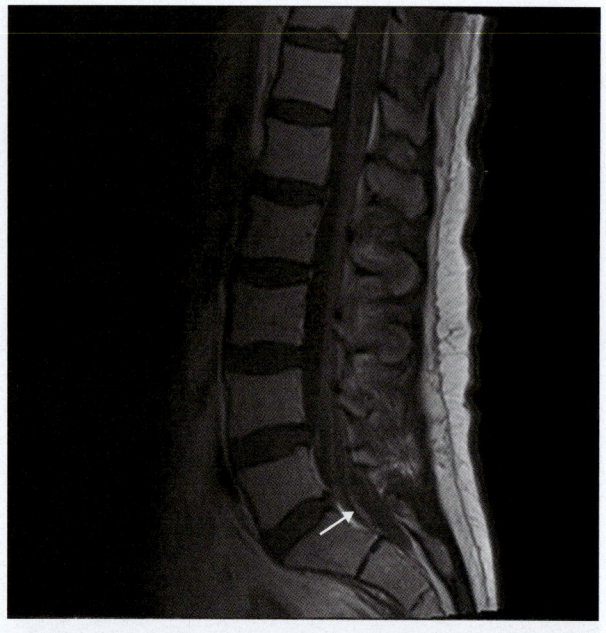
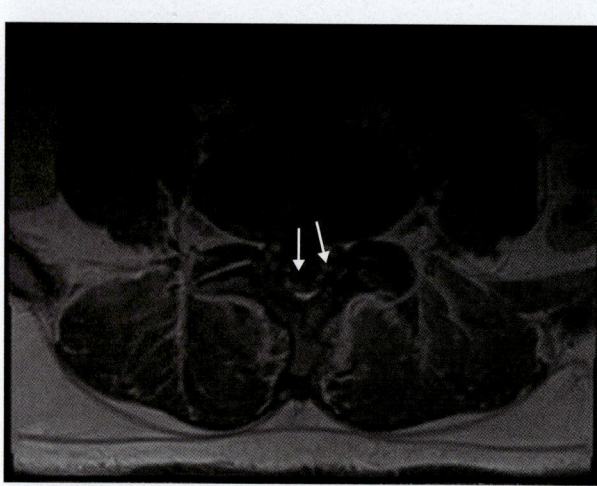

Figure 19-4. Lumbosacral MRI (T1 with contrast) demonstrates enhancement of roots in sagittal (A) and axial sections (B) in a patient with lymphomatous polyradiculopathy.

confusion. After confirmatory diagnosis, patients do frequently respond to irradiation, systemic chemotherapy, or intrathecal chemotherapy. While in the short-term these treatments may lead to improvement in symptoms and neurologic deficits, the long-term outcomes in these patients are often poor.[65,66,68]

▶ PLEXOPATHY IN PATIENTS WITH CANCER

Brachial or lumbosacral plexopathy may result from regional spread of a local tumor (i.e., Pancoast tumor), metastases, or radiation-induced injury. Clinical features and findings on imaging or electrodiagnostic testing can help distinguish between these possibilities.

BRACHIAL PLEXOPATHY

Metastatic disease is responsible for most causes of brachial plexopathy in cancer patients, 78% in one large series.[81] Lung and breast cancers are the most common culprits. The tumors most often spread via the lymphatics to the lateral

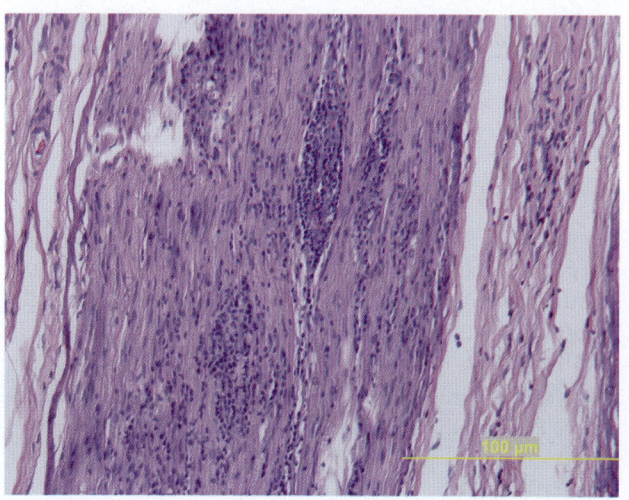
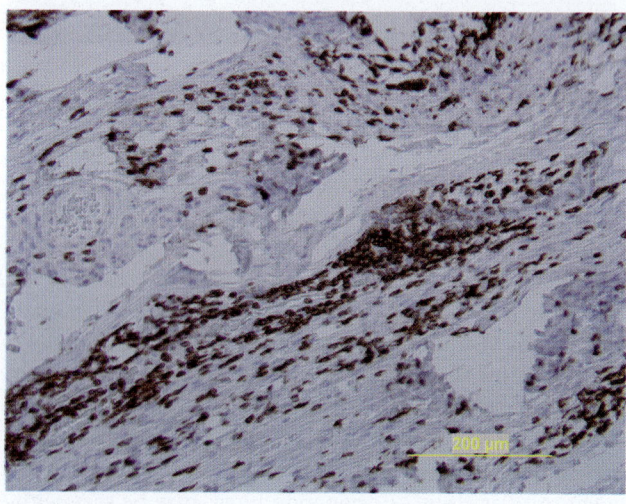

Figure 19-5. Lymphoma. Sural nerve biopsy demonstrates perivascular and endoneurial infiltration of lymphomatous cells on routine H&E (A) and immunoperoxidase stain using CD3 antibody (B).

group of axillary lymph nodes, where divisions of the lower trunk of the brachial plexus are located. Lung cancers in the apices of the lungs may also invade the paravertebral space, the extraspinal C8–T3 mixed spinal nerves, the sympathetic chain, and the stellate ganglia.

Most patients complain of pain in the shoulder area radiating down the arm into the fingers, in particular the fourth and fifth digits. Sensory loss and weakness usually conform to the distribution of the lower trunk, and Horner syndrome may be seen due to involvement of the superior cervical sympathetic ganglion. The arm may appear swollen because of associated lymphedema. Signs and symptoms attributable to involvement of the upper and middle trunk of the brachial plexus are much less common and, when present, suggest epidural extension of the tumor or radiation-induced injury.

Radiation plexitis is usually associated with doses greater than 6,000 rads and can present 3 months to 26 years (mean 6 years) following radiation treatment to the region.[81] Paresthesias and lymphedema of the affected arm are common. Pain occurs in only 15% of patients and is usually not severe, which may help distinguish radiation-induced plexitis from tumor invasion. Further, the upper plexus is involved in 77% and diffuse plexus involvement occurs in 23% of patients with radiation plexitis. Some studies note that the entire plexus is more commonly involved than just the upper trunk.

Imaging studies may demonstrate malignant invasion of the plexus and perhaps extension to the epidural space (Fig. 19-3). Motor and sensory NCSs reveal reduced amplitudes of involved nerves. Myokymic discharges may be appreciated on EMG and, when seen, are highly suggestive of radiation-induced damage. However, the absence of myokymia does not exclude radiation plexopathy. When noninvasive testing cannot differentiate between metastatic and radiation diseases, surgical exploration and biopsy may be required for definitive diagnosis.

Neoplastic invasion of the brachial plexus can be treated with radiation therapy. Pain may be improved but the prognosis for return of motor function is poor. Treatment of the pain with transcutaneous stimulation, sympathetic blockage, and dorsal rhizotomies has been disappointing.

LUMBOSACRAL PLEXOPATHY

The lumbosacral plexus may be invaded by local extension of intraabdominal tumors (73%) or metastasis of distant neoplasms (27%).[82] Colorectal, cervical, and breast cancers, lymphoma and sarcoma are the most common associated malignancies. The lumbar plexus is involved in 31%, lumbosacral trunk in 51%, and the entire lumbosacral plexus in 18% of patients with malignant invasion of the plexus.[82,83] Patients usually complain of an insidious onset of pain, numbness, weakness, and edema of the lower limb. Approximately 25% of patients have involvement of both legs. Fewer than 10% of patients develop bowel or bladder incontinence or impotence.

Radiation-induced lumbosacral plexopathy can develop 1–31 years (mean 5 years) after completion of treatment. It usually manifests as slowly progressive weakness, and, unlike plexopathy secondary to tumor invasion, pain is present in only half the patients and typically is not as severe. Typically, there is symmetrical involvement of both legs, with the distal muscles being more affected than proximal muscles. Bowel and bladder incontinence may occur secondary to nerve injury or due to radiation-induced proctitis or cystitis.

MRI or CT of the lumbosacral spine and pelvis can demonstrate the tumor invading the lumbosacral plexus and perhaps extension into the epidural space. On EMG, fibrillation potentials and positive sharp waves are found in the paraspinal muscles in approximately 50% of patients with radiation-induced damage, suggesting that the disorder is more appropriately termed a radiation-induced radiculoplexopathy. Myokymic discharges are seen on EMG in over 50% of patients with radiation-induced lumbosacral radiculoplexopathy.

▶ PARAPROTEINEMIC NEUROPATHIES

There is increased incidence of monoclonal gammopathies in patients with peripheral neuropathy, and neuropathies may be more frequent in patients with monoclonal gammopathies than in the general population.[84] Approximately 10% of patients with otherwise idiopathic peripheral neuropathies have monoclonal proteins compared to 2.5% of patients with peripheral neuropathies secondary to other diseases.[85,86] The incidence of neuropathy and paraproteinemia both increase with age, however, so the detection of both in a patient may at times be coincidental. Further complicating matters, multiple distinct types of neuropathy may be seen in association with the various categories of hematologic illness associated with paraproteinemia. A causal relationship of demyelinating sensorimotor polyneuropathy and monoclonal IgM has been established (see Chapter 14, and discussion on DADS neuropathy).[86,87] Antibodies directed against myelin-associated glycoprotein (MAG) are present in at least 50% of these patients. By contrast, what relationship IgA and IgG monoclonal gammopathies have to the pathogenesis of axonal peripheral neuropathies remains less clear. Unlike IgM-associated demyelinating neuropathies, IgA and IgG immunoglobulin deposition is generally not seen on nerve sheaths in patients with neuropathies and concurrent IgA or IgG monoclonal gammopathy.

We test all patients with peripheral neuropathies for the presence of monoclonal gammopathies in the serum and urine. The combination of serum protein electrophoresis (SPEP), immunofixation (IFE), and assessment of serum free light chains is recommended to maximize sensitivity. When amyloidosis is specifically suspected, a 24-hour urine collection is advised to also perform urine protein electrophoresis and IFE. When a monoclonal gammopathy is identified, we perform a workup to determine what, if any, underlying hematologic condition is present. Although most patients with monoclonal gammopathies have no underlying malignancy, there is a 1% risk per year of patients subsequently developing myeloma, lymphoma, leukemia, amyloidosis, or plasmacytoma.[86,88–92] We ensure a complete blood count and serum chemistries including calcium have been recently performed, and order a radiologic skeletal survey to assess for osteolytic or sclerotic lesions. A hematology consultation is typically advised to consider a bone marrow biopsy or additional workup. When the serum monoclonal protein burden is low (<3 mg/dL), there is less than 10% involvement of the bone marrow by plasma cells, and there is no evidence of end-organ damage related to the paraprotein, the patient can be deemed to have monoclonal gammopathy of uncertain significance (MGUS). Ultimately, determining the precise phenotype of the neuropathy and the underlying hematologic process can help determine whether there is a link between them and thus guide the appropriate management. When a hematologic malignancy or amyloidosis is identified, treatment of the neuropathy depends on treatment of the malignancy.

MULTIPLE MYELOMA

Multiple myeloma usually presents in the fifth to seventh decades of life with fatigue, bone pain, anemia, and sometimes hypercalcemia. Clinical signs and symptoms of peripheral neuropathies develop in 3%–13% of patients,[85,89–91] while NCS demonstrates that as many as 40% of patients have a subclinical peripheral neuropathy.[91] The most common pattern is that of a distal, axonal, sensory, or sensorimotor polyneuropathy.[90,91] Less frequently, a chronic demyelinating polyneuropathy may develop.[90] Multiple myeloma can also be complicated by amyloid polyneuropathy, which should be considered in patients with painful paresthesias, loss of pinprick and temperature discrimination, and autonomic dysfunction (suggestive of a small fiber neuropathy) and/or patients who develop atypically rapid and severe carpal tunnel syndrome (CTS). Expanding plasmacytomas can compress cranial nerves and spinal roots as well.

Laboratory Features

Multiple myeloma is the most common hematologic malignancy associated with a monoclonal gammopathy. Anemia and hypercalcemia are common. Skeletal survey typically reveals osteolytic lesions. Diagnosis of multiple myeloma requires the demonstration of at least 10% plasma cells on a bone marrow biopsy. Motor and sensory NCSs usually reveal reduced amplitudes with normal or only mildly abnormal distal latencies and conduction velocities.[90,91] Superimposed median neuropathy at the wrist is common.

Histopathology

Abdominal fat-pad, rectal, or sural nerve biopsy can be performed to look for amyloid deposition. Nerve biopsies usually reveal axonal degeneration along with mild segmental demyelination.[91] Amyloid deposition is seen in approximately two-thirds of nerve biopsies.[90] In CTS, amyloid may be deposited in the flexor retinaculum of the wrist, which is worthwhile biopsying if a patient with suspected amyloidosis undergoes carpal tunnel release surgery.

Pathogenesis

The mechanism of the neuropathy in multiple myeloma is multifactorial. The neuropathy may be related to primary amyloidosis with infiltration of the nerves. Other mechanisms of neuropathy may be due to the systemic consequences of multiple myeloma (e.g., cytokines) or amyloidosis (e.g., renal failure). Chemotherapies employed to treat multiple myeloma (e.g., bortezomib and thalidomide) are commonly associated with neuropathy.

Treatment

Unfortunately, treatment of the underlying multiple myeloma does not usually affect the course of the neuropathy.

PRIMARY OR AL AMYLOIDOSIS

Clinical Features

Amyloid comprises 10–20 nm, nonbranching protein fibrils, which aggregate to form three-dimensional β-pleated sheets that are resistant to proteolytic decomposition.[92,93] Amyloidosis can be hereditary or acquired and is associated with systemic proteinaceous deposition in multiple organs (e.g., kidney, liver, heart, and GI tract) including peripheral nerves and muscle. In primary or AL amyloidosis, the abnormal protein deposition is composed of immunoglobulin light chains. AL amyloidosis occurs in the setting of multiple myeloma, Waldenström macroglobulinemia (WM), lymphoma, other plasmacytomas or lymphoproliferative disorders, or in the absence of another identifiable disease.

Patients with primary (AL) amyloidosis can be present with nephrotic syndrome, congestive heart failure, cardiac arrhythmia, purpura, bruises, sicca syndrome, and dyspnea due to pleural effusions, gastrointestinal dysmotility (nausea/constipation/diarrhea/pain), splenomegaly, hepatomegaly, lymphadenopathy, fatigue, weight loss, myopathy, CTS, or polyneuropathy.[94,95] It is more common in men over 50 years of age, which may help distinguish AL from familial amyloidosis, which usually presents earlier in adult life. However, AL amyloidosis can develop in people in their 30s and hereditary amyloidosis can present later in life.

Polyneuropathy develops in as many as 30% of patients with AL amyloidosis and can be the presenting manifestation.[92,95–97] There is an early predilection for small fiber modalities resulting in painful dysesthesias and burning sensations along with diminished pain and temperature sensation and allodynia on examination. The legs are usually affected in a symmetric, length-dependent fashion; however, the trunk can be involved and as many as 20% or more present asymmetrically in a multifocal neuropathy pattern. CTS occurs in 25% of patients and may be the initial complication. Cranial nerves may be affected. The neuropathy is slowly progressive, and eventually weakness develops along with large fiber sensory loss. Generalized proximal and distal weakness can develop such that it resembles CIDP.[96] Most patients develop autonomic involvement with postural hypertension, syncope, impotence, bowel and bladder incontinence, constipation, and impaired sweating. Occasionally, enlarged peripheral nerves are appreciated by an astute clinician. The general physical examination can demonstrate limb edema, hoarse voice, hepatomegaly, and macroglossia. Mortality is typically related to systemic illness (renal failure and cardiac disease).

Laboratory Features

The monoclonal protein can be composed of IgG, IgA, IgM, or only free light chain. Lambda (λ) is more common than κ light chain (>2:1) in AL amyloidosis, in contrast to multiple myeloma in which κ light chains are more common. Immunoelectrophoresis (IEP) or IFE of the serum and urine is more sensitive in identifying monoclonal proteins than serum or urine protein electrophoresis (SPEP or UPEP); but serum free light-chain assay is even more sensitive and thus should be performed on patients with possible amyloid neuropathy. Hypogammaglobulinemia, anemia, renal failure, proteinuria, and transaminitis due to liver involvement may be seen. The serum CK levels can also be elevated in patients with concurrent amyloid myopathy. The CSF protein is often increased (with normal cell count), and thus the neuropathy may be mistaken for CIDP.[96]

Sensory nerve action amplitudes are usually reduced or absent in involved nerves. When obtainable, the distal sensory latencies can be normal or only moderately prolonged and the conduction velocities are similarly normal or moderately slow. Motor conductions are less involved than the sensory conduction but, nonetheless, are frequently abnormal. Motor NCVs can be normal or moderately reduced.[92,95–101] The distal motor latencies are normal or only moderately prolonged in the upper limbs and usually prolonged in the lower limbs. CMAP amplitudes are normal or only mildly reduced during the early course of the disease and not as severely affected as the SNAP. The motor and sensory conduction abnormalities are usually symmetric but can be asymmetric in patients with multifocal neuropathies.[102] Electrophysiological evidence of superimposed median neuropathy at the wrist (CTS) is common.

Needle EMG examination usually reveals positive sharp waves and fibrillation potentials along with reduced recruitment of long-duration, high-amplitude, polyphasic MUAPs in affected muscles. Myotonic discharges and myopathic MUAPs, particularly in more proximal muscles, may be seen in patients with superimposed amyloid myopathy.

Histopathology

Nerve biopsies reveal axonal degeneration and severe loss of small myelinated and unmyelinated fibers. There is a less pronounced but obvious degeneration of the large myelinated nerve fibers as well. Amyloid deposits have a characteristic apple-green birefringence when stained with Congo red and observed under polarized light and bright red under rhodamine fluorescence. Amyloid is also metachromatic when stained with methyl violet or crystal violet and also stains with Alcian blue. Amyloid deposition in a globular or diffuse pattern may be demonstrated in the endoneurium, perineurium, or epineurium and around blood vessels (Fig. 19-6).[103] Chronic inflammatory cell infiltrate may be appreciated. Concomitant muscle biopsy may also reveal amyloid deposits encasing muscle fibers or around blood vessels. Of note, the appearance of the Congo red or metachromatic staining does not distinguish between the various subtypes of amyloidosis. Approximately 10% of patients with a presumptive diagnosis of systemic AL amyloidosis actually have hereditary amyloidosis with genetic testing.[104] Immunohistochemistry using antibodies directed against light chains, apolipoprotein A, gelsolin, and TTR and genetic testing is required to distinguish between the various forms of amyloidosis. Proteomic analysis of nerve tissue using laser microdissection (LMD) and mass spectrometric (MS)-based proteomic analysis can distinguish specific types of amyloid independent of clinical information.[105] Although often not necessary, electron microscopy (EM) can also confirm the presence of amyloid fibrils (Fig. 19-7).

Amyloid deposition can also be demonstrated in the sympathetic and dorsal root ganglion. Because of the patchy, multifocal pattern of amyloid deposition, biopsies are not always diagnostic. Abdominal fat pad biopsies are a sensitive method to detect amyloid deposits and these are abnormal in 50%–85% of patients.[106,107] Other sites commonly biopsied include the bone marrow, kidney, rectal mucosa, stomach, salivary glands, muscle, and skin.

Pathogenesis

The pathogenic basis for the neuropathy associated with amyloidosis is unclear and may be multifactorial. Amyloid deposition in the epineurial and endoneurial connective tissue may lead to compression of nerve fibers with focal demyelination and axonal degeneration. Deposition around blood vessels might cause ischemic damage to nerve fibers.[108] Transport of nutrients into and waste products out of the nerves may also be affected by amyloid deposition within the endoneurium and epineurium and around blood vessels.

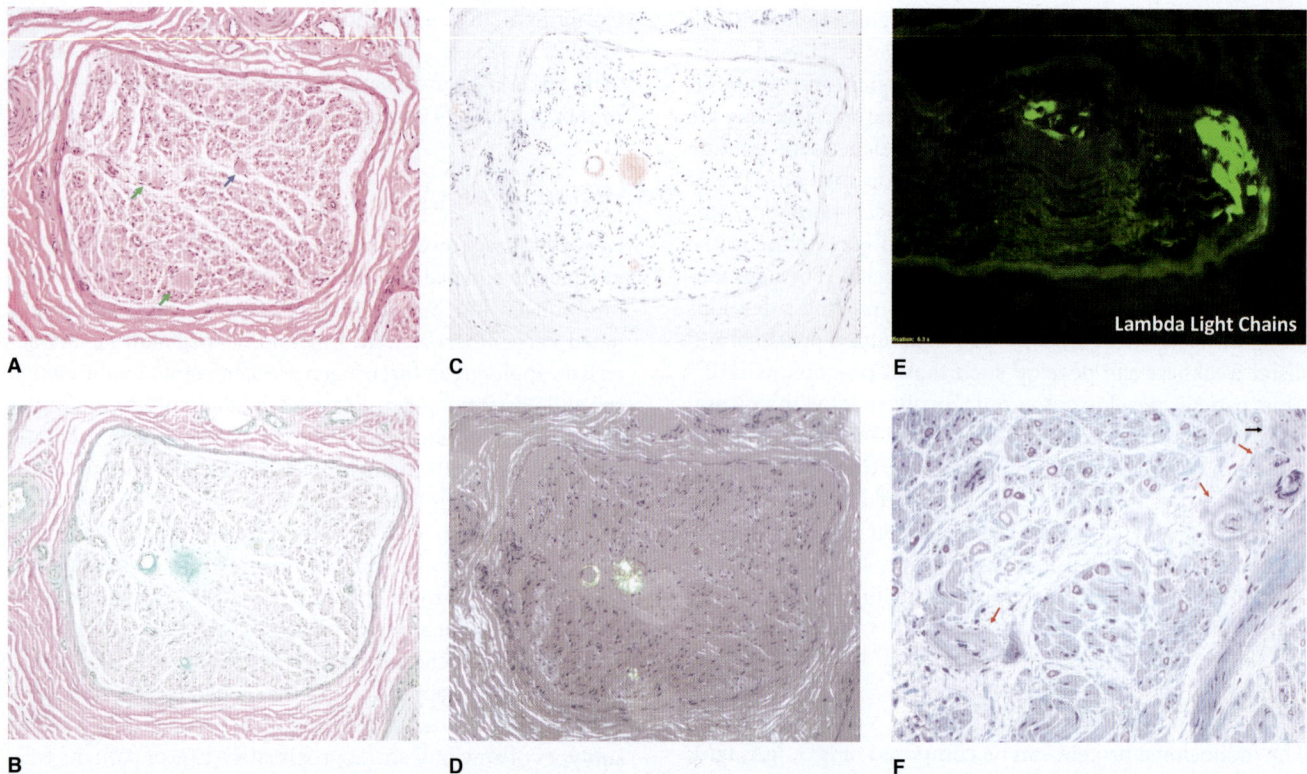

Figure 19-6. Sural nerve biopsy (**A–D**, paraffin sections and **E,** immunofluorescence, and **F**, epoxy sections). Serial paraffin cross sections show (**A**, hematoxylin and eosin stain) areas of eosinophilic amorphous endoneural and perivascular deposits. In (**B**), sulfated alcian blue stain highlights these deposits of amyloid in blue. The deposits stain salmon-pink on Congo red stain (**C**), and, when viewed under polarized light (**D**), show apple-green birefringence in the areas of amorphous material. Immunofluorescence (**E**) demonstrates that the deposits react strongly for lambda light chains but not for kappa light chains (not shown). The plastic-embedded, toluidine blue-stained semithin sections (**F**) show depletion of large and small myelinated fibers and occasional degenerating axons. The same amorphous deposits are again seen. These findings are diagnostic of primary amyloidosis from a lambda light chain.

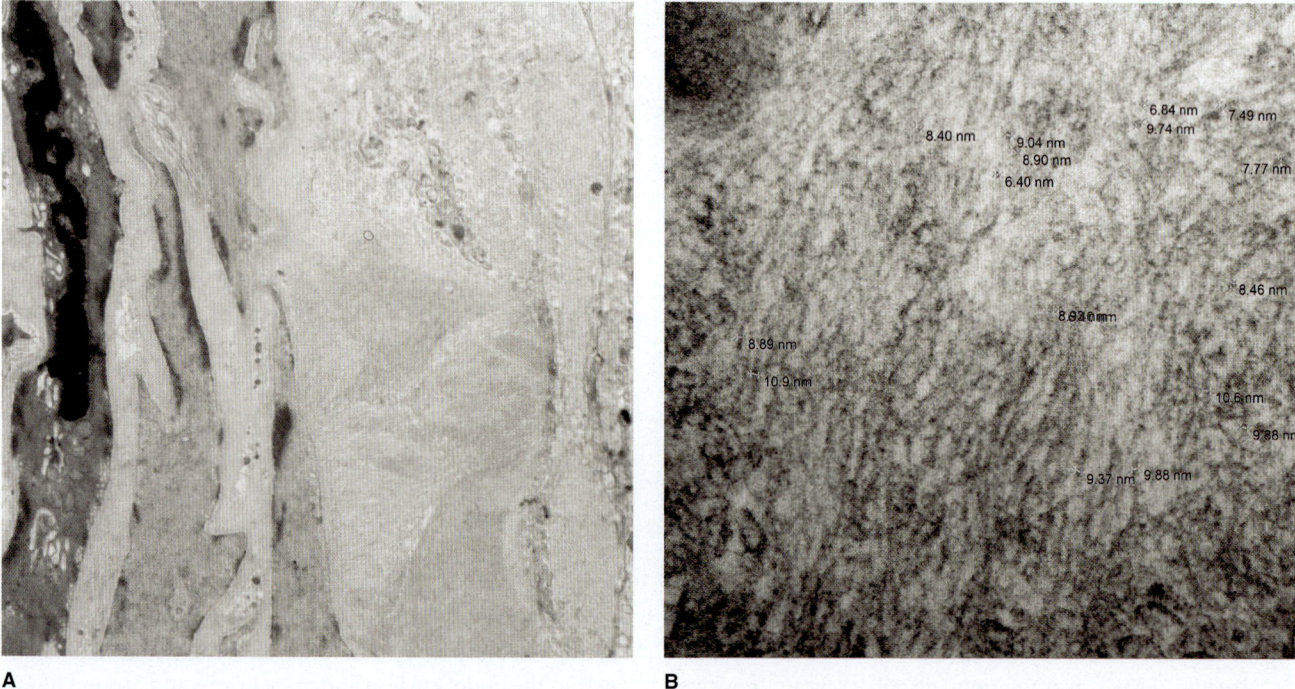

Figure 19-7. Sural nerve biopsy, electron microscopy, in a patient with AL amyloidosis associated with an IgG lambda paraprotein. Panel (**A**) shows bundles of amyloid fibrils haphazardly arranged "haystacks." Amyloid deposits can also be seen within the interstitium. In (**B**), the diameter of amyloid fibrils is quantified. The expected diameter is 7.5–10 nm.

Treatment

Chemotherapy with melphalan, prednisone, colchicine that reduces the concentration of monoclonal proteins, and autologous stem cell transplantation (SCT) may prolong survival and improve neuropathy.[109–111] The severity of baseline cardiac and renal involvement, number of organs involved, and presence of autonomic neuropathy may be independent, adverse determinants of survival in these patients.

OSTEOSCLEROTIC MYELOMA (POEMS SYNDROME)

Clinical Features

Osteosclerotic myeloma is rare and is responsible for less than 3% of myelomas. Symptomatic polyneuropathy develops in near 50% of patients with osteosclerotic myeloma and often is the presenting feature.[112] The acronym POEMS syndrome (originally known as Crow–Fukase syndrome) is used to describe the common constellation of associated systemic features in this rare paraneoplastic disorder: Polyneuropathy, Organomegaly, Endocrinopathy, Monoclonal protein, and Skin changes.[89,112–119] While by definition all patients with POEMS must have both polyneuropathy and a monoclonal plasma cell disorder, not every patient will display all the other features of POEMS syndrome. Most individuals with POEMS syndrome have osteosclerotic myeloma, but the syndrome can also occur with Castleman disease (angiofollicular lymphoid hyperplasia), or rarely extramedullary plasmacytomas, WM, and solitary lytic plasmacytoma. Some patients have no identifiable malignancy at initial workup.

About 50%–63% have organomegaly: hepatomegaly, splenomegaly, and/or lymphadenopathy. Nearly two-thirds have some endocrinopathy; hypothyroidism is most common, but adrenal insufficiency, gynecomastia, testicular atrophy with impotence in men, amenorrhea in women, and diabetes mellitus can all be seen. Hyperpigmentation or acrocyanosis are the most common skin change noted; hypertrichosis is also frequent. Although not in the acronym, volume overload leading to edema, pericardial, and pleural effusions occurs in more than half.[91,115–121]

The neuropathy of POEMS syndrome usually presents as symmetric pain, tingling, and numbness in the feet followed by weakness that progress in a length-dependent manner. Because progression is typically subacute and the weakness can become quite severe and disabling, misdiagnosis of CIDP is common.[119] Rarely, the onset may be acute such that it resembles Guillain–Barré syndrome (GBS).[116] Muscle stretch reflexes are reduced or absent. The cranial nerves and respiratory muscles can be affected, and papilledema is evident in 29%–55% of patients, findings that are uncommon in idiopathic CIDP.[118,121] Patients can also develop a myopathy secondary to associated hypothyroidism or rarely an inflammatory myopathy.[117]

Castleman disease or angiofollicular lymph node hyperplasia is characterized by lymphoid hyperplasia associated with capillary proliferation and can be also be associated with POEMS syndrome in the absence of the osteosclerotic lesions.[120] The angiofollicular lymph node hyperplasia and neuropathy may be related to increases in serum cytokine levels and vascular endothelial growth factor (VEGF), which are associated with the disorder.

Laboratory Features

POEMS is almost universally associated with monoclonal gammopathy that has a lambda light-chain component; the heavy chain is typically IgG or IgA.[121] Because the amount of monoclonal protein can be small, IEP and IFE are much more sensitive than protein electrophoresis; testing the urine is useful for the minority of cases in which the paraprotein is not detectable in the serum.[115,118] CSF protein levels are often markedly elevated, contributing to the frequent confusion with idiopathic CIDP.[119] POEMS syndrome is associated with high levels of serum VEGF and, conversely, low levels of serum erythropoietin.[122,123] Serum levels of VEGF and erythropoietin normalize with a response to therapy.[122]

Skeletal survey typically reveals characteristic sclerotic or mixed sclerotic and lytic bony lesions usually in the vertebral bodies, pelvis, or ribs (Fig. 19-8). In 50% of cases, these skeletal lesions are multiple and represent focal plasmacytomas.

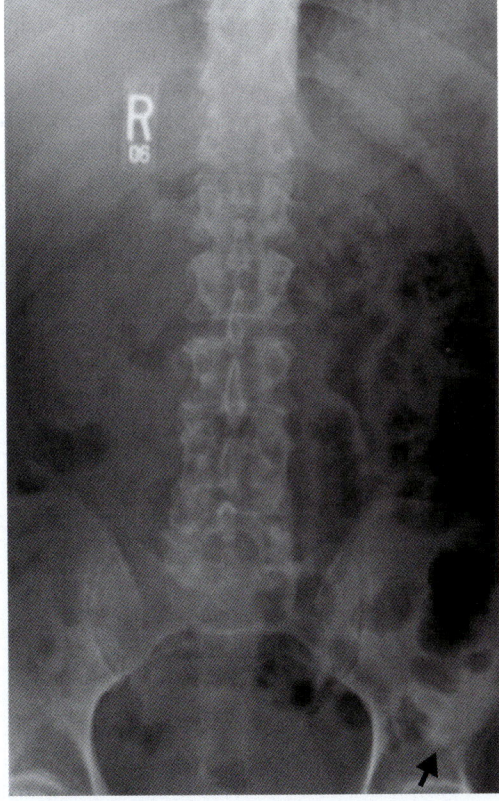

Figure 19-8. POEMS. Pelvic x-ray demonstrates a large osteosclerotic lesion (*arrow*) in the left iliac crest.

Bony lesions may be absent in patients with associated Castleman disease.

NCS/EMG typically demonstrates features of a severe, length-dependent sensorimotor polyneuropathy with both axonal and primary demyelinating features.[90,91,112,114,120,121,124,125] Conduction block and temporal dispersion are much less common in POEMS as compared to idiopathic CIDP. Features of axonal loss are also more prominent than idiopathic CIDP, with reduction of CMAP amplitudes and robust fibrillation potentials distally. Unlike in idiopathic CIDP, the "sural sparing" pattern of sensory amplitude reduction is not typically seen, more consistent with a length-dependent process.

Histopathology

Nerve biopsies usually reveal a combination of segmental demyelination and axonal degeneration.[114,126] A few endomysial or perivascular inflammatory cells may be seen. VEGF is highly expressed in blood vessels and some non–myelin-forming Schwann cells in nerve biopsies of patients with POEMS.[122] Light microscopy reveals an increased thickness of the basal lamina and a narrowing of the lumina of endoneurial vessels, while EM demonstrates proliferation of endothelial cells and opening of tight junctions.[122] EM may also reveal uncompacted myelin.[126]

Pathogenesis

The pathogenesis of POEMS syndrome is not clear, but likely autoimmune in nature. Various cytokines including VEGF and matrix metalloproteinases are elevated in patients with POEMS syndrome and appear to correlate with the severity of the neuropathy.[122,123,127,128] Over expression of VEGF may increase nerve microvascular permeability, thereby inducing endoneurial edema and allowing neurotoxic cytokines and other chemicals access to the nerve parenchyma, which leads to demyelination and secondary axonal degeneration.[116]

Treatment

POEMS syndrome is typically treated with chemotherapy. Patients can improve, especially if treatment is initiated closer to the onset of symptoms. The neuropathy can occasionally improve with usual treatment given to patients with idiopathic CIDP (e.g., corticosteroids). However, the neuropathy is more refractory to treatment than typical CIDP, and POEMS needs to be suspected and reevaluated for in all cases of refractory CIDP with repeated serum and urine IFE/IEP and skeletal surveys. Autologous peripheral blood SCT has been associated with prolonged progression-free survival compared with chemotherapy.[119,123,128]

WALDENSTRÖM MACROGLOBULINEMIA

WM is a lymphoplasmacytic lymphoma of the bone marrow associated with the production of an IgM monoclonal protein, usually with a κ light chain.[89,129–133] It most commonly occurs between the ages of 50 and 70 years and may present with an insidious onset of progressive fatigue, weight loss, lymphadenopathy, hemorrhages (especially nose bleeds), anemia, and/or weakness. The symptoms of WM can be caused either by infiltration of lymphoma cells into tissue or by the effects of the related IgM monoclonal protein. WM can evolve from a patient with prior IgM MGUS.

Symptoms of neuropathy are present in about 20% of WM patients at diagnosis and nearly 50% will have symptoms or signs of neuropathy at some point in their course of illness.[134,135] The clinical spectrum of neuropathies seen with WM and with IgM MGUS is similar, so hematologic workup is essential to determine the proper underlying diagnosis. Neurologic symptoms in WM may alternatively relate to serum hyperviscosity. Typical symptoms include headache, dizziness, ataxia, blurry vision, diplopia, tinnitus, or hearing loss. This is more likely when serum IgM levels are very high (>6,000 mg/dL).

Clinical Features

Multiple phenotypes of neuropathy have been described among patients with WM.[130,133–138] Most commonly, patients initially complain of distal, symmetric numbness and paresthesias beginning in the feet. Gradually, symptoms progress into the legs and eventually the hands. Axonal, demyelinating, or mixed features on electrodiagnostic studies have described in WM patients presenting with such symptoms.

Patients with demyelinating features frequently have anti-MAG antibodies detectable in serum and clinically develop a phenotype consistent with distal acquired demyelinating symmetric neuropathy (DADS; described in additional detail in Chapter 14). These patients can develop difficulty in walking and loss of fine motor control of the fingers due to prominent sensory ataxia. Distal strength (e.g., toe extension) becomes impaired with time. Areflexia is typically more prominent in these patients than those with axonal forms.

A small fraction of patients will instead present with an asymmetric, multifocal phenotype of neuropathy resembling either mononeuropathy multiplex or a polyradiculopathy. Cases resembling idiopathic multifocal acquired demyelinating sensory and motor neuropathy (MADSAM) or multifocal motor neuropathy (MMN) have been described.[139] This multifocal pattern, however, may indicate infiltration of nerves by lymphoplasmacytic lymphoma cells. WM can also rarely directly invade the CNS and leptomeninges, known as Bing–Neel syndrome. Weakness and/or sensory symptoms can result from either brain parenchymal damage or from nerve root involvement in these cases, so workup in these cases may require CNS imaging. Alternatively, this pattern can result from a secondary vasculitis provoked by WM. A minority of patients will develop **cryoglobulinemia** as a complication of WM.[140–143] Cryoglobulins are abnormal proteins that precipitate out of the serum at colder temperatures. Symptoms result from the occlusion of smaller blood vessels and/or secondary inflammation, particularly in the limbs where temperatures are cooler. WM can lead to either type I cryoglobulinemia (in which the cryoglobulin is comprised solely of monoclonal proteins) or type II cryoglobulinemia (in which the monoclonal protein actually targets a component of other immunoglobulins, such as the Fc fragment of IgG, leading to the cryoglobulin containing both an IgM monoclonal protein and a polyclonal component). Skin involvement is more prominent in type I cryoglobulinemia. Neuropathy can occur in either, but is more frequent with type II. Mononeuropathy multiplex is the most common pattern of neuropathy seen, with greater sensory involvement than motor involvement. Occasionally, a pure sensory distal neuropathy can result. Pain is a prominent feature, so this can be an important clue in the distal sensory cases.

Predominantly small fiber sensory neuropathy has also been described, though its pathologic association with WM is less well established. A workup to exclude AL amyloidosis and cryoglobulinemia should be considered, as both can present with painful distal sensory symptoms early in their course.

Laboratory Findings

Anti-MAG antibodies are detectable in the serum in some patients with WM and neuropathy. Many, but not all, of these patients will have a classic DADS phenotype.[134,144,145] Neither the titer of the anti-MAG antibodies nor the total serum IgM levels correlate well with the severity of the neuropathy.[135] Occasionally, IgM antibodies to other neural antigens (including GD1a, GD1b, GM1, GM2) can be found. Whereas a clear pathogenic link has been established between anti-MAG antibodies and the development of neuropathy, the causal association for these other ganglioside antibodies is less clear. Testing for these antibodies is therefore most useful in patients with a compelling clinical phenotype—a patient suspected to have MMN, for example, which can be seen in association with IgM anti-GM1 antibodies. Likewise, IgM anti-GD1b antibodies can be seen in association with the unique phenotypes of CANOMAD or CANDA (see "Neuropathies associated with MGUS" below), so their identification can help more definitively link the monoclonal gammopathy to the neuropathy in such cases.

CSF analysis is most useful for patients with a multifocal clinical presentation, since an infiltrative pathophysiology is more important to consider in these cases. Cytology and/or flow cytometry may detect lymphoma cells in cases of Bing–Neel syndrome. The MYD88^{L265P} mutation is seen very commonly within the clonal population of malignant lymphocytes in WM. Detection of this mutation in a CSF sample can also help establish a diagnosis of Bing–Neel syndrome, though the introduction of peripheral blood lymphocytes into the CSF via a traumatic lumbar puncture could lead to false positives.[146] Patients with DADS frequently have high CSF protein without pleocytosis, similar to idiopathic CIDP.

Among patients with a distal symmetric sensory-predominant presentation, NCS/EMG can demonstrate features of either an axonal or a demyelinating sensorimotor polyneuropathy. Occasionally, NCS/EMG will be normal, suggesting a small fiber neuropathy. Patients with anti-MAG antibodies and a classic DADS phenotype more frequently have demyelinating features. The specific electrodiagnostic features seen in DADS are described in Chapter 14.[89,129–133]

Histopathology

In cases of demyelinating neuropathy with MAG antibodies, nerve biopsies may show prominent demyelination and IgM deposition on the outer myelin membranes and occasionally in the periaxonal space but not on compact myelin.[133] A related characteristic feature on EM is separation of myelin lamella. Deposition of light chains in the endoneurium and epineurium resulting in massive fascicular hyalinosis and epineural arteries disruption has also been reported.[147]

Treatment

The presence of peripheral neuropathy due to WM is an established indication to begin oncologic treatment of the WM.[134,136,145] A critical first step, however, is determining whether the patient's neuropathy is indeed related to WM. This is straightforward in cases of DADS with anti-MAG neuropathy. In cases with an axonal pathophysiology, clinical judgment is required and it is essential that adequate workup to exclude alternative causes is performed. Evidence is not yet available to determine whether patients with concurrent WM and small fiber neuropathy benefit from oncologic treatment. Treatment regimens utilized include rituximab alone, rituximab in combination with bendamustine or other traditional forms of chemotherapy, and bruton tyrosine kinase inhibitors such as ibrutinib. The choice of therapy should be determined by an oncologist. Patients with a very high serum IgM who are treated with rituximab-containing regimens are at risk for paradoxical worsening of the associated neuropathy, deemed an "IgM flare".[148] Either delaying the start of rituximab for the initial cycles or treatment with plasma exchange prior to starting treatment may lower the risk.

NEUROPATHIES ASSOCIATED WITH MGUS

Clinical Features

Neuropathy in patients with MGUS is heterogeneous in clinical, laboratory, and electrophysiologic features.[86,134,138,145,149–153] Neuropathy is both more common and more likely to be definitively related to the monoclonal protein in cases of IgM MGUS. Neuropathy is seen in 15%–50% of patients with an IgM monoclonal protein, but only in approximately 5% of patients with IgG and at most 15% of patients with IgA monoclonal protein. Because there is no oncologic indication to treat MGUS in and of itself, management of these patients will be solely guided by the specific phenotype of neuropathy identified; careful classification is therefore essential.

Both axonal and demyelinating neuropathies are seen in association with MGUS. Patients with an axonal neuropathy usually present with sensory symptoms in a length-dependent fashion. This is most common among patients with IgG or IgA MGUS. Their clinical, laboratory, histopathology, and electrophysiologic features are indistinguishable from idiopathic sensory or sensorimotor polyneuropathies. Amyloidosis and cryoglobulinemia remain important considerations in such patients with apparent MGUS, since the associated neuropathy can be distal and sensory predominant early in the course.

Neuropathies associated with an IgM monoclonal protein are more likely to be demyelinating. The DADS phenotype is most common, frequently in association with anti-MAG antibodies. The clinical and electrodiagnostic phenotype is indistinguishable from DADS seen in WM patients (see WM section above, as well as Chapter 14).[135] Patients may alternatively present with symmetric proximal and distal weakness typical of idiopathic CIDP; this is more common with IgG and IgA MGUS. Aside from monitoring the MGUS, the management of these patients need not differ from idiopathic CIDP.

Very rarely, a unique phenotype of neuropathy can be seen in patients with IgM MGUS in association with disialosyl antibodies.[102,154,155] Affected patients present with distal numbness and gait imbalance due to sensory ataxia. Uniquely, there is evidence of cranial nerve involvement, most commonly ophthalmoplegia. Bulbar weakness and/or facial numbness can also be seen. This syndrome is akin to a chronic form of Miller Fisher syndrome and has been called **Chronic Ataxic Neuropathy, Ophthalmoplegia, IgM paraprotein, cold Agglutinins, and Disialosyl antibodies (CANOMAD).** A separate acronym has been used to describe similar patients without the cranial nerve involvement: **Chronic Ataxic Neuropathy with Disialosyl Antibodies (CANDA).**

Laboratory Features

About 50% of the patients with IgM-MGUS neuropathy have antibodies directed against MAG.[86,156,157] However, patients without detectable anti-MAG antibodies who otherwise have a clinical and electrodiagnostic profile consistent with DADS have a similar course and should be managed the same. Elevated CSF levels are common in patients with a demyelinating neuropathy. NCS in patients with IgG- and IgA-MGUS neuropathies can be either axonal or demyelinating in nature. The IgM-MGUS neuropathies are typically demyelinating with markedly prolonged distal latencies and moderately slow conduction velocities as is typical of DADS. Motor NCS reveals markedly prolonged distal latencies with moderate slowing of conduction velocities, but there is usually no evidence of temporal dispersion or conduction block.[150,156-159]

Patients with CANOMAD or CANDA usually have IgM antibodies in the serum that target GD1b or other disialosyl gangliosides. About 50% also have cold agglutinins. NCS/EMG shows a mixed axonal-demyelinating pattern.

Pathogenesis

Endoneurial injection or passive transfer of serum from patients with IgM-MAG antibodies to animals leads to conduction block and demyelination. Except for cases of amyloid neuropathy, there is no pathogenically proven causal relationship of monoclonal gammopathy and axonal sensorimotor polyneuropathy.

Treatment

Patients with MGUS neuropathy who fulfill clinical and electrophysiologic criteria for typical CIDP with proximal and distal weakness can improve with immunotherapy, similar to idiopathic CIDP (discussed in Chapter 14).[156,157] In contrast, DADS/anti-MAG demyelinating neuropathies with predominantly sensory symptoms and only distal weakness are typically refractory to typical treatments for CIDP. For example, IVIg has been reported to be effective in 16% to 25% of cases,[160-162] PLEX in 40%,[162] and cyclophosphamide in 36%.[162] None of these benefits have been demonstrated to be either durable or achieve statistical significance.[163] Some patients may respond to rituximab.[164-170] A small subset of patients treated with rituximab may instead have worsening neuropathy symptoms, often but not always transient, upon initiation of therapy.[171-173] This may be similar to the "IgM flare" phenomenon that can be seen in rituximab-treated patients with WM.[148] Because of the slowly progressive nature of this disorder, we do not treat all patients with anti-MAG neuropathy. Instead, we engage in shared decision making with the patient regarding the risks of treatment, the chance of benefit, and the expected progression of this disorder over time. We are more likely to recommend treatment in patients with significant disability or a faster disease trajectory.[174]

Patients with CANOMAD/CANDA have responded to IVIG or rituximab treatment.[102,154] There is no strong evidence that treating the MGUS in patients has any impact on axonal neuropathies. Importantly, patients with MGUS and neuropathy may be at a higher risk of transformation to a later hematologic malignancy, with IgM MGUS carrying the highest rate of transformation.[175,176] Regardless of whether treatment for the neuropathy is pursued, ongoing monitoring of the monoclonal gammopathy is therefore paramount.

▶ NEUROPATHY AS A COMPLICATION OF HEMATOPOIETIC STEM CELL TRANSPLANTATION/GRAFT-VERSUS-HOST DISEASE

Neuropathies may develop in patients who undergo autologous or allogenic SCT because of toxic effects of chemotherapy, radiation, infection, or an autoimmune response directed against the peripheral nerves.[41,177,178] Symptoms of neuropathy are more common among those patients with a history of chronic graft-versus-host disease (GVHD). Painful muscle cramps are particularly common among affected patients.[179]

Chronic GVHD shares many features with a variety of autoimmune disorders, and it is possible that an immune-mediated response can be directed against peripheral nerves. Patients with chronic GVHD may develop cranial neuropathies including loss of olfactory and gustatory sensation,[180] sensorimotor polyneuropathy, multifocal neuropathy/multiple mononeuropathies, and severe generalized peripheral neuropathy resembling GBS[177,181,182] or CIDP.[183] Myositis, myasthenia gravis, and LEMS can also complicate GVHD. In patients with neuropathy, NCS may demonstrate primarily axonal, demyelinating, or mixed features. Some cases of GBS have been attributed to chemotherapy, cytomegalovirus, or *Campylobacter jejuni* infections and have improved with plasma exchange[181] or IVIg. The neuropathy may also improve with increased immunotherapy and resolution of the GVHD.[41]

▶ TOXIC NEUROPATHIES SECONDARY TO CHEMOTHERAPY

Many of the commonly used chemotherapy agents can cause a toxic neuropathy (Table 19-3).[1] The mechanisms by which these agents cause toxic neuropathies vary, as can the specific type of neuropathy. The risk of developing a toxic neuropathy or more severe neuropathy appears to be greater in patients with a preexisting neuropathy (e.g., Charcot–Marie–Tooth disease and diabetes) and in those who concomitantly take more than one neurotoxic drug (e.g., nitrofurantoin, isoniazid, disulfiram, pyridoxine, etc.). Chemotherapeutic agents usually cause a sensory greater than motor length-dependent axonal neuropathy or SN/ganglionopathy.

PLATINUM-BASED ANTINEOPLASTIC MEDICATIONS

Clinical Features

Cisplatin is used for a variety of cancers and can cause a dose-related predominantly sensory neuropathy (ganglionopathy), usually at cumulative doses of 225–500 mg/m^2.[184–192] There is a predilection for involvement of large-myelinated nerve fibers leading to paresthesia, hypesthesia, loss of vibratory perception and proprioception, often resulting in gait ataxia and pseudoathetoid movements. Muscle stretch reflexes are reduced or absent throughout. Interestingly, as many as 40% of patients can develop Lhermitte sign, perhaps due to demyelination and edema of the posterior columns. Only a few patients (approximately 2%) develop weakness.[186] Onset of symptoms can appear as late as 8 weeks after the drug has been stopped and may progress up to 6 months following discontinuation of cisplatin, a phenomenon known as coasting.

Carboplatin can similarly cause a dose-related neuropathy, though is overall less neurotoxic than cisplatin. Oxaliplatin is a third-generation platin derivative used mainly for the treatment of colorectal cancer. Like other platinum-based agents, oxaliplatin can cause a chronic sensory neuropathy. Early symptoms may be worse in the hands than in the feet, whereas symptoms in the feet are more persistent.[193–197] Oxaliplatin has also been uniquely associated with an acute, transient form of peripheral nerve hyperexcitability in the 24–48 hours following each infusion of the medication.[194] Affected patients may note cold-induced paresthesias, throat and jaw tightness and cold sensitivity, and even focal weakness. Interestingly, patients with more severe symptoms of acute hyperexcitability experience more chronic sensory neuropathy.

Laboratory Features

NCSs demonstrate low-amplitude or absent SNAPs with normal or only slightly prolonged distal latencies and slow sensory conduction velocities.[188–190] Vibratory perception is usually impaired on quantitative sensory testing. Motor NCSs and needle EMG are usually normal.

Histopathology

Sural nerve biopsies reveal a predominant loss of large myelinated nerve fibers with axonal degeneration, segmental demyelination, and regenerating axonal sprouts.[185,187,188] Degeneration of neurons in the dorsal root ganglion and secondary axonal degeneration on both central and peripheral nerve processes are seen in rats given toxic doses of cisplatin.[189]

Pathogenesis

Cisplatin covalently binds DNA creating inter- and intrastrand cross-links. Pathologic and electrophysiologic studies suggest that neurons in the dorsal root ganglion are preferentially affected. Binding of the drug to neuronal DNA may inhibit transcription of important proteins and impair axonal transport.

VINCA ALKALOIDS

Clinical Features

Vincristine is commonly associated with a toxic sensorimotor and autonomic neuropathy.[198–200] Affected patients develop paresthesias and numbness, which can at times occur in the fingers before the toes. The loss of ankle jerks often precedes the subjective loss of sensation. Weakness of the hands and feet may occur in 25%–35% of patients with increased dosage. Autonomic neuropathy characterized by constipation, urinary retention, impotence, and orthostatic hypotension may occur as well. Cranial neuropathies are uncommon, but optic neuropathy, oculomotor palsies, facial weakness, hearing loss, and laryngeal paralysis have been described. Neuropathic symptoms and signs are more prominent after a cumulative dose of 12 mg of vincristine.[157] However, neuropathy can develop as early as 2 weeks following a single 2 mg/m^2 dose. A coasting effect can be seen such that 24%–30% of

TABLE 19-3. TOXIC NEUROPATHIES SECONDARY TO CHEMOTHERAPY

Drug	Mechanism of Neurotoxicity	Clinical Features	Nerve Histopathology	EMG/NCS
Cisplatin	Preferential damage to dorsal root ganglia: • binds to and cross-links DNA • inhibits protein synthesis • impairs axonal transport	Predominant large fiber sensory neuronopathy; sensory ataxia	Loss of large > small myelinated and unmyelinated fibers; axonal degeneration with small clusters of regenerating fibers; secondary segmental demyelination	Low-amplitude or unobtainable SNAPs with normal CMAPs and EMG; abnormal QST, particularly vibratory perception
Vinca alkaloids (vincristine, vinorelbine)	Interfere with axonal microtubule assembly; impairs axonal transport	Symmetric, S-M, large/small fiber PN; autonomic symptoms common; infrequent cranial neuropathies	Axonal degeneration of myelinated and unmyelinated fibers; regenerating clusters, minimal segmental demyelination	Axonal sensorimotor PN; distal denervation on EMG; abnormal QST, particularly vibratory perception
Etoposide (VP-16)	Unknown; • selective dorsal root ganglia toxicity	Length-dependent, sensory predominant PN; autonomic neuropathy	None described	Abnormalities consistent with an axonal S-M PN
Taxanes (paclitaxel, docetaxel)	Promotes axonal microtubule assembly; interferes with axonal transport	Symmetric, predominantly sensory, PN; large fiber modalities affected more than small fiber	Loss of large > small myelinated and unmyelinated fibers; axonal degeneration with small clusters of regenerating fibers; secondary segmental demyelination	Axonal sensorimotor PN; distal denervation on EMG; abnormal QST, particularly vibratory perception
Ixabepilone and eribulin	Both interfere with microtubule function, but with different mechanisms	Symmetric S-M PN	None described	Not well described
Suramin				
Axonal PN	Unknown; • inhibition of neurotrophic growth factor binding; • neuronal lysosomal storage	Symmetric, length-dependent, sensory-predominant, PN	None described	Abnormalities consistent with an axonal S-M PN
Demyelinating PN	Unknown; • immunomodulating effects	Subacute, S-M PN with diffuse proximal and distal weakness; areflexia; increased CSF protein	Loss of large and small myelinated fibers with primary demyelination and secondary axonal degeneration; occasional epi- and endoneurial inflammatory cell infiltrates	Features suggestive of an acquired demyelinating sensorimotor PN (e.g., slow CVs, prolonged distal latencies and F-wave latencies, conduction block, and temporal dispersion)

Drug	Mechanism	Clinical features	Pathology	Electrodiagnostic findings
ARA-C	Unknown; • selective Schwann cell toxicity • immunomodulating effects	GBS-like syndrome; pure sensory neuropathy; brachial plexopathy	Loss of myelinated nerve fibers; axonal degeneration; segmental demyelination; no inflammation	Axonal, demyelinating, or mixed S-M PN; denervation on EMG
Proteosome inhibitors (bortezomib, carfilzomib, and ixazomib)	Unknown	Length-dependent, sensory, predominantly small fiber PN	Not described	Abnormalities consistent with an axonal sensory neuropathy with early small fiber involvement (abnormal autonomic studies or abnormal epidermal nerve fiber density on skin biopsy)
Thalidomide and lenalidomide	Unknown	Symmetric, length-dependent sensory predominant PN. Pain is common	Loss of large-diameter myelinated fibers, axonal degeneration	Low-amplitude or unobtainable SNAPs with normal or reduced CMAP amplitudes
Antibody-drug conjugates (e.g., brentuximab vedotin, trastuzumab emtansine)	The chemotherapy payload in these drugs acts as either a tubulin binder or has antimitotic properties	Symmetric, length-dependent sensory predominant PN. Numbness may also affect hands early with brentuximab vedotin	Not described	Axonal PN, with sensory fibers affected more than motor fibers
Immune checkpoint inhibitors (PD-1 inhibitors, PD-L1 inhibitors, and CTLA-4 inhibitors)	By removing inhibitory signals against T cells, the immune system is upregulated and off-target autoimmunity can occur	An extremely diverse array of clinical phenotypes has been described. Acute to subacute polyradiculoneuropathy is the most common of these	Infiltration of nerve, nerve root, or dorsal root ganglia with T cells	Diverse findings depending on the clinical phenotype, with both demyelinating and axonal S-M PN patterns described

S-M, sensorimotor; PN, polyneuropathy; EMG, electromyography; NCS, nerve conduction study; QST, quantitative sensory testing; GBS, Guillain–Barré syndrome; CMAP, compound muscle action potential; SNAP, sensory nerve action potential.

Modified with permission from Amato AA, Collins MP. Neuropathies associated with malignancy. *Semin Neurol.* 1998;18(1):125–144.

patients continue to worsen the first month after discontinuation of vincristine.[198] The median duration of symptoms after stopping the medication is around 3 months.[198] Vincristine should be avoided in patients with Charcot–Marie–Tooth hereditary neuropathy, as it has been associated with the development of severe, disabling neuropathy even in those who were asymptomatic before treatment.[201]

Vinorelbine is a semisynthetic vinca alkaloid that causes a dose-related peripheral neuropathy in 20%–50% of patients.[202–204] It is less neurotoxic than vincristine, and the associated neuropathy is severe in only 1% of cases. Patients present with distal sensory loss and paresthesia, and motor weakness can occur after 3–6 months of treatment. After 12 cycles of vinorelbine, most patients have reduced or absent muscle stretch reflexes at the ankles.[204] As with vincristine, symptoms and signs of autonomic neuropathy may develop but are less common.

Laboratory Features

Sensory and motor NCSs reveal diminished amplitudes or absent responses with normal or only mildly prolonged distal latencies and slow conduction velocities.[198,205] The SNAP and CMAP amplitudes improve usually following discontinuation, but do not usually return to pretreatment levels. Active denervation in the form of fibrillation potentials and positive sharp waves may be seen on EMG in distal muscles.

Histopathology

Nerve biopsies demonstrate axonal degeneration and loss of myelinated and unmyelinated nerve fibers and clusters of regenerating axonal sprouts.

Pathogenesis

Vinca alkaloids inhibit microtubule formation by binding to tubulin. This, in turn, impairs axoplasmic transport and leads to cytoskeletal disarray and axonal degeneration.[206]

ETOPOSIDE

Etoposide is a semisynthetic derivative of podophyllotoxin, which causes a moderate-to-severe predominantly sensory axonal neuropathy or ganglionopathy in 4%–10% of patients.[207] Severe autonomic neuropathy can develop, leading to orthostatic hypotension and gastroparesis. The neuropathy gradually improves over several weeks or months following discontinuation.

In mice, etoposide causes degeneration of the cell bodies within the dorsal root ganglion.[207] However, histopathology has not been well described in humans with the neuropathy. Etoposide inhibits microtubule function, and the pathogenic basis of the neuropathy is probably similar to vincristine and vinorelbine.

TAXANES

Clinical Features

Paclitaxel (Taxol) is used as adjuvant treatment of breast cancer and has been associated with a dose-dependent, predominantly sensory neuropathy.[208–217] A subclinical or mild neuropathy develops in up to 85% of patients after three to seven cycles of taxol at doses of 135–200 mg/m^2. A severe neuropathy occurs in 2% of patients at this lower dose range. As many as 70% of patients have a severe neuropathy after high-dose paclitaxel with cumulative doses above 1,500 mg/m^2.[210,211] Paclitaxel can also be associated with an acute pain syndrome, with aching pain in the extremities occurring within 24 hours of infusion.[218] Preexisting neuropathy and prior or concurrent exposure to neurotoxic agents are additional risk factors for developing a severe neuropathy.[211]

Docetaxel (Taxotere), a semisynthetic analogue of taxol, is also associated with a dose-dependent, predominantly sensory neuropathy. Neuropathies are less frequent and less severe than those seen with Taxol.[219–223] Patients describe pain in the hands and feet and also may have a Lhermitte sign. On examination, large fiber sensory modalities are preferentially affected and most patients have reduced or absent muscle stretch reflexes at the ankles. Mild proximal and distal weakness is evident in 5%–19% of patients. Most patients improve 1–2 months after cessation of the chemotherapy; however, neuropathic symptoms can continue to worsen for several months after discontinuation of the docetaxel.

Laboratory Features

Sensory and motor NCSs demonstrate reduced SNAP and CMAP amplitudes, which correlate with the cumulative dose of taxol.[208–217,219–225] Distal latencies and conduction velocities are usually normal, although demyelinating features have been described.[209,213] NCS abnormalities may predate the occurrence of neuropathic symptoms.[217] Quantitative sensory testing reveals impairment of vibratory perception more often than abnormal thermal thresholds.[208,214] Needle EMG may reveal fibrillation potentials in distal limb muscles.[209,212]

Histopathology

Sural nerve biopsies reveal a preferential loss of large myelinated nerve fibers along with axonal degeneration with secondary demyelination and remyelination.[212,213] Regenerating axonal sprouts are uncommon. On EM, one may find accumulation of tubular and membranous structures within the axons.[212,224]

Pathogenesis

Taxol may have a toxic effect on the neuronal cell body, the axon, or both. In contrast to the vinca alkaloids, which disassemble microtubules, the taxanes (taxol and taxotere) promote microtubule assembly by increasing tubulin polymerization. The subsequent aggregation and accumulation of abnormal bundles of microtubules in dorsal root ganglia, axons, and Schwann cells impair axoplasmic transport.[224]

IXABEPILONE

Ixabepilone acts as a microtubule stabilizer, similar to taxanes, and is used in the treatment of refractory breast cancer. Like taxanes, it can also cause a dose-dependent sensorimotor polyneuropathy.[226] Preexisting peripheral neuropathy and prior chemotherapy exposure are added risk factors. The resulting neuropathy seems to be reversible, as many patients report resolution of symptoms after treatment. Dose reduction alone can be quite effective at reversing symptoms during ongoing treatment.

ERIBULIN

Eribulin is also used in the treatment of refractory breast cancer, as well as for liposarcomas. It too is a microtubular inhibitor, but with a mechanism of action distinct from the vinca alkaloids etc. Sensorimotor polyneuropathy is similarly a common adverse effect. The incidence of neuropathy has been shown to be similar to ixabepilone, but fewer patients required treatment discontinuation and the onset of neuropathy with eribulin tends to occur later in treatment than with ixabepilone.[227]

SURAMIN

Clinical Features

Suramin is a hexasulfonated naphthylurea that causes a peripheral neuropathy in 25%–90% treated patients.[225,228,229] Neurotoxicity is the dose-limiting side effect, and there appears to be two distinct types of toxic neuropathy: (1) a dose-dependent, distal, axonal sensorimotor polyneuropathy and (2) a subacute demyelinating polyradiculoneuropathy.

The distal axonopathy is more common and manifests with distal numbness and paresthesias.[225,229] Examination reveals reduced light touch, pain, and vibratory perception; mild weakness of the distal limbs (e.g., toe extensors); and diminished ankle reflexes. This neuropathy is reversible upon suramin discontinuation.

A subacute sensorimotor demyelinating polyradiculoneuropathy is more severe and develops in 10%–20% of patients after 1–5 months of treatment.[225,228,229] It is associated with peak plasma concentrations of over 300 µg/L, exposure to greater than 200 µg/L for more than 25 days per month, or cumulative dose of 40,000 mg/L. Patients present with numbness and paresthesias of the distal limbs or face, followed by symmetric, proximal greater than distal weakness. Muscle stretch reflexes are decreased or absent throughout.

The weakness is insidiously progressive and can involve the respiratory muscles. Up to 25% of affected patients become bedridden and require mechanical ventilation. The neuropathy can continue to progress for 1 month following suramin discontinuation. It can take several months for patients to recover, and there frequently are residual numbness and weakness. Plasma exchange has been tried in an uncontrolled fashion with mixed results.

Laboratory Features

CSF protein may be elevated in patients with subacute demyelinating polyradiculoneuropathy.[225,229] NCSs in the more common distal sensorimotor polyneuropathy reveal decreased amplitudes of SNAPs and CMAPs with relatively preserved distal latencies and conduction velocities.[225,229] Abnormal vibratory and cooling thresholds are seen with quantitative sensory testing.[225] Needle EMG may reveal fibrillation potentials and neurogenic MUAPs in distal muscles.

Electrodiagnostic studies in the subacute sensorimotor polyradiculoneuropathy reveal features of demyelination: prolonged distal latencies and F-waves, slow conduction velocities, temporal dispersion, and conduction block.[225,228,229] As in the distal axonopathy, quantitative sensory testing shows increased vibratory and cooling thresholds.[225] EMG demonstrates decreased recruitment of MUAPs in proximal and distal muscles and occasional fibrillation potentials.

Histopathology

Sural nerve biopsies in patients with the subacute demyelinating polyradiculoneuropathy demonstrate loss of large and small myelinated nerve fibers, demyelination and remyelination, and secondary axonal degeneration.[225,228,229] Epi- and endoneurial mononuclear inflammatory infiltrates may be seen. In animal models, suramin induces a length-, dose-, and time-dependent axonal sensorimotor polyneuropathy associated with axonal degeneration, atrophy, and accumulation of glycolipid lysosomal inclusions.[230]

Pathogenesis

The mechanism of neurotoxicity is unknown. Suramin may inhibit the interaction of neurotrophic factors with its peripheral nerve receptors[231] or induce a form of lysosomal storage disease. The demyelinating neuropathy may be immune mediated, related to the immunomodulating effects of suramin.[232]

CYTOSINE ARABINOSIDE

Clinical Features

Cytosine arabinoside (ARA-C) is an antimetabolite used in the treatment of leukemia and lymphoma. Sensory neuropathy and severe sensorimotor polyneuropathy resembling

GBS[233–238] have been reported with cumulative doses ranging from 60 mg/m^2 to 36 g/m^2. These neuropathies can begin within hours or weeks following treatment.

Laboratory Features

Patients with a GBS-like neuropathy have increased CSF protein.[236] EMG and NCS can be compatible with a primary axonal[237] or an acquired demyelinating sensorimotor polyneuropathy.[234]

Histopathology

Sural nerve biopsies may reveal demyelination or axonal degeneration.[233,236,237]

Pathogenesis

The pathophysiologic mechanism(s) for the neuropathies are not known. The antimetabolite action of ARA-C may inhibit proteins necessary for myelin production, axonal structure, or axonal transport. Alternatively, the immunomodulating effects of ARA-C may predispose patients to an immune attack against the peripheral nerves.

IFOSFAMIDE

Ifosfamide, a cyclophosphamide analog, has been associated with polyneuropathy with total doses of 14 g/m^2 or more.[239] Patients manifest numbness, and painful paresthesias that begin in the hands and feet 10–14 days after treatment and gradually resolve but recur if they are rechallenged with the chemotherapy. Electrodiagnostic and histopathologic data are lacking, but the occasional onset beginning in the hands rather than the feet is suggestive of a ganglionopathy.

PROTEOSOME INHIBITORS

Clinical Features

Bortezomib (Velcade), a selective, reversible inhibitor of the proteasome, has been instrumental for the treatment of multiple myeloma.[240] Treatment-emergent neuropathy or symptomatic worsening of a preexistent neuropathy developed in a third to two-thirds of myeloma patients in treatment trials.[233,240–244] The risk of neuropathy correlates with the cumulative dose of bortezomib. Less frequent administration or subcutaneous administration rather than the traditional intravenous route has been shown to lower the incidence of neuropathy.[245] Patients usually complain of paresthesia, pain, and numbness in a length-dependent distribution. The neuropathy usually improves when the dose is reduced or drug is discontinued.[232,234]

Second-generation proteosome inhibitors—carfilzomib and ixazomib—have since been developed and are associated with a lower risk of neuropathy compared with bortezomib.[246] Many of the patients enrolled in clinical trials for these agents had preexisting neuropathy and had to stop prior chemotherapy medications due to neuropathy. Despite this, dose modifications or discontinuations for neuropathy were rare. The pooled rate of reported peripheral neuropathy in four phase II carfilzomib trials was 13.9%.[247] In the initial phase III trial for ixazomib, the rate of peripheral neuropathy for lenalidomide/dexamethasone alone was 22% compared with a rate of 27% for lenalidomide/dexamethasone/ixazomib.[248]

Laboratory Features

NCS may demonstrate a reduction or loss of amplitudes of SNAPs in a length-dependent pattern.[241,244] Motor studies are usually spared and EMG is typically normal. Autonomic studies, in particular, quantitative sweat testing may be abnormal. The absence of electrophysiologic changes in some patients with symptoms of burning and dysesthesias in their feet suggests involvement of small-diameter nerve fibers (i.e., a small fiber neuropathy) as well.

Histopathology

Skin biopsies have shown a reduction in intraepidermal nerve fiber density.[244,249] Nerve biopsies of patients with the characteristic toxic neuropathy have not been reported. However, in Wistar rats, pathologic examination reported shows a dose-dependent axonopathy of the unmyelinated fibers in nerves of treated animals.[250] In mice, histopathologic findings have demonstrated a mild reduction of myelinated and unmyelinated fibers, mostly involving large and C fibers, with abnormal vesicular inclusion bodies in unmyelinated axons.[251] In addition, degeneration of dorsal root ganglia has been observed in mice treated with bortezomib.[252]

Pathogenesis

The pathophysiologic mechanism is not known. Bortezomib may block the ubiquitin–proteasome pathway, possibly causing a "toxic" buildup of proteins that should be degraded by the proteasome, resulting in impairment of neuronal function, initially in the dorsal root ganglia, and then leading to a retrograde (or "dying-back") axonopathy of small nerve fibers followed by larger nerve fibers.

THALIDOMIDE AND ANALOGS

Clinical Features

Thalidomide is an immunomodulating agent used to treat multiple myeloma, GVHD, leprosy, and other autoimmune disorders. Thalidomide is associated with severe teratogenic effects as well as peripheral neuropathy, which can be dose limiting.[253–257] The neuropathy is dose dependent, with patients who develop the neuropathy typically having received a cumulative dose of at least 20 g of thalidomide. Patients complain of numbness, painful tingling, burning discomfort in the feet and hands, and less commonly, muscle weakness and atrophy. Even after stopping the drug for 4–6 years, as many as 50% of patients continue to have significant symptoms. Physical examination demonstrates a reduction in vibration and position sense, hypo- or areflexia, and occasionally proximal and distal weakness.

Lenalidomide and pomalidomide are newer analogs of thalidomide and both are also associated with a sensory-predominant axonal neuropathy. The severity and rate of neuropathy with these agents thus far appears lower than with thalidomide.[258–260] Interestingly, the development of neuropathy with lenalidomide has not been shown to be dose dependent.[260]

Laboratory Features

NCSs demonstrate reduced amplitudes or complete absence of the SNAPs with preserved conduction velocities when obtainable. Motor NCSs are usually normal.

Histopathology

Nerve biopsies reveal a loss of large-diameter myelinated fibers and axonal degeneration. Degeneration of dorsal root ganglion cells has been appreciated on autopsies.

Pathogenesis

The pathogenic basis of the neuropathy is not known.

ANTIBODY-DRUG CONJUGATES

Antibody-drug conjugates deliver a potent chemotherapeutic agent directly to cancer cells by linking them to a monoclonal antibody that targets a relevant antigen on the cancer cells. This mechanism allows for delivery of a chemotherapy payload that would otherwise be too neurotoxic to be given systemically. Brentuximab vedotin is a commonly used example, combining a humanized IgG monoclonal antibody directed against CD30 with an antimitotic agent [monomethylauristatin E (MMAE)]. Brentuximab is used in the treatment of hematologic malignancies including anaplastic large-cell lymphomas, T-cell lymphomas, and Hodgkin lymphoma.

Brentuximab has been shown to cause a dose-related, sensory-predominant axonal peripheral neuropathy.[261] In clinical trials utilizing brentuximab, 30%–69% of patients developed neuropathy.[262,263] However, treated patients often had relapsed disease or a prior hematologic stem cell transplant, so they may have already received prior neurotoxic chemotherapies. Symptoms are frequently mild, however, with distal numbness being the most frequent symptom and weakness being uncommon. Vibratory sensation loss is the most frequent abnormality on physical examination. Some patients will have numbness in both the hands and the feet. NCSs typically show axonal neuropathy, with sensory responses affected more than motor responses. The majority of affected patients will improve after treatment stops; in one phase II trial, 67% of affected patients had complete resolution of symptoms.[264]

Additional agents using MMAE as their payload have been developed more recently and may be similarly associated with neuropathy. Tisotumab vedotin is used for cervical cancer and binds to tissue factor.[265] Polatuzumab vedotin is used for the treatment of relapsed/refractory diffuse large B cell lymphoma (DLBCL) and binds to CD79b.[266] Enfortumab vedotin is used for urothelial cancer and binds to nectin-4.[267]

Other payloads have been developed over time. For example, mirvetuximab soravtansine combines a folate receptor alpha binding antibody with maytansinoid DM4—a tubulin-binder. This was recently approved for treatment of platinum-resistant ovarian cancer; 26.7% of patients in the phase III trial developed peripheral neuropathy, typically mild.[268] Trastuzumab emtansine is a conjugate of a monoclonal antibody against HER2 and the cytotoxic agent DM1, which binds tubulin. It is accordingly used in the treatment of HER2-positive breast and gastrointestinal cancers. A sensory-predominant neuropathy has developed in some treated patients.[269] In the treatment of breast cancer, the risk of all-grade neuropathy is lower with trastuzumab compared with taxane-based regimens—between 4% and 18.6% in phase II trials.[270] Notably, many regimens actually combine trastuzumab and paclitaxel.[271]

IMMUNE CHECKPOINT INHIBITORS

Clinical Features

Immune checkpoint inhibitors (ICIs) are a novel class of medications that target mechanisms used by cancer to evade destruction by the immune system. Three major classes have reached clinical practice: anti-cytotoxic T-lymphocyte-associated antigen-4 (anti-CTLA4: ipilimumab and tremelimumab), anti-programmed cell death-1 receptor (anti-PD1: nivolumab, pembrolizumab, cemiplimab, dostarlimab), and anti-programmed death-ligand 1 (anti-PDL1: atezolizumab, avelumab, durvalumab). These medications exert their antineoplastic effect by removing inhibitory signals against T cells, allowing a more robust response against cancer cells. This effect is not antigen specific, however, and can therefore lead to off-target immune-related adverse events (irAEs) throughout the body, including the nervous system. In one review including 9,208 ICI-treated patients, the overall incidence of neurologic irAEs was 3.8% in patients receiving anti–CTLA-4 antibodies, 6.1% in patients receiving anti–PD-1 antibodies, and 12.0% in patients receiving both.[272] A wide spectrum of both CNS and PNS disorders have been described as irAEs, but to date, neuromuscular complications have been reported more frequently than CNS disorders.[273] Myositis, sometimes in combination with myocarditis and/or myasthenia gravis, is one of the more frequent neurologic irAEs and is covered in Chapter 35.

In one meta-analysis, the incidence of peripheral neuropathy following PD-1 or PD-L1 inhibitor treatment was 1.2%, of which 0.3% was severe.[274] Importantly, this compared quite favorably to the incidence of peripheral neuropathy following traditional chemotherapeutic agents (8.6%, of which 1.1% were severe). The clinical phenotype of neuropathy seen in association with ICIs, however, is more diverse and overall quite different than what is typically seen with traditional chemotherapy. The most commonly observed phenotype is an acute or subacute non–length-dependent polyradiculoneuropathy.[273,275-277] Many of these cases clinically mimic forms of GBS; individual cases in the literature have been labeled as AIDP, AMSAN, and even Miller Fisher syndrome. Cranial nerve involvement including bulbar weakness can occur. Weakness in some patients can be very severe and include respiratory muscle weakness. Significant dysautonomia has also been reported in some cases. Accordingly, the mortality of GBS-like cases was 11% in one review.[273]

The spectrum is even broader as more slowly progressive varieties more closely mimicking CIDP have also been reported. Moreover, some patients have more asymmetric or focal weakness and sensory loss than would be expected with typical GBS or CIDP; thus some cases of ICI-related neuropathy in the literature have been best labeled as plexopathy, radiculoplexopathy, or polyradiculitis. Isolated cranial neuropathies without limb weakness are relatively frequent, with the facial nerve being most commonly affected. Finally, rare cases of small fiber neuropathy, autonomic neuropathy, enteric neuropathy, phrenic neuropathy, and vasculitis leading to a mononeuropathy multiplex pattern have all been described. Despite this broad constellation, there are some laboratory and imaging features that may help unify these conditions and aid in diagnosis (see below).

There is also a frequent overlap between ICI-related neuropathy and other irAEs. In one case series of 28 patients, 5 patients (18%) had a concurrent CNS syndrome (e.g., encephalitis) and 19 patients (68%) had a concurrent nonneurologic irAE (e.g., enterocolitis, pneumonitis, myocarditis, thyroiditis, or vitiligo).[276] The median onset of neuropathy symptoms is after 3 or 4 cycles of treatment in the reported cases, but a wide range has been reported (1–104 weeks after treatment initiation).[276-278]

Laboratory Findings

CSF analysis is often prudent, since an important alternative diagnostic consideration is radiculitis from leptomeningeal spread of the cancer. The CSF is frequently abnormal in patients with ICI-related neuropathy, an estimated 89% of patients.[273] Fifty-five percent to 84% of patients will have an elevated CSF protein. In contrast to typical GBS, 39%–63% will also have a lymphocytic pleocytosis (typically 10–20 cells/μL, range 0–130 cells/μL).[273,277] Approximately 50% of patients will have abnormal leptomeningeal enhancement on MRI of the brain and/or spinal cord. Enhancement of spinal nerve roots is the most common abnormality seen (24%) whereas 10% of patients have cranial nerve enhancement.

A range of abnormalities have been reported on electrodiagnostic studies, even within a specific clinical phenotype. For example, both demyelinating and axonal forms of acute polyradiculoneuropathy have been reported. In a case series of 14 patients with diverse clinical phenotypes from a single institution, 21% had features of demyelination on NCS and 50% had features of motor and sensory axon loss.[277] In the larger literature review, among 94 cases with NCS/EMG data reported 46% had a demyelinating pattern and 34% had an axonal pattern.[273]

Histopathology

Nerve biopsy is typically not necessary if the time course, electrodiagnostic findings, and CSF analysis are typical. In cases reported in the literature, however, infiltration of T lymphocytes in nerves, nerve roots, or the dorsal root ganglion has been demonstrated.[273,275-277] Epineurial perivascular inflammatory collections of T cells have also been seen (see Fig. 19-9).

Pathogenesis

Regulatory T cells are essential for maintaining the immune system's tolerance of self—these are direct targets of ICIs. While it is understandable that autoimmunity is more likely in treated patients, why a *specific* clinical syndrome arises in a given patient is less clear. One plausible mechanism is that there may be cross-reactivity between antigens expressed on tumor cells and similar epitopes on normal human cells. Melanocytes and peripheral nerve myelin, for example, share protein epitopes and CIDP has been described in melanoma patients even outside the context of ICI treatment.[279] Another possibility is that the immune-mediated destruction of tissue around the tumor may also release nontumor antigens and spur on a secondary autoimmune response.[280] Finally, some patients may have had an autoimmune or paraneoplastic process that was subclinical or mild prior to the ICI therapy and then unleashed by the increased immune system activity.[281] Testing pretreatment serum that had been banked from patients in clinical trials has demonstrated that some affected patients indeed had detectable autoantibodies and such patients were at higher risk of developing irAEs. This may be particularly relevant in patients who develop sensory ganglionopathy, for example.

Management

In acute cases akin to GBS, the first step is to stop the checkpoint inhibitor immediately.[282] Since severe generalized

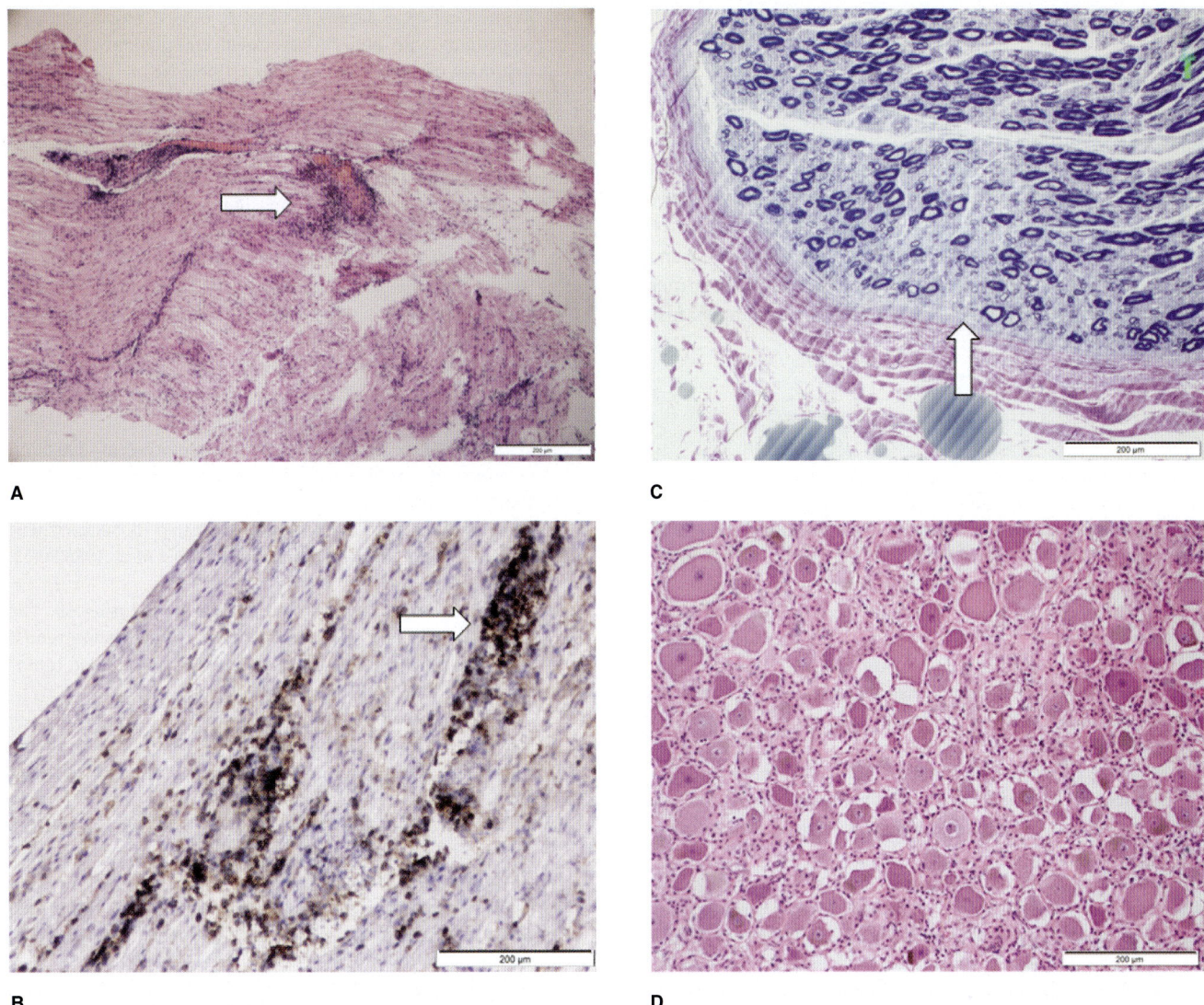

Figure 19-9. Pathologic findings in immune checkpoint inhibitor-associated neuropathy. In a patient with an acquired demyelinating polyradiculoneuropathy: (**A**, **B**), hematoxylin and eosin–stained sections of dorsal T12 nerve root demonstrate severe lymphocytic inflammation (**A**, *arrow*) composed of CD3-positive T lymphocytes (**B**, *arrow*). In a patient with non–length-dependent sensory and motor polyneuropathy with axonal features on NCS/EMG: (**C**, **D**), plastic sections of peripheral show patchy loss of large myelinated fibers (*arrow*, **C**) and hematoxylin and eosin–stained sections of (**D**) dorsal root ganglion demonstrate inflammatory infiltrate surrounding ganglion cells consistent with sensory ganglionitis. (Reproduced with permission from Dubey D, David WS, Amato AA, et al. Varied phenotypes and management of immune checkpoint inhibitor-associated neuropathies. *Neurology.* 2019;93(11):e1093–e1103. Figure 3, p. e1097.)

weakness and respiratory weakness have been described, hospital admission for observation is reasonable. IVIg is typically used, similar to idiopathic GBS. Unlikely idiopathic GBS, however, a trial of corticosteroids alongside IVIg is also reasonable. In general, corticosteroids are a mainstay of treatment of irAEs. Among 69 patients with a GBS-like acute neuropathy treated with corticosteroids either alone or with another treatment (usually IVIg or plasma exchange), 59 (86%) improved.[273] Recommended dosing strategies have included either a pulse of methylprednisolone 1 g daily for 5 days or methylprednisolone PO 2–4 mg/kg/day; in either case, this is followed by an oral taper over 4–6 weeks.[282] In more subacute to chronic cases, the severity of the neuropathy will guide treatment decisions. In mild cases, it may be reasonable to simply hold the checkpoint inhibitor and monitor closely. Overall, a partial or full recovery has been described in a majority of patients (77%).

Development of an irAE of any kind may complicate ongoing treatment of the cancer. It can be reasonable to retrial a different class of ICI in patients with a prior irAE, especially if it was a milder case. Very close monitoring and careful patient counseling are clearly warranted. Fifteen out of 94 patients (16%) retrialed on another ICI had a relapse of symptoms in one reported review.[273]

SUMMARY

Neuropathy is not an uncommon complication in a cancer patient. Although a paraneoplastic etiology is often considered, most neuropathies in the setting of cancer are not the result of a remote, immune-mediated effect of cancer. The neuropathy is more commonly due to a direct, adverse side effect of chemotherapeutic agents (toxic neuropathy), or as a consequence of nutritional deficiency. In some cases, it may be due to compression or infiltration of the tumor. Treatment and prognosis are dependent on the etiology and mechanism of the neuropathy.

REFERENCES

1. Briemberg HR, Amato AA. Neuromuscular complications of cancer. *Neurol Clin.* 2003;21(1):141–165.
2. Amato AA, Collins MP. Neuropathies associated with malignancy. *Semin Neurol.* 1998;18(01):125–144.
3. Campbell MJ, Paty DW. Carcinomatous neuromyopathy: 1. Electrophysiological studies: an electrophysiological and immunological study of patients with carcinoma of the lung. *J Neurol Neurosurg Psychiatry.* 1974;37(2):131–141.
4. Denny-Brown D. Primary sensory neuropathy with muscular changes associated with carcinoma. *J Neurol Neurosurg Psychiatry.* 1948;11(2):73–87.
5. Dalmau J, Graus F, Rosenblum M K, Posner JB. Anti-Hu-associated paraneoplastic encephalomyelitis/sensory neuronopathy a clinical study of 71 patients. *Medicine (Baltimore).* 1992;71(2):59–72.
6. Lucchinetti CF, Kimmel DW, Lennon VA. Paraneoplastic and oncologic profiles of patients seropositive for type 1 antineuronal nuclear autoantibodies. *Neurology.* 1998;50(3):652–657.
7. Molinuevo JL, Graus F, Serrano C, Reñe R, Guerrero A, Illa I. Utility of anti-Hu antibodies in the diagnosis of paraneoplastic sensory neuropathy. *Ann Neurol.* 1998;44(6):976–980.
8. Graus F, Elkon KB, Lloberes P, et al. Neuronal antinuclear antibody (anti-Hu) in paraneoplastic encephalomyelitis simulating acute polyneuritis. *Acta Neurol Scand.* 1987;75(4):249–252.
9. Wanschitz J, Hainfellner JA, Kristoferitsch W, Drlicek M, Budka H. Ganglionitis in paraneoplastic subacute sensory neuronopathy: a morphologic study. *Neurology.* 1997;49(4):1156–1159.
10. Jean WC, Dalmau J, Ho A, Posner JB. Analysis of the IgG subclass distribution and inflammatory infiltrates in patients with anti-Hu-associated paraneoplastic encephalomyelitis. *Neurology.* 1994;44(1):140–147.
11. Rosenblum MK. Paraneoplasia and autoimmunologic injury of the nervous system: the anti-Hu syndrome. *Brain Pathology.* 1993;3(3):199–212.
12. Benyahia B, Liblau R, Merle-Beral H, Tourani JM, Dalmau J, Delattre JY. Cell-mediated autoimmunity in paraneoplastic neurological syndromes with anti-Hu antibodies. *Ann Neurol.* 1999;45(2):162–167.
13. Voltz R, Dalmau J, Posner JB, Rosenfeld MR. T-cell receptor analysis in anti-Hu associated paraneoplastic encephalomyelitis. *Neurology.* 1998;51(4):1146–1150.
14. Keime-Guibert F, Graus F, Broet P, et al. Clinical outcome of patients with anti-Hu-associated encephalomyelitis after treatment of the tumor. *Neurology.* 1999;53(8):1719–1723.
15. Graus F, Vega F, Delattre JY, et al. Plasmapheresis and antineoplastic treatment in CNS paraneoplastic syndromes with antineuronal autoantibodies. *Neurology.* 1992;42(3):536–536.
16. Antoine JC, Mosnier JF, Honnorat J, et al. Paraneoplastic demyelinating neuropathy, subacute sensory neuropathy, and anti-hu antibodies: clinicopathological study of an autopsy case. *Muscle Nerve.* 1998;21(7):850–857.
17. Sancho Saldaña A, Mahdi-Rogers M, Hadden RD. Sensory neuronopathies: a case series and literature review. *J Peripher Nerv Syst.* 2021;26(1):66–74.
18. Graus F, Keime-Guibert F, Rene R, et al. Anti-Hu-associated paraneoplastic encephalomyelitis: analysis of 200 patients. *Brain.* 2001;124(6):1138–1148.
19. Wilkinson PC, Zeromski J. Immunofluorescent detection of antibodies in sensory carcinomatous neuropathy. *Brain.* 1965;88(3):529–538.
20. Graus F, Elkon KB, Cordon-Cardo C, Posner JB. Sensory neuronopathy and small cell lung cancer. *Am J Med.* 1986;80(1):45–52.
21. Dalmau J, Furneaux HM, Cordon-Cardo C, Posner JB. The expression of the Hu (paraneoplastic encephalomyelitis/sensory neuronopathy) antigen in human normal and tumor tissues. *Am J Pathol.* 1992;141(4):881–886.
22. Dalmau J, Furneaux HM, Gralla RJ, Kris MG, Posner JB. Detection of the anti-Hu antibody in the serum of patients with small cell lung cancer? A quantitative western blot analysis. *Ann Neurol.* 1990;27(5):544–552.
23. Dubey D, Lennon VA, Gadoth A, et al. Autoimmune CRMP5 neuropathy phenotype and outcome defined from 105 cases. *Neurology.* 2018;90(2):e103–e110.
24. Dubey D, Jitprapaikulsan J, Bi H, et al. Amphiphysin-IgG autoimmune neuropathy: a recognizable clinicopathologic syndrome. *Neurology.* 2019;93(20):E1873–E1880.
25. Totland C, Haugen M, Vedeler C. CRMP5 Antibodies—Diagnostic Challenges. *Front Neurol.* 2021;12:729075.
26. Birnbaum J, Lalji A, Piccione EA, Izbudak I. Magnetic resonance imaging of the spinal cord in the evaluation of 3 patients with sensory neuronopathies: Diagnostic assessment, indications of treatment response, and impact of autoimmunity: A case report. *Medicine (Baltimore).* 2017;96(49):e8483.
27. Amato AA, Sanelli PC, Anderson MP. Case records of the Massachusetts General Hospital. Weekly clinicopathological exercises. Case 38-2001. A 51-year-old woman with lung cancer and neuropsychiatric abnormalities. *N Engl J Med.* 2001;345(24):1758–1765.
28. Vega F, Graus F, Chen QM, Poisson M, Schuller E, Delattre JY. Intrathecal synthesis of the anti-Hu antibody in patients with paraneoplastic encephalomyelitis or sensory neuronopathy: clinical-immunologic correlation. *Neurology.* 1994;44(11):2145–2147.
29. Dalmau J, Furneaux HM, Rosenblum MK, Graus F, Posner JB. Detection of the anti-Hu antibody in specific regions of the nervous system and tumor from patients with paraneoplastic encephalomyelitis/sensory neuronopathy. *Neurology.* 1991;41(11):1757–1764.
30. Auger RG. Role of the masseter reflex in the assessment of subacute sensory neuropathy. *Muscle Nerve.* 1998;21(6):800–801.

31. Auger RG, Windebank AJ, Lucchinetti CF, Chalk CH. Role of the blink reflex in the evaluation of sensory neuronopathy. *Neurology.* 1999;53(2):407–408.
32. Lennon VA, Sas DF, Busk MF, et al. Enteric neuronal autoantibodies in pseudoobstruction with small-cell lung carcinoma. *Gastroenterology.* 1991;100(1):137–142.
33. Altermatt HJ, Rodriguez M, Scheithauer BW, Lennon VA. Paraneoplastic anti-Purkinje and type I anti-neuronal nuclear autoantibodies bind selectively to central, peripheral, and autonomic nervous system cells. *Lab Invest.* 1991;65(4):412–420.
34. Sillevis Smith P, Manley GT, Posner JB. Immunization with the paraneoplastic encephalomyelitis antigen HuD does not cause neurologic disease in mice. *Neurology.* 1995;45(10):1873–1878.
35. Panegyrest PK, Reading MC, Esiri MM. The inflammatory reaction of paraneoplastic ganglionitis and encephalitis: an immunohistochemical study. *J Neurol.* 1993;240(2):93–97.
36. Antoine JC, Camdessanché JP. Treatment options in paraneoplastic disorders of the peripheral nervous system. *Curr Treat Options Neurol.* 2013;15(2):210–223.
37. Antoine JC, Robert-Varvat F, Maisonobe T, et al. Identifying a therapeutic window in acute and subacute inflammatory sensory neuronopathies. *J Neurol Sci.* 2016;361:187–191.
38. Yu Z, Kryzer TJ, Griesmann GE, Kim K, Benarroch EE, Lennon VA. CRMP-5 neuronal autoantibody: marker of lung cancer and thymoma-related autoimmunity. *Ann Neurol.* 2001;49(2):146–154.
39. Honnorat J, Cartalat-Carel S, Ricard D, et al. Onco-neural antibodies and tumour type determine survival and neurological symptoms in paraneoplastic neurological syndromes with Hu or CV2/CRMP5 antibodies. *J Neurol Neurosurg Psychiatry.* 2009;80(4):412–416.
40. Shah S, Vazquez Do Campo R, Kumar N, et al. Paraneoplastic myeloneuropathies: clinical, oncologic, and serologic accompaniments. *Neurology.* 2021;96(4):e632–e639.
41. Amato AA, Barohn RJ, Sahenk Z, Tutschka PJ, Mendell JR. Polyneuropathy complicating bone marrow and solid organ transplantation. *Neurology.* 1993;43(8):1513–1518.
42. Gabriel SE, Conn DL, Phyliky RL, Pittelkow MR, Scott RE. Vasculitis in hairy cell leukemia: review of literature and consideration of possible pathogenic mechanisms. *J Rheumatol.* 1986;13(6):1167–1172.
43. Hasler P, Kistler H, Gerber H. Vasculitides in hairy cell leukemia. *Semin Arthritis Rheum.* 1995;25(2):134–142.
44. Johnson PC, Rolak LA, Hamilton RH, Laguna JF. Paraneoplastic vasculitis of nerve: a remote effect of cancer. *Ann Neurol.* 1979;5(5):437–444.
45. Kurzrock R, Cohen PR, Markowitz A. Clinical manifestations of vasculitis in patients with solid tumors. A case report and review of the literature. *Arch Intern Med.* 1994;154(3):334–340.
46. Oh SJ, Slaughter R, Harrell L. Paraneoplastic vasculitic neuropathy: a treatable neuropathy. *Muscle Nerve.* 1991;14(2):152–156.
47. Bird SJ, Brown MJ, Shy ME, Scherer SS. Chronic inflammatory demyelinating polyneuropathy associated with malignant melanoma. *Neurology.* 1996;46(3):822–824.
48. Weiss MD, Luciano CA, Semino-Mora C, Dalakas MC, Quarles RH. Molecular mimicry in chronic inflammatory demyelinating polyneuropathy and melanoma. *Neurology.* 1998;51(6):1738–1741.
49. Levin KH, Lutz G. Angiotropic large-cell lymphoma with peripheral nerve and skeletal muscle involvement: early diagnosis and treatment. *Neurology.* 1996;47(4):1009–1011.
50. Grisold W, Piza-Katzer H, Jahn R, Herczeg E. Intraneural nerve metastasis with multiple mononeuropathies. *J Peripher Nerv Syst.* 2000;5(3):163–167.
51. Oei ME, Kraft GH, Sarnat HB. Intravascular lymphomatosis. *Muscle Nerve.* 2002;25(5):742–746.
52. Kelly JJ, Karcher DS. Lymphoma and peripheral neuropathy: a clinical review. *Muscle Nerve.* 2005;31(3):301–313.
53. Bobker DH, Deloughery TG. Natural killer cell leukemia presenting with a peripheral neuropathy. *Neurology.* 1993;43(9):1853–1854.
54. Borit A, Altrocchi PH. Recurrent polyneuropathy and neurolymphomatosis. *Arch Neurol.* 1971;24(1):40–49.
55. Krendel DA, Stahl RL, Chan WC. Lymphomatous polyneuropathy. Biopsy of clinically involved nerve and successful treatment. *Arch Neurol.* 1991;48(3):330–332.
56. Thomas FP, Vallejos U, Foitl DR, et al. B cell small lymphocytic lymphoma and chronic lymphocytic leukemia with peripheral neuropathy: two cases with neuropathological findings and lymphocyte marker analysis. *Acta Neuropathol.* 1990;80(2):198–203.
57. Aregawi DG, Sherman JH, Douvas MG, Burns TM, Schiff D. Neuroleukemiosis: case report of leukemic nerve infiltration in acute lymphoblastic leukemia. *Muscle Nerve.* 2008;38(3):1196–1200.
58. Créange A, Théodorou I, Sabourin JC, Vital C, Farcet JP, Gherardi RK. Inflammatory neuromuscular disorders associated with chronic lymphoid leukemia: evidence for clonal B cells within muscle and nerve. *J Neurol Sci.* 1996;137(1):35–41.
59. Krendel DA, Albright RE, Graham DG. Infiltrative polyneuropathy due to acute monoblastic leukemia in hematologic remission. *Neurology.* 1987;37(3):474–477.
60. Sumi SM, Farrell DF, Knauss TA. Lymphoma and leukemia manifested by steroid-responsive polyneuropathy. *Arch Neurol.* 1983;40(9):577–582.
61. Vital C, Bonnaud E, Arne L, Barrat M, Leblanc M. Polyneuritis in chronic lymphoid leukemia. Ultrastructural study of the peripheral nerve. *Acta Neuropathol.* 1975;32(2):169–172.
62. Cameron DG, Howell DA, Hutchison JL. Acute peripheral neuropathy in Hodgkin's disease: report of a fatal case with histologic features of allergic neuritis. *Neurology.* 1958;8(7):575–577.
63. Lisak RP, Mitchell M, Zweiman B, Orrechio E, Asbury AK. Guillain-Barré syndrome and Hodgkin's disease: three cases with immunological studies. *Ann Neurol.* 1977;1(1):72–78.
64. Flanagan EP, Sandroni P, Pittock Sean J, Inwards DJ, Jones LK. Paraneoplastic lower motor neuronopathy associated with Hodgkin lymphoma. *Muscle Nerve.* 2012;46(5):823–827.
65. Baehring JM, Batchelor TT. Diagnosis and management of neurolymphomatosis. *Cancer J.* 2012;18(5):463–468.
66. Grisariu S, Avni B, Batchelor TT, et al. Neurolymphomatosis: an International Primary CNS Lymphoma Collaborative Group report. *Blood.* 2010;115(24):5005–5011.
67. Kamiya-Matsuoka C, Shroff S, Gildersleeve K, Hormozdi B, Manning JT, Woodman KH. Neurolymphomatosis: a case series of clinical manifestations, treatments, and outcomes. *J Neurol Sci.* 2014;343(1–2):144–148.
68. Keddie S, Nagendran A, Cox T, et al. Peripheral nerve neurolymphomatosis: clinical features, treatment, and outcomes. *Muscle Nerve.* 2020;62(5):617–625.

69. Tomita M, Koike H, Kawagashira Y, et al. Clinicopathological features of neuropathy associated with lymphoma. *Brain*. 2013;136(8):2563-2578.
70. Vital C, Heraud A, Vital A, Coquet M, Julien M, Maupetit J. Acute mononeuropathy with angiotropic lymphoma. *Acta Neuropathol*. 1989;78(1):105-107.
71. Dubas F, Saint-Andre JP, Pouplard-Barthelaix A, Delestre F, Emile J. Intravascular malignant lymphomatosis (so-called malignant angioendotheliomatosis): a case confined to the lumbosacral spinal cord and nerve roots. *Clin Neuropathol*. 1990;9(3):115-120.
72. Glass J, Hochberg FH, Miller DC. Intravascular lymphomatosis a systemic disease with neurologic manifestations. *Cancer*. 1993;71(10):3156-3164.
73. Wilson WH, Kingma DW, Raffeld M, Wittes RE, Jaffe ES. Association of lymphomatoid granulomatosis with Epstein-Barr viral infection of B lymphocytes and response to interferon-alpha 2b. *Blood*. 1996;87(11):4531-4537.
74. Calatayud T, Vallejo AR, Dominguez L, Sotelo T, Peña P, Jimenez M. Lymphomatoid granulomatosis manifesting as a subacute polyradiculoneuropathy. *Eur Neurol*. 1980;19(4):213-223.
75. Katzenstein ALA, Carrington CB, Liebow AA. Lymphomatoid granulomatosis. A clinicopathologic study of 152 cases. *Cancer*. 1979;43(1):360-373.
76. Liebow AA, Carrington CR, Friedman PJ. Lymphomatoid granulomatosis. *Hum Pathol*. 1972;3(4):457-558.
77. Kasamon YL, Nguyen TN, Chan JA, Nascimento AF. EBV-associated lymphoma and chronic inflammatory demyelinating polyneuropathy in an adult without overt immunodeficiency. *Am J Hematol*. 2002;69(4):289-293.
78. Kinoshita H, Yamakado H, Kitano T, et al. Diagnostic utility of FDG-PET in neurolymphomatosis: report of five cases. *J Neurol*. 2016;263(9):1719-1726.
79. Vijayan J, Chan YC, Therimadasamy A, Einar B, Wilder-Smith P. Role of combined B-mode and Doppler sonography in evaluating neurolymphomatosis. *Neurology*. 2015;85(9):752-755.
80. Walsh JC. Neuropathy associated with lymphoma. *J Neurol Neurosurg Psychiatry*. 1971;34(1):42-50.
81. Kori SH, Foley KM, Posner JB. Brachial plexus lesions in patients with cancer = 100 cases. *Neurology*. 1981;31(1):45-50.
82. Jaeckle KA, Young DF, Foley KM. The natural history of lumbosacral plexopathy in cancer. *Neurology*. 1985;35(1):8-15.
83. Evans RJ, Walton CPN. Lumbosacral plexopathy in cancer patients. *Neurology*. 1985;35(9):1392-1393.
84. Vrethem M, Cruz M, Wen-Xin H, Malm C, Holmgren H, Ernerudh J. Clinical, neurophysiological and immunological evidence of polyneuropathy in patients with monoclonal gammopathies. *J Neurol Sci*. 1993;114(2):193-199.
85. Kelly JJ, Kyle RA, O'Brien PC, Dyck PJ. Prevalence of monoclonal protein in peripheral neuropathy. *Neurology*. 1981;31(11):1480-1480.
86. Latov N. Prognosis of neuropathy with monoclonal gammopathy. *Muscle Nerve*. 2000;23(2):150-152.
87. Latov N, Sherman WH, Nemni R, et al. Plasma-cell dyscrasia and peripheral neuropathy with a monoclonal antibody to peripheral-nerve myelin. *N Engl J Med*. 1980;303(11):618-621.
88. Kyle RA, Larson DR, Therneau TM, et al. Long-term follow-up of monoclonal gammopathy of undetermined significance. *N Engl J Med*. 2018;378(3):241-249.
89. Kissel JT, Mendell JR. Neuropathies associated with monoclonal gammopathies. *Neuromuscular Disorders*. 1996;6(1):3-18.
90. Kelly JJ, Kyle RA, Miles JM, O'Brien PC, Dyck PJ. The spectrum of peripheral neuropathy in myeloma. *Neurology*. 1981;31(1):24-24.
91. Walsh JC. The neuropathy of multiple myeloma. *Arch Neurol*. 1971;25(5):404-414.
92. Kyle RA, Greipp PR. Amyloidosis (AL). Clinical and laboratory features in 229 cases. *Mayo Clin Proc*. 1983;58(10):665-683.
93. Rukavina JG, Block WD, Jackson CE, Falls HF, Carey JH, Curtis AC. Primary systemic amyloidosis: a review and an experimental, genetic, and clinical study of 29 cases with particular emphasis on the familial form. *Medicine*. 1956;35(3):239-334.
94. Duston MA, Skinner M, Anderson J, Cohen AS. Peripheral neuropathy as an early marker of AL amyloidosis. *Arch Intern Med*. 1989;149(2):358-360.
95. Kelly JJ, Kyle RA, O'Brien PC, Dyck PJ. The natural history of peripheral neuropathy in primary systemic amyloidosis. *Ann Neurol*. 1979;6(1):1-7.
96. Vucic S, Chong PST, Cros D. Atypical presentations of primary amyloid neuropathy. *Muscle Nerve*. 2003;28(6):696-702.
97. Tracy JA, Dyck PJ, Dyck PJB. Primary amyloidosis presenting as upper limb multiple mononeuropathies. *Muscle Nerve*. 2010;41(5):710-715.
98. Mathis S, Magy L, Diallo L, Boukhris S, Vallat JM. Amyloid neuropathy mimicking chronic inflammatory demyelinating polyneuropathy. *Muscle Nerve*. 2012;45(1):26-31.
99. Andersson R, Blom S. Neurophysiological studies in hereditary amyloidosis with polyneuropathy. *Acta Med Scand*. 1972;191(3):233-239.
100. Dyck PJ, Lambert EH. Dissociated sensation in amyloidosis: compound action potential, quantitative histologic and teased-fiber, and electron microscopic studies of sural nerve biopsies. *Arch Neurol*. 1969;20(5):490-507.
101. Thomas PK, King RH. Peripheral nerve changes in amyloid neuropathy. *Brain*. 1974;97(2):395-406.
102. Garcia-Santibanez R, Zaidman CM, Sommerville RB, et al. CANOMAD and other chronic ataxic neuropathies with disialosyl antibodies (CANDA). *J Neurol*. 2018;265(6):1402-1409.
103. Rajani B, Rajani V, Prayson RA. Peripheral nerve amyloidosis in sural nerve biopsies: a clinicopathologic analysis of 13 cases. *Arch Pathol Lab Med*. 2000;124(1):114-118.
104. Lachmann HJ, Booth DR, Booth SE, et al. Misdiagnosis of hereditary amyloidosis as AL (primary) amyloidosis. *N Engl J Med*. 2002;346(23):1786-1791.
105. Klein CJ, Vrana JA, Theis JD, et al. Mass spectrometric-based proteomic analysis of amyloid neuropathy type in nerve tissue. *Arch Neurol*. 2011;68(2):195-199.
106. Duston MA, Skinner M, Shirahama T, Cohen AS. Diagnosis of amyloidosis by abdominal fat aspiration. Analysis of four years' experience. *Am J Med*. 1987;82(3):412-414.
107. Garcia Y, Collins AB, Stone JR. Abdominal fat pad excisional biopsy for the diagnosis and typing of systemic amyloidosis. *Hum Pathol*. 2018;72:71-79.
108. Berghoff M, Kathpal M, Khan F, Skinner M, Falk R, Freeman R. Endothelial dysfunction precedes C-fiber abnormalities in primary (AL) amyloidosis. *Ann Neurol*. 2003;53(6):725-730.
109. Skinner M, Sanchorawala V, Seldin DC, et al. High-dose melphalan and autologous stem-cell transplantation in patients

with AL amyloidosis: an 8-year study. *Ann Intern Med.* 2004; 140(2):85–93.
110. Dispenzieri A, Kyle RA, Lacy MQ, et al. Superior survival in primary systemic amyloidosis patients undergoing peripheral blood stem cell transplantation: a case-control study. *Blood.* 2004;103(10):3960–3963.
111. Dingli D, Tan TS, Kumar SK, et al. Stem cell transplantation in patients with autonomic neuropathy due to primary (AL) amyloidosis. *Neurology.* 2010;74(11):913–918.
112. Kelly JJ, Kyle RA, Miles JM, Dyck PJ. Osteosclerotic myeloma and peripheral neuropathy. *Neurology.* 1983;33(2):202–210.
113. Nakanishi T, Sobue I, Toyokura Y, et al. The Crow-Fukase syndrome: a study of 102 cases in Japan. *Neurology.* 1984;34(6): 712–720.
114. Ohi T, Kyle RA, Dyck PJ. Axonal attenuation and secondary segmental demyelination in myeloma neuropathies. *Ann Neurol.* 1985;17(3):255–261.
115. Dispenzieri A. POEMS syndrome: 2011 update on diagnosis, risk-stratification, and management. *Am J Hematol.* 2011; 86(7):591–601.
116. Isose S, Misawa S, Kanai K, et al. POEMS syndrome with Guillan-Barre syndrome-like acute onset: a case report and review of neurological progression in 30 cases. *J Neurol Neurosurg Psychiatry.* 2011;82(6):678–680.
117. Goebels N, Walther EU, Schaller M, Pongratz D, Mueller-Felber W. Inflammatory myopathy in POEMS syndrome. *Neurology.* 2000;55(9):1413–1414.
118. Dispenzieri A, Kyle RA, Lacy MQ, et al. POEMS syndrome: definitions and long-term outcome. *Blood.* 2003;101(7): 2496–2506.
119. Keddie S, Foldes D, Caimari F, et al. Clinical characteristics, risk factors, and outcomes of POEMS syndrome: a longitudinal cohort study. *Neurology.* 2020;95(3):e268–e279.
120. Donaghy M, Hall P, Gawler J, et al. Peripheral neuropathy associated with Castleman's disease. *J Neurol Sci.* 1989;89(2-3): 253–267.
121. Mauermann ML, Sorenson EJ, Dispenzieri A, et al. Uniform demyelination and more severe axonal loss distinguish POEMS syndrome from CIDP. *J Neurol Neurosurg Psychiatry.* 2012;83(5):480–486.
122. Scarlato M, Previtali SC, Carpo M, et al. Polyneuropathy in POEMS syndrome: role of angiogenic factors in the pathogenesis. *Brain.* 2005;128(8):1911–1920.
123. Kuwabara S, Misawa S, Kanai K, et al. Autologous peripheral blood stem cell transplantation for POEMS syndrome. *Neurology.* 2006;66(1):105–107.
124. Donofrio PD, Albers JW, Greenberg HS, Mitchell BS. Peripheral neuropathy in osteosclerotic myeloma: clinical and electrodiagnostic improvement with chemotherapy. *Muscle Nerve.* 1984;7(2):137–141.
125. Sung JY, Kuwabara S, Ogawara K, Kanai K, Hattori T. Patterns of nerve conduction abnormalities in POEMS syndrome. *Muscle Nerve.* 2002;26(2):189–193.
126. Vital C, Vital A, Ferrer X, et al. Crow-Fukase (POEMS) syndrome: a study of peripheral nerve biopsy in five new cases. *J Peripher Nerv Syst.* 2003;8(3):136–144.
127. Michizono K, Umehara F, Hashiguchi T, et al. Circulating levels of MMP-1, -2, -3, -9, and TIMP-1 are increased in POEMS syndrome. *Neurology.* 2001;56(6):807–810.
128. Dyck PJ, Engelstad J, Dispenzieri A. Vascular endothelial growth factor and POEMS. *Neurology.* 2006;66(1):10–12.
129. Gotham JE, Wein H, Meyer JS. Clinical studies of neuropathy due to macroglobulinemia (Waldenstroem's syndrome). *Can Med Assoc J.* 1963;89(16):806–809.
130. Iwashita H, Argyrakis A, Lowitzsch K, Spaar FW. Polyneuropathy in Waldenström's macroglobulinaemia. *J Neurol Sci.* 1974;21(3):341–354.
131. Propp RP, Means E, Deibel R, Sherer G, Barron K. Waldenstrom's macroglobulinemia and neuropathy: deposition of M-component on myelin sheaths. *Neurology.* 1975;25(10): 980–988.
132. Vital C, Vallat JM, Deminiere C, Loubet A, Leboutet MJ. Peripheral nerve damage during multiple myeloma and Waldenstrom's macroglobulinemia. An ultrastructural and immunopathologic study. *Cancer.* 1982;50(8):1491–1497.
133. Levine T, Pestronk A, Lopate G. Peripheral neuropathies in Waldenstrom's macroglobulinaemia. *J Neurol Neurosurg Psychiatry.* 2006;77(2):224–228.
134. Bardel B, Molinier-Frenkel V, Le Bras F, et al. Revisiting the spectrum of IgM-related neuropathies in a large cohort of IgM monoclonal gammopathy. *J Neurol.* 2022;269(9): 4955–4960.
135. Galassi G, Tondelli M, Ariatti A, Benuzzi F, Nichelli P, Valzania F. Long-term disability and prognostic factors in polyneuropathy associated with anti-myelin-associated glycoprotein (MAG) antibodies. *Int J Neurosci.* 2017;127(5):439–447.
136. D'Sa S, Kersten MJ, Castillo JJ, et al. Investigation and management of IgM and Waldenström-associated peripheral neuropathies: recommendations from the IWWM-8 consensus panel. *Br J Haematol.* 2017;176(5):728–742.
137. Klein CJ, Moon JS, Mauermann ML, et al. The neuropathies of Waldenström's macroglobulinemia (WM) and IgM-MGUS. *Can J Neurol Sci.* 2011;38(2):289–295.
138. Rison RA, Beydoun SR. Paraproteinemic neuropathy: a practical review. *BMC Neurol.* 2016;16(1):1–14.
139. Shelly S, Mills JR, Martinez-Thompson JM, et al. IgM-gammopathy strongly favours immune treatable MMN and MADSAM over ALS. *J Neurol Neurosurg Psychiatry.* 2020;91(3): 324–326.
140. Ferri C, La Civita L, Cirafisi C, et al. Peripheral neuropathy in mixed cryoglobulinemia: clinical and electrophysiologic investigations. *J Rheumatol.* 1992;19(6):889–895.
141. Zhang LL, Cao XX, Shen KN, et al. Clinical characteristics and treatment outcome of type I cryoglobulinemia in Chinese patients: a single-center study of 45 patients. *Ann Hematol.* 2020;99(8):1735–1740.
142. Gemignani F, Brindani F, Alfieri S, et al. Clinical spectrum of cryoglobulinaemic neuropathy. *J Neurol Neurosurg Psychiatry.* 2005;76(10):1410–1414.
143. Khwaja J, D'Sa S, Minnema MC, Kersten MJ, Wechalekar A, Vos JM. IgM monoclonal gammopathies of clinical significance: diagnosis and management. *Haematologica.* 2022;107(9):2037–2050.
144. Magy L, Kaboré R, Mathis S, et al. Heterogeneity of polyneuropathy associated with anti-MAG antibodies. *J Immunol Res.* 2015;2015:450391.
145. Svahn J, Petiot P, Antoine JC, et al. Anti-MAG antibodies in 202 patients: clinicopathological and therapeutic features. *J Neurol Neurosurg Psychiatry.* 2018;89(5):499–505.
146. Poulain S, Boyle EM, Roumier C, et al. MYD88 L265P mutation contributes to the diagnosis of Bing Neel syndrome. *Br J Haematol.* 2014;167(4):506–513.

147. Luigetti M, Frisullo G, Laurenti L, et al. Light chain deposition in peripheral nerve as a cause of mononeuritis multiplex in Waldenström's macroglobulinaemia. *J Neurol Sci.* 2010;291(1–2):89–91.
148. Ghobrial IM, Fonseca R, Greipp PR, et al. Initial immunoglobulin M "flare" after rituximab therapy in patients diagnosed with Waldenstrom macroglobulinemia: an Eastern Cooperative Oncology Group Study. *Cancer.* 2004;101(11):2593–2598.
149. Gosselin S, Kyle RA, Dyck PJ. Neuropathy associated with monoclonal gammopathies of undetermined significance. *Ann Neurol.* 1991;30(1):54–61.
150. Suarez GA, Kelly JJ. Polyneuropathy associated with monoclonal gammopathy of undetermined significance. *Neurology.* 1993;43(7):1304–1308.
151. Nobile-Orazio E, Marmiroli P, Baldini L, et al. Peripheral neuropathy in macroglobulinemia: incidence and antigen-specificity of M proteins. *Neurology.* 1987;37(9):1506–1514.
152. Naddaf E, Mauermann ML. Peripheral neuropathies associated with monoclonal gammopathies. *Continuum (Minneap Minn).* 2020;26(5):1369–1383.
153. Niermeijer JMF, Fischer K, Eurelings M, Franssen H, Wokke JHJ, Notermans NC. Prognosis of polyneuropathy due to IgM monoclonal gammopathy: a prospective cohort study. *Neurology.* 2010;74(5):406–412.
154. Attarian S, Boucraut J, Hubert AM, et al. Chronic ataxic neuropathies associated with anti-GD1b IgM antibodies: response to IVIg therapy. *J Neurol Neurosurg Psychiatry.* 2010;81(1):61–64.
155. Willison HJ, Renaud S, Thomas PK, et al. The clinical and laboratory features of chronic sensory ataxic neuropathy with anti-disialosyl IgM antibodies. *Brain.* 2001;124(10):1968–1977.
156. Katz JS, Saperstein DS, Gronseth G, Amato AA, Barohn RJ. Distal acquired demyelinating symmetric neuropathy. *Neurology.* 2000;54(3):615–620.
157. Saperstein DS, Katz JS, Amato AA, Barohn RJ. Clinical spectrum of chronic acquired demyelinating polyneuropathies. *Muscle Nerve.* 2001;24(3):311–324.
158. Kelly JJ. The electrodiagnostic findings in peripheral neuropathy associated with monoclonal gammopathy. *Muscle Nerve.* 1983;6(7):504–509.
159. Donofrio PD, Kelly JJ. AAEE case report #17: peripheral neuropathy in monoclonal gammopathy of undetermined significance. *Muscle Nerve.* 1989;12(1):1–8.
160. Ellie E, Vital A, Steck A, Boiron JM, Vital C, Julien J. Neuropathy associated with "benign" anti-myelin-associated glycoprotein IgM gammopathy: clinical, immunological, neurophysiological pathological findings and response to treatment in 33 cases. *J Neurol.* 1995;243(1):34–43.
161. Cook D, Dalakas M, Galdi A, Biondi D, Porter H. High-dose intravenous immunoglobulins in the treatment of demyelinating neuropathy associated with monoclonal gammopathy. *Neurology.* 1990;40(2):212–214.
162. Gorson KC, Ropper AH, Weinberg DH, Weinstein R. Treatment experience in patients with anti-myelin-associated glycoprotein neuropathy. *Muscle Nerve.* 2001;24(6):778–786.
163. Lunn MP, Nobile-Orazio E. Immunotherapy for IgM anti-myelin-associated glycoprotein paraprotein-associated peripheral neuropathies. In: Lunn MP, ed. *Cochrane Database of Systematic Reviews.* John Wiley & Sons, Ltd; 2016.
164. Niermeijer JMF, Eurelings M, Lokhorst HL, et al. Rituximab for polyneuropathy with IgM monoclonal gammopathy. *J Neurol Neurosurg Psychiatry.* 2009;80(9):1036–1039.
165. Dalakas MC, Rakocevic G, Salajegheh M, et al. Placebo-controlled trial of rituximab in IgM anti-myelin-associated glycoprotein antibody demyelinating neuropathy. *Ann Neurol.* 2009;65(3):286–293.
166. Lunn MP, Nobile-Orazio E. Immunotherapy for IgM anti-myelin-associated glycoprotein paraprotein-associated peripheral neuropathies. *Cochrane Database of Systematic Reviews.* 2016;2016(10):CD002827.
167. Leger JM, Viala K, Nicolas G, et al. Placebo-controlled trial of rituximab in IgM anti-myelin-associated glycoprotein neuropathy. *Neurology.* 2013;80(24):2217–2225.
168. Benedetti L, Briani C, Franciotta D, et al. Long-term effect of rituximab in anti-mag polyneuropathy. *Neurology.* 2008;71(21):1742–1744.
169. Benedetti L, Briani C, Grandis M, et al. Predictors of response to rituximab in patients with neuropathy and anti-myelin associated glycoprotein immunoglobulin M. *J Peripher Nerv Syst.* 2007;12(2):102–107.
170. Souayah N, Noopur R, Tick-Chong PS. Beneficial effects of Rituximab in patients with anti-MAG (myelin-associated glycoprotein) neuropathy: case reports. *Immunopharmacol Immunotoxicol.* 2013;35(5):622–624.
171. Sala E, Robert-Varvat F, Paul S, Camdessanché JP, Antoine JC. Acute neurological worsening after rituximab treatment in patients with anti-MAG neuropathy. *J Neurol Sci.* 2014;345(1–2):224–227.
172. Broglio L, Lauria G. Worsening after rituximab treatment in anti-mag neuropathy. *Muscle Nerve.* 2005;32(3):378–379.
173. Noronha V, Fynan TM, Duffy T. Flare in neuropathy following rituximab therapy for Waldenstrom's macroglobulinemia. *J Clin Oncol.* 2006;24(1):e3.
174. Gazzola S, Delmont E, Franques J, et al. Predictive factors of efficacy of rituximab in patients with anti-MAG neuropathy. *J Neurol Sci.* 2017;377:144–148.
175. Eurelings M, Lokhorst HM, Kalmijn S, Wokke JHJ, Notermans NC. Malignant transformation in polyneuropathy associated with monoclonal gammopathy. *Neurology.* 2005;64(12):2079–2084.
176. Kyle RA, Larson DR, Therneau TM, et al. Long-term follow-up of monoclonal gammopathy of undetermined significance. *New England Journal of Medicine.* 2018;378(3):241–249.
177. Eliashiv S, Brenner T, Abramsky O, et al. Acute inflammatory demyelinating polyneuropathy following bone marrow transplantation. *Bone Marrow Transplant.* 1991;8(4):315–317.
178. Openshaw H, Hinton DR, Slatkin NE, Bierman PJ, Hoffman FM, Snyder DS. Exacerbation of inflammatory demyelinating polyneuropathy after bone marrow transplantation. *Bone Marrow Transplant.* 1991;7(5):411–414.
179. Lehky T, Fernandez IP, Krakow EF, et al. Neuropathy and muscle cramps in autologous and allogeneic hematopoietic cell transplantation survivors. *Transplant Cell Ther.* 2022;28(9):608.e1–608.e9.
180. Greenspan A, Deeg HJ, Cottler-Fox M, Sirdofski M, Spitzer TR, Kattah J. Incapacitating peripheral neuropathy as a manifestation of chronic graft-versus-host disease. *Bone Marrow Transplant.* 1990;5(5):349–352.
181. Bashir RM, Bierman P, McComb R. Inflammatory peripheral neuropathy following high dose chemotherapy and autologous bone marrow transplantation. *Bone Marrow Transplant.* 1992;10(3):305–306.

182. Myers SE, Williams SF, Iverson T, Treleaven J, Powles R. Guillain-Barré syndrome after autologous bone marrow transplantation for breast cancer: report of two cases. *Bone Marrow Transplant*. 1994;13(3):341–344.
183. Cocito D, Romagnolo A, Rosso M, Peci E, Lopiano L, Merola A. CIDP-like neuropathies in graft versus host disease. *J Peripher Nerv Syst*. 2015;20(1):1–6.
184. Ashraf M, Scotchel PL, Krall JM, Flink EB. cis-Platinum-induced hypomagnesemia and peripheral neuropathy. *Gynecol Oncol*. 1983;16(3):309–318.
185. Barajon I, Bersani M, Quartu M, et al. Neuropeptides and morphological changes in cisplatin-induced dorsal root ganglion neuronopathy. *Exp Neurol*. 1996;138(1):93–104.
186. Cersosimo RJ. Cisplatin neurotoxicity. *Cancer Treat Rev*. 1989;16(4):195–211.
187. Gregg RW, Molepo JM, Monpetit VJ, et al. Cisplatin neurotoxicity: the relationship between dosage, time, and platinum concentration in neurologic tissues, and morphologic evidence of toxicity. *J Clin Oncol*. 1992;10(5):795–803.
188. Krarup-Hansen A, Fugleholm K, Helweg-Larsen S, et al. Examination of distal involvement in cisplatin-induced neuropathy in man. *Brain*. 1993;116(5):1017–1041.
189. LoMonaco M, Milone M, Batocchi AP, Padua L, Restuccia D, Tonali P. Cisplatin neuropathy: clinical course and neurophysiological findings. *J Neurol*. 1992;239(4):199–204.
190. Mollman JE, Hogan WM, Glover DJ, McCluskey LF. Unusual presentation of cis-platinum neuropathy. *Neurology*. 1988;38(3):488–490.
191. Mollman JE, Glover DJ, Hogan WM, Furman RE. Cisplatin neuropathy. Risk factors, prognosis, and protection by WR-2721. *Cancer*. 1988;61(11):2192–2195.
192. Russell JW, Windebank AJ, McNiven MA, Brat DJ, Brimijoin WS. Effect of cisplatin and ACTH4-9 on neural transport in cisplatin induced neurotoxicity. *Brain Res*. 1995;676(2):258–267.
193. Pachman DR, Qin R, Seisler DK, et al. Clinical course of oxaliplatin-induced neuropathy: results from the randomized phase III trial N08CB (Alliance). *J Clin Oncol*. 2015;33(30):3416–3422.
194. Lehky TJ, Leonard GD, Wilson RH, Grem JL, Floeter MK. Oxaliplatin-induced neurotoxicity: acute hyperexcitability and chronic neuropathy. *Muscle Nerve*. 2004;29(3):387–392.
195. Grothey A. Oxaliplatin-safety profile: neurotoxicity. *Semin Oncol*. 2003;30:5–13.
196. Burakgazi AZ, Messersmith W, Vaidya D, Hauer P, Hoke A, Polydefkis M. Longitudinal assessment of oxaliplatin-induced neuropathy. *Neurology*. 2011;77(10):980–986.
197. Brouwers EEM, Huitema ADR, Boogerd W, Beijnen JH, Schellens JHM. Persistent neuropathy after treatment with cisplatin and oxaliplatin. *Acta Oncol*. 2009;48(6):832–841.
198. Verstappen CCP, Koeppen S, Heimans JJ, et al. Dose-related vincristine-induced peripheral neuropathy with unexpected off-therapy worsening. *Neurology*. 2005;64(6):1076–1077.
199. Casey EB, Jellife AM, le Quense PM, Millett YL. Vincristine Neuropathy. *Brain*. 1973;96(1):69–86.
200. Legha SS. Vincristine neurotoxicity. *Med Toxicol*. 1986;1(6):421–427.
201. Hildebrandt G, Holler E, Woenkhaus M, et al. Acute deterioration of Charcot-Marie-Tooth disease IA (CMTIA) following 2 mg of vincristine chemotherapy. *Ann Oncol*. 2000;11(6):743–747.
202. Goa KL, Faulds D. Vinorelbine. *Drugs Aging*. 1994;5(3):200–234.
203. O'Reilly S, Kennedy MJ, Rowinsky EK, Donehower RC. Vinorelbine and the topoisomerase 1 inhibitors: current and potential roles in breast cancer chemotherapy. *Breast Cancer Res Treat*. 1995;33(1):1–17.
204. Pace A, Bove L, Nistico C, et al. Vinorelbine neurotoxicity: clinical and neurophysiological findings in 23 patients. *J Neurol Neurosurg Psychiatry*. 1996;61(4):409–411.
205. Pal PK. Clinical and electrophysiological studies in vincristine induced neuropathy. *Electromyogr Clin Neurophysiol*. 1999;39(6):323–330.
206. Sahenk Z, Brady ST, Mendell JR. Studies on the pathogenesis of vincristine-induced neuropathy. *Muscle Nerve*. 1987;10(1):80–84.
207. Bregman CL, Buroker RA, Hirth RS, Crosswell AR, Durham SK. Etoposide- and BMY-40481-induced sensory neuropathy in mice. *Toxicol Pathol*. 1994;22(5):528–535.
208. Forsyth P A, Balmaceda C, Peterson K, Seidman AD, Brasher P, Deangelis LM. Prospective study of paclitaxel-induced peripheral neuropathy with quantitative sensory testing. *J Neurooncol*. 1997;35(1):47–53.
209. Lipton RB, Apfel SC, Dutcher JP, et al. Taxol produces a predominantly sensory neuropathy. *Neurology*. 1989;39(3):368–373.
210. Postma TJ, Vermorken JB, Liefting AJ, Pinedo HM, Heimans JJ. Paclitaxel-induced neuropathy. *Ann Oncol*. 1995;6(5):489–494.
211. Rowinsky EK, Chaudhry V, Forastiere AA, et al. Phase I and pharmacologic study of paclitaxel and cisplatin with granulocyte colony-stimulating factor: neuromuscular toxicity is dose-limiting. *J Clin Oncol*. 1993;11(10):2010–2020.
212. Sahenk Z, Barohn R, New P, Mendell J. Taxol neuropathy. *Arch Neurol*. 1994;51(7):726–729.
213. van den Bent MJ, van Raaij-van den Aarssen VJ, Verweij J, Doorn PA, Sillevis Smitt PA. Progression of paclitaxel-induced neuropathy following discontinuation of treatment. *Muscle Nerve*. 1997;20(6):750–752.
214. van Gerven JM, Moll JW, van den Bent MJ, et al. Paclitaxel (Taxol) induces cumulative mild neurotoxicity. *Eur J Cancer*. 1994;30A(8):1074–1077.
215. Kuroi K, Shimozuma K. Neurotoxicity of taxanes: symptoms and quality of life assessment. *Breast Cancer*. 2004;11(1):92–99.
216. Makino H. Treatment and care of neurotoxicity from taxane anticancer agents. *Breast Cancer*. 2004;11(1):100–104.
217. Park SB, Lin CSY, Krishnan AV, Friedlander ML, Lewis CR, Kiernan MC. Early, progressive, and sustained dysfunction of sensory axons underlies paclitaxel-induced neuropathy. *Muscle Nerve*. 2011;43(3):367–374.
218. Pachman DR, Qin R, Seisler D, et al. Comparison of oxaliplatin and paclitaxel-induced neuropathy (Alliance A151505). *Support Care Cancer*. 2016;24(12):5059–5068.
219. Freilich RJ, Balmaceda C, Seidman AD, Rubin M, DeAngelis LM. Motor neuropathy due to docetaxel and paclitaxel. *Neurology*. 1996;47(1):115–118.
220. Hilkens PH, Verweij J, Stoter G, Vecht CJ, van Putten WLJ, van den Bent MJ. Peripheral neurotoxicity induced by docetaxel. *Neurology*. 1996;46(1):104–108.
221. New PZ, Jackson CE, Rinaldi D, Burris H, Barohn RJ. Peripheral neuropathy secondary to docetaxel (Taxotere). *Neurology*. 1996;46(1):108–111.

222. Hsu Y, Sood AK, Sorosky JI. Docetaxel versus paclitaxel for adjuvant treatment of ovarian cancer. *Am J Clin Oncol.* 2004;27(1):14–18.
223. Guastalla III JP, Diéras V. The taxanes: toxicity and quality of life considerations in advanced ovarian cancer. *Br J Cancer.* 2003;89(S3):S16–S22.
224. Röyttä M, Raine CS. Taxol-induced neuropathy: chronic effects of local injection. *J Neurocytol.* 1986;15(4):483–496.
225. Chaudhry V, Eisenberger MA, Sinibaldi VJ, Sheikh K, Griffin JW, Cornblath DR. A prospective study of suramin-induced peripheral neuropathy. *Brain.* 1996;119(6):2039–2052.
226. Vahdat LT, Thomas ES, Roché HH, et al. Ixabepilone-associated peripheral neuropathy: data from across the phase II and III clinical trials. *Support Care Cancer.* 2012;20(11):2661–2668.
227. Vahdat LT, Garcia AA, Vogel C, et al. Eribulin mesylate versus ixabepilone in patients with metastatic breast cancer: a randomized Phase II study comparing the incidence of peripheral neuropathy. *Breast Cancer Res Treat.* 2013;140(2):341–351.
228. La Rocca RV, Meer J, Gilliatt RW, et al. Suramin-induced polyneuropathy. *Neurology.* 1990;40(6):954–954.
229. Soliven B, Dhand UK, Kobayashi K, et al. Evaluation of neuropathy in patients on suramin treatment. *Muscle Nerve.* 1997;20(1):83–91.
230. Russell JW, Gill JS, Sorenson EJ, Schultz DA, Windebank AJ. Suramin-induced neuropathy in an animal model. *J Neurol Sci.* 2001;192(1–2):71–80.
231. Sullivan KA, Kim B, Buzdon M, Feldman EL. Suramin disrupts insulin-like growth factor-II (IGF-II) mediated autocrine growth in human SH-SY5Y neuroblastoma cells. *Brain Res.* 1997;744(2):199–206.
232. Czernin S, Gessl A, Wilfing A, et al. Suramin affects human peripheral blood mononuclear cells in vitro: inhibition of T cell growth and modulation of cytokine secretion. *Int Arch Allergy Immunol.* 1993;101(3):240–246.
233. Borgeat A, Stalder M, de Muralt B. Peripheral neuropathy associated with high-dose Ara-C therapy. *Cancer.* 1986;58(4):852–854.
234. Johnson NT, Crawford SW, Sargur M. Acute acquired demyelinating polyneuropathy with respiratory failure following high-dose systemic cytosine arabinoside and marrow transplantation. *Bone Marrow Transplant.* 1987;2(2):203–207.
235. Nevill TJ, Benstead TJ, McCormick CW, Hayne OA. Horner's syndrome and demyelinating peripheral neuropathy caused by high-dose cytosine arabinoside. *Am J Hematol.* 1989;32(4):314–315.
236. Openshaw H, Slatkin NE, Stein AS, Hinton DR, Forman SJ. Acute polyneuropathy after high dose cytosine arabinoside in patients with leukemia. *Cancer.* 1996;78(9):1899–1905.
237. Paul M, Joshua D, Rahme N, et al. Fatal peripheral neuropathy associated with high-dose cytosine arabinoside in acute leukemia. *Br J Haematol.* 1991;79(3):521–523.
238. Russell JA, Powles RL. Letter: neuropathy due to cytosine arabinoside. *BMJ.* 1974;4(5945):652–653.
239. Patel SR, Forman AD, Benjamin RS. High-dose ifosfamide-induced exacerbation of peripheral neuropathy. *J Natl Cancer Inst.* 1994;86(4):305–306.
240. Richardson PG, Barlogie B, Berenson J, et al. A phase 2 study of bortezomib in relapsed, refractory myeloma. *N Engl J Med.* 2003;348(26):2609–2617.
241. Richardson PG, Briemberg H, Jagannath S, et al. Frequency, characteristics, and reversibility of peripheral neuropathy during treatment of advanced multiple myeloma with bortezomib. *J Clin Oncol.* 2006;24(19):3113–3120.
242. Davis NB, Taber DA, Ansari RH, et al. Phase II trial of PS-341 in patients with renal cell cancer: A University of Chicago Phase II Consortium Study. *J Clin Oncol.* 2004;22(1):115–119.
243. Stubblefield MD, Slovin S, MacGregor-Cortelli B, et al. An electrodiagnostic evaluation of the effect of pre-existing peripheral nervous system disorders in patients treated with the novel proteasome inhibitor bortezomib. *Clin Oncol.* 2006;18(5):410–418.
244. Richardson PG, Xie W, Mitsiades C, et al. Single-agent Bortezomib in previously untreated multiple myeloma: efficacy, characterization of peripheral neuropathy, and molecular correlations with response and neuropathy. *J Clin Oncol.* 2009;27(21):3518–3525.
245. Sidana S, Narkhede M, Elson P, et al. Neuropathy and efficacy of once weekly subcutaneous bortezomib in multiple myeloma and light chain (AL) amyloidosis. *PLoS One.* 2017;12(3):e0172996.
246. Mina SA, Muhsen IN, Burns EA, et al. Post-marketing analysis of peripheral neuropathy burden with newer generation proteasome inhibitors using the FDA Adverse Event Reporting System. *Turk J Haematol.* 2021;38(3):218–221.
247. Siegel D, Martin T, Nooka A, et al. Integrated safety profile of single-agent carfilzomib: experience from 526 patients enrolled in 4 phase II clinical studies. *Haematologica.* 2013;98(11):1753–1761.
248. Moreau P, Masszi T, Grzasko N, et al. Oral ixazomib, lenalidomide, and dexamethasone for multiple myeloma. *N Engl J Med.* 2016;374(17):1621–1634.
249. Giannoccaro MP, Donadio V, Gomis Pèrez C, Borsini W, di Stasi V, Liguori R. Somatic and autonomic small fiber neuropathy induced by bortezomib therapy: an immunofluorescence study. *Neurol Sci.* 2011;32(2):361–363.
250. Meregalli C, Canta A, Carozzi VA, et al. Bortezomib-induced painful neuropathy in rats: a behavioral, neurophysiological and pathological study in rats. *Eur J Pain.* 2010;14(4):343–350.
251. Bruna J, Udina E, Alé A, et al. Neurophysiological, histological and immunohistochemical characterization of bortezomib-induced neuropathy in mice. *Exp Neurol.* 2010;223(2):599–608.
252. Carozzi VA, Canta A, Oggioni N, et al. Neurophysiological and neuropathological characterization of new murine models of chemotherapy-induced chronic peripheral neuropathies. *Exp Neurol.* 2010;226(2):301–309.
253. Fullerton PM, O'Sullivan DJ. Thalidomide neuropathy: a clinical electrophysiological, and histological follow-up study. *J Neurol Neurosurg Psychiatry.* 1968;31(6):543–551.
254. Lagueny A, Rommel A, Vignolly B, et al. Thalidomide neuropathy: an electrophysiologic study. *Muscle Nerve.* 1986;9(9):837–844.
255. Cavaletti G, Beronio A, Reni L, et al. Thalidomide sensory neurotoxicity: a clinical and neurophysiologic study. *Neurology.* 2004;62(12):2291–2293.
256. Chaudhry V, Cornblath DR, Corse A, Freimer M, Simmons-O'Brien E, Vogelsang G. Thalidomide-induced neuropathy. *Neurology.* 2002;59(12):1872–1875.
257. Plasmati R, Pastorelli F, Cavo M, et al. Neuropathy in multiple myeloma treated with thalidomide: a prospective study. *Neurology.* 2007;69(6):573–581.
258. Miguel JS, Weisel K, Moreau P, et al. Pomalidomide plus low-dose dexamethasone versus high-dose dexamethasone alone

for patients with relapsed and refractory multiple myeloma (MM-003): a randomised, open-label, phase 3 trial. *Lancet Oncol.* 2013;14(11):1055–1066.
259. Richardson PG, Siegel DS, Vij R, et al. Pomalidomide alone or in combination with low-dose dexamethasone in relapsed and refractory multiple myeloma: a randomized phase 2 study. *Blood.* 2014;123(12):1826–1832.
260. Dalla Torre C, Zambello R, Cacciavillani M, et al. Lenalidomide long-term neurotoxicity. *Neurology.* 2016;87(11):1161–1166.
261. van der Weyden C, Dickinson M, Whisstock J, Prince HM. Brentuximab vedotin in T-cell lymphoma. *Expert Rev Hematol.* 2019;12(1):5–19.
262. Gopal AK, Ramchandren R, O'Connor OA, et al. Safety and efficacy of brentuximab vedotin for Hodgkin lymphoma recurring after allogeneic stem cell transplantation. *Blood.* 2012;120(3):560–568.
263. Corbin ZA, Nguyen-Lin A, Li S, et al. Characterization of the peripheral neuropathy associated with brentuximab vedotin treatment of Mycosis fungoides and Sézary syndrome. *J Neurooncol.* 2017;132(3):439–446.
264. Pro B, Advani R, Brice P, et al. Five-year results of brentuximab vedotin in patients with relapsed or refractory systemic anaplastic large cell lymphoma. *Blood.* 2017;130(25):2709–2717.
265. Coleman RL, Lorusso D, Gennigens C, et al. Efficacy and safety of tisotumab vedotin in previously treated recurrent or metastatic cervical cancer (innovaTV 204/GOG-3023/ENGOT-cx6): a multicentre, open-label, single-arm, phase 2 study. *Lancet Oncol.* 2021;22(5):609–619.
266. Lu D, Gillespie WR, Girish S, et al. Time-to-event analysis of polatuzumab vedotin-induced peripheral neuropathy to assist in the comparison of clinical dosing regimens. *CPT Pharmacometrics Syst Pharmacol.* 2017;6(6):401–408.
267. Rosenberg JE, O'Donnell PH, Balar AV, et al. Pivotal trial of enfortumab vedotin in urothelial carcinoma after platinum and anti-programmed death 1/programmed death ligand 1 therapy. *J Clin Oncol.* 2019;37(29):2592–2600.
268. Moore KN, Oza AM, Colombo N, et al. Phase III, randomized trial of mirvetuximab soravtansine versus chemotherapy in patients with platinum-resistant ovarian cancer: primary analysis of FORWARD I. *Ann Oncol.* 2021;32(6):757–765.
269. Liu K, Li YH, Zhang X, et al. Incidence and risk of severe adverse events associated with trastuzumab emtansine (T-DM1) in the treatment of breast cancer: an up-to-date systematic review and meta-analysis of randomized controlled clinical trials. *Expert Rev Clin Pharmacol.* 2022;15(11):1343–1350.
270. Jahan N, Rehman S, Khan R, Jones C. Relative risk of peripheral neuropathy with ado-trastuzumab emtansine (T-DM1) compared to taxane-based regimens in human epidermal growth factor receptor 2 (HER2)-positive cancers: a systematic review and meta-analysis. *Cureus.* 2021;13(5):e15282.
271. Krop IE, Modi S, LoRusso PM, et al. Phase 1b/2a study of trastuzumab emtansine (T-DM1), paclitaxel, and pertuzumab in HER2-positive metastatic breast cancer. *Breast Cancer Res.* 2016;18(1):34.
272. Cuzzubbo S, Javeri F, Tissier M, et al. Neurological adverse events associated with immune checkpoint inhibitors: review of the literature. *Eur J Cancer.* 2017;73:1–8.
273. Marini A, Bernardini A, Gigli GL, et al. Neurologic adverse events of immune checkpoint inhibitors: a systematic review. *Neurology.* 2021;96(16):754–766.
274. Nishijima TF, Shachar SS, Nyrop KA, Muss HB. Safety and tolerability of PD-1/PD-L1 inhibitors compared with chemotherapy in patients with advanced cancer: a meta-analysis. *Oncologist.* 2017;22(4):470–479.
275. Psimaras D, Velasco R, Birzu C, et al. Immune checkpoint inhibitors-induced neuromuscular toxicity: from pathogenesis to treatment. *J Peripher Nerv Syst.* 2019;24(S2):S74–S85.
276. Dubey D, David WS, Reynolds KL, et al. Severe neurological toxicity of immune checkpoint inhibitors: growing spectrum. *Ann Neurol.* 2020;87(5):659–669.
277. Dubey D, David WS, Amato AA, et al. Varied phenotypes and management of immune checkpoint inhibitor-associated neuropathies. *Neurology.* 2019;93(11):e1093–e1103.
278. Reynolds KL, Guidon AC. Diagnosis and management of immune checkpoint inhibitor-associated neurologic toxicity: illustrative case and review of the literature. *Oncologist.* 2019;24(4):435–443.
279. Bird SJ, Brown MJ, Shy ME, Scherer SS. Chronic inflammatory demyelinating polyneuropathy associated with malignant melanoma. *Neurology.* 1996;46(3):822–824.
280. June CH, Warshauer JT, Bluestone JA. Corrigendum: is autoimmunity the Achilles' heel of cancer immunotherapy? *Nat Med.* 2017;23(8):1004.
281. Manson G, Maria ATJ, Poizeau F, et al. Worsening and newly diagnosed paraneoplastic syndromes following anti-PD-1 or anti-PD-L1 immunotherapies, a descriptive study. *J Immunother Cancer.* 2019;7(1):337.
282. Schneider BJ, Naidoo J, Santomasso BD, et al. Management of immune-related adverse events in patients treated with immune checkpoint inhibitor therapy: ASCO guideline update. *J Clin Oncol.* 2021;39(36):4073–4126.

CHAPTER 20

Toxic Neuropathies

This chapter reviews neuropathies associated with various drugs (Table 20-1) and other environmental exposures (Tables 20-2 and 20-3). Toxic neuropathies due to chemotherapeutic agents are discussed in Chapter 19. The associated neuropathy for most of these is an axonal, length-dependent predominantly sensory neuropathy. While a high degree of suspicion may be required to identify some toxic insults to nerves, oftentimes the proximity of symptom onset to the exposure and/or the recognition of concurrent involvement of other organ systems can serve as helpful clues to help identify the toxic cause. Although we mention features that have been reported on nerve biopsy, this is generally not recommended to secure a diagnosis since in most cases the abnormalities found are nonspecific.

▶ TOXIC NEUROPATHIES ASSOCIATED WITH MEDICATIONS

ANTI-INFECTIVES

Metronidazole

Metronidazole is used to treat a variety of bacterial and protozoan infections and Crohn disease.[1-8] Metronidazole is a member of the nitroimidazole group and has been associated with hyperalgesia and hypesthesia in a length-dependent pattern. Autonomic dysfunction may develop as well. Motor strength is typically normal. The cumulative dose at which neuropathy occurs is wide, ranging from 3.6 to 228 g. Although there is no clear dose effect, neuropathy appears to occur more frequently in patients receiving greater than 1.5 g daily of metronidazole for 30 or more days. Metronidazole toxicity can also cause encephalopathy, seizures, and/or optic neuropathy. Brain MRI in such patients frequently demonstrates lesions in the splenium of the corpus callosum or the bilateral dentate nuclei of the cerebellum.[9] The incidence of developing central nervous system (CNS) or peripheral nervous system (PNS) events was estimated at 0.25% in a case-control study.[10] Neuropathy symptoms usually improve upon discontinuation of the drug, but there can be a coasting effect such that the symptoms may continue to worsen for several weeks. Some patients are left with residual sensory symptoms. Misonidazole, a related compound used as an adjuvant agent in the treatment of various malignancies, can similarly cause neuropathy.[11-14]

Nerve conduction studies (NCSs) may be normal, as typical of a small fiber neuropathy, or reveal reduced amplitudes or absent sensory nerve action potentials (SNAPs) in the legs worse than in the arms. Motor conduction studies are usually normal. Nerve biopsies are not routinely performed for this but have demonstrated loss of myelinated nerve fibers.

The pathogenic basis of the neuropathy is not known. Some have found that metronidazole binds to DNA and/or RNA, which could lead to breaks and impair transcription or translation to normal proteins.[7,8] Others have speculated that toxicity may arise from the production of nitro radical anions that bind and disrupt normal protein/enzyme function.[8] Furthermore, the histological abnormalities in metronidazole-treated rodents and abnormalities on brain MRI scans in patients with metronidazole-associated encephalopathy resemble thiamine (vitamin B1) deficiency. It has been postulated that there may be enzymatic conversion of metronidazole to an analog of thiamine, which may act as a B1 antagonist.[15]

Nitrofurantoin

Nitrofurantoin is an antibiotic most often used to treat urinary tract infections and may cause an acute and severe sensorimotor polyneuropathy[16-19] or a non–length-dependent small fiber neuropathy/ganglionopathy.[20] Patients may develop numbness, painful paresthesia, and sometimes quadriparesis. Elderly patients and those with baseline renal insufficiency are most at risk. Physical examination most often reveals decrease of all sensory modalities (except in cases of small fiber neuronopathy) in the distal regions of the upper and lower limbs. Muscle stretch reflexes are reduced or absent. Most patients slowly improve following discontinuation of the drug.

NCSs may demonstrate reduced amplitudes or absent SNAPs and compound muscle action potentials (CMAPs) suggestive of an axonopathy[17,18] or may be normal in cases of a small fiber neuropathy/ganglionopathy.[20] Sural nerve biopsy may reveal loss of large myelinated fibers with signs of active Wallerian degeneration.[17] Skin biopsies in patients with small fiber sensory neuropathy/ganglionopathy have shown distinctive morphologic changes with clustered terminal nerve swellings without a reduction in density.[20]

The pathogenic basis of the neuropathy is not known.

Fluoroquinolones

The fluoroquinolones are wide-spectrum antibiotics that have been associated with the rare development of peripheral neuropathy.[21-23] While two case-control studies have demonstrated an elevated relative incidence of peripheral

▶ TABLE 20-1. TOXIC NEUROPATHIES RELATED TO MEDICATIONS

Drug	Mechanism of Neurotoxicity	Clinical Features	Nerve Histopathology	Diagnostic Testing
Anti-Infectives				
Metronidazole	Unknown	Pain and paresthesias. Length-dependent loss of large + small sensory > motor function. Encephalopathy, seizures, and optic neuropathy may also occur	Axonal degeneration	Low-amplitude or unobtainable SNAPs with normal CMAP. Abnormalities on brain MRI, including splenial lesions in corpus callosum, may be seen in patients with CNS symptoms
Nitrofurantoin	Unknown	Acute, severe sensorimotor polyneuropathy resembling GBS. Or, non–length-dependent small fiber neuropathy. Often painful	Axonal degeneration; autopsy studies reveal degeneration of dorsal root ganglia and anterior horn cells. Skin biopsy with cluster terminal nerve swellings	Low-amplitude or unobtainable SNAPs with normal or reduced CMAP amplitudes
Fluoroquinolones	Unknown	Axonal sensory and motor neuropathies of varying severity have been reported; consistent clinical phenotype not yet clarified	Not well described	Not well described
Linezolid	Mitochondrial dysfunction suspected	Painful length-dependent sensorimotor polyneuropathy. Allodynia common. Optic neuropathy can occur	Not well described	Low-amplitude or unobtainable SNAPs, with or without reduced CMAP amplitudes. Reduced ENFD on skin biopsy
Dapsone	Unknown	Distal weakness that may progress to proximal muscles; sensory loss	Axonal degeneration and segmental demyelination	Low-amplitude or unobtainable CMAPs with normal or reduced SNAP amplitudes
Chloroquine and hydroxychloroquine	Amphiphilic properties may lead to drug–lipid complexes that are indigestible and result in accumulation of autophagic vacuoles	Length-dependent sensorimotor neuropathy. Superimposed myopathy may lead to proximal weakness	Axonal degeneration with autophagic vacuoles in nerves as well as muscle fibers	Low-amplitude or unobtainable SNAPs with normal or reduced CMAP amplitudes; distal denervation on EMG; irritability and myopathic-appearing MUAPs proximally in patients with superimposed toxic myopathy
Isoniazid	Inhibit pyridoxal phosphokinase leading to pyridoxine deficiency	Dysesthesia and sensory ataxia; impaired large fiber sensory modalities on examination	Marked loss of sensory axons and cell bodies in dorsal root ganglia and degeneration of the dorsal columns	Reduced amplitudes or absent SNAPs and to a lesser extent CMAPs
Ethambutol	Unknown	Numbness with loss of large fiber modalities on examination	Axonal degeneration	Reduced amplitudes or absent SNAPs
Nucleoside reverse transcriptase inhibitors	Mitochondrial dysfunction; acetyl-carnitine deficiency may also contribute	Dysesthesia and sensory ataxia; impaired large fiber sensory modalities on examination	Axonal degeneration	Reduced amplitudes or absent SNAPs

(continued)

TABLE 20-1. (CONTINUED)

Drug	Mechanism of Neurotoxicity	Clinical Features	Nerve Histopathology	Diagnostic Testing
Cardiac Medications				
Amiodarone	Amphiphilic properties may lead to drug–lipid complexes that are indigestible and result in accumulation of autophagic vacuoles	Painful length-dependent sensorimotor polyneuropathy. Superimposed myopathy may lead to proximal weakness	Axonal degeneration and segmental demyelination with myeloid inclusions in nerves and muscle fibers	Low-amplitude or unobtainable SNAPs with normal or reduced CMAP amplitudes; can also have prominent slowing of CVs; distal denervation on EMG; irritability and myopathic-appearing MUAPs proximally in patients with superimposed toxic myopathy
Rheumatologic/Immunomodulatory Medications				
Colchicine	Inhibits polymerization of tubulin in microtubules and impairs axoplasmic flow	Primarily length-dependent large fiber sensory polyneuropathy. Superimposed myopathy may lead to proximal in addition to distal weakness	Nerve biopsies demonstrate axonal degeneration; muscle biopsies reveal fibers with vacuoles	Low-amplitude or unobtainable SNAPs with normal or reduced CMAP amplitudes; irritability and myopathic-appearing MUAPs proximally in patients with superimposed toxic myopathy
Leflunomide	Unknown	Paresthesias and numbness in a length-dependent pattern	Not well described	Low-amplitude or unobtainable SNAPs with normal or reduced CMAP amplitudes
TNF-α inhibitors	Uncertain	Diverse clinical phenotypes have been reported including AIDP, CIDP, MMN, and generalized sensory neuropathies	Not well described	Reported cases have been highly variable
CNS-Acting Medications				
Phenytoin	Unknown	Numbness with loss of large fiber modalities on examination	Axonal degeneration and segmental demyelination	Low-amplitude or unobtainable SNAPs with normal or reduced CMAP amplitudes
Lithium	Unknown	Numbness with loss of large fiber modalities on examination	Axonal degeneration	Low-amplitude or unobtainable SNAPs with normal or reduced CMAP amplitudes
Disulfiram	Accumulation of neurofilaments and impaired axoplasmic flow	Numbness, tingling, and burning pain in a length-dependent pattern	Axonal degeneration with accumulation of neurofilaments in the axons	Low-amplitude or unobtainable SNAPs with normal or reduced CMAP amplitudes
Other				
Pyridoxine (vitamin B6) toxicity	Unknown	Dysesthesia and sensory ataxia; impaired large fiber sensory modalities on examination	Marked loss of sensory axons and cell bodies in dorsal root ganglia	Reduced amplitudes or absent SNAPs
Podophylin	Binds to microtubules and impairs axoplasmic flow	Sensory loss, tingling, muscle weakness, and diminished muscle stretch reflexes in length-dependent pattern; autonomic neuropathy	Axonal degeneration	Low-amplitude or unobtainable SNAPs with normal or reduced CMAP amplitudes

AIDP, acute inflammatory demyelinating polyneuropathy; CIDP, chronic inflammatory demyelinating polyneuropathy; CMAP, compound muscle action potential; CV, conduction velocity; EMG, electromyography; ENFD, epidermal nerve fiber density; GBS, Guillain–Barré syndrome; MMN, multifocal motor neuropathy; MUAPs, motor unit action potentials; NCS, nerve conduction study; SNAP, sensory nerve action potential.

neuropathy among patients given fluoroquinolones, the absolute risk is low. In a UK study, the absolute risk was 2.4 per 10,000 patients per year of use, equating to a number needed to harm with a standard 10-day course of 152,083 patients. A consistent clinical and electrodiagnostic phenotype has yet to be well described. In one review, onset of adverse events was described as usually being rapid, with 33% of patients developing symptoms within 24 hours of initiating treatment, 58% within 72 hours, and 84% within one week.[21] One case-control study identified increasing incidence with each additional day of ongoing use, however, suggesting that prolonged use is a potential risk factor. There also has been a report that fluoroquinolones might unmask previously unrecognized hereditary neuropathy.[24] Many of the reported cases did not resolve after discontinuation of the fluoroquinolone.[24,25]

Linezolid

Linezolid is an oxazolidinone antibiotic used to treat infections caused by gram-positive bacteria that are resistant to other antibiotics, including methicillin-resistant *Staphylococcus aureus* (MRSA) or vancomycin-resistant *Enterococcus* (VRE) infections. It is also increasingly being used in regimens against multidrug-resistant or extensively drug-resistant tuberculosis (MDR-TB, XDR-TB), nocardiosis, or actinomycosis.[26] With prolonged use, typically over 28 days, linezolid can lead to a painful, length-dependent sensorimotor polyneuropathy.[27–29] In one review of 22 cases, symptoms of peripheral neuropathy began at a median of 4 months; the earliest onset was 10 days.[30] In another series of 796 patients treated with linezolid, only 3 (1%) developed neuropathy but only one-third of the cohort were treated longer than 28 days.[31] Weakness is typically not seen on examination, but distal loss of both small and large fiber sensory functions and diminished muscle stretch reflexes are common. Allodynia is also common. Two cases of isolated painful small fiber sensory neuropathy have been published.[32,33] Optic neuropathy can also occur, either in isolation or together with peripheral neuropathy. With discontinuation of the drug, neuropathic pain frequently improves but some sensory loss typically persists.

NCS/electromyography (EMG) in most reported cases demonstrate a pattern of length-dependent, symmetric, axonal sensorimotor polyneuropathy. One case showed only absence or severe reduction in SNAP amplitudes, raising the possibility of sensory ganglionopathy.[34]

Mitochondrial dysfunction has been implicated in the pathogenesis of linezolid-induced neuropathy.[35,36] *In vitro* exposure of rodent sensory neurons to linezolid has been shown to lead to mitochondrial dysfunction.[37] Some affected patients develop lactic acidosis, and pathologic samples from a single patient who developed optic neuropathy, encephalopathy, skeletal myopathy, lactic acidosis, and renal failure after prolonged use of linezolid also demonstrated decreased mitochondrial respiratory chain enzyme activity.[38]

Dapsone

Dapsone is used primarily for the treatment of leprosy and for various dermatologic conditions. A primarily motor neuropathy can develop from 5 days to 5 years after starting the drug.[39–43] Weakness initially involves the hands and feet and over time progresses to affect more proximal muscles. Occasionally, patients complain of sensory symptoms without weakness.

Motor and sensory NCSs usually demonstrate reduced amplitudes with normal or only slightly slow conduction velocities.[39–43] The NCSs usually improve after the dapsone is discontinued. Biopsy of the motor nerve terminal at the extensor brevis muscle has demonstrated axonal atrophy and Wallerian degeneration of the distal motor nerve terminals.[43] Sural nerve biopsy may reveal a loss of myelinated nerve fibers. The pathogenic basis of the neuropathy is not known.

Chloroquine

Chloroquine is used in the treatment of malaria, sarcoidosis, systemic lupus erythematosus, scleroderma, and rheumatoid arthritis (RA). Chloroquine is associated with a toxic myopathy characterized by slowly progressive, painless, proximal weakness and atrophy, which is worse in the legs than in the arms (discussed in Chapter 35).[44–46] A neuropathy can also develop with or without the myopathy, leading to sensory loss, distal weakness, and reduced muscle stretch reflexes. The "neuromyopathy" usually appears in patients taking 500 mg/day for a year or more but has been reported with doses as low as 200 mg/day. The signs and symptoms of the neuropathy and myopathy are usually reversible following discontinuation of chloroquine.

Serum creatine kinase (CK) levels are usually elevated due to the superimposed myopathy. NCSs reveal mild slowing of motor and sensory nerve conduction velocities (NCVs) with a mild-to-moderate reduction in the amplitudes. NCSs may be normal in patients with only the myopathy. EMG demonstrates myopathic motor unit action potentials (MUAPs), increased insertional activity in the form of positive sharp waves, fibrillation potentials, and occasionally myotonic potentials, particularly in the proximal muscles. Neurogenic MUAPs and reduced recruitment are found in more distal muscles.

Nerve biopsies demonstrate autophagic vacuoles and inclusions within Schwann cells. Vacuoles may also be evident in muscle biopsies.

The pathogenic basis of the neuropathy is not known but may be related to the amphiphilic properties of the drug. Chloroquine contains both hydrophobic and hydrophilic regions that allow chloroquine to interact with the anionic phospholipids of cell membranes and organelles. This drug–lipid complex may be resistant to digestion by lysosomal enzymes, leading to the formation of autophagic vacuoles filled with myeloid debris that may, in turn, cause degeneration of nerves and muscle fibers.

Hydroxychloroquine

Hydroxychloroquine, also used in the treatment of rheumatologic disorders, is structurally similar to chloroquine. The incidence of associated toxic neuromyopathy is much lower, however.[47] Weakness and histological abnormalities are usually not as severe either.[48] Vacuoles are typically absent on biopsy, but EM still may demonstrate abnormal accumulation of myeloid and curvilinear bodies.

Isoniazid

Isoniazid (INH) is used for the treatment of tuberculosis. One of the most common side effects of INH is peripheral neuropathy.[49–51] Standard doses of INH (3–5 mg/kg/day) are associated with a 2% incidence of neuropathy, while neuropathy develops in at least 17% of patients taking in excess of 6 mg/kg/day of INH. INH inhibits pyridoxal phosphokinase resulting in pyridoxine deficiency. Because INH is metabolized by acetylation, individuals who are slow acetylators (an autosomal-recessive trait) maintain a higher serum concentration of INH and are more at risk of developing the neuropathy than people with rapid acetylation. Acetylation can also slow with age. The elderly, malnourished, and "slow acetylators" are therefore at increased risk of developing the neuropathy.

Patients present with numbness and tingling in their hands and feet. The neuropathy usually develops after 6 months in patients receiving smaller doses but can begin within a few weeks in patients on large doses. The neuropathic symptoms resolve after a few days or weeks upon stopping the INH, if done early. However, if the medication is continued, the neuropathy may evolve with more proximal numbness as well as distal weakness. Recovery at this stage can take months and may be incomplete. Examination reveals loss of all sensory modalities, distal muscle atrophy and weakness, reduced muscle stretch reflexes, and occasionally sensory ataxia. Prophylactic administration of pyridoxine 100 mg/day can prevent the neuropathy from developing.

NCSs reveal decreased amplitudes of the SNAPs. Sural nerve biopsies reveal axonal degeneration and loss of both myelinated and unmyelinated nerve fibers.[50] Autopsy studies have demonstrated degeneration of the dorsal columns.

Ethambutol

Ethambutol is also used to treat tuberculosis and has been associated with a sensory neuropathy and a severe optic neuropathy in patients receiving prolonged doses in excess of 20 mg/kg/day.[52,53] Patients develop numbness in the hands and feet without significant weakness. Examination reveals a loss of large fiber modalities and reduced muscle stretch reflexes distally. The peripheral neuropathy gradually improves after stopping of the medication; however, recovery of the optic neuropathy is more variable.

NCSs reveal decreased amplitudes of the SNAPs with normal sensory distal latencies and conduction velocities. Motor conduction studies are usually normal. A decreased number of myelinated nerve fibers due to axonal degeneration has been noted on nerve biopsies and animal studies.[54] The pathogenic basis of the neuropathy is not known.

Nucleoside Analog Neuropathies

The nucleoside analogs zalcitabine (dideoxycytidine or ddC), didanosine (dideoxyinosine or ddI), stavudine (d4T), and lamivudine (3TC) are antiretroviral nucleoside reverse transcriptase inhibitor used to treat HIV infection. One of the major dose-limiting side effects of these medications is a predominantly sensory, length-dependent, symmetrically painful neuropathy.[55–59] ddC is the most extensively studied nucleoside analog and at doses greater than 0.18 mg/kg/day, is associated with a subacute onset of severe burning and lancinating pains in the feet and hands. One-third of patients on lower doses of ddC (0.03 mg/kg/day) develop a neuropathy within 1 week to a year (mean of 16 weeks) after starting the medication. The cumulative dose of these medications increases the risk of developing neuropathy.[60] On examination, hyperpathia, reduced pinprick, and temperature sensation, and to a lesser degree impaired touch and vibratory perception are found. Muscle stretch reflexes are diminished, particularly at the ankles. Occasionally, mild weakness of the ankles and of foot intrinsics is appreciated. Because of a "coasting effect," patients can continue to worsen even 2–3 weeks after stopping the medication. However, improvement in the neuropathy is seen in most patients following dose reduction after several months (mean time about 10 weeks). While protease inhibitors may be associated with a small increased risk,[61,62] most newer classes of antiretroviral therapy (ART) are not associated with neuropathy.

Because peripheral neuropathy has been associated with HIV infection itself, it can be challenging to isolate the unique pathophysiology of ART-associated neuropathy. One study, for example, suggests that the nucleoside analogs preferentially affect small sensory nerve fibers, leading to reduced intraepidermal nerve fiber density (IENFD) on skin biopsy.[63] Sensory NCSs can reveal decreased amplitudes or absent responses with normal distal latencies and conduction velocities (CVs).[55–58] Motor NCSs are usually normal. Uncontrolled HIV, by contrast, may be more damaging to myelinated nerve fibers and therefore lead to some reduction in NCVs.[55]

These nucleoside analogs inhibit mitochondrial DNA polymerase, which is the suspected pathogenic basis for the neuropathy. Acetyl-carnitine deficiency may also contribute to the neurotoxicity of these nucleoside analogs.

CARDIAC MEDICATIONS

Amiodarone

Amiodarone is an antiarrhythmic medication that is also associated with a neuromyopathy similar to chloroquine.[64–69] Severe proximal and distal weakness can develop in the legs worse than in the arms, combined with distal sensory loss, tingling, and burning pain. In addition, amiodarone is also associated with tremor, thyroid dysfunction, keratitis, pigmentary skin changes, hepatitis, pulmonary fibrosis, and parotid gland hypertrophy. The neuromyopathy typically appears after patients have taken the medication for 2–3 years. Physical examination demonstrates arm and leg weakness, reduced sensation to all modalities, and diminished muscle stretch reflexes. The neuromyopathy usually improves following discontinuation of the drug.

Sensory NCSs reveal markedly reduced amplitudes and, when obtainable, mild-to-moderately slow conduction velocities and prolonged distal latencies.[65,67,68] Motor NCSs may also be abnormal, but usually not to the same degree as seen in sensory studies. EMG demonstrates fibrillation potentials, positive sharp waves, and occasionally myotonic discharges with a mixture of myopathic and neurogenic-appearing MUAPs.

Muscle biopsies demonstrate neurogenic atrophy, particularly in distal muscles, and autophagic vacuoles with myeloid and dense inclusions on EM. Sural nerve biopsies demonstrate a combination of segmental demyelination and axonal loss. EM reveals lamellar or dense inclusions in Schwann cells, pericytes, and endothelial cells. The inclusions in muscle and nerve biopsies have persisted as long as 2 years following discontinuation of the medication.

The pathogenesis is presumably similar to other amphiphilic medications (e.g., chloroquine).[70–73]

RHEUMATOLOGIC/IMMUNOMODULATORY MEDICATIONS

Colchicine

Colchicine is used primarily to treat patients with gout and is also associated with a toxic neuropathy and myopathy.[74–76] Affected individuals usually present with proximal weakness along with numbness and tingling in the distal extremities. Reduced sensation to touch, vibration, position sense, and diminished muscle stretch reflexes are found on examination.

Motor and sensory NCSs demonstrate reduced amplitudes.[74–76] The distal motor and sensory latencies can be normal or slightly prolonged and conduction velocities are normal or mildly slow. EMG demonstrates fibrillation potentials and positive sharp waves along with short-duration, low-amplitude MUAPs in the proximal limb muscles and long-duration, large-amplitude MUAPs distally. Muscle biopsies reveal a vacuolar myopathy, while sensory nerve biopsies demonstrate axonal degeneration.

Colchicine inhibits the polymerization of tubulin into microtubules. The disruption of the microtubules probably leads to defective intracellular movement of important proteins, nutrients, and waste products in muscles and nerves.[75]

Leflunomide

Leflunomide is used for the treatment of RA. It is a prodrug for an active metabolite that reversibly inhibits dihydroorotate dehydrogenase. This enzyme catalyzes the rate-limiting step in the de novo synthesis of pyrimidines that are necessary for lymphocyte production. There have been several reports of patients treated with leflunomide who developed distal numbness and paresthesia.[77–82] The median duration of treatment at the onset of neuropathy was 7.5 months (range 3 weeks to 29 months) in one large study.[79]

NCSs may demonstrate features of a primarily axonal, sensorimotor polyneuropathy.[77–82] More commonly, the NCSs are normal and do not correlate with symptoms, which suggests that leflunomide may cause a small fiber neuropathy.[81] In this regard, a study of leflunomide treatment in patients with RA revealed abnormal cold detection on quantitative sensory testing compared to controls; vibratory thresholds were normal.[82] The neuropathy usually improves after withdrawal of the medication.

Tumor Necrosis Factor Alpha (TNF-α) Antagonists

TNF-α antagonists are used to treat rheumatologic conditions such as RA and include etanercept, infliximab, adalimumab, golimumab, and certolizumab. Infrequent occurrences of both CNS and PNS demyelinating events have been reported in patients on these medications.[83–89] Because of both the rarity and the heterogeneity of these events, an etiologic link with the medications remains uncertain. Reduction in TNF-α levels has been speculated to lead to failed regression of myelin-specific T-cell reactivity and prolonged survival of activated T cells, however, which could promote an autoimmune response.[84]

A wide spectrum of neuropathy phenotypes has been reported in association with TNF-α antagonists, including acute inflammatory demyelinating polyneuropathy (AIDP), chronic inflammatory demyelinating polyneuropathy (CIDP), Miller Fisher variant Guillain–Barré syndrome (GBS), multifocal motor neuropathy, mononeuropathy or mononeuropathy multiplex, and generalized sensory predominant neuropathies. The onset of symptoms has ranged from 2 weeks to 60 months in reported cases. In addition to the cases resembling AIDP or CIDP, many of the other reported cases were suspected to share an immune-mediated pathogenesis based on elevated cerebrospinal fluid (CSF) protein, MRI demonstrating T2 hyperintensity in affected nerve segments, or an associated multisystemic vasculitis. Regardless of the phenotype, these events are rare. An estimated 0.4 cases of neuropathy per 1,000 person-years occurred in one single-center study.[86] In a survey of 1,800 rheumatologists and internists over a 3-year period, nine cases of CIDP and two cases of AIDP were reported.[87] In a registry study that utilized comprehensive literature review to identify complications from TNF-α antagonist therapy, 233 total cases of any secondary autoimmune diseases developed during treatment.[83] The authors estimated that these cases were drawn from a treated population of over 1 million patients. Among these, 6 patients had an isolated neuropathy; another 113 developed some form of vasculitis, 16% of which involved the peripheral nerves. In most cases, patients improved after withdrawal of the TNF-α antagonist with or without immunomodulatory therapy such as intravenous immune globulin. Two patients with CIDP did have relapse when an alternative TNF-α antagonist was tried after they initially improved.[87]

CNS-ACTING MEDICATIONS

Phenytoin

Phenytoin is a commonly used antiepileptic medication. A rare side effect of phenytoin is a mild, primarily sensory neuropathy associated with reduced light touch, proprioception, and vibration as well as diminished or absent muscle stretch reflexes at the ankles.[90–94] Mild distal weakness may be seen. The neuropathy improves on discontinuation of the medication.

NCSs reveal decreased amplitudes of the SNAPs with normal sensory distal latencies and conduction velocities. NCSs demonstrate slightly reduced amplitudes and slow CVs in about 20% of patients taking only phenytoin. Motor NCSs are usually normal. Sural nerve biopsy has reportedly demonstrated a loss of the large myelinated axons along with segmental demyelination and remyelination.[94]

Lithium

Lithium is more often associated with CNS toxicity (tremor, dysarthria, confusion, obtundation, sweating, and seizures), but some patients have developed sensorimotor peripheral neuropathies (distal motor and sensory loss and reduced muscle stretch reflexes).[95–97]

NCSs reveal decreased amplitudes of the SNAPs with normal sensory distal latencies and conduction velocities. NCSs demonstrate reduced amplitudes or absent SNAPs and CMAPs. Nerve biopsies have demonstrated a loss of large myelinated fibers.

Disulfiram

Disulfiram is used in the treatment of alcohol use disorder. It is metabolized to carbon disulfide, which is a neurotoxin and can have adverse effects on both the PNS and the CNS.[98–104] A neuropathy with distal weakness (e.g., foot drop) and sensory loss may develop as early as 10 days to as long as 18 months after starting the drug.

NCSs are suggestive of an axonal sensorimotor polyneuropathy with reduced amplitudes or absent SNAPs and CMAPs with normal or only moderately slow conduction velocities.[98,101,102] Needle EMG reveals fibrillation potentials and positive sharp waves in distal muscles along with decreased recruitment of neurogenic-appearing MUAPs.

Sural nerve biopsy has demonstrated axonal degeneration and segmental demyelination with a loss of predominately large-diameter fibers, although small-diameter fibers can be affected as well.[98–101] On EM, swollen axonal due to the accumulation of neurofilamentous debris within the myelinated and unmyelinated axons may be appreciated.

The neuropathy may be secondary to carbon disulfide, which is a metabolite of disulfiram. A similar axonal neuropathy characterized by accumulation of neurofilaments occurs with carbon disulfide toxicity.

OTHER MEDICATIONS AND SUPPLEMENTS

Pyridoxine (Vitamin B6) Toxicity

Pyridoxine is an essential vitamin that serves as a coenzyme for transamination and decarboxylation. The recommended daily allowance in adults is 2–4 mg. However, at high doses (116 mg/day) patients can develop a severe sensory neuropathy with dysesthesia and sensory ataxia.[105–109] Some patients also complain of a Lhermitte sign. There is one report of a patient taking 9.6-g pyridoxine per day who developed weakness as well.[110] Neurological examination reveals marked impaired vibratory perception and proprioception. Sensory loss can begin and be more severe in the upper than in the lower limbs. Muscle strength is usually normal, although there may be loss of fine motor control. Gait is wide based and unsteady secondary to the sensory ataxia. Muscle stretch reflexes are reduced or absent.

NCSs usually reveal absent or markedly reduced SNAP amplitudes with relatively preserved CMAPs,[105–109] although one case with severe weakness reported reduced CMAP amplitudes and moderately slowing of CVs.[110]

Nerve biopsies have shown loss of axons of all fiber diameters.[108,109] Reduced numbers of dorsal root ganglion cells and subsequent degeneration of both the peripheral and the central sensory tracts have been appreciated in animal models. The pathogenic basis for the neuropathy associated with pyridoxine toxicity is not known.

Podophyllin

Podophyllin is a topical agent used to treat condylomata acuminata. Systemic side effects include pancytopenia and liver and renal dysfunction. Podophyllin is also potentially toxic to both the CNS and the PNS, leading to psychosis, altered consciousness, and polyneuropathy.[111,112] The neuropathy is characterized by slowly progressive sensory loss, paresthesias, muscle weakness, and diminished muscle stretch reflexes in a length-dependent pattern. Autonomic neuropathy with nausea, vomiting, gastrointestinal paresis, urinary retention, orthostatic hypotension, and tachycardia may also occur. The signs and symptoms of this toxic neuropathy can progress for a couple of months even after stopping the medication. The neuropathy gradually improves with discontinuation of the podophyllin, but it can take several months to over a year and residual deficits may remain.

CSF protein levels can be elevated. Laboratory evaluation may also demonstrate pancytopenia, liver function abnormalities, and renal insufficiency. Sensory NCSs reveal absent SNAPs or their reduced amplitudes. Motor NCSs are less affected but can demonstrate reduced amplitudes. Nerve biopsies demonstrate axonal degeneration. Podophyllin binds to microtubules similar to colchicine and probably inhibits axoplasmic flow leading to axonal degeneration.[113]

TOXIC NEUROPATHIES ASSOCIATED WITH INDUSTRIAL AGENTS

ACRYLAMIDE

Clinical Features

Acrylamide, a vinyl monomer, is an important industrial agent used as a flocculating and grouting agent. It can be absorbed through the skin, ingested (following exposure to contaminated well water due to acrylamide grouting of the wells) or inhaled into the lungs. Following exposure, affected individuals may develop a distal sensorimotor polyneuropathy characterized by a loss of large fiber function.[114–118] Pain and paresthesia are uncommon. Some patients have ataxia and dysarthria; increasing irritability may also be seen. Chronic low-level exposure may cause

▶ TABLE 20-2. **TOXIC NEUROPATHIES RELATED TO INDUSTRIAL AGENTS**

Substance	Mechanism of Neurotoxicity	Clinical Features— Neuropathy	Clinical Features— Nonneuropathy	Diagnostic Testing
Acrylamide	Unknown; may be caused by impaired axonal transport	Numbness with loss of large fiber modalities on examination; sensory ataxia; mild distal weakness	Dysarthria and ataxia, hallucinations, confusion, urinary incontinence. Contact dermatitis	Low-amplitude or unobtainable SNAPs with normal or reduced CMAP amplitudes
Carbon disulfide	Unknown	Length-dependent numbness and tingling with mild distal weakness	Psychosis	Low-amplitude or unobtainable SNAPs with normal or reduced CMAP amplitudes
Ethylene oxide	Unknown; may act as alkylating agent and bind DNA	Length-dependent numbness and tingling; may have mild distal weakness	Nausea and vomiting Confusion Dermatitis, mucous membrane irritation	Low-amplitude or unobtainable SNAPs with normal or reduced CMAP amplitudes
Organophosphates	Binds and inhibits neuropathy target esterase	Early features are those of neuromuscular blockade with generalized weakness, including fasciculations; later axonal sensorimotor PN ensues. Pathologic evidence suggests concurrent damage to corticospinal tracts and dorsal columns	Anxiety, emotional lability, confusion or impaired consciousness; ataxia Seizures Nausea, vomiting, diarrhea Bradycardia Pulmonary edema	Early: repetitive firing of CMAPs and decrement with repetitive nerve stimulation. Late: axonal sensorimotor PN
Hexacarbons	Unknown; may lead to covalent cross-linking between neurofilaments	Acute, severe sensorimotor PN that may resemble GBS	Encephalopathy and hallucinations	Features of a mixed axonal and/or demyelinating sensorimotor axonal PN-reduced amplitudes, prolonged distal latencies, conduction block, and slowing of CVs. On nerve biopsy, giant axons swollen with neurofilaments may be seen
Vinyl benzene	Unknown	Pain and paresthesias; primarily small fiber sensory dysfunction	n/a	CMAP CVs may be mildly reduced

CMAP, compound muscle action potential; CV, conduction velocity; GBS, Guillain–Barré syndrome; PN, peripheral neuropathy; SNAP, sensory nerve action potential.

mental confusion and hallucinations in addition to weakness, gait difficulties, and occasionally urinary incontinence. Exposure to the skin is associated with contact dermatitis.

On examination, there is a loss of vibration and proprioception with relatively good preservation of touch, pain, and temperature sensation. Patients may be ataxic and demonstrate a positive Romberg sign. Muscle stretch reflexes are reduced. Mild distal muscle atrophy and weakness may be appreciated. Patients with only low levels of exposure usually make a good recovery; however, those exposed to large amounts can take a year or more for significant improvement to occur and may not completely recover.

Laboratory Features

NCSs reveal decreased amplitudes of the SNAPs with normal sensory distal latencies and conduction velocities. NCSs reveal absent or markedly reduced amplitude in the SNAPs.[114–118] The CMAP amplitudes are normal or only slightly reduced, but temporal dispersion of the CMAPs may be observed in patients exposed to high levels of the substance.

Histopathology

Sural nerve biopsies reveal axonal degeneration with loss of the large myelinated fibers. The earliest histological abnormality in animals exposed to acrylamide is paranodal accumulation of 10-nm neurofilaments at the distal ends of the peripheral nerves. Subsequently, the distal axons enlarge and degenerate as can the posterior columns, spinocerebellar tracts, optic tracts, mammillary bodies, and the corticospinal tracts.

Pathogenesis

The exact pathogenic basis for the toxic neuropathy is unknown but is felt that acrylamide impairs fast bidirectional axonal transport as well as slow antegrade transport.

CARBON DISULFIDE

Clinical Features

Carbon disulfide is used to make rayon and cellophane and can be inhaled or absorbed through the skin. Acute exposure to high levels of carbon disulfide may lead to CNS abnormalities (e.g., psychosis), which resolve with elimination of exposure. Chronic low-level exposure to carbon disulfide has also been associated with a toxic peripheral neuropathy characterized by length-dependent numbness and tingling.[119] Examination reveals a loss of all sensory modalities and diminished muscle stretch reflexes. Mild muscle atrophy and weakness may be evident distally.

Laboratory Features

NCSs reveal slowing of sensory and perhaps motor CVs.

Histopathology

Detailed descriptions of the histopathology in humans are lacking. However, experimental studies in animals have shown accumulation of 10-nm neurofilaments and axonal swellings similar to that seen in acrylamide and hexacarbon toxicity.

Pathogenesis

The pathogenic basis for the neuropathy is not known.

ETHYLENE OXIDE

Clinical Features

Ethylene oxide may be used to sterilize heat-sensitive materials, and exposure to ethylene oxide usually is associated with dermatologic lesions, mucosal membrane irritation, nausea, vomiting, and altered mentation. Exposure to high levels can lead to a severe sensorimotor peripheral neuropathy characterized by distal numbness and paresthesia.[120,121] Examination demonstrates a loss of all sensory modalities and occasionally distal weakness. Dysmetria due to a sensory ataxia, unsteady gait, and diminished muscle stretch reflexes are also seen.

Laboratory Features

NCSs demonstrate reduced amplitudes or absent SNAPs and CMAPs.

Histopathology

Sensory nerve biopsies reveal the loss of primarily, but not exclusively, the large myelinated fibers.

Pathogenesis

The pathogenic basis of the neuropathy is not known. Ethylene oxide can act as an alkylating agent and can bind with many organic molecules, including DNA.

ORGANOPHOSPHATE POISONING

Clinical Features

The organophosphates are used in the production of insecticides, plastics, petroleum products, and as toxic nerve agents for biological warfare. Exposure to organophosphates can lead to severe neurological CNS and PNS side effects.[122–127] These compounds inhibit acetylcholinesterase and result in the accumulation of acetylcholine at cholinergic synapses. Thus, toxic exposure to organophosphate esters may produce acute clinical symptoms and signs referable to peripheral muscarinic and nicotinic receptors as well as in the CNS. The CNS side effects include anxiety, emotional lability, ataxia, altered mental status, unconsciousness, and seizures. The muscarinic effects can cause nausea, vomiting, abdominal cramping, diarrhea, pulmonary edema, and bradycardia. Side effects at nicotinic synapses at the neuromuscular junction result in generalized weakness and fasciculations.

Some patients with acute organophosphate toxicity later develop a distal sensorimotor peripheral neuropathy [organophosphate-induced delayed polyneuropathy (OPIDP)].[122–127] OPIDP evolves after several weeks following exposure and maximizes within several weeks. Cramping in the calf muscles, burning or tingling in the feet, and distal weakness are early symptoms. Symptoms and signs may then progress to involve the hands. Increased tone and hyperreflexia may be seen because of superimposed CNS dysfunction. The prognosis is good in patients with mild peripheral neuropathy. However, those individuals with severe peripheral and CNS insults generally do not fully recover and are left with significant residual deficits.

Laboratory Features

In the acute and subacute stages of toxic exposure, there is electrophysiological evidence of neuromuscular dysfunction secondary to compromise of acetylcholinesterase.[122–127] Motor NCSs may demonstrate repetitive firing of the CMAPs following a single nerve stimulus. On low rates of repetitive stimulation, a decrementing response is seen, and this can persist for about 4–11 days. At both low (2–5 Hz) and high (20 Hz) rates of repetitive stimulation, the CMAP amplitudes initially decrement but then recover—approaching the baseline amplitudes. In OPIDP, NCSs reveal decreased amplitudes of SNAPs and CMAPs consistent with an axonal sensorimotor polyneuropathy.

Histopathology

Autopsy studies have demonstrated a distal axonopathy and degeneration of the gracile fasciculus and the corticospinal tract. In addition, marked loss of both myelinated and unmyelinated nerve fibers in the sural nerve and a moderate loss of nerve fibers in the sciatic nerve were observed on autopsy of a patient who died from exposure to sarin gas.[122]

Pathogenesis

The pathogenic basis for OPIDP is not clear. Organophosphates bind to and inhibit an enzyme called neuropathy target esterase (NTE).[125] However, inhibition of NTE is not sufficient for the development of OPIDP. The organophosphate—NTE complex must age, whereby a lateral side chain of NTE is cleaved. Downstream this leads to the degeneration of nerves.

HEXACARBONS (n-HEXANE, METHYL n-BUTYL KETONE)

Clinical Features

n-Hexane and methyl n-butyl ketone are water-insoluble industrial organic solvents, which are also present in some glues. Exposure through inhalation, accidentally or intentionally (glue sniffing), or through skin absorption can lead to a profound subacute sensorimotor polyneuropathy progressing over the course of 4–6 weeks.[128–133] The neuropathy presents with numbness and tingling in the feet and later involves the proximal legs and arms. Progressive weakness also develops. Ventilatory muscles are usually spared.

Laboratory Features

NCSs demonstrate decreased amplitudes of the SNAPs and CMAPs with slightly slow CVs.[128,131,132] Partial conduction block has also been appreciated in motor conduction studies in some patients.[104]

Histopathology

Nerve biopsy has revealed a loss of myelinated nerve fibers and the presence of giant axons (Fig. 20-1).[129] Segmental demyelination may be seen. EM reveals that the swollen axons are filled with 10-nm neurofilaments.

Pathogenesis

The exact mechanism by which hexacarbons cause a toxic neuropathy is not known. Hexacarbon exposure may lead to covalent cross-linking between axonal neurofilaments, which results in their aggregation, impaired axonal transport, swelling of the axons, and eventual axonal degeneration.

VINYL BENZENE (STYRENE)

Vinyl benzene or styrene is used to make some plastics and synthetic rubber. Toxic exposure leads to a primarily sensory neuropathy with burning pain and paresthesia in the legs.[134] Neurological examination demonstrates a reduction in pain and temperature, with relatively good preservation of proprioception, vibration sense, and muscle stretch reflexes. Strength is normal. NCSs demonstrate a mild reduction in motor conduction velocities in the lower limbs.

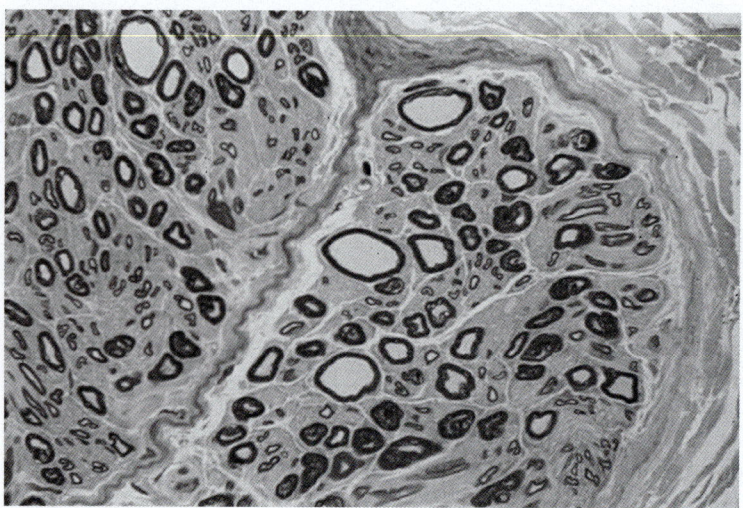

Figure 20-1. Hexacarbon toxicity. Giant axons are appreciated on this nerve biopsy in an individual who developed a severe neuropathy associated with chronic glue sniffing. (Reproduced with permission from Amato AA, Dumitru D. Acquired neuropathies. In: Dumitru D, Amato AA, Swartz MJ, eds. *Electrodiagnostic Medicine*, 2nd ed. Philadelphia, PA: Hanley & Belfus, 2002.)

▶ NEUROPATHIES ASSOCIATED WITH HEAVY METAL INTOXICATION

Heavy metal toxicity can be associated with axonal polyneuropathy. The severity of the neuropathy is usually related to the amount of metal that entered the patient's system either acutely or chronically. Clinical improvement is dependent on cessation of the exposure and supportive measures. Multiple organ systems can be involved besides the PNS, which can serve as an important clue to the specific toxic exposure.

LEAD

Clinical Features

Lead neuropathy is uncommon, but it can be seen in children who accidentally ingest lead-based paints in older buildings or in industrial workers exposed to lead-containing products. The most common presentation of lead poisoning is an encephalopathy, but symptoms and signs of a primarily motor neuropathy can also occur.[135–141] The neuropathy is characterized by an insidious and progressive onset of weakness usually beginning in the arms, particularly involving the wrist/finger extensor muscles such that it resembles a radial neuropathy. Foot drop can be seen. Weakness can be asymmetric. Sensation is generally preserved; however, the autonomic nervous system can be affected, leading to constipation. Muscle stretch reflexes are diminished and plantar responses are flexor. Bluish black discoloration of gums near the teeth may be appreciated.

Laboratory Features

Laboratory investigation can reveal microcytic/hypochromic anemia with basophilic stippling of erythrocytes and an elevated serum coproporphyrin level. A 24-hour urine collection may demonstrate elevated levels of lead excretion. The NCSs typically reveal reduced CMAP amplitudes, while the SNAPs are usually normal.

Histopathology

Nerve biopsy may show a loss of large myelinated axons.

Pathogenesis

The pathogenic mechanism of nerve injury is unclear but may be related to abnormal porphyrin metabolism (see Chapter 12). It is not known if the primary target of the toxic insult is the anterior horn cell or more distally in the peripheral nerve.

Treatment

The most important treatment is removing the source of the exposure. Chelation therapy with calcium disodium ethylenediaminetetraacetate, British anti-Lewisite, and penicillamine has been tried with variable success.

MERCURY

Clinical Features

Mercury toxicity may occur as a result of exposure to either organic or inorganic mercurials. The organic form of mercury is usually found in methyl or ethyl mercury; ingestion of seafood, especially large predatory fish, is a common source of exposure. Organic mercury poisoning presents with paresthesias in hands and feet, which progress

▶ TABLE 20-3. TOXIC NEUROPATHIES RELATED TO HEAVY METALS

Substance	Clinical Features—Neurological	Clinical Features—Nonneurologic	NCS/EMG Findings	Detection
Lead	Motor neuropathy (often resembles radial neuropathy with wrist and finger drop); Autonomic neuropathy	Encephalopathy; Bluish-black discoloration of gums	Reduction of CMAP amplitudes with active denervation on EMG	24-hour urine collection for lead excretion; elevated serum coproporphyrin. Microcytic anemia with basophilic stippling may also be a clue
Mercury	Organic mercury: paresthesias in hands and feet, ataxia. Encephalopathy. Inorganic mercury: sensorimotor PN	Inorganic: Abdominal pain, Nephrotic syndrome, bronchitis or pneumonitis	Low-amplitude or unobtainable SNAPs with normal or reduced CMAP amplitudes	24-hour urine collection for detection inorganic mercury; organic mercury much harder to diagnose
Thallium	Encephalopathy with thirst and psychosis; painful sensory symptoms; mild loss of vibration; distal or generalized weakness may also develop; autonomic neuropathy	Abdominal pain and vomiting often first symptoms; pigmentation of hair; acne-like malar rash; alopecia; anemia; renal insufficiency; Mee's lines at base of nails	Low-amplitude or unobtainable SNAPs with normal or reduced CMAP amplitudes	Thallium levels typically elevated in both serum and urine
Arsenic	Burning pain, and paresthesia; generalized weakness; autonomic insufficiency; can resemble GBS. Encephalopathy is common	Abdominal discomfort, nausea, vomiting, and diarrhea precede the neuropathy. Change in skin pigmentation. Anemia. Mee's lines at base of nails	Low-amplitude or unobtainable SNAPs with normal or reduced CMAP amplitudes may have demyelinating features: prolonged distal latencies and slowing of CVs	Serum testing unreliable. Test urine, hair, or fingernails
Gold	Distal paresthesia and reduction of all sensory modalities	Rash and pruritus	Low-amplitude or unobtainable SNAPs	Reliable testing not available

CMAP, compound muscle action potential; CV, conduction velocity; GBS, Guillain–Barré syndrome; PN, peripheral neuropathy; SNAP, sensory nerve action potential; EMG, electromyography; NCS, nerve conduction study.

proximally and may involve the face and tongue.[142–147] The CNS is also affected, so patients may have dysarthria, ataxia, reduced mentation, and visual and hearing loss.

The inorganic mercury compounds are primarily used for industrial purposes and consist of various mercury salts. Toxicity may arise from ingestion or inhalation of the compounds. Gastrointestinal symptoms and nephrotic syndrome are the primary clinical features associated with acute toxicity with inorganic mercury, but encephalopathy and sensorimotor polyneuropathy can also develop.

Laboratory Features

Organic mercury intoxication is difficult to diagnose because the metal is highly lipid soluble and thus remains in the body, so urinary excretion can be scant. Inorganic mercury is more readily excreted and a 24-hour urine collection can reveal an increased concentration of this metal. Sensory NCSs may reveal low-amplitude SNAPs and borderline CVs.[142,144–147] Motor conductions are normal or show borderline CVs. Somatosensory-evoked potentials of the median nerve demonstrate absent cortical but present peripheral potentials.[147] Needle EMG is usually normal, but occasionally, there is abnormal spontaneous activity in the form of positive sharp waves and fibrillation potentials.

Histopathology

Autopsies of patients with organic mercury toxicity through eating contaminated fish in Minimata Bay demonstrated degeneration of the calcarine aspect of the cerebral cortex, cerebellum, and axons in the sural nerves and lumbar dorsal roots that likely account for the visual loss, ataxia, and polyneuropathy.

Pathogenesis

Mercury may bind to sulfhydryl groups of enzymatic or structural proteins, thereby impairing their proper function and leading to degeneration of the neurons. The primary site of neuromuscular pathology appears to be the dorsal root ganglia.

Treatment

The mainstay of treatment is removing the source of exposure. Too few patients have been treated with chelating agents such as penicillamine to adequately assess efficacy.

THALLIUM

Clinical Features

Thallium can exist in a monovalent or trivalent form and is primarily used as a rodenticide. Thallium poisoning usually manifests as burning paresthesias of the feet, abdominal pain, and vomiting.[148–151] Increased thirst, sleep disturbances, and psychotic behavior may be noted. Within the first week, patients develop pigmentation of the hair, an acne-like rash in the malar area of the face, and hyperreflexia. By the second and third weeks, autonomic instability with labile heart rate and blood pressure may be seen in addition. Hyporeflexia and alopecia also occur but may not be evident until the third or fourth week following exposure.

On examination, there is a reduction in pain and temperature sensation along with a mild decrease in vibratory perception and proprioception. Muscle stretch reflexes are reduced distally but generally preserved proximally. Distal muscle atrophy and weakness gradually ensue. With severe intoxication, proximal weakness and involvement of the cranial nerves can occur. Some patients require mechanical ventilation due to respiratory muscle involvement. The lethal dose of thallium is variable, ranging from 8 to 15 mg/kg of body weight. Death can result in less than 48 hours following a particularly large dose.

Laboratory Features

Serum and urine levels of thallium are increased. Routine laboratory testing can reveal anemia, renal insufficiency, and abnormal liver function tests. CSF protein levels are also elevated. NCSs demonstrate features of a primarily axonal, sensorimotor polyneuropathy.[148–151] Within the first few days of intoxication NCSs can be normal. After 1–2 weeks, the SNAPs and CMAPs in the legs have reduced amplitudes and H-reflexes are lost.

Histopathology

Autopsy studies and nerve biopsies demonstrate chromatolysis of cranial and spinal motor nuclei, dorsal spinal ganglia, and axonal degeneration of motor and sensory nerves.[148–151]

Pathogenesis

The pathogenic basis for the toxicity is not known.

Treatment

With acute intoxication, potassium ferric ferrocyanide II may be effective in preventing absorption of thallium from the gut. However, there may be no benefit once thallium has been absorbed. Unfortunately, chelating agents are not very efficacious. Adequate diuresis is essential to help eliminate thallium from the body without increasing tissue availability from the serum.

ARSENIC

Clinical Features

Arsenic is another heavy metal that is associated with a toxic sensorimotor polyneuropathy.[152–156] The neuropathy manifests 5–10 days after ingestion of arsenic and progresses for several weeks and can mimic GBS clinically. The presenting symptoms are typically an abrupt onset of abdominal discomfort, nausea, vomiting, pain, and diarrhea, followed, within several days, by burning pain in the feet and hands. Subsequently, distal weakness ensues, and, with severe intoxication, proximal muscles and the cranial nerves are also affected. Muscle stretch reflexes are reduced. Some patients require mechanical ventilation because of ventilatory muscle involvement. Increased morbidity and mortality are associated with ventilatory muscle weakness and autonomic instability. Some patients appear confused due to a superimposed encephalopathy.

Examination of the skin can be helpful in diagnosing arsenic poisoning. The loss of the superficial epidermal layer results in patchy regions of increased or decreased pigmentation on the skin several weeks after an acute exposure or with chronic low levels of ingestion. Mee's lines, which are transverse lines at the base of fingernails and toenails, do not become evident until 1 or 2 months after exposure. Multiple Mee's lines may be appreciated in patients with long fingernails with more chronic exposure to arsenic. Mee's lines are not specific for arsenic toxicity, as these can also be seen following thallium poisoning. These arise from transient episodes of growth arrest.

Laboratory Features

Because arsenic is cleared from blood rapidly, assessing serum concentration of arsenic is not a reliable method to diagnose toxicity. However, arsenic levels are increased in the urine, hair, or fingernails of patients exposed to arsenic. Anemia with stippling of erythrocytes is common and occasionally pancytopenia and aplastic anemia can develop. Increased CSF protein levels without pleocytosis can be seen, which again can lead to a misdiagnosis of

Guillain–Barré syndrome. NCSs are usually more suggestive of an axonal sensorimotor polyneuropathy; however, demyelinating features can be present.[152–156] Sensory NCSs reveal low-amplitude or absent SNAPs with relatively preserved distal latencies and CVs. Motor conduction studies may demonstrate possible conduction block and prolongation of F-wave latencies. Serial studies may show progressive deterioration of the CMAP amplitudes to distal stimulation associated with slowing of the conduction velocities. Needle EMG reveals positive sharp waves and fibrillation potentials with reduced numbers of motor units in the distal muscles progressing proximally in patients exposed to significant amounts of arsenic.

Histopathology

Nerve biopsies demonstrate axonal degeneration, reduced large- and small-diameter myelinated fibers, and occasionally onion-bulb formations. Autopsy studies have revealed a loss of anterior horn cells.

Pathogenesis

The pathogenic basis of arsenic toxicity is not known. Arsenic may react with sulfhydryl groups of enzymatic (e.g., pyruvate dehydrogenase complex) and structural proteins in the neurons leading to their degeneration.

Treatment

Chelation therapy with British anti-Lewisite has yielded inconsistent results and its effect is not dramatic; therefore, it is not generally recommended.

GOLD

Clinical Features

Gold therapy (e.g., sodium aurothiomalate) was used in the past to treat RA. Some patients treated with gold salts develop a sensorimotor neuropathy several months following drug initiation manifesting as distal paresthesias in the hands and feet and occasionally mild weakness.[157,158] In addition, a systemic reaction (e.g., rash and pruritus) to the gold usually accompanies the neuropathic symptoms. Examination reveals reduced sensation to all modalities and diminished muscle stretch reflexes. Fasciculations or myokymia may be evident on examination. It may be impossible to distinguish the toxic neuropathy related to gold to the other more common neuropathies associated with RA (see Chapter 16).

Laboratory Features

NCSs reveal reduced amplitudes of SNAPs with relative preservation of motor studies.

Histopathology

Nerve biopsies demonstrate axonal degeneration and segmental demyelination.

Pathogenesis

The pathogenic basis for the neuropathy is not known. It may be related to an immunological reaction triggered by the gold therapy.

Treatment

Treatment consists of stopping the gold therapy. British anti-Lewisite has been tried as well in a few patients, but it is unclear if this therapy is effective.

▶ NEUROPATHY ASSOCIATED WITH ALCOHOL USE DISORDER

Alcohol-related peripheral neuropathy had at one time been assumed to be the result of nutritional deficiency, based on observations made decades ago that the neuropathy seemed to be similar to that observed with thiamine deficiency (see Chapter 18).[159] Over time, however, evidence has mounted that alcohol exerts a direct toxic effect on nerves.[160,161] When careful laboratory testing is used to exclude thiamine deficiency, not only does an association between neuropathy and alcohol use remain, a distinct phenotype emerges.[162,163] Patients with alcohol-related neuropathy *without* nutritional deficiency develop a small fiber predominant sensory axonopathy. Pain and burning discomfort distally in the feet are the most common presenting symptoms. Progression is chronic over months to years, with numbness and pain reaching higher up the legs. About half of patients develop some mild distal weakness; autonomic symptoms are sparse. Small fiber sensory modalities are most affected on neurologic examination, but the Achilles reflexes are reduced or absent in 86% of patients. By contrast, weakness and deficits in large fiber sensory modalities are more prominent among patients with thiamine deficiency, and the onset is often acute.

Electrodiagnostic testing in patients with alcohol-related neuropathy is consistent with sensory > motor axonal degeneration. While mild-to-moderate reduction in the motor and sensory NCVs may be seen, it is typically commensurate with the reduction in response amplitudes. Similarly, sural nerve biopsies have demonstrated histopathological findings consistent with a small fiber sensory axonopathy, with more prominent loss of unmyelinated axons. Segmental demyelination and remyelination resulting from widening of consecutive nodes of Ranvier has also been reported.

The cumulative lifetime dose of ethanol seems to be the most important risk factor for the development of neuropathy.[164–166] It has been estimated that an intake of 100 mL of pure ethanol—the equivalent of 3 L of beer or 300 mL of spirits—per day for 3 years is the minimum required for the development of neuropathy.[163] In another study, 41% of patients with a lifetime consumption of more than 15 kg of ethanol per kilogram of body weight had developed neuropathy.[166] The exclusive consumption of wine may be associated with an even greater risk of neuropathy, perhaps due to impurities such as lead.

Clinicians should screen carefully for alcohol use among patients presenting with a new diagnosis of neuropathy, as patients may underreport use. In some cohorts of patients being worked up for the cause of their polyneuropathy, alcohol is found to play an etiologic role in 5%-10% of cases.[164] Occasionally, routine blood work may disclose clues—elevated liver function tests, for example, or macrocytosis of red blood cells. Cessation of alcohol use can lead to slow, partial improvement of the neuropathy. Even in patients with another underlying cause, it is prudent to advise that alcohol be used only in moderation to avoid further damage.

► SUMMARY

Many drugs and environmental exposures have been associated with a toxic neuropathy, and thus the need for taking extensive medication and exposure history in any patient being evaluated for a neuromuscular disorder. The mechanisms by which these agents cause neuropathy are variable. These may have a primary effect on the neuronal cell body (ganglionopathy, the Schwann cells and myelin sheath, or axons). Most of the time, the neuropathies stabilize and improve after discontinuing the offending agent. However, there can be a coasting effect such that the neuropathy clinically worsens for a few months even after stopping the medication.

REFERENCES

1. Coxon A, Pallis CA. Metronidazole neuropathy. *J Neurol Neurosurg Psychiatry*. 1976;39(4):403–405.
2. Takeuchi H, Yamada A, Touge T, Miki H, Nishioka M, Hashimoto S. Metronidazole neuropathy: a case report. *Psychiatry Clin Neurosci*. 1988;42(2):291–295.
3. Zivkovic S, Lacomis D, Guiliani M. Sensory neuropathy associated with metronidazole: report of four cases and review of the literature. *J Clin Neuromuscul Dis*. 2001;3(1):8–12.
4. Gondim FAA, Brannagan TH III, Sander HW, Chin RL, Latov N. Peripheral neuropathy in patients with inflammatory bowel disease. *Brain*. 2005;128(4):867–879.
5. Tan CH, Chen YF, Chen CC, Chao CC, Liou HH, Hsieh ST. Painful neuropathy due to skin denervation after metronidazole-induced neurotoxicity. *J Neurol Neurosurg Psychiatry*. 2011;82(4):462–466.
6. Hobson-Webb LD, Roach ES, Donofrio PD. Metronidazole: newly recognized cause of autonomic neuropathy. *J Child Neurol*. 2006;21(5):429–431.
7. Bradley WG, Karlsson IJ, Rassol CG. Metronidazole neuropathy. *Br Med J*. 1977;2(6087):610–611.
8. Leitsch D, Kolarich D, Binder M, Stadlmann J, Altmann F, Duchêne M. Trichomonas vaginalis: metronidazole and other nitroimidazole drugs are reduced by the flavin enzyme thioredoxin reductase and disrupt the cellular redox system. Implications for nitroimidazole toxicity and resistance. *Mol Microbiol*. 2009;72(2):518–536.
9. Seok JI, Yi H, Song YM, Lee WY. Metronidazole-induced encephalopathy and inferior olivary hypertrophy: lesion analysis with diffusion-weighted imaging and apparent diffusion coefficient maps. *Arch Neurol*. 2003;60(12):1796.
10. Daneman N, Cheng Y, Gomes T, et al. Metronidazole-associated neurologic events: a nested case-control study. *Clin Infect Dis*. 2021;72(12):2095–2100.
11. Melgaard B, Hansen HS, Kamieniecka Z, et al. Misonidazole neuropathy: a clinical, electrophysiological, and histological study. *Ann Neurol*. 1982;12(1):10–17.
12. Walker MD, Strike TA. Misonidazole peripheral neuropathy: its relationship to plasma concentration and other drugs. *Cancer Clin Trials*. 1980;3(2):105–109.
13. Mamoli B, Wessely P, Kogelnik HD, Müller M, Rathkolb O. Electroneurographic investigations of misonidazole polyneuropathy. *Eur Neurol*. 1979;18(6):405–414.
14. Paulson OB, Melgaard B, Hansen HS, et al. Misonidazole neuropathy. *Acta Neurol Scand Suppl*. 1984;100:133–136.
15. Alston TA, Abeles RH. Enzymatic conversion of the antibiotic metronidazole to an analog of thiamine. *Arch Biochem Biophys*. 1987;257(2):357–362.
16. de Olivarius BF. Polyneuropathy due to nitrofurantoin therapy. *Ugeskr Laeger*. 1956;118(26):753–755.
17. Yiannikas C, Pollard JD, McLeod JG. Nitrofurantoin neuropathy. *Aust N Z J Med*. 1981;11(3):400–405.
18. Toole JF, Parrish ML. Nitrofurantoin polyneuropathy. *Neurology*. 1973;23(5):554–554.
19. Kammire LD, Donofrio PD. Nitrofurantoin neuropathy: a forgotten adverse. *Obstet Gynecol*. 2007;110(2):510–512.
20. Tan IL, Polydefkis M, Ebenezer G, Hauer P, McArthur J. Peripheral nerve toxic effects of nitrofurantoin. *Arch Neurol*. 2012;69(2):265–268.
21. Cohen JS. Peripheral neuropathy associated with fluoroquinolones. *Ann Pharmacother*. 2001;35(12):1540–1547.
22. Etminan M, Brophy JM, Samii A. Oral fluoroquinolone use and risk of peripheral neuropathy: a pharmacoepidemiologic study. *Neurology*. 2014;83(14):1261–1263.
23. Morales D, Pacurariu A, Slattery J, Pinheiro L, McGettigan P, Kurz X. Association between peripheral neuropathy and exposure to oral fluoroquinolone or amoxicillin-clavulanate therapy. *JAMA Neurol*. 2019;76(7):827–833.
24. Panas M, Karadima G, Kalfakis N, Vassilopoulos D. Hereditary neuropathy unmasked by levofloxacin. *Ann Pharmacother*. 2011;45(10):1312–1313.
25. Huruba M, Farcas A, Leucuta DC, Bucsa C, Mogosan C. A VigiBase descriptive study of fluoroquinolone-associated peripheral nervous system disorders. *Pharmaceuticals*. 2022;15(2):143.
26. Conradie F, Bagdasaryan TR, Borisov S, et al; ZeNix Trial Team. Bedaquiline-pretomanid-linezolid regimens for drug-resistant tuberculosis. *N Engl J Med*. 2022;387(9):810–823.
27. Legout L, Senneville E, Gomel JJ, Yazdanpanah Y, Mouton Y. Linezolid-induced neuropathy. *Clin Infect Dis*. 2004;38(5):767–768.
28. Rho JP, Sia IG, Crum BA, Dekutoski MB, Trousdale RT. Linezolid-associated peripheral neuropathy. *Mayo Clin Proc*. 2004;79(7):927–930.

29. Bressler AM, Zimmer SM, Gilmore JL, Somani J. Peripheral neuropathy associated with prolonged use of linezolid. *Lancet Infect Dis.* 2004;4(8):528–531.
30. Narita M, Tsuji BT, Yu VL. Linezolid-associated peripheral and optic neuropathy, lactic acidosis, and serotonin syndrome. *Pharmacotherapy.* 2007;27(8):1189–1197.
31. Birmingham MC, Rayner CR, Meagher AK, Flavin SM, Batts DH, Schentag JJ. Linezolid for the treatment of multidrug-resistant, gram-positive infections: experience from a compassionate-use program. *Clin Infect Dis.* 2003;36(2):159–168.
32. Chao CC, Sun HY, Chang YC, Hsieh ST. Painful neuropathy with skin denervation after prolonged use of linezolid. *J Neurol Neurosurg Psychiatry.* 2008;79(1):97–99.
33. Heckmann JG, Dütsch M, Schwab S. Linezolid-associated small-fiber neuropathy. *J Peripher Nerv Syst.* 2008;13(2):157–158.
34. Zivkovic SA, Lacomis D. Severe sensory neuropathy associated with long-term linezolid use. *Neurology.* 2005;64(5):926–927.
35. Lee E, Burger S, Shah J, et al. Linezolid-associated toxic optic neuropathy: a report of 2 cases. *Clin Infect Dis.* 2003;37(10):1389–1391.
36. Apodaca AA, Rakita RM. Linezolid-induced lactic acidosis. *N Engl J Med.* 2003;348(1):86–87.
37. Bobylev I, Maru H, Joshi AR, Lehmann HC. Toxicity to sensory neurons and Schwann cells in experimental linezolid-induced peripheral neuropathy. *J Antimicrob Chemother.* 2016;71(3):685–691.
38. de Vriese AS, Coster RV, Smet J, et al. Linezolid-induced inhibition of mitochondrial protein synthesis. *Clin Infect Dis.* 2006;42(8):1111–1117.
39. Navarro JC, Rosales RL, Ordinario AT, Izumo S, Osame M. Letter to the editor. *Muscle Nerve.* 1989;12(7):604–606.
40. Ahrens EM, Meckler RJ, Callen JP. Dapsone-induced peripheral neuropathy. *Int J Dermatol.* 1986;25(5):314–316.
41. Gutmann L, Martin JD, Welton W. Dapsone motor neuropathy—an axonal disease. *Neurology.* 1976;26(6):514–514.
42. Rapoport AM, Guss SB. Dapsone-induced peripheral neuropathy. *Arch Neurol.* 1972;27(2):184–185.
43. Sirsat AM, Lalitha VS, Pandya SS. Dapsone neuropathy-report of three cases and pathologic features of a motor nerve. *Int J Lepr Other Mycobact Dis.* 1987;55(1):23–29.
44. Estes ML, Ewing-Wilson D, Chou SM, et al. Chloroquine neuromyotoxicity. Clinical and pathologic perspective. *Am J Med.* 1987;82(3):447–455.
45. Mastaglia FL, Papadimitriou JM, Dawkins RL, Beveridge B. Vacuolar myopathy associated with chloroquine, lupus erythematosus and thymoma. *J Neurol Sci.* 1977;34(3):315–328.
46. Wasay M, Wolfe GI, Herrold JM, Burns DK, Barohn RJ. Chloroquine myopathy and neuropathy with elevated CSF protein. *Neurology.* 1998;51(4):1226–1227.
47. Stein M, Bell MJ, Ang LC. Hydroxychloroquine neuromyotoxicity. *J Rheumatol.* 2000;27(12):2927–2931.
48. Papazisis G, Siafis S, Cepaytye D, et al. Safety profile of chloroquine and hydroxychloroquine: a disproportionality analysis of the FDA Adverse Event Reporting System database. *Eur Rev Med Pharmacol Sci.* 2021;25(19):6003–6012.
49. Jones WA, Jones GP. Peripheral neuropathy due to isoniazid report of two cases. *The Lancet.* 1953;261(6770):1073–1074.
50. Ochoa J. Isoniazid neuropathy in man: quantitative electron microscope study. *Brain.* 1970;93(4):831–850.
51. Ohnishi A, Chua CL, Kuroiwa Y. Axonal degeneration distal to the site of accumulation of vesicular profiles in the myelinated fiber axon in experimental isoniazid neuropathy. *Acta Neuropathol.* 1985;67(3–4):195–200.
52. Tugwell P, James SL. Peripheral neuropathy with ethambutol. *Postgrad Med J.* 1972;48(565):667–670.
53. Nair VS, LeBrun M, Kass I. Peripheral neuropathy associated with ethambutol. *Chest.* 1980;77(1):98–100.
54. Matsuoka Y, Takayanagi T, Sobue I. Experimental ethambutol neuropathy in rats. *J Neurol Sci.* 1981;51(1):89–99.
55. Berger AR, Arezzo JC, Schaumburg HH, et al. 2′,3′-dideoxycytidine (ddC) toxic neuropathy: a study of 52 patients. *Neurology.* 1993;43(2):358–362.
56. Blum AS, Dal Pan GJ, Feinberg J, et al. Low-dose zalcitabine-related toxic neuropathy: frequency, natural history, and risk factors. *Neurology.* 1996;46(4):999–1003.
57. Dubinsky RM, Yarchoan R, Dalakas M, Broder S. Reversible axonal neuropathy from the treatment of AIDS and related disorders with 2′,3′-dideoxycytidine (ddc). *Muscle Nerve.* 1989;12(10):856–860.
58. Verma A, Schein RMH, Jayaweera DT, Kett DH. Fulminant neuropathy and lactic acidosis associated with nucleoside analog therapy. *Neurology.* 1999;53(6):1365–1365.
59. Julian T, Rekatsina M, Shafique F, Zis P. Human immunodeficiency virus–related peripheral neuropathy: a systematic review and meta-analysis. *Eur J Neurol.* 2021;28(4):1420–1431.
60. Lambert JS, Seidlin M, Reichman RC, et al. 2′,3′-dideoxyinosine (ddI) in patients with the acquired immunodeficiency syndrome or AIDS-related complex. A phase I trial. *N Engl J Med.* 1990;322(19):1333–1340.
61. Crabb C. Protease inhibitors and risk of developing HIV-related sensory neuropathy. *AIDS.* 2004;18(14):N9–N11.
62. Ellis RJ, Marquie-Beck J, Delaney P, et al. Human immunodeficiency virus protease inhibitors and risk for peripheral neuropathy. *Ann Neurol.* 2008;64(5):566–572.
63. Kokotis P, Schmelz M, Papadimas GK, et al. Polyneuropathy induced by HIV disease and antiretroviral therapy. *Clin Neurophysiol.* 2013;124(1):176–182.
64. Charness ME, Morady F, Scheinman MM. Frequent neurologic toxicity associated with amiodarone therapy. *Neurology.* 1984;34(5):669–669.
65. Fraser AG, McQueen IN, Watt AH, Stephens MR. Peripheral neuropathy during longterm high-dose amiodarone therapy. *J Neurol Neurosurg Psychiatry.* 1985;48(6):576–578.
66. Jacobs JM, Costa-Jussa FR. The pathology of amiodarone neurotoxicity. II. Peripheral neuropathy in man. *Brain.* 1985;108(3):753–769.
67. Meier C, Kauer B, Müller U, Ludin HP. Neuromyopathy during chronic amiodarone treatment. A case report. *J Neurol.* 1979;220(4):231–239.
68. Pellissier JF, Pouget J, Cros D, de Victor B, Serratrice G, Toga M. Peripheral neuropathy induced by amiodarone chlorhydrate. A clinicopathological study. *J Neurol Sci.* 1984;63(2):251–266.
69. Orr CF, Ahlskog JE. Frequency, characteristics, and risk factors for amiodarone neurotoxicity. *Arch Neurol.* 2009;66(7):865–869.
70. Chong PH, Boskovich A, Stevkovic N, Bartt RE. Statin-associated peripheral neuropathy: review of the literature. *Pharmacotherapy.* 2004;24(9):1194–1203.
71. Gaist D, Jeppesen U, Andersen M, García Rodríguez LA, Hallas J, Sindrup SH. Statins and risk of polyneuropathy: a case-control study. *Neurology.* 2002;58(9):1333–1337.

72. Corrao G, Zambon A, Bertù L, Botteri E, Leoni O, Contiero P. Lipid lowering drugs prescription and the risk of peripheral neuropathy: an exploratory case-control study using automated databases. *J Epidemiol Community Health (1978)*. 2004;58(12):1047–1051.
73. Tierney EF, Thurman DJ, Beckles GL, Cadwell BL. Association of statin use with peripheral neuropathy in the US population 40 years of age or older. *J Diabetes*. 2013;5(2):207–215.
74. Kuncl RW, Cornblath DR, Avila O, Duncan G. Electrodiagnosis of human colchicine myoneuropathy. *Muscle Nerve*. 1989;12(5):360–364.
75. Kuncl RW, Duncan G, Watson D, Alderson K, Rogawski MA, Peper M. Colchicine myopathy and neuropathy. *N Engl J Med*. 1987;316(25):1562–1568.
76. Riggs JE, Schochet SS, Gutmann L, Crosby TW, DiBartolomeo AG. Chronic human colchicine neuropathy and myopathy. *Arch Neurol*. 1986;43(5):521–523.
77. Gabelle A, Antoine JC, Hillaire-Buys D, Coudeyre E, Camu W. Neuropathie axonale sévère et léflunomide. *Rev Neurol (Paris)*. 2005;161(11):1106–1109.
78. Kho LK, Kermode AG. Leflunomide-induced peripheral neuropathy. *J Clin Neurosci*. 2007;14(2):179–181.
79. Martin K, Bentaberry F, Dumoulin C, et al. Neuropathy associated with leflunomide: a case series. *Ann Rheum Dis*. 2005;64(4):649–650.
80. Metzler C, Arlt AC, Gross WL, Brandt J. Peripheral neuropathy in patients with systemic rheumatic diseases treated with leflunomide. *Ann Rheum Dis*. 2005;64(12):1798–1800.
81. Richards BL, Spies J, McGill N, et al. Effect of leflunomide on the peripheral nerves in rheumatoid arthritis. *Intern Med J*. 2007;37(2):101–107.
82. Kim HK, Park SB, Park JW, et al. The effect of leflunomide on cold and vibratory sensation in patients with rheumatoid arthritis. *Ann Rehabil Med*. 2012;36(2):207–212.
83. Ramos-Casals M, Brito-Zerón P, Muñoz S, et al. Autoimmune diseases induced by TNF-targeted therapies: analysis of 233 cases. *Medicine*. 2007;86(4):242–251.
84. Stübgen JP. Tumor necrosis factor-α antagonists and neuropathy. *Muscle Nerve*. 2008;37(3):281–292.
85. Kunchok A, Aksamit AJ, Davis JM, et al. Association between tumor necrosis factor inhibitor exposure and inflammatory central nervous system events. *JAMA Neurol*. 2020;77(8):937–946.
86. Tsouni P, Bill O, Truffert A, et al. Anti-TNF alpha medications and neuropathy. *J Peripher Nerv Syst*. 2015;20(4):397–402.
87. Seror R, Richez C, Sordet C, et al. Pattern of demyelination occurring during anti-TNF-α therapy: a French national survey. *Rheumatology (Oxford)*. 2013;52(5):868–874.
88. Lozeron P, Denier C, Lacroix C, Adams D. Long-term course of demyelinating neuropathies occurring during tumor necrosis factor-alpha-blocker therapy. *Arch Neurol*. 2009;66(4):490–497.
89. Richez C, Blanco P, Lagueny A, Schaeverbeke T, Dehais J. Neuropathy resembling CIDP in patients receiving tumor necrosis factor-alpha blockers. *Neurology*. 2005;64(8):1468–1470.
90. Dobkin BH. Reversible subacute peripheral neuropathy induced by phenytoin. *Arch Neurol*. 1977;34(3):189–190.
91. Chokroverty S, Sayeed ZA. Motor nerve conduction study in patients on diphenylhydantoin therapy. *J Neurol Neurosurg Psychiatry*. 1975;38(12):1235–1239.
92. Lovelace RE, Horwitz SJ. Peripheral neuropathy in long-term diphenylhydantoin therapy. *Arch Neurol*. 1968;18(1):69–77.
93. Shorvon SD, Reynolds EH. Anticonvulsant peripheral neuropathy: a clinical and electrophysiological study of patients on single drug treatment with phenytoin, carbamazepine or barbiturates. *J Neurol Neurosurg Psychiatry*. 1982;45(7):620–626.
94. Ramirez JA, Mendell JR, Warmolts JR, Griggs RC. Phenytoin neuropathy: structural changes in the sural nerve. *Ann Neurol*. 1986;19(2):162–167.
95. Brust JCM, Hammer JS, Challenor Y, Healton EB, Lesser RP. Acute generalized polyneuropathy accompanying lithium poisoning. *Ann Neurol*. 1979;6(4):360–362.
96. Pamphlett RS, Mackenzie RA. Severe peripheral neuropathy due to lithium intoxication. *J Neurol Neurosurg Psychiatry*. 1982;45(7):656.
97. Johnston SR, Burn D, Brooks DJ. Peripheral neuropathy associated with lithium toxicity. *J Neurol Neurosurg Psychiatry*. 1991;54(11):1019–1020.
98. Ansbacher LE, Bosch EP, Cancilla PA. Disulfiram neuropathy: a neurofilamentous distal axonopathy. *Neurology*. 1982;32(4):424–424.
99. Bergouignan FX, Vital C, Henry P, Eschapasse P. Disulfiram neuropathy. *J Neurol*. 1988;235(6):382–383.
100. Borrett D, Ashby P, Bilbao J, Carlen P. Reversible, late-onset disulfiram-induced neuropathy and encephalopathy. *Ann Neurol*. 1985;17(4):396–399.
101. Mokri B, Ohnishi A, Dyck PJ. Disulfiram neuropathy. *Neurology*. 1981;31(6):730.
102. Palliyath SK, Schwartz BD, Gant L. Peripheral nerve functions in chronic alcoholic patients on disulfiram: a six month follow up. *J Neurol Neurosurg Psychiatry*. 1990;53(3):227–230.
103. Olney RK, Miller RG. Peripheral neuropathy associated with disulfiram administration. *Muscle Nerve*. 1980;3(2):172–175.
104. Filosto M, Tentorio M, Broglio L, et al. Disulfiram neuropathy: two cases of distal axonopathy. *Clin Toxicol*. 2008;46(4):314–316.
105. Dalton K, Dalton MJT. Characteristics of pyridoxine overdose neuropathy syndrome. *Acta Neurol Scand*. 1987;76(1):8–11.
106. Albin RL, Albers JW. Long-term follow-up of pyridoxine-induced acute sensory neuropathy-neuronopathy. *Neurology*. 1990;40(8):1319.
107. Albin RL, Albers JW, Greenberg HS, et al. Acute sensory neuropathy-neuronopathy from pyridoxine overdose. *Neurology*. 1987;37(11):1729–1729.
108. Schaumburg H, Kaplan J, Windebank A, et al. Sensory neuropathy from pyridoxine abuse. *N Eng J Med*. 1983;309(8):445–448.
109. Parry GJ, Bredesen DE. Sensory neuropathy with low-dose pyridoxine. *Neurology*. 1985;35(10):1466–1466.
110. Gdynia HJ, Müller T, Sperfeld A-D, et al. Severe sensorimotor neuropathy after intake of highest dosages of vitamin B6. *Neuromuscul Disord*. 2008;18(2):156–158.
111. Filley CM, Graff-Radford NR, Lacy JR, Heitner MA, Earnest MP. Neurologic manifestations of podophyllin toxicity. *Neurology*. 1982;32(3):308–311.
112. Campbell AN. Accidental poisoning with podophyllin. *The Lancet*. 1980;315(8161):206–207.
113. Paulson JC, McClure WO. Microtubules and axoplasmic transport. Inhibition of transport by podophyllotoxin: an interaction with microtubule protein. *J Cell Biol*. 1975;67(2):461–467.
114. Leswing RJ, Ribelin WE. Physiologic and pathologic changes in acrylamide neuropathy. *Arch Environ Health*. 1969;18(1):23–29.
115. Davenport JG, Farrell DF, Sumi SM. "Giant axonal neuropathy" caused by industrial chemicals: neurofilamentous axonal masses in man. *Neurology*. 1976;26(10):919–923.

116. Sumner AJ, Asbury AK. Acrylamide neuropathy: selective vulnerability of sensory fibers. *Trans Am Neurol Assoc.* 1974; 99:79–83.
117. LoPachin RM, Balaban CD, Ross JF. Acrylamide axonopathy revisited. *Toxicol Appl Pharmacol.* 2003;188(3):135–153.
118. Kjuus H, Goffeng LO, Heier MS, et al. Effects on the peripheral nervous system of tunnel workers exposed to acrylamide and N-methylolacrylamide. *Scand J Work Environ Health.* 2004;30(1):21–29.
119. Corsi G, Maestrelli P, Picotti G, Manzoni S, Negrin P. Chronic peripheral neuropathy in workers with previous exposure to carbon disulphide. *Br J Ind Med.* 1983;40(2):209–211.
120. Finelli PF, Morgan TF, Yaar I, Granger CV. Ethylene oxide-induced polyneuropathy. *Arch Neurol.* 1983;40(7):419–421.
121. Kuzuhara S, Kanazawa I, Nakanishi T, Egashira T. Ethylene oxide polyneuropathy. *Neurology.* 1983;33(3):377–380.
122. Himuro K, Murayama S, Nishiyama K, et al. Distal sensory axonopathy after sarin intoxication. *Neurology.* 1998;51(4):1195–1197.
123. Besser R, Gutmann L, Dillmann U, Weilemann LS, Hopf HC. End-plate dysfunction in acute organophosphate intoxication. *Neurology.* 1989;39(4):561–567.
124. de Jager AEJ, van Weerden TW, Houthoff HJ, de Monchy JGR. Polyneuropathy after massive exposure to parathion. *Neurology.* 1981;31(5):603–605.
125. Lotti M, Becker CE, Aminoff MJ. Organophosphate polyneuropathy: pathogenesis and prevention. *Neurology.* 1984;34(5):658–662.
126. Vasilescu C, Alexianu M, Dan A. Delayed neuropathy after organophosphorus insecticide (Dipterex) poisoning: a clinical, electrophysiological and nerve biopsy study. *J Neurol Neurosurg Psychiatry.* 1984;47(5):543–548.
127. Wadia RS, Chitra S, Amin RB, Kiwalkar RS, Sardesai H V. Electrophysiological studies in acute organophosphate poisoning. *J Neurol Neurosurg Psychiatry.* 1987;50(11):1442–1448.
128. Korobkin R, Asbury AK, Sumner AJ, Nielsen SL. Glue-sniffing neuropathy. *Arch Neurol.* 1975;32(3):158–162.
129. Towfighi J, Gonatas NK, Pleasure D, Cooper HS, McCree L. Glue sniffer's neuropathy. *Neurology.* 1976;26(3):238–238.
130. Spencer PS, Schaumburg HH, Raleigh RL, Terhaar CJ. Nervous system degeneration produced by the industrial solvent methyl n-butyl ketone. *Arch Neurol.* 1975;32(4):219–222.
131. Allen N, Mendell J, Billmaier D, Fontaine R, O'Neill J. Toxic polyneuropathy due to methyl n-butyl ketone. An industrial outbreak. *Arch Neurol.* 1975;32(4):209–218.
132. King PJL, Morris JGL, Pollard JD. Glue Sniffing Neuropathy. *Aust N Z J Med.* 1985;15(3):293–299.
133. Pastore C, Izura V, Marhuenda D, Prieto MJ, Roel J, Cardona A. Partial conduction blocks in N-hexane neuropathy. *Muscle Nerve.* 2002;26(1):132–135.
134. Behari M, Choudhary C, Roy S, Maheshwari MC. Styrene-induced peripheral neuropathy. *Eur Neurol.* 1986;25(6):424–427.
135. Feldman RG, Hayes MK, Younes R, Aldrich FD. Lead neuropathy in adults and children. *Arch Neurol.* 1977;34(8):481–488.
136. Feldman RG, Haddow J, Kopito L, Schwachman H. Altered peripheral nerve conduction velocity. *Am J Dis Child.* 1973;125(1):39–41.
137. Jeyaratnam J, Devathasan G, Ong CN, Phoon W-O, Wong PK. Neurophysiological studies on workers exposed to lead. *Occup Environ Med.* 1985;42(3):173–177.
138. Seppäläinen AM, Hernberg S. Sensitive technique for detecting subclinical lead neuropathy. *Occup Environ Med.* 1972;29(4):443–449.
139. Seppäläinen AM, Tola S, Hernberg S, Kock B. Subclinical neuropathy at "safe" levels of lead exposure. *Arch Environ Health.* 1975;30(4):180–183.
140. Seto DS, Freeman J. Lead neuropathy in childhood. *Am J Dis Child.* 1964;107(4):337–342.
141. Simpson JA, Seaton DA, Adams JF. Response to treatment with chelating agents of anaemia, chronic encephalopathy, and myelopathy due to lead poisoning. *J Neurol Neurosurg Psychiatry.* 1964;27(6):536–541.
142. Albers JW, Cavender GD, Levine SP, Langolf GD. Asymptomatic sensorimotor polyneuropathy in workers exposed to elemental mercury. *Neurology.* 1982;32(10):1168–1168.
143. Adams CR, Ziegler DK, Lin JT. Mercury intoxication simulating amyotrophic lateral sclerosis. *JAMA.* 1983;250(5):642–643.
144. Iyer K, Goodgold J, Eberstein A, Berg P. Mercury poisoning in a dentist. *Arch Neurol.* 1976;33(11):788–790.
145. Shapiro Irving M, Sumner Austin J, Spitz Lawrence K, et al. Neurophysiological and neuropsychological function in mercury-exposed dentists. *Lancet.* 1982;319(8282):1147–1150.
146. le Quesne PM, Damluji SF, Rustam H. Electrophysiological studies of peripheral nerves in patients with organic mercury poisoning. *J Neurol Neurosurg Psychiatry.* 1974;37(3):333–339.
147. Tokuomi H, Uchino M, Imamura S, Yamanaga H, Nakanishi R, Ideta T. Minamata disease (organic mercury poisoning): neuroradiologic and electrophysiologic studies. *Neurology.* 1982;32(12):1369–1369.
148. Dumitru D, Kalantri A. Electrophysiologic investigation of thallium poisoning. *Muscle Nerve.* 1990;13(5):433–437.
149. Bank WJ, Pleasure DE, Suzuki K, Nigro M, Katz R. Thallium poisoning. *Arch Neurol.* 1972;26(5):456–464.
150. Limos LC, Ohnishi A, Suzuki N, et al. Axonal degeneration and focal muscle fiber necrosis in human thallotoxicosis: histopathological studies of nerve and muscle. *Muscle Nerve.* 1982;5(9):698–706.
151. Davis LE, Standefer JC, Kornfeld M, Abercrombie DM, Butler C. Acute thallium poisoning: toxicological and morphological studies of the nervous system. *Ann Neurol.* 1981;10(1):38–44.
152. Donofrio PD, Wilbourn AJ, Albers JW, Do LR, Salanga V, Greenberg HS. Acute arsenic intoxication presenting as Guillain–Barré-like syndrome. *Muscle Nerve.* 1987;10(2):114–120.
153. Goddard MJ, Tanhehco JL, Dau PC. Chronic arsenic poisoning masquerading as Landry-Guillain-Barré syndrome. *Electromyogr Clin Neurophysiol.* 1992;32(9):419–423.
154. Murphy MJ, Lyon LW, Taylor JW. Subacute arsenic neuropathy: clinical and electrophysiological observations. *J Neurol Neurosurg Psychiatry.* 1981;44(10):896–900.
155. Oh SJ. Electrophysiological profile in arsenic neuropathy. *J Neurol Neurosurg Psychiatry.* 1991;54(12):1103–1105.
156. Greenberg S. Acute demyelinating polyneuropathy with arsenic ingestion. *Muscle Nerve.* 1996;19(12):1611–1613.
157. Katrak SM, Pollock M, Brien CPO, et al. Clinical and morphological features of gold neuropathy. *Brain.* 1980;103(3):671–693.
158. Mitsumoto H, Wilbourn AJ, Subramony SH. Generalized myokymia and gold therapy. *Arch Neurol.* 1982;39(7):449–450.

159. Mellion M, Gilchrist JM, de La Monte S. Alcohol-related peripheral neuropathy: nutritional, toxic, or both? *Muscle Nerve*. 2011;43(3):309–316.
160. Bosch EP, Pelham RW, Rasool CG, et al. Animal models of alcoholic neuropathy: morphologic, electrophysiologic, and biochemical findings. *Muscle Nerve*. 1979;2(2):133–144.
161. Mellion ML, Nguyen V, Tong M, Gilchrist J, de La Monte S. Experimental model of alcohol-related peripheral neuropathy. *Muscle Nerve*. 2013;48(2):204–211.
162. Koike H, Iijima M, Sugiura M, et al. Alcoholic neuropathy is clinicopathologically distinct from thiamine-deficiency neuropathy. *Ann Neurol*. 2003;54(1):19–29.
163. Behse F, Buchthal F. Alcoholic neuropathy: clinical, electrophysiological, and biopsy findings. *Ann Neurol*. 1977;2(2):95–110.
164. Julian T, Glascow N, Syeed R, Zis P. Alcohol-related peripheral neuropathy: a systematic review and meta-analysis. *J Neurol*. 2019;266(12):2907–2919.
165. Vittadini G, Buonocore M, Colli G, Terzi M, Fonte R, Biscaldi G. Alcoholic polyneuropathy: a clinical and epidemiological study. *Alcohol Alcohol*. 2001;36(5):393–400.
166. Monforte R, Estruch R, Valls-Solé J, Nicolás J, Villalta J, Urbano-Marquez A. Autonomic and peripheral neuropathies in patients with chronic alcoholism. A dose-related toxic effect of alcohol. *Arch Neurol*. 1995;52(1):45–51.

CHAPTER 21

Neuropathies Associated with Endocrinopathies

Various peripheral neuropathies are associated with the different endocrinopathies (Table 21-1). In particular, peripheral neuropathy associated with diabetes mellitus (DM) is one of the most common causes worldwide.

▶ DIABETIC NEUROPATHY

DM is the most common endocrinopathy and can be separated into two major subtypes: (1) insulin-dependent DM (IDDM or type 1 DM) and (2) non–insulin-dependent DM (NIDDM or type 2 DM). DM is the most common cause of peripheral neuropathy in developed countries. DM is associated with several types of polyneuropathies: distal symmetric sensory or sensorimotor polyneuropathy, autonomic neuropathy, treatment-induced diabetic neuropathy (TIND), diabetic neuropathic cachexia (DNC), radiculoplexus neuropathies, cranial neuropathies, and other mononeuropathies (Table 21-1).[1-6] Nearly half of patients with type 1 or type 2 diabetes, including children and adults, develop a neuropathy.[3,6,7]

Long-standing, poorly controlled DM, and the presence of retinopathy and nephropathy are risk factors for the development of peripheral neuropathy in diabetic patients.[8] In a large community-based study, 1.3% of the population had DM (27% type 1 DM and 73% type 2 DM).[8] Of these, approximately 66% of individuals with type 1 DM had some form of neuropathy: generalized polyneuropathy, 54%; asymptomatic median neuropathy at the wrist, 22%; symptomatic carpal tunnel syndrome, 11%; autonomic neuropathy, 7%; and various other mononeuropathies alone or in combination (3%) such as ulnar neuropathy, peroneal neuropathy, lateral femoral cutaneous neuropathy, and diabetic polyradiculoneuropathy. In the type 2 DM group, 45% had generalized polyneuropathy, 29% had asymptomatic median neuropathy at the wrist, 6% had symptomatic carpal tunnel syndrome, 5% had autonomic neuropathy, and 3% had other mononeuropathies/multiple mononeuropathies. Considering all forms of DM, 66% of patients had some objective signs of neuropathy, but only 20% of patients with DM were symptomatic from neuropathy.

DIABETIC DISTAL SYMMETRIC SENSORY AND SENSORIMOTOR POLYNEUROPATHY

Clinical Features

Distal symmetric sensory polyneuropathy (DSPN) is the most common form of diabetic neuropathy.[1-6] It is a length-dependent neuropathy in which affected individuals develop sensory loss beginning in the toes, which gradually progresses over time up the legs and into the fingers and arms.[6,7] When severe, a patient may also develop sensory loss in the trunk (chest and abdomen) in the midline that spreads out laterally toward the spine. There is a predilection for earlier involvement of small myelinated and unmyelinated nerve fibers lead to paresthesia, lancinating pains, burning, or a deep aching discomfort in 40%–60% of patients.[1,9] A severe loss of sensation can lead to increased risk of infection, ulceration, and Charcot joints. Patients with small fiber neuropathy can also develop symptoms and signs of an autonomic dysfunction, as the autonomic nervous system is mediated by small myelinated and unmyelinated nerve fibers. Poor control of DM and the presence of nephropathy correlate with an increased risk of developing or worsening of DSPN.[3,8]

Neurological examination reveals loss of small fiber function (pain and temperature sensation) only or pan-modality sensory loss. Those individuals with large fiber sensory loss have reduced muscle stretch reflexes, particularly at the ankles, but reflexes can be normal in patients with only small fiber involvement or in patients whose neuropathy has not ascended far enough proximally to affect the reflex arc of the Achilles deep tendon reflex. Muscle strength and function are typically normal, although mild atrophy and weakness of foot intrinsics and ankle dorsiflexors may be detected. Because patients without motor symptoms or signs on clinical examination often still have electrophysiological evidence of subclinical motor involvement, the term "distal symmetric or length-dependent sensorimotor peripheral neuropathy" is also appropriate.[10]

Laboratory Features

DSPN can be the presenting manifestation of DM as many patients may be unaware of their abnormal glucose metabolism.

▶ **TABLE 21-1. NEUROPATHIES ASSOCIATED WITH ENDOCRINOPATHIES**

Diabetes Mellitus
    Distal symmetric sensory and sensorimotor polyneuropathy
    Autonomic neuropathy
    Diabetic neuropathic cachexia
    Polyradiculoplexus neuropathy
    Mononeuropathy/multiple mononeuropathies
    Acute treatment–induced painful neuropathy
Metabolic Syndrome
Hypoglycemia/Hyperinsulinemia
    Generalized sensory or sensorimotor polyneuropathy
Acromegaly
    Generalized sensory or sensorimotor polyneuropathy
    Carpal tunnel syndrome
Hypothyroidism
    Carpal tunnel syndrome
    Generalized sensory or sensorimotor polyneuropathy

There may be an increased risk of impaired glucose tolerance (IGT) on oral glucose tolerance test even in those individuals with normal fasting blood sugars (FBS) and hemoglobin A1C levels. Some studies report IGT (defined as 2-hour glucose of >140 and <200 mg/dL) in as many as 36% and DM (defined as 2-hour glucose of >200 mg/dL or FBS of >126 mg/dL) in up to 31% of patients with sensory neuropathy.[11-13] In patients with painful sensory neuropathy, the incidence of IGT or DM may be even higher. Although we have been impressed with the prevalence of IGT in our patients with burning feet, the linkage of IGT with DSPN remains controversial as other authorities have not found an association.[14,15]

Up to 50% of patients with DM have reduced sensory nerve action potential (SNAP) amplitudes and slow conduction velocities of the sural or plantar nerves, while up to 80% of symptomatic individuals have abnormal sensory nerve conduction studies (NCSs).[1,16,17,18] Quantitative sensory testing (QST) may reveal reduced vibratory and thermal perception. Autonomic testing may also be abnormal, in particular quantitative sweat testing.[19]

Motor NCSs are less severely affected than the sensory studies but still are frequently abnormal with low amplitudes and normal or only slightly prolonged distal latencies and slow nerve conduction velocities (NCVs).[1,15,16] Rarely, the NCV slowing can be within the "demyelinating range" (e.g., <30% below the lower limit of normal); however, conduction block and temporal dispersion are not usually appreciated.[16,17] Needle electromyography (EMG) examination may demonstrate fibrillation potentials, positive sharp waves, and large motor unit action potentials (MUAPs) in the distal muscles.

Histopathology

Nerve biopsies are not routinely done in patients with DSPN. In part, this is because of the nonspecific nature of the nerve pathology and the potential for poor wound healing in diabetics. If performed, nerve biopsy can reveal axonal degeneration, clusters of small, regenerated axons, and segmental demyelination that is more pronounced distally, as expected in a length-dependent process (Fig. 21-1).[19] An asymmetric loss of axons between and within nerve fascicles may be appreciated. There is often endothelial hyperplasia of epi- and endoneurial arterioles and capillaries along with redundant basement membranes around these small blood vessels and thickening of the basement membrane of the perineurial cells (Fig. 21-2).[20] In addition, perivascular infiltrate consisting predominantly of CD8+ T cells can sometimes be seen.

Nerve biopsies may appear normal in patients with pure small fiber neuropathy. However, skin biopsies can demonstrate

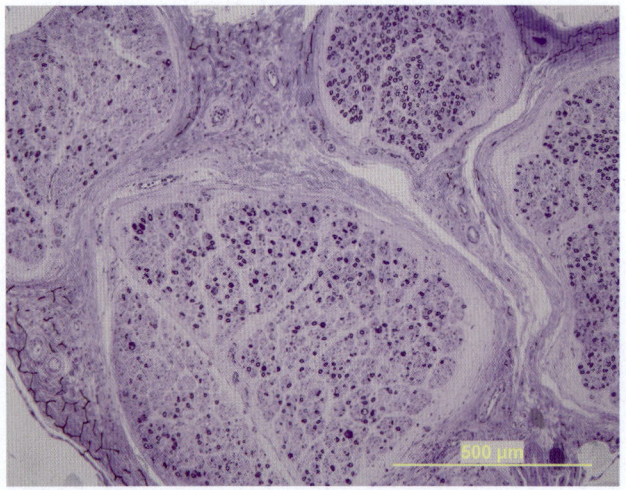
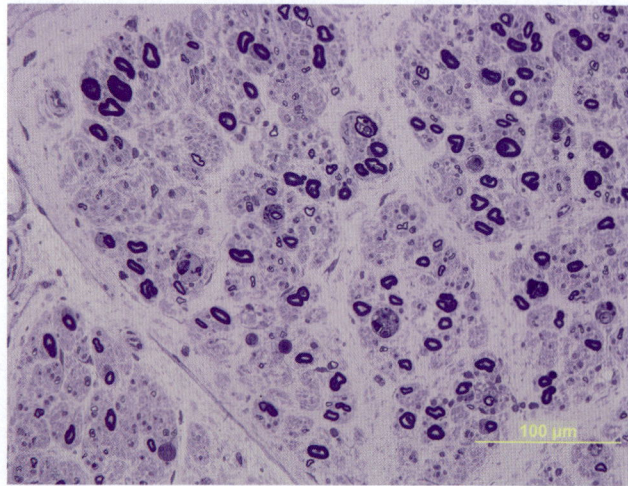

Figure 21-1. Diabetic neuropathy. Sural nerve biopsy demonstrates asymmetric loss of myelinated nerve fibers between and within nerve fascicles (**A**). Higher power reveals loss of large and small fibers and active axonal degeneration (**B**). Plastic sections stained with toluidine blue.

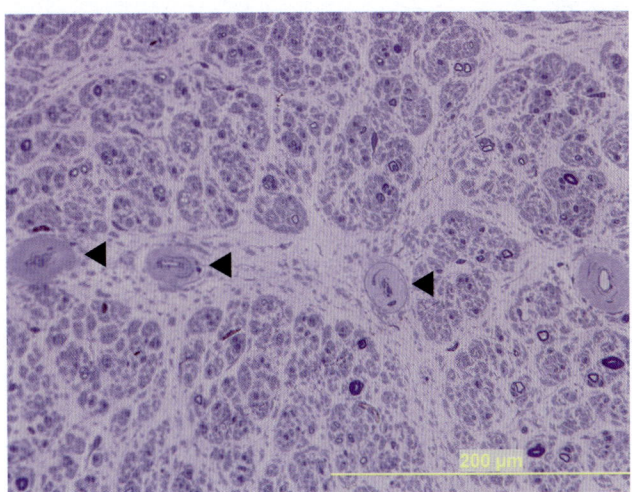

Figure 21-2. Diabetic neuropathy. Sural nerve biopsy demonstrates marked loss of myelinated nerve fibers and blood vessels with markedly thickened basement membrane (*arrowheads*). Plastic sections stained with toluidine blue.

a reduction of small myelinated intraepidermal nerve fibers in such cases.[21–23] Reduced intraepidermal nerve fiber densities correlate with impaired temperature thresholds on QST and the duration of the DM.[23] Patients with IGT are more likely to have a predominantly small fiber neuropathy, compared to patients with DM, who have more involvement of large nerve fibers.[13]

Pathogenesis

The exact pathogenic basis for DSPN is unknown. Notably, glycemic control prevents DPN development in type 1 diabetes, however, glycemic control has modest or no benefit in individuals with type 2 diabetes.[6,24] Thus, some surmise that DSPN has different pathogenic mechanisms in type 1 and type 2 diabetes, with the former being more related to hyperglycemia and the later from other complications of metabolic syndrome.[24]

Suspected pathogenic mechanisms of DSPN include abnormalities in various metabolic processes, microangiopathic ischemia, and inflammation (Fig. 21-3).[1,24–29] In regard to aberrant metabolism, diabetes is associated with hyperglycemia, dyslipidemia, and impaired insulin signaling. Increased intracellular glucose may damage neurons by causing excessive glycolysis that overloads mitochondria, resulting in the production of reactive oxygen species (ROS).[1,6,24,30] Furthermore, polyol pathway activity may be increased leading to hyperosmolarity and oxidative stress.[6] Hyperglycemia is also associated with glycosylation of reactive carbohydrate groups to various proteins, lipids, nucleic acids, and the so-called advanced glycation end products (AGEs), which impair their normal function.[1,6] Also, these AGEs may bind to a receptor (RAGE), which in turn, leads to activation of inflammatory cascades and oxidative stress. Increased free fatty acids and triglycerides bind to receptors on neurons and Schwann cells leading to increased oxidative stress and inflammation. Diminished insulin production (seen in type 1 DM) and insulin resistance (seen in type 2 DM) may be associated with abnormal neurotrophic effects.[1]

Treatment

The mainstay of treatment and prevention of DSPN in type 1 diabetes is tight control of glucose, as studies have shown that this can reduce the risk of developing neuropathy or improve the underlying neuropathy.[6,24,31–34] As mentioned previously though tight control of glycemia does not appear to have a similar benefit in type 2 diabetes.[6,24] Pancreatic transplantation may stabilize or slightly improve sensory, motor, and autonomic function in severe type 1 diabetes, but this is not a pragmatic solution for most patients.[19,33] A few small studies have suggested alpha-lipoic acid, an antioxidant, at doses of 400–600 mg a day may improve neuropathic sensory symptoms such as pain and several other neuropathic end points.[35,36] A recent meta-analysis reported that exercise may be beneficial in treating DSPN.[37] Most guidelines recommend antidepressants (tricyclic or serotonin uptake inhibitors), gabapentinoids (pregabalin or gabapentin), and/or sodium channel blockers as initial analgesic treatment for DSPN (Table 21-2).[38–49] A recent study comparing amitriptyline plus pregabalin, pregabalin plus amitriptyline, duloxetine plus pregabalin, and monotherapies of each for initial treatment of diabetic peripheral neuropathic pain found that all three combination treatments and monotherapies had similar analgesic efficacy.[48]

In patients with just distal leg pain, we often try lidoderm patches on the feet, as this is associated with fewer systemic side effects. If this is insufficient or patients have more generalized pain, we often start gabapentin at a dose of 300 mg TID or pregabalin (50 mg TID). We typically go with gabapentin initially because it is less expensive. We gradually increase the dosage as tolerated and necessary. If this is still ineffective, we usually add an antidepressant medication: duloxetine (30–120 mg daily), venlafaxine (37.5–225 mg daily), or a tricyclic antidepressant medication (amitriptyline 25–100 mg every night), again starting at a low dose and gradually increasing as tolerated. For breakthrough pain, we have prescribed tramadol 50 mg every 6 hours.[42] In general though we try to avoid opioids. There is little evidence that oxcarbazepine, lamotrigine, topiramate, lacosamide, mexiletine, magnets, or Reiki therapy are of any significant benefit.[1,38,39]

DIABETIC AUTONOMIC NEUROPATHY

Clinical Features

Autonomic neuropathy typically is seen in combination with DSPN and only rarely in isolation.[1,4–6,50–52] The autonomic neuropathy can manifest as abnormal sweating, dry feet, dysfunctional thermoregulation, dry eyes and mouth, pupillary abnormalities, cardiac arrhythmias, postural hypotension, gastrointestinal abnormalities (e.g., gastroparesis, postprandial bloating, chronic diarrhea, or constipation), and genitourinary dysfunction (e.g., impotence, retrograde ejaculation,

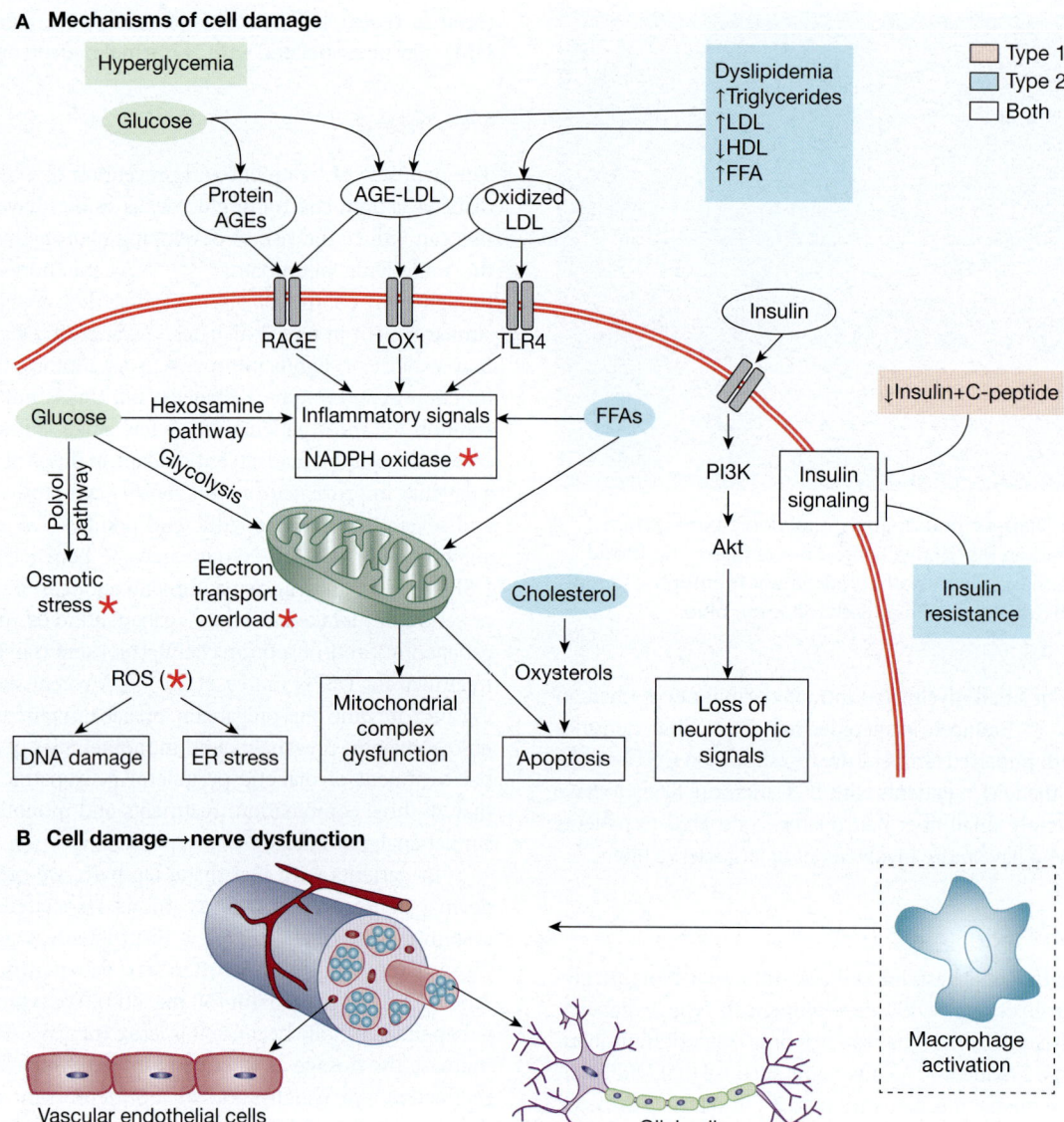

Figure 21-3. Mechanisms of diabetic neuropathy. Factors linked to type 1 diabetes (*orange*), type 2 diabetes (*blue*), and both (*green*) cause DNA damage, endoplasmic reticulum stress, mitochondrial complex dysfunction, apoptosis, and loss of neurotrophic signaling (**A**). This cell damage can occur in neurons, glial cells, and vascular endothelial cells, as well as trigger macrophage activation, all of which can lead to nerve dysfunction and neuropathy (**B**). The relative importance of the pathways in this network will vary with cell type, disease profile, and time. AGE, advanced glycation end products; LDL, low-density lipoprotein; HDL, high-density lipoprotein; FFA, free fatty acids; ROS, reactive oxygen species (*red star*); ER, endoplasmic reticulum; PI3 K, phosphatidylinositol-3-kinase; LOX1, oxidized LDL receptor 1; RAGE, receptor for advanced glycation end products; TLR4, toll-like receptor 4. (Reproduced with permission from Callaghan BC, Cheng HT, Stables CL, et al. Diabetic neuropathy: Clinical manifestations and current treatments. *Lancet Neurol.* 2012;11(6):521–534.)

and incontinence). Importantly, the presence of autonomic neuropathy doubles the risk of mortality.[53]

Laboratory Features

Tests of autonomic function are generally abnormal, including impaired heart rate variability on deep breathing, blood pressure and heart rate on Valsalva maneuver, and reduction on sweat production on sudomotor testing (see section regarding Autonomic Testing in Chapter 2).[50–52] Sensory and motor NCSs generally demonstrate the same features described above with DSPN.

Histopathology

Degeneration of sympathetic and parasympathetic neurons along with inflammatory infiltrates within the ganglia has been appreciated.[54]

▶ TABLE 21-2. TREATMENT OF PAINFUL SENSORY NEUROPATHIES

Therapy	Route	Dose	Side Effects
First Line			
Pregabalin	PO	50–200 mg TID	Cognitive changes, sedation
Gabapentin	PO	300–1,200 mg TID	Cognitive changes, sedation
Serotonin-norepinephrine reuptake inhibitors (e.g., duloxetine, venlafaxine)	PO	Duloxetine, 30–120 mg daily Venlafaxine, 37.5–225 mg daily	Cognitive changes, sedation
Tricyclic antidepressants (e.g., amitriptyline)	PO	10–100 mg qhs	Cognitive changes, sedation, dry eyes and mouth, urinary retention, constipation
Second Line			
Tramadol	PO	50–100 mg QID	Cognitive changes, sedation, GI upset, addiction
Opioids (oxycodone, morphine)	PO	10–120 mg daily	Cognitive changes, sedation, GI upset, addiction
Dextromethorphan	PO	400 mg daily	Drowsiness, dizziness, nausea, vomiting
Other agents			
Lidocaine, 2.5%/pylocaine, 2.5% cream	Apply cutaneously	QID	Local irritation
Lidoderm, 5% patch	Apply to painful area	Up to three patches daily for 12 hours at a time	Local irritation
Capsaicin, 0.025–0.075% cream	Apply cutaneously	QID	Painful burning skin

Pathogenesis

The pathogenic basis for autonomic neuropathy is unknown but may be similar to DSPN.

Treatment

Pancreatic transplantation may stabilize or slightly improve autonomic function.[19] In patients with symptomatic orthostatic hypotension, we try as many nonpharmacologic treatments as possible, including pressure stockings, small frequent meals, raising the head of the bed at night, and avoidance of alcohol. When drug treatment is required, we initiate treatment with fludrocortisone (starting at 0.1 mg BID) or midodrine (10 mg TID).[51] Pyridostigmine may also be helpful. It is important to note that asymptomatic standing time, rather than improvement in standing blood pressure, is the most important parameter to monitor. Nonsteroidal anti-inflammatory agents may also be of benefit. Metoclopramide is used to treat diabetic gastroparesis, while clonidine may help with persistent diarrhea. Sildenafil and other similar medications are used to treat erectile dysfunction.

DIABETIC NEUROPATHIC CACHEXIA

Clinical Features

DNC is very rare but can be the presenting manifestation of DM.[55–58] This form of diabetic neuropathy is more common in men (usually associated with type 2 DM) than in women (most cases associated with type 1 DM) and generally occurs in their sixth or seventh decade of life. Patients with DNC develop an abrupt onset of severe generalized painful paresthesias involving the trunk and all four limbs, usually setting off significant precipitous weight loss. Mild sensory loss may be detected on examination along with reduced muscle stretch reflexes. Weakness and atrophy are evident in some patients. DNC tends to gradually improve spontaneously, usually preceded by recovery of the weight loss. Rarely, DNC can recur.

Laboratory Features

Cerebrospinal fluid (CSF) protein may be increased. SNAPs may be absent or have very low amplitudes.[55,56] Normal or slightly diminished compound muscle action potential (CMAP) amplitudes with mild slowing of conduction velocities can also be observed. Needle EMG typically demonstrates evidence of active denervation in the form of fibrillation potentials and positive waves in affected muscles.

Histopathology

Nerve biopsies demonstrate severe loss of large, myelinated axons with relative sparing of small myelinated and unmyelinated fibers.[56]

Pathogenesis

The pathogenic basis for the disorder is not known.

Treatment

Most patients improve spontaneously, with control over the DM within 1–3 years. Symptomatic treatment of the painful paresthesias is the same as that described for DSPN.

DIABETIC POLYRADICULOPATHY OR RADICULOPLEXUS NEUROPATHY

Two categories of diabetic radiculoplexus neuropathy can be made on the basis of clinical differences: (1) the more common asymmetric, painful, radiculoplexus neuropathy (i.e., diabetic amyotrophy) and (2) the rare symmetric, relatively painless, radiculoplexus neuropathy.[52] The latter form is controversial. It may represent chronic inflammatory demyelinating polyneuropathy (CIDP) in a patient with diabetes, a distinct form of diabetic neuropathy, or may just fall within the spectrum of diabetic amyotrophy.

ASYMMETRIC, PAINFUL DIABETIC POLYRADICULOPATHY OR RADICULOPLEXUS NEUROPATHY (DIABETIC AMYOTROPHY)

Clinical Features

This is the most common form of polyradiculopathy or radiculoplexus neuropathy associated with DM (also known as diabetic amyotrophy, Bruns–Garland syndrome, diabetic lumbosacral radiculoplexopathy, and proximal diabetic neuropathy).[59–68] It more commonly affects older patients with DM type 2, but it can affect type 1 diabetic patients. It can be the presenting manifestation of DM in approximately one-third of patients. Typically, patients present with severe pain in the low back, hip, and thigh in one leg. Rarely, the diabetic polyradiculoneuropathy begins in both legs at the same time. Nevertheless, in such cases nerve involvement is generally asymmetric. About 50% of patients also complain of numbness and paresthesia. Atrophy and weakness of proximal and distal muscles in the affected leg become apparent within a few days or weeks. The term "proximal diabetic neuropathy" stems from the observation that muscles innervated by the L2–L4 myotomes are the most commonly affected, producing weakness of hip flexion, hip adduction, and knee extension. The knee jerk on the affected side is virtually always diminished or lost in many cases. However, any leg muscle may be affected.[60] In fact, we have seen cases with L5 or S1 monoradiculopathy patterns of pain and weakness in newly diagnosed diabetics without compressive lesions. Conversely and unfortunately, we have seen many patients undergo unnecessary laminectomies because of incidental magnetic resonance imaging (MRI) findings in the presence of severe radicular pain and weakness suggesting structural impingement. Although the onset is typically unilateral, it is not uncommon for the contralateral leg to become affected several weeks or months later. As with DNC, the polyradiculoneuropathy is often accompanied or heralded by severe weight loss. Weakness progresses gradually or in a stepwise fashion, usually over several weeks or months, but can continue to progress for 18 months or more.[60] Most patients usually have underlying DSPN. Eventually, the disorder stabilizes, and slow recovery ensues over 1–3 years. However, in many cases there is significant residual weakness, sensory loss, and pain.

Rather than the more typical lumbosacral radiculoplexus neuropathy, some patients develop thoracic radiculopathy.[65,69] Patients describe pain radiating from the posterolateral chest wall anteriorly to the abdominal region, with associated loss of sensation anterolaterally. Weakness of the abdominal wall may lead to herniations of the viscera. A cervical variant of diabetic radicular plexus neuropathy manifesting as acute pain, weakness, and sensory loss in one or both upper limbs can rarely occur as well.[62,63]

Laboratory Features

Lumbar puncture usually reveals an elevated CSF protein with a normal cell count. Erythrocyte sedimentation rate is often increased. MRI scans of the nerve roots and plexus can reveal enhancement.[60,64] NCSs reveal features suggestive of multifocal axonal damage to the roots and plexus with reduced or low amplitudes of SNAPs and CMAPs.[60–62,65,67] Conduction velocities in the affected limbs are normal or mildly slow. Autonomic studies may be abnormal as well.[62,65] Needle EMG reveals positive sharp waves and fibrillation potentials and reduced recruitment of affected proximal and distal muscles in the affected limbs and paraspinal muscles in keeping with the radiculoplexus localization. Large-amplitude, long-duration, polyphasic MUAPs are seen after 3–6 months as reinnervation occurs.

Histopathology

Sural, superficial peroneal, and lateral femoral cutaneous nerve biopsies, if performed, reveal loss of myelinated nerve fibers, which is often asymmetric between and within nerve fascicles.[60,62,66,70–74] Active axonal degeneration and clusters of small, thinly myelinated regenerating fibers are appreciated. Mild perivascular inflammation and, less commonly, vasculitis with fibrinoid necrosis involving epineurial and perineurial blood vessels have been noted on some nerve biopsies (Fig. 21-4).[62,66,67] Again, nerve biopsy is not recommended in the vast majority of cases.

Pathogenesis

Some authorities have speculated that diabetic radiculoplexus neuropathy is an immune-mediated microangiopathy; however, the exact pathogenic mechanism is unclear.[66,70,75]

Treatment

Small retrospective studies have reported that intravenous immunoglobulin (IVIG), prednisone, and other forms of immunosuppressive therapy might be helpful in some patients with diabetic amyotrophy.[59,65–68,70] We have seen that short courses of corticosteroids ease the pain associated with the severe radiculoplexus neuropathy; this can allow the patients to undergo physical therapy. However, the natural history of this neuropathy is gradual improvement, so the

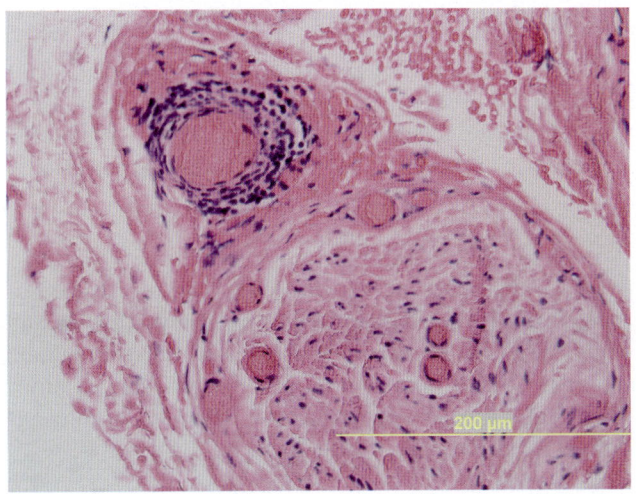

Figure 21-4. Lumbosacral radiculoplexus neuropathy. Superficial peroneal nerve biopsy reveals perivascular inflammation of a small epineurial vessel. H&E stain.

actual effect, if any, of these immunotherapies on the radiculoplexus neuropathy is not known. Prospective, double-blind, placebo-controlled trials are necessary to define the role of various immunotherapies in this disorder.

SYMMETRIC, PAINLESS, DIABETIC POLYRADICULOPATHY OR RADICULOPLEXUS NEUROPATHY

Clinical Features

The second major group of diabetic polyradiculopathy or radiculoplexus neuropathy manifests as progressive, relatively painless, symmetrical proximal and distal weakness that typically evolves over weeks to months, such that it clinically resembles CIDP.[62,65,70,73,74,76–81] Whether this neuropathy represents the coincidental occurrence of CIDP in a patient with DM, or this is a distinct form of diabetic neuropathy, is unclear and controversial.[81] This type of neuropathy occurs in both type 1 and type 2 DM.

The pattern of weakness resembles CIDP in that there is symmetric distal and proximal weakness affecting the legs more than the arms. Distal muscles are more affected than proximal muscles. In our experience there is usually distal arm weakness, but proximal arm involvement is often less noticeable than that seen in patients with idiopathic CIDP. Unlike the more common "diabetic amyotrophy" discussed in the previous section, the onset of weakness is not heralded or accompanied by such severe back and proximal leg pain, and the motor weakness is relatively symmetric. However, distal dysesthesias, perhaps secondary to a superimposed DSPN, are occasionally present.

Laboratory Features

CSF protein concentration is often increased. NCSs demonstrate mixed axonal and demyelinating features, with absent or reduced SNAP and CMAP amplitudes combined with slowing of NCVs, prolongation of distal latencies, and absent or prolonged latencies of F waves.[62,70,73,76,78,81] Rarely, conduction block and temporal dispersion are found.[62,73,77] Occasionally, the electrophysiological features can fulfill research criteria for demyelination, but these patients generally have patterns that are more axonal in nature than seen in idiopathic CIDP.[73,74,77] EMG reveals fibrillation potentials and positive sharp waves diffusely, including multiple levels of the paraspinal musculature. Autonomic studies may demonstrate abnormalities in sudomotor, cardiovagal, and adrenergic functions.[62,65]

Histopathology

Sural nerve biopsies, if performed, demonstrate a loss of large and small myelinated nerve fibers with axonal degeneration and clusters of small regenerating fibers as well as perivascular inflammation or the so-called "microvasculitis."[62,65,70,73,76,81] Nerve biopsies may show immunoreactivity for matrix metalloproteinase-9 as seen in idiopathic CIDP.[80] A study out of the Mayo Clinic compared pathological features of nerve biopsies of this painless, symmetric, diabetic radiculoplexus neuropathy to the more typical painful, asymmetric, diabetic radiculoplexus neuropathy and to 25 CIDP biopsies.[81] Nerve biopsies of two types of diabetic radiculoplexus neuropathies were similar, showing features of ischemic injury (multifocal fiber loss), perineurial thickening, injury neuroma, neovascularization, and microvasculitis (epineurial perivascular inflammation, prior bleeding, vessel wall inflammation). In contrast, CIDP biopsies did not show ischemic injury or microvasculitis but revealed demyelination and onion bulbs. However, the study did not include any biopsies of patients who may have had diabetes and coincidental CIDP that was responsive to immunotherapy.

Pathogenesis

The pathogenic basis for this form of polyradiculoneuropathy is unknown and perhaps is multifactorial. This neuropathy may represent part of the spectrum of diabetic amyotrophy, believed by some to result from microvasculitis.[81] We suspect that rare cases represent CIDP occurring coincidentally in patients with DM, as some appear to improve with various immunotherapies. However, this apparent response does not imply that the patients have CIDP, because these patients can improve spontaneously without treatment and because microvasculitis may be responsive to immunotherapies as well.[62,65] Alternatively, the disorder in some patients may represent a distinct form of diabetic neuropathy caused by associated metabolic disturbances, such as uremia.

Treatment

As noted, some patients improve with immunotherapy [i.e., IVIG, plasma exchange (PE), and corticosteroids], suggesting that this type of diabetic neuropathy may be immune mediated.[62,65,70,73,76,78] We often perform lumbar puncture on these patients. If the CSF protein is normal, then we would not proceed with immunotherapy, as it is highly unlikely that the patient has CIDP. If the CSF protein is elevated, one does not know if the patient has CIDP or the protein is elevated because of the diabetes. In these cases, we give a trial of plasmapheresis or IVIG in these patients.

DIABETIC MONONEUROPATHIES OR MULTIPLE MONONEUROPATHIES

Diabetic patients are vulnerable to developing mononeuropathies and multiple mononeuropathies, including cranial neuropathies.[1,82-84] Most of the time patients have underlying DSPN. The mononeuropathies are usually insidious in onset and presumably mechanical in nature due to entrapment or compressive mechanisms. Mononeuropathies that have an abrupt onset and a presumed ischemic mechanism (e.g., a diabetic third nerve palsy), are more likely to occur in individuals not yet identified as being diabetic. The most common neuropathies are median neuropathy at the wrist and ulnar neuropathy at the elbow, but peroneal neuropathy at the fibular head and sciatic, lateral femoral cutaneous, and cranial neuropathies also occur. In regard to cranial mononeuropathies, a seventh nerve palsy is most common, followed by third, sixth, and, less frequently, fourth nerve palsies. The multiple mononeuropathies, perhaps in combination with a radiculoplexus neuropathy, may give the appearance of a mononeuropathy multiplex pattern.

TREATMENT-INDUCED PAINFUL NEUROPATHY

Clinical Features

As mentioned previously, chronic painful neuropathies are common in diabetic patients. However, some patients suffer from severe acute neuropathic pain. This may occur in the setting of DNC or anorexia associated with severe weight loss. Rarely, severe pain develops soon after starting intensive glycemic treatment with rapid control of the glycemia, the so-called treatment-induced neuropathy or insulin neuritis.[75,85-90] This can occur in patients with type 1 or type 2 diabetes following treatment with insulin or oral hypoglycemic agents. The pain is usually in a length-dependent distribution but can be diffuse. Many patients, particularly those with type 1 DM, suffer from autonomic symptoms (orthostatic lightheadedness, nausea, vomiting, diarrhea, early satiety, and erectile dysfunction in men). Worsening retinopathy also parallels the course of the neuropathic pain. On examination, pain and temperature sensation are reduced, while most patients have hyperalgesia and allodynia. Muscle strength is not impaired.

Laboratory Features

NCSs may be normal or abnormal, similar to DSPN. Autonomic testing usually reveals abnormal heart rate response to deep breathing and abnormal Valsalva ratio with diminished variability in the heart rate as well as orthostatic hypotension.[85]

Histopathology

When performed, sural nerve biopsies have revealed variable loss of myelinated fibers, acute axonal degeneration, and some clusters of regenerating myelinated fibers which are indistinguishable from other forms of diabetic neuropathy.[73] Skin biopsies usually demonstrate a reduction in intraepidermal nerve fiber density.[85]

Pathogenesis

The pathogenic basis of acute treatment–induced neuropathy is not known, but the phenotype suggests diffuse damage to the unmyelinated and lightly myelinated nerve fibers.[85]

Treatment

The pain associated with this neuropathy is very difficult to control. Fortunately, it is a spontaneously reversible disorder, and typically patients report pain improvement after many months of continued glucose control.

NEUROPATHIES ASSOCIATED WITH METABOLIC SYNDROME

There is an increased risk of neuropathy in patients who are "prediabetic" or who have metabolic syndrome. The most common presentation is DSPN with an early involvement of small fibers, and it is indistinguishable from that seen in patients with type 2 diabetes.[6,91-99] There also appears to be a risk of autonomic neuropathy and radiculoplexus neuropathy as well. As mentioned in the Pathogenesis section in regard to diabetic DSPN, the mechanism of DSPN in type 2 diabetes may be related to metabolic syndrome.

▶ NEUROPATHIES ASSOCIATED WITH OTHER ENDOCRINOPATHIES

HYPOGLYCEMIA/HYPERINSULINEMIA

Clinical Features

Polyneuropathy has been associated with persistent hypoglycemia secondary to an islet cell tumor of the pancreas, hyperinsulinemia, or in early stages of treatment of DM.[100,101,102] The neuropathy is characterized by progressive numbness and paresthesias in the hands and feet. Over time, distal motor weakness and atrophy may develop. Muscle stretch reflexes are generally reduced in a length-dependent fashion.

With correction of the hypoglycemia, the sensory symptoms usually improve; however, muscle atrophy and weakness often remain to some extent.

Laboratory Features

NCSs reveal SNAPs that are reduced in amplitude or absent.[101] The CMAP amplitudes are slightly decreased, while the conduction velocities are normal or only mildly reduced. Needle EMG may demonstrate fibrillation potentials, positive sharp waves, and reduced recruitment of large polyphasic MUAPs in the distal limb muscles.[100–102]

Histopathology

Very few nerve biopsies have been performed on individuals with this disorder, but axonal loss primarily affecting the large, myelinated fibers has been reported.[101]

Pathogenesis

The basis for the polyneuropathy is not known but is felt to be directly attributable to reduced glucose levels in peripheral nerves. A rat model of recurrent episodes of severe hypoglycemia was associated with early vascular anomalies in endoneurial microvessels in rat sciatic nerves without any observable changes in nerve fibers.[103] Other studies demonstrated that acute lowering of glucose levels under hypoxic conditions in rats leads to apoptosis of dorsal root ganglia neurons.[104] Hypoxia-induced cell death was decreased when dorsal root ganglia neurons were maintained in high-glucose medium, suggesting that high levels of substrate protected against hypoxia. Apoptosis was completely prevented by increasing the concentration of nerve growth factor.

Treatment

Patients should be treated for the underlying cause of the hyperinsulinemia.

ACROMEGALY

Clinical Features

Acromegaly can be associated with several types of neuropathy, in addition to myopathy.[105–109] Carpal tunnel syndrome is the most common neuropathy complicating acromegaly.[105,107] A generalized sensorimotor peripheral neuropathy, characterized by numbness, paresthesias, and mild distal weakness beginning in the feet and progressing to the hands, is less frequent. Clinical or electrophysiological evidence of carpal tunnel syndrome has been demonstrated in 82% of patients and a generalized sensorimotor peripheral neuropathy in 73% of patients with acromegaly.[105] In addition, the bony overgrowth in or about the spinal canal and neural foramina can result in spinal cord compression or polyradiculopathies.

Laboratory Features

NCSs in patients with generalized polyneuropathy demonstrate reduced amplitudes of SNAPs with prolonged distal latencies and slow CVs.[105] The CMAPs are usually normal, but there may be slightly reduced amplitudes, prolonged distal latencies, and slow motor conduction velocities.

Histopathology

Nerve biopsies in patients with acromegaly and generalized polyneuropathy may reveal an increase in endoneurial and subperineurial connective tissue and an overall increase in the fascicular area, combined with a loss of myelinated and unmyelinated nerve fibers.[105,109]

Pathogenesis

The pathogenic basis of the polyneuropathy associated with acromegaly is unknown. The neuropathy may be related to superimposed DM in some cases. Increased growth hormone and upregulation of insulin-like growth factor receptors may result in proliferation of endoneurial and subperineurial connective tissue, which could make the nerve fibers more vulnerable to pressure and trauma.

Treatment

It is unclear at this time if the polyneuropathy improves with treatment of this endocrinopathy.

HYPOTHYROIDISM

Clinical Features

Hypothyroidism is more commonly associated with a proximal myopathy, but patients are predisposed to develop carpal tunnel syndrome.[110–115] Rarely, a generalized sensory polyneuropathy, characterized by painful paresthesias and numbness in both the hands and the legs, also complicates hypothyroidism.[111,112,116]

Laboratory Features

NCS features suggestive of carpal tunnel syndrome are most common, but a generalized sensorimotor polyneuropathy may be demonstrated.[110–112] In patients with a generalized neuropathy, the SNAP amplitudes are reduced and distal latencies may be slightly prolonged.[113,114] CMAPs reveal normal or slightly reduced amplitudes, mild-to-moderate slowing of CVs, and slight prolongation of motor distal latencies.

Histopathology

Nerve biopsies, when performed, have revealed a loss of myelinated nerve fibers, mild degrees of active axonal degeneration, and segmental demyelination with small onion-bulb formations.[89,92] Skin biopsies have shown reduced intraepidermal nerve fiber density in patients with hypothyroid neuropathy, but also in patients with asymptomatic hypothyroidism.[116,117]

Pathogenesis

Carpal tunnel syndrome is most likely the result of reduced space within the flexor retinaculum as a result of associated edematous changes. The etiology of the generalized neuropathy associated with hypothyroidism is not known.

Treatment

Correction of the hypothyroidism usually at least halts further progression of the polyneuropathy, and in some cases leads to improvement.

▶ SUMMARY

DM is the most common etiology of neuropathy (at least in industrialized nations) when the cause of the neuropathy is found. There are several types of neuropathy associated with DM as discussed. Treatment is aimed at control of the blood sugar and symptomatic management of pain. Aside from diabetic neuropathies, the endocrine-related neuropathies are relatively uncommon, although hyperinsulinemia, hypothyroidism, and acromegaly have also been associated with neuropathy.

REFERENCES

1. Callaghan BC, Cheng HT, Stables CL, Smith AL, Feldman EL. Diabetic neuropathy: clinical manifestations and current treatments. *Lancet Neurol*. 2012;11:521–534.
2. Podwall D, Gooch C. Diabetic neuropathy: clinical features, etiology, and therapy. *Curr Neurol Neurosci Rep*. 2004;4(1):55–61.
3. Partanen J, Niskanen L, Lehtinen J, Mervaala E, Siitonen O, Uusitupa M. Natural history of peripheral neuropathy in patients with non-insulin-dependent diabetes mellitus. *N Engl J Med*. 1995;333:89–94.
4. Patel K, Horak H, Tiryaki E. Diabetic neuropathies. *Muscle Nerve*. 2021;63(1):22–30.
5. Sasaki H, Kawamura N, Dyck PJ, Dyck PJB, Kihara M, Low PA. Spectrum of diabetic neuropathies. *Diabetol Int*. 2020;11(2):87–96.
6. Elafros MA, Andersen H, Bennett DL, et al. Towards prevention of diabetic peripheral neuropathy: clinical presentation, pathogenesis, and new treatments. *Lancet Neurol*. 2022;21(10):922–936.
7. Bao XH, Wong V, Wang Q, Low LC. Prevalence of peripheral neuropathy with insulin-dependent diabetes mellitus. *Pediatr Neurol*. 1999;20:204–209.
8. Dyck PJ, Kratz KM, Litchy WJ, et al. The prevalence by staged severity of various types of diabetic neuropathy, retinopathy, and nephropathy in a population-based cohort: The Rochester diabetic neuropathy study. *Neurology*. 1993;43:817–824.
9. Boulton AJ, Knight G, Drury J, Ward JD. The prevalence of symptomatic diabetic neuropathy in an insulin-treated population. *Diabetes Care*. 1985;8:125–128.
10. Dyck PJ, Karnes JL, O'Brien PC, et al. The Rochester diabetes neuropathy study: reassessment of tests and criteria for diagnosis and stages severity. *Neurology*. 1992;42:1164–1170.
11. Singleton JR, Smith AG, Bromberg MB. Painful sensory polyneuropathy associated with impaired glucose tolerance test. *Muscle Nerve*. 2001;24:1225–1228.
12. Novella SP, Inzucchi SE, Goldstein JM. The frequency of undiagnosed diabetes and impaired glucose tolerance in patients with idiopathic sensory neuropathy. *Muscle Nerve*. 2001;24:1229–1231.
13. Sumner CJ, Seth S, Griffin JW, Cornblath DR, Polyswdkia M. The spectrum of neuropathy in diabetes and impaired glucose tolerance. *Neurology*. 2003;60:108–111.
14. Hughes RA, Umapathi T, Gray IA, et al. A controlled investigation of the cause of chronic idiopathic axonal polyneuropathy. *Brain*. 2004;127:1723–1730.
15. Dyck PJ, Overland CJ, Davies JL, et al. Does impaired glycemia cause polyneuropathy and other diabetic complications? *J Peripheral Nervous Soc*. 2011;16(suppl 3):30–31.
16. Wilson JR, Stittsworth JD Jr, Kadir A, Fisher MA. Conduction velocity versus amplitude analysis: evidence for demyelination in diabetic neuropathy. *Muscle Nerve*. 1998;21:1228–1230.
17. Abu-Shukra SR, Cornblath DR, Avila OL, et al. Conduction block in diabetic neuropathy. *Muscle Nerve*. 1991;14:858–862.
18. Krarup C. An update on electrophysiological studies in neuropathy. *Curr Opin Neurol*. 2003;16:603–612.
19. Navarro X, Sutherland DE, Kennedy WR. Long-term effects of pancreatic transplantation on diabetic neuropathy. *Ann Neurol*. 1997;42:727–736.
20. Hill RE, Williams PE. Perineurial cell basement membrane thickening and myelinated nerve fibre loss in diabetic and non-diabetic peripheral nerve. *J Neurol Sci*. 2004;217(2):157–163.
21. Herrman DN, Griffin JW, Hauer P, Cornblath DR, McArthur JC. Intraepidermal nerve fiber density, sural nerve morphometry and electrodiagnosis in peripheral neuropathies. *Neurology*. 1999;53:1634–1640.
22. Polydefkis M, Griffin JW, McArthur J. New insights into diabetic polyneuropathy. *JAMA*. 2003;290:1371–1376.
23. Shun CT, Chang YC, Wu HP, et al. Skin denervation in type 2 diabetes: correlations with diabetic duration and functional impairments. *Brain*. 2004;127:1593–1605.
24. Feldman EL, Nave KA, Jensen TS, Bennett DLH. New Horizons in Diabetic Neuropathy: Mechanisms, Bioenergetics, and Pain. *Neuron*. 2017;93(6):1296–1313.
25. Dyck PJ, Sherman WR, Halcher LM, et al. Human diabetic endoneurial sorbitol, fructose, and myo-inositol related to sural nerve morphometry. *Ann Neurol*. 1980;8:590–596.
26. Gillon KR, Hawthorne JN, Tomlinson DR. Myo-inositol and sorbitol metabolism in relation to peripheral nerve function in experimental diabetes in the rat: effect of aldose reductase inhibition. *Diabetologia*. 1983;25:365–371.
27. Vlassara H. Recent progress in advanced glycosylation end products and diabetic complications. *Diabetes*. 1997;46:S19–S25.
28. Dyck PJ, Zimmerman BR, Vilen TH, et al. Nerve glucose, fructose, sorbitol, myo-inositol, and fiber degeneration and regeneration in diabetic neuropathy. *N Engl J Med*. 1998;319:542–548.

29. Sima AA. New insights into the metabolic and molecular basis for diabetic neuropathy. *Cell Mol Life Sci*. 2003;60: 2445–2464.
30. Sanaye MM, Kavishwar SA. Diabetic neuropathy: review on molecular mechanisms. *Curr Mol Med*. 2023;23(2):97–110.
31. Diabetes Control and Complications Trial Research Group. The effect of diabetes on the development and progression of long-term complications in insulin-dependent diabetes mellitus. *N Engl J Med*. 1993;329:977–986.
32. Diabetes Control and Complications Trial. Effect of intensive diabetes treatment on nerve conduction in the diabetes control and complications trial. *Ann Neurol*. 1995;38:869–880.
33. Kennedy WR, Navarro X, Goetz FC. Sutherland DE, Najarian JS. Effects of pancreatic transplantation on diabetic neuropathy. *N Engl J Med*. 1990;322:1031–1037.
34. Writing Team for the Diabetes Control and Complications Trial/Epidemiology of Diabetes Interventions and Complications Research Group. Effect of intensive therapy on the microvascular complications of type 1 diabetes mellitus. *JAMA*. 2002;287(19):2563–2569.
35. Jeffrey S, Samraj PI, Raj BS. The role of alpha-lipoic acid supplementation in the prevention of diabetes complications: a comprehensive review of clinical trials. *Curr Diabetes Rev*. 2021;17(9):e011821190404.
36. Ametov AS, Barinov A, Dyck PJ, et al; SYDNEY Trial Study Group. The sensory symptoms of diabetic polyneuropathy are improved with alpha-lipoic acid: The SYDNEY trial. *Diabetes Care*. 2003;26:770–776.
37. Streckmann F, Balke M, Cavaletti G, et al. Exercise and neuropathy: systematic review with meta-analysis. *Sports Med*. 2022;52(5):1043–1065.
38. Attal N, Cruccu G, Baron R, et al. EFNS guidelines on the pharmacological treatment of neuropathic pain: 2010 revision. *Eur J Neurol*. 2010;17:1113-e88.
39. Bril V, England J, Franklin GM, et al. American Academy of Neurology; American Association of Neuromuscular and Electrodiagnostic Medicine; American Academy of Physical Medicine and Rehabilitation. Evidence-based guideline: Treatment of painful diabetic neuropathy: Report of the American Academy of Neurology, the American Association of Neuromuscular and Electrodiagnostic Medicine, and the American academy of Physical Medicine and Rehabilitation. *Neurology*. 2011;76:1758–1765.
40. Backonja M, Beydoun A, Edwards KR, et al. Gabapentin for the symptomatic treatment of painful neuropathy in patients with diabetes mellitus: a randomized control trial. *JAMA*. 1998;280:1831–1836.
41. The Capsaicin Study Group. Treatment of painful diabetic peripheral neuropathy with topical capsaicin: a multi-center, double-blind, vehicle-controlled study. *Arch Intern Med*. 1991; 151:2225–2229.
42. Harati Y, Gooch C, Swenson M, et al. Double-blind randomized trial of tramadol for the treatment of the pain of diabetic neuropathy. *Neurology*. 1998;50:1842–1846.
43. Max MB, Lynch SA, Muir J, et al. Effects of desipramine, amitriptyline, and fluoxetine on pain in diabetic neuropathy. *N Engl J Med*. 1992;326:1250–1256.
44. Morello CM, Leckband SG, Stoner CP, Morhouse DF, Sahagian GA. Randomized double-blind study comparing the efficacy of gabapentin with amitriptyline on diabetic neuropathy pain. *Arch Intern Med*. 1999;159:1931–1937.
45. Wolfe GI, Trivedi JR. Painful peripheral neuropathy and its nonsurgical treatment. *Muscle Nerve*. 2004;30:3–19.
46. Kochar DK, Rawat N, Agrawal RP, et al. Sodium valproate for painful diabetic neuropathy: a randomized double-blind placebo-controlled study. *QJM*. 2004;97:33–38.
47. Price R, Smith D, Franklin G, et al. Oral and topical treatment of painful diabetic polyneuropathy: Practice Guideline Update Summary: Report of the AAN Guideline Subcommittee. *Neurology*. 2022;98(1):31–43.
48. Tesfaye S, Sloan G, Petrie J, et al. Comparison of amitriptyline supplemented with pregabalin, pregabalin supplemented with amitriptyline, and duloxetine supplemented with pregabalin for the treatment of diabetic peripheral neuropathic pain (OPTION-DM): a multicentre, double-blind, randomised crossover trial. *Lancet*. 2022;400(10353):680–690.
49. Elafros MA, Callaghan BC. Effective treatment pathways exist for DPNP. *Lancet*. 2022;400(10353):639–641.
50. Cohen JA, Jeffers BW, Faldut D, Marcoux M, Schrier RW. Risks for sensorimotor peripheral neuropathy and autonomic neuropathy in non-insulin-dependent diabetes mellitus (NIDDM). *Muscle Nerve*. 1998;21:72–80.
51. Vinik AI, Freeman R, Erbas T. Diabetic autonomic neuropathy. *Semin Neurol*. 2003;23(4):365–372.
52. Freeman R. Autonomic peripheral neuropathy. *Continuum (Minneap Minn)*. 2020;26(1):58–71.
53. Soedamah-Muthu SS, Chaturvedi N, Witte DR, et al. Relationship between risk factors and mortality in type 1 diabetic patients in Europe: The EURODIAB Prospective Complications Study (PCS). *Diabetes Care*. 2008;31:1360–1366.
54. Duchen LW, Anjorin A, Watkins PJ, Mackay JD. Pathology of autonomic neuropathy in diabetes mellitus. *Ann Intern Med*. 1980;92:301–303.
55. Godil A, Berriman D, Knapik S, Normal M, Godil F, Firek AF. Diabetic neuropathic cachexia. *West J Med*. 1996;165:882–885.
56. Jackson CE, Barohn RJ. Diabetic neuropathic cachexia: report of a recurrent case. *J Neurol Neurosurg Psychiatry*. 1998;64: 785–787.
57. Neal JM. Diabetic neuropathic cachexia: a rare manifestation of diabetic neuropathy. *South Med J*. 2009;102:327–329.
58. Bellelli A, Santi D, Simoni M, Greco C. Diabetic neuropathic cachexia: a clinical case and review of literature. *Life (Basel)*. 2022;12(5):680.
59. Amato AA, Barohn RJ. Diabetic lumbosacral radiculoneuropathies. *Curr Treat Options Neurol*. 2001;3:139–146.
60. Barohn RJ, Sahenk Z, Warmolts JR, Mendell JR. The Bruns–Garland syndrome (diabetic amyotrophy): revisited 100 years later. *Arch Neurol*. 1991;48:1130–1135.
61. Stewart JD. Diabetic truncal neuropathy: topography of the sensory deficit. *Ann Neurol*. 1989;25:233–238.
62. Pascoe MK, Low PA, Windebank AJ, Litchy WJ. Subacute diabetic proximal neuropathy. *Mayo Clin Proc*. 1997;72:1123–1132.
63. Katz JS, Saperstein DS, Wolfe G, et al. Cervicobrachial involvement in diabetic radiculoplexopathy. *Muscle Nerve*. 2001;24:794–798.
64. O'Neil BJ, Flanders AE, Escandon S, Tahmoush AJ. Treatable lumbosacral polyradiculitis masquerading as diabetic amyotrophy. *J Neurol Sci*. 1997;151:223–225.
65. Jaradeh SS, Prieto TE, Lobeck LJ. Progressive polyradiculoneuropathy in diabetes: correlation with variables and clinical outcome after immunotherapy. *J Neurol Neurosurg Psychiatry*. 1999;67:607–612.

66. Dyck PJ, Norell JE, Dyck PJ. Microvasculitis and ischemia in diabetic lumbosacral radiculoplexus neuropathy. *Neurology.* 1999;53:2113–2121.
67. Dyck PJ, Windebank AJ. Diabetic and nondiabetic lumbosacral radiculoplexus neuropathies: new insights into pathophysiology and treatment. *Muscle Nerve.* 2002;25:477–491.
68. Pinto MV, Ng PS, Howe BM, et al. Lumbosacral radiculoplexus neuropathy: neurologic outcomes and survival in a population-based study. *Neurology.* 2021;96(16):e2098–e2108.
69. Ellenberg M. Diabetic truncal mononeuropathy—A new clinical syndrome. *Diabetes Care.* 1978;1:10–13.
70. Krendel DA, Costigan DA, Hopkins LC. Successful treatment of neuropathies in patients with diabetes mellitus. *Arch Neurol.* 1995;52:1053–1061.
71. Said G, Goulon-Goeau C, Lacroix C, Moulonguet A. Nerve biopsy findings in different patterns of proximal diabetic neuropathy. *Ann Neurol.* 1994;35:559–569.
72. Said G, Elgrably F, Lacroix C, et al. Painful proximal diabetic neuropathy: inflammatory nerve lesions and spontaneous favorable outcome. *Ann Neurol.* 1997;41:762–770.
73. Gorson KC, Ropper AH, Adelman LS, Weinberg DH. Influence of diabetes mellitus on chronic inflammatory demyelinating polyneuropathy. *Muscle Nerve.* 2000;23:37–43.
74. Riley DE, Shields RE. Diabetic amyotrophy with upper limb involvement. *Neurology.* 1984;34(suppl 1):173.
75. Vital C, Vital A, Dupon M, Gin H, Rouanet-Larriviere M, Lacut JY. Acute painful diabetic neuropathy: two patients with recent insulin-dependent diabetes mellitus. *J Peripher Nerv Syst.* 1997;2:151–154.
76. Stewart JD, Mckelvey R, Durcan L, Carpenter S, Karpati G. Chronic inflammatory demyelinating polyneuropathy (CIDP) in diabetics. *J Neurol Sci.* 1996;142:59–64.
77. Sharma KR, Cross J, Farronay O, Ayyar DR, Shebert RT, Bradley WG. Demyelinating neuropathy in diabetes mellitus. *Arch Neurol.* 2002;59:758–765.
78. Sharma KR, Cross J, Ayyar DR, Martinez-Arizala A, Bradley WG. Diabetic demyelinating polyneuropathy responsive to intravenous immunoglobulin therapy. *Arch Neurol.* 2002;59:751–757.
79. Haq RU, Pendlebury WW, Fries TJ, Tandan R. Chronic inflammatory demyelinating polyradiculoneuropathy in diabetic patients. *Muscle Nerve.* 2003;27:465–470.
80. Jann S, Bramerio MA, Beretta S, et al. Diagnostic value of sural nerve matrix metalloproteinase-9 in diabetic patients with CIDP. *Neurology.* 2003;61:1607–1610.
81. Garces-Sanchez M, Laughlin RS, Dyck PJ, Engelstad JK, Norell JE, Dyck PJ. Painless diabetic motor neuropathy: a variant of diabetic lumbosacral radiculoplexus neuropathy? *Ann Neurol.* 2011;69:1043–1054.
82. Albers JW, Brown MB, Sima AA, Greene DA. Frequency of median mononeuropathy in patients with mild diabetic neuropathy in the early diabetes intervention trial (EDIT). *Muscle Nerve.* 1996;19:140–146.
83. Zimmerman M, Gottsäter A, Dahlin LB. Carpal tunnel syndrome and diabetes—a comprehensive review. *J Clin Med.* 2022;11(6):1674.
84. Gündüz A, Candan F, Asan F, et al. Ulnar neuropathy at elbow in patients with type 2 diabetes mellitus. *J Clin Neurophysiol.* 2020;37(3):220–224.
85. Gibbons CH, Freeman R. Treatment-induced diabetic neuropathy: a reversible painful autonomic neuropathy. *Ann Neurol.* 2010;67:534–541.
86. Caravati CM. Insulin neuritis: a case report. *VA Med Monthly.* 1933;59:745–746.
87. Tesfaye S, Malik R, Harris N, et al. Arterio-venous shunting and proliferating new vessels in acute painful neuropathy of rapid glycaemic control (insulin neuritis). *Diabetologia.* 1996;39:329–335.
88. Dabby R, Sadeh M, Lampl Y, Gilad R, Watemberg N. Acute painful neuropathy induced by rapid correction of serum glucose levels in diabetic patients. *Biomed Pharmacother.* 2009;63:707–709.
89. Siddique N, Durcan R, Smyth S, Tun TK, Sreenan S, McDermott JH. Acute diabetic neuropathy following improved glycaemic control: a case series and review. *Endocrinol Diabetes Metab Case Rep.* 2020;2020:19-0140.
90. Quiroz-Aldave JE, Del Carmen Durand-Vásquez M, Puelles-León SL, Concepción-Urteaga LA, Concepción-Zavaleta MJ. Treatment-induced neuropathy of diabetes: an underdiagnosed entity. *Lancet Neurol.* 2023;22(3):201–202.
91. Kazamel M, Stino AM, Smith AG. Metabolic syndrome and peripheral neuropathy. *Muscle Nerve.* 2021;63(3):285–293.
92. Stino AM, Smith AG. Peripheral neuropathy in prediabetes and the metabolic syndrome. *J Diabetes Investig.* 2017;8(5):646–655
93. Franklin GM, Kahn LB, Baxter J, et al. Sensory neuropathy in non-insulin-dependent diabetes mellitus: The San Luis Valley Diabetes Study. *Am J Epidemiol.* 1990;131:633–643.
94. Ziegler D, Rathmann W, Dickhaus T, et al. Neuropathic pain in diabetes, prediabetes and normal glucose tolerance: The MONICA/KORA Augsburg Surveys S2 and S3. *Pain Med.* 2009;10:393–400.
95. Lee CC, Perkins BA, Kayaniyil S, et al. Peripheral neuropathy and nerve dysfunction in individuals at high risk for type 2 diabetes: the PROMISE cohort. *Diabetes Care.* 2015;38:793–800.
96. Novella SP, Inzucchi SE, Goldstein JM. The frequency of undiagnosed diabetes and impaired glucose tolerance in patients with idiopathic sensory neuropathy. *Muscle Nerve.* 2001;24:1229–1331.
97. Sumner CJ, Sheth S, Griffin JW, et al. The spectrum of neuropathy in diabetes and impaired glucose tolerance. *Neurology.* 2003;60:108–111.
98. Visser NA, Vrancken AF, Van Der Schouw YT, et al. Chronic idiopathic axonal polyneuropathy is associated with the metabolic syndrome. *Diabetes Care.* 2013;36:817–822.
99. Smith AG, Rose K, Singleton JR. Idiopathic neuropathy patients are at high risk for metabolic syndrome. *J Neurol Sci.* 2008;273:25–28.
100. Danta G. Hypoglycemic peripheral neuropathy. *Arch Neurol.* 1969;21:121–132.
101. Jaspan JB, Wollman RL, Berstein L, Rubenstein AH. Hypoglycemic peripheral neuropathy in association with insulinoma: implication of glucopenia rather than hyperinsulinism. *Medicine (Baltimore).* 1982;61:33–44.
102. Mulder DW, Bastron JA, Lambert EH. Hyperinsulin neuronopathy. *Neurology.* 1956;6:627–635.
103. Ohshima J, Nukada H. Hypoglycaemic neuropathy: microvascular changes due to recurrent hypoglycaemic episodes in rat sciatic nerve. *Brain Res.* 2002;947:84–89.
104. Honma H, Podratz JL, Windebank AJ. Acute glucose deprivation leads to apoptosis in a cell model of acute diabetic neuropathy. *J Peripher Nerv Syst.* 2003;8(2):65–74.
105. Low PA, McLeod JG, Turtle JR, et al. Peripheral neuropathy in acromegaly. *Brain.* 1974;97:139–152.

106. Khaleeli AA, Levy RD, Edwards RH. The neuromuscular features of acromegaly: a clinical and pathological study. *J Neurol Neurosurg Psychiatry*. 1984;47:1009–1015.
107. Pickett JBE, Layzer RB, Levin SR, Scheider V, Campbell MJ, Sumner AJ. Neuromuscular complications of acromegaly. *Neurology*. 1975;25:638–645.
108. Dinn JJ, Dinn EI. Natural history of acromegalic peripheral neuropathy. *Q J Med*. 1985;57:833–842.
109. Dinn JJ. Schwann cell dysfunction in acromegaly. *J Clin Endocrinol*. 1970;31:140–143.
110. Martin J, Tomkin GH, Hutchinson M. Peripheral neuropathy in hypothyroidism—an association with spurious polycythemia (Gaisbock's syndrome). *J R Soc Med*. 1983;76:187–189.
111. Meier C, Bischoff A. Polyneuropathy in hypothyroidism. *J Neurol*. 1977;215:103–114.
112. Nemni R, Bottacchi E, Fazio R, et al. Polyneuropathy in hypothyroidism: clinical, electrophysiologic and morphologic findings in four cases. *J Neurol Neurosurg Psychiatry*. 1987;50:1454–1460.
113. Dyck PJ, Lambert EH. Polyneuropathy associated with hypothyroidism. *J Neuropathol Exp Neurol*. 1970;29:631–658.
114. Fincham RW, Cape CA. Neuropathy in myxedema. *Arch Neurol*. 1968;19:464–466.
115. Eslamian F, Bahrami A, Aghamohammadzadeh N, Niafar M, Salekzamani Y, Behkamrad K. Electrophysiologic changes in patients with untreated primary hypothyroidism. *J Clin Neurophysiol*. 2011;28:323–328.
116. Penza P, Lombardi R, Camozzi F, Ciano C, Lauria G. Painful neuropathy in subclinical hypothyroidism: clinical and neuropathological recovery after hormone replacement therapy. *Neurol Sci*. 2009;30:149–151.
117. Magri F, Buonocore M, Oliviero A, et al. Intraepidermal nerve fiber density reduction as a marker of preclinical asymptomatic small-fiber sensory neuropathy in hypothyroid patients. *Eur J Endocrinol*. 2010;163:279–284.

CHAPTER 22

Idiopathic Polyneuropathy

Chapters 1 and 2 discuss how we diagnostically approach patients with possible polyneuropathies. However, in our experience and others, a cause for neuropathy will not be found in as many as 50% of cases despite an extensive workup.[1-11] The chronic idiopathic polyneuropathies are likely a heterogeneous group of neuropathies. With advances in genetics, some may be found to have a genetic basis. Most individuals have only sensory symptoms, but some may have mild weakness (e.g., toe extension) or slight abnormalities on motor conduction studies. The neuropathy may affect large- and/or small-diameter nerve fibers. As the etiology is unknown, only symptomatic management of the neuropathic pain is available.

▶ CHRONIC, IDIOPATHIC OR CRYPTOGENIC, LENGTH-DEPENDENT SENSORY OR SENSORIMOTOR POLYNEUROPATHY

CLINICAL FEATURES

Most individuals present with numbness, tingling, or pain (e.g., sharp stabbing paresthesias, burning, or deep aching sensation) in the feet between the ages of 45 and 70 years.[1-13] This is a common problem occurring in approximately 3% of adults as they age. In a large series of 93 patients with idiopathic sensory polyneuropathy, 63% presented with numbness and paresthesia along with pain, 24% with numbness or paresthesia without pain, and 10% with pain alone.[9] Eventually, 65%–80% of affected individuals develop neuropathic pain.[6,9-13] Sensory symptoms are first noted in the toes and slowly progress up the legs and later into the arms. The average time to involvement of the hands is approximately 5 years.[6,9]

Neurological examination reveals the typical length-dependent pattern of sensory loss.[6,7,9,11-13] Vibratory perception is reduced in 80%–100%, proprioception is impaired in 20%–30%, pinprick sensation is diminished in 75%–85%, and light touch is decreased in 54%–92% of those with the neuropathy. Strength is usually normal, although mild distal weakness and atrophy involving toe muscles may be appreciated in 40%–75% of cases, and rarely of ankle dorsiflexors and plantar flexors.[6,9,11-13] However, upper limb strength, including the hand intrinsics, should be normal. Muscle stretch reflexes are usually absent at the ankle and diminished at the knees and arms. Generalized areflexia though is less common and would point to a hereditary or acquired demyelinating neuropathy.

Within the category of idiopathic sensory or sensorimotor polyneuropathies are those cases of isolated small fiber neuropathy.[2,3,7,9,13-20] A recent study from the Mayo Clinic reported an incidence of small fiber neuropathy of 13.3 per 100,000 in Olmsted County, MN of which 70% were idiopathic in nature following extensive evaluation.[15] The mean onset age was 54 years (range 14–83 years). Notably, large fiber involvement subsequently developed in 36%, on average 5.3 years (range 0.2–14.3 years) from the onset of small fiber neuropathy symptoms and signs. By definition, these individuals with small fiber neuropathy should have normal nerve conduction studies (NCSs). Nerve biopsies are not recommended, but if performed, demonstrate a relatively normal density of large, myelinated nerve fibers. Most individuals with small fiber neuropathy (approximately 80%) complain of burning pain in the feet, while 40%–60% describe sharp, lancinating pain; paresthesias; or just numbness. Symptoms may involve the distal upper extremities. Rarely, the neuropathy is restricted to the arms and face or involves the autonomic nervous system.[2,3] Examination reveals reduced pinprick or temperature sensation in almost all patients, while vibratory perception is impaired in half. Muscle strength is preserved. Likewise, muscle stretch reflexes are also usually normal, but a few patients have reduced reflexes at the ankles.

LABORATORY FEATURES

The diagnosis of chronic idiopathic polyneuropathy is one of exclusion. Laboratory testing should include fasting blood glucose (FBS), hemoglobin A1C (HgbA1C), anti-Ro and anti-La antibodies (SSA and SSB), erythrocyte sedimentation rate, vitamin B12 (and methylmalonic acid when the B12 level is borderline), serum and urine immunoelectrophoresis/immunofixation, free light chain analysis, and thyroid, liver, and renal function tests.[21,22] If the FBS and HgbA1C are normal, we typically order an oral glucose tolerance test (GTT). The most common abnormality found in patients with sensory neuropathy is diabetes or impaired glucose tolerance (IGT). IGT (defined as glucose of >140 and <200 mg/dL on 2-hour GTT) is seen in 17%–61% and frank diabetes mellitus (DM) (defined as 2-hour glucose of >200 mg/dL on GTT or FBS of >126 mg/dL) in 20%–31% of patients with sensory neuropathy (Table 22-1).[23-28] In patients with painful sensory symptoms (not just numbness), the likelihood of IGT or DM is even higher. However, some authorities have not found increased

▶ TABLE 22-1. RESULTS OF GLUCOSE TOLERANCE TESTING IN OTHERWISE IDIOPATHIC POLYNEUROPATHY[23–25]

Authors (References)	No. of Patients	Mean Age (Range)	Total With Abnormal Glucose Metabolism	Impaired Glucose Tolerance	Diabetes Mellitus
Singleton et al.	89 (total)	64 years (44–92 years)	43/89 (56%)	15/89 (25%)	28/89 (31%)
	33 (painful sensory neuropathy)		20/33 (60%)	7/33 (21%)	13/33 (39%)
Novella et al.	48 (total)	64 years (41–82 years)	24/48 (50%)	13/48 (27%)	11/48 (23%)
	24 (painful sensory neuropathy)		18/28 (65%)	10/28 (36%)	8/28 (29%)
Sumner et al.	73 (total)	61 years (44–91 years)	41/73 (56%)	26/73 (36%)	15/73 (20%)
Harris et al.	National survey of 18,825 adults with or without previous diagnosis of DM of whom 2,884 were 40–74 years of age without a prior history of DM who underwent fasting blood glucose and oral glucose tolerance test		14.0% in patients aged 40–74 years	15.6% in patients aged 40–74 years 20.7% in patients 60–74 years	18–20% in patients 60–74 years

Haroutounian S, Todorovic MS, Leinders M, et al. Diagnostic criteria for idiopathic small fiber neuropathy: A systematic review. *Muscle Nerve.* 2021;63(2):170–177.
Johnson SA, Shouman K, Shelly S, et al. Small fiber neuropathy incidence, prevalence, longitudinal impairments, and disability. *Neurology.* 2021;97(22):e2236–e2247.
Finsterer J, Scorza FA. Small fiber neuropathy. *Acta Neurol Scand.* 2022;145(5):493–503.
Bitzi LM, Lehnick D, Wilder-Smith EP. Small fiber neuropathy: Swiss cohort characterization. *Muscle Nerve.* 2021;64(3):293–300.

risk of IGT in their patients with idiopathic neuropathy compared to age-matched controls.[29] Thus, although the risk of both previously undetected DM and IGT may be increased in patients with sensory neuropathy, this is still controversial and a causal relationship has not been firmly established.[30,31]

About 10% of patients with chronic idiopathic sensory or sensorimotor polyneuropathy have a monoclonal protein detected in the serum or urine, but this is not much higher than the age-matched normal controls.[32] Furthermore, the relationship of these monoclonal proteins to the pathogenesis of most neuropathies is unclear. There is a strong pathogenic relationship established in people with demyelinating sensorimotor polyneuropathies with IgM monoclonal proteins, half of whom have myelin-associated glycoprotein (MAG) antibodies (discussed in Chapters 14 and 19). However, most individuals with chronic idiopathic sensory or sensorimotor polyneuropathy have axonal neuropathies both histologically and electrophysiologically. Light chain amyloidosis is the other condition in which a pathogenic relationship between the neuropathy and the monoclonal protein is clear. Thus, amyloid neuropathy needs to be excluded in patients with a monoclonal gammopathy before concluding that the neuropathy is idiopathic in nature (see Chapter 19). This may require a fat pad, rectal, bone marrow, or nerve biopsy.

Although some studies have suggested that antisulfatide, trisulfated heparan disaccharide (TS-HDS), or fibroblast growth factor receptor-3 (FGF3) antibodies are common with painful small fiber neuropathy,[33–35] subsequent reports suggest that these antibodies have a very low sensitivity and poor specificity.[6,10,36] We do not order them as we have found them to be of little use clinically, and a pathogenic relationship has never been demonstrated. That is, the presence of these antibodies does not imply that the patients have an immune-mediated neuropathy and that they may respond to treatment with immunotherapy. We also feel that there is no role for screening various antiganglioside and other antinerve antibodies (e.g., GM1 and Hu antibodies) in the workup of patients with chronic, indolent, sensory predominant, length-dependent polyneuropathies. CSF examination is usually normal and is also unwarranted.

In people with a large fiber polyneuropathy, the sensory NCSs reveal either absent or reduced amplitudes that are worse in the legs.[1,3,4,6–13,21] Sensory nerve conduction velocities (NCVs) are normal or only mildly slow. Quantitative sensory testing (QST) demonstrates abnormal thermal and vibratory perception in as many as 85% of patients.[7,9,37] In addition, autonomic testing [e.g., quantitative sudomotor axon reflex testing (QSART) and heart rate (HR) testing with deep breathing (DB) or Valsalva] is abnormal in some patients. Despite the fact that sensory symptoms predominate, motor NCSs are often abnormal. Wolfe et al.[9] reported that 60% of their patients with idiopathic polyneuropathy had abnormal motor NCSs. The most common motor abnormalities are reduced peroneal and posterior tibialis compound muscle action potential (CMAP) amplitudes, while distal latencies and conduction velocities of the peroneal and posterior tibial CMAPs are normal or only slightly impaired. Abnormalities of median and ulnar CMAPs are much less common. Fibrillation potentials and positive waves on needle EMG may be found in intrinsic foot muscles as a further indicator of frequently subclinical motor involvement.

In patients with pure small fiber polyneuropathies, motor and sensory NCSs are, by definition, normal. Diagnosis utilizing a combination of symptoms, examination findings, intraepidermal nerve fiber density (IENFD) on skin punch biopsy, and QST is recommended with a suggested sensitivity up to 94%.[19,20,38] Diagnostic criteria using these suggest a diagnosis of *possible* small fiber neuropathy when symptoms are present along with at least two clinical signs, a diagnosis of *probable* small fiber neuropathy if subsequent NCSs are normal, and a diagnosis of definite small fiber neuropathy when decreased IENFD and/or abnormal QST are also evident.[19] As the peripheral autonomic nervous system is often affected in small fiber neuropathies autonomic testing can be useful.[22,39–42] The QSART can be performed in the distal and proximal aspects of the legs and arms (Fig. 22-1). Sweat glands are innervated by small nerve fibers, and impaired QSART is moderately specific and sensitive for small fiber damage, with 59%–80% of patients having an abnormal study.[39–42] Other autonomic tests (e.g., HR variability with DB or Valsalva maneuver) may also be abnormal in affected individuals.[7] In this regard, assessments include variability of HR to DB (Fig. 22-2) and response of the HR and blood pressure to Valsalva maneuvers and positional changes (e.g., response to tilt table or supine to standing position).

Abnormal thermal and vibratory perception thresholds may be demonstrated using QST.[19,20,29] Unlike NCSs that only assess the physiology of large-diameter sensory fibers, QST of heat and cold perception can evaluate small fiber function. Abnormal QST has been reported in 60%–85% of patients with predominantly painful sensory neuropathy.[9,40,43,44] However, QST depends on patient attention and

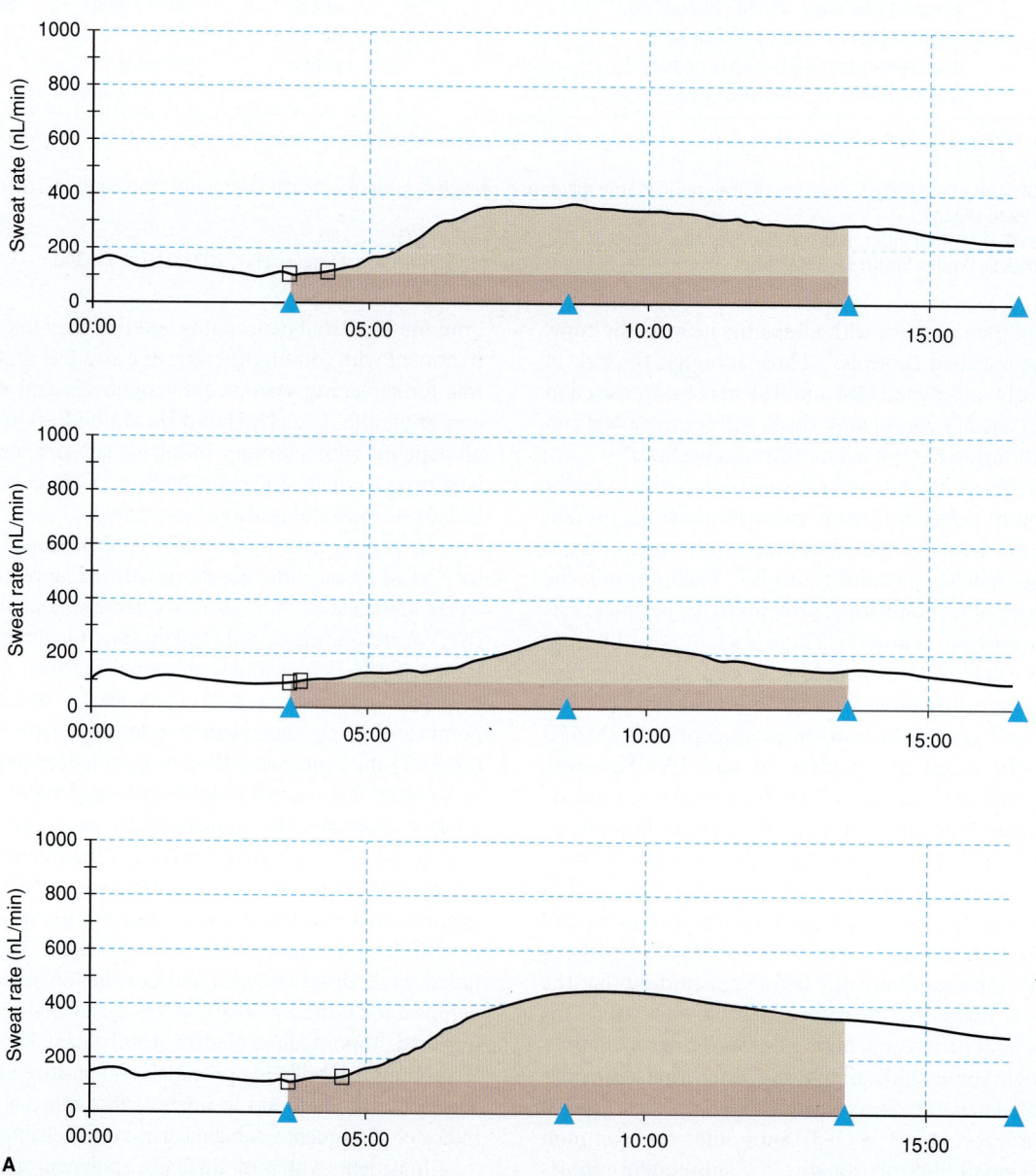

Figure 22-1. Quantitative sudomotor axon reflex test (QSART). Sudomotor function can be quantitated by measuring the amount of sweat produced in the distal and proximal aspects of the legs and arms. In (**A**), a normal response is seen (lower panel recorded from foot, middle panel for shin, and upper panel from thigh). Individuals with small fiber neuropathy may have reduced cumulative sweat. In length-dependent process, the QSART is worse distally [e.g., at the foot compared to more proximally (**B**), lower panel recorded from foot, middle panel for shin, and upper panel from thigh].

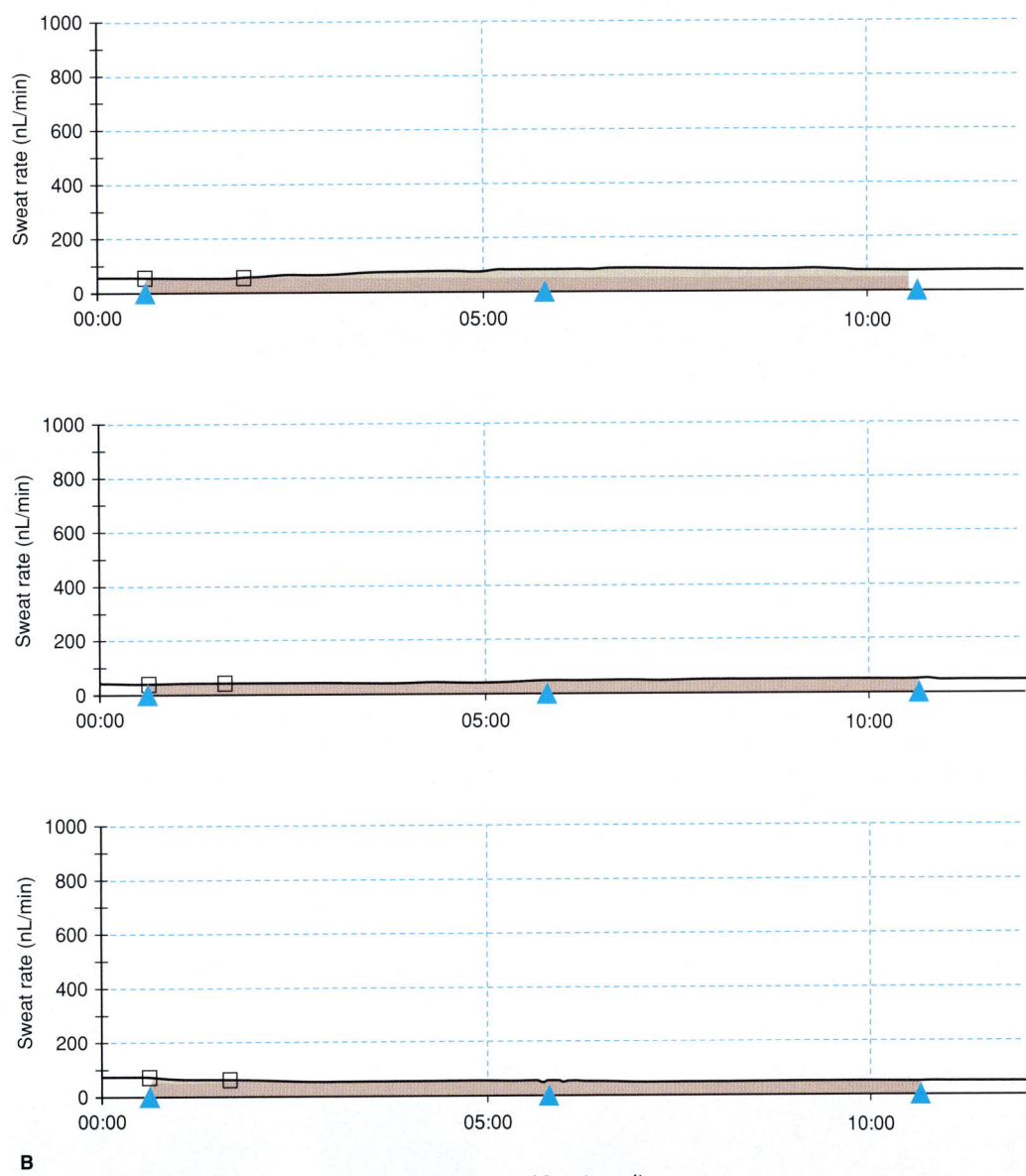

Figure 22-1. *(Continued)*

cooperation; it cannot differentiate between simulated sensory loss and sensory neuropathy. Furthermore, the sensitivity and specificity of QST are lower than QSART and skin biopsies.[45,46]

HISTOPATHOLOGY

Nerve biopsies in patients with chronic, sensory predominant, length-dependent neuropathies may reveal axonal degeneration, regenerating axonal sprouts, or axonal atrophy with or without secondary demyelination.[5–7,9,47] Quantitative morphometry may reveal loss of large- and small-diameter myelinated fibers and small unmyelinated fibers. Occasionally, scattered perivascular and endoneurial lymphocytes may be seen on nerve biopsy,[47,48] although necrotizing vasculitis is not a feature. A clonal restriction of the variable T-cell receptor γ-chain gene has been demonstrated by one group of researchers.[49] Basal lamina area thickness, endoneurial cell area, and number of endothelial cell nuclei may be increased. However, the abnormalities on nerve biopsy are nonspecific and are generally not helpful in finding an etiology for the neuropathy. There, we do recommend nerve biopsies on all patients with unexplained polyneuropathies. We consider doing a biopsy in people with autonomic sign or monoclonal gammopathies to assess for amyloidosis and those with multiple mononeuropathies in whom we suspect an inflammatory neuropathy or vasculitis (e.g., connective tissue disorders, cryoglobulinemia, and hepatitis B or C).

Nerve biopsies in individuals with small fiber neuropathies may show selective loss of small myelinated nerves and unmyelinated nerve fibers, but this requires quantitative analysis by electron microscopy (Fig. 22-3).[22] A more sensitive and less invasive means of assessing these small fiber neuropathies

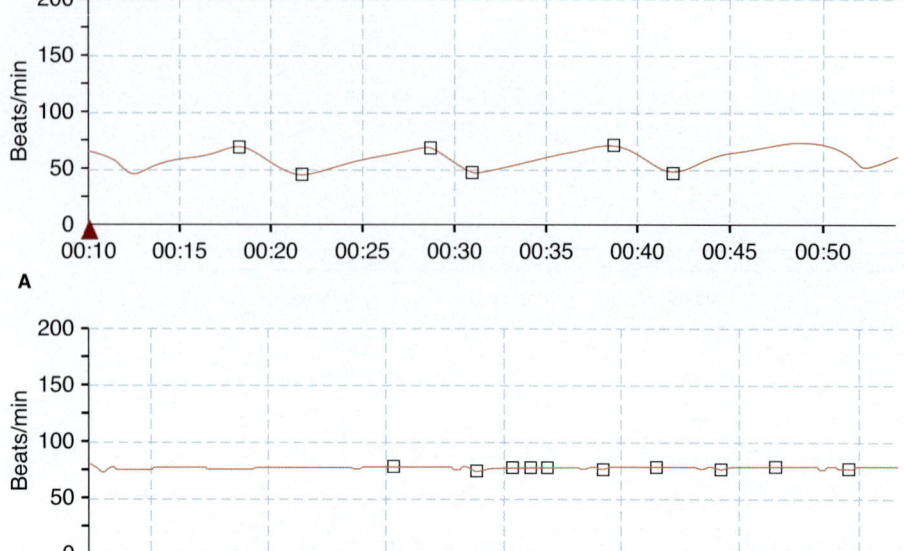

Figure 22-2. Heart rate variability. Normally, the heart rate varies with respiration (**A**). Some individuals with small fiber involvement have an autonomic neuropathy with cardiovagal abnormalities, as demonstrated by reduced heart rate variability with deep breathing (**B**).

histopathologically is by measuring IENFD on skin biopsies (Fig. 22-4).[3,7,13–20,43,50–55] Assessment of IENFD also appears to be more sensitive in identifying patients with small fiber neuropathies than sural nerve biopsies, NCSs, or QST. A punch biopsy of the skin can be obtained at the foot, calf, and/or thigh, and immunohistochemistry using antibodies directed against protein gene product 9.5 (PGP 9.5) is used to stain small intraepidermal fibers. IENFs arising entirely from the dorsal root ganglia represent the terminals of C and Aδ nociceptors. The density of these nerve fibers is reduced in patients with small fiber neuropathies, in which NCSs, QST, and routine nerve biopsies are often normal. In at least a third of people with painful sensory neuropathies, IENFD on skin biopsies represents the only objective abnormality present following extensive evaluation.[7] Furthermore, IENFD can be normal in patients with symptoms and signs of a small fiber neuropathy. Thus, it can be argued as well that skin biopsies are not required for a clinical diagnosis of small fiber neuropathy but are a useful tool for research studies. A skin biopsy is certainly not necessary in patients with abnormal sensory NCS.

One recent large study of patients with small fiber polyneuropathy reported two clinical signs and abnormal QST

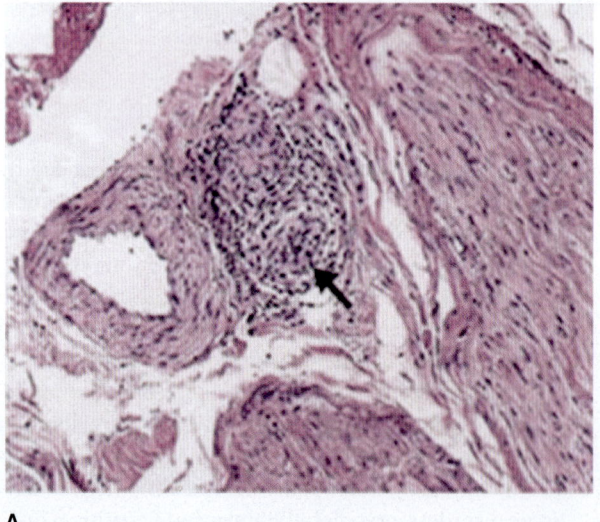
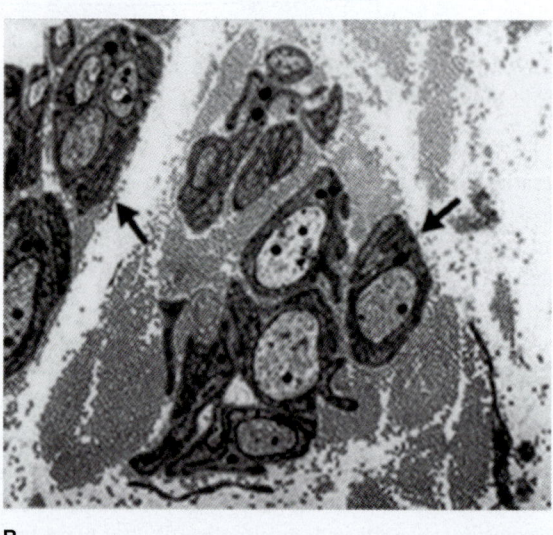

Figure 22-3. Specimen from a sural nerve biopsy. The nerve is morphologically normal on light microscopy (**A**). There is a focal perivascular lymphocytic infiltrate, and in one small perineurial vessel (*arrow*) the infiltrate extends through the wall (hematoxylin and eosin, ×125). There is no necrosis or other evidence of vasculitis or intraneural inflammation. An electron micrograph (**B**) shows empty Schwann-cell processes (*arrows*) that are consistent with the loss of small, unmyelinated fibers (×8,000). (Used with permission of Doctors Lawrence Hayward and Thomas Smith, University of Massachusetts Medical School, Worcester, MA.)

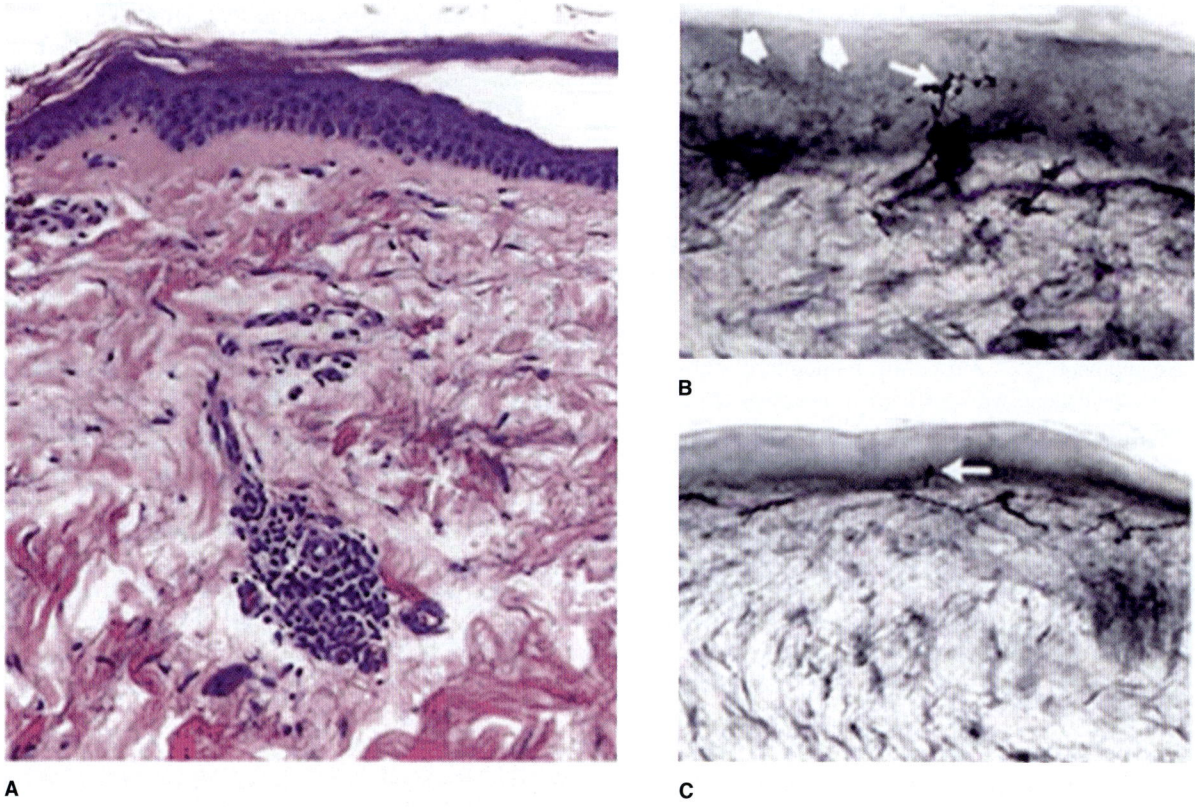

Figure 22-4. Specimens from skin-punch biopsies. A specimen obtained at the time of the patient's first evaluation at this hospital (**A**) shows a focal perivascular lymphocytic infiltrate (hematoxylin and eosin, ×125). A section immunolabeled against protein gene product 9.5 to reveal neural processes or axons (*thick arrows*) (**B**) shows an epidermal neurite with axonal swellings, which are abnormal (*thin arrow*). The density of nerve fibers is greater than normal (immunoperoxidase, ×500). A specimen obtained 11 months later (**C**) shows marked reduction in neurite density and axonal swelling (*arrow*) in a remaining neurite (×300). (Reproduced with permission from Amato AA, Oaklander AL. Case 162004: A 76-year-old woman with numbness and pain in the feet and legs. *N Engl J Med.* 2004;350:2181–2189. Figure 2, p. 2187.)

and IENFD in 69.1%, abnormal QST alone in 5.4%, abnormal IENFD alone in 20.1%, while only 5.4% had abnormal QST and IENFD but no clinical signs.[19] Notably, some patients had sensory symptoms but had a normal clinical exam. Of those, 89.4% had normal QST and IENFD, 10.5% had abnormal QST and normal IENFD, and none had only abnormal IENFD. Their conclusion was that the combination of clinical signs and abnormal QST and/or IENFD findings was more reliable than the combination of abnormal QST and IENFD findings in the absence of clinical signs in diagnosing small fiber polyneuropathy.

PATHOGENESIS

As the name implies, the pathogenic basis of chronic, idiopathic, length-dependent sensory or sensorimotor polyneuropathy is unknown, but is likely multifactorial in etiology. Some may have a primary degenerative or immunologic basis. Prediabetes is part of the metabolic syndrome, which also includes hypertension, hyperlipidemia, and obesity. Individual aspects of the metabolic syndrome influence risk and progression of diabetic neuropathy and may play a causative role in neuropathy for those with both prediabetes and otherwise idiopathic neuropathy.

A number of studies have shown that some cases of "idiopathic" or "cryptogenic" sensorimotor polyneuropathies subsequently were demonstrated to a genetic etiology.[56–64] Prominent distal weakness in addition to sensory abnormalities should prompt investigation for hereditary neuropathies as most idiopathic neuropathies are primarily sensory. A recent study of that assessed patients with otherwise idiopathic polyneuropathy found 18% had causal variants in various genes known to cause Charcot–Marie–Tooth disease (CMT)—the most frequent being in *MME* that encodes for the metalloprotease neprilysin.[57] Others have found that biallelic mutations in the sorbitol dehydrogenase gene (*SORD*) is the most frequent recessive form of hereditary neuropathy.[58] This mutation is not picked up on routine next-generation sequencing panels and require more advance testing such as long read sequencing.[59] Pathogenic sequence variants in the replication factor complex subunit 1 gene, *RFC1*, usually cause the autosomal recessive cerebellar ataxia, neuropathy, vestibular areflexia (CANVAS) syndrome (see Chapter 12). However, patients can present with only sensory symptoms and signs.[60,61] In regard to small fiber neuropathies, at least 80 pathogenic mutations have been reported in a variety of different sodium channel genes, the most common of which include SCN7A, SCN9A, SCN10A, and SCN11A (see Chapter 11).[62-64]

TREATMENT

Unfortunately, there is no treatment for slowing the progression or reversing the "numbness" or lack of sensation. Therapies are aimed at symptomatic management of neuropathic pain and reducing the risk of falling through the use of durable medical equipment.[8,9,65-69] Most of the randomized controlled trials addressed patients with postherpetic neuralgia or painful neuropathy mainly caused by diabetes. A large number of such class I trials provide level A evidence for the efficacy of tricyclic antidepressants, gabapentin, pregabalin, and opioids followed by topical lidocaine (in postherpetic neuralgia) and newer antidepressants such as venlafaxine and duloxetine (in painful neuropathy).[68] A recent adaptive trial in which participants were randomized to receive nortriptyline ($n = 134$), duloxetine ($n = 126$), pregabalin ($n = 73$), or mexiletine ($n = 69$) demonstrated that none of these medications were clearly superior, though nortriptyline and duloxetine appeared to be better than pregabalin and mexiletine when pain reduction and undesirable adverse effects were combined as a single endpoint.[69] Randomized, placebo-controlled trials have failed to demonstrate efficacy of IVIG in treatment of patients with small fiber polyneuropathy with our without various autoantibodies (i.e., anti–TS-HDS and FGFR-3).[70,71]

Our approach to treating the painful paresthesias and burning sensation associated with chronic idiopathic sensory neuropathy is uniform regardless of etiology (e.g., painful sensory neuropathies related to DM, HIV infection, and herpes zoster infection) (Table 22-2).[72-78] We often start off with lidocaine 5% patches to the feet, as this treatment is associated with less systemic side effects. If this does not suffice (and it usually does not), our next step is to add a medication from one of four classes of medications that have been shown to be effective for neuropathic pain: (1) gabapentin/pregabalin, (2) tricyclic antidepressants (TCA), (3) serotonin/norepinephrine reuptake inhibitors (SNRIs), (4) sodium-channel blockers (e.g., oxcarbazepine). There is no evidence that any one class is more efficacious than the others, so the choice of medication should be individualized based on patient preference and other comorbidities. A patient with concurrent depression, for example, might benefit from a TCA or SNRI; a patient with epilepsy might benefit from oxcarbazepine. We usually start at a low dose and gradually increase as necessary and as tolerated. A combination of an antiepileptic and antidepressant medication should be tried if monotherapy leads to an insufficient response. Chronic opiate treatment, including the use of tramadol, should be avoided. Asking patients about concurrent mood disorders or sleep disorders and managing them accordingly can be a helpful adjunct in managing neuropathic pain, as well.

▶ IDIOPATHIC SENSORY NEURONOPATHY/GANGLIONOPATHY

There are a number of known etiologies for sensory neuropathy/ganglionopathy.[79-81] Most cases are believed to be caused by an autoimmune attack directed against the dorsal root ganglia. These include a paraneoplastic syndrome, which is typically associated with anti-Hu antibodies, a sensory

▶ **TABLE 22-2. TREATMENT OF PAINFUL SENSORY NEUROPATHIES**

Therapy	Route	Dose	Side Effects
Lidoderm 5% patch	Apply cutaneously	Up to three patches daily for 12 hours at a time	Local irritation
Capsaicin 0.025–0.075% cream	Apply cutaneously	QID	Painful burning skin
Gabapentin	p.o.	300–1,200 mg TID	Cognitive changes and sedation
Pregabalin	p.o.	300–600 mg total daily dose, divided into BID or TID	Cognitive changes and sedation
Tricyclic antidepressants (e.g., amitriptyline and nortriptyline)	p.o.	10–100 mg qhs	Cognitive changes, sedation, dry eyes and mouth, urinary retention, and constipation
Duloxetine	p.o.	30–60 mg daily	Cognitive changes, dizziness, sedation, insomnia, nausea, and constipation
Venlafaxine	p.o.	75–150 mg daily	Asthenia, sweating, nausea, constipation, anorexia, vomiting, somnolence, dry mouth, dizziness, nervousness, anxiety, tremor, and blurred vision as well as abnormal ejaculation/orgasm and impotence
Oxcarbazepine	p.o.	150–900 mg BID	Cognitive changes, dizziness, hyponatremia, leukopenia or thrombocytopenia, rare risk of Stevens-Johnson syndrome

GI, gastrointestinal.

ganglionitis related to Sjögren syndrome, and celiac disease. The acute cases may represent a variant of GBS, although the onset can be insidiously in nature and slowly progressive. Certain medications or toxins (e.g., various chemotherapies, vitamin B6), infectious agents (e.g., HIV), and other systemic disorders are also associated with a sensory neuronopathy. Less common are genetic disorders [e.g., cerebellar ataxia, neuropathy, and vestibular areflexia syndrome (CANVAS), hereditary vitamin E deficiency, and rare mitochondria neuropathies]. Despite extensive evaluation, many cases of sensory neuronopathy have no clear etiology, the so-called idiopathic sensory neuronopathy.

CLINICAL FEATURES

Idiopathic sensory neuronopathy is a rare disorder that usually presents in adulthood (mean age of onset 49 years, with range 18–81 years) and has a slight female predominance.[79–88] Symptoms can develop over a few hours or evolve more insidiously over several months or years, and the course can be monophasic with a stable or remitting deficit, chronic progressive, or chronic relapsing. Unlike typical GBS, only rare patients report a recent antecedent infection. The presenting complaint is numbness and tingling face, trunk, or limbs, which can be painful. Symptoms begin asymmetrically and in the upper limbs in nearly half of the patients, suggesting a ganglionopathy as opposed to a length-dependent process. Usually, the sensory symptoms become generalized, but they can remain asymmetric. Patients also describe clumsiness of the hands and gait instability. Severe autonomic symptoms develop in some.[82,88]

On examination, marked reduction in vibration and proprioception are found, while pain and temperature sensations are less affected. Manual muscle testing is usually normal. Some muscle groups may appear weak, but this is usually secondary to impaired modulation of motor activity due to the proprioceptive defect. Most patients have sensory ataxia, which can be readily demonstrated by having the patient perform the finger–nose–finger test with their eyes open and then closed. Patients may have only mild dysmetria with their eyes open, but when their eyes are closed, they consistently miss their nose and the examiner's stationed finger. Pseudoathetoid movements of the extremities may also be appreciated. Patients exhibit a positive Romberg sign and, not surprisingly, describe more gait instability in the dark or with their eyes closed while in the shower. Muscle stretch reflexes are decreased or absent, while plantar reflexes are flexor.

A detailed history and examination are essential to exclude a toxic neuronopathy, paraneoplastic syndrome, or disorder related to a connective tissue disease (i.e., Sjögren syndrome). Importantly, the sensory neuronopathy can precede the onset of malignancy or Sicca symptoms (i.e., dry eyes and mouth); therefore, these disorders should always be kept in mind. Pertinent laboratory and malignancy workup should be ordered. A rose bengal stain or Schirmer's test may be abnormal in patients with sicca symptoms. A lip or parotid gland biopsy likewise can be abnormal revealing inflammatory cell infiltration and destruction of the glands. Subacute sensory neuronopathy has also been associated with recent Epstein–Barr virus infection.[89]

LABORATORY FEATURES

The CSF protein is normal or only slightly elevated in most patients. However, the CSF protein can be markedly elevated (reportedly as high as 300 mg/dL) when examined within a few days in cases with a hyperacute onset. Only rare patients exhibit CSF pleocytosis. MRI scan can reveal gadolinium enhancement of the posterior spinal roots or increased signal abnormalities on T2-weighted images in the posterior columns of the spinal cord.[88,90] Some patients have a monoclonal gammopathy (IgM, IgG, or IgA). Ganglioside antibodies, particularly GD1b antibodies, have been demonstrated in some cases of idiopathic sensory neuronopathy associated with IgM monoclonal gammopathy.[91]

Antineuronal nuclear antibodies (e.g., anti-Hu antibodies) should be assayed in all individuals with sensory neuronopathy to evaluate for a paraneoplastic syndrome. Likewise, antinuclear, SSA, and SSB antibodies should be ordered to look for evidence of Sjögren syndrome, which can also present with a sensory neuronopathy.

The characteristic NCS finding is low-amplitude or absent sensory nerve action potentials (SNAPs) in the arms, while the SNAPs in the legs may be normal,[84,85,87,90] a pattern that can also be seen in sensory nerve conductions in acquired inflammatory demyelinating neuropathy. In the either case, this pattern indicates the non–length-dependent nature of these disorders. However, some patients can present with distal symmetric lower extremity symptoms, signs, and SNAP abnormalities mimicking a length-dependent process.[92] When SNAPs are obtainable, the distal sensory latencies and NCVs are normal or only mildly abnormal. In contrast, motor NCSs either are normal or reveal only mild abnormalities. In addition, H reflexes and blink reflexes are typically be unobtainable.[93] An abnormal blink reflex favors a nonparaneoplastic etiology for a sensory neuronopathy but does not exclude an underlying malignancy.[94] The masseter reflex or jaw jerk is abnormal in patients with sensory neuropathy but is usually preserved in patients with sensory neuronopathy.[93] The masseter reflex is unique among the stretch reflexes in that the cell bodies of the afferent limb lie in the mesencephalic nucleus within the CNS. This differs from the sensory cell bodies innervating the limbs, which reside in the dorsal root ganglia of the PNS. The blink reflex can be impaired in sensory ganglionopathies because the afferent cell bodies lie in the gasserian ganglia that are outside the CNS.

HISTOPATHOLOGY

Sensory nerve biopsies may reveal a preferential loss of large myelinated or small unmyelinated fibers. Mild perivascular inflammation may be seen, but prominent endoneurial infiltrate is not appreciated. There is no evidence of segmental demyelination.

Autopsies performed in a couple of patients with acute idiopathic sensory neuronopathy have revealed widespread inflammation involving sensory and autonomic ganglia, with loss of associated neurons and wallerian degeneration of the posterior nerve roots and dorsal columns being evident in one.[83] The motor neurons and roots were normal. Immunohistochemistry suggested a CD8+ T-cell mediated attach directed against sensory ganglia. In another autopsy, there was severe neuronal cell loss in the thoracic sympathetic and dorsal root ganglia, and Auerbach's plexus with well-preserved anterior horn cells.[88] Myelinated fibers in the anterior spinal root were preserved, while those in the posterior spinal root and the posterior column of the spinal cord were depleted.

PATHOGENESIS

In some cases, the sensory neuronopathies may be caused by an autoimmune attack directed against the dorsal root ganglia. Serum from affected patients immunostain dorsal root ganglia cells in culture and inhibits neurite formation.[95] The neuronal epitope is unknown, but some authors have hypothesized that ganglioside GD1b might be target antigen in some cases.[91] GD1b localizes to neurons in the dorsal root ganglia, and antibodies directed against this ganglioside have been detected in some patients with idiopathic sensory neuronopathy.[83] Furthermore, rabbits immunized with purified GD1b develop ataxic sensory neuropathy associated with loss of the cell bodies in the dorsal root ganglia and axonal degeneration of the dorsal column of the spinal cord but without demyelination or an inflammatory infiltrate.

TREATMENT

Various modes of immunotherapy have been tried, including corticosteroids, plasma exchange (PE), and intravenous immune globulin (IVIG).[88,90] However, there have been no prospective, double-blind, placebo-controlled trials. Occasionally, patients appear to improve with therapy; however, some improve spontaneously and many stabilize without treatment. In our experience, most patients have not experienced a dramatic improvement following treatment. Perhaps, this is because once the cell body of the sensory neuron is destroyed, it will not regenerate. However, in patients seen in the acute setting or those who have a chronic progressive deficit, a trial of immunotherapy may be warranted.

▶ IDIOPATHIC SMALL FIBER SENSORY NEURONOPATHY/GANGLIONOPATHY

This may represent a subtype of sensory neuropathy/ganglionopathy discussed in the preceding section that clinically only involves small fiber neurons.

CLINICAL FEATURES

Most patients with small fiber neuropathy present insidiously with slowly progressive burning pain and paresthesia in a length-dependent fashion beginning in the feet. Such cases are often idiopathic in nature, but DM, amyloidosis, Sjögren syndrome, and hereditary sensory and autonomic neuropathy need to be excluded. However, some individuals present with symptoms suggestive of a small fiber neuropathy that are not length-dependent.[80,96–101] Often this type of neuropathy begins acutely and an antecedent infection is common. Affected individuals often describe numbness, tingling, or burning pain in the face, trunk, or arms before or more severe than in the distal lower extremities. Patients with non–length-dependent small fiber neuronopathy may more often report an "itchy" quality and allodynia to light touch.[100] Neurological examination discloses normal muscle strength and a non–length-dependent sensory loss for pain or temperature. Proprioception, vibratory perception, and reflexes are normal. The burning dysesthesia usually disappears within 4 months; however, the numbness and objective sensory loss tended to persist longer.

LABORATORY FEATURES

CSF examination may reveal albuminocytological dissociation. Motor and sensory conduction studies that primarily assess large fiber function are normal. Autonomic testing may be abnormal.

HISTOPATHOLOGY

In an autopsy case, there was severe neuronal cell loss in the thoracic sympathetic and dorsal root ganglia, and Auerbach's plexus with well-preserved anterior horn cells.[88] Myelinated fibers in the anterior spinal root were preserved, while those in the posterior spinal root and the posterior column of the spinal cord were depleted. Skin biopsies in some patients have shown reduced nerve fiber density that is not length-dependent (i.e., loss is worse in the thigh compared to calf).[99,102,103]

PATHOGENESIS

The acute clinical presentation often following an infection and CSF findings suggests an autoimmune variant, perhaps a rare variant of GBS. A recent retrospective multicentric case-control study screened 132 patients with small fiber neuropathy, 301 with other polyneuropathies, 274 with other autoimmune diseases, and 116 healthy controls for antibodies targeting Argonaute (AGO) proteins, a family of 4 RNA-binding proteins.[104] They reported AGO antibodies in 12.9% of patients with small fiber neuropathy, 3.7% with other neuropathies, and those with 5.8% of those with other autoimmune diseases.

TREATMENT

Those patients with chronic, slowly progressive idiopathic small fiber neuropathy can be managed symptomatically in a similar fashion to idiopathic sensory or sensorimotor polyneuropathy. If a patient is diagnosed with an acute, non-length-dependent form of small fiber neuropathy resembling a GBS variant, a trial of IVIG could be considered during the acute progressive phase though the evidence base for this is sparse. Importantly, a non-length-dependent pattern in patients with chronic small fiber neuropathy does not automatically equate to an autoimmune etiology. Evidence from randomized control trials does not suggest that these patients benefit from chronic, maintenance immunomodulatory therapy. Patients with non-length-dependent small fiber neuropathy do, however, have a higher frequency of underlying autoimmune disorders so laboratory work-up should generally be more thorough in these patients.[105–108]

▶ FACIAL ONSET SENSORY AND MOTOR NEURONOPATHY

This is a non–length-dependent neuronopathy/ganglionopathy that starts with loss of facial sensation and overtime also involves motor neurons.

CLINICAL FEATURES

Patients usually developed paraesthesia and numbness initially in a trigeminal nerve distribution that slowly progresses to involve sensory neurons innervating the scalp, neck, upper trunk, and upper limbs in a descending pattern.[109–113] Over 5–10 years, dysphagia and dysarthria occur along with cramps, fasciculations and weakness, and atrophy in the arms due to slowly progressive lower motor neuron involvement. Ventilatory failure may also develop. Upper motor neuron signs do not typically appear.

LABORATORY FEATURES

NCSs typically reveal reduced amplitudes or absent SNAPs in arms, while SNAPs are normal in the legs. Blink reflexes are abnormal. Subsequently, CMAP amplitudes may diminish and active denervation is apparent on EMG. MRI scans may demonstrate mild atrophy of the brainstem and spinal cord. Some patients have been reported with antisulfatide or GD1b antibodies.[65]

HISTOPATHOLOGY

Autopsy in one patient disclosed loss of motor neurons in the hypoglossal nucleus and cervical anterior horns, along with loss of sensory neurons in the main trigeminal sensory nucleus and dorsal root ganglia.[65]

PATHOGENESIS

The pathogenic basis of facial onset sensory and motor neuronopathy (FOSMN) is unknown. Those patients harboring autoantibodies have suggested a possible autoimmune basis. However, treatment with a variety of immunotherapies has not resulted in improvement or halt of progression, a finding which suggesting FOSMN is a primary neurodegenerative disorder. Rare patients have been found to have mutations in genes that can cause familial motor neuron disease, including *SOD1*, *TARDBP*, *SQSTM1*, *VCP*, and *CHCHD10* that support that FOSMN is likely a neurogenic disorder of oligogenetic etiology.[114–117]

TREATMENT

Treatment at this time is supportive therapy.

▶ SUMMARY

Chronic idiopathic/cryptogenic polyneuropathies are quite common in clinical practice despite extensive laboratory evaluation. A standard laboratory workup, including NCSs, is important to perform before concluding that the neuropathy is idiopathic in nature. Many of the patients may have IGT, particularly those with a small fiber phenotype, if an oral GTT is performed, even if they have normal FBS and HgbA1C levels. Nerve biopsies are generally not indicated. Although skin biopsy may be informative by showing reduced epidermal nerve fibers when other studies (e.g., NCSs, QST, and autonomic studies) are normal, they do not define etiology and often do tell us nothing that we don't already know based on the history and clinical examination. That is, persons with burning and tingling pain in their feet with normal reflexes and NCSs probably have a small fiber neuropathy, regardless of what the skin biopsy shows. Patients need reassurance that it is not all that unusual for an etiology of neuropathy to be undetermined despite workup. Primary treatment is directed and symptomatic management of their pain.

REFERENCES

1. Amato AA, Oaklander AL. Case records of the Massachusetts general hospital. Weekly clinicopathological exercises. Case16-2004. A 76-year-old woman with numbness and pain in the feet and legs. *N Engl J Med*. 2004;350(21):2181–2189.
2. Gorson KC, Ropper AH. Idiopathic distal sensory small fiber neuropathy. *Acta Neurol Scand*. 1995;92(5):376–382.
3. Holland NR, Crawford TO, Hauer P, Cornblath DR, Griffin JW, McArthur JC. Small-fiber sensory neuropathies: clinical course and neuropathology of idiopathic cases. *Ann Neurol*. 1998;44(1):47–59.
4. Lacomis D. Small-fiber neuropathy. *Muscle Nerve*. 2002; 26(2):173–188.

5. McLeod JG, Tuck RR, Pollard JD, Cameron J, Walsh JC. Chronic polyneuropathy of undetermined cause. *J Neurol Neurosurg Psychiatry*. 1984;47(5):530–535.
6. Notermans NC, Wokke JH, Franssen H, et al. Chronic idiopathic polyneuropathy presenting in middle or old age: a clinical and electrophysiological study of 75 patients. *J Neurol Neurosurg Psychiatry*. 1993;56(10):1066–1071.
7. Periquet MI, Novak V, Collins MP, et al. Painful sensory neuropathy: prospective evaluation of painful feet using electrodiagnosis and skin biopsy. *Neurology*. 1999;53(8):1641–1647.
8. Wolfe GI, Barohn RJ. Cryptogenic sensory and sensorimotor polyneuropathies. *Semin Neurol*. 1998;18(1):105–111.
9. Wolfe GI, Baker NS, Amato AA, et al. Chronic cryptogenic sensory polyneuropathy: clinical and laboratory characteristics. *Arch Neurol*. 1999;56(5):540–547.
10. Grahmann F, Winterholler M, Neundörfer B. Cryptogenic polyneuropathies: an out-patient follow-up study. *Acta Neurol Scand*. 1991;84(3):221–225.
11. Notermans NC, Wokke JH, van den Berg LH, et al. Chronic idiopathic axonal polyneuropathy. Comparison of patients with and without monoclonal gammopathy. *Brain*. 1996;119(pt 2):421–427.
12. Zis P, Sarrigiannis PG, Rao DG, Hewamadduma C, Hadjivassiliou M. Chronic idiopathic axonal polyneuropathy: a systematic review. *J Neurol*. 2016;263(10):1903–1910.
13. Freeman R, Gewandter JS, Faber CG, et al. Idiopathic distal sensory polyneuropathy: ACTTION diagnostic criteria. *Neurology*. 2020;95(22):1005–1014.
14. Haroutounian S, Todorovic MS, Leinders M, et al. Diagnostic criteria for idiopathic small fiber neuropathy: a systematic review. *Muscle Nerve*. 2021;63(2):170–177.
15. Johnson SA, Shouman K, Shelly S, et al. Small fiber neuropathy incidence, prevalence, longitudinal impairments, and disability. *Neurology*. 2021;97(22):e2236–e2247.
16. Finsterer J, Scorza FA. Small fiber neuropathy. *Acta Neurol Scand*. 2022;145(5):493–503.
17. Bitzi LM, Lehnick D, Wilder-Smith EP. Small fiber neuropathy: Swiss cohort characterization. *Muscle Nerve*. 2021;64(3):293–300.
18. Terkelsen AJ, Karlsson P, Lauria G, Freeman R, Finnerup NB, Jensen TS. The diagnostic challenge of small fibre neuropathy: clinical presentations, evaluations, and causes. *Lancet Neurol*. 2017;16(11):934–944.
19. Devigili G, Rinaldo S, Lombardi R, et al. Diagnostic criteria for small fibre neuropathy in clinical practice and research. *Brain*. 2019;142(12):3728–3736.
20. Devigili G, Tugnoli V, Penza P, et al. The diagnostic criteria for small fibre neuropathy: from symptoms to neuropathology. *Brain*. 2008;131(7):1912–1925.
21. England JD, Gronseth GS, Franklin G, et al. Evaluation of distal symmetric polyneuropathy: the role of laboratory and genetic testing (an evidence-based review). *Muscle Nerve*. 2009;39(1):116–125.
22. England JD, Gronseth GS, Franklin G, et al. Evaluation of distal symmetric polyneuropathy: the role of autonomic testing, nerve biopsy, and skin biopsy (an evidence-based review). *Muscle Nerve*. 2009;39(1):106–115.
23. Singleton JR, Smith AG, Bromberg MB. Painful sensory polyneuropathy associated with impaired glucose tolerance test. *Muscle Nerve*. 2001;24(9):1225–1228.
24. Novella SP, Inzucchi SE, Goldstein JM. The frequency of undiagnosed diabetes and impaired glucose tolerance in patients with idiopathic sensory neuropathy. *Muscle Nerve*. 2001;24(9):1229–1231.
25. Sumner CJ, Sheth S, Griffin JW, Cornblath DR, Polyswdkia M. The spectrum of neuropathy in diabetes and impaired glucose tolerance. *Neurology*. 2003;60(1):108–111.
26. Harris MI, Flegal KM, Cowie CC, et al. Prevalence of diabetes, impaired fasting glucose, and impaired glucose tolerance in U.S. adults. The third national health and nutrition examination survey, 1988–1994. *Diabetes Care*. 1998;21(4):518–524.
27. Smith AG, Singleton JR. The diagnostic yield of a standardized approach to idiopathic sensory-predominant neuropathy. *Arch Intern Med*. 2004;164(9):1021–1025.
28. Gordon Smith A, Robinson Singleton J. Idiopathic neuropathy, prediabetes and the metabolic syndrome. *J Neurol Sci*. 2006;242(1–2):9–14.
29. Hughes RAC, Umapathi T, Gray IA, et al. A controlled investigation of the cause of chronic idiopathic axonal polyneuropathy. *Brain*. 2004;127(Pt 8):1723–1730.
30. Russell JW, Feldman EL. Impaired glucose tolerance—does it cause neuropathy? *Muscle Nerve*. 2001;24(9):1109–1112.
31. Dyck PJ, Dyck PJB, Klein CJ, Weigand SD. Does impaired glucose metabolism cause polyneuropathy? Review of previous studies and design of a prospective controlled population-based study. *Muscle Nerve*. 2007;36(4):536–541.
32. Kissel JT, Mendell JR. Neuropathies associated with monoclonal gammopathies. *Neuromuscul Disord*. 1996;6(1):3–18.
33. Nemni R, Fazio R, Quattrini A, Lorenzetti I, Mamoli D, Canal N. Antibodies to sulfatide and to chondroitin sulfate C in patients with chronic sensory neuropathy. *J Neuroimmunol*. 1993;43(1–2):79–85.
34. Pestronk A, Li F, Griffin J, et al. Polyneuropathy syndromes associated with serum antibodies to sulfatide and myelin-associated glycoprotein. *Neurology*. 1991;41(3):357–362.
35. Levine TD, Kafaie J, Zeidman LA, et al. Cryptogenic small-fiber neuropathies: serum autoantibody binding to trisulfated heparan disaccharide and fibroblast growth factor receptor-3. *Muscle Nerve*. 2020;61(4):512–515.
36. Chompoopong P, Rezk M, Mirman I, et al. TS-HDS autoantibody: clinical characterization and utility from real-world tertiary care center experience. *J Neurol*. 2023;270(9):4523–4528.
37. Dyck PJ, O'Brien PC. Quantitative sensory testing in epidemiological and therapeutic studies of peripheral neuropathy. *Muscle Nerve*. 1999;22(6):659–662.
38. Verdugo RJ, Matamala JM, Inui K, et al. Review of techniques useful for the assessment of 406 sensory small fiber neuropathies: report from an IFCN expert group. *Clin Neurophysiol*. 2022;136:13–38.
39. Stewart JD, Low PA, Fealy RD. Distal small fiber neuropathy: results of tests of sweating and autonomic cardiovascular reflexes. *Muscle Nerve*. 1992;15(6):661–665.
40. Novak V, Freimer ML, Kissel JT, et al. Autonomic impairment in painful neuropathy. *Neurology*. 2001;56(7):861–868.
41. Tobkin K, Guiliani MJ, Lacomis D. Comparison of different modalities for detection of small fiber neuropathy. *Clin Neurophysiol*. 1999;110(11):1909–1912.
42. Low VA, Sandroni P, Fealey RD, Low PA. Detection of small-fiber neuropathy by sudomotor testing. *Muscle Nerve*. 2006;34(1):57–61.
43. Holland NR, Stocks A, Hauer P, Cornblath DR, Griffin JW, McArthur JC. Intraepidermal nerve fiber density in patients with painful sensory neuropathy. *Neurology*. 1997;48(3):708–711.
44. Smith AG, Raachandran P, Tripp S, Singleton JR. Epidermal nerve innervation in impaired glucose tolerance and diabetes-associated neuropathy. *Neurology*. 2001;57(9):1701–1704.

45. Mendell JR, Sahenk Z. Painful sensory neuropathy. *N Engl J Med*. 2003;348(13):1243–1255.
46. Freeman R, Chase KP, Risk MR. Quantitative sensory testing cannot differentiate simulated sensory loss from sensory neuropathy. *Neurology*. 2003;60(3):465–470.
47. Kelkar P, McDermott WR, Parry GJ. Sensory-predominant, painful, idiopathic neuropathy: inflammatory changes in sural nerves. *Muscle Nerve*. 2002;26:413–416.
48. Bosboom WM, Van den Berg LH, De Boer L, et al. The diagnostic value of sural nerve T cells in chronic inflammatory demyelinating polyneuropathy. *Neurology*. 1999;53(4):837–845.
49. Gherardi RK, Farcet J-P, Créange A, et al. Dominant T-cell clones of unknown significance in patients with idiopathic sensory neuropathies. *Neurology*. 1998;51(2):384–389.
50. Vlcková-Moravcová E, Bednařík J, Dusek L, Toyka KV, Sommer C. Diagnostic validity of epidermal nerve fiber densities in painful sensory neuropathies. *Muscle Nerve*. 2008;37(1):50–60.
51. Herrmann DN, Griffin JW, Hauer P, Cornblath DR, McArthur JC. Epidermal nerve fiber density, sural nerve morphometry and electrodiagnosis in peripheral neuropathies. *Neurology*. 1999;53(8):1634–1640.
52. McCarthy BG, Hseih ST, Stocks A, et al. Cutaneous innervation in sensory neuropathies: evaluation by skin biopsy. *Neurology*. 1995;45(10):1848–1855.
53. Wendelschafer-Crabb G, Kennedy WR, Walk D. Morphological features of nerves in skin biopsies. *J Neurol Sci*. 2006;242(1–2):15–21.
54. Hays AP. Utility of skin biopsy to evaluate peripheral neuropathy. *Curr Neurol Neurosci Rep*. 2010;10(2):101–107.
55. Walk D, Wendelschafer-Crabb G, Davey C, Kennedy WR. Concordance between epidermal nerve fiber density and sensory examination in patients with symptoms of idiopathic small fiber neuropathy. *J Neurol Sci*. 2007;255(1–2):23–26.
56. Shy ME. Genetics and adult-onset chronic idiopathic axonal neuropathy. *Neurology*. 2020;95(24):1071–1073.
57. Senderek J, Lassuthova P, Kabzińska D, et al. The genetic landscape of axonal neuropathies in the middle-aged and elderly: focus on MME. *Neurology*. 2020;95:e3163–e3179.
58. Cortese A, Zhu Y, Rebelo AP, et al. Biallelic mutations in SORD cause a common and potentially treatable hereditary neuropathy with implications for diabetes. *Nat Genet*. 2020;52(5):473–481.
59. Grosz BR, Stevanovski I, Negri S, et al. Long read sequencing overcomes challenges in the diagnosis of SORD neuropathy. *J Peripher Nerv Syst*. 2022;27(2):120–126.
60. Currò R, Salvalaggio A, Tozza S, et al. RFC1 expansions are a common cause of idiopathic sensory neuropathy. *Brain*. 2021;144(5):1542–1550.
61. Tagliapietra M, Cardellini D, Ferrarini M, et al. RFC1 AAGGG repeat expansion masquerading as chronic idiopathic axonal polyneuropathy. *J Neurol*. 2021;268(11):4280–4290.
62. Chan ACY, Kumar S, Tan G, et al. Expanding the genetic causes of small-fiber neuropathy: SCN genes and beyond. *Muscle Nerve*. 2023;67(4):259–271.
63. Eijkenboom I, Sopacua M, Hoeijmakers JGJ, et al. Yield of peripheral sodium channels gene screening in pure small fibre neuropathy. *J Neurol Neurosurg Psychiatry*. 2019;90(3):342–352.
64. Almomani R, Sopacua M, Marchi M, et al. Genetic profiling of sodium channels in diabetic painful and painless and idiopathic painful and painless neuropathies. *Int J Mol Sci*. 2023;24(9):8278.
65. Wolfe GI, Trivedi JR. Painful peripheral neuropathy and its non-surgical treatment. *Muscle Nerve*. 2004;30(1):3–19.
66. Gilron I, Bailey JM, Dongsheng T, Holderen RR, Weaver DF, Houlden RL. Morphine, gabapentin, or other combination for neuropathic pain. *N Engl J Med*. 2005;352(13):1324–1334.
67. Singleton JR. Evaluation and treatment of painful peripheral polyneuropathy. *Semin Neurol*. 2005;25(2):185–195.
68. Attal N, Cruccu G, Haanpaa M, et al. EFNS guidelines on pharmacological treatment of neuropathic pain. *Eur J Neurol*. 2006;13(11):1153–1169.
69. Barohn RJ, Gajewski B, Pasnoor M, et al. Patient assisted intervention for neuropathy: comparison of treatment in real life situations (PAIN-CONTRoLS): Bayesian Adaptive Comparative Effectiveness Randomized Trial. *JAMA Neurol*. 2021;78(1):68–76.
70. Geerts M, de Greef BTA, Sopacua M, et al. Intravenous immunoglobulin therapy in patients with painful idiopathic small fiber neuropathy. *Neurology*. 2021;96(20):e2534–e2545.
71. Gibbons CH, Rajan S, Senechal K, Hendry E, McCallister B, Levine TD. A double-blind placebo-controlled pilot study of immunoglobulin for small fiber neuropathy associated with TS-HDS and FGFR-3 autoantibodies. *Muscle Nerve*. 2023;67(5):363–370.
72. Attal N, Cruccu G, Baron R, et al. EFNS guidelines on the pharmacological treatment of neuropathic pain: 2010 revision. *Eur J Neurol*. 2010;17(9):1113–e88.
73. Finnerup NB, Attal N, Haroutounian S, et al. Pharmacotherapy for neuropathic pain in adults: systematic review, meta-analysis and updated NeuPSIG recommendations. *Lancet Neurol*. 2015;14(2):162–173.
74. Griebeler ML, Morey-Vargas OL, Brito JP, et al. Pharmacologic interventions for painful diabetic neuropathy: an umbrella systematic review and comparative effectiveness network meta-analysis. *Ann Intern Med*. 2014;161(9):639–649.
75. Hoffman EM, Watson JC, St Sauver J, Staff NP, Klein CJ. Association of long-term opioid therapy with functional status, adverse outcomes, and mortality among patients with polyneuropathy. *JAMA Neurol*. 2017;74(7):773–779.
76. Tesfaye S, Sloan G, Petrie J, et al. Comparison of amitriptyline supplemented with pregabalin, pregabalin supplemented with amitriptyline, and duloxetine supplemented with pregabalin for the treatment of diabetic peripheral neuropathic pain (OPTIONDM): a multicentre, double-blind, randomised crossover trial. *Lancet*. 2022;400(10353):680–690.
77. Price R, Smith D, Franklin G, et al. Oral and topical treatment of painful diabetic polyneuropathy: practice guideline update summary: Report of the AAN Guideline Subcommittee. *Neurology*. 2022;98(1):31–43.
78. Barohn RJ, Gajewski B, Pasnoor M, et al. Patient assisted intervention for neuropathy: comparison of treatment in real life situations (PAIN-CONTRoLS): Bayesian Adaptive Comparative Effectiveness Randomized Trial. *JAMA Neurol*. 2021;78(1):68–76. Erratum in: *JAMA Neurol*. 2020;77(11):1453.
79. Gwathmey KG. Sensory neuronopathies. *Muscle Nerve*. 2016;53(1):8–19.
80. Amato AA, Ropper AH. Sensory ganglionopathy. *N Engl J Med*. 2020;383(17):1657–1662.
81. Sancho Saldaña A, Mahdi-Rogers M, Hadden RD. Sensory neuronopathies: a case series and literature review. *J Peripher Nerv Syst*. 2021;26(1):66–74.
82. Gutierrez J, Palma JA, Kaufmann H. Acute sensory and autonomic neuronopathy: a devastating disorder affecting

sensory and autonomic ganglia. *Semin Neurol.* 2020;40(5): 580–590.
83. Hainfellner JA, Kristferitsch W, Lassmann H, et al. T cell-mediated ganglionitis associated with acute sensory neuronopathy. *Ann Neurol.* 1996;39(4):543–547.
84. Knazan M, Bohlega S, Berry K, Eisen A. Acute sensory neuronopathy with preserved SEPs and long-latency reflexes. *Muscle Nerve.* 1990;13(5):381–384.
85. Sterman AB, Schaumburg HH, Asbury AK. The acute sensory neuronopathy syndrome: a distinct clinical entity. *Ann Neurol.* 1980;7(4):354–358.
86. Kuntzer T, Atoine JC, Steck AJ. Clinical features and pathophysiological basis of sensory neuronopathies (ganglionopathies). *Muscle Nerve.* 2004;30(3):255–268.
87. Camdessanché JP, Jousserand G, Ferraud K, et al. The pattern and diagnostic criteria of sensory neuronopathy: a case-control study. *Brain.* 2009;132(pt 7):1723–1733.
88. Koike H, Atsuta N, Adachi H, et al. Clinicopathological features of acute autonomic and sensory neuropathy. *Brain.* 2010;133(10):2881–2896.
89. Rubin D, Daube JR. Subacute sensory neuropathy associated with Epstein–Barr virus. *Muscle Nerve.* 1999;22(11):1607–1610.
90. Wada M, Kato T, Yuki N, et al. Gadolinium-enhancement of the spinal posterior roots in acute sensory ataxic neuropathy. *Neurology.* 1997;49(5):1470–1471.
91. Dalakas MC. Autoimmune ataxic neuropathies (sensory ganglionopathies): are glycolipids the responsible autoantigens? *Ann Neurol.* 1996;39(4):419–422.
92. Davalos L, Nowacek DG, London ZN. Distal symmetric polyneuropathy phenotype in patients with sensory neuronopathy at the time of electrodiagnosis. *Muscle Nerve.* 2022;65(4):456–459.
93. Auger RG. The role of the masseter reflex in the assessment of subacute sensory neuropathy. *Muscle Nerve.* 1998;21(6):800–801.
94. Auger RG, Windebank AJ, Lucchinetti CF, Chalk CH. Role of the blink reflex in the evaluation of sensory neuronopathy. *Neurology.* 1999;53(2):407–408.
95. Van Dijk GW, Wokke JH, Notermans NC, van den Berg LH, Bär PR. Indications for an immune-mediated etiology of idiopathic sensory neuronopathy. *J Neuroimmunol.* 1997;74(1–2):165–172.
96. Gemignani F, Bellanova MF, Saccani E, Pavesi G. Non-length-dependent small fiber neuropathy: not a matter of stockings and gloves. *Muscle Nerve.* 2022;65(1):10–28.
97. Khoshnoodi MA, Truelove S, Burakgazi A, Hoke A, Mammen AL, Polydefkis M. Longitudinal assessment of small fiber neuropathy: evidence of a non-length-dependent distal axonopathy. *JAMA Neurol.* 2016;73(6):684–690.
98. Seneviratne U, Gunasekera S. Acute small fibre sensory neuropathy: another variant of Guillain–Barre syndrome? *J Neurol Neurosurg Psychiatry.* 2002;72(4):540–542.
99. Gorson KC, Herrmann DN, Thiagarajan R, et al. Non-length dependent small fibre neuropathy/ganglionopathy. *J Neurol Neurosurg Psychiatry.* 2008;79(2):163–169.
100. Gemignani F, Giovanelli M, Vitetta F, et al. Non-length dependent small fiber neuropathy. A prospective case series. *J Peripher Nerv Syst.* 2010;15(1):57–62.
101. Koike H, Sobue G. Small neurons may be preferentially affected in ganglionopathy. *J Neurol Neurosurg Psychiatry.* 2008;79(2):113.
102. Provitera V, Gibbons CH, Wendelschafer-Crabb G, et al. The role of skin biopsy in differentiating small-fiber neuropathy from ganglionopathy. *Eur J Neurol.* 2018;25:848–853.
103. Lauria G, Sghirlanzoni A, Lombardi R, Pareyson D. Epidermal nerve fiber density in sensory ganglionopathies: clinical and neurophysiologic correlations. *Muscle Nerve.* 2001;24:1034–1039.
104. Moritz CP, Tholance Y, Vallayer PB, et al. Anti-AGO1 antibodies identify a subset of autoimmune sensory neuronopathy. *Neurol Neuroimmunol Neuroinflamm.* 2023;10(3):e200105.
105. Khan S, Zhou L. Characterization of non-length-dependent small-fiber sensory neuropathy. *Muscle Nerve.* 2012;45(1):86–91.
106. Provitera V, Gibbons CH, Wendelschafer-Crabb G, et al. The role of skin biopsy in differentiating small-fiber neuropathy from ganglionopathy. *Eur J Neurol.* 2018;25(6):848–853. Erratum in: *Eur J Neurol.* 2019;26(1):202.
107. Geerts M, de Greef BTA, Sopacua M, et al. Intravenous immunoglobulin therapy in patients with painful idiopathic small fiber neuropathy. *Neurology.* 2021;96(20):e2534–e2545.
108. Gibbons CH, Rajan S, Senechal K, Hendry E, McCallister B, Levine TD. A double-blind placebo-controlled pilot study of immunoglobulin for small fiber neuropathy associated with TS-HDS and FGFR-3 autoantibodies. *Muscle Nerve.* 2023;67(5):363–370.
109. Hu N, Zhang L, Yang X, Fu H, Cui L, Liu M. Facial onset sensory and motor neuronopathy (FOSMN syndrome): cases series and systematic review. *Neurol Sci.* 2023;44(6):1969–1978.
110. Vucic S, Tian D, Chong PS, Cudkowicz ME, Hedley-Whyte ET, Cros D. Facial onset sensory and motor neuronopathy (FOSMN syndrome): a novel syndrome in neurology. *Brain.* 2006;129(pt 2):3384–3390.
111. Isoardo G, Troni W. Sporadic bulopsinal muscle atrophy with facial-onset sensory neuropathy. *Muscle Nerve.* 2008;37(5):659–662.
112. Hokonohara T, Shigeto H, Kawano Y, Ohyagi Y, Uehara M, Kira J. Facial onset sensory and motor neuronopathy (FOSMN) syndrome responding to immunotherapies. *J Neurol Sci.* 2008;275(1–2):157–158.
113. Fluchere F, Verschueren A, Cintas P, et al. Clinical features and follow-up of four new cases of facial-onset sensory and motor neuronopathy. *Muscle Nerve.* 2011;43(1):136–140.
114. Dalla Bella E, Rigamonti A, Mantero V, et al. Heterozygous D90A-SOD1 mutation in a patient with facial onset sensory motor neuronopathy (FOSMN) syndrome: a bridge to amyotrophic lateral sclerosis. *J Neurol Neurosurg Psychiatry.* 2014;85(9):1009–1011.
115. Vázquez-Costa JF, Pedrola Vidal L, Moreau-Le Lan S, et al. Facial onset sensory and motor neuronopathy: a motor neuron disease with an oligogenic origin? *Amyotroph Lateral Scler Frontotemporal Degener.* 2019;20(3–4):172–175.
116. Amy Pinto WBVR, Naylor FGM, Chieia MAT, de Souza PVS, Oliveira ASB. New findings in facial-onset sensory and motor neuronopathy (FOSMN) syndrome. *Rev Neurol (Paris).* 2019;175(4):238–246.
117. Zhang Q, Cao B, Chen Y, et al. Facial onset motor and sensory neuronopathy syndrome with a novel TARDBP mutation. *Neurologist.* 2019;24(1):22–25.

CHAPTER 23

Focal Processes Affecting the Upper Extremity and Trunk: Radiculopathies, Brachial Plexopathies, and Mononeuropathies

Numbness, pain, and/or weakness involving one or both arms are common reasons for referral to the neuromuscular clinician. These symptoms may be due to radiculopathy, brachial plexopathy, or one or more mononeuropathies. Some systemic etiologies for these focal neuropathic disorders have been discussed in preceding chapters (e.g., Lyme disease, vasculitis, and diabetes mellitus). This chapter will focus mainly on radiculopathies secondary to compression (e.g., degenerative joint disease and herniated discs), brachial plexitis, traumatic plexopathies, and focal mononeuropathies related to compression or entrapment. Before discussing the evaluation and management of these disorders, a review of the normal anatomy is needed.

▶ ANATOMY

SPINAL NERVES

Recall that there are seven cervical vertebrae, the first of which, the atlas, articulates with the skull's occipital condyles. The orientation of this joint allows primarily for flexion and extension movements. The second cervical vertebra, the axis, has a superiorly directed bony prominence, the dens, which articulates with the atlas and allows for rotational movements of the head and neck. The third through seventh cervical vertebrae are composed of the vertebral bodies themselves as well as short pedicles giving rise to laminae, which end in comparatively short and often bifid spinous processes. The transverse processes arise near the junctional zone of the pedicle and lamina. Between the transverse processes at each vertebral level lies a sulcus for the spinal nerves.

The spinal nerves are composed of a dorsal root and a ventral root (Fig. 23-1). The dorsal root consists of sensory fibers emanating from the dorsal root ganglia (DRG) that lie outside the spinal cord. These dorsal root fibers enter the posterolateral aspect of the spinal cord and into the dorsal horn. Along the anterior aspect of the spinal cord, 2 or as many as 12 individual rootlets called fila radicularis, which arise from anterior horn cells, fuse to form the ventral root. Just distal to the DRG, the ventral and dorsal roots merge to form the spinal nerve. In the cervical region, there are eight cervical spinal roots on each side but only seven cervical vertebrae. The first cervical spine nerve arises between the skull and atlas. As a result, each numbered cervical nerve root is related to the bony level immediately inferior to it down to the T1 vertebra. For example, the fifth cervical nerve root exits the spinal column just superior to the fifth cervical vertebrae. The eighth cervical nerve root exits the spinal column superior to the first thoracic vertebra.

At the intervertebral foramina, spinal nerves are joined by gray rami from the cervical sympathetic chain ganglia (Fig. 23-1). The superior cervical ganglion communicates with C1–4 spinal roots, the middle cervical ganglion with C5 and C6 spinal nerves, and the inferior cervical ganglion with C8 and T1 spinal roots. Importantly, sympathetic nerves to the head and neck arise from the first thoracic segment. Thus, injuries to the T1 nerve root may result in ipsilateral Horner syndrome (ptosis, miosis, and anhidrosis). Just distal to the entry point of the gray rami, cervical spinal nerves branch to form an anterior and posterior primary ramus. Nerve fibers in the posterior primary ramus innervate paraspinal muscles, while anterior primary rami of C5–T1 cervical spinal nerves form the brachial plexus (Fig. 23-2).

A dermatome refers to the cutaneous region supplied by a specific spinal nerve root segment (Fig. 23-3). Notably, there is some overlap of the cutaneous innervation by individual spinal nerves. Motor fibers emanating from the anterior horn cells, which course through the ventral root, spinal root, brachial plexus, and finally individual nerves, innervate specific muscle groups. Most muscles are supplied by motor nerves arising from at least two spinal cord segments (e.g., the deltoid muscle is innervated by motor fibers originating within the C5 and C6 spinal roots).

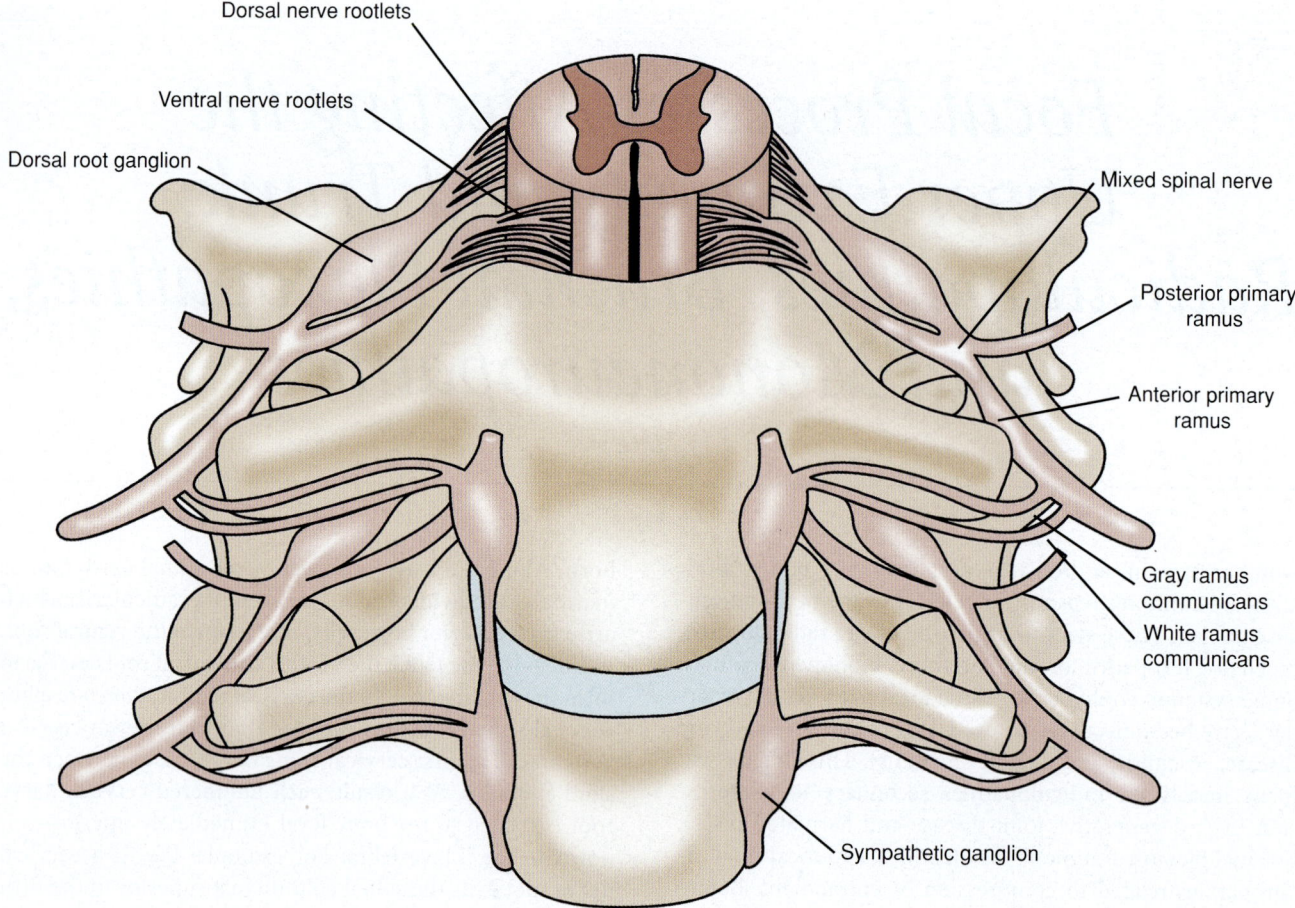

Figure 23-1. The spinal cord is depicted with multiple ventral and dorsal rootlets joining to form the mixed spinal nerve root. Communications between the sympathetic ganglia and the spinal nerves are appreciated, and the gray and white rami are seen as well. (Reproduced with permission from Ferrante MA. Brachial plexopathies: classification, causes, and consequences. *Muscle Nerve*. 2004;30(5):547–568.)

BRACHIAL PLEXUS

The brachial plexus is composed of three trunks (upper, middle, and lower), with two divisions (anterior and posterior) per trunk. Subsequently, the three trunks then divide into three cords (medial, lateral, and posterior), and from these arise multiple terminal nerves innervating the arm and hand (Table 23-1, Fig. 23-2).[1-3] More specifically, the anterior primary rami of C5 and C6 fuse to form the upper trunk, the anterior rami of C8 and T1 join to form the lower trunk, and the anterior primary ramus of C7 continues as the middle trunk. Some normal anatomic variation has been noted in anatomic dissections and during explorations in patients with trauma. In approximately 62% of anatomic dissections of the brachial plexus, the C4 spinal nerve contributes to the upper trunk.[1,4] In this situation, the brachial plexus is said to be a "prefixed plexus," in which all spinal nerve contributions are shifted up one level. As a result, the T1 spinal segment may contribute minimally to the lower trunk of the brachial plexus. In contrast, in approximately 7% of anatomic dissections of the brachial plexus, C5 contributes minimally and the plexus is called "postfixed."[1] In the latter case, spinal nerve contributions may be shifted down by one level; C7 would contribute to the upper trunk and T2 to the lower trunk. Based on surgical explorations in patients following trauma, however, the exact frequency of contributions of C4 and T2 to the brachial plexus remains controversial.[1,5]

The anterior divisions of the upper and middle trunks fuse to form the lateral cord, while the anterior division of the lower trunk continues as the medial cord. The three posterior divisions of the upper, middle, and lower trunks join to form the posterior cord. The cords constitute the longest subsection of the brachial plexus.[6] Their designation "medial, lateral, or posterior" refers to the cord's anatomic position relative to the axillary artery. Again, anatomic variation exists and nerve fibers may run between the different cords. For example, nerve fibers sometimes exit the lateral cord to join the medial cord. In those cases, the ulnar nerve would receive contribution from the C7 spinal nerve.

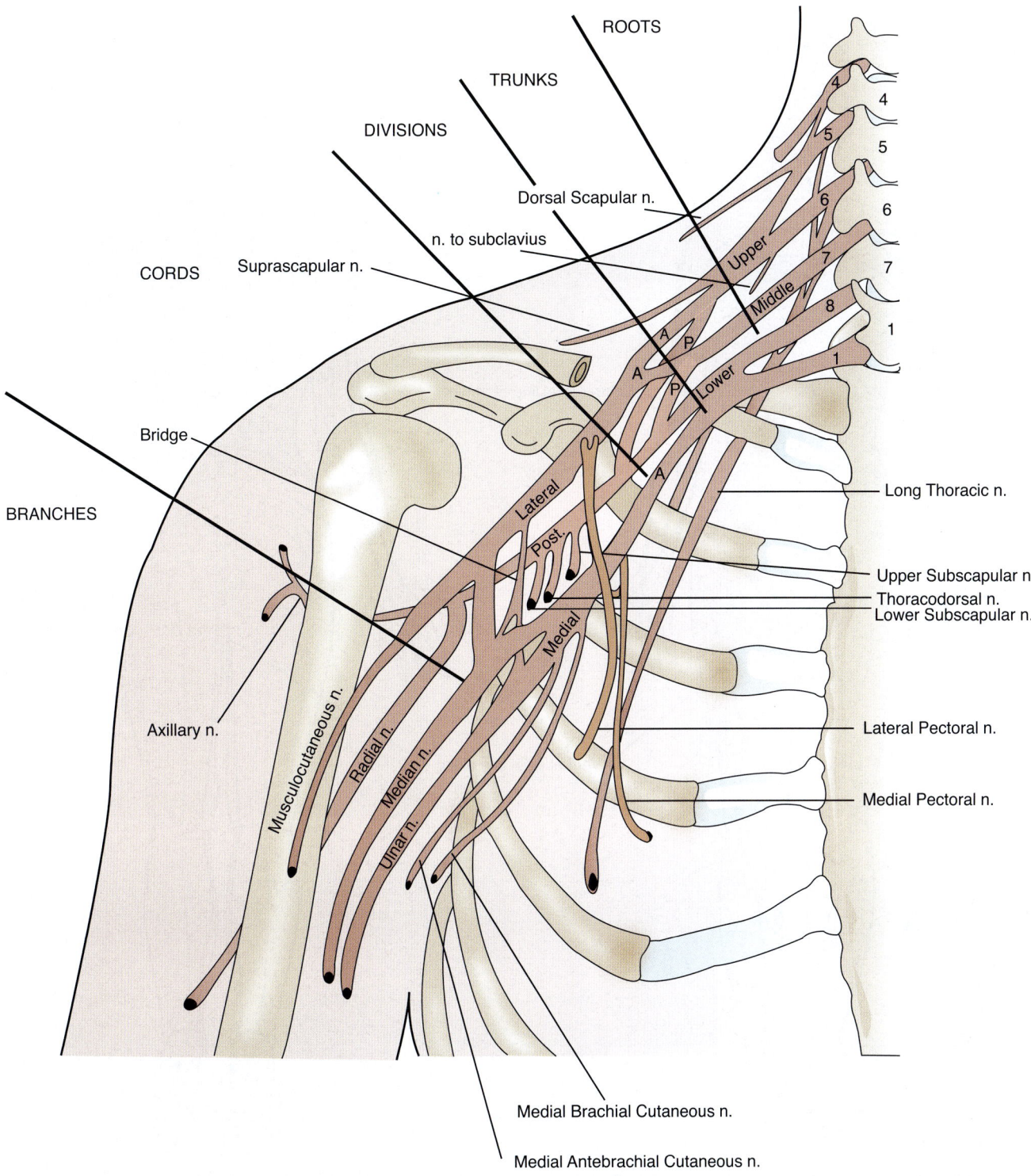

Figure 23-2. Diagrammatic representation of the brachial plexus (trunks, cords, and divisions) as well as its terminal nerves is depicted. A, anterior division; P, posterior division; n, nerve. (Reproduced with permission from Dumitru D, Zwarts MJ. Brachial plexopathies and proximal mononeuropathies. *Electrodiagnostic Medicine*. 2nd ed. Hanley & Belfus; 2002.)

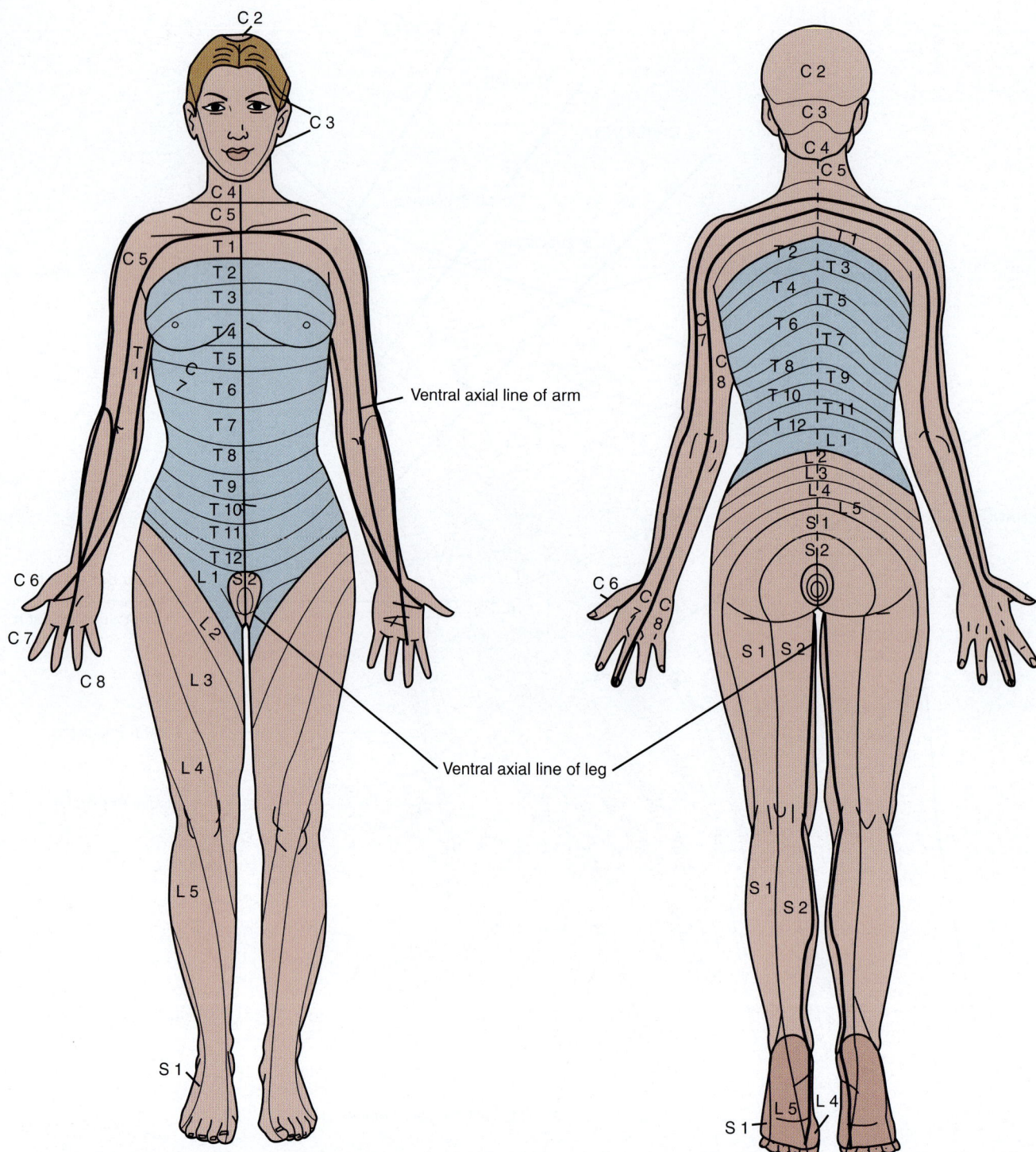

Figure 23-3. Dermatomal representation. (Reproduced with permission from Keegan JJ, Garret FD. Segmental distribution of the cutaneous nerves in the limbs of man. *Anat Rec.* 1948;102(4):409–437.)

TABLE 23-1. INNERVATION OF MUSCLES OF THE UPPER EXTREMITY

Muscle	Root(s)	Trunk	Cord	Nerve
Trapezius				Spinal accessory (cranial nerve XI)
Rhomboid major and minor	(C4), C5			Dorsal scapular
Serratus anterior	C5, C6, C7			Long thoracic
Supraspinatus/infraspinatus	C5, C6	Upper		Suprascapular
Pectoralis major	C5, C6	Upper/middle	Lateral	Lateral pectoral
Pectoralis major and minor	C7, C8, T1	Lower	Medial	Medial pectoral
Latissimus dorsi	C6, C7, C8	Upper/middle/lower	Posterior	Thoracodorsal
Teres major	C5, C6, C7	Upper/middle	Posterior	Lower subscapular
Teres minor	C5, C6	Upper	Posterior	Axillary
Deltoid	C5, C6	Upper	Posterior	Axillary
Brachioradialis	C5, C6	Upper	Posterior	Radial
Biceps brachii	C5, C6	Upper	Lateral	Musculocutaneous
Brachialis	C5, C6	Upper	Lateral/(posterior)	Musculocutaneous/(radial)
Triceps	C6, C7, C8	Upper/middle/lower	Posterior	Radial
Anconeus	C7, C8	Middle/lower	Posterior	Radial
Supinator	C7, C8	Middle/lower	Posterior	Posterior interosseous
Extensor carpi radialis	C6, C7	Middle/lower	Posterior	Radial
Extensor carpi ulnaris	C6, C7, C8	Upper/middle/lower	Posterior	Posterior interosseous
Extensor digitorum communis	C7, C8	Middle/lower	Posterior	Posterior interosseous
Extensor indicis proprius	C7, C8	Middle/lower	Posterior	Posterior interosseous
Extensor pollicis	C7, C8	Middle/lower	Posterior	Posterior interosseous
Pronator teres	C6, C7	Middle/lower	Lateral/medial	Median
Flexor digitorum superficialis	C7, C8, T1	Middle/lower	Lateral/medial	Median
Flexor digitorum profundus digit II and III	C7, C8, T1	Middle/lower	Lateral/medial	Anterior interosseous (median)
Flexor digitorum profundus digit IV and V	C7, C8, T1	Middle/lower	Lateral/medial	Ulnar
Flexor carpi radialis	C6, C7, (C8)	Middle/lower	Lateral/medial	Median
Flexor carpi ulnaris	C7, C8, T1	(Middle)/lower	(Lateral)/medial	Ulnar
Flexor pollicis longus	(C7), C8, T1	(Middle)/lower	(Lateral)/medial	Anterior interosseous (median)
Pronator quadratus	C8, T1	Lower	Medial	Anterior interosseous (median)
Abductor pollicis brevis	C8, T1	Lower	Medial	Median
Adductor pollicis	C8, T1	Lower	Medial	Ulnar
Opponens pollicis	C8, T1	Lower	Medial	Median
Abductor digiti minimi	C8, T1	Lower	Medial	Ulnar
Dorsal and volar interossei	C8, T1	Lower	Medial	Ulnar
First and 2nd lumbrical	C8, T1	Lower	Medial	Median
Third and 4th lumbrical	C8, T1	Lower	Medial	Ulnar

In parentheses are roots, trunks, cords, or nerves that may have mild contribution to innervation of the muscle group in some patients.

TERMINAL NERVES

Terminal nerves arise from the brachial plexus and may be purely sensory, motor, or mixed sensory and motor (Fig. 23-2). The dorsal scapular nerve, long thoracic nerve, and a branch to the phrenic nerve arise directly from spinal roots. The only two terminal nerves which arise from trunks are the subclavian and suprascapular nerves, and both branch off the upper trunk. No terminal nerves come directly from the middle or lower trunk. The upper and lower subscapular and thoracodorsal nerves depart from the posterior cord, while the posterior cord terminates as the axillary and radial nerves. From the proximal medial cord arises a single motor branch innervating pectoral muscles called the medial pectoral nerve. The purely sensory medial brachial and medial antebrachial cutaneous nerves originate from the distal aspect of the medial cord. The medial cord terminates by sending a medial branch to the median nerve with the remnant continuing as the ulnar nerve. The lateral pectoral nerve comes off the proximal portion of the lateral cord. The lateral cord terminates as the musculocutaneous nerve and a lateral branch that joins a branch from the medial cord to form the median nerve. Individual terminal nerves are discussed in more detail below.

Spinal Accessory Nerve

Although it does not arise from brachial plexus, the spinal accessory nerve (SAN), or cranial nerve XI, courses through the neck and shoulder region and is often affected in brachial plexus injuries. The SAN consists of a bulbar or "accessory" component that arises from the medulla and a "spinal" portion that arises from anterior horn cells in the cervical cord down to C6. The nerves from the bulbar origin supply the soft palate and contribute to the recurrent laryngeal nerve. Parasympathetic fibers possibly then merge into the vagal nerve to the heart. The spinal component ascends between the ligamentum denticulatum and posterior spinal nerve roots, enters the cranium through the foramen magnum, and then exits the skull via the jugular foramen. The nerve descends posterior to the digastric and stylohyoid muscles to innervate sternocleidomastoid and finally trapezius, where it terminates.

Terminal Nerves Arising from Cervical Roots

Phrenic Nerve
The phrenic nerve is derived primarily from the C4 spinal nerve, but the C3 and C5 roots also contribute (Fig. 23-2). The phrenic nerve crosses the anterior scalene and enters the thorax, where it innervates the diaphragm.

Dorsal Scapular Nerve
The dorsal scapular nerve usually arises directly from the C5 spinal nerve shortly after it exits the intervertebral foramen. The nerve then courses between the middle and posterior scalenes. It innervates the rhomboid major and minor muscles and the levator scapulae.

Long Thoracic Nerve
Branches of C5, C6, and C7 spinal roots join to form the long thoracic nerve which descends along the lateral chest wall, where it innervates the serratus anterior muscle.

Terminal Nerves Arising from Trunks

Suprascapular Nerve
The suprascapular nerve arises from the upper trunk shortly after it is formed (Fig. 23-2). The nerve descends posteriorly between the omohyoid and the trapezius muscles. In the posterior shoulder, it courses through the suprascapular notch under the scapula's superior transverse ligament to innervate the supraspinatus muscle, then through the spinoglenoid notch to innervate the infraspinatus muscle.

Nerve to the Subclavius
This is a small nerve that arises from the C5 root or upper trunk, which innervates the small subclavius muscle that runs between the clavicle and first rib.

Terminal Nerves Arising from Cords

Medial Pectoral Nerves
The medial pectoral nerve arises from the medial trunk (Fig. 23-2). This nerve innervates both the pectoralis major and the pectoralis minor muscles. The major spinal contributions to this nerve are C8 and T1.

Lateral Pectoral Nerves
The lateral pectoral nerve innervates the pectoralis major. It usually comes from the lateral cord, but occasionally arises from the anterior division of the upper and middle trunks just prior to the formation of the lateral cord. This anatomic variation may explain the observation that in plexus injuries affecting the medial and lateral cords resulting in a flail arm, the strength of the pectoralis major muscle may be relatively preserved. The major spinal contributions of this nerve are C5–7.

Subscapular Nerves
The upper and lower subscapular nerves originate from the posterior cord in the axilla. The upper subscapular nerve innervates the subscapularis muscle, while the lower subscapular nerve supplies subscapularis and the teres major muscle. The major spinal contributions to this nerve are from C5 and C6.

Thoracodorsal Nerve
The thoracodorsal nerve, also known as the middle subscapular nerve, comes off the posterior cord and innervates the latissimus dorsi muscle. This nerve can also arise in some cases from the radial or axillary nerves.[4] The major spinal nerves contributing to the thoracodorsal nerve are C5–7, particularly C7.

Medial Cutaneous Nerve of the Arm
The medial cutaneous nerve of the arm (medial brachial cutaneous nerve) originates from the medial cord and supplies sensation to the medial aspect of the arm. Its primary contribution comes from the C8 and T1 spinal nerves.

Medial Cutaneous Nerve of the Forearm
The medial cutaneous nerve of the forearm (medial antebrachial cutaneous nerve) usually projects from the medial cord, but it may arise from the medial cutaneous nerve of the arm.[4] The nerve supplies sensation from the medial forearm and also originates from the C8 and T1 spinal nerves.

Musculocutaneous Nerve
The lateral cord terminates as a bifurcation resulting in the musculocutaneous nerve and a lateral branch that combines with a branch from the medial cord to form the median nerve. In about 5% of individuals, the musculocutaneous nerve originates from the anterior division of the upper trunk, in which case the lateral root to the median nerve arises from the middle trunk only.[4] The major spinal nerves contributing to the musculocutaneous nerve are C5 and C6. In addition, C7 contributes to this nerve in at least half but less than two-thirds of cadavers examined.[4] The musculocutaneous nerve innervates the coracobrachialis, biceps brachii, and brachialis muscles. It terminates as the lateral cutaneous nerve of the forearm, supplying sensation to the lateral aspect of the volar surface of the forearm.

Axillary Nerve
The axillary nerve contains portions of the spinal nerves arising from C5 and C6 and is one of the two terminal branches of the posterior cord. The nerve usually originates near the

subscapularis muscle posterior to the pectoralis minor muscle and then traverses the quadrangular or quadrilateral space formed inferiorly by teres major, laterally by the long head of the triceps brachii, medially by the humerus, and superiorly by the teres minor. Upon exiting this space, the axillary nerve innervates the teres minor and deltoid muscles. The axillary nerve also sends cutaneous branches that supply sensation to the lateral aspect of the proximal arm overlying the deltoid muscle.

Radial Nerve

The radial nerve contains contributions from mainly C5–8 (as well as T1 in approximately 10% of individuals) and is a continuation of the posterior cord after the axillary nerve branches off.[1,7] While still in the axillary region, a posterior cutaneous nerve branches off the radial nerve to provide sensation to the posterior aspect of the upper arm to the level of the elbow. In the proximal arm, the radial nerve travels medial to the humerus and descends between the medial and long heads of the triceps muscle along the spiral groove. In the proximal arm, the radial nerve innervates the long, medial, and lateral heads of the triceps brachii and the anconeus muscles. Upon leaving the spiral groove in the mid to distal portion of the upper arm, the radial nerve courses down to the lateral aspect of the arm and innervates the brachioradialis and extensor carpi radialis longus as well as a small branch to the brachialis muscle, the latter receiving its main contribution from the musculocutaneous nerve. An additional branch, the posterior antebrachial cutaneous nerve, separates from the radial nerve in the midarm region and descends to supply sensation to the posterior aspect of the forearm.

In the elbow region, the radial nerve splits to form the purely sensory superficial radial nerve and the purely motor posterior interosseous nerve (PIN). This area is referred to as the "radial tunnel." Its boundaries are the radius, the capsule of the radiocapitellar joint, the brachialis and biceps brachii tendons (forming the medial walls), and the brachioradialis, extensor carpi radialis, and extensor carpi ulnaris muscles (forming the lateral and anterior walls). The radial tunnel ends at the fibrous band around the superficial head of the supinator muscle, which is known as the arcade of Fröhse. The superficial radial nerve travels on the undersurface of the brachioradialis, outside the radial tunnel, into the forearm. Around the midforearm, the nerve moves more superficially and travels along the extensor aspect of the distal forearm. After the superficial radial nerve passes the wrist, it supplies sensation to the lateral, extensor surface of the hand and fingers, analogous to the median distribution on the palmar surface (except the distal aspects of the fingertips on the dorsal surface which are supplied by the median nerve). The PIN traverses the radial tunnel and then descends under the arcade of Fröhse. The PIN continues down the extensor aspect of the forearm. Along the way, it innervates the extensor carpi radialis brevis, supinator, extensor digitorum communis, extensor digiti minimi, extensor carpi ulnaris, abductor pollicis longus, extensor pollicis longus and brevis, and the extensor indicis proprius.

Median Nerve

The median nerve is formed by the fusion of branches from the lateral and medial cords. Spinal nerve contributions from C6 to T1 form the median nerve. Motor fibers arise from C6 to T1 spinal segments, while sensory fibers are derived primarily from the C6 and C7 segments. Occasionally, C5 can also contribute to the median nerve.[1] The sensory fibers travel through the upper and middle trunks to the lateral cord into the median nerve. In contrast, the median nerve's motor fibers pass through all the trunks as well as the medial and lateral cords.

The median nerve descends in the anterior compartment of the arm on the medial side to the antecubital fossa region. Past the elbow, the median nerve courses through the two heads of the pronator teres muscle and then between the flexor digitorum superficialis and profundus muscles to the wrist. In the forearm, the median nerve innervates the pronator teres, flexor carpi radialis, palmaris longus, and flexor digitorum superficialis muscles. In the upper to midforearm level, the anterior interosseous nerve (AIN) branches from the main median nerve. This is a pure motor nerve that supplies the flexor digitorum profundus to digits 2 and 3, flexor pollicis longus, and pronator quadratus muscles. The main median nerve trunk continues distally down the forearm to the wrist. Just before entering the carpal tunnel, the palmar cutaneous branch arises and supplies sensation to the thenar eminence. The nerve then enters the carpal tunnel which is the space bounded by the roof-like transverse ligament and the carpal bones forming the floor. Also, within the carpal tunnel lie the nine flexor tendons to the fingers. Within or just distal to the carpal tunnel, the recurrent branch of the median nerve arises and innervates the abductor pollicis brevis, opponens pollicis, and the superficial head of the flexor pollicis brevis. The terminal branches of the median nerve supply the first and second lumbrical muscles, while the digital branches provide sensation to the volar aspects (and the tips of the dorsal aspects) of the thumb, index, and middle fingers, and the lateral half of the forth finger.

Ulnar Nerve

The ulnar nerve arises at the termination of the medial cord distal to the medial cutaneous nerves of the arm and forearm and the medial branch of the median nerve. The spinal nerve contributions are mainly C8 and T1, but C7 fibers may also be present in 43%–92% of cases, as suggested by brachial plexus dissections.[1,4] The C7 contribution derives from a branch of the lateral cord and innervates the flexor carpi ulnaris muscle. The ulnar nerve descends anterior to the teres major and latissimus dorsi muscles into the arm. Then the nerve travels down the posterior compartment of the upper arm to the retroepicondylar ulnar groove at the elbow. The ulnar groove is formed by the medial epicondyle of the humerus and the olecranon process of the ulna, with the ulnar collateral ligament serving as the floor. Approximately 1.0–2.5 cm distal to the ulnar groove, the nerve traverses under a fibrous aponeurotic arch connecting the humeral and ulnar heads of the flexor carpi ulnaris muscle. The area encompassing the ulnar groove and aponeurotic arch is commonly referred to as either the cubital tunnel or the humeroulnar arcade. Of note, the ulnar nerve yields no branches in the arm proximal to the elbow.

Distal to the elbow, the ulnar nerve descends to the wrist between the flexor carpi ulnaris and flexor digitorum profundus muscles. In the forearm, it innervates the flexor carpi ulnaris and the flexor digitorum profundus to digits 4 and 5. The dorsal ulnar cutaneous nerve originates in the mid or distal forearm to provide sensation to the dorsum of the medial aspect of the hand and fourth and fifth digits. Just before entering Guyon's canal at the wrist, the palmar branch arises to provide sensation to the hypothenar eminence and motor innervation to the palmaris brevis muscle. The remaining components of the ulnar nerve travel into Guyon's canal, formed by the hook of the hamate bone (on the radial aspect), the pisiform bone (on the ulnar aspect), the pisohamate ligament (serves as the floor), and the transverse carpal ligament (serves as the roof). Within or just distal to Guyon's canal, the ulnar nerve splits into its terminal branches. A superficial terminal branch supplies sensation to the palmar aspect of the little finger and half of the ring finger, plus some of the distal aspects of these digits dorsally. A deep motor branch innervates the hypothenar muscles and then turns and continues across the hand to innervate the third and fourth lumbricals, interossei, adductor pollicis, and deep head of the flexor pollicis brevis muscle.

▶ PATHOPHYSIOLOGY OF RADICULOPATHIES, PLEXOPATHIES, AND MONONEUROPATHIES

Before discussing the approach to patients with focal nerve lesions in the arm, it is important to understand the pathophysiologic basis of these neuropathies. Clinicians need to be aware of types of nerve injury which include demyelination, conduction block, and axonal degeneration. Also, the mechanisms (e.g., gunshot wound to upper arm, prolonged hyperextension of the arm during surgery, or falling asleep on the arm) often provide insight into the underlying pathophysiology. This knowledge helps clinicians plan and interpret electrodiagnostic (EDX) studies, assess prognosis and offer best treatments.

TYPES OF NERVE FIBER DAMAGE

Neuropraxia

The term "neuropraxia," also known as first-degree injury, refers to neuronal dysfunction due to transient conduction block.[1,8–10] Neuropraxia may arise from nerve ischemia or demyelination. Compression of a nerve can result in segmental ischemia. If the compression is short-lived, physiologic conduction block is typically rapidly reversible, lasting only minutes to hours. However, experimental studies suggest that pressure related to nerve compression can sometimes result in distortion of the underlying nerve segment with paranodal and then segmental demyelination.[11] Neuropraxia due to demyelination typically resolves after several weeks following remyelination of the nerve segment. Thus, prognosis is excellent in lesions associated with only conduction block resulting from mechanical demyelination (as opposed to immune-mediated or radiation) mechanisms and without secondary axonal loss.

Axonotmesis

Axonotmesis or second-degree injury refers to nerve injuries in which the axon is interrupted but the epineurium is intact.[1,8–10] Following this type of nerve injury, the axon distal to the lesion, now separated from its cell body, degenerates over 7–10 days. Subsequently, regenerating nerve sprouts emerge from the proximal stump of the sectioned nerve to attempt reinnervation of previously denervated tissues (e.g., muscle or skin). Because the endoneurium is preserved, the regenerating axons are more likely to grow back and reinnervate denervated tissues than in neurotmesis described below. Axons grow back at a rate of 1 mm/day. Depending on the site of the lesion and length of the nerve, restoration of function can take several months to more than a year.

Neurotmesis

Neurotmesis refers to severe, often penetrating nerve injuries, in which axons and supporting epineurium are interrupted (i.e., nerve transaction).[1,8–10] Present technology precludes distinction between axonotmesis and neurotmesis without exploratory surgery and direct inspection of the nerve. Because endoneurium is also interrupted, regenerating nerve sprouts have more difficulty reinnervating target tissues. Scarring secondary to disruption of overlying connective tissue can also impede reinnervation. Regenerating nerves can become entwined with scar tissue and form a neuroma. Thus, prognosis for spontaneous recovery following this type of lesion is poor.

▶ APPROACH TO PATIENTS

As with other neuromuscular disorders, the most important first step is trying to localize the site of the lesion based on the history and physical examination. Following this, EDX studies are performed to confirm localization and to describe chronicity and severity of the focal or generalized process. Often radiologic studies further assist in identifying the site and possible etiology of the lesion. Next, we'll discuss the approach to such patients with a review of EDX studies that can be helpful.

ELECTRODIAGNOSTIC STUDIES

Evaluation of the arm for possible cervical radiculopathy, brachial plexopathy, or mononeuropathy(ies) requires performing sensory, motor, and mixed sensorimotor nerve conduction studies (NCSs) along with electromyography (EMG) (Table 23-2). This text is not meant to be a "how-to" book on NCSs and EMG, and for this, we refer the reader to several excellent reference books regarding EDX medicine (a more detailed discussion can also be found in Chapter 2 of this book).[6,12–15] However, clinicians taking care of patients with neuromuscular disorders need to be aware of the utility and limitations of EDX studies. EDX studies also must be tailored to individual patients depending on their clinical history and physical examination. Importantly, EDX data are analyzed in real time by the electromyographer, who can further modify the study based on the data being generated to answer the clinical question.

Sensory NCSs

Sensory nerve action potential (SNAP) evaluation is essential to distinguish radiculopathy from a more distal process. In most radiculopathies, the lesion lies proximal to the DRG. Because cell bodies and distal axons are intact in cervical radiculopathies, SNAPs should be normal. In contrast, SNAPs are typically abnormal in brachial plexopathies and mononeuropathies (affecting those nerves with sensory fibers) where the lesion is distal to the DRG. If there has been axonal injury, one sees reduced SNAP amplitudes in the distribution of the affected nerve. In demyelinating lesions which cause conduction block (neuropraxic injuries), SNAPs distal to the lesion site are typically normal.

Timing of the EDX study relative to the injury is critical in interpreting the data. It takes several days from the time of the injury for Wallerian degeneration of axons to occur distally. Thus, even if a nerve were completely severed, it would take approximately 7–14 days for the SNAPs to disappear. After this time window, one can more reliably distinguish pathophysiology (axonal vs. demyelinating) and localization (pre vs. postganglionic). However, an abnormal SNAP does not necessarily imply that the spinal root is normal. For example, in traumatic brachial plexopathies, avulsion of nerve roots may occur concurrently with injury to the peripheral nerve distal to the DRG.

Comparison of SNAPs in the affected arm to the analogous nerves in the contralateral arm is important in certain situations. SNAP amplitude(s) in an affected arm may fall "within the reference values" for that EDX laboratory and be "normal" even if injured. An asymptomatic limb sometimes provides better normative data for that individual than does normative data derived from populations, particularly in unilateral processes such as trauma. Like most electromyographers, we consider SNAP amplitude(s) less than half of

▶ TABLE 23-2. NERVE CONDUCTION STUDIES

	Sensory Studies		
	Brachial Plexus		
Spinal Root	Trunk	Cord	Peripheral Nerve
C6	Upper	Lateral	Lateral antebrachial cut.
C6	Upper	Lateral	Median to first/second digit
C6	Upper	Posterior	Radial to base of first digit
C6	Upper	Lateral	Median to second digit
C7	Middle	Lateral	Median to third digit
C8	Lower	Medial	Ulnar to fifth digit
C8	Lower	Medial	Dorsal ulnar cut.
T1	Lower	Medial	Medial antebrachial cut.

	Motor Studies			
	Brachial Plexus			
Spinal Root	Trunk	Cord	Peripheral Nerve	Muscle
C5, C6	Upper	Lateral	Musculocutaneous	Biceps
C5, C6	Upper	Posterior	Axillary	Deltoid
C5, C6	Upper		Suprascapular	SS, IS
C7, C8	Middle/Lower	Posterior	Radial	EIP
C8, T1	Lower	Medial	Median	APB
C8, T1	Lower	Medial	Ulnar	ADM, FDI

cut., cutaneous; SS, supraspinatus; IS, infraspinatus; EIP, extensor indicis proprius; ABP, abductor pollicis brevis; FDI, first dorsal interosseous; ADM, abductor digiti minimi.

those obtained from the analogous nerve in an asymptomatic limb to be abnormal in most cases. Side to side comparison is much less informative if symptoms are bilateral.

The selection of sensory studies for EDX depends on the suspected location of abnormality (Table 23-2).[13] For example, when patients present with thumb numbness, the differential includes C6 radiculopathy, upper trunk or lateral cord lesions, or mononeuropathies of the median or radial nerves. The most high-yield sensory studies to include to localize this lesion are a median SNAP from the thumb or index finger, a superficial radial SNAP, and perhaps a lateral antebrachial cutaneous SNAP. In addition, the median and ulnar mixed nerve palmar studies are helpful to look for carpal tunnel syndrome (CTS). As with all EDX evaluations, it is important to define the boundaries of abnormality by identifying a normal response in a nerve that is not felt to be clinically affected (e.g., an ulnar SNAP in this case). This "bracketing of abnormality with normality" is a key concept in EDX medicine. If a patient has symptoms involving the fourth digit, the studies performed must distinguish a C8/T1 radiculopathy from a lower trunk or medial cord lesion, or isolated ulnar neuropathy.

Motor NCSs

Evaluation of individual motor nerves is performed by stimulating the nerve at several locations and recording the compound muscle action potential (CMAP) generated from an accessible muscle belly, as discussed in Chapter 2 (Table 23-2).[13] As with sensory studies, most accessible motor stimulation sites are remote from proximally located lesions associated with radiculopathy or plexopathy. Thus, it is technically difficult to assess for abnormality at these proximal sites. Further, most EDX laboratories routinely perform median, ulnar, and radial motor conductions recording from muscles that are innervated primarily by the C8–T1 segments. These motor studies are most useful to assess for lower trunk and medial cord pathology as well as median, ulnar, or radial neuropathies. They will typically be normal in C5–7 radiculopathy or portions of the brachial plexus through which these fibers descend. Motor conduction studies can assist in localizing the site and nature of the lesion (e.g., axonal or demyelinating) involving easily testable nerves. Again, it's important to be aware of the limitations of motor NCSs. Following complete axonal lesions, CMAP amplitudes take 3–5 days to reach their nadir and for Wallerian degeneration to occur. Note that this is less time than the 7–14 days it takes for sensory responses to maximally drop. To identify demyelinating lesions, one must stimulate the motor nerve proximal and distal to the site of the lesion to demonstrate conduction block and/or conduction velocity slowing.

Axillary or musculocutaneous CMAPs recorded from the deltoid or biceps brachii muscles, respectively are technically more difficult to perform and interpret. CMAPs of these deeply positioned nerves are frequently limited by patient movement and intolerance of the high-intensity stimulus required to achieve a supramaximal CMAP. As such, for proximal nerves, side-to-side CMAP comparison is informative if the contralateral side is asymptomatic. Radiculopathies are not usually associated with abnormal CMAPs, unless there has been severe end-stage neurogenic atrophy of the muscle. This is a product of most muscles being innervated by more than one nerve root, and by the difficulty of identifying conduction block at the root level. Thus, detecting reduced CMAP amplitudes in cervical radiculopathies is uncommon unless it is severe or there are multiple roots affected.

F-Waves

F-wave studies have limited value in the evaluation of most radiculopathies and focal neuropathies. The reason for this is clear if one understands the pathogenesis of most of these focal neuropathies and the limitations inherent in F-wave assessment. The length of a possible compressive/demyelinating lesion is small in most radiculopathies and even mononeuropathies due to entrapment/compression (e.g., ulnar neuropathy at the elbow or median neuropathy at the wrist). Remember, the F-wave latency includes the time for the stimulus to travel retrograde through the motor nerve toward the spinal cord, stimulate a pool of anterior horn cells, and then travel back down the motor axon to stimulate the muscle. Thus, even if there were focal slowing across a small site of demyelination, this may be obscured by the normal conduction to and from the spine across most of the nerve. Further, most criteria regarding F-wave assessment use minimum onset latency of multiple responses to define reference values. If there is one normally functioning axon, the F-wave minimum latency can be normal. Finally, amplitude measurement, the most important parameter obtained in NCS, cannot be reliably assessed in F-wave studies. However, if one is looking for a large proximal demyelinating lesion, as can be seen in some forms of acquired inflammatory demyelinating neuropathies which affect the nerve roots, then F-waves can be valuable.

H-Reflex

The only reliable H-reflex in the arm is that obtained by recording from the flexor carpi radialis muscle following median nerve stimulation at the antecubital fossa.[16] This study is not routinely performed, as it usually does not assist in localization beyond clinical examination and routine EDX studies. Nevertheless, the H-reflex for the flexor carpi radialis muscle may be abnormal in C6 or C7 radiculopathies, upper or middle trunk plexopathies, lateral cord lesions, or proximal median neuropathies. The primary contribution of the H-reflex in the upper extremities occurs when H-reflexes are recognized during routine NCS. This implicates the presence of pyramidal tract pathology affecting that limb and may shift the investigation of the patient's complaints from the peripheral to central nervous system.[17]

Somatosensory-Evoked Potentials

Somatosensory-evoked potentials (SSEPs) have limited utility in evaluation of radiculopathies and most neuropathies for the same reasons as discussed with F-waves. However, SSEPs can add value to assessment of brachial plexopathies because routine sensory NCSs will not detect demyelination or conduction block in the plexus.[16,18,19]

Needle EMG

Needle EMG is essential in the evaluation of patients for radiculopathy, plexopathy, and mononeuropathy. Combined with the clinical examination and carefully performed motor and sensory NCS, EMG of muscles supplied by different spinal roots, trunks, divisions, and cords of the brachial plexus, and different terminal nerves solidifies the localization of the site of the lesion. As discussed in Chapter 2, with EMG we assess the presence of abnormal insertional and spontaneous activity, the morphology of motor unit action potentials (MUAPs), and the recruitment properties and firing rates of these units. Abnormal insertional or spontaneous activity in the form of positive sharp waves or fibrillation potentials implies muscle membrane instability, which in neurogenic processes is typically due to axonal degeneration. Other abnormal spontaneous activity generated at the level of muscle includes myotonia and complex repetitive discharges. Irritation of the nerve with or without axonal degeneration may result in fasciculation potentials, myokymic discharges, neuromyotonia, and cramps. The detection of myokymic discharges in a patient with history of cancer and radiation presenting with new weakness would strongly suggest radiation-induced injury to the roots or plexus. However, radiation-induced injury can coexist with tumor infiltration of the nerve and the presence of myokymia does not exclude the need to evaluate both processes.[20,21] The demonstration of abnormal spontaneous activity in the paraspinal muscles suggests that there is at least some injury to the anterior horn cells or spinal nerves but also does not exclude an injury more distally (e.g., double crush).

Importantly, fibrillation potentials and positive sharp waves may not be present for up to 1 week in paraspinal muscles and up to 3 weeks in limb muscles following axonal injury to a nerve root. However, voluntary recruitment of MUAPs is affected immediately. Thus, any injury to the nerve that results in a significant loss of muscle strength should be accompanied by reduced recruitment (e.g., fast-firing) of MUAPs. In neuropraxic injuries in which there is demyelination or conduction block without axonal degeneration, fibrillation potentials and positive sharp waves are not seen and the only abnormality apparent on the EMG is reduced recruitment of MUAPs. Reduced recruitment in the absence of abnormal spontaneous activity, NCS abnormalities, and morphological change in MUAPs more than 3 weeks after symptom onset implicates conduction block.

Following axonal injury, if reinnervation of muscle fibers is complete and the denervating process has ceased, fibrillation potentials and positive sharp waves disappear. Reinnervation is more complete in muscles closer to the site of axonal injury (e.g., paraspinal muscles in a radiculopathy). If reinnervation occurs by successful axonal regrowth, then re-establishment of a near-normal number of motor units and innervation ratio is possible. MUAP morphology may appear normal again. In contrast, if reinnervation takes place via collateral sprouting, the motor units of an affected muscle will remain chronically reduced in number and increased in size, even if strength is reestablished. Muscle groups more distal to the site of the lesion (e.g., hand intrinsic muscles in a cervical radiculopathy) are less likely to be completely reinnervated, and thus fibrillation potentials and positive sharp waves may persist indefinitely.

Another important point is that because of fascicular arrangement of axons running through various segments of the nerve trunk from the spine to the target muscle, an incomplete nerve injury may not necessarily demonstrate abnormality in every muscle innervated by an affected spinal nerve root, trunk, cord, or terminal nerve. Therefore, some redundancy in myotomes when selecting muscles to examine for needle EMG can be important.

RADIOLOGICAL STUDIES

Imaging studies such as magnetic resonance imaging (MRI) of the cervical spine, brachial plexus, and peripheral nerve are critical pieces of the evaluation. They complement the clinical and EDX evaluations. MRI has, for the most part, replaced myelogram and computerized axial tomographic (CT) scans except in individuals in whom MRI is contraindicated (e.g., those with magnetic or metal implants, some pacemakers and spinal cord stimulators for evaluation of radiculopathies). CT scans, particularly with contrast within the subarachnoid space, can be useful[22] but high-resolution MRI is much more sensitive for radiculopathies, plexopathies, and focal neuropathies (Figs. 23-4 to 23-6).[23-29] Ultrasound complements EDX studies in atypical cases, nerve transection, when EDX studies are normal or when abnormalities are non-localizing.[30-33]

▶ SPECIFIC DISORDERS

CERVICAL RADICULOPATHIES

Recall the disparity between the number of cervical vertebrae (seven) and nerve roots (eight). As a result, each numbered cervical nerve root is related to the bony level immediately inferior to it. For example, the C5 spinal root exits the spinal column between the fourth and fifth cervical vertebrae, and it is vulnerable to compression from a herniated disc (herniated nucleus pulposus or HNP) between C4 and C5. The C6 spinal root exits the spinal column between the fifth and the sixth cervical vertebrae and may be injured from an HNP between C5 and C6. In the same manner, an HNP between C6 and C7 levels may damage the C7 root, while an HNP between the C7 and T1 vertebrae may impinge the C8 nerve root. The T1 spinal nerve exists between the T1 and T2 vertebrae and may be damaged by an HNP at this level. Cervical

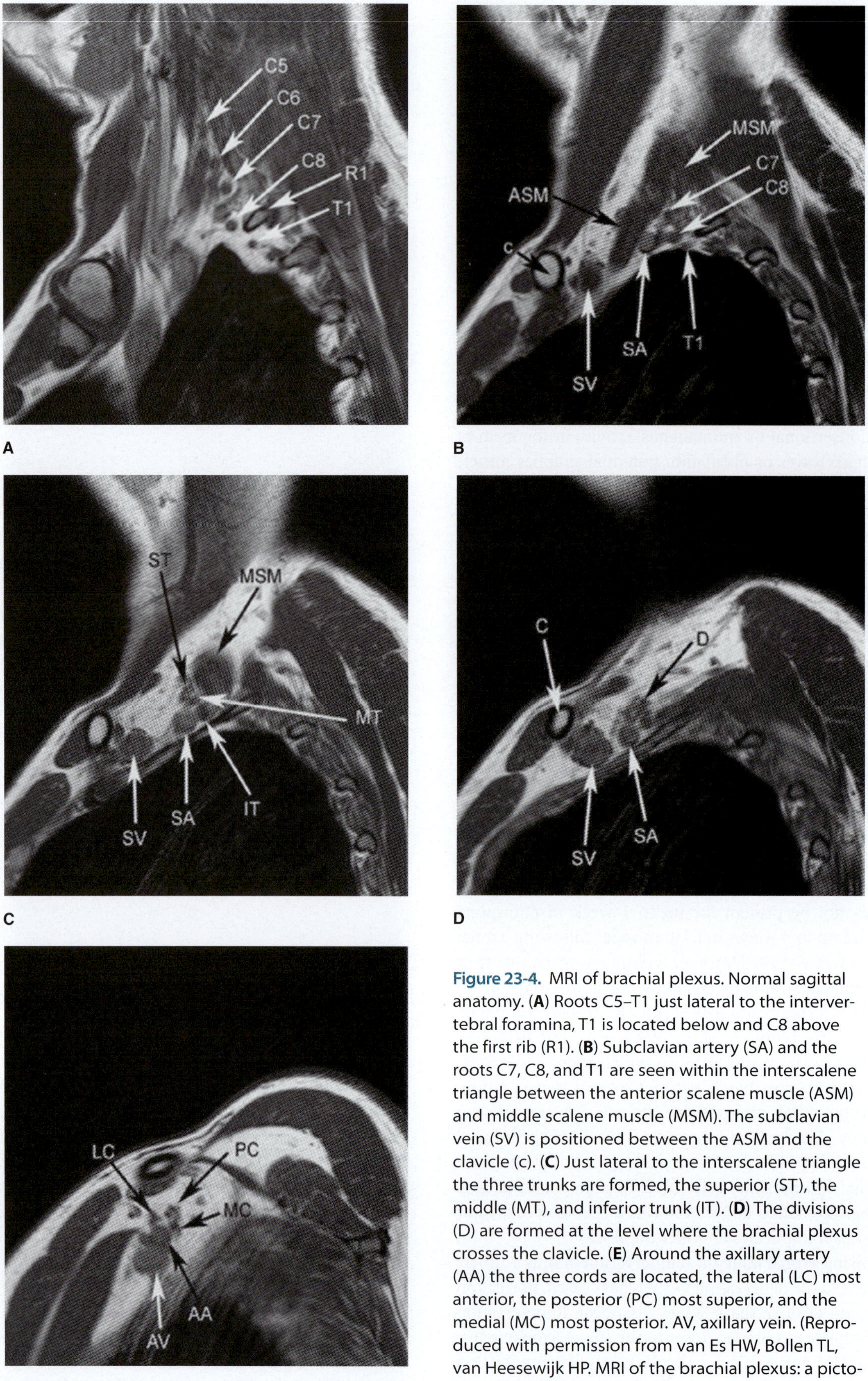

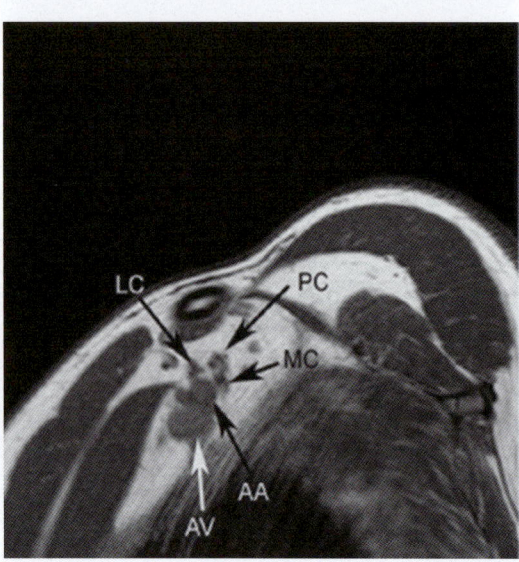

Figure 23-4. MRI of brachial plexus. Normal sagittal anatomy. (**A**) Roots C5–T1 just lateral to the intervertebral foramina, T1 is located below and C8 above the first rib (R1). (**B**) Subclavian artery (SA) and the roots C7, C8, and T1 are seen within the interscalene triangle between the anterior scalene muscle (ASM) and middle scalene muscle (MSM). The subclavian vein (SV) is positioned between the ASM and the clavicle (c). (**C**) Just lateral to the interscalene triangle the three trunks are formed, the superior (ST), the middle (MT), and inferior trunk (IT). (**D**) The divisions (D) are formed at the level where the brachial plexus crosses the clavicle. (**E**) Around the axillary artery (AA) the three cords are located, the lateral (LC) most anterior, the posterior (PC) most superior, and the medial (MC) most posterior. AV, axillary vein. (Reproduced with permission from van Es HW, Bollen TL, van Heesewijk HP. MRI of the brachial plexus: a pictorial review. *Eur J Radiol.* 2010;74(2):391–402. Figure 1.)

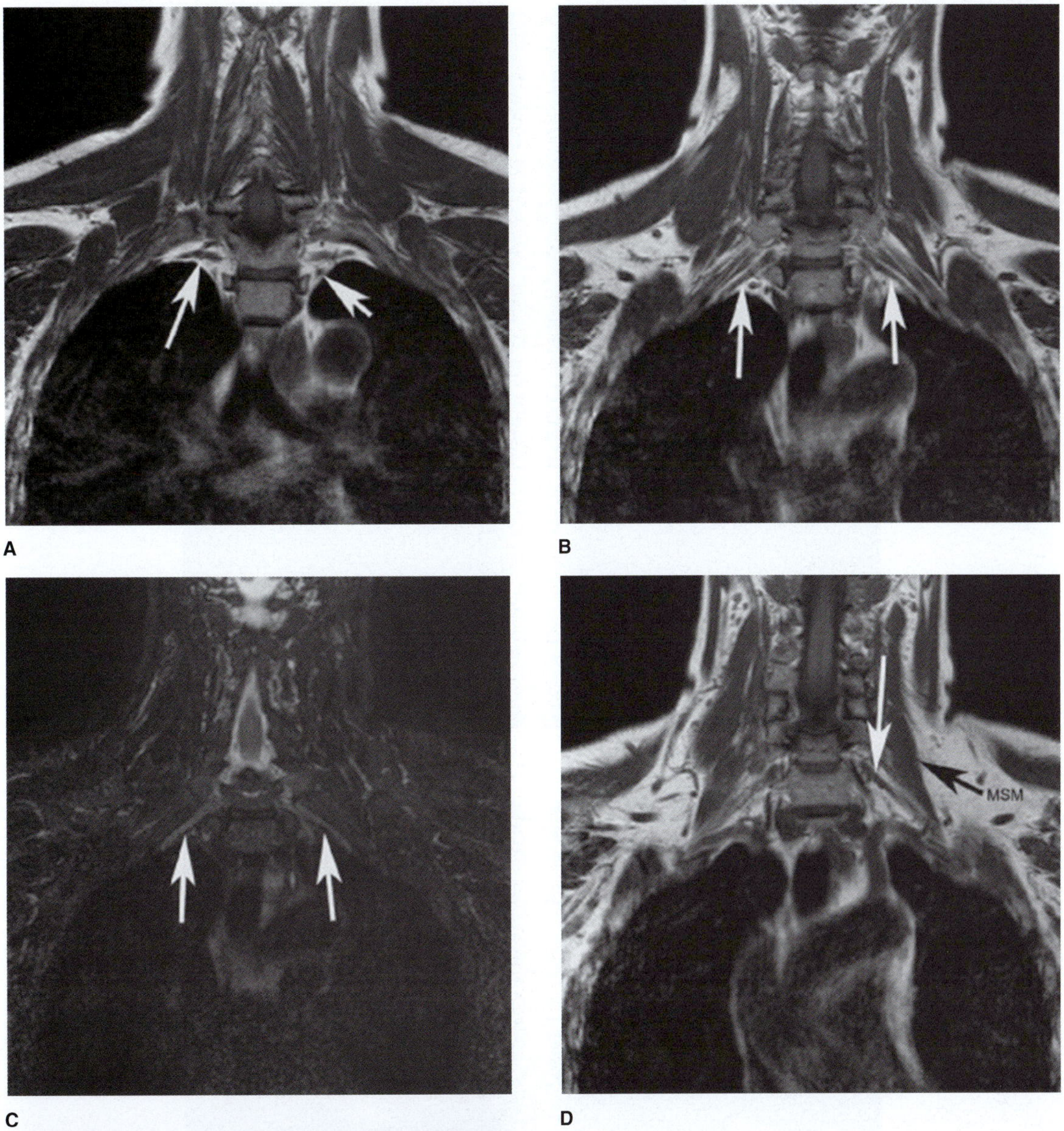

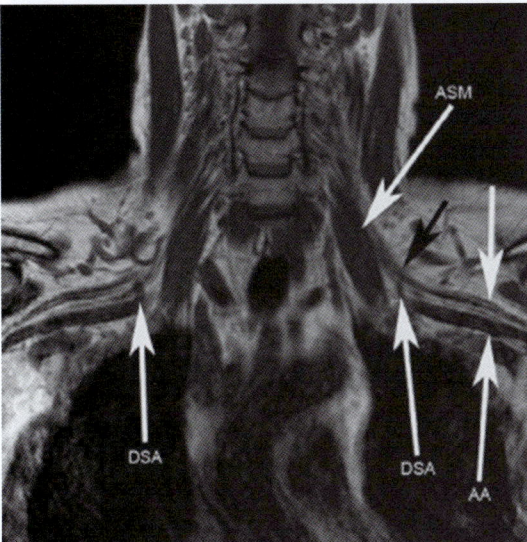

Figure 23-5. MRI of brachial plexus. Normal coronal anatomy. (A) Most posterior image with the horizontal course of the T1 nerve root (*long arrow*), very close to the lung apex. Short arrow points to the stellate ganglion. (B) Image just anterior to (A) with the C8 nerve roots (*arrows*). (C) T2-STIR image at the same level as (B) shows the slightly increased signal intensity of the normal C8 nerve roots (*arrows*). (D) *Arrow* points to the C7 nerve root. MSM, middle scalene muscle. (E) The cords (*white arrow*) are seen as linear structures above the axillary artery (AA). The dorsal scapular artery (DSA) courses between the trunks of the brachial plexus, *black arrow* points to the superior trunk. ASM, anterior scalene muscle. (Reproduced with permission from van Es HW, Bollen TL, van Heesewijk HP. MRI of the brachial plexus: a pictorial review. *Eur J Radiol*. 2010;74(2):391–402. Figure 2.)

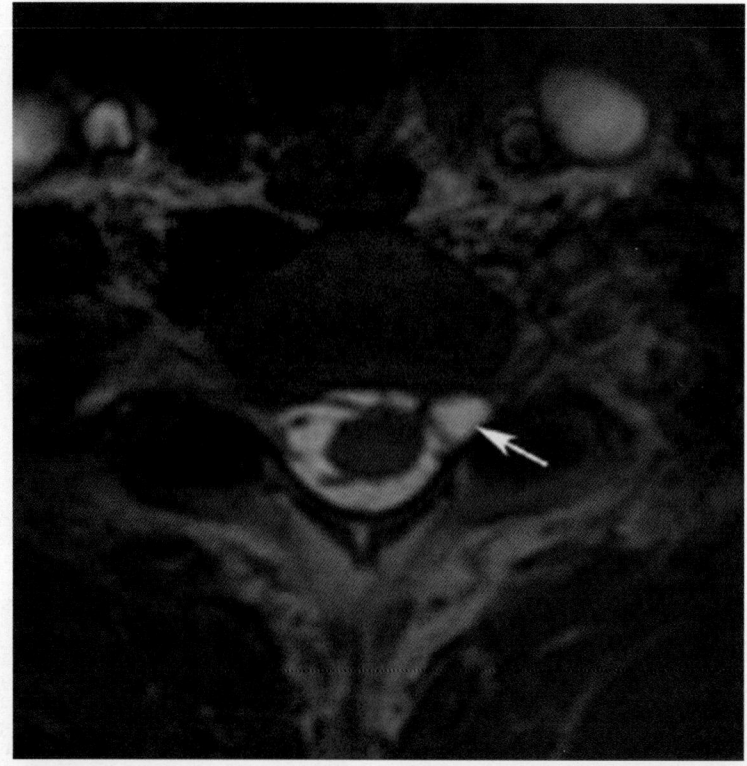

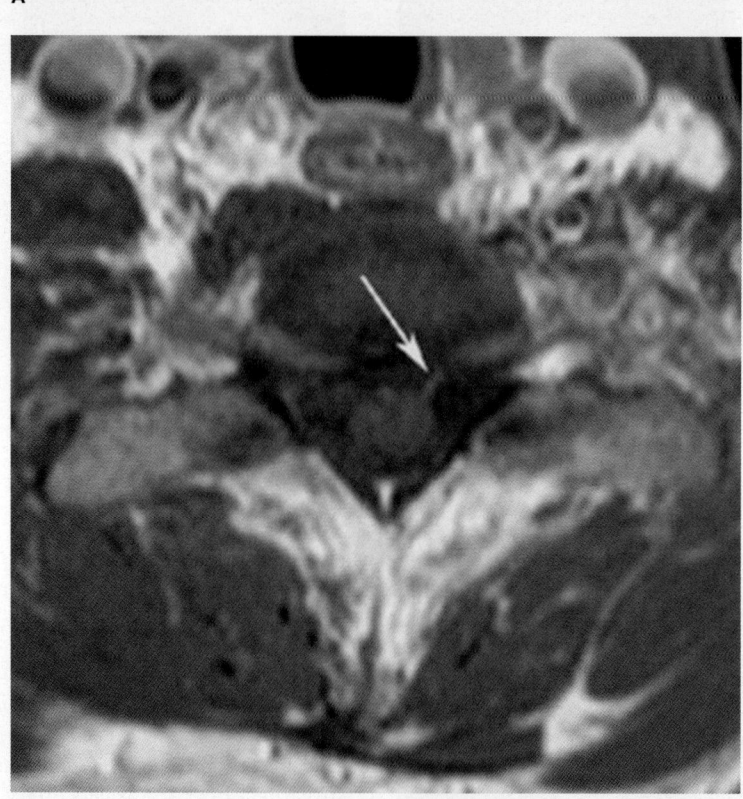

Figure 23-6. MRI of cervical spine. Traumatic nerve root avulsion. (**A**) Axial balanced fast field echo (FFE) image demonstrates a traumatic pseudomeningocele (*arrow*). (**B**) Axial T1-weighted image with intravenous gadolinium shows the enhancement of an avulsed nerve root (*arrow*). (Reproduced with permission from van Es HW, Bollen TL, van Heesewijk HP. MRI of the brachial plexus: a pictorial review. *Eur J Radiol*. 2010;74(2):391–402. Figure 14.)

TABLE 23-3. CAUSES OF RADICULOPATHY

Herniated nucleus proposus
Degenerative joint disease
Rheumatoid arthritis
Trauma
Vertebral body compression fracture
Pott disease
Compression by extradural mass (e.g., meningioma, metastatic tumor, hematoma, abscess)
Primary nerve tumor (e.g., neurofibroma, schwannoma, neuroma)
Carcinomatous meningitis
Perineural spread of tumor (e.g., prostate cancer)
Acute inflammatory demyelinating polyradiculopathy
Chronic inflammatory demyelinating polyradiculopathy
Acute or chronic immune-mediated axonal polyradiculoneuropathy
Sarcoidosis
Amyloidoma
Diabetic radiculopathy
Infection (e.g., Lyme disease, herpes zoster, cytomegalovirus, syphilis, strongyloides)

nerve roots become impinged by two main mechanisms: HNP or bony hypertrophy either at the uncovertebral joint or facet joint.[34]

Most cervical radiculopathies involve C5–8 spinal nerve roots (C7 in 31%–81%, C6 in 19%–25%, C8 in 4%–10%, and C5 in 2%–10%).[13,35–39] Causes of cervical radiculopathy are multiple (Table 23-3), and most commonly involve compression of nerve root by an HNP or osteophytes in the case of degenerative spine disease. Individuals with a cervical radiculopathy typically present with neck or posterior shoulder pain in the scapular region that radiates down the affected arm. Lateral flexion of the neck toward the painful arm and neck extension, can narrow the neural foramen further compressing the nerve root and thus exacerbating the pain, as can downward pressure on the affected individual's head. This is called the Spurling maneuver.[34] The patient may have weakness in the distribution of the affected myotome and sensory loss in the dermatome that is involved. The deep tendon reflexes of affected segment may also be reduced. Because there is much overlap in the territories supplied by individual spinal roots, symptoms and signs can mimic a plexopathy or focal neuropathy. Therefore, as previously discussed, EMG and NCSs combined with imaging studies are extremely valuable in localization. Imaging studies are also important to assess structural etiology (e.g., HNP, osteophyte impinging on root, tumor of the nerve or extrinsic tumor/mass compression of the nerve, or inflammatory process). Further, nerve root avulsion may accompany nearly 80% of severe brachial plexopathies due to trauma.

C5 Radiculopathy

The presentation of C5 radiculopathy may include weakness of shoulder abduction (deltoid, supraspinatus) and external rotation (infraspinatus), scapular winging (rhomboid), elbow flexion (biceps and brachioradialis), and supination of the forearm (supinator). Sensory loss is absent in many cases but, if present, involves a portion of the lateral shoulder and proximal arm. The biceps brachii and brachioradialis deep tendon reflexes may be asymmetrically reduced compared to the unaffected arm. Routine median and ulnar motor and sensory NCSs are normal, as these do not carry any nerve fibers originating in the C5 spinal root. EDX localization is dependent on the EMG examination (Table 23-1). Abnormalities in midcervical paraspinal muscles, supraspinatus, infraspinatus, deltoid, biceps brachii, supinator, and brachioradialis muscles can be seen in C5 radiculopathies. However, these muscles are also innervated by C6. The rhomboids are primarily innervated by C5. Therefore, abnormalities in this muscle strongly support a C5 radiculopathy. Further, if one sees abnormal spontaneous activity or neurogenic changes in motor unit potential morphology or recruitment in the triceps, pronator teres, extensor carpi radialis, or flexor carpi radialis that are innervated by C6, but not by C5, the C6 nerve root is likely also involved.

It's important to remember musculoskeletal mimics in the differential. Just like C5 radiculopathy, rotator cuff injury, can also produce shoulder pain and weakness in shoulder abduction and external rotation. Rotator cuff injuries are distinguished by reproducing discomfort through passive shoulder movement, instead of neck movement, and by preserved biceps strength and reflexes. Other differential diagnostic considerations not related to trauma or degenerative spine disease include brachial plexopathy, diseases that may present as multifocal neuropathies, and in the absence of pain or sensory symptoms, motor neuron disease.

C6 Radiculopathy

In many ways, C6 radiculopathy can present like a C5 radiculopathy. However, rhomboid strength is normal but weakness may also involve elbow extension (triceps), forearm pronation (pronator teres), and wrist extension (extensor carpi radialis). Patients often describe a "numb thumb" with or without sensory symptoms more proximally in the C6 dermatome. In patients with suspected C6 radiculopathy, it is important to consider and to evaluate for brachial plexopathy (upper trunk and lateral cords) and focal neuropathies involving the median or radial nerves. Therefore, at the very least, we usually perform median and radial SNAPs and a median CMAP. In addition, we obtain lateral antebrachial cutaneous SNAPs, if we are suspicious for brachial plexopathy affecting the upper trunk or lateral cord. As discussed, these NCSs should be normal in C6 radiculopathy. We do not routinely perform H-reflex recording from the flexor carpi radialis but it may be abnormal. Localization primarily hinges on the needle EMG examination (Table 23-1). Not surprisingly, there is significant overlap of abnormalities in C6 with C5 and C7 radiculopathies. Needle EMG may demonstrate abnormalities in mid to lower cervical paraspinals, supraspinatus, infraspinatus, deltoid, biceps brachii, triceps brachii, pronator teres, brachioradialis, supinator, extensor carpi radialis, and flexor carpi radialis muscles. Rotator cuff injury, multifocal neuropathies, and brachial plexus neuritis are likely to be the most common differential diagnostic considerations unrelated to trauma or degenerative joint disease of the cervical spine.

C7 Radiculopathy

C7 radiculopathy often presents with pain radiating into the scapula and down the arm and numbness and paresthesias of digit III. Weakness of elbow extension and wrist or finger extension may be evident along with a diminished triceps reflex. In patients with suspected C7 radiculopathy, the median CMAP and median and superficial radial SNAPs are performed at a minimum to assess for a more distal lesion. But again, one expects these routine NCSs to be normal in C7 radiculopathy, except for possibly the flexor carpi radialis H-reflex which is not routinely studied. On needle EMG, abnormalities may be detected particularly in the triceps brachii, pronator teres, flexor carpi radialis, extensor digitorum communis, and less commonly the extensor digitorum indicis, extensor pollicis longus and brevis, and flexor pollicis longus muscles (Table 23-1). The differential diagnosis of C7 radiculopathy is limited. The most likely mimic is a radial mononeuropathy. Most radial neuropathies occur at or distal to the spiral groove, resulting in sparing of the triceps and with prominent weakness of wrist and finger extension. On the other hand, C7 radiculopathies typically affect the triceps, but rarely produce severe weakness of wrist extension and finger extension.

C8/T1 Radiculopathy

It is often difficult to distinguish C8 from T1 radiculopathies, and so these are combined for discussion. Individuals with C8/T1 radiculopathy describe sensory disturbance affecting the medial aspect of the hand and forearm along with hand weakness, typically in both median, ulnar, and radial innervated hand and forearm muscles. Differential diagnosis includes brachial plexopathy (lower trunk or medial cord), ulnar neuropathy, and in the absence of pain and sensory symptoms, motor neuron disease. In cases of ulnar neuropathy, the site of the lesion may be at the wrist, elbow, or elsewhere.

At minimum, we perform ulnar and median CMAPs and SNAPs and often a medial antebrachial cutaneous SNAP to exclude a plexus lesion (Table 23-2). The SNAPs should be normal in a radiculopathy, but in a lower trunk or medial cord injury, the ulnar and medial antebrachial cutaneous SNAP amplitudes may be reduced, particularly in comparison to the unaffected side. A reduction in the median CMAP amplitude with a normal median SNAP further supports a lower trunk or medial cord abnormality (Table 23-2). On needle EMG, one may see abnormalities in any of the median- or ulnar-innervated muscles innervated by C8 and T1 spinal roots (Table 23-1). The thenar eminence is predominantly innervated by T1, so the median CMAP amplitude may be disproportionately reduced compared to the ulnar CMAP in a T1 radiculopathy. Most of the radial-innervated muscles supplying the fingers originate from the C7 and C8 spinal segments but not T1. Therefore, EMG of these muscle groups can help distinguish a C8 from a T1 radiculopathy. In the case of a lower trunk lesion, muscles innervating radial muscles via the C8 nerve root will be affected as well as intrinsic hand muscles, whereas this will not be the case in medial cord lesions.

Multiple Cervical Radiculopathies

Most cervical radiculopathies involve only one root, but approximately 12%–30% involve multiple levels.[36,38] If multilevel involvement exists, CMAP amplitudes are more likely to be reduced although SNAPs will remain spared. The presence of needle EMG abnormalities suggesting a polyradiculopathy must raise the suspicion of other diseases, particularly motor neuron disease. In such cases, it is important to study the lower extremity, thoracic paraspinals, and even selected muscles innervated by cranial nerves (e.g., tongue and sternocleidomastoid).

THORACIC RADICULOPATHIES

Although they remain uncommon, we will briefly discuss thoracic radiculopathies for completeness. HNPs in the thoracic region account for only 0.22%–5.3% of all disc protrusions.[40–43] Approximately 75% of symptomatic thoracic radiculopathies occur between T8 and T12, with most occurring between T11 and T12. Central and centrolateral HNPs can compress the spinal cord, leading to symptoms and signs of a myelopathy. Patients may present with circumferential chest or abdominal pain and/or paresthesias, leg pain or weakness, or bowel or bladder difficulties (e.g., constipation, urinary retention, and incontinence). At the T11–12 region, the conus medullaris or cauda equina may be affected with ensuing bowel/bladder and lower extremity deficits.

Trauma is the most common cause of a herniated thoracic disc accounting for 14%–63% of cases.[44,45] Degenerative changes of the spine account for a minority of cases. Other structural causes for thoracic radiculopathies that need to be considered include compression due to metastatic disease, vertebral collapse, Pott disease, and primary nerve tumors. Perhaps, the most common etiology of thoracic radiculopathy is diabetes mellitus (e.g., diabetic radiculoneuropathy). Additional nonstructural (e.g., inflammatory, infiltrative, infectious) causes of thoracic radiculopathies include Lyme disease, herpes zoster, cytomegalovirus, sarcoidosis, and carcinomatous meningitis. Of note, thoracic disc herniations incidentally noted on imaging are far more common than causally related clinical syndromes, and clinicians need to be cautious before attributing nonspecific clinical symptoms to an imaging abnormality.

The EDX evaluation of thoracic radiculopathies is limited. NCSs are not helpful because they cannot directly assess thoracic roots. Needle EMG of thoracic paraspinal muscle may demonstrate abnormal insertional and spontaneous activity. Care must be taken to insert the needle using correct landmarks and not too deep or laterally. Pneumothorax is a rare complication but is infrequently encountered. EMG of abdominal muscles may be of value, as one can also assess for MUAP morphology and recruitment abnormalities.

TREATMENT OF RADICULOPATHIES

Treatment is dependent on the etiology of the radiculopathy. For the sake of discussion, we will focus here on treatment of radiculopathies related to HNPs or spondylotic disease, as radiculoneuropathies related to other entities (e.g., Lyme disease, diabetes) are discussed in other chapters in this book. It is difficult to make evidence-based medical decisions regarding the best therapeutic approach to patients with cervical radiculopathies due to the lack of well-designed, prospective, controlled, and blinded trials. That said, it is important to realize that the natural history of radiculopathies related to compression from HNPs is favorable. In a large series of patients with cervical radiculopathy followed for up to 5 years, 90% were asymptomatic or had only slight pain at last follow-up; however, 26% of all patients underwent surgery.[46]

Treatment of acute cervical radiculopathy is focused first on ruling out red flags, then on relieving pain and then on reassurance. Red flags which would be concerning for malignancy, myelopathy, or spinal abscess include fever, shaking chills, weight loss, immunocompromise, IV drug use, clumsiness, or urinary urgency/incontinence. Red flags on exam would include hyperreflexia, clonus, Hoffman or Babinski signs, new gait disturbance, and/or difficulty with coordination. MRI is the preferred imaging modality for patients with complex cervical radiculopathy (i.e., any red flag sign or symptom) or patients who have no improvement after 4–6 weeks of nonoperative management or progression of neurologic deficit. MRI is typically of less utility outside of this population as approximately 57% of patients older than 64 years who do not have symptoms of cervical radiculopathy have evidence of disk herniation and 26% have spinal cord impingement.[47] Physical therapy with stretching combined with strengthening can be beneficial in acute cervical radiculopathy.[48] Most patients will improve with any nonsurgical modality used among physical therapy, home exercise, nonsteroidal anti-inflammatories, muscle relaxants and massage, and there is no strong evidence for efficacy of any modality. Steroid injections can be considered for patients whose symptoms persist after 4–6 weeks. Commonly used medications for neuropathic pain such as antiepileptic agents or tricyclic antidepressants can be tried. Opioid analgesia is not recommended given the risk of addiction and the lack of benefit compared to placebo in a recent large randomized controlled trial.[49] In patients with intractable pain or those with significant weakness, decompressive surgery may be warranted. Small trials assessing the effects of surgery versus conservative management for cervical spondylotic radiculopathy or myelopathy have shown little or no difference in the long-term, though there was quicker pain relief in the surgical group.[50,51] Despite many years of calls for additional evidence to guide decision making regarding who might benefit from surgery, these data are still lacking.[52]

BRACHIAL PLEXOPATHY

Brachial plexopathies can be classified based on the nature of the injury (i.e., an open or closed brachial plexopathy), the anatomic location of the lesion, or the mechanism of injury (Table 23-2).[1-3] MRI can be helpful in identifying both the site and cause of the lesion because the anatomical resolution of the roots, trunks, divisions, and cords is very well depicted due to the inherent contrast differences between the nerves and surrounding fat (Figs. 23-3 and 23-4).[25] However, MRI is not always feasible and usually we can make an accurate diagnosis on the basis of clinical examination, supplemented when necessary by EDX studies at least as to localization. Therefore, we will begin by reviewing clinical and EDX features that one may expect to see with lesions affecting various trunks and cords of the brachial plexus.

Upper Trunk

Individuals with upper trunk lesions have weakness in the deltoid, biceps brachii, and brachioradialis muscles (Fig. 23-2). Therefore, they commonly complain of difficulty lifting their arm above their head or lifting objects which require bending the elbow. Sensory loss involves the lateral arm and forearm down to the lateral aspect of the hand and fingers. The biceps brachii and brachioradialis reflexes are typically reduced. Upper trunk injuries in isolation are relatively common when compared to isolated middle or lower trunk lesions.

EMG and NCSs are useful in differentiating upper trunk lesions from C5 or C6 radiculopathies. In upper trunk lesions, the posterior primary rami and nerve branches to the rhomboid and serratus anterior muscles are spared whereas they are involved in C5/C6 radiculopathies. Because trunk lesions, by definition, occur distal to the DRG, relevant sensory responses will generally be abnormal. If the injury is axonal damage and not just neuropraxia (i.e., conduction block and/or demyelination), the superficial radial, median recording from the thumb and possibly from digit 2, and lateral antebrachial cutaneous SNAPs may have reduced amplitudes, particularly when compared to the asymptomatic contralateral arm (Table 23-2). These SNAPs would be normal in a cervical radiculopathy or in a purely neuropraxic or demyelinating process affecting the trunk. Routine median and ulnar CMAPs are performed to exclude involvement of other trunks or nerves. Needle EMG is further localizing in combination with these sensory and motor studies. Recall that the posterior primary rami to paraspinal muscles, the dorsal scapular nerve to rhomboid, and the long thoracic nerve to serratus anterior take off from cervical roots before the formation of the upper trunk. EMG of these muscles may show evidence of denervation in a C5 or C6 radiculopathies, but would be spared if the lesion was confined to the upper trunk. Performing needle EMG not only of muscles in the upper trunk and in C5/C6 myotomes, but also of muscles supplied by the middle and lower trunks, will ensure that abnormalities are indeed restricted muscles innervated by the upper trunk (Table 23-1).

Middle Trunk

Isolated middle trunk lesions are extremely rare and most often occur in combination with other plexus lesions (Fig. 23-2). Symptoms and signs resemble a C7 radiculopathy. Affected individuals may experience weakness of elbow, wrist, and finger extension. Sensory loss and/or pain may occur in the posterior forearm and the dorsal and palmar aspects of the third finger. The triceps reflex is often reduced.

Provided the injury is axonal, the median-D3 SNAP amplitude may be reduced as the cutaneous fibers that supply this finger usually traverse the middle trunk (Table 23-2). Also, the radial CMAP recorded from extensor indicis proprius may have reduced amplitude, if there is sufficient axon loss. However, needle EMG is most important in delineating the extent of motor involvement. Remember that the middle trunk contains the C7 spinal nerves, which, after passing through the middle trunk, diverge and traverse the posterior and lateral cords (Table 23-1, Fig. 23-2). Thus, most muscles innervated by the radial nerve and its posterior interosseous branch are affected by middle trunk lesions. The brachioradialis muscle which is supplied by the upper trunk is a notable exception. Additionally, some median-innervated forearm muscles with C6 and C7 and lateral cord innervation will also be affected. Although less commonly studied, EMG abnormalities may also be appreciated in the pectoralis major, latissimus dorsi, and teres major muscles, as these muscles are partially innervated by C7 spinal nerves and the middle trunk via the medial and posterior cords. However, the serratus anterior muscle, which has C7 innervation in common but not the middle trunk, would be spared with a middle trunk lesion (recall the long thoracic nerve branches directly off the roots). There are no nerve branches arising directly from the middle trunk, and so it can be difficult to distinguish a lesion involving the middle trunk from those affecting portions of the lateral and posterior cords.

Lower Trunk

Lesions affecting the lower trunk present similarly to C8/T1 radiculopathies, medial cord plexopathies, and ulnar neuropathies (Fig. 23-2). Affected individuals have sensory loss of the medial aspect of the forearm and hand, and weakness of ulnar-, median-, and radial nerve–innervated wrist and intrinsic hand muscles. Involvement of radial nerve and posterior cord–innervated C8/T1 muscles puts the lesion more proximal than the medial cord.

NCSs are valuable in localizing the lesion (Table 23-2). With axonal lesions, one would expect to see reduced amplitudes of ulnar and medial antebrachial cutaneous SNAPs in both lower trunk and medial cord lesions, but not in C8 or T1 radiculopathies. Reduced ulnar and median CMAP amplitudes may be seen. The median CMAP is usually more affected than the ulnar CMAP. C8/T1 radiculopathies can also reduce the median and ulnar CMAPs but the degree of reduction is typically less and the amplitude drops in only moderate to severe radiculopathy. EMG likely will show signs of neurogenic change in radial-, median-, and ulnar-innervated distal upper extremity and hand muscles, as the nerves supplying these muscles all course through the lower trunk (Table 23-1). However, lower cervical paraspinal muscles are expected to be normal in brachial plexus lesions. Compared to other plexus injuries, the prognosis for recovery is comparatively poor because of the long distance a regenerating nerve must cover to reinnervate the muscles in the distal arm.[1]

Posterior Cord

The nerves originating from the posterior cord include the thoracodorsal, the upper and lower subscapular, axillary, and radial nerves (Fig. 23-2). Depending on the lesion's location within the posterior cord, affected individuals may have weakness of shoulder abduction or extension, forearm supination, and elbow/wrist/finger extension. Sensory disturbance and/or pain may exist in the shoulder area, posterior arm and forearm, and the dorsum of the hand.

Provided the posterior cord lesion is axonal, both superficial radial and posterior cutaneous nerve of the forearm SNAP amplitudes may be reduced (Table 23-2). However, the lateral antebrachial cutaneous SNAP would be normal. It also receives supply from the upper trunk but instead of the posterior cord, it receives fibers from the lateral cord. The radial-EIP CMAP will likely have reduced amplitude compared to the contralateral unaffected side when significant axonal loss involving the C7 and C8 spinal nerve fibers coursing through the posterior cord has occurred. EMG would be expected to demonstrate abnormalities of the deltoid, radial-innervated muscles, latissimus dorsi, and teres major and minor (Table 23-1).

Lateral Cord

The lateral cord is the continuation of the anterior division of the upper trunk (Fig. 23-2). Individuals with a lateral cord lesion may experience weakness of shoulder flexion and abduction, elbow flexion and pronation, and wrist flexion. In addition, sensory disturbance would involve the lateral, volar aspect of the upper arm and forearm along with the lateral and palmar aspect of the hand and fingers. The biceps brachii reflex should be reduced with sparing of the brachioradialis reflex.

Median SNAPs to the first three digits, superficial radial nerve to the thumb, and the lateral antebrachial cutaneous nerve should be studied to help localize pathology to the lateral cord (Table 23-3). With axonal lesions to the lateral cord, the median and lateral antebrachial SNAPs are expected to have decreased amplitude, but the radial SNAP should be normal as this arises from the posterior cord. A musculocutaneous CMAP recording from the biceps brachii muscles may have reduced amplitude. EMG can demonstrate evidence of denervation in the biceps brachii, pronator teres, flexor carpi radialis muscles, and perhaps the infraclavicular and midsternal fibers of the pectoralis major (Table 23-1). These findings coupled with normal EMG of the cervical paraspinal, supraspinatus, infraspinatus, deltoid, and triceps muscles localize the lesion distal to the upper trunk and out of the territory of the posterior cord.

Medial Cord

The medial cord is a continuation of the anterior division of the lower trunk (Fig. 23-2). A medial cord injury clinically resembles a lower trunk lesion except that radial nerve–innervated C8/T1 wrist/hand muscles (e.g., extensor indicis proprius and extensor digitorum communis) would be spared. Remember that nerves to radial-innervated muscles in the forearm course through the lower trunk and then enter the posterior cord rather than the medial cord. Therefore, the ulnar-, median-, and radial-innervated muscles to the digits are affected in a lower trunk lesion, only the ulnar- and median-innervated muscles will be abnormal with medial cord damage.

The medial antebrachial cutaneous and ulnar SNAPs may be reduced in amplitude provided there is axonal injury, but this does not help distinguish a medial cord from a lower trunk lesion (Table 23-2). The medial antebrachial cutaneous response is disproportionately reduced in comparison to the ulnar SNAP in neurogenic thoracic outlet syndrome, however, presumably due to a larger component from the T1 spinal nerve. Conversely, the ulnar SNAP is typically more affected from poststernotomy plexopathies as the C8 spinal nerve appears to be the primary structure injured. Decreased amplitudes of median and ulnar CMAPs recording from thenar and hypothenar muscles do not discriminate between injury to the lower trunk and medial cord. One way to try to differentiate a medial cord from a lower trunk lesion would be by assessing the radial CMAP recorded from the extensor indicis proprius muscles. EMG is more helpful in distinguishing between lower trunk and medial cord lesions. Again, if EMG demonstrates signs of denervation in C8/T1 radial- as well as median- and ulnar-innervated musculature, then a lower trunk as opposed to medial cord injury should be considered (Table 23-1).

SPECIFIC BRACHIAL PLEXUS DISORDERS

In the following section, we will go into more detail about the common types of brachial plexopathies (Table 23-4).

Immune-Mediated Brachial Plexus Neuropathy

Immune-mediated brachial plexus neuropathy (IBPN) goes by various terminologies, including acute brachial plexitis or neuritis, neuralgic amyotrophy, and Parsonage–Turner syndrome.[2,3,53-55] IBPN usually presents with the acute, often nocturnal, onset of severe pain in the shoulder region. The pain is frequently described like a hot poker jammed into the upper arm, so severe that patients often seek urgent medical attention. Sometimes the pain involves the forearm or may be restricted to this segment of the arm (as seen in individuals with anterior interosseous syndrome, a forme fruste of IBPN). The pain is often exacerbated by movement of the arm. The intense pain usually lasts several days to a few weeks, but a dull ache can persist for 3 years or more. Individuals who are affected may not initially appreciate weakness because pain limits movement. However, as the pain dissipates, weakness and often, a lesser degree sensory loss are appreciated. Imaging advances have shed light on the distribution of nerve involvement and led to recommendations for standardized imaging protocols.[56,57] Attacks can occasionally recur.[53,58] This disorder is usually clinically unilateral, but the opposite arm can occasionally be affected occasionally to a lesser degree.

▶ **TABLE 23-4. BRACHIAL PLEXUS CLASSIFICATION: NATURE OF INJURY**

Closed	Open
Idiopathic brachial plexus neuropathy	Trauma
Traction injuries (obstetric, postsurgical)	(e.g., gunshot
Closed trauma	wound,
Radiation related	shrapnel,
Tumor (primary/secondary)	lacerations)
Neurogenic thoracic outlet syndrome	
Rucksack palsy	
Genetic (HNA, HNPP)	

HNA, hereditary neuralgia amyotrophy; HNPP, hereditary neuropathy with liability to pressure palsy.
Modified from Wilbourn AJ. Brachial plexus disorders. In: Dyck PJ, Thomas PK, Griffin JU, et al., eds. *Peripheral Neuropathy*. 3rd ed. W.B. Saunders; 1992.

Clinical findings are dependent on the distribution of involvement which is often patchy. This patchiness distinguishes IBPN from a structural brachial plexopathy. Occasionally, mild abnormalities of the cerebrospinal fluid (increased protein or pleocytosis) are found indicative of a presumed inflammatory process also extending to the roots.[59] One large study suggested that 36% of patients recovered most function within 1 year, 75% by the end of year 2, and 89% by the end of year 3.[59] However, another large study of 246 cases found that approximately two-thirds of patients still had persistent pain and weakness after 3 years and <8% had a full recovery.[53] Mild paresis was still evident in 69%, with severe weakness in 3%. Proximally located muscles are more likely to regain strength than the more distal hand muscles. Persistent deficits relate to reduced endurance and altered patterns of movement.[58]

The most common pattern of IBPN involves the upper trunk or a single or multiple mononeuropathies. The suprascapular, long thoracic and axillary are the most common single nerves affected.[53,60] Additionally, the phrenic nerve is involved in approximately 8% of patients with IBPN.[61] In addition, the AIN[62,63] and PIN are commonly affected.[58,61] Any of these nerves may also be affected in isolation as a variant of IBPN. In most IBPNs, the paraspinal muscles are normal on EMG, suggesting that the lesion is distal to the root/spinal nerve level, but occasionally signs of active denervation are apparent, suggesting root involvement. Rarely, multiple cranial nerves (IX, X, XI, and XII) may be involved.[64] In this regard, an isolated spinal accessory neuropathy presenting as acute unilateral suboccipital and neck pain and weakness of the trapezius muscle may also represent a type of IBPN.[65]

The pathogenic basis of IBPN is unknown but presumed to be immunologic. Circumstantial evidence of an inflammatory basis is that IBPN may develop following immunologic challenge by infection, vaccination, surgery, or following treatment with immune-modulating agents (e.g., interferons, interleukin-2, and tumor necrosis-alpha blockers).[66–69] In addition, some series have reported antibodies directed against peripheral nerve myelin and soluble terminal complement complexes.[70] Biopsies of the brachial plexus are not typically performed for IBPN, but there are few descriptions of such biopsies revealing perivascular epineurial and endoneurial inflammatory cell infiltrates. The antigen(s) towards which the autoimmune attack is directed are unknown, but the EDX abnormalities suggest a primary insult against the axons of the nerves as opposed to the myelin.

The EDX findings are dependent on the site(s) of involvement and can be rather multifocal.[59,71] The upper trunk is primarily involved in most patients. Thus, not surprisingly, median and ulnar motor studies are abnormal in only about 15% of patients with IBPN.[60] Median, lateral antebrachial cutaneous, and radial SNAPs are more likely to be abnormal. Also, CMAPs recorded from the deltoid and biceps muscles can demonstrate abnormalities. Other laboratory abnormalities include slightly increased cerebrospinal fluid protein with or without mild pleocytosis in a little over 10% of patients however CSF is not needed for diagnosis in most cases.[53,59] MRI of the brachial plexus may demonstrate increased T2 signal in the nerve suggestive of inflammation or edema.[24,29,53]

We often treat patients presenting acutely who continue to have severe pain with a short course of corticosteroids (e.g., prednisone 50–60 mg daily tapering by 10 mg every 4–5 days), although there are very few evidence-based studies that have demonstrated efficacy. However, in our anecdotal experience, corticosteroids help alleviate pain, which helps the patient proceed with physical therapy and reduces impact on upper extremity function. Corticosteroids do not expedite return of strength. If pain has already resolved by the time patients present to us for medical attention, we do not treat with corticosteroids. The mainstay of treatment is physical and occupational therapy to prevent contractures in an immobilized arm, improve function, and maintain strength in unaffected muscles.

Other Immune-Mediated Neuropathies

Rarely, a painful or painless brachial plexopathy may be the sole manifestation of an asymmetric form of chronic inflammatory demyelinating neuropathy, multifocal acquired motor and sensory demyelinating neuropathy, or multifocal motor neuropathy.[72] Diagnosis of these entities requires demonstration of conduction block or focal slowing localized to the brachial plexus, which is often technically difficult. The importance of identifying multifocal acquired motor and sensory demyelinating neuropathy or multifocal motor neuropathy is their potential responsiveness to immunotherapy as is discussed in Chapter 14.

Obstetrically Related Plexopathies

The annual incidence of obstetrically related plexus injuries ranges between 0.38 and 2.0 per 1,000 live births.[73–78] Three types of brachial plexus injury complicate childbirth: (1) diffuse plexopathy, (2) upper trunk plexopathy (Erb palsy), or (3) lower trunk plexopathy (Klumpke palsy/paralysis). The plexus can be damaged during childbirth due to traction on the arm which then stretches the brachial plexus. Increased risk is associated with heavy birth weight of the infant, mothers with short stature, breech presentation, long and difficult labor, and heavily sedated mothers (resulting in diminished muscle tone during delivery).[78–83] In addition, forceful downward traction applied to the head after the fetal third rotation is a risk factor of obstetric brachial plexus palsy in vaginal deliveries in cephalic presentation.[81]

Erb palsy, the most common type of obstetric paralysis, results from stretch of the nerves of the upper trunk of the brachial plexus.[75,82] Severe traction injury may also lead to avulsion of the C5 or C6 spinal nerves. Traction of the upper trunk can occur with shoulder dystocia in a vertex presentation or difficulty delivering head in a breech presentation. An upper trunk lesion leads to weakness of supra- and infraspinatus, deltoid, biceps brachii, teres minor, brachioradialis, extensor carpi radialis longus/brevis, and supinator muscles. An infant with Erb palsy lies in a typical position with the shoulder adducted and internally rotated (unopposed pull of the sternal portion of the pectoralis major and latissimus dorsi muscles), elbow extended and forearm pronated (unopposed triceps and pronator teres/quadratus muscles), and wrist/fingers flexed (weak wrist extensors—the so-called "waiter's tip position").[1] Diaphragmatic or serratus anterior weakness suggests the possibility of root avulsion, as the nerves to these muscles (phrenic and long thoracic, respectively) arise proximal to the upper trunk.

Rarely, the lower trunk or C8 or T1 roots are injured during childbirth (Klumpke paralysis).[83] These usually occur in the setting of face presentation and hyperextension of the neck but can also complicate breech deliveries with hyperabduction of the arm. Infants will have good proximal arm strength, but weakness of hand muscles is evident. Finally, the entire plexus can also be affected to varying degrees.[84,85]

Radiological imaging is essential to assess for the possibility of associated humeral or clavicular fractures as well as diaphragmatic paralysis. In addition, MRI should be done to assess for nerve root avulsion.[2,86,87]

EDX studies are useful to determine the site and severity of injury, prognosis, and to decide about the appropriateness and timing of any operative intervention.[1,2,74,75,84,87] Abnormalities in SNAPs and CMAPs may be evident in 7–10 days. EDX studies are typically performed 4–6 weeks following delivery, as it can take this long for active signs of denervation to be evident on EMG. However, detection of voluntary MUAPs at any time, even before the 4- to 6-week period, demonstrates that there is at least partial continuity between the anterior horn cells and the target muscle. SNAPs are typically more vulnerable to injury than CMAPs. When SNAP amplitude(s) are low, but CMAP amplitude(s) are disproportionately reduced suggests pathology both proximal and distal to the level of the DRG and raises the possibility of avulsion. Prognosis is better if the nerve is not completely severed. If SNAPs or CMAPs are low or absent and no MUAPs are present on initial testing, serial studies can be performed every 6–8 weeks to assess for evidence of reinnervation.

The natural history is not well defined, but patients with upper trunk lesions often have significant improvement within 3 months. Those with lower trunk lesions are more likely to have a more prolonged course and incomplete recovery. Unfortunately, there is no chance for regeneration of the nerves following a root avulsion. Reconstructive surgical procedures may be employed to help restore elbow flexion and shoulder abduction in patients with severe axonal injury.[88–90]

Neurogenic Thoracic Outlet Syndrome

The term "thoracic outlet syndrome" has been ascribed to both neurogenic and vascular disorders attributed to compromise of blood vessels between the base of the neck and the axilla.[3,21] Our discussion is limited to the rare neurogenic form of thoracic outlet syndrome, which is a lower trunk brachial plexopathy.[91] Most individuals with true neurogenic thoracic outlet syndrome are women with a prominent C7 transverse process or a cervical rib that can be appreciated on plain films of the cervical spine (Fig. 23-7). These cases are often associated with a sharp fibrous band extending from the tip of the elongated C7 transverse process or cervical rib to the first thoracic rib. This band usually cannot be visualized on imaging studies, including MRI scans. Its presence is however suggested by demonstration of the bony anomalies described above. The proximal aspect of the lower trunk becomes angulated or stretched as it passes over this fibrous band. The T1 fibers, which lie below the C8 fibers, become distorted and thus are more likely to be damaged in this condition. Thus, affected individuals have muscle atrophy and weakness that is often greater in the thenar muscles, which have more T1 innervation than the hypothenar muscles, which have more C8 innervation. In addition, patients describe numbness, paresthesias, and pain along the medial aspect of the arm, forearm, and hand. On NCS, the median CMAP and medial antebrachial cutaneous SNAP amplitudes are reduced to a greater extent than the ulnar SNAP and CMAP, because the former studies primarily assess T1 fibers, while ulnar studies primarily assess C8 fibers.[2,92–95] Similarly, needle EMG of the abductor pollicis brevis is typically more abnormal than the first dorsal interosseous muscle for the same reason. Neurogenic thoracic outlet syndrome is typically treated by surgical resection of the taut band. In our experience, surgery may relieve pain and arrest progression of weakness but rarely would restore bulk or strength of hand muscles.

Plexopathies Associated With Neoplasms

Neoplasms involving the brachial plexus include primary nerve tumors, local invasion from nearby cancers (e.g., Pancoast lung tumor or lymphoma), and metastatic cancer.[96,97] Primary brachial plexus tumors, which are less common than secondary tumors, include schwannomas and neurofibromas.[24,98,99] These primary tumors may present as mass lesions in the supraclavicular fossa or axilla. Pain and paresthesias are early symptoms as the tumor initially distorts nerve fibers. Motor and sensory loss occur later as conduction block, demyelination, and/or axonal loss develops.

Schwannomas are commonly benign and well encapsulated. They affect proximal segments of the plexus and may be surgically removed with minimal damage to nearby nerve fibers (Fig. 23-8).[98–101] Neurofibromas are the most common form of peripheral nerve tumor and are typically benign. The exception is when neurofibromas occur in the context of neurofibromatosis. These neurofibromas typically occur in multiples and affect a larger portion of the brachial plexus.[98] Additionally, neurofibromas interdigitate more with nerve fibers and within each nerve fascicle and are more commonly associated with neurological

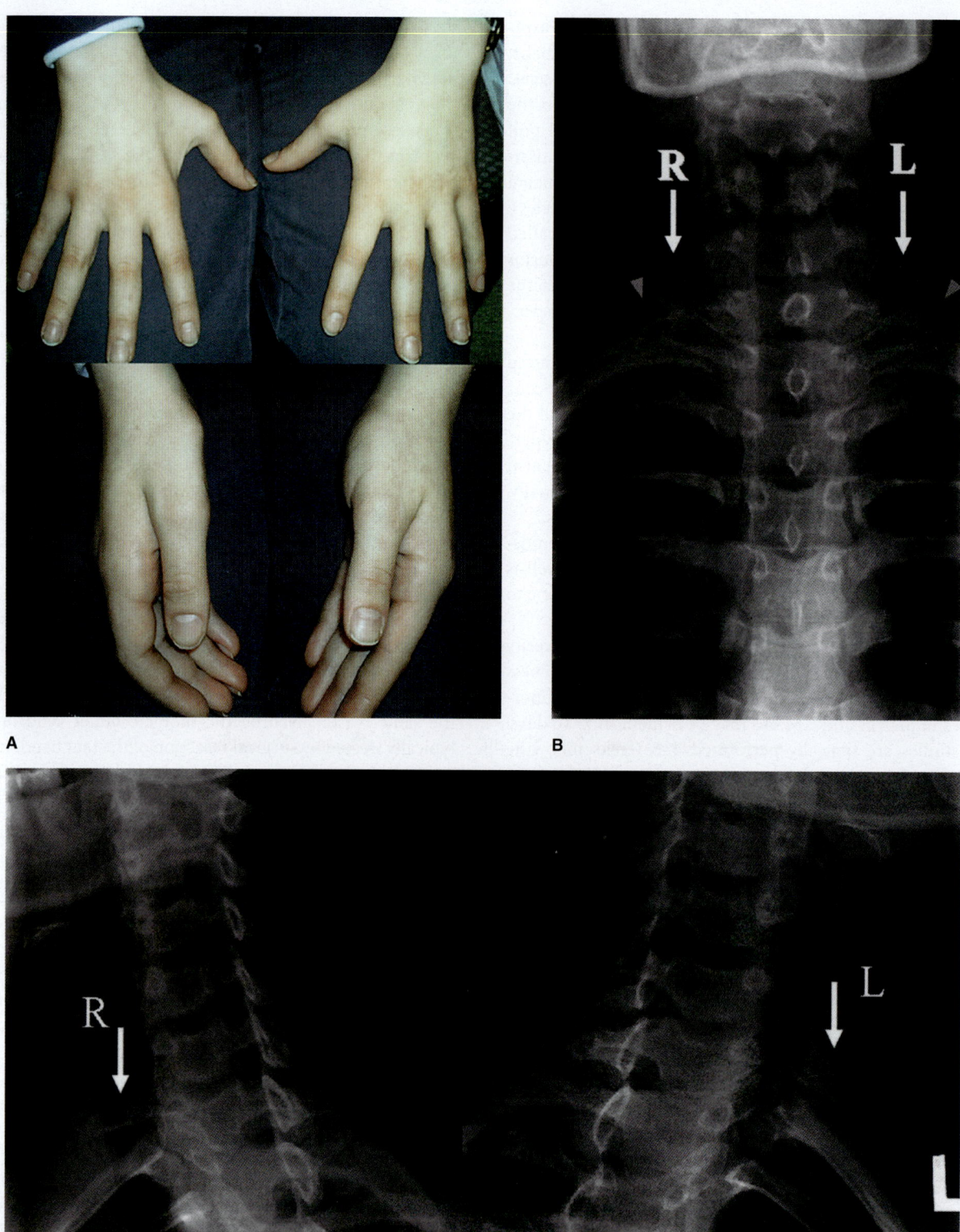

Figure 23-7. Neurogenic thoracic outlet syndrome. Atrophy of the right thenar eminence and first dorsal interosseous muscles are evident (**A**). Plain cervical spine films demonstrate small cervical ribs (*arrows*) bilaterally on AP view (**B**) and oblique view (**C**). (Reproduced with permission from of Steven A. Greenberg, MD. Reproduced with permission from Greenberg SA, Amato AA. *EMG Pearls*. Hanley & Belfus; 2004. Figure 3, p. 50 and Figure 1AB, p. 46.)

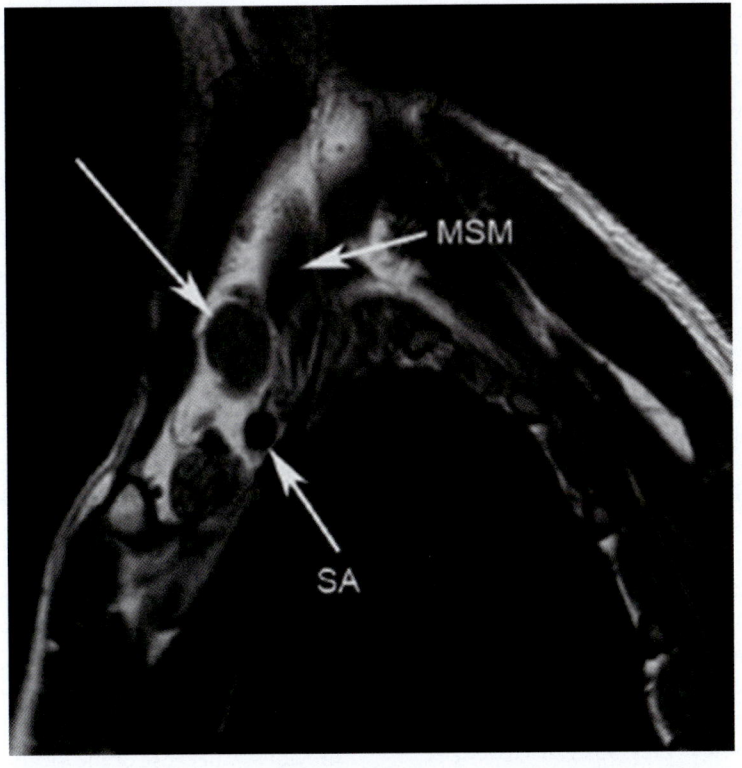
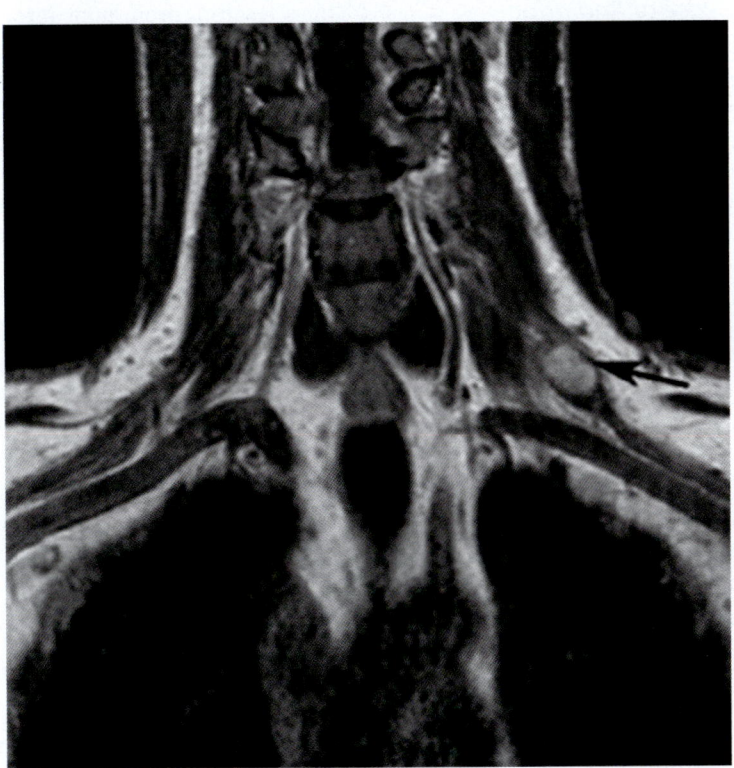

Figure 23-8. MRI of brachial plexus. Schwannoma of the superior trunk. (**A**) Sagittal T1-weighted image, *arrows* point to the tumor which is located in the superior trunk just lateral to the interscalene triangle and above the subclavian artery (SA). MSM, middle scalene muscle. (**B**) Coronal T1-weighted image with intravenous gadolinium shows the enhancing tumor (*arrow*). (Reproduced with permission from van Es HW, Bollen TL, van Heesewijk HP. MRI of the brachial plexus: a pictorial review. *Eur J Radiol.* 2010;74(2):391–402. Fig 3.)

deficits than schwannomas. Because of this interdigitation, it is difficult to remove them surgically without damaging the affected nerve. These tumors can also convert to a more malignant form, particularly in neurofibromatosis.[102]

Secondary tumors affecting the brachial plexus are more common and are always malignant. First, these may arise from local tumors expanding into the plexus. For example, a Pancoast tumor of the upper lobe of the lung may invade or compress the lower trunk of the brachial plexus. Pancoast tumors typically present as an insidious onset of pain in the upper arm, sensory disturbance in the medial aspect of the forearm and hand, and weakness and atrophy of the intrinsic hand muscles along with an ipsilateral Horner syndrome. Chest CT scans or MRI can demonstrate extension of the tumor into the brachial plexus. Second, a primary lymphoma arising from cervical or axillary lymph nodes may also infiltrate the plexus.[96,97] Last, metastatic involvement of the brachial plexus may occur with spread of breast cancer into the axillary lymph nodes and the nearby nerves (Fig. 23-9). Pain and widespread paresthesias are usually the presenting manifestation due to spread of the cancer into the plexus. Weakness and sensory loss conform to the distribution of the affected nerves. Likewise, EDX abnormalities are dependent on the nerves that are involved as previously discussed.[14,20]

Recurrent Neoplastic Disease or Radiation

Treatment for various malignancies (e.g., lung, breast, and lymphoma) often involves radiation therapy, the field of which may include parts of the brachial plexus. It can be difficult in such situations to determine if a new brachial plexopathy is related to tumor within the plexus or from radiation-induced nerve damage. Radiation can be associated with microvascular abnormalities and fibrosis of surrounding tissues, which can damage the axons and the Schwann cells.[1,103] Radiation-induced plexopathy is dose dependent. It is typically delayed, developing sometimes months, but more commonly years, following therapy.[7,96]

Tumor invasion is usually painful and more commonly affects the lower trunk, while radiation injury is often painless and affects the upper trunk.[96] Imaging studies such as MRI and CT scans are useful but can be insensitive in detecting microscopic invasion of the plexus. EMG can be informative, if myokymic discharges are appreciated, as this finding strongly suggests radiation-induced damage. However, absence of myokymic discharges does not rule out radiation as the cause of the plexopathy. Although, the presence of myokymic discharges demonstrates that radiation injury is likely present, but it does not confirm that the cause of the plexopathy is the radiation (e.g., there may still be invasion or compression by tumor).

Backpack or Rucksack Palsy

This condition refers to paresis of the arm or arms occurring in soldiers or civilians wearing heavy backpacks or rucksacks strapped around the shoulders.[1,2,104,105] Motor and sensory losses most typically are in the distribution of the upper trunk but can be more widespread. The injury is usually neuropraxic in nature, although secondary axonal degeneration may occur. If one sees electrophysiological features of multifocal demyelination at common compression sites (e.g., at the carpal tunnel, across the elbow, and across the fibular head) then hereditary neuropathy with liability to pressure palsy (HNPP) needs to be considered as an underlying condition predisposing the patient to developing rucksack palsy.

Perioperative Plexopathies (Median Sternotomy)

The most common surgical procedures associated with brachial plexopathy as a complication are those that involve median sternotomies (e.g., open-heart surgeries, some thymectomies and thoracotomies). Brachial plexopathies occur in as many as 5% of patients following a median sternotomy and typically affects the spinal nerve of the C8 root.[106–108] Thus, individuals manifest with sensory disturbance affecting the medial aspect of forearm and hand along with weakness of the intrinsic hand muscles, as discussed previously. Because of the location of the sensory symptoms, these lesions are often incorrectly blamed on ulnar neuropathies resulting from poor intraoperative elbow positioning or padding. The mechanism of this plexopathy is felt to be related to the stretch of the spinal nerve of the C8 root. These injuries are usually neuropraxic in nature, so most individuals who are affected recover in a few months.[107,109] However, some patients with significant axon loss may have a longer and incomplete recovery. Neurophysiological features are those previously discussed for lower trunk lesions.

Burners/Stingers

Burners and stingers refer to brachial plexus injuries caused by impact to shoulder region usually in the course of contact sports (e.g., football).[21] Usually, the affected athlete notes severe pain and sensory disturbance in the arms without any motor deficits. Symptoms typically resolve after a few minutes. The mechanism is unclear, but the rapid recovery in most cases suggests a neuropraxic injury to the cervical roots or plexus, particularly the upper trunk.

Hereditary Neuropathies Manifesting as Brachial Plexopathy

Hereditary neuralgic amyotrophy (HNA) is an autosomal-dominant disorder characterized by recurrent attacks of pain, weakness, and sensory loss in the distribution of the brachial plexus, often beginning in childhood.[53,110] The clinical and electrophysiological features of HNA resemble those of IBPN. HNA should be considered in patients with recurrent attacks of brachial plexitis. Rare patients may present without pain.[53] Some individuals with HNA have characteristic facial

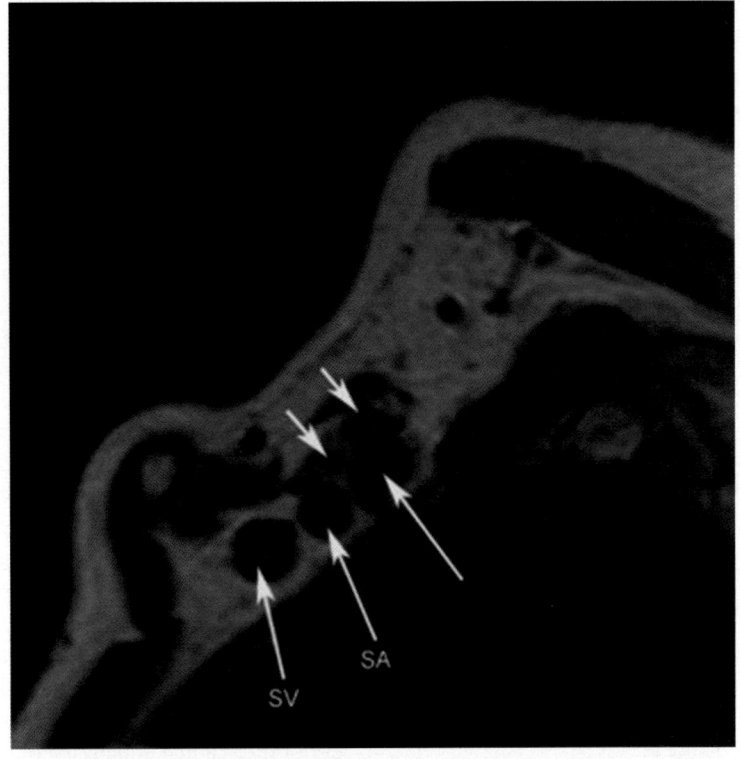
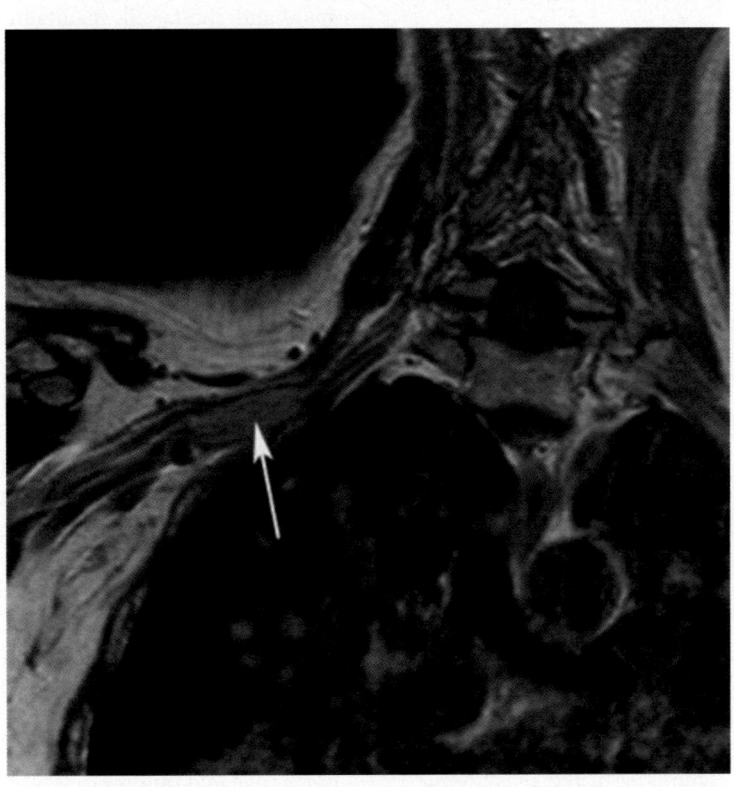

Figure 23-9. MRI of brachial plexus. Metastatic plexopathy of breast carcinoma. (**A**) Sagittal T1-weighted image shows a mass at the level of the divisions of the brachial plexus (*long arrows*). Note the normal neighboring nerves of the brachial plexus (*short arrows*). SA, subclavian artery; SV, subclavian vein. (**B**) Coronal T1-weighted image with intravenous gadolinium demonstrates the enhancement of the metastasis (*arrow*). (Reproduced with permission from van Es HW, Bollen TL, van Heesewijk HP. MRI of the brachial plexus: a pictorial review. *Eur J Radiol.* 2010;74(2):391–402. Fig 12.)

features including a long, slender face and narrow, close-set eyes slanting upward and unusual skin or scalp folds.[111,112] This facial appearance has been compared to a style favored in portraits by the early 20th-century Italian painter Amedeo Modigliani.[111] HNA can be caused by mutations in the gene encoding septin 9 (SEPT9) located on chromosome 17.[113] In contrast to HNA, HNPP is a generalized or multifocal process, which is demyelinating in nature. HNPP is usually caused by deletions in chromosome 17p11.2, resulting in a loss of function of peripheral myelin protein 22 (PMP-22). See Chapter 11 regarding "Charcot–Marie–Tooth Disease and Related Disorders" for more details.

SURGICAL TREATMENT OF BRACHIAL PLEXOPATHIES

The treatment of traumatic brachial plexopathies and timing of any surgical intervention are dependent on the type and severity of the injury, the location, and the timeframe.[90] Most closed injuries result in neuropraxis or axonotmesis that may recover spontaneously. As a result, they are initially treated conservatively with physical and occupational therapies. Patients are followed closely with serial clinical and EDX assessments to assess for recovery. If patients show no signs of recovery after 2–3 months in upper trunk lesions or 4–5 months for middle or lower trunk lesions, then surgical intervention is often considered.[114] Injuries associated with high-energy trauma or those associated with near-total paralysis may be observed for a shorter period of time (2 weeks to 3 months) prior to surgery.[115–117] Injuries associated with sharp penetrating trauma are more likely associated with severing of nerves and should be repaired within 72 hours, if possible.[118] Worsening neurological function, hematoma formation, concomitant bone or vascular injuries, and compartment syndrome are other indications for more acute surgical intervention.[90] Various surgical techniques including neurolysis, nerve grafting, neurotization, and free muscle transfer are performed in order to assist in regaining shoulder abduction and elbow flexion and some use of the hand function.[115,118–120]

▶ TERMINAL NERVE LESIONS

In this section, we discuss mononeuropathies of the upper limb mainly due to trauma, compression, or entrapment, or those that are idiopathic in nature. Any of these nerves may be affected alone or in combination with other nerve lesions in other settings such as vasculitis (isolated or systemic), infection (e.g., Lyme disease, leprosy, HIV, cytomegalovirus, and hepatitis), immune-mediated demyelination (e.g., multifocal motor neuropathy and multifocal acquired demyelinating motor and sensory neuropathy), and other inflammatory neuropathies (e.g., perineuritis and sarcoidosis), as discussed in other chapters in this book.

SPINAL ACCESSORY

As discussed previously, the SAN does not arise from the brachial plexus. Since it is often damaged with trauma to the neck and shoulder region with or without brachial plexus involvement, we discuss spinal accessory neuropathy in this chapter. Lymph node biopsy and other surgical procedures in the posterior triangle are common etiologies for spinal accessory neuropathies. The nerve can also be involved in IBPN. Injury of the nerve is often painful, presumably due to the mechanical effects from the dropped shoulder it produces. The shoulder drop is best observed from behind the patient. An accessory nerve palsy often results in scapular winging as well and a reduced capability of flexing the arm fully at the shoulder in the sagittal plane (Fig. 23-10). Winging from a SAN lesion is distinguished from winging from rhomboid and serratus anterior weakness by a number of observations and provocative maneuvers. Winging from trapezius weakness is accentuated by resisted external rotation of the arm at the shoulder. This occurs as the trapezius normally acts to hold the entire medial border of the scapula against the chest wall to provide the resistance necessary for effective external rotation. The winging typically affects the entire medial border of the scapula equally, so the inferior angle and posterior angle tend to be at near-equivalent distances from both the spine and chest wall, maintaining the medial scapular border in a vertical orientation. Trapezius weakness can also be detected and distinguished from serratus anterior weakness by maximum winging present with the shoulder abducted whereas maximal winging in serratus anterior weakness occurs when performing forward flexion of the arm. This maneuver results in compensatory lumbar hyperlordosis and producing the triangle sign (the three sides of the triangle being the table, anterior chest wall, and undersurface of the arm with the axilla being the apex).[121,122] Most lesions are distal to the innervation of the sternocleidomastoid muscles; however, proximal damage may result in weakness of turning the head to the contralateral side. CMAPs recorded from the trapezius muscle may demonstrate reduced amplitude compared to the contralateral side, but electrodiagnosis usually relies on demonstrating denervation changes in this muscle.

DORSAL SCAPULAR NERVE

The dorsal scapular nerve arises mainly from the C5 spinal root but may also receive contributions from the C4 segment. The nerve innervates the rhomboid major and minor, which assist in scapular retraction (drawing its medial border closer to rib cage and midline), elevation, and medial inferior angle rotation of the scapula. Therefore, damage to the dorsal scapular nerve leads to scapular winging, with the inferior angle rotated laterally. Elevation of the arm overhead will accentuate the scapular winging. It is very unusual to have an isolated dorsal scapular nerve injury.[9] NCSs are not particularly helpful but are performed to exclude other etiologies of scapular

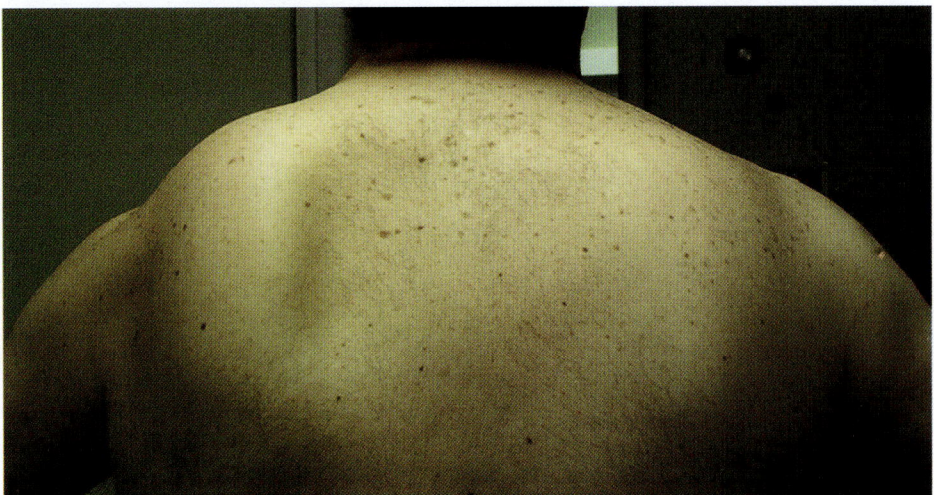

Figure 23-10. Spinal accessory neuropathy. Winging of the left scapula is appreciated and is brought out by abduction of the shoulder. (Reproduced with permission from of Steven A. Greenberg, MD. Reproduced with permission from Greenberg SA, Amato AA. *EMG Pearls.* Hanley & Belfus; 2004. Figure 1A, p. 37.)

winging. EDX confirmation requires demonstration of EMG abnormalities isolated to the rhomboid muscles.

LONG THORACIC NERVE

The long thoracic nerve originates from the fusion of branches from the C5, C6, and often C7 spinal roots, and it innervates the serratus anterior muscle (Fig. 23-2). This muscle stabilizes the scapula and holds it tight against the chest wall during movement of the shoulder girdle. In addition, it assists in rotating the scapula laterally to allow for full elevation of the arm as the glenohumeral joint provides for only 90 degrees of arm flexion and abduction at the shoulder. A long thoracic neuropathy manifests as scapular winging, a reduction in the ability to elevate the arm in a sagittal and coronal plane, and with reduced strength in pushing activities. The whole scapula is winged. As the muscle originates from the bottom half of the scapula, the inferior angle of the scapula tends to be more affected than the superior angle resulting in the inferior angle to be rotated toward the spine and to be farther off the chest wall than the superior angle (Fig. 23-11). This winging is accentuated by having the patient flex the arm forward at the shoulder against resistance.

The long thoracic nerve may be damaged from trauma or during surgical procedures, particularly mastectomies and thoracotomies (Table 23-5).[123–126] Most often, we see long thoracic neuropathies either isolated or in combination with other neuropathies in the setting of IBPN.[53] Motor NCS of the long thoracic nerve is not typically performed, and EDX confirmation of a long thoracic neuropathy requires demonstration of EMG abnormalities isolated to the serratus anterior muscle. Needle EMG of this muscle should be done cautiously due to risk of pneumothorax.

Long thoracic neuropathies are usually managed conservatively. Open injuries due to trauma may require surgery but otherwise these neuropathies are typically managed conservatively. We typically start with physical and occupational therapy along with bracing. Scapulothoracic stabilization braces can be used to help keep the shoulder abutted against

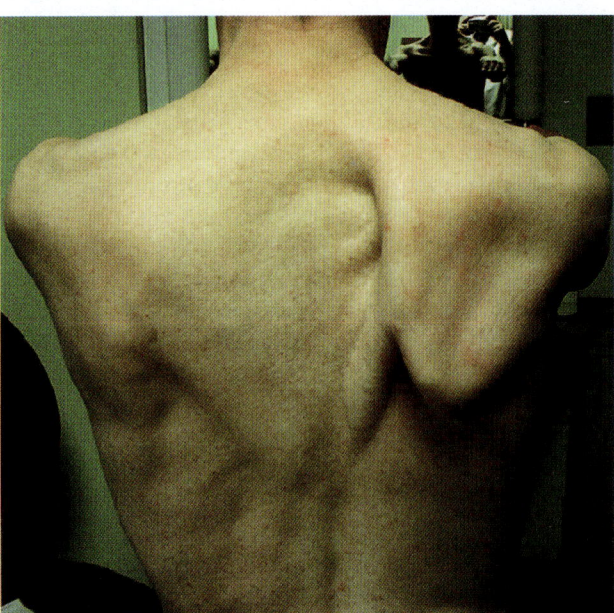

Figure 23-11. Long thoracic neuropathy. Winging of the right scapula is appreciated and is enhanced by having the patient flex the arm forward at the shoulder. There is also atrophy of the infraspinatus secondary to a superimposed suprascapular nerve injury. (Reproduced with permission from of Steven A. Greenberg, MD. Reproduced with permission from Greenberg SA, Amato AA. *EMG Pearls.* Philadelphia, PA: Hanley & Belfus; 2004. Fig 1B p. 42.)

> **TABLE 23-5. CONDITIONS ASSOCIATED WITH PROXIMAL LONG THORACIC NEUROPATHY**

Trauma
Surgical injury (postthoracotomy, radical mastectomy, axillary surgery, rib resection)
Immune-mediated brachial plexus neuropathy/neuralgic amyotrophy

the thorax. If the shoulder function does not improve over time, surgery can be considered to stabilize the scapula.[127,128]

SUPRASCAPULAR NERVE

The suprascapular nerve arises from the upper trunk and innervates the supraspinatus and infraspinatus muscles. The supraspinatus muscle assists the deltoid in the first 15 degrees of shoulder abduction, while the infraspinatus muscle is used to externally rotate the arm at the shoulder. Thus, these movements are limited, depending on the location of the suprascapular nerve injury.

The nerve may be damaged with trauma to the shoulder region, particularly if there is a dislocation or fracture of the shoulder.[129–132] The nerve may be injured at the suprascapular notch affecting both muscles, or rarely in the spinoglenoid notch with weakness confined to the infraspinatus.[133,134] More commonly, this suprascapular nerve is affected in the setting of IBPN and involvement may be isolated to this nerve.[53,135]

Motor conduction studies to this nerve are of limited utility, and therefore electrodiagnosis relies on EMG demonstration of neurogenic abnormalities in supraspinatus and/or infraspinatus muscles.

Management depends on etiology of the neuropathy. Surgery is warranted for open lesions related to trauma, otherwise conservative therapy with pain control is recommended. Local injections of corticosteroids can be tried if the cause is felt to be related to compression of the nerve in the suprascapular or supraglenoid notch, and some even advocate surgery; however, entrapment of the nerves at this site remains a controversial topic and nonsurgical options including treatment for IBPN are often pursued initially.[136–139]

MEDIAL AND LATERAL PECTORAL NERVES

Medial and lateral pectoral nerves are discussed together as they both innervate the pectoralis major and minor muscles (Fig. 23-2). The large pectoralis major muscle assists in internal rotation, anterior flexion, and adduction of the arm at the shoulder. The pectoralis minor assists in scapula stabilization during arm extension at the shoulder. These nerves are rarely injured, usually during surgical procedures in the anterior chest and axillary region. Again, motor conduction studies of these nerves are not routinely performed, and EDX confirmation requires demonstration of neurogenic EMG abnormalities in the pectoralis major and minor muscles.

SUBSCAPULAR NERVE

The subscapular nerves include the upper subscapular, middle subscapular (thoracodorsal), and lower subscapular nerves which include two branches. The upper subscapular nerve innervates the upper portion of the subscapularis muscle, the thoracodorsal nerve innervates the latissimus dorsi and the lower portion innervates the lower portion of the subscapularis muscle and the teres major. Injury to the subscapular nerves rarely occurs in isolation and therefore has not been described in detail. It may be involved in a more generalized plexopathy. As the lower subscapular nerve innervates the teres major muscle, damage to this nerve may result in weakness of internal rotation and adduction of the arm at the shoulder. There are no motor NCSs for this nerve, and needle EMG of the muscle is difficult given its deep location.

THORACODORSAL NERVE

The thoracodorsal nerve arises from the posterior cord and innervates the latissimus dorsi muscle (Fig. 23-2). Weakness of this muscle results in impaired ability to adduct, internally rotate, and extend the arm at the shoulder. Slight winging of the inferior margin of the scapula may be observed when the patient is asked to place the dorsum of the hand of the affected arm on the buttock.[10,126]

The nerve is usually affected in association with posterior cord or more proximal brachial plexus injuries. NCSs are not routinely done on this nerve, but EMG of the latissimus dorsi muscle is easy to perform and helps in localizing the lesion to C5–7 nerve fibers at or proximal to the posterior cord.

MUSCULOCUTANEOUS NERVE

The musculocutaneous nerve represents a continuation of the lateral cord and innervates the coracobrachialis, biceps brachii, and to some extent the brachialis. After innervating these muscles, it terminates as the lateral antebrachial cutaneous nerve to supply sensation to the lateral aspect of the forearm from the elbow to the wrist. Damage to the musculocutaneous nerve may therefore result in sensory loss in this distribution and weakness of elbow flexion accompanied by a reduced deep tendon reflex of the biceps brachii. The musculocutaneous nerve may be damaged by anterior dislocations of the shoulder and prolonged hyperextension of the arm, secondary to weightlifting (perhaps compressed within hypertrophic muscle) (Table 23-6).[8,126,140–142] It also can be affected in IBPN.[53]

The lateral antebrachial cutaneous SNAP is easy to obtain and is expected to be reduced in axonal lesions affecting the musculocutaneous nerve (Table 23-2). This is nonlocalizing as an isolated finding as the SNAP could also be reduced with lateral cord or upper trunk lesions; it would,

▶ **TABLE 23-6. CONDITIONS ASSOCIATED WITH MUSCULOCUTANEOUS NEUROPATHY**

Trauma (fracture or dislocation of shoulder, fracture of humerus, missile injuries, stab wounds, blunt force injuries)
Injection injury
Immune-mediated brachial plexus neuropathy/neuralgic amyotrophy
Soft tissue or peripheral nerve tumor
Ischemia (e.g., vasculitis)
Multifocal motor neuropathy or multifocal acquired demyelinating motor and sensory neuropathy
Compression within hypertrophied biceps brachii muscle after vigorous exercise
Compression by sharp free margin of biceps aponeurosis

▶ **TABLE 23-7. CONDITIONS ASSOCIATED WITH AXILLARY NEUROPATHY**

Trauma (e.g., fracture or dislocation of shoulder, fracture of humerus, missile injuries, stab wounds, blunt force injuries)
Stretch injury (e.g., hyperabduction during sleep, surgery)
Injection injury
Immune-mediated brachial plexus neuropathy
Soft tissue or peripheral nerve tumor
Ischemia (e.g., vasculitis)
Multifocal motor neuropathy or multifocal acquired demyelinating motor and sensory neuropathy

however, be normal in C6 radiculopathy. A musculocutaneous CMAP can be obtained by stimulating the brachial plexus in the supraclavicular fossa and recording from the biceps brachii and in conjunction with needle EMG findings can provide valuable prognostic information. Comparing the CMAP amplitude if greater than 10 days have passed since the injury to the opposite side can provide an estimate of the degree of axon loss with lower comparative amplitudes having a worse prognosis. EMG may show denervation abnormalities in the coracobrachialis, biceps brachii, and brachialis muscles (Table 23-1). Again abnormalities in the supraspinatus, deltoid, biceps brachii, and pronator teres muscles, but not in serratus anterior, rhomboids, or paraspinal regions, would imply an upper trunk injury, while denervation changes in the latter three regions would suggest a radiculopathy or anterior horn cell disease. Alternatively, finding abnormalities in only the biceps brachii and pronator teres, sparing deltoid, is more consistent with a lateral cord injury.

Initial management depends on the etiology of the mononeuropathy. Those caused by severe trauma, particularly when the nerve is not in continuity, may require surgical treatment. However, in most cases a conservative approach is warranted.

AXILLARY NERVE

The axillary nerve originates from the posterior cord and innervates the teres minor and deltoid muscles. In addition, the lateral cutaneous nerve of the arm arises from the axillary nerve. Thus, axillary neuropathies may manifest with weakness of abduction of the arm and sensory loss in the region of skin overlying the deltoid muscle.

Axillary neuropathies may occur in the setting of IBPN, trauma to the shoulder, fractures of the upper humerus, or stretch injury (Table 23-7).[8,9,126,142–145] Axillary CMAPs may be recorded from the deltoid muscle following supraclavicular stimulation of the brachial plexus to see if there is asymmetrical loss of amplitude on the affected side. A superficial radial SNAP is normal in axillary neuropathy but expected to be affected in posterior cord lesion or upper trunk lesions (Table 23-2). Furthermore, needle EMG should show evidence of denervation in the deltoid and teres minor muscles with sparing of radial or posterior interosseous innervated muscles in an isolated axillary neuropathy (Table 23-1). In addition, a normal EMG of the supraspinatus, infraspinatus, rhomboids, biceps brachii, pronator teres, and brachioradialis suggests that the lesion is distal to the C5/C6 roots or upper trunk when combined with denervation of the deltoid.

Axillary neuropathies related to penetrating injuries should be surgically explored. Otherwise, they are managed conservatively with pain management and physical and occupational therapy. If there is no improvement within 6 months, surgical treatment and grafting can be considered.[146]

RADIAL NERVE

The radial nerve, the other major terminal branch of the posterior cord, is composed of fibers from spinal segments C5–8, and occasionally contains T1 fibers. The radial nerve is long and provides innervation to upper arm and forearm muscles, as well as for cutaneous sensation of large portions of the arm. The clinical and EDX features of radial neuropathies depend on the site of the lesion. The superficial radial SNAP should be abnormal, if there is significant axonal nerve injury, except with PIN damage, as this is a purely motor nerve. A radial CMAP to the radial-innervated muscles such as the extensor indicis proprius can be performed with short incremental stimulation of the radial nerve through the spinal groove to assess for focal conduction block and/or slowing across this site. With significant axonal injury, the CMAP amplitude should be reduced regardless of stimulation site. EMG is more helpful in localizing the site of the lesion with axonal injury. Evidence of active denervation in the form of fibrillation potentials and positive sharp waves is expected in axonal nerve injuries, provided there has been sufficient time for Wallerian degeneration to occur. In a pure neuropraxic injury, only reduced recruitment of MUAPs would be appreciated on needle EMG of affected muscles, although many predominantly demyelinating injuries may have some element of axon loss. A few fibrillation potentials do not preclude a good recovery as they may originate from a very small number of injured axons.

► **TABLE 23-8. CONDITIONS ASSOCIATED WITH PROXIMAL RADIAL NEUROPATHY**

Trauma
Fracture of humerus
Improper use of crutches (e.g., compression in axilla)
Stretch injury (e.g., hyperabduction of arm during surgery, sleep)
Saturday night palsy (external compression by arm being compressed against firm edge at the spiral groove—usually in individuals with reduced level of consciousness due to alcohol or sedating drugs)
Other external compression (partner falling asleep on arm)
Immune-mediated brachial plexus neuropathy/neuralgic amyotrophy
Soft tissue or peripheral nerve tumor
Ischemia (e.g., A-V fistulas, vasculitis)
Multifocal motor neuropathy or multifocal acquired demyelinating motor and sensory neuropathy

► **TABLE 23-9. CONDITIONS ASSOCIATED WITH POSTERIOR INTEROSSEOUS NEUROPATHY**

Immune-mediated brachial plexus neuropathy/neuralgic amyotrophy
Trauma
Compression by tumors, ganglion cysts, lipoma, bursitis
Compression by the arcade of Fröhse
Compression by facial bands connecting the brachialis to the brachioradialis muscle at the radial head
Compression by edge or fibrous bands within the supinator muscle
Compression by a bifid extensor carpi radialis brevis muscle
Rheumatoid arthritis
Soft tissue or peripheral nerve tumor
Ischemia (e.g., A-V fistulas, vasculitis)
Multifocal motor neuropathy or multifocal acquired demyelinating motor and sensory neuropathy

Proximal Radial Neuropathy

Damage to the nerve in the axilla or proximal arm is uncommon but can result from compression (e.g., crutches, intoxicated patients who fall asleep with outstretched arm pressed against a hard surface, missile injuries, and other trauma to the axilla) (Table 23-8).[7–9] Of course, a radial neuropathy can also occur in the setting of a more widespread multifocal process (e.g., vasculitis, IBPN). Proximal radial nerve injuries can result in weakness of elbow, wrist, and finger extension as well as supination of the forearm. In addition, sensory disturbance may be evident in the posterior aspect of the forearm and dorsum of the hand and fingers. Provided there is sufficient axon loss, the superficial radial SNAP and radial CMAP recorded from the extensor indicis proprius may have reduced amplitudes (Table 23-2). EMG should demonstrate signs of denervation in the triceps as well as more distal radial-innervated forearm muscles (Table 23-1).

Radial neuropathy in the arm distal to the branches innervating the triceps arises from various mechanisms. One of the most common radial neuropathies is the so-called "Saturday night palsy" and is usually the result of prolonged compression of the radial nerve in the spiral groove in an individual who is under the influence of alcohol or sedating medications such as opioids and/or benzodiazepines. Another common cause is radius shaft bone fracture. Proximal radial nerve lesions have also been speculated to be the result of anomalous fibrous band of the lateral head of the triceps and subsequent nerve compression with elbow flexion and extension.[147,148] On clinical examination, one would expect to find weakness of the radial-innervated muscles distal to the triceps in addition to sensory loss in the posterior aspect of the forearm and dorsum of the hand and fingers. Again, a superficial radial SNAP and a radial CMAP may have reduced amplitudes, if the injury is axonal. EMG should demonstrate signs of denervation of radial-innervated forearm muscles, with sparing of the more proximal triceps muscles, unless the mechanism is conduction block in isolation.

Proximal radial neuropathies caused by penetrating trauma should be surgically explored and treated with end-to-end anastomosis or grafting. Closed traumas, including humeral fractures, are often due to neuropraxia and recover gradually on their own. A trial of conservative therapy is employed prior to any surgery. Proximal radial neuropathies related to pressure or stretch injuries (e.g., Saturday night palsy) or IBPN are also treated conservatively. Finger and wrist splints, pain control, and physical and occupational therapy are employed.

Posterior Interosseous Neuropathy

Damage to the PIN will result in weakness of wrist and finger extensors with sparing of sensation. The PIN can be damaged from multiple mechanisms (Table 23-9). Although some have speculated that the nerve can be entrapped within the supinator muscle (arcade of Fröhse), this is quite rare in our opinion. Many such cases probably represent a forme fruste of an IBPN or another immune-mediated neuropathy (e.g., multifocal motor neuropathy or MADSAM) (Fig. 23-12). On NCSs, the superficial radial SNAP should be normal, but the radial CMAP recorded from the extensor indicis proprius may reveal a reduction in amplitude, provided there is significant axon loss (Table 23-2). EMG should demonstrate signs of denervation in muscles innervated by the PIN.

Unless the posterior interosseous neuropathy is related to open trauma, it is managed conservatively as discussed with proximal radial neuropathies. Rare cases of the so-called radial tunnel syndrome with compression of the PIN may improve with surgery.[149] Again, we feel that such entrapment is quite rare and its existence is controversial.

Superficial Radial Neuropathy

The superficial radial nerve is a pure sensory branch of the radial nerve that provides sensation to the dorsum of the hand. It can be damaged by various means (Table 23-10). In particular, compression by tight bands, watches, and handcuffs or

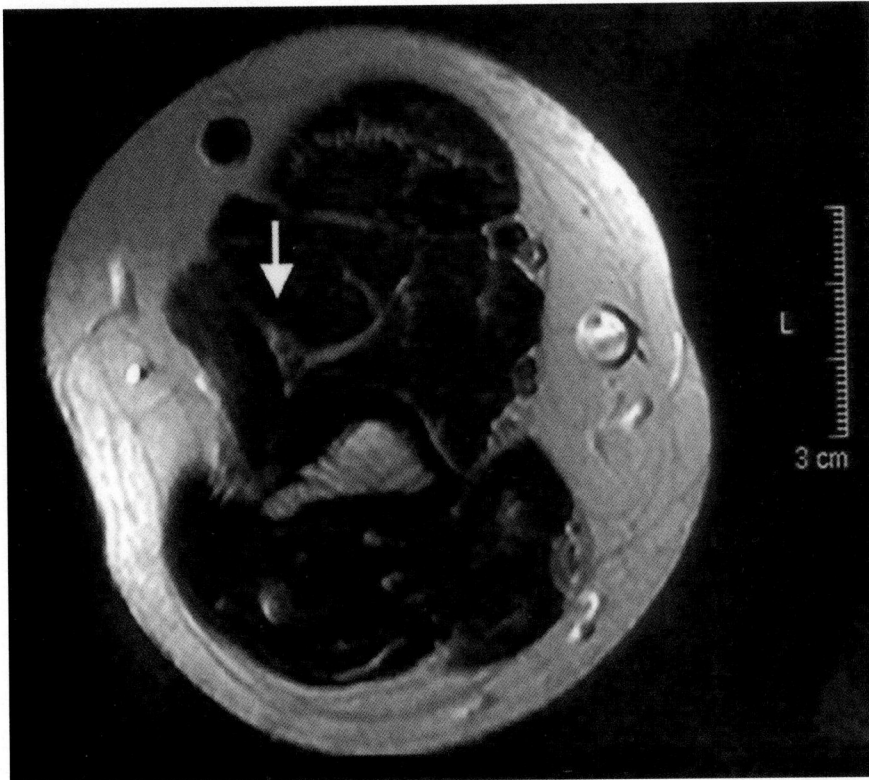

Right radial nerve

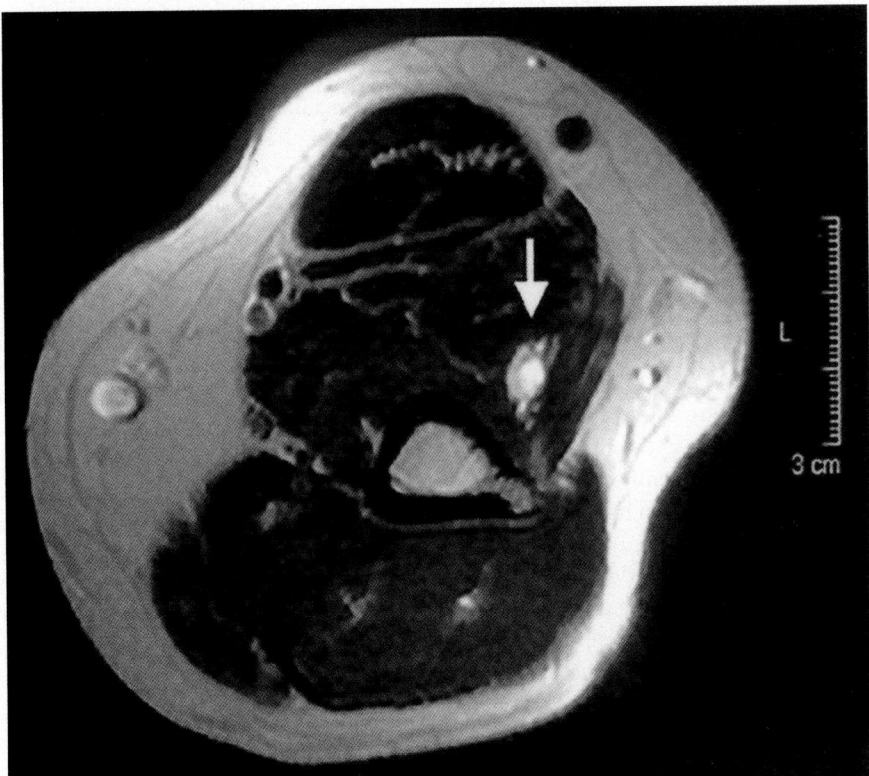

Left radial nerve

Figure 23-12. MRI of (T2) forearms in a patient with multifocal motor neuropathy affecting the left radial nerve demonstrates focal enlargement and enhancement of the radial nerve (*arrows*) in the forearm on the left side. (Reproduced with permission from of Steven A. Greenberg, MD. Reproduced with permission from Greenberg SA, Amato AA. *EMG Pearls.* Hanley & Belfus; 2004. Figure 2, p. 208.)

► **TABLE 23-10. CONDITIONS ASSOCIATED WITH SUPERFICIAL RADIAL NEUROPATHY**

External compression (handcuffs, tight wrist bands, casts)
De Quervain tenosynovitis
Trauma
Peripheral intravenous catheter placement
Soft tissue or peripheral nerve tumor

► **TABLE 23-11. CONDITIONS ASSOCIATED WITH PROXIMAL MEDIAN NEUROPATHY**

Improper use of crutches (e.g., compression in axilla)
Trauma (e.g., dislocation of shoulder, fracture of humerus, missile injuries, stab wounds, tourniquets)
Compression by ligament of Struthers
Pronator teres syndrome
   Thickened lacertus fibrosus
   Fibrous arch of the flexor digitorum superficialis
   Tendinous band or hypertrophied pronator teres muscle
Sleep palsies
Compartment syndrome
Ischemia (e.g., A-V fistulas, vasculitis)
Immune-mediated brachial plexus neuropathy/neuralgic amyotrophy
Soft tissue or peripheral nerve tumor
Multifocal motor neuropathy or multifocal acquired demyelinating motor and sensory neuropathy

direct injury from a peripheral intravenous catheter can lead to a superficial radial neuropathy. The superficial radial SNAP is usually decreased in amplitude, while motor studies and EMG would be normal. This type of neuropathy is usually due to neuropraxia and improves spontaneously. Cases related to nerve laceration or other trauma may require surgery.

MEDIAN NERVE

As previously discussed, the median nerve contains fibers originating from spinal segments C6–T1, which then course through all three trunks and the medial and lateral cords. The median nerve is formed by the merging of branches from the medial and lateral cords. Axons from spinal segments C5–7 that course through the upper and middle trunks and lateral cords are responsible for providing cutaneous sensation to the palmar aspect of the hand and digits 1 to 3 and usually the lateral half of digit 4. In addition, these segments also innervate several forearm muscles, primarily the pronator teres and flexor carpi radialis. On the other hand, C8 and T1 nerve fibers course through the lower trunk and medial cord and innervate muscles controlling finger movements and provide no sensory input.

Proximal Median Neuropathy

Proximal median neuropathies in the axilla, upper arm, and forearm may result from misuse of crutches, missile injuries, and laceration of the nerve by trauma (Table 23-11, Fig. 23-13).[8,9,150,151] Compression of the nerve can also occur due to an awkward sleeping position—often in individuals who are intoxicated. Ischemic damage to the median nerve can occur as a complication of nerve ischemia due to arterial diversion resulting from creation of shunts of fistulas for renal dialysis.[152] The median nerve can be affected as well in the setting of IBPN. Proximal median neuropathies have been reported to be caused by compression by the ligament of Struthers, but this is controversial.[147–150,153–156] Compression by the lacertus fibrosus, which is the bicipital aponeurosis distal to the elbow, has also been implicated as a possible etiology.[114]

Individuals with proximal median neuropathies present with weakness of the median-innervated forearm and hand muscles and reduced sensation in the palmar aspect of the hand, digits 1 to 3, and the lateral aspect of digit 4. In our experience, it is not uncommon for proximal median neuropathies to clinically manifest as predominantly anterior interosseous syndromes, even though electrodiagnosis suggests that the entire nerve is affected. In these cases, median SNAPs to any of these digits would be expected to show reduced amplitudes again, provided there is sufficient axonal injury. The distal latency or conduction velocity of the median SNAP would be expected to be normal or only slightly impaired compared to the loss of amplitude. Similarly, the median CMAP amplitude recorded from the abductor pollicis studies may be reduced. It is important in these proximal median neuropathies to look for evidence of slowing of CV, temporal dispersion, or focal conduction block. EMG would be expected to demonstrate abnormalities in median-innervated muscles in the forearm and hand (Table 23-1).

A controversial entity is the so-called pronator teres syndrome. In this disorder, the median nerve is thought to be compressed where it passes under the fibrous arch connecting the two heads of the pronator teres muscle. The major clinical manifestation is pain and tenderness in the volar aspect of the forearm and paresthesias in the distribution of the median nerve. These symptoms are exacerbated by having the patient actively trying to pronate the forearm against resistance. We remain rather skeptical of this diagnosis, as there is usually no objective clinical or electrodiagnostical evidence of median nerve injury.

Proximal median neuropathies carry a poor prognosis if there is significant axonal degeneration. The reason is the long distance the nerve must grow in order for complete reinnervation to occur. If voluntary MUAPs in the forearm and hand muscles are present, potential for recovery exists.

The proximal median neuropathies are usually treated conservatively unless trauma is involved. Decompression surgeries have not been adequately studied in a scientific fashion, owing in part to the rarity of proximal median compressive neuropathies.

Anterior Interosseous Syndrome

The AIN can be damaged from multiple mechanisms (Table 23-12). Most commonly, in our experience, an anterior

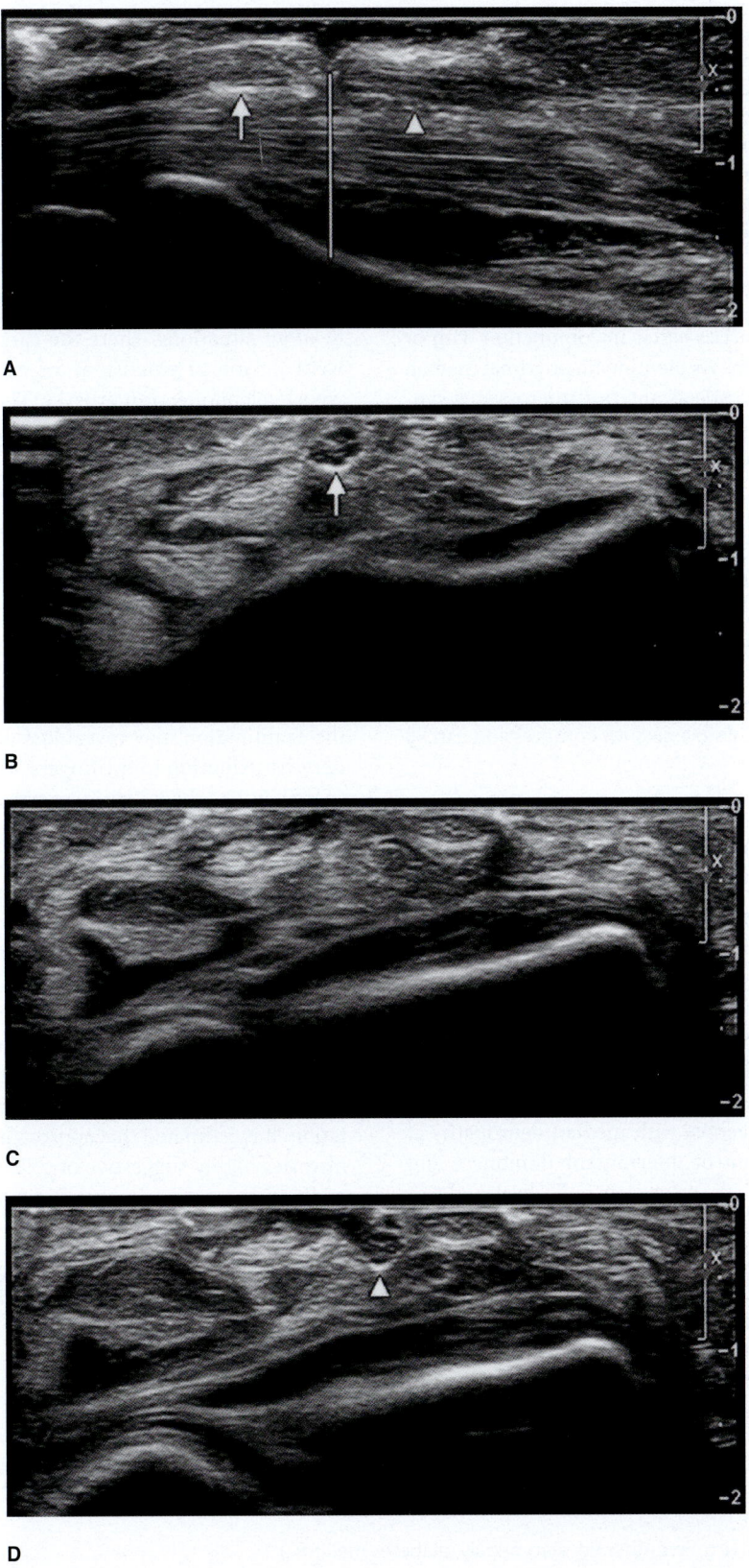

Figure 23-13. Ultrasound images depicting transection of the median nerve in the forearm. (**A**) Sagittal view showing the distal nerve stump (*arrow*), proximal stump (*arrowhead*), and the transection (*line*). Cross-sectional views at the level of the distal nerve (**B**), site of transection (**C**), and proximal nerve (**D**). The median nerve is seen in images (**B**) and (**D**), but it is not present in image (**C**) at the site of transection. (Reproduced with permission from Cartwright MS, Chloros GD, Walker FO, Wiesler ER, William W, Campbell WW. Diagnostic ultrasound for nerve transaction. *Muscle Nerve.* 2007;796–799. Fig 1.)

▶ **TABLE 23-12.** CAUSES OF ANTERIOR INTEROSSEOUS NEUROPATHY

Immune-mediated brachial plexus neuropathy/neuralgic amyotrophy
Trauma
Fibrous band within the pronator teres
Compartment syndrome
Soft tissue or peripheral nerve tumor
Ischemia (e.g., A-V fistulas, vasculitis)
Multifocal motor neuropathy and multifocal acquired motor and sensory neuropathy

interosseous neuropathy arises either in conjunction with or as a forme fruste of an IBPN. As mentioned, proximal median neuropathies may masquerade as anterior interosseous syndrome. As the AIN is a pure motor nerve, patients do not have sensory loss. However, severe pain in the forearm for several days or weeks is typical in cases related to IBPN. Individuals have weakness in the flexor digitorum profundus I and II, flexor hallucis longus, and pronator quadratus muscles. This leads to difficulty with pinching maneuvers or forming the letter "O" with their thumb and index or middle fingers, as they have weakness of flexion of the distal aspects of these digits. Most cases should be managed conservatively. However, if there is no improvement in function after 4–6 months, surgical exploration to assess for compression can be considered.[157,158]

Median Neuropathy at the Wrist or Carpal Tunnel Syndrome

Median neuropathy at the wrist or CTS is the most common mononeuropathy. There are multiple causes of median neuropathy at the wrist, although the vast majority are thought to be related to tenosynovitis of the flexor tendons which also occupy the carpal tunnel along with the median nerve (Table 23-13).[8,126] Some clinicians restrict the term "CTS" only to those median neuropathies at the wrist caused by tenosynovitis. People with median neuropathy at the wrist usually complain of intermittent numbness and tingling of their fingers. This occurs particularly at night or in other situations where the carpal tunnel is narrowed by wrist flexion or extension, for example, holding a steering wheel, telephone, or hairdryer. The numbness, tingling, and pain patients describe often extend beyond the territory of the median nerve. Patents frequently describe sensory symptoms in the fifth digit and aching in the forearm as well. The symptoms may be exacerbated by repetitive activity. However, discomfort often occurs at rest. The painful paresthesias may be briefly alleviated by shaking out the hands, the so-called "flick sign."[159]

Clinical examination is frequently normal when the nerve is predominantly irritated, not injured. When axon loss occurs, patients may develop constant numbness and the examination may reveal loss of sensation in the median nerve distribution to the fingers. Motor function is generally spared, unless the injury is severe at which point weakness of atrophy of the thenar muscles is appreciated. Tapping over the median nerve at the wrist (Tinel sign) or having the person flex both wrists against one another and hold the posture (Phalen sign) may exacerbate the uncomfortable paresthesias in the fingers. Phalen sign is more specific for CTS.[160]

Despite over 30 years of study, there is no consensus on a single protocol for diagnosis and management of CTS. Several NCSs are performed to confirm the clinical impression of a median neuropathy at the wrist. Like all tests, NCSs are imperfect, in part because they test for nerve injury, not irritation. It is estimated that approximately 10% of patients with histories highly suggestive of CTS will have normal NCS. In addition to performing median sensory and motor studies,

▶ **TABLE 23-13.** CONDITIONS ASSOCIATED WITH MEDIAN NEUROPATHY AT THE WRIST

Idiopathic
Flexor tenosynovitis
Degenerative joint disease
Rheumatoid arthritis
Sarcoidosis
Space occupying lesions (e.g., ganglion cysts, lipomas, hemangiomas, giant cell tumors, osteomas)
Trauma (e.g., Colles fracture, dislocation/fracture of carpal bones)
Pregnancy
Endocrine (e.g., hypothyroid, acromegaly, diabetes mellitus[a])
Amyloidosis (familial and primary)
Hereditary neuropathy with liability to pressure palsies
Soft tissue or peripheral nerve tumor

[a]It is unclear if individuals with typical generalized diabetic polyneuropathy may be predisposed to focal mononeuropathies related to compression.

it is essential to include sensory and motor studies of other nerves (e.g., ulnar or radial) to ensure that any neuropathy is not more generalized. Studies are tailored according to the individual's symptoms. If a patient complains of sensory disturbance mainly in the third digit, then a median SNAP to the third digit could be performed as opposed to doing the median SNAP to the thumb or second digit. Median SNAPs are more sensitive than CMAPs in detecting abnormalities associated with CTS. Mixed compound nerve action potentials (CNAPs), which are obtained by stimulating the median and ulnar mixed nerves in the palm and recording over the respective nerves at the wrist, are often even more sensitive as they are usually performed across a shorter distance. Significantly prolonged distal latencies of the median palmar mixed CNAP compared to the ulnar study would support the clinical impression of CTS. In addition to stimulating at the wrist and recording at the digit, it is sometimes useful to do a mid-palm stimulation (halfway between site of wrist stimulation and the recording electrodes) when performing the median SNAPs. If one sees a prolonged distal latency/slow CV and reduced amplitude following wrist stimulation, this should be compared to latency/CV and amplitude after stimulation in the palm to see if there was more focal slowing or conduction block across the wrist. This is particularly valuable in people who have a coexisting generalized polyneuropathy to see if there is a superimposed median neuropathy at the wrist.

The earliest EDX abnormalities on NCSs in CTS are prolonged distal latencies or slowing of the median SNAP or palmar mixed CNAP across the palm. Subsequently, there may be a reduction in SNAP or mixed CNAP amplitude due to either axon loss or conduction block. Subsequently, distal latencies of the median CMAP become prolonged. Amplitudes of the median CMAP are usually affected much later in the course. In severe cases of CTS, median SNAPs and median CMAPs recorded from the abductor pollicis brevis may be unobtainable. Thus, from an NCS standpoint, one cannot localize the site of the median neuropathy, as a lesion may be anywhere from the hand to the origin of the median nerve in the plexus. In such cases, it is useful to perform median CMAP to the second lumbrical and ulnar CMAP to the second interosseous muscles while stimulating the median and ulnar nerves, respectively, at the wrist. The reason is that the median CMAP from the second lumbrical is often less affected in CTS than the CMAP from the APB. Therefore, a CMAP from this muscle may be obtained when one from the APB cannot. Thus, a prolonged distal latency and reduced amplitude of the median CMAP (second lumbrical) compared to the ulnar CMAP (second interosseous) may be appreciated and confirm the localization of the lesion to the wrist. EMG is often done to further assess the degree of axonal damage and assess the localization of the lesion. Often the EMG is normal in mild CTS. Reduced recruitment of normal appearing MUAPs suggests conduction block. Given its chronic nature, enlarged MUAPs in the APB commonly occur. Signs of active denervation (e.g., fibrillation potentials) are less common but may become evident in rapidly progressive or severe cases.

Sonography of the median nerve at the wrist in CTS may demonstrate swelling and deformation (e.g., flattening or hourglass shape) of the median nerve at the wrist at the level of the transverse carpal ligament (Fig. 23-14). Sensitivity and specificity of NCSs (median sensory peak latency) and ultrasound for CTS diagnosis are 75/93% and 77.6/86.8%, respectively.[161,162] A recent Delphi panel reached consensus that the combination of EDX and ultrasound are better than either one alone in the evaluation of CTS. Ultrasound has an important localizing role for very severe CTS, atypical CTS, patients with symptoms of CTS with normal NCS, failed CTS surgery, polyneuropathy, and CTS suspected to be secondary to a structural pathology.[163-165] Ultrasound cannot determined severity of CTS and EDX studies must be performed at the same time for that purpose and to rule out concurrent processes which can influence presentation (e.g., ulnar neuropathy, cervical radiculopathy, polyneuropathy). MRI of the wrist may show reduction of the cross-sectional diameter of the carpal tunnel.[27,28] Swelling of the tendons, bony and cystic lesions, as well as compression of the nerve may be visualized by MRI. The major drawback of MRI is high cost. Given more widespread availability and lower cost, MRI imaging of the carpal tunnel is not routinely used by most clinicians.

The treatment of CTS has been the subject of several reviews.[162,166] Treatments of CTS include modification of activities, splinting of the wrist, corticosteroid injections, nonsteroidal anti-inflammatory drugs, diuretics, and surgery. Among surgery, there are various techniques that can be employed (e.g., standard open surgery with exploration and release vs. minimally invasive endoscopic approach). Unfortunately, most studies of CTS have lacked scientific rigor, and thus recommendations for the best therapeutic approach are debatable.

Twenty to 70% of patients with CTS treated nonsurgically improve to some extent.[166] Corticosteroid injection is superior to wrists splints for symptom control in mild to moderate CTS.[167] Corticosteroid injections into the carpal tunnel have become an increasingly used alternative to surgery. Risks include cutaneous atrophy, depigmentation, and inadvertent puncture of the median nerve, blood vessels, or tendons within the carpal tunnel.[166] Median nerve injury and tendon rupture are the most severe complications, but each occurs in <0.1% of injections. Approximately 30% of patients have no or only mild improvement following local corticosteroid injection, while 70% have a very good response (complete relief or only minor residual symptoms).[166,168] A study comparing corticosteroid injection versus surgery demonstrated similar short-term efficacy of both treatments, but the relapse rate was common in the injection group and rare in the surgical group after 1 year.[101,169] In this regard, there are no good studies assessing the safety and efficacy of repeated corticosteroid injections. A randomized trial comparing surgery to conservative management with wrist

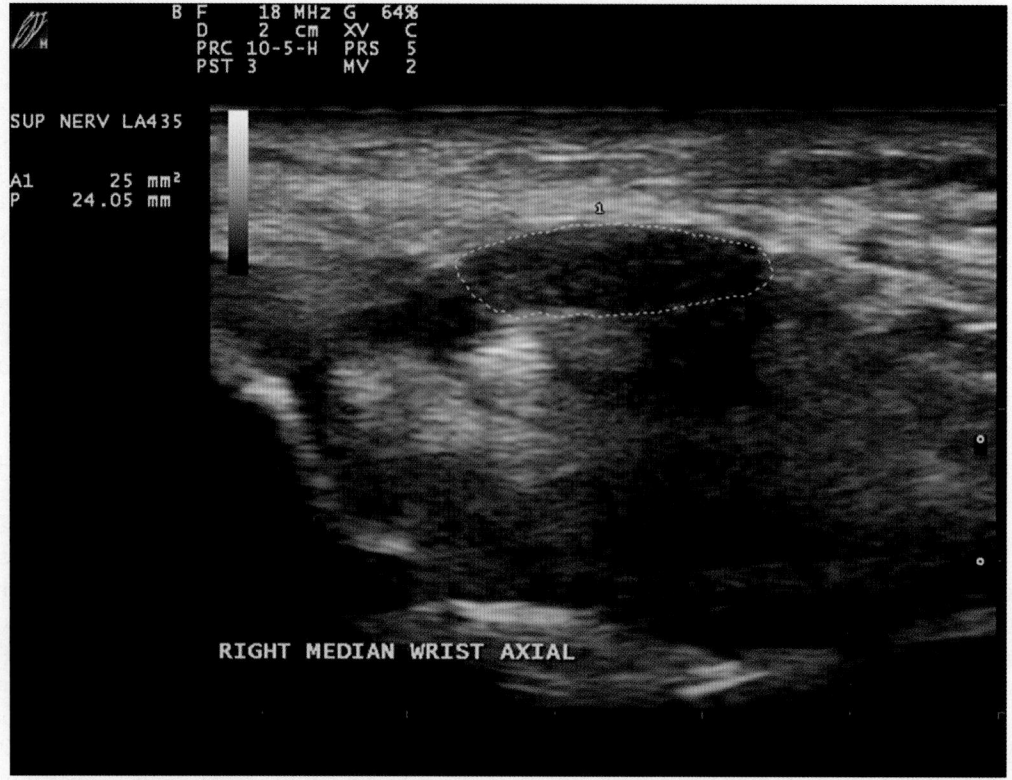

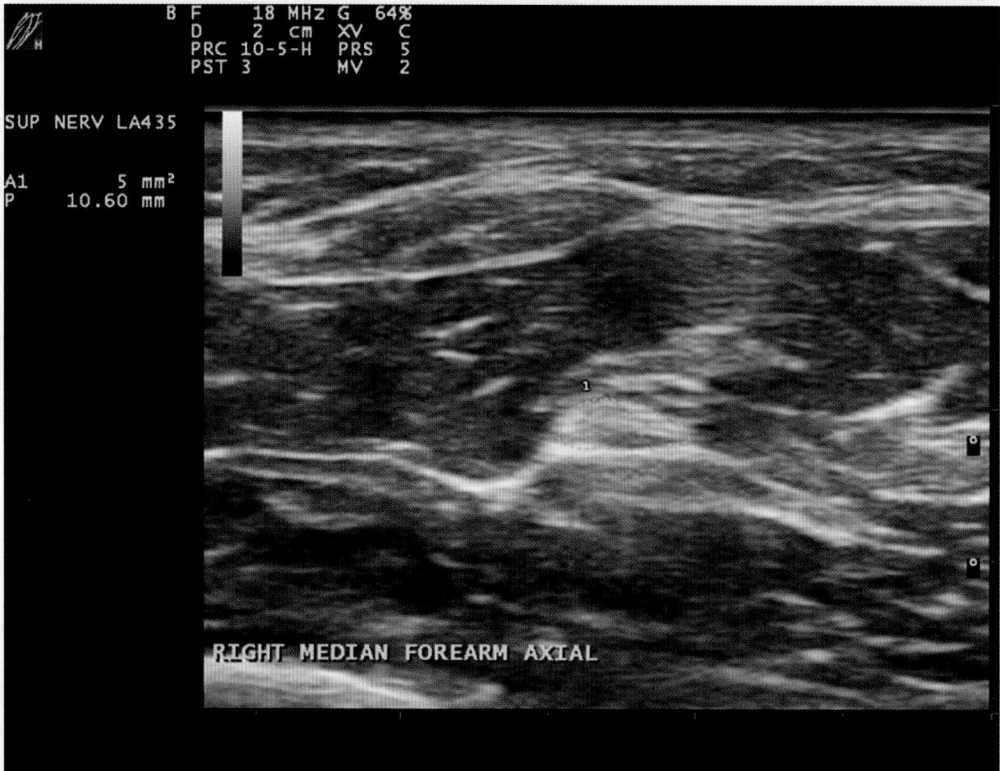

Figure 23-14. Sonograms of a patient with symptomatic right carpal tunnel syndrome. The right median nerve had a markedly increased cross-sectional area (CSA) of 25 mm² at the distal wrist crease (normal <12 mm²) (**A**), and 5 mm² in the forearm (**B**), as outlined by the green dashes resulting in an increased wrist/forearm CSA ratio of 5 (normal <1.5).

splints and nonsteroidal medications demonstrated a modest benefit of unclear clinical significance with surgery.[170]

The average success rate from surgery is approximately 75% (range 27%–100%), but 8% of patients worsen.[166] Failure rates may relate to patients being operated on who do not actually have CTS. In this regard, improvement following surgery is noted in only half of patients who had normal EDX testing prior surgery, while success rates are much higher in those with NCSs that were abnormal. Another common cause of failed surgery is incomplete division of the transverse carpal ligament, perhaps owing to poor choice of incision and inadequate exposure.[166] Another reason for failed surgery is such end-stage denervation resulting from delayed treatment that the window for recovery has closed. There may be a <50% success rate for surgery in patients with marked thenar atrophy and weakness, no recordable median CMAPs and SNAPs, and active denervation on EMG.[166,168] In our opinion, CTS surgery in this population should only be considered for reasons of pain relief, not with the expectation that strength or sensation will return in any meaningful way.

Complications of surgery occur in 1%–2% of cases and include injury to the recurrent motor and cutaneous branches of the median nerve, lesions of the main trunk of the median nerve, the main trunk and deep motor branch of the ulnar nerve, postoperative hematoma, wound infection, scarring, and complex regional pain syndrome type II.[166]

With the above caveats, we initially try conservative management with neutral angle wrists. In patients with objective motor deficits, we still try a short trial of wrist splints along with corticosteroid injections. However, we refer them for surgery if there is no benefit after a couple of months. We usually do not recommend surgery when NCSs are normal.

ULNAR NERVE

The ulnar nerve is the anatomic continuation of the medial cord and contains nerve fibers originating from the C8 and T1 spinal roots, which course through the lower trunk and then medial cord. As previously discussed, there may also be a contribution from C7 in some individuals. This is a long nerve and lesions may occur anywhere along its course. Therefore, the clinical and electrophysiological findings are dependent on the site and nature of the lesion.

Proximal Ulnar Neuropathy (Axilla to Upper Elbow Region)

Similar mechanisms that cause proximal median and radial neuropathies can cause a proximal ulnar neuropathy (Table 23-14).[8,9] There are no ulnar-innervated muscles in the upper arm; therefore, any proximal lesion will clinically resemble those caused by more common ulnar neuropathy at the elbow (discussed in next section). Ulnar neuropathies in the upper arm related to open trauma usually require surgical repair.

▶ **TABLE 23-14. CONDITIONS ASSOCIATED WITH PROXIMAL ULNAR NEUROPATHY**

Trauma
Compression during sleep
Soft tissue or peripheral nerve tumor
Ischemia (e.g., A-V fistulas, vasculitis)
Multifocal motor neuropathy or multifocal acquired demyelinating motor and sensory neuropathy

Provided significant axonal loss has had time to occur, the ulnar and dorsal ulnar cutaneous SNAPs will have reduced amplitudes, while the medial antebrachial cutaneous SNAP will be normal. The ulnar CMAP may demonstrate reduced amplitude without focal slowing or conduction block across the elbow. EMG should show abnormalities confined to ulnar-innervated muscles in the hand and forearm (Table 23-1). However, these SNAPs and EMG alterations do not distinguish a proximal ulnar neuropathy in the upper arm from one across the elbow. Electrophysiologically, the only way to localize an ulnar neuropathy to the proximal upper arm is by demonstrating focal conduction block or slowing of ulnar CV between the axilla and above elbow stimulation sites. Due to challenges with accurate measurements, this is typically unreliable for localization.

Ulnar Neuropathy at the Elbow

Ulnar neuropathy at the elbow, the second most common mononeuropathy after CTS, is usually the result of compression at one or both sites of compression at the elbow. As the nerve is superficial around the ulnar groove, it is more susceptible to extrinsic compression (e.g., from leaning on the elbow). There are numerous intrinsic mechanisms by which the ulnar nerve may be injured in this region (Table 23-15).[8,9] The term "tardy ulnar palsy" is applied to ulnar neuropathies that occur on a delayed basis following bone injuries at the

▶ **TABLE 23-15. CONDITIONS ASSOCIATED WITH ULNAR NEUROPATHY AT THE ELBOW**

Tardy ulnar palsy (due to deformities of elbow related to previous fractures of humerus or other trauma to the joint)
Subluxation of the ulnar nerve
Compression by arcade of Struthers (medial intramuscular septum)
Compression by aponeurotic band between heads of flexor carpi ulnaris
Compression by ligament/band (retrocondylar)
Trauma
Soft tissue tumor or masses
Leprosy
Diabetes mellitus[a]

[a]It is unclear if individuals with typical generalized diabetic polyneuropathy may be predisposed to focal mononeuropathies related to compression.

elbow. It is speculated that the nerve may become stretched or compressed by exuberant callus formation or altered angle of the elbow joint. The nerve may also become entrapped or compressed by the humeroulnar aponeurotic retinaculum or by other anatomic structural variants in and around the ulnar groove and cubital tunnel. Also, the nerve can occasionally prolapse out of the ulnar groove although this happens in many normal individuals and should not be assumed to be pathologic.

Regardless of etiology, the clinical signs and symptoms of an ulnar neuropathy at the elbow are similar. Affected individuals often describe of discomfort and tenderness to palpation around the medial elbow. They typically describe numbness and tingling in the medial aspect of the hand and the fifth and medial portion of the fourth digits (both palmar and dorsal aspects). Tapping the nerve in the elbow often exacerbates these symptoms (e.g., positive Tinel sign). Weakness may involve any or all ulnar-innervated muscles in the hand and forearm. This can lead to decreased grip strength, finger abduction and adduction, and deep finger and wrist flexion. Typically, hand weakness is more noticeable than forearm weakness. Testing for weakness of the flexion of the distal interphalangeal joint of digits 4 and 5 is the most reliable means by which to detect ulnar forearm muscle weakness when present. With axonal degeneration, atrophy of the hypothenar and interossei muscles may be seen (most notably appreciated in the first dorsal interosseous). While weakness may be present, it is important to realize that most compressive ulnar neuropathies present with sensory symptoms. Compressive or entrapment ulnar neuropathies presenting with purely motor signs and symptoms are extremely rare and alternate localizations and noncompressive etiologies should be considered.

Ulnar and dorsal ulnar cutaneous SNAP amplitudes should be reduced if there is significant axonal damage at or near the elbow. However, if there is only a neuropraxic or demyelinating lesion in the elbow these SNAPs are typically normal, as these do not assess slowing of conduction across the elbow. Localization is dependent on the ulnar motor conductions and EMG.[6,171–174] We usually perform ulnar motor conductions recording from both the first dorsal interosseous and the abductor digiti minimi muscles with stimulation sites at the wrist, below the elbow, and above the elbow. Because of the fascicular arrangement of nerves destined to innervate these muscles, one may find abnormalities in one but not the other muscle. Most of the lesions in the elbow initially lead to demyelination in this segment. One would expect to see normal distal latencies, amplitudes, and CV between the wrist and below-elbow stimulation sites. However, mild slowing of CV may be appreciated between the below- and above-elbow sites.[172] As the size of the demyelinating lesion may be small, the shorter the distance between the below- and above-elbow sites, the more likely one will be able to demonstrate focal slowing (we try to keep the distance at most 8–10 cm). In addition, conduction block may be appreciated between these sites of stimulation. Inching studies can further localize the lesion to a site within the elbow segment. Perhaps, a more appropriate term is "centimetering" as the nerve is stimulated every 1–2 cm, beginning 5 cm below to 5 cm above the elbow.[171,173] In most patients with focal demyelinating lesions in this location detected with this technique, both an abrupt latency shift and change in CMAP morphology can be reproducibly demonstrated. Assessing for slowing of the ulnar CNAPs across the elbow may be informative in some patients.[173] If secondary axonal degeneration has occurred, focal CV slowing or conduction block may no longer be apparent. In such cases, the ulnar CMAP does not help differentiate ulnar neuropathy at the wrist from a more proximal lesion. An abnormal dorsal ulnar cutaneous SNAP, however, implies a lesion proximal to the wrist, which can be further supported by EMG abnormalities in ulnar-innervated forearm muscles (e.g., flexor carpi ulnararis and flexor digitorum profundus III and IV). Unfortunately, in many cases with severe axonal lesions degeneration, the site of the lesion cannot be precisely localized. Ulnar nerve ultrasound can assist in localization, particularly in such circumstances[171] (Fig. 23-15). Again, in neuropraxic or demyelinating lesions, the EMG may only demonstrate reduced recruitment of MUAPs. One unique pitfall in assessment of ulnar neuropathies is the demonstration of a greater than 20% drop in ulnar CMAP amplitude comparing below elbow to wrist stimulation. Although this could implicate a demyelinating ulnar neuropathy in the forearm, a Martin-Gruber anastomosis provides another common and plausible explanation which must be excluded.

Recently, there was a meta-analysis published comparing outcomes patients who underwent ulnar nerve surgery thought various techniques. Randomized, controlled prospective studies aimed at assessing the efficacy of various treatments of the more common treatments of ulnar neuropathy at the elbow are lacking.[167] Most studies have been retrospective and subject to bias. Individuals with intermittent sensory symptoms may respond to conservative measures. Nonsurgical measures include elbow pads, avoidance of leaning on the elbow, splinting the elbow in extension at night, and nonsteroidal anti-inflammatory drugs. Surgical procedures may be more beneficial in patients who have motor signs and symptoms, more constant symptoms, and who have not had trauma at this elbow. But still not everyone improves. There are various surgical approaches (e.g., simple decompression, medial epicondylectomy, and nerve transposition).[175] There may be increased theoretical risks with nerve transposition including infarction due to devascularization of the nerve and increased scarring. We are particularly reluctant to recommend this procedure to diabetics with their increased risk of microvasculopathy.

Ulnar Neuropathy in the Hand

The ulnar nerve can be damaged at various locations within the wrist or hand and by different mechanisms (Table 23-16). One of the most common etiologies is a compression by a

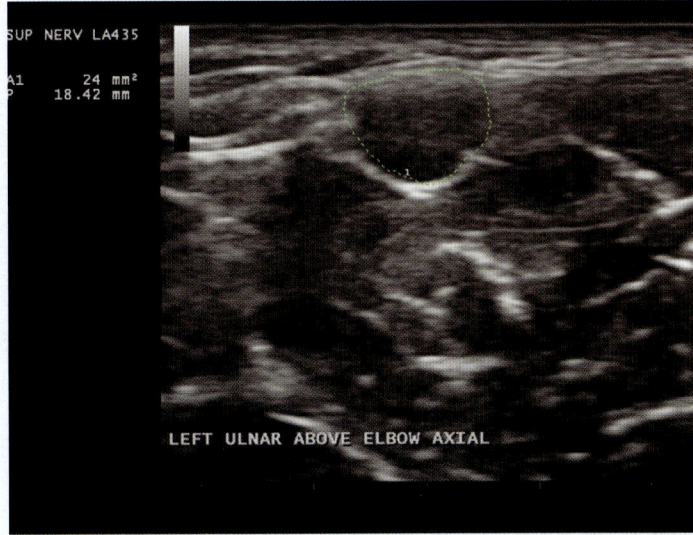

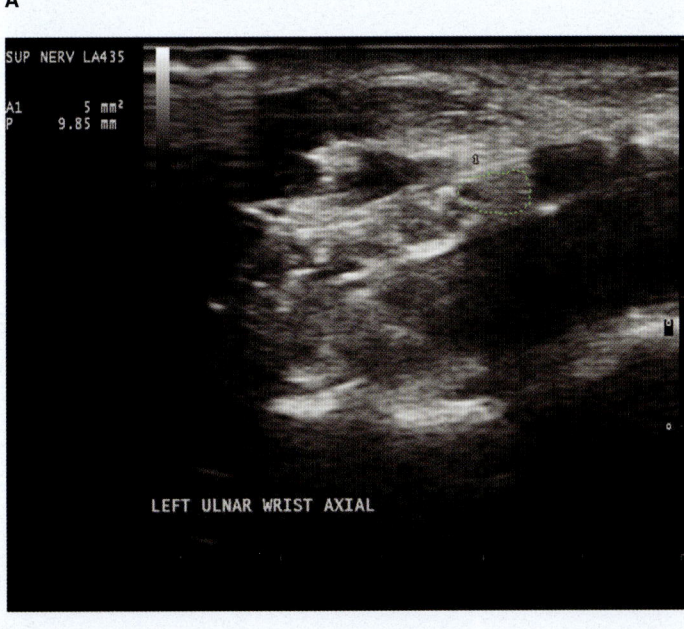

Figure 23-15. Ultrasound of ulnar nerve reveals marked increase in area above the elbow of 24 mm² (normal ≤10 mm²) and normal area at the wrist of 5 mm² (normal ≤6 mm²) resulting in an increased elbow/wrist ratio of 4.8 (normal <2).

▶ **TABLE 23-16. CONDITIONS ASSOCIATED WITH ULNAR NEUROPATHY AT THE WRIST**

External compression (e.g., bicyclist)
Space occupying lesions (e.g., ganglion cysts, lipoma, nerve sheath tumors)
Trauma (fracture to metacarpals, pisiform, hamate, dislocation of distal ulna, laceration)
Degenerative arthritis
Rheumatoid arthritis
Diabetes mellitus[a]

[a]It is unclear if individuals with typical generalized diabetic polyneuropathy may be predisposed to focal mononeuropathies related to compression.

ganglion cyst, which can easily be seen on MRI (Fig. 23-16) or ultrasound of the hand.[35] The ulnar nerve can be damaged in one of four sites within the hand, and the clinical and electrophysiological findings are dependent on the site and nature of the lesion (Fig. 23-17).

1. The entire nerve may be damaged just proximal to or within Guyon canal. This type of lesion affects the superficial sensory and deep motor branches of the distal ulnar nerve, resulting in sensory loss of the volar aspect of the fifth digit and usually the medial half of the fifth digit and weakness of all ulnar-innervated hand muscles. In contrast to more proximal ulnar lesions (e.g., ulnar neuropathy at the

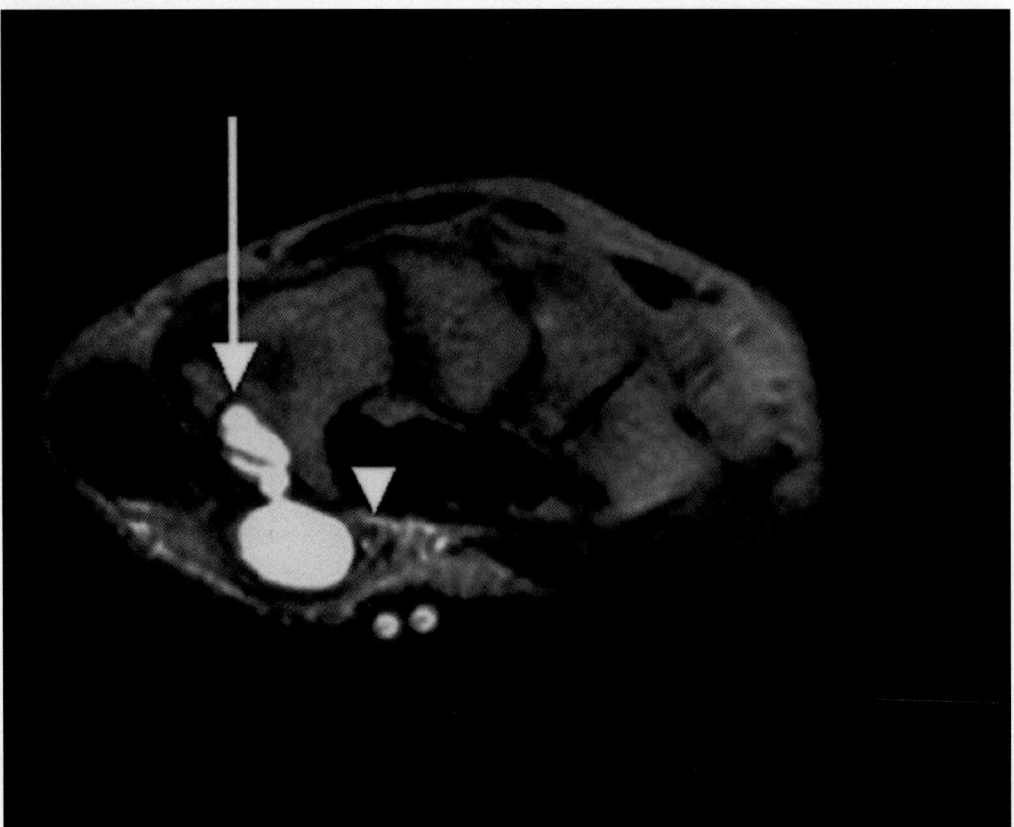
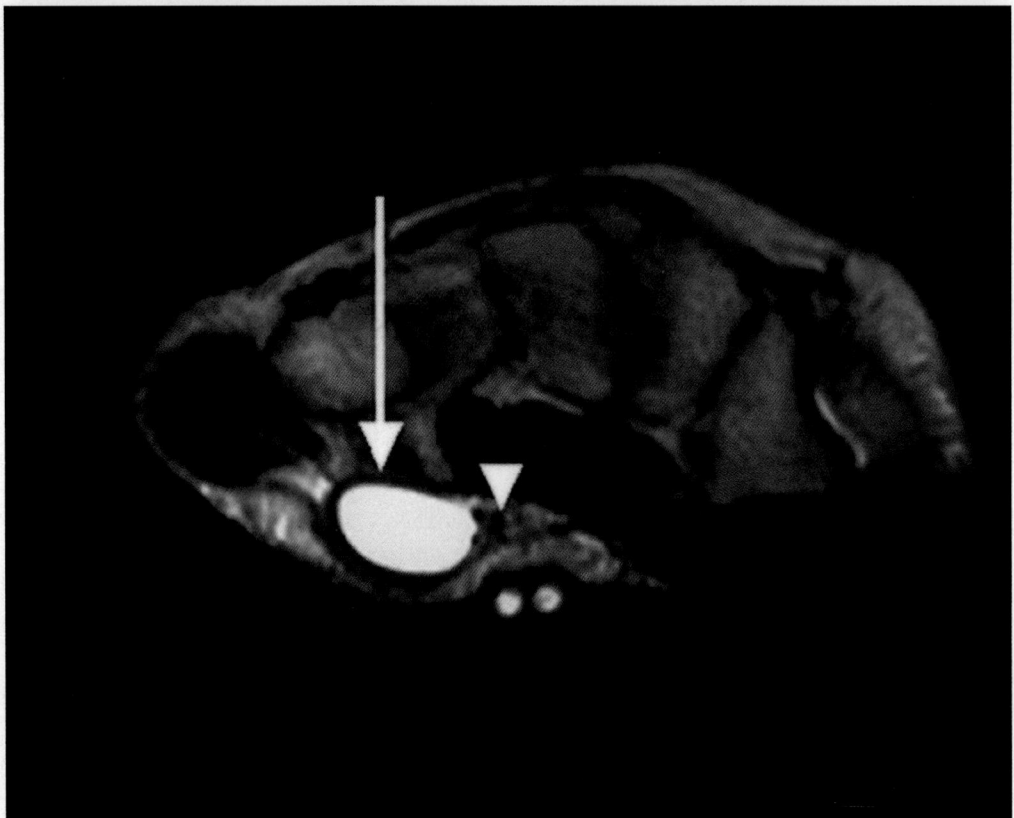

Figure 23-16. MRI of the wrist in a patient with ulnar neuropathy. MRI reveals a ganglionic cyst (*arrow*) adjacent to the hamate in Guyon canal that is displacing the ulnar nerve and artery (*arrowhead*). (Reproduced with permission from of Steven A. Greenberg, MD. Reproduced with permission from: Greenberg SA, Amato AA. *EMG Pearls*. Philadelphia, PA: Hanley & Belfus, Inc; 2004. Fig 2 p. 30.)

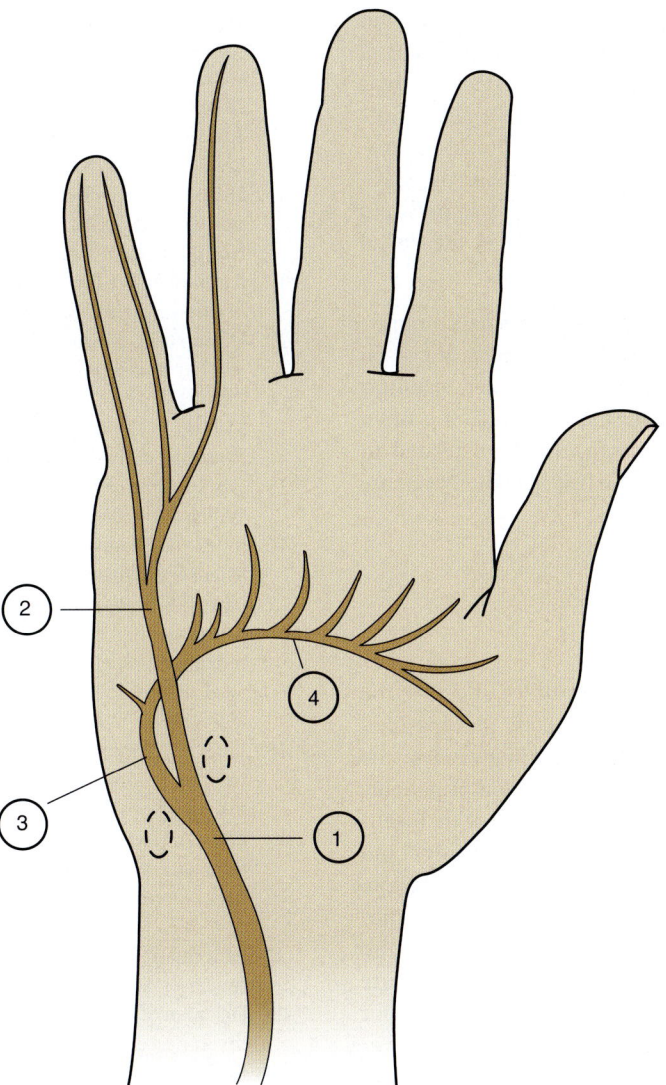

Figure 23-17. There are four main areas in which the ulnar nerve can be damaged at the wrist, and each leads to different clinical and electrophysiological abnormalities as discussed in the text. (Reproduced with permission from Stewart JD. *Focal Peripheral Neuropathies*. Elsevier; 1987.)

elbow), the dorsal ulnar cutaneous nerve is spared; thus, individuals have normal sensation of the dorsum of the ulnar aspect of the hand. In addition, there is normal strength of the flexor carpi ulnaris and flexor digitorum profundus IV and V. The ulnar SNAP may demonstrate prolonged distal latency or reduced amplitude depending on the degree of axon loss, while the dorsal ulnar cutaneous SNAP should be normal. The ulnar CMAP recorded from both the abductor digiti minimi and the first dorsal interosseous may show prolonged distal latencies or reduced amplitudes, again dependent on the nature and severity of the lesion. EMG may demonstrate evidence of denervation in the first dorsal interosseous and abductor digiti minimi but the flexor carpi ulnaris and flexor digitorum profundus IV and V should be normal.

2. The nerve may be compressed just outside Guyon canal such that only the superficial sensory branch is affected. In this case, sensation is decreased but all motor functions are spared. EDX studies would only show abnormalities of the ulnar SNAP.

3. The nerve may be damaged distal to the take-off of the superficial sensory branch and affect only the deep motor branch. In such cases, sensation is spared, but motor function affecting any or all of the ulnar hand intrinsic muscles in the hand may be affected. The ulnar SNAPs would be normal, but ulnar CMAPs to both the first dorsal interosseous and the abductor digiti minimi should be abnormal, as would EMG of these muscles.

4. Finally, the nerve may be compressed distal to the branch innervating the hypothenar eminence. Thus, only the interossei and adductor pollicis muscles are

affected. A lesion may be even more distal such that only the adductor pollicis or perhaps the first dorsal interosseous are abnormal. Ulnar SNAPs and ulnar CMAPs to the abductor digiti minimi would be normal. Only the ulnar CMAP from the dorsal interosseous would show abnormalities. Likewise, on EMG, the abductor digiti minimi would be spared and denervation may be appreciated only in the dorsal interossei and adductor pollicis muscles.

Ulnar neuropathy in the hand due to external compression (e.g., bicyclist) may be treated conservatively. If caused by a fracture of the hamate or pisiform bones, exploratory surgery with decompression and neurolysis are often required. Also, ulnar neuropathies in the hand related to open trauma or internal compression (e.g., ganglion cyst) are usually managed with surgery.

▶ CONCLUSION

The multiple etiologies of focal neuropathies affecting the upper extremity (including radiculopathies, plexopathies, and mononeuropathies) can be quite daunting even to the experienced clinician. The key to the evaluation of patients with these types of focal neuropathies begins with localization. This is accomplished by a thorough history and hypothesis-driven physical examination and by extension, EDX study. Other studies such as various modes of radiological imaging can assist in localizing and identifying an etiology. Prognosis is dependent on the cause and nature of the neuropathy. Neuropraxic lesions secondary to minor compression or stretch usually of the nerve tend to recover well; however, those associated with severe axonal degeneration take much longer to regenerate and recover. Treatment likewise is dependent on the nature of the nerve injury. Most focal neuropathies are initially managed conservatively, but severe nerve injuries may require surgical intervention.

REFERENCES

1. Dumitru D, Zwarts MJ. Brachial plexopathies and proximal mononeuropathies. In: Dumutru D, Amato A, Zwarts MJ, eds. *Electrodiagnostic Medicine.* Hanley & Belfus; 2002:777–836.
2. Ferrante MA. Brachial plexopathies: classification, causes, and consequences. *Muscle Nerve.* 2004;30:547–568.
3. Wilbourn AJ. Plexopathies. *Neurol Clin.* 2007;25:139–171.
4. Kerr AT. The brachial plexus of nerves in man, the variations in its formation and branches. *Am J Anat.* 1918;23:285–395.
5. Millesi H. Brachial plexus injuries. Management and results. *Clin Plast Surg.* 1984;11:115–120.
6. Greenberg SA, Amato AA. Focal neuropathies. In: *EMG Pearls.* Elsevier; 2004;1–68.
7. Haymaker W, Lindgreen M. Nerve disturbances following exposure to ionizing radiation. In: Vinken PJ, Bruyn GW, eds. *Handbook of Clinical Neurology.* vol. 7. 1970:338.
8. Dawson DM, Hallett M, Wilbourn A, et al. *Entrapment Neuropathies.* 3rd ed. Lippincott-Raven; 1999:134–135.
9. Stewart JD. *Focal Peripheral Neuropathies.* 4th ed. JBJ Publishing; 2010:196–198.
10. Sunderland S. *Nerve and Nerve Injuries.* 2nd ed. Churchill-Livingstone; 1978.
11. Ochoa J. Nerve fiber pathology in acute and chronic compression. In: Omer GE, Spinner M, eds. *Management of Peripheral Nerve Problems.* Saunders; 1980:487.
12. Aminoff MJ. Clinical electromyography. In: *Electrodiagnosis in Clinical Neurology.* Churchill Livingstone; 1986:231–263.
13. Dumitru D, Amato AA, Swartz MJ. Nerve conduction studies. *Electrodiagnostic Medicine.* 2nd ed. Hanley & Belfus; 2002: 159–223.
14. Kimura J. *Electrodiagnosis of Diseases of Nerve and Muscle: Principles and Practice.* FA Davis; 2013.
15. Oh SJ. *Clinical Electromyography. Nerve Conduction Studies.* William & Wilkins; 2004.
16. Jones SJ. Diagnostic value of peripheral and spinal somatosensory evoked potentials in traction lesions of the brachial plexus. *Clin Plast Surg.* 1984;11:167–172.
17. Schimsheimer RJ, de Visser BW, Kemp B. The flexor carpi radialis H-reflex in lesions of the sixth and seventh cervical nerve roots. *J Neurol Neurosurg Psychiatr.* 1985;48: 445–449.
18. Jones SJ, Parry CB, Landi A. Diagnosis of brachial plexus traction lesions by sensory nerve action potentials and somatosensory evoked potentials. *Injury.* 1981;12:376–382.
19. Eisen A, Hoirch M. Electrodiagnostic evaluation of radiculopathies and plexopathies using somatosensory evoked potentials. *Electroencephalogr Clin Neurophysiol Suppl.* 1982;36: 349–357.
20. Lederman RJ, Wilbourn AJ. Brachial plexopathy: recurrent cancer or radiation? *Neurology.* 1984;34:1331–1335.
21. Delanian S, Lefaix JL, Pradat PF. Radiation-induced neuropathy in cancer survivors. *Radiother Oncol.* 2012;105:273–282.
22. Rapoport S, Blair DN, McCarthy SM, Desser TS, Hammers LW, Sostman HD. Brachial plexus: correlation of MR imaging with CT and pathologic findings. *Radiology.* 1988;167:161–165.
23. Wittenberg KH, Adkins MC. MR imaging of nontraumatic brachial plexopathies: frequency and spectrum of findings. *Radiographics.* 2000;20:1023–1032.
24. Gilcrease-Garcia BM, Deshmukh SD, Parsons MS. Anatomy, imaging, and pathologic conditions of the brachial plexus. *Radiographics.* 2020;40:1686–1714.
25. van Es HW, Bollen TL, van Heesewijk HPM. MRI of the brachial plexus: a pictorial review. *Eur J Radiol.* 2010;74:391–402.
26. Dailey AT, Tsuruda JS, Filler AG, Maravilla KR, Goodkin R, Kliot M. Magnetic resonance neurography of peripheral nerve degeneration and regeneration. *Lancet.* 1997;350:1221–1222.
27. Filler AG, Maravilla KR, Tsuruda JS. MR neurography and muscle MR imaging for image diagnosis of disorders affecting the peripheral nerves and musculature. *Neurol Clin.* 2004; 22:643–682, vi.
28. Grant GA, Britz GW, Goodkin R, Jarvik JG, Maravilla K, Kliot M. The utility of magnetic resonance imaging in evaluating peripheral nerve disorders. *Muscle Nerve.* 2002;25:314–331.
29. Gupta RK, Mehta VS, Banerji AK, Jain RK. MR evaluation of brachial plexus injuries. *Neuroradiology.* 1989;31:377–381.
30. Hobson-Webb LD, Padua L. Ultrasound of focal neuropathies. *J Clin Neurophysiol.* 2016;33:94–102.

31. Gonzalez NL, Hobson-Webb LD. Neuromuscular ultrasound in clinical practice: a review. *Clin Neurophysiol Pract*. 2019;4:148–163.
32. Cartwright MS, Chloros GD, Walker FO, Wiesler ER, Campbell WW. Diagnostic ultrasound for nerve transection. *Muscle Nerve*. 2007;35:796–799.
33. Strakowski JA. Ultrasound evaluation of peripheral nerves. In: *Ultrasound Evaluation of Peripheral Nerves and Focal Neuropathies*. 2nd ed. Springer; 2021:51–77.
34. Childress MA, Becker BA. Nonoperative management of cervical radiculopathy. *Am Fam Physician*. 2016;93:746–754.
35. Kelsey JL, Githens PB, Walter SD, et al. An epidemiological study of acute prolapsed cervical intervertebral disc. *J Bone Joint Surg Am*. 1984;66:907–914.
36. Lunsford LD, Bissonette DJ, Jannetta PJ, Sheptak PE, Zorub DS. Anterior surgery for cervical disc disease. Part 1: treatment of lateral cervical disc herniation in 253 cases. *J Neurosurg*. 1980;53:1–11.
37. Martins AN. Anterior cervical discectomy with and without interbody bone graft. *J Neurosurg*. 1976;44:290–295.
38. Negrin P, Lelli S, Fardin P. Contribution of electromyography to the diagnosis, treatment and prognosis of cervical disc disease: a study of 114 patients. *Electromyogr Clin Neurophysiol*. 1991;31:173–179.
39. Scoville WB, Dohrmann GJ, Corkill G. Late results of cervical disc surgery. *J Neurosurg*. 1976;45:203–210.
40. Abbott KH, Retter RH. Protrusions of thoracic intervertebral disks. *Neurology*. 1956;6:1–10.
41. Arce CA, Dohrmann GJ. Herniated thoracic disks. *Neurol Clin*. 1985;3:383–392.
42. Arseni C, Nash F. Thoracic intervertebral disc protrusion: a clinical study. *J Neurosurg*. 1960;17:418–430.
43. Otani K, Yoshida M, Fujii E, Nakai S, Shibasaki K. Thoracic disc herniation. Surgical treatment in 23 patients. *Spine*. 1988;13:1262–1267.
44. Bohlman HH, Zdeblick TA. Anterior excision of herniated thoracic discs. *J Bone Joint Surg Am*. 1988;70:1038–1047.
45. Benson MK, Byrnes DP. The clinical syndromes and surgical treatment of thoracic intervertebral disc prolapse. *J Bone Joint Surg Br*. 1975;57:471–477.
46. Radhakrishnan K, Litchy WJ, O'Fallon WM, Kurland LT. Epidemiology of cervical radiculopathy. A population-based study from Rochester, Minnesota, 1976 through 1990. *Brain*. 1994;117(Pt 2):325–335.
47. Teresi LM, Lufkin RB, Reicher MA, et al. Asymptomatic degenerative disk disease and spondylosis of the cervical spine: MR imaging. *Radiology*. 1987;164:83–88.
48. Gross A, Gross A, Goldsmith C, et al; Cervical Overview Group. Exercises for mechanical neck disorders. *Cochrane Database Syst Rev*. 2015;1:CD004250.
49. Jones CMP, Day RO, Koes BW, et al; OPAL Investigators Coordinator. Opioid analgesia for acute low back pain and neck pain (the OPAL trial): a randomised placebo-controlled trial. *Lancet*. 2023;402:304–312.
50. Persson LC, Carlsson CA, Carlsson JY. Long-lasting cervical radicular pain managed with surgery, physiotherapy, or a cervical collar. A prospective, randomized study. *Spine*. 1997;22:751–758.
51. Nikolaidis I, Fouyas IP, Sandercock PA, Statham PF. Surgery for cervical radiculopathy or myelopathy. *Cochrane Database Syst Rev*. 2010;2010(1):CD001466.
52. Carette S, Fehlings MG. Clinical practice. Cervical radiculopathy. *N Engl J Med*. 2005;353:392–399.
53. van Alfen N, van Engelen BGM. The clinical spectrum of neuralgic amyotrophy in 246 cases. *Brain*. 2006;129:438–450.
54. Parsonage MJ, Turner JWA. Neuralgic amyotrophy; the shoulder-girdle syndrome. *Lancet*. 1948;1:973–978.
55. Turner JWA, Parsonage MJ. Neuralgic amyotrophy (paralytic brachial neuritis); with special reference to prognosis. *Lancet*. 1957;273:209–212.
56. Cignetti NE, Cox RS, Baute V, et al. A standardized ultrasound approach in neuralgic amyotrophy. *Muscle Nerve*. 2023;67:3–11.
57. Ripellino P, Arányi Z, van Alfen N, et al. Imaging of neuralgic amyotrophy in the acute phase. *Muscle Nerve*. 2022;66:709–714.
58. IJspeert J, Janssen RMJ, van Alfen N. Neuralgic amyotrophy. *Curr Opin Neurol*. 2021;34:605–612.
59. Tsairis P, Dyck PJ, Mulder DW. Natural history of brachial plexus neuropathy. Report on 99 patients. *Arch Neurol*. 1972;27:109–117.
60. Flaggman PD, Kelly JJ. Brachial plexus neuropathy. An electrophysiologic evaluation. *Arch Neurol*. 1980;37:160–164.
61. van Alfen N, Doorduin J, van Rosmalen MHJ, et al. Phrenic neuropathy and diaphragm dysfunction in neuralgic amyotrophy. *Neurology*. 2018;91:e843–e849.
62. Kiloh LG, Nevin S. Isolated neuritis of the anterior interosseous nerve. *Br Med J*. 1952;1:850–851.
63. Rennels GD, Ochoa J. Neuralgic amyotrophy manifesting as anterior interosseous nerve palsy. *Muscle Nerve*. 1980;3:160–164.
64. Pierre PA, Laterre CE, Van den Bergh PY. Neuralgic amyotrophy with involvement of cranial nerves IX, X, XI and XII. *Muscle Nerve*. 1990;13:704–707.
65. Eisen A, Bertrand G. Isolated accessory nerve palsy of spontaneous origin. A clinical and electromyographic study. *Arch Neurol*. 1972;27:496–502.
66. Kiwit JC. Neuralgic amyotrophy after administration of tetanus toxoid. *J Neurol Neurosurg Psychiatr*. 1984;47:320.
67. Loh FL, Herskovitz S, Berger AR, Swerdlow ML. Brachial plexopathy associated with interleukin-2 therapy. *Neurology*. 1992;42:462–463.
68. Weintraub MI, Chia DT. Paralytic brachial neuritis after swine flu vaccination. *Arch Neurol*. 1977;34:518.
69. Bernsen PL, Wong Chung RE, Vingerhoets HM, Janssen JT. Bilateral neuralgic amyotrophy induced by interferon treatment. *Arch Neurol*. 1988;45:449–451.
70. Vriesendorp FJ, Dmytrenko GS, Dietrich T, Koski CL. Anti-peripheral nerve myelin antibodies and terminal activation products of complement in serum of patients with acute brachial plexus neuropathy. *Arch Neurol*. 1993;50:1301–1303.
71. England JD, Sumner AJ. Neuralgic amyotrophy: an increasingly diverse entity. *Muscle Nerve*. 1987;10:60–68.
72. Amato AA, Jackson CE, Kim JY, Worley KL. Chronic relapsing brachial plexus neuropathy with persistent conduction block. *Muscle Nerve*. 1997;20:1303–1307.
73. Adler JB, Patterson RL. Erb's palsy. Long-term results of treatment in eighty-eight cases. *J Bone Joint Surg Am*. 1967;49:1052–1064.
74. Eng GD, Koch B, Smokvina MD. Brachial plexus palsy in neonates and children. *Arch Phys Med Rehabil*. 1978;59:458–464.
75. Eng GD. Brachial plexus palsy in newborn infants. *Pediatrics*. 1971;48:18–28.
76. Greenwald AG, Schute PC, Shiveley JL. Brachial plexus birth palsy: a 10-year report on the incidence and prognosis. *J Pediatr Orthop*. 1984;4:689–692.

77. Specht EE. Brachial plexus palsy in the newborn. Incidence and prognosis. *Clin Orthop Relat Res.* 1975;(110):32–34.
78. Johnson EW, Alexander MA, Koenig WC. Infantile Erb's palsy (Smellie's palsy). *Arch Phys Med Rehabil.* 1977;58:175–178.
79. McFarland LV, Raskin M, Daling JR, Benedetti TJ. Erb/Duchenne's palsy: a consequence of fetal macrosomia and method of delivery. *Obstet Gynecol.* 1986;68:784–788.
80. Meyer RD. Treatment of adult and obstetrical brachial plexus injuries. *Orthopedics.* 1986;9:899–903.
81. Mollberg M, Wennergren M, Bager B, Ladfors L, Hagberg H. Obstetric brachial plexus palsy: a prospective study on risk factors related to manual assistance during the second stage of labor. *Acta Obstet Gynecol Scand.* 2007;86:198–204.
82. Erb W. Ueber eine eigenthumliche localisation von lähmungen im plexus brachialis. *Verhandl d Naturhist-Med Heidelberg.* 1874;2:130–137.
83. Klumpkee A. Contribution a l'etude des paralysies radiculaires du plexus brachial: paralysies radiculaires totals: paralysies radiculaires inférieures: de la participation des filest sympathiques oculo-pupillaires dans ces paralysies. *Rev Med.* 1885;5:591.
84. Boome RS, Kaye JC. Obstetric traction injuries of the brachial plexus. Natural history, indications for surgical repair and results. *J Bone Joint Surg Br.* 1988;70:571–576.
85. Rossi LN, Vassella F, Mumenthaler M. Obstetrical lesions of the brachial plexus. Natural history in 34 personal cases. *Eur Neurol.* 1982;21:1–7.
86. Kneeland JB, Kellman GM, Middleton WD, et al. Diagnosis of diseases of the supraclavicular region by use of MR imaging. *AJR Am J Roentgenol.* 1987;148:1149–1151.
87. Popovich MJ, Taylor FC, Helmer E. MR imaging of birth-related brachial plexus avulsion. *AJNR Am J Neuroradiol.* 1989;10:S98.
88. Kline DG. Surgical repair of peripheral nerve injury. *Muscle Nerve.* 1990;13:843–852.
89. Kline DG. Hudson AR. *Nerve Injuries. Operative Results from Major Nerve Injuries, Entrapments, and Tumors.* W. B. Saunders Company; 1995:596.
90. Spinner RJ, Kline DG. Surgery for peripheral nerve and brachial plexus injuries or other nerve lesions. *Muscle Nerve.* 2000;23:680–695.
91. Ferrante MA, Ferrante ND. The thoracic outlet syndromes: Part 1. Overview of the thoracic outlet syndromes and review of true neurogenic thoracic outlet syndrome. *Muscle Nerve.* 2017;55:782–793.
92. Aminoff MJ, Olney RK, Parry GJ, Raskin NH. Relative utility of different electrophysiologic techniques in the evaluation of brachial plexopathies. *Neurology.* 1988;38:546–550.
93. Cuetter AC, Bartoszek DM. The thoracic outlet syndrome: controversies, overdiagnosis, overtreatment, and recommendations for management. *Muscle Nerve.* 1989;12:410–419.
94. Gilliatt RW, Le Quesne PM, Logue V, Sumner AJ. Wasting of the hand associated with a cervical rib or band. *J Neurol Neurosurg Psychiatr.* 1970;33:615–624.
95. Gilliatt RW, Willison RG, Dietz V, Williams IR. Peripheral nerve conduction in patients with a cervical rib and band. *Ann Neurol.* 1978;4:124–129.
96. Kori SH, Foley KM, Posner JB. Brachial plexus lesions in patients with cancer: 100 cases. *Neurology.* 1981;31:45–50.
97. Jaeckle KA. Nerve plexus metastases. *Neurol Clin.* 1991;9:857–866.
98. Lusk MD, Kline DG, Garcia CA. Tumors of the brachial plexus. *Neurosurgery.* 1987;21:439–453.
99. Sell PJ, Semple JC. Primary nerve tumours of the brachial plexus. *Br J Surg.* 1987;74:73–74.
100. Dubuisson A, Reuter G, Kaschten B, et al. Management of benign nerve sheath tumors of the brachial plexus: relevant diagnostic and surgical features. About a series of 17 patients (19 tumors) and review of the literature. *Acta Neurol Belg.* 2021;121:125–131.
101. Godwin JT. Encapsulated neurilemoma (schwannoma) of the brachial plexus; report of eleven cases. *Cancer.* 1952;5:708–720.
102. Donaldson EK, Winter JM, Chandler RM, Clark TA, Giuffre JL. Malignant peripheral nerve sheath tumors of the brachial plexus: a single-center experience on diagnosis, management, and outcomes. *Ann Plast Surg.* 2023;90:339–342.
103. Harper CM, Thomas JE, Cascino TL, Litchy WJ. Distinction between neoplastic and radiation-induced brachial plexopathy, with emphasis on the role of EMG. *Neurology.* 1989;39:502–506.
104. Daube JR. Rucksack paralysis. *JAMA.* 1969;208:2447–2452.
105. Corkill G, Lieberman JS, Taylor RG. Pack palsy in backpackers. *West J Med.* 1980;132:569–572.
106. Graham JG, Pye IF, McQueen IN. Brachial plexus injury after median sternotomy. *J Neurol Neurosurg Psychiatr.* 1981;44:621–625.
107. Hanson MR, Breuer AC, Furlan AJ, et al. Mechanism and frequency of brachial plexus injury in open-heart surgery: a prospective analysis. *Ann Thorac Surg.* 1983;36:675–679.
108. Morin JE, Long R, Elleker MG, Eisen AA, Wynands E, Ralphs-Thibodeau S. Upper extremity neuropathies following median sternotomy. *Ann Thorac Surg.* 1982;34:181–185.
109. Seyfer AE, Grammer NY, Bogumill GP, Provost JM, Chandry U. Upper extremity neuropathies after cardiac surgery. *J Hand Surg Am.* 1985;10:16–19.
110. Chance PF, Lensch MW, Lipe H, Brown RH Sr, Brown RH Jr, Bird TD. Hereditary neuralgic amyotrophy and hereditary neuropathy with liability to pressure palsies: two distinct genetic disorders. *Neurology.* 1994;44:2253–2257.
111. Jeannet PY, Watts GD, Bird TD, Chance PF. Craniofacial and cutaneous findings expand the phenotype of hereditary neuralgic amyotrophy. *Neurology.* 2001;57:1963–1968.
112. Laccone F, Hannibal MC, Neesen J, Grisold W, Chance PF, Rehder H. Dysmorphic syndrome of hereditary neuralgic amyotrophy associated with a SEPT9 gene mutation—a family study. *Clin Genet.* 2008;74:279–283.
113. Kuhlenbäumer G, Hannibal MC, Nelis E, et al. Mutations in SEPT9 cause hereditary neuralgic amyotrophy. *Nat Genet.* 2005;37:1044–1046.
114. Spinner RJ, Carmichael SW, Spinner M. Partial median nerve entrapment in the distal arm because of an accessory bicipital aponeurosis. *J Hand Surg Am.* 1991;16:236–244.
115. Hentz VR. Is microsurgical treatment of brachial plexus palsy better than conventional treatment? *Hand Clin.* 2007;23:83–89.
116. Sulaiman OAR, Kim DD, Burkett C, Kline DG. Nerve transfer surgery for adult brachial plexus injury: a 10-year experience at Louisiana State University. *Neurosurgery.* 2009;65:A55–A62.
117. Pondaag W, van Driest FY, Groen JL, Malessy MJA. Early nerve repair in traumatic brachial plexus injuries in adults: treatment algorithm and first experiences. *J Neurosurg.* 2018;130:172–178.

118. Shin AY, Spinner RJ, Steinmann SP, Bishop AT. Adult traumatic brachial plexus injuries. *J Am Acad Orthop Surg.* 2005;13:382–396.
119. Terzis JK, Kostopoulos VK. The surgical treatment of brachial plexus injuries in adults. *Plast Reconstr Surg.* 2007;119:73e–92e.
120. Terzis JK, Kostas I, Soucacos PN. Restoration of shoulder function with nerve transfers in traumatic brachial plexus palsy patients. *Microsurgery.* 2006;26:316–324.
121. Levy O, Relwani JG, Mullett H, Haddo O, Even T. The active elevation lag sign and the triangle sign: new clinical signs of trapezius palsy. *J Shoulder Elbow Surg.* 2009;18:573–576.
122. Chan PKH, Hems TEJ. Clinical signs of accessory nerve palsy. *J Trauma.* 2006;60:1142–1144.
123. Goodman CE, Kenrick MM, Blum MV. Long thoracic nerve palsy: a follow-up study. *Arch Phys Med Rehabil.* 1975;56:352–358.
124. Johnson JT, Kendall HO. Isolated paralysis of the serratus anterior muscle. *J Bone Joint Surg Am.* 1955;37-A:567–574.
125. Kaplan PE. Electrodiagnostic confirmation of long thoracic nerve palsy. *J Neurol Neurosurg Psychiatr.* 1980;43:50–52.
126. Haymaker W, Woodhall B. *Peripheral Nerve Injuries: Principles of Diagnosis.* 2nd ed. American Association of Neurological Surgeons; 2005.
127. Warner JJ, Navarro RA. Serratus anterior dysfunction. Recognition and treatment. *Clin Orthop Relat Res.* 1998;(349):139–148.
128. Wiater JM, Flatow EL. Long thoracic nerve injury. *Clin Orthop Relat Res.* 1999;(368):17–27.
129. Clein LJ. Suprascapular entrapment neuropathy. *J Neurosurg.* 1975;43:337–342.
130. Swafford AR, Lichtman DH. Suprascapular nerve entrapment—case report. *J Hand Surg Am.* 1982;7:57–60.
131. Zoltan JD. Injury to the suprascapular nerve associated with anterior dislocation of the shoulder: case report and review of the literature. *J Trauma.* 1979;19:203–206.
132. Bozzi F, Alabau-Rodriguez S, Barrera-Ochoa S, et al. Suprascapular neuropathy around the shoulder: a current concept review. *J Clin Med.* 2020;9(8):2331.
133. Aiello I, Serra G, Traina GC, Tugnoli V. Entrapment of the suprascapular nerve at the spinoglenoid notch. *Ann Neurol.* 1982;12:314–316.
134. Piasecki DP, Romeo AA, Bach BR Jr, Nicholson GP. Suprascapular neuropathy. *J Am Acad Orthop Surg.* 2009;17:665–676.
135. Le Hanneur M, Maldonado AA, Howe BM, Mauermann ML, Spinner RJ. "Isolated" suprascapular neuropathy: compression, traction, or inflammation? *Neurosurgery.* 2019;84:404–412.
136. Antoniadis G, Richter HP, Rath S, Braun V, Moese G. Suprascapular nerve entrapment: experience with 28 cases. *J Neurosurg.* 1996;85:1020–1025.
137. Antoniou J, Tae SK, Williams GR, Bird S, Ramsey ML, Iannotti JP. Suprascapular neuropathy. Variability in the diagnosis, treatment, and outcome. *Clin Orthop Relat Res.* 2001;(386):131–138.
138. Strauss EJ, Kingery MT, Klein D, Manjunath AK. The evaluation and management of suprascapular neuropathy. *J Am Acad Orthop Surg.* 2020;28:617–627.
139. van Alfen N, van Engelen BGM, Hughes RAC. Treatment for idiopathic and hereditary neuralgic amyotrophy (brachial neuritis). *Cochrane Database Syst Rev.* 2009;2009:CD006976.
140. Braddom RL, Wolfe C. Musculocutaneous nerve injury after heavy exercise. *Arch Phys Med Rehabil.* 1978;59:290–293.
141. Kim SM, Goodrich JA. Isolated proximal musculocutaneous nerve palsy: case report. *Arch Phys Med Rehabil.* 1984;65:735–736.
142. Liveson JA. Nerve lesions associated with shoulder dislocation; an electrodiagnostic study of 11 cases. *J Neurol Neurosurg Psychiatr.* 1984;47:742–744.
143. Aita JF. An unusual compressive neuropathy. *Arch Neurol.* 1984;41:341.
144. Berry H, Bril V. Axillary nerve palsy following blunt trauma to the shoulder region: a clinical and electrophysiological review. *J Neurol Neurosurg Psychiatr.* 1982;45:1027–1032.
145. Kirby JF, Kraft GH. Entrapment neuropathy of anterior branch of axillary nerve: report of case. *Arch Phys Med Rehabil.* 1972;53:338–340.
146. Steinmann SP, Moran EA. Axillary nerve injury: diagnosis and treatment. *J Am Acad Orthop Surg.* 2001;9:328–335.
147. Lotem M, Fried A, Levy M, Solzi P, Najenson T, Nathan H. Radial palsy following muscular effort. A nerve compression syndrome possibly related to a fibrous arch of the lateral head of the triceps. *J Bone Joint Surg Br.* 1971;53:500–506.
148. Patino JM, Fernandez A, Mondino NP. Severe apraxia due to entrapment of the radial nerve in the arm: "lotem syndrome." *Rev Assoc Argent Ortop Traumatol.* 2022;87:534–539.
149. Kim DH, Murovic JA, Kim Y-Y, Kline DG. Surgical treatment and outcomes in 45 cases of posterior interosseous nerve entrapments and injuries. *J Neurosurg.* 2006;104:766–777.
150. Boswick JA, Stromberg WB. Isolated injury to the median nerve above the elbow. A review of thirteen cases. *J Bone Joint Surg Am.* 1967;49:653–658.
151. Staal A, van Voorthuisen AE, van Dijk LM. Neurological complications following arterial catheterisation by the axillary approach. *BJR.* 1966;39:115–116.
152. Bolton CF, Driedger AA, Lindsay RM. Ischaemic neuropathy in uraemic patients caused by bovine arteriovenous shunt. *J Neurol Neurosurg Psychiatr.* 1979;42:810–814.
153. al-Naib I. Humeral supracondylar spur and Struthers' ligament. A rare cause of neurovascular entrapment in the upper limb. *Int Orthop.* 1994;18:393–394.
154. Aydinlioglu A, Cirak B, Akpinar F, Tosun N, Dogan A. Bilateral median nerve compression at the level of Struthers' ligament. Case report. *J Neurosurg.* 2000;92:693–696.
155. Bilge T, Yalaman O, Bilge S, Cokneşeli B, Barut S. Entrapment neuropathy of the median nerve at the level of the ligament of Struthers. *Neurosurgery.* 1990;27:787–789.
156. Schrader PA, Reina CR. Struthers' ligament neuropathy in a juvenile. *Orthopedics.* 1994;17:723–725.
157. Kodama N, Ando K, Takemura Y, Imai S. Treatment of spontaneous anterior interosseous nerve palsy. *J Neurosurg.* 2020;132:1243–1248.
158. Schantz K, Riegels-Nielsen P. The anterior interosseous nerve syndrome. *J Hand Surg Br.* 1992;17:510–512.
159. Pryse-Phillips WE. Validation of a diagnostic sign in carpal tunnel syndrome. *J Neurol Neurosurg Psychiatr.* 1984;47:870–872.
160. Kuschner SH, Ebramzadeh E, Johnson D, Brien WW, Sherman R. Tinel's sign and Phalen's test in carpal tunnel syndrome. *Orthopedics.* 1992;15:1297–1302.
161. Fowler JR, Gaughan JP, Ilyas AM. The sensitivity and specificity of ultrasound for the diagnosis of carpal tunnel syndrome: a meta-analysis. *Clin Orthop Relat Res.* 2011;469:1089–1094.
162. Padua L, Cuccagna C, Giovannini S, et al. Carpal tunnel syndrome: updated evidence and new questions. *Lancet Neurol.* 2023;22:255–267.
163. Pelosi L, Arányi Z, Beekman R, et al. Expert consensus on the combined investigation of carpal tunnel syndrome with

electrodiagnostic tests and neuromuscular ultrasound. *Clin Neurophysiol.* 2022;135:107–116.
164. Iyer V. Role of ultrasonography in severe distal median nerve neuropathy. *J Clin Neurophysiol.* 2019;36:312–315.
165. Chen J, Fowler JR. Ultrasound findings in patients with normal nerve conduction despite clinical signs and symptoms consistent with carpal tunnel syndrome. *Plast Reconstr Surg.* 2022;150:1025e–1032e.
166. Bland JDP. Treatment of carpal tunnel syndrome. *Muscle Nerve.* 2007;36:167–171.
167. Chesterton LS, Blagojevic-Bucknall M, Burton C, et al. The clinical and cost-effectiveness of corticosteroid injection versus night splints for carpal tunnel syndrome (INSTINCTS trial): an open-label, parallel group, randomised controlled trial. *Lancet.* 2018;392:1423–1433.
168. Bland JD. Do nerve conduction studies predict the outcome of carpal tunnel decompression? *Muscle Nerve.* 2001;24:935–940.
169. Ly-Pen D, Andréu J-L, de Blas G, Sánchez-Olaso A, Millán I. Surgical decompression versus local steroid injection in carpal tunnel syndrome: a one-year, prospective, randomized, open, controlled clinical trial. *Arthritis Rheum.* 2005;52:612–619.
170. Jarvik JG, Comstock BA, Kliot M, et al. Surgery versus nonsurgical therapy for carpal tunnel syndrome: a randomised parallel-group trial. *Lancet.* 2009;374:1074–1081.
171. Practice parameter for electrodiagnostic studies in ulnar neuropathy at the elbow: summary statement. American Association of Electrodiagnostic Medicine, American Academy of Physical Medicine and Rehabilitation, American Academy of Neurology. *Arch Phys Med Rehabil.* 1999;80:357–359.
172. Kincaid JC, Phillips LH, Daube JR. The evaluation of suspected ulnar neuropathy at the elbow. Normal conduction study values. *Arch Neurol.* 1986;43:44–47.
173. Visser LH, Beekman R, Franssen H. Short-segment nerve conduction studies in ulnar neuropathy at the elbow. *Muscle Nerve.* 2005;31:331–338.
174. Raynor EM, Shefner JM, Preston DC, Logigian EL. Sensory and mixed nerve conduction studies in the evaluation of ulnar neuropathy at the elbow. *Muscle Nerve.* 1994;17:785–792.
175. Macadam SA, Gandhi R, Bezuhly M, Lefaivre KA. Simple decompression versus anterior subcutaneous and submuscular transposition of the ulnar nerve for cubital tunnel syndrome: a meta-analysis. *J Hand Surg Am.* 2008;33:1314.e1–1314.e12.

CHAPTER 24

Focal Neuropathies of the Lower Extremities: Radiculopathies, Plexopathies, and Mononeuropathies

Limb pain, diminished sensation (numbness), altered sensory perception (paresthesias and dysesthesias), and impaired function due to weakness are exceedingly common complaints in the practice of medicine. Distinguishing neuromuscular from musculoskeletal pathologies can be challenging, particularly when pain is the predominant symptom. Complicating this distinction, some patients with musculoskeletal problems also report intermittent sensory symptoms, which do not adhere to anatomical distributions, or a perception of weakness that may result from limitations imposed by pain. Not uncommonly, however, patients with lower extremity pain, sensory symptoms, and altered function will have focal nerve injuries affecting the lumbosacral nerve roots or plexus, or individual peripheral nerves of the lower extremities.

The purpose of this chapter is to provide a conceptual framework by which to evaluate and manage patients with these focal lower limb symptoms, and specifically, focal nerve pathologies. This process begins by distinguishing these pathologies from the musculoskeletal causes of monomelic symptoms described in Chapter 36. Subsequently, as with all neurologic problem-solving exercises, we attempt to localize the symptom-causing abnormality to nerve root(s), plexus or one or more individual peripheral nerves. This process facilitates generating a differential diagnosis and ultimately a final diagnosis to guide management. Consideration of symptom time-course, risk factors, and comorbid conditions aids in generating a differential diagnosis for each patient.

This chapter will mirror the format of the analogous upper extremity chapter. We refer the reader to Chapter 23 regarding relevant anatomy, pathophysiology, and electrodiagnostic (EDX) evaluation. To avoid redundancy, these subjects will only be revisited here when there are relevant differences between the upper and lower extremities. A detailed review of the clinical features, etiologies, evaluation, and management of individual focal neuropathies of the lower extremities will be provided. As in other chapters in this book, descriptions will rest on a foundation of published data, but will be expanded upon by the personal experiences of the authors.

▶ ANATOMY

LUMBOSACRAL NERVE ROOTS

Several clinically relevant differences in anatomy and nomenclature between the upper and lower limbs are worth reviewing at the outset. The organization of nerve roots in the lumbosacral spine is identical in many ways to that in the cervical spine. One notable exception is that dorsal root ganglia may reside in an intraspinal location within the lumbosacral spine. In some cases, this results in mechanical nerve root compression distal, rather than proximal, to the dorsal root ganglion, producing a potentially confusing pattern of EDX findings to those unfamiliar with this anatomical variant.[1]

In the lumbosacral spinal cord, nerve roots descend more obliquely than their cervical counterparts. This occurs because the length of the spinal cord differs from the length of the vertebral column (Fig. 24-1). Nerve roots arise from the conus medullaris, form the cauda equina and then descend in the spinal canal before they exit through their designated foramen. Nerve roots begin to separate from the cauda equina and move to the lateral portion of the spinal canal called the lateral recess, one level above where they will exit. This "traversing" nerve root is vulnerable to compression from disc herniations and facet hypertrophy.[2] Logically, the traversing nerve root exits the foramen from the most rostral position within the foramen possible, immediately beneath the pedicle of the vertebral body with the same numerical designation. This exit route is typically superior to the plane in which disc material extrudes, or spondylitic protrusions are most likely to develop. As such, the root compressed at any level is typically the next nerve root, which has not yet exited the spinal column, and the one corresponding to the lower of the two vertebrae constituting that foramen.

For example, the L5 nerve root traverses between the L4 and L5 vertebrae where it is susceptible to pathology of the L4–5 disc. The nerve then exists through the foramen between the L5 and S1 vertebrae.[2] Additionally, as the descending lumbosacral nerve roots traverse the disc

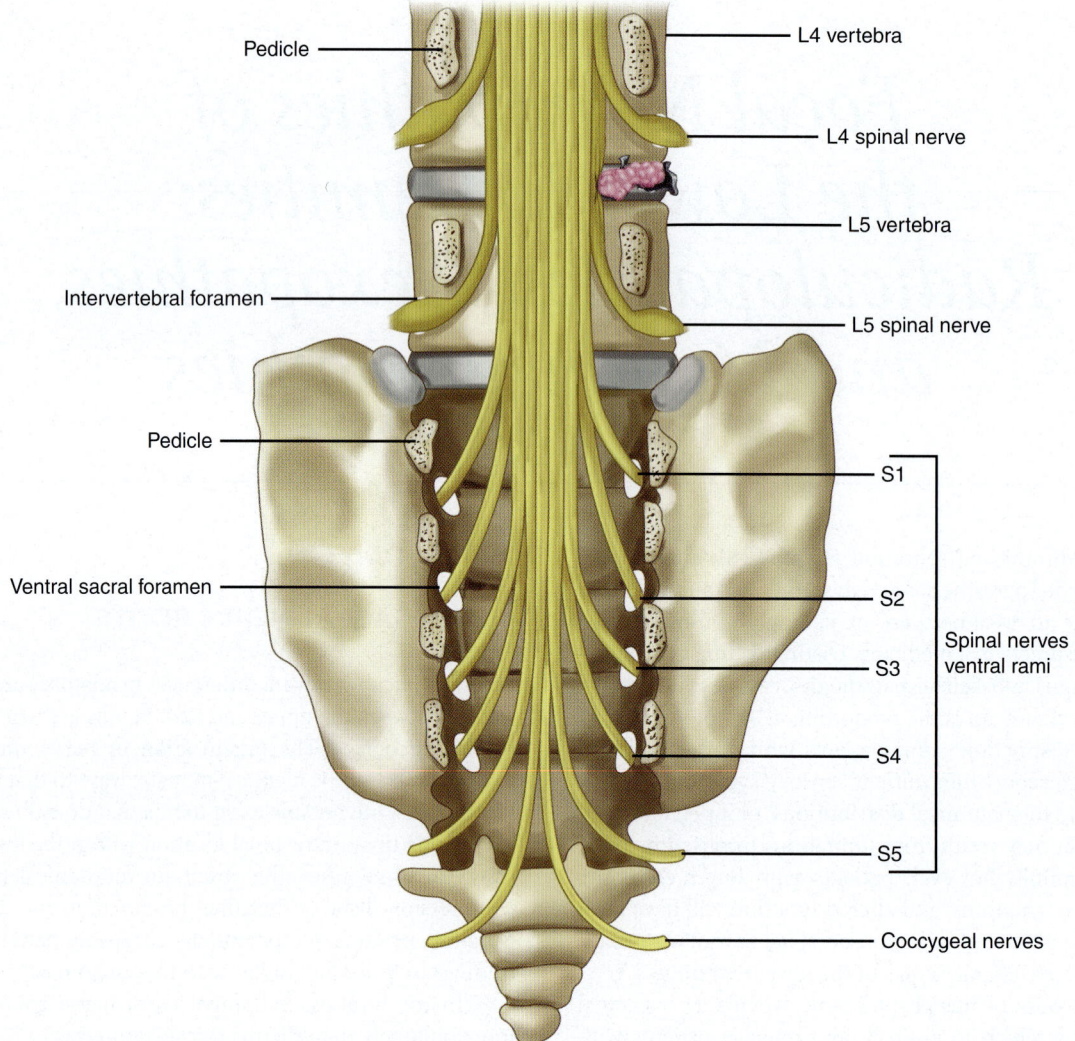

Figure 24-1. Anatomic correlations between disc herniation and affected nerve root in the lumbosacral spine.

perpendicularly, the nerve root that is preferentially compressed is related to how far medial or lateral the disc material protrudes. For example, disc herniation at L4–5 near the midline preferentially compresses a more medially positioned S1 or other sacral nerve root. Alternatively, the more typical posterior–lateral disc herniation, which occurs lateral to the posterior longitudinal ligament, may preferentially affect the L5 root. A very far lateral herniation may compress the laterally situated L4 root against its pedicle or overlying lamina (Fig. 24-1). To recall, in the cervical spine, the C5–6 disc pathology preferentially affects the C6 root, as their courses parallel one other.

Two potential variations from typical compressive radiculopathy should be recognized. Segmental patterns of injury do not necessarily originate from pathology of nerve roots, but rather from injury to the analogous segments of the spinal cord. This is particularly relevant if the pathology affects the cell bodies in the anterior horns but spares the centrifugally located descending motor and ascending sensory tracts. These segmental deficits may also result from compressive cord injury, sometimes at a level more rostral than the clinical deficits. Hypothetically, this results from an ischemic mechanism like that in neoplastic spinal cord compression. Lower motor neuron deficits resulting from presumed ischemic anterior horn cell injury has been described in injury from both cervical spondylitic myelopathy and dural arteriovenous fistula.[3,4] It is also true that radiculopathy can be obscured by myelopathy, particularly in the cervical and thoracic regions. A spondylitic bar encroaching on the spinal canal in the neck is more likely to manifest with tract rather than segmental signs and symptoms. In contrast, this same bar in the lumbosacral spine would result in a radiculopathic but not myelopathic presentation.

Mechanical causes underlie approximately 97% of cases of lower back pain, among which musculoskeletal syndromes of lower back strain or sprain are the most common.[5] Degenerative processes of the discs or facet joints including herniated discs and spinal stenosis account for approximately 10% of cases.[5] General approaches to lower back pain have been reviewed.[5–8] Physical exam maneuvers to help diagnose the cause of low back pain are also outlined.[9]

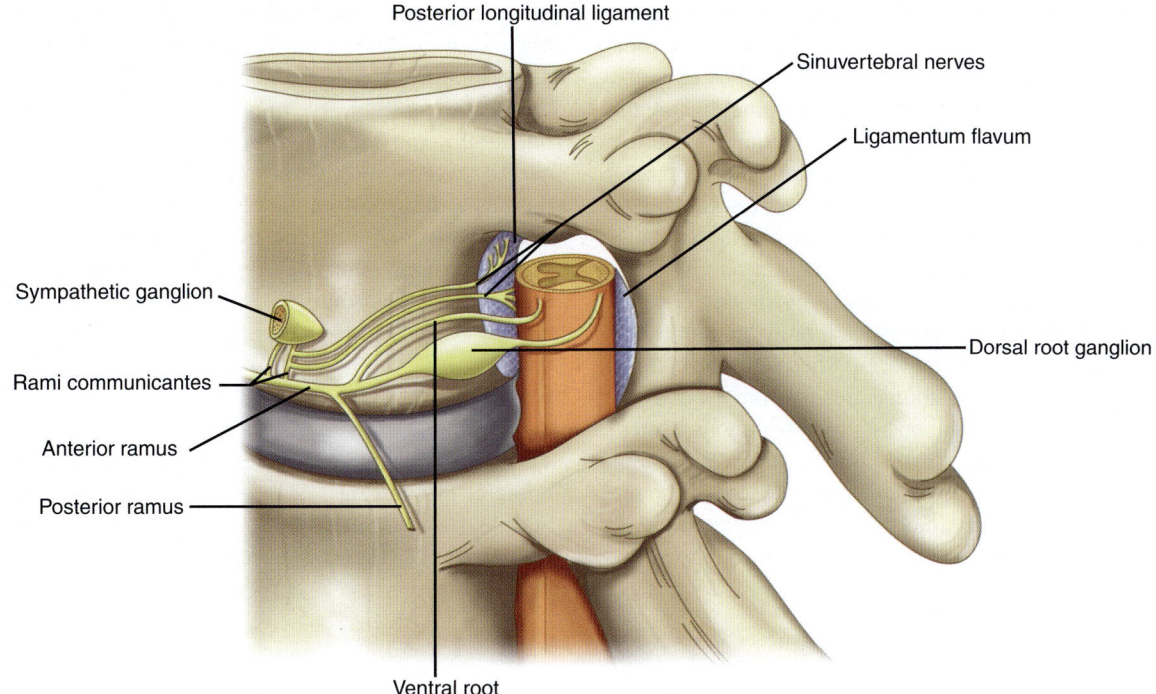

Figure 24-2. Anatomy of the spine.

This chapter will focus on radicular syndromes and pain. Understanding the neurologic presentation of radiculopathy requires a basic understanding of lumbosacral spine anatomy (Fig. 24-2).[5,9] Articular surfaces contribute to both the mobility and stability of the spine. These include the intervertebral discs and two pairs of synovial joints at each spinal level, which are called "facet" or zygapophyseal joints. Together, the pair forms the articular connections between contiguous vertebrae, the uncovertebral joints. Facet joints are comprised of extensions of two contiguous vertebral laminae and are innervated by branches of the posterior rami of spinal nerves. Diseases affecting these structures are some of the many potential sources of nonradiating back pain. Spinal nerve roots exit the spinal canal through neural foramina. Each foramen is bordered anteriorly by the intervertebral disc and adjacent vertebral body surfaces, posteriorly by the facet joint, and superiorly and inferiorly by pedicles.[9]

Two major ligamentous structures exist within the spinal canal: the posterior longitudinal ligament and the ligamentum flavum. Both are oriented longitudinally, the former running along the anterior aspect of the central canal just posterior to the vertebral bodies and disc spaces. The latter runs along the posterior aspect of the spinal canal just underneath the spinous processes. The posterior longitudinal ligament is half the width of its cervical counterpart in the lumbar spinal canal. This may add to an increased risk of paramedian disc herniation with potential consequence related to bowel and bladder control. The posterior longitudinal ligament is innervated by the sinuvertebral (recurrent meningeal or recurrent nerves of Luschka) nerves that arise from the rami communicantes outside the neural foramina. These travel posteriorly to innervate the dura, annulus fibrosis, the walls of intraspinal blood vessels as well as the posterior longitudinal ligaments (Fig. 24-2). The ligamentum flavum contains few nociceptive fibers. Its major clinical significance may be to contribute to canal stenosis by its tendency to hypertrophy as part of the spondylotic process. The diameter of the central canal averages 18 mm in most normal adults with a range of between 15 and 23 mm. As in the cervical canal, it widens by a few millimeters when the patient bends forward.

Although this is a text on neuromuscular disorders, it is appropriate to mention other potential sources of back, buttock, thigh, and leg pain. It is safe to say that isolated back pain without radicular pain or neurologic signs or symptoms may occur as the initial symptom of disorders which may eventually have neurologic consequences. It is equally safe to say that it may be difficult to initially distinguish common nonneurologic and often musculoskeletal causes of back pain from less common ones that have or may develop neurologic consequences. In the former category, potential anatomic sources of back pain include many spinal structures, such as the posterior longitudinal and other ligaments, capsules of the facet and sacroiliac joints, vertebral periosteum, dura, the paravertebral musculature and fascia, blood vessels, annulus fibrosus, spinal nerve roots, epidural veins and arterioles, and epidural fibroadipose tissue.[5] Identifying the anatomic source of back pain in an individual patient is an extremely difficult undertaking. Due to their lack or relative lack of nociceptive nerve endings, neither the nucleus pulposus nor the ligamentum flavum appear to be likely culprits.[9]

Degenerative spine disease (i.e., spondylosis) affects several different structures, which individually or collectively may narrow the diameter of the neural foramen or the central canal of the spinal column.[5] Consequently, nerve root integrity may be compromised in either location by enlargement of normal anatomic structures. Intraspinal ligaments may hypertrophy. Degeneration of the facet joints promotes osteophyte formation and space-occupying joint enlargement. Degeneration of the intervertebral disc results in bulging of the annular ring and loss of its vertical height, reducing interpedicular distances and contributing to foraminal narrowing. If both spondylolysis and resulting spondylolisthesis, which is the shifting of one vertebral body on another in an anterior–posterior direction, occur, then both the central canal and foraminal cross-sectional area are compromised.[5]

The intervertebral disc consists of a gelatinous center, the nucleus pulposus, and a cartilaginous margin, the annulus fibrosis. As mentioned, the concept of discogenic pain is somewhat nebulous in that there are few nociceptive pain fibers innervating the outer annulus and none within the nucleus pulposus itself. Although the pain and pathophysiology of nerve root disease are typically attributed to direct compression of the nerve root and the inflammation that accompanies it, it is important to remember that other potentially pain-sensitive structures such as the sinuvertebral nerves traverse the neural foramina as well.[10–12] Although there is a rich anastomotic blood supply to the spinal cord and nerve roots, ischemic injury resulting from radicular vascular compression may represent an alternative mechanism of nerve root injury.

LUMBOSACRAL PLEXUS

There is considerable variation in the anatomy of the lumbosacral plexus (Figs. 24-3 and 24-4). It may have contributions from as many as 11 spinal nerves but is typically composed of 8 (L1–S3). The lumbar plexus is predominantly

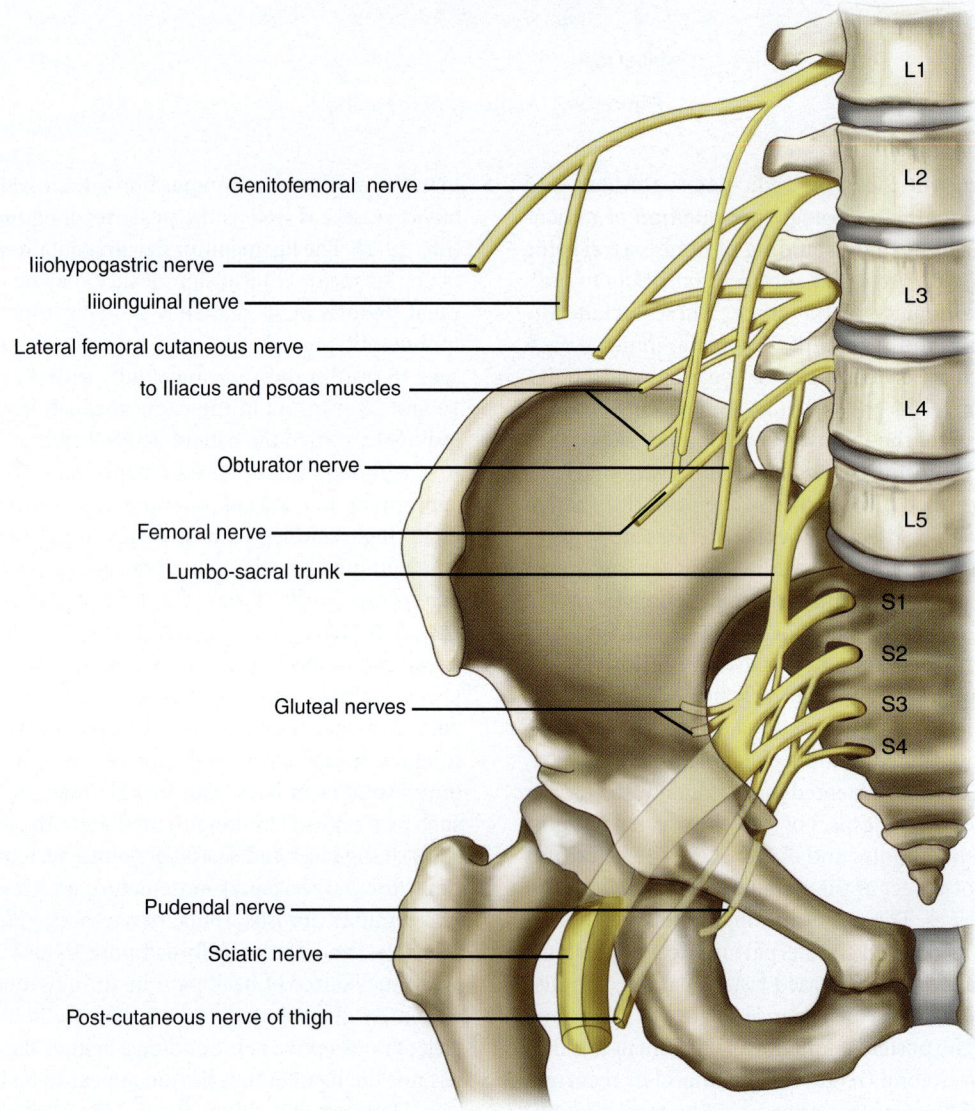

Figure 24-3. Lumbosacral plexus.

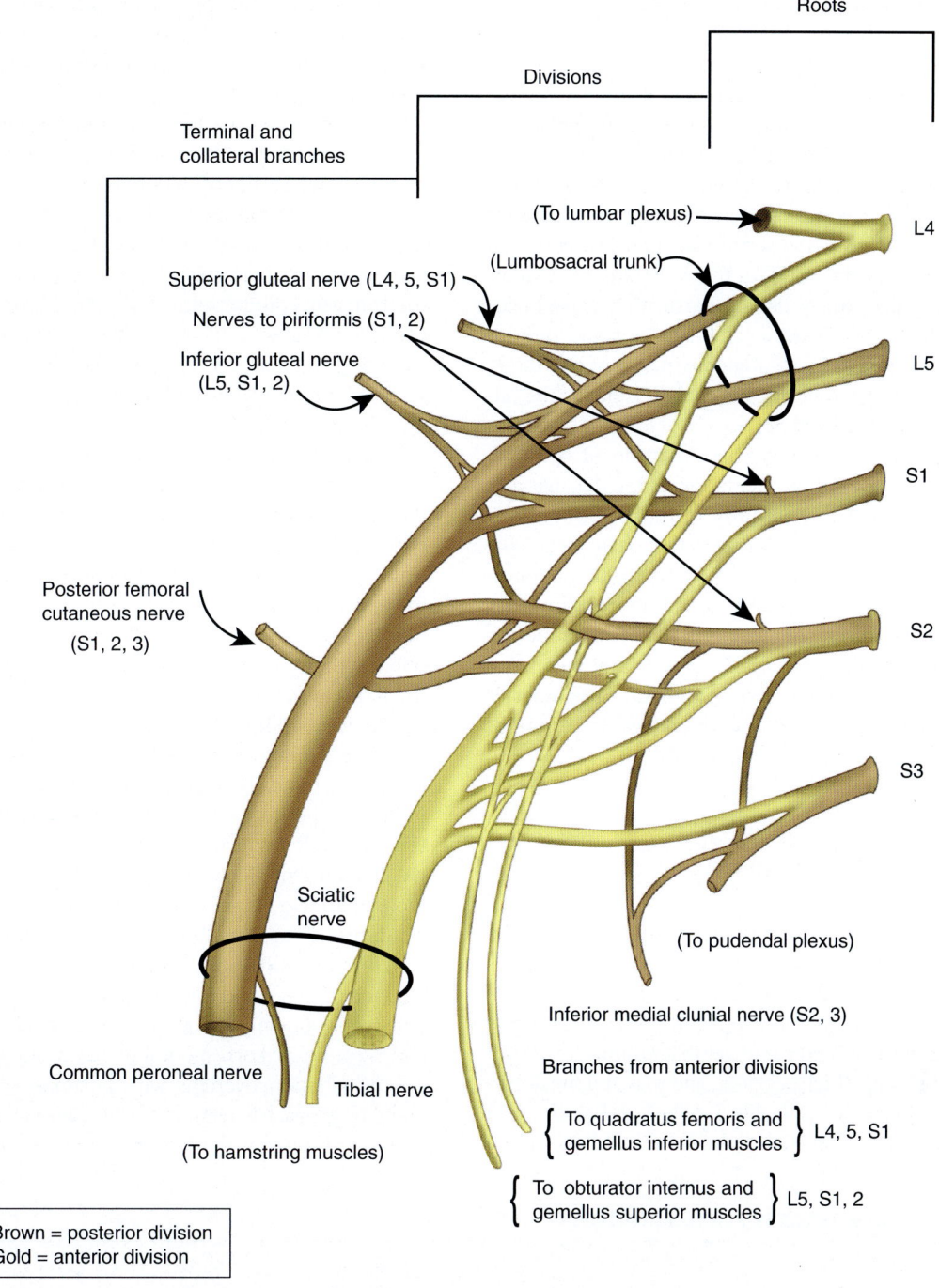

Figure 24-4. Lumbosacral trunk, sacral plexus, and sciatic nerve.

composed of branches from L1–L4, with variable contributions from T11, T12, and L5. Typically, the majority of L4 fibers travel with the lumbar plexus, with a much smaller contribution from L4 joining with L5 to form the lumbosacral trunk. In a "prefixed" plexus, the plexus shifts downward so that there is more of an L1 contribution to the lumbar plexus, the femoral and obturator nerves become comprised of L2–3 rather than L3–4 segmental contributions and the majority of L4 fibers end up in the sacral plexus. In the so-called "postfixed" plexus, the plexus is shifted upward so that virtually all of L4 and some of L5 are now confined within the lumbar rather than sacral plexuses.

The lumbar plexus is formed in the retroperitoneum, just inferior to the kidney and just behind the psoas muscle. Its blood supply originates from the internal iliac artery. Ischemic injury may occur from distal aortic or internal iliac arterial occlusion. The major branches of the upper lumbar plexus are the ilioinguinal, genitofemoral, and lateral femoral cutaneous nerve (LFCN) or lateral cutaneous nerve of the thigh. The femoral, obturator, and lumbosacral trunks are the major components of the lower aspect of the lumbar plexus.

The sacral plexus is formed within the concavity of the ventral surface of the sacrum, behind and lateral to the rectum. The L4 and L5 contributions to the sacral plexus and to the sciatic nerve are provided by the lumbosacral trunk, the conduit between the lumbar and the sacral plexuses. The lumbosacral trunk traverses the pelvic brim at the posterior aspect of the pelvis, over the sacral alae, and just lateral to the sacroiliac joints (Fig. 24-3). In this location, it is vulnerable to compressive injury during parturition. The major branches of the sacral plexus are the superior and inferior gluteal nerves, the posterior cutaneous nerve of the thigh, the fibular (formerly peroneal) and tibial divisions of the sciatic nerve, and the pudendal nerve.

As mentioned, the embryologic rotation of the limb results not only in the spiral orientation of the dermatomes and hip ligaments but in relocation of muscles from their original anatomic positions. Muscles that were originally located on the posterior surface of the lower limb are innervated by the posterior branches of the lumbosacral plexus, for example, femoral, fibular (formerly peroneal), superior, and inferior gluteal nerves as well as the lateral cutaneous nerve of the thigh. Muscles that were originally in an anterior location are innervated by anterior branches, for example, genitofemoral, obturator, and tibial nerves.

INDIVIDUAL PERIPHERAL NERVES OF THE LOWER EXTREMITIES

Identification of lower extremity mononeuropathies relies upon recognizing patterns of muscle weakness, sensory symptoms and loss of deep tendon reflexes, if applicable. As the pattern of muscle weakness provides the most objective localizing information, knowledge of the muscles that promote the major movements of the hip, thigh, leg, foot, and toes and the nerves that innervate them is invaluable (Tables 24-1 and 24-2). Determination of potential etiology however is enhanced by a detailed understanding of the relationship between the nerves and contiguous anatomic structures. The following paragraphs summarize the relevant lower extremity peripheral nerve anatomy.

The iliohypogastric nerve is primarily an extension of the L1 nerve root with some contribution from T12. It exits on the lateral border of the psoas muscle in proximity to the lower pole of the kidney and traverses the ventral surface of the quadratus lumborum muscle. It exits the abdominal wall superior to the iliac crest. It provides partial innervation to the transverse abdominus and internal oblique muscles of the abdominal wall. There are two cutaneous branches, one overlying the iliac crest in the posterior axillary line and a second innervating a small transverse patch above the pubic symphysis (Fig. 24-5).

The ilioinguinal nerve has a similar L1 segmental origin and anatomic course. Its course is parallel but caudal to the iliohypogastric nerve along the upper border of the iliac crest. Its course is retrocolic along the posterior abdominal wall. The nerve passes through the superficial inguinal ring to supply the skin overlying the inguinal ligament, extending to the regions just above the genitals and just below the pubic symphysis (Fig. 24-5). Like the iliohypogastric nerve, the ilioinguinal nerve innervates the transverse abdominus and internal oblique muscles.

The genitofemoral nerve has near equal contributions from the L1 and L2 segments. It penetrates the psoas muscle in the retroperitoneum and descends vertically along its ventral surface. It lies near the external iliac artery, ureters, terminal ileum on the right, and sigmoid colon on the left. Like the iliohypogastric nerve, it has two separate sensory branches. The larger of the two, the femoral branch, innervates the anterior, proximal thigh in the midline, just distal to the inguinal ligament. The second, smaller genital branch, supplies a small cutaneous zone on the lateral aspect of the root of the penis and scrotum or corresponding area of the labia. Its cutaneous distribution overlaps with portions of the ilioinguinal and iliohypogastric territories (Figs. 24-3 and 24-5). The only muscular branch is the cremaster muscle which controls the

▶ **TABLE 24-1. LUMBOSACRAL PLEXUS ANATOMY**

Muscles Innervated	Cutaneous Distribution	Segmental Contribution	Plexus	Nerve
Transverse abdominus and internal oblique	Superior iliac crest at the posterior axillary line and small patch above the pubic symphysis	T12, L1	Lumbar	Iliohypogastric
Transverse abdominus and internal oblique	Skin overlying the inguinal ligament extending to the base of penis	L1	Lumbar	Ilioinguinal
Cremaster	Anterior proximal thigh in midline just caudal to the inguinal ligament and the scrotum, labia majora, and adjacent thigh	L1, L2	Lumbar—anterior	Genitofemoral

▶ TABLE 24-1. (CONTINUED)

Muscles Innervated	Cutaneous Distribution	Segmental Contribution	Plexus	Nerve
None (sensory nerve)	Anterolateral thigh	L2–3	Lumbar—posterior	Lateral cutaneous nerve of the thigh
Psoas minor	None	L1–2–3	Lumbar	Branches of lumbar plexus and femoral
Iliacus and psoas major	None	L2–3–4	Lumbar	Branches of lumbar plexus and femoral
Sartorius	Anterior thigh	L2–3–4	Lumbar—posterior	Femoral
Rectus femoris, vastus lateralis–medialis–intermedius, and pectineus	Anterior thigh	L2–3–4	Lumbar	Femoral
None (sensory nerve)	Medial leg	L4	Lumbar	Saphenous
Gracilis, adductor magnus–longus–brevis, and obturator internus	Small patch of medial thigh	L2–3–4	Lumbar—anterior	Obturator (dual innervation from sciatic nerve to adductor magnus)
None (sensory nerve)	Posterior thigh, inferior buttock, lateral perineum, proximal medial thigh	S1–2–3	Sacral	Posterior cutaneous nerve of the thigh
Gluteus medius-minimus, and tensor fascia lata	None	L4–5, S1	Lumbosacral trunk Sacral—posterior	Superior gluteal
Gluteus maximus	None	L5, S1–2	Lumbosacral trunk Sacral—posterior	Inferior gluteal
External anal sphincter	Distal anal canal and perianal skin	S2–3–4	Sacral	Pudendal—inferior rectal
Muscles of the pelvic floor, external urethral sphincter, and the erectile tissue of the penis	Perineum ventral to the rectum as well as the scrotum and labia	S2–3–4	Sacral	Pudendal—perineal
None (sensory nerve)	Penis or labia	S2–3–4	Sacral	Pudendal—dorsal nerve of the penis/labia
Semimembranosus/semitendinosus	NA	L5, S1–2	Lumbosacral trunk Sacral—anterior	Sciatic—tibial
Long head of biceps femoris	NA	L5, S1–2	Lumbosacral trunk Sacral—anterior	Sciatic—tibial
Short head of biceps femoris	NA	L5, S1–2	Lumbosacral trunk Sacral—posterior	Sciatic—common fibular (peroneal)
Tibialis anterior, extensor digitorum longus and brevis, and extensor hallucis longus	Interspace between first and second digits	L4–5, S1	Lumbosacral trunk Sacral—posterior	Common fibular—deep fibular (peroneal)
Peroneus longus and brevis	Distal-lateral leg and dorsum of foot	L4–5, S1	Lumbosacral trunk Sacral—posterior	Common fibular—superficial fibular (peroneal)
Flexor hallucis longus, flexor digitorum longus, and tibialis posterior	NA	L5, S1	Lumbosacral trunk Sacral—anterior	Tibial
Medial and lateral gastrocnemius, soleus, plantaris, and popliteus	NA	S1–2	Sacral—anterior	Tibial
None (sensory nerve)	Lateral surface of foot	S1	Sacral	Sural
Intrinsic foot muscles (toe flexors–adductors–abductors)	Sole of the foot	S1–2	Sacral—anterior	Tibial—medial and lateral plantar nerves, calcaneal nerve

▶ TABLE 24-2. MUSCLES CONTRIBUTING TO SPECIFIC LOWER EXTREMITY MOVEMENTS

Hip						Knee		Ankle			
Flexion	Extension	Abduction	Adduction	External Rotation	Internal Rotation	Extension	Flexion	Dorsiflexion	Plantar Flexion	Inversion	Eversion
Iliopsoas	Gluteus maximus	Gluteus medius	Adductor magnus	Sartorius	Tensor fascia lata	Vastus medialis	Semimembranosus	Tibialis anterior	Medial gastrocnemius	Tibialis posterior	Peroneus longus
Rectus femoris	Adductor magnus	Gluteus minimus	Adductor longus	Iliopsoas	Gluteus medius	Vastus lateralis	Semitendinosus	Extensor digitorum longus	Lateral gastrocnemius	Tibialis anterior	Peroneus brevis
Sartorius	Long head of biceps femoris	Tensor fascia lata	Adductor brevis	Pectineus	Gluteus minimus	Vastus intermedius	Short head of biceps femoris	Extensor hallucis longus	Soleus	Flexor digitorum longus	Extensor digitorum longus
Pectineus	Semitendinosus	Piriformis	Gracilis	Adductor longus		Rectus femoris	Long head of biceps femoris		Peroneus longus	Flexor hallucis longus	Extensor hallucis longus
Adductor longus	Semimembranosus	Obturator internus	Iliopsoas	Adductor magnus			Sartorius		Peroneus brevis		
Adductor magnus		Gemelli	Pectineus	Gluteus maximus			Gracilis		Plantaris		
Tensor fascia lata				Gluteus medius			Popliteus		Flexor hallucis longus		
				Piriformis			Gastrocnemius		Flexor digitorum longus		
				Obturator internus			Plantaris		Tibialis posterior		
				Gemelli							
				Obturator externus							
				Quadratus femoris							

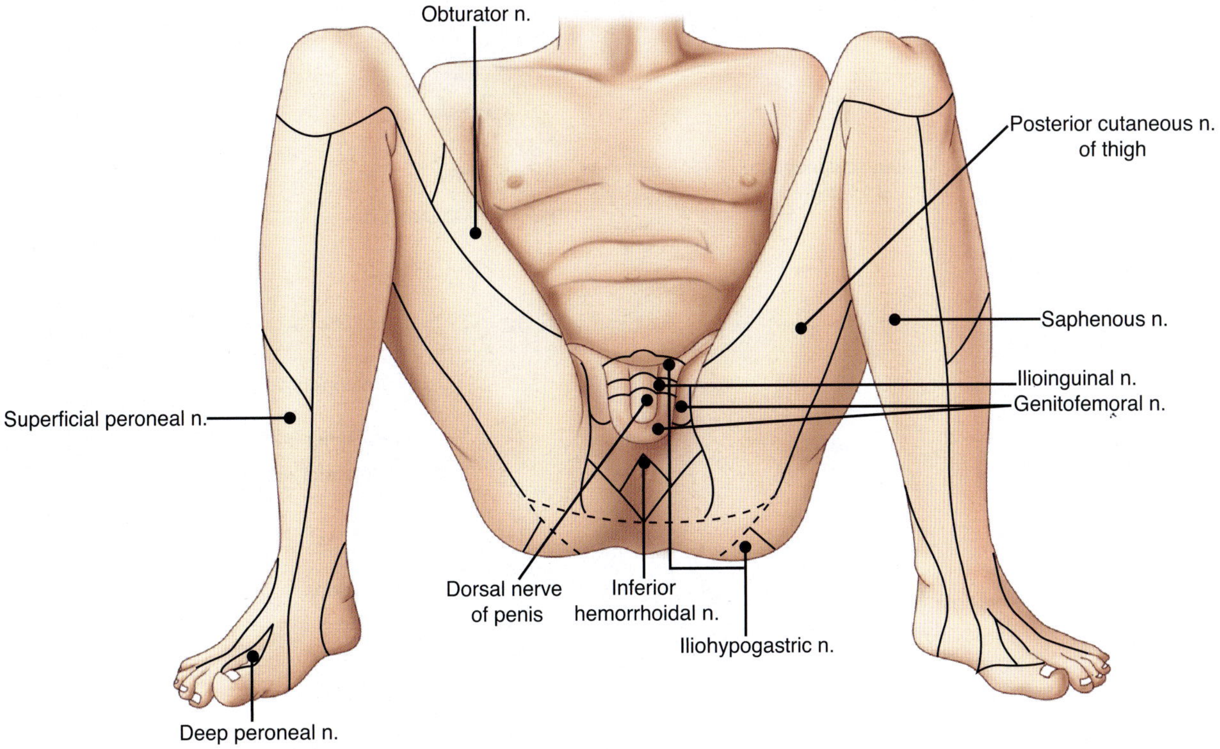

Figure 24-5. Cutaneous innervation of the groin, perineum, and genitals.

ascent/descent of the testes to maintain spermatic temperature homeostasis.

The obturator nerve receives contributions from the second through fourth lumbar segments (Figs. 24-3, 24-5 to 24-7). It emerges from the medial border of the psoas muscle just rostral to the pelvic brim and descends through the pelvis vertically, medial to the course of the femoral nerve, to exit the pelvis through the obturator foramen. It innervates the adductor longus, brevis, and a portion of the adductor magnus muscle, as well as the gracilis, and obturator externus muscles. The major function of these muscles is to adduct the thigh with contributions to thigh flexion and external rotation. Cutaneous sensation is supplied to a small patch on the inner thigh.

The femoral nerve is also an extension of the L2–4 segments (Figs. 24-3 and 24-7). It arises in a retroperitoneal location and passes between the psoas and the iliacus muscles before traveling under the iliacus fascia in the lateral pelvis, where it is vulnerable to an iliacus compartment syndrome. It exits the pelvis below the inguinal ligament and lateral to the femoral artery. From a motor perspective, the femoral nerve innervates the psoas and the iliacus muscles in the pelvis and six muscles in the thigh, including the four components of the quadriceps (the rectus femoris, and vastus lateralis, intermedius, and medialis), the sartorius, and the pectineus muscles. The primary function of most of these muscles is to extend the leg at the knee joint. In addition, the iliopsoas, sartorius, pectineus, and the rectus femoris all contribute to hip flexion. The rectus femoris is the only quadriceps muscle that originates from the pelvis and is therefore the only one of the quadriceps capable of contributing to hip flexion. The sartorius contributes to external rotation at the hip joint, flexion at the knee joint, and hip flexion is notable for two reasons. First, it is the longest muscle in the body and second, its actions move one's leg into the working position of a "tailor," from which its name is derived in Latin. The pectineus muscle contributes both to external rotation and adduction of the thigh. From a sensory perspective, the femoral nerve supplies sensation to the anterior surface of the thigh and the medial aspect of the leg through its terminal sensory branch, the saphenous nerve.

The LFCN is an extension of the second and third lumbar nerve roots (Figs. 24-3 and 24-6). It also emerges from the lateral border of the psoas and traverses the lateral pelvis deep to the iliacus fascia. It exits the pelvis at the anterior superior iliac spine, often penetrating the lateral margin of the inguinal ligament. It has no motor function and provides cutaneous innervation to the anterolateral thigh as well as the underlying fascia.

Prior to the actual formation of the sciatic nerve, there are four nerves originating from the upper sacral segments. The pudendal nerve is the more proximate of these, originating from the S2–4 segments. In a slightly more caudal location, the posterior cutaneous nerve of the thigh is formed by two or more S1–3 segments before these segments merge with the lumbosacral trunk to form the sciatic nerve which occurs just lateral and anterior to the sacrum. The last branches departing the sacral plexus prior to the formation of the sciatic nerve are the superior and inferior gluteal nerves. They are comprised of the L4–S1 and L5–S2

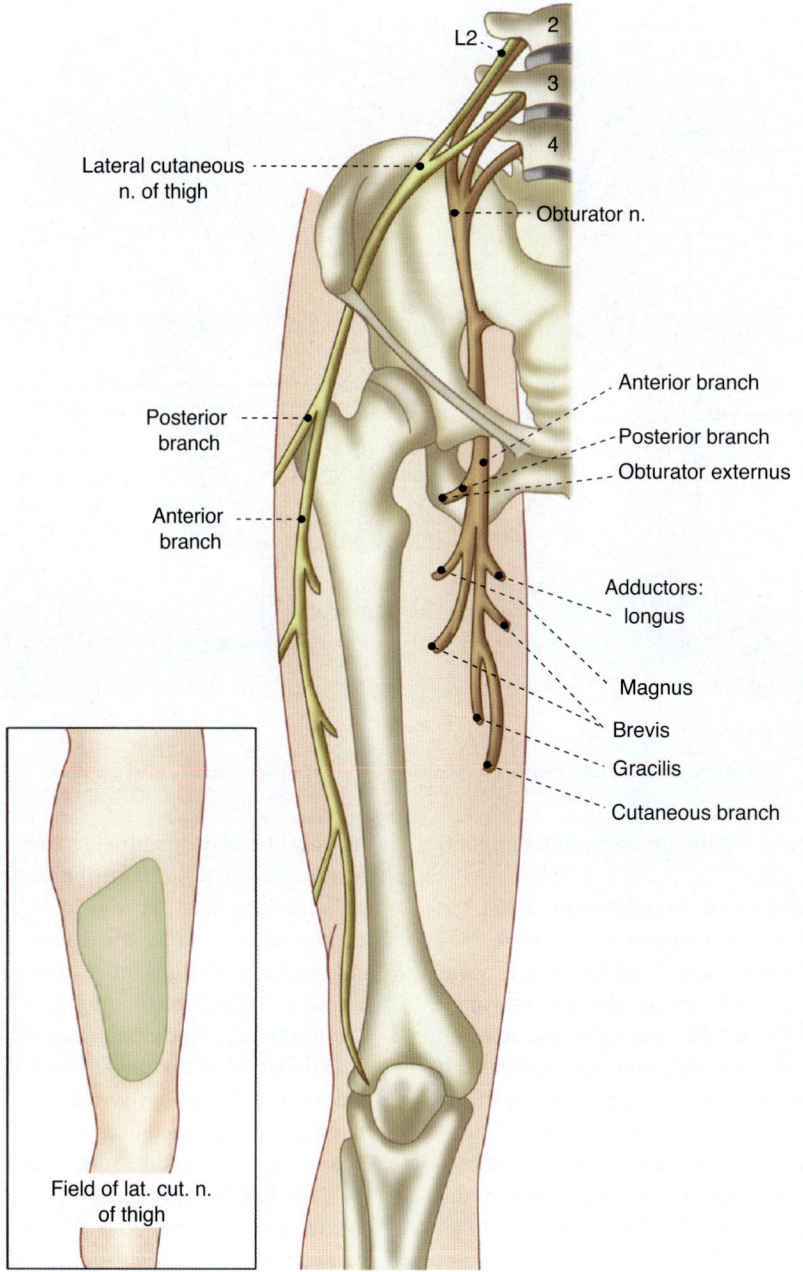

Figure 24-6. Obturator and lateral femoral cutaneous nerves. Cut, cutaneous.

segments, respectively. The superior gluteal nerve is typically the only nerve to exit the sciatic notch above the piriformis muscle, the sciatic, inferior gluteal, pudendal, and posterior cutaneous nerves of the thigh all typically exiting the sciatic notch caudal to this horizontally oriented muscle. Intramuscular injections are avoided in the inferior, medial quadrant of the buttocks, to avoid injury to these nerves which travel deep through this topographical location. The superior gluteal nerve innervates the gluteus medius, gluteus minimus, and tensor fascia lata muscles. Thigh abduction at the hip is their major action. All contribute to internal rotation of the thigh as well. The gluteus minimus provides a minor contribution to hip flexion, and the posterior aspect of the gluteus medius contributes partially to external rotation of the thigh. The inferior gluteal nerve innervates the gluteus maximus, which is the primary hip extensor, but also provides a minor contribution to external rotation. Neither gluteal nerve has a sensory component or cutaneous representation.

The sciatic nerve receives contributions from the last two lumbar roots via the lumbosacral trunk and the first three sacral segments (Figs. 24-3 and 24-4). In fact, the sciatic nerve is comprised of two nerves that are conjoined, the tibial and the fibular (formerly peroneal) nerves. This is a helpful concept to keep in mind as many sciatic neuropathies preferentially affect the fibular nerve and may mimic a fibular neuropathy at a more distal location. The segmental

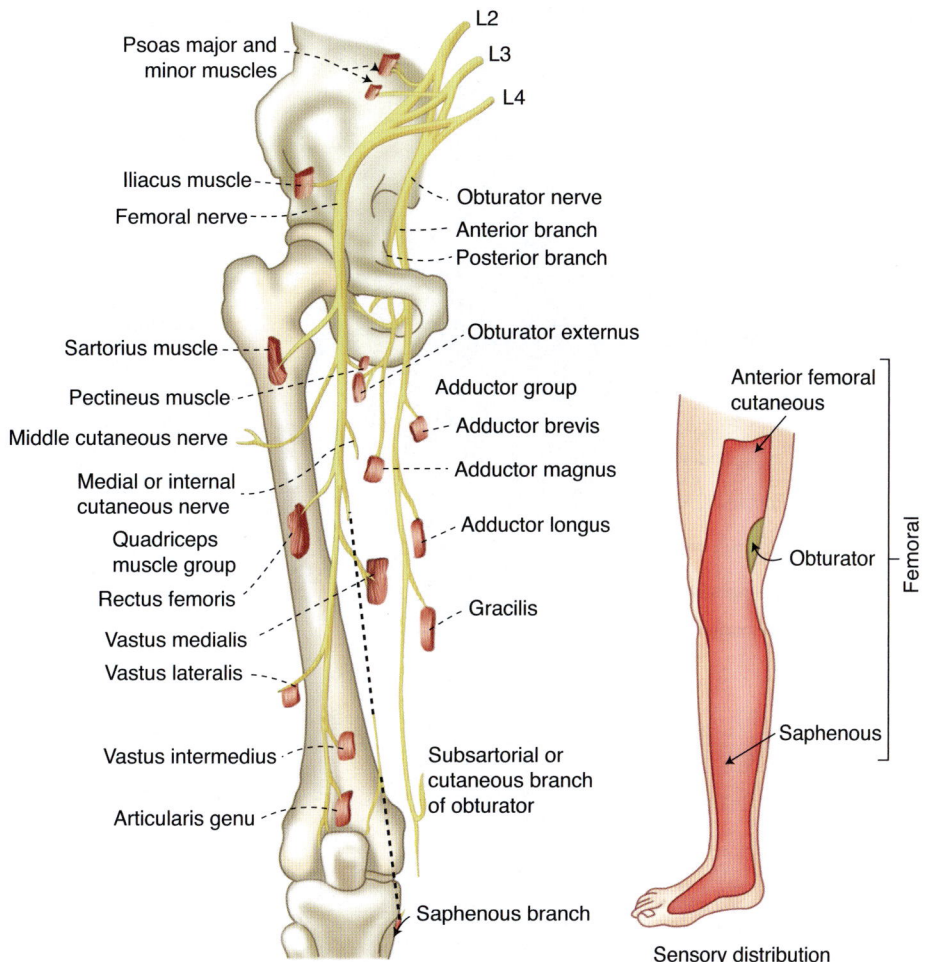

Figure 24-7. Femoral and obturator nerves.

contribution to these two nerves is also different. The peroneal nerve contains few, if any, S3 fibers, whereas there is no meaningful L4 contribution to the tibial nerve in most individuals. The sciatic nerve exits the pelvis through the sciatic notch, typically beneath the piriformis muscle, but at times traversing through or above it. The former provides the anatomic basis for the controversial piriformis syndrome. The sciatic nerve descends lateral to the ischial tuberosity of the pelvis and medial to the greater trochanter of the proximal femur, where it is potentially vulnerable not only to misplaced injections but also to displaced hip fractures or inadvertent injury during arthroplasty.[13–14]

In the thigh, the sciatic nerve innervates the hamstrings. The short head of the biceps femoris is innervated by the lateral trunk or fibular (peroneal) portion of the nerve. The short head of the biceps femoris is the most proximal fibular innervated muscle and the only one proximal to the fibular head. The three remaining hamstring muscles (semitendinosus, semimembranosus, and long head of the biceps femoris) are innervated by the medial trunk of the sciatic nerve which is the tibial division. The lateral two muscles are largely S1-innervated whereas the medial two muscles (semitendinosus and semimembranosus) are predominantly L5. In addition, the adductor magnus may receive partial innervation by the sciatic nerve, providing a potential source of EDX confusion for the unwary. A lesion of the sciatic nerve proximal to the knee will produce a pattern of sensory symptoms or sensory loss that includes the entire foot and the distal half of the lateral surface of the leg, sparing the L4/saphenous innervated medial leg. The blood supply to the sciatic nerve originates predominantly from branches of the inferior gluteal artery and popliteal arteries. This creates a watershed at mid-thigh level, which has been proposed as an explanation for both the location and prevalence of sciatic neuropathies in vasculitis.[15–16]

The posterior cutaneous nerve of the thigh exits the pelvis through the lower sciatic notch, medial to the sciatic nerve, and lateral to the pudendal nerve. Like the sciatic nerve, it may travel through the piriformis muscle in some individuals. It travels deep to the gluteus maximus which protects it. At the level of the gluteal crease, cluneal branches exit and ascend to supply the skin of the buttocks. There are perineal branches as well, which supply the skin and fascia of the lateral perineum, the proximal medial thigh, and the posterolateral aspect of the scrotum/labia as well as the root

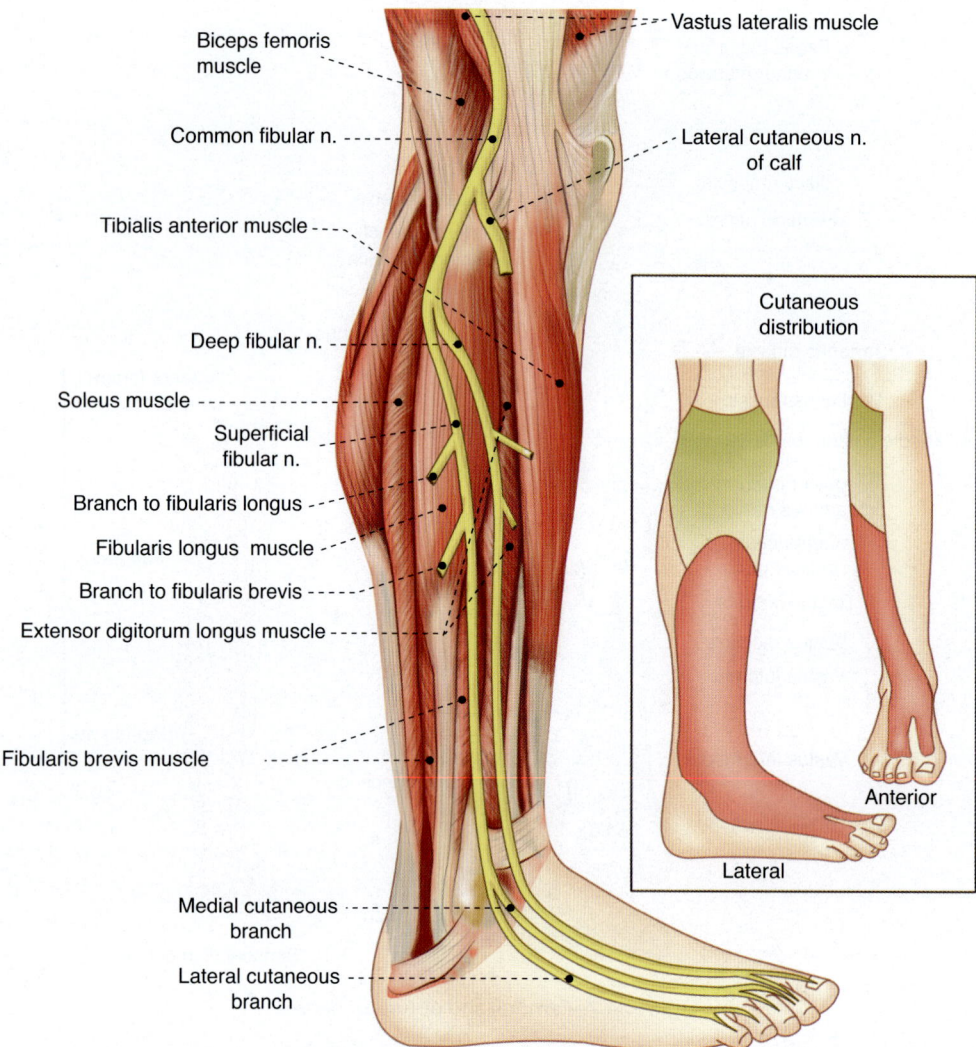

Figure 24-8. Fibular (peroneal) nerve.

of the penis/clitoris. The terminal branch descends vertically to provide sensory capability to the posterior thigh and often proximal aspect of the posterior calf. The posterior cutaneous nerve of the thigh has no motor function.

In the leg, the common fibular nerve bifurcates below the level of the fibular head into its deep fibular (peroneal) and superficial fibular divisions (Figs. 24-4 and 24-8). The deep fibular nerve innervates the muscles of the anterior compartment: the tibialis anterior (TA), the extensor hallucis, the extensor digitorum longus, and the peroneus tertius. In the foot, the deep fibular nerve innervates only one muscle, the extensor digitorum brevis (EDB). Collectively, the major function of these muscles is to dorsiflex the foot at the ankle and to extend the toes at the metatarsal–phalangeal joints. Notably, however, the peroneus tertius also contributes to ankle eversion. The superficial fibular (peroneal) nerve innervates the lateral compartment of the leg, including the peroneus longus and brevis muscles. The major function of these muscles is to evert the foot at the ankle. The deep fibular nerve has a predominantly motor function with a very small cutaneous contribution to the webspace between the first and second toes. The superficial fibular nerve innervates the skin of the dorsal surface of the foot and the lateral portion of the lower leg.

The tibial nerve receives contributions from L5–S3 nerve roots and is the continuation of the medial portion of the sciatic nerve (Figs. 24-4 and 24-9). It physically separates itself from its fibular (peroneal) counterpart in the distal thigh, just proximal to or at the knee. It then passes through the popliteal fossa and courses between the medial and lateral gastrocnemius muscles. As previously mentioned, tibial branches of the sciatic nerve innervate three of the four hamstring muscles in the thigh. In the leg, the tibial nerve proper supplies the posterior compartment including the two heads of the gastrocnemius, soleus, tibialis posterior, flexor digitorum longus, and flexor hallucis longus muscles. In the foot, it supplies all intrinsic foot muscles except the EDB. Its primary functions are to flex the leg at the knee, to plantar flex and invert the foot at the ankle, and to flex, abduct, and adduct the toes. The three cutaneous branches of the tibial nerve all

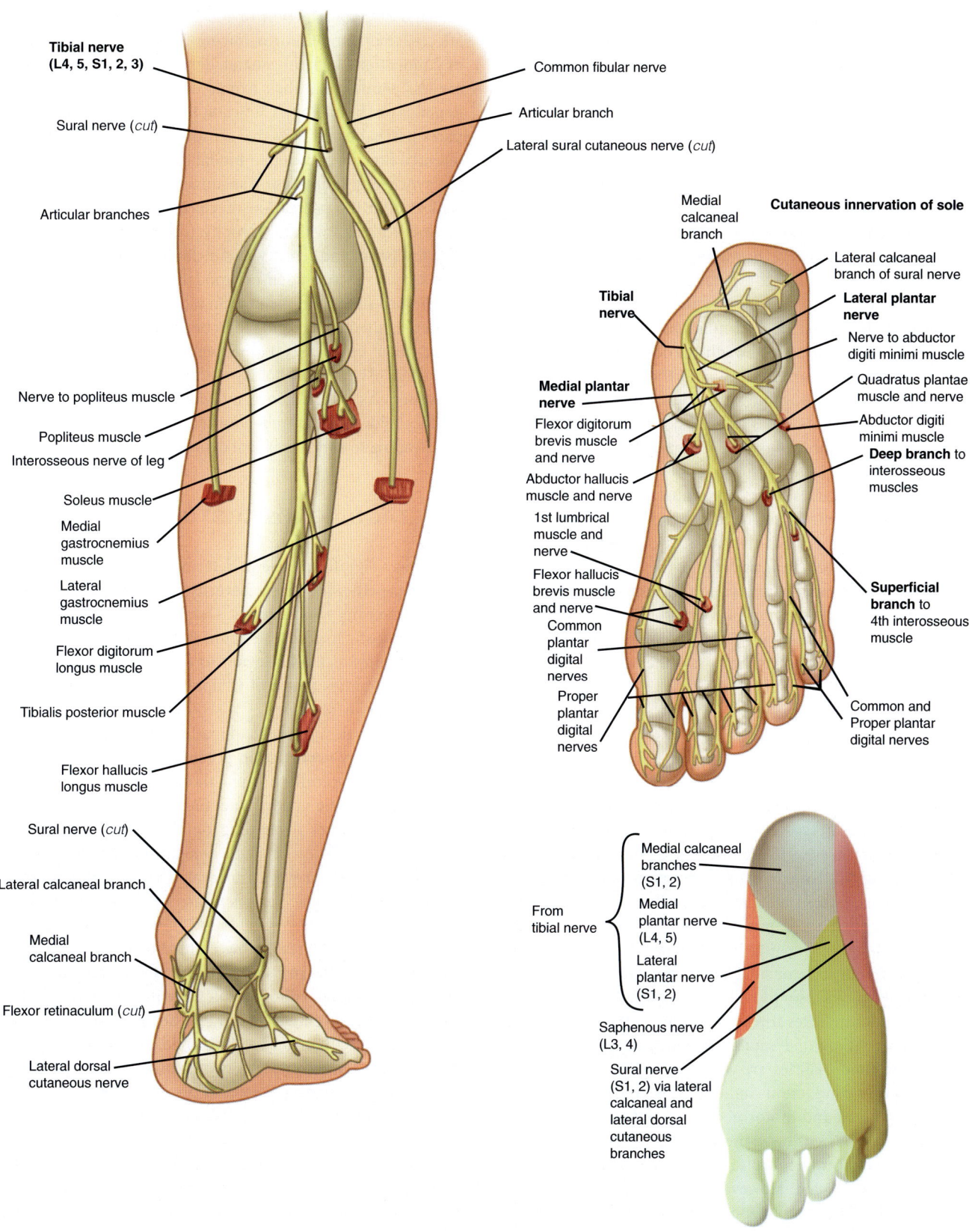

Figure 24-9. Tibial nerve. Cut, cutaneous.

branch at the level of the medial malleolus and include the medial and lateral plantar and calcaneal nerves. These provide the cutaneous innervation for the medial sole, lateral sole, and heel surface, respectively.

The sural nerve is formed in the popliteal fossa by anastomotic contributions from the common fibular and tibial nerves. It is derived primarily from the S1 nerve root. It descends in a superficial, posterior position in the calf, moving laterally as it courses posterior to the lateral malleolus. It provides cutaneous innervation to the lateral foot.

The pudendal nerve has a convoluted course. It first exits the pelvis through the greater gluteal foramen only to re-enter through a narrow aperture and potential site of entrapment between the sacrotuberous and sacrospinous ligaments. It then passes through Alcock canal created by the obturator muscle posteriorly and the ischial tuberosity anteriorly before exiting the pelvis permanently just below the pubis symphysis.[17] It has three major branches: the inferior rectal (or hemorrhoidal), the perineal, and the dorsal nerve of the penis/clitoris (Figs. 24-3 to 24-5). The inferior rectal nerve innervates the external anal sphincter and supplies sensation to the distal anal canal and perianal skin. The perineal nerve innervates the muscles of the pelvic floor, the external urethral sphincter, and the erectile tissue of the penis. Its cutaneous innervation includes the perineum anterior to the rectum as well as the scrotum and labia. The dorsal nerve of the penis is a purely sensory branch whose cutaneous representation is the skin of the penis and labia.

PATHOPHYSIOLOGY

The pathophysiology of peripheral nerve injury has been described in detail in Chapters 2 and 3. Axon loss with Wallerian degeneration typically results from disorders that infiltrate or infarct nerves. It can also result from when nerves are sufficiently inflamed or mechanically injured by compression or stretch of adequate intensity and/or duration. Axon loss is often accompanied by pain, typically described as deep, aching, or burning in character. Pain is common, particularly with acute or subacute pathologic. Muscle weakness and atrophy, sensory loss that affects all modalities, loss of deep tendon reflexes if relevant to the nerve injured, and even manifestations of dysautonomia including sweating and vasomotor abnormalities are anticipated. Electrodiagnostically, on nerve conduction studies (NCSs), the amplitudes of involved sensory and motor nerves are reduced once sufficient time has passed to see these changes. Acutely, reduced recruitment of normal morphology motor unit action potentials (MUAPs) is seen. However, as the weeks and months pass, fibrillation potentials/positive sharp waves and then reinnervation changes in MUAP morphology emerge.

Many experimental models of nerve compression support the belief that myelin is preferentially damaged in the early stages of external compression or internal entrapment. Electrodiagnostically, this myelin dysfunction can manifest through any combination of focal and uniform slowing of affected fibers, nonuniform slowing (i.e., temporal dispersion), or conduction block. In general, demyelinating nerve injuries are less painful than their axonal counterparts, but this also depends on the etiology. Clinically, focal slowing may produce paresthesias but no objective sensory or motor deficits. Differential slowing may impair modalities that are dependent on the synchrony of impulse transmission such as deep tendon reflexes and the perception of vibration. Conduction block causes weakness without atrophy (other than that attributable to disuse) and sensory loss including vibration and position sense as these are sensory modalities dependent on large, myelinated fibers. Needle examination of muscles innervated by nerves affected by conduction block demonstrates reduced recruitment of MUAPs but neither fibrillation potentials nor abnormal MUAP morphology as there is no axon loss or reinnervation. As implied above, individual fibers may be affected by focal slowing, demyelinating conduction block, or axon loss, leading to a mixed axonal demyelinating EDX pattern.

ELECTRODIAGNOSTIC STUDIES

EDX has a significant role in determination of the existence, location, pathophysiology, severity, and prognosis of focal lower extremity neuropathies. Detailed description of EDX as a diagnostic tool can be found in Chapter 2 and many of the principles of EDX relevant to focal neuropathies of the upper extremities found in Chapter 23 and in the previous section apply here as well.

In general, monoradiculopathies are characterized by normal sensory nerve action potentials (SNAPs) in relevant dermatomes, typically normal though sometimes reduced compound muscle action potential amplitudes (CMAP) in relevant myotomes depending on the degree and type of injury, and evidence of acute denervation and/or chronic reinnervation in muscles innervated by a single segment but by more than one peripheral nerve. Denervation is frequently, but not universally, found in analogous paraspinal muscle segments. Presumably, failure to demonstrate paraspinal denervation in radiculopathy reflects sampling error, and demyelinating pathophysiology or in more longstanding cases, successful reinnervation. Practically speaking, monoradiculopathies that can be confirmed electrodiagnostically have at least some components of axon loss as the ability to identify demyelinating lesions in proximal locations is limited by anatomic and other considerations.

For example, the EDX pattern of an L5 radiculopathy would include a normal superficial peroneal SNAP and typically normal, and less commonly reduced, CMAP amplitude recording from the peroneal-EDB or TA muscles. There would be evidence of denervation in muscles such as TA, tibialis posterior, flexor digitorum longus, tensor fascia lata as well as lumbosacral paraspinal muscles. These share L5 segmental innervation but are innervated by multiple peripheral nerves. Like the clinical examination however, not all muscles innervated by the L5 segment will be denervated in every patient, and because of fascicular involvement and reinnervation, not all muscles will be denervated to the same degree.[18]

Polyradiculopathy has a similar EDX pattern. The major exception is the pattern of denervation and/or reinnervation on needle EMG, which, by definition, is found in multiple myotomal segments and may even be bilateral. The major distinction between polyradiculopathy and multifocal neuropathy or plexopathy is the sparing of SNAPs in polyradiculopathy. However, variables such as advanced age, intraspinal positioning of the dorsal root ganglia (L5 radiculopathy), lower extremity edema, or concomitant but unrelated polyneuropathy, which may be confounding. In addition, particularly in chronic polyradiculopathies such as lumbar spinal stenosis, denervation may take on a pseudo-length–dependent pattern, which is more commonly seen in polyneuropathy.[19] CMAP amplitudes are also more likely to be reduced as the protection offered to individual muscles by multisegmental innervation is less robust.

Polyradiculoneuropathy or radiculoplexus neuropathy is a pattern that is arguably more relevant to the lower extremities in view of the predilection for diabetes to affect lumbar nerve roots and contiguous plexus and nerve elements. It is a pattern that may also occur with acquired, inflammatory demyelinating neuropathies, but these are usually easily distinguished both by phenotype and by characteristic demyelinating features on NCSs. In general, polyradiculoneuropathies are electrodiagnostically defined by concomitant paraspinal denervation and abnormal SNAPs.

Plexopathies are typically monomelic but may affect the contralateral limb concomitantly or sequentially, depending on etiology. Both clinically and electrodiagnostically, the pattern is typically one of both motor and sensory involvement involving multiple peripheral nerve and nerve root distributions. Relevant SNAP and CMAP amplitudes are reduced. Denervation will be found in proximal as well as distal limb muscles innervated by the same elements of the plexus. For example, both the tensor fascia lata and the TA would be affected in a lumbosacral trunk lesion. However, abnormalities should not occur in the representative areas of the lumbosacral paraspinal muscles. Demyelinating features may occur in plexopathies but are again often obscured by the proximal location of the pathology, which is difficult to assess on routine NCSs. Uncommonly focal, acquired demyelinating neuropathies such as multifocal acquired demyelinating sensory and motor neuropathy (MADSAM or Lewis–Sumner syndrome) may initially occur in a pattern that is both clinically and electrodiagnostically suggestive of plexopathy, although MADSAM more commonly affects the upper extremities.[17]

In mononeuropathies which result in axon loss, reduced SNAP and CMAP amplitudes are expected, assuming EDX are performed late enough to have allowed completion of Wallerian degeneration. Mild degrees of axon loss may be more readily detected by comparing the amplitude of the affected to the unaffected side rather than to population reference values. This is particularly true for SNAPs. Most electrodiagnosticians consider an amplitude of less than 50% of the unaffected side to be abnormal. Denervation on needle examination would be confined to muscles innervated by the peripheral nerve in question but may be limited by site of injury along the length of the nerve as well as by selective fascicular involvement. As an example, denervation would occur in the TA, but not in the peroneus longus muscle in a deep peroneal neuropathy with associated axonal loss. The same pattern of denervation, however, could conceivably be observed in more proximal neuropathies affecting the common peroneal or even sciatic nerves, due to selective fascicular involvement. Fibers destined to innervate specific muscles may be sequestered to specific nerve fascicles. Therefore, a partial nerve injury in a proximal location may result in selective fascicular injury resulting in an incomplete pattern of denervation.[20,21]

The EDX pattern in primarily demyelinating mononeuropathies differs considerably from their axonal counterparts. Again, by definition, the pattern of abnormalities would be confined to a singular nerve distribution. Sensory nerve conductions should be normal unless there is an axonal component to the injury or there is conduction block that exists between the stimulation and recording sites. Demyelination will have no effect on the conductive properties of a nerve if the lesion is either proximal or distal (as opposed to within) the tested segment of nerve. For example, with a demyelinating common fibular neuropathy at the fibular head, the superficial fibular SNAP amplitude obtained from a location distal to the site of pathology will be normal. Similarly, the CMAP amplitude will be normal if the stimulation site is below the demyelinated segment. For that reason, in any suspected demyelinating mononeuropathy, an attempt should be made if technically possible to stimulate the nerve in question above, and if possible, across the affected site. This allows not only for identification of the abnormality, but also for precise localization and prognostic information. Needle EMG in a demyelinating mononeuropathy may be normal or consist of reduced recruitment of normal-appearing MUAPs if there is a conduction block. Focal slowing and temporal dispersion are not associated with abnormalities on needle examination. As many nerve injuries include demyelinating and axonal components, it is not uncommon to identify EDX features associated with both types of injuries.

IMAGING

Historically, x-rays of the lumbosacral spine were performed routinely in patients with back or radicular pain. In consideration of radiation exposure and their very limited yield in this clinical context, we agree with those who would utilize routine back x-rays for those with significant trauma, those with symptoms or at high risk for systemic disease, or those with histories suggesting recent compression fracture.[5]

When indicated and when feasible, magnetic resonance imaging (MRI) is the imaging procedure of choice for suspected mono- or polyradiculopathy. Although we have a low threshold for ordering MRIs in individuals with radiculopathy and neurologic deficits, we do not consider it mandatory. We are comfortable following someone clinically when all information points to a routine compressive radiculopathy due to disc herniation, if improvement with subsequent evaluations can be demonstrated and red flags are absent. Key red flags include fever, systemic infection, history of cancer, trauma, use of chronic corticosteroids, osteoporosis, or bowel or bladder symptoms. Information gleaned from imaging studies requires careful clinical correlation as incidental findings are exceedingly frequent. Depending on age, herniated discs are identifiable in 20%–40% of asymptomatic individuals and bulging discs in 80%.[5] The decision to utilize gadolinium is individualized. It provides limited benefit in typical discogenic or spondylotic disease and poses some risk, particularly in those with reduced glomerular filtration. Gadolinium is most likely to be helpful in those with prior back surgery, or if there is suspicion of systemic disease (i.e., malignancy, infection, inflammatory polyradiculoneuropathy) as the cause of radiculopathy. If MRI is precluded for any reason, postmyelographic CT scans provide an excellent imaging surrogate for nerve root disease. Although ultrasound has other roles in the evaluation of neuromuscular disorders, it has limited or no utility in the evaluation of radiculopathy.[22]

MRI has become the modality of choice for evaluation of lumbosacral plexopathy or radiculoplexopathy as well, particularly utilizing 3 Tesla or higher neurography techniques.[23] It is valuable not only with structural pathology of nerve-like neurofibromatosis, but also in presumed inflammatory or ischemic injury, in disorders such as nondiabetic lumbosacral radiculoplexus neuropathy (non-DLRPN).[23,24] Its resolution is superior to CT, and it provides the added benefit of readily providing axial, sagittal, and coronal viewing planes. Gadolinium is often of value, as neoplastic and inflammatory conditions are both relatively common causes of plexopathy, whose identification and characterization will be enhanced with the addition of gadolinium.[25]

Imaging of mononeuropathies in the lower extremities, particularly in proximal locations, is rendered difficult not only by the small diameter and circuitous course of the nerves, but also by the complex regional anatomy. MRI and/or ultrasound imaging of at least seven nerves (femoral, lateral femoral cutaneous, obturator, sciatic, superior and inferior gluteal, and pudendal) are feasible and warranted in the case of unexplained or progressive neuropathies identified by clinical and/or EDX means.[17] The imaging may allow for identification of focal T2 signal abnormalities at sites of compression, nerve enlargement and enhancement from neural tumors, enhancement from focal inflammatory lesions, or external compression from any contiguous mass.[23] Imaging may also have a therapeutic application, allowing, for example, more precise application of steroid injections in obese individuals with meralgia paresthetica (MP) in whom normal anatomic landmarks may be difficult to identify.[17] Diffusion tensor imaging has been utilized to detect axonal changes in patients with peripheral neuropathy. Conceivably, this or similar technologies could allow for imaging and monitoring of axonal regeneration after injury and/or therapeutic intervention.[26]

▶ SPECIFIC DISORDERS

MONORADICULOPATHIES

Lumbosacral radiculopathies are more prevalent than their cervical or thoracic counterparts. They typically result from mechanical compression from some aspect of spondyloarthropathy: narrowing of the central canal or lateral recesses, and/or neural foramina by disc material, osteophyte, hypertrophied ligament, or some combination thereof. Less commonly, they may result from compression from a hematoma, abscess, benign or malignant neoplasm, or infectious and inflammatory disorders with predilection for nerve roots or meninges (Table 24-3 and Fig. 24-10). A heightened index of suspicion is required for these less common causes. The primary symptom of monoradiculopathy is pain, colloquially

▶ **TABLE 24-3. MONORADICULOPATHIES: PATTERNS OF CLINICAL INVOLVEMENT**

Nerve Root	Muscle Action Most Commonly Weak	Other Muscle Actions That May Be Weak	Characteristic Areas of Sensory Symptoms/Sensory Loss	Reflex Loss
L2	Hip flexion	NA	Anterior thigh	Cremasteric
L3	Knee extension (one leg partial squat)	Hip flexion and adduction	Medial knee	Quadriceps reflex
L4	Knee extension (one leg partial squat)	Hip flexion and adduction	Medial leg	Quadriceps reflex
L5	Great toe dorsiflexion	Dorsiflexion of digits II–V and foot, ankle inversion and eversion, knee flexion, and hip abduction	Great toe, dorsum of foot, and distal-lateral leg	+/− Internal hamstring
S1	Foot plantar flexion (single leg heel lift)	Toe and knee flexion and hip extension	Digits IV and V, lateral foot, and heel and plantar surface	Achilles reflex

CHAPTER 24 FOCAL NEUROPATHIES OF THE LOWER EXTREMITIES 579

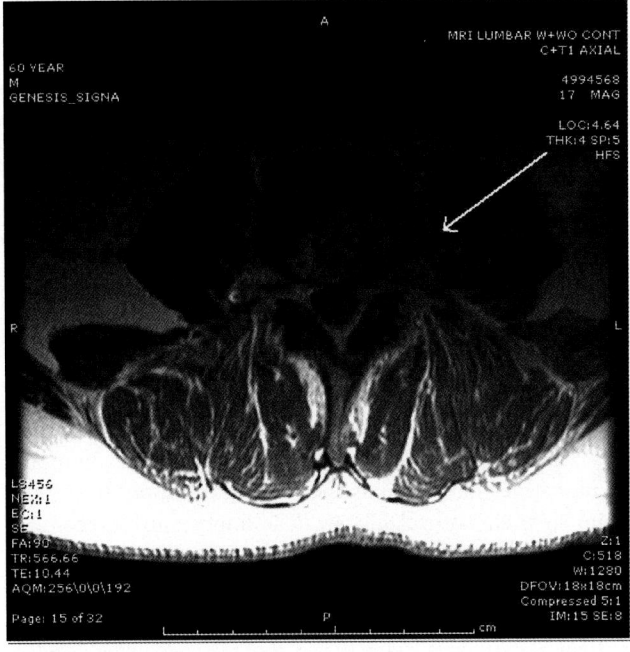 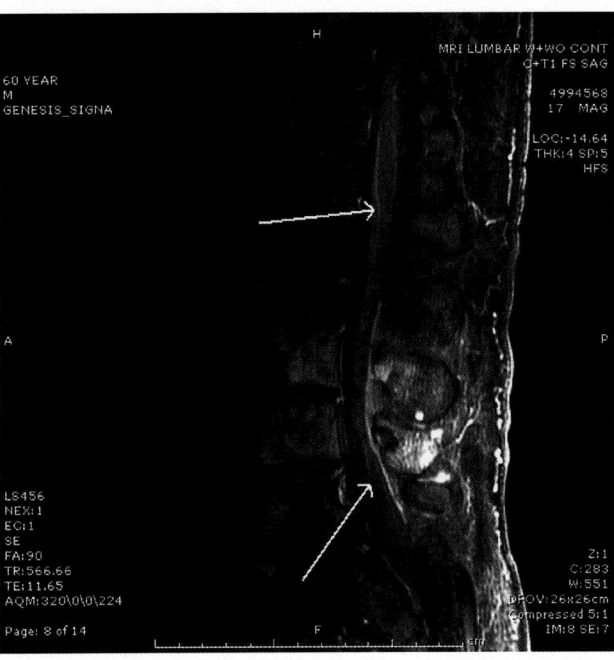

Figure 24-10. Gadolinium-enhanced T1 (**A**) axial and (**B**) sagittal MR images of the lumbar spine in a 60-year-old male with atypical, progressive left L3–L4 radiculopathy demonstrating abnormal enhancement of multiple vertebral bodies, epidural space, cauda equina, and left L2–3, 3–4, and 4–5 neural foramina resulting from previously asymptomatic B-cell lymphoma.

described as "sciatica" due to its linear trajectory following the course of the sciatic nerve in most cases. It has been estimated that disc herniations associated with objective neurologic deficits occur in the complete absence of pain in only 1/1,000 patients.[5]

Radicular pain in the lower extremity often occurs in the absence of significant back pain and often begins in the sacroiliac or gluteal regions. Although the pain commonly follows a continuous path, it also may be interrupted, for example, affecting the buttock and anterior leg but skipping the thigh. The pain is often positional depending on the exact site and vector of compression, often related to specific back postures which may increase or decrease the cross-sectional area of the central canal or neural foramina. Limb pain that is aggravated by side-bending toward the affected side or by straight leg raising of the ipsilateral or contralateral leg is likely to be due to nerve root compression. Radicular pain induced by straight leg raising of less than 60 degrees is a sensitive but nonspecific sign estimated to occur in 90% of patients with radiculopathy secondary to disc herniation.[27] Conversely, reproduction of ipsilateral radicular pain by raising the opposite limb (i.e., "the reverse straight leg test") is a highly specific but fairly insensitive provocative test.[5] In upper lumbar disc disease, pain may be reproduced by reverse straight raising, that is, by passively extending rather than flexing the thigh at the hip joint.[28] Provocative physical exam maneuvers have been nicely reviewed.[29]

Pain may also be increased by increased pressure within the intraspinal canal. The latter is frequently provoked by maneuvers that increase intrathoracic pressure resulting in increased volume of the epidural venous plexus. Pain radiating down the leg provoked by straining or coughing is therefore a helpful, although inconsistent, clinical clue.

Several notable generalities are important to keep in mind when performing a physical exam to evaluate neurologic symptoms in the lower extremity compared to the upper extremity. The lower extremity has fewer testable muscles and actions than the upper extremity. For example, there is no pronation or supination at the knee, and the testable movements of the toes are limited in comparison to the fingers. In the lower extremities, there may be greater difficulty in distinguishing a nerve from a nerve root lesion as there is greater overlap in both the motor and sensory functions of specific nerves and nerve roots. For example, there are more similarities than differences in the motor, sensory, and reflex findings in an L3–4 radiculopathy and femoral neuropathy. One advantage that the lower extremity holds over the upper extremity, however, both clinically and electrodiagnostically, is that that muscles belonging to the same myotome can be found in both proximal and distal locations. For example, the L5 segment contributes significantly to both toe extension and hip abduction, whereas the C5 segment has no meaningful contribution to distal upper extremity functions such as wrist or finger movement.

It is also important for a clinician to recognize that clinically evident motor deficits in monoradiculopathy may be subtle, if evident at all, due to the typical multisegmental innervation of virtually all muscles. As a corollary of this, weakness from monoradiculopathy when present

▶ TABLE 24-4. MONORADICULOPATHY: ETIOLOGIES

Herniated nucleus pulposus
Spondylosis (e.g., osteophyte formation and ligamentous hypertrophy)
Nerve sheath tumors
Diabetes (rare)
Herpes zoster
Initial manifestation of eventual polyradiculopathy (see Table 24-5)

should not produce complete paralysis of any muscle. It is also important to recognize that the pattern of weakness in monoradiculopathy although segmental, typically does not affect all muscles innervated by a single myotome to the same extent (Table 24-4). This is particularly true for muscles that are more proximally located in each segment. For example, the weakness in an L5 radiculopathy may be confined to great toe extension and is less frequently detected in hip abduction. Relevant deep tendon reflexes in monoradiculopathies are typically reduced or are absent in the affected segment.

As previously emphasized, sensory symptoms in monoradiculopathy, like many neurologic diseases, are a more sensitive indicator of sensory involvement than sensory signs. Practically speaking, this means that some patients with radiculopathy have sensory symptoms, but their objective sensory exam is normal. Again, with suspected L5 radiculopathy, subjective big toe numbness should be considered as a robust symptom of the radiculopathy even in the absence of objective sensory deficits on examination. In addition, paresthesias and sensory loss often persist long after radicular pain and demonstrable weakness have resolved. Another potential source of error in the interpretation of radicular sensory involvement is the failure to recognize that the topographical area of sensory involvement described by the patient or demonstrable on examination is typically far smaller than predicted based on commonly published dermatomal maps (Fig. 24-11).

Although the vast majority of compressive monoradiculopathies have pain as their cardinal symptom at some point in their natural history, it is important to recognize that exceptions exist. Patients may have either dermatomal sensory symptoms or myotomal motor signs in the absence or relative absence of pain. On occasion, patients will have radicular pain with paresthesia that will abruptly resolve, only to be replaced by weakness in a segmental pattern. It has been hypothesized that this may occur because of disc sequestration and migration.[30,31]

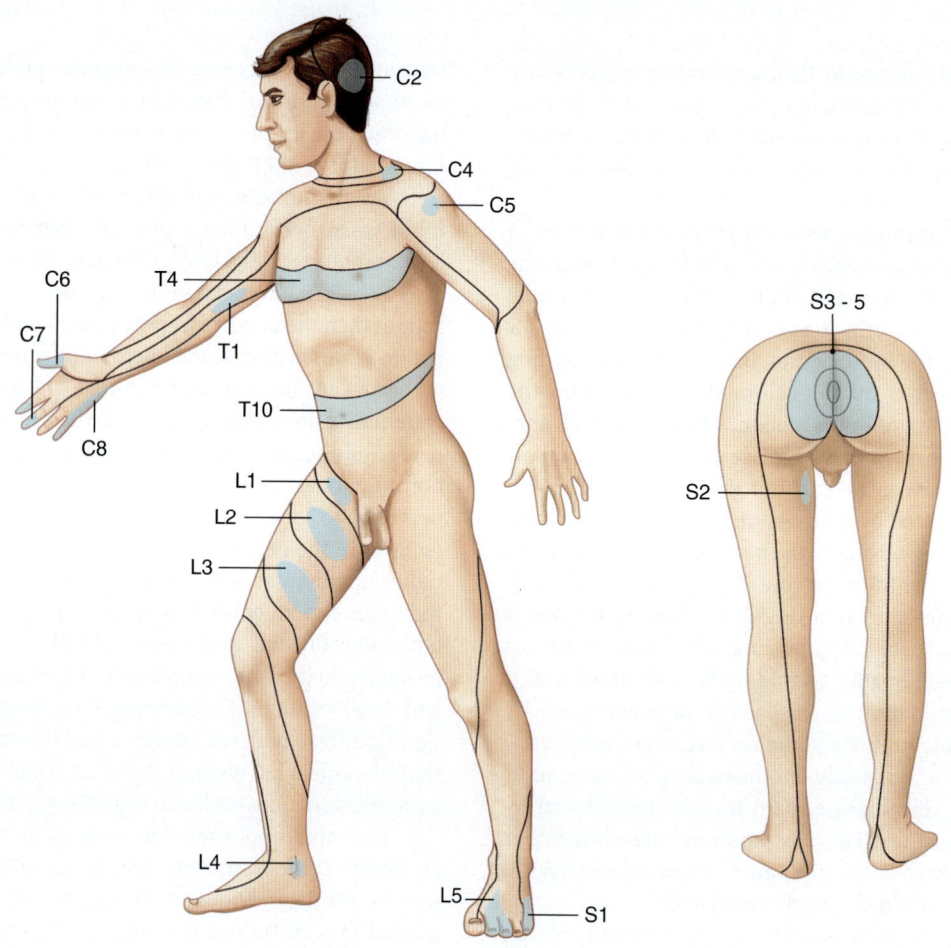

Figure 24-11. Clinical dermatome map.

L1–2

Monoradiculopathies affecting these roots are uncommon and typically present with pain referred into the inguinal region and sometimes the proximal, anterior thigh. Pain in this region, however is uncommonly neurogenic in nature. Other than L1–2 radiculopathies, neurogenic pain with this topographic distribution may result from mononeuropathies of the ilioinguinal or genitofemoral nerves. Although discogenic L1/L2 radiculopathy may occur, suspected L1/L2 radiculopathy should generate an increased level of suspicion for an unusual etiology of root disease (Fig. 24-12). Paresthesias occur in the trochanteric and/or upper groin regions in L1 lesions and the anterior thigh in L2. Weakness is uncommon but may be detectable in hip flexion with L2 root disease. The ipsilateral cremasteric reflex may be lost.

L3–4

L3–4 monoradiculopathies have the potential for substantial morbidity if quadriceps weakness occurs. Pain and sensory symptoms of the thigh and medial knee imply L3 involvement, whereas involvement of the medial lower leg implicates the L4 root. Either lesion may lead to a diminished or absent knee jerk and weakness of hip flexion and adduction in addition to the critical function of knee extension. As the quadriceps is a particularly strong muscle, mild weakness in particularly fit individuals may only be detectable by asking the patient to get up from a chair on one leg at a time without using the arms. Alternatively, mild weakness may be detected by asking the patient to do a partial squat while weight bearing on one leg alone. Both tests should be applied cautiously and only after sufficient strength to do these maneuvers safely has been demonstrated through routine manual muscle testing. In either case, the examiner must position themselves in such a manner and be confident that they can support the patient and prevent a fall should one occur with either maneuver. Many texts suggest that the TA receives partial innervation through the L4 segment. In the authors' experience and in the published experience of others, weakness of foot dorsiflexion and denervation of the TA rarely occur in documented L4 monoradiculopathies.[19] The differential diagnosis of L3–4 radiculopathy includes femoral mononeuropathies, lumbar plexopathies, and radiculoplexus neuropathies. Clinical and EDX sparing of hip adductors distinguishes a femoral mononeuropathy from any of the other disorders. The more difficult distinction is from lumbar radiculoplexus neuropathies or plexopathies which may share a similar pattern of pain, sensory involvement, weakness, and denervation. A combination of imaging of the back and retroperitoneum, EDX, and the clinical contextual features may be required to resolve this differential diagnostic dilemma.

L5

L5 is the most common lower extremity monoradiculopathy. The pain typically extends from buttock to posterolateral

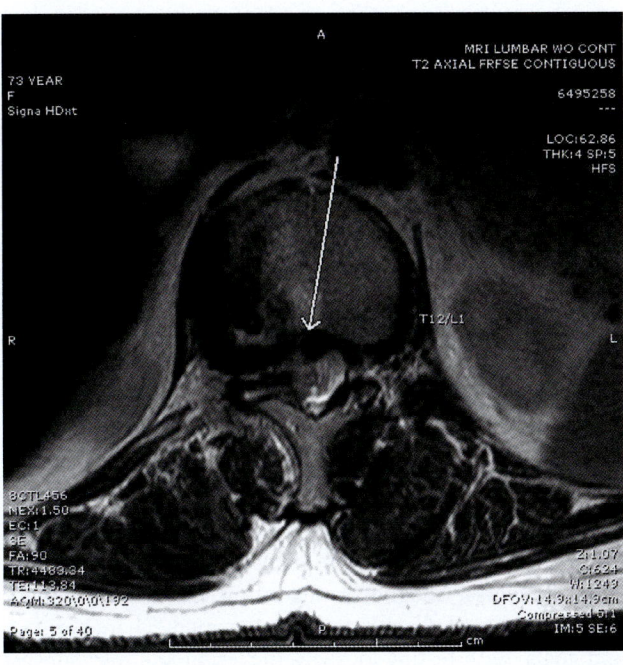
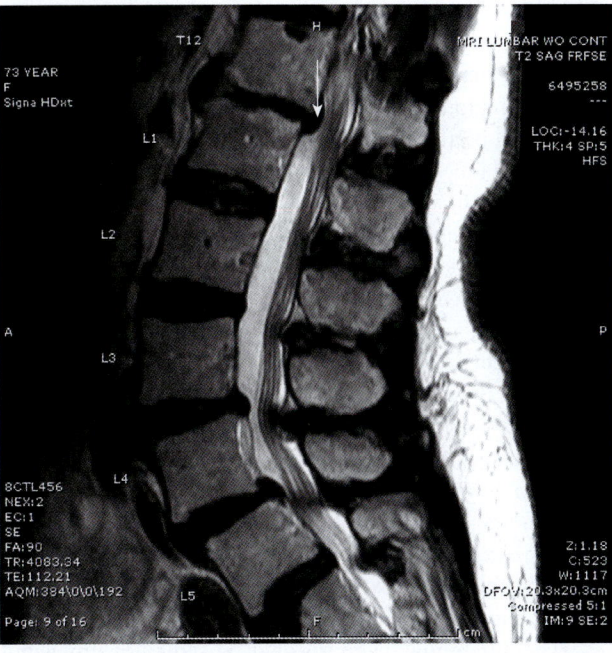

Figure 24-12. T2 (**A**) axial and (**B**) sagittal MR images of the lumbar spine demonstrating right T12–L1 disc herniation in a patient with ipsilateral neuropathic groin pain.

thigh to anterolateral leg. Sensory symptoms affect the lateral leg, instep, dorsum of the foot, and particularly in the big toe. In most people, weakness will be most commonly and readily detected in great toe extension. Weakness of ankle dorsiflexion and inversion may occur as well. Eversion weakness can also be present though to a lesser degree. Weakness of knee flexion and hip abduction are less frequent and/or are more difficult to detect. The differential diagnosis of L5 radiculopathies is essentially the differential diagnosis of foot drop. As many causes of polyneuropathy, motor neuron disease, and even myopathy have a predilection to affect foot dorsiflexion, this differential diagnosis is expansive. As the most common etiology of foot drop is a common fibular neuropathy, it is critically important to assess the strength of ankle inversion which should not be affected in a common fibular (peroneal) neuropathy.

As suggested, a diagnosis of L5 monoradiculopathy should be made cautiously in the absence of pain and/or sensory symptoms. Additionally, when foot drop is greater than, or without toe drop, distal myopathy, myasthenia gravis, or upper motor neuron disease must be considered. Weakness in distal myopathies is often bilateral and symmetric. An absent ankle jerk should not occur in an L5 monoradiculopathy. This finding suggests more proximal pathology of the sciatic nerve or concomitant involvement of the S1 nerve root.

S1

This is the second most common lower extremity monoradiculopathy. The radicular or "sciatic" pain of S1 root disease typically extends from the buttock down the posterior thigh and leg into the heel and at times into the lateral foot/toes. "Sciatica" is of course a common description but a misnomer for S1 radicular pain because the sciatic nerve is not involved. Sensory symptoms are most pronounced in the posterior lateral leg and particularly in the lateral and plantar surfaces of the foot and little toe. Muscle weakness, if present, most commonly occurs in ankle plantar flexion. Detection of S1 weakness may be hampered by the considerable baseline strength of foot plantar flexion, knee flexion, and hip extension. Like with hip flexion, functional testing is helpful to demonstrate weakness when mild or even moderate. This is performed by having the patient do a one-legged calf raise (i.e., elevating the heel fully off the floor while standing on one leg and the knee fully extended is helpful). As this is meant to be a test of strength and not balance, this maneuver is typically performed with the patient holding onto a sturdy, immobile object or a nearby wall or doorframe for balance. Detectable weakness in S1-innervated hip extension is uncommon and is most rigorously tested by having the patient extend the thigh at the hip while lying prone. A suppressed or absent Achilles reflex is also expected.

The differential diagnosis of an S1 radiculopathy is not as extensive as its L5 counterpart. Tibial, sural, and plantar neuropathies are uncommon. Sciatic neuropathies are more common however are typically dominated by the deficits arising from its fibular division. Sacral plexopathies are usually readily distinguished from S1 root disease by their more widespread pattern of weakness and sensory loss.

▶ ETIOLOGIES OF MONORADICULOPATHIES

Table 24-4 lists the more common causes of monoradiculopathies. Herniation of intervertebral discs causes the vast majority of monoradiculopathies in those younger than 50 years. Spondylosis is a far more common cause of root disease in older adults. Typically, the clinical deficits are more evident in a monoradiculopathy caused by disc herniation than in spondylosis, presumably due to its relative acuity. Spondylotic disease is typically more insidious in its development and commonly affects multiple levels bilaterally in an older population, a pattern that may be evident only through EDX evaluation. Contrary to common belief, disc herniations rarely result from traumas such as motor vehicle accidents. Nonspondylotic causes of monoradiculopathy deserve a higher index of suspicion in individuals at risk (e.g., individuals who are immunosuppressed or with prior history of malignancy); those with fever, weight loss, or other symptoms of systemic disease; or those whose neurologic deficits are progressive.

The differential diagnosis of monoradiculopathy is limited. Neoplasms, either nerve sheath tumors or malignancies affecting vertebrae or meninges, are one cause of nondiscogenic/spondylotic monoradiculopathy (Fig. 24-10). Any slowly progressive monoradiculopathy should prompt a careful discussion of family history and search for neurocutaneous stigmata, including subcutaneous and Lisch nodules, café-au-lait spots, and axillary freckles. Diabetes is not commonly considered as a cause of monoradiculopathy, but self-limited monoradiculopathies will occasionally occur in diabetics in the absence of other apparent causes. Herpes zoster (shingles) is a fairly common cause of radicular pain and sensory loss but on occasion can produce "zoster motor paresis" in approximately 5% of affected individuals, presumably due to retrograde viral movement from the dorsal root ganglia into the anterior horn.[32–34] Other disorders with an affinity for nerve roots may occasionally present as a monoradiculopathy as an initial manifestation of an evolving polyradiculopathy (Table 24-5).

▶ EVALUATION OF SUSPECTED MONORADICULOPATHIES

Imaging and EDX play complementary roles in the evaluation of monoradiculopathies of the lower extremity. There is no universal diagnostic algorithm. Clinical judgment should be blended with individual patient characteristics and goals. EDX testing localizes the lesion and may suggest the etiology though frequently ancillary imaging, or CSF or laboratory studies are needed for confirmation. As previously mentioned, the significance of imaging abnormalities

▶ **TABLE 24-5. POLYRADICULOPATHY: ETIOLOGIES**

Arachnoiditis
Degenerative
    Spondylosis (spinal stenosis)
    Central disc herniation
    Epidural lipomatosis
Diabetes (polyradiculoplexus neuropathy)
Iatrogenic (epidural and caudal anesthesia)
Ischemic
    Dural vascular malformations
    Spinal cord infarction
    Nonsystemic vasculitic neuropathy
Infectious
    CMV
    HIV (CMV, herpes simplex, syphilis, *Cryptococcus*, and
        atypical mycobacteria)
    Lyme disease
    Schistosomiasis
    Spinal epidural abscess
Inflammatory
    Sarcoidosis
Neoplastic
    Meningitis
    Primary spinal cord tumors—ependymomas, lipomas, dermoid, epidermoid, hemangioblastoma, paraganglioma, and ganglioneuroma
    Primary nerve sheath tumors—neurofibromas and schwannomas
    Primary vertebral tumors—cordomas, multiple myeloma, and osteoma
    Primary paravertebral tumors—lymphomas
    Metastatic vertebral tumors—breast, lung, and prostate
    Intravascular tumors—lymphoma
Osseous
    Paget disease
    Inflammatory spondyloarthropathies, e.g., ankylosing spondylitis
Radiation

CMV, cytomegalovirus.

is hampered by the frequent occurrence of clinically irrelevant anatomic abnormalities as approximately one-third of asymptomatic individuals have evidence of structural spine disease on imaging. These findings are not predictive of current low back pain. Also, they are also not predictive of the development of low back pain within several years.[35–37] Imaging is also limited in its ability to identify causes of nonstructural radiculopathy.

EDX, on the other hand, is a physiologic test, capable of detecting disordered nerve function in the absence of imaging abnormalities. Like imaging, it often detects abnormalities irrelevant to the presenting symptoms, which may result from preexisting nerve pathology or be related to normal changes which occur with advanced age (i.e., incidental reduction of SNAP amplitudes). As such, we use EDX to provide further evidence for the pathogenicity of imaging findings or when there is a lack of concordance between clinical and imaging data. As alluded to, we are comfortable following a patient with a typical presentation of a discogenic monoradiculopathy clinically, initially without ancillary testing. If patients fail to improve, worsen, develop symptoms of systemic disease or symptoms last more than 6 weeks despite conservative measures such as PT, imaging and frequently EDX should be obtained. We also consider imaging to be a mandatory predecessor to any surgical procedure. Other diagnostic modalities have been described in the evaluation of lumbosacral radiculopathy such as somatosensory-evoked potentials and lumbar puncture. In general, they add little to the evaluation for most patients.

▶ **MANAGEMENT OF MONORADICULOPATHY**

First and foremost, the management of lumbosacral monoradiculopathy requires understanding its natural history. Approximately 90% of patients with symptomatic radiculopathy associated with imaging-confirmed disc herniations have symptom improvement with time and/or conservative measures.[5,38] Clinical improvement seems to correlate with MR evidence of disc involution or regression, which occurs in two-thirds of patients within 6 months. Despite these favorable statistics, evidence to support individual "conservative" treatment modalities is often limited. Many recommendations are consensus-based in the setting of either low-quality or insufficient evidence.[39] A recent paper nicely reviewed the evidence for prevention and management of acute and chronic low back pain in general, including low back pain due to radiculopathy.[38] This review summarized the UK, European, and US guidelines.[38,40] The goal of treatment of acute LBP is to reduce pain and prevent transition to chronic LBP. Typically exercise and education are recommended for prevention of primary low back pain or progression from acute to chronic symptoms.[38]

Recommendations for treatment of radicular pain are like those for nonspecific back pain, as long as no red flag symptoms are present. Prolonged bedrest is no longer recommended and patients are encouraged to stay active and remain at work, as long as their work activities mirror daily living.[38,40,41] Prolonged bedrest may actually have a deleterious effect on functional recovery compared to short periods of immobilization.[42,43] Currently, most physicians favor maintaining activity, except those which involve heavy lifting, repetitive torsion, or prolonged axial loading of the trunk, such as prolonged sitting for the short term. Manual therapies, including physical therapy, structured exercise, and manipulative therapy by osteopathic and chiropractic technique may provide short-term symptomatic relief in mild to moderate radiculopathies.[39] We are more comfortable with manipulative therapy in the musculoskeletal back pain population than we are in individuals with acute disc herniations. In the latter group, we have observed the abrupt onset of neurologic deficits, such as foot drop, chronologically linked to back manipulation. Short courses of nonsteroidal anti-inflammatories may also be recommended in addition to hot compresses. A meta-analysis evaluating the efficacy of anticonvulsant medications (gabapentin, pregabalin, and topiramate) for the treatment of radicular back pain showed no benefit and had a higher risk of adverse events.[44] In general, anticonvulsant and antidepressant medications are not recommended. NSAIDs and muscle relaxants are used with caution in selected patients.[38] Opioids are typically avoided. Muscle relaxants have the potential to be most beneficial in musculoskeletal and nonradicular causes of pack pain. Although widely used, systemic glucocorticoids are not recommended.[38]

Epidural and facet joint steroid injections are also treatment options in selected patients for short-term pain reduction.[45–47] There is no evidence that would indicate a reduction in the duration of functional impairment, the need for surgery, or the incidence of pain beyond 3 months.[45,48] Other techniques such as fluoroscopically guided blockade of selective nerve roots or facet joints or transcutaneous nerve stimulation appear to have limited if any benefit.[46,47,49,50] Although predominantly of historical interest, chymopapain injections and lumbar traction are mentioned here for the sake of completeness as treatments whose time has come and gone.

The decision to proceed to surgical intervention is dependent on the demonstration of surgically amenable pathology that is anatomically concordant with the patient's phenotype. The typical indication is a patient with refractory pain despite a reasonable trial of conservative therapy. The primary goal of surgery in these situations is to provide accelerated pain relief which appears to be supported by current evidence.[51] Patients with surgical intervention however, do not return to work faster than those treated conservatively.[5] Surgical outcomes appear comparable between microdiscectomy and the more traditional open discectomy technique.[51] Decision making may be confounded however by the recognition that some patients will experience the paradoxical dissipation of pain at the same time their neurologic deficits are worsening.[52] Most clinicians would also consider it prudent to move rapidly to surgical decompression in the less common situations where acute–subacute involvement of multiple nerve roots with genitourinary dysfunction occurs (cauda equina syndrome) or with particularly severe (MRC 3/5 or less) weakness. Although there is no evidence basis to support early surgical intervention in these less common situations, it remains the recommended approach by most neurologists and neurosurgeons.[52] Although it is hoped that early surgical intervention will favorably alter the natural history and outcome in these situations, available studies,[53] although not specifically addressing the more severe phenotypes of acute cauda equina syndrome or severe limb weakness, suggest that the eventual outcome relevant to both pain and neurologic deficit are independent of whether surgical or conservative treatment is applied.[54] Microdiscectomy and standard discectomy results in similar outcomes. Similarly, less extensive decompressions for spinal stenosis appear to result in similar outcomes compared to their more extensive counterparts.[55]

POLYRADICULOPATHIES

Clinically apparent polyradiculopathy occurs more commonly in the lumbosacral than cervical region. The most common cause is spinal stenosis resulting from degenerative spondylotic disease and/or congenital narrowing of the central spinal canal and/or neural foramina. As a result, compression of the cauda equina may occur, the symptoms of which are often positional.[52,56,57] The signs and symptoms of spinal stenosis are limited to the back and lower extremities and occasionally to bowel, bladder, and sexual function. Onset is typically insidious and protean in nature with nonspecific low back discomfort and morning stiffness, relieved by activity. The most recognizable symptomatic expression of spinal stenosis is neurogenic claudication (i.e., pain), numbness and the perception of weakness in the back, buttocks, or legs that is often bilateral and typically exacerbated by back extension, standing, or walking.[52] Symptoms are typically diminished by sitting, lying down, or assuming a flexed lumbar posture. The patient may report relief of claudication symptoms when walking behind a shopping cart or walker which promotes this positioning. This same effect may be noted by the relative ease of ascending rather than descending stairs and by activities that encourage lumbar spine flexion (e.g., riding an exercise bicycle) in comparison to those that do not (e.g., walking).

The clinical examination of a patient with symptomatic spinal stenosis is normal in most cases.[52] Straight leg raising does not reproduce symptoms. Although it may be possible to elicit abnormal findings on the neurologic examination after the patient is rendered symptomatic by walking, the yield of this strategy is low in our experience. Although less well recognized and somewhat controversial, it has been suggested that sensory symptoms or even weakness occurring without significant pain may be the dominant initial symptoms of this disorder.[19,58] The former may mimic a length-dependent polyneuropathy, presumably due to the more successful reinnervation process in proximal limb locations. Paradoxically, unilateral calf hypertrophy has also been reported to occur in lumbosacral spinal stenosis often in the setting of muscle cramps or fasciculation in the hypertrophic calf.[59,60] Our personal experience would support the validity of these uncommon presentations (Fig. 24-13).

Alternatively, polyradiculopathy may result from harm to nerve roots because of meningeal-based pathology. In these cases, cervical and thoracic roots and cranial nerves may be affected as well as their lumbosacral counterparts. Most of these disorders are painful and are commonly associated with systemic disorders that produce constitutional or other symptoms indicative of nonneurologic end-organ involvement. These are most readily recognized by the sequential development of motor, sensory, and reflex deficits,

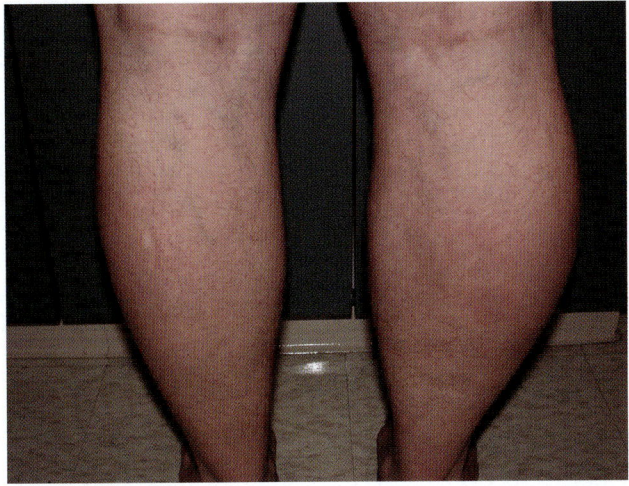 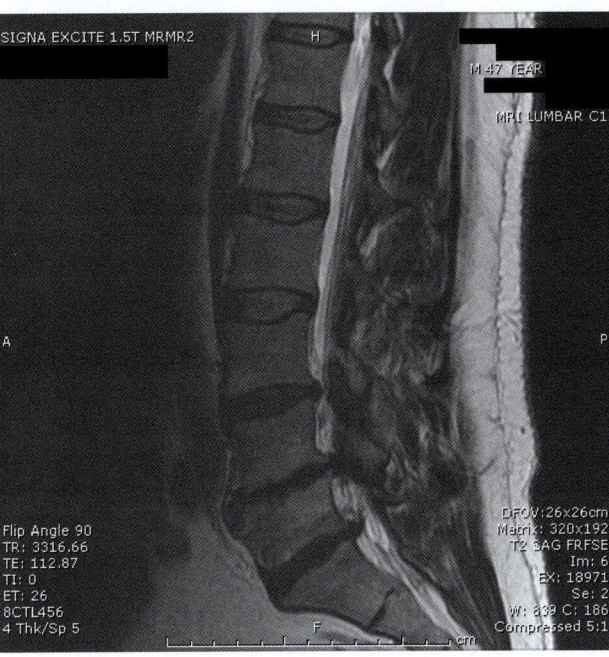

Figure 24-13. (**A**) Right Calf hypertrophy in a 47-year-old male with neurogenic claudication with (**B**) T2 MR sagittal imaging demonstrating spinal stenosis (gastrocnemius muscle biopsy not shown demonstrating neurogenic atrophy).

which are segmental in their pattern and often asymmetric and haphazard in their distribution. Eventually, these deficits may become confluent and with their localization becoming less recognizable unless the history can be recalled in a detailed and chronologic fashion.

The differential diagnosis of lumbosacral polyradiculopathy includes disorders of the conus medullaris, multifocal neuropathy, plexopathy, and radiculoplexopathy. Multifocal neuropathies are potentially distinguished by their nerve rather than segmental distribution of symptoms, with a tendency to spare the trunk and cranial nerves. Lumbosacral plexopathies commonly affect either the lumbar or sacral portions of the plexus individually and are often unilateral in presentation. Disorders of the lower spinal cord parenchyma (i.e., the conus medullaris syndrome) may produce motor and sensory deficits typically confined to the lower extremities, which appear segmental in nature, in addition to the common and often initial symptoms of bowel, bladder, and sexual dysfunction. Because of their intraparenchymal location, pain is typically less of an issue than in cauda equina syndromes which it may otherwise closely mimic. For the most part, unlike polyradiculopathy from systemic disease and multifocal neuropathy, signs and symptoms would be expected to remain confined to the lower extremities and genitourinary function.

ETIOLOGIES OF POLYRADICULOPATHY

The potential etiologies of lumbosacral polyradiculopathy are more extensive than monoradiculopathy (Table 24-5).[61]

The time course of symptom onset aids in narrowing the differential diagnosis. Acute polyradiculopathies develop over hours to days to weeks whereas chronic radiculopathies typically develop over several months. The more notable etiologies will be elaborated on here.

Spondylosis producing the syndrome of spinal stenosis is far and away the most common cause of lumbosacral polyradiculopathy, estimated to occur with a prevalence of 5 in every 1,000 Americans older than 50 years.[29] Spinal stenosis may be congenital in nature as well which may synergistically predispose to symptomatic disease with acquired spondylosis later in life. Conversely, the syndrome may be created by a normal canal size with hypertrophic nerve roots in chronic inflammatory demyelinating polyneuropathy or Charcot–Marie–Tooth disease (Fig. 24-14).[62] Some patients have both structural and inflammatory causes of polyradiculopathy which coexist (Fig. 24-15). Large, midline disc herniations may produce an acute or subacute cauda equina syndrome but are relatively uncommon, presumably due to the protective nature of the posterior longitudinal ligament.

There are numerous, less common causes of polyradiculopathy or conus medullaris lesions that may mimic polyradiculopathy by anterior horn cell loss produced by intramedullary ischemic change. Some of these disorders may present as monoradiculopathies that subsequently evolve. Increased suspicion for these secondary causes should occur with acute to subacute symptom onset or disease progression, concurrence of constitutional symptoms or other clues of potential systemic disease, or unusual pain patterns such as worsening at night suggesting neoplastic, infectious, or inflammatory disease.[5]

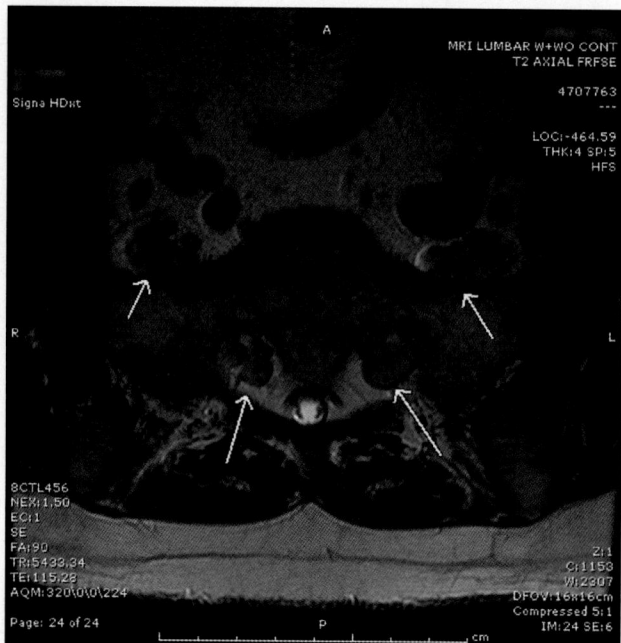

Figure 24-14. T2 MRI axial images of hypertrophied sacral nerve roots extending into the sacral plexus in a patient with Charcot–Marie–Tooth disease.

Considerations for secondary causes of polyradiculopathy (or conus medullaris syndrome) include primary neoplasms of the spine or spinal cord, metastatic disease to the spine with secondary cauda equina compression, or meningeal-based disease-causing neoplastic meningitis.[63] Primary tumors with an affinity for lower spine or spinal cord include glioma, ependymoma, chordoma, schwannomas, neurofibromas, meningiomas, hemangioblastomas, or dermoid tumors. Prostate, myeloma, breast, and lung cancers are the more common causes of tumors with an affinity to metastasize to bone. Back pain as a presenting feature of malignancy is rare. Less than 1% of individuals presenting with back pain in one large series were found to have cancer. Older age, an elevated sedimentation rate and anemia were helpful diagnostic clues in this series.[64] Leukemia, non-Hodgkin lymphoma, breast, lung, melanoma, and gastroesophageal malignancies are the most common causes of neoplastic meningitis.

Ischemic disorders of the lower spinal cord and nerve roots may cause or mimic polyradiculopathy.[3] Causes include occlusive diseases of the aorta and its different branches[65,124] and spinal arteriovenous vascular malformations. Acute aortic occlusions often present with the sudden onset of sensory or motor deficits in the legs, accompanied by skin mottling and asymmetric lower extremity pulses.[65] Dural vascular malformations commonly present with the stepwise progression of lower extremity sensory and motor signs and symptoms, gait dysfunction, with or without signs and symptoms of genitourinary tract involvement.[3] Technically, they should be classified as myeloradiculopathy, as both spinal cord parenchyma and nerve roots are vulnerable to the ischemic change. Symptoms may initiate with some traumatic event and may be noted to intensify with either the upright position or the Valsalva maneuver. Approximately half of patients experience pain. Although both upper and lower motor neuron features typically occur, approximately 30% of patients with dural malformations will have motor features that are predominantly or exclusively lower motor neuron in character. If imaging is focused on the lower lumbar spine, the enlarged, edematous conus characteristic of this disorder may be overlooked (Fig. 24-16). At times, the sensory signs and symptoms created by dural malformations are minor and may be overlooked. In this situation, both the clinical and the EDX patterns may suggest motor neuron disease. There is typically a delay to diagnosis of these vascular

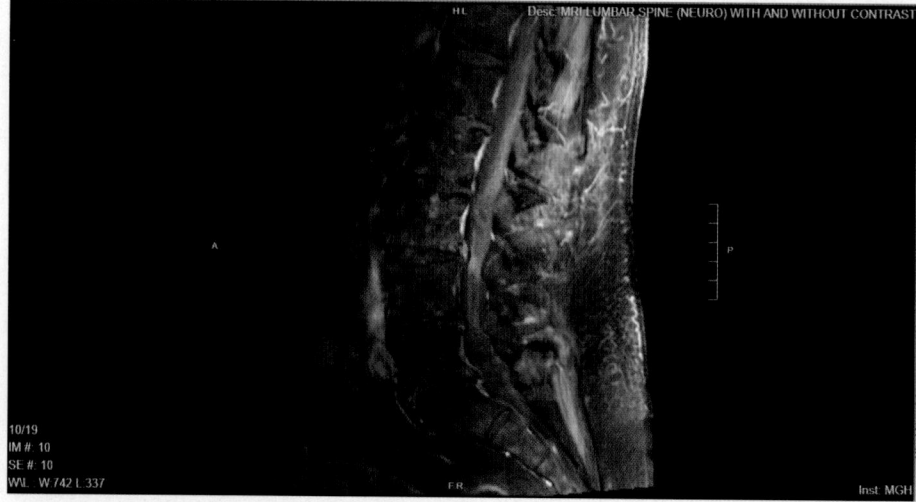

Figure 24-15. MRI sagittal T1 postcontrast images in a 76-year-old man with both degenerative spinal disease and CIDP demonstrating spinal stenosis at the L3–4 and L4–5 levels. The combination of spinal stenosis with an enlarged and enhancing cauda equina results in increased binding and compression of the cauda equina.

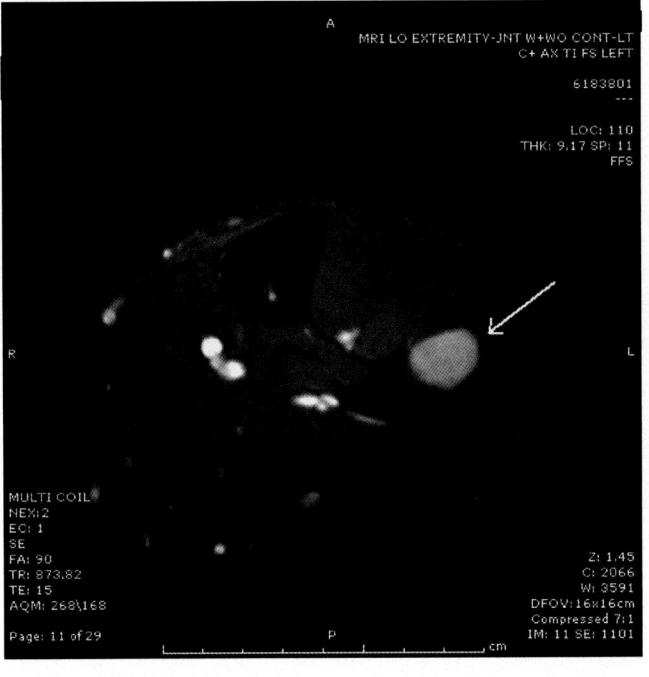 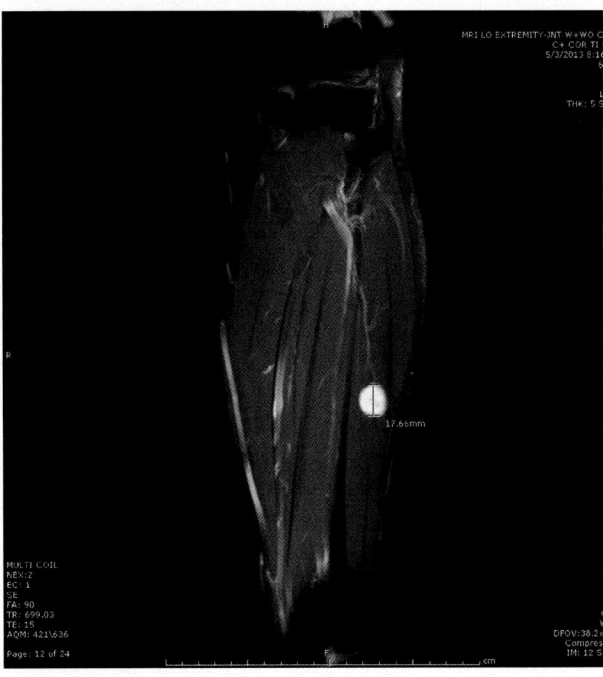

Figure 24-16. (A) Axial and (B) coronal gadolinium-enhanced T1 MR images demonstrating a schwannoma in a 47-year-old male who would experience a Tinel sign every time his lateral left leg was touched.

disorders and initial incorrect diagnoses often include inflammatory or structural causes of myelopathy and/or polyradiculopathy.[3,66,67]

Numerous infectious disorders have a predilection for lumbosacral nerve roots including HIV, cytomegalovirus (CMV), herpes simplex, varicella zoster virus (VZV), atypical mycobacteria, cryptococcus, and treponemal agents, tuberculosis, hepatitis C, Lyme disease, and schistosomiasis.[61,68] Spinal epidural abscesses, most commonly caused by *Staphylococcus aureus*, may also present as a monoradiculopathy evolving into polyradiculopathy.[69] Suspicion should be heightened in context of fever or other constitutional symptoms, intravenous drug abuse or indwelling catheters, percussion tenderness of the spine, or recent bacteremia. Severe acute pain is the most common presenting symptom of the triad of pain, fever, and neurologic deficits characteristic of spinal epidural abscess.[69,70]

Polyradiculopathy is also one of the numerous HIV-related neurologic and neuromuscular syndromes.[71,72] It is typically related to infection with CMV affecting the cauda equina nerve roots, and less commonly due to neurolymphomatosis, VZV, or an idiopathic, inflammatory form.[72] It is estimated to affect approximately 2% of patients who are infected, typically patients with established acquired immunodeficiency syndrome (AIDS) and CD4 counts <100 cell/μL.[73] It may present as a pure motor syndrome.[74] Polyradiculopathy may also result from infections with herpes simplex, atypical mycobacteria, cryptococcus, and treponemal agents in this or any severely immunocompromised patient population.[73,75]

Polyradiculopathy is one of the more common neurologic manifestations of Lyme disease, affecting approximately half of infected patients with peripheral nerve involvement.[76–79] Dermatomal sensory loss and pain are the most common symptoms. Segmental weakness occurs, but is less prevalent.[80] Lyme polyradiculopathy typically occurs within days to weeks of the characteristic rash, seemingly linked to the hematogenous dissemination of the organism. In addition to the meninges and nerve roots, the joints, peripheral nerves, and cardiac conduction system are the end organs at particular risk. Potential or known exposure risk to the transmitting *Ixodes* tick species, seasonal predilection, prior rash, arthralgias, truncal pain secondary to thoracic and upper abdominal root involvement, and/or facial neuropathy are helpful diagnostic clues.[78]

In addition to infections, inflammatory disorders, including sarcoidosis, frequently have an affinity for the lumbosacral nerve roots.[81–83] Sarcoidosis has diverse phenotypic manifestations that may affect the peripheral and central nervous systems (CNS) in addition to other potential end-organ involvement. It is estimated that 5% of individuals will have symptomatic nervous system involvement. In one series of sarcoidosis associated with a focal neuropathy, polyradiculopathy was the most common pattern affecting 22 of 57 reported patients.[81] The cauda equina is at particular risk.[82,83] Other neuropathic patterns that may result from sarcoidosis include radiculoplexus neuropathy, multifocal neuropathy, or length-dependent polyneuropathy. Sarcoidosis can also cause a distal myopathy that can be confused with a radiculopathy in a patient with ankle dorsiflexion weakness. Pain and sensory symptoms occur more frequently than motor signs in most cases, being typically multifocal and non-length dependent in distribution and monophasic in their chronologic course. Constitutional symptoms as well as symptoms referable to other end organs frequently affected by this disease are commonplace. Although many publications about neurosarcoidosis emphasize that neurologic manifestations typically occur in patients with established disease, our experience is that many neurologists are the first to suspect sarcoid based on a consistent neurologic presentation.

Vasculitis is another inflammatory disorder which can present as a polyradiculopathy. Although more commonly associated with a multifocal or length-dependent neuropathy pattern, a polyradiculopathy phenotype has been reported with nonsystemic vasculitis or vasculitis secondary to rheumatologic disorders.[84,85]

Nondegenerative structural disorders may cause or mimic polyradiculopathy. These may include occult myelodysplasia with or without syringomyelia[86] or epidural lipomatosis.[87] Lumbosacral polyradiculopathy may also result from adhesive arachnoiditis. This is a syndrome in which the pia mater becomes thickened, scarred, and adherent with presumed secondary ischemic consequences to nerve roots.[88] Historically, the syndrome has been most closely linked to the use of myelographic contrast agents.[88] Arachnoiditis may also be iatrogenic, either as a side effect of intentional intrathecal injection of therapeutic agents (e.g., chemotherapy) or due to unintended intrathecal injection of potentially toxic agents (e.g., epidural anesthetics during childbirth).[88] Other causes of adhesive arachnoiditis include infection or postoperative or postsubarachnoid hemorrhage inflammatory changes. MRI is the most sensitive imaging modality and has characteristics findings.[89]

Radiation-induced nerve injury, also discussed in Chapter 9, may result in a lumbosacral polyradiculopathy.[90] Symptom onset is typically delayed by an average of 9 years after exposure. The range, however, is exceedingly broad, with onset latency varying between 4 months and 25 years. It most commonly occurs in the context of treatment of testicular cancer or lymphoma. Radiation doses typically exceed 4,000 cGY.[90] As postirradiation neuropathy is frequently a pure motor syndrome, the actual localization of nerve injury has been in dispute. Less than a third of patients have notable sensory symptoms or signs. Whether the pathology preferentially occurs in the anterior horn cells of the conus medullaris, the ventral roots, the lumbosacral plexus, or a combination of any of the elements is uncertain.[91] Current evidence, including reports of root enhancement on MRI in some patients, favors localization to the nerve roots.[92-94] Typically the deficits are bilateral and asymmetric, although monomelic presentations do occur.[95] Any segment may be affected, with L5 and S1 deficits being the most frequent. Pain may occur but typically follows the development of weakness and is usually not a major issue. Nodular enhancement of nerve roots and the conus medullaris with MRI resulting from radiation effect have been reported.[93] Understandable confusion with polyradiculopathy secondary to neoplastic meningitis will occur when enhancement is nodular. Polyradiculopathy has also been reported as an iatrogenic complication of epidural injections for both analgesic and anesthetic purposes.[96] Patients with preexisting spinal stenosis would appear to be at greater risk of this apparently rare and unintended consequence of a common procedure.

▶ EVALUATION OF SUSPECTED POLYRADICULOPATHY

In patients with suspected polyradiculopathy, the evaluation, as always is dictated by clinical context and likely differential diagnostic considerations. Imaging, preferably with MRI is the first step. It is imperative however that imaging be correlated with clinical findings. We take the approach that decisions regarding spinal stenosis surgery should be based on the total clinical presentation rather than the imaging appearance alone, in consideration of the significant incidence of asymptomatic stenosis.[97] Asymptomatic spinal stenosis is estimated to occur in 65% of asymptomatic volunteers, particularly in an older population.[98,99] As neurologic examinations in patients with spondylotic spinal stenosis are commonly normal, EDX can be very useful in identifying subclinical denervation in a characteristic pattern with signs of chronic denervation and reinnervation, and in some cases ongoing denervation. Studies have suggested that there is a strong correlation between abnormal EDX studies, imaging findings, and characteristic symptoms of spinal stenosis, a correlation that does not exist with severity of imaging findings alone without symptoms. EDX confirmation of symptomatic spinal stenosis has been identified to occur in 50%–93% of individuals.[99,100] The EDX pattern of polyradiculopathy is not specific for spinal stenosis however as it can be seen with any condition affecting multiple nerve roots or with anterior horn cell disease.[101,102] For this reason, EDX studies should be interpreted cautiously in patients with a polyradiculopathy pattern in the absence of pain or sensory symptoms, and generalized disorders of motor neurons should be considered.

The threshold for lumbar puncture performance is much lower in polyradiculopathy as opposed to monoradiculopathy and is typically performed in anyone with concern for systemic disease, particularly in patients who have clinically evident polyradiculopathy without proportionate structural pathology on imaging. In these cases, routine CSF analysis for white cells, protein, and glucose should be obtained in addition to cytologic analysis and appropriate additional testing for disorders such as sarcoid, Lyme, CMV, and HIV among others. Cytology and flow cytometry is important. If cord enlargement with T2 signal changes over multiple segments on MR images within the conus is identified, consideration of imaging of the proximal spinal cord in consideration of spinal dural malformation should be considered. The diagnosis of spinal dural arteriovenous fistulas requires a high index of suspicion. A more specific, although less commonly seen, feature is the presence of serpiginous flow voids representing engorged venous structures typically located dorsal to the spinal cord.

MANAGEMENT OF POLYRADICULOPATHY

Optimal management of spinal stenosis in each individual patient is hampered by the variable natural history of the disorder. It is an indolent disorder for the most part. It is estimated that over 4 years, 15% will improve, an equal number will worsen, and 70% will remain the same.[5] Conservative measures are largely supported by anecdotal evidence.[100] Abdominal and back strengthening exercises benefit some patients. Durable medical equipment including rolling walkers which encourage favorable postures often improve the duration and distance of comfortable ambulation. Epidural injections may provide short-term although rarely durable relief.[45] The current weight of evidence favors, but does not mandate an operative approach. In the majority of cases, there is no urgency to intervene and an initial conservative course is reasonable, particularly in patients with minimal clinical deficits.[56] It is estimated that 75%–85% of well-selected individuals will experience significant improvement of lower extremity symptoms that may last for years with 10%–15% of patients experiencing complications.[52] Considerable controversy persists relating to the nature of the surgical procedure, a discussion of which is beyond the scope of this chapter. Many patients require intervention at multiple levels. There is no consensus regarding the relative benefits of fusion versus decompression alone, and whether fusion should include the introduction of costly hardware. One less invasive surgical procedure potentially performed under local anesthesia involves the placement of an intralaminar spacing device in individuals who experience positional relief of symptoms. The device mechanically limits extension and promotes a posture of relative lumbar flexion. Reports suggest a beneficial effect on symptom relief in a significant proportion of selected individuals.[103]

Spinal dural arteriovenous fistulas are typically managed by a combination of selective catheterization and embolization of feeding arterial structures and surgical decompression, assuming that the diagnosis is made prior to complete and permanent ischemic injury to the spinal cord. As it is associated with abnormal CSF findings, implying CNS involvement, current recommendations for the treatment of Lyme polyradiculopathy are to treat with parenteral antibiotics, typically a cephalosporin.[78,104] Symptomatic sarcoidosis is typically treated with corticosteroids or other immunomodulating agents. Neoplastic meningitis may be treated with local radiation or intrathecal chemotherapy. Aggressive treatment is most likely undertaken with the hope of preserving rather than reclaiming a good quality of life. An extensive disease burden and significant morbidity typically warrant a more palliative approach in consideration of the poor natural history of the disease even with aggressive treatment regimens.

▶ PLEXOPATHIES AND RADICULOPLEXUS NEUROPATHIES

Plexopathies are typically recognized when motor, sensory, and, if applicable, reflex deficits occur in multiple nerve and segmental distributions confined to one extremity. Although lumbar plexopathies may be bilateral, they rarely occur concurrently, involvement of the second limb typically occurring in a chronologically dissociated manner. Sacral plexopathies however are more likely to manifest bilaterally due to the more proximate anatomic relationship between the left- and right-sided nerve elements. Radiculoplexus neuropathies have a near identical phenotype to plexopathies. As the name implies, the distinction is based upon pathology that involves nerve roots as well as plexus elements. This may be demonstrable by imaging but is much more likely to be identified electrodiagnostically where concomitant denervation in lumbosacral paraspinal muscles and abnormalities of anatomically analogous SNAPs implicates both root and spinal nerve/plexus involvement. In the author's opinion, the concept of radiculoplexus neuropathy has value as it is very disease specific. The pattern was likely coined in response to the almost unique tendency of diabetes to affect the peripheral nervous system in this way.[105]

The differential diagnosis of plexopathy includes disorders of the conus medullaris and cauda equina (polyradiculopathy). If there is a paucity of pain and sensory involvement, motor neuron disease needs to be considered as well. In general, intraspinal causes of lumbosacral radiculopathy affecting the conus medullaris or cauda equina are more likely to be bilateral than causes of lumbosacral plexopathy. Exceptions are frequent enough, however, to diminish the value of this rule in the evaluation of the individual patient. Otherwise, patterns of pain, sensory symptoms, weakness, and reflex loss may overlap considerably. At times, the clinical context may be helpful but imaging and EDX evaluation are often necessary to sort out anatomic localization in individual cases.

ETIOLOGIES OF LUMBOSACRAL PLEXOPATHY OR RADICULOPLEXUS NEUROPATHY

The numerous causes of lumbosacral plexopathies and radiculoplexus neuropathies are listed in Table 24-6. Diabetes is the strongest risk factor for lumbosacral radiculoplexus neuropathy (DLRPN), however, comorbid autoimmune diseases, history of stroke and higher BMI also increase risk and likely account for the increased mortality observed in

▶ TABLE 24-6. LUMBOSACRAL PLEXOPATHIES AND RADICULOPLEXUS NEUROPATHIES

Retroperitoneal hematoma
Psoas abscess
Malignant neoplasm
Benign neoplasm
Radiation
Amyloid
Diabetic radiculoplexus neuropathy
Idiopathic radiculoplexus neuropathy
Postinfectious radiculoplexus neuropathy
Sarcoidosis
Aortic occlusion/surgery
Lithotomy positioning
Hip arthroplasty
Pelvic fracture
Obstetric injury

this group.[106,107] Currently, lumbosacral radiculoplexus neuropathy is divided into diabetic and nondiabetic forms for classification.[108] DLRPN has been historically referred to by many names, including diabetic amyotrophy, diabetic femoral neuropathy, and the Bruns–Garland syndrome among others.[105,109-111] Current thinking implicates that DLRPN is a spectrum disorder both clinically and pathophysiologically related to both inflammatory and metabolic factors.[106,111] Most recently, COVID-19 has been reported to cause a postinfectious LRPN with features of vasculitis responsive to pulsed high-dose IV steroids.[112]

Acute to subacute onset of severe unilateral hip and/or thigh pain as the initial symptom, followed within days by awareness of ipsilateral leg weakness is the typically clinical presentation. Adjectives such as aching, stabbing, lancinating, and burning have all been used. The exact onset of weakness may be obscured by pain. The syndrome evolves over weeks to months in most cases. DLRPN may become bilateral in a substantial proportion of individuals who are affected, usually with an interval of weeks to months.

The weakness of DLRPN is typically restricted to muscles innervated by the lumbar plexus, affecting hip flexion, adduction, and particularly knee extension. The latter is a considerable source of morbidity. There is a frequent need for durable equipment to minimize fall risk, particularly walkers or crutches, and in some cases knee–ankle–foot orthoses, or even wheelchairs. Two-thirds of individuals will have weakness in the L5 myotome and half in the S1 dermatome in addition to the muscles innervated by the L2–4 roots.[105] L5 and S1 myotomal weakness may occur without concomitant involvement of proximal myotomes. The reference to diabetic monoradiculopathies earlier in this chapter probably represents a limited expression of this disorder. Paresthesias and sensory loss may occur but are typically overshadowed by pain and weakness. A small percentage will have a concurrent or chronologically proximate truncal neuropathy, which is a helpful clue in support of a diabetic etiology. Weight loss, the so-called diabetic cachexia, is a common comorbidity and the onset of symptoms often occurs when average blood glucose is falling rapidly. Approximately half of individuals who are afflicted will have signs and symptoms attributable to dysautonomia if queried, including orthostatic intolerance, urinary dysfunction, constipation and diarrhea, tachycardia, and impotence.[109] Concurrent, sensory predominant, length-dependent, and symmetric polyneuropathy occurs frequently based on clinical and EDX assessments but may be absent.

Less frequently, a radiculoplexus neuropathy occurs in diabetics that differs from the classic form in that it is symmetric in distribution, more insidious in onset, and predominantly motor in its manifestations with limited pain and sensory symptomatology.[111] Like DLRPN, lower extremity muscles bear the brunt of the disease. Unlike the classic syndrome, the weakness typically begins distally rather than proximally and can affect the arms in some cases. In consideration of these clinical features, it has been suggested that this syndrome may represent chronic inflammatory demyelinating polyradiculoneuropathy (CIDP) rather than DLRPN. Data provided through EDX, biopsy of peripheral nerve, and the natural history of the disease, however, suggest that this phenotype is part of the DLRPN spectrum and distinctive from CIDP.[111] In addition, there appears to be no increased incidence of classical CIDP in the diabetic population.[113]

DLRPN, like other focal diabetic neuropathies, but in contrast to the more common length-dependent symmetric diabetic polyneuropathy, is not clearly related to disease duration or control and appears to have a more favorable natural history.[114] It is not rare for the onset of DLRPN to lead to the discovery of impaired glucose tolerance or diabetes.[115] It has been reported that impaired glucose tolerance may be identified in approximately two-thirds of individuals with apparent idiopathic lumbosacral plexopathy.[115] The typical natural history is for pain to relent within weeks to months. Eventual improvement in strength and significant functional recovery occurs in the majority of patients over the course of months to a year or two although many will have some residual weakness and/or disability.[107] As in most neuropathies in which proximal and distal muscle weakness occurs, return of function occurs most successfully in proximal muscles.

The preponderance of evidence suggests that DLRPN occurs as a result of an inflammatory disorder, directed at the microvasculature resulting in ischemic nerve injury.[109,111,116] Peripheral nerve biopsies demonstrate in about 80% of classic asymmetric DLRPN and 50% of the motor predominant symmetric phenotype evidence of multifocal nerve fiber degeneration within or between fascicles, strongly implicating an ischemic mechanism.[111] Other common pathologic findings include infiltrates of lymphocytes (CD45) and macrophages (CD68) most commonly surrounding epineurial arterioles, venules, and capillaries but at times infiltrating vessel walls (microvasculitis) with occasional evidence of prior hemorrhage.[111]

A similar, perhaps identical, phenotype has been described as an idiopathic condition.[110,117–120] Again, the lumbar plexus appears to be predominantly affected in most cases, although both sacral plexopathies and panplexopathies may occur as well. As in its diabetic counterpart, delayed involvement of the opposite side may occur. The disorder is also monophasic in most individuals but can be relapsing or progressive in some.[120,121] As in its brachial plexus analog, an antecedent immunization or infection may have been present. This phenomenon appears to be more common in children than in adults.[122] Nerve pathology in apparent idiopathic lumbosacral radiculoplexus neuropathy appears to be similar if not identical to DLRPN.[116,119]

Acute lower extremity monoplegia has been reported as a rare presenting manifestation of acute aortic occlusion.[123] The localization of nerve injury in this condition is uncertain but is classified here as a plexopathy due to its phenotype.[124] Lumbar plexopathies are a well-recognized complication of retroperitoneal hemorrhage.[125,126] Various primary and metastatic malignancies can affect the lumbosacral plexus as well as treatment with radiation and interarterial chemotherapy.[127] Primary tumors known to infiltrate the plexus include those originating from the cervix, endometrium, ovary, testes, prostate, bone, and colon as well as hematologic malignancies such as myeloma, lymphoma, and acute myelogenous leukemia.[128–130] Radiation of cervical and endometrial cancer is a recognized cause of lumbar plexopathy.[94,128,131] Other reported etiologies include psoas abscess, intraneural spread of amyloid, pelvic fracture, benign tumors such uterine leiomyoma, sarcoidosis, lithotomy positioning, and hip arthroplasty.[130,132–135] Obstetrical injury often associates with a phenotype that approximates a lumbosacral trunk injury, both clinically and electrodiagnostically. Women of short stature seem to be at particular risk.

EVALUATION OF SUSPECTED LUMBOSACRAL PLEXOPATHIES OR RADICULOPLEXUS NEUROPATHIES

Most patients with plexopathies will undergo both imaging and EDX evaluations. It is logical to begin with EDX to localize pathology and focus imaging. Again, the absence of paraspinal denervation and abnormalities of anatomically relevant SNAPs serve to distinguish plexopathies from radiculopathies.[136] However, the presence of abnormal spontaneous activity is a more robust finding than the absence in distinguishing radiculopathy from plexopathy. Distinction of plexopathies from mononeuropathies is more dependent on the pattern of abnormalities on needle examination and less on the pattern of nerve conductions. For example, sacral plexopathies are distinguished from sciatic neuropathies by denervation of muscles innervated by the superior and inferior gluteal nerves which would not occur with sciatic neuropathies. Although the yield of imaging in DLRPN is extremely low, we feel obligated to image these patients nonetheless to exclude other causes.[23,24] Although the clinical syndrome is fairly distinctive, particularly in patients with concomitant paraspinal denervation, the tendency for the weakness to progress over weeks to months makes both patient and physician uncomfortable with a watch-and-wait approach, without the reassurance provided by imaging that is either normal or consistent with idiopathic or diabetic LRPN.[24] As with all suspected diabetic neuropathies, we do not advocate for the routine use of nerve biopsy in plexopathy or radiculoplexus neuropathy unless there are clinical, imaging, or laboratory features that would suggest a disorder capable of infiltrating the nerves in which a nerve biopsy would be diagnostic, for example, amyloid, sarcoid, or lymphoma. We also do not advocate for the routine use of CSF evaluation in cases where plexus localization can be confidently made through clinical, EDX, or imaging means.

▶ MANAGEMENT OF LUMBOSACRAL PLEXOPATHY OR RADICULOPLEXUS NEUROPATHY

There are no known effective treatments for either the idiopathic or the diabetic forms of lumbosacral radiculoplexus neuropathy. Various immunomodulating agents such as corticosteroids, intravenous immunoglobulin (IVIG), plasma exchange, and cyclophosphamide have been used both in diabetic and in idiopathic forms of radiculoplexus neuropathy.[110,122,137] A suggested benefit has been suggested, in some, but not all reports.[137,138] Case reports suggest a benefit of IVIG in idiopathic lumbosacral radiculoplexus neuropathy.[139] This suggested benefit is described more as a tendency to arrest progression and to treat pain rather than to result in immediate improvement. A handful of small observational and one randomized controlled trial, which was published only as an abstract, have been performed, and are summarized in the 2017 update to the original 2009 Cochrane Review.[140,141] In our practice, we will typically try a course of pulse, high-dose IV corticosteroids or IVIG.

With retroperitoneal hemorrhage, it is not known whether surgical decompression alters the natural history of the condition. If surgery is to be done, it is rational to do it expeditiously rather than on a delayed basis after axon loss is more likely to have occurred. Similarly, there are no known effective treatments for radiation-induced nerve injury. Many patients with plexopathy or radiculoplexus neuropathies will benefit from evaluation by a physiatrist or physical therapist, particularly if there is significant quadriceps weakness. Consideration should be given to relevant orthotic devices such as knee–ankle–foot orthoses and/or durable medical equipment such as canes, crutches, or walkers as discussed in Chapter 5. Neuropathic pain should be treated with medications that may have an acceptable benefit to side effect ratio such as tricyclic antidepressants, anticonvulsants such as carbamazepine, gabapentin or pregabalin, or serotonin norepinephrine reuptake inhibitors such as duloxetine or venlafaxine.

MONONEUROPATHIES AND MONOMELIC POLYNEUROPATHIES

Mononeuropathies are usually the result of compression or entrapment. For purposes of this discussion, we will consider compression as a force that originates outside of the body that irritates or injures a nerve structure. In contrast, we will consider entrapment to represent an internal force created by altered anatomy of a normal structure. The mechanism of compressive injury may result from direct stretch and distortion of nerve elements, indirect injury from concussive effects from, for example, a bomb blast, or ischemic injury resulting from the concomitant compression of blood supply to nerves. It is suspected that there are several conditions that make nerve more susceptible to pressure injury. Hereditary neuropathy with liability to pressure palsy (HNPP) is perhaps the best-established example of this. Both diabetes and prior radiation are also suspected to render peripheral nerves more susceptible to mechanical injury, presumably as both are thought to compromise the vasa nervorum and the blood supply of peripheral nerves.[142] Although the vast majority of mononeuropathies occur from mechanical injury, mononeuropathy may uncommonly occur due to alternative mechanisms. Specifically, mononeuropathy may be the first manifestation of a systemic disorder with a predilection to infarct, inflame, or infiltrate peripheral nerve which then commonly evolves into a multifocal neuropathy pattern.

Mononeuropathies may be painful or painless, depending on multiple factors such as the etiology, acuity, and pathophysiology of the injury. The presence of motor or sensory symptoms, typically the reason why nerve injury is suspected, is largely dependent on the makeup of the nerve. For example, meralgia paresthetica, one of the more common lower extremity mononeuropathies may produce pain, paresthesias, and sensory loss but would not cause motor weakness. Like all nerve injuries, the pattern of weakness, usually the most objective means to determine the existence and localization of nerve injury either clinically or electrodiagnostically, may not always precisely localize the nerve injury site. As previously mentioned, certain fascicles and therefore certain muscles may be spared with a given injury, falsely localizing the problem to a more distal location than is the actual localization.[20,21] Reflex loss is dependent on the nerve affected, being the norm in femoral and sciatic neuropathies but unexpected in any other lower extremity mononeuropathy. Table 24-7 provides a list of many of the reported causes of the common lower extremity mononeuropathies.

▶ EVALUATION OF SUSPECTED MONONEUROPATHIES

EDX of suspected mononeuropathies has numerous potential benefits. Needle electromyography may demonstrate abnormalities in muscles that are not clinically weak, aiding both in localizing the process to an individual nerve and point within that nerve. This is particularly true with axon loss injury. For example, in patients with an apparent fibular (peroneal neuropathy) denervation of the short head of the biceps implicates a sciatic neuropathy rather than the more common fibular (peroneal) neuropathy at the fibular head. Nerve conductions may not only help to confirm localization to a single nerve but will even more precisely localize a nerve injury if focal demyelination in any of its forms can be demonstrated. For example, 45% of common peroneal neuropathies can be localized to the fibular head region because of demyelinating features identified by sequential, segmental stimulation in this region.[143] Identifying a predominantly demyelinating injury is also beneficial for prognostic reasons, a predominantly demyelinating injury typically having a much quicker and complete recovery than its predominantly axonal counterpart. Finally NCSs may provide additional insights. The demonstration of a focal demyelinating lesion at a location where compression or entrapment does not typically occur may suggest that an apparent mononeuropathy may be the first manifestation of an imminent multifocal neuropathy, for example, MADSAM. Also, nerve conductions may reveal evidence of a more widespread polyneuropathy in a patient with a demyelinating polyneuropathy at a typical compression site, suggesting the possibility of a hereditary disorder like HNPP.

The use of imaging in the evaluation of lower extremity mononeuropathies has expanded considerably.[17,23,144–148] It provides a far greater probability for an etiologic diagnosis than EDX. Generally, we consider imaging in patients with apparent mononeuropathies occurring in the absence of a clear compression/entrapment mechanism, in a clinical context that would suggest a noncompressive/entrapment cause, or in the setting of unexplained progression. We also image nerves in compression neuropathies particularly when the etiology is unknown.

With MRI, increased T2 signal within nerve is thought to correlate with the lesion site in acute axonal injury.[148] MRI with the addition of gadolinium is the test of choice to identify a suspected nerve sheath tumor (Fig. 22-16). MRI may also be used to identify an abnormal structure that is compressing and injuring a peripheral nerve such as an osteochondroma of the fibular head or a Baker cyst within the popliteal fossa. MRI can also provide indirect evidence of nerve injury by demonstrating abnormal signal change in muscles.[144] For example, the presence of increased T2 signal (suggesting edema) or increased T1 signal (suggesting fatty infiltration) confined to the gluteus medius, minimus, and tensor fascia lata would strongly implicate a superior gluteal mononeuropathy. MRI can demonstrate muscle enlargement and signal change in each anatomic compartment that help to define a compartment syndrome. Finally, MRI may demonstrate focal nerve swelling and increased T2 signal in nerve, particularly within the brachial plexus, that may be helpful in the diagnosis of multifocal neuropathy syndromes such as multifocal motor neuropathy that may present as mononeuropathies and be initially diagnostically elusive.[149]

► TABLE 24-7. **MONONEUROPATHIES: ETIOLOGIES**

Iliohypogastric
    Lower quadrant surgery—appendectomy and nephrectomy
    Retroperitoneal tumor
Ilioinguinal
    Surgery—herniorrhaphies, suprapubic (Pfannenstiel), nephrectomy, and appendectomy incisions
    Parturition
    Bone harvesting from the iliac crest
    Abdominal wall entrapment syndrome
Genitofemoral
    Surgery—herniorrhaphy and appendectomy
    Psoas abscess
Obturator
    Tumor—transitional cell carcinoma of the bladder, cervical carcinoma, lymphoma, prostate carcinoma and sarcoma, histologically undefinable
    Parturition
    Prolonged lithotomy position
    Hip arthroplasty
    Surgical tourniquets
    Myositis ossifications
    Obturator hernias
    Pelvic surgery including those done laparoscopically
    Pelvic fracture
Femoral
    Retroperitoneal or iliacus hematoma
    Lithotomy positioning
    Hip arthroplasty or dislocation
    Iliac artery occlusion
    Femoral arterial procedures—diagnostic or therapeutic
    Femoral artery aneurysms or pseudoaneurysms
    Infiltration by hematogenous malignancies
    Penetrating groin trauma
    Pelvic surgery
    Idiopathic
    Mechanical pressure clamp on the femoral artery
Lateral cutaneous nerve of the thigh
    Meralgia paresthetica
    Bone graft harvesting
    Retrocecal appendectomy
    Hip arthroplasty
    Cesarean section
    Pelvic fracture
    Aortobifemoral bypass surgery
Sciatic
    Gluteal compartment syndrome from hematoma and "toilet seat" neuropathy
    Hip arthroplasty and fracture—dislocation
    Femoral fracture
    Groin injury including gunshot wound
    Infarction due to vasculitis or vascular surgical procedures of the lower extremity
    Lithotomy positioning
    Gluteal injection injury
    Immobilization with impaired consciousness
    Intraoperative thigh tourniquet
    Infiltration by lymphoma
    Endometriosis
    Gluteal artery aneurysms
    Gluteal varicosities
    Compression from lipoma or nerve sheath tumor
    Umbilical artery injections in neonates
    Persistent sciatic artery
    Cardiac surgery
    Compression from prominent lesser trochanter
    Piriformis syndrome
Fibular (Peroneal)
    External compression—stockings, casts, leg crossing, weight loss
    Stretch—bungee jumping, acute plantar flexion/inversion, and prolonged knee flexion during childbirth
    Prolonged squatting
    Cysts and tumors of the tibiofibular joint
    Postoperative
    Closed or open trauma
    Fibular fractures
    Dislocated knees
    Surgery in the popliteal fossa
    Vasculitis
    Baker cyst
    Acute occlusion of femoral or popliteal arteries
Tibial
    Trauma—compression from casts or tourniquets, hip arthroplasty, gunshot and other penetrating wounds, tibial plateau fracture/dislocations, and gluteal injections
    Ischemia—acute large artery occlusive disease or posterior Compartment syndrome
    Tumor—neurofibroma, neurosarcoma, osteochondroma, and lymphoma
    Miscellaneous—ruptured Baker cyst, popliteal hemorrhage, sclerosing treatment of varicose veins, and repetitive foot plantar flexion occupations
    Tarsal tunnel syndrome
Sural
    Ankle injury
    Vein stripping procedures
    Schwannomas
    Ganglionic cysts
    Baker cyst or surgery
    Fracture of the base of the fifth metatarsal
    Compression from the hard upper edges of ski boots
    Vasculitis
    Calf muscle biopsy
    Arthroscopic surgery
    Idiopathic

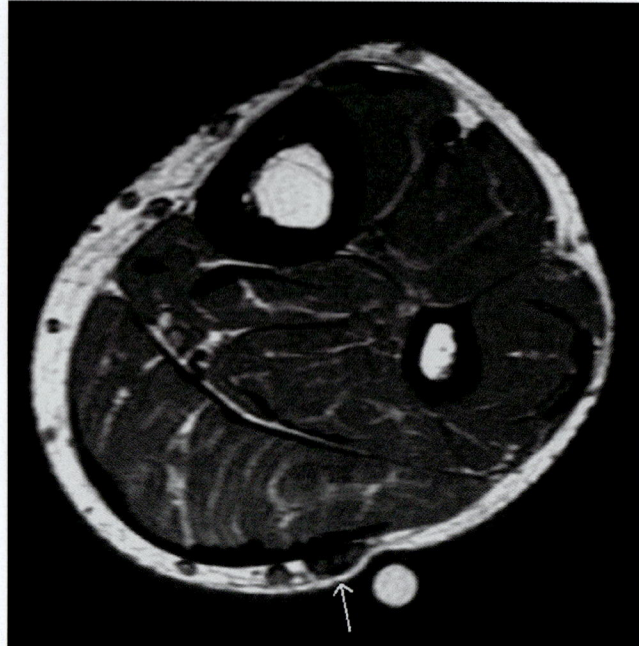 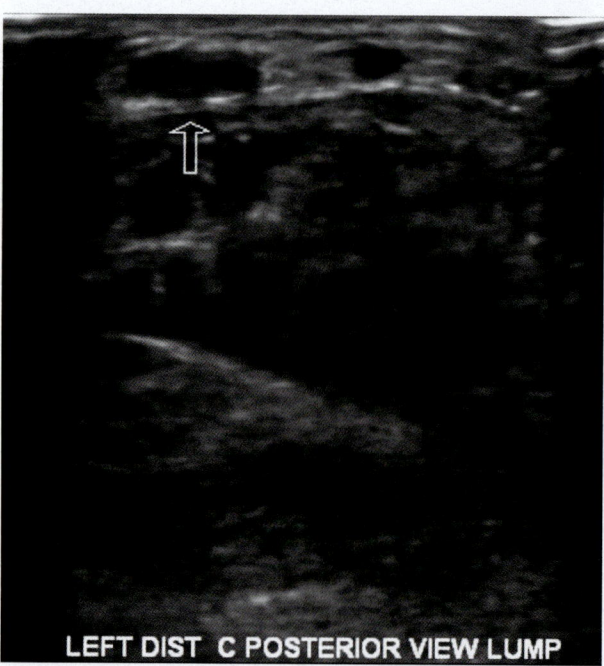

Figure 24-17. T1 MR (**left**) and ultrasound (**right**) images of nodular enlargement of cutaneous nerves, as indicated by the thin and thick *arrows* in Hansen's disease.

Ultrasonography of nerve and muscle disease is also an expanding field. The information that it provides overlaps considerably with that provided by MRI although it has both benefits and limitations (Fig. 24-17).[145–147,150] It can be difficult to utilize when nerves are deeply situated in regions with complex anatomy.[17] Conversely, it is often easier to track a nerve along its longitudinal course with ultrasound compared to MRI. Ultrasound is obviously more portable than MRI and does not have the limitations imposed by pacemakers and other devices. We do not routinely obtain blood work in mononeuropathy patients unless the clinical context directs us to do so.

▶ MANAGEMENT OF MONONEUROPATHIES

Management is dependent on the etiology, location, severity, and duration of nerve injury.[151] With rare exception, monophasic compressive nerve injuries are treated conservatively. If it can be determined that a nerve injury is progressive and due to a definable cause of external compression, the source of compression should be surgically altered or removed. Surgical intervention in diabetics with mononeuropathies should be undertaken cautiously, as the already potentially compromised microvasculature may be further injured with nerve manipulation or transposition.

In case of trauma from "clean" penetrating injuries such as knife or glass wounds in which complete loss of function implicates potential nerve transaction, immediate exploration with attempted primary reanastomosis is considered. If potential nerve transaction occurs from trauma associated with considerably surrounding tissue damage such as a gunshot wound, exploration is typically delayed for a month or more, assuming that there is no suggestion of recovery from either a clinical or an EDX perspective. If the nerve is transected, nerve grafting will be required if anastomosis is attempted, as the retraction of the severed ends will prevent primary reanastomosis on a delayed basis. If the nature of the injury makes nerve transaction unlikely, even in the setting of complete or near-complete nerve injury, surgical exploration is usually not attempted for at least 6 months. If there is partial but convincing improvement measured either clinically or electrically, it is unlikely that surgical intervention will improve outcome. If there is no evidence of improvement, exploration may be considered. The goals in this case would be to perform nerve grafting if the nerve is transected, to identify and remove any external source of nerve compression (external neurolysis), and to potentially perform internal neurolysis. The latter is considered if the epineurium is intact, but intraoperative nerve conductions indicate that there is no impulse transmission through the injured segment. The intent is to dissect out individual fascicles and to potentially free them from any scarring that has taken place within the confines of the epineurial sheath. Alternatively, if upon dissection, all fascicles are anatomically discontinuous despite preservation of epineural continuity, a predictably rare event, nerve grafting may be attempted.[152]

The outcome of surgical intervention for peripheral nerve injury is often disappointing. The age of the patient, comorbid illnesses, and the distance between injury and reinnervating target are key variables. In general, muscles in proximity to axon loss lesions are more likely to recover meaningful function than those at a distance, regardless of whether surgical intervention takes place or not.

As discussed in the plexopathy section, bracing and other forms of durable equipment may improve both mobility and safety. With common peroneal or sciatic neuropathies, custom-fitted ankle–foot orthoses (AFO) are recommended if patients "catch their toes" and trip. Some patients benefit from AFOs by improving their gait as well as by diminishing their risk of falling. Selected patients with femoral neuropathies may benefit from a knee–ankle–foot orthoses. In addition, a cane, walker, or even wheelchair may be necessary, depending on the severity of quadriceps weakness and the strength of unaffected muscles. Patients with quadriceps weakness may also benefit from raised chairs and toilet seats, lift chairs, which will aid them in getting to their feet, and stair lifts if access to second floors or basements in their homes or places of work is required and cannot be accomplished by some other means.

▶ INDIVIDUAL MONONEUROPATHIES OF THE LOWER EXTREMITIES

- Ilioinguinal neuropathy

  Clinical recognition of an ilioinguinal mononeuropathy is based on sensory complaints in the appropriate topographic area, typically occurring in a postoperative context.[153] The ilioinguinal nerve provides cutaneous innervation most reliably to the base of penis (mons pubis, labia majora) as well as along the inguinal ligament or in the most proximal aspect of the anteromedial thigh. Either reduced or heightened sensibility may be found on tactile stimulation of these areas. The most problematic symptom is "neuralgic" pain along the inguinal ligament, medial groin, scrotum, or labia that often has burning or lancinating characteristics. This pain is typically reproducible by groin pressure or by extending the thigh at the hip. As a result, patients often maintain a flexed posture while walking. The ilioinguinal nerve also provides motor branches to the transverse abdominus and internal oblique muscles of the lower abdominal wall. Paresis in the ipsilateral lower abdominal musculature may be demonstrable by having the patient contract the abdominal wall by attempting a sit up. Involvement of the abdominal musculature may be more readily detected by needle electromyography, particularly in those with an endomorphic body habitus. The differential diagnosis is largely that of L1 radiculopathies, iliohypogastric or genitofemoral mononeuropathies, and nonneurologic causes of groin pain.

  The prevalence of ilioinguinal neuropathy probably relates to the frequency of potentially causative surgical procedures. Hernia repair surgeries, through both laproscopic and open methods, are the most common cause with an incidence reported as high as 10%.[153–155] When explored, the mechanism of neuropathy appears to be nerve transaction, entrapment, or traumatic neuroma.[155] Other pelvic procedures including suprapubic (Pfannenstiel) incision, nephrectomy, femoral catheter placement, hysterectomy, orchiectomy, and appendectomy have been associated with this injury as well. Ilioinguinal neuropathy has been rarely described as a complication of parturition, bone harvesting from the iliac crest, and presumed tearing of the external oblique aponeurosis in hockey players. Spontaneously and idiopathically occurring ilioinguinal neuropathies have also been described, attributed to anatomic variation in anatomy and presumed entrapment from surrounding musculoaponeurotic structures.[153]

  Diagnosis may be aided by reproduction of the typical pain pattern by palpation (Tinel sign) or hip extension, EDX demonstration of denervation confined to abdominal wall muscles, and/or by pain relief achieved by nerve block with local anesthetic. With nerve percussion, the pain typically radiates into the medial thigh and/or genitalia. Treatment may involve pharmacologic attempts at neuropathic pain relief with drugs such as gabapentin, nerve blocks with steroids and local anesthetics, or unproven noninvasive measures such as transcutaneous nerve stimulation or pulsed radiofrequency therapy to the upper lumbar roots. Surgical interventions for intractable cases including neurectomy have been favorably reported.[156–158]

- Iliohypogastric neuropathy

  Iliohypogastric neuropathies are far less common than their ilioinguinal counterparts.[151,155] The nerve has anterior and lateral branches. The lateral branch provides sensation to a vertically oriented patch that descends from the superior margin of the iliac crest in the posterior axillary line to a position just posterior to the head of the trochanter. The anterior branch supplies a small area just rostral to the symphysis pubis. Like the ilioinguinal nerve, it provides motor branches to the transverse abdominus and internal oblique muscles of the lower abdominal wall. There is considerable overlap in the signs and symptoms of ilioinguinal and iliohypogastric nerve injury and they may be indistinguishable from one another.

  Iliohypogastric neuropathies typically result from surgery in the lower quadrants including appendectomy, hysterectomy, inguinal herniorrhaphy, and nephrectomy or from pathology in the retroperitoneum. They may occur in the third trimester or because of sports injury. Diagnostic strategies and treatment options are identical to ilioinguinal nerve injury.[157]

- Genitofemoral neuropathy

  The phenotype of genitofemoral neuropathy is like ilioinguinal and iliohypogastric neuropathies.[151] If distinction is to be made, it is most likely to occur as a result of the topographic area that is affected. Sensory loss or hyperesthesia in genitofemoral neuropathies occurs in a small zone in the anterior thigh just inferior to the mid-inguinal ligament (femoral branch) and immediately lateral to part of the cutaneous distribution of the ilioinguinal nerve. The sensory distribution of the genital branch includes the labia majora and scrotum and is probably indistinguishable in this location from ilioinguinal and iliohypogastric nerve injury. The phenotype usually consists of sensory complaints in medial groin, exacerbated by walking, rotation of the hip joint, or by tactile stimulation of the nerve. The loss of the cremasteric reflex on the symptomatic side provides diagnostic support but inexplicably is not invariably lost with injuries to this nerve.

Once again, the most likely cause is a complication of a preceding lower abdominal surgery including herniorrhaphy, appendectomy, biopsy, cesarean section, or as a complication of retroperitoneal hematoma or pregnancy. Fortunately, these injuries are rare. Anesthetic block of the L1–L2 roots is reported to reliably predict a good response to surgical intervention if required. When required, neurectomy is the procedure of choice and has been reported to be very effective in selected patients.[157,158]

- Superior and inferior gluteal neuropathies

    The superior and inferior gluteal nerves are virtually never affected in isolation. They have been reported after hip arthroplasty either due to direct injury from instrumentation or indirectly from stretch. It has been suggested that these nerves may be compressed by pelvic osteophytes and posttraumatic bone spurs as well.[17] There have been reports of superior gluteal nerve injuries in response to injection injuries and inferior gluteal nerve injuries with pelvic malignancy. The latter usually occurs with concurrent injury to the sciatic, pudendal, and/or posterior cutaneous nerve of the thigh. Posterior cutaneous nerve of the thigh injuries has been reported to occur with injection injuries, lacerations, and prolonged bike riding. Recognition is based on sensory complaints/loss of the posterior thigh and inferior buttock. An intermittent neuralgia of this nerve has been reported.[159]

- Lateral femoral cutaneous neuropathy (LFCN)/ "meralgia paresthetica"

    One of the first documented and certainly more eloquent descriptions of MP was by Sigmund Freud regarding his personal experience. He described a "furry sensation, a feeling of alien skin almost imperceptible at rest but exacerbated by walking, frequently accompanied by painful short, pricking at right angles to the skin as well as a disagreeable sensitivity to the rubbing of underclothes."[160] Like Freud, many patients experience pain, often burning in character. Typically, there is either a diminished or increased response to tactile stimulus in the anterior lateral thigh, typically in an area analogous to the positioning of a hand in a pants' pocket.[161] In most individuals, symptoms are unilateral. In the 10% whose symptoms are bilateral, there is still unilateral dominance.[162] Patellar reflexes and strength, particularly of hip flexion and adduction, and knee extension, are normal.

    The diagnosis of MP is largely clinical and a diagnosis of exclusion.[163] It has been suggested that placing a patient in the lateral recumbent position with the asymptomatic side downward and placing pressure on the symptomatic iliac crest for 45 seconds will relieve the symptoms of MP in 95% of cases with similar specificity.[151] EDX may be helpful if the LFCN SNAP is reduced in amplitude or absent on the symptomatic side. Unfortunately, it is not uncommon for the response to be absent bilaterally, which may be related to technical factors such as patient body habitus or bilateral pathology. In some cases, the LFCN SNAP may be normal bilaterally in the setting of a convincing clinical diagnosis.[162] Presumably, this is a consequence of a predominantly demyelinating lesion at the inguinal ligament, proximal to both the stimulation and recording site. The differential diagnosis of MP includes L2–L3 radiculopathy, lumbar plexopathy, femoral neuropathy, or a nonneuropathic cause of thigh pain, for example, hip joint disease.

    MP is most attributed to entrapment or injury to the nerve as it passes through the lateral portion of the inguinal ligament, just medial to the anterior superior iliac spine. This is supported by observations made during therapeutic neurectomy in patients with chronic, intractable meralgia.[162] This is a common disorder with an estimated age and sex-adjusted incidence of 32.6 per 100,000 patient years.[161] Diabetes mellitus (DM) increases the risk of MP sevenfold, and people with MP were more likely to have or develop DM and to have elevated BMI. The incidence appears to climb with increasing age, and peaks between ages 55 and 65 at approximately double the population's rate.[161] Additionally, wearing tight clothes like jeans or work belts which compress the nerve also can cause symptoms. The disorder seems to be most commonly idiopathic. Identifiable causes that have been reported include retrocecal appendectomy, hip surgery, cesarean section, pelvic fracture, seat belt injury, iliac crest bone marrow harvesting, prone positioning during spinal surgery, and aortobifemoral bypass grafting.[164,165]

    The natural history of the disorder is variable.[163] The disorder can be self-limited or persist chronically. There are no controlled trials that we are aware of that identify the effect of weight loss on the natural history, but this is typically the first step we recommend for management in additional to medications to treat neuropathic pain if present. Other uncommonly used paradigms for refractory and severe symptoms include injection in proximity of the presumed site of entrapment at the lateral aspect of inguinal ligament at the anterior superior iliac spine, or neurolysis or neurectomy in chronic, intractable cases. Surgical intervention has favorable outcomes in small case series, but we have not used this in our clinical practice.[162,164–166] At the time of neurectomy, four of seven resected nerves demonstrated focal indentation of the nerve at the inguinal ligament, a finding not demonstrable in control individuals. Nonetheless, a Cochrane review concludes that no intervention has proven benefit over the natural history of the disease.[167] Pathologic examination of the nerve demonstrated findings described in animal models of chronic nerve compression with multifocal nerve fiber loss. In addition, there was evidence of inflammation in most cases.[162]

- Femoral neuropathy

  The phenotype of a femoral mononeuropathy phenotype is typically dominated by weakness of knee extension, and depending on the location, weakness of hip flexion as well. Hip adduction which is primary controlled by the obturator nerve is normal. Sensory symptoms occurring on either the anterior thigh and/or the medial leg occur in only half of reported cases. A prominent painful component is the exception rather than the rule. It may be delayed and is often self-limited in nature. Preservation of the quadriceps (patellar) reflex would be unusual and call the diagnosis into question.[168]

  The diagnosis is typically made by clinical examination supported by EDX findings. Imaging of the pelvis is recommended if a readily available cause is not apparent. This is particularly true if the deficits are progressive or if the clinical context suggests an increased risk of hematoma or abscess. The EDX evaluation may include motor conduction studies of the femoral nerve although we do not find them particularly helpful in most cases. The diagnosis is supported by an abnormal saphenous SNAP with preservation of the other ipsilateral sensory responses. As the saphenous SNAP may be technically difficult to obtain, we do not place a great deal of weight on a low amplitude or absent response unless it is readily acquired on the opposite side. Depending on how proximal or distal the lesion, needle EMG findings should be confined to some or all the eight femoral innervated muscles if tested. The differential diagnosis of femoral neuropathies consists of lumbar plexopathies and radiculoplexus neuropathies, L3/L4 radiculopathies and nonneurogenic causes of pelvic, hip or thigh pain in which there may be perceived weakness resulting from pain.

  The reported causes of femoral mononeuropathies are varied but are most commonly related in one large series to compressive (40%), perioperative stretch (35%), and inflammatory (6%) etiologies.[169] Compressive etiologies included labor and anticoagulated-associated femoral neuropathies including retroperitoneal or iliacus hematomas.[169] Also included are femoral neuropathies related to prolonged immobilization which we have seen increasingly in the setting of opioid and other sedating drug use, either in prone or supine positions.[170] Presentation typically includes weakness, sensory loss in the anterior thigh and less commonly, pain.[169]

  Management is largely determined by etiology but is conservative in most cases. Pain management and physical therapy are the primary therapeutic modalities. As described in Chapter 5, bracing such as knee–ankle–foot orthoses and durable medical equipment such as canes, crutches, walkers, or even wheelchairs may allow for independent mobility associated with a diminished risk of falling, which is a particular risk for these patients.

- Saphenous neuropathy

  The saphenous nerve is the terminal sensory branch of the femoral nerve, passing through Hunter canal on the medial surface of the knee after innervating the anteromedial surface of the leg, the medial malleolar region, and the medial surface of the foot. This is the only region of the lower extremity below the knee innervated by nonsciatic nerve branches. Patients with saphenous neuropathy have pain and paresthesias in this region. There may be a Tinel sign at the most common entrapment point at the medial knee.[151,171] Saphenous neuropathy has been reported to occur as a result of a ganglion cyst or following surgery in the popliteal fossa.[172–175] Many patients respond to conservative treatment or to nerve block although success with neurectomy may occur as well. As expected, the latter procedure results in residual sensory loss in the medial leg and ankle.

- Obturator neuropathy

  Obturator mononeuropathy typically presents with pain in the groin, anterior, and/or medial thigh which is the initial symptom in most patients. Paresthesias in the medial thigh occur but are often obscured by pain. Weakness may not be evident clinically, and EDX evidence of denervation confined to obturator-innervated muscles may be required. Weakness occurs predominantly in hip adduction, although weakness in hip flexion may coexist.[176] Ipsilateral leg edema may occur. The differential diagnosis is largely that of lumbar plexopathy or radiculoplexus neuropathy in addition to nonneurologic causes of pelvic and thigh pain. In the author's as well as others' experience, diabetic radiculoplexus neuropathy may occasionally mimic an obturator mononeuropathy with apparent clinical and EDX sparing of the quadriceps.[177] The clinical diagnosis of obturator neuropathy is confirmed electrodiagnostically.[177] Imaging of the pelvis is recommended if the etiology is not apparent.[17]

These mononeuropathies occur infrequently. Etiologies include pelvic instrumentation, occult, or previously recognized malignancy.[176,177] Reported malignancies include transitional cell carcinoma of the bladder, cervical carcinoma, lymphoma, prostatic carcinoma and sarcoma, or tumors that are histologically undefinable. Most cases are related to mechanical injury. Reported causes are like femoral mononeuropathies and include childbirth, osteitis pubis, acetabular labral cysts, the prolonged lithotomy position, total hip arthroplasty, surgical tourniquets, myositis ossifications, obturator hernias, pelvic surgery including those done laparoscopically, and pelvic fracture.[17,177] Prognosis is in large part determined by etiology and is favorable with neuropathies that occur acutely.[177]

- Sciatic neuropathies

    Sciatic neuropathies are often painful and may lead to a causalgia syndrome. Sensory complaints and sensory loss occur in the entire foot and the distal-lateral leg. The ankle jerk and, on occasion, the internal hamstring reflex are diminished or absent on the affected side. Ambulation is significantly impaired. A severe sciatic neuropathy results in weakness involving all motions of the ankle and toes as well as flexion of the leg at the knee. Abduction and extension of the thigh at the hip should be spared. As previously mentioned, the peroneal functions of the sciatic nerve are typically involved disproportionately to their tibial counterparts.[178,179] Misdiagnosis of a common peroneal neuropathy may occur with incomplete sciatic neuropathies which may be the most common differential diagnostic consideration. Other considerations include length-dependent monomelic polyneuropathies from lower extremity arterial occlusion, sacral plexopathy, or lumbosacral polyradiculopathy. Distinction between sciatic mononeuropathy and these entities can usually be easily made by careful EDX evaluation. If the cause of sciatic neuropathy is remains unknown from the history, MRI with gadolinium from sciatic notch to popliteal fossa is suggested.

    Sciatic neuropathies are most commonly traumatic, most notably related to hip arthroplasty or fracture/dislocations.[178-181] There are numerous other diverse causes including penetrating trauma, intramuscular injections, hemorrhage into the piriformis region, aneurysm of the inferior gluteal artery, prolonged lithotomy positioning, vasculitis, endometrial implants leading to catamenial sciatica, prolonged immobility leading to a gluteal compartment syndrome sometimes resulting from sitting on a hard surface, also known as "toilet seat" neuropathy, infiltration by lymphoma, intraoperative thigh tourniquet, persistent sciatic arteries, gluteal varicosities, and nerve sheath tumors.[182-186] Sciatic neuropathy has been reported to occur in association with cardiac surgery, presumably due to an ischemic mechanism related to intra-arterial balloon placement or concomitant peripheral vascular disease.[187] Sciatic neuropathies in children have different causes including inadvertent injection into the umbilical artery in a newborn.[188]

    A potential and controversial cause of sciatic nerve entrapment is the piriformis syndrome.[189-192] Symptoms consist of buttock and posterior thigh pain reproduced by maneuvers that stretch the sciatic nerve. Provocative diagnostic maneuvers such as tenderness to palpation in the inferior medial quadrant of the buttock, or exacerbation of pain by passively internally rotating, adducting and flexing the thigh while the patient is in supine position, actively abducting the thigh against resistance in the seated position, or abducting the thigh of the symptomatic side while in the left lateral recumbent positions have been reported.[190] Objective clinical and EDX evidence of nerve injury are notable for their absence. We do not perform this clinically however a prolonged H reflex latency in the symptomatic leg when the thigh is maintained in a flexed, internally rotated, and adducted position is a reported but unvalidated means by which to support the diagnosis.[190] It has been reported that ipsilateral evidence of piriformis enlargement coupled with MR evidence of nerve edema has a 93% specificity and 64% sensitivity in identifying this syndrome as determined by surgical outcome.[193] Conversely, the piriformis has been reported to be atrophied ipsilaterally in chronic cases. The proposed mechanism for the piriformis syndrome is sciatic nerve compression by an abnormal piriformis muscle or an abnormal relationship between nerve and muscle as the nerve exits the pelvis at the sciatic notch. The nerve typically exits below the muscle, but on occasion exits above or traverses through it.

    We favor conservative therapy with stretching or targeted injections with local anesthetics and corticosteroids.[190,194] Recently, injection with botulinum toxin utilized to relax the piriformis muscle and relieve pressure on the sciatic nerve has been reported with benefit.[190] We avoid any consideration of exploration in the absence of objective, clinical, EDX, or convincing imaging abnormalities.

- Common fibular neuropathy

    Common fibular mononeuropathies along with MP are the most commonly occurring lower extremity mononeuropathies. Fibular neuropathies often occur with a paucity of pain, present in only a fifth of patients.[143] Sensory symptoms are often minimal or absent and correspondingly the superficial peroneal nerve may be unaffected on NCS either due to a demyelinating pathophysiology or fascicular involvement.[195] As a result, recognition is commonly prompted by the development of foot drop. The pattern of weakness is distinctive, affecting foot and toe dorsiflexion and foot eversion alone, thus distinguishing it from other causes of foot drop. Like all partial nerve injuries, there may be either diminished sensation or hypersensitivity. This tends to be subtle and found on the distal-lateral leg and/or the dorsum of the foot. Deep tendon reflexes are spared in the absence of a second confounding problem. The differential diagnosis includes an L5 radiculopathy, a partial sciatic neuropathy, a lumbosacral trunk lesion, motor neuron disease, distal weakness in myasthenia gravis or a distal myopathy if foot drop is bilateral.

Causes of common fibular neuropathy include structural pathology of the fibular head including cysts of the tibiofibular joint,[196] external compression particularly following weight loss (termed "slimmer's palsy")[197] or habitual leg crossing. Other sources of external compression include casts or compression stockings, surgery, closed or open trauma, prolonged squatting, fibular fractures, dislocated knees, surgery in the popliteal fossa, vasculitis, fibular tumors, Baker cysts, stretch injuries from acute plantar flexion/inversion or prolonged knee flexion during childbirth, and acute occlusion of femoral or popliteal arteries.[143,198] Thirteen of 103 patients in one series were diabetic, representing a possible predisposition to compressive injury.[143] Peroneal neuropathies occur in childhood as well.[199]

- Tibial neuropathy

    Tibial neuropathies proximal to the ankle are uncommon. The pattern of weakness of a tibial mononeuropathy in isolation varies by location. Knee flexion is weak with a lesion near or proximal to the hip joint but is spared with lesions located distal to the proximal thigh. Lesions in the distal thigh or proximal leg are typically associated with weakness of foot plantar flexion and inversion, toe flexion, and, if detectable, toe abduction. Sensory symptoms and sensory loss are confined to the sole of the foot and the very distal aspect of the dorsal surface of the toes. Depression or loss of the ankle jerk is invariable. Tibial mononeuropathies are most confused with S1 monoradiculopathies.

    Tibial neuropathies typically result from trauma, tumor, or ischemia. Traumatic causes account for approximately half of all cases. The nature of the trauma is variable and may include compression from casts or tourniquets, hip arthroplasty, gunshot and other penetrating wounds, tibial fractures, and gluteal injections. Acute limb ischemia was the most common nontraumatic cause in one series affecting approximately 20% of patients (see monomelic neuropathy below).[200] Coexistent fibular neuropathies may occur in both traumatic and ischemic etiologies. Rare causes include idiopathic hypertrophic nerve lesions, ruptured Baker cysts, and hematoma formation in the popliteal fossa.

    Tarsal tunnel syndrome is a controversial entity most closely associated with external compression from tight-fitting footwear or prior ankle injury.[201-204] Arguably, it is associated with symptoms more than signs. In a manner analogous to carpal tunnel syndrome, patients may be typically plagued by pain in the ankle and foot and dysesthesias often burning in of the sole that are intermittent and worse nocturnally. As weakness of tibial innervated intrinsic foot muscles may be difficult to clinically detect, objective motor deficits are uncommon. Due to the frequent calloused condition of the sole of the foot, examination for sensory loss may be technically limited. The validity of a Tinel sign over the distal tibial nerve at the flexor retinaculum is uncertain. A minority of patients referred to neurologists with suspected tarsal tunnel syndrome will receive that diagnosis when subjected to careful clinical and EDX scrutiny and rather will be diagnosed with plantar fasciitis, polyneuropathy, or an S1 lumbosacral radiculopathy.

- Sural neuropathy

    They are uncommon and most frequently caused by nerve biopsy. They present with some combination of numbness, pain, or paresthesias on the lateral foot in the cutaneous distribution of the nerve. Sural neuropathies are otherwise most commonly traumatic in etiology associated with ankle injury, surgery, or vein stripping procedures. Schwannomas, ganglionic cysts, Baker cysts or their surgery, fracture of the base of the fifth metatarsal, arthroscopic knee surgery, muscle biopsy of the calf, compression from the hard upper edges of ski boots, vasculitis, and idiopathic are other recognized causes.[205,206] EDX confirmation is readily obtained unless confounded by comorbidity such as polyneuropathy.

- Pudendal neuropathy

    Pudendal neuropathy typically presents with chronic perineal pain. It is typically aggravated by sitting, relieved by standing, and resolves when supine or sitting without pressure placed on the perineum, for example, when sitting on a donut hole "pillow" or a toilet seat.[17] Distinguishing pudendal neuropathy from the more common indeterminate causes of perineal pain may be aided by the concomitant description of numbness or other sensory symptoms of the penis, scrotum, labia majora, and perineum. If bilateral, disturbances in micturition, defecation, erection, and ejaculation may occur.[207]

Pudendal neuropathy may result from pelvic and hip fractures, injection injuries, hemorrhage into piriformis, neoplastic invasion, surgical procedures, childbirth, or prolonged or inordinate pressure on perineum from ill-fitting bicycle seats or pressure devices that may be used to reduce hip dislocations.[207–209] Predisposition to entrapment or compression is thought to be facilitated by the relationship of the pudendal nerve with the sacrotuberous and sacrospinous ligaments or the ischial tuberosity as the nerve exits the pelvis through Alcock canal where fibrosis of the obturator internus muscle has been described.[17,209]

The diagnosis of pudendal neuropathy is challenging as there are limited objective findings to distinguish true neuropathy from the seemingly far more prevalent cases of undefined perineal and genital pain and sensory symptoms such as vulvodynia and proctalgia fugax that may defy objective diagnosis. Some of these have been attributed to pudendal neuralgia presumed but unproven to represent an entrapment syndrome.[210] A number of EDX techniques have been applied to the evaluation of the pudendal nerves including NCSs but we have limited confidence in either their sensitivity or specificity in the identification of pudendal nerve injury.[211] Identifying evidence of denervation confined to the external anal sphincter would provide strong supportive evidence of axon loss injury to the pudendal nerve. MRI is of value in selective cases.[17] Relief of symptoms with pudendal nerve block would serve both a diagnostic and therapeutic purpose.[212] Surgical intervention should be undertaken judiciously and is recommended only in those cases with significant morbidity and definable pathology.[213]

▶ MONOMELIC NEUROPATHIES

The monomelic neuropathies are relatively uncommon disorders that typically directly or indirectly result from acute limb ischemia. Occlusion of major limb vessels such as the aortic bifurcation, external iliac, or superficial femoral artery resulting from embolus or instrumentation such as intra-aortic balloon pumping or arterial cannulation associated with coronary bypass grafting are the typical causes in the lower extremities.[16,214–216] Implicit in the description of this syndrome is the belief that nerve is either more readily injured or less readily recoverable with acute limb ischemia than are other limb tissues. Chronic limb ischemia has been reported to associate with EDX findings, suggesting length-dependent axon loss.[214,215,217–219] Whether this ever translates into a clinically evident neuropathy in the absence of other tissue damage is a matter of controversy.

Most disorders that affect multiple nerves or multiple nerve roots are systemic disorders that typically affect more than one extremity. Monomelic neuropathies bear resemblance to plexopathies in that both motor and sensory deficits occur, affecting more than one nerve distribution but confined to a single extremity. The dominant feature is deep, persistent, burning pain in the foot associated with cutaneous hypersensitivity. The distribution of motor and sensory deficits is typically length dependent, affecting all nerves below the knee and typically below mid-calf. Muscle innervated by those same nerves and segments more proximally located are spared.[16] Although motor deficits occur, like length-dependent axonal polyneuropathies, these are typically less evident from a clinical perspective. Part of this stems from the clinical difficulty in clinically assessing the most severely affected intrinsic foot muscles. From an EDX standpoint, this syndrome may resemble a sciatic neuropathy. Notable differences are that the hamstring muscles tend to be spared and the saphenous sensory response will be abnormal in monomelic polyneuropathy if it can be reliably contrasted to the uninvolved opposite limb. The EDX pattern of monomelic polyneuropathy is unique in that it is a multifocal neuropathy, but one that is both length dependent and confined to one limb as the name implies in most cases.

Compartment syndromes refer to ischemic tissue damage within confined anatomic spaces typically bordered by taut fascial membranes. Peripheral nerves are at risk from the cycle of ischemia that is created by increased compartmental pressure. Typically, an initial injury promotes edema and increased compartment pressure. This impairs compartment perfusion and promotes further ischemic injury and, as a result, further swelling. A vicious positive feedback cycle is thus created. Pressure blisters, a swollen limb, and/or myoglobinuria are potentially associated clinical features that may warn of impending nerve injury or aid to clarify the mechanism of nerve injury.[220,221] Many of the mononeuropathies previously mentioned in this chapter are a risk from immobilization, either due to a direct pressure or in association with nerve injury occurring from more diffuse compartmental pressure. Recognized compartment syndromes in the lower extremity include sciatic neuropathy from the gluteal compartment or posterior compartment of the thigh syndromes, femoral neuropathy from the iliacus compartment or within the anterior thigh, and a peroneal neuropathy resulting from an anterior compartment syndrome in the leg.[221,222]

Imaging of the involved area will typically identify swelling and signal changes within the muscle of that compartment. Manometric measurements may confirm elevated pressure within that compartment, pressures as low as 30 mm Hg being potentially injurious to nerve.[220] A compartment syndrome is a surgical emergency that requires decompression and potentially debulking of the involved anatomic compartment(s).

► SUMMARY

Focal neuropathies of the lower extremities are common neurologic problems that are frequently caused by compressive mechanisms. Clinically directed localization supplemented by EDX testing (when required) provides the foundation for the evaluation of these disorders. When the neuropathy cannot be readily attributed to a common compressive mechanism, imaging rationally directed by the localization process facilitates identification of less commonly occurring secondary causes of individual nerve injury.

Focal neuropathies are potentially more amenable to surgical intervention than are most disorders described elsewhere in this text. Many of these disorders will have natural histories that are self-limited and a decision to surgically intervene should not be based solely on EDX or imaging data. Once again, the skilled and judicious neuromuscular clinician is in a unique position to provide both accurate disease identification and optimal management.

REFERENCES

1. Levin KH. L5 radiculopathy with reduced superficial peroneal sensory responses: intraspinal and extraspinal causes. *Muscle Nerve*. 1998;21(1):3–7.
2. Klein JP. A practical approach to spine imaging. *Continuum (Minneap Minn)*. 2015;21(1 Spinal Cord Disorders):36–51.
3. Jellema K, Tijssen CC, van Gijn J. Spinal dural arteriovenous fistulas: a congestive myelopathy that initially mimics a peripheral nerve disorder. *Brain*. 2006;129(Pt 12):3150–3164.
4. Mathews JA. Wasting of the small hand muscles in upper and mid-cervical cord lesions. *QJM*. 1998;91(10):691–700.
5. Deyo RA, Weinstein JN. Low back pain. *N Engl J Med*. 2001;344(5):363–370.
6. Koes BW, van Tulder MW, Thomas S. Diagnosis and treatment of low back pain. *BMJ*. 2006;332(7555):1430–1434.
7. Carragee EJ. Clinical practice. Persistent low back pain. *N Engl J Med*. 2005;352(18):1891–1898.
8. Chiarotto A, Koes BW. Nonspecific low back pain. *N Engl J Med*. 2022;386(18):1732–1740.
9. Devereaux MW. Anatomy and examination of the spine. *Neurol Clin*. 2007;25(2):331–351.
10. Furusawa N, Baba H, Miyoshi N, et al. Herniation of cervical intervertebral disc: immunohistochemical examination and measurement of nitric oxide production. *Spine (Phila Pa 1976)*. 2001;26(10):1110–1116.
11. Kang JD, Georgescu HI, McIntyre-Larkin L, Stefanovic-Racic M, Evans CH. Herniated cervical intervertebral discs spontaneously produce matrix metalloproteinases, nitric oxide, interleukin-6, and prostaglandin E2. *Spine (Phila Pa 1976)*. 1995;20(22):2373–2378.
12. Kang JD, Stefanovic-Racic M, McIntyre LA, Georgescu HI, Evans CH. Toward a biochemical understanding of human intervertebral disc degeneration and herniation. Contributions of nitric oxide, interleukins, prostaglandin E2, and matrix metalloproteinases. *Spine (Phila Pa 1976)*. 1997;22(10):1065–1073.
13. Kline DG, Kim D, Midha R, Harsh C, Tiel R. Management and results of sciatic nerve injuries: a 24-year experience. *J Neurosurg*. 1998;89(1):13–23.
14. Liu Z, Tao F, Xu W, et al. Incidence of traumatic sciatic nerve injury in patients with acetabular fractures and factors affecting recovery: a retrospective study. *J Orthop Surg Res*. 2023;18:35.
15. Richards RL. Ischaemic lesions of peripheral nerves: a review. *J Neurol Neurosurg Psychiatry*. 1951;14:76–87.
16. Wilbourn AJ, Furlan AJ, Hulley W, Ruschhaupt W. Ischemic monomelic neuropathy. *Neurology*. 1983;33(4):447–451.
17. Martinoli C, Miguel-Perez M, Padua L, Gandolfo N, Zicca A, Tagliafico A. Imaging of neuropathies about the hip. *Eur J Radiol*. 2013;82(1):17–26.
18. Burakgazi AZ, Kelly JJ, Richardson P. The electrodiagnostic sensitivity of proximal lower extremity muscles in the diagnosis of L5 radiculopathy. *Muscle Nerve*. 2012;45(6):891–893.
19. Rutkove SB, Nardin RA, Raynor EM, Levy ML, Landrio MA. Lumbosacral polyradiculopathy mimicking distal polyneuropathy. *J Clin Neuromuscul Dis*. 2000;2(2):65–69.
20. Stewart JD. Magnificent MRI and fascinating selective nerve fascicle damage. *Neurology*. 2014;82(7):554–555.
21. Pham M, Bäumer P, Meinck H-M, et al. Anterior interosseous nerve syndrome: fascicular motor lesions of median nerve trunk. *Neurology*. 2014;82(7):598–606.
22. American Academy of Neurology's Therapeutics; Technology Assessment Subcommittee. Review of the literature on spinal ultrasound for the evaluation of back pain and radicular disorders: report of the Therapeutics and Technology Assessment Subcommittee of the American Academy of Neurology. *Neurology*. 1998;51(2):343–344.
23. Delaney H, Bencardino J, Rosenberg ZS. Magnetic resonance neurography of the pelvis and lumbosacral plexus. *Neuroimaging Clin N Am*. 2014;24(1):127–250.
24. Filosto M, Pari E, Cotelli M, et al. MR neurography in diagnosing nondiabetic lumbosacral radiculoplexus neuropathy. *J Neuroimaging*. 2013;23(4):543–544.
25. Ishii K, Tamaoka A, Shoji S. MRI of idiopathic lumbosacral plexopathy. *Neurology*. 2004;63(2):E6.
26. Mathys C, Aissa J, Meyer Zu Hörste G, et al. Peripheral neuropathy: assessment of proximal nerve integrity by diffusion tensor imaging. *Muscle Nerve*. 2013;48(6):889–896.
27. Sprangfort E. Lasègue's sign in patients with lumbar disc herniation. *Acta Orthop Scand*. 1971;42(5):459.
28. Dyck P. The femoral nerve traction test with lumbar disc protrusions. *Surg Neurol*. 1976;(3):163–166.
29. Tavee JO, Levin KH. Low back pain. *Continuum (Minneap Minn)*. 2017;23(2, Selected Topics in Outpatient Neurology):467–486.
30. Bozzao A, Gallucci M, Masciocchi C, Aprile I, Barile A, Passariello R. Lumbar disk herniation: MR imaging assessment of natural history in patients treated without surgery. *Radiology*. 1992;185(1):135–141.
31. Delauche-Cavallier MC, Budet C, Laredo JD, et al. Lumbar disc herniation. Computed tomography scan changes after conservative treatment of nerve root compression. *Spine (Phila Pa 1976)*. 1992;17(8):927–933.
32. Tilki HE, Mutluer N, Selçuki D, Stålberg E. Zoster paresis. *Electromyogr Clin Neurophysiol*. 2003;43(4):231–234.
33. Cockerell OC, Ormerod IE. Focal weakness following herpes zoster. *J Neurol Neurosurg Psychiatr*. 1993;56(9):1001–1003.

34. Bahadir C, Kalpakcioglu AB, Kurtulus D. Unilateral diaphragmatic paralysis and segmental motor paresis following herpes zoster. *Muscle Nerve*. 2008;38(2):1070–1073.
35. Jensen MC, Brant-Zawadzki MN, Obuchowski N, Modic MT, Malkasian D, Ross JS. Magnetic resonance imaging of the lumbar spine in people without back pain. *N Engl J Med*. 1994;331(2):69–73.
36. Boden SD, Davis DO, Dina TS, Patronas NJ, Wiesel SW. Abnormal magnetic-resonance scans of the lumbar spine in asymptomatic subjects. A prospective investigation. *J Bone Joint Surg Am*. 1990;72(3):403–408.
37. Borenstein DG, O'Mara JW, Boden SD, et al. The value of magnetic resonance imaging of the lumbar spine to predict low-back pain in asymptomatic subjects : a seven-year follow-up study. *J Bone Joint Surg Am*. 2001;83(9):1306–1311.
38. Foster NE, Anema JR, Cherkin D, et al. Prevention and treatment of low back pain: evidence, challenges, and promising directions. *Lancet*. 2018;391(10137):2368–2383.
39. Kreiner DS, Hwang SW, Easa JE, et al. An evidence-based clinical guideline for the diagnosis and treatment of lumbar disc herniation with radiculopathy. *Spine J*. 2014;14(1):180–191.
40. Qaseem A, Wilt TJ, McLean RM, et al; Clinical Guidelines Committee of the American College of Physicians. Noninvasive treatments for acute, subacute, and chronic low back pain: a clinical practice guideline from the American College of Physicians. *Ann Intern Med*. 2017;166(7):514–530.
41. Rozenberg S, Delval C, Rezvani Y, et al. Bed rest or normal activity for patients with acute low back pain: a randomized controlled trial. *Spine (Phila Pa 1976)*. 2002;27(14):1487–1493.
42. Deyo RA, Diehl AK, Rosenthal M. How many days of bed rest for acute low back pain? A randomized clinical trial. *N Engl J Med*. 1986;315(17):1064–1070.
43. Malmivaara A, Häkkinen U, Aro T, et al. The treatment of acute low back pain—bed rest, exercises, or ordinary activity? *N Engl J Med*. 1995;332(6):351–355.
44. Enke O, New HA, New CH, et al. Anticonvulsants in the treatment of low back pain and lumbar radicular pain: a systematic review and meta-analysis. *CMAJ*. 2018;190(26):E786–E793.
45. Armon C, Argoff CE, Samuels J, Backonja M-M; Therapeutics and Technology Assessment Subcommittee of the American Academy of Neurology. Assessment: use of epidural steroid injections to treat radicular lumbosacral pain: report of the Therapeutics and Technology Assessment Subcommittee of the American Academy of Neurology. *Neurology*. 2007;68(10):723–729.
46. Carette S, Marcoux S, Truchon R, et al. A controlled trial of corticosteroid injections into facet joints for chronic low back pain. *N Engl J Med*. 1991;325(14):1002–1007.
47. MacVicar J, King W, Landers MH, Bogduk N. The effectiveness of lumbar transforaminal injection of steroids: a comprehensive review with systematic analysis of the published data. *Pain Med*. 2013;14(1):14–28.
48. Carette S, Leclaire R, Marcoux S, et al. Epidural corticosteroid injections for sciatica due to herniated nucleus pulposus. *N Engl J Med*. 1997;336(23):1634–1640.
49. Deyo RA, Walsh NE, Martin DC, Schoenfeld LS, Ramamurthy S. A controlled trial of transcutaneous electrical nerve stimulation (TENS) and exercise for chronic low back pain. *N Engl J Med*. 1990;322(23):1627–1634.
50. Beurskens AJ, de Vet HC, Köke AJ, et al. Efficacy of traction for nonspecific low back pain. 12-week and 6-month results of a randomized clinical trial. *Spine (Phila Pa 1976)*. 1997;22(23):2756–2762.
51. Gibson JNA, Waddell G. Surgical interventions for lumbar disc prolapse. *Cochrane Database Syst Rev*. 2007;2007(1):CD001350.
52. Hall S, Bartleson JD, Onofrio BM, Baker HL Jr, Okazaki H, O'Duffy JD. Lumbar spinal stenosis. Clinical features, diagnostic procedures, and results of surgical treatment in 68 patients. *Ann Intern Med*. 1985;103(2):271–275.
53. Jordan J, Konstantinou K, O'Dowd J. Herniated lumbar disc. *BMJ Clin Evid*. 2011;2011:1118.
54. Weber H. Lumbar disc herniation. A controlled, prospective study with ten years of observation. *Spine*. 1983;8(2):131–140.
55. Hermansen E, Myklebust TÅ, Weber C, et al. Postoperative dural sac cross-sectional area as an association for outcome after surgery for lumbar spinal stenosis: clinical and radiological results from the NORDSTEN-spinal stenosis trial. *Spine*. 2023;48(10):688–694.
56. Chad DA. Lumbar spinal stenosis. *Neurol Clin*. 2007;25(2):407–418.
57. Katz JN, Harris MB. Clinical practice. Lumbar spinal stenosis. *N Engl J Med*. 2008;358(8):818–825.
58. Guigui P, Benoist M, Delecourt C, Delhoume J, Deburge A. Motor deficit in lumbar spinal stenosis: a retrospective study of a series of 50 patients. *J Spinal Disord*. 1998;11(4):283–288.
59. Montagna P, Martinelli P, Rasi F, Cirignotta F, Govoni E, Lugaresi E. Muscular hypertrophy after chronic radiculopathy. *Arch Neurol*. 1984;41(4):397–398.
60. Swartz KR, Fee DB, Trost GR, Waclawik AJ. Unilateral calf hypertrophy seen in lumbosacral stenosis: case report and review of the literature. *Spine*. 2002;27(18):E406–E409.
61. Rubin DI. Acute and chronic polyradiculopathies. *Continuum (Minneap Minn)*. 2011;17(4):831–854.
62. Liao JP, Waclawik AJ. Nerve root hypertrophy in CMT type 1A. *Neurology*. 2004;62(5):783.
63. Bennett SJ, Katzman GL, Roos RP, Mehta AS, Ali S. Neoplastic cauda equina syndrome: a neuroimaging-based review. *Pract Neurol*. 2016;16(1):35–41.
64. Deyo RA, Diehl AK. Cancer as a cause of back pain: frequency, clinical presentation, and diagnostic strategies. *J Gen Intern Med*. 1988;3(3):230–238.
65. Crawford JD, Perrone KH, Wong VW, et al. A modern series of acute aortic occlusion. *J Vasc Surg*. 2014;59(4):1044–1050.
66. Chiang S, Pet DB, Talbott JF, LaHue SC, Douglas VC, Rosendale N. Spinal epidural arteriovenous fistula with nerve root enhancement mimicking myeloradiculitis: a case report. *BMC Neurol*. 2023;23(1):62.
67. Ehresman J, Catapano JS, Baranoski JF, Jadhav AP, Ducruet AF, Albuquerque FC. Treatment of spinal arteriovenous malformation and fistula. *Neurosurg Clin N Am*. 2022;33(2):193–206.
68. Carod Artal FJ, Vargas AP, Horan TA, Marinho PB, Coelho Costa PH. Schistosoma mansoni myelopathy: clinical and pathologic findings. *Neurology*. 2004;63(2):388–391.
69. Mackenzie AR, Laing RB, Smith CC, Kaar GF, Smith FW. Spinal epidural abscess: the importance of early diagnosis and treatment. *J Neurol Neurosurg Psychiatr*. 1998;65(2):209–212.

70. Tetsuka S, Suzuki T, Ogawa T, Hashimoto R, Kato H. Spinal epidural abscess: a review highlighting early diagnosis and management. *JMA J.* 2020;3(1):29–40.
71. Grill MF. Neurologic complications of human immunodeficiency virus. *Continuum (Minneap Minn).* 2021;27(4):963–991.
72. Robinson-Papp J, Simpson DM. Neuromuscular diseases associated with HIV-1 infection. *Muscle Nerve.* 2009;40(6):1043–1053.
73. Corral I, Quereda C, Casado JL, et al. Acute polyradiculopathies in HIV-infected patients. *J Neurol.* 1997;244(8):499–504.
74. Benatar MG, Eastman RW. Human immunodeficiency virus-associated pure motor lumbosacral polyradiculopathy. *Arch Neurol.* 2000;57(7):1034–1039.
75. So YT, Olney RK. Acute lumbosacral polyradiculopathy in acquired immunodeficiency syndrome: experience in 23 patients. *Ann Neurol.* 1994;35(1):53–58.
76. Thaisetthawatkul P, Logigian EL. Peripheral nervous system manifestations of Lyme borreliosis. *J Clin Neuromuscul Dis.* 2002;3(4):165–171.
77. Logigian EL, Steere AC. Clinical and electrophysiologic findings in chronic neuropathy of Lyme disease. *Neurology.* 1992;42(2):303–311.
78. Halperin JJ. Lyme disease and the peripheral nervous system. *Muscle Nerve.* 2003;28(2):133–143.
79. Lantos PM, Rumbaugh J, Bockenstedt LK, et al. Clinical practice guidelines by the Infectious Diseases Society of America, American Academy of Neurology, and American College of Rheumatology: 2020 guidelines for the prevention, diagnosis, and treatment of Lyme disease. *Neurology.* 2021;96(6):262–273.
80. Scelsa SN, Herskovitz S, Berger AR. A predominantly motor polyradiculopathy of Lyme disease. *Muscle Nerve.* 1996;19(6):780–783.
81. Burns TM, Dyck PJB, Aksamit AJ, Dyck PJ. The natural history and long-term outcome of 57 limb sarcoidosis neuropathy cases. *J Neurol Sci.* 2006;244(1–2):77–87.
82. Koffman B, Junck L, Elias SB, Feit HW, Levine SR. Polyradiculopathy in sarcoidosis. *Muscle Nerve.* 1999;22(5):608–613.
83. Verma KK, Forman AD, Fuller GN, Dimachkie MM, Vriesendorp FJ. Cauda equina syndrome as the isolated presentation of sarcoidosis. *J Neurol.* 2000;247(7):573–574.
84. Stefurak TL, Midroni G, Bilbao JM. Vasculitic polyradiculopathy in systemic lupus erythematosus. *J Neurol Neurosurg Psychiatr.* 1999;66(5):658–661.
85. Molyneux PD, Barker R, Thomas PK, King RH, Miller DH. Non-systemic vasculitic neuropathy presenting with a painful polyradiculopathy: a case report. *J Neurol.* 2000;247(8):645–646.
86. Muhn N, Baker SK, Hollenberg RD, Meaney BF, Tarnopolsky MA. Syringomyelia presenting as rapidly progressive foot drop. *J Clin Neuromuscul Dis.* 2002;3(3):133–134.
87. Miller DW, Katirji B, Preston DC. Idiopathic epidural lipomatosis. *J Clin Neuromuscul Dis.* 2005;6(3):144–146.
88. Bourne IH. Lumbo-sacral adhesive arachnoiditis: a review. *J R Soc Med.* 1990;83(4):262–265.
89. Anderson TL, Morris JM, Wald JT, Kotsenas AL. Imaging appearance of advanced chronic adhesive arachnoiditis: a retrospective review. *AJR Am J Roentgenol.* 2017;209(3):648–655.
90. Abraham A, Drory VE. Postradiation lower motor neuron syndrome: case series and literature review. *J Neurol.* 2013;260(7):1802–1806.
91. Bowen J, Gregory R, Squier M, Donaghy M. The post-irradiation lower motor neuron syndrome neuronopathy or radiculopathy? *Brain.* 1996;119(Pt 5):1429–1439.
92. Feistner H, Weissenborn K, Münte TF, Heinze HJ, Malin JP. Post-irradiation lesions of the caudal roots. *Acta Neurol Scand.* 1989;80(4):277–281.
93. Hsia AW, Katz JS, Hancock SL, Peterson K. Post-irradiation polyradiculopathy mimics leptomeningeal tumor on MRI. *Neurology.* 2003;60(10):1694–1696.
94. Greenfield MM, Stark FM. Post-irradiation neuropathy. *Am J Roentgenol Radium Ther.* 1948;60(5):617–622.
95. Lamy C, Mas JL, Varet B, Ziegler M, de Recondo J. Postradiation lower motor neuron syndrome presenting as monomelic amyotrophy. *J Neurol Neurosurg Psychiatr.* 1991;54(7):648–649.
96. Yuen EC, Layzer RB, Weitz SR, Olney RK. Neurologic complications of lumbar epidural anesthesia and analgesia. *Neurology.* 1995;45(10):1795–1801.
97. Beyer F, Prasse T, Eysel P, Bredow J. Quality of life in lumbar spinal stenosis: does it correlate with magnetic resonance imaging and spinopelvic parameters? *J Orthop.* 2024;47:67–71.
98. Tomkins-Lane C, Melloh M, Lurie J, et al. ISSLS prize winner: consensus on the clinical diagnosis of lumbar spinal stenosis: results of an international Delphi study. *Spine (Phila Pa 1976).* 2016;41(15):1239–1246.
99. Haig AJ, Tong HC, Yamakawa KS, et al. Spinal stenosis, back pain, or no symptoms at all? A masked study comparing radiologic and electrodiagnostic diagnoses to the clinical impression. *Arch Phys Med Rehabil.* 2006;87(7):897–903.
100. Haig AJ, Tomkins CC. Diagnosis and management of lumbar spinal stenosis. *JAMA.* 2010;303(1):71–72.
101. Dillingham TR, Annaswamy TM, Plastaras CT. Evaluation of persons with suspected lumbosacral and cervical radiculopathy: electrodiagnostic assessment and implications for treatment and outcomes (Part I). *Muscle Nerve.* 2020;62(4):462–473.
102. Dillingham TR, Annaswamy TM, Plastaras CT. Evaluation of persons with suspected lumbosacral and cervical radiculopathy: electrodiagnostic assessment and implications for treatment and outcomes (Part II). *Muscle Nerve.* 2020;62(4):474–484.
103. Kuchta J, Sobottke R, Eysel P, Simons P. Two-year results of interspinous spacer (X-Stop) implantation in 175 patients with neurologic intermittent claudication due to lumbar spinal stenosis. *Eur Spine J.* 2009;18(6):823–829.
104. Halperin JJ, Shapiro ED, Logigian E, et al. Practice parameter: treatment of nervous system Lyme disease (an evidence-based review): report of the Quality Standards Subcommittee of the American Academy of Neurology. *Neurology.* 2007;69(1):91–102.
105. Bastron JA, Thomas JE. Diabetic polyradiculopathy: clinical and electromyographic findings in 105 patients. *Mayo Clin Proc.* 1981;56(12):725–732.
106. Pinto MV, Ng P-S, Laughlin RS, et al. Risk factors for lumbosacral radiculoplexus neuropathy. *Muscle Nerve.* 2022;65(5):593–598.
107. Pinto MV, Ng P-S, Howe BM, et al. Lumbosacral radiculoplexus neuropathy: neurologic outcomes and survival in a population-based study. *Neurology.* 2021;96(16):e2098–e2108.
108. Ng PS, Dyck PJ, Laughlin RS, Thapa P, Pinto MV, Dyck PJB. Lumbosacral radiculoplexus neuropathy: incidence and the association with diabetes mellitus. *Neurology.* 2019;92(11):e1188–e1194.

109. Dyck PJ, Norell JE, Dyck PJ. Microvasculitis and ischemia in diabetic lumbosacral radiculoplexus neuropathy. *Neurology.* 1999;53(9):2113–2121.
110. Dyck PJB, Windebank AJ. Diabetic and nondiabetic lumbosacral radiculoplexus neuropathies: new insights into pathophysiology and treatment. *Muscle Nerve.* 2002;25(4):477–491.
111. Garces-Sanchez M, Laughlin RS, Dyck PJ, Engelstad JK, Norell JE, Dyck PJB. Painless diabetic motor neuropathy: a variant of diabetic lumbosacral radiculoplexus neuropathy? *Ann Neurol.* 2011;69(6):1043–1054.
112. Aragon Pinto C, Pinto MV, Engelstad JK, Dyck PJB. Lumbosacral radiculoplexus neuropathy after COVID-19. *Neurologist.* 2023;28(4):273–276.
113. Laughlin RS, Dyck PJ, Melton LJ, Leibson C, Ransom J, Dyck PJB. Incidence and prevalence of CIDP and the association of diabetes mellitus. *Neurology.* 2009;73(1):39–45.
114. Sumner CJ, Sheth S, Griffin JW, Cornblath DR, Polydefkis M. The spectrum of neuropathy in diabetes and impaired glucose tolerance. *Neurology.* 2003;60(1):108–111.
115. Kelkar P, Hammer-White S. Impaired glucose tolerance in nondiabetic lumbosacral radiculoplexus neuropathy. *Muscle Nerve.* 2005;31(2):273–274.
116. Said G, Elgrably F, Lacroix C, et al. Painful proximal diabetic neuropathy: inflammatory nerve lesions and spontaneous favorable outcome. *Ann Neurol.* 1997;41(6):762–770.
117. Bradley WG, Chad D, Verghese JP, et al. Painful lumbosacral plexopathy with elevated erythrocyte sedimentation rate: a treatable inflammatory syndrome. *Ann Neurol.* 1984;15(5):457–464.
118. Sander JE, Sharp FR. Lumbosacral plexus neuritis. *Neurology.* 1981;31(4):470–473.
119. Dyck PJ, Engelstad J, Norell J, Dyck PJ. Microvasculitis in nondiabetic lumbosacral radiculoplexus neuropathy (LSRPN): similarity to the diabetic variety (DLSRPN). *J Neuropathol Exp Neurol.* 2000;59(6):525–538.
120. Yee T. Recurrent idiopathic lumbosacral plexopathy. *Muscle Nerve.* 2000;23(9):1439–1442.
121. Dyck PJ, Norell JE, Dyck PJ. Non-diabetic lumbosacral radiculoplexus neuropathy: natural history, outcome and comparison with the diabetic variety. *Brain.* 2001;124(Pt 6):1197–1207.
122. Tarulli A, Rutkove SB. Lumbosacral plexitis. *J Clin Neuromuscul Dis.* 2005;7(2):72–78.
123. Gloviczki P, Cross SA, Stanson AW, et al. Ischemic injury to the spinal cord or lumbosacral plexus after aorto-iliac reconstruction. *Am J Surg.* 1991;162(2):131–136.
124. Lee SB, Hall CW, Wijdicks EFM. Monoplegia due to acute aortic occlusion. *Muscle Nerve.* 2005;32(5):686–687.
125. Emery S, Ochoa J. Lumbar plexus neuropathy resulting from retroperitoneal hemorrhage. *Muscle Nerve.* 1978;1(4):330–334.
126. Chiu WS. The syndrome of retroperitoneal hemorrhage and lumbar plexus neuropathy during anticoagulant therapy. *South Med J.* 1976;69(5):595–599.
127. Pettigrew LC, Glass JP, Maor M, Zornoza J. Diagnosis and treatment of lumbosacral plexopathies in patients with cancer. *Arch Neurol.* 1984;41(12):1282–1285.
128. Thomas JE, Cascino TL, Earle JD. Differential diagnosis between radiation and tumor plexopathy of the pelvis. *Neurology.* 1985;35(1):1–7.
129. Jaeckle KA, Young DF, Foley KM. The natural history of lumbosacral plexopathy in cancer. *Neurology.* 1985;35(1):8–15.
130. Ladha SS, Spinner RJ, Suarez GA, Amrami KK, Dyck PJB. Neoplastic lumbosacral radiculoplexopathy in prostate cancer by direct perineural spread: an unusual entity. *Muscle Nerve.* 2006;34(5):659–665.
131. Aho K, Sainio K. Late irradiation-induced lesions of the lumbosacral plexus. *Neurology.* 1983;33(7):953–955.
132. Ladha SS, Dyck PJB, Spinner RJ, et al. Isolated amyloidosis presenting with lumbosacral radiculoplexopathy: description of two cases and pathogenic review. *J Peripher Nerv Syst.* 2006;11(4):346–352.
133. Kutsy RL, Robinson LR, Routt ML. Lumbosacral plexopathy in pelvic trauma. *Muscle Nerve.* 2000;23(11):1757–1760.
134. Felice KJ, Donaldson JO. Lumbosacral plexopathy due to benign uterine leiomyoma. *Neurology.* 1995;45(10):1943–1944.
135. Zuniga G, Ropper AH, Frank J. Sarcoid peripheral neuropathy. *Neurology.* 1991;41(10):1558–1561.
136. Levin KH. Approach to the patient with suspected radiculopathy. *Neurol Clin.* 2012;30(2):581–604.
137. Dyck PJ, Norell JE, Dyck PJ. Methylprednisolone may improve lumbosacral radiculoplexus neuropathy. *Can J Neurol Sci.* 2001;28(3):224–227.
138. Zochodne DW, Isaac D, Jones C. Failure of immunotherapy to prevent, arrest or reverse diabetic lumbosacral plexopathy. *Acta Neurol Scand.* 2003;107(4):299–301.
139. Kawagashira Y, Watanabe H, Oki Y, et al. Intravenous immunoglobulin therapy markedly ameliorates muscle weakness and severe pain in proximal diabetic neuropathy. *J Neurol Neurosurg Psychiatr.* 2007;78(8):899–901.
140. Kilfoyle D, Kelkar P, Parry GJ. Pulsed methylprednisolone is a safe and effective treatment for diabetic amyotrophy. *J Clin Neuromuscul Dis.* 2003;4(4):168–170.
141. Chan YC, Lo YL, Chan ES. Immunotherapy for diabetic amyotrophy. *Cochrane Database Syst Rev.* 2017;7(7):CD006521.
142. Pradat P-F, Bouche P, Delanian S. Sciatic nerve moneuropathy: an unusual late effect of radiotherapy. *Muscle Nerve.* 2009;40(5):872–874.
143. Katirji MB, Wilbourn AJ. Common peroneal mononeuropathy: a clinical and electrophysiologic study of 116 lesions. *Neurology.* 1988;38(11):1723–1728.
144. Grant GA, Britz GW, Goodkin R, Jarvik JG, Maravilla K, Kliot M. The utility of magnetic resonance imaging in evaluating peripheral nerve disorders. *Muscle Nerve.* 2002;25(3):314–331.
145. Halford H, Graves A, Bertorini T. Muscle and nerve imaging techniques in neuromuscular diseases. *J Clin Neuromuscul Dis.* 2000;2(1):41–51.
146. Walker FO, Cartwright MS, Wiesler ER, Caress J. Ultrasound of nerve and muscle. *Clin Neurophysiol.* 2004;115(3):495–507.
147. Cartwright MS, Chloros GD, Walker FO, Wiesler ER, Campbell WW. Diagnostic ultrasound for nerve transection. *Muscle Nerve.* 2007;35(6):796–799.
148. Koltzenburg M, Bendszus M. Imaging of peripheral nerve lesions. *Curr Opin Neurol.* 2004;17(5):621–626.
149. Briani C, Cacciavillani M, Lucchetta M, Cecchin D, Gasparotti R. MR neurography findings in axonal multifocal motor neuropathy. *J Neurol.* 2013;260(9):2420–2422.
150. Gonzalez NL, Hobson-Webb LD. Neuromuscular ultrasound in clinical practice: a review. *Clin Neurophysiol Pract.* 2019;4:148–163.
151. Toussaint CP, Perry EC, Pisansky MT, Anderson DE. What's new in the diagnosis and treatment of peripheral nerve entrapment neuropathies. *Neurol Clin.* 2010;28(4):979–1004.

152. Robinson LR. Traumatic injury to peripheral nerves. *Muscle Nerve*. 2000;23(6):863–873.
153. Miller JP, Acar F, Kaimaktchiev VB, Gultekin SH, Burchiel KJ. Pathology of ilioinguinal neuropathy produced by mesh entrapment: case report and literature review. *Hernia*. 2008;12(2):213–216.
154. Ndiaye A, Diop M, Ndoye JM, et al. Anatomical basis of neuropathies and damage to the ilioinguinal nerve during repairs of groin hernias. (about 100 dissections). *Surg Radiol Anat*. 2007;29(8):675–681.
155. Vuilleumier H, Hübner M, Demartines N. Neuropathy after herniorrhaphy: indication for surgical treatment and outcome. *World J Surg*. 2009;33(4):841–845.
156. Hahn L. Clinical findings and results of operative treatment in ilioinguinal nerve entrapment syndrome. *Br J Obstet Gynaecol*. 1989;96(9):1080–1083.
157. Lee CH, Dellon LA. Surgical management of groin pain of neural origin1. *J Am Coll Surg*. 2000;191(2):137–142.
158. Murovic JA, Kim DH, Tiel RL, Kline DG. Surgical management of 10 genitofemoral neuralgias at the Louisiana State University Health Sciences Center. *Neurosurgery*. 2005;56(2):298–303; discussion 298.
159. Chutkow JG. Posterior femoral cutaneous neuralgia. *Muscle Nerve*. 1988;11(11):1146–1148.
160. Schiller F. Sigmund Freud's meralgia paresthetica. *Neurology*. 1985;35(4):557–558.
161. Parisi TJ, Mandrekar J, Dyck PJB, Klein CJ. Meralgia paresthetica: relation to obesity, advanced age, and diabetes mellitus. *Neurology*. 2011;77(16):1538–1542.
162. Berini SE, Spinner RJ, Jentoft ME, et al. Chronic meralgia paresthetica and neurectomy: a clinical pathologic study. *Neurology*. 2014;82(17):1551–1555.
163. Seror P, Seror R. Meralgia paresthetica: clinical and electrophysiological diagnosis in 120 cases. *Muscle Nerve*. 2006;33(5):650–654.
164. Nahabedian MY, Dellon AL. Meralgia paresthetica: etiology, diagnosis, and outcome of surgical decompression. *Ann Plast Surg*. 1995;35(6):590–594.
165. Grossman MG, Ducey SA, Nadler SS, Levy AS. Meralgia paresthetica: diagnosis and treatment. *J Am Acad Orthop Surg*. 2001;9(5):336–344.
166. Nahabedian MY, Dellon AL. Outcome of the operative management of nerve injuries in the ilioinguinal region. *J Am Coll Surg*. 1997;184(3):265–268.
167. Khalil N, Nicotra A, Rakowicz W. Treatment for meralgia paraesthetica. *Cochrane Database Syst Rev*. 2012;12(12):CD004159.
168. Kuntzer T, van Melle G, Regli F. Clinical and prognostic features in unilateral femoral neuropathies. *Muscle Nerve*. 1997;20(2):205–211.
169. Santilli AR, Martinez-Thompson JM, Speelziek SJA, Staff NP, Laughlin RS. Femoral neuropathy: a clinical and electrodiagnostic review. *Muscle Nerve*. 2024;69(1):64–71.
170. Tsiptsios D, Daud D, Tsamakis K, Rizos E, Anastadiadis A, Cassidy A. Bilateral femoral neuropathy: a rare complication of drug overdose due to prolonged posturing in lithotomy position. *Case Rep Neurol Med*. 2020;2020:2352850.
171. Romanoff ME, Cory PC, Kalenak A, Keyser GC, Marshall WK. Saphenous nerve entrapment at the adductor canal. *Am J Sports Med*. 1989;17(4):478–481.
172. Sole JS, Pingree MJ, Spinner RJ, Murthy NS, Sellon JL. Saphenous neuropathy secondary to extraneural ganglion cyst 15 years after reconstruction of the anterior cruciate ligament. *PM R*. 2014;6(5):451–455.
173. Shenoy AM, Wiesman J. Saphenous mononeuropathy after popliteal vein aneurysm repair. *Neurologist*. 2010;16(1):47–49.
174. Mountney J, Wilkinson GA. Saphenous neuralgia after coronary artery bypass grafting. *Eur J Cardiothorac Surg*. 1999;16(4):440–443.
175. Hakim SM, Narouze SN. Risk factors for chronic saphenous neuralgia following coronary artery bypass graft surgery utilizing saphenous vein grafts. *Pain Pract*. 2015;15(8):720–729.
176. Rogers LR, Borkowski GP, Albers JW, Levin KH, Barohn RJ, Mitsumoto H. Obturator mononeuropathy caused by pelvic cancer: six cases. *Neurology*. 1993;43(8):1489–1492.
177. Sorenson EJ, Chen JJ, Daube JR. Obturator neuropathy: causes and outcome. *Muscle Nerve*. 2002;25(4):605–607.
178. Yuen EC, Olney RK, So YT. Sciatic neuropathy: clinical and prognostic features in 73 patients. *Neurology*. 1994;44(9):1669–1674.
179. Yuen EC, So YT, Olney RK. The electrophysiologic features of sciatic neuropathy in 100 patients. *Muscle Nerve*. 1995;18(4):414–420.
180. Goldberg G, Goldstein H. AAEM case report 32: nerve injury associated with hip arthroplasty. *Muscle Nerve*. 1998;21(4):519–527.
181. Nercessian OA, Macaulay W, Stinchfield FE. Peripheral neuropathies following total hip arthroplasty. *J Arthroplasty*. 1994;9(6):645–651.
182. Salazar-Grueso E, Roos R. Sciatic endometriosis: a treatable sensorimotor mononeuropathy. *Neurology*. 1986;36(10):1360–1363.
183. Holland NR, Schwartz-Williams L, Blotzer JW. "Toilet seat" sciatic neuropathy. *Arch Neurol*. 1999;56(1):116.
184. Kornetzky L, Linden D, Berlit P. Bilateral sciatic nerve "Saturday night palsy." *J Neurol*. 2001;248(5):425.
185. Preston DC, Shapiro BE. Lymphoma of the sciatic nerve. *J Clin Neuromuscul Dis*. 2001;2(4):227–228.
186. Gasecki AP, Ebers GC, Vellet AD, Buchan A. Sciatic neuropathy associated with persistent sciatic artery. *Arch Neurol*. 1992;49(9):967–968.
187. McManis PG. Sciatic nerve lesions during cardiac surgery. *Neurology*. 1994;44(4):684–687.
188. Srinivasan J, Ryan MM, Escolar DM, Darras B, Jones HR. Pediatric sciatic neuropathies: a 30-year prospective study. *Neurology*. 2011;76(11):976–980.
189. Probst D, Stout A, Hunt D. Piriformis syndrome: a narrative review of the anatomy, diagnosis, and treatment. *PM R*. 2019;11(Suppl 1):S54–S63.
190. Kirschner JS, Foye PM, Cole JL. Piriformis syndrome, diagnosis and treatment. *Muscle Nerve*. 2009;40(1):10–18.
191. Fishman LM, Schaefer MP. The piriformis syndrome is underdiagnosed. *Muscle Nerve*. 2003;28(5):646–649.
192. Stewart JD. The piriformis syndrome is overdiagnosed. *Muscle Nerve*. 2003;28(5):644–646.
193. Filler AG, Haynes J, Jordan SE, et al. Sciatica of nondisc origin and piriformis syndrome: diagnosis by magnetic resonance neurography and interventional magnetic resonance imaging with outcome study of resulting treatment. *J Neurosurg Spine*. 2005;2(2):99–115.
194. Vij N, Kiernan H, Bisht R, et al. Surgical and non-surgical treatment options for piriformis syndrome: a literature review. *Anesth Pain Med*. 2021;11(1):e112825.
195. Kang PB, Preston DC, Raynor EM. Involvement of superficial peroneal sensory nerve in common peroneal neuropathy. *Muscle Nerve*. 2005;31(6):725–729.

196. Iverson DJ. MRI detection of cysts of the knee causing common peroneal neuropathy. *Neurology*. 2005;65(11):1829–1831.
197. Sotaniemi KA. Slimmer's paralysis–peroneal neuropathy during weight reduction. *J Neurol Neurosurg Psychiatr*. 1984;47(5):564–566.
198. Campellone JV. Peroneal neuropathy from antithrombotic stockings. *J Clin Neuromuscul Dis*. 1999;1(1):14–16.
199. Jones HR, Felice KJ, Gross PT. Pediatric peroneal mononeuropathy: a clinical and electromyographic study. *Muscle Nerve*. 1993;16(11):1167–1173.
200. Drees C, Wilbourn AJ, Stevens GHJ. Main trunk tibial neuropathies. *Neurology*. 2002;59(7):1082–1084.
201. DeLisa JA, Saeed MA. The tarsal tunnel syndrome. *Muscle Nerve*. 1983;6(9):664–670.
202. Goodgold J, Kopell HP, Spielholz NI. The tarsal-tunnel syndrome. Objective diagnostic criteria. *N Engl J Med*. 1965;273(14):742–745.
203. Oh SJ, Sarala PK, Kuba T, Elmore RS. Tarsal tunnel syndrome: electrophysiological study. *Ann Neurol*. 1979;5(4):327–330.
204. Campbell WW, Landau ME. Controversial entrapment neuropathies. *Neurosurg Clin N Am*. 2008;19(4):597–608, vi.
205. Yuebing L, Lederman RJ. Sural mononeuropathy: a report of 36 cases. *Muscle Nerve*. 2014;49(3):443–445.
206. Stickler DE, Morley KN, Massey EW. Sural neuropathy: etiologies and predisposing factors. *Muscle Nerve*. 2006;34(4):482–484.
207. Silbert PL, Dunne JW, Edis RH, Stewart-Wynne EG. Bicycling induced pudendal nerve pressure neuropathy. *Clin Exp Neurol*. 1991;28:191–196.
208. Andersen KV, Bovim G. Impotence and nerve entrapment in long distance amateur cyclists. *Acta Neurol Scand*. 1997;95(4):233–240.
209. Insola A, Granata G, Padua L. Alcock canal syndrome due to obturator internus muscle fibrosis. *Muscle Nerve*. 2010;42(3):431–432.
210. Stav K, Dwyer PL, Roberts L. Pudendal neuralgia. Fact or fiction? *Obstet Gynecol Surv*. 2009;64(3):190–199.
211. O'Brien C, O'Herlihy C, O'Connell PR. Pudendal neuropathy is best determined by full neurophysiologic assessment. *Am J Obstet Gynecol*. 2004;191(5):1836.
212. Hough DM, Wittenberg KH, Pawlina W, et al. Chronic perineal pain caused by pudendal nerve entrapment: anatomy and CT-guided perineural injection technique. *AJR Am J Roentgenol*. 2003;181(2):561–567.
213. Hruby S, Dellon L, Ebmer J, Höltl W, Aszmann OC. Sensory recovery after decompression of the distal pudendal nerve: anatomical review and quantitative neurosensory data of a prospective clinical study. *Microsurgery*. 2009;29(4):270–274.
214. Levin KH. AAEE case report #19: ischemic monomelic neuropathy. *Muscle Nerve*. 1989;12(10):791–795.
215. Weinberg DH, Simovic D, Isner J, Ropper AH. Chronic ischemic monomelic neuropathy from critical limb ischemia. *Neurology*. 2001;57(6):1008–1012.
216. Lachance DH, Daube JR. Acute peripheral arterial occlusion: electrophysiologic study of 32 cases. *Muscle Nerve*. 1991;14(7):633–639.
217. Weber F, Ziegler A. Axonal neuropathy in chronic peripheral arterial occlusive disease. *Muscle Nerve*. 2002;26(4):471–476.
218. Nukada H, van Rij AM, Packer SG, McMorran PD. Pathology of acute and chronic ischaemic neuropathy in atherosclerotic peripheral vascular disease. *Brain*. 1996;119 (Pt 5):1449–1460.
219. England JD, Ferguson MA, Hiatt WR, Regensteiner JG. Progression of neuropathy in peripheral arterial disease. *Muscle Nerve*. 1995;18(4):380–387.
220. Shields RW, Root KE, Wilbourn AJ. Compartment syndromes and compression neuropathies in coma. *Neurology*. 1986;36(10):1370–1374.
221. Farrell CM, Rubin DI, Haidukewych GJ. Acute compartment syndrome of the leg following diagnostic electromyography. *Muscle Nerve*. 2003;27(3):374–377.
222. Poppi M, Giuliani G, Gambari PI, Acciarri N, Gaist G, Calbucci F. A hazard of craniotomy in the sitting position: the posterior compartment syndrome of the thigh. Case report. *J Neurosurg*. 1989;71(4):618–619.

CHAPTER 25

Autoimmune Myasthenia Gravis

▶ INTRODUCTION

Myasthenia gravis (MG) represents one of medicine's most notable translational successes in bringing basic science to the bedside. MG was the first antibody-mediated neurologic disorder identified and has since served as a model for the identification of pathophysiology and targeted therapeutic development. Neuromuscular junction (NMJ) disorders can be conceptualized and categorized as adversely affecting neuromuscular transmission (NMT) at the presynaptic, synaptic, or postsynaptic levels. This chapter will focus on acquired, autoimmune MG, a postsynaptic disorder representing the prototypical disorder of neuromuscular transmission (DNMT). Chapter 26 will discuss Lambert-Eaton myasthenic syndrome, and the less frequently occurring infectious/toxic and genetic DNMTs [i.e., congenital myasthenic syndromes (CMS)].

▶ PIVOTAL EVENTS IN THE HISTORY OF MYASTHENIA GRAVIS

The clinical description of MG followed by an understanding of its neurophysiology unfolded over centuries.[1] The first description of a woman with likely MG was made in 1672 by British physician Thomas Willis in his book *De Anima Brutorum*, which described this presentation among other clinical syndromes. He described a woman with a chronic paralytic disorder which affected her limbs and tongue. He wrote, "she speaks freely and readily enough for a while, but after a long period of speech ... she is not able to speak a word and is as mute as a fish. Her voice does not return for one or two hours."[2] Two centuries later, Erb and Goldflam, after whom the disease was initially named, described the fatigue, the fluctuating nature of symptoms, and the tendency for relapses and remissions over time, which distinguished the condition from progressive bulbar palsy.[3,4] In 1895, Jolly was the first to demonstrate that repetitive stimulation of motor nerves produces decreasing muscle contraction in MG patients, which accounted for weakness and fatigue. He called this "myasthenia gravis pseudoparalytica (myo = muscle; asthenia = weakness; gravis = severe)."[5] By 1901, 118 cases had been described by two papers in the literature.[6,7] In 1921, Loewi demonstrated that NMT had a chemical basis, and Dale showed that this depended on the release of acetylcholine (ACh) from motor nerve terminals.[8,9] In 1936, British physician Mary Walker first described that MG could be improved by acetylcholinesterase inhibitors (AChEIs). Her discovery was extrapolated from her observations related to the similarities between MG and curare toxicity.[1] In the 1930s and 1940s, Blalock, a cardiothoracic surgeon in the United States, performed thymectomy first for a patient with MG and a thymic tumor[10] and then, having seen clinical improvement in that first case, for a series of patients with MG but without thymoma.[11] This predated the known role of the thymus in the pathophysiology of MG. The sequences of all five AChR subunits that make up the adult and fetal isoforms of human AChR were unknown until the 1990s.[12]

In the mid-20th century, proof for an autoimmune basis of MG was discovered next, along with additional details about the nature of disordered NMT.[1] In 1960, Simpson hypothesized an autoimmune basis for MG after he observed increased MG prevalence in young women and in individuals with other autoimmune diseases.[13] At the same time, the following occurred: (1) support for MG as a DNMT was provided by the in vitro electrophysiological demonstration that miniature end plate potential (EPP) amplitudes in MG were reduced, and (2) the concept of MG as a postsynaptic DNMT was solidified by demonstrating loss of acetylcholine receptors (AChR) in MG patients through α-bungarotoxin labeling techniques.[1] Then in 1973, Patrick and Lindstrom confirmed the autoimmune nature of MG with the development of an experimental MG model in rabbits who became weak when immunized with AChR.[14] In 1976, Lindstrom et al. published a seminal article describing the value of AChR autoantibody testing in the diagnosis of myasthenia and a radioimmunoprecipitation assay (RIPA) was developed.[15] Marked clinical benefit was demonstrated in MG patients with plasma exchange (PLEX).[16] In the 1980s, disease heterogeneity in terms of serum autoantibodies, age of onset and thymic pathology, and role in AChR production was beginning to be recognized. Additionally, the role of T cells in pathophysiology was first described.[17,18]

In 2001, Hoch et al. reported the association between MG and autoantibodies directed against muscle-specific tyrosine kinase (MuSK).[19] In 2008, unnamed autoantibodies directed at clustered AChRs were found in low titer in the serum of approximately two-thirds of AChR and MuSK seronegative patients.[20,21] In 2011, patients with autoantibodies directed at the lipoprotein receptor protein 4 (LPR4) were identified as a third MG serotype.[22] The discovery of easily measurable MG-specific antibodies, development of disease-specific outcomes measures, and design of clinical research standards facilitated clinical trials in MG.[23,24] At the same time, gaps in evidence-based practice were recognized and international task forces developed consensus guidance statements, pending generation of additional evidence.[25,26] In 2016, Wolfe et al. published results from the randomized controlled trial of thymectomy in myasthenia gravis (MGTX RCT) which demonstrated the benefit of thymectomy in early-onset AChR antibody (ab) positive MG.[27] In 2017, Howard et al. published REGAIN, the first phase III trial of a drug targeted toward a MG disease-specific mechanism.[28] These two landmark studies ushered in the contemporary era in MG, which has been termed the "golden age" of clinical trials.[29] Despite the advanced knowledge of the pathophysiology of MG compared to many other autoimmune diseases, improvement in survival and outcomes has ironically come mostly from advances in general medical care (i.e., mechanical ventilation, critical care, antibiotics to treat concurrent infection), and corticosteroids (CS) and immunosuppressants adapted from transplant medicine.[30] This current era of targeted therapy will usher in discoveries and treatments which do not replace, but rather build on the prior. Both eras would not have been possible without the painstaking work and careful observations of the individuals named and many others in prior decades and centuries.

▶ STRUCTURE AND FUNCTION OF THE NORMAL NEUROMUSCULAR JUNCTION

Each motor axon interacts with a muscle fiber through a synapse called the NMJ. NMT is a tightly regulated process that depends on several events happening sequentially. First, presynaptic voltage-gated calcium channels (VGCCs) open (Fig. 25-1). Then, ACh is released across the synaptic cleft

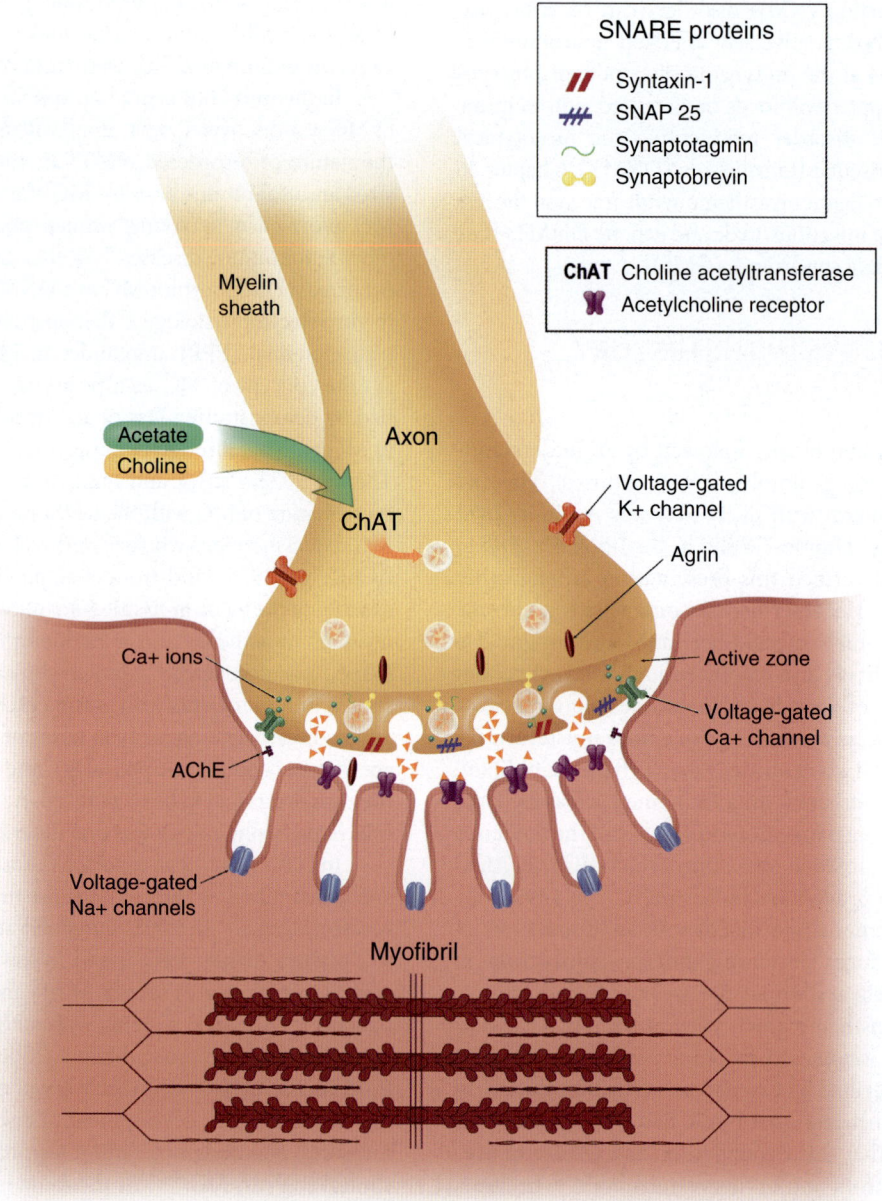

Figure 25-1. Normal presynaptic structures at the neuromuscular junction.

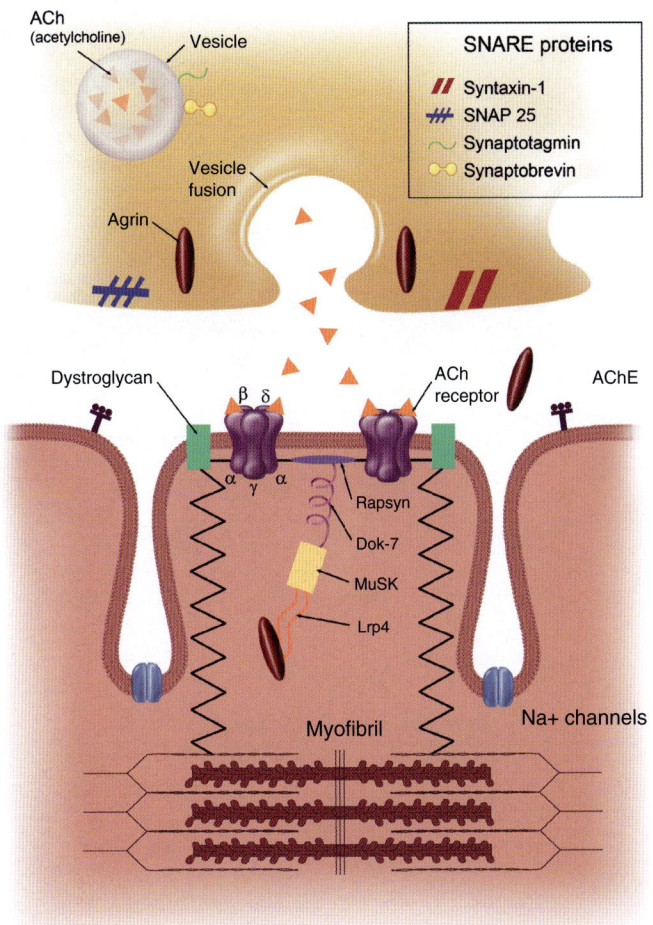

Figure 25-2. Normal postsynaptic structures at the neuromuscular junction.

and binds to the AChRs, which are packed together on the folded, postsynaptic membrane, and this binding triggers AChR opening (Fig. 25-2).[31] A single action potential (AP) causes simultaneous release of approximately 30 quanta of ACh which produces an EPP of approximately 20–30 mV.[32] This exceeds the muscle fiber's firing threshold by a comfortable margin to trigger a postsynaptic AP and therefore, contraction of the muscle fiber occurs.[32] ACh's action is terminated when it is hydrolyzed by acetylcholinesterase in the synaptic cleft.

▶ PATHOPHYSIOLOGY OF MYASTHENIA GRAVIS

In MG, the safety factor of NMT (the amount by which EPP exceeds the muscle fiber's firing threshold) becomes reduced. During sustained or repeated muscle contraction, ACh availability is further diminished, thereby lowering the EPP amplitude. In MG, the combination of a low safety factor to start and further reduction of the EPP amplitude with exercise results in failure of muscle fiber AP generation and contraction, and thus muscle weakness.[32]

Postsynaptic mechanisms maintain the NMJ and are primarily directed at clustering AChR.[31] First, MuSK, which is a postsynaptic transmembrane protein, acts locally to stabilize postsynaptic clusters of AChRs.[33] Agrin, a protein released presynaptically, binds low-density lipoprotein receptor-related protein 4 (LRP4), and then forms a complex with, and activates MuSK. This facilitates recruitment of cytoplasmic proteins including downstream of tyrosine kinase 7 (Dok-7) and rapsyn, to assist in clustering AChRs.[34] Some of these mechanisms provide positive feedback on the presynaptic nerve terminal to further promote this process.[35,36]

Turnover of AChR is a normal part of dynamic processes of the NMJ. Half-life of AChRs in the postsynaptic muscle membrane is about 8–10 days.[37] Senescent AChRs are internalized through endocytosis and transported to lysosomes for degradation through an intricate network of intracellular tubules. Cross-linking of channels with AChR autoantibodies in MG accelerates this process up to three times faster than in normal individuals.[38] Synthesis of AChRs remains unchanged and therefore, a net reduction of 70%–90% AChRs per NMJ results.[39,40] AChRs are not recycled. They are replaced by newly synthesized receptors. This is one reason why MG can be more quickly responsive to treatment compared to other

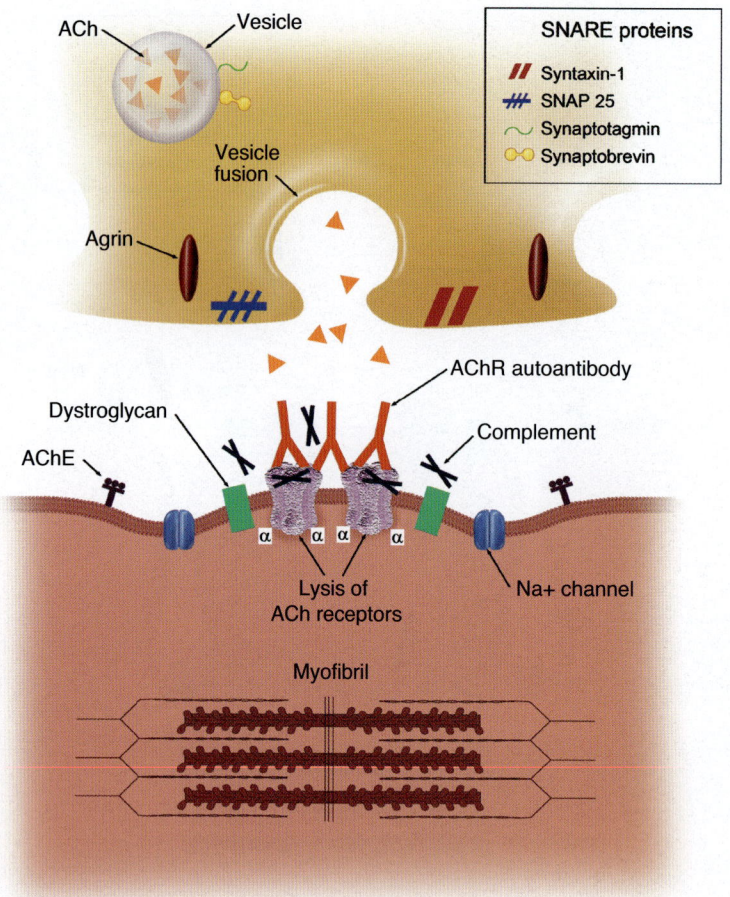

Figure 25-3. Neuromuscular junction in AChR ab positive MG.

neuromuscular disorders in which damaged components are not as readily restored, even if the disease process is arrested.

Integral to the pathogenesis of AChR ab positive MG is the reduction of AChRs at the end plate, as initially demonstrated through radiolabeled α-bungarotoxin techniques.[40] Pathogenic AChR autoantibodies are IgG1 and IgG3 subtypes and bind predominantly to the main immunogenic regions of the AChR, which exist on two alpha subunits of the channel.[41–44] Once bound to the AChR, these antibodies initiate several irreversible processes directed at the AChR and postsynaptic membrane, including activation of complement and steric hindrance. During the latter, autoantibodies physically block ACh-binding sites on adjacent channels and/or prevent the conformational change resulting in opening of the ion pore.[45] Complement activation also reduces the number of voltage-gated sodium channels that are clustered at the depths of the end plate folds and further increases the threshold for muscle fiber AP generation (Fig. 25-3).[38,46,47]

ROLE OF COMPLEMENT

In AChR ab positive MG, complement activation is a key part of the pathophysiology which results in impaired NMT. AChR antibodies bound with AChRs activate the complement cascade, which leads to formation of membrane attack complex (MAC). This is outlined nicely in more detail elsewhere[48] and is summarized here.

The complement system is a tightly regulated, sequential cascade of more than 30 proteins located in plasma and on cell surfaces. It forms a link between innate and adaptive immunity by enhancing antibody responses. The complement cascade protects the host by recognizing and eliminating infectious organisms. It is activated by three pathways [classical (antigen/antibody), lectin and alternative] and results in the formation of C3, which is the product of the "proximal complement" system and the last step before C5 formation. All proteins upstream (i.e., "proximal") to C5 are critical for microbial opsonization and immune complex clearance. Next, C5 is cleaved into C5a and C5b. This generates molecules with proinflammatory and cell-lytic properties including MAC, which an eventual product of C5b. MAC is involved in cell lysis, cell signaling, and clearance of encapsulated bacteria including *Neisseria*.[48,49]

The key role of complement in pathogenesis had been shown extensively in AChR ab positive MG, from preclinical animal models of experimental autoimmune myasthenia gravis (EAMG) to phase III interventional drug trials of complement inhibitors. Engel and others in the 1970s hypothesized the role of complement in MG after observing AChR antibodies, C3, and MAC bound to debris at the postsynaptic membrane in MG patients.[50] EAMG studies suggest that induction of the classical complement pathway, and particularly formation of the MAC, are required for induction of MG symptoms. Conversely, inhibiting MAC formation improves MG symptoms in animal models. Mice without complement factors (C3, C4, C5, or C6) are resistant to EAMG. In contrast, mice without protective regulators, DAF1 and CD59a, are more prone to developing EAMG.

MG WITH MuSK ANTIBODIES

MuSK ab positive MG has a pathophysiology which is distinct from AChR ab positive MG.[19] Disease-causing MuSK antibodies are of the IgG4 subtype, and as such, do not activate complement. They have low affinity for activating Fc receptors on immune cells and are generally considered "anti-inflammatory."[51,52] MuSK antibodies exert their pathogenic effect by directly inhibiting binding between MuSK and LRP4, leading to loss of AChRs, and other functions of MuSK.[53] It is possible that MuSK antibody valency and isotype may influence pathogenicity and ultimate MG severity.[54] MuSK antibodies also likely disrupt the interaction between MuSK and collagen Q,[55] which anchors acetylcholinesterase.[56] Unmooring of acetylcholinesterase could explain the hypersensitivity to AChEI therapy experienced by some patients with MuSK ab positive MG.[31]

MG WITH LRP4 ANTIBODIES AND SERONEGATIVE MG

Approximately 2% of individuals diagnosed with double seronegative generalized MG have low-density LRP4 antibodies (anti-LRP4 ab), which are primarily of the IgG1 subclass.[57] LRP4 ab are pathogenic by causing complement-mediated destruction similar to AChR ab, and possibly interrupting agrin-induced MuSK activation.[55,58] It is not clear from current evidence that antibodies to agrin in isolation are pathogenic and disease-causing in MG.[59,60] Pathophysiology of seronegative MG is thought to be most like AChR ab positive disease. A proportion of seronegative patients have low-affinity antibodies, which cannot be detected by routine radioimmunoassays (RIAs) and but can be detected by specific assays such as cell-based assays (CBAs).[61,62]

▶ PERIPHERAL IMMUNE DYSREGULATION

Although AChR MG is conceptually a disorder mediated by autoantibodies, a significant T-cell–mediated, CD4 lymphocyte component also contributes to the pathophysiology. In MG, T-cell abnormalities involve both T-regulatory (Treg) cells and conventional T cells.

In understanding the pathophysiology of MG, it is helpful to briefly summarize how normal immune tolerance is established. Immune tolerance to self occurs during thymic development through the process of clonal deletion of potentially autoreactive T cells. The thymus generates responsive T cells from the immature precursors called thymocytes, which become critical components of the adaptive immune system. In short, it provides a critical environment for the differentiation and selection of T cells, which shapes an individual's adaptive immunity. It also serves a role in preventing autoimmune diseases through negative selection, which deletes most autoreactive T cells.[63] Recently a study used single-cell RNA sequencing to create an atlas of human thymic cells across development and compare findings to the mouse thymus.[64]

In normal individuals, some of these pathogenic antigenic cells, including those with reactivity to AChR, survive clonal deletion. In individuals without MG, disease does not develop because these survival cells are kept in check by peripheral tolerance mechanisms, particularly Treg cells, which are a specialized subset of CD4+ T cells.[65,66] Treg cells play a critical role in immune system homeostasis and self-tolerance by suppressing activation of other immune cells, including those T cells which escaped negative selection in the thymus and exited to the periphery.[65] These mechanisms of self-tolerance require multiple cell types within the thymus including thymic epithelial cells (TECs), dendritic cells (DCs), and B cells. They also involve several anatomic locations within the thymus, namely the cortex, medulla, and perivascular spaces (PVSs).[63]

The thymus is the primary source of Treg cells which constitute approximately 5%–10% of the peripheral CD4+ T-cell population.[65] Treg cells also suppress the activation and proliferation of cytokine production from effector autoreactive T cells that arise de novo or escape thymic deletion.[65] Deficiency or dysfunction of Treg cells contributes to the pathogenesis not only of MG but also of many autoimmune diseases.[67] In MG to date, there is more evidence for dysfunction than deficiency of Treg cells.[68] Recent work has shed light on how medullary TECs facilitate self-tolerization of maturing T cells. In short, they are thought to repurpose the lineage-defining transcription factors of various extrathymic cell types to create cellular mimics of extrathymic tissue types (i.e., peripheral-tissue antigens) within the thymus.[69] The transcription factor autoimmune regulator (AIRE) and, in some circumstances, the coinhibitory receptor cytotoxic T-lymphocyte–associated protein 4 (CTLA-4) are expressed by TECs and regulate this process.[70] This may be one mechanism behind why immune checkpoint inhibitor (ICI) drugs, which further remove the inhibitory T-cell signals in the periphery including by inhibiting CTLA-4 on tumor tissues, can be associated with fatal immune-related adverse events (irAEs) including overlapping MG, myositis, and myocarditis in patients with thymoma.[71]

The upregulation of CD4+ T cells which results from loss of immune tolerance, leads to the release of proinflammatory cytokines (e.g., IL-2, IL-4 and IL-6, IL-17, IFN-gamma).[68] These cytokines stimulate B cells which results in antibody production. In the mouse model of AChR positive MG, AChR ab generation by B cells was shown to be dependent on IL-17 production by CD4+ T cells. This illustrates how IL-17–expressing CD4+ T helper 17 (Th17) cells are involved in inducing a classical antibody-mediated disease such as MG.[72] This has since been shown to be relevant in humans and acts as a positive feedback cycle, stimulating further activation of mature T and B lymphocytes in the thymus gland. Further activation of T cells results in more secretion of proinflammatory cytokines, increasing the imbalance between abnormal Treg cells and hyperactivated Th17 cells, and further amplifying antibody production in MG. Additionally, Th17 cells are considered to be critical regulators of thymic inflammation and hyperplasia in AChR MG patients.[73] Circulating Th1/Th17 cells may be a marker of disease severity in AChR ab positive patients.[74]

T-cell abnormalities are not limited to AChR ab positive MG. In MuSK MG, frequencies of Th1 and Th17 cytokines were shown to be higher than healthy controls, along with an increase in T-cell polyfunctionality.[75] The link between T-cell abnormality and antibody production was described when Tfh17 cells, a subset of Tfh cells important for B-cell–mediated antibody production, was shown to be enhanced in MuSK MG patients.[76] While total numbers of Tfh17 cells were normal, which is not surprising given lack of thymic abnormalities in MuSK MG, a higher Tfh:Tfr ratio was seen. This suggests insufficient regulation of the Tfh cells. MuSK MG patients also have higher frequencies of CD4 T cells producing IL-17, IFNγ, and IL-21.[76]

▶ GENETIC CONTRIBUTIONS TO AUTOIMMUNE MG

Autoimmune MG is not a hereditary disease and does not follow a classic Mendelian inheritance pattern. However, several studies have demonstrated an increased chance of family members also developing MG compared to the general population.[77-79] A North American study of 1,032 AChR ab positive MG patients identified a family history of MG retrospectively in 58 (5.6%). Notably, approximately a quarter of these patients also had a personal and family history of autoimmune disease besides MG.[79] Additionally, a 35% concordance rate in monozygotic twins and 5% in dizygotic twins has been reported, suggesting both a genetic and environmental contribution to MG pathogenesis.[78] Genetic susceptibility to MG also associates with specific HLA alleles and haplotypes at the class I and II regions in different populations. These associations are different for early- and late-onset MG different MG subtypes.[80]

Non-HLA genes have also been associated with MG.[81] Two large genome-wide association (GWAS) studies have been performed with AChR ab positive MG patients of European descent compared to healthy individuals to identify disease-associated genetic risk loci.[82,83] Replication of the discovered loci was performed in an independent cohort from the UK Biobank as well as transcriptome-wide association study (TWAS) using expression data from muscle, blood, and nerve to test effects of disease-associated polymorphisms on gene expression.[83] The Renton et al. GWAS study[82] identified association signals at CTLA4 and HLA-DQAI which were replicated in an independent cohort of Italian cases and control individuals. HLA-DQA1 was replicated in the Chia et al. study,[83] but CTLA4 was not, perhaps due to a different population or sample size limitations. However, Chia et al. further replicated the finding of distinct genetic susceptibly in early- and late-onset MG.[83] Second, genetic evidence was found linking MG with other autoimmune diseases, including rheumatoid arthritis, multiple sclerosis, type 1 diabetes, and ulcerative colitis, supporting many previous clinical observations. Third, and most importantly, associations were found in two genes encoding AChR subunits: (1) GWAS signal in the cholinergic receptor nicotinic alpha 1 subunit (CHRNA1) gene, and (2) TWAS association with the cholinergic receptor nicotinic beta 1 subunit (CHRNB1) gene. These were both replicated in the UK biobank cohort. These susceptibility loci are feasible from a mechanistic sense as mutations in both AChR subunits are implicated as etiologies of CMS. In addition to providing insight into what might trigger MG, these studies, if replicated in more diverse patient populations, may provide targets for future therapeutic interventions.

THYMIC PATHOPHYSIOLOGY IN EARLY-ONSET AND THYMOMA-ASSOCIATED MG

The hallmark thymic pathology of early-onset AChR ab positive MG is thymic follicular hyperplasia (TFH). An abnormal abundance of TFH can result in a grossly enlarged, "hyperplastic" thymus (Fig. 25-4A). TFH describes ectopic lymphoid follicles in PVSs merging with the thymic medulla (Fig. 25-4B,C). The trigger for TFH is unknown. A proportion of healthy individuals have AChR-reactive T cells circulating in blood as part of their normal T-cell repertoire for unknown reasons. These T cells return to the thymus and then become activated by an unknown trigger. The T cells are subsequently primed by medullary thymic epithelial cells (mTECs) expressing MHC/AChR-peptide complexes. The primed T cells activate thymic B cells to produce low affinity anti-AChR antibodies which bind to thymic myoid cells (TMCs) expressing AChRs. Binding triggers complement activation which induces the release of AChR/ab complexes from TMCs for processing by adjacent DCs. These DCs bind to follicular dendritic cells (FDCs) in a reaction located in thymic germinal centers, which yields plasma cells (PCs) producing high-affinity anti-AChR autoantibodies. MG self-perpetuates even after removal of

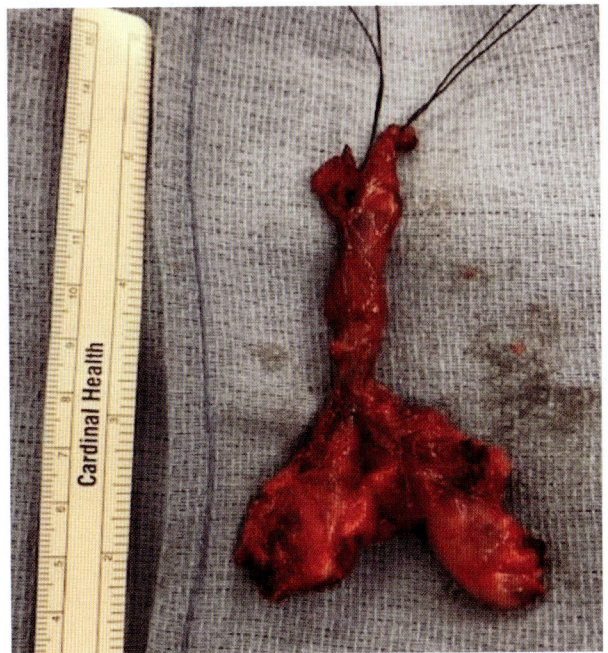
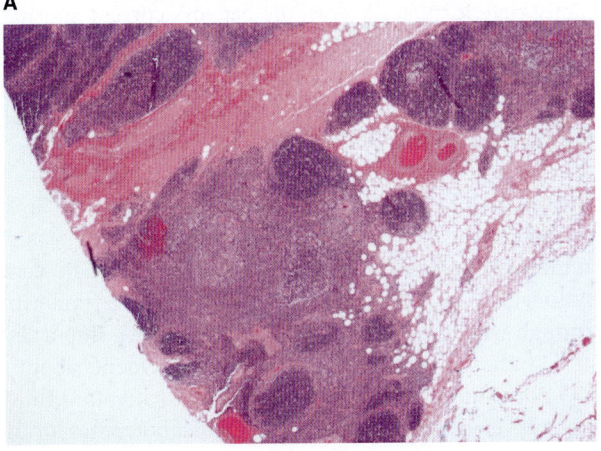
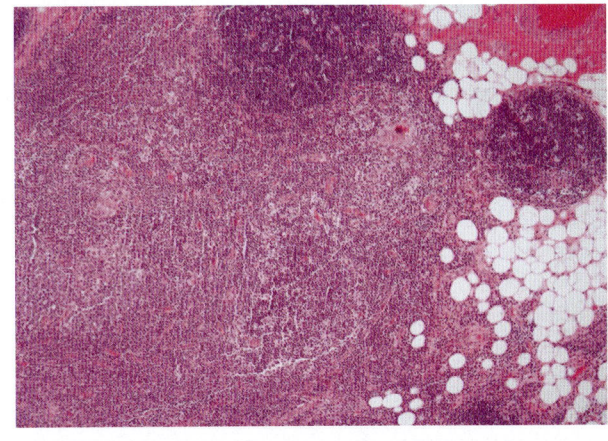

Figure 25-4. A 28-year-old woman with AChR-positive gMG without thymoma who underwent thymectomy. Gross pathology revealed a hyperplastic 26-g thymus (**A**) with marked follicular hyperplasia on low-power (**B**) and high-power (**C**) fields.

the thymus hypothetically due to the flow of skeletal muscle-derived AChR/ab complexes to regional lymph nodes and functionally impaired Treg cells.[63]

Thymoma-associated MG (TAMG) has differences in pathophysiology compared to nonthymoma-associated early- and late-onset MG.[63,84] It is unknown whether thymoma lives on the same spectrum as thymic hyperplasia. Triggers for the development of thymoma and then for associated MG in 30% of those patients are unknown.

▶ CONNECTION BETWEEN PHENOTYPE AND PATHOPHYSIOLOGY

The questions of why certain MG subtypes preferentially involve certain muscles more commonly, and why the muscles affected in the same subtype differ between patients or over the course of disease are longstanding and yet largely unresolved question.[31] Differences in pathologic features of various muscles and their NMJs have been hypothesized. Possible factors include (1) access of the pathogenic IgG to NMJs,[85] (2) characteristics, density, and turnover rate of antigenic proteins at NMJs, (3) magnitude of the safety factor of NMT greater in type 2 versus type 1 muscles,[86] (4) variable level of protection against complement activation [particularly low in extraocular muscles (EOMs)],[87] (5) greater concentration of fetal-type AChR in EOMs which are disproportionately susceptible to AChR ab,[38] and (6) patient or muscle-specific differences in muscle regeneration.[88,89]

▶ EPIDEMIOLOGY

The epidemiology of autoimmune MG has been studied for many decades and may be changing over time. The

▶ TABLE 25-1. EPIDEMIOLOGY OF MG AND SUBTYPES

Category	Annual Incidence	Prevalence	Comments
Overall	6.3–29/million	100–361/million	Incidence in very late-onset disease is increasing
Juvenile	1/1,000,000-1/200,000		
Early onset	4.2/million		
Late onset	19/million		
Very late onset	—		
Thymoma	1.3–2.6/million	—	Rate of MG associated with thymoma likely underestimated. Rate of thymoma in MG is approximately 10%.
MG in patients with thymoma	—	30% of thymoma	
Generalized			Prevalence of MuSK depends on geography—rare in Scandinavian countries
AChR	8.5–18.4/million	AChR 85% of gMG	
MuSK		MuSk 0–40% of AChR neg gMG	
LRP4		LRP4 Rare	
Ocular	—	15% overall of MG	
AChR	—	50% of ocular MG	
MuSK	—	Rare	
LRP4	—	Unknown	

incidence, prevalence, and subtype distribution of MG vary with geography and ethnicity. Initial studies were performed primarily in Europe and to a lesser degree in the southeast United States. In the past 5–10 years, there has been additional epidemiologic work in Canada and South America, Asia, and a handful of studies from Africa, the Middle East, and Australia. Incidence and prevalence may be easier to measure in certain health systems and this could account for some of the differences in incidence and prevalence instead of actual differences between populations (Table 25-1).

The overall incidence of thymoma is approximately 0.13–0.26 per 100,000 people, which has a higher incidence in Black and Asian/Pacific Islander populations.[90] MG is the most common paraneoplastic disorder occurring in approximately 30% of patients with thymoma. Others neurologic and non-neurologic paraneoplastic disorders such as cerebellar ataxia, autonomic dysfunction, myositis, neuromyotonia, encephalitis, dysgeusia, and intestinal pseudo-obstruction may present.[91,92]

Traditionally, the epidemiology of MG considers the heterogeneity of disease. Autoimmune MG is divided into juvenile MG, early-onset MG, late-onset MG, and thymoma-associated MG. More recently, very late–onset MG has been termed. MG has traditionally been a disease of younger women and older men with incidence in women equal to that of men in middle age. However, recent data point to the possibility that overall, the average age of onset is increasing, driven by increased incidence and/or recognition in the very late-onset population, the majority of whom are men. Another way of phenotyping MG and studying epidemiology is by antibody status and distribution of muscle weakness. Patients are described as having ocular MG (OMG) or generalized MG. These phenotypes and their approximate frequencies are outlined in Table 25-1. When speaking of an individual patient, it is important to describe antibody status, whether disease is ocular or generalized, and whether the patient has a thymoma and/or underwent thymectomy. In this disease snapshot, we also describe the date of diagnosis (or symptom onset, if more appropriate for that patient), the patient's current and maximum severity, and current treatments.

NATURAL HISTORY

The natural history of MG refers to outcomes of a MG patient cohort that has received the standard care available in the location and at the time it was studied. Single-center, multicenter, and national registries are effective frameworks through which to study natural history in MG. Importantly, such studies allow us to make general statements about the MG population, or specific subgroups of patients with MG. It is still very difficult, however, to predict outcomes for individual patients. This uncertainty is a limitation which likely sometimes leads to over- and undertreatment of MG. Newer therapies can be compared to one another, or sometimes, to outcomes of historical controls, though using historical controls is an uncommon practice to date in MG.

Treatment standards for MG have changed dramatically in the past two decades. Serial natural history studies starting in the 1950s, then the 1980s, and finally 2008, are some of the most cited. They illustrate the evolution of the disease and its changing outcomes through the decades.[93–95] The last in this series includes some of the most widely cited natural history data in MG. However, this paper included data from studies performed prior to the availability of current therapeutic options, and therefore likely does not reflect outcomes with current standard of care management. More recently, data from the registry of a single academic medical in the United States has been published. This study outlines both historical and more contemporary natural history, albeit still prior to the advent of newer biologic therapies.[96,97]

Currently, there is a multicenter biomarker and contemporary natural history study underway in the United States called EXPLORE-MG2 which will likely yield additional useful data. Importantly, this includes patient-reported and physician-measured outcome data. However, this includes patients only from MG clinics at academic centers in the United States and may not be generalizable to the general population in the United States or the global population of patients with MG.[98] Additionally, registries with patient-reported data have been developed in the past decade in MG like in other rare diseases. Debate remains about the utility of patient-reported data in MG when the accuracy of diagnosis and disease subtype are not validated.[99] No single type of natural history study is perfect methodologically in MG, and in general, several are needed to complement one another.

CLINICAL COURSE OF MG

Although we cannot predict the clinical course of MG in any one patient with certainty, it is important to discuss natural history and to set expectations regarding possible course of MG at diagnosis. Myasthenia's course is variable, but the disease usually worsens in severity and involves additional areas of weakness during the first 1–2 years.[95] In the beginning, patients may notice that symptoms resolve completely for days to months at a time, but then return.[100] Reassuringly, approximately two-thirds of patients will have reached their maximum severity by the end of their first year.[95] Without treatment, severely weak muscles may become atrophic, however, this is uncommon in the contemporary era. "Fixed weakness," which has no potential to respond to therapy, is exceedingly uncommon, if it exists at all in MG. Rarely, patients have early very focal, muscle atrophy.[100] However, with advances in treatment, persistent muscle atrophy is rare. Muscle atrophy in general is more common in MuSK ab positive MG, however early treatment with rituximab makes even this unlikely.

Several additional important MG natural history outcomes are important to measure given their medical significance and importance to patients. These include the (1) chance that MG will remain ocular and the contrary risk of generalization, (2) risk of MG crisis or death from MG, and (3) likelihood that MG will go into a state of quiescence either on or off medications. MG quiescence has several forms—complete stable remission (CSR) off medications, pharmacologic remission (PR) on medications, and minimal manifestations (MMs) of disease—which will be discussed in the section of this chapter about MG outcome measures. All three are considered desirable treatment goals (Table 25-2).[101]

Several studies have suggested that immunomodulating treatment may diminish the risk of ocular manifestations of MG evolving into generalized disease. This concept, while likely true anecdotally, is difficult to study and prove, and therefore is not broadly accepted.[36,37] Recently, efforts have been made to predict outcomes on the individual patient level in MG both for risk of MG crisis perioperatively[105] and after thymectomy.[106] A prognostic score to determine the risk of

▶ **TABLE 25-2. RELEVANT NATURAL HISTORY OUTCOMES IN MG TREATED HISTORICALLY PRIOR TO INCLUSION OF NEWER BIOLOGICS**

Patients remaining with ocular only MG after 12 years of follow-up	10%–16%[102]
Lifetime risk of MG crisis (respiratory failure from MG)	15%[103]
Risk of death from MG	a. 1900—70% (MV only) b. 1950s—30% (MV + CEI)[104] c. Present—1.2%–5% (MV, CEI + immunomodulatory therapies)[13,23,38]
Likelihood of minimal manifestations or better on or off medications	72% by 2 years[97] 80% by 5 years[97]
Median time to achieve MM or better	Approximately 2 years[97]

CEI, cholinesterase inhibitor; MV, mechanical ventilation.

generalization in patients who first present with ocular disease has been developed though not tested prospectively or applied to a validation cohort.[107] EXPLORE MG2's focus on immunophenotyping of MG is to develop predictive serum biomarkers for severe disease, impending MG exacerbation, and response to specific therapies.[98] In general, MG subtype-specific tools applied at diagnosis to predict disease status at 6–12 months could stratify patients at risk of severe MG. This could identify patients who would likely benefit from more intensive treatments up front while potentially sparing other patients at lower risk.

Thymomatous MG is generally more severe at onset and has a worse prognosis than nonthymomatous MG.[92,108] This manifests as lower CSR rate, higher frequency of generalized disease with bulbar signs at onset and at maximum severity, and higher frequency of immunosuppressive treatment. The large natural history studies have occurred in Europe and include patient data prior to 2006.[92,108] Thus, the generalizability to other populations and the contemporary treatment era is unknown. Because this is a MG subgroup which experiences more refractory disease and has been excluded from many clinical trials, contemporary natural history studies to inform clinical trials of targeted therapies are needed.

CLINICAL PRESENTATION OF MG

Myasthenia is unique in neurology in that one can take a history, do a physical examination, perform electrodiagnostic (EDX) testing to confirm diagnosis, start treatment, and see improvement in the patient's symptoms, all within the time it requires to take these steps and administer a dose of pyridostigmine. This provides unique intellectual and professional gratification for the practitioner to see near immediate benefit to the patient from one's efforts. It also highlights how critical it is to make an early, accurate diagnosis. The typical and atypical clinical features must be recognized so that appropriate and timely therapy can be instituted.

The two primary phenotypic features of MG are its characteristic patterns of skeletal muscle weakness and the tendency of the severity of this weakness to fluctuate. However, "common" neuromuscular disorders can present atypically, and MG should be considered in any patient with painless weakness without sensory symptoms, even if the weakness is focal. There are theories about why certain muscles are selectively vulnerable and more likely to be weak in MG which will be addressed in the pathophysiology section of this chapter. The fluctuating nature of myasthenic symptoms is related to the dynamic biology of the NMJ.[109] It is a quality of the disease that may be a dominant feature of the patient's history or may be overlooked. MG patients recognize that their symptoms may vary on a minute-to-minute, diurnal, or week-to-week basis. For example, patients frequently describe normal articulation at the onset of a telephone conversation and may have unintelligible speech 5 minutes later. Patients may observe normal eyelid position upon awakening and then develop ptosis as the day wears on. Fluctuation may not be simply diurnal, and patients may have symptoms 1 month which seem to improve the following month without apparent explanation. Fluctuations may also occur in response to identifiable variables such as temperature/season, systemic infection, medications, menses, anxiety, emotional stress, and pregnancy.[110–115]

MG SYMPTOMS

Blurred vision, diplopia, eyelid ptosis, or a combination of these is the sole initial presenting symptom in about 60% of patients with MG and presents in combination in about 70%.[96,102] The next most common presenting symptom, reported by about 15% of patients, is "bulbar" weakness, which refers to dysarthria, dysphagia, or difficulty chewing. Up to about 22% report this in combination with other areas of weakness as an initial presentation. Isolated limb or axial muscle weakness is the third most common single presenting symptom in approximately 5% of patients. Generalized fatigue or isolated dysphagia (without other bulbar symptoms) or shortness of breath (SOB) in the absence of symptoms of more widespread ocular, bulbar, or limb/axial weakness are very uncommon presentations of myasthenia.[96,102]

Weakness in MG can begin insidiously or seem to start rather abruptly. Upon careful questioning, patients might recall symptoms which they recognize only in hindsight as myasthenia. Common examples are: changes in the appearance of one's face due to facial weakness (e.g., trouble smiling, or a "sad," "angry," "expressionless," or "sleepy" appearance), or frequently buying new prescription glasses in an unsuccessful attempt to correct blurred vision.[100]

While ocular weakness can begin insidiously, most patients remember the day or window of several days during which symptoms began. Sometimes these ocular symptoms are initially brief and infrequent, but then become more prolonged and regular, or even constant. Eyelid ptosis usually begins unilaterally, but then often becomes bilateral. The initial side often remains the more severely ptotic lid, but not always. Alternating ptosis is essentially pathognomonic for MG. Diplopia is always painless and binocular. Overt diplopia may be preceded by nonspecific visual blurring when ocular malalignment is minimal and insufficient to produce two distinct images. The presence of other signs and symptoms of myasthenia and/or the resolution of blurring by covering either eye supports that ocular malalignment is causing the blurring.[100] Some patients report a sensation of "dizziness" with their diplopia. It is important to clarify this further. If diplopia is from MG, this typically involves feeling off balance due to double vision and that it takes extra effort for activities which require use of the eyes as a result. Specifically, diplopia from MG should not be accompanied by vertigo, incoordination, or lightheadedness.

Common upper extremity symptoms may include weakness with activities such as washing or blow-drying hair, unloading a dishwasher, painting a wall, kneading bread, vacuuming, or transferring a gallon of milk into a refrigerator or the equivalent. These movements require repeated or sustained contraction of proximal arm and shoulder muscles, which are commonly affected in MG. They are also repeated frequently and so can be used as a barometer to measure change over time. Lower extremity symptoms may involve trouble standing up from a chair, climbing stairs or walking long distances. Patients describe axial weakness as difficulty holding up the head or trouble maintaining an upright posture (i.e., "slumping" or "slouching") when sitting or walking, often seeking creative ways to support their heads. Common strategies include leaning back on a wall or a couch, supporting the chin from below with a hand or wearing a soft collar. When assessing possible axial and limb weakness, it is critical to understand the patient's baseline activity level and any medical comorbidities which may influence function. For example, symptom description will be affected by common musculoskeletal disorders such as osteoarthritis, spinal stenosis, or cardiopulmonary disease, which can also cause reduced endurance. One must try to tease out the contribution from MG to symptoms.

In addition to knowing the patient's baseline, another way of distinguishing what symptoms might be MG-related is to understand what symptoms are variable and fatigable. The hallmark of MG is fatigable weakness, which is caused by abnormal NMT. Fatiguability of ocular and bulbar symptoms is most specific for MG as many patients with neuromuscular diseases of all kinds causing weakness report some diurnal worsening of symptoms as the day progresses.[100]

In MG, ptosis and diplopia are typically worse at the end of the day, after prolonged use of the eyes, with fatigue and in bright light. Ocular symptoms are better upon awakening in the morning and after a period of rest such as a nap or even just closing the eyes for 30 seconds. For some, wearing sunglasses is helpful in reducing eye fatigue and therefore, lessens symptoms.[100] Slurred speech in myasthenia can worsen with prolonged speaking. Speech may be adversely affected in several ways.[116] Patients may describe hypophonia (vocal cord paresis or expiratory muscle weakness), a nasal quality (palatal insufficiency and nasal air leak), slurring (weakness of the lips, tongue, or cheeks) or hoarseness (laryngeal weakness).[117] Nasal regurgitation of food and liquid, difficulty manipulating food due to tongue weakness, as well as ineffective sniffing, coughing, nose blowing, or throat clearing may be reported. When nasal regurgitation is severe, patients will describe "holding their nose" to swallow. Because of weakness of muscles of mastication, fatigue with chewing may occur, particularly with tough foods like steak or hard bread.[118] Meals take longer to complete as chewing becomes more and more difficult as the meal progresses. Manipulating food in the mouth can be difficult due tongue weakness. Salad greens are challenging for many. Food can become immobile in the back of the throat and trigger coughing, throat clearing, or choking after eating. As a result of these problems, patients may eat less, or eat more earlier in the day when feeling stronger. Patients often lose weight if bulbar weakness is moderate to severe.

In addition to dysarthria, symptoms of facial weakness may include difficulty whistling, inflating a balloon, or drinking from a straw. If facial weakness is very severe, patients may experience trouble puckering their lips to give a kiss or drooling while awake.[100,119] Drooling in MG is uncommon in the absence of very severe facial weakness. Respiratory muscle weakness in MG will often be described as either SOB with rest or with exertion. SOB from MG will often be worse supine. Importantly, SOB from MG typically does not exist in isolation and will most often be accompanied by other signs and symptoms of myasthenic weakness.[120]

UNCOMMON MG SYMPTOMS

At times, MG presents with an uncommon manifestation or patients describe a common symptom of MG in an atypical manner. Distal upper or lower extremity weakness can occur in myasthenia though is uncommon.[121-124] When present, weakness typically involves ankle dorsiflexion and wrist/finger extension. Symptoms include tripping while walking and difficulty with grip or with typing/texting. Rarely, patients have axial weakness which presents as difficulty moving in bed or with sit-ups due to neck flexion and abdominal muscle weakness. Severe neck extension weakness with "dropped head" can be accompanied by focal neck pain due to prolonged musculoskeletal strain.[125] Pain in general is not a feature of MG. Weakness of upper facial muscles is as common as lower facial weakness but less likely to be symptomatic. Occasionally, patients may complain of visual blurring due to lower eyelid weakness resulting in pooling of tears.[100] Patients sometimes describe weakness as "numbness," labeling dysarthria as "tongue numbness," and facial weakness as "facial numbness." It is important to clarify whether "numbness" refers to sensory abnormality or a loss of strength or power.

MG PHYSICAL EXAMINATION FINDINGS

The examination of the suspected or established MG patient starts with a complete general neurologic examination which is then tailored. Several components must be added to detect variable weakness and to assess muscles most frequently affected by myasthenia.

GENERAL NEUROLOGIC EXAMINATION

Mental status should be normal if there are no secondary metabolic or cardiopulmonary disturbances. This also means that much of the history is typically obtained from the patient directly unless limited by severe dysarthria or other comorbidities. Similarly, sensation, coordination, and deep tendon reflexes are typically normal. If very severe weakness exists, corresponding reflexes may be reduced focally (i.e., severe triceps weakness and reduced triceps reflex). Gait is also typically normal.[100,115] However, patients with (1) severe quadriceps weakness may lock out their knees, (2) ankle dorsiflexion weakness may have steppage gait, (3) hip-girdle weakness may have a Trendelenburg gait,[126] and (4) axial weakness may have fatigable head drop or camptocormia with ambulation. If diplopia interferes with the coordination and gait exams, these sections can be performed with one eye closed.

OCULAR MUSCLE EXAMINATION

Key features of the ocular muscle examination in MG are outlined in Table 25-3. As ptosis is such a common manifestation of MG, documentation of the baseline upper and lower lid positions in relationship to the pupil is recommended prior to provocative testing. Distinguish ptosis from squinting, both of which narrow the palpebral fissure.[100] When ptosis is moderate to severe, and partially to completely covers the pupil, vision will be obstructed.

In MG, pupil function is spared, although physiological anisocoria is common enough to provide a potentially

▶ **TABLE 25-3. KEY FEATURES OF THE OCULAR EXAMINATION IN MG**

Ptosis and extraocular muscle weakness are typically asymmetric
Variability and/or fatigability can be demonstrated (observe ptosis severity throughout the entire encounter)
Findings do not confirm to lesions of single or multiple individual cranial nerves
Pupillary responses are normal

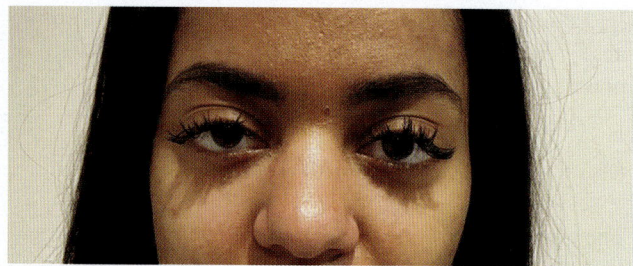

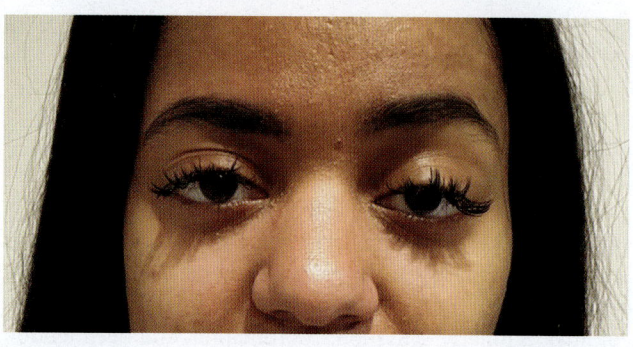

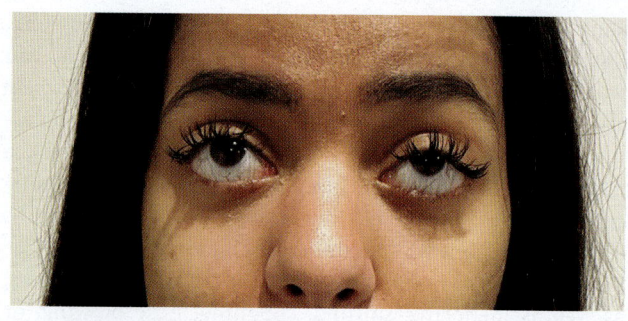

Figure 25-5. (A–C) Patient with ocular manifestations of myasthenia with fatigable alternating ptosis and disconjugate gaze. (A) Mild right > left ptosis, (B) 30 seconds into sustained upgaze, ptosis alternates and is more severe on the left. Notice disconjugate gaze develop with impaired upgaze and exophoria of the right eye, and (C) after completion of 1 minute of upgaze demonstrating left > right ptosis. Notice the elevation of the left eyebrow with contraction of the frontalis muscle to compensate for left ptosis (e.g., a frontalis sign).

confounding feature. Fundoscopic examination is normal. To unmask or exacerbate ptosis or EOM weakness, the patients is asked to sustain either upgaze or lateral gaze for 1 minute, while limiting blinking as much as possible (Fig. 25-5A–C).[127] Any drifting of lid or eyeball position is noted. Cogan lid twitch is another sign which is relatively specific, although not necessarily sensitive, for MG. With this maneuver, the patient is first asked to look down and then rapidly saccade to reassume primary gaze. Normally the eyelid moves synchronously with the eyeball. A positive sign is defined by the eyelid overshooting the eyeball position leading to a transient scleral exposure and upper lid oscillation.[128,129]

Another maneuver with potential diagnostic benefit has been referred to as a curtain's sign or enhanced ptosis.[130] More frequently described in patients with bilateral asymmetric ptosis, it is also valuable in unilateral ptosis. In this maneuver, the clinician manually elevates the most affected eyelid, which may result in the appearance or exacerbation of ptosis on the opposite side. The proposed explanation for this phenomenon is Herring's law of equal innervation. Theoretically, with manual lid elevation, there is less need for supranuclear stimulation of the levator subnucleus of the oculomotor nerve. As this is a single midline nucleus which innervates both levator palpebrae muscles, lifting the more severely affected lid reduces the need for supranuclear stimulation of this subnucleus affecting the contralateral as well as ipsilateral levator palpebrae.[130]

The last bedside maneuver relative to the evaluation of ptosis is the icepack test which relies on the recognized physiological enhancement of NMT by cooling.[112] In this rapid bedside test, an ice pack is applied to a closed eyelid for 2 minutes. Ptosis is measured with a ruler before and after cooling. A lid rise (i.e., reduction of ptosis) of 2 mm is a positive result. As the icepack is potentially uncomfortable, exposure can be first limited to a minute if the patient has difficulty tolerating it.[131] A positive icepack test should be confirmed by other diagnostic methods, given the diagnostic possibilities for ptosis and the potential for false-positive testing.[132]

The most frequently affected EOM in MG is the medial rectus. When weak, horizontal diplopia develops upon lateral gaze to the opposite side. The eyes diverge more with upgaze as the medial rectus cannot adequately resist the lateral pull of the superior rectus. Therefore, diplopia referable to the right medial rectus is worst when looking left and up. The second most common muscle affected is the superior rectus. This yields vertical diplopia elicited or worsened by upgaze. Most commonly, patterns are more complex as multiple EOMs are weak. Red lens testing and single cover and then alternative cover–uncover testing can help delineate the patterns of EOM weakness.[100]

There are several potential pitfalls in the ocular examination for MG. First, if the extraocular motility abnormality is very severe and the eyes are widely divergent, if visual acuity is poor in one eye, or the extraocular motility abnormality is very chronic, patients may suppress the image from one eye and report a single image. Second, a severely ptotic lid which covers the pupil will block vision. In that circumstance, the patient (or examiner) must hold up the eyelid while assessing extraocular motility to allow for testing of binocular vision.[133] Third, simultaneous weakness of medial rectus and contralateral lateral rectus in MG can mimic intranuclear ophthalmoplegia (INO). An INO, often seen in multiple sclerosis, occurs with lesions of the medial longitudinal fasciculus in the dorsomedial brainstem tegmentum of either the pons or the midbrain. It causes adduction weakness of the ipsilateral eye and a contralateral abduction nystagmus. In MG, this is called a pseudo-INO because the same pattern of weakness occurs, but in the absence of a central nervous system lesion.[134,135] Fourth, dermatochalasis, which is loose or redundant eyelid skin, may develop with age, creating "hoods" over the lids. This can give the appearance of ptosis or be present in conjunction with ptosis. Ptosis is measured from the position of the eyelid, not the hood, which sometimes droops lower. Additionally, prolonged activation of any weak EOM can result in nystagmus-like movements in the direction of gaze, the more the muscle fatigues.[100] Finally, if the patient does not relax the forehead and eliminate all contraction of the frontalis muscle (i.e., the "frontalis sign"), ptosis can be missed, or its severity underestimated.[133]

FACIAL AND OROPHARYNGEAL MUSCLE EXAMINATION

Nearly all patients with MG have weakness of orbicularis oculi and therefore, forced eye closure can be overcome. Examiners can learn how to test eye closure and calibrate what is normal and abnormal eye closure strength by testing for patients of all ages with and without MG. Weakness of the orbicularis oculi typically persists even when patients are in remission and all other weakness has resolved. The frontalis muscle can also be weak, manifesting as reduced contraction/movement of the forehead with attempted eyebrow elevation. Both orbicularis oculi and frontalis weakness are typically asymptomatic. Lower facial weakness is tested by attempts to smile which may reveal incomplete muscle activation and a "snarl." Patients are then asked to keep their cheeks inflated with air against gentle resistance. Normal strength is demonstrated by ability to hold air in the inflated cheeks and maintain a normal "O" seal to the lips without the lips becoming horizontal or "transverse." Jaw closure weakness, which can be testing by trying to open the mouth while the patient clenches the teeth, may be affected in MG. Jaw opening is typically normal. The tongue typically has normal bulk, speed of movement, and be without fasciculations. Tongue strength is assessed by asking the patient to push the tongue against the inside of the ipsilateral cheek while the examiner applies pressure to the outside of the cheek. Placing a thumb on the patient's chin and index and middle finger on the tongue protrusion in the cheek usually creates sufficient force for testing. Like testing eye closure, this requires some training as an examiner and calibration of "normal" strength. Untreated severe weakness tongue weakness in MuSK and very uncommonly in AChR ab positive disease can result in tongue atrophy, typically with a triple furrowed appearance.[136] This atrophy is reversible in some cases.[137] Histopathology of atrophic muscles can appear either neurogenic or myopathic.[138] In MuSK MG, atrophy of facial muscles can occur early in disease or with chronic, severe weakness.[139] If safe to do so, the patient can be observed taking a sip of water and monitored for coughing afterward to evaluate swallowing function at the bedside.[127]

Speech is assessed from the beginning of the encounter when the patient is providing a history. Focused bedside assessment includes sustained "ahhhh" phonation which tests palatal elevation as well as diaphragmatic strength. Laryngeal strength is measured by the presence or absence of hoarseness and sustained high-pitched "eeeee" sound.[100] Counting from 1 to 50 at a rate of 1 per second assesses fatigable dysarthria.[140] A summary of findings on the ocular and bulbar examination is outlined in Table 25-4.

AXIAL AND LIMB MUSCLE EXAMINATION

Testing of neck strength is a critical part of the MG-specific neurologic examination. Neck (and bulbar) strength correlate closely with strength of respiratory muscles.[141] Neck flexor muscles are typically weaker on confrontational testing than

▶ TABLE 25-4. NOTABLE ADDITIONAL PHYSICAL EXAMINATION FINDINGS IN MG

Cogan lid twitch sign or the "lid twitch sign"	Quick lid retraction after refixation to the primary position from sustained downgaze OR one or more twitches of the upper eyelid when the eyes are directed downward and then returned to primary gaze.
Curtain sign	Passive elevation of each eyelid one after the other exaggerates ptosis in the contralateral eyelid.
Frontalis sign	Contraction of the ipsilateral frontalis muscle to elevate the eyelid and reduce the severity of ptosis which concurrently elevates the ipsilateral eyelid. Patient often unaware of contraction and therefore relaxation of the eyelid to assess ptosis requires coaching by examiner.
Peek sign	Inability to bury eyelashes completely during sustained forced eye closure. After 30 seconds, unable to keep the lids fully closed.
Ice pack test	Improvement in eyelid ptosis when an ice pack is placed on the ptotic eyelid for 2 minutes.
Pseudointernuclear ophthalmoplegia (INO)	Simultaneous weakness of medial rectus and contralateral lateral rectus.
Myasthenic "Sneer" or "Snarl"	Mid-portion of the upper lip elevates without elevation of the corners of the mouth during an attempted smile.
Triple furrow	Atrophy of the tongue in the midline and on both lateral edges producing a triple furrowed appearance.

neck extensors. However, neck extensor weakness causes more symptoms related to head drop and related neck strain. The optimal position for testing neck flexion is supine and for neck extension, prone. If this positioning is not feasible, having the patient sit in a low-backed chair or supported if needed on the examination table is second best.[142] Paraspinal muscle atrophy in weak muscles appreciable by visual inspection is very unusual. Severe muscle atrophy of paraspinal muscles would prompt consideration of alternative diagnostic possibilities.

Limb weakness in MG is typically asymmetric, but not unilateral. Proximal muscles are generally more affected, with preferential involvement of the triceps and hip flexors. Finger extension and ankle dorsiflexion are the most affected distal deficits.[100] Unless very severe and chronic, muscle bulk is typically normal. Several exceptions are patients with a phenotype of marked focal triceps atrophy.[143] Other focal muscle involvement in MG has included shoulder-girdle, masseter, and finger flexor muscles.[144,145]

RESPIRATORY MUSCLE EXAMINATION

In addition to standard lung auscultation and observation of work of breathing, several additional maneuvers can assess respiratory status in MG patients. A single breath count (SBC) estimates vital capacity. The SBC involves having the patient count as high as they can at a rate of 2 counts per second on a single inhalation following complete exhalation. SBC > 20–30 indicates that pulmonary function is generally adequate. This can be confounded by many factors including bulbar weakness, other cardiopulmonary disease, and effort.[141,146] Asking the patient to cough forcefully assesses laryngeal and diaphragm muscle function and to sniff sharply, negative inspiratory force (NIF). Oxygen saturation, blood gasses, bedside NIF and forced vital capacity (FVC) and full formal pulmonary function testing (including supine testing) can be helpful in certain circumstances.[100]

DIAGNOSIS OF MYASTHENIA GRAVIS

Suspecting MG is often the biggest hurdle to and most important part of making the diagnosis of MG and distinguishing MG from mimics outlined in Table 25-5.

Patients typically see optometrists, ophthalmologists, primary care providers, otolaryngologists, or emergency medicine physicians initially with MG symptoms. Nonneurologists initially suspecting MG is critical for a timely and accurate diagnosis. In one study, MG was the first diagnosis received in about 50% of patients. The next most common initial diagnoses were cerebrovascular disease, cranial nerve or EOM abnormalities, other eye problems, and psychosomatic. Men were more often diagnosed with cerebrovascular disease and women with psychosomatic disorders.[96] There can also be diagnostic delay, at least 2 years in 34% of women and 10% of men in one cohort.[147] MG should be considered in any patient with painless weakness

▶ **TABLE 25-5. DIFFERENTIAL DIAGNOSIS OF MG**

Brain/Cranial Nerves
  Abnormality of brainstem nuclei due to inflammatory or neoplastic etiology[a]
  Chronic meningitis[a]
  Wernicke encephalopathy[a]
  Rabies[a]
  Cerebral aneurysm[a]
  Cavernous sinus thrombosis[a]
Anterior horn cell
  ALS
  Kennedy syndrome[a]
  Spinal muscular atrophy[a]
  Enterovirus or West Nile Virus infection[a]
Root/nerve
  Chronic meningitis[a]
  Miller Fisher syndrome[a]
  Diphtheria[a]
  Immune-mediated polyradiculopathies[a]
NMJ
  Congenital myasthenic syndromes
  Lambert–Eaton myasthenic syndrome
  Botulism (including iatrogenic botulinum toxin)
  Tick paralysis
Muscle
  Oculopharyngeal muscular dystrophy (OPMD)
  Myotonic muscular dystrophy[a]
  Mitochondrial myopathy
  Congenital myopathy[a]
  Inflammatory myopathy[a]
  Immune checkpoint inhibitor-related myositis
  Orbital myositis
Miscellaneous
  Depression[a]
  Chronic fatigue syndrome[a]
  Dysthyroid ophthalmopathy
  Orbital pseudotumor[a]
  Blepharospasm
  Levator muscle dehiscense

[a]Unlikely source of diagnostic confusion.

without sensory symptoms, even if focal in onset, and particularly if ocular or bulbar weakness is present. The likelihood of MG increases with objective demonstration of fatigable weakness, particularly in an oculobulbar distribution. Primary differential diagnostic considerations include other DNMT, MND, and myopathies. Clinical features of LEMS are distinct from MG and are discussed in Chapter 26. Both MND and MG can present with dysarthria, dysphagia, head drop, and weakness of limb, axial and respiratory muscles. Lack of fasciculations, muscle atrophy, and upper motor neuron signs, and the presence of ocular weakness favor MG. Thyroid eye disease can cause limited extraocular motility and proptosis. Mitochondrial myopathy and resultant chronic progressive external ophthalmoplegia (CPEO) typically cause chronic, gradually progressive, symmetric ptosis, and severe ophthalmoparesis without diplopia. Oculopharyngeal muscular dystrophy (OPMD) causes eye closure, swallowing, neck flexion, and EOM muscle weakness. Blepharospasm can mimic ptosis but involves a forced contraction of both the upper and lower lid causing narrowing of the palpebral fissure instead of the lid drooping of MG. In most cases, the diagnosis is suspected by the astute clinician by the conclusion of a detailed history and tailored physical examination as has been reviewed earlier in the chapter. To support the clinical diagnosis, at least one of the following is needed:

- Abnormal titers of AChR binding or MuSK antibodies OR
- Unequivocal response to AChEI (pyridostigmine, neostigmine, or edrophonium) as measured by both the patient and practitioner—ptosis is typically the parameter measured OR
- EDX studies showing a primary DNMT—good quality, abnormal, slow repetitive nerve stimulation (RNS) and/or single-fiber electromyography (SFEMG). Importantly, there is also no evidence for an underlying process which could account for the abnormality (e.g., motor neuron disease, focal neurogenic abnormality, history of botulinum toxin injections, etc.).

▶ LABORATORY FEATURES

The reader is referred to Chapter 2 where the testing modalities used to support an MG diagnosis are reviewed. In this section, we will briefly review the serological, EDX, pharmacological, and imaging methods available to aid in the diagnosis and management of myasthenic patients, with a focus on strengths and weaknesses. The relative sensitivities of different tests used to support the clinical diagnosis of MG have been estimated and are summarized in Table 25-6.

Diagnostic strategies in MG undoubtedly vary between clinicians and institutions due to preference, test availability, and relevant differential diagnostic considerations for individual patients. Even in the most clinically straightforward cases, however, it is critical to pursue diagnostic confirmation, particularly if immunomodulating therapy or thymectomy is contemplated.

SEROLOGICAL TESTING

Identification of AChR-binding or MuSK autoantibodies in a clinical scenario consistent with MG confirms the diagnosis. Several types of AChR autoantibodies exist. AChR-binding antibody is the principal pathogenic and diagnostic antibody. It will be considered synonymous with AChR autoantibodies throughout this chapter unless otherwise specified.

From a practical standpoint, in the outpatient setting, we typically send AChR-binding and modulating antibodies initially with a reflex to MuSK ab testing, if AChR ab testing is negative. Differences between radioimmunoprecipitation assay (RIPA), enzyme-linked immunosorbent assay (ELISA) and cell-based assay (CBA) have been reviewed elsewhere.[149] RIPA is the most used test. If this antibody testing is negative, we perform EDX testing. Sending LRP4 ab can be useful on a case-by-case basis.[57] Given the low specificity of LRP4 antibodies for MG, we typically perform EDX studies in these patients to further confirm the diagnosis. If weakness is severe, treatment must begin immediately or if the patient is hospitalized, we send antibodies and perform EDX studies simultaneously; therefore, we have the results from the EDX to support the diagnosis to begin treatment while the antibody results are pending. In other scenarios, we send antibody testing first and only if negative, proceed to EDX testing.

If AChR antibodies are positive, routine testing for other autoantibodies is unnecessary as AChR/MuSK or AChR/VGCC ab overlaps, for example are exceedingly rare.[150,151] As mentioned, the sensitivity of AChR antibodies is estimated at approximately 50%–60% in OMG, 85%–90% in generalized MG, and 70%–85% in all MG patients.[149,152,153] However, they are highly specific for MG. False positives may rarely occur in patients with other autoimmune diseases such as systemic lupus, rheumatoid arthritis, hepatitis, thymoma without MG, inflammatory neuropathy, motor neuron disease, 13% of patients with LEMS, 3% of patients with lung cancer without an apparent neurological disorder and in some asymptomatic relatives of MG patients.[154]

The value of AChR antibodies is to establish initial diagnosis. Although titers typically decline with immunomodulatory or immunosuppressive treatment and thymectomy, the titer does not definitely correlate with disease severity, response to treatment, or predict remission or relapse.[155–157] Unlike many other tests used in everyday practice, even mild elevations in the AChR autoantibody titer are typically diagnostic. Reference range varies according to the laboratory used. Conversely, patients without AChR autoantibodies may have a different disease, harbor a different MG autoantibody, have seronegative MG, or on occasion have a false-negative result. This latter situation may arise with testing that has been done very early in the course of disease, or in

▶ TABLE 25-6. DIAGNOSTIC YIELD OF TESTS USED IN THE DIAGNOSIS OF AUTOIMMUNE MG[148]

MG Type	Ice Pack (sensitivity/specificity)	AChR-Binding Ab (sensitivity/specificity)	RNS (sensitivity/specificity)	SFEMG Frontalis (sensitivity/specificity)	SFEMG Orb Oculi (sensitivity/specificity)	CN-SFEMG Frontalis (sensitivity/specificity)
Ocular	0.94/0.97	0.44–0.66/0.99	0.29/0.94	0.86/0.73	0.97/0.92	0.62/0.92
Generalized	0.82/0.96	0.90/0.99	0.79/0.97	0.97/0.97 (EDC)	—	0.75/0.96

CN-SFEMG, concentric needle single-fiber EMG; EDC, extensor digitorum communis; RNS, repetitive nerve stimulation; SFEMG, single-fiber EMG.

an individual in whom autoantibody formation has been suppressed by immunomodulating treatment or thymectomy. For these reasons, testing prior to the initiation of immunomodulating treatment or most certainly before thymectomy is ideal. As initially seronegative patients may develop AChR measurable autoantibodies over time, repeat testing at least once 6–12 months after initial negative testing, and/or at the time of generalization in the appropriate clinical context may be considered.

AChR-modulating and AChR-blocking autoantibodies are also commercially available but play a less significant clinical role. AChR-modulating autoantibodies measure degradation of the AChR in cultured human myotubes.[158] Both autoantibodies are most likely to coexist in individuals who are AChR-binding autoantibody seropositive and are unlikely to occur in isolation. In one report, AChR-modulating autoantibodies were found in 75% of patients with AChR-binding autoantibodies but in only 5% of AChR-binding ab negative patients.[159] High titers of AChR-modulating autoantibodies also play a potential role in the detection of thymoma. Seventy-three percent of patients afflicted with both thymoma and MG harbor AChR-modulating autoantibodies producing a >90% receptor loss.[160]

AChR-blocking autoantibodies bind to the same site as ACh or α-bungarotoxin, close to but distinct from the main immunogenic region on the extracellular domain of the ACh channel.[158] They are found in approximately half of patients with generalized MG, but in only 30% of patients with ocular disease.[154] In one study, these autoantibodies were found in 30% of MG patients seropositive for AChR-binding autoantibodies, but in no seronegative MG patients.[158] Because the blocking antibody test has a low sensitivity, we find the assay to have limited clinical value and do not routinely perform it.

An estimated 40%–70% of AChR ab negative patients with generalized MG will have MuSK autoantibodies. Prevalence varies based on geographic region.[19,161,162] Unlike AChR ab, a correlation exists between anti-MuSK titers, disease severity, and treatment effect, making it a useful biomarker for treatment response.[163,164] Usually, treatment effect in MuSK is obvious but we repeat antibody titers in selected cases as an additional way to monitor disease status.

Striated muscle antibodies are against intracellular components of skeletal muscle including titin, the ryanodine receptor, myosin, and α-actinin. Importantly, they are not disease causing, and their presence does not confirm the diagnosis of MG.[165] These are found primarily in young patients with thymomatous MG, patients with thymoma or autoimmune disorders without MG, and many older patients.[165] Given their limited utility and potential misinterpretation of positive results, to our knowledge, striated muscle antibodies have been removed from most MG autoantibody testing panels.

Several additional laboratory studies may be required at diagnosis. We routinely obtain a thyroid-stimulating hormone level and sometimes anti-thyroid peroxidase (TPO) ab particularly if disease is purely or predominantly ocular.

The prevalence of hypo- or hyperthyroidism is high in MG patients and a failure to recognize dysthyroidism may affect treatment efficacy. Additionally, thyroid eye disease can coexist with MG.[166] It is not uncommon for other autoantibodies to coexist with MG and/or thymoma such as ganglionic AChR antibodies, voltage-gated potassium channel antibodies, and anti-collapsin response mediator protein (CRMP)-5 autoantibodies.[160,167] We do not routinely test for autoantibodies more closely related to other autoimmune diseases in MG patients unless there is clinical suspicion to do so. If immunosuppression is considered, testing for hepatitis B and C, tuberculosis, and HIV may be required. Baseline complete blood counts with differential, metabolic panels with liver function tests and treatment-specific testing (i.e., hemoglobin A1c before starting maintenance CS) are important to consider.

ELECTRODIAGNOSTIC TESTING

EDX testing has an essential role in the evaluation of possible MG. The technical performance of repetitive stimulation studies and SFEMG are discussed in greater detail in Chapter 2. In this section, we will focus on the strategies in the EDX evaluation of suspected MG, interpretation of results, characteristic patterns of abnormalities and potential pitfalls encountered.[168]

In normal NMT, compound muscle action potentials (CMAPs) reflect the spatial and temporal summation of muscle fiber action potentials (MFAPs) following stimulation of the motor nerve. In MG, when NMT is impaired, the fall in EPP size ("depression") that normally occurs following repeated motor nerve activation may not exceed the threshold to generate an MFAP. Therefore, impulse failure occurs and results in reduced CMAP amplitude and area. This underlies the fatigable weakness seen clinically in MG. This impulse failure may occur at baseline or only after exercise when impairment of NMT is milder.[168,169]

When the EPP size is decreased and end plates are blocked, maximal voluntary exercise for 10 seconds and high-frequency RNS (10–50 Hz if the patient in unable to exercise) both increase ACh quantal release. This results in CMAP amplitude facilitation and "repair" of the decrement. Increased CMAP amplitude occurs because, during maximum voluntary contraction, calcium accumulates in the extracellular space around the nerve terminal and diffuses into the nerve terminal faster than it diffuses out. This increases the number of quanta of ACh released with each nerve stimulation. "Decrement" is partially counteracted by increased mobilization of ACh. The amplitude of the CMAPs recorded during RNS represents the net result of these two opposing processes.[168,169]

SFEMG can be performed either through voluntary activation of a tested muscle or by electrical stimulation of a motor nerve branch innervating that muscle. Each method has benefits and drawbacks. One strength of stimulated SFEMG is that it is less reliant on patient cooperation than voluntary SFEMG, making it the technique of choice in infants, patients who may not be able to steadily sustain a minimal level of muscle activation, or any potentially uncooperative individual.[170–173] Stimulated SFEMG is typically faster to perform than voluntary SFEMG, providing an additional advantage. Its major disadvantage occurs when a muscle rather than nerve fiber is stimulated leading to a falsely reduced jitter value. We perform voluntary SFEMG.

As described in Chapter 2, SFEMG assesses NMT by comparing the discharge intervals of time-locked muscle fiber action potentials (MFAPs) belonging to the same motor unit. This is technically accomplished by limiting the recording radius of the EMG needle. Historically, this was accomplished both by raising the low-frequency filter settings of the EMG machine and by using a special single-fiber needle with a limited recording radius.[174–176] These needles were expensive and reusable, necessitating sterilization after each use as well as periodic sharpening. For practical reasons, many institutions now use disposable, concentric needles with a small recording radius which are adequate surrogates providing acceptable accuracy if attention is paid to detail during performance and interpretation. Normal values are different for concentric EMG and have been devised.[175] Disposable SFEMG needles have recently also become available and provide the advantages of single-fiber EMG without the logistical hurdles of the historical reusable needles.

Two parameters are typically measured in SFEMG assessment. Jitter refers to the variation in the interval between the two single MFAPs, as mentioned above. When recording with a concentric electrode, these are called "apparent" single MFAPs. Because of the normal variation in EPP amplitude, jitter is a property of normal muscle, typically falling in the 15–45 μs range depending on age, the muscle studied, and type of electrode used.[177–179] Jitter becomes abnormal only when it is either smaller or in the case of MG, larger than normal (Fig. 25-6A,B). Increased jitter reflects abnormal or delayed NMT, but not NMT failure. As a result, abnormal jitter does not translate to weakness. With an increase in jitter values to 80–100 μs or above, however, NMT becomes tenuous and begins to intermittently fail. As a result, blocking, which is the equivalent of a decremental response to repetitive stimulation, and clinical weakness, becomes manifest (Fig. 25-6B).

In most cases, EDX testing is not required to diagnose MG if AChR or MuSK antibodies are present, and the clinical scenario is consistent with MG. When antibody positive, EDX may be used to identify or exclude abnormalities suggestive of an alternative cause of weakness (i.e., motor neuron disease, myopathy, or a focal concurrent disorder, such as L5 radiculopathy causing foot drop). Repetitive nerve conduction studies (NCSs) are not typically used after diagnosis to monitor disease status in MG. If the electromyographer is sufficiently trained, SFEMG can be used in addition to the physical examination as another way of monitoring disease severity, both in clinic and as an outcome measure in clinical trials.[180,181] Unfortunately, this is not feasible for most practitioners in clinic or trials, as additional quantitative data reflective of the degree of abnormality of NMT is a useful quantifiable outcome measure.

The EDX evaluation of patients with suspected MG begins with routine NCSs. Typically, in patients with generalized symptoms, we obtain one sensory and one motor conduction from an upper and lower limb. We would expect these to be normal in a postsynaptic DNMT. If the CMAP amplitudes are reduced in a patient with a phenotype resembling MG, motor neuron disease, or a presynaptic DNMT, such as Lambert–Eaton myasthenic syndrome (LEMS) or botulism, should be considered. If CMAP amplitudes are reduced, we exercise the muscle the CMAP is being recorded from for 10 seconds, then relax the muscle completely, and immediately follow with a second, supramaximal stimulus. The percent CMAP amplitude facilitation is calculated by the following formula: %Facilitation = ((Potential$_N$/Potential$_1$) − 1) ×100%.[182,183]

We then proceed to RNS testing at 2–3 Hz. Selection of muscles to study depends on the patient's pattern of weakness; ideally, RNS is performed in weak muscles, as neuromuscular blockade is the reason for both clinical weakness and CMAP decrement in MG (Fig. 25-7).[169] While RNS of ulnar-abductor digiti minimi is easily performed and well

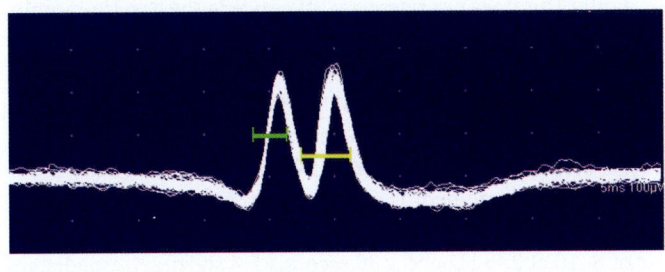

A

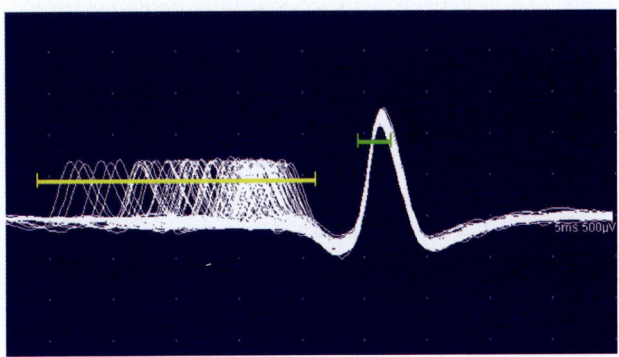

B

Figure 25-6. Single-fiber electromyography of the frontalis muscle demonstrating a normal recording with normal jitter of 20 microseconds (**A**) and abnormal recording with severely increased jitter of 150 microseconds with blocking (**B**) from a patient with MG.

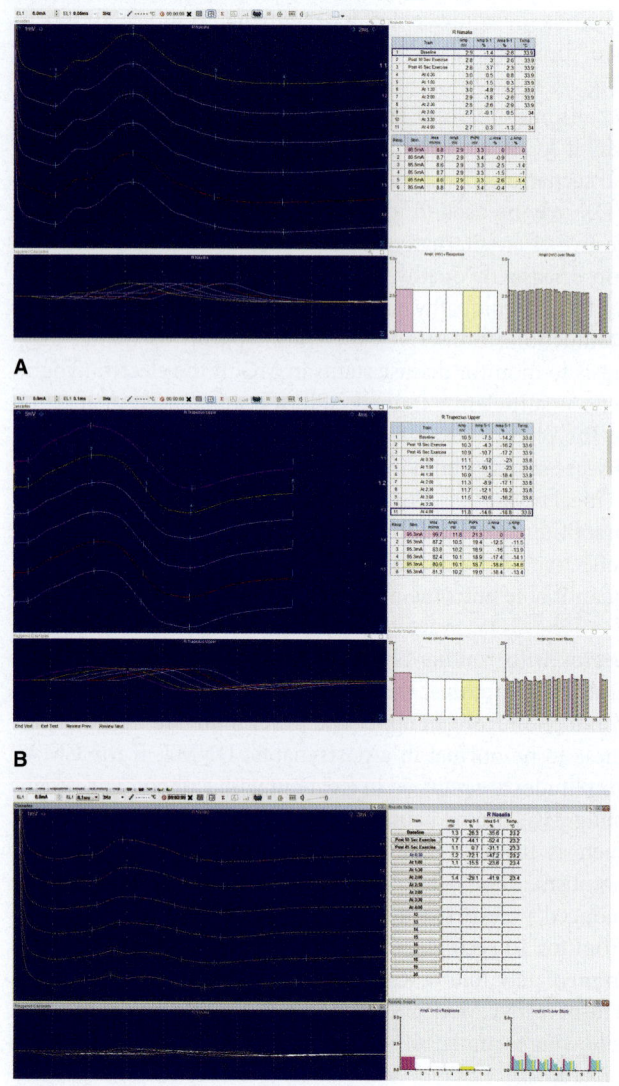

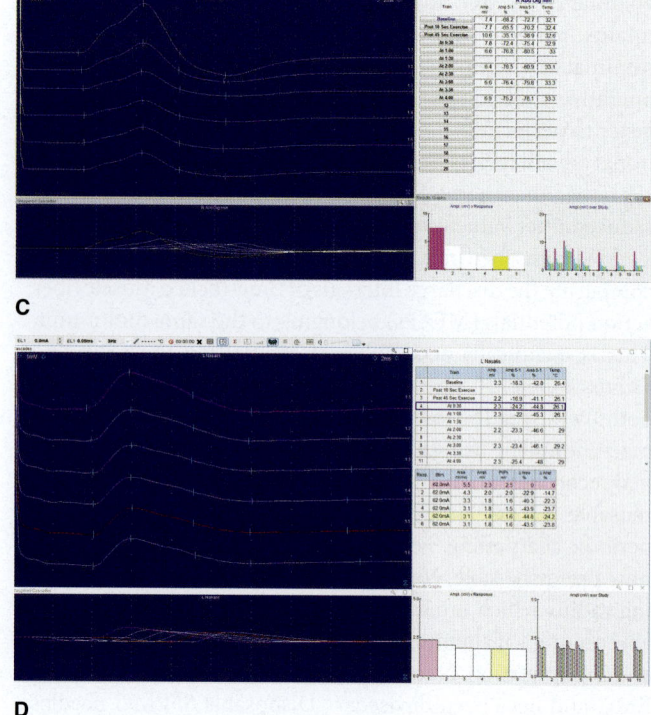

Figure 25-7. Typical pattern of "slow" (2–3 Hz) repetitive nerve stimulation which is normal of nasalis (**A**), shows mild decrement with saddle shape of trapezius (**B**), shows severe decrement with saddle shape of abductor digiti minimi (**C**), and mild decrement without saddle shape in nasalis in patient with MuSK Ab positive MG (**D**). Part **E** is RNS contaminated by movement artifact and cannot be interpreted. Notice decrement which varies drastically from train to train, inconsistent baseline amplitude, changing waveform morphology and inconsistent cursor placement on the CMAP.

tolerated, it is frequently normal as finger abduction is typically unaffected in MG. If MG is suspected, we typically study the facial-nasalis first in patients with facial or bulbar predominant weakness and the spinal accessory-trapezius nerve first in patients with an axial-limb predominant pattern of weakness. If a third RNS is needed, we then examine the ulnar-ADM.[184] If LEMS is higher on the differential, we choose more distal muscles (e.g., ulnar-ADM, median-abductor pollicis brevis, and peroneal-extensor digitorum brevis) as these have higher sensitivity for abnormality in LEMS, as discussed further in Chapter 26.[182] It is most convincing for diagnosis if abnormal decrement is seen in two nerve–muscle combinations. If seen in only one, ensuring that the RNS is free from adverse technical factors and that the decrement has characteristics, which make it consistent with physiologic decrement. If there is still doubt, we repeat the abnormal nerve–muscle combination after a period of several minutes of rest. Any abnormal physiologic decrement should be reproducible after a period of rest.

"Decrement" refers to the percentage of change in the amplitude between the first and fourth/fifth stimulus in a train of 6–10 stimuli. It can be calculated from the formula: % Decrement = $(1 - (Potential_N/Potential_1)) \times 100\%$. Importantly, this does not refer to a difference in the baseline amplitudes of the first stimulus of sequential trains. If RNS reveals abnormal decrement, we repeat the pre-exercise baseline train to ensure reproducibility. We then attempt to "repair the decrement" (if present) by exercising the muscle for 10 seconds and then repeating the RNS. However, if no abnormal decrement is seen, we exercise the muscle instead for 60 seconds and then repeat repetitive stimulation in trains of 6–10 at 2–3 Hz every 30 seconds × 3 starting immediately postexercise and then every minute for up to 5 minutes, looking for postexercise exhaustion. An amplitude decrement of ≥10% is abnormal.[185] Some data suggest a 7%–8% decrement threshold could be used for facial-nasalis to increase sensitivity, without sacrificing specificity if technically of high quality, though this is not universally accepted.[186]

Although RNS testing is performed widely, it is the more technically fraught procedure in the EMG lab and subject to many artifacts. Quality control and attention to detail are essential to avoid pitfalls that may give the impression of abnormal decrement when it is not present. Examples of pitfalls include movement of the stimulator, patient or recording electrodes, submaximal stimulation, cool temperature, or CMAP marker placement inconsistencies (Fig. 25-7E). Failure to minimize and/or recognize these factors can lead to the misdiagnosis of MG. Additionally, RNS can be abnormal in motor neuron disease, myopathy, or any focal process affecting the nerve–muscle combination chosen (i.e., C8 radiculopathy for ulnar-ADM RNS).

Given this potential lack of specificity of abnormal RNS, concentric needle EMG studies should accompany any abnormal RNS studies. EMG evaluates for motor unit potential instability as evidence of a DNMT, or features of other possible neuromuscular disorders that may mimic MG (e.g., myopathy, motor neuron disease) or result in abnormal RNS.[187,188] If both repetitive stimulation and concentric needle EMG do not show a DNMT and are nondiagnostic for an alternative explanation for symptoms, we proceed to SFEMG. This testing order is based on the knowledge that SFEMG is more sensitive than RNS but not specific.[189] The one exception to this order is in the diagnostic evaluation of patients with symptoms and weakness confined to ocular muscles. In these patients, we begin with SFEMG. If SFEMG is normal and the pretest suspicion for MG is low to moderate, we stop. If SFEMG is abnormal, then we do routine NCSs and EMG and sometimes limited RNS.

The choice of muscle(s) for SFEMG depends on the patient's pattern of weakness. Most patients in whom SFEMG is performed in our laboratories have isolated ocular symptoms for which the referring physician wishes to exclude MG after negative MG ab testing. We typically study either frontalis or orbicularis oculi muscles in these cases. However, each patient should be individually assessed with the choice based on clinical evaluation. Diagnostic yield will always be highest in a clinically weak muscle. If suspicion for MG is high and the frontalis is normal, we then study the orbicularis oculi. Again, failure to demonstrate a decremental response, increased jitter, and neuromuscular blockade in a clinically weak muscle implicates a diagnosis other than MG.

Several additional factors can affect the results of RNS and SFEMG testing for suspected MG. Temperature changes affect NMT. Warming the limbs to at least 34°C minimizes the chance of cool temperatures enhancing NMT, and in turn, masking decrement and causing a false-negative RNS study.[190] Cholinesterase inhibitors (ChEIs) may also mask SFEMG abnormalities in mild MG.[191] Pyridostigmine should be held if feasible to do so for at least 12, and ideally 24 hours prior to the SFEMG study to lessen the possibility of a false-negative result. However, if the patient still has moderate to severe myasthenic weakness despite taking pyridostigmine, SFEMG is still expected to be abnormal. Botulinum toxin, for medical or cosmetic purposes, will result in increased jitter based on the intended effect of presynaptic NMT blockade and the utility of SFEMG is lessened as a diagnostic tool.[192] For example, receiving botulinum toxin for migraine headaches or blepharospasm will cause SFEMG of the frontalis and orbicularis oculi to be abnormal, for years, and possibly indefinitely. Additionally, due to spread of the toxin, increased jitter can be seen in limb muscles related to the botulinum toxin even if injections were only performed in the facial muscles.[193] Therefore, a normal limb SFEMG is helpful in making MG less likely, but an abnormal limb SFEMG has less diagnostic certainty for a primary disorder of NMT. We typically perform a concentric EMG of the frontalis and extensor digitorum communis (EDC) in these patients. Then we perform a limited SFEMG of the frontalis and complete SFEMG of the EDC. If needle EMG is normal of the trapezius and ADM, abnormal RNS can also be helpful and lean toward an MG diagnosis in the appropriate clinical setting. Ideally, potential MG patients should be tested in the EMG lab prior to exposure to any medication that might significantly affect the disease, particularly through interference with NMT (Table 25-7). Pyridostigmine and botulinum toxin are the primary medications of note which influence NMT and therefore DNMT EDX assessment directly. While the history of botulinum toxin is critical to obtain, we have also seen many patients whose MG presented in the context of botulinum toxin use and so MG may coexist.

False positives are an even larger potential pitfall than false-negative studies. The most common cause of a false-positive examination is undoubtedly technical, particularly with repetitive stimulation testing. As discussed above, movement artifact and other factors can result in "pseudo-decrement" (Fig. 25-7E). Unwanted movement resulting in a changing baseline CMAP amplitude and morphology is a particular problem both in large proximal muscles like the trapezius and in the face. The latter often occurs from grimacing in response to facial nerve stimulation or the undesired coactivation of other facial innervated muscles.

Given these technical challenges, close inspection of the RNS waveform for quality is the first step in interpretation and normal RNS is shown in Figure 25-7A. Criteria include: (1) normal and consistent baseline CMAP amplitude and morphology, (2) amplitude nadir that occurs at the fourth or fifth response of a 6–10-stimulus train, (3) greatest decrease in CMAP amplitude between the first and second stimuli in each train, and (4) similar and progressive amount of decrement in previous and subsequent trains. Take the example of amplitude decrement which jumps from −5% to −15% and then to −1% on successive trains. In this case, one would suspect that the decrement of −15% is due to technical artifact. If confirmed to be technical, and this is the only "abnormal decrement" in the study, the study should not be interpreted as abnormal. As stated earlier, if results of testing remain unclear, the RNS study can be repeated after a sufficient period of rest for clarification.

Possible immediate postexercise decrement repair and postexercise exhaustion where the decrement is maximal

▶ **TABLE 25-7. DRUGS TO AVOID OR USE WITH CAUTION IN MG**[25,26,194]

✓ **Avoid**
- Telithromycin: antibiotic for community-acquired pneumonia. "Black box" warning for use in MG.
- Botulinum toxin: for cosmetic or medical use (e.g., migraine, spasticity)
- D-penicillamine: for Wilson disease/rarely for rheumatoid arthritis. Associated with causing MG.

✓ **Avoid or use with caution if no reasonable alternative, benefit outweighs risk**
- Fluoroquinolones (e.g., ciprofloxacin, moxifloxacin, and levofloxacin): broad-spectrum antibiotics associated with worsening MG. "Black box" warning for use in MG.
- Magnesium: may worsen MG if given intravenously, i.e., for eclampsia during late pregnancy or for hypomagnesemia. Use only if no alternative and observe for worsening.
- Quinine: occasionally used for leg cramps. Use prohibited except in malaria in the United States.
- Macrolides (e.g., erythromycin, azithromycin, clarithromycin): antibiotics for gram-positive infections.
- Aminoglycosides (e.g., gentamycin, neomycin, tobramycin): antibiotics for gram-negative infections.
- Immune checkpoint Inhibitors for cancer such as anti-PD1 and CTLA-4 agents (e.g., pembrolizumab, ipilimumab, nivolumab, atezolimumab, etc.)
- Live or live-attenuated vaccines: avoid for patients on immunosuppressive therapy due to concern for development of active infection. Not associated with MG disease worsening.

✓ **May worsen MG—use with caution and observe**[a]
- Corticosteroids: standard treatment for MG, may cause transient worsening within the first 2 weeks. Monitor for this possibility and do not discontinue if worsening occurs.
- Procainamide: antiarrhythmic.
- Deferoxamine: Chelating agent used for hemochromatosis.
- Beta-blockers: used hypertension, heart disease, migraine, and tremor. Risk primarily with new starts of higher doses, intravenously.
- Chloroquine and hydroxychloroquine: used to treat malaria and some autoimmune diseases.
- Statins (e.g., atorvastatin, simvastatin etc.): used to reduce serum cholesterol.
- Iodine contrast dye: older varieties.
- Neuromuscular blocking agents: MG patients sensitive to nondepolarizing NMBA and resistant to succinylcholine (depolarizing NMBA).

[a]Many other drugs have been rarely associated with worsening of MG which may be coincidental. Clinical judgment and assessment of risk:benefit ratio needed.

---

at 3–4 minutes are anticipated. Another typical feature of postsynaptic DNMT is a rise in the CMAP amplitude after the fourth or fifth response that allows the CMAP amplitude to approach but not achieve that of the first response, producing a "U-shaped" or "saddle shape" train envelope (Fig. 25-7A–C). In MG, this saddle shape occurs due to mobilization of the secondary stores of ACh once the primary stores have been depleted. This "saddle shape" is helpful when present in providing reassurance that decrement seen is truly physiologic, but its absence does not necessarily indicate technical problems if other criteria for quality control are satisfied. This saddle shape is more commonly seen in AChR positive MG and less commonly in MuSK and LEMS due to the presynaptic abnormality in the latter two (including MuSK) which precludes mobilization of the secondary stores (Fig. 25-7D).[195–197]

The other false-positive scenario is assigning EDX abnormalities to MG, when the abnormal DNMT is due to a different disease process, such as ALS or myopathy. In MG, RNS and SFEMG are abnormal because of a primary DNMT. In ALS and myopathy, a secondary DNMT results in abnormal decrement on RNS and increased jitter on SFEMG. The secondary DNMT is thought to stem from immature NMJ occurring because of reinnervation.[198–202] From the routine concentric needle EMG, motor neuronopathy is typically evident. However, myopathy can be more difficult to distinguish from MG on needle examination given similarities in motor unit action potential (MUAP) morphology. Additionally, while neither increased insertional activity nor abnormal spontaneous activity is typically present in MG, fibrillation potentials and positive waves may occur, particularly in paraspinal, bulbar, and proximal muscles. Presumably, they result from severe end plate destruction and effective denervation. In support of this, their prevalence appears to correlate with patients who are more severely affected by generalized disease.[203] Abundant spontaneous activity (in the absence of signs of motor neuronopathy), particularly in the setting MG with thymoma, should prompt consideration of a concurrent inflammatory myositis.

Two types of abnormal MUAP changes may occur in MG. Short-duration, low-amplitude MUAPs with or without early recruitment may occur. This pattern results from an effective reduction in the number of functional myofibers within a given motor unit, analogous to what may occur with myopathies.[188] Short-duration, low-amplitude MUAPs have been reported in MuSK MG as well, also consistent with a reduced number of normally functioning muscle fibers per motor unit resulting from either neuromuscular blockade, or muscle fiber loss and/or atrophy.[204]

A more sensitive and valuable needle EMG finding, however, is MUAP instability, which is typically seen as variation in amplitude (Fig. 25-8). One can think of MUAP instability as the EMG analog of variable clinical weakness, a decremental response with repetitive stimulation, or increased jitter with blocking on SFEMG. It represents NMT failure of one or more single-fiber components to the MUAP that is typically intermittent, resulting in constant variation in the size, shape, and sound produced by an isolated MUAP. Unstable MUAPs are readily identified by the trained ear and visualized by triggering on individual MUAPs. They provide additional evidence of abnormal NMT in muscles not easily studied by repetitive stimulation and separate from SFEMG examination.[183]

The EDX yield in MG varies depending on the serotype, severity, the EDX technique chosen, and the nerve/muscle

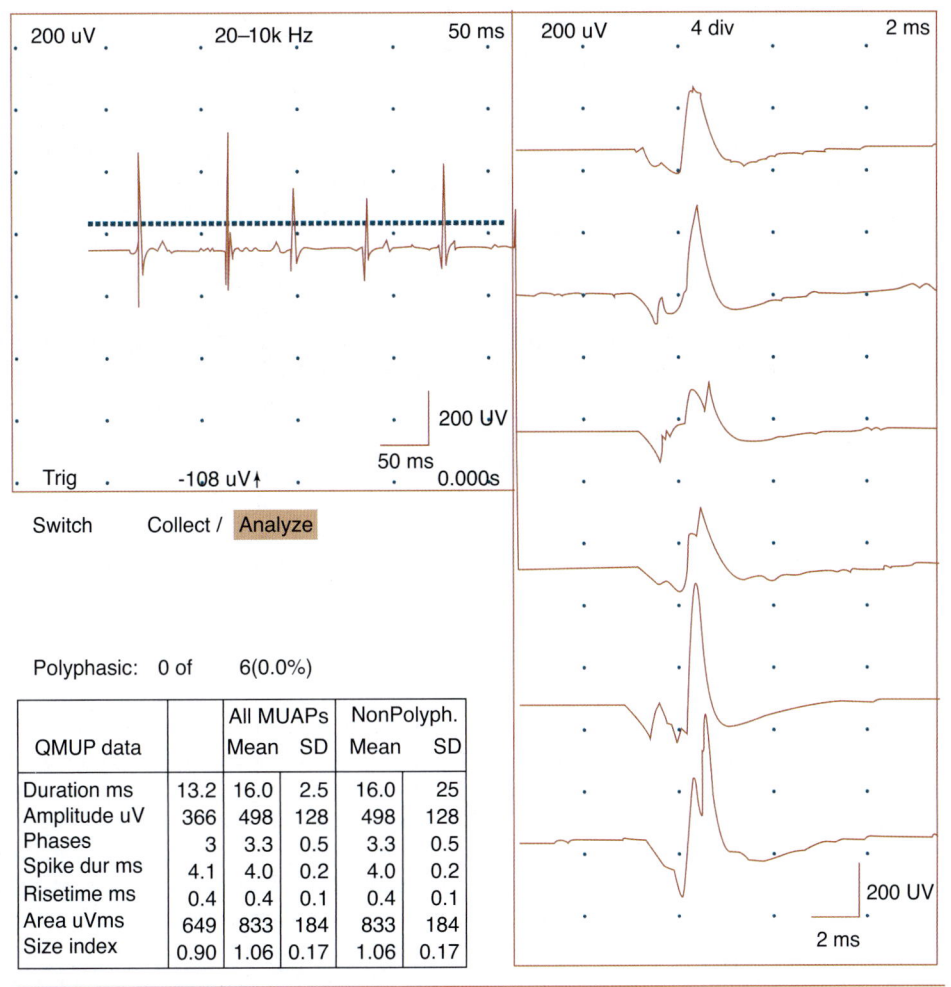

Figure 25-8. Motor unit potential instability (e.g., variable MUAP morphology with consecutive firings).

studied. SFEMG is a sensitive diagnostic tool for DNMT with sensitivity approximately 98%, however the specificity is much lower ≤70%.[205] Specifically, the sensitivity of SFEMG is estimated at 97% if both a limb and a facial muscle are studied. SFEMG abnormalities are found in the frontalis or orbicularis oculi in 87%–99% of patients with oculobulbar weakness.[206] One prospective study of SFEMG (orbicularis oculi muscle) in patients with OMG found an overall sensitivity of 79% and a specificity of 80%. Sensitivity was higher for patients with ptosis than in those who had isolated diplopia.[207] It is still important to remember that an abnormal SFEMG is not diagnostic of MG in isolation, but rather results must always be interpreted in the context of the clinical presentation.

PHARMACOLOGIC TESTING

Edrophonium (i.e., Tensilon) is a parenteral AChEI which has a rapid onset and a short duration of action. Like pyridostigmine, which has the same mechanism of action, it results in a transient increase in ACh availability at the NMJ and amplifies the EPP. The "Tensilon test" was frequently used as a supportive diagnostic test for MG starting in the 1930s though gradually became less commonly used after the 2000s. The test is no longer in widespread clinical use. The US Food and Drug Administration (FDA) withdrew approval for diagnostic use of edrophonium in 2018. The risk of side effects plus the more widespread availability of antibody testing for diagnosis also make it less favored globally.[81]

The test is well described and important in the understanding of the evolution of diagnostic tools in MG.[208] Additionally, the basis of diagnosis for some patients is a historical edrophonium test. After administration of edrophonium in a graded and systematic way, while measuring for response after each partial dose, the examiner observes for improvement in MG. The weakness chosen as a yardstick for the MG must be indisputable. Ptosis or moderate to severe ophthalmoparesis is typically used. Improvement after edrophonium was consistent with diagnosis of a DNMT. The sensitivity of edrophonium testing in MG was reported to be 86% for ocular and 95% for generalized MG.[209] Like repetitive stimulation and SFEMG, an abnormal test signified abnormal NMT but did not define a singular cause. False-positive responses have been reported in LEMS, ALS, CMS, botulism, Guillain–Barré syndrome, dysthyroid ophthalmopathy, and brainstem tumors.[37,210–213] Edrophonium testing had less utility in MuSK MG with a reported sensitivity of 50%–70%, and more side effects.[78,82] Edrophonium testing was not without some risk. Historically, these were office-based procedures, performed without incident in most cases though with parenteral atropine available in the event of bradycardia. Some patients would experience transient, disquieting, but harmless symptoms such as nausea, vomiting, increased tearing, lacrimation, fasciculations, borborygmi, and eructation. Rarely, however, serious reactions including bradycardia or heart block would occur. As such, the test required to have atropine readily available if needed.

THYMIC ABNORMALITIES AND THYMOMA

Pathological thymic abnormalities are found in >80% of patients with generalized MG who harbor AChR antibodies.[214] These abnormalities include follicular or diffuse hyperplasia in approximately 50%, thymic involution, thymoma, or thymic carcinoma. In early-onset MG, hyperplasia is the most common alteration. In late-onset MG, thymoma and involuted thymus predominate. MuSK positive patients have minimal histological alterations of the thymus, and the thymus typically resembles that from age-matched controls.[215] Thymoma would be very uncommon in MuSK positive or AChR ab negative MG. This is supported by a study of serum autoantibody profiles of 201 patients with thymoma in which none of the MG patients were AChR ab negative or MuSK positive.[167] Seronegative patients may or may not show hyperplastic changes.[214] In a minority yet still substantial number of patients with MG estimated between 10% and 30%, a thymoma or thymic carcinoma is discovered.[216] Noninvasive thymomas are fully encapsulated, however, 15%–40% are invasive and extend beyond the capsule.[214] Invasive thymoma first spreads to adjacent mediastinal fat and then pleura, pericardium, lung, or mediastinal vessels.[216] MG often triggers diagnosis of thymoma and vice versa. Conversely, approximately 30% of patients with thymoma have myasthenia, present at the time of thymoma diagnosis.[217]

Thymomas, thymic carcinomas, and thymic neuroendocrine tumors (NETs) are all types of thymic epithelial tumors (TETs). While accounting for more than 50% of tumors anterior/prevascular mediastinum, they are still rare, accounting for <1% of all tumors.[90,218] A basic understanding of the subtype and stage classification system is useful in caring for MG patients with thymoma or thymic carcinoma. The possible subtypes of thymoma based on the World Health Organization's 5th Edition Classification include: Type A, type AB and type B1, B2, B3, and other rare subtypes.[219] From type A to type B3 is a continuum of abnormality in terms of both the degree of invasion of lymphocytes into the tumor and how abnormal the thymus cells appear. Type A has normal-looking thymus cells and no lymphocytes whereas type B3 has the fewest normal thymus cells and the most lymphocyte invasion. Between type A and B3 there is more invasion of lymphocytes into the thymoma itself, and prognosis worsens. B2 is the most common subtype.[218] Thymic carcinoma has very abnormal thymic cells and almost no lymphocytes. It is a more aggressive tumor with a poorer prognosis.[219] In addition to this classification, thymic tumors are staged. The staging system was initially the Masaoka-Kaga system and then Tumor, Node, Metastasis (TNM) system looking at tumor size, node status, and the presence or absence of metastases was proposed. Both are in use today.[220] These systems combine to determine the level of risk and "malignancy" of the thymoma, and to guide treatment.[217] Whenever feasible, complete resection is the initial and primary aim of management because it has the greatest impact on reduction of recurrence and increased overall survival.[217]

THYMIC IMAGING

Thymic imaging occurs in three clinical scenarios in patients with MG. First, patients have chest imaging done for another reason (e.g., trauma, lung cancer screening, pneumonia, etc.) and a mediastinal mass is discovered incidentally, prompting a workup which leads to diagnosis of thymoma and MG. This is not uncommon. Approximately 30% of patients with thymoma are completely asymptomatic from the tumor, particularly if completely encapsulated. Some patients may have nonspecific symptoms such as cough, chest pain, hoarseness, or dyspnea and they have chest imaging to evaluate these nonspecific symptoms.[221] In both scenarios, patients are likely to have either an x-ray or CT of the chest. The second scenario is patients newly diagnosed with MG who require chest imaging to rule in or rule out a thymoma, and for presurgical planning if the patient will undergo thymectomy. For most patients, serial chest imaging is not needed if initial workup shows no thymoma at MG diagnosis. The third scenario is serial chest imaging following thymoma resection which monitors for recurrence.

In the past, the standard imaging evaluation has been stepwise, beginning with CT and then advancing to MRI if initial results were inconclusive.[222] However, the American College of Radiology Guidance on Thoracic Imaging recently published updated guidance for imaging of mediastinal masses, which does not always recommend this sequential process.[223] CT and MRI are both "usually appropriate" first-line diagnostic modalities for initial imaging both for clinically suspected mediastinal mass or as the next imaging study for indeterminate mass on radiography. For any indeterminate lesion on CT, MRI is the next appropriate imaging study.[223] Additionally, some advocate for MRI as superior in the initial diagnostic evaluation of the chest and mediastinum for thymoma, which is the most common prevascular mediastinal lesion accounting for 28% of such masses, followed by benign cyst (20%) and then lymphoma (16%).[224]

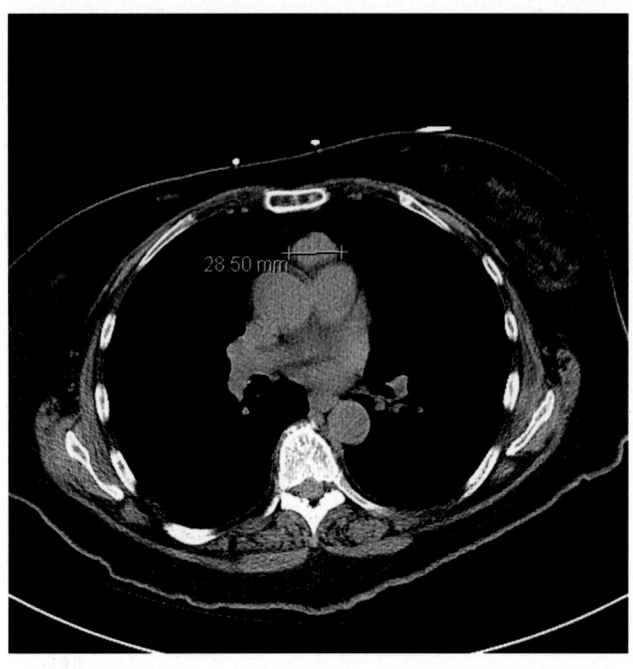 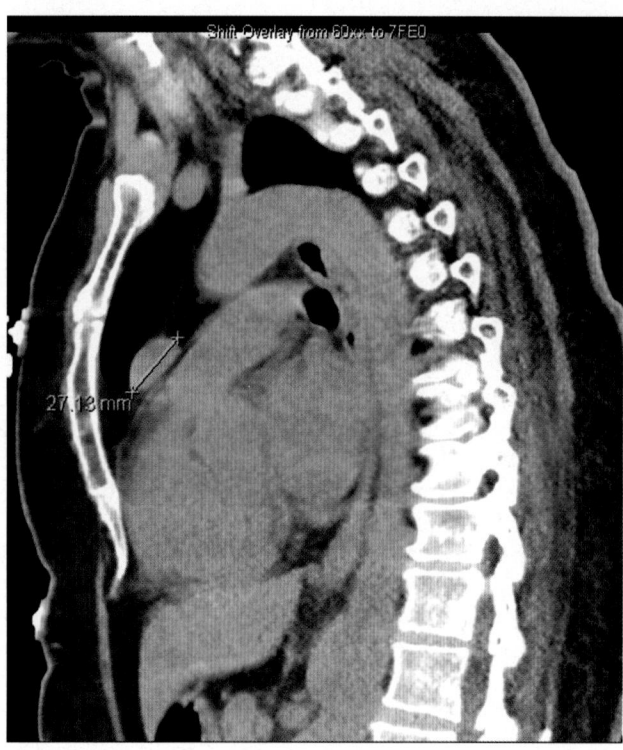

Figure 25-9. CT scan of the chest in axial (**A**) and sagittal (**B**) orientation revealing small thymoma in an MG patient.

Normal thymus is homogeneous on CT, with attenuation characteristics like muscle. It shrinks with age, as fatty replacement occurs. In fact, the gland loses its appearance as a discreet structure between 25 and 40 years of age.[216] Normal child and early adult thymus on MRI are also homogeneous and have signal characteristics between muscle and fat. On both CT and MRI, normal parameters exist for thymic size and shape. Either overall enlargement or focal contour abnormality raises suspicion for an underlying neoplasm.

Thymic hyperplasia has normal attenuation properties on CT. In slightly more than 50% of cases, the gland appears abnormal because of overall enlargement or, in some cases, a focal mass.[216] Thymoma on CT appears as sharply demarcated round or lobulated masses, commonly associated with low attenuation components which represent cysts, hemorrhage, or necrosis (Fig. 25-9A,B). Calcifications can occur but do not distinguish between invasive and noninvasive tumors (Fig. 25-10A).[216] MRI of normal and pathologic

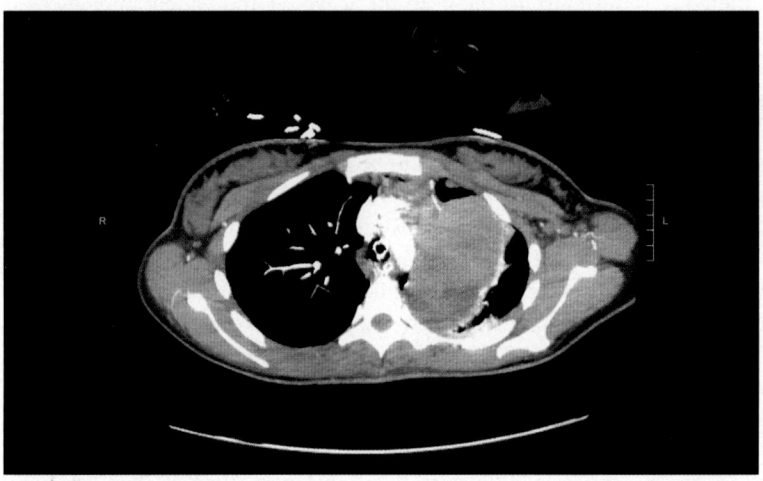 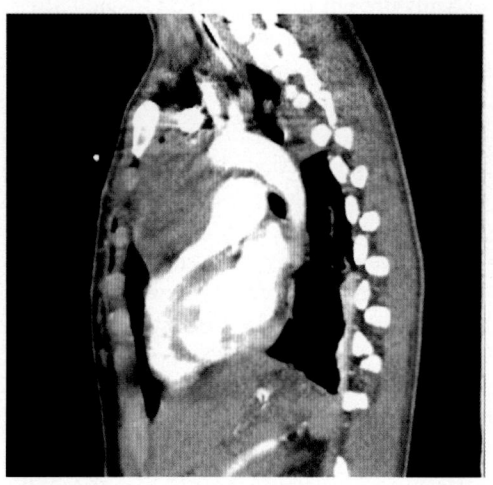

Figure 25-10. CT scan of the chest in axial (**A**) and sagittal (**B**) orientation revealing a large heterogeneous 13.0 × 11.1 × 7.3 cm mass with internal vascularity within the mass with scattered calcifications with mass effect.

thymus have different imaging features. Thymic hyperplasia typically manifests as gland enlargement with normal signal characteristics. Thymoma appears as a round, oval, or lobulated mass which is incorporated into the thymus gland.[216] Large thymomas can cause mass effect in the anterior mediastinum (Fig. 25-10A,B). Like muscle, signal intensity is low on T1-weighted images and high on T2-weighted images.

MRI has several potential advantages over CT when imaging the thymus.[224] MRI can:

1. Illustrate the cystic nature of an indeterminate, non–water attenuating thymic mass on CT, potentially preventing biopsy and thymectomy.
2. Detect microscopic fat, which potentially distinguishes normal and hyperplastic thymus from thymic tumors and lymphoma [by chemical shift MRI in adults or by DWI with apparent diffusion coefficient (ADC) mapping in all ages].
3. Help differentiate low-risk, from high-risk thymomas, thymic carcinoma, and lymphoma by the dynamic contract enhancement (DCE) pattern of these lesions and by diffusion-weighted imaging (DWI).
4. Detect invasion of masses across tissue planes, better than CT, including chest wall and diaphragm, fat planes, and neurovascular structures.
5. Assess movement of the mass relative to adjacent structures during free breathing or cardiac gating. Potential paradoxical or lack of movement could indicate phrenic nerve involvement by the mass.

Importantly, in terms of appropriateness, MRI with or without contrast or CT with or without contrast is appropriate as initial imaging. In our practice, we typically perform MRI of the chest without contrast as initial imaging in the following outpatient groups: (1) young individuals, (2) older individuals who can undergo MRI, and (3) those who require follow-up imaging when CT is inconclusive. If patients present to care with a CT chest already completed which was conclusively negative for thymoma, we typically do not repeat the imaging with MRI. For patients admitted to the hospital, CT is often the most feasible imaging modality.

Although the thymus is located in the anterior mediastinum, thymic tissue may exist ectopically in the neck or other regions of the chest.[216] Ectopic thymus occurs because of defective pathways of the embryologic descent of thymus. Ectopic thymus can occur anywhere along the path of the thymopharyngeal duct. One systematic review estimated ectopic thymic tissue in 58% of patients undergoing thymectomy for MG with or without thymoma, most commonly in the anterior mediastinal fat (33.2%), pericardiophrenic angles (13.6%), the aortopulmonary window (10.4%), the cervical region (pretracheal fat) (7.5%), and others.[225] For this reason, for initial screening, we perform an MRI chest (instead of the more limited MRI thymus/mediastinum) and specify to include images extending from the supraclavicular region to the costophrenic angles. A retrospective study of 106 patients with MG who had imaging and pathology data showed that routine chest CT and MRI can both effectively identify a thymoma (sensitivity 90% and specificity 95%). In this study, both modalities had a low sensitivity for correctly identifying hyperplasia compared to normal thymus. CT with and without contrast had the same sensitivity for thymoma, and therefore, contrast is typically unnecessary for these routine screening CTs.[226] Although there was great concern historically for worsening of MG with iodine contrast, this risk is low with modern contrast agents.[227]

MEASURING DISEASE SEVERITY, DESCRIBING HETEROGENEITY, AND QUANTIFYING OUTCOMES

There are many factors from both a patient's and practitioner's perspective as to whether a patient's MG is doing "better" or "worse" and whether the MG is "mild," "moderate," or "severe." These factors relate to degree and distribution of weakness, burden and side effects of treatment, and general expectations regarding health and daily function. Clear, standardized language to express disease heterogeneity and change within an individual patient is necessary for research and medical decision-making. This next section discusses the vocabulary, rating systems, and scales which have been developed to quantify and communicate disease severity and impact.

Outcome measures have been developed to evaluate patients with MG.[228] Among these outcome measures exists a range of what is measured, how the information is reported and how data are used. The first MG-specific scales were the physician-measured, quantitative myasthenia gravis (QMG) score and patient-reported MG activities of daily living profile (ADLs) developed in the late 1980s and 1990s, respectively. In 2000, a consensus statement was published in response to the need for accepted and widely implemented MG disease classifications, grading systems, and methods of analysis for patients undergoing treatment.[23] At that time, the primary motivation was for research, and particularly clinical trials, however recognition existed that these classification systems would be useful for clinical care as well. The Myasthenia Gravis Foundation of America (MGFA) Severity Classification was developed through this consensus group. It aimed to identify subgroups of patients with MG who shared distinct clinical features or disease severity that could indicate different prognoses or responses to therapy (Table 25-8). Several points are important to note. First, it was not designed to be used as an outcome measure. Second, it distinguishes between ocular and generalized MG. Patients are considered to have generalized MG if they have any weakness outside of the eyes, even if that weakness involves exclusively facial and bulbar muscles and spares the limbs. Class V is MG crisis, which is defined as requiring intubation or noninvasive ventilation to avoid intubation.[25]

▶ TABLE 25-8. MGFA SEVERITY CLASS

Class I	Any ocular muscle weakness; may have weakness of eye closure. All other muscle strength is normal
Class II	*Mild* generalized weakness +/− ocular weakness of any severity
	IIA: *Mild* weakness predominantly affecting limb or axial muscles, or both
	IIB: *Mild* weakness predominantly affecting oropharyngeal or respiratory muscles, or both
Class III	*Moderate* generalized weakness +/− ocular weakness of any severity
	IIIA: *Moderate* weakness predominantly affecting limb or axial muscles, or both
	IIIB: *Moderate* weakness predominantly affecting oropharyngeal or respiratory muscles, or both
Class IV	*Severe* generalized weakness +/− ocular weakness of any severity
	IVA: *Moderate* weakness predominantly affecting limb or axial muscles, or both
	IVB: *Moderate* weakness predominantly affecting oropharyngeal or respiratory muscles, or both
	Use of a feeding tube without intubation is IVB
Class V[b]	*Intubation or noninvasive ventilation* to avoid intubation due to worsening MG weakness (except when these measures are employed during routine postoperative management)

[a]Adapted from Jaretzki A, Barohn RJ, Ernstoff RM, et al. Myasthenia gravis: recommendations for clinical research standards. Task Force of the Medical Scientific Advisory Board of the Myasthenia Gravis Foundation of America. *Ann Thorac Surg.* 2000;70(1):327.[23]

[b]Updated by the consensus guidance statements from 2016. Sanders DB, Wolfe GI, Benatar M, et al. International consensus guidance for management of myasthenia gravis: executive summary. *Neurology.* 2016;87(4):419–425.[25]

OMG includes any eye weakness (ptosis, diplopia, eye closure weakness). To be ocular only, strength in all other facial, bulbar, and limb muscles must be normal. Some patients report "fatigue" when strength testing is normal. The physician's judgment is used as to whether to attribute this fatigue to MG and if it signifies generalized disease in the absence of objective, nonocular weakness.

The MGFA Postintervention Status (PIS) was established by the same consensus process to complement the MGFA severity class (Table 25-9).[23] It is an outcome measure to assess the clinical state of MG patients at any time after initiation of treatment for MG. "Improved," "unchanged," and "worse" include both consideration of symptoms and also changes in treatment intensity (i.e., medication doses/number of therapies).[23]

MG outcome measures are either patient-reported, physician-reported, or a hybrid. Two entirely patient-reported outcome measures are the MGADL[229,230] and the revised MG quality-of-life scale (MGQOL15r).[231] Both have been translated into and validated in many languages. The MGADL is an eight-item patient-reported outcome measure that assesses MG-specific symptoms and their impact on daily activities. It was initially designed to be physician-administered but now is accepted to be patient-reported with a recall period of symptoms over the previous 7 days.[142,232] The MGADL has been used as a secondary, and increasingly, a primary outcome measure in clinical trials. Items can be scored with information from the history obtained from patients in routine clinical care. A notable limitation is that it does not assess effects of axial weakness on ADLs. The MGQOL15r is patient-reported with a recall period of the previous 4 weeks. The QMG[127,233] and the manual muscle test (MMT)[234] are entirely physician-reported. Clarifications to the MMT

▶ TABLE 25-9. POSTINTERVENTION STATUS (PIS)

Complete Stable Remission (CSR)	No signs or symptoms of MG for at least 1 year (during which patient has received no therapy for MG). No weakness on careful examination by someone skilled in the evaluation of neuromuscular disease (isolated weakness of eyelid closure is accepted).
Pharmacologic Remission (PR)	Same criteria as CSR, except patient continues to take MG therapy.
Minimal Manifestations (MM)	No symptoms or functional limitations from MG, but weakness on examination of some muscles. Recognizes that some patients who otherwise meet the definition of CSR or PR do have weakness only detectable by careful examination.
Improved (I)	*Substantial decrease* in pretreatment clinical manifestations or sustained substantial reduction in MG medications, sometimes predefined in research protocol.
Unchanged (U)	*No substantial change* in pretreatment manifestations or reduction in MG medications, sometimes predefined in research protocol.
Worse (W)	*Substantial increase* in pretreatment clinical manifestations or substantial increase in MG, sometimes predefined in research protocol.
Exacerbation (E)	Patients who fulfilled criteria of CSR, PR, or MM but subsequently developed clinical findings greater than permitted by these criteria.
Died of MG (D of MG)	Patients who died of MG, of complications of MG therapy, or within 30 days after thymectomy.

Reproduced with permission from Jaretzki A, Barohn RJ, Ernstoff RM, et al. Myasthenia gravis: recommendations for clinical research standards. Task Force of the Medical Scientific Advisory Board of the Myasthenia Gravis Foundation of America. *Ann Thorac Surg.* 2000;70(1):327.

which defined MRC 4+ as mild weakness, 4 as moderate, and 3 or less as severe weakness were later published.[142] The MG Composite[235] and MG Impairment Index (MGII)[236] are both hybrid scales which combine patient- and physician-reported elements. Global clinical impression scales, such as the MG patient-acceptable symptom state (MG PASS)[237] or the single simple question[238] can be subject to bias but provide an overall impression which can be missed by the more detailed instruments. Newer outcome measures designed for virtual patient assessment over telemedicine are in various phases of development.[239–241] Placebo response[242] has been a major factor in MG clinical trials prompting calls for use of more objective outcome measures, such as single-fiber EMG,[181,243] and further outcome development. Consensus on outcome measures and other guidance for clinical trials was outlined in 2012 and, along with disease-specific outcomes, facilitated performance of subsequent clinical trials.[24]

Patients understandably hope that treatment will "cure" MG or drive it into "remission." To date, unfortunately there is no cure for MG. However, prolonged, and even life-long remissions may occur. The definition of remission is that the patient has no symptoms or signs of MG on examination. Weakness of eyelid closure is the only residual deficit accepted for "remission," but weakness of any other muscle may not be present on careful examination. Patients taking ChEIs everyday with symptomatic benefit are excluded from remission status.[25] CSR or PR may be attainable for some patients and not others. However, remission is not the only treatment goal. MM is also considered to be a desirable patient outcome in MG.[97] For MMs, favorable MG status can also be paired with measures of treatment intensity[244] or minimal side effects of MG therapy including no more than a CTCAE (Common Terminology Criteria for Adverse Events) grade 1 medication side effects (i.e., asymptomatic or only mild side effects which do not require intervention). The adverse event unit (AEU) has now been studied in MG.[245] Minimal symptom expression (MSE)[246,247] which incorporates the MGADL scale and the MG PASS question have also been used to determine whether goals of care have been met.[237]

Refractory MG has been defined variably. Having valid and reliable criteria for refractory disease helps select patients in whom more aggressive treatments may be needed.[248] The international consensus definitions outlined refractory as PIS unchanged or worse after CS and at least two other immunosuppressive agents, used in adequate doses for adequate durations, with persistent symptoms or side effects that limit functioning, as defined by patient and physician.[25] This is one of the most stringent and restrictive definitions of refractory disease when compared to others in the literature.[248]

In summary, newer outcome measures have undergone more rigorous psychometric analysis and generally are geared toward incorporating more patient input. Measures in clinical care are ideally brief and straightforward to administer within the usual clinic workflow. In clinical trials, comprehensive and overlapping assessments are selected for some intentional redundancy, to demonstrate the effect of the intervention under investigation. Minimal clinically important differences can help to inform clinical trial design and sample size estimation. Unfortunately, knowledge of minimally clinically important differences are available for only a few of the outcome measures in MG.[249] Standardization of outcome measure performance is critical across examiners within clinical trial settings to prevent confusion and variability in clinical trial data. Some of the most utilized outcomes have undergone reassessment for areas of potential variable interpretation and rigorous attempts at clarification.[142]

MG "Snapshot" Summary of Disease

Several key disease characteristics are important to include in clinical communications to present a clear "snapshot" of an individual's MG. This list will change over time as more understanding about disease heterogeneity emerges and treatment becomes even more personalized. For now, these elements are listed in Table 25-10.

Current State of Treatment Paradigm

The approach to treatment of MG is at a crossroads. Now more than ever, patients and clinicians are incredibly fortunate to have more options for MG treatment.[250,251] Even with "traditional" treatment paradigms, which have been largely unchanged for decades, MG outcomes were favorable, particularly when patients are treated according to the principles of the international consensus guidance statements.[97,252] However, newer therapies have the potential to reach treatment goals sooner, with less burden of disease and fewer side effects. These comparative efficacy and tolerability data are still lacking; safety and efficacy of newer therapies have not been compared prospectively to one another, or to traditional therapies. Furthermore, data about which patients will benefit from which therapies are lacking.[243] A nice chronology of all 62 drug studies in AChR ab positive MG is presented in a recent review.[253] As expected, these

▶ **TABLE 25-10. CLINICAL CHARACTERISTICS OF AN INDIVIDUAL'S MG COURSE—MG "SNAPSHOT"**

Determined at Diagnosis	Dynamic
• Month/year of symptom onset + diagnosis	• Maximum severity (MGFA class)
• Distribution at initial presentation (ocular, bulbar, axial, limb, or combination)	• Current severity (MGFA class)
• Antibody status	• +/− thymectomy
• +/− thymoma	• Prior MG medications (list)
	• Current MG medications and doses (list)

new therapies were initially conceived to be utilized in the 10%–15% of patients with refractory MG, given the high burden of disease in this subset.[254] However, having seen the potential for benefit in these refractory patients, the question has arisen as to whether their use requires other treatment failures or whether there is a potential benefit to using them earlier in disease, or in nonrefractory patients. From recent clinical trials, it has been observed that, as anticipated, not every patient will benefit from every new therapy, and in fact, about 25% typically are nonresponders. Therefore, to reap the full therapeutic potential of these newer treatments, we will simultaneously need to define the immunologic or other phenotypic characteristics of patients most likely to be "responders" and select treatments accordingly.[243]

General Approach

Treating a patient with myasthenia requires understanding the best evidence- and consensus-based recommendations and consideration of patient-specific and disease-specific variables outlined in Table 25-11. The strategies suggested in this chapter represent our approach, based on the teaching of our mentors and personal experience, heavily blended with evidence from the literature. Our approach is intended to provide guidance but not to be dogmatic or inflexible in its application. Access and cost may be barriers which limit the use of some therapies.

Therapeutic strategies in MG include using symptomatic therapies (ChEIs), removing a potential contributor to disease pathogenesis (thymectomy in early-onset AChR positive disease or thymoma), suppressing, removing, or inhibiting components of disease immunopathogenesis [immunomodulation through the use of immunosuppressant therapies, complement inhibition, neonatal Fc receptor (FcRn) antagonism, intravenous immunoglobulin (IVIG), or PLEX], preventing and addressing potential exacerbating factors (e.g., avoidance of drugs with potential to worsen weakness in MG, treating intercurrent infections and comorbidities such as dysthyroidism), and potentially preventing the escalation from mild to more severe disease. As discussed in Chapter 4 about immunotherapy in general, it is critical in MG to understand the risk-to-benefit ratio of treatments. A large part of this is clinicians' understanding of the natural history of MG as well as the properties of therapies themselves. The latency between treatment and clinical response, magnitude and duration of benefit, and amount of time the patient will require therapy must also be considered. These elements are typically dependent on the pharmacology of the immunomodulating agents used and the pathophysiology of MG. This information must be clearly communicated to the patient in advance of starting immunotherapy. Mutual expectations are set, and anticipatory guidance given. Patients require education on what to look for which would indicate possible MG worsening or medication side effects.

SYMPTOMATIC TREATMENT

Acetylcholinesterase Inhibitors

AChEIs are used as part of the initial treatment in most MG patients. They are fast-acting, safe, and free of long-term side effects. In patients with mild ocular symptoms or mild nonfunctionally limiting, stable, generalized weakness, they may suffice as monotherapy. However, AChEIs by themselves will rarely, if ever, treat moderate to severe generalized weakness. They will not prevent worsening in impending myasthenic crisis, or rescue patients from crisis once it occurs. Most patients will have a partial response at best.

Pyridostigmine bromide is the AChEI of choice because it has the most favorable duration of action and side effect profile compared to other drugs in its class. The initial oral dose is typically 30–60 mg three to four times a day with meals and at bedtime. To ensure tolerability first, we prefer to start on the low end of the range, at 30 mg three times daily for several days, and then increase to 60 mg three times daily and add the bedtime dose if needed. If the desired therapeutic effect is not achieved by a total daily dose of 360–480 mg, in our experience, patients are unlikely to benefit by further dose escalation. Patients should not awaken from sleep to take a dose. In MuSK MG, 30 mg twice daily might be tried initially with a slower uptitration, as MuSK ab positive patients are less likely to experience benefit and more likely to have side effects. Doses on the high end of the range are rarely used in this population. The onset of benefit occurs within 30–45 minutes of taking the drug and typically wears off in a few hours, before taking the next dose. Noticing less benefit from individual doses of pyridostigmine and being able to taper the dose usually indicates that other concomitant therapies are working. In general, very high AChEI doses are typically avoided in the contemporary era, and thus, cholinergic crisis is a disorder largely of historical interest.

▶ **TABLE 25-11. PATIENT AND MG-SPECIFIC FACTORS WHICH AFFECT TREATMENT SELECTION**

Patient-Specific Factors	MG-Specific Variables
• Age and baseline functional status	• Antibody status
• Sex and childbearing potential	• +/− Thymoma
• Medical comorbidities	• Current and maximum MG severity
• Preferences regarding types of therapies (e.g., oral, intravenous, subcutaneous and, when applicable, surgical)	• Time since MG onset and tempo of disease worsening
• Effect of MG on ADLs, occupation, and hobbies -> patient expectations	• Distribution of weakness
• Social support for obtaining treatments and medication cost and access	• Prior treatment successes, failures, and side effects

Short-term side effects are relatively common, particularly upon initiation. They occur due to the increased concentration of ACh at nicotinic receptors (skeletal muscle) and muscarinic synapses (smooth muscle and autonomic glands). Nicotinic side effects consist of muscle fasciculations and cramping. The most common muscarinic side effects are abdominal cramps, nausea, diarrhea, flatulence, fecal urgency, increased lacrimation, salivation, and sweating, and rarely, bradycardia. Gastrointestinal side effects can be minimized by taking the medication with food. As these symptoms are not nicotinic side effects, they may be treated with anticholinergic drugs without adversely affecting the beneficial effects on nicotinic NMT. Glycopyrrolate can reduce excess secretions if bothersome, while hyoscyamine and loperamide treat diarrhea and bowel frequency.

Over time, most patients self-adjust pyridostigmine dosing and timing within parameters established with the prescriber. A daily maximum dose of 480 mg daily and instructions not to take more than 120 mg every 3–4 hours is typically effective guidance. For dysphagia or chewing fatigue, pyridostigmine can be taken 30 minutes before meals. Additionally, some patients take an extra dose as needed before certain activities which they know will worsen their fatigable weakness such as public speaking, playing sports, social outings where prolonged smiling is anticipated, singing or long driving trips which tax ocular strength. For patients who think pyridostigmine helps them function in the mornings, taking a dose before bedtime can be helpful in addition to a dose first thing upon awakening in the morning, before getting out of bed.

AChEIs come in several other forms besides immediate-release pyridostigmine tablets. Pyridostigmine is also available in 180 mg Timespan capsules, utilized primarily for treatment of nocturnal symptoms or symptoms which limit functioning immediately upon awakening. This extended-release formulation is rarely used in other ways due to its variable absorption. Pyridostigmine is also available as a liquid (60 mg/5 mL) which can be used for children. We typically start at 0.5–1 mg/kg taken three to four times daily. Maximum pediatric dose is 1.5 mg/kg five times daily, up to 450 mg/daily.[255] Intravenous pyridostigmine should not be used as it is associated with cardiac arrhythmias. If patients are strictly NPO before a procedure and cannot receive medications orally, it is typically better to skip the dose of pyridostigmine that to give it parentally. Neostigmine is another short-acting AChEI that is usually started at 15 mg orally every 4 hours at 0.5–2.5 mg IV, IM, or SC every 1–3 hours. The maximum adult dose is 10 mg/day, while standard pediatric dosing is 2 mg/kg/day, divided into doses administered every 3–4 hours. In our practice, we do not use neostigmine.

Pyridostigmine is typically one of the last medications tapered unless patients are having side effects, in which case it can be the first. We typically do not try to stop pyridostigmine unless patients experience no benefit from it and until patients have tapered down to a low dose of oral prednisone. If they still appreciate benefit, or do not wish to taper, there is typically no harm in continuing. Sometimes, patients will have come completely off pyridostigmine, but use a dose occasionally as needed for certain activities or breakthrough symptoms.

IMMUNOMODULATORY AND IMMUNOSUPPRESSIVE TREATMENTS

General Principles

Immunotherapies can be categorized by many different criteria. The mechanism of action of each therapy has been reviewed earlier in Chapter 4, though we will review in more detail here the newer MG-specific treatments. When choosing the initial immunomodulatory therapy in MG, important considerations are MG subtypes, time to benefit, duration of benefit, anticipated efficacy, and side effects. Choice of initial therapy in MG is important because it can set the trajectory of the disease, but it can also be challenging, particularly in the outpatient setting. The MG may not have declared its maximum severity. Moreover, patients are receiving a new diagnosis, and it may be difficult for them to understand the details of different treatment options. The practitioner is also learning about each patient's MG, comorbidities, and preferences.

Several general principles of immunotherapy management in MG are: (1) Make one medication change at a time and allow enough time to pass to see the effect of the change, (2) Do not start and stop medications abruptly, particularly prednisone, tapering prednisone too quickly or stopping abruptly is a known cause of MG exacerbation or crisis, (3) If high-dose prednisone is started, particularly in patients more likely to develop side effects, consider starting a steroid-sparing agent at the same time or shortly thereafter, (4) Check TB testing, hepatitis B serologies (HepB surface ab, surface antigen, core ab) before starting immunosuppressive therapies (ISTs) and before IVIG if using. IVIG can cause false-positive HepB core ab through passive transfer which can be problematic if the patient later requires rituximab, and (5) Symptoms/areas of weakness which are the least severe or most recent in onset will improve first and other areas will take longer. Extraocular motility tends to be one of the last areas to improve.

Rapid Onset of Benefit/"Rescue Therapies"

IVIG and PLEX are mostly used as short-term, "rescue" therapies in MG and less commonly for maintenance, particularly with the availability of newer drugs. They are particularly effective in patients with severe or life-threatening MG such as respiratory insufficiency, dysphagia, or when rapid improvement in strength is needed. Other uses are in preparation for thymectomy or other surgery for patients with significant weakness (particularly bulbar). IVIG or PLEX can also be necessary prior to corticosteroid (CS) initiation for moderate to severe weakness to prevent possible early steroid-associated exacerbation.[256] Choosing between IVIG and PLEX depends on several factors. The first is availability, as PLEX is less widely available. The second is venous access. Because side effects of PLEX are related to the access method, peripheral venous access should be used whenever possible.[257] If peripheral access is not possible, and/or if placement of central venous pheresis catheter will delay the initiation of treatment, IVIG may be favored. IVIG and PLEX are probably equally effective for treatment of severe generalized MG, however, PLEX is likely more effective in MuSK MG.[258] Additionally, the timing of onset of benefit after PLEX is more predictable than IVIG, typically most noticeable between the third and fourth exchange. PLEX can also be repeated in short succession postoperatively should MG worsening occur. The benefit of a series of 5–6 exchanges typically lasts 4–6 weeks patients typically notice a gradual wearing off with return of symptoms if the bridge therapy has not yet taken full effect. PLEX is contraindicated in patients with sepsis and caution is advised in fully anticoagulated patients. IVIG should not be used in patients with renal insufficiency/failure (unless dialysis dependent and coordinated with the renal team).

Typically, in moderate to severe disease, rapid benefit is needed to prevent manifest MG crises or another adverse outcome from severe weakness. To achieve this, multiple therapies are added up front and then gradually pulled off one by one once clinical improvement is seen. If MG is mild to moderate, we might just start bridge therapy and/or maintenance and await the benefit. This approach is illustrated in Table 25-12.

Bridge Therapies With Intermediate Onset of Benefit

Prednisone has traditionally been the bridge therapy used in MG to provide a relatively quick onset of benefit, typically within 2–3 weeks. For patients with severe MG, early initial follow-up, at 4–6 weeks, either by phone, telemedicine, or ideally in person is needed to assess the efficacy and side effects of medications. During this time, one continues bridge therapy until the patient's functionally limiting symptoms have resolved. If functionally limiting symptoms have resolved and the physical examination has significantly improved, one can begin to lower the prednisone. For patients on high-dose prednisone, taper generally begins at 4–8 weeks to prevent accumulation of side effects. If the response to high-dose prednisone has been incomplete, one

▶ **TABLE 25-12. CHOOSING INITIAL THERAPY IN GENERALIZED MG**

MGFA Severity Class V: See Section on "Myasthenic Crisis"	
MGFA Severity Class IIIb, IVa/b (Moderate to Severe MG)	
AChR Ab positive, LRP4 Ab positive or Double Seronegative **Rescue:** IVIG or PLEX (PLEX preferred if antibody status unknown) Note: Class IV (and some class III) typically admitted to the hospital. **Bridge:** Prednisone (moderate to high starting dose) and/or FcRn antagonist[b] or complement inhibitor (if AChR ab positive) or rituximab or maintenance IVIG **Note:** Frequently need prednisone + another bridge therapy simultaneously for severe MG unless prednisone contraindicated or not tolerated **Maintenance**: Nonsteroidal immunosuppressive therapy azathioprine (AZA) or mycophenolate mofetil (MMF)/mycophenolenic acid[a] or rituximab. Thymectomy (if <50–65 years old and AChR ab positive) Note: Thymectomy can be used with another maintenance therapy or as the sole maintenance therapy, depending on the individual circumstance	**MuSK Ab Positive** **Rescue:** PLEX Note: Preferred over IVIG in MuSK Note: Class IV (and some class III) typically admitted to the hospital • **Bridge:** Rituximab and/or prednisone (moderate to high starting dose) FcRn antagonist[b] • **Maintenance:** Rituximab Nonsteroidal immunosuppressive therapy (if needed) MMF (if needed)[a] AZA • Cyclosporin
MGFA Severity Class IIa/b, IIIa (Mild to Moderate MG)	
AChR Ab positive, LRP4 Ab positive or seronegative • **Rescue**: Consider IVIG for class IIIa if functionally limiting: none typically needed for class IIa/b **Bridge**: Same as class V, IVa/b, IIIb except consider moderate prednisone starting dose Note: Typically requires one bridge therapy—either prednisone OR another bridge therapy • **Maintenance**: Same as class V, IVa/b, IIIb	**MuSK Ab positive** • **Rescue:** Consider IVIG or PLEX for class IIIa if functionally limiting; none typically needed for class IIa/b • **Bridge:** Same as class V, IVa/b, IIIb except consider moderate prednisone starting dose • **Maintenance:** Same as class V, IVa/b, IIIb
MGFA Severity Class I: See Section on "Ocular MG"	

[a]Consider alternative if patient is female of child-bearing potential.
[b]Safety of FcRn antagonist in pregnancy is unknown; therefore, consider alternative if patient is female of child-bearing potential and planning pregnancy or pregnant.

either needs to increase the dose, if feasible, and/or add a different bridge therapy. If all goes smoothly without return of symptoms during the prednisone taper, most patients will be able to attain a dose of approximately 15 mg by 6 months. At that time, the oral IST is likely beginning to have onset of benefit. Then from month 6–18 the steroids can likely be further tapered, and the oral IST will reach maximum benefit. If there is a return of symptoms, the steroid taper is halted, the steroids are increased back to the last effective dose or slightly higher, and then retapered.

Complement Inhibitors

Traditionally, therapies in MG have targeted autoantibody production. None have targeted complement except IVIG which acts via multiple mechanisms.[259] As a therapeutic drug target, C5 was appealing because inhibiting it would not interfere with the essential functions of the proximal complement cascade. Additionally, the C5 inhibitor eculizumab had already received regulatory approval for complement-mediated hemolysis associated with paroxysmal nocturnal hemoglobinuria (PNH) and atypical hemolytic uremic syndrome (aHUS).[259] Clinical studies in patients with generalized AChR ab positive MG have shown that inhibiting the cleavage of C5 by treating with eculizumab,[28] ravulizumab,[260] or zilucoplan,[261] which are all "terminal" C5 complement inhibitors, can lead to significant, often rapid, improvement in symptoms in most patients.

Currently three complement inhibitors have a label indication for AChR ab positive generalized MG. The first, eculizumab, was approved by the FDA in 2017 based on the positive phase III study REGAIN.[28,262] Ravulizumab, Eculizumab's longer-acting cousin, was FDA approved in 2021 based on the CHAMPION study. Zilucoplan is the latest complement inhibitor, approved in 2023, based on the RAISE study. Key similarities and differences are summarized in Table 25-13. The primary outcome in each phase III double-blinded RCT was the proportion of patients in each treatment group to have a significant reduction in the MGADL score. Secondary outcomes included whether reductions in the QMG, MGQOL15, and the myasthenia gravis composite (MGC) scores were reduced in the intervention group and whether this change was statistically significant.

In general, across trials, complement inhibitors have improved ADLs, muscle strength, functional ability, QOL, and fatigue in patients with MG.[28,260,261] Reductions in exacerbations and rescue therapies and ability to taper prednisone and maintenance IVIG/PLEX therapies have resulted. These benefits have been maintained at the end of 3 years in most patients who remained on therapy.[262,264,265] Most patients who will improve on C5 inhibitors will do so within the first 12 weeks and in fact, many noticed improvement within the

▶ **TABLE 25-13. COMPARISON OF COMPLEMENT INHIBITORS FOR gMG**

Drug/Mechanism	Trial(s)	FDA-Approved Dosing	Clinical Trial Population	Notes
Eculizumab (humanized monoclonal ab anti-C5, inhibits terminal complement/MAC activation)	Phase II[263] REGAIN[28]–26 weeks REGAIN OLE[262]–22.7 months (median), up to 3 years	Loading: 900 mg IV weekly × 4 Maintenance: 1,200 mg IV on week 5 then Q2 weeks	AChR ab + gMG (class II–IV) Refractory (at least 2 NSISTs or at least 1 NSIST and PLEX/IVIG) MGADL score ≥6	Did not reach statistical significance for primary MGADL endpoint. Reached significance for multiple secondary endpoints.
Ravulizumab (humanized monoclonal ab anti-C5, inhibits terminal complement/MAC activation)	Phase II CHAMPION MG[260]–26 weeks CHAMPION MG OLE[264]	Actual body weight-based dosing. Loading: 40–<60 kg: 2,400 mg IV; 60–<100 kg: 2,700 mg IV; ≥100 kg: 3,000 mg IV. Maintenance (14 days after loading and then Q8weeks): 40–<60 kg: 3,000 mg IV; 60–<100 kg: 3,300 mg IV; ≥100 kg: 3,600 mg IV	Adults with AChR ab + gMG (class II–IV) MGADL score ≥6	
Zilucoplan (synthetic macrocyclic peptide targeting C5/C5b, inhibits terminal complement/MAC activation)	Phase II RAISE[261]–12 weeks RAISE-XT OLE[265]	Phase III dosing 0.3 mg/kg SC daily. Label dosing (prefilled syringes): Actual body weight-based daily SC injections: <56 kg—16.6 mg daily: 56 kg–<77kg—23 mg: 77 kg or above—32.4 mg	Adults with AChR ab + gMG (class II–IV) MGADL score ≥ 6 QMG ≥ 12	Interim analysis from OLE published

first 1–4 weeks. A subset of later responders, however, does exist in clinical trials.

Early responders to eculizumab had not only reduced complement levels, but also experienced changes in adaptive immunity. This expands our understanding of the potential effects of the class in MG patients.[266] In the eculizumab trials, by week 12 and conclusion of the open label extension (OLE), MGADL response had been achieved at some point by 67.3% and 84.7% of patients, respectively, and QMG response by 56.1% and 71.4%, respectively.[267] More eculizumab-treated patients achieved "minimal symptom expression" versus placebo defined as MGADL total score of 0–1 or MGQOL15 total score of 0–3. [MGADL: 21.4% vs. 1.7%; difference 19.8%; 95% confidence interval (CI) 8.5, 31.0; $P = .0007$; MGQOL15: 16.1% vs. 1.7%; difference 14.4%; 95% CI 4.3, 24.6; $P = .0069$].[247]

The safety profiles of complement inhibitors have been favorable in trials. To date, clinical use has not demonstrated new safety signals. Risk of infusion reaction is very low. Most common adverse events in REGAIN and its OLE were headache, upper respiratory tract infection, nasopharyngitis.[28] Susceptibility to encapsulated bacteria, especially life-threatening Neisserial infections, such as *Neisseria meningitidis*, but also *Streptococcus pneumoniae*, *Haemophilus influenzae*, and to a lesser degree *Neisseria gonorrhoeae*, is the main serious risk of complement inhibitor use. Complement inhibition is associated with a 1,000- to 2,000-fold increase in the incidence of meningococcal illness, however, the absolute risk remains very low. In a 10-year pharmacovigilance study of eculizumab in PNH and aHUS which included 28,518 person-years (PY) of exposure, 76 meningococcal infections were reported with 8 fatal cases. This corresponds to a rate of 0.25 per 100 PYs for any infection and 0.03 per 100 PYs for fatal infection.[268] These were individuals vaccinated against meningococcal infection. In comparison, the risk of being struck by lightning in the United States is an average of approximately 0.00008 per 100 PYs.[269] Vaccination reduces but does not eliminate the risk of meningitis. Physicians must enroll in drug-specific risk evaluation and mitigation strategy (REMS) programs for all complement inhibitors and counsel patients regarding the risk and signs and symptoms of meningitis. Patients are recommended to carry a safety/alert wallet card. Current AICP guidance recommends that patients complete vaccination with quadrivalent and serotype B meningococcal (Men B) vaccines at least 2 weeks before the first dose of complement inhibitors, with a second round of both vaccines 1–2 months later.[270] Brands of the Men B vaccine are not interchangeable and vaccination must continue with the same brand. Both Bexsero (two doses) and Trumenba (two or three doses) require more than one shot in the initial series. Men B boosters are recommended at year 1 and then every 2–3 years while on therapy. Quadrivalent boosters are recommended every 5 years while on therapy. If urgent complement inhibitor treatment is needed, prophylactic antibiotics can be used until initial vaccination is complete.[259] This typically consists of penicillin VK 250–500 mg every 12 hours with alternative choices for penicillin-allergic patients.[259]

Case series at single centers in the United States and a postmarketing study in Japan demonstrated that safety and efficacy of eculizumab appears to be similar to that demonstrated in REGAIN and the REGAIN OLE.[271–273] Notably the patients with generalized MG treated were similar to the clinical trial populations of mostly refractory patients. Use of eculizumab primarily allowed for tapering of CS and/or IVIG/PLEX with concurrent disease improvement and fewer exacerbations. Tapering of nonsteroidal ISTs was not typically undertaken or reported. Postanalysis has suggested ability to taper concomitant nonsteroidal immunosuppressive therapies (NSISTs),[274] however, understanding actual success rates would benefit from additional experience from the clinical environment. Notably, the Japanese series include 15 patients (37%) with a history of thymoma and efficacy was similar in the thymoma versus nonthymoma patients.[272] In practice, we typically reassess efficacy at 12 weeks on C5 inhibitors and decide whether to continue treatment.

The most recently approved complement inhibitor, zilucoplan, is a synthetic macrocyclic peptide which binds to a different site than eculizumab on C5. Because it is not a monoclonal antibody like eculizumab and ravulizumab, it could be administered with PLEX, IVIG, or FcRn antagonists. Zilucoplan also acts further down the complement cascade and inhibits MAC formation through two mechanisms: (1) binding to C5, and blocking its cleavage to C5a and C5b; and (2) directly inhibiting the first step of MAC assembly (i.e., C5b–C6 binding).[259] As a review, C5a is involved in leukocyte recruitment and activation, activation of T cells and APCs and tissue regeneration. C5b activates MAC and C5b–9 are involved in cell lysis and apoptosis.[259]

Patients self-administer zilucoplan via a prefilled syringe. Dosing in the phase III RAISE trial was 0.3 mg/kg of body weight injected subcutaneously daily. The package insert instructions however have weight-based dosing by range.[275] Medication can stay unrefrigerated for up to 3 months which is desirable for some patients particularly who travel. Some patients, including those with poor IV access, prefer to be able to self-inject instead of relying on infusions. Efficacy compared to eculizumab has not been studied however a phase IIIb study to evaluate safety and efficacy of switching to zilucoplan in patients previously on an intravenous C5 inhibitor is underway (NCT05514873). A similar study evaluating transition from eculizumab to ravulizumab has not been performed to date.

Meningococcal vaccination requirements are the same for zilucoplan as for the IV C5 inhibitors. It is recommended that amylase and lipase are checked once at baseline prior to starting zilucoplan, given a higher rate of elevations in the RAISE trial, which were generally asymptomatic. Current recommendations do not have specific guidance regarding starting zilucoplan if baseline levels or elevated or whether levels should be followed. We currently will start the drug with mild to moderate amylase and lipase and do not recheck levels unless signs and symptoms of pancreatitis develop. Pancreatic cysts were also diagnosed in trial patients. This was thought to be of unlikely relationship to the drug and unrelated to high amylase or lipase.

Nonresponse to Complement Inhibition

A proportion of patients have a rapid and robust response to complement inhibitor therapies which begins even after one dose. Nonresponse however is an issue, prompting the questions of (1) why an estimated 25% of patients with generalized MG demonstrate no clinical improvement with complement inhibitors,[28] and (2) whether this lack of improvement could be predicted a priori. Reasons for nonresponse to complement (and other therapies for MG) are unknown and additional investigation is needed. One possibility is that AChR antibodies are heterogeneous in their ability to activate complement, resulting in a dissociation between autoantibody binding and MAC formation.[276] The assay implemented in this study has not yet to our knowledge been used to prospectively as a predictive tool. Another possibility is a genetic mutation in C5, like one which has been described in Japanese patients with PNH which prevents binding and blockade by eculizumab, while retaining the functional capacity of the mutant C5.[277]

Neonatal Fc Receptor (FcRn) Antagonists

Neonatal Fc receptors (FcRn) salvage IgG and albumin from degradation by lysosomes, leading to longer IgG half-lives. This IgG recycling accounts for the short-term humoral immunity that is provided passively in utero from mother to fetus.[278] Blocking the FcRn is a treatment strategy for antibody-mediated disorders because it leads to catabolism of IgG, thereby reducing IgG (and pathogenic antibody) levels. The end result is like that of PLEX.[278-280] The potential benefits over PLEX include the ease of administration, increased availability and reduced risk in patients with coagulopathies or limited peripheral venous access. Several FcRn antagonists are either approved for gMG or under development as outlined in Table 25-14.

In 2021, efgartigimod was the first FcRn antagonist approved for use and gMG as the first indication. Like complement inhibitors, FcRn antagonists improve QOL, ADLs, and muscle strength in MG. All FcRn trials have had either percent of ADL responders or change in ADL from baseline as the primary endpoints.[282,283,285] Batoclimab also incorporates sustained ADL response as an outcome.[289] One potential benefit of FcRn antagonists over complement inhibitors is that guidance from clinical trials exists on how to ramp up or ramp down administration frequency based on clinical response. By extension, therapy can be tapered off in this way over time. Tapering or discontinuing complement inhibitors has not been similarly studied.

Efgartigimod IV and SC and rozanolixizumab are now approved for clinical use. Batoclimab has a phase III trial recently published and nipocalimab has phase III underway. Each drug has slightly different routes and schedules of administration, and side effect profiles. To date they are approved in adults with AChR ab positive gMG (efgartigimod, rozanolixizumab) and MuSK positive MG (rozanolixizumab). For the later population, it is important to note that safety of co-administration or administration within 6 months of rituximab has not been established. Comparative efficacy between FcRn antagonists cannot be readily ascertained with existing clinical trial data.

Side effects are somewhat variable between the FcRn drugs though serious side effects are rare, with the highest rate in the efgartigimod phase III trial at 5%. All the FcRns with published phase III data have been associated with an increased rate of respiratory and/or urinary tract infections compared to the placebo group (efgartigimod URI 11% vs. 5% and UTI 10% vs. 5%; rozanolixizumab URI 30% vs. 19%; batoclimab URI 35.8% vs. 21.5% and UTI 19.4% vs. 15.4%).[279,282,285,289] Because FcRn also prevents lysosomes from degrading albumin, the class of inhibitors may be associated with hypoalbuminemia.[278] Rozanolixizumab and batoclimab are associated with hypoalbuminemia, with the latter causing a mean reduction in albumin of 31%.[289] Peripheral edema occurred in 38.8% of the batoclimab compared to 3% of the placebo group. Headache is seen more frequently with rozanolixizumab (up to 38%–45%, with aseptic meningitis rarely reported), nipocalimab and efgartigimod, but in only 6% in the batoclimab group which was not increased from placebo.[282,285,286] Total cholesterol increased in 10% of the batoclimab group compared to 1% of placebo and returned to 90% of baseline within 4 weeks after the last dose.[289] GI side effects (diarrhea and/or nausea) are more common in trials of rozanolixizumab and nipocalimab than placebo.[285,286] Efgartigimod may transiently lower titers of protective antibodies though they remain above the protective threshold in most. The ability to mount a response to vaccines appears to remain intact despite treatment.[290]

Two small single center cohort studies of patients treated clinically with efgartigimod have been published.[291,292] It is being used in patients with incomplete response to or side effects from other therapies or in whom at least one other therapy had been tried, and in those in whom more rapid benefit was needed. In a population like ADAPT except with the addition of a patient each with active cancer, anti-PD1 associated MG and thymoma, 5 of 17 patients (29.4%) discontinued treatment after an average of 5 months. Four patients stopped due to poor response. There were no serious infectious side effects, and headache was not treatment-limiting. Similarly, 6/22 (27%) of patients in the second series had non-response. 8/10 patients on prednisone were able to taper the dose. There were no series side effects except one death from respiratory failure in a patient with asthma which was poorly characterized to understand whether infectious etiologies or MG were contributing factors.[292]

The primary role currently of complement inhibitors and FcRn antagonists is to be able to transition patients off IVIG or PLEX, as bridge therapies or to taper prednisone while awaiting the onset of benefit of an NSIST. Although the CHAMPION, RAISE, ADAPT, and MycarinG studies did not specify that patients had to be refractory, the mean disease durations at entry were like REGAIN at approximately 9–10 years.

▶ **TABLE 25-14. COMPARISON OF FCRN ANTAGONISTS FOR gMG**

Drug	Trial(s)	Dosing	Trial Population	Notes
Efgartigimod IV/SQ (Human anti-FcRn IgG1 Fc fragment; reduces autoantibody levels and IgG recycling)	Phase II[281] ADAPT[282]– 26 weeks ADAPT OLE[283]—up to 3 years ADAPT-SC noninferiority study—open label parallel group—12 weeks with OLE	Weight-based IV: 10 mg/kg IV (up to 1,200 mg) weekly × 4 = 1 cycle. Fixed dose S.C.: 1,008 mg SC weekly × 4 = 1 cycle	Adults with gMG regardless of ab status, MGADL at least 5 with 50% nonocular	ADAPT was designed to observe wearing off—cycles repeated return of symptoms and no sooner than every 8 weeks. Number of infusions per cycle and time between cycles can be individualized (as was done in the OLE). Efgartigimod SC is not currently approved for self-injection—health care provider administered; refrigeration required
Rozanolixizumab (human anti-FcRn IgG4 monoclonal antibody; reduces autoantibody levels and IgG recycling)	Phase II,[284] MycarinG[285]—18 weeks, OLE completed	Phase III included 7 and 10 mg/kg given as a subcutaneous infusion weekly for 6 weeks followed by 8 weeks off. Patients averaged 4 treatment cycles per year (range 1–7) Clinical dosing: <50 kg—420 mg; 50 to <100 kg—560 mg; ≥100 kg—840 mg given as a weekly health care provider administered subcutaneous infusion for 6 weeks (1 cycle)	Adults with AChR or MuSK ab + gMG (11% of participants) MG- ADL score ≥3 QMG score ≥11	Headache occurred in 38%–45% of treatment group and 19% of placebo, including rare aseptic meningitis infection rate higher in 10 mg/kg dosing group—efficacy equivalent. Shorter mean disease duration than other phase III trials (5–6 years)
Nipocalimab (human deglycosylated anti-FcRn IG1 monoclonal ab; reduces autoantibody levels and IgG recycling**)**	Phase II[286] VIVACITY-MG (NCT04951622)[287]—24 weeks; OLE—up to 2 years	Phase II: multiple doses. Phase III: 30 mg/kg at first infusion, 15 mg/kg thereafter Q2weeks for 24 weeks	Adults with gMG; MGADL score ≥6 at baseline	Phase III currently enrolling
Batoclimab (human anti-FcRn IG1 monoclonal ab; reduces autoantibody levels and IgG recycling**)**	Phase II[288]	680 mg SC weekly × 6 weeks then 4 weeks observation, repeat cycle if needed—2 cycles maximum	Adults with AChR or MuSK ab + gMG	Primary outcome = sustained ADL improvement ≥3 points over 4 weeks; Novel secondary outcomes met (sustained QMG improvement, duration of MGADL improvement and minimal symptom expression). Outcome of early ADL response within 2 weeks not met.

B-Cell Directed Therapies

Cytokines and helper T tells influence B-cell differentiation in the thymus into memory B cells, plasmablasts, and plasma cells (PCs) in thymic germinal centers. A key function of plasmablasts and PCs is secreting autoantibodies. B-cell subpopulations are classified based on the molecules expressed on the surface (e.g., CD19, CD20), which allows for drugs to target specific populations. B-cell targeting therapies are used widely in rheumatology and oncology in addition to other areas of neurology including the treatment of multiple sclerosis and neuromyelitis optica spectrum disorder (NMOSD).[293] Rituximab is an anti-CD monoclonal antibody which targets CD20-expressing B cells, but spares B cells in the bone marrow and lymph nodes, as well as stem cells, pro-B cells, and long-lived PCs and plasmablasts. Its use has been increasing in MG since the early 2000s. Rituximab is highly efficacious in MuSK ab positive MG often with years-long durable remissions achieved, as discussed in the section on treatment of MuSK MG.[244,294-299] Evidence in support of efficacy in AChR ab positive patients has not been shown in a large randomized controlled trial though multiple retrospective studies and systematic reviews show benefit.[298,300,301] The BEAT-MG phase II trial did not meet its futility steroid sparing endpoint and therefore support for performing a phase III trial was unfortunately not present.[210] However, rituximab may be particularly safe and effective in certain clinical scenarios for non-MuSK MG such as early on in disease at a single low dose[211] or in younger[212] or older MG patients[213,302] (Table 25-15).

Details of prescribing including risks and benefits are outlined in a recent review[303] and in Chapter 2. We typically prescribe at doses of 1,000 mg IV on day 1 and day 15 instead of body surface area (BSA) dosing, given that two infusions per cycle are generally more desirable for patients than four. However, consideration for BSA dosing instead should be given to patients whose BSA dose is much higher or lower than the fixed dose. Cycles typically can be repeated every 6 months if needed. If PLEX is used, rituximab dosing is best to follow the last exchange so that it is not removed. Patients are routinely premedicated for each rituximab infusion with solumedrol 125 mg IV once, oral and IV diphenhydramine, and acetaminophen to minimize allergic reactions. Patients who have infusion reactions can undergo desensitization if treatment must be continued.[304] Importantly, hepatitis B must be excluded prior to initiation. If a history of prior HepB is present, viral suppression can be used to prevent reactivation. For complicated cases or signs of ongoing infection, we typically work closely with infectious disease colleagues.

Decisions regarding timing of redosing can be challenging though is generally guided by the clinical history and exam. Some clinicians choose also to follow percent of CD20 B cells present in rituximab-treated patients though this is not required. Near complete or complete reduction of CD20 positive B cells in serum is expected when therapeutic effect is maximal. Main potential serious side effects are infusion reaction and infection including very rarely progressive multifocal leukoencephalopathy (PML).[300] Hypogammaglobulinemia which can result from rituximab increases the risk of serious infection.[300,305] Patients who develop hypogammaglobulinemia can be treated with supplemental immunoglobulin therapy.

▶ **TABLE 25-15. COMPARISON OF B-CELL DIRECTED THERAPIES FOR gMG**

Drug (Mechanism)	Trial(s)	Dosing	Trial Population	Outcomes
Rituximab (chimeric anti-CD20 IgG1, targets CD20-expressing B cells)	Phase II—futility design—Beat MG[210]	One cycle Q 6 months (each cycle with 375 mg/m² for 4 consecutive weeks) vs. placebo	Ages 21–90 years old with AChR ab + gMG Prednisone ≥15 mg/day	52 weeks. Primary outcomes. 1. Safety endpoints met. 2. Steroid sparing endpoint not met (≥75% reduction in mean daily prednisone dose with clinical improvement or no significant worsening)
	RINOMAX[211]	Single 500 mg IV infusion at baseline vs. placebo	Adults with onset of generalized symptoms ≤12 months prior QMG score ≥6 No history of thymoma or thymectomy; NSISTs or high-dose CS: 45/47 patients AChR ab positive	16 weeks Primary outcome met: Rituximab group had a significantly greater chance of reaching minimal manifestations at 16 weeks (QMG score ≤4) or less with prednisone ≤10 mg/day, and no rescue treatment
Mezagitamab/TAK-079 (anti-CD38 monoclonal antibody)	Phase II— NCT04159805	Weekly injections 300 mg or 600 mg SC for 8 weeks	Adults with AChR or MuSK ab positive gMG (MGADL) total score of 6 or greater at screening, with at least 4 points attributed to nonocular items	Enrollment complete but unpublished
Inebilizumab (humanized monoclonal ab; targets CD19-expressing B cells including plasma cells and plasmablasts)	MINT (Phase III)— NCT04524273— currently enrolling	Infusion on days 1, 15, and 6 months later	Adults with AChR ab or MuSK ab + gMG. MGADL score ≥6 with >50% non-ocular. QMG ≥11	26 weeks plus OLE. Primary outcome is change in ADL from baseline

Other next-generation anti–B-cell therapies (e.g., ocrelizumab, obinutuzumab, ublituximab, veltuzumab, and ofatumumab) have not been trialed in MG. However, the phase III MINT study is underway in AChR ab positive gMG of the anti-CD19 agent inebilizumab, which targets a broader range of B cells than rituximab.[306] Inebilizumab received FDA approval in NMOSD after the positive NMO-mentum trial in which it reduced attack frequency even in patients with prior incomplete disease control on rituximab.[307,308]

Oral Nonsteroidal Immunosuppressive Therapies

NSISTs remain a cornerstone in the management of MG. Newer therapies have not replaced these medications which have as benefits the ease of administration, relatively low side-effect burden, and ability to drive the disease into PR as monotherapy. Maintenance IVIG/PLEX, complement inhibitors, and FcRn antagonists have not yet been evaluated in this capacity to induce PR as monotherapy. Starting an NSIST is recommended in the setting of need for high-dose CS, side effects from CS or to facilitate weaning bridge therapies (IVIG, PLEX, or complement or FcRn antagonists).

Selection of the specific NSIST depends in large part on regional/national practice patterns and whether the patient is a woman of childbearing potential, trying to avoid potentially teratogenic medications. Some consensus and randomized control trial (RCT) data exist to support use of azathioprine (AZA) first line.[25,309,310] In the United States and Europe, mycophenolate mofetil (MMF) is typically used as a second-line NSIST,[25,309] despite some controversy regarding efficacy.[311] MMF has been studied in MG, though mycophenolic acid, which is used to prevent organ rejection in transplant recipients, can be substituted and sometimes is associated with fewer GI side effects. RCTs in the early 2000s failed to demonstrate the benefit of MMF in MG likely due to a short follow-up period (3 months) and more benefit from prednisone therapy alone in the comparison group than was expected.[312–315] A large retrospective study of MMF in MG subsequently found the onset of benefit around 6 months both in combination with prednisone and as monotherapy.[316] Additionally, disease worsening has been studied and present when tapering in patients in PR or with MM of disease, further supporting its efficacy.[315–317] Most recently, PROMISE-MG, a comparative effectiveness study between MMF and AZA found them equally efficacious in newly diagnosed patients. In this study, just over 50% of patients in each group had improved QOL on the medication at 1 year.[318] Additionally, side effect rate was lower in the MMF group compared to AZA. MMF was more often associated with GI side effects like diarrhea and AZA more often with hepatotoxicity. The study suggested that lower-than-expected doses of AZA may be sufficient to maintain disease control and minimize toxicity.[318]

Details of safe prescribing and required laboratory monitoring for AZA and MMF have been described in Chapter 2 and elsewhere.[319,320] It is critical to counsel patients regarding the 10% risk of an idiosyncratic, flu-like reaction to AZA within the first month of therapy, which necessitates stopping the drug and typically resolves within 24–48 hours of doing so. The reaction will recur with rechallenge. In terms of dosing, we typically start patients on AZA 50 mg PO daily and increase weekly by 50 mg to a target dose of 150 mg PO daily (or approximately 2 mg/kg of actual body weight if lower). Activity of the enzyme thiopurine methyl transferase (TPMT) influences the risk of side effects and can be tested. Some recommend testing and avoiding therapy in patients with low activity.[321] Lab monitoring is similarly required in patients with high or low TPMT activity, and therefore we do not routinely check this lab before starting AZA though many practitioners do.

The precise lab monitoring schedule on AZA or MMF must be tailored to the patient. In general, we follow CBC with differential and liver enzymes every other week for the first 8 weeks and then monthly for the next 4 months and then approximately every 3 months up to 2 years to ensure that leukopenia/lymphopenia and/or transaminitis do not develop. Patients with a history of fatty liver disease, low baseline total lymphocyte counts or who take other medications which have similar side effects or interact with AZA (e.g., allopurinol) often need more frequent monitoring. A mild macrocytic anemia is expected, though if significant, screening for other contributing factors (e.g., B12/folate deficiency) is recommended. Mild to moderate macrocytosis and lymphopenia are desired and indicate that AZA is appropriately dosed. If CBC and hepatic function testing are acceptable at the 3-month mark, we may increase the dose to 175 mg and then 200 mg for patients weighing more than 90–100 kg. Otherwise, we continue the dose of 150 mg PO daily. It takes approximately 6–9 months to potentially start seeing benefit, a full 12–18 months to see maximum benefit of the starting dose and about 3–6 months to see the full benefit of subsequent dose increases.

In some patients, we choose to start MMF over AZA and vice versa. Anecdotally, patients with a history of diverticular disease or chronic diarrhea may have dose-limiting GI side effects from MMF. We typically start MMF at 500 mg PO BID and increase to 1,000 mg PO BID after 1 week. If possible, MMF should be taken on an empty stomach and separately from proton pump inhibitors or H2 blockers to maximize absorption. There is a REMS program for MMF in women of childbearing potential. Lab abnormalities (lymphopenia and leukopenia) are less common in MMF than in AZA and hepatotoxicity is not a concern. Therefore, for patients who anticipate challenges adhering to a frequent lab monitoring schedule, we often prefer using MMF and follow CBC with differential monthly for the first 3 months then every 3 months for the first year and then space out further. Diarrhea if present may owe to pyridostigmine, MMF, or the combination and so elimination of each sequentially is often recommended before complete discontinuation. Patients do not typically achieve more benefit from doses of MMF higher than 1,500 mg PO BID.

While methotrexate (MTX) is used frequently in rheumatologic disorders, its use is less common in MG in the contemporary era, particularly given its teratogenicity. However, because the cost of AZA or MMF can be prohibitive, it may be an appealing lower-cost alternative in financially constrained health systems,[322,323] and by some consensus is a second-line NSIST.[321] A 2016 RCT of MTX 20 mg PO weekly in 50 patients in the United States with AChR ab positive MG showed that MTX was well tolerated over the 1-year study period but failed to meet its primary outcome which was steroid-sparing effect between 4 and 12 months.[324] Another trial of steroid sparing and safety was performed of MTX versus AZA in South Africa. Twenty-four recently diagnosed gMG patients, 17 out of 24 of whom had AChR antibodies with or without thymoma, were randomized to 17.5 mg/week MTX or 2.5 mg/kg/day of AZA.[322] In this study, MTX was an effective steroid-sparing agent and had similar safety and efficacy as AZA. The most recent study, an open-label, randomized trial of 35 patients with MGFA severity class II and III compared safety and efficacy of MTX 10 mg PO weekly plus prednisone versus prednisone monotherapy.[325] In this study, MTX demonstrated a significant steroid sparing effect with comparable safety and efficacy as prednisone alone at 6 and 9–18 months. The international consensus guidance statements update in 2020 concluded that: "although evidence from RCTs is lacking, oral MTX may be considered as a steroid-sparing agent in patients with generalized MG who have not tolerated or responded to steroid-sparing agents that are better supported by RCT data."[26] Safety monitoring includes lab monitoring and daily folic acid supplementation and is discussed in Chapter 2.

Tacrolimus (FK506) and cyclosporin are both calcineurin inhibitors are used in a variety of autoimmune disorders and in preventing organ rejection after transplantation.[326] Cyclosporin has RCT-level data to support efficacy in MG and has a more rapid onset of benefit than either AZA or MMF.[327–329] However, its potential for serious side effects, including hypertension and nephrotoxicity, and its many drug–drug interactions, preclude use in most patients.[25] Tacrolimus is more potent and associated with fewer side effects than cyclosporin and therefore recommended by consensus, along with MTX, as a possible second-line IST, and is used frequently in Asia.[321] By inhibiting calcineurin activity and interfering with transcription of IL-2, tacrolimus suppresses T-cell responses and lessens antibody production from B cells.[330] The suspected pathophysiologic underpinnings of the beneficial effects in AChR and MuSK ab positive MG have been described.[331,332] Prior studies including a large RCT have demonstrated safety and efficacy as a steroid-sparing agent in MG.[333] However, a recent retrospective study also showed equivalent efficacy of monotherapy in the reduction of MG-related weakness, impairment in QOL, and improved likelihood of reaching MM status as monotherapy with fewer side effects compared to oral glucocorticoid monotherapy.[334] Although other NSISTs like MMFs are sometimes used as monotherapy, they have not been studied in MG in this way. Tacrolimus was dosed starting at 2 mg/day and adjusted based on clinical efficacy, side effects, and to keep a trough concentration of 2.8–10 ng/mL. Steroids were dosed and tapered according to a standard protocol. As early as 9 months, and definitely by 12 months, the tacrolimus group had an equivalent 75% likelihood of achieving MMs as the steroid group. The number of patients with adverse events (12 vs. 25, $P = .002$) and the total number of adverse events (13 vs. 44) was less in the propensity score matched tacrolimus group compared to the steroid group. Rates of drug discontinuation due to AEs were not significantly different between groups (3 vs. 4, $P > .99$).[334] Another prospective study also supported safety and efficacy as monotherapy starting at 3 mg/day with approximately half showing a rapid significant response in the QMG and MGADL within 3 weeks.[326] In summary, tacrolimus is a reasonable second-line oral agent for monotherapy in mild to moderate gMG to achieve a more rapid response without steroids or as a steroid-sparing IST. Data from rheumatologic disorders and the transplant population inform assessment of safety during pregnancy and lactation.[335] Additional details regarding prescribing and monitoring are outlined.[319]

Anti-Interleukin 6 Therapy

Upregulation of IL-6 occurs in AChR ab positive MG and levels track with disease activity. In animal models, anti–IL-6 treatment has led to clinical improvement. Tocilizumab is a monoclonal antibody directed at IL-6. Small open label trials and case series suggest improvement in MG.[336–338] Satralizumab, another IL-6 inhibitor which was approved for use in 2020 for NMOSD completed a phase III trial (LUMINESCE) in AChR, MuSK, or LRP4 ab positive adults and adolescents with gMG (NCT04963270). Enrollment is complete but results have not yet been published.

Chimeric Antigen Receptor (CAR)T-Cell Therapy

T cells which have been engineered to target specific cells via chimeric antigen receptors (CARs) were initially developed to treat B-cell malignancies such as lymphoma.[339,340] The T cells are termed "chimeric" to reflect the different origins of the CAR components including an extracellular antigen recognition domain derived from antibodies, a transmembrane domain, and an intracellular activation domain derived from T cells. Another technology is chimeric autoantibody receptor T (CAART) cell therapy. Both CART and CAART therapies are in clinical trials for MG and other autoimmune disorders (Table 25-16).

Traditionally, B-cell depletion has been possible through treatment with monoclonal antibodies (e.g., rituximab and others). However, several limitations exist with this approach. First, the beneficial clinical effect may be incomplete and/or wear off. Second, the resulting IgG depletion increases risk of severe infection. Third, monoclonal antibodies target circulating B cells, but depletion of tissue-resident memory B cells is often incomplete. Lastly, the best antigen to target is

▶ TABLE 25-16. COMPARISON OF CART/CAART FOR gMG

Drug (Mechanism)	Trial(s)	Dosing	Trial Population	Outcome Measures
Descartes-08 CART	Phase Ia/IIa/IIb study—Autologous T-cells expressing A chimeric antigen receptor directed to B-cell maturation antigen (BCMA)	Dose escalation, expansion and RCT	30 adults with gMG (seropositive and seronegative)	Safety and preliminary efficacy (MGADL = primary outcome)
MuSK-CAART	Phase I, open-label, safety and dose-finding study of autologous MuSK-CAART	Dose-finding study, cyclophosphamide with or without fludarabine	24 adults with MuSK ab positive MG—MGFA severity class I-IVa	Safety outcomes

CAART, chimeric autoantibody receptor T; CART, chimeric antigen receptor T.

unknown. Anti-CD20 agents do not deplete PCs or plasmablasts and therefore different antigenic targets such as anti-CD38 PCs have been developed. CART cell therapy promises a more durable immune "reset" with fewer off-target effects which would potentially allow patients to stop immunosuppressive therapies.[340]

It is helpful to understand the process of CART cell therapy corresponding mechanism of action/benefit.[340] First, apheresis collects leukocytes from the patient's peripheral circulation. Then, lymphocytes are transfected with a lentiviral vector which encodes the CAR and then undergo in vitro expansion. CARs against specific surface antigens [e.g., CD19, CD20, B-cell maturation antigen (BCMA)] on B cells throughout their lineage are used for autoimmune indications.[340] Patients then have chemotherapy to deplete lymphocytes, typically consisting of a combination of cyclophosphamide and fludarabine. The CART cells are reinfused into the patients where they undergo expansion to lyse B cells which express the target antigen (e.g., CD19) and direct cell differentiation into long-lasting memory CART cells. This targeted approach spares CD19 negative B cells including long-lived PCs in bone marrow. Potential side effects of CART cell therapies are immune effector cell-associated neurotoxicity syndrome (ICANS) and cytokine release syndromes caused by proinflammatory cytokines such as IL-6. These toxicities have limited their use to patients without advanced cancers or very severe, refractory autoimmune disease (e.g., NMOSD and lupus).

More targeted CARs with fewer side effects have allowed for greater expansion of use into autoimmune diseases. In 2023, the first phase Ib/IIa trial of Descartes-08 CAR therapy in MG, using RNA engineering rather than the usual DNA approach to target BCMA, was published.[341] With the RNA approach, none of the 14 patients had ICANs or cytokine release syndrome, and the therapy was safe and generally well tolerated. Additionally, improvements in disease severity were seen and maintained at 9 months when the study ended. A phase IIb study to evaluate the safety and preliminary efficacy of Descartes-08 CART cells in patients with gMG has started. It aims to recruit 30 adults with gMG including seronegative patients (NCT04146051).

Additional cell-based therapies are in development for MG. Data support that autoantibodies in MuSK MG are produced by short-lived PCs.[342] BCMA is found on the surface of PCs but not immature or mature B cells. Therefore, targeted depletion of anti-MuSK B cell receptor positive B cells by MuSK CAART could prevent replenishment of the PCs producing anti-MuSK autoantibodies, while retaining healthy B cells. A phase I dose-finding and safety trials of MuSK CAART is currently ongoing and aims to enroll 24 patients with MuSK MG (NCT05451212).

Symptomatic Therapies in Development

Oral symptomatic therapies are lacking for MG and an unmet need for patients who do not respond to or tolerate pyridostigmine. Proof of concept work regarding the beneficial effects of chloride channel (ClC-1) inhibitors on NMT led to a phase I and small phase II trial which was positive and supports further development.[343,344] Amifampridine phosphate has been studied in MG populations besides LEMS and CMS. A phase IIb study showed that amifampridine phosphate was safe and effective in MuSK MG but the phase III RCT in MuSK, which has not yet been published, was negative. A subsequent open-label trial however did show benefit.[345,346]

Thymectomy

Thymectomy is a therapeutic option for those with AChR ab positive MG without thymoma, who are 18–65 years old. The MGTX trial showed that thymectomy afforded significant benefit in nonthymomatous MG compared to prednisone alone at 3 and 5 years.[27,347] Patients in the thymectomy group required less prednisone, had fewer hospitalizations for MG, needed less AZA, and had lower treatment-related side effects and distress. Benefit is most clear for patients less than 50 years old.[26] While benefit may be greater if performed early in disease, we do recommend thymectomy in selected patients with longer disease durations if they are symptomatic and/or still require high-intensity treatment.

Thymectomy should be performed when the MG is well controlled to minimize risk of postoperative failure to extubate or MG exacerbation. We use IVIG or PLEX preoperatively in patients with moderate weakness and in some patients with mild weakness if they have bulbar symptoms and/or history of severe disease. Surgery is scheduled approximately 1 week after completing IVIG or several days after the final exchange.

Though MGTX employed a transsternal surgical approach, minimally invasive techniques [transcervical and video-assisted thoracoscopic surgery (VATS)] are increasingly used to reduce perioperative risk, even in patients with thymoma.[348] Thymectomy considerations are different for patients with thymoma. With rare exceptions, these patients undergo complete thymectomy for tumor removal as soon as possible after appropriate pretreatment and MG stabilization, with oncologic evaluation to consider adjuvant therapy if indicated.[25] Medical MG therapy is frequently required postoperatively for both thymomatous and nonthymomatous MG.

Myasthenic Crisis

Myasthenic crisis is a serious, life-threatening, rapid worsening of MG with airway compromise from ventilatory or bulbar dysfunction.[25] Any other "worsening" of MG which does not involve impending or manifest respiratory failure is termed an "exacerbation." In the 2016 International Consensus Guidance Statements, "impending MG crisis" was also defined to recognize that there is often a window of time prior to crisis. This is clinical worsening of MG that, in the opinion of the treating physician, could lead to crisis in days to weeks.[25] Signs of impending MG crisis are worsening neck and/or bulbar muscle weakness, orthopnea, use of accessory muscles to breathe and hypercapnia. Hypoxia is a late sign of MG crisis and normal oxygen saturation does not reassure against the possibility of impending crisis. Historical data suggest that MG crisis occurs at least once in approximately 15% of all patients with MG and can be the presenting manifestation of MG.[103] Triggers can include illness, surgery including thymectomy, medication changes, pregnancy/postpartum or sometimes no trigger is identified. Contemporary mortality where intensive care is available is less than 5% and full recovery is possible.[103,349]

Management of MG crisis continues to be IVIG or PLEX and supportive care.[103] Importantly, high-dose CS in regimens such as IV methylprednisolone 1,000 mg daily for 1–5 days has never shown benefit in MG and can instead cause acute worsening of MG. Although discussed in some literature as part of the management of MG crisis, this is not evidence-based and high-dose IV steroids do not typically have a routine place in the care of patients with MG crisis. This makes management distinctly different than management of other neurologic autoimmune disorders in the inpatient setting. If patients cannot take their regular PO CS, and gastric tube access is not available, an IV equivalent of the patient's oral prednisone can be given IV. MG crisis management as not been significantly changed to date by the influx of new biologic therapies to date. None has been studied yet for MG crisis and cost has made availability limited for routine care in most inpatient settings.

Challenges in the management of crisis include knowing when it is safe to extubate patients and avoid the need for reintubation.[349–351] Most patients with MG are intubated for 6–14 days before successful extubation.[351] If patients require reintubation, a tracheostomy and PEG are more likely. Noninvasive ventilation such as BiPAP can be used to avoid mechanical ventilation can be used in very selected circumstances. This is most likely to be successful if patients have intact mental status, younger age, have minimal cardiac or pulmonary comorbidities, nonsevere bulbar muscle weakness and can be monitored closely in an intensive care setting.[352,353] A postdischarge plan for longer-term MG treatment (e.g., starting new treatments or adjusting current medications) is critical as part of the in-hospital treatment for MG crisis.

MG SUBTYPES

Ocular MG

OMG involves weakness restricted to ocular muscles and manifests as ptosis, diplopia, and/or eye closure weakness.[128] While most patients initially present with ocular weakness, a majority will generalize, typically within 2–3 years, while a smaller proportion will have exclusively ocular manifestations for the duration of their disease. Approximately 15% of patients have MG confined to the eyes after 3 years. Diagnosis can be more challenging as half of patients with OMG are antibody negative. Key differential diagnostic considerations and an algorithm for evaluation are outlined.[128] Thyroid eye disease in particular must be considered and excluded.[166] Single-fiber EMG studies and the icepack test have a larger role in diagnosis of OMG.[128,354] MuSK ab positive OMG is very rare.[355,356]

Biomarkers to predict generalization are lacking. Debate exists as to whether early treatment with prednisone or other immunosuppressant drugs could prevent generalization. Small case-control studies support that risk of generalization is lower in treated groups.[357–359] A study of 147 patients with OMG found that prednisone reduced the incidence of generalization at 2 years from 36% to 7%.[360] A risk score to predict generalization has been created, however, has not been validated. Antibody positivity, thymic hyperplasia (as determined by imaging, which has limitations), and concurrent autoimmune diagnoses are risk factors for generalization in this score.[107] Unfortunately, despite standard-of-care treatment with prednisone and AChEIs, almost 40% of patients have persistent symptoms within 2–3 years. Although this is considered the mildest form of MG, OMG results in significant impairment of QOL.[361] Initial severity of ocular symptoms is predictive of ongoing disease burden despite treatment.[358]

RCT data to support treatment approaches to OMG are lacking. However, guidelines provide support for various approaches to treatment.[362,363] Additionally, the EPITOME trial, which evaluated efficacy of prednisone in OMG outlines an approach to prednisone dosing which can be replicated.[364] Our typical approach is to start with pyridostigmine and uptitrate the dose. Within a week or two, if symptoms persist, we start prednisone at approximately 15–20 mg PO daily or the equivalent 30–40 mg PO every other day. This dose is continued for 2–4 weeks and then increased or decreased depending on improvement in MG or dose-limiting side effects. If high doses of steroids are needed, the patient is unable to taper prednisone without worsening, or has side effects to prednisone which limit efficacy, we start an NSIST (e.g., AZA or MMF). Sometimes, if symptoms are bothersome but not functionally limiting, we will start an NSIST, usually MMF, as monotherapy with pyridostigmine. Thymoma is rare in patients with OMG however needs to be evaluated for and removed if present. The role for thymectomy for treatment of nonthymomatous OMG is controversial.[362]

Some patients with MG have reported improvement in ptosis with oxymetazoline hydrochloride ophthalmic solution 0.1%, which is a nonselective alpha-adrenergic agonist that stimulates alpha-1 and alpha-2 receptors, including those found in the Müller muscle of the eyelid. The US FDA approved its use for acquired ptosis in July 2020.[365] If utilized, we recommend occasional usage though daily usage has been reported without side effects in case reports of patients with MG.[365]

Several nonpharmacologic therapies exist for managing ocular weakness in MG. Eye crutches or tacking up the lids with soft medical tape can be used to temporarily reduce ptosis. Keeping the eyes moist with artificial tears is important to prevent keratopathy. The most immediate way to improve diplopia is to block vision from one eye. This can be done with an eye patch, opaque contact lenses or placing a strip of occlusive tape across the diameter horizontally of one eyeglass lens. Strabismus surgery for extraocular motility abnormality is not typically recommended. It is likely to be ineffective due to variable weakness. We do consider surgery in very limited circumstances, namely if disease duration is long, the pattern/severity of weakness is stable over a year and fixed despite maximal medical management, and custom prisms are ineffective. Blepharoplasty to correct ptosis is typically not recommended due to the same reason that weakness often fluctuates. Sometimes patients with both dermatochalasis and ptosis will appreciate improved vision and ptosis with surgical removal of the redundant eyelid skin.

MuSK Antibody Positive MG

MuSK ab positive MG can be clinically identical to AChR ab positive MG or present with prominent bulbar, axial, and respiratory weakness.[215,258,366–368] Before rituximab was used more widely after approximately 2005–2015,[294] MuSK was often more refractory and associated with more severe disease than other MG subtypes.[299] Like in other IgG4 mediated diseases, rituximab is highly effective.[68,163] The mainstays of therapy are currently PLEX, prednisone and rituximab.

Pyridostigmine is typically started initially, however, has a minimal role in treatment of MuSK. Most patients experience intolerable side effects including excessive muscle twitching/cramping, diarrhea, and salivation, without substantial benefit. We will try a low dose of pyridostigmine 30 mg PO daily to start and increase by 30 mg increments. For mild to moderate disease, we typically start prednisone with rituximab. Increasingly, however, if patients are stable and disease is mild (class IIA or IIB), we use rituximab as monotherapy as a first-line alternative to prednisone, given durable benefit in most patients.[244,294,299] For class IIIA/B moderate disease, we use rituximab plus prednisone. If rituximab does not allow or provide enough steroid-sparing benefit and/or marked improvement within 6 weeks, we typically add MMF. Rituximab can be started immediately after completing a cycle of PLEX. MuSK ab positive patients tend to be less responsive to IVIG, AZA, and no benefit from thymectomy has been demonstrated.[258,369,370] Some patients require rituximab every 6 months and others only every 1–3 years. MuSK antibody level is a biomarker of disease activity. MuSK antibody levels can be followed selectively in patients who we are considering redosing rituximab as this can sometimes help in decision-making regarding timing of redosing rituximab.[163,164]

As would be anticipated based on the mechanism of action, FcRn antagonists are effective in MuSK MG. After the MycarinG trial, rozanolixizumab was FDA approved for MuSK MG.[285] At this time, experience and data are insufficient to guide how this will fit into the treatment paradigm with rituximab. Using an FcRn in place of PLEX around diagnosis in moderate to severe disease and following this with rituximab could be a possibility in the future. Additional B-cell depleting therapies (inebilizumab) and CART cells are in clinical trials (NCT04524273) for MuSK MG.

Double Seronegative and LRP4 Antibody Positive MG

AChR ab/MuSK ab negative ("double seronegative") and LRP4 ab positive MG are treated similarly (Table 25-12). The disease phenotype and pathophysiology are like AChR ab positive disease.[55,57] Therefore, these subtypes are managed like AChR positive MG except for use of complement inhibitors and FcRn antagonists. Small numbers of seronegative patients were included in clinical trials, if included at all, and therefore efficacy data are limited. Additional clinical trials are anticipated for double seronegative patients. Ensuring accurate diagnosis in these patients and excluding CMS in atypical or treatment refractory cases is critical.

MG With Thymoma

Understanding the standard of oncologic care for thymoma helps clinicians best manage coincident MG. While thymoma-associated MG can be more refractory, the oncologic prognosis for thymoma is good with a 5-year survival rate of about 90%. It is generally a slow growing tumor which infrequently spreads to adjacent mediastinal structures and metastasizes to lung. By comparison, only 55% of patients with thymic carcinoma and between 28% and 75% of patients with thymic NETs survive for 5 years.[90] To date, targeted treatments for thymoma have been limited despite growing understanding of their heterogeneous molecular genetic underpinnings.[371] The current standard of care is first thymectomy with attempt to achieve clear surgical margins.[372,373] Completeness of resection is the most impactful prognostic factor. If the thymoma is encapsulated or invasion is limited, surgery is frequently curative. In large thymomas or those with significant invasion into mediastinum structures, neoadjuvant platinum-based chemotherapy may be given to shrink the tumor prior to surgery. Postoperative radiation therapy with or without adjuvant chemotherapy is used for patients with poorer prognosis.[372,373] Immunotherapy has potential for efficacy in TETs but its use outside of the clinical trial setting has been limited by severe irAEs.[374] In those rare patients with nonoperative tumors, typically in the setting of advanced age, radiation with or without chemotherapy can be used.[375]

Treatment for patients with MG associated with thymoma has essentially been the same as that for AChR positive MG but there are several key considerations. The most pressing is deciding when the patient is medically optimized for thymectomy. The goal is to minimize the risk of postoperative MG exacerbation or crisis.[376] There is more urgency to perform thymectomy in patients with thymoma compared to patients with nonthymomatous MG, both for oncologic reasons and also because for many, MG control can be difficult to achieve preresection. However, because thymomas are slow growing tumors, MG treatment before thymectomy should be prioritized. Typically, either IVIG or PLEX are used preoperatively and CS can be initiated. A benefit to PLEX is that additional exchanges are readily possible if needed postoperatively, should MG worsening occur. Preoperative efgartigimod has been reported and it is likely that its use in this setting with increase.[377] Complement inhibitors have also been used in patients with thymoma though reports of preoperative use are lacking.[378] Recent clinical trials have excluded patients with recent thymectomy, thymectomy planned during the duration of the clinical trial or active thymoma/thymic carcinoma.[260,285,282] Approximately 25% of the study population in the phase III RAISE study had a history of resected thymoma.[261,378]

Additional considerations in TAMG are consideration of total burden of immunosuppression inclusive of chemotherapies and the possibility of concurrent Good syndrome, which is adult-onset hypogammaglobulinemia.[379,380] How to best screen for or adjust MG therapies for Good syndrome or other immunologic abnormalities is unknown.[381] Clinical trials of FcRn antagonists included patients with IgG levels in an essentially normal range.[285,282] To date, we generally use the same treatment approach as nonthymomatous AChR ab positive gMG and screen for Good syndrome with input from immunology colleagues in the event of recurrent infections.

Juvenile MG

Juvenile MG is autoimmune MG with onset in children younger than 18 years of age. Management, particularly of postpubertal teens, is similar to adults however there are several key differences.[382–384] Before puberty, there is no gender predominance, more patients are seronegative and frequently, MG is purely ocular.[385] Spontaneous remissions of ocular symptoms are common. However, in young children with generalized MG, weakness can be severe.[384]

Symptomatic therapy with pyridostigmine is the mainstay of treatment of ocular disease. IVIG and PLEX are employed for more severe disease. Immunosuppression with prednisone and AZA can be used. Attempts are made to delay prednisone use until after puberty and growth is complete. A small cohort showed that rituximab is safe and effective in moderate to severe juvenile MG.[212] Eculizumab is approved for expanded use globally in Japan and the European Union for example for children and adolescents 6–17 years old with refractory AChR ab positive MG.[386] A trial is underway for efgartigimod in juvenile MG (ADAPT Jr).[387] Thymoma is rare in children and even more rare in juvenile MG.[388] Thymectomy is utilized to treat MG in older teens who have AChR ab positive nonthymomatous MG. Given the active role of the thymus in immune system development in younger children, waiting at least until after puberty and preferably the later teenage years to perform thymectomy is preferred.[255]

MG and Pregnancy

MG frequently affects women during childbearing years and can even first present during pregnancy or postpartum. Anticipating pregnancy and counseling women about childbearing from the time of diagnosis and throughout their disease, so that they can make informed reproductive decisions, is critical. Pregnancy can be supported in MG through expert multidisciplinary care resulting in favorable maternal and fetal outcomes. Therefore, women with MG should not be discouraged from childbearing. Guidance for best management of MG during pregnancy have been established by workgroups and presented in reviews.[389–395]

Approximately two-thirds of patients have either unchanged or improved MG during pregnancy.[394,396] However, medications frequently need to be adjusted in advance of pregnancy both to optimize MG control and to minimize any potential fetal risks.[25] IVIG, PLEX, and pyridostigmine have been the mainstays of treatment during pregnancy. Prednisone can be started or continued during pregnancy with doses lower than 20 mg daily preferred.[395] AZA can be continued during pregnancy at the lowest possible dose if the patient is already on stable therapy. MMF cannot be used in pregnancy due to teratogenicity. There is a REMS program for MMF use and prescribing must be accompanied by two forms of birth control in women of childbearing potential if used in this population at all. MTX and cyclophosphamide are avoided as they are teratogenic. Prescribing guidance from the manufacturer recommends avoiding rituximab for 12 months prior to pregnancy.[395] However, consensus guidance supports rituximab use even while trying to conceive.[397] For this reason, it can be an appealing option in this age group, particularly with MuSK

MG.[398] If timing allows, we try to have women with AChR ab positive generalized MG undergo thymectomy well in advance of pregnancy as this increases the likelihood that they could be in remission (or well controlled) on fewer or no medications during pregnancy.[27,347] There are few to no data regarding safety of other newer biologic therapies or zilucoplan in pregnancy or breastfeeding. The exception is eculizumab where pregnancy data exist from the PNH population, and outcomes are favorable.[268,399,400] There are selected case reports of use during pregnancy in MG.[401,402] Eculizumab can be used if absolutely necessary during pregnancy. There are no published data to date on FcRn antagonists such as efgartigimod or rozanolixizumab in pregnancy. They will reduce IgG concentrations in the newborn, which would likely lower passive protection received from the mother against infections during the first weeks after birth.

Delivery at a facility with neonatal intensive care is recommended given the approximately 10% risk of infants being born with transient neonatal MG. This results from passive transfer of pathogenic antibodies to the newborn and is a treatable disorder. Affected infants have temporary feeding and sometimes breathing problems after birth.[395] This typically manifests within the first 48 hours after delivery. Therefore, if both mother and newborn are healthy, they typically leave the hospital together and the newborn does not typically require additional in-hospital observation. Intravenous magnesium should be avoided if possible in mothers with MG and therefore alternative treatments are typically recommended in the event of pre-eclampsia or eclampsia.[395] Women should be encouraged to deliver vaginally unless there is an obstetric indication for cesarean section.

MG and Immune Checkpoint Inhibitor Therapy for Cancer

MG is an uncommon complication of ICI therapy for cancer and termed, immune-related MG (irMG).[403,404] ICIs approved for use in clinical practice target various components of the checkpoint pathway (e.g., CTLA-4, PD-1/PD-L1, or LAG-3) which are receptor-ligand pairings that modulate T-cell activity. Likely, some cases represent de novo disease onset and others exacerbation of preexisting diagnosed or undiagnosed disease.[405] Ocular, bulbar, neck, and respiratory weakness typically presents within the first 1–4 cycles of ICI therapy (Fig. 25-11A,B,C,D). Dysphonia is more common than dysarthria however dysphagia is common and often severe. Compared to idiopathic MG, irMG is more likely to be seronegative,[406] and overlap with myositis and myocarditis. Some cases may be paraneoplastic and antibody mediated, however some are likely inflammatory.[407] Fatality is approximately 20%.[408,409] It's critical to remember that ICI-related myositis (irMyositis), which is more common than irMG, can resemble MG clinically, with prominent or exclusively ocular weakness but without evidence for a DNMT on EDX testing of the NMJ. Guidance regarding how to differentiate between junctional and muscle disease are outlined.[410] Interestingly, AChR antibodies have been reported in irMyositis without definite evidence for a DNMT.[411] Thus, the pathogenicity of AChR antibodies in these patients is unknown at this time.[412,413] Understanding of the pathophysiology of myocarditis and myositis will be key toward targeted treatments for irMG.[412,413]

The mainstay of treatment for irMG is CS, including IV solumedrol which differs from idiopathic MG, with

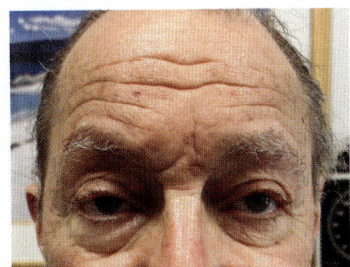
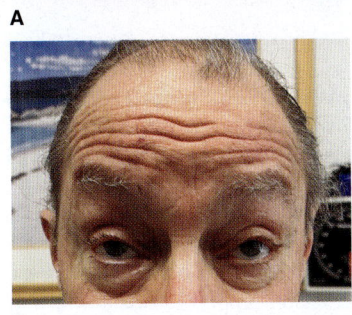
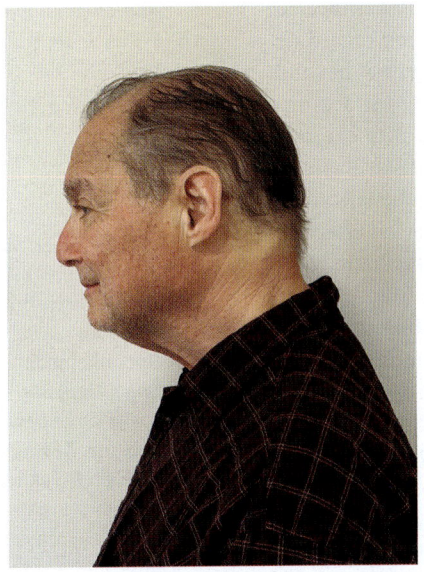
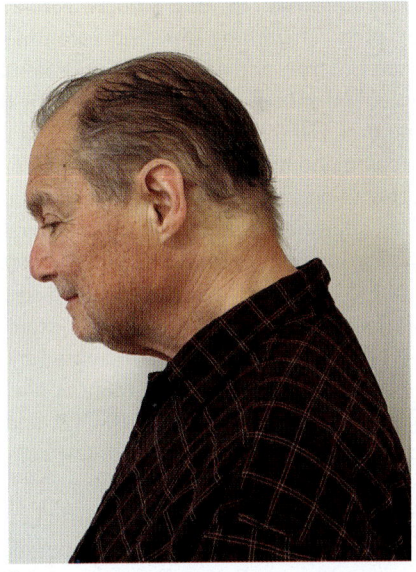

Figure 25-11. Patient with new onset AChR antibody positive MG with myositis and myocarditis after immune checkpoint inhibitor therapy. Notice bilateral ptosis and frontalis signs with disconjugate gaze at baseline (**A**); the enhanced frontalis contraction and limited upward eye movement with attempted upgaze in the context of the head bowing forward due to neck weakness (**B**); mild forward neck flexion/head drop (**C**); fatigable neck extension weakness after 10 seconds of standing (**D**).

PLEX added for severe weakness or crisis.[414] Typically, the myocarditis is the most severe complications and therefore immunosuppressive therapy is typically targeted toward that indication. Recent reports suggest a possible role for complement inhibitors acutely[415,416] or to prevent exacerbation in patients with known MG being treated with ICIs.[405,417] Understanding the pathophysiology of this new NMTD will likely usher in new understanding of and treatments for idiopathic MG.

Exercise and MG

Patients and clinicians often ask the question about safety and possible benefits of exercise in MG. Theoretical concern exists about over-fatiguing muscles and possible inflammation that muscle breakdown after exercise might trigger. Benefits can include, counteracting adverse metabolic effects of prednisone, reduced depression, anxiety and fatigue, improving strength and endurance, and potential favorable immunomodulatory benefits.[321,418] The primary barrier to exercise, in mild to moderate MG, often more than weakness, is fatigue.[419] Some patients with MG describe profound fatigue which is poorly understood. Because the fatigue exists in ocular and well-controlled generalized MG, its etiology is hypothesized to be distinct from the etiology of weakness in MG.[420] Exercise has been proposed as a possible antidote to fatigue.

Research on exercise in MG has been limited but there have been several recent notable additions to the literature. A systematic review in 2021 evaluated 10 interventional studies which included 159 patients with mild to moderate generalized MG regarding the effect of physical training, three of them on respiratory muscles.[419] In summary, the programs were safe, and muscle strength, daily function, and QOL improved, in most studies. Fatigue was less impacted by physical training. Specific recommendations regarding exercise type and intensity could not be derived beyond a general mix of aerobic and strength training for a minimum of 150 minutes per week. This is in line with exercise recommendations for general health for adults.[421] Exercise prior to elective thymectomy was particularly beneficial.[419] Two additional studies on exercise were published after the systematic review. In the RESTOREX trial, 20 patients with mild to moderate MG were assigned to either 30 minutes of walking daily or rest. Notably, the exercise group started at 10 minutes of walking and increased by 10 minutes weekly to the full 30 minutes. At 3 months, the walking group had significant improvement in MGQOL and walking efficacy as measured by the 6 minute walk test compared to the rest.[422] Second, in a prospective randomized controlled trial, 45 patients received usual care or usual care plus instruction to complete 3 times weekly unsupervised 40-minute rowing machine exercise sessions in their homes. There was no health-related quality of life change in the intervention group but also no safety issues occurred. Several methodologic issues may have accounted for these findings including drop out, type of exercise, lack of supervision with exercise, and unequal baseline characteristics of the two groups.[418]

Routine Medical and Dental Care

Maintenance of primary and routine medical care in patients with MG is critical. Dental work and routine screenings such as colonoscopy are often a source of concern for patients and providers. Most patients with well-controlled or even mild to moderate generalized MG weakness can typically undergo these safely. Jaw or neck fatigue and dysphagia/management of secretions must be considered with dental work. Age-appropriate and seasonal vaccinations including the influenza, COVID-19, Shingrix, and pneumovax are recommended and the risk of MG worsening is very low with administration.[423,424]

▶ SUMMARY

Autoimmune MG is a clinically and biologically heterogeneous DNMT which affects patients of all ages. Early diagnosis, careful disease monitoring, and definitive management tailored to the patient and disease severity are paramount. Mortality is low though contemporary natural history data are needed. Most patients improve with treatment. Response or nonresponse to therapy, however, cannot be reliably predicted, and biomarkers of disease activity are limited. Additionally, side effects of treatment are common may limit efficacy or adversely affect quality of life. The pipeline of drug development with associated increased understanding of disease pathophysiology is robust. As a result, treatment paradigms are likely to change significantly over the next decade.

REFERENCES

1. Vincent A. Unravelling the pathogenesis of myasthenia gravis. *Nat Rev Immunol.* 2002;2(10):797–804.
2. Willis T. *De Anima Brutorum (Oxonii Theatro Sheldoniano).* 1672:404–407.
3. Erb W. Zur casuistik der bulbären lähmungen. *Arch Psychiatr Nervenkr.* 1879;9:336–350.
4. Goldflam S. Uebereinen scheinbar heilbaren bulbär paralytischen Symptomencomplex mitBetheiligung der Extremiten. *DtschZ Nervenheilkd.* 1893;4:312–352.
5. Jolly F. Ueber Myasthenia gravis pseudoparalytica. *Berl Klin Wochenschr.* 1895;32:1–7.
6. Campbell H, Bramwell E. Myasthenia gravis. *Brain.* 1900;23:277–336.
7. Oppenheim H. *Die Myasthenische Paralyse (Bulbarparalyse Ohne Anatomischen Befund.* JHH Karger; 1901.
8. Loewi O. Über humorale Übertragbarkeit der Herznervenwirkung. *Pflügers Arch ges Physiol.* 1921;189:239–242.
9. Dale HH, Feldburg W, Vogt M. Release of acetylcholine at voluntary motor nerve endings. *J Physiol.* 1936:353–380.
10. Blalock A, Mason MF, Morgan HJ, Riven SS. Myasthenia gravis and tumors of the thymic region: report of a case in which the tumor was removed. *Ann Surg.* 1939;110(4):544–561.
11. Blalock A, Harvey AM, Ford FR, Lilienthal JL. The treatment of myasthenia gravis by removal of the thymus gland. *JAMA.* 1941;117(18):1529.
12. Beeson D, Brydson M, Betty M, et al. Primary structure of the human muscle acetylcholine receptor. cDNA cloning of

the gamma and epsilon subunits. *Eur J Biochem.* 1993;215(2): 229–238.
13. Simpson JA. Myasthenia gravis: a new hypothesis. *Scott Med J.* 1960;5(10):419–436.
14. Patrick J, Lindstrom J. Autoimmune response to acetylcholine receptor. *Science.* 1973;180(4088):871–872.
15. Lindstrom JM, Seybold ME, Lennon VA, Whittingham S, Duane DD. Antibody to acetylcholine receptor in myasthenia gravis. Prevalence, clinical correlates, and diagnostic value. *Neurology.* 1976;26(11):1054–1059.
16. Pinching AJ, Peters DK. Remission of myasthenia gravis following plasma-exchange. *Lancet.* 1976;2(8000):1373–1376.
17. Scadding GK, Vincent A, Newsom-Davis J, Henry K. Acetylcholine receptor antibody synthesis by thymic lymphocytes: correlation with thymic histology. *Neurology.* 1981;31(8):935–943.
18. Hohlfeld R, Toyka KV, Heininger K, Grosse-Wilde H, Kalies I. Autoimmune human T lymphocytes specific for acetylcholine receptor. *Nature.* 1984;310(5974):244–246.
19. Hoch W, McConville J, Helms S, Newsom-Davis J, Melms A, Vincent A. Auto-antibodies to the receptor tyrosine kinase MuSK in patients with myasthenia gravis without acetylcholine receptor antibodies. *Nat Med.* 2001;7(3):365–368.
20. Leite MI, Jacob S, Viegas S, et al. IgG1 antibodies to acetylcholine receptors in "seronegative" myasthenia gravis. *Brain.* 2008;131(Pt 7):1940–1952.
21. Jacob S, Viegas S, Leite MI, et al. Presence and pathogenic relevance of antibodies to clustered acetylcholine receptor in ocular and generalized myasthenia gravis. *Arch Neurol.* 2012;69(8):994–1001.
22. Higuchi O, Hamuro J, Motomura M, Yamanashi Y. Autoantibodies to low-density lipoprotein receptor-related protein 4 in myasthenia gravis. *Ann Neurol.* 2011;69(2):418–422.
23. Jaretzki A, Barohn RJ, Ernstoff RM, et al. Myasthenia gravis: recommendations for clinical research standards. Task Force of the Medical Scientific Advisory Board of the Myasthenia Gravis Foundation of America. *Ann Thorac Surg.* 2000;70(1):327–334.
24. Benatar M, Sanders DB, Burns TM, et al. Recommendations for myasthenia gravis clinical trials. *Muscle Nerve.* 2012;45(6):909–917.
25. Sanders DB, Wolfe GI, Benatar M, et al. International consensus guidance for management of myasthenia gravis: executive summary. *Neurology.* 2016;87(4):419–425.
26. Narayanaswami P, Sanders DB, Wolfe G, et al. International consensus guidance for management of myasthenia gravis: 2020 update. *Neurology.* 2021;96(3):114–122.
27. Wolfe GI, Kaminski HJ, Aban IB, et al; MGTX Study Group. Randomized trial of thymectomy in myasthenia gravis. *N Engl J Med.* 2016;375(6):511–522.
28. Howard JF, Utsugisawa K, Benatar M, et al. Safety and efficacy of eculizumab in anti-acetylcholine receptor antibody-positive refractory generalised myasthenia gravis (REGAIN): a phase 3, randomised, double-blind, placebo-controlled, multicentre study. *Lancet Neurol.* 2017;16(12):976–986.
29. Nguyen-Cao TM, Gelinas D, Griffin R, Mondou E. Myasthenia gravis: historical achievements and the "golden age" of clinical trials. *J Neurol Sci.* 2019;406:116428.
30. Keesey JC. A history of treatments for myasthenia gravis. *Semin Neurol.* 2004;24(1):5–16.
31. Huijbers MG, Marx A, Plomp JJ, Le Panse R, Phillips WD. Advances in the understanding of disease mechanisms of autoimmune neuromuscular junction disorders. *Lancet Neurol.* 2022;21(2):163–175.
32. Plomp JJ, Morsch M, Phillips WD, Verschuuren JJGM. Electrophysiological analysis of neuromuscular synaptic function in myasthenia gravis patients and animal models. *Exp Neurol.* 2015;270:41–54.
33. Kim N, Burden SJ. MuSK controls where motor axons grow and form synapses. *Nat Neurosci.* 2008;11(1):19–27.
34. Cetin H, Webster R, Liu WW, et al. Myasthenia gravis AChR antibodies inhibit function of rapsyn-clustered AChRs. *J Neurol Neurosurg Psychiatr.* 2020;91(5):526–532.
35. Yumoto N, Kim N, Burden SJ. Lrp4 is a retrograde signal for presynaptic differentiation at neuromuscular synapses. *Nature.* 2012;489(7416):438–442.
36. Zhu H, Bhattacharyya BJ, Lin H, Gomez CM. Skeletal muscle IP3R1 receptors amplify physiological and pathological synaptic calcium signals. *J Neurosci.* 2011;31(43):15269–15283.
37. Salpeter MM, Harris R. Distribution and turnover rate of acetylcholine receptors throughout the junction folds at a vertebrate neuromuscular junction. *J Cell Biol.* 1983;96(6):1781–1785.
38. Kaminski HJ, Suarez JI, Ruff RL. Neuromuscular junction physiology in myasthenia gravis: isoforms of the acetylcholine receptor in extraocular muscle and the contribution of sodium channels to the safety factor. *Neurology.* 1997;48(Supplement 5):8S–17S.
39. Kao I, Drachman DB. Myasthenic immunoglobulin accelerates acetylcholine receptor degradation. *Science.* 1977;196(4289):527–529.
40. Fambrough DM, Drachman DB, Satyamurti S. Neuromuscular junction in myasthenia gravis: decreased acetylcholine receptors. *Science.* 1973;182(4109):293–295.
41. Lindstrom J. What initiates the autoimmune response to muscle AChRs in myasthenia gravis? *Neurology.* 2012;79(4):304–305.
42. Tzartos SJ, Seybold ME, Lindstrom JM. Specificities of antibodies to acetylcholine receptors in sera from myasthenia gravis patients measured by monoclonal antibodies. *Proc Natl Acad Sci U S A.* 1982;79(1):188–192.
43. Bray JJ, Drachman DB. Binding affinities of anti-acetylcholine receptor autoantibodies in myasthenia gravis. *J Immunol.* 1982;128(1):105–110.
44. Masuda T, Motomura M, Utsugisawa K, et al. Antibodies against the main immunogenic region of the acetylcholine receptor correlate with disease severity in myasthenia gravis. *J Neurol Neurosurg Psychiatr.* 2012;83(9):935–940.
45. Schönbeck S, Chrestel S, Hohlfeld R. Myasthenia gravis: prototype of the antireceptor autoimmune diseases. In: *International Review of Neurobiology.* Vol 32. Elsevier; 1990:175–200.
46. Ruff RL, Lennon VA. End-plate voltage-gated sodium channels are lost in clinical and experimental myasthenia gravis. *Ann Neurol.* 1998;43(3):370–379.
47. Ruff RL. Endplate contributions to the safety factor for neuromuscular transmission. *Muscle Nerve.* 2011;44(6):854–861.
48. Howard JF. Myasthenia gravis: the role of complement at the neuromuscular junction. *Ann N Y Acad Sci.* 2018;1412(1):113–128.
49. Albazli K, Kaminski HJ, Howard JF. Complement inhibitor therapy for myasthenia gravis. *Front Immunol.* 2020;11:917.
50. Engel AG, Lambert EH, Howard FM. Immune complexes (IgG and C3) at the motor end-plate in myasthenia gravis: ultrastructural and light microscopic localization and electrophysiologic correlations. *Mayo Clin Proc.* 1977;52(5):267–280.
51. Klooster R, Plomp JJ, Huijbers MG, et al. Muscle-specific kinase myasthenia gravis IgG4 autoantibodies cause severe neuromuscular junction dysfunction in mice. *Brain.* 2012;135(Pt 4):1081–1101.

52. Rispens T, Huijbers MG. The unique properties of IgG4 and its roles in health and disease. *Nat Rev Immunol.* 2023;23(11):763–778.
53. Huijbers MG, Zhang W, Klooster R, et al. MuSK IgG4 autoantibodies cause myasthenia gravis by inhibiting binding between MuSK and Lrp4. *Proc Natl Acad Sci U S A.* 2013;110(51):20783–20788.
54. Vergoossen DLE, Plomp JJ, Gstöttner C, et al. Functional monovalency amplifies the pathogenicity of anti-MuSK IgG4 in myasthenia gravis. *Proc Natl Acad Sci U S A.* 2021;118(13):e2020635118.
55. Rivner MH, Quarles BM, Pan J-X, et al. Clinical features of LRP4/agrin-antibody-positive myasthenia gravis: a multicenter study. *Muscle Nerve.* 2020;62(3):333–343.
56. Kawakami Y, Ito M, Hirayama M, et al. Anti-MuSK autoantibodies block binding of collagen Q to MuSK. *Neurology.* 2011;77(20):1819–1826.
57. Zisimopoulou P, Evangelakou P, Tzartos J, et al. A comprehensive analysis of the epidemiology and clinical characteristics of anti-LRP4 in myasthenia gravis. *J Autoimmun.* 2014;52:139–145.
58. Shen C, Lu Y, Zhang B, et al. Antibodies against low-density lipoprotein receptor-related protein 4 induce myasthenia gravis. *J Clin Invest.* 2013;123(12):5190–5202.
59. Lisak RP. Antibodies to LRP4 and agrin are pathogenic in myasthenia gravis: at the junction where it happens. *Neurology.* 2021;97(10):463–464.
60. Yu Z, Zhang M, Jing H, et al. Characterization of lrp4/agrin antibodies from a patient with myasthenia gravis. *Neurology.* 2021;97(10):e975–e987.
61. Rodríguez Cruz PM, Al-Hajjar M, Huda S, et al. Clinical features and diagnostic usefulness of antibodies to clustered acetylcholine receptors in the diagnosis of seronegative myasthenia gravis. *JAMA Neurol.* 2015;72(6):642–649.
62. Masi G, Li Y, Karatz T, et al. The clinical need for clustered AChR cell-based assay testing of seronegative MG. *J Neuroimmunol.* 2022;367:577850.
63. Marx A, Yamada Y, Simon-Keller K, et al. Thymus and autoimmunity. *Semin Immunopathol.* 2021;43(1):45–64.
64. Park J-E, Botting RA, Domínguez Conde C, et al. A cell atlas of human thymic development defines T cell repertoire formation. *Science.* 2020;367(6480):eaay3224.
65. Workman CJ, Szymczak-Workman AL, Collison LW, Pillai MR, Vignali DAA. The development and function of regulatory T cells. *Cell Mol Life Sci.* 2009;66(16):2603–2622.
66. Dzhagalov I, Phee H. How to find your way through the thymus: a practical guide for aspiring T cells. *Cell Mol Life Sci.* 2012;69(5):663–682.
67. Baecher-Allan C, Hafler DA. Human regulatory T cells and their role in autoimmune disease. *Immunol Rev.* 2006;212:203–216.
68. Berrih-Aknin S, Le Panse R. Myasthenia gravis: a comprehensive review of immune dysregulation and etiological mechanisms. *J Autoimmun.* 2014;52:90–100.
69. Michelson DA, Hase K, Kaisho T, Benoist C, Mathis D. Thymic epithelial cells co-opt lineage-defining transcription factors to eliminate autoreactive T cells. *Cell.* 2022;185(14):2542–2558.e18.
70. Michelson DA, Benoist C, Mathis D. CTLA-4 on thymic epithelial cells complements Aire for T cell central tolerance. *Proc Natl Acad Sci U S A.* 2022;119(48):e2215474119.
71. Mammen AL, Rajan A, Pak K, et al. Pre-existing antiacetylcholine receptor autoantibodies and B cell lymphopaenia are associated with the development of myositis in patients with thymoma treated with avelumab, an immune checkpoint inhibitor targeting programmed death-ligand 1. *Ann Rheum Dis.* 2019;78(1):150–152.
72. Schaffert H, Pelz A, Saxena A, et al. IL-17-producing CD4(+) T cells contribute to the loss of B-cell tolerance in experimental autoimmune myasthenia gravis. *Eur J Immunol.* 2015;45(5):1339–1347.
73. Villegas JA, Bayer AC, Ider K, et al. Il-23/Th17 cell pathway: a promising target to alleviate thymic inflammation maintenance in myasthenia gravis. *J Autoimmun.* 2019;98:59–73.
74. Ma Q, Ran H, Li Y, et al. Circulating Th1/17 cells serve as a biomarker of disease severity and a target for early intervention in AChR-MG patients. *Clin Immunol.* 2020;218:108492.
75. Yi JS, Guidon A, Sparks S, et al. Characterization of CD4 and CD8 T cell responses in MuSK myasthenia gravis. *J Autoimmun.* 2014;52:130–138.
76. Li Y, Guptill JT, Russo MA, et al. Imbalance in T follicular helper cells producing IL-17 promotes pro-inflammatory responses in MuSK antibody positive myasthenia gravis. *J Neuroimmunol.* 2020;345:577279.
77. Liu F-C, Kuo C-F, See L-C, Tsai H-I, Yu H-P. Familial aggregation of myasthenia gravis in affected families: a population-based study. *Clin Epidemiol.* 2017;9:527–535.
78. Ramanujam R, Pirskanen R, Ramanujam S, Hammarström L. Utilizing twins concordance rates to infer the predisposition to myasthenia gravis. *Twin Res Hum Genet.* 2011;14(2):129–136.
79. Green JD, Barohn RJ, Bartoccion E, et al. Epidemiological evidence for a hereditary contribution to myasthenia gravis: a retrospective cohort study of patients from North America. *BMJ Open.* 2020;10(9):e037909.
80. Creary LE, Gangavarapu S, Caillier SJ, et al. Next-generation sequencing identifies extended HLA class I and II haplotypes associated with early-onset and late-onset myasthenia gravis in Italian, Norwegian, and Swedish populations. *Front Immunol.* 2021;12:667336.
81. Punga AR, Maddison P, Heckmann JM, Guptill JT, Evoli A. Epidemiology, diagnostics, and biomarkers of autoimmune neuromuscular junction disorders. *Lancet Neurol.* 2022;21(2):176–188.
82. Renton AE, Pliner HA, Provenzano C, et al. A genome-wide association study of myasthenia gravis. *JAMA Neurol.* 2015;72(4):396–404.
83. Chia R, Saez-Atienzar S, Murphy N, et al. Identification of genetic risk loci and prioritization of genes and pathways for myasthenia gravis: a genome-wide association study. *Proc Natl Acad Sci U S A.* 2022;119(5):e2108672119.
84. Marx A, Porubsky S, Belharazem D, et al. Thymoma related myasthenia gravis in humans and potential animal models. *Exp Neurol.* 2015;270:55–65.
85. Eigenmann MJ, Karlsen TV, Krippendorff B-F, et al. Interstitial IgG antibody pharmacokinetics assessed by combined in vivo- and physiologically-based pharmacokinetic modelling approaches. *J Physiol (Lond).* 2017;595(24):7311–7330.
86. Reid B, Martinov VN, Njå A, Lømo T, Bewick GS. Activity-dependent plasticity of transmitter release from nerve terminals in rat fast and slow muscles. *J Neurosci.* 2003;23(28):9340–9348.
87. Kusner LL, Halperin JA, Kaminski HJ. Cell surface complement regulators moderate experimental myasthenia gravis pathology. *Muscle Nerve.* 2013;47(1):33–40.

88. Attia M, Maurer M, Robinet M, et al. Muscle satellite cells are functionally impaired in myasthenia gravis: consequences on muscle regeneration. *Acta Neuropathol*. 2017;134(6):869–888.
89. Vilquin J-T, Bayer AC, Le Panse R, Berrih-Aknin S. The muscle is not a passive target in myasthenia gravis. *Front Neurol*. 2019;10:1343.
90. Hsu C-H, Chan JK, Yin C-H, Lee C-C, Chern C-U, Liao C-I. Trends in the incidence of thymoma, thymic carcinoma, and thymic neuroendocrine tumor in the United States. *PLoS ONE*. 2019;14(12):e0227197.
91. Iorio R, Lennon VA. Paraneoplastic autoimmune neurologic disorders associated with thymoma. *Handb Clin Neurol*. 2024;200:385–396.
92. Maggi L, Andreetta F, Antozzi C, et al. Thymoma-associated myasthenia gravis: outcome, clinical and pathological correlations in 197 patients on a 20-year experience. *J Neuroimmunol*. 2008;201-202:237–244.
93. Grob D. Course and management of myasthenia gravis. *J Am Med Assoc*. 1953;153(6):529–532.
94. Grob D, Arsura EL, Brunner NG, Namba T. The course of myasthenia gravis and therapies affecting outcome. *Ann N Y Acad Sci*. 1987;505:472–499.
95. Grob D, Brunner N, Namba T, Pagala M. Lifetime course of myasthenia gravis. *Muscle Nerve*. 2008;37(2):141–149.
96. Sanders DB, Raja SM, Guptill JT, Hobson-Webb LD, Juel VC, Massey JM. The Duke myasthenia gravis clinic registry: I. Description and demographics. *Muscle Nerve*. 2021;63(2):209–216.
97. Sanders DB, Lutz MW, Raja SM, et al. The Duke myasthenia gravis clinic registry: II. Analysis of outcomes. *Muscle Nerve*. 2023;67(4):291–296.
98. Guptill J, Nowak R, Guidon A, et al. A prospective natural history study and biorepository for patients with myasthenia gravis (EXPLORE-MG2) (P6-13.005). *Neurology*. 2022;98(18 Suppl):2269.
99. Ruiter AM, Strijbos E, de Meel RHP, et al. Accuracy of patient-reported data for an online patient registry of autoimmune myasthenia gravis and Lambert-Eaton myasthenic syndrome. *Neuromuscul Disord*. 2021;31(7):622–632.
100. Sanders D, Massey J. Clinical features of myasthenia gravis. In: Engel A, ed. *Neuromuscular Junction Disorders. Handbook of Clinical Neurology*. Vol 91. Elsevier B.V.; 2009:229–252.
101. Wartmann H, Hoffmann S, Ruck T, Nelke C, Deiters B, Vollmer T. Incidence, prevalence, hospitalization rates and treatment patterns in myasthenia gravis: a 10-year real-world data analysis of German claims data. *Neuroepidemiology*. 2023;57(2):121–128.
102. Grob D, Brunner NG, Namba T. The natural course of myasthenia gravis and effect of therapeutic measures. *Ann N Y Acad Sci*. 1981;377:652–669.
103. Claytor B, Cho S-M, Li Y. Myasthenic crisis. *Muscle Nerve*. 2023;68(1):8–19.
104. Oosterhuis HJ. The natural course of myasthenia gravis: a long term follow up study. *J Neurol Neurosurg Psychiatr*. 1989;52(10):1121–1127.
105. Akaishi T, Motomura M, Shiraishi H, et al. Preoperative risks of post-operative myasthenic crisis (POMC): a meta-analysis. *J Neurol Sci*. 2019;407:116530.
106. Liu C, Liu P, Zhang XJ, Li WQ, Qi G. Assessment of the risks of a myasthenic crisis after thymectomy in patients with myasthenia gravis: a systematic review and meta-analysis of 25 studies. *J Cardiothorac Surg*. 2020;15(1):270.
107. Wong SH, Petrie A, Plant GT. Ocular myasthenia gravis: toward a risk of generalization score and sample size calculation for a randomized controlled trial of disease modification. *J Neuroophthalmol*. 2016;36(3):252–258.
108. Evoli A, Minisci C, Di Schino C, et al. Thymoma in patients with MG: characteristics and long-term outcome. *Neurology*. 2002;59(12):1844–1850.
109. Keesey JC. Clinical evaluation and management of myasthenia gravis. *Muscle Nerve*. 2004;29(4):484–505.
110. Mitchell PJ, Bebbington M. Myasthenia gravis in pregnancy. *Obstet Gynecol*. 1992;80(2):178–181.
111. Borenstein S, Desmedt JE. Temperature and weather correlates of myasthenic fatigue. *Lancet*. 1974;2(7872):63–66.
112. Borenstein S, Desmedt JE. Local cooling in myasthenia. Improvement of neuromuscular failure. *Arch Neurol*. 1975;32(3):152–157.
113. Gutmann L. Heat-induced myasthenic crisis. *Arch Neurol*. 1980;37(10):671–672.
114. Osserman KE, Genkins G. Studies in myasthenia gravis: review of a twenty-year experience in over 1200 patients. *Mt Sinai J Med*. 1971;38(6):497–537.
115. Gilhus NE. Myasthenia gravis. *N Engl J Med*. 2016;375(26):2570–2581.
116. Maher J, Grand'Maison F, Nicolle MW, Strong MJ, Bolton CF. Diagnostic difficulties in myasthenia gravis. *Muscle Nerve*. 1998;21(5):577–583.
117. Mao VH, Abaza M, Spiegel JR, et al. Laryngeal myasthenia gravis: report of 40 cases. *J Voice*. 2001;15(1):122–130.
118. Pal S, Sanyal D. Jaw muscle weakness: a differential indicator of neuromuscular weakness—preliminary observations. *Muscle Nerve*. 2011;43(6):807–811.
119. Farrugia ME, Robson MD, Clover L, et al. MRI and clinical studies of facial and bulbar muscle involvement in MuSK antibody-associated myasthenia gravis. *Brain*. 2006;129(Pt 6):1481–1492.
120. Keenan SP, Alexander D, Road JD, Ryan CF, Oger J, Wilcox PG. Ventilatory muscle strength and endurance in myasthenia gravis. *Eur Respir J*. 1995;8(7):1130–1135.
121. Gilad R, Sadeh M. Bilateral foot drop as a manifestation of myasthenia gravis. *J Clin Neuromuscul Dis*. 2000;2(1):23.
122. Nicolle MW. Wrist and finger drop in myasthenia gravis. *J Clin Neuromuscul Dis*. 2006;8(2):65–69.
123. Janssen JC, Larner AJ, Harris J, Sheean GL, Rossor MN. Myasthenic hand. *Neurology*. 1998;51(3):913–914.
124. Karacostas D, Mavromatis I, Georgakoudas G, Artemis N, Milonas I. Isolated distal hand weakness as the only presenting symptom of myasthenia gravis. *Eur J Neurol*. 2002;9(4):429–430.
125. Puruckherr M, Pooyan P, Dube D, Byrd RP, Roy TM. The dropped head sign: an unusual presenting feature of myasthenia gravis. *Neuromuscul Disord*. 2004;14(6):378–379.
126. Rodolico C, Toscano A, Autunno M, et al. Limb-girdle myasthenia: clinical, electrophysiological and morphological features in familial and autoimmune cases. *Neuromuscul Disord*. 2002;12(10):964–969.
127. Bedlack RS, Simel DL, Bosworth H, Samsa G, Tucker-Lipscomb B, Sanders DB. Quantitative myasthenia gravis score: assessment of responsiveness and longitudinal validity. *Neurology*. 2005;64(11):1968–1970.
128. O'Hare M, Doughty C. Update on ocular myasthenia gravis. *Semin Neurol*. 2019;39(6):749–760.

129. Cogan DG. Myasthenia gravis: a review of the disease and a description of lid twitch as a characteristic sign. *Arch Ophthalmol*. 1965;74:217–221.
130. Gorelick PB, Rosenberg M, Pagano RJ. Enhanced ptosis in myasthenia gravis. *Arch Neurol*. 1981;38(8):531.
131. Giannoccaro MP, Paolucci M, Zenesini C, et al. Comparison of ice pack test and single-fiber EMG diagnostic accuracy in patients referred for myasthenic ptosis. *Neurology*. 2020;95(13):e1800–e1806.
132. Yadegari S. Approach to a patient with blepharoptosis. *Neurol Sci*. 2016;37(10):1589–1596.
133. Juel VC, Massey JM. Myasthenia gravis. *Orphanet J Rare Dis*. 2007;2:44.
134. Argyriou AA, Karanasios P, Potsios C, et al. Myasthenia gravis initially presenting with pseudo-internuclear ophthalmoplegia. *Neurol Sci*. 2009;30(5):387–388.
135. Nijsse B, Bettink MW, Neuteboom RF. Pseudointernuclear ophthalmoplegia as a presenting feature of ocular myasthenia gravis. *BMJ Case Rep*. 2014;2014.
136. Shiba H, Furukawa K, Tamaki S, Takahashi M. Triple-furrowed tongue in myasthenia gravis. *QJM*. 2023;116(7):534–535.
137. Kitamura E, Takiyama Y, Nakamura M, Iizuka T, Nishiyama K. Reversible tongue muscle atrophy accelerated by early initiation of immunotherapy in anti-MuSK myasthenia gravis: a case report. *J Neurol Sci*. 2016;360:10–12.
138. Brownell B, Oppenheimer DR, Spalding JM. Neurogenic muscle atrophy in myasthenia gravis. *J Neurol Neurosurg Psychiatr*. 1972;35(3):311–322.
139. Zouvelou V, Rentzos M, Toulas P, Evdokimidis I. MRI evidence of early muscle atrophy in MuSK positive myasthenia gravis. *J Neuroimaging*. 2011;21(3):303–305.
140. Muppidi S. Outcome measures in myasthenia gravis: incorporation into clinical practice. *J Clin Neuromuscul Dis*. 2017;18(3):135–146.
141. Elsheikh B, Arnold WD, Gharibshahi S, Reynolds J, Freimer M, Kissel JT. Correlation of single-breath count test and neck flexor muscle strength with spirometry in myasthenia gravis. *Muscle Nerve*. 2016;53(1):134–136.
142. Guptill JT, Benatar M, Granit V, et al; MGNet Clinical Trial Outcome Measure Working Group. Addressing outcome measure variability in myasthenia gravis clinical trials. *Neurology*. 2023;101(10):442–451.
143. Domingo CA, Landau ME, Campbell WW. Selective triceps muscle weakness in myasthenia gravis is under-recognized. *J Clin Neuromuscul Dis*. 2016;18(2):103–104.
144. Alanazy MH, Alkhalidi H. Finger flexor weakness in myasthenia gravis. *J Coll Physicians Surg Pak*. 2022;32(12):SS168–SS170.
145. Oosterhuis H, Bethlem J. Neurogenic muscle involvement in myasthenia gravis. A clinical and histopathological study. *J Neurol Neurosurg Psychiatr*. 1973;36(2):244–254.
146. Dishnica N, Vuong A, Xiong L, et al. Single count breath test for the evaluation of respiratory function in myasthenia gravis: a systematic review. *J Clin Neurosci*. 2023;112:58–63.
147. Beekman R, Kuks JB, Oosterhuis HJ. Myasthenia gravis: diagnosis and follow-up of 100 consecutive patients. *J Neurol*. 1997;244(2):112–118.
148. Benatar M. A systematic review of diagnostic studies in myasthenia gravis. *Neuromuscul Disord*. 2006;16(7):459–467.
149. Li Y, Peng Y, Yang H. Serological diagnosis of myasthenia gravis and its clinical significance. *Ann Transl Med*. 2023;11(7):290.
150. Oh SJ. Myasthenia gravis Lambert-Eaton overlap syndrome. *Muscle Nerve*. 2016;53(1):20–26.
151. Zouvelou V, Kyriazi S, Rentzos M, et al. Double-seropositive myasthenia gravis. *Muscle Nerve*. 2013;47(3):465–466.
152. Vincent A, Newsom-Davis J. Acetylcholine receptor antibody as a diagnostic test for myasthenia gravis: results in 153 validated cases and 2967 diagnostic assays. *J Neurol Neurosurg Psychiatr*. 1985;48(12):1246–1252.
153. Peeler CE, De Lott LB, Nagia L, Lemos J, Eggenberger ER, Cornblath WT. Clinical utility of acetylcholine receptor antibody testing in ocular myasthenia gravis. *JAMA Neurol*. 2015;72(10):1170–1174.
154. Lennon VA. Serologic profile of myasthenia gravis and distinction from the Lambert-Eaton myasthenic syndrome. *Neurology*. 1997;48(Supplement 5):23S–27S.
155. Vincent A, Newsom-Davis J, Newton P, Beck N. Acetylcholine receptor antibody and clinical response to thymectomy in myasthenia gravis. *Neurology*. 1983;33(10):1276–1282.
156. Heldal AT, Eide GE, Romi F, Owe JF, Gilhus NE. Repeated acetylcholine receptor antibody-concentrations and association to clinical myasthenia gravis development. *PLoS ONE*. 2014;9(12):e114060.
157. Sanders DB, Burns TM, Cutter GR, et al. Does change in acetylcholine receptor antibody level correlate with clinical change in myasthenia gravis? *Muscle Nerve*. 2014;49(4):483–486.
158. Howard FM, Lennon VA, Finley J, Matsumoto J, Elveback LR. Clinical correlations of antibodies that bind, block, or modulate human acetylcholine receptors in myasthenia gravis. *Ann N Y Acad Sci*. 1987;505:526–538.
159. Sanders DB, Ian Andrews P, Howard JF, Massey JM. Seronegative myasthenia gravis. *Neurology*. 1997;48(Supplement 5):40S–45S.
160. Vernino S, Lennon VA. Ion channel and striational antibodies define a continuum of autoimmune neuromuscular hyperexcitability. *Muscle Nerve*. 2002;26(5):702–707.
161. Ohta K, Shigemoto K, Kubo S, et al. MuSK antibodies in AChR Ab-seropositive MG vs AChR Ab-seronegative MG. *Neurology*. 2004;62(11):2132–2133.
162. Zhou L, McConville J, Chaudhry V, et al. Clinical comparison of muscle-specific tyrosine kinase (MuSK) antibody-positive and -negative myasthenic patients. *Muscle Nerve*. 2004;30(1):55–60.
163. Niks EH, van Leeuwen Y, Leite MI, et al. Clinical fluctuations in MuSK myasthenia gravis are related to antigen-specific IgG4 instead of IgG1. *J Neuroimmunol*. 2008;195(1-2):151–156.
164. Bartoccioni E, Scuderi F, Minicuci GM, Marino M, Ciaraffa F, Evoli A. Anti-MuSK antibodies: correlation with myasthenia gravis severity. *Neurology*. 2006;67(3):505–507.
165. Meriggioli MN, Sanders DB. Muscle autoantibodies in myasthenia gravis: beyond diagnosis? *Expert Rev Clin Immunol*. 2012;8(5):427–438.
166. Claytor B, Li Y. Challenges in diagnosing coexisting ocular myasthenia gravis and thyroid eye disease. *Muscle Nerve*. 2021;63(5):631–639.
167. Vernino S, Lennon VA. Autoantibody profiles and neurological correlations of thymoma. *Clin Cancer Res*. 2004;10(21):7270–7275.
168. Juel VC. Evaluation of neuromuscular junction disorders in the electromyography laboratory. *Neurol Clin*. 2012;30(2):621–639.
169. Juel VC. Repetitive nerve stimulation testing in myasthenic crisis. *Muscle Nerve*. 2019;59(5):528–530.

170. Trontelj JV, Mihelin M, Fernandez JM, Stålberg E. Axonal stimulation for end-plate jitter studies. *J Neurol Neurosurg Psychiatr*. 1986;49(6):677–685.
171. Trontelj JV, Khuraibet A, Mihelin M. The jitter in stimulated orbicularis oculi muscle: technique and normal values. *J Neurol Neurosurg Psychiatr*. 1988;51(6):814–819.
172. Trontelj JV, Stålberg E, Mihelin M, Khuraibet A. Jitter of the stimulated motor axon. *Muscle Nerve*. 1992;15(4):449–454.
173. Jabre JF, Chirico-Post J, Weiner M. Stimulation SFEMG in myasthenia gravis. *Muscle Nerve*. 1989;12(1):38–42.
174. Stålberg E, Ekstedt J, Broman A. Neuromuscular transmission in myasthenia gravis studied with single fibre electromyography. *J Neurol Neurosurg Psychiatr*. 1974;37(5):540–547.
175. Sanders DB, Kouyoumdjian JA, Stålberg EV. Single fiber electromyography and measuring jitter with concentric needle electrodes. *Muscle Nerve*. 2022;66(2):118–130.
176. Stålberg E, Sanders DB, Kouyoumdjian JA. Pitfalls and errors in measuring jitter. *Clin Neurophysiol*. 2017;128(11):2233–2241.
177. Single fiber EMG reference values: a collaborative effort. Ad Hoc Committee of the AAEM Special Interest Group on Single Fiber EMG. *Muscle Nerve*. 1992;15(2):151–161.
178. Farrugia ME, Weir AI, Cleary M, Cooper S, Metcalfe R, Mallik A. Concentric and single fiber needle electrodes yield comparable jitter results in myasthenia gravis. *Muscle Nerve*. 2009;39(5):579–585.
179. Stålberg E, Sanders DB, Ali S, et al. Reference values for jitter recorded by concentric needle electrodes in healthy controls: a multicenter study. *Muscle Nerve*. 2016;53(3):351–362.
180. Sanders DB, Massey JM. Does change in neuromuscular jitter predict or correlate with clinical change in MG? *Muscle Nerve*. 2017;56(1):45–50.
181. Juel VC, Sanders DB, Hobson-Webb LD, et al. Marked clinical and jitter improvement after eculizumab in refractory myasthenia. *Muscle Nerve*. 2017;56(3):E16–E18.
182. Sanders DB. Lambert-Eaton myasthenic syndrome: diagnosis and treatment. *Ann N Y Acad Sci*. 2003;998:500–508.
183. Howard JF, Sanders DB, Massey JM. The electrodiagnosis of myasthenia gravis and the Lambert-Eaton myasthenic syndrome. *Neurol Clin*. 1994;12(2):305–330.
184. Costa J, Evangelista T, Conceição I, de Carvalho M. Repetitive nerve stimulation in myasthenia gravis—relative sensitivity of different muscles. *Clin Neurophysiol*. 2004;115(12):2776–2782.
185. AAEM Quality Assurance Committee; American Association of Electrodiagnostic Medicine. Literature review of the usefulness of repetitive nerve stimulation and single fiber EMG in the electrodiagnostic evaluation of patients with suspected myasthenia gravis or Lambert-Eaton myasthenic syndrome. *Muscle Nerve*. 2001;24(9):1239–1247.
186. Abraham A, Alabdali M, Alsulaiman A, et al. Repetitive nerve stimulation cutoff values for the diagnosis of myasthenia gravis. *Muscle Nerve*. 2017;55(2):166–170.
187. Lamb CJ, Rubin DI. Sensitivity and specificity of repetitive nerve stimulation with lower cutoffs for abnormal decrement in myasthenia gravis. *Muscle Nerve*. 2020;62(3):381–385.
188. Stalberg E. Clinical electrophysiology in myasthenia gravis. *J Neurol Neurosurg Psychiatr*. 1980;43(7):622–633.
189. Gilchrist JM, Massey JM, Sanders DB. Single fiber EMG and repetitive stimulation of the same muscle in myasthenia gravis. *Muscle Nerve*. 1994;17(2):171–175.
190. Rutkove SB. Effects of temperature on neuromuscular electrophysiology. *Muscle Nerve*. 2001;24(7):867–882.
191. Massey JM, Sanders DB, Howard JF. The effect of cholinesterase inhibitors of SFEMG in myasthenia gravis. *Muscle Nerve*. 1989;12(2):154–155.
192. Punga AR, Liik M. Botulinum toxin injections associated with suspected myasthenia gravis: an underappreciated cause of MG-like clinical presentation. *Clin Neurophysiol Pract*. 2020;5:46–49.
193. Sanders DB, Massey EW, Buckley EG. Botulinum toxin for blepharospasm: single-fiber EMG studies. *Neurology*. 1986;36(4):545–547.
194. Barra ME, Webb AJ, Roberts RJ, et al. Implementation of a myasthenia gravis drug-disease interaction clinical decision support tool reduces prescribing of high-risk medications. *Muscle Nerve*. 2023;67(4):284–290.
195. Amandusson Å, Elf K, Grindlund ME, Punga AR. Diagnostic utility of repetitive nerve stimulation in a large cohort of patients with myasthenia gravis. *J Clin Neurophysiol*. 2017;34(5):400–407.
196. Sanders DB, Cao L, Massey JM, Juel VC, Hobson-Webb L, Guptill JT. Is the decremental pattern in Lambert-Eaton syndrome different from that in myasthenia gravis? *Clin Neurophysiol*. 2014;125(6):1274–1277.
197. Baslo MB, Deymeer F, Serdaroglu P, Parman Y, Ozdemir C, Cuttini M. Decrement pattern in Lambert-Eaton myasthenic syndrome is different from myasthenia gravis. *Neuromuscul Disord*. 2006;16(7):454–458.
198. Daube JR. Electrodiagnostic studies in amyotrophic lateral sclerosis and other motor neuron disorders. *Muscle Nerve*. 2000;23(10):1488–1502.
199. Maselli RA, Wollman RL, Leung C, et al. Neuromuscular transmission in amyotrophic lateral sclerosis. *Muscle Nerve*. 1993;16(11):1193–1203.
200. Wang FC, De Pasqua V, Gérard P, Delwaide PJ. Prognostic value of decremental responses to repetitive nerve stimulation in ALS patients. *Neurology*. 2001;57(5):897–899.
201. Caldas VM, Heise CO, Kouyoumdjian JA, et al. Electrophysiological study of neuromuscular junction in congenital myasthenic syndromes, congenital myopathies, and chronic progressive external ophthalmoplegia. *Neuromuscul Disord*. 2020;30(11):897–903.
202. Elahi B, Laughlin RS, Litchy WJ, Milone M, Liewluck T. Neuromuscular transmission defects in myopathies: Rare but worth searching for. *Muscle Nerve*. 2019;59(4):475–478.
203. Kannaditharayil D, Napier F, Granit V, Bieri P, Herskovitz S. Abnormal spontaneous activity on needle electromyography in myasthenia gravis. *Muscle Nerve*. 2017;56(2):E11–E12.
204. Farrugia ME, Kennett RP, Hilton-Jones D, Newsom-Davis J, Vincent A. Quantitative EMG of facial muscles in myasthenia patients with MuSK antibodies. *Clin Neurophysiol*. 2007;118(2):269–277.
205. Padua L, Caliandro P, Di Iasi G, Pazzaglia C, Ciaraffa F, Evoli A. Reliability of SFEMG in diagnosing myasthenia gravis: sensitivity and specificity calculated on 100 prospective cases. *Clin Neurophysiol*. 2014;125(6):1270–1273.
206. Sanders DB. Clinical impact of single-fiber electromyography. *Muscle Nerve Suppl*. 2002;11:S15–S20.
207. Giannoccaro MP, Di Stasi V, Zanesini C, Donadio V, Avoni P, Liguori R. Sensitivity and specificity of single-fibre EMG in the diagnosis of ocular myasthenia varies accordingly to clinical presentation. *J Neurol*. 2020;267(3):739–745.
208. Pascuzzi RM. The edrophonium test. *Semin Neurol*. 2003;23(1):83–88.

209. Phillips LH, Melnick PA. Diagnosis of myasthenia gravis in the 1990s. *Semin Neurol.* 1990;10(1):62–69.
210. Nowak RJ, Coffey CS, Goldstein JM, et al. Phase 2 trial of rituximab in acetylcholine receptor antibody-positive generalized myasthenia gravis: The BeatMG Study. *Neurology.* 2022;98(4):e376–e389.
211. Piehl F, Eriksson-Dufva A, Budzianowska A, et al. Efficacy and safety of rituximab for new-onset generalized myasthenia gravis: the RINOMAX randomized clinical trial. *JAMA Neurol.* 2022;79(11):1105–1112.
212. Ramdas S, Della Marina A, Ryan MM, et al. Rituximab in juvenile myasthenia gravis—an international cohort study and literature review. *Eur J Paediatr Neurol.* 2022;40:5–10.
213. Doughty CT, Suh J, David WS, Amato AA, Guidon AC. Retrospective analysis of safety and outcomes of rituximab for myasthenia gravis in patients ≥65 years old. *Muscle Nerve.* 2021;64(6):651–656.
214. Cavalcante P, Le Panse R, Berrih-Aknin S, et al. The thymus in myasthenia gravis: Site of "innate autoimmunity"? *Muscle Nerve.* 2011;44(4):467–484.
215. Evoli A, Tonali PA, Padua L, et al. Clinical correlates with anti-MuSK antibodies in generalized seronegative myasthenia gravis. *Brain.* 2003;126(Pt 10):2304–2311.
216. Takahashi K, Al-Janabi NJ. Computed tomography and magnetic resonance imaging of mediastinal tumors. *J Magn Reson Imaging.* 2010;32(6):1325–1339.
217. Marx A, Willcox N, Leite MI, et al. Thymoma and paraneoplastic myasthenia gravis. *Autoimmunity.* 2010;43(5-6):413–427.
218. Weis C-A, Yao X, Deng Y, et al. The impact of thymoma histotype on prognosis in a worldwide database. *J Thorac Oncol.* 2015;10(2):367–372.
219. Marx A, Chan JKC, Chalabreysse L, et al. The 2021 WHO classification of tumors of the thymus and mediastinum: what is new in thymic epithelial, germ cell, and mesenchymal tumors? *J Thorac Oncol.* 2022;17(2):200–213.
220. Markowiak T, Hofmann H-S, Ried M. Classification and staging of thymoma. *J Thorac Dis.* 2020;12(12):7607–7612.
221. Minervini F, Kocher GJ. When to suspect a thymoma: clinical point of view. *J Thorac Dis.* 2020;12(12):7613–7618.
222. Nicolaou S, Müller NL, Li DK, Oger JJ. Thymus in myasthenia gravis: comparison of CT and pathologic findings and clinical outcome after thymectomy. *Radiology.* 1996;201(2):471–474.
223. Expert Panel on Thoracic Imaging; Ackman JB, Chung JH, Walker CM, et al. ACR appropriateness criteria® imaging of mediastinal masses. *J Am Coll Radiol.* 2021;18(5S):S37–S51.
224. Heeger AP, Ackman JB. Added value of magnetic resonance imaging for the evaluation of mediastinal lesions. *Radiol Clin North Am.* 2021;59(2):251–277.
225. Li F, Tao Y, Bauer G, et al. Unraveling the role of ectopic thymic tissue in patients undergoing thymectomy for myasthenia gravis. *J Thorac Dis.* 2019;11(9):4039–4048.
226. Klimiec E, Quirke M, Leite MI, Hilton-Jones D. Thymus imaging in myasthenia gravis: the relevance in clinical practice. *Muscle Nerve.* 2018.
227. Rath J, Mauritz M, Zulehner G, et al. Iodinated contrast agents in patients with myasthenia gravis: a retrospective cohort study. *J Neurol.* 2017;264(6):1209–1217.
228. Burns TM. History of outcome measures for myasthenia gravis. *Muscle Nerve.* 2010;42(1):5–13.
229. Muppidi S, Silvestri NJ, Tan R, Riggs K, Leighton T, Phillips GA. Utilization of MG-ADL in myasthenia gravis clinical research and care. *Muscle Nerve.* 2022;65(6):630–639.
230. Wolfe GI, Herbelin L, Nations SP, Foster B, Bryan WW, Barohn RJ. Myasthenia gravis activities of daily living profile. *Neurology.* 1999;52(7):1487–1489.
231. Burns TM, Sadjadi R, Utsugisawa K, et al. International clinimetric evaluation of the MG-QOL15, resulting in slight revision and subsequent validation of the MG-QOL15r. *Muscle Nerve.* 2016;54(6):1015–1022.
232. Lee HL, Min J-H, Seok JM, et al. Physician- and self-assessed myasthenia gravis activities of daily living score. *Muscle Nerve.* 2018;57(3):419–422.
233. Barohn RJ, McIntire D, Herbelin L, Wolfe GI, Nations S, Bryan WW. Reliability testing of the quantitative myasthenia gravis score. *Ann N Y Acad Sci.* 1998;841:769–772.
234. Sanders DB, Tucker-Lipscomb B, Massey JM. A simple manual muscle test for myasthenia gravis: validation and comparison with the QMG score. *Ann N Y Acad Sci.* 2003;998:440–444.
235. Burns TM, Conaway MR, Cutter GR, Sanders DB; Muscle Study Group. Construction of an efficient evaluative instrument for myasthenia gravis: the MG composite. *Muscle Nerve.* 2008;38(6):1553–1562.
236. Barnett C, Bril V, Kapral M, Kulkarni AV, Davis AM. Myasthenia gravis impairment index: responsiveness, meaningful change, and relative efficiency. *Neurology.* 2017;89(23):2357–2364.
237. Mendoza M, Tran C, Bril V, Katzberg HD, Barnett C. Patient-acceptable symptom states in myasthenia gravis. *Neurology.* 2020;95(12):e1617–e1628.
238. Menon D, Barnett C, Bril V. Comparison of the single simple question and the patient acceptable symptom state in myasthenia gravis. *Eur J Neurol.* 2020;27(11):2286–2291.
239. Guidon AC, Muppidi S, Nowak RJ, et al. Telemedicine visits in myasthenia gravis: expert guidance and the Myasthenia Gravis Core Exam (MG-CE). *Muscle Nerve.* 2021;64(3):270–276.
240. Ricciardi D, Casagrande S, Iodice F, et al. Myasthenia gravis and telemedicine: a lesson from COVID-19 pandemic. *Neurol Sci.* 2021;42(12):4889–4892.
241. Pasqualin F, Guidoni SV, Albertini E, et al. Development and validation of the Myasthenia Gravis TeleScore (MGTS). *Neurol Sci.* 2022;43(7):4503–4509.
242. Frisaldi E, Shaibani A, Vollert J, et al. The placebo response in myasthenia gravis assessed by quantitative myasthenia gravis score: a meta-analysis. *Muscle Nerve.* 2019;59(6):671–678.
243. Sanders DB. Advancing research in autoimmune neuromuscular disorders. *Lancet Neurol.* 2022;21(2):108–110.
244. Hehir MK, Hobson-Webb LD, Benatar M, et al. Rituximab as treatment for anti-MuSK myasthenia gravis: multicenter blinded prospective review. *Neurology.* 2017;89(10):1069–1077.
245. Hehir MK, Conaway M, Clark EM, et al. The Adverse Event Unit (AEU): a novel metric to measure the burden of treatment adverse events. *PLoS ONE.* 2022;17(2):e0262109.
246. Uzawa A, Ozawa Y, Yasuda M, Onishi Y, Akamine H, Kuwabara S. Minimal symptom expression achievement over time in generalized myasthenia gravis. *Acta Neurol Belg.* 2023;123(3):979–982.
247. Vissing J, Jacob S, Fujita KP, O'Brien F, Howard JF; REGAIN study group. "Minimal symptom expression" in patients with acetylcholine receptor antibody-positive refractory generalized myasthenia gravis treated with eculizumab. *J Neurol.* 2020;267(7):1991–2001.

248. Tran C, Biswas A, Mendoza M, Katzberg H, Bril V, Barnett C. Performance of different criteria for refractory myasthenia gravis. *Eur J Neurol.* 2021;28(4):1375–1384.
249. Barnett C, Herbelin L, Dimachkie MM, Barohn RJ. Measuring clinical treatment response in myasthenia gravis. *Neurol Clin.* 2018;36(2):339–353.
250. Menon D, Bril V. Pharmacotherapy of generalized myasthenia gravis with special emphasis on newer biologicals. *Drugs.* 2022;82(8):865–887.
251. Iorio R. Myasthenia gravis: the changing treatment landscape in the era of molecular therapies. *Nat Rev Neurol.* 2024;20(2):84–98.
252. Andersen JB, Gilhus NE, Sanders DB. Factors affecting outcome in myasthenia gravis. *Muscle Nerve.* 2016;54(6):1041–1049.
253. Verschuuren JJ, Palace J, Murai H, Tannemaat MR, Kaminski HJ, Bril V. Advances and ongoing research in the treatment of autoimmune neuromuscular junction disorders. *Lancet Neurol.* 2022;21(2):189–202.
254. Engel-Nitz NM, Boscoe A, Wolbeck R, Johnson J, Silvestri NJ. Burden of illness in patients with treatment refractory myasthenia gravis. *Muscle Nerve.* 2018;58.
255. O'Connell K, Ramdas S, Palace J. Management of juvenile myasthenia gravis. *Front Neurol.* 2020;11:743.
256. Bae JS, Go SM, Kim BJ. Clinical predictors of steroid-induced exacerbation in myasthenia gravis. *J Clin Neurosci.* 2006;13(10):1006–1010.
257. Guptill JT, Oakley D, Kuchibhatla M, et al. A retrospective study of complications of therapeutic plasma exchange in myasthenia. *Muscle Nerve.* 2013;47(2):170–176.
258. Guptill JT, Sanders DB, Evoli A. Anti-MuSK antibody myasthenia gravis: clinical findings and response to treatment in two large cohorts. *Muscle Nerve.* 2011;44(1):36–40.
259. Waheed W, Newman E, Aboukhatwa M, Moin M, Tandan R. Practical management for use of Eculizumab in the treatment of severe, refractory, non-thymomatous, AChR + generalized myasthenia gravis: a systematic review. *Ther Clin Risk Manag.* 2022;18:699–719.
260. Vu T, Meisel A, Mantegazza R, et al. Terminal complement inhibitor Ravulizumab in generalized myasthenia gravis. *NEJM Evid.* 2022;1(5):EVIDoa2100066.
261. Howard JF, Bresch S, Genge A, et al. Safety and efficacy of zilucoplan in patients with generalised myasthenia gravis (RAISE): a randomised, double-blind, placebo-controlled, phase 3 study. *Lancet Neurol.* 2023;22(5):395–406.
262. Muppidi S, Utsugisawa K, Benatar M, et al; Regain Study Group. Long-term safety and efficacy of eculizumab in generalized myasthenia gravis. *Muscle Nerve.* 2019;60(1):14–24.
263. Howard JF, Barohn RJ, Cutter GR, et al. A randomized, double-blind, placebo-controlled phase II study of eculizumab in patients with refractory generalized myasthenia gravis. *Muscle Nerve.* 2013;48(1):76–84.
264. Meisel A, Annane D, Vu T, et al. Long-term efficacy and safety of ravulizumab in adults with anti-acetylcholine receptor antibody-positive generalized myasthenia gravis: results from the phase 3 CHAMPION MG open-label extension. *J Neurol.* 2023;270(8):3862–3875.
265. Freimer M, Leite MI, Genge A, et al. RAISE-XT: an interim analysis of safety and efficacy in an open-label extension study of zilucoplan in patients with myasthenia gravis (P1-5.007). *Neurology.* 2023;100(17_supplement_2).
266. Li Y, Yi JS, Howard JF, Chopra M, Russo MA, Guptill JT. Cellular changes in eculizumab early responders with generalized myasthenia gravis. *Clin Immunol.* 2021;231:108830.
267. Howard JF, Karam C, Yountz M, O'Brien FL, Mozaffar T; REGAIN Study Group. Long-term efficacy of eculizumab in refractory generalized myasthenia gravis: responder analyses. *Ann Clin Transl Neurol.* 2021;8(7):1398–1407.
268. Socié G, Caby-Tosi M-P, Marantz JL, et al. Eculizumab in paroxysmal nocturnal haemoglobinuria and atypical haemolytic uraemic syndrome: 10-year pharmacovigilance analysis. *Br J Haematol.* 2019;185(2):297–310.
269. How Dangerous is Lightning? Accessed April 1, 2024. https://www.weather.gov/safety/lightning-odds
270. Mbaeyi SA, Bozio CH, Duffy J, et al. Meningococcal vaccination: recommendations of the advisory committee on immunization practices, United States, 2020. *MMWR Recomm Rep.* 2020;69(9):1–41.
271. Suh J, Clarke V, Amato AA, Guidon AC. Safety and outcomes of eculizumab for acetylcholine receptor-positive generalized myasthenia gravis in clinical practice. *Muscle Nerve.* 2022;66(3):348–353.
272. Murai H, Suzuki S, Hasebe M, Fukamizu Y, Rodrigues E, Utsugisawa K. Safety and effectiveness of eculizumab in Japanese patients with generalized myasthenia gravis: interim analysis of post-marketing surveillance. *Ther Adv Neurol Disord.* 2021;14:17562864211001996.
273. Katyal N, Narula N, Govindarajan R. Clinical experience with eculizumab in treatment-refractory acetylcholine receptor antibody-positive generalized myasthenia gravis. *J Neuromuscul Dis.* 2021;8(2):287–294.
274. Nowak RJ, Muppidi S, Beydoun SR, O'Brien FL, Yountz M, Howard JF. Concomitant immunosuppressive therapy use in eculizumab-treated adults with generalized myasthenia gravis during the REGAIN open-label extension study. *Front Neurol.* 2020;11:556104.
275. ZILBRYSQ® (zilucoplan) Injection For gMG Treatment. Accessed March 31, 2024. https://www.zilbrysq.com/?utm_source=google&utm_medium=cpc&utm_campaign=2024_Zilbrysq+DTC_gMG_Branded%3BS%3BPH%3BBR%3BIMM%3BDTC%3BBR&utm_content=Branded+Generic&utm_term=zilucoplan&gclid=Cj0KCQjwk6SwBhDPARIsAJ59Gwcj_FlAGHdc0v28OvEVypa0SGcXWawM4JEw4uEdA_s4HIVaxLAwh48aAqPUEALw_wcB&gclsrc=aw.ds
276. Obaid AH, Zografou C, Vadysirisack DD, et al. Heterogeneity of acetylcholine receptor autoantibody-mediated complement activity in patients with myasthenia gravis. *Neurol Neuroimmunol Neuroinflamm.* 2022;9(4):e1169.
277. Nishimura J, Yamamoto M, Hayashi S, et al. Genetic variants in C5 and poor response to eculizumab. *N Engl J Med.* 2014;370(7):632–639.
278. Gable KL, Guptill JT. Antagonism of the neonatal fc receptor as an emerging treatment for myasthenia gravis. *Front Immunol.* 2019;10:3052.
279. Bhandari V, Bril V. FcRN receptor antagonists in the management of myasthenia gravis. *Front Neurol.* 2023;14:1229112.
280. Guptill JT, Juel VC, Massey JM, et al. Effect of therapeutic plasma exchange on immunoglobulins in myasthenia gravis. *Autoimmunity.* 2016;49(7):472–479.
281. Howard JF, Bril V, Burns TM, et al. Randomized phase 2 study of FcRn antagonist efgartigimod in generalized myasthenia gravis. *Neurology.* 2019;92(23):e2661–e2673.

282. Howard JF, Bril V, Vu T, et al. Safety, efficacy, and tolerability of efgartigimod in patients with generalised myasthenia gravis (ADAPT): a multicentre, randomised, placebo-controlled, phase 3 trial. *Lancet Neurol.* 2021;20(7):526–536.
283. Howard JF, Bril V, Vu T, et al. Long-term safety, tolerability, and efficacy of efgartigimod (ADAPT+): interim results from a phase 3 open-label extension study in participants with generalized myasthenia gravis. *Front Neurol.* 2023;14:1284444.
284. Bril V, Benatar M, Andersen H, et al; MG0002 Investigators. Efficacy and safety of rozanolixizumab in moderate to severe generalized myasthenia gravis: a phase 2 randomized control trial. *Neurology.* 2021;96(6):e853–e865.
285. Bril V, Drużdż A, Grosskreutz J, et al. Safety and efficacy of rozanolixizumab in patients with generalised myasthenia gravis (MycarinG): a randomised, double-blind, placebo-controlled, adaptive phase 3 study. *Lancet Neurol.* 2023;22(5):383–394.
286. Antozzi C, Guptill J, Bril V, et al. Safety and efficacy of nipocalimab in patients with generalized myasthenia gravis: results from the randomized phase 2 vivacity-MG study. *Neurology.* 2024;102(2):e207937.
287. Ramchandren S, Sanga P, Burcklen M, Sun H. Vivacity MG phase 3 study: clinical trial of nipocalimab administered to adults with generalized myasthenia gravis. *Neurology.* 2022;99(23_Supplement_2).
288. Yan C, Duan R-S, Yang H, et al. Therapeutic effects of batoclimab in Chinese patients with generalized myasthenia gravis: a double-blinded, randomized, placebo-controlled phase II study. *Neurol Ther.* 2022;11(2):815–834.
289. Yan C, Yue Y, Guan Y, et al. Batoclimab vs placebo for generalized myasthenia gravis: a randomized clinical trial. *JAMA Neurol.* 2024.
290. Guptill JT, Sleasman JW, Steeland S, et al. Effect of FcRn antagonism on protective antibodies and to vaccines in IgG-mediated autoimmune diseases pemphigus and generalised myasthenia gravis. *Autoimmunity.* 2022;55(8):620–631.
291. Singer M, Khella S, Bird S, et al. Single institution experience with efgartigimod in patients with myasthenia gravis: patient selection, dosing schedules, treatment response, and adverse events. *Muscle Nerve.* 2024;69(1):87–92.
292. Fuchs L, Shelly S, Vigiser I, et al. Real-World experience with efgartigimod in patients with myasthenia gravis. *J Neurol.* 2024.
293. Dalakas MC. IgG4-mediated neurologic autoimmunities: understanding the pathogenicity of IgG4, ineffectiveness of IVIg, and long-lasting benefits of anti-B cell therapies. *Neurol Neuroimmunol Neuroinflamm.* 2022;9(1):e1116.
294. Díaz-Manera J, Martínez-Hernández E, Querol L, et al. Long-lasting treatment effect of rituximab in MuSK myasthenia. *Neurology.* 2012;78(3):189–193.
295. Keung B, Robeson KR, DiCapua DB, et al. Long-term benefit of rituximab in MuSK autoantibody myasthenia gravis patients. *J Neurol Neurosurg Psychiatr.* 2013;84(12):1407–1409.
296. Hain B, Jordan K, Deschauer M, Zierz S. Successful treatment of MuSK antibody-positive myasthenia gravis with rituximab. *Muscle Nerve.* 2006;33(4):575–580.
297. Yi JS, Decroos EC, Sanders DB, Weinhold KJ, Guptill JT. Prolonged B-cell depletion in MuSK myasthenia gravis following rituximab treatment. *Muscle Nerve.* 2013;48(6):992–993.
298. Tandan R, Hehir MK, Waheed W, Howard DB. Rituximab treatment of myasthenia gravis: a systematic review. *Muscle Nerve.* 2017;56(2):185–196.
299. Morren J, Li Y. Myasthenia gravis with muscle-specific tyrosine kinase antibodies: a narrative review. *Muscle Nerve.* 2018;58(3):344–358.
300. Caballero-Ávila M, Álvarez-Velasco R, Moga E, et al. Rituximab in myasthenia gravis: efficacy, associated infections and risk of induced hypogammaglobulinemia. *Neuromuscul Disord.* 2022;32(8):664–671.
301. Zhao C, Pu M, Chen D, et al. Effectiveness and safety of rituximab for refractory myasthenia gravis: a systematic review and single-arm meta-analysis. *Front Neurol.* 2021;12:736190.
302. Sahai SK, Maghzi AH, Lewis RA. Rituximab in late-onset myasthenia gravis is safe and effective. *Muscle Nerve.* 2020;62(3):377–380.
303. Farmakidis C, Dimachkie MM, Pasnoor M, Barohn RJ. Immunosuppressive and immunomodulatory therapies for neuromuscular diseases. Part II: New and novel agents. *Muscle Nerve.* 2020;61(1):17–25.
304. Suh J, Slawski BR, Long AA, Guidon AC. Rituximab desensitization in two patients with muscle-specific kinase myasthenia gravis. *Muscle Nerve.* 2019;60(5):E35–E37.
305. Szepanowski F, Warnke C, Meyer Zu Hörste G, et al. Secondary immunodeficiency and risk of infection following immune therapies in neurology. *CNS Drugs.* 2021;35(11):1173–1188.
306. Forsthuber TG, Cimbora DM, Ratchford JN, Katz E, Stüve O. B cell-based therapies in CNS autoimmunity: differentiating CD19 and CD20 as therapeutic targets. *Ther Adv Neurol Disord.* 2018;11:1756286418761697.
307. Cree BAC, Bennett JL, Kim HJ, et al. Inebilizumab for the treatment of neuromyelitis optica spectrum disorder (N-MOmentum): a double-blind, randomised placebo-controlled phase 2/3 trial. *Lancet.* 2019;394(10206):1352–1363.
308. Flanagan EP, Levy M, Katz E, et al. Inebilizumab for treatment of neuromyelitis optica spectrum disorder in patients with prior rituximab use from the N-MOmentum Study. *Mult Scler Relat Disord.* 2022;57:103352.
309. Wiendl H, Abicht A, Chan A, et al. Guideline for the management of myasthenic syndromes. *Ther Adv Neurol Disord.* 2023;16:17562864231213240.
310. Palace J, Newsom-Davis J, Lecky B. A randomized double-blind trial of prednisolone alone or with azathioprine in myasthenia gravis. Myasthenia Gravis Study Group. *Neurology.* 1998;50(6):1778–1783.
311. Heatwole C, Ciafaloni E. Mycophenolate mofetil for myasthenia gravis: a clear and present controversy. *Neuropsychiatr Dis Treat.* 2008;4(6):1203–1209.
312. Meriggioli MN, Ciafaloni E, Al-Hayk KA, et al. Mycophenolate mofetil for myasthenia gravis: an analysis of efficacy, safety, and tolerability. *Neurology.* 2003;61(10):1438–1440.
313. Meriggioli MN, Rowin J, Richman JG, Leurgans S. Mycophenolate mofetil for myasthenia gravis: a double-blind, placebo-controlled pilot study. *Ann N Y Acad Sci.* 2003;998:494–499.
314. Muscle Study Group. A trial of mycophenolate mofetil with prednisone as initial immunotherapy in myasthenia gravis. *Neurology.* 2008;71(6):394–399.
315. Sanders DB, Hart IK, Mantegazza R, et al. An international, phase III, randomized trial of mycophenolate mofetil in myasthenia gravis. *Neurology.* 2008;71(6):400–406.

316. Hehir MK, Burns TM, Alpers J, Conaway MR, Sawa M, Sanders DB. Mycophenolate mofetil in AChR-antibody-positive myasthenia gravis: outcomes in 102 patients. *Muscle Nerve*. 2010;41(5):593–598.
317. Hobson-Webb LD, Hehir M, Crum B, Visser A, Sanders D, Burns TM. Can mycophenolate mofetil be tapered safely in myasthenia gravis? A retrospective, multicenter analysis. *Muscle Nerve*. 2015;52(2):211–215.
318. Narayanaswami P, Sanders DB, Thomas L, et al. Comparative effectiveness of azathioprine and mycophenolate mofetil for myasthenia gravis (PROMISE-MG): a prospective cohort study. *Lancet Neurol*. 2024;23(3):267–276.
319. Farmakidis C, Dimachkie MM, Pasnoor M, Barohn RJ. Immunosuppressive and immunomodulatory therapies for neuromuscular diseases. Part I: traditional agents. *Muscle Nerve*. 2020;61(1):5–16.
320. Jack KL, Koopman WJ, Hulley D, Nicolle MW. A Review of azathioprine-associated hepatotoxicity and myelosuppression in myasthenia gravis. *J Clin Neuromuscul Dis*. 2016;18(1):12–20.
321. Gilhus NE, Andersen H, Andersen LK, et al. Generalized myasthenia gravis with acetylcholine receptor antibodies: a guidance for treatment. *Eur J Neurol*. 2024;31(5):e16229.
322. Heckmann JM, Rawoot A, Bateman K, Renison R, Badri M. A single-blinded trial of methotrexate versus azathioprine as steroid-sparing agents in generalized myasthenia gravis. *BMC Neurol*. 2011;11:97.
323. Prado MB, Adiao KJB. Methotrexate in generalized myasthenia gravis: a systematic review. *Acta Neurol Belg*. 2023;123(5):1679–1691.
324. Pasnoor M, He J, Herbelin L, et al. A randomized controlled trial of methotrexate for patients with generalized myasthenia gravis. *Neurology*. 2016;87(1):57–64.
325. Di L, Shen F, Wen X, et al. A randomized open-labeled trial of methotrexate as a steroid-sparing agent for patients with generalized myasthenia gravis. *Front Immunol*. 2022;13:839075.
326. Itani K, Nakamura M, Wate R, et al. Efficacy and safety of tacrolimus as long-term monotherapy for myasthenia gravis. *Neuromuscul Disord*. 2021;31(6):512–518.
327. Tindall RS, Phillips JT, Rollins JA, Wells L, Hall K. A clinical therapeutic trial of cyclosporine in myasthenia gravis. *Ann N Y Acad Sci*. 1993;681:539–551.
328. Tindall RS, Rollins JA, Phillips JT, Greenlee RG, Wells L, Belendiuk G. Preliminary results of a double-blind, randomized, placebo-controlled trial of cyclosporine in myasthenia gravis. *N Engl J Med*. 1987;316(12):719–724.
329. Ciafaloni E, Nikhar NK, Massey JM, Sanders DB. Retrospective analysis of the use of cyclosporine in myasthenia gravis. *Neurology*. 2000;55(3):448–450.
330. Furukawa Y, Yoshikawa H, Iwasa K, Yamada M. Clinical efficacy and cytokine network-modulating effects of tacrolimus in myasthenia gravis. *J Neuroimmunol*. 2008;195(1-2):108–115.
331. Li Y, Guptill JT, Russo MA, et al. Tacrolimus inhibits Th1 and Th17 responses in MuSK-antibody positive myasthenia gravis patients. *Exp Neurol*. 2019;312:43–50.
332. Wu H, Wang Z, Xi J, et al. Therapeutic and immunoregulatory effects of tacrolimus in patients with refractory generalized myasthenia gravis. *Eur Neurol*. 2020;83(5):500–507.
333. Yoshikawa H, Kiuchi T, Saida T, Takamori M. Randomised, double-blind, placebo-controlled study of tacrolimus in myasthenia gravis. *J Neurol Neurosurg Psychiatr*. 2011;82(9):970–977.
334. Fan Z, Lei L, Su S, et al. Comparison between mono-tacrolimus and mono-glucocorticoid in the treatment of myasthenia gravis. *Ann Clin Transl Neurol*. 2023;10(4):589–598.
335. Hiramatsu Y, Yoshida S, Kotani T, et al. Changes in the blood level, efficacy, and safety of tacrolimus in pregnancy and the lactation period in patients with systemic lupus erythematosus. *Lupus*. 2018;27(14):2245–2252.
336. Yang T-T, Wang Z-Y, Fan Z-X, et al. A pilot study on tocilizumab in very-late-onset myasthenia gravis. *J Inflamm Res*. 2023;16:5835–5843.
337. Jia D, Zhang F, Li H, et al. Responsiveness to tocilizumab in anti-acetylcholine receptor-positive generalized myasthenia gravis. *Aging Dis*. 2024;15(2):824–830.
338. Jonsson DI, Pirskanen R, Piehl F. Beneficial effect of tocilizumab in myasthenia gravis refractory to rituximab. *Neuromuscul Disord*. 2017;27(6):565–568.
339. Oh S, Payne AS. Engineering cell therapies for autoimmune diseases: from preclinical to clinical proof of concept. *Immune Netw*. 2022;22(5):e37.
340. Schett G, Mackensen A, Mougiakakos D. CAR T-cell therapy in autoimmune diseases. *Lancet*. 2023;402(10416):2034–2044.
341. Granit V, Benatar M, Kurtoglu M, et al. Safety and clinical activity of autologous RNA chimeric antigen receptor T-cell therapy in myasthenia gravis (MG-001): a prospective, multicentre, open-label, non-randomised phase 1b/2a study. *Lancet Neurol*. 2023;22(7):578–590.
342. Stathopoulos P, Kumar A, Nowak RJ, O'Connor KC. Autoantibody-producing plasmablasts after B cell depletion identified in muscle-specific kinase myasthenia gravis. *JCI Insight*. 2017;2(17):e94263.
343. Pedersen TH, Macdonald WA, Broch-Lips M, Halldorsdottir O, Baekgaard Nielsen O. Chloride channel inhibition improves neuromuscular function under conditions mimicking neuromuscular disorders. *Acta Physiol (Oxf)*. 2021;233(2):e13690.
344. Skov M, Ruijs TQ, Grønnebæk TS, et al. The ClC-1 chloride channel inhibitor NMD670 improves skeletal muscle function in rat models and patients with myasthenia gravis. *Sci Transl Med*. 2024;16(739):eadk9109.
345. Bonanno S, Pasanisi MB, Frangiamore R, et al. Amifampridine phosphate in the treatment of muscle-specific kinase myasthenia gravis: a phase IIb, randomized, double-blind, placebo-controlled, double crossover study. *SAGE Open Med*. 2018;6:2050312118819013.
346. Ceccanti M, Libonati L, Ruffolo G, et al. Effects of 3,4-diaminopyridine on myasthenia gravis: preliminary results of an open-label study. *Front Pharmacol*. 2022;13:982434.
347. Wolfe GI, Kaminski HJ, Aban IB, et al. Long-term effect of thymectomy plus prednisone versus prednisone alone in patients with non-thymomatous myasthenia gravis: 2-year extension of the MGTX randomised trial. *Lancet Neurol*. 2019;18(3):259–268.
348. Raja SM, Guptill JT, McConnell A, Al-Khalidi HR, Hartwig MG, Klapper JA. Perioperative outcomes of thymectomy in myasthenia gravis: a thoracic surgery database analysis. *Ann Thorac Surg*. 2022;113(3):904–910.
349. Alshekhlee A, Miles JD, Katirji B, Preston DC, Kaminski HJ. Incidence and mortality rates of myasthenia gravis and myasthenic crisis in US hospitals. *Neurology*. 2009;72(18):1548–1554.
350. Thomas CE, Mayer SA, Gungor Y, et al. Myasthenic crisis: clinical features, mortality, complications, and risk factors for prolonged intubation. *Neurology*. 1997;48(5):1253–1260.

351. Neumann B, Angstwurm K, Mergenthaler P, et al. Myasthenic crisis demanding mechanical ventilation: a multicenter analysis of 250 cases. *Neurology.* 2020;94(3):e299–e313.
352. Iori E, Mazzoli M, Ariatti A, et al. Predictors of outcome in patients with myasthenic crisis undergoing non-invasive mechanical ventilation: a retrospective 20 year longitudinal cohort study from a single Italian center. *Neuromuscul Disord.* 2021;31(12):1241–1250.
353. Costanzo DD, Mazza M, Esquinas A. Non-invasive mechanical ventilation in myasthenic crisis outside intensive care unit setting: a safe step? *Neuromuscul Disord.* 2022;32(6):539.
354. Proudman W, Kleinig O, Lam L, et al. The icepack test in the diagnosis of myasthenia gravis with ocular features: a systematic review of diagnostic accuracy, technique, and economic utility. *Semin Ophthalmol.* 2023;38(7):679–685.
355. Ricciardi D, Todisco V, Tedeschi G, Cirillo G. Anti-MuSK ocular myasthenia with extrinsic ocular muscle atrophy: a new clinical phenotype? *Neurol Sci.* 2020;41(1):221–223.
356. Caress JB, Hunt CH, Batish SD. Anti-MuSK myasthenia gravis presenting with purely ocular findings. *Arch Neurol.* 2005;62(6):1002–1003.
357. Nagia L, Lemos J, Abusamra K, Cornblath WT, Eggenberger ER. Prognosis of ocular myasthenia gravis: retrospective multicenter analysis. *Ophthalmology.* 2015;122(7):1517–1521.
358. Mee J, Paine M, Byrne E, King J, Reardon K, O'Day J. Immunotherapy of ocular myasthenia gravis reduces conversion to generalized myasthenia gravis. *J Neuroophthalmol.* 2003;23(4):251–255.
359. Li M, Ge F, Guo R, et al. Do early prednisolone and other immunosuppressant therapies prevent generalization in ocular myasthenia gravis in Western populations: a systematic review and meta-analysis. *Ther Adv Neurol Disord.* 2019;12:1756286419876521.
360. Kupersmith MJ, Latkany R, Homel P. Development of generalized disease at 2 years in patients with ocular myasthenia gravis. *Arch Neurol.* 2003;60(2):243–248.
361. Suzuki S, Murai H, Imai T, et al. Quality of life in purely ocular myasthenia in Japan. *BMC Neurol.* 2014;14:142.
362. Kerty E, Elsais A, Argov Z, Evoli A, Gilhus NE. EFNS/ENS Guidelines for the treatment of ocular myasthenia. *Eur J Neurol.* 2014;21(5):687–693.
363. Benatar M, Kaminski HJ; Quality Standards Subcommittee of the American Academy of Neurology. Evidence report: the medical treatment of ocular myasthenia (an evidence-based review): report of the Quality Standards Subcommittee of the American Academy of Neurology. *Neurology.* 2007;68(24):2144–2149.
364. Benatar M, Mcdermott MP, Sanders DB, et al. Efficacy of prednisone for the treatment of ocular myasthenia (EPITOME): a randomized, controlled trial. *Muscle Nerve.* 2016;53(3):363–369.
365. Taha M, Li Y, Morren J. Oxymetazoline hydrochloride eye-drops as treatment for myasthenia gravis-related ptosis: a description of two cases. *Cureus.* 2023;15(3):e36351.
366. Sanders DB, El-Salem K, Massey JM, McConville J, Vincent A. Clinical aspects of MuSK antibody positive seronegative MG. *Neurology.* 2003;60(12):1978–1980.
367. Lavrnic D, Losen M, Vujic A, et al. The features of myasthenia gravis with autoantibodies to MuSK. *J Neurol Neurosurg Psychiatr.* 2005;76(8):1099–1102.
368. Gilhus NE, Tzartos S, Evoli A, Palace J, Burns TM, Verschuuren JJGM. Myasthenia gravis. *Nat Rev Dis Primers.* 2019;5(1):30.
369. Clifford KM, Hobson-Webb LD, Benatar M, et al. Thymectomy may not be associated with clinical improvement in MuSK myasthenia gravis. *Muscle Nerve.* 2019;59(4):404–410.
370. Leite MI, Ströbel P, Jones M, et al. Fewer thymic changes in MuSK antibody-positive than in MuSK antibody-negative MG. *Ann Neurol.* 2005;57(3):444–448.
371. Suster DI, Basu MK, Mackinnon AC. Molecular pathology of thymoma and thymic carcinoma. *JCMT.* 2022;8(5):19.
372. Falkson CB, Vella ET, Ellis PM, Maziak DE, Ung YC, Yu E. Surgical, radiation, and systemic treatments of patients with thymic epithelial tumors: a systematic review. *J Thorac Oncol.* 2023;18(3):299–312.
373. Conforti F, Marino M, Vitolo V, et al. Clinical management of patients with thymic epithelial tumors: the recommendations endorsed by the Italian Association of Medical Oncology (AIOM). *ESMO Open.* 2021;6(4):100188.
374. Maniar R, Loehrer PJ. Understanding the landscape of immunotherapy in thymic epithelial tumors. *Cancer.* 2023;129(8):1162–1172.
375. Falkson CB, Bezjak A, Darling G, et al. The management of thymoma: a systematic review and practice guideline. *J Thorac Oncol.* 2009;4(7):911–919.
376. Xue L, Wang L, Dong J, et al. Risk factors of myasthenic crisis after thymectomy for thymoma patients with myasthenia gravis. *Eur J Cardiothorac Surg.* 2017;52(4):692–697.
377. Wang S, Wang Q, Jin L, Dong J, Ding J. Efgartigimod is a new option for the treatment of thymoma associated myasthenia gravis: a case report. *Int J Surg Case Rep.* 2024;115:109241.
378. Vélez-Santamaría V, Nedkova V, Díez L, Homedes C, Alberti MA, Casasnovas C. Eculizumab as a promising treatment in thymoma-associated myasthenia gravis. *Ther Adv Neurol Disord.* 2020;13:1756286420932035.
379. Guevara-Hoyer K, Fuentes-Antrás J, Calatayud Gastardi J, Sánchez-Ramón S. Immunodeficiency and thymoma in Good syndrome: two sides of the same coin. *Immunol Lett.* 2021;231:11–17.
380. Bernard C, Frih H, Pasquet F, et al. Thymoma associated with autoimmune diseases: 85 cases and literature review. *Autoimmun Rev.* 2016;15(1):82–92.
381. Ishizuchi K, Takizawa T, Ohnuki Y, et al. Immunodeficiency in patients with thymoma-associated myasthenia gravis. *J Neuroimmunol.* 2022;371:577950.
382. Lin Y, Kuang Q, Li H, et al. Outcome and clinical features in juvenile myasthenia gravis: a systematic review and meta-analysis. *Front Neurol.* 2023;14:1119294.
383. Lindner A, Schalke B, Toyka KV. Outcome in juvenile-onset myasthenia gravis: a retrospective study with long-term follow-up of 79 patients. *J Neurol.* 1997;244(8):515–520.
384. Evoli A, Batocchi AP, Bartoccioni E, Lino MM, Minisci C, Tonali P. Juvenile myasthenia gravis with prepubertal onset. *Neuromuscul Disord.* 1998;8(8):561–567.
385. Fisher K, Shah V. Pediatric ocular myasthenia gravis. *Curr Treat Options Neurol.* 2019;21(10):46.
386. Brandsema JF, Ginsberg M, Hoshino H, et al. A phase 3, open-label, multicenter study to evaluate eculizumab in adolescents with refractory generalized myasthenia gravis (S5.009). *Neurology.* 2023;100(17_supplement_2).
387. Abstracts from Myasthenia Gravis Foundation of America's 14th International Conference on Myasthenia Gravis and Related Disorders. May 10–12, 2022 in Miami, Florida: *Muscle & Nerve*: Vol 65, No S1. Accessed March 30, 2024. https://onlinelibrary.wiley.com/toc/10974598/2022/65/S1

388. Rossi C, Zanelli M, Sanguedolce F, et al. Pediatric thymoma: A review and update of the literature. *Diagnostics (Basel)*. 2022;12(9):2205.
389. Norwood F, Dhanjal M, Hill M, et al. Myasthenia in pregnancy: best practice guidelines from a U.K. multispecialty working group. *J Neurol Neurosurg Psychiatr*. 2014;85(5):538–543.
390. Hamel J, Ciafaloni E. An update: myasthenia gravis and pregnancy. *Neurol Clin*. 2018;36(2):355–365.
391. Waters J. Management of myasthenia gravis in pregnancy. *Neurol Clin*. 2019;37(1):113–120.
392. Hoff JM, Daltveit AK, Gilhus NE. Myasthenia gravis: consequences for pregnancy, delivery, and the newborn. *Neurology*. 2003;61(10):1362–1366.
393. Massey JM, Gable KL. Neuromuscular disorders and pregnancy. *Continuum (Minneap Minn)*. 2022;28(1):55–71.
394. Massey JM, De Jesus-Acosta C. Pregnancy and myasthenia gravis. *Continuum (Minneap Minn)*. 2014;20(1 Neurology of Pregnancy):115–127.
395. Gilhus NE. Treatment considerations in myasthenia gravis for the pregnant patient. *Expert Rev Neurother*. 2023;23(2):169–177.
396. Batocchi AP, Majolini L, Evoli A, Lino MM, Minisci C, Tonali P. Course and treatment of myasthenia gravis during pregnancy. *Neurology*. 1999;52(3):447–452.
397. Dobson R, Rog D, Ovadia C, et al. Anti-CD20 therapies in pregnancy and breast feeding: a review and ABN guidelines. *Pract Neurol*. 2023;23(1):6–14.
398. Harada Y, Bettin M, Juel VC, et al. Pregnancy in MuSK-positive myasthenia gravis: a single-center case series. *Muscle Nerve*. 2023;68(1):85–90.
399. Kelly RJ, Höchsmann B, Szer J, et al. Eculizumab in pregnant patients with paroxysmal nocturnal hemoglobinuria. *N Engl J Med*. 2015;373(11):1032–1039.
400. Hallstensen RF, Bergseth G, Foss S, et al. Eculizumab treatment during pregnancy does not affect the complement system activity of the newborn. *Immunobiology*. 2015;220(4):452–459.
401. Vu T, Harvey B, Suresh N, Farias J, Gooch C. Eculizumab during pregnancy in a patient with treatment-refractory myasthenia gravis: a case report. *Case Rep Neurol*. 2021;13(1):65–72.
402. Li X, Mehrabyan A. Managing myasthenia gravis with eculizumab monotherapy through pregnancy. *Can J Neurol Sci*. 2023;50(5):803–805.
403. Zhang P, Lao D, Chen H, et al. Neuromuscular junction dysfunctions due to immune checkpoint inhibitors therapy: An analysis of FAERS data in the past 15 years. *Front Immunol*. 2022;13:778635.
404. Johansen A, Christensen SJ, Scheie D, Højgaard JLS, Kondziella D. Neuromuscular adverse events associated with anti-PD-1 monoclonal antibodies: systematic review. *Neurology*. 2019;92(14):663–674.
405. Snavely A, Pérez-Torres EJ, Weber JS, Sandigursky S, Thawani SP. Immune checkpoint inhibition in patients with inactive pre-existing neuromuscular autoimmune diseases. *J Neurol Sci*. 2022;438:120275.
406. Müller-Jensen L, Knauss S, Ginesta Roque L, et al. Autoantibody profiles in patients with immune checkpoint inhibitor-induced neurological immune related adverse events. *Front Immunol*. 2023;14:1108116.
407. Farina A, Villagrán-García M, Vogrig A, et al. Neurological adverse events of immune checkpoint inhibitors and the development of paraneoplastic neurological syndromes. *Lancet Neurol*. 2024;23(1):81–94.
408. Farina A, Birzu C, Elsensohn M-H, et al. Neurological outcomes in immune checkpoint inhibitor-related neurotoxicity. *Brain Commun*. 2023;5(3):fcad169.
409. Sher AF, Golshani GM, Wu S. Fatal Adverse Events Associated with Pembrolizumab in Cancer Patients: a meta-analysis. *Cancer Invest*. 2020;38(2):130–138.
410. Guidon AC, Burton LB, Chwalisz BK, et al. Consensus disease definitions for neurologic immune-related adverse events of immune checkpoint inhibitors. *J Immunother Cancer*. 2021;9(7):e002890.
411. Masi G, Pham MC, Karatz T, et al. Clinicoserological insights into patients with immune checkpoint inhibitor-induced myasthenia gravis. *Ann Clin Transl Neurol*. 2023;10(5):825–831.
412. Blum SM, Zlotoff DA, Smith NP, et al. Immune responses in checkpoint myocarditis across heart, blood, and tumor. *BioRxiv*. 2023;2023.09.15.557794.
413. Gong J, Neilan TG, Zlotoff DA. Mediators and mechanisms of immune checkpoint inhibitor-associated myocarditis: insights from mouse and human. *Immunol Rev*. 2023;318(1):70–80.
414. Haanen J, Obeid M, Spain L, et al. Management of toxicities from immunotherapy: ESMO clinical practice guideline for diagnosis, treatment and follow-up. *Ann Oncol*. 2022;33(12):1217–1238.
415. Nelke C, Pawlitzki M, Kerkhoff R, et al. Immune checkpoint inhibition-related myasthenia-myositis-myocarditis responsive to complement blockade. *Neurol Neuroimmunol Neuroinflamm*. 2024;11(1):e200177.
416. Zadeh S, Price H, Drews R, Bouffard MA, Young LH, Narayanaswami P. Novel uses of complement inhibitors in myasthenia gravis—Two case reports. *Muscle Nerve*. 2024;69(3):368–372.
417. Lee C, Drobni ZD, Zafar A, et al. Pre-existing autoimmune disease increases the risk of cardiovascular and noncardiovascular events after immunotherapy. *JACC Cardio Oncol*. 2022;4(5):660–669.
418. Birnbaum S, Porcher R, Portero P, et al. Home-based exercise in autoimmune myasthenia gravis: a randomized controlled trial. *Neuromuscul Disord*. 2021;31(8):726–735.
419. Gilhus NE. Physical training and exercise in myasthenia gravis. *Neuromuscul Disord*. 2021;31(3):169–173.
420. Ruiter AM, Verschuuren JJGM, Tannemaat MR. Fatigue in patients with myasthenia gravis. A systematic review of the literature. *Neuromuscul Disord*. 2020;30(8):631–639.
421. Piercy KL, Troiano RP, Ballard RM, et al. The physical activity guidelines for Americans. *JAMA*. 2018;320(19):2020–2028.
422. Misra UK, Kalita J, Singh VK, Kapoor A, Tripathi A, Mishra P. Rest or 30-min walk as exercise intervention (RESTOREX) in myasthenia gravis: a randomized controlled trial. *Eur Neurol*. 2021;84(3):168–174.
423. Alnaimat F, Sweis JJG, Jansz J, et al. Vaccination in the era of immunosuppression. *Vaccines (Basel)*. 2023;11(9):1446.
424. Alcantara M, Koh M, Park AL, Bril V, Barnett C. Outcomes of COVID-19 infection and vaccination among individuals with myasthenia gravis. *JAMA Netw Open*. 2023;6(4):e239834.

CHAPTER 26

Other Disorders of Neuromuscular Transmission

This chapter describes disorders of neuromuscular transmission (DNMT) other than autoimmune myasthenia gravis (MG) (Table 26-1). The neuromuscular junction (NMJ) is a physiologically complex structure. Its ability to function optimally requires integration of numerous proteins including ion channels that are correctly configured and distributed. These become potential sites of vulnerability and DNMTs may result. Autoimmune, genetic, or toxic mechanisms can disrupt the ultrastructure or physiology of the NMJ, and thus, interfere with NMT.

► LAMBERT–EATON MYASTHENIC SYNDROME

CLINICAL FEATURES

The Lambert–Eaton myasthenic syndrome (LEMS) can be conceptualized as an acquired, presynaptic DNMT. The classical clinical triad includes fluctuating proximal lower extremity weakness/gait abnormalities, hyporeflexia, and autonomic dysfunction. Although first described by Anderson and colleagues in 1953, its eponym is credited to Edward Lambert (neurophysiologist) and Lee Eaton (clinical neurologist) from the Mayo Clinic.[1,2] Their 1956 paper with Edward Rooke described the electrophysiological and clinical characteristics of the disorder in six patients.[2]

LEMS is a rare disease which is about 20 times less common than acetylcholine receptor (AChR) antibody-positive MG. Incidence is estimated at 0.17–0.4 per 1 million people per year and prevalence at 2.3–3.5 per million based on large population studies in the United States and the Netherlands.[3–5] LEMS primarily affects adults 40–70 years of age and mean age of onset is 60.[6,7] Rare pediatric cases have been described, both as an acquired autoimmune condition and as a congenital myasthenic syndrome (CMS).[8] Although paraneoplastic in two-thirds of patients, LEMS can be a primary autoimmune disorder, without underlying cancer. The epidemiology of cancer-associated (CA) and non-CA LEMS is different. Incidence of CA, paraneoplastic LEMS peaks at age 60 and two-thirds of those affected are men who commonly have a history of tobacco use.[9] Non-CA LEMS more commonly affects younger women in their 40s and 50s who commonly have a history of other autoimmune disorders.[7,10,11]

Small-cell carcinoma of the lung (SCLC), a neuroendocrine tumor, is the underlying malignancy in approximately 90% of CA LEMS and presents in 50%–60% of all LEMS patients overall.[12,13] The Dutch-English LEMS Tumor Association Prediction (DELTA-P) score can predict likelihood of association with small cell lung cancer at the time of LEMS diagnosis.[14,15] Thymic tumors, non-SCLC lung cancers, lymphoproliferative disorders, and prostate cancers are the next most common associations, while Wilms tumor, and pancreatic, breast, and ovarian cancer may represent chance associations.[9] Conversely, between 0.5% and 4% of all SCLC patients will develop clinical features of LEMS and approximately 8% will develop voltage-gated calcium channel (VGCC) autoantibodies without LEMS clinically.[16,17] LEMS symptoms usually precede tumor recognition. Historically, cancer, if present, is detected within a year of LEMS symptom onset. A more recent study reported data from 100 LEMS patients followed for a minimum of 3 and a median of 8 years. Ninety-one percent of SCLC cancers had been identified within 3 months and 96% by 1 year, with some added value for FDG-PET in early detection.[13]

The phenotypic and electrophysiological characteristics of paraneoplastic and nonparaneoplastic LEMS are mostly indistinguishable in any one individual.[18] However, suspicion for an underlying malignancy should increase if the patient is older than 50 years, has a history of tobacco use, progresses rapidly, or develops weight loss, erectile dysfunction, or bulbar symptoms within 3 months of symptom onset.[9] A person with all six of these characteristics has a greater than 90% chance of harboring an underlying malignancy.[19] In adult LEMS, detectable autoantibodies are directed against presynaptic P/Q type VGCC in nearly 100% of CA LEMS and approximately 90% of cases overall.[20] LEMS may coexist with other paraneoplastic disorders which, if present, would also increase the probability of underlying malignancy. In general, paraneoplastic LEMS becomes more severe more rapidly, typically over several months, than its non-CA counterpart which often has a more insidious presentation.[21] Other autoimmune diseases such as rheumatoid arthritis, thyroiditis, systemic lupus erythematosus, inflammatory bowel disease, primary biliary cirrhosis, vitiligo, celiac disease, or even MG occur in approximately 25% of cases. Their presence favors a non-CA form of the disease.[11,12] Patients with non-CA LEMS have a normal life expectancy and most

▶ TABLE 26-1. DISORDERS OF NEUROMUSCULAR TRANSMISSION OTHER THAN AUTOIMMUNE MYASTHENIA GRAVIS

Presynaptic
- Lambert–Eaton myasthenic syndrome (LEMS)
- Botulism and botulinum toxin
- Tick paralysis
- Congenital myasthenia gravis
    - Choline acetyltransferase deficiency (ChAT)
    - Mitochondrial citrate carrier SLC25A1
    - Vesicular acetylcholine transported (VACHT)
    - PREPL
    - Sodium-dependent high-affinity choline transporter 1 (CHT1/SLC5A7)
    - Paucity of synaptic vesicles
    - Congenital LEMS
- Toxins
    - Envenomation
        - Elapid snake species (kraits, mambas, coral snakes)
        - Arthropods (black and brown widow spiders, scorpions)
        - Marine species (cone snails, sea snakes)
- Drugs
    - Aminoglycosides and other antibiotics
    - Calcium channel blocking agents (minor)
    - Aminopyridines
    - Corticosteroids
    - Hemicholinium-3

Synaptic/basal lamina
- Congenital myasthenic syndromes
    - Acetylcholine esterase deficiency (COLQ)
    - Laminin β2 (LAMB2)
- Drugs and toxins
    - Reversible cholinesterase inhibitors—edrophonium, pyridostigmine, and neostigmine
    - Irreversible—organophosphates and carbamates

Postsynaptic
- Drug-induced myasthenia gravis
    - Penicillamine
    - Alpha-interferon
- Congenital myasthenic syndromes
    - Agrin deficiency (AGRN)
    - LRP4 Deficiency (LRP4)
    - AChR (subunit) deficiency with or without kinetic defect [slow (opening) or fast (opening) channel syndromes]
        - εAChR subunit (CHRNE)
        - αAChR subunit (CHRNA1)
        - βAChR subunit (CHRNB1)
        - δAChR subunit (CHRND)
        - γAChR subunit (Escobar syndrome)
    - AChR—structural or organizational defects
        - Dok-7 deficiency (Dok-7)
        - MuSK deficiency (MuSK)
        - Rapsyn deficiency (RAPSN)
            - AChR mutations with or without plectin deficiency (PLEC)
    - Sodium channel myasthenia (SCN4A)
    - Glutamine-fructose-6-phosphate transaminase 1 MG (GFPT1)
    - Dolichyl-phosphate N-acetylglucosamine-phosphotransferase 1 MG (DPAGT1)
- Drugs and toxins
    - d-Tubocurarine, vecuronium, and other Nondepolarizing blocking agents
    - Succinylcholine, decamethonium, and other Depolarizing blocking agents
    - Tetracyclines, lincomycin, and other antibiotics

---

have a relatively stable disease course after diagnosis and treatment, remaining or becoming independent for self-care after treatment. Health-related quality of life (QOL), however, is lower than the general population and comparable to MG. Overall survival is longer in patients with small cell lung CA LEMS than the general population of patients with small cell lung cancer, regardless of cancer stage.[22]

Lower extremity weakness resulting in trouble standing from a chair, climbing stairs, or walking is the most common presenting syptom.[23,24] We agree with the common observation that disability/morbidity caused by symptoms usually seems to far exceed objective weakness. This discordance may contribute to initial diagnostic suspicion for psychogenic or functional neurologic disorders, particularly in young women. A potential explanation for discordance between patient-reported symptom severity and muscle strength measured objectively on manual muscle testing may lie in disease pathophysiology. As brief exercise can transiently enhance neuromuscular transmission in presynaptic disorders, muscle strength should be assessed at the initiation of contraction, not several seconds later after facilitation may have already occurred. This transient improvement in strength usually dissipates with sustained muscle contraction. Initial facilitation followed by postexercise diminution of strength is most easy to demonstrate in hip and shoulder girdle muscles. Repetitive squatting or repeated sit-to-stand movements show this phenomenon. Exercise may temporarily lessen ptosis severity with sustained upgaze in a manner opposite to MG.[25]

Symptomatic weakness in LEMS typically affects functions which require proximal, extremity muscles, particularly hip girdle, and leg muscles. This is noted in approximately 80% of patients during the illness. A third of patients complains of muscle aching and stiffness during or following physical exertion. Approximately 20% of patients note that their weakness and fatigue are exacerbated by hot weather or bathing in warm water. Ocular and bulbar symptoms are less common and severe than in MG but can occur. They typically develop later in the disease and are rarely the sole or initial manifestation.[26,27] Symptomatic diplopia without overt ophthalmoparesis is typically transient and mild when it occurs. Ptosis is more common in our experience and is estimated to occur in a third to a half of cases. In those with cranial muscle involvement, neck flexor, extensor, and facial muscles are among the most affected. Head drop has been reported as a presenting manifestation.[28] Some patients develop dysarthria or dysphagia. Ventilatory muscle involvement is rare, although breathing issues related to smoking, chronic lung disease, and lung cancer are common in SCLC-associated LEMS. Ventilatory failure as a very rare presenting manifestation of LEMS has been described.[29–31]

In contrast to MG, as a presynaptic DNMT, LEMS frequently affects both nicotinic and muscarinic function with resultant cholinergic dysautonomia. This manifests as blurred vision (impaired accommodation), xerostomia, xerophthalmia, constipation, hypohidrosis, and/or impotence.[20,32] Xerostomia may contribute to dysphagia and dysarthria. Cholinergic dysfunction is heralded by sluggish pupillary responses to light and reduced sweating. Descriptions of an unpleasant metallic taste in the mouth are common. Patients with LEMS may have coexistent paraneoplastic syndromes such as sensory neuronopathy, cerebellar ataxia, and/or limbic encephalitis with frequently coexistent Hu autoantibodies.[33]

Typical of DNMTs, muscle bulk in LEMS tends to be preserved. In contrast to MG, worsening weakness and atrophy does not typically occur with prolonged untreated disease since LEMS patients typically present with their maximum disease severity. Deep tendon reflexes are typically diminished or absent in LEMS. Clinical deep tendon and electrophysiologic H-reflexes may facilitate in LEMS after 10 seconds of maximal exercise. However, this is less common than one might expect and is present in about half of patients. As such, reflex facilitation is a helpful clinical sign when present, but its absence does not exclude LEMS.[34,35] Like assessments of strength, this phenomenon may be obscured if manual muscle testing is done prior to deep tendon reflex assessment. For this reason, we recommend testing deep tendon reflexes (DTRs) prior to manual muscle testing and then observe for augmentation of the DTR immediately following 10 seconds of sustained contraction of the corresponding muscle.

MG/LEMS overlap syndrome can exist but is rare.[36] Most MG cases overlapping with LEMS are based on the presence of AChR antibodies in patients who otherwise appear to have LEMS on a clinical and electrophysiological basis, but double seropositivity can exist.[37,38] As many as 13% of patients with LEMS have AChR-binding autoantibodies.[37] The AChR autoantibodies may be epiphenomenal rather than pathogenic in at least some LEMS patients. Nonetheless, rare patients may exhibit clinical features of both LEMS and MG.[36,37,39,40]

DIAGNOSIS AND DIFFERENTIAL DIAGNOSIS

As a disorder characterized by a subacute limb-girdle weakness and fatigue, the primary differential diagnostic considerations for LEMS are limb-girdle myopathies and MG. MG may readily be confused with LEMS, particularly if signs and symptoms of oculobulbar weakness are readily evident with LEMS or if they are inapparent in MG. While rare exceptions exist, oculobulbar signs occur early and prominently in MG and tend to be less frequent, less severe, and occur later in the disease course in LEMS.[9,27] As another presynaptic disorder of neuromuscular transmission, it is not surprising that botulism shares some clinical and electrodiagnostic (EDX) features with LEMS including the presence of cholinergic dysautonomia. However, botulism typically presents with descending weakness with acute onset, which is the usual discriminating factor. CMSs deserve consideration in any LEMS suspect as well as LEMS can present in childhood and CMS may first manifest itself in adulthood. Motor neuron diseases that produce a limb-girdle pattern of weakness such as Kennedy disease are distinguished by their chronicity, and the presence of atrophy and fasciculations, among other features. The pattern and evolution of weakness produced by multifocal motor neuropathy are, as the name implies, usually distinctive from LEMS. Motor predominant forms of acute inflammatory demyelinating polyradiculoneuropathy (AIDP) or chronic inflammatory demyelinating polyradiculoneuropathy (CIDP) may represent a very relevant diagnostic consideration in a LEMS suspect, particularly as both abolish deep tendon reflexes and affect the autonomic nervous system. Most of these disorders, however, are readily distinguished from LEMS by EDX testing.

Electrodiagnostic Testing

Diagnostic confirmation of LEMS is obtained by electrophysiological testing with or without positive P/Q VGCC antibodies. EDX plays a key role in the diagnosis and the electromyographer may be the first clinician to suspect LEMS. As with all DNMTs, sensory conductions are normal unless paraneoplastic sensory neuronopathy, chemotherapy-induced polyneuropathy, or other confounding disorders coexist. On occasion, the EDX pattern in LEMS may be confused with that in MG, but distinguishing features exist. In LEMS and other presynaptic DNMTs, the baseline compound muscle action potential (CMAP) amplitudes are usually reduced in a widespread in the distribution in the arms and legs, but less commonly in proximal muscles such nasalis or trapezius. In one study with 73 LEMS patients (42% with lung cancer), the CMAP amplitude was reduced in the abductor digiti minimi (ADM) in 95%, abductor pollicis brevis (APB) in 85%, extensor digitorum brevis (EDB) in 80%, and trapezius in only 55% of cases.[41] This diffuse pattern of reduced CMAP amplitudes in the presence of normal sensory nerve action potentials (SNAPs) may provide the initial suspicion for LEMS. The CMAP response to exercise and/or repetitive stimulation along with serological testing provide confirmation. Some patients with LEMS, however, have baseline CMAP amplitudes may fall within population norms. In this situation, the incremental response characteristic of a presynaptic deficit may not be evident or further explored. Therefore, a high index of suspicion for LEMS as well as performing slow 2–3 Hz repetitive nerve stimulation (RNS) is critical. To avoid influence of prior routine CMAP testing and evaluation for facilitation, waiting 150 seconds for active recovery is recommended between assessing for postexercise facilitation and RNS.[42]

In an awake and cooperative patient, testing to facilitation can be rapidly and easily performed with brief voluntary exercise. A supramaximal baseline CMAP is obtained after suitable hand or foot warming. The muscle tested is then subjected to 10 seconds of isometric resistance. Immediately thereafter, a second, supramaximal electrical stimulus is applied. In normal individuals, there may be a mild increase in CMAP amplitude (<40%) associated with a shorter duration and similar area under the curve (pseudofacilitation). The actual basis of this phenomenon is poorly understood. It has been postulated to represent improved motor unit synchronization due to a disproportionate increase in the conduction velocity of the slowest conducting muscle fibers. In most patients with LEMS, brief exercise will produce a 100%–400% increase in CMAP amplitude. Recently, the cut-off of abnormal facilitation has been lowered to 60% without sacrificing specificity.[43] In individuals who cannot perform with isometric exercise for whatever reason, "fast" repetitive stimulation of 10–20 Hz or higher represents a feasible but more uncomfortable means by which to demonstrate the characteristic increment.

In addition to CMAP amplitude facilitation after brief exercise and CMAP increment with fast RNS, LEMS patients also have CMAP decrement following slow RNS (Fig. 26-1A–D).[41,44] Of course this decrement with slow RNS is characteristic of

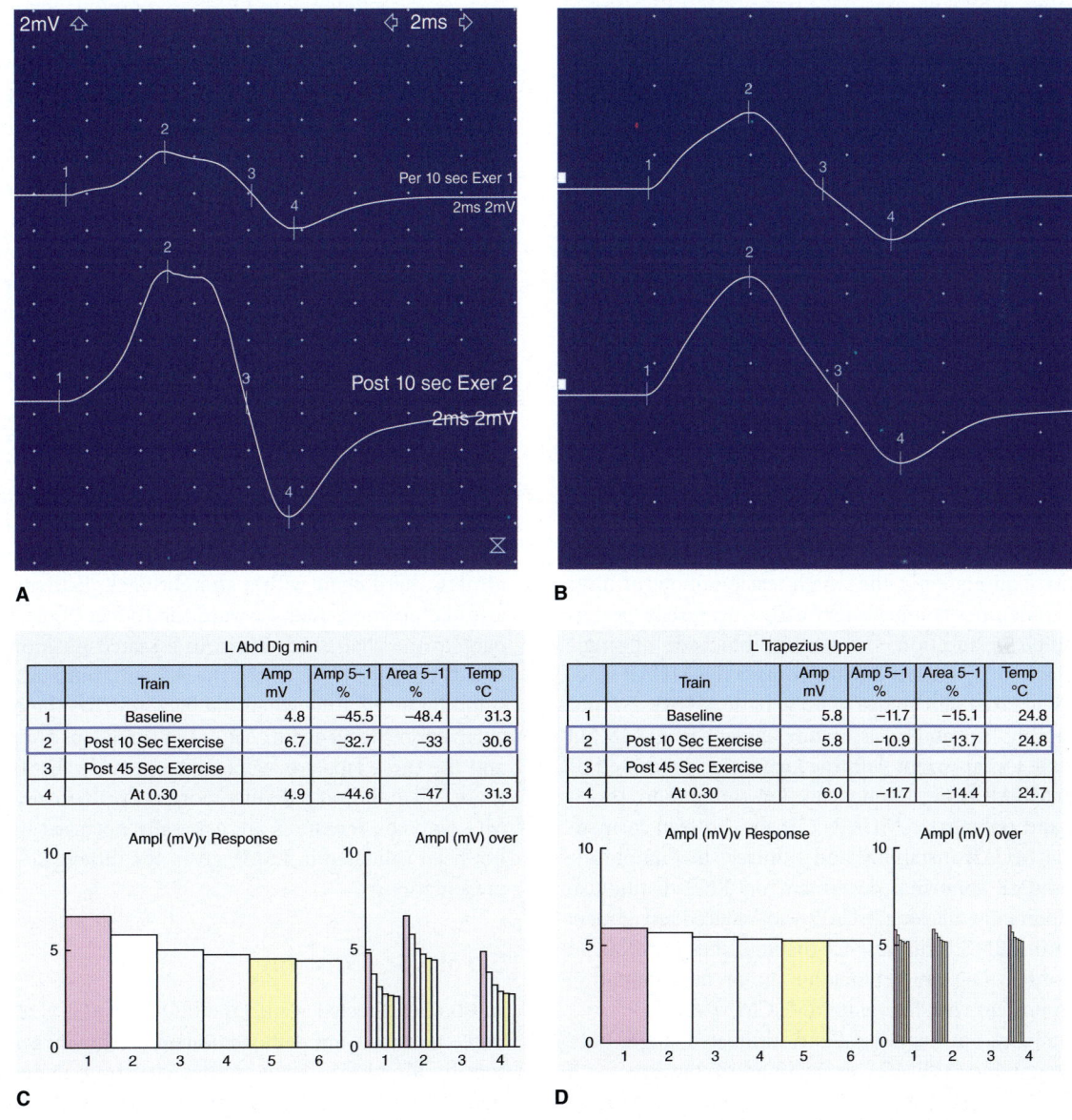

Figure 26-1. Amplitude facilitation of the ulnar-ADM CMAP after 10 seconds of exercise in LEMS from (A) 2.3–7.1 mV and (B) 5.5–8.4 mV. (C) Abnormal decrement and postexercise facilitation in 3 Hz RNS of the ulnar-ADM in LEMS and (D) Lesser decrement without postexercise facilitation in the SAN-trapezius. Note the lack of the saddle shape in the trains of stimuli typically seen in MG.

both LEMS and MG. This decremental pattern in LEMS is similar although not necessarily identical to that described in MG.

In MG, following the initial decrement between the 1st and 4th/5th stimuli, there is an increase in CMAP amplitude between the 4th/5th and 10th stimuli. This creates the classily seen "saddle shape" pattern of decrement. In LEMS [and also sometimes in muscle-specific kinase (MuSK) MG], the CMAP amplitudes plateau or continue to decline between the 4th/5th and 10th responses[45,46] (Fig. 26-1C and D). Decrement to 3 Hz RNS is the most sensitive EDX feature in LEMS, and may be present even when baseline CMAPs are normal and CMAP amplitude facilitation with brief exercise is not present.

In LEMS, decrement in response to 3-Hz stimulation is present in the ADM in 98%, APB in 98%, EDB in 84%, and trapezius in 89% of cases.[41] We typically test RNS in the ulnar-ADM, median-APB, and peroneal-EDB nerve–muscle combinations when LEMS is suspected. Decrement in at least one of these sites is nearly 100% sensitive for LEMS.[41] Decreasing muscle temperature results in an improvement in the CMAP amplitude at rest, reduces the magnitude of decrement at low rates of stimulation, and prolongs the duration of postactivation facilitation. Like MG, the yield of EDX testing will be increased not only by ensuring that limbs are adequately warm but also by discontinuing cholinesterase inhibitors 24 hours before testing.

Abnormal insertional and spontaneous activity on needle examination such as fibrillation potentials and/or positive sharp waves are typically absent in LEMS. Abnormalities of motor unit action potential (MUAP) morphology are apparent in weak muscles but can be subtle. Neuromuscular blockade at individual myoneural junctions effectively reduces the number of single-fiber action potentials contributing to the MUAP, resulting in shorter duration and lower-amplitude waveforms. Consequently, the twitch tension of motor units declines. Sometimes compensatory early (increased) recruitment results. In addition, the random blockade of single myofiber action potentials desynchronizes the MUAP leading to an increased percentage of polyphasic MUAPs. Motor unit variability (instability) is readily evident in LEMS but may become less apparent with the facilitation promoted by increased MUAP firing frequencies. Low-amplitude, short-duration and polyphasic MUAPs can also be seen in myopathy. The MUAP instability and diffusely low-amplitude CMAPs and/or abnormal decrement on RNS distinguish LEMS. Importantly, tall, long MUAPs with reduced recruitment are absent in LEMS. This absence distinguishes LEMS from other disorders (e.g., radiculopathy, motor neuronopathy) which can present with low-amplitude CMAPs.[47–49]

Predictably, both volitional and stimulated single-fiber electromyography (SFEMG) evaluations of patients with LEMS yield abnormal results.[50–52] Jitter values in patients with LEMS are significantly elevated and statistically exceed those observed in MG. In essentially all NMJs examined, irrespective of the muscle chosen, markedly abnormal jitter values are evident. This is disparate from MG where a spectrum of jitter values from normal to highly abnormal exists within and between individual muscles. Unlike MG, the jitter in patients with LEMS is not dependent on the degree of weakness in a particular muscle. Blocking is often more prevalent and severe in LEMS in comparison to MG. Some of the highest percentages of blocked potentials occur in LEMS. Frequency-dependent alterations in jitter and blocking are also observed in LEMS if sought for as implied in the previous statements regarding frequency-dependent MUAP variability (instability). Specifically, at low rates of voluntary firing, jitter and blocking can be quite impressive. Further increase in the duration of muscle activation or rate of individual MUAP firing will result in reduced jitter and blocking.[52,53] These observations can be quantitated by using stimulated SFEMG.[52]

As dysautonomia in LEMS is common, abnormal autonomic nervous system testing is anticipated. In a series of 30 patients with LEMS, autonomic testing revealed abnormalities of sudomotor function in 83% of patients, abnormal cardiovagal reflexes in 75%, decreased salivation in 44%, and abnormal adrenergic function in 37% of tested individuals. This is in keeping with the predominantly cholinergic dysautonomia of the disease.[54,55] We do not routinely perform autonomic testing unless the patient has symptoms of dysautonomia.

EDX parameters are also responsive to clinical change. Jitter increases with increasing disease severity and magnitude of decrement on RNS in LEMS, and reduces with clinical improvement.[51,56] However, a practical and reliable measure, which was used in various ways in the 3,4-DAP trials, is the baseline CMAP amplitude, which is typically averaged.[57,58] Another non-EDX measure of disease severity, which is responsive to change in disease severity, is the Triple Timed-Up-and-Go (Triple TUG). This is performed with a 10-foot-long space to walk and a standard-height, armless, hard chair with a straight back. Patients rise from a seated position, walk forward for 10 feet (3 m), turn, walk back to the chair, and return to a seated position. One lap equals the time from which the patients' buttocks rise when standing to the time when the back touches the back of the chair upon sitting again. A total of three laps are performed and the three laps are averaged to provide the Triple TUG score.[32,59] Standard patient-reported or physician-measured MG outcome measures are generally not used in and have not been validated in LEMS given the differences in disease presentations.

Serological Testing

Antibodies directed against the P/Q-type VGCC of the motor nerve terminals are pathogenic and are highly sensitive and specific for LEMS. They are detected by immunoprecipitation of VGCC from human brain, labeled with ω-conotoxin derived from the fish-eating Conus species of snails, incubated with serum from LEMS patients.[60–62] These antibodies are detectable in the serum in 98% or more of paraneoplastic and >80% of nonparaneoplastic LEMS patients.[18,20,37]

Conversely, as previously mentioned, it is estimated that 4% of patients with SCLC will have VGCC autoantibodies.[63,64] In addition, antibodies directed against the N-type VGCCs, which are located on autonomic and peripheral nerves as well as cerebellar, cortical, and spinal neurons, are present in 74% of patients with paraneoplastic LEMS and 40% of nonparaneoplastic LEMS patients, but are nonspecific and not diagnostic for LEMS.[20,65,66]

LEMS patients may harbor other autoantibodies. The SOX1 antigen was originally found because of antiglial nuclear antibodies cross reacting with Bergmann glia of the Purkinje cell layer of rat cerebellum. The SOX1 antigen also plays a role in the development of airway epithelia and is found in SCLC. SOX autoantibodies are of potential clinical value as they are highly specific for LEMS and SCLC. They are found in two-thirds of LEMS patients with SCLC, 12% of SCLC without LEMS, and <5% of LEMS without cancer.[64,67] Despite the cerebellar location of the antigen, no consistent association with paraneoplastic cerebellar degeneration or other paraneoplastic disorders has been demonstrated. These antibodies are commercially available as antiglial nuclear antibodies as part of the Mayo Clinic's paraneoplastic antibody panel. As previously mentioned, some patients with paraneoplastic LEMS will also harbor Hu autoantibodies associated with sensory ganglionopathy, cerebellar degeneration, and/or limbic encephalitis.[20,33,37] Autoantibodies against the presynaptic protein synaptotagmin have also been described in LEMS patients, but have no current clinical applications.[9] Plasma from patients with LEMS contains antibodies that bind to the synaptic vesicle protein synaptotagmin. Synaptotagmin associates with calcium channels and appeared to regulate synaptic vesicle docking at the plasma membrane prior to neurotransmitter release.[68] However, further work then suggested that large-molecular–weight proteins (Ca^{2+} channel subunits) rather than syntaxin and synaptotagmin were the targets of LEMS autoantibodies. Interestingly, however, synaptotagmin-2 mutations have since been associated with autosomal dominant form of LEMS with motor neuropathy.[69]

Serological testing for VGCC and AChR autoantibodies usually discriminates between LEMS and MG when there is phenotypic overlap. Nonetheless, as previously mentioned, overlap can exit. AChR-binding antibodies are found in as many as 13% of patients with LEMS[37] and P/Q VGCC antibodies in <5% of patients who have the phenotypic and electrophysiological characteristics of MG.[37,38] The concurrence of both antibodies is thought to be epiphenomenal in most cases.[37] Given the potential for VGCC without symptoms of LEMS, we typically perform EDX studies for confirmation of a disorder of neuromuscular transmission, even for patients with positive VGCC.

Pharmacological Testing

Edrophonium testing in LEMS produces variable results and is not utilized.

Imaging

Surveillance for a potential underlying neoplasm should be undertaken in any patient with LEMS, regardless of age or antibody status. Published guidance directs how extensive the initial evaluation for neoplasm should be, and how frequently to repeat imaging if the initial evaluation is negative.[70] The DELTA-P risk score to predict the presence of SCLC in a patient with LEMS at the time of diagnosis was created and then used successfully in a validation cohort.[14,15] This gives a pretest probability for malignancy, which is helpful in tailoring screening and interpreting testing results.

The malignancy evaluation begins with chest imaging. Chest x-ray is an insufficiently sensitive imaging procedure in this context. CT of the chest (followed by FDG-PET if negative) or integrated FDG-PET/CT is recommended in addition to age and medical history–appropriate screenings.[70,71] In an older patient with a smoking history, CT of the thorax will detect most tumors detectable upon LEMS presentation. FDG-PET is likely the most sensitive means by which to detect an underlying malignancy though issues with access still exist. Regarding subsequent surveillance in individuals in whom no tumor is initially detected, evaluation has been suggested at 6-month intervals for 2 years in LEMS. If clinical suspicion for cancer is high, the first repeat imaging is recommended at 3–4 months. If small pulmonary nodules are detected in a current or former smoker, we typically pursue biopsy up front if feasible instead of observation, given the high likelihood for malignancy.

HISTOPATHOLOGY

Performing EDX in patients with limb-girdle patterns of weakness can distinguish LEMS from myopathy and avoid muscle biopsy in these patients. While unnecessary for diagnosis, if a biopsy were performed in LEMS, histopathology typically shows nonspecific type II fiber atrophy. On quantitative electron microscopic analysis, nerve terminals appear normal in both their size and the number of synaptic vesicles they contain. Similarly, the postsynaptic membrane is intact, but with an increase in the postsynaptic fold area and number of secondary synaptic clefts, presumably as a compensatory mechanism in response to reduced quantal release of ACh. The total number and activation properties of individual AChRs appear normal. Freeze-fracture analysis of the presynaptic membrane demonstrates a marked decrease in the number of intramembranous proteinaceous particles, which are assumed to be P/Q VGCC. These presumptive channels are disorganized and aggregated in clumps.[72,73]

PATHOGENESIS

LEMS is a disorder of impaired presynaptic ACh release resulting from autoantibody-mediated–VGCC dysfunction.

The mechanism is downregulation and endocytosis of VGCC channels rather than mechanical blockade.[74] As a consequence of this autoimmune assault, reduced presynaptic calcium ion concentrations occur in response to a motor nerve action potential.[20,37] The number of active ACh vesicles or "quanta" released in response to a nerve action potential is reduced and therefore, neuromuscular transmission is compromised.[12,20,75,76]

Presynaptic functions at the nerve terminal include concentrating and storing ACh within vesicles and facilitating their movement to active release zones where they dock and fuse.[77] This maintenance activity allows ready ACh release into the synaptic cleft in response to a motor nerve action potential. The migration, docking, and fusion with the presynaptic plasma membrane and subsequent exocytosis into the synaptic cleft are all dependent on the complex interaction of an extensive number of proteins. Some of the more notable constituents of this complex neuromuscular transmission process include synaptobrevin and synaptotagmin (associated with the synaptic vesicles), NSF (*N*-ethylamide sensitive ATPase) and α-SNAP (both found in the cytosol), syntaxin and SNAP-25 (synaptic vesicle–associated 25-kDa protein), and membrane-bound VGCCs.[77] Synaptobrevin, syntaxin, and SNAP-25 are collectively known as SNARE (SNAP receptor) proteins. The known specificity of tetanus and botulism toxins for SNARE proteins and the impaired ACh release that results from their exposure to the NMJ illustrate the essential function of SNARE proteins in presynaptic vesicular exocytosis.

In normal individuals, a motor nerve action potential transiently opens presynaptic VGCCs, increasing the intracellular calcium concentration in motor nerve termina. The effect does not achieve the magnitude it potentially could; the <1 ms duration of the nerve action potential undershoots the activation time constant of the VGCC (1.3 ms).[78] It is important for understanding of RNS data to know that intracellular calcium concentration peaks by 200 microsec and persistents for approximately 800 microsec following nerve action potential. An intracellular calcium concentration of 200–300 μM is achieved under normal circumstances. Approximately 60 VGCCs must open to allow the influx of the approximately 13,000 calcium ions required for exocytosis of a single vesicle of ACh. In mammalian systems, the normal response to a motor nerve action potential is a quantal content of 50–300. In LEMS, however, the mean is roughly 8 (3.3–15).[78] Similar reductions in quantal content can also be achieved by reducing calcium or increasing magnesium concentrations in the extracellular fluid bathing the nerve terminal.[77]

To begin the process which ends in exocytosis of ACh vesicles, calcium first binds to synaptotagmin, then syntaxin and SNAP-25, and eventually, to synaptobrevin. This calcium plays an essential role in cleaving the bonds holding ACh vesicles to the intraneural cytoskeletal framework, which is largely composed of actin and microtubules. This framework exists to prevent the vesicle from fusing or docking with recognition proteins at the active zones (AZs) before this is desired.[62,77]

Six types of VGCCs, distinguished by their pharmacological and biophysical properties, exist in mammalian systems (L, N, P, Q, R, T). The predominant channel in mammalian NMJs is the P/Q channel. The P/Q channel is composed of a pore-forming α_{1a} subunit as well as $\alpha 2\delta$, γ, and β_{4a} subunits. These VGCCs are controlled by presynaptic voltage-gated potassium channels (VGKCs). Opening of VGKCs keeps VGCC in their desired closed position. Failure of VGCC channels to close promptly results in prolonged depolarization, and certain disorders of neuromuscular hyperactivity described in Chapter 32.

In normal individuals, these P/Q-type VGCCs are present on both the granule and Purkinje cells of the cerebellum and in presynaptic motor nerve terminals. They exist as well on small-cell carcinoma cells, providing a logical substrate for an autoimmune, paraneoplastic mechanism. In support of this, autoantibodies reacting with the P/Q-type VGCCs are found in 90% of patients with LEMS.

Autoantibody binding appears to specify the α_{1a} subunit of the VGCC. Consequently, a downregulation in the number of calcium channels results in less total current flow, without a reduction of current flow in individual channels. Complement does not appear to play a role in this process. The nerve terminal maintains a grossly normal appearance without evidence of lytic destruction.[79] A causative role for these autoantibodies is supported by the induction of all of the electrophysiological, morphological, and clinical manifestations of LEMS by passive transfer of IgG from patients with paraneoplastic and nonparaneoplastic LEMS to animals, or from mother to fetus.[18,76,80,81] In addition, similar results utilizing the serum of seronegative patients supports an autoimmune mechanism in this group as well.

Increasingly, attention has focused on additional mechanisms of pathophysiology beyond the VGCC and that disease requires more than just VGCC antibody. A recent computational model of the active zone (AZ) in the NMJ in mammals has suggested that there is disruption of a normally organized transmitter release sites. Abnormal presynaptic AZ organization and protein content (particularly synaptotagmin) play an important role in LEMS pathophysiology, in addition to the simple removal of presynaptic calcium channels.[82] In mouse models, removal of VGCC alone does not cause disease.[83] Additionally, most patients have a mixture of antibodies both to VGCC and other proteins.

As in many autoimmune disorders, the trigger for patients to develop disease is unknown. In patients with cancer, it is speculated that molecular mimicry results in the presynaptic motor nerve terminal becoming the innocent bystander in an immune response initially targeted at the neoplasm.[75,78,84] As LEMS occurs in only a small proportion of patients harboring SCLC, a genetic predisposition is hypothesized.[85] Sixty-five percent of LEMS patients have the HLA haplotype HLA-B8-DR3, lending some support for this hypothesis although its prevalence appears greatest in the younger, nonneoplastic cohort.[86–88]

TREATMENT

Identification and treatment of an underlying neoplasm, if present, is the foundation of LEMS treatment. If the tumor can be treated successfully, the morbidity of LEMS can often be substantially reduced with concomitant improvement in electrophysiological studies.[84,89] The chemotherapy typically used to treat SCLC has additional immunosuppressive effects. Symptomatic therapy, IVIg or plasma exchange, and corticosteroids can be used when tumor status remains unknown. During this period, however, holding off on starting long-term immunosuppressants is recommended.[90] Immunomodulatory and immunosuppressive therapies could potentially adversely affect cancer outcomes or be contraindicated for use in combination with concurrent anticancer treatments. If the patient remains symptomatic, with or without successful tumor treatment, therapies that either enhance neuromuscular transmission, manage autonomic symptoms, or address autoimmunity can be utilized.[9,32,90-93] Like myasthenia, the treatment regimen should be individually tailored to disease severity and burden, as well as numerous other contextual features including availability and relevant comorbidities. Like in MG, cautious use or avoidance altogether of drugs with known neuromuscular blocking properties is recommended. Most relevant in LEMS patients are neuromuscular blocking anesthetic agents, certain antibiotics (macrolides, aminoglycosides, and fluoroquinolones), intravenous magnesium, and immune checkpoint inhibitors for cancer.[94]

Symptomatic therapy for LEMS consists mainly of anticholinesterase and 3,4-diaminopyridine (3,4-DAP) medications. Anticholinesterase medications can be used in a manner identical to patients with MG. Analogous to MG, pyridostigmine provides symptomatic treatment without addressing the root cause of the disease. In our experience, the drug is effective although the improvement in strength is often minimal. It is typically insufficient in controlling the morbidity of the disease as monotherapy. We use it primarily to augment the effect of aminopyridines and to treat autonomic symptoms. It can be taken at the same time as 3,4-DAP or staggered throughout the day.

As a class, the aminopyridines (3,4-DAP/amifampridine) block voltage-dependent potassium channel conductance and thereby increase the concentration of calcium presynaptically. This increases synaptic transmission by increasing neurotransmission release in both the central nervous system (CNS) and peripheral nervous system (PNS). At the motor nerve terminal, this effect increases the number of ACh quanta released per nerve impulse which ameliorates presynaptic abnormality seen in LEMS. Base and phosphate salt forms of amifampridine exist. Amifampridine is not a new drug. The first study of 3,4-DAP which showed benefit in LEMS was performed in the 1980s[95] and the most recent in 2018.[57] Several prospective, randomized placebo-controlled trial of 3,4-DAP in LEMS patients (paraneoplastic and nonparaneoplastic) identified improvements in multiple outcome measures including strength, quantitative myasthenic scales, and CMAP amplitudes.[58,95-98] The phosphate salt formulation (Firdapse) was approved for clinical use in Europe in 2009 and in the United States with a label indication for LEMS in 2018.[99] Amifampridine is highly effective. A study with 70 patients showed that amifampridine monotherapy or in combination with pyridostigmine resulting in near-normal function in 45% and an additional 34% reported improvement in ADLs.[41] The route to approval and the postapproval period have been controversial.[19,100] Drug costs for patients with LEMS in the United States are now substantially higher than previously, and substantially higher than in other countries where amifampridine is available.

Like pyridostigmine, the clinical effect of amifampridine occurs approximately 20–30 minutes after an oral dose and lasts for approximately 4 hours. We typically start with a dose of 10 mg TID and increase gradually to symptom relief or a maximum dose of 20 mg QID. Since the benefit of any dose may not be seen fully for several days, we typically increase the dose every 5–7 days. The medication is generally well tolerated, with a few patients experiencing perioral and acral paresthesias. Worsening of reactive airway disease and diarrhea can also occur. Bothersome side effects can be addressed by lowering the dose. Caution is recommended if patients have a history of seizures or an abnormal EKG at baseline given the possibility of QTc prolongation. No EKG changes have been reported in patients taking less than 100 mg per daily. We perform an electrocardiogram (EKG) at baseline, once patients reach a steady dose and periodically afterward, particularly if they start taking other medications which can prolong QTc.

In addition to 3,4-DAP which indirectly increases the number of VGCC open at any one time by acting on potassium channels, direct calcium channel agonists have been highlighted as a potential additional therapeutic avenue.[101] GV-58 is a direct calcium channel agonist which increases the mean open time of calcium channels regardless of the nature of the presynaptic abnormality. These could potentially be used as monotherapy or in combination with 3,4-DAP.[102]

If patients have more severe weakness, plasma exchange, or intravenous immunoglobulin can be used acutely.[103] A single crossover trial of IVIg demonstrated a benefit in strength and a decline in VGCC autoantibody titers but failed to demonstrate a statistically significant improvement in CMAP amplitudes.[103] Plasma exchange has been reported to have a clinical and electrical benefit in LEMS but has never been subjected to a prospective clinical trial.[104,105] Improvements in CMAP amplitudes at rest, following exercise, or in response to high rates of repetitive stimulation following plasmapheresis may be seen.[104,105] The peak response is observed about 2 weeks after the treatment, with a diminution in effectiveness by the end of 3–4 weeks. There are no controlled trials in LEMS of any of the commonly used immunomodulating agents, though they are commonly used, particularly when amifampridine is not available.[3] The most common regimen used in LEMS is probably a combination of prednisone and azathioprine which has been shown to induce clinical remission in some patients.[103,106] It may improve CMAP amplitudes as well as patient strength and stamina. Mycophenolate has also been used.[3] Case reports have suggested a benefit from rituximab.[107,108] Symptoms of autonomic dysfunction often improve and worsen in tandem with other symptoms of LEMS in response to immunotherapy. Orthostatic hypotension, constipation, erectile dysfunction, and sicca symptoms should all be addressed symptomatically.[32]

One theoretical concern with LEMS or any other paraneoplastic neuromuscular disorder is the potential risk that suppressing the patient's immune system will have adverse effects on tumor control. One hypothesis as to why LEMS often precedes tumor detection is that the same immune response that produces LEMS simultaneously limits tumor growth. Limited data, however, suggest that immunomodulation can be utilized in LEMS without an adverse effect on tumor control.[84]

▶ CONGENITAL MYASTHENIC SYNDROMES

CLINICAL FEATURES

CMSs are uncommon, inherited DNMTs which do not have an autoimmune etiology. Rather, genetic mutations cause abnormalities of one or more proteins, whose normal functions are requisite to successful neuromuscular transmission.[77,109–112] Pathologic germline variants have been reported in at least 35 genes.[113] Many new CMSs have been recognized over the past decade with the advent of next-generation sequencing, combined with increased diagnostic awareness.[110] Disorders are characterized based on the anatomic location or function of the impaired protein. These include disorders of presynaptic, synaptic, or postsynaptic locations and of protein glycosylation or NMJ development and maintenance. Over half of these disorders occur at the postsynaptic region. Mutations in AChR, rapsyn, Acetylcholine esterase (AChE), and downstream of tyrosine kinase 7 (Dok-7) account for over 85% of CMS patients.[110,112] Treatment strategy depends on the type of CMS.

The prevalence of genetically identifiable CMS is estimated at 25–125 per 1 million.[114] CMSs typically become evident at birth, in infancy, or in childhood but adult-onset cases do occur and are characteristic of specific genotypes (Tables 26-2 and 26-3).[115–119] It is not uncommon for early-onset cases to go undiagnosed until later life, often misdiagnosed as seronegative myasthenia, myopathy, or spinal muscular atrophy.[116,117] A family history may be absent or go unrecognized, since most CMSs are inherited in a recessive fashion. The exception to this inheritance pattern is slow-channel syndrome (SCCMS), which is inherited in an autosomal dominant fashion. Others with AD inheritance are SNAP25, PURA, and about a third of patients with SYT2 CMS.[113] Recognition of recessive inheritance patterns and/or parenteral consanguinity are supportive diagnostic clues for CMS, although in small or fragmented families, cases may appear to be sporadic. A family history of sudden infant death syndrome (SIDS) or scoliosis/contractures would raise suspicion for CMS.

Most CMSs are related to proteins unique to the NMJ, resulting in a purely neuromuscular syndrome. A few CMSs, however, are related to proteins affecting other organ systems including cardiac and smooth muscle, skin, and kidney.[120] Rarely, there may be CNS involvement with microcephaly, seizures, developmental delay, and ocular and/or auditory abnormalities. Connective tissue involvement with skeletal deformities or contractures occur in some cases most notably in rapsyn deficiency, AChR γ deficiency (Escobar syndrome) and some of the more recently described, later-onset, limb-girdle syndromes associated with abnormal glycosylation.[115,121–125]

CMSs are phenotypically heterogeneous, even within neonates and children. This heterogeneity exists both within and between different CMS genotypes, likely due to the variety of proteins affected. The CMSs result from the disordered structure of nerve terminals, individual AChRs, abnormal AChR distribution, or abnormal NMT physiology at either the presynaptic, synaptic, or postsynaptic level. Manifestations of CMS serve both to suggest not only a CMS, but also in some cases implicating one or more specific CMS genotypes. These features are outlined in Tables 26-2 and 26-3 and further described below.

Cardinal clinical features include muscle weakness and fatigue, muscle hypotrophy, and skeletal abnormalities such as low-set ears, high-arched palate, scoliosis, and contractures. Importantly, many patients do not report fluctuations in weakness. Additionally, given the chronicity of extraocular motility abnormalities, severity of ophthalmoplegia, when present, often exceeds symptoms of diplopia. Episodic apneas may occur, particularly in choline acetyltransferase (ChAT), COLQ, and SCN4A CMS. CMS may become evident in utero with recognition of reduced fetal movement. This phenotype is most associated with AChR γ subunit gene mutations and to a lesser extent with mutations of the α, β, and δ subunits, Dok-7, and rapsyn genes.[126] More commonly, CMSs present at birth or during infancy. As "floppy infants," patients have neonatal hypotonia in combination with a poor suck and weak cry, or apneic episodes. Contractures are another potential neonatal manifestation and have been reported in rapsyn deficiency (associated with facial deformities), AChR deficiency (particularly the γ and fetal γ subunits), GFPT1, ALG2, and ALG14 deficiencies.[122–125,127]

When present, ptosis and diplopia help distinguish CMS from other causes of weakness in all age groups (Fig. 26-2).[128] Ptosis in CMS is typically, but not universally, symmetric and diurnally variable. However, in some patients, particularly those with later-onset, limb-girdle weakness may predominate with relative sparing of oculobulbar musculature. Historically, this was referred to as limb-girdle MG.[109,129–131] This nomenclature has been supplanted by classification based on genotype as mutations correlating with this phenotype

TABLE 26-2. CONGENITAL MYASTHENIC SYNDROMES

CMS Subtype	Gene/Protein Deficiency	Clinical Features	Electrophysiological Features	Response to AChE Inhibitors	Treatment
Presynaptic disorder					
CMS with paucity of ACh release	ChAT	AR; early onset; respiratory failure at birth; episodic apnea; improvement with age	Decremental response with RNS	Improve	AChE inhibitors; 3,4-DAP
Synaptic disorder					
AChE deficiency	COLQ	AR; early onset; variable severity; axial weakness with scoliosis; apnea; ±EOM involvement, slow or absent pupillary responses	Afterdischarges on nerve stimulation and decrement with RNS	Worsen	Albuterol; ephedrine; 3,4-DAP; avoid AChE inhibitors
Postsynaptic disorders involving AChR deficiency or kinetics					
Primary AChR deficiency	AChR subunit genes	AR; early onset; variable severity; fatigue; typical MG features	Decremental response with RNS	Improve	AChE inhibitors; 3,4-DAP
AChR kinetic disorder: slow-channel syndrome	AChR subunit genes	AD; onset childhood to early adult; weak forearm extensors and neck; respiratory weakness; variable severity	Afterdischarges on nerve stimulation and decrement with RNS	Worsen	Fluoxetine and Quinidine; avoid AChE inhibitors
AChR kinetic disorder: fast-channel syndrome	AChR subunit genes	AR; onset early; mild to severe; ptosis, EOM involvement; weakness and fatigue	Decremental response with RNS	Improve	AChE inhibitors; caution with 3,4-DAP
Postsynaptic disorders involving abnormal clustering/function of AChR					
	Dok-7	AR; limb-girdle weakness with ptosis but no EOM involvement	Decremental response with RNS	Variable	Albuterol; ephedrine; may worsen with AChE inhibitors
	Rapsyn	AR; early onset with hypotonia, respiratory failure, and arthrogryposis at birth to early adult onset resembling MG	Decremental response with RNS	Variable	Albuterol
	Agrin	AR; limb-girdle or distal weakness; apnea	Decremental response with RNS	Variable	Albuterol; may worsen with AChE inhibitors
	MuSK	AR; congenital or childhood onset of ptosis, EOM land progressive limb-girdle weakness	Decremental response with RNS	Variable	Variable response to AChE inhibitors and 3,4-DAP; positive response to albuterol
	LPR4	AR; congenital onset with hypotonia; ventilatory failure; mild ptosis and EOM weakness, proximal weakness	Decremental response with RNS	Worsen	Worsen with AChE inhibitors
Other postsynaptic disorders					
Limb-girdle CMS with tubular aggregates	GFPT1; DPAGT1; ALG2; ALG14	AR; limb-girdle weakness usually without ptosis or EOM weakness; onset in infancy or early adult	Decremental response with RNS	Variable	Albuterol; ephedrine; variable response to AChE inhibitors and 3,4-DAP; albuterol
Congenital muscular dystrophy with myasthenia	Plectin	AR; infantile or childhood onset of generalized weakness including ptosis and EOM; epidermolysis bullosa simplex; elevated CK	Decremental response with RNS	Variable	No response to AChE and 3,4-DAP

AD, autosomal dominant; AR, autosomal recessive; ChAT, choline acetyl transferase; CMS, congenital myasthenic syndrome; COLQ, collaginic tail of end-plate acetylcholinesterase; Dok-7, downstream of tyrosine kinase 7; DPAGT1, UDP-N-acetylglucosamine-dolichyl-phosphate N-acetylglucosamine phosphotransferase; GFPT1, glutamine-fructose-6-phosphate amidotransferase 1; LRP4, lipoprotein receptor-related protein 4; MuSK, muscle-specific kinase; RNS, repetitive nerve stimulation; 3,4-DAP, 3,4-diaminopyridine.

TABLE 26-3. DIAGNOSTIC CLUES USED TO IDENTIFY AND CLASSIFY CONGENITAL MYASTHENIC SYNDROMES

General clues (relative, not absolute)
- Early onset (in utero, neonatal, or infantile)
- Consanguinity, affected relatives suggesting an AR pedigree
- Seronegativity for autoimmune MG
- Refractoriness to cholinesterase inhibitors
- Failure to respond to immunomodulating agents
- Nonspecific light microscopic changes in muscle (if performed)

Epidemiology
- Ethnicity
  - German, Western/Central Europe
    - Dok-7, Rapsyn deficiencies
  - Brazil, Portugal, Spain, Tunisia, Algeria
    - AChR ε deficiency—CHRNE
  - Near-Eastern Jewish
    - Rapsyn deficiency
- Age of onset
  - Severe, lethal, akinetic syndrome
    - AChR γ deficiency
    - AChR α, β, δ subunit deficiencies
    - Rapsyn deficiency
    - Dok-7 deficiency
  - Typical onset—birth or infancy
    - ChAT deficiency
    - AChE deficiency
    - AChR subunit deficiencies
    - AChR deficiency with kinetic defect—fast-channel syndrome
    - Rapsyn deficiency
    - LRP4
  - Variable including potential late onset
    - Rapsyn deficiency (some cases)
    - Dok-7 deficiency
    - GFPT1 myasthenia (some cases)
    - DPAGT1 myasthenia
    - AChR (subunit) deficiency with kinetic defect—slow-channel syndrome
    - MuSK deficiency
    - ALG2 and ALG14
- Symptoms worsened by cold
  - AChE deficiency
- Periodic exacerbations
  - Intercurrent infection
    - Rapsyn deficiency
    - ChAT deficiency
    - AChR (subunit) deficiency and fast-channel syndrome
  - Pregnancy and menstruation
    - Dok-7
    - MuSK deficiency
  - Indeterminate reasons
    - DPAGT1 MG
- Dominant inheritance
  - AChR deficiency—kinetic disorder—slow channel
  - SNAP25
  - PURA
  - SYT2 (1/3 of patients)

Electrophysiology
- Afterdischarges
  - AChE deficiency (not universal)
  - AChR deficiency—kinetic disorder—slow channel
  - Agrin deficiency
- CMAP incremental response
  - Congenital LEMS
- Decremental response to repetitive stimulation at 2–5 Hz
  - AChR (subunit) deficiency
  - Dok-7
  - ChAT deficiency (some cases)
  - AChE deficiency
  - Congenital LEMS
  - DPAGT1 CMS
  - GFPT1 CMS
  - ALG2/ALG14 CMS
  - LRP4 CMS
- CMAP decremental response to variable rates
  - ChAT deficiency (10 Hz RNS for 5 minutes)

Muscle histology
- End-plate myopathy
  - AChR deficiency—kinetic disorder—slow channel
  - AChE deficiency
- Tubular aggregates
  - GFPT1 CMS
  - DPAGT1 CMS
  - ALG2/ALG14 CMS

Response to treatment
- Refractory to or exacerbated by cholinesterase inhibitors
  - AChE deficiency (COLQ) (relative contraindication)
  - Laminin β2 myasthenia (relative contraindication)
  - AChR (subunit)—kinetic disorder—slow-channel syndrome
  - Dok-7 deficiency
  - Agrin deficiency
  - Rapsyn deficiency
  - Plectin
  - LRP4 CMS
- Responsive to cholinesterase inhibitors
  - Laminin β2 myasthenia
  - GFPT1 myasthenia
  - DPAGT1 myasthenia
  - ChAT deficiency (variable)
  - AChR (subunit) deficiency or fast-channel syndrome (partial)
  - CMS with a paucity of synaptic vesicles
  - MuSK deficiency (partial)
  - Congenital LEMS
- Refractory to 3,4-DAP
  - AChE deficiency
  - Congenital LEMS
  - Agrin defect
  - AChR deficiency—kinetic disorder—slow channel
  - AChR deficiency—kinetic disorder—fast-channel syndrome (relatively contraindicated)
  - Dok-7 deficiency
- Responsive to 3,4-DAP
  - ChAT deficiency (variable)
  - AChR (subunit) deficiency
  - Rapsyn deficiency
  - Agrin deficiency
  - MuSK deficiency (limited)
  - Congenital LEMS
  - GFPT1 myasthenia

TABLE 26-3. (CONTINUED)

- **Responsive to sympathomimetic amines (albuterol, ephedrine, salbutamol)**
    - AChR deficiency—kinetic disorder—slow channel
    - AChE deficiency (some cases)
    - Agrin deficiency
    - MuSK deficiency
    - Dok-7 deficiency (some cases)
    - Laminin β2 myasthenia
    - DPAGT1 MG
- **Responsive to open-channel blockers (quinidine, quinine, fluoxetine)**
    - Slow-channel syndrome
- **Responsive to guanidine**
    - Congenital LEMS

Phenotype
- **Pattern of weakness**
    - Typical oculobulbar pattern
        - CMS with a paucity of synaptic vesicles
        - ACh receptor deficiency
        - MuSK deficiency
    - Ophthalmoparesis limited or absent
        - AChR deficiency with kinetic defect—slow-channel syndrome
        - Dok-7 myasthenia
        - GFPT1 deficiency
        - Rapsyn deficiency
        - ChAT deficiency
        - Congenital LEMS
        - Agrin deficiency
        - ALG2/ALG14 CMS
    - Significant involvement of limb and axial muscles
        - ACh receptor deficiency
        - Dok-7 deficiency
        - GFPT1 MG
        - DPAGT1 MG
        - Rapsyn (some cases)
        - Agrin deficiency (some cases)
        - MuSK deficiency
        - ALG2/ALG14
    - Preferential involvement of distal muscles or distinctive muscle groups
        - Rapsyn (late-onset) (foot drop)
        - AChR deficiency—kinetic disorder—slow channel (cervical muscles, wrist/finger drop)
        - Agrin deficiency
        - GFPT1 myasthenia (scapular winging, foot drop, wrist/finger drop)
        - DPAGT1 MG (foot drop, wrist/finger drop)
    - Stridor/vocal cord paralysis
        - Dok-7 deficiency
    - Infantile hypotonia
        - ChAT deficiency
        - AChR deficiency
        - LRP4
    - Episodic apnea
        - ChAT deficiency
        - Na—channel myasthenia
        - Rapsyn deficiency
        - AChE deficiency
        - Dok-7 deficiency
        - MuSK deficiency
        - GFPT1
- **Contractures or dysmorphic features**
    - Rapsyn deficiency (facial deformities)
    - ACh receptor deficiency (particularly the gamma and fetal γ subunit)
    - GFPT1 myasthenia
    - ALG2/ALG14 CMS
- **Delayed pupillary light reflex**
    - Acetylcholinesterase deficiency
    - Laminin β2 myasthenia
- **Systemic features**
    - Nephrotic syndrome, ocular abnormalities
        - Laminin β2 myasthenia
    - Epidermolysis bullosa simplex
        - Plectin deficiency

continue to be identified. Currently, Dok-7, GFPT1, DPAGT1, ALG2, and ALG14 deficiencies are the most frequent causes of this syndrome.[113]

Other distinct patterns of weakness include scapular winging, wrist/finger drop, and foot drop. The finger drop may affect some digits more than others and suggest an increased likelihood of specific CMS genotypes in the appropriate context (Tables 26-2 and 26-3; Figs. 26-3 and 26-4). Despite NMJ localization, muscle atrophy or hypotrophy is sometimes seen. In older individuals, limited stamina and prominent fatigue may be the primary sources of morbidity.

Both diurnal variation and periodic exacerbation of CMS may occur, the latter commonly resulting from typical potential triggers of all disorders of NMT: fever or intercurrent illness, pregnancy, menstruation, medications which impair neuromuscular transmission or stress.[120,126,127] Involvement of other end organs with certain CMS genotypes may produce recognizable syndromes providing an additional source of diagnostic information. Cardiac and smooth muscle, however, are uncommonly involved in most syndromes[132] (Tables 26-2 and 26-3). We are unaware of significant dysautonomia occurring in these disorders. Natural history of CMS is quite variable. Delayed motor milestones are the norm in affected infants. Some individuals have a static course whereas insidious disease progression is anticipated in some subtypes.

As rare disorders, CMSs are often not initially considered in the differential diagnosis of a weak patient. Predictably, this pitfall is more likely to be encountered in older individuals, particularly in those with predominantly limb-girdle patterns of weakness. Even in an older individual with a typical MG phenotype, CMSs should be given consideration in any patient with suspected seronegative myasthenia, myopathy of indeterminate cause, or other proximal weakness. The following summarizes the notable clinical features of

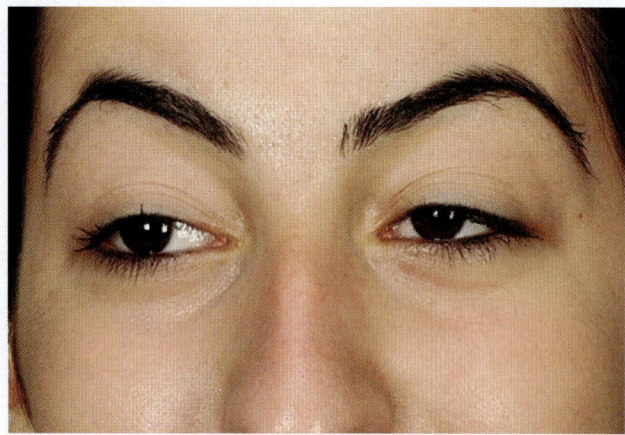

Figure 26-2. Ptosis, compensatory frontalis contraction, and partial ophthalmoparesis in a 15-year-old female with epsilon subunit deficiency. (Used with permission from Prof. Feza Deymeer, University of Istanbul, Istanbul, Turkey.)

specific CMS. Associated genes are listed in parentheses after each disorder heading (Tables 26-2 and 26-3). Five CMS disorders account for approximately 90% of CMS. These include primary AChR deficiency or kinetic abnormality/CHRNE (50%), rapsyn deficiency (15%–20%), AChE deficiency/COLQ (10%–15%), Dok-7 (10%–15%), and ChAT (4%–5%). We will focus our discussion on these syndromes.

Presynaptic CMS (Approximately 5%)

Choline Acetyltransferase Deficiency

Disorder of ACh synthesis, and specifically ChAT deficiency, is the most common subtype of presynaptic CMS. As a review, ChAT catalyzes transfer of an acetyl group from acetyl coenzyme A (AcCoA) to choline in the formation of ACh in cholinergic neurons.[133] Thus, ChAT deficiency results in impaired ACh synthesis. This disorder characteristically manifests as a distinctive phenotype of bulbar weakness with a weak cry and

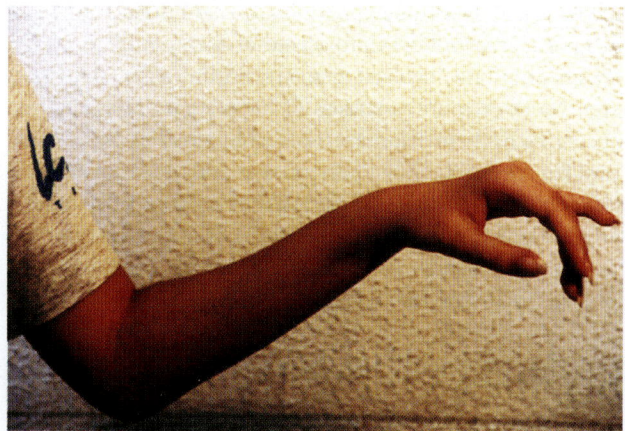

Figure 26-3. Weakness of wrist and finger extension in slow-channel syndrome. (Used with permission from Prof. Feza Deymeer, University of Istanbul, Istanbul, Turkey.)

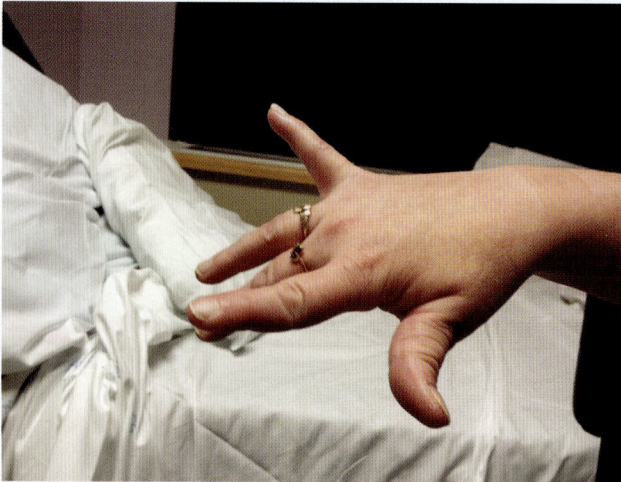

Figure 26-4. Weakness of finger extension in adult female with neonatal dysphagia and apneic episodes attributed to nonspecific myopathy. Became ventilator dependent following scoliosis surgery at age 11 and walked unassisted until age 15. Developed unilateral ptosis in adulthood. Diagnosed with CMS secondary to agrin deficiency at age 43.

poor sucking capability. Ventilatory distress with episodic and unpredictable apnea is the most troublesome manifestation. Ptosis is common, but ophthalmoparesis is rare. The natural history is variable. Apneic episodes may begin in the neonatal period, infancy, or childhood and may be lethal. They may resolve or recur episodically even into adult life. Exacerbations can be triggered by intercurrent infection or other stress.[120,133–137]

Congenital LEMS

Rare cases of congenital LEMS like CMS have been described, predominantly recognized by the characteristic presynaptic EDX pattern described in the diagnostic section. The two described cases involved a severely affected neonate with hypotonia, bulbar weakness, and ventilator dependency and a young child with less-severe manifestations including delayed motor milestones without eye movement or other distinctive abnormalities.[110,138] LEMS like CMS can be related to abnormality in SNARE proteins and calcium sensors. Mutations involving the mutations in the following proteins have been associated with congenital LEMS: AGRN, SYT2, VAMP1, SNAP25B and MUNC13-1, LAMA5.[139,140]

Other Presynaptic CMS Subtypes

Several additional less common presynaptic disorders have been identified. Mutations in the presynaptic sodium-dependent high-affinity choline transporter 1 (CHT1/SLC5A7) are associated with severe phenotypes of CMS, often with respiratory crises.[141–143] Case reports of patients with paucity of synaptic vesicles describe a phenotype of ptosis, ophthalmoparesis, facial weakness, and generalized fatigable weakness of the extremities that began in infancy.[126,136,144,145] The molecular basis of this disorder is unknown. Recently identified defects in vesicular acetylcholine transporter (VACHT)[146,147] are associated with a severe CMS. Mutation in mitochondrial citrate carrier SLC25A1[148] and PREPL deficiency[149] cause a presynaptic CMS.[150]

Synaptic CMS (Approximately 15%)

End-Plate Acetylcholine Esterase Deficiency/COLQ

This deficiency is the most common synaptic CMS and is inherited in a recessive fashion. Despite the name, end-plate AChE deficiency is caused by recessive mutations in the COLQ gene encoding the collagenic tail subunit; it is not caused by mutations in the AChE gene encoding the catalytic subunit.[113,115,119,151,152] Due to the absence of AChE, ACh has a prolonged lifetime in the synaptic space. This increases the duration of the end-plate current making it outlast the refractory period of the muscle fiber.[153–155] This is the basis of excitation of a second, repetitive CMAP which can be seen on routine NCS.

Natural history is again variable. Most have a typical neonatal disorder with severe morbidity and a smaller group has later-onset cases with a more indolent course. Early-onset cases tend to be dominated by hypotonia and delayed motor milestones, ventilatory and bulbar difficulties, associated with ptosis and ophthalmoparesis in some cases. Slow pupillary responses to light are reported as a distinctive although not necessarily unique feature of this genotype. In later life, limb weakness, muscle atrophy, and skeletal deformities, particularly involving the spine may become apparent. Survival into adulthood is the norm.

Laminin β2 Deficiency

This is a rare, severe form of synaptic CMS. As the β2 chain of laminin is found in other tissues, LAMβ2 gene mutations may also result in Pierson syndrome with associated congenital nephrotic syndrome and ocular defects. The described phenotype includes delayed motor milestones, and facial and limb-girdle weakness. Ptosis, ophthalmoparesis, pupillary and macular abnormalities and ventilatory muscle weakness may occur.[152,156,157]

Postsynaptic CMS (Approximately 80%)

Postsynaptic disorders comprise approximately 80% of CMS cases and are divided into CMS with reduced AChR expression (with or without minor kinetic abnormality) or AChR kinetic abnormality (some with mildly reduced AChR expression). CMS related to reduced AChR expression include those with mutations in Dok-7, rapsyn, MuSK, and AChR mutations with or without plectin deficiency.

AChR Deficiency: Structural or Organizational

Dok-7 Deficiency[121,158–164]

Dok-7 deficiency typically manifests with delayed onset in childhood, but may present as late as the third decade, with a variable phenotype. Although infantile onset can occur, normal motor milestones are commonly achieved before deterioration begins. Disease severity is variable, ranging from the mildly to severely symptomatic individuals. A progressive course is the most common. The typical phenotype is a limb-girdle pattern of weakness with ambulatory difficulties during childhood. Ptosis may occur in later life. Ophthalmoparesis is infrequent and typically mild. Facial weakness is common. Significant bulbar symptoms including vocal cord paralysis, stridor, and poor feeding may occur in infancy. Severe disability including ventilatory failure may occur by the third decade in some cases. Worsening during pregnancy has been described.[165]

Rapsyn Deficiency[122,166–170]

This is one of the more common CMS, constituting approximately 15%–20% of cases. The phenotype including age of onset is variable. Most cases present at birth or at infancy although cases presenting as late as the third decade have occured. Neonatal arthrogryposis is common. Prognathism and high-arched palate can occur. Crises may be precipitated by intercurrent infection. Ptosis, facial, jaw, and neck weakness are common whereas ophthalmoparesis is rare. Limb weakness is more common in later-onset cases. Although often proximal and symmetric, foot drop in late-onset cases is well recognized. If children survive the neonatal period, improvement with aging is not uncommon and the subsequent course is often benign.

MuSK Deficiency[160,161,171–173]

The few reported cases of this disorder describe onset variability ranging from the neonatal period to later life. There is variability in disease severity as well. Ptosis, partial ophthalmoparesis, and mild facial weakness are commonplace. Weakness affecting proximal limbs, particularly shoulder abductors and ventilatory muscles occur in some but not all individuals.

AChR Mutations with or without Plectin Deficiency[113,174,175]

Plectin is a protein that links cytoskeletal elements to target organelles in different body tissues. It provides crucial support for the junctional folds of the NMJ. As a result, the phenotype includes the potential for multiorgan involvement including skin [epidermolysis bullosa simplex (EBS)], skeletal muscle (muscular dystrophy), smooth muscle (esophageal atresia), and cardiac muscle (cardiomyopathy). The phenotype typically begins in infancy as EBS and evolves into a disorder producing ptosis and ophthalmoparesis, dysphagia, facial, and limb weakness associated with a decremental response to slow repetitive stimulation. Modest CK elevations may occur.

AChR Kinetic Abnormalities

Acetylcholine Receptor (AChR) (Subunit Deficiency), With or Without Kinetic Defect [i.e., Slow (Closing) Channel Syndrome or Fast (Closing) Channel Syndrome] (CHRNA1, CHRNB1, CHRND0, and CHRNE)[133–135,176–179]

Subunit mutations are the most common forms of the postsynaptic CMS. The ACh channel typically consists of two α subunits, one β, one δ, and one ε, the latter which normally supplants the fetal γ subunit late in gestation. Adult subunits are encoded by the individual genes listed above. The ε subunit gene (CHRNE) is the most common subunit deficiency and the most common CMS in most series.[126] This mutation tends to be more benign than other CMS as the ε subunit deficiency may be buffered to some extent by persistent fetal γ subunit function. This compensatory mechanism is not possible for other subunit mutations. Subunit mutations may adversely affect neuromuscular transmission by at least two mechanisms which occur independently or concurrently. They either reduce subunit expression and consequently receptor function and/or alter ACh channel kinetic properties. Kinetic alterations produce either a slow-channel (i.e., slow to close resulting in increased ionic passage) or fast-channel (i.e., fast to close resulting in truncation of normal ionic passage) syndrome. The channel of interest connects the extracellular to intracellular compartments. As previously implied, impaired NMT may result from either subunit deficiency and/or abnormal kinetic function and are not mutually exclusive.

The phenotype of AChR subunit mutations is again variable though more likely to be static than progressive. As described, mutations in the AChR ε subunit gene with reduced subunit expression typically correlate with a mild phenotype. Affected patients tend to have a nonprogressive phenotype typically manifesting as feeding problems and ptosis at birth or in infancy. Ophthalmoparesis is common although may not be present at birth (Fig. 26-2). Limb weakness occurs but ventilatory muscle involvement is rare. In contrast, non-ε AChR subunit gene mutations typically correlate with a more severe phenotype with ventilatory crises precipitated by choking and shortening of life expectancy. EDX patterns of fast-channel syndrome do not have the same characteristic features of slow-channel syndrome (Fig. 26-5).

With a kinetic defect producing a slow-channel syndrome, the clinical course is typically indolent, often sparing cranial musculature, and frequently affecting cervical muscles as well as wrist/finger extensors (Figs. 26-3 and 26-4). Spinal deformities may develop later in life. The fast-channel syndrome tends to arise from the mutations in the α, δ, and ε subunit genes.[180] Neonatal onset is the norm with a severe phenotype incorporating ptosis and ophthalmoparesis, bulbar, and ventilatory weakness.

The Escobar syndrome results from mutations in the fetal γ subunit. As the contributions of the fetal subunit are largely dissipated by 33 weeks of gestation, neonates born with γ subunit mutations are typically born with arthrogryposis and ventilatory difficulties and do not develop a typical CMS phenotype.

Agrin Deficiency[176,181–187]

Despite the presynaptic site of its synthesis, the major role of agrin is to initiate AChR clustering by binding to lipoprotein receptor-related protein 4 (LRP4) resulting in phosphorylation of MuSK.[182,188,189] Activated MuSK interacts in

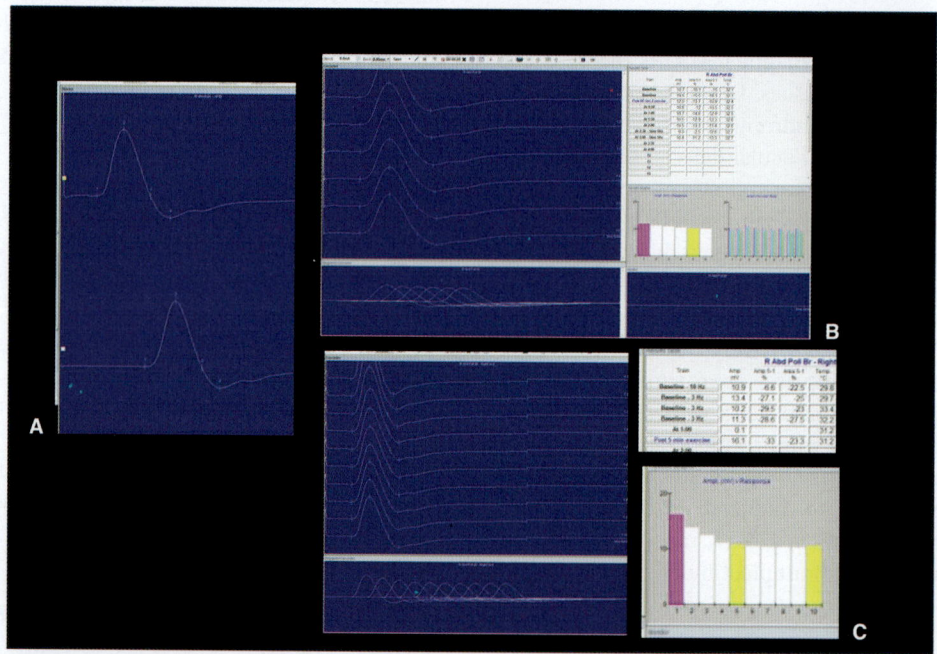

Figure 26-5. A 16-year-old girl with ptosis, ophthalmoplegia, facial weakness, hypophonia and distal UE > LE weakness with prominent wrist and finger drop. Deletion in CHRNB1. Responsive to pyridostigmine and 3,4 DAP. (**A**) Normal median-APB CMAP amplitude without repetitive CMAPs. (**B**) 16.1% decrement in 3 Hz RNS of median-APB at baseline with partial repair after exercise and no increase in decrement with 5 Hz RNS. (**C**) No additional decrement after 5 minutes of exercise.

turn with Dok-7 and rapsyn to promote AChR aggregation. Agrin CMS is rarely reported, with a mild phenotype characterized by ptosis, delayed motor milestones, and mild proximal weakness. We have seen prominent head drop and wrist and finger drop when the diagnosis was delayed until adulthood.[190,191] Ophthalmoparesis is an inconsistent feature. Facial and ventilatory muscle weakness occurs in some cases.

LPR4 Deficiency[113,184,192–194]

LPR4 gene mutation has been described to cause CMS. The phenotype includes hypotonia at birth with ventilatory and feeding difficulties. Motor milestones can be delayed. Prominent fatigue with proximal greater than distal extremity weakness can become evident along with mild ptosis and ophthalmoparesis.

Sodium Channel CMS[195–201]

Several dozen mutations of SCN4A encoding the Nav1.4 sodium channel in skeletal muscles have been identified and linked with a spectrum of neuromuscular disorders. The most notable are myotonic disorders/periodic paralysis, which manifest with a gain of function mutation. Recently, loss of function mutations has been associated with CMS and congenital myopathy.[202] Reported cases are uncommon but typically severe, present in infancy, and are associated with recurrent attacks of apnea.[195,196] Interestingly, recent work has demonstrated SCN4A variants which alter Nav1.4 function in infants who have died from SIDS.[197]

Glutamine-Fructose-6-Phosphate Transaminase 1 Deficiency (GFPT1)[123,198]

Like many of the CMS, this genotype has phenotypic heterogeneity. The onset of reported cases ranges from in-utero recognition to 19 years of age. The course is typically slowly progressive. Neonatal cases may be arthrogrypotic, with poor bulbar function and apneic episodes. A later-onset syndrome dominated by a proximal > distal pattern of weakness is the most common phenotype. The distal muscles most involved include forearm extensors, intrinsic hand muscles, and the anterior compartment of the leg. Serum CK values are elevated in 50% of cases. RNS is abnormal without unique features (Fig. 26-6).

Dolichyl-Phosphate N-Acetylglucosamine-Phosphotransferase 1 Deficiency (DPAGT1)[125,199,200]

Like GFPT1, DPAGT1 is an enzyme thought to be necessary for the glycosylation of the nicotinic AChR and integral to the assembly and insertion of the channel into the postsynaptic membrane. It shares other features with GFPT1 CMS including a propensity to begin beyond the neonatal period and to produce a limb-girdle pattern of weakness. Life expectancy is not typically altered and individuals in their sixth decade have been reported. Other features common to GFPT1 and DPAGT1 CMS are tubular aggregates on muscle biopsy, decremental responses to slow repetitive stimulation, and responsiveness to cholinesterase inhibitors, and 3,4-DAP. Unlike GFPT1 CMS, CK values are reported to be normal. Consistent with DPAGT1's role in glycosylation in locations

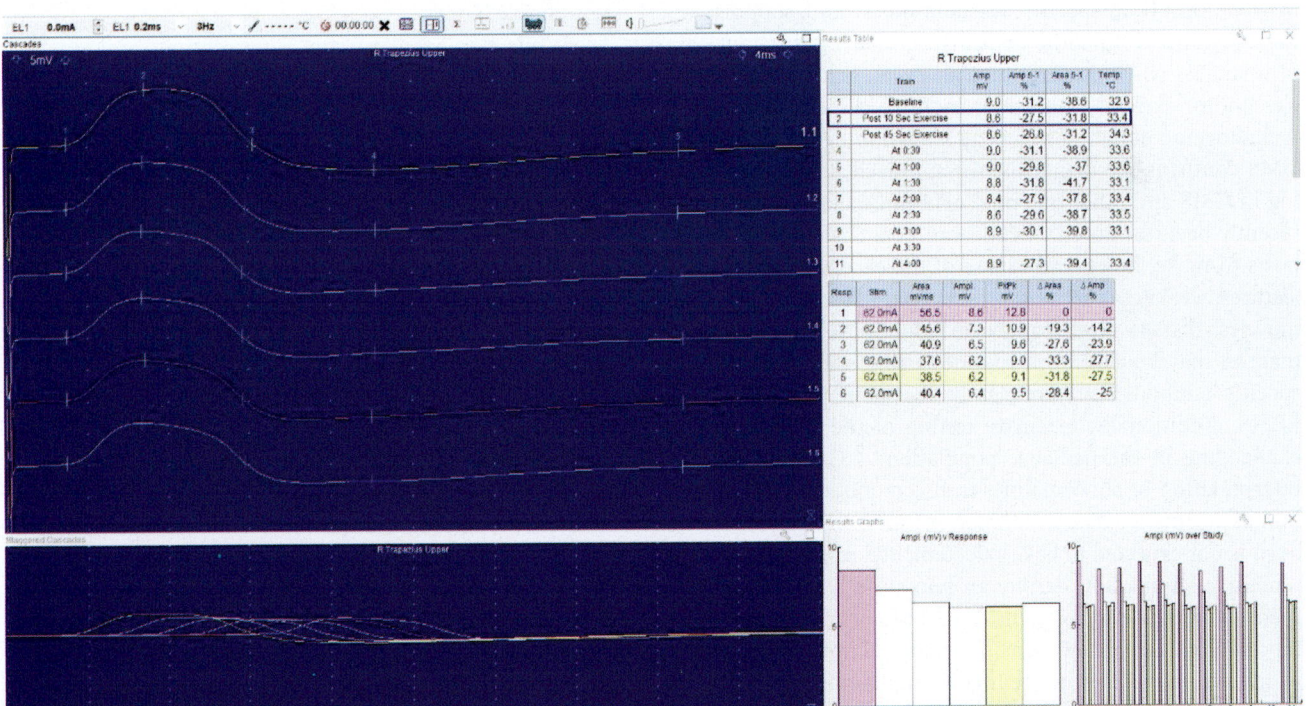

Figure 26-6. Abnormal slow RNS of the SAN-trapezius in a 35-year-old with GFPT1 CMS. Note lack of postexercise facilitation or repair of the decrement and lack of postexercise exhaustion in this patient.

other than the NMJ, mutations of this gene may also produce a severe, neonatal multisystem disorder referred to as type 2 which may include seizures, microcephaly, ventilatory distress, hypotonia, and behavioral abnormalities. Phenotype appears to be determined by the location of the mutation.

ALG2 and ALG14 CMS[124,201]

Asparagine-related glycosylation plays a critical role in protein folding, transport, localization, and folding. Recessively inherited mutations in these two genes that contribute to this process have been recently reported to result in CMS that bear many similarities to DPAGT1 and GFPT1 CMS. Most affected individuals reported to date have had a limb-girdle phenotype affecting limb muscles preferentially, typically symmetrically with proximal predominance. Contractures are common, and scapular winging and high-arched palate may occur. While facial weakness may be present, extraocular muscle involvement is not a typical feature of the disease. Learning disability may occur. Onset age ranges from infancy with hypotonia to adulthood, although initial symptoms in the late first decade are the norm. Wheelchair dependency may or may not occur. A decremental response to slow repetitive stimulation and responsiveness to cholinesterase inhibitors are typical. Tubular aggregates may be found on muscle biopsy. CK is usually normal but may be minimally elevated.

DIAGNOSIS AND DIFFERENTIAL DIAGNOSIS

A diagnosis of CMS is suspected when there is a clinical phenotype of weakness, often fatigable, the absence of MG- or LEMS-specific autoantibodies, and supportive EDX features.[119] Infantile or pediatric onset, a distribution of weakness which includes ocular, facial, and bulbar muscles and/or skeletal deformities increase clinical suspicion. A pathogenic mutation in a gene known to be causative for CMS confirms the diagnosis. An approach to genetic testing in CMS and other potential neuromuscular mimics has recently been proposed.[203] CMS can be a challenging diagnosis to make, however, because of the exceptions to these features: weakness can be static and spare facial and cranial muscles, disease onset can be in adulthood, EDX abnormalities may be absent on routine testing and MG/LEMS-specific antibodies are frequently absent in juvenile MG/LEMS. Additionally, extensive testing of the NMJ can be challenging in the pediatric population.[119] Caution in the interpretation of abnormalities is also required as there are limited normative data in infancy. A full-term normal newborn is not expected to have a decremental response to slow repetitive stimulation despite an immature NMJ. A decrement in response to frequencies of 5 Hz or more has been reported in normal newborns. Therefore, abnormalities seen using techniques that utilize higher stimulation frequencies including stimulated SFEMG must be interpreted with caution in this population.[204–206] Notably, patients with myopathies can rarely exhibit decrement on RNS.[207]

Identification of pathogenic mutations from benign polymorphisms is another challenge. This process involves detailed clinical phenotyping and EDX studies, ultrastructural analysis of NMJs and in vitro physiological testing of NMT to prove pathogenicity.[78,110] Mutational analysis is also incapable of defining a kinetic defect in association with an identified subunit mutation. Kinetic defects, important in therapeutic decision making, are identified only with the use of in vitro microelectrode or single-channel patch clamp recordings.[166] Successful genotyping can occur in half to as many as 90% of CMS cases.[126,127,176] Next-generation sequencing has changed the approach to genetic testing which was previously targeted to single genes based on phenotype and likelihood/frequency (Tables 26-2 and 26-3).

The differential diagnosis of CMS in the neonatal period is largely that of the floppy infant (Table 1-2). Clinical features may be nonspecific and involve only feeding problems, weak cry and suck, hypotonia, and arthrogryposis.[119] In the presence of ptosis and ophthalmoparesis, consideration should be given to the possibility of transient neonatal MG due to passive transfer of maternal antibodies, certain congenital myopathies, mitochondrial myopathy, and myotonic dystrophy (Table 1-8). Later in infancy, infantile botulism may be considered, particularly with an acute to subacute onset, and symptoms of cholinergic dysautonomia, such as sluggish pupils and constipation. In childhood, autoimmune MG and rarely autoimmune LEMS require consideration. When the phenotype is a limb-girdle pattern of weakness, myopathy (numerous) and spinal muscular atrophy are primary considerations. The latter may be suspected by the presence of fasciculations and a neurogenic pattern on EDX, or if necessary, muscle biopsy.

While important to complete, routine serologic testing is of limited diagnostic value in CMS. MG and LEMS autoantibodies should be checked to exclude an autoimmune etiology. Serum CK levels are characteristically normal or modestly elevated similar to other neuromuscular disorders with which CMS might be confused.[208] CPK testing may be helpful in distinguishing between DPAGT1 and GFPT1, which have similar phenotypes, but CPK is normal in the former but it is elevated in approximately 50% of the latter group.[208] Muscle biopsy is typically unnecessary when next-generation sequencing can be performed.

Several features characterize EDX studies in CMS.[205] Repetitive CMAPs are typically identified in only three forms of CMS: AChE deficiency, agrin, and AChR receptor (associated with the slow-channel syndrome) deficiency. In all three, the afterdischarges represent prolonged postsynaptic depolarization and undergo early decrement before the primary CMAP on RNS. Afterdischarges may also occur with neuromyotonia, envenomation with K^+ channel poisons, intoxication with organophosphate or other anticholinesterase agents, and certain muscle channelopathies. Decremental response may be present with slow-frequency RNS or after prolonged exercise. MUAPs may be variable and SFEMG abnormal.

As described below and summarized in Tables 26-2 and 26-3, however, not all CMS may be identified by abnormal EDX testing. Repetitive stimulation at various frequencies and stimulated SFEMG are the most frequently used techniques in the pediatric age group.[205]

Decremental responses to repetitive stimulation have been described in all forms of CMS. As with autoimmune MG, a decremental response in CMS is expected in clinically weak muscles and in some, but not necessarily all, clinically unaffected muscles, but may not always be present.[204] Standard RNS protocols at 2–3 Hz may have to be modified to identify abnormal NMT in some CMS syndromes. For example, certain forms (e.g., ChAT deficiency) require prolonged stimulation for up to 5 minutes at higher rates (10 Hz) to bring out the decrement, which is followed by a slow recovery of CMAP amplitude (Fig. 26-6).[120,123,124,127,194,201] Additionally, the magnitude of decrement in AChE deficiency and slow-channel syndrome typically becomes greater with faster rates of stimulation, thereby demonstrating "rate-dependent decrement."[127]

Interestingly, in contrast to autoimmune LEMS where pathology always exists at the VGCC, some but not all presynaptic CMS demonstrate CMAP facilitation after brief exercise or fast RNS.[204] This likely owes to the heterogeneity of proteins affected by presynaptic gene mutations with functions in acetylcholine synthesis, packaging into vesicles, and vesicle docking and release from the presynaptic nerve terminal.[204] Synaptobrevin-1-CMS, MUNC-13-1-CMS, synaptotagmin-2-CMS, laminin alpha5-CMS, and agrin-CMS have facilitation.[204]

MUAPs that are polyphasic and smaller in both amplitude and duration may occur in CMS because of at least two mechanisms. Neuromuscular blockade at individual NMJs may reduce the number of single-fiber action potentials that contribute to the normal MUAP size and configuration. In addition, in AChE deficiency-CMS and SCS-CMS, an end-plate myopathy may develop because of excessive end-plate stimulation resulting also in lower-amplitude and shorter duration MUAPs.[133]

HISTOPATHOLOGY

Light microscopic examination of muscle biopsy is of limited value in CMS but is often performed early in the patient's workup for evaluation of myopathy, particularly if the patient presents as an older individual. Perhaps the most specific potential finding is the presence of tubular aggregates. Although neither sensitive nor specific for CMS,[209] tubular aggregates are seen in some limb-girdle phenotypes of CMS including most commonly GFPT1 but also DPAGT1, and ALG2/ALG14.[123–125,200,210–214] Otherwise, light microscopic findings are of limited benefit. In most cases, they neither distinguish CMS from other neuromuscular diseases, nor aid in defining a specific CMS subtype.

Several nonspecific, largely myopathic findings have been described in muscle biopsy specimens from CMS patients. Type 1 fiber predominance is perhaps the most common of these and has been described in rapsyn, Dok-7, GFPT1, and MuSK CMS.[121,122,158,161,198] Additional features described in other CMS including Dok-7, GFPT1, plectin, and MuSK include type 2 fiber atrophy/hypotrophy, isolated myofiber necrosis and regeneration, diminished oxidative stain uptake, ragged red fibers, increased frequency of internal nuclei, fiber splitting, and subsarcolemmal nuclear chains.[121,158,161,198,121] Autophagic vacuoles that may stain with acid phosphatase and may contain glycogen have been described in DPAGT1 and GFPT1 CMS.[123,125] Neurogenic features of small-grouped atrophy and target formations have been described.[123,125,138,198]

Ultrastructural abnormalities of the NMJ occur in most CMS.[110] They are not CMS subtype specific. Simplified junctional folds appear to be the most common abnormality in some, but not all, end plates in many CMS and are frequently associated with reduced numbers of AChRs.[123,175] This finding has been reported in a number of syndromes including the slow-channel AChR kinetic disorder, and the AChE, LAMB2, rapsyn, plectin, MuSK, LRP4, GFPT1, and Dok-7 forms of CMS.[122,123,126,161,175,194] The pattern of simplification of the junctional folds is focal in synaptic disorders and diffuse in many postsynaptic disorders such as AChR ε subunit or rapsyn deficiency.[152] In synaptic CMS (e.g., LAMB2, agrin, and AChE deficiency, as well as in MuSK CMS), ultrastructural findings may include reduction of the axon terminal size, partial encasement of the nerve endings by Schwann cells, widening of the primary synaptic cleft, and invasion of the synaptic cleft by the processes of Schwann cells in addition to focal simplification of postsynaptic folds.[152] This observation of abnormal presynaptic morphology in a synaptic disorder reflects that the pathophysiology of individual CMS may extend beyond the primary site of involvement. In Dok-7 myasthenia, myeloid structures may populate the junctional cytoplasm. Nerve terminals ending as growth cones without AChR contact has been described in MuSK CMS.[172]

In AChE deficiency and the slow-channel syndrome, prolonged end-plate current produces postsynaptic cationic overloading resulting in an end-plate myopathy.[152] Resultant histological features are subsynaptic degenerative abnormalities, autophagic vacuoles, dilated sarcotubular elements, increased lipid droplets, and apoptosis of junctional nuclei occurring. In the presynaptic disorder of CMS with a paucity of synaptic vesicles, electron microscopy demonstrates the feature that defines the condition.[133] However, ultrastructural abnormalities do not occur routinely in all CMS. In agrin deficiency, congenital LEMS, and the fast-channel kinetic syndrome of AChR deficiency, the postsynaptic regions are ultrastructurally normal.[135]

PATHOGENESIS

Efficiency of NMT depends on many interrelated factors. The first steps are adequate synthesis and packaging of ACh, and optimal positioning of synaptic vesicles at AZs of presynaptic nerve terminals. Equally important are adequate quantal content (e.g., the number of vesicles released following a nerve action potential) and amplitude and duration of current that the vesicular–end-plate interaction produces. Just the right amount of synaptic metabolism of ACh is needed to optimize this vesicular–end-plate interaction. Normal positioning, clustering, and kinetics of both the ACh and Na$^+$ channels on the peaks and troughs of the end-plate folds, respectively, is the last critical factor.

As we have discussed earlier in the chapter, single-gene mutations resulting in abnormal structure or function in one or more of these components of NMT cause CMS. In each CMS subtype, there is altered end-plate current, impaired generation of myofiber action potentials, and consequently, reduced strength and stamina of voluntary muscles. With most genotypes, a reduction in end-plate current occurs. In two of these disorders, however, AChE deficiency and the slow-channel kinetic disorder of the AChR, the current is excessively prolonged.[215] While adverse pathophysiological events typically occurring in a single presynaptic, synaptic, or postsynaptic region, many CMSs have secondary consequences which involve additional loci of the NMJ.

In ChAT deficiency, impaired resynthesis of ACh compromises NMT by progressively depleting quantal content. As such, miniature end-plate potential (MEPP) and end-plate potential (EPP) amplitude are normal at rest but decline with repetitive stimulation at 10 Hz for 5 minutes with subsequent gradual recovery.[135] CMS with a paucity of synaptic vesicles is associated with a reduced density of synaptic vesicles at the AZs. The probability of quantal release, however, meaning the proportion of vesicles released per nerve action potential, is normal.[126] Conversely, in the LEMS variant of CMS, both reduced quantal content and lower probability of quantal release contribute to impairing NMT.[126]

With AChE deficiency, the most common synaptic disorder, the absence of AChE prolongs the life of ACh in the synaptic space and therefore, the duration of the MEPP and EPP. As a result, the duration of synaptic current outlasts the refractory period of the muscle fiber, which overstimulates the postsynaptic region. Neuromuscular transmission is thus impaired by desensitization from ACh overexposure. In addition, there are presynaptic effects with the small and often Schwann cell–encased nerve terminals associated with reduced quantal release. The resulting excessive stimulation promotes cationic overloading, causing an end-plate myopathy.

Laminin is an integral component of the basal lamina, which plays a key role in the creation and configuration of motor end plates. Therefore, LAMB2 deficiency adversely affects the development of complex end-plate anatomy.[133] LAMB2 deficiency also associates with abnormal nerve terminals that are both small and encased by Schwann cells. Widening of the synaptic space and junctional folds, and decreased MEPP are additional consequences.[126,135] Agrin is bound to laminin on the synaptic basement membrane. Therefore, agrin deficiency (described below) likely has a synaptic as well as postsynaptic pathogenesis.[134]

The most common postsynaptic disorders involve mutations of AChR subunits, most commonly ε. Again, mutations may produce a deficiency of AChR and/or a kinetic disorder. With receptor deficiency, as the name implies, the distribution of AChRs at NMJs is patchy and the number reduced. This causes a proportionate reduction in end-plate current.[126,215] The pathophysiology of the AChR mutations resulting in kinetic disorders differs depending on whether the problem is one of delayed (slow-channel) or premature (fast-channel) AChR closure, after the generation of an initial muscle fiber action potential. The pathophysiology of the slow-channel syndrome is like AChE deficiency, including depolarization block and the development of an end-plate myopathy from excessive stimulation.[126] The pathophysiology of the fast-channel syndrome includes reduced ACh affinity for the AChR, shortened duration of the EPP, and consequently, diminished Na$^+$ activation.[215] AChR density on the postsynaptic fold is normal.[216]

Many of the CMSs relate to mutations of genes that produce proteins integral to the proper placement and aggregation of AChRs on the postsynaptic membrane. Agrin is one such protein critical for NMT. It is secreted by the distal motor nerve terminal and binds to LRP4. The LRP4–agrin complex activates MuSK which then, with Dok-7, stimulates rapsyn to concentrate and anchor AChR at the NMJ.[134]

CMSs due to LPR4, MuSK, rapsyn, and Dok-7 can all be conceptualized as disrupting NMT through impaired AChR clustering. In CMS due to rapsyn deficiency, AChR clustering is impaired, the number of AChRs per end plate is reduced, and as a consequence, the amplitude of the MEPPs is also reduced.[217,218] Impaired NMT in MuSK CMS is due to the failure of normal MuSK to bind LPR4 and promote agrin-induced AChR clustering.[110] In CMS related to Dok-7 mutations, AChR loss occurs from degenerating postsynaptic folds.[121] Na$^+$ channels are also reduced in number. Consequently, MEPP and predictably EPP amplitudes are reduced in most but not all patients.[160] There are presynaptic effects as well including encasement of nerve terminals with Schwann cell processes resulting in reduced quantal content in some cases.[160] Recent work in mouse models has further illustrated the pathophysiology of Dok-7 CMS as involving deficiency in phosphorylation not of Dok-7 but of MuSK.[164] DPAGT1, GFPT1, and ALG2/ALG14 play roles in AChR subunit glycosylation.[123–125,219] All have been hypothesized to adversely affect NMT by impeding the normal assembly and transport of AChRs into the postsynaptic membrane resulting in simplified postsynaptic membranes with decreased end-plate AChR density.[133,201,220]

Plectin is a versatile protein that links cytoskeletal proteins in different locations resulting in multisystem pathologies including at the NMJ. The mechanism of impaired NMT is uncertain but is associated with reduced MEPP amplitudes. Morphological changes in muscle may correlate with the limb-girdle dystrophic pattern that occurs in some patients.[110] Na$^+$ channel CMS is a rare disorder that understandably diminishes the end-plate current because of SCN4A mutations affecting Nav1.4 channel function.[110]

TREATMENT

Most CMS will respond to pharmacological treatment (Tables 26-2 and 26-3). For many years AChE inhibitors such as pyridostigmine were the mainstay in the treatment of CMS. Blocking the action of AChE prolongs the presence of ACh within the synapse and therefore, there is a greater probability of reaching the depolarization threshold for muscle action potential generation.[221] Pyridostigmine is effective for many CMS subtypes but provides no benefit or even can lead to harm in others. In children, the typical dose of liquid pyridostigmine is 1 mg/kg given four to six times per day orally with the maximum dose being 7 mg/kg/day or, as like for, adults, 480 mg/day.[133] Therefore, CMSs are unlike autoimmune MG where pyridostigmine is usually tried first in all patients. Even some patients with autoimmune MuSK antibody positive MG may have some benefit and at worst, the excessive sensitivity/side effects do not typically result in worsening weakness and are short lived. This is not the case in CMS and a critical benefit of accurate CMS genotyping is the ability to choose appropriate treatment and specifically, to first exclude CMS due to end-plate AChR deficiency due to mutations in COLQ before starting pyridostigmine. Pyridostigmine worsens the already present deficit in AChE function which characterizes the pathophysiology of the disorder. Similarly, for slow-channel syndrome, increasing the amount and longevity of AChE in the synaptic cleft worsens symptoms.

Dok-7 CMS does not typically worsen with pyridostigmine but is unlikely to improve. Oral albuterol or ephedrine are first-line treatments for Dok-7 and AChE deficiency CMS.[222] 3,4-DAP may also be used for Dok-7.[223] For slow-channel syndrome, fluoxetine, an AChR open-channel blocker, is first line with quinidine second.[224] For AChR deficiency, rapsyn, fast-channel syndrome, ChAT, and defects of glycosylation, pyridostigmine is used first with 3,4-DAP added shortly thereafter.[127] In AChR deficiency due to CHRNE mutations where the benefit of pyridostigmine can wane, oral albuterol and ephedrine can improve strength.[225] CMS due to abnormalities in the Agrin–LRP4–MuSK–Dok-7 signaling pathway for clustering AChR responds well to β2-agonists (oral albuterol) although the response for AGRN CMS tends to be less pronounced.[223]

In general, 3,4-DAP has potential positive effects in CMS related to mutations in ChAT, AChR subunit, rapsyn, agrin, and MuSK, as well as GFPT1 and DPAGT1 deficiency. Patients with AChE deficiency, both the slow- and fast-channel syndrome, congenital LEMS, and agrin deficiency do not typically respond favorably. Patients with Dok-7 deficiency may benefit in some, but not all cases.[226] The recommended dose of 3,4-DAP is up to 1 mg/kg/day in divided doses up to a maximum of 80 mg/day.

Sympathomimetic amines such as albuterol and ephedrine are effective in selected CMS, particularly those which are refractory to 3,4-DAP and cholinesterase inhibitors.[220,222] These include the slow-channel syndrome, some cases of AChE, agrin, MuSK, and Dok-7 deficiency, and DPAGT1 and LAMB2 CMS. Oral albuterol is typically given in divided doses of 4–18 mg/day.[180] Additionally, slow-channel syndrome may respond to open-channel blockers including quinidine, quinine, or fluoxetine.[224]

In the future, treatment for CMS will likely include gene therapy. Significant preclinical development of adeno-associated virus (AAV) vector gene therapy for Dok-7 and ChAT is underway with early success in mouse models.[164,227,228] Gene therapy which results in overexpression of Dok-7 in skeletal muscle conceivably could be applied to CMS caused by mutations in agrin, LRP4, and MuSK and even to other neuromuscular disorders, which would benefit from enhanced neuromuscular transmission.[164,229] Gene therapy will likely be used in addition to symptomatic treatment.

Like most neuromuscular diseases, supportive treatments are typically also a key piece of therapy. Parents with children with CMS associated with episodic ventilatory crises require apnea and oxygen saturation monitors, and breathing aids such as Ambu bags along with the training necessary for their proper use. In addition, patient counseling to avoid drugs that might further impair neuromuscular transmission is advised (Table 26-3). If anesthesia is required for any purpose, neuromuscular blocking agents should be avoided. Gastrostomy tubes may be required in individual patients with severe feeding difficulties. Skeletal deformities, in particular, scoliosis should be addressed.

▶ BOTULISM

The disease we know as botulism was named following an 18th-century outbreak caused by improper preparation of sausage (*botulus*—Latin). Botulism is a relatively unique disease by virtue of the diversity of mechanisms by which it can be acquired in multiple clinical contexts. In general, the disease occurs either as an infection, when spores are inadvertently ingested (infant botulism) or as an intoxication with a preformed toxin (adults). The latter often results because of improperly prepared foods or beverages. The organisms also may incubate in wounds that facilitate growth under anaerobic conditions, particularly in the setting of parenteral drug abuse. In view of its potency, botulism is a potential weapon in the arsenal of bioterrorists. Inadvertent toxic effects may also occur as the unintended, iatrogenic consequence of toxin used as a cosmetic or therapeutic agent for multiple indications.[230]

CLINICAL FEATURES

In adults, botulism is most often acquired as a foodborne illness or through wounds. Foodborne botulism is a rare disease, with a median of 19 cases annually in the United States. These cases are mostly in men in middle age and fatality is 5%, mainly in older individuals.[231] Infantile botulism is more prevalent, with 80–100 cases estimated to occur annually in the United States.[232] The highest incidence rate in the United

States is in California where there are 6.5 cases/100,000 live-births/year.[233] In Canada, there were 205 foodborne cases reported in a 10-year span for an annual incidence of 0.03×10^5.[234] Infant botulism typically occurs before 6 months of age, and usually between 2 and 4 months. Breastfed infants tend to present later in this age range than those who are formula-fed.[233] The commercial preparation of food and the typically adverse conditions for spore formation within the adult GI tract are the primary reasons for this low incidence. Reported cases are often related to regional or cultural food preparation or storage practices. Even in foodborne botulism, most reported cases are sporadic making outbreaks of more than two to three people unusual.[232]

The morbidity of botulism is considerable. In several series, 30%–67% of patients require intubation.[234,235] Hospitalization of infants is nearly 100% in the United States.[233] Mortality, however, has dropped considerably from historically quoted rates and is estimated at 5%, primarily in older adults. Supportive care in intensive care units and the availability of the heptavalent antitoxin likely account for these improved outcomes.[232,234] Although an uncontrolled study, one report described a statistically significant reduction in the length of hospital stay for patients receiving antitoxin compared to those who did not.[234] Mortality rates for infantile botulism are even lower. With appropriate intensive care and use of the human source antitoxin, infant survival rate is nearly 100%.[232] Although the effects of botulinum toxin are permanent once bound to peripheral nerve terminals, recovery occurs with adequate support, presumably from growth of new nerve terminals. This recovery takes months for motor nerves and even longer for autonomic functions. Length of recovery may also be dependent on serotype, with type A toxin having the most protracted effect.[236] Full recovery is estimated to occur in 95% of individuals if adequately supported.[232] Of interest, three children born to women who developed botulism during pregnancy were unaffected by the disease however, maternal mortality is not insignificant and infants may be preterm.[230,237]

Botulism is commonly categorized by one of five different mechanisms of intoxication or infection (i.e., foodborne, infantile, wound, iatrogenic, and bioterrorism). The clinical presentation of botulism is similar, regardless of the mechanism of inoculation.[238-240] Foodborne botulism in adults is the classic form, first recognized in 1897, with symptoms typically occurring within 2–72 hours of ingestion of food contaminated with the preformed toxin. Patients typically present to the hospital within 48 hours of illness onset and most patients requiring intubation were intubated within the first 2 days of hospitalization. Thus, respiratory failure is not a late event in botulism and may occur with a relative scarcity of other symptoms and weakness.[241]

Clinical suspicion is the cornerstone of diagnosis and several helpful checklists have been developed to aid in recognition and diagnosis.[242-244] Initial symptoms are typically related to impaired GI motility and may include constipation, emesis, abdominal cramping, and/or diarrhea. Neurological impairment follows in short order. The severity of the illness is thought to be related largely to the amount of toxin ingestion. Signs and symptoms referable to motor functions of cranial nerves are typically the initial neurological manifestation. Dysautonomia, particularly of cholinergic function, soon follows. For purposes of easy recall, the clinical manifestations have been referred to as the "dozen Ds." They include dry mouth, diplopia, dilated pupils, droopy eyelids, droopy face, diminished gag reflex, dysphagia, dysarthria, dysphonia, difficulty lifting the head, descending paralysis, and dyspnea related to diaphragmatic paralysis. Importantly, symptoms can exist in various combinations and typically, not all are present.[241]

Manifestations of dysautonomia may include blurred vision from impaired accommodation, urinary retention, ileus, and postural hypotension. The latter is presumably related to impaired cholinergic release at vasomotor, preganglionic sympathetic neurons. Of potential symptoms, xerostomia, diplopia, and dysphagia are the most frequent and occur in over 90% of reported cases. Dyspnea and ventilatory muscle weakness occur in a large proportion of patients, with respiratory failure requiring mechanical ventilation in 32%–81%.[240,241] Duration of required mechanical ventilation is dependent on the severity of the illness and serotype of the infecting organism, with a mean of 58 days for type A and 26 days for type B botulism.[240] Careful observation suggests that ventilatory muscle weakness precedes the recognition of limb and trunk weakness. The latter is common, typically occurring in a descending pattern affecting arms before legs, and typically although not always symmetric in distribution.[239] Deep tendon reflexes may be normal or diminished initially, with progression to complete loss in severely affected individuals. The sensorium and sensory system are unaffected unless CO_2 retention from ventilatory muscle weakness ensues.

Infantile botulism was first described in 1976. It is the most common form of botulism in the United States with an incidence that is approximately twice that of foodborne disease. Unlike foodborne intoxication in adults, infant botulism is an infection as the organisms colonize the vulnerable intestine of the infant. It typically affects children in the first 6 months of life, typically between 2–4 months of life, and is strongly related to the use of honey, which has been shown to harbor clostridial spores (particularly type B) in up to 25% of products.[233,239] Only 20% of infantile cases, however, are attributable to honey ingestion.[232] As expected, given variability in the child's maturational age, clinical manifestations can be more protean than in adults, and disease severity is quite variable. Constipation is usually the first, and sometimes only, manifestation. Children typically develop a weak cry, poor suck, and swallowing dysfunction. Excessive drooling accompanied by a weak cry is particularly worrisome. Ptosis and "smoothing" of facial expression may be noted. Hypotonia, particularly of the neck, occurs in the more severe cases. Tachycardia and urinary retention are additional manifestations of dysautonomia.[241]

Like infantile botulism, wound botulism represents an infection rather than an intoxication. Between 2010 and 2019, 206 laboratory-confirmed cases of wound botulism were reported in the United States, of which 78% were in California.[245] First described in 1943 because of trauma or surgery, it presumably relates to the anaerobic environment created by necrotic tissue. Ironically, in some cases, it may have been related to the use of honey, which has been applied to wounds to facilitate healing through its bactericidal and hygroscopic properties. However, wound botulism is now most associated with recreational drug use, commonly subcutaneous ("skin popping") or intramuscular injection of black tar heroin, but also subcutaneous injection of cocaine.[232,246] This may occur as a result of abscess formation at injection sites which can be quite subtle and appear as no more than a furuncle or small area of cellulitis. As the toxin can penetrate mucous membranes as well disrupted skin, botulism has also resulted from inhalation of cocaine.[239] The clinical manifestations of wound botulism are like foodborne botulism except that gastrointestinal complaints are less common. Wound botulism is more likely to affect individuals as opposed to groups, as is anticipated in foodborne disease, though sharing of a drug supply may occur. The incubation period of 4–14 days is longer in wound botulism than the hours for toxin or spore ingestion.[247,248]

"Hidden" botulism was first described in 1977 and can be conceptualized as the adult variant of infantile botulism. The acidic milieu of the normal adult gastrointestinal tract is not normally conducive to the proliferation of the *Clostridium botulinum* organism once introduced. However, adults with abnormal gastrointestinal tracts due to surgery, inflammatory bowel disease, antimicrobial use, or achlorhydria may be at risk for bacterial colonization.[249] The diagnosis in these cases is often rendered more challenging as there is no history of the more common forms of contact with either the spores or the toxin, that is, suspicious food ingestion or drug use.[239]

Iatrogenic botulism, first described in 1997, refers largely to the unintentional consequences of botulinum toxin used for cosmetic or therapeutic indications (e.g., dystonia, spasticity, migraine, sialorrhea, etc.).[250] This practice may, in some cases, result in inadvertent weakness of nearby muscles or more widespread weakness. Systemic effects of local intramuscular injections have been reported as well. If this occurs, it is important to consider whether an underlying disorder of neuromuscular transmission such as MG may also be present and have made the patient more susceptible to develop weakness following injections. This systemic spread is typically occult and measurable only through SFEMG. Rarely, however, actual botulism has resulted from injection of doses well within therapeutic ranges. An additional inadvertent mechanism of botulism is through aerosolization and inhalation of the toxin, as has been reported in laboratory workers where the organism is stored and studied.[239]

Botulinum toxin as an instrument of terrorists would be most likely delivered as a contaminant of food preparations or in an aerosolized form. As the toxin rapidly denatures with exposure to sunlight or chlorine, contamination of public water supplies would be an unlikely strategy.[251]

DIAGNOSIS AND DIFFERENTIAL DIAGNOSIS

Practically speaking, botulism remains a clinical diagnosis.[242,252] As soon as the diagnosis is suspected, the clinician should contact the 24-hour Centers for Disease Control (CDC) hotline for additional guidance in the United States or follow local national guidelines elsewhere.[230] The diagnosis should be strongly suspected with the acute onset of multiple cranial nerve abnormalities confined to the motor domain, particularly when preceded by gastrointestinal symptoms and accompanied by signs and symptoms of dysautonomia, impaired ventilation, and a descending pattern of limb weakness. The CDC's criteria for diagnosis of foodborne botulism require this phenotype plus identification of the toxin or the cultured organism. As identification of the organism or the toxin takes time and is imperfect, a heightened clinical index of suspicion is key. When suspected, a detailed history of potential exposures early in the course is essential as the opportunity to obtain this information may be quickly lost if intubation is required. Even when the diagnosis is strongly supported or confirmed by ancillary testing, treatment decisions are typically required prior to the identification of toxin or organism based on clinical suspicion of the diagnosis as confirmation by ancillary testing is often not available for several days, if at all. The recent detailed clinical guidance for diagnosis and treatment of botulism is invaluable.[230]

Confirmation of foodborne botulism can be achieved by detection of the neurotoxin and identification of its subtype in serum, stool, gastric aspirate, or samples of ingested food. However, the opportunity diminishes rapidly with passing time, as the positive yield of sample testing declines to <30% after 2 days. Samples also need to be obtained before the administration of antitoxin which nullifies the result of the mouse bioassay.[251] In all forms of botulism (except iatrogenic), the focus is on isolating the organism, not the toxin. In infantile or hidden botulism, the intent is to culture *C. botulinum* from fecal material or gastric aspirate/vomitus.[234] The sensitivity of stool cultures is estimated at 60% but declines to 36% after 3 days.[239] The presence of the bacillus is considered de facto evidence of botulism, as they are virtually never found in healthy individuals. In cases of suspected wound botulism, the integument should be carefully searched, not only for gross disruption and wound contamination, but also for minor bruising with or without signs of infection. Culture of these areas should be performed for anaerobic organisms. The nasal mucosa should be visualized and nasal swabs with anaerobic culture media utilized. Diagnostic criteria allow for a definite diagnosis to be made in someone with a characteristic phenotype, who is epidemiologically linked to one or more other infected individuals with laboratory confirmation. This may occur in foodborne disease but is essentially nonexistent in wound botulism and other forms of the disease.

Differential diagnosis for botulism includes other acute–subacute disorders that result in multiple cranial nerve deficits.[230,251] If more than one case were to occur simultaneously, the likelihood of botulism would be significantly increased, as most differential diagnostic considerations would be less apt to cluster. An outbreak of carbamate (insecticide) toxicity used on watermelons, although a somewhat different phenotype, represents a notable potential exception.[253] Based on its prevalence alone, stroke is probably the primary mimic diagnosed upon initial presentation to the emergency department.[254] Guillain–Barré syndrome (GBS) variants, tick paralysis, neuropathy related to marine intoxications, and MG are the most likely other considerations. This is particularly true in consideration of the motor predominance with a cranial nerve predilection initially. Additional dysautonomia can be present in GBS and its variants.[255] Any acute to subacute cause of cranial and limb weakness, including disorders with an affinity for the meninges, including viral infections like polio and West Nile virus, neoplastic meningitis, sarcoidosis, marine intoxications, and Lyme disease should also be considered. Many will have sensory rather than motor symptoms and are more likely to affect the limb rather than cranial nerve function. Although characterized by pharyngitis and a swollen neck, the local penetration of the diphtheria exotoxin can produce palatal paralysis, dysphonia, and dysphagia as well as a demyelinating polyneuropathy. The red, painful throat that may accompany the xerostomia of botulism may serve to confound the distinction between the two conditions. CMS would have to be considered in children although the time course should be distinctive from botulism in most cases. LEMS is also a potential consideration given that it produces muscle weakness in concert with a cholinergic dysautonomia. Cranial nerve findings are less prevalent in LEMS and the clinical context is usually different, thus allowing confident distinction from botulism in most cases.

LABORATORY FEATURES

EDX evaluation typically provides strong diagnostic support in the appropriate context.[239,256–259] The pattern is typical of a presynaptic DNMT in many but not all cases. Sensory nerve conduction studies are normal. CMAP amplitudes are frequently reduced in 85% of tested nerves. A decremental response to slow repetitive stimulation (2–5 Hz) and an incremental response to fast repetitive stimulation (10–50 Hz) are frequent but not invariable findings.[260] It is generally accepted that rates of 20 Hz or higher have greater diagnostic yields. At times, however, either the decremental or incremental response may be elusive. EDX abnormalities in limb muscles including reduced CMAP amplitudes may be less commonly encountered in individuals whose phenotype is restricted to cranial nerve signs and symptoms. Conversely, the inability to convincingly demonstrate an incremental response also appears to correlate with very low amplitude or even absent CMAPs at baseline.[259] In keeping with this, the incremental response, when present, tends to be of lesser magnitude than that in LEMS. To distinguish this increment from a physiological increment, it should achieve a maximal amplitude of greater than 40% of baseline. In botulism, the increment is commonly less than 100% as opposed to LEMS in which facilitation typically exceeds 100% of baseline CMAP amplitude in any given muscle.[239] The duration of the increment is brief, often in the 30–60 second range when subsequent, single stimuli are delivered. It is estimated that incremental responses are demonstrable in only 60% of patients.[239] Needle examination findings are often abnormal, but not specific. With needle electromyography, low amplitude, short duration, polyphasic MUAPs with early/increased recruitment, and fibrillation potentials may be demonstrable. Increased jitter values with blocking on SFEMG are to be expected, but again indicate only the existence of a neuromuscular transmission abnormality, not the etiology. Over time, once reinnervation has begun to occur, MUPs go through the standard evolution of reinnervated MUPs.

Demonstration of toxin or organism in appropriately symptomatic individuals confirms the diagnosis of botulism.[230] Currently, the gold standard for the detection of botulinum toxin in foodborne botulism is the mouse bioassay, which is performed by designated BSL-3 containment facilities. It is traditionally used to confirm the presence of toxin in serum, gastric content, stool, or the suspected food source of the inoculum. Unfortunately, its sensitivity is insufficient to detect low toxin levels. No more than 45% of patients will test positive. Positivity rate depends on factors such as how rapidly the specimen is obtained and the specific serotype.[232,261] The duration of toxin detection is limited and declines rapidly following exposure. Detection of botulinum toxin type B may be possible for up to 12 days, while type A which persists 4 days or less.[235] In general, specimens obtained more than 7 days postexposure are unlikely to be positive.[232] In addition, results of the assay typically require at least 24 hours and sometimes up to 4 days to return. Methodologies utilizing functional dual coating (FDC) and polymerase chain reaction (PCR) technologies promise higher diagnostic yield.[262,263] Specimens obtained for purposes of toxin identification should be refrigerated, not frozen, until they can be shipped to the CDC, or the limited number of state laboratories in the United States equipped to perform the assays.[230]

The diagnostic test of choice in infantile and hidden botulism is stool culture. In wound botulism, anaerobic culture of the abscess site is performed. As many patients will be constipated due to autonomic dysfunction from botulism, acquisition of stool with the administration of a sterile water enema may be required. Cultures of nasal swabs may be helpful in rare inhalational cases related to vocational exposures or cocaine use. Other testing is of limited diagnostic value in suspected botulism. Cerebrospinal fluid (CSF) is often obtained to exclude infectious or inflammatory mimics in the differential diagnosis. Cell count and protein are normal in botulism.[232] Although of limited diagnostic value, assessment of forced vital capacity or negative inspiratory force are important tools for purposes of disease management.[230]

HISTOPATHOLOGY

There is no role for either nerve or muscle biopsy in botulism in most if not all cases. In one autopsied case, the findings in muscle were degenerating muscle fibers and scattered angular atrophic fibers. As expected, sural and peroneal nerves displayed no significant histopathology in this individual.[264]

PATHOGENESIS

Botulinum toxin is an exotoxin produced by the anaerobic, spore-forming bacillus C. botulinum in most cases. C. butyricum and C. baratii are also reported neurotoxigenic in India and China.[232] The toxin exists in seven currently recognized serotypes, designated A to G, that have similar but not identical biological properties. In North America, disease is associated with toxin types A, B, E, and to a lesser extent type F. Type E is the most common strain causing foodborne disease in North America.[232,241] Botulinum toxicity is substantial, rivaled by few other substances. Parenteral exposure requires a far smaller inoculum than inhalational exposure, which is more potent in turn than ingestion.[232,241]

Foodborne disease has been linked to a long list of food types or food preparation practices that may be both geographically and culturally based.[234,265] One of the more interesting and contemporary forms of foodborne botulism are outbreaks that have occurred in prison populations attributed to the production and ingestion of an illicit fermented beverage known as "pruno."[231,266] Despite the name, it is likely that the botulinum spores in reported outbreaks of pruno ingestion originated from potato. The C. botulinum bacillus reverts to a spore form under stress. Ideal conditions for spore germination include an anaerobic milieu, nonacidic pH, and low salt and sugar content.[232] These conditions occur with home canning procedures which are inadequate due to insufficient duration and/or degree of high temperatures. Outbreaks of foodborne botulism are also reported in cultures where fermentation or smoking preparations are common.[232,234] Although spores are susceptible to heat, their elimination requires temperatures (85°C) that may be difficult to attain and maintain at higher altitudes. Outbreaks of foodborne disease appear to be more common with home canning in higher altitude.[239] Poorly prepared or stored root vegetables such as potatoes or mushrooms are frequent culprits due to their significant soil exposure where the clostridial organisms are ubiquitous.[266] In view of that, it is not surprising that ingestion of botulism spores may occur commonly without causing disease. In adults, either a large inoculum (poorly prepared or stored food) or gut conditions conducive to spore germination (achlorhydria) are required for foodborne botulism to occur. Unlike the spores, the botulinum toxin itself is readily denatured by heat.[230]

Botulinum toxin can be absorbed through inhalation. Toxin cannot traverse unbroken skin but is bound to and can be transported across the membranes of epithelial cells. This includes nasal mucosa during cocaine inhalation, or aerosolization in laboratories or a bioterrorist attack.[239,267] It can also be introduced through broken skin via inadvertent wounds, or through recreational (heroin) or therapeutic (botox) injections. Once absorbed, the toxin migrates to the perineuronal microcompartment in the vicinity of vulnerable cholinergic nerve endings. Only these cells can selectively accumulate the molecule, and do so by receptor-mediated endocytosis and translocator mechanisms.[267] The toxins then interfere with the release of ACh through slightly different mechanisms affecting the SNARE protein complex. They all gain entrance to the presynaptic terminal through endocytosis via synaptic vesicles, a "Trojan horse" effect. Once in the presynaptic terminal, botulinum toxin serotypes A, C, and E target SNAP-25 whereas botulinum toxin B, D, F, and G cleave VAMP/synaptobrevin. The net effect in both cases is disruption of quantal release. In vitro electrophysiological studies indicate a significant reduction in the EPP amplitude occurs, far below the 7–20 mV necessary to bring the myofiber from its resting membrane potential to action potential threshold. Intuitively, the frequency of MEPPs is reduced, but not MEPP amplitude.[268,269]

TREATMENT

Botulism treatment involves early acquisition of diagnostic specimens and the earliest possible administration of botulinum antitoxin.[230,252] It is important to have a high diagnostic suspicion of botulism in any case of acute polycranial neuropathy particularly if preceded by gastrointestinal symptoms. Botulism may represent the most important reason to obtain emergent EDX testing. Other than antitoxin administration, intensive care support, when necessary, is the other critical component of successful botulism treatment. Because of potential public health implications, every case of botulism must be reported to public health officials, who may also aid the physician in the necessary epidemiological investigation.

Consensus opinion is that heptavalent botulinum antitoxin (HBAT), which binds to circulating toxin and addresses multiple subtypes, should be administered expeditiously, prior to availability of any supportive or confirmatory testing results.[230] Antitoxin, particularly when given early, significantly reduces mortality.[270] Specifically, equine-derived HBAT, which was licensed in 2013 and is the only available treatment for noninfant botulism in the United States, reduces hospital and intensive care length of stay when given within 2 days, and is generally safe.[271] Baby botulism immune globulin (BIG) is used to treat botulism in infants less than 12 months old. Ordering BIG-IV is a multistep and multidisciplinary process. In the Unites States, treating physicians discuss any suspicious case with the Infant Botulism Treatment and Prevention Program (IBTPP), which is a branch of the California Department of Public Health.[230,272] In one study, baby BIG reduced the average length of hospitalization from 6–3 weeks in infants.[232]

Local measures may be employed with specific botulism mechanisms. In suspected foodborne botulism, gastric lavage, or enemas may be employed if ingestion is recent to remove as much unabsorbed toxin from the gastrointestinal tract as possible. With wound botulism, it is recommended that any potential abscess be debrided and cultured with antimicrobials administered as required to address other potential, concomitant infections.[230]

Pharmacologically, both pyridostigmine, guanidine, and 3,4-DAP have been used in the treatment of botulism.[273] They appear to have limited, transient benefit and have not been recommended for routine use. Avoidance of any drugs with significant NMJ-blocking properties is strongly recommended (Table 26-3). Newer approaches which have completed phase I studies involve monoclonal antibodies as treatment for various strains instead of antitoxin.[274–276]

▶ TOXINS/ENVENOMATIONS

Many environmental intoxications or envenomations exist whose morbidity result largely from disordered neuromuscular transmission. Many are rare and exotic. Categories include tick paralysis, organophosphate and carbamate poisoning, snake envenomation, latrodectism (from black widow spider bites), drugs, and electrolyte abnormalities. This section will review some of the more notable examples. Table 26-1 provides a list of the more well-known neuromuscular toxins and attempts to categorize them by their presumed site of action as pre-, post-, or synaptic disorders.

TICK PARALYSIS

Tick paralysis is a caused by exposure to the saliva of the Ixodid (hard-shelled) tick family. Its history is colorful and entertaining.[277] The first presumed cases were reported in southeastern Australia in 1824.[277,278] It is a disease that affects multiple animal species including dogs, cats, and cattle in addition to humans.[277] In Australia, its prevalence in domestic animals makes it a disease of considerable economic consequence.[277] Of the two major endemic regions in North America, *Dermacentor andersoni* (Rocky Mountain wood tick) is the most common vector in the Pacific Northwest and Canada. *Dermacentor variabilis* (dog tick) is the predominant vector in the Southeastern United States where the disease is less frequently identified (Fig. 26-7). Other less common vectors include *Amblyomma americanum* and *maculatum*, and *Ixodes scapularis* and *pacificus* in the United States, and *I. holocyclus*, the major vector in Australia.[279] Like botulism, tick paralysis usually presents as isolated cases, but

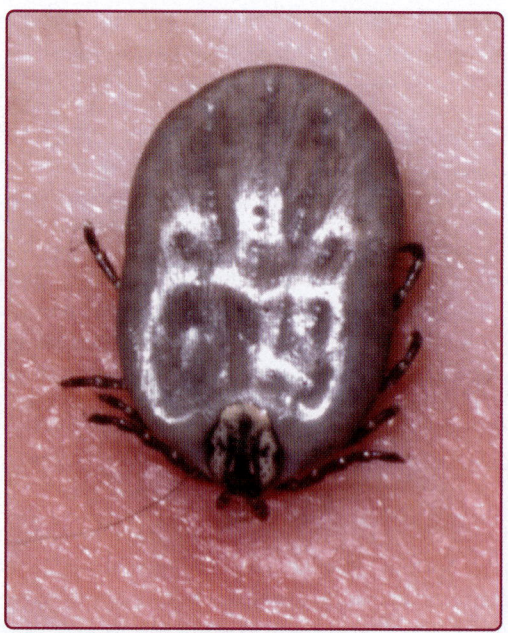

Figure 26-7. *Dermacentor variabilis* feeding. The tick has been attached for 24 hours. (Reproduced from Goldsmith LA, Katz SI, Gilchrest BA, Paller AS, Leffell DJ, Wolff K. *Fitzpatrick's Dermatology in General Medicine*. 8th ed. McGraw-Hill; 2012. Figure 210-6.)

may present with clusters as well.[279] Tick paralysis is believed to be a DNMT in which the predominant effect of the toxin is to impair the presynaptic release of ACh.[280,281]

Clinical Features

The phenotype of tick paralysis is strikingly like GBS. As the time of the tick attachment is often uncertain, the time between tick attachment and symptom onset is usually imprecise, but is estimated at a mean of 5 days, although experiments in sheep suggest that feeding for a week by a gravid female tick is typical.[277,279] After symptoms develop, the disorder moves rapidly with the nadir occurring on an average of 1.5 days after initial symptoms.[278,279,282–289] Once the tick is identified and removed, full neurological recovery takes place at an average of 1.5 days in North America, but is more protracted in Australia where tick paralysis is a more severe disease.[278,279,290]

Affected individuals, particularly children, characteristically experience a prodrome of irritability, somnolence, myalgias, asthenia, and ataxia.[277,291] The ataxia may be so prominent in some cases that it resembles a cerebellar syndrome. Despite the "flu-like" prodrome, fever is not a part of the illness. Diarrhea may occur, but unlike botulism, gastrointestinal symptoms are otherwise limited. Paresthesias or dysesthesia may precede the development of weakness, affecting the hands and feet, in keeping with a non–length-dependent neuropathy. Paresthesias may have a pruritic or burning quality, although significant pain is uncharacteristic.[277] Despite these sensory symptoms, objective sensory loss is mild, if evident at all.

Like in GBS, sensory symptoms are rapidly overshadowed by the evolution of flaccid weakness. This weakness typically ascends over hours to days, affecting legs before arms, and therefore opposite the descending pattern of botulism.[277] Cranial nerve and autonomic function are typically affected after development of limb weakness. Bulbar involvement including hoarseness, dysphagia, and sialorrhea occur as does bifacial weakness.[278] Both internal (mid-position, unreactive pupils) and external ophthalmoparesis including ptosis occur, particularly in the more severe, Australian form of the disease.[278,290] Ventilatory muscle weakness, with the need for assisted mechanical ventilation, is estimated to occur in 10% of patients.[279] Patients are typically areflexic, but like GBS, this finding is not always present early in the disease.[277,292] The mortality of tick paralysis is reported between 6% and 11%, but since most of these cases occurred in the pre-ICU era, contemporary mortality is likely lower.[279]

As previously mentioned, tick paralysis in Australia appears to be a more severe disease.[277,278,293,294] An atypical pattern of focal weakness, mimicking Bell's palsy or a brachial plexopathy has been reported in Australian, but not North American cases.[277,290,295] Pupillary involvement occurs commonly in Australian cases, but is rare in North Americans and should prompt consideration of botulism or Miller Fisher syndrome.[277] Hypertension is also a common manifestation of tick paralysis in Australia but not in North America. Worsening paralysis may continue following removal of the *I. holocyclus* tick for up to 48 hours but continued progression following tick removal is unusual in the United States where dramatic improvement within hours may occur. Prolonged need for mechanical ventilation for a week or more is not uncommon in Australia, but uncharacteristic in the United States.[278,290]

Diagnosis and Differential Diagnosis

Tick paralysis may be unique in that the mechanisms for both the diagnosis and treatment are identical (i.e., identification and removal of the tick). The definitive diagnosis simple involves clinical improvement of the characteristic syndrome following tick removal. In that spirit, the key to diagnosis is a heightened index of suspicion for tick paralysis in patients with apparent GBS, particularly in the spring and summer months, and in children with a history of outdoor exposure in endemic areas.[279,291] Unfortunately, the diagnosis may be impeded if the tick may has completed feeding and detached itself prior to its identification.[277] None of these epidemiological features are absolute, however, as tick paralysis has been reported in adults in 20% of cases and in nonendemic regions including urban areas, and at attachment sites other than the scalp, behind the ears, neck, and groin.[277,279,296]

The major differential diagnostic consideration for tick paralysis is GBS for which tick paralysis is often misdiagnosed.[277] There are relative, but no absolute differences, between the two disorders. Tick paralysis tends to evolve more rapidly, has few if any demyelinating features on motor nerve conduction studies, spares SNAPs, is less likely to be painful, and is accompanied by a normal CSF profile. Again, in consideration with this sizeable overlap, is imperative that any GBS suspect undergoes a thorough body search particularly of the scalp. Other causes of acute motor weakness require consideration as well. These include acute myelopathies such as transverse myelitis, poliomyelitis, and other enteroviral infections, botulism, myasthenia, diphtheria, porphyria, metabolic disturbances such as severe hypokalemia or hypophosphatemia and potentially other intoxications or envenomations discussed in this chapter and other chapters affecting nerve, NMJ, or muscle.

Laboratory Features

Spinal fluid analysis is of potential value in tick paralysis as it is characteristically normal, unlike GBS or many of the other differential diagnostic considerations.[277,278] As CSF protein may be normal in early GBS as well, it is not an absolute discriminator for these two diseases. Although atypical for DNMT, elevated CK has been reported in some cases.[278] Acetylcholinesterase inhibitors are felt to have no effect on the weakness produced by tick paralysis.[277,278,292]

The major EDX finding in tick paralysis is a reduction in CMAP amplitudes with normal SNAPs.[278,292,297-301] This nerve conduction pattern is not pathognomonic, however, and can be seen with any presynaptic DNMT, or disorder of anterior horn cells, ventral roots, or motor nerves. Although minor slowing of motor conduction velocities has been reported in North American cases, they are not of any apparent diagnostic or clinical significance.[277] It may become evident however with sequential testing before and after tick removal that distal latencies may be mildly affected by the disease.[292,297] Theoretically, this may reflect disordered neuromuscular transmission time or potentially slowed conduction in terminal nerve twigs. Features suggesting acquired demyelination such as CMAP temporal dispersion or conduction block, as occurs often in GBS, are not described.[292,297] We are aware of one report of proximal nerve inexcitability with normal motor conduction parameters on distal stimulation.[295] This has been attributed to sodium channel dysfunction within nerve in a manner similar to certain marine toxins or the acute motor axonal neuropathy form of GBS. Neither repetitive stimulation at either low and high frequency nor exercise either brief or prolonged seems to affect CMAP amplitudes in tick paralysis in contrast to other DNMT.[292,297] Needle electromyographic results are normal other than for one extreme case of a child with more than 50 attached ticks in which fibrillation potentials were identified.[299]

Histopathology

There is no apparent role for muscle or peripheral nerve biopsy.

Pathogenesis

Children, particularly girls, are three times as likely to be afflicted with tick paralysis as are adults.[278,282–284,302] One hypothesis for this discrepancy is that children's short stature makes their head more accessible to ticks. In addition, long hair, found more frequently in girls, is hypothesized to provide a covert location for the protracted feeding necessary to cause disease.[277] Other considerations potentially relevant to the increased incidence in children are that (1) the toxin load is diluted in adults with larger body sizes than children and, (2) adults are more likely to find and remove the tick at an earlier stage.[277]

Tick paralysis, at least that produced by *I. holocyclus*, results from holocyclotoxin that is secreted from the salivary glands of the offending vector.[277] The toxin's concentration increases as the tick feeds, explaining in part the latency between tick attachment and symptom onset. North American ticks are presumed to have a slightly different toxin with a similar mechanism of action. However, in both Northern and Southern hemisphere disease, the toxin interferes with presynaptic release of ACh from nerve terminals of NMJs and presumably autonomic neurons as well, although pupillary abnormalities are the only common autonomic manifestation of the disease.[277,280,281] In addition, experimental evidence implicates an additional effect on nerve conduction, hypothetically via sodium channel dysfunction, providing a potential explanation for the sensory symptoms or prolonged motor distal latencies which sometimes accompany the disease.[277,295] Regardless of mechanism, tick paralysis is unlikely to be associated with any structural injury as electrophysiological recovery can begin within hours of tick removal.[295]

Treatment

Treatment strategies include prevention, supportive care, and tick removal. When outdoors in endemic areas, limiting exposed skin surfaces, utilizing light clothing to improve tick detection, and spraying or impregnating clothing with insect repellants such as those containing pyrethrin/pyrethroid are deterrent strategies.[295] Supportive care is like any paralyzing neuromuscular illness including prophylaxis against deep vein thrombosis, skin breakdown, nerve compression, and surveillance for, and when necessary, treatment of dysautonomia and ventilatory failure.

The most important aspect of care is the identification and removal of the offending tick. Historical cases in which the tick was found postmortem emphasize this point.[288] It is strongly recommended that ticks be removed with slow and steady pressure applied with tweezers placed as close to the skin as possible, to ensure removal of mouth parts.[279] In addition, as individual ticks can harbor multiple different pathogenic organisms, it is important to avoid the expression of further material into the wound by fingertip pressure.[278] Testing for Lyme disease should ensure. Heating or covering the tick with Vaseline or similar substances impervious to air is not generally recommended.[277]

A polyclonal antitoxin is available for the treatment of *I. holocyclus*. It is a canine derivative and is associated with a high incidence of adverse allergic responses including serum sickness and anaphylaxis.[277,278] It is only used in severe cases. No antitoxin exists for North American disease nor would it be recommended due to the typical rapid clinical improvement following tick removal.[277] Antitoxin also must be utilized rapidly to provide any benefit. Advances in development of a vaccine for tick paralysis in Australia have seen success in the laboratory.[293,303,304] However, we are unaware of either the availability or effectiveness of a vaccine for humans.

ACUTE ORGANOPHOSPHATE AND CARBAMATE POISONING

Organophosphates and carbamates are chemicals that respectively irreversibly or reversibly inactivate AChE. They are used as insecticides or as instruments of homicide, suicide, or chemical warfare.[305] Incidence of inadvertent exposure is highest in the developing world. The World Health Organization estimates that the majority of the more than 200,000 deaths that occur globally each year are self-inflicted, a problem particularly prevalent in Sri Lanka.[306–308] Mortality is estimated at 15%–30% or more, particularly in regions where intensive care is not readily available.[307]

CLINICAL FEATURES

Organophosphate toxicity produces both an acute and a delayed neurological syndrome with different mechanisms of action and different phenotypes. The neuropathy, referred to as organophosphate-induced delayed polyneuropathy or OPIDP, develops as a delayed response to toxic exposure through a mechanism unrelated to AChE inhibition. It is discussed in Chapter 20. This section will focus exclusively on the manifestations of acute exposure. Unlike most of the disorders in this and the preceding chapter, the effects of acute organophosphate or carbamate exposure enhance rather than impair the effects of ACh at the NMJs and autonomic synapses. This occurs initially through irreversible inhibition of AChE. Over time, however, the clinical features often evolve into manifestations of synaptic exhaustion. The phenotype of acute organophosphate toxicity is distinctive from other DNMT for two reasons. One is the initial manifestations of cholinergic excess. The other relates to the ability of organophosphates to cross the blood–brain barrier producing CNS as well as PNS cholinergic disruption.

Acute organophosphate toxicity manifests within 24 hours of exposure, typically less. Some of the more notable symptoms pertain largely to the autonomic manifestations of the disease and are referred to by the acronym SLUDGE. This stands for salivation, lacrimation, urination, defecation, increased gastrointestinal motility, and emesis.[307] One report identified that 75% of affected patients have miotic pupils and

CNS symptoms.[309] CNS side effects more commonly occur in organophosphates than in carbamates which have less-effective CNS penetration. CNS manifestations may include agitated delirium and potentially coma, with or without seizures. Two-thirds of patients in the aforementioned series of 47 patients were noted to have hypersalivation and roughly half-experienced agitation and muscle fasciculations.[309] Other muscarinic symptoms include bronchospasm, bronchorrhea, and bradycardia. Both hypotension and hypertension may occur, attributed to overstimulation of muscarinic parasympathetic and nicotinic sympathetic neurons, respectively.[307] Diaphoresis may also occur. Muscarinic symptoms may dissipate with the development of large pupils in some cases presumably due to cholinergic bombardment and postsynaptic exhaustion in a manner like succinylcholine effect. Muscle weakness is presumably related to the same mechanism.

In addition to limb paresis, ophthalmoparesis and ventilatory muscle weakness requiring mechanical ventilation and intensive care may occur.[310] In one study, approximately 20% of intoxicants required mechanical ventilation.[309] Death most commonly results from respiratory or ventilatory failure that stems from a combination of impaired CNS ventilatory drive plus excessive pulmonary secretions, and diaphragmatic or intercostal muscle weakness.[307] The term "intermediate syndrome" has been coined to describe ventilatory failure that may suddenly occur from diaphragmatic and intercostal muscle weakness after the patient has been treated and stabilized relating to the initial symptoms of muscarinic excess.[307] As in other NMTD, patients' ability to lift their head off the bed (neck flexion) has been suggested as a means of indirectly monitoring ventilatory muscle weakness.[307]

DIAGNOSIS AND DIFFERENTIAL DIAGNOSIS

A diagnosis of organophosphate toxicity is typically based on clinical suspicion with supportive data. Clinical suspicion is generated by recognition of characteristic clinical signs and symptoms and possibly a smell of pesticides or solvents on the patient. The initial clinical presentation commonly includes miotic pupils, excessive sweating, and altered level of consciousness with hypoventilation.[307] Characteristic EDX features described below and reduced butyrylcholinesterase or AChE activity in the blood are supportive features for diagnosis.[307] The major differential diagnosis of organophosphate toxicity is carbamate toxicity.[253,307] Any acute disorder producing signs and symptoms of both muscle weakness and dysautonomia such as GBS, botulism, tick paralysis, and other phenotypically similar intoxications/envenomations should be considered.

LABORATORY FEATURES

Unlike presynaptic disorders of NMT, CMAP amplitudes at rest are typically normal in acute organophosphate poisoning.[310] Repetitive stimulation at both low and high frequencies results in a decremental response.[310] Like two forms of CMS, the slow-channel syndrome and AChE deficiency, nerve conduction studies in organophosphate toxicity are distinctive from most DNMT in that CMAP afterdischarges occur in response to a single supramaximal stimulus (Fig. 26-4) in an estimated 60% of intoxicated individuals.[310] The afterdischarge, like the parent CMAP, decrements with repetitive stimulation.[310]

Inhibition of plasma butyrylcholinesterase, also known as pseudocholinesterase or plasma cholinesterase, aids in determining the existence, but not severity of organophosphate effect. A decline in the degree of butyrylcholinesterase inhibition may signify the elimination of organophosphate from the body. As mentioned, AChE exists on red cells as well as at cholinergic synapses. Red cell cholinesterase levels measured in whole blood provide an additional means by which to determine not only organophosphate exposure, but also severity of AChE inhibition.[307] The accuracy of both assays is highly dependent on technical considerations, specifically the need to cool the patient's blood immediately after acquisition. Methodology also exists for the detection of organophosphates in air and water samples as well as on the clothing of exposed individuals.

HISTOLOGY

There is no role for nerve or muscle biopsy in acute organophosphate toxicity.

PATHOGENESIS

Organophosphates gain access to the human body through ingestion (usually intentional) or through inhalation or dermal exposure, either of which could be intentional or accidental.[305] They adversely affect AChE at synapses and on red cell membranes and additionally inhibit butyrylcholinesterase in plasma. The latter effect appears to have little or no associated morbidity.[307] Organophosphates work by irreversibly preventing the ability of an AChE molecule from metabolizing ACh, by depositing a phosphoryl group at the active serine hydroxyl site of AChE at both nicotinic and muscarinic synapses.[308] OPIDP is due to inhibition of a different enzyme, neurotoxic esterase.

TREATMENT

Like all acutely paralyzing diseases capable of resulting in ventilatory failure, ICU care is integral to the care of many acutely intoxicated patients.[307] When toxin has been ingested, gastric lavage with or without activated charcoal is routinely utilized in an attempt to reduce the toxin burden.[306,307] Intravenous fluids, usually normal saline, are delivered to maintaining systolic blood pressure above 80 mm Hg and urine output above 0.5 mL/kg/h.[307] Nasal oxygen is commonly administered. Positioning patients on their left side may aid in secretion clearance, reduce risk of aspiration, and decrease pyloric emptying and toxin absorption in patients who have ingested the toxin.[307]

Intravenous atropine, which can also cross the blood–brain barrier, is used to lessen adverse muscarinic and CNS morbidity. Various regimens have been recommended. An initial IV bolus of 1–3 mg is suggested.[307] A second bolus, double the original, is recommended if the pupil size, blood pressure, pulse, breath sounds, or sweat production do not improve within 5 minutes of the first dose. Alternative regimens include either continuous IV infusion of atropine at an initial rate of 0.02–0.08 mg/kg or intermittent intravenous injections of 4 mg every 15 minutes until secretions control has been achieved.[309] Use of intravenous β- or calcium channel blockers are typically used for cardioprotection if heart rates exceed 130 bpm.[309] Benzodiazepines provide benefit for agitation in addition to their routine use for intubated patients and in treatment of seizures. Magnesium sulfate, α2-adrenergic agonists such as clonidine, sodium bicarbonate, butyrylcholinesterase, hemodialysis/hemofiltration and bacterially derived phosphotriesterases, or hydrolases that break down organophosphates enzymatically are also suggested treatments but have unproven benefit.[307,311]

Pralidoxime is the most used agent of the oxime class. Its utility is relevant only in organophosphate toxicity and to treat severe weakness. It has no effect on the toxicity of other carbamylated cholinesterases such as physostigmine or neostigmine. It reactivates AChE by binding the cholinesterase molecule and, by doing so, induces a conformational change in the organophosphate molecule attached to the other end of AChE. This allows for dissociation of the otherwise irreversible bond between AChE and organophosphate.[308] Unlike atropine, pralidoxime does not cross the blood–brain barrier and does not benefit CNS manifestations. The World Health Organization recommended regimen is a 30 mg/kg pralidoxime chloride bolus followed by an 8 mg/kg/h infusion.[306] An alternative regimen employed in Asia is 1 g of pralidoxime every 4–6 hours for 1–3 days.[311] Despite evidence of benefit in animals, however, benefit for humans remains unproven with some reports actually suggesting a deleterious effect.[306,309,311] There are numerous proposed hypotheses as to why a disparity exists between in vitro and in vivo effects.[309]

Numerous species of venomous arthropods, snakes, and marine species whose bite or less commonly, ingestion may produce weakness or other symptoms referable to the neuromuscular system.[312–316] Although uncommon in North America, it is estimated that there are more than 150,000 envenomation deaths from bites annually worldwide.[314] The land and surrounding waters of Australia and Southeast Asia are the home to many of the implicated species. Although these toxins typically have systemic effects as well as direct effects on peripheral nerve and muscle, the morbidity typically owes to their adverse effects on neuromuscular transmission. As many of these disorders indirectly affect neuromuscular transmission by affecting sodium or potassium channels on presynaptic nerve terminals, separating envenomations considered as neuropathic from those whose mechanisms of action appear to be focused on NMT alone is somewhat arbitrary and artificial. As neuropathies caused by envenomations often produce sensory as well as motor consequences, this separation has some clinical relevance, and will be maintained throughout this text. This section, although not intended to be comprehensive, will highlight some of the more noteworthy toxins that produce neuromuscular disorders largely attributable to disordered NMT.

SNAKES

Serpents belonging to some but not all of the Elapid species (cobras, kraits, mambas, coral snakes, sea snakes, and a number of terrestrial Australian) produce venom that adversely affects NMT at either the presynaptic or postsynaptic level.[313,317] Kraits (*Bungarus* sp.) secrete both presynaptic toxins referred to as β-neurotoxins and postsynaptic α- or γ-neurotoxins that have curare-like effects.[313,316] These pre- and postsynaptic actions are not mutually exclusive, although it is the β-neurotoxin that is felt to be the predominant source of morbidity.[316] The β-neurotoxin is a phospholipase that causes loss of synaptophysin and reduced numbers of synaptic vesicles.

Eastern Green Mambas (*Dendroaspis* sp.) release two toxins, dendrotoxin and fasciculin. The former specifically binds neuronal potassium channels and prolongs depolarization in nerve terminals, thus facilitating ACh release. The latter is a cholinesterase inhibitor. Cobras (*Naja* sp.) secrete cobrotoxin that inhibits binding of ACh at nicotinic receptors (κ-neurotoxin).[316] *Micrurus* sp., the only Elapids indigenous to the United States, secrete an α-neurotoxin (postsynaptic).[318] Envenomation from vipers and rattlesnake (*Crotalid* sp.) may have neurological consequences (e.g., generalized myokymia from rattlesnakes), but does not typically affect neuromuscular transmission.

Snake envenomation, regardless of species, often affects other organ systems due to additional toxic components, particularly those that incite inflammation with a prominent local wound reaction or that have either pro or anticoagulant effects. Snake venom does not cross the blood–brain barrier, but can adversely affect the CNS through thrombotic or hemorrhagic complications.[313] Optic neuritis, cerebellar syndromes and encephalomyelitis are rare delayed complications of venomous snake bites.[313] The mechanism is unknown but may represent a hypersensitivity reaction to antivenom.

Risk for local reaction depends on snake species and constituents of the venom. With krait and coral snakes, local reactions tend to be negligible. Systemic symptoms typically begin within 1–4 hours but may be delayed for up to 12 hours. Initial symptoms are nonspecific and may include chest and abdominal discomfort and tightness, myalgias, and nausea. CNS symptoms are thought to result from hypoxia or hypotension as these toxins do not cross the blood–brain barrier. While DNMTs occur exclusively with Elapid species, such disorders do not occur with every envenomation.[313] Symptoms referable to cholinergic excess, such as fasciculations and hypersalivation, may or may not occur. When weakness does occur, the prototypical pattern, like botulism, is descending. Ptosis and ophthalmoparesis typically precede facial weakness. Neck flexor weakness is a harbinger of ventilatory muscle involvement. Arm weakness typically precedes leg weakness.[313,315] A direct myotoxic effect of neurotoxins resulting in rhabdomyolysis may occur. Rhabdomyolysis is typically associated with β-neurotoxicity but also has been reported with α-neurotoxicity.[316,318] Mortality rates vary but are high without adequate medical care, and death may occur within 48 hours of envenomation.[316] During the Vietnam War, American soldiers referred to the multibanded krait as the "two-step snake" due to the legend that death occurred within two steps of being bitten. With Mamba envenomation, local swelling and nausea precede descending paralysis which includes cranial nerve palsies, ventilatory muscle and limb weakness. EDX evaluations have been rarely reported in Elapid envenomation.[315,317] The pattern is one of reduced CMAP amplitudes at baseline with a mild decremental response with slow repetitive stimulation.

Treatment considerations are individualized.[313,319] In general, the involved limb should be immobilized and kept in a dependent position to limit toxin dissemination. Intubation and mechanical ventilation are instituted early, with any indication of breathing difficulties. If shock or allergic reaction to antivenin, volume repletion, antihistamines, corticosteroids, and epinephrine are considered. Monitoring for adverse procoagulant or anticoagulant effects is important. If bleeding occurs, use of fresh frozen plasma, cryoprecipitates, and human fibrinogen concentrates is indicated. Monitoring for compartment syndrome in the vicinity of the wound is important. Fasciotomy should be undertaken cautiously, however, due to considerations of hemostatic difficulties that these patients may experience. Monitoring CK levels in anticipation of possible rhabdomyolysis and myoglobinuric renal failure is recommended.[316] Wound debridement may be required if local tissue necrosis ensues. If there is doubt of the patient's vaccination status, tetanus toxoid should be provided. Cholinesterase inhibitors may be considered if the species of snake is known, and the venom recognized to be an α-neurotoxin with reversible postsynaptic blocking properties. Antivenom, delivered as soon as possible, is recommended, and is felt to reduce the mortality rates of envenomation significantly. Antivenoms exist in the preferable monovalent (species specific) or polyvalent forms.[320–322] Elapid envenomation is rare in North America, but does rarely occur in natural habits in the southern United States and Latin America from Coral snakes or exotic species in pet owners and zoo employees.[318,323] Antivenoms for Elapids may be difficult to obtain, particularly in the United States. Valuable resources include the poison center hotline[324] and the Association of Zoological Parks and Aquariums.[325] As antivenoms are developed in nonhuman species, risk of allergic reactions is significant in humans and requires close monitoring for with rapid treatment.

ARTHROPODS

A-Latrotoxin is the active constituent of black widow and brown widow spider venom.[312,313,326] The venom stimulates the release of several neurotransmitters including norepinephrine, dopamine, and acetylcholine, resulting in vesicle depletion.[327] The mechanism of ACh depletion at presynaptic terminals at the NMJ appears to be independent of normal calcium dependent ACh-release mechanisms. Both the PNS and CNS are affected. The syndrome differs from most DNMT described in this chapter, as it results in symptoms of neuromuscular hyperactivity instead of weakness. Local pain is a characteristic symptom of the spider bite. Initial symptoms are those of overstimulation with autonomic overactivity including vasoconstriction, hypertension, diaphoresis, and neuromuscular overactivity, including painful muscle rigidity and cramping, which typically begin at the bite site and spread centrifugally. Spasms of the abdominal wall may mimic a surgical abdomen. Not surprisingly, serum CK values may be elevated. Headache, dyspnea secondary to bronchoconstriction, emesis, priapism, lethargy, irritability, tremor, fasciculations, and/or ataxia are other common manifestations.[313] Myocarditis is a reported and potentially fatal manifestation.[328] Treatment includes antivenom which should be used judiciously, and with prophylactic antihistamines and epinephrine, in light of high rates of allergic reactions including anaphylaxis. As always, airway management is a priority. Symptomatic use of benzodiazepines, infusions of calcium gluconate to address cramping, atropine and tetanus immunization may be considered.

Scorpion intoxication also manifests through an increase in presynaptic ACh release as well as a direct effect on muscle, both due to impaired inactivation of sodium channels.[327] The clinical picture of scorpion envenomation is dominated by muscle weakness associated with arterial hypertension, cardiac arrhythmias, myocarditis, and/or pulmonary edema. These latter manifestations result from catecholamine release or direct cardiac toxicity.[313] Treatment with vasodilators can counteract these hyperadrenergic sequelae.

MARINE ENVENOMATIONS

Numerous marine species transmit toxins to humans. The transmission may occur through bites, stings, or ingestion. Only a few of these toxins impair NMT as their primary mechanism of action.[329,330]

Sea snakes formerly considered members of the Hydrophiidae family but now classified as Elapids, share many of the toxic properties described above.[331] They reside almost exclusively in the warm waters of the South Pacific, Indian Ocean, and Costal California. Symptom onset is usually 1–6 hours after the bite. Local reactions are limited. Morbidity stems from both direct myotoxic effects and disordered NMT. Myotoxic effects include movement-aggravated myalgias, trismus, and rhabdomyolysis, which carry risk of myoglobinuric renal failure. Disordered NMT causes dysphagia, ptosis, and ophthalmoplegia, and ascending paralysis. Seizures, coma, and potentially death from ventilatory failure may occur. Identification of a specific sea snake species among 52 types is less likely to occur than with bites of their terrestrial cousins. Fortunately, sea snake antivenom appears equally effective regardless of species. The availability is very limited in the Western hemisphere. The Long Beach California aquarium can facilitate the dispensing. Risk of allergic reaction needs to be taken into consideration and patients typically require premedication. Management is otherwise like that recommended for terrestrial Elapid envenomations.[331]

The cone snail resides in habits like sea snakes.[330] A dart-like barb, coated in toxin, can be fired from between the edges of its shell if handled. Envenomation with conotoxin, intended to paralyze its prey, has resulted in numerous human deaths. The conotoxins have affinity for nicotinic AChRs, neuronal calcium channels, muscle sodium channels, vasopressin receptors, and N-methyl-D-aspartate receptors. Presumably, its affinity for presynaptic calcium channels is the mechanism for the paralysis it causes.[332,333] A local reaction to snail envenomation produces variable degrees of discomfort followed or accompanied by local swelling and numbness, blanching, cyanosis, and necrosis. Systemically patients may experience nausea and pruritus in addition to dysphagia, blurred vision, paralysis, and in severe cases, ventilatory failure and cardiovascular collapse. Without support, death may occur as rapidly as 2 hours after envenomation. No antivenom exists for the cone snail.

DRUGS AND METABOLIC DISTURBANCES

There are multiple drugs and notable metabolic disturbances that can affect neuromuscular transmission, and multiple mechanisms by which they can do so. These effects occur at either a presynaptic, synaptic, or postsynaptic location.[327,334–338] Those that are capable of augmenting neuromuscular transmission may be therapeutically useful in DNMT. Guanidine, rarely used now because of side effects, but used historically in the treatment of LEMS, enhances NMT by inhibiting calcium egress from the presynaptic terminal and thereby increasing the probability of ACh vesicle fusion and quantal release. Pyridostigmine, edrophonium, neostigmine, and physostigmine are helpful both diagnostically and therapeutically to enhance NMT via reversible cholinesterase inhibition. Physostigmine, which crosses the blood–brain barrier, be used as a treatment for the CNS toxicity of drugs with anticholinergic properties.

When drugs that augment cholinergic function are used in normal individuals where NMT is already optimal, they may cause symptoms of cholinergic excess at muscarinic, nicotinic, and CNS synapses, if able to penetrate the blood–brain barrier. Conversely, with certain drugs such as succinylcholine, this effect at sufficient magnitude exhausts the NMJ and results in paralysis. This effect is used therapeutically to ensure immobility during surgery and/or to reduce resistance to mechanical ventilation. This same therapeutic paralytic effect can also be obtained by nondepolarizing neuromuscular blockers whose mechanism of action is post, rather than presynaptic. The most notorious of these nondepolarizing neuromuscular blocking agents is curare, which is a naturally occurring derivative of the plant *Strychnos toxifera*. Although first utilized as a toxin in hunting and war, like botulinum toxin, it can be used therapeutically as a paralyzing agent (d-tubocurarine). It was once used to augment the diagnostic yield of repetitive stimulation testing in patients with suspected MG.

Many other drugs have neuromuscular blocking properties that vary in degree even though their primary therapeutic target is not the NMJ. These drugs may have little or no effect on people with a full neuromuscular reserve but may worsen weakness individual with a preexisting DNMT such as myasthenia. Finally, there are drugs, most notably penicillamine and α-interferon, that can induce autoimmune myasthenia.[339–354] The reader is referred to Table 26-3 for list of agents known to adversely affect neuromuscular transmission.

The release of ACh at presynaptic terminals is calcium dependent, an effect theoretically compromised by increased concentrations of magnesium, its competing cation. A paucity of information, however, exists that either hypocalcemia or hypermagnesemia have significant impact on neuromuscular transmission in most individuals. Autoantibodies (VGCC autoantibodies in LEMS) and environmental toxins (conotoxin in Cone snails) that specifically react with presynaptic VGCCs impair NMT and produce weakness. Despite this, tetany rather than weakness, is the typical effect of hypocalcemia, and appears to result from its effect on muscle sarcoplasmic reticulum, not on the NMJ. In addition, drugs with calcium channel blocking properties seem to have little, if any, significant adverse clinical or electrophysiological effects on NMT. Conversely, hypermagnesemia has rarely been reported as a cause of significant neuromuscular weakness by competitively inhibiting calcium entry into the nerve terminal.[294,355,356] Serum levels of >5 mEq/L may abolish deep tendon reflexes, with generalized weakness typically present with levels >9–10 mEq/L. The EDX pattern, when reported, is consistent with a presynaptic DNMT, namely reduced CMAP amplitude at rest, a decremental response to slow (2–5 Hz) repetitive stimulation and an incremental response to brief exercise or more rapid stimulation frequencies (10–50 Hz).[294]

► SUMMARY

Neuromuscular transmission is a complex physiological event that can be readily disrupted by numerous acquired or heritable conditions affecting one or more of its presynaptic, synaptic, or postsynaptic components. Autoimmune MG is the most common of these disorders. This chapter describes less common DNMT in individuals presenting with painless weakness, which therefore require a high index of suspicion. This is particularly true when the history reveals a clinical context predisposing to one of these disorders, or when weakness is accompanied by symptoms referable to autonomic or CNS cholinergic dysfunction.

REFERENCES

1. Anderson HJ, Churchill-Davidson HC, Richardson AT. Bronchial neoplasm with myasthenia; prolonged apnoea after administration of succinylcholine. *Lancet.* 1953;265:1291–1293.
2. Lambert EH. Defect of neuromuscular conduction associated with malignant neoplasm. *Am J Physiol.* 1956;187:612–613.
3. Abenroth DC, Smith AG, Greenlee JE, Austin SD, Clardy SL. Lambert-Eaton myasthenic syndrome: epidemiology and therapeutic response in the national veterans affairs population. *Muscle Nerve.* 2017;56:421–426.
4. Wirtz PW, van Dijk JG, van Doorn PA, et al. The epidemiology of the Lambert-Eaton myasthenic syndrome in the Netherlands. *Neurology.* 2004;63:397–398.
5. Punga AR, Maddison P, Heckmann JM, Guptill JT, Evoli A. Epidemiology, diagnostics, and biomarkers of autoimmune neuromuscular junction disorders. *Lancet Neurol.* 2022;21:176–188.
6. Pascuzzi RM, Bodkin CL. Myasthenia gravis and Lambert-Eaton myasthenic syndrome: new developments in diagnosis and treatment. *Neuropsychiatr Dis Treat.* 2022;18:3001–3022.
7. Ruiter AM, Strijbos E, de Meel RHP, et al. Accuracy of patient-reported data for an online patient registry of autoimmune myasthenia gravis and Lambert-Eaton myasthenic syndrome. *Neuromuscul Disord.* 2021;31:622–632.
8. Morgan-Followell B, de Los Reyes E. Child neurology: diagnosis of Lambert-Eaton myasthenic syndrome in children. *Neurology.* 2013;80:e220–e222.
9. Titulaer MJ, Lang B, Verschuuren JJ. Lambert-Eaton myasthenic syndrome: from clinical characteristics to therapeutic strategies. *Lancet Neurol.* 2011;10:1098–1107.
10. Schoser B, Eymard B, Datt J, Mantegazza R. Lambert-Eaton myasthenic syndrome (LEMS): a rare autoimmune presynaptic disorder often associated with cancer. *J Neurol.* 2017;264:1854–1863.
11. Wirtz PW, Bradshaw J, Wintzen AR, Verschuuren JJ. Associated autoimmune diseases in patients with the Lambert-Eaton myasthenic syndrome and their families. *J Neurol.* 2004;251:1255–1259.
12. Lang B, Newsom-Davis J, Wray D, Vincent A, Murray N. Autoimmune aetiology for myasthenic (Eaton-Lambert) syndrome. *Lancet.* 1981;2:224–226.
13. Titulaer MJ, Wirtz PW, Willems LNA, van Kralingen KW, Smitt PAES, Verschuuren JJGM. Screening for small-cell lung cancer: a follow-up study of patients with Lambert-Eaton myasthenic syndrome. *J Clin Oncol.* 2008;26:4276–4281.
14. Titulaer MJ, Maddison P, Sont JK, et al. Clinical Dutch-English Lambert-Eaton myasthenic syndrome (LEMS) tumor association prediction score accurately predicts small-cell lung cancer in the LEMS. *J Clin Oncol.* 2011;29:902–908.
15. Maddison P, Lipka AF, Gozzard P, et al. Lung cancer prediction in Lambert-Eaton myasthenic syndrome in a prospective cohort. *Sci Rep.* 2020;10:10546.
16. Maddison P, Newsom-Davis J, Mills KR, Souhami RL. Favourable prognosis in Lambert-Eaton myasthenic syndrome and small-cell lung carcinoma. *Lancet.* 1999;353:117–118.
17. Wirtz PW, Lang B, Graus F, et al. P/Q-type calcium channel antibodies, Lambert-Eaton myasthenic syndrome and survival in small cell lung cancer. *J Neuroimmunol.* 2005;164:161–165.
18. Nakao YK, Motomura M, Fukudome T, et al. Seronegative Lambert-Eaton myasthenic syndrome: study of 110 Japanese patients. *Neurology.* 2002;59:1773–1775.
19. Burns TM, Smith GA, Allen JA, et al. Editorial by concerned physicians: unintended effect of the orphan drug act on the potential cost of 3,4-diaminopyridine. *Muscle Nerve.* 2016;53:165–168.
20. Lennon VA, Kryzer TJ, Griesmann GE, et al. Calcium-channel antibodies in the Lambert-Eaton syndrome and other paraneoplastic syndromes. *N Engl J Med.* 1995;332:1467–1474.
21. Wirtz PW, Wintzen AR, Verschuuren JJ. Lambert-Eaton myasthenic syndrome has a more progressive course in patients with lung cancer. *Muscle Nerve.* 2005;32:226–229.
22. Lipka AF, Boldingh MI, van Zwet EW, et al. Long-term follow-up, quality of life, and survival of patients with Lambert-Eaton myasthenic syndrome. *Neurology.* 2020;94:e511–e520.
23. Juel VC, Sanders DB. The Lambert-Eaton myasthenic syndrome. In: Engel AG, ed. *Myasthenia Gravis and Myasthenic Disorders.* Oxford University Press; 2012:156–172.
24. O'Neill JH, Murray NM, Newsom-Davis J. The Lambert-Eaton myasthenic syndrome. A review of 50 cases. *Brain.* 1988;111(Pt 3):577–596.
25. Breen LA, Gutmann L, Brick JF, Riggs JR. Paradoxical lid elevation with sustained upgaze: a sign of Lambert-Eaton syndrome. *Muscle Nerve.* 1991;14:863–866.
26. Rudnicki SA. Lambert-Eaton myasthenic syndrome with pure ocular weakness. *Neurology.* 2007;68:1863–1864.
27. Wirtz PW, Sotodeh M, Nijnuis M, et al. Difference in distribution of muscle weakness between myasthenia gravis and the Lambert-Eaton myasthenic syndrome. *J Neurol Neurosurg Psychiatr.* 2002;73:766–768.
28. Rácz A, Giede-Jeppe A, Schramm A, Schwab S, Maihöfner C. Lambert-Eaton myasthenic syndrome presenting with a "dropped head syndrome" and associated with antibodies against N-type calcium channels. *Neurol Sci.* 2013;34:1253–1254.
29. Smith AG, Wald J. Acute ventilatory failure in Lambert-Eaton myasthenic syndrome and its response to 3,4-diaminopyridine. *Neurology.* 1996;46:1143–1145.
30. Barr CW, Claussen G, Thomas D, Fesenmeier JT, Pearlman RL, Oh SJ. Primary respiratory failure as the presenting symptom in Lambert-Eaton myasthenic syndrome. *Muscle Nerve.* 1993;16:712–715.
31. Nicolle MW, Stewart DJ, Remtulla H, Chen R, Bolton CF. Lambert-Eaton myasthenic syndrome presenting with severe respiratory failure. *Muscle Nerve.* 1996;19:1328–1333.

32. Raja SM. Lambert-Eaton myasthenic syndrome and botulism. *Continuum (Minneap Minn)*. 2022;28:1596–1614.
33. Mason WP, Graus F, Lang B, et al. Small-cell lung cancer, paraneoplastic cerebellar degeneration and the Lambert-Eaton myasthenic syndrome. *Brain*. 1997;120(Pt 8):1279–1300.
34. Poh M, Ming YC, Yanni PC, et al. Postexercise reflex facilitation in Lambert-Eaton myasthenic syndrome. *Pract Neurol*. 2024:pn-2023-004032.
35. Odabasi Z, Demirci M, Kim DS, et al. Postexercise facilitation of reflexes is not common in Lambert-Eaton myasthenic syndrome. *Neurology*. 2002;59:1085–1087.
36. Oh SJ. Myasthenia gravis Lambert-Eaton overlap syndrome. *Muscle Nerve*. 2016;53:20–26.
37. Lennon VA. Serologic profile of myasthenia gravis and distinction from the Lambert-Eaton myasthenic syndrome. *Neurology*. 1997;48:23S–27S.
38. Katz JS, Wolfe GI, Bryan WW, Tintner R, Barohn RJ. Acetylcholine receptor antibodies in the Lambert-Eaton myasthenic syndrome. *Neurology*. 1998;50:470–475.
39. Oh SJ, Dwyer DS, Bradley RJ. Overlap myasthenic syndrome: combined myasthenia gravis and Eaton-Lambert syndrome. *Neurology*. 1987;37:1411–1414.
40. Newsom-Davis J, Leys K, Vincent A, Ferguson I, Modi G, Mills K. Immunological evidence for the co-existence of the Lambert-Eaton myasthenic syndrome and myasthenia gravis in two patients. *J Neurol Neurosurg Psychiatr*. 1991;54:452–453.
41. Tim RW, Massey JM, Sanders DB. Lambert-Eaton myasthenic syndrome: electrodiagnostic findings and response to treatment. *Neurology*. 2000;54:2176–2178.
42. Oh SJ. Assessment of the compound muscle action potential amplitude return time between exercises or tests in the repetitive nerve stimulation test for Lambert-Eaton myasthenic syndrome. *Muscle Nerve*. 2020;62:742–745.
43. Lipka AF, Titulaer MJ, Tannemaat MR, Verschuuren JJGM. Lowering the cutoff value for increment increases the sensitivity for the diagnosis of Lambert-Eaton myasthenic syndrome. *Muscle Nerve*. 2020;62:111–114.
44. Tim RW, Massey JM, Sanders DB. Lambert-Eaton myasthenic syndrome (LEMS). Clinical and electrodiagnostic features and response to therapy in 59 patients. *Ann N Y Acad Sci*. 1998;841:823–826.
45. Sanders DB, Cao L, Massey JM, Juel VC, Hobson-Webb L, Guptill JT. Is the decremental pattern in Lambert-Eaton syndrome different from that in myasthenia gravis? *Clin Neurophysiol*. 2014;125:1274–1277.
46. Baslo MB, Deymeer F, Serdaroglu P, Parman Y, Ozdemir C, Cuttini M. Decrement pattern in Lambert-Eaton myasthenic syndrome is different from myasthenia gravis. *Neuromuscul Disord*. 2006;16:454–458.
47. Howard JF Jr, Sanders DB, Massey JM. The electrodiagnosis of myasthenia gravis and the Lambert-Eaton myasthenic syndrome. *Neurol Clin*. 1994;12:305–330.
48. Juel VC. Clinical neurophysiology of neuromuscular junction disease. *Handb Clin Neurol*. 2019;161:291–303.
49. Juel VC. Evaluation of neuromuscular junction disorders in the electromyography laboratory. *Neurol Clin*. 2012;30:621–639.
50. Sanders DB, Arimura K, Cui L, et al. Guidelines for single fiber EMG. *Clin Neurophysiol*. 2019;130:1417–1439.
51. Oh SJ, Ohira M. Single-fiber EMG and clinical correlation in Lambert-Eaton myasthenic syndrome. *Muscle Nerve*. 2013;47:664–667.
52. Todisco V, Cirillo G, Capuano R, d'Ambrosio A, Tedeschi G, Gallo A. Stimulated single-fiber electromyography (sSFEMG) in Lambert-Eaton syndrome. *Clin Neurophysiol Pract*. 2018;3:148–150.
53. Trontelj JV, Stålberg E. Single motor end-plates in myasthenia gravis and LEMS at different firing rates. *Muscle Nerve*. 1991;14:226–232.
54. Rubenstein AE, Horowitz SH, Bender AN. Cholinergic dysautonomia and Eaton-Lambert syndrome. *Neurology*. 1979;29:720–723.
55. O'Suilleabhain P, Low PA, Lennon VA. Autonomic dysfunction in the Lambert-Eaton myasthenic syndrome: serologic and clinical correlates. *Neurology*. 1998;50:88–93.
56. Kim DS, Claussen GC, Oh SJ. Single-fiber electromyography improvement with 3,4-diaminopyridine in Lambert-Eaton myasthenic syndrome. *Muscle Nerve*. 1998;21:1107–1108.
57. Sanders DB, Juel VC, Harati Y, et al. 3,4-diaminopyridine base effectively treats the weakness of Lambert-Eaton myasthenia. *Muscle Nerve*. 2018;57:561–568.
58. Sanders DB, Massey JM, Sanders LL, Edwards LJ. A randomized trial of 3,4-diaminopyridine in Lambert-Eaton myasthenic syndrome. *Neurology*. 2000;54:603–607.
59. Raja SM, Sanders DB, Juel VC, et al. Validation of the triple timed up-and-go test in Lambert-Eaton myasthenia. *Muscle Nerve*. 2019;60:292–298.
60. Leys K, Lang B, Johnston I, Newsom-Davis J. Calcium channel autoantibodies in the Lambert-Eaton myasthenic syndrome. *Ann Neurol*. 1991;29:307–314.
61. Pinto A, Iwasa K, Newland C, Newsom-Davis J, Lang B. The action of Lambert-Eaton myasthenic syndrome immunoglobulin G on cloned human voltage-gated calcium channels. *Muscle Nerve*. 2002;25:715–724.
62. Leveque C, Hoshino T, David P, et al. The synaptic vesicle protein synaptotagmin associates with calcium channels and is a putative Lambert-Eaton myasthenic syndrome antigen. *Proc Natl Acad Sci U S A*. 1992;89:3625–3629.
63. Titulaer MJ, Klooster R, Potman M, et al. SOX antibodies in small-cell lung cancer and Lambert-Eaton myasthenic syndrome: frequency and relation with survival. *J Clin Oncol*. 2009;27:4260–4267.
64. Sabater L, Titulaer M, Saiz A, Verschuuren J, Güre AO, Graus F. SOX1 antibodies are markers of paraneoplastic Lambert-Eaton myasthenic syndrome. *Neurology*. 2008;70:924–928.
65. Bekircan-Kurt CE, Derle Çiftçi E, Kurne AT, Anlar B. Voltage gated calcium channel antibody-related neurological diseases. *World J Clin Cases*. 2015;3:293–300.
66. Zalewski NL, Lennon VA, Lachance DH, Klein CJ, Pittock SJ, McKeon A. P/Q- and N-type calcium-channel antibodies: oncological, neurological, and serological accompaniments. *Muscle Nerve*. 2016;54:220–227.
67. Lipka AF, Verschuuren JJGM, Titulaer MJ. SOX1 antibodies in Lambert-Eaton myasthenic syndrome and screening for small cell lung carcinoma. *Ann N Y Acad Sci*. 2012;1275:70–77.
68. David P, Martin-Moutot N, Leveque C, el Far O, Takahashi M, Seagar MJ. Interaction of synaptotagmin with voltage gated calcium channels: a role in Lambert-Eaton myasthenic syndrome? *Neuromuscul Disord*. 1993;3:451–454.
69. Herrmann DN, Horvath R, Sowden JE, et al. Synaptotagmin 2 mutations cause an autosomal-dominant form of Lambert-Eaton myasthenic syndrome and nonprogressive motor neuropathy. *Am J Hum Genet*. 2014;95:332–339.

70. Titulaer MJ, Soffietti R, Dalmau J, et al. Screening for tumours in paraneoplastic syndromes: report of an EFNS task force. *Eur J Neurol.* 2011;18:19-e3.
71. Sundermann B, Schröder JB, Warnecke T, et al. Imaging workup of suspected classical paraneoplastic neurological syndromes: a systematic review and retrospective analysis of 18F-FDG-PET-CT. *Acad Radiol.* 2017;24:1195–1202.
72. Fukuoka T, Engel AG, Lang B, Newsom-Davis J, Prior C, Wray DW. Lambert-Eaton myasthenic syndrome: I. Early morphological effects of IgG on the presynaptic membrane active zones. *Ann Neurol.* 1987;22:193–199.
73. Fukuoka T, Engel AG, Lang B, Newsom-Davis J, Vincent A. Lambert-Eaton myasthenic syndrome: II. Immunoelectron microscopy localization of IgG at the mouse motor end-plate. *Ann Neurol.* 1987;22:200–211.
74. Gutmann L, Crosby TW, Takamori M, Martin JD. The Eaton-Lambert syndrome and autoimmune disorders. *Am J Med.* 1972;53:354–356.
75. Fukunaga H, Engel AG, Lang B, Newsom-Davis J, Vincent A. Passive transfer of Lambert-Eaton myasthenic syndrome with IgG from man to mouse depletes the presynaptic membrane active zones. *Proc Natl Acad Sci U S A.* 1983;80:7636–7640.
76. Kim YI. Passively transferred Lambert-Eaton syndrome in mice receiving purified IgG. *Muscle Nerve.* 1986;9:523–530.
77. Engel AG. The neuromuscular junction. *Handb Clin Neurol.* 2008;91:103–148.
78. Hughes BW, Kusner LL, Kaminski HJ. Molecular architecture of the neuromuscular junction. *Muscle Nerve.* 2006;33:445–461.
79. Engel AG. Review of evidence for loss of motor nerve terminal calcium channels in Lambert-Eaton myasthenic syndrome. *Ann N Y Acad Sci.* 1991;635:246–258.
80. Reuner U, Kamin G, Ramantani G, Reichmann H, Dinger J. Transient neonatal Lambert-Eaton syndrome. *J Neurol.* 2008;255:1827–1828.
81. Lecky BRF. Transient neonatal Lambert-Eaton syndrome. *J Neurol Neurosurg Psychiatr.* 2006;77:1094.
82. Ginebaugh SP, Badawi Y, Tarr TB, Meriney SD. Neuromuscular active zone structure and function in healthy and Lambert-Eaton myasthenic syndrome states. *Biomolecules.* 2022;12(6):740.
83. Ginebaugh SP, Badawi Y, Laghaei R, et al. Simulations of active zone structure and function at mammalian NMJs predict that loss of calcium channels alone is not sufficient to replicate LEMS effects. *J Neurophysiol.* 2023;129:1259–1277.
84. Chalk CH, Murray NM, Newsom-Davis J, O'Neill JH, Spiro SG. Response of the Lambert-Eaton myasthenic syndrome to treatment of associated small-cell lung carcinoma. *Neurology.* 1990;40:1552–1556.
85. De Aizpurua HJ, Lambert EH, Griesmann GE, Olivera BM, Lennon VA. Antagonism of voltage-gated calcium channels in small cell carcinomas of patients with and without Lambert-Eaton myasthenic syndrome by autoantibodies omega-conotoxin and adenosine. *Cancer Res.* 1988;48:4719–4724.
86. Wirtz PW, Willcox N, van der Slik AR, et al. HLA and smoking in prediction and prognosis of small cell lung cancer in autoimmune Lambert-Eaton myasthenic syndrome. *J Neuroimmunol.* 2005;159:230–237.
87. Wirtz PW, Roep BO, Schreuder GM, et al. HLA class I and II in Lambert-Eaton myasthenic syndrome without associated tumor. *Hum Immunol.* 2001;62:809–813.
88. Muñiz-Castrillo S, Vogrig A, Honnorat J. Associations between HLA and autoimmune neurological diseases with autoantibodies. *Auto Immun Highlights.* 2020;11(1):2.
89. Jenkyn LR, Brooks PL, Forcier RJ, Maurer LH, Ochoa J. Remission of the Lambert-Eaton syndrome and small cell anaplastic carcinoma of the lung induced by chemotherapy and radiotherapy. *Cancer.* 1980;46:1123–1127.
90. Skeie GO, Apostolski S, Evoli A, et al. Guidelines for treatment of autoimmune neuromuscular transmission disorders. *Eur J Neurol.* 2010;17:893–902.
91. Keogh M, Sedehizadeh S, Maddison P. Treatment for Lambert-Eaton myasthenic syndrome. *Cochrane Database Syst Rev.* 2011;2011:CD003279.
92. Verschuuren JJ, Palace J, Murai H, Tannemaat MR, Kaminski HJ, Bril V. Advances and ongoing research in the treatment of autoimmune neuromuscular junction disorders. *Lancet Neurol.* 2022;21:189–202.
93. Evoli A, Liguori R, Romani A, et al. Italian recommendations for Lambert-Eaton myasthenic syndrome (LEMS) management. *Neurol Sci.* 2014;35:515–520.
94. Narayanaswami P, Sanders DB, Wolfe G, et al. International consensus guidance for management of myasthenia gravis: 2020 update. *Neurology.* 2021;96:114–122.
95. Lundh H, Nilsson O, Rosén I. Treatment of Lambert-Eaton syndrome: 3,4-diaminopyridine and pyridostigmine. *Neurology.* 1984;34:1324–1330.
96. Oh SJ, Claussen GG, Hatanaka Y, Morgan MB. 3,4-Diaminopyridine is more effective than placebo in a randomized, double-blind, cross-over drug study in LEMS. *Muscle Nerve.* 2009;40:795–800.
97. McEvoy KM, Windebank AJ, Daube JR, Low PA. 3,4-Diaminopyridine in the treatment of Lambert-Eaton myasthenic syndrome. *N Engl J Med.* 1989;321:1567–1571.
98. Wirtz PW, Verschuuren JJ, van Dijk JG, et al. Efficacy of 3,4-diaminopyridine and pyridostigmine in the treatment of Lambert-Eaton myasthenic syndrome: a randomized, double-blind, placebo-controlled, crossover study. *Clin Pharmacol Ther.* 2009;86:44–48.
99. Shieh P, Sharma K, Kohrman B, Oh SJ. Amifampridine phosphate (firdapse) is effective in a confirmatory phase 3 clinical trial in LEMS. *J Clin Neuromuscul Dis.* 2019;20:111–119.
100. Burns TM, Crowell JL, Smith AG. A crisis in US drug pricing: consequences for patients with neuromuscular diseases, physicians, and society, part 2. *Muscle Nerve.* 2020;62:573–578.
101. Tarr TB, Wipf P, Meriney SD. Synaptic pathophysiology and treatment of Lambert-Eaton myasthenic syndrome. *Mol Neurobiol.* 2015;52:456–463.
102. Tarr TB, Lacomis D, Reddel SW, et al. Complete reversal of Lambert-Eaton myasthenic syndrome synaptic impairment by the combined use of a K+ channel blocker and a Ca2+ channel agonist. *J Physiol (Lond).* 2014;592:3687–3696.
103. Newsom-Davis J, Murray NM. Plasma exchange and immunosuppressive drug treatment in the Lambert-Eaton myasthenic syndrome. *Neurology.* 1984;34:480–485.
104. Bain PG, Motomura M, Newsom-Davis J, et al. Effects of intravenous immunoglobulin on muscle weakness and calcium-channel autoantibodies in the Lambert-Eaton myasthenic syndrome. *Neurology.* 1996;47:678–683.
105. Dau PC, Denys EH. Plasmapheresis and immunosuppressive drug therapy in the Eaton-Lambert syndrome. *Ann Neurol.* 1982;11:570–575.

106. Maddison P. Treatment in Lambert-Eaton myasthenic syndrome. *Ann N Y Acad Sci.* 2012;1275:78–84.
107. Maddison P, McConville J, Farrugia ME, et al. The use of rituximab in myasthenia gravis and Lambert-Eaton myasthenic syndrome. *J Neurol Neurosurg Psychiatr.* 2011;82:671–673.
108. Pellkofer HL, Voltz R, Kuempfel T. Favorable response to rituximab in a patient with anti-VGCC-positive Lambert-Eaton myasthenic syndrome and cerebellar dysfunction. *Muscle Nerve.* 2009;40:305–308.
109. McQuillen MP. Familial limb-girdle myasthenia. *Brain.* 1966;89:121–132.
110. Engel AG. Congenital myasthenic syndromes in 2018. *Curr Neurol Neurosci Rep.* 2018;18:46.
111. Engel AG. Genetic basis and phenotypic features of congenital myasthenic syndromes. *Handb Clin Neurol.* 2018;148:565–589.
112. Engel AG, Shen X-M, Selcen D. The unfolding landscape of the congenital myasthenic syndromes. *Ann N Y Acad Sci.* 2018;1413:25–34.
113. Ohno K, Ohkawara B, Shen X-M, Selcen D, Engel AG. Clinical and pathologic features of congenital myasthenic syndromes caused by 35 genes—A comprehensive review. *Int J Mol Sci.* 2023;24(4):3730.
114. Finsterer J. Congenital myasthenic syndromes. *Orphanet J Rare Dis.* 2019;14:57.
115. Engel AG, Shen XM, Selcen D, Sine SM. Congenital myasthenic syndromes: pathogenesis, diagnosis, and treatment. *Lancet Neurol.* 2015;14(5):461.
116. Kao JC, Milone M, Selcen D, Shen XM, Engel AG, Liewluck T. Congenital myasthenic syndromes in adult neurology clinic: a long road to diagnosis and therapy. *Neurology.* 2018;91:e1770–e1777.
117. Garg N, Yiannikas C, Hardy TA, et al. Late presentations of congenital myasthenic syndromes: how many do we miss? *Muscle Nerve.* 2016;54:721–727.
118. Gilhus NE. Myasthenia gravis and congenital myasthenic syndromes. *Handb Clin Neurol.* 2023;195:635–652.
119. Estephan EP, Zambon AA, Thompson R, et al. Congenital myasthenic syndrome: correlation between clinical features and molecular diagnosis. *Eur J Neurol.* 2022;29:833–842.
120. Barišić N, Chaouch A, Müller JS, Lochmüller H. Genetic heterogeneity and pathophysiological mechanisms in congenital myasthenic syndromes. *Eur J Paediatr Neurol.* 2011;15:189–196.
121. Selcen D, Milone M, Shen XM, et al. Dok-7 myasthenia: phenotypic and molecular genetic studies in 16 patients. *Ann Neurol.* 2008;64:71–87.
122. Milone M, Shen XM, Selcen D, et al. Myasthenic syndrome due to defects in rapsyn: clinical and molecular findings in 39 patients. *Neurology.* 2009;73:228–235.
123. Selcen D, Shen XM, Milone M, et al. GFPT1-myasthenia: clinical, structural, and electrophysiologic heterogeneity. *Neurology.* 2013;81:370–378.
124. Cossins J, Belaya K, Hicks D, et al. Congenital myasthenic syndromes due to mutations in ALG2 and ALG14. *Brain.* 2013;136:944–956.
125. Finlayson S, Palace J, Belaya K, et al. Clinical features of congenital myasthenic syndrome due to mutations in DPAGT1. *J Neurol Neurosurg Psychiatr.* 2013;84:1119–1125.
126. Engel AG. Current status of the congenital myasthenic syndromes. *Neuromuscul Disord.* 2012;22:99–111.
127. Finlayson S, Beeson D, Palace J. Congenital myasthenic syndromes: an update. *Pract Neurol.* 2013;13:80–91.
128. Beeson D, Hantaï D, Lochmüller H, Engel AG. 126th International Workshop: congenital myasthenic syndromes, 24-26 September 2004, Naarden, the Netherlands. *Neuromuscul Disord.* 2005;15:498–512.
129. Dobkin BH, Verity MA. Familial neuromuscular disease with type 1 fiber hypoplasia, tubular aggregates, cardiomyopathy, and myasthenic features. *Neurology.* 1978;28:1135–1140.
130. Furui E, Fukushima K, Sakashita T, Sakato S, Matsubara S, Takamori M. Familial limb-girdle myasthenia with tubular aggregates. *Muscle Nerve.* 1997;20:599–603.
131. Johns TR, Crowley WJ, Miller JQ, Campa JF. The syndrome of myasthenia and polymyositis with comments on therapy. *Ann N Y Acad Sci.* 1971;183:64–71.
132. Schara U, Della Marina A, Abicht A. Congenital myasthenic syndromes: current diagnostic and therapeutic approaches. *Neuropediatrics.* 2012;43:184–193.
133. Lorenzoni PJ, Scola RH, Kay CSK, Werneck LC. Congenital myasthenic syndrome: a brief review. *Pediatr Neurol.* 2012;46:141–148.
134. Punga AR, Ruegg MA. Signaling and aging at the neuromuscular synapse: lessons learnt from neuromuscular diseases. *Curr Opin Pharmacol.* 2012;12:340–346.
135. Engel AG, Shen X-M, Selcen D, Sine SM. What have we learned from the congenital myasthenic syndromes. *J Mol Neurosci.* 2010;40:143–153.
136. Walls TJ, Engel AG, Nagel AS, Harper CM, Trastek VF. Congenital myasthenic syndrome associated with paucity of synaptic vesicles and reduced quantal release. *Ann N Y Acad Sci.* 1993;681:461–468.
137. Arredondo J, Lara M, Gospe SM Jr, et al. Choline acetyltransferase mutations causing congenital myasthenic syndrome: molecular findings and genotype-phenotype correlations. *Hum Mutat.* 2015;36:881–893.
138. Bady B, Chauplannaz G, Carrier H. Congenital Lambert-Eaton myasthenic syndrome. *J Neurol Neurosurg Psychiatr.* 1987;50:476–478.
139. Lorenzoni PJ, Scola RH, Kay CSK, Werneck LC, Horvath R, Lochmüller H. How to spot congenital myasthenic syndromes resembling the Lambert-Eaton myasthenic syndrome? A brief review of clinical, electrophysiological, and genetics features. *Neuromolecular Med.* 2018;20:205–214.
140. Shen X-M, Selcen D, Brengman J, Engel AG. Mutant SNAP25B causes myasthenia, cortical hyperexcitability, ataxia, and intellectual disability. *Neurology.* 2014;83:2247–2255.
141. McMacken G, Whittaker RG, Evangelista T, Abicht A, Dusl M, Lochmüller H. Congenital myasthenic syndrome with episodic apnoea: clinical, neurophysiological and genetic features in the long-term follow-up of 19 patients. *J Neurol.* 2018;265:194–203.
142. Bauché S, O'Regan S, Azuma Y, et al. Impaired presynaptic high-affinity choline transporter causes a congenital myasthenic syndrome with episodic apnea. *Am J Hum Genet.* 2016;99:753–761.
143. Banerjee M, Arutyunov D, Brandwein D, et al. The novel p.Ser263Phe mutation in the human high-affinity choline transporter 1 (CHT1/SLC5A7) causes a lethal form of fetal akinesia syndrome. *Hum Mutat.* 2019;40:1676–1683.
144. Engel AG, Walls TJ, Nagel A, Uchitel O. Newly recognized congenital myasthenic syndromes: I. Congenital paucity of

synaptic vesicles and reduced quantal release. II. High-conductance fast-channel syndrome. III. Abnormal acetylcholine receptor (AChR) interaction with acetylcholine. IV. AChR deficiency and short channel-open time. *Prog Brain Res.* 1990;84:125–137.

145. Maselli RA, Kong DZ, Bowe CM, et al. Presynaptic congenital myasthenic syndrome due to quantal release deficiency. *Neurology.* 2001;57:279–289.

146. Aran A, Segel R, Kaneshige K, et al. Vesicular acetylcholine transporter defect underlies devastating congenital myasthenia syndrome. *Neurology.* 2017;88:1021–1028.

147. Magalhães-Gomes MPS, Motta-Santos D, Schetino LPL, et al. Fast and slow-twitching muscles are differentially affected by reduced cholinergic transmission in mice deficient for VAChT: a mouse model for congenital myasthenia. *Neurochem Int.* 2018;120:1–12.

148. Chaouch A, Porcelli V, Cox D, et al. Mutations in the mitochondrial citrate carrier SLC25A1 are associated with impaired neuromuscular transmission. *J Neuromuscul Dis.* 2014;1:75–90.

149. Régal L, Shen XM, Selcen D, et al. PREPL deficiency with or without cystinuria causes a novel myasthenic syndrome. *Neurology.* 2014;82:1254–1260.

150. Prior DE, Ghosh PS. Congenital myasthenic syndrome from a single center: phenotypic and genotypic features. *J Child Neurol.* 2021;36:610–617.

151. Mihaylova V, Müller JS, Vilchez JJ, et al. Clinical and molecular genetic findings in COLQ-mutant congenital myasthenic syndromes. *Brain.* 2008;131:747–759.

152. Maselli RA, Arredondo J, Ferns MJ, Wollmann RL. Synaptic basal lamina-associated congenital myasthenic syndromes. *Ann N Y Acad Sci.* 2012;1275:36–48.

153. Engel AG, Lambert EH, Mulder DM, et al. Recently recognized congenital myasthenic syndromes: (a) end-plate acetylcholine (ACh) esterase deficiency (b) putative abnormality of the ACh induced ion channel (c) putative defect of ACh resynthesis or mobilization – clinical features, ultrastructure and cytochemistry. *Ann N Y Acad Sci.* 1981;377:614–639.

154. Engel AG, Lambert EH, Gomez MR. A new myasthenic syndrome with end-plate acetylcholinesterase deficiency, small nerve terminals, and reduced acetylcholine release. *Ann Neurol.* 1977;1:315–330.

155. Hutchinson DO, Walls TJ, Nakano S, et al. Congenital endplate acetylcholinesterase deficiency. *Brain.* 1993;116(Pt 3):633–653.

156. Maselli RA, Ng JJ, Anderson JA, et al. Mutations in LAMB2 causing a severe form of synaptic congenital myasthenic syndrome. *J Med Genet.* 2009;46:203–208.

157. Takamori M. Myasthenia gravis: from the viewpoint of pathogenicity focusing on acetylcholine receptor clustering, trans-synaptic homeostasis and synaptic stability. *Front Mol Neurosci.* 2020;13:86.

158. Müller JS, Herczegfalvi A, Vilchez JJ, et al. Phenotypical spectrum of DOK7 mutations in congenital myasthenic syndromes. *Brain.* 2007;130:1497–1506.

159. Palace J, Lashley D, Newsom-Davis J, et al. Clinical features of the DOK7 neuromuscular junction synaptopathy. *Brain.* 2007;130:1507–1515.

160. Anderson JA, Ng JJ, Bowe C, et al. Variable phenotypes associated with mutations in DOK7. *Muscle Nerve.* 2008;37:448–456.

161. Maselli RA, Arredondo J, Cagney O, et al. Mutations in MUSK causing congenital myasthenic syndrome impair MuSK-Dok-7 interaction. *Hum Mol Genet.* 2010;19:2370–2379.

162. Beeson D, Higuchi O, Palace J, et al. Dok-7 mutations underlie a neuromuscular junction synaptopathy. *Science.* 2006;313:1975–1978.

163. Selcen D, Milone M, Shen XM, et al. NMP040 Dok-7 myasthenia: clinical spectrum, endplate (EP) electrophysiology and morphology, 12 novel DNA rearrangements, and genotype-phenotype relations in a mayo cohort of 13 patients. *Eur J Paediatr Neurol.* 2007;11:116.

164. Oury J, Zhang W, Leloup N, et al. Mechanism of disease and therapeutic rescue of Dok7 congenital myasthenia. *Nature.* 2021;595:404–408.

165. Fernandes M, Caetano A, Pinto M, Medeiros E, Santos L. Diagnosis of DOK7 congenital myasthenic syndrome during pregnancy: a case report and literature review. *Clin Neurol Neurosurg.* 2021;203:106591.

166. Liao X, Wang Y, Lai X, Wang S. The role of Rapsyn in neuromuscular junction and congenital myasthenic syndrome. *Biomol Biomed.* 2023;23:772–784.

167. Xing G, Xiong W-C, Mei L. Rapsyn as a signaling and scaffolding molecule in neuromuscular junction formation and maintenance. *Neurosci Lett.* 2020;731:135013.

168. Gillespie SK, Balasubramanian S, Fung ET, Huganir RL. Rapsyn clusters and activates the synapse-specific receptor tyrosine kinase MuSK. *Neuron.* 1996;16:953–962.

169. Burke G, Cossins J, Maxwell S, et al. Rapsyn mutations in hereditary myasthenia: distinct early- and late-onset phenotypes. *Neurology.* 2003;61:826–828.

170. Saito M, Ogasawara M, Inaba Y, et al. Successful treatment of congenital myasthenic syndrome caused by a novel compound heterozygous variant in RAPSN. *Brain Dev.* 2022;44:50–55.

171. Mihaylova V, Salih MA, Mukhtar MM, et al. Refinement of the clinical phenotype in musk-related congenital myasthenic syndromes. *Neurology.* 2009;73:1926–1928.

172. Chevessier F, Faraut B, Ravel-Chapuis A, et al. MUSK, a new target for mutations causing congenital myasthenic syndrome. *Hum Mol Genet.* 2004;13:3229–3240.

173. Murali C, Li D, Grand K, Hakonarson H, Bhoj E. Isolated vocal cord paralysis in two siblings with compound heterozygous variants in MUSK: expanding the phenotypic spectrum. *Am J Med Genet A.* 2019;179:655–658.

174. Mroczek M, Durmus H, Töpf A, Parman Y, Straub V. Four individuals with a homozygous mutation in exon 1f of the PLEC gene and associated myasthenic features. *Genes.* 2020;11:716.

175. Selcen D, Juel VC, Hobson-Webb LD, et al. Myasthenic syndrome caused by plectinopathy. *Neurology.* 2011;76:327–336.

176. Maselli RA, Fernandez JM, Arredondo J, et al. LG2 agrin mutation causing severe congenital myasthenic syndrome mimics functional characteristics of non-neural (z-) agrin. *Hum Genet.* 2012;131:1123–1135.

177. Engel AG, Ohno K, Milone M, et al. New mutations in acetylcholine receptor subunit genes reveal heterogeneity in the slow-channel congenital myasthenic syndrome. *Hum Mol Genet.* 1996;5:1217–1227.

178. Engel AG, Lambert EH, Mulder DM, et al. A newly recognized congenital myasthenic syndrome attributed to a prolonged open time of the acetylcholine-induced ion channel. *Ann Neurol.* 1982;11:553–569.

179. Burke G, Cossins J, Maxwell S, et al. Distinct phenotypes of congenital acetylcholine receptor deficiency. *Neuromuscul Disord*. 2004;14:356–364.
180. Shen XM, Ohno K, Fukudome T, et al. Congenital myasthenic syndrome caused by low-expressor fast-channel AChR delta subunit mutation. *Neurology*. 2002;59:1881–1888.
181. Huzé C, Bauché S, Richard P, et al. Identification of an agrin mutation that causes congenital myasthenia and affects synapse function. *Am J Hum Genet*. 2009;85:155–167.
182. Bogdanik LP, Burgess RW. A valid mouse model of AGRIN-associated congenital myasthenic syndrome. *Hum Mol Genet*. 2011;20:4617–4633.
183. Xi J, Yan C, Liu WW, et al. Novel SEA and LG2 Agrin mutations causing congenital Myasthenic syndrome. *Orphanet J Rare Dis*. 2017;12:182.
184. Rudell JB, Maselli RA, Yarov-Yarovoy V, Ferns MJ. Pathogenic effects of agrin V1727F mutation are isoform specific and decrease its expression and affinity for HSPGs and LRP4. *Hum Mol Genet*. 2019;28:2648–2658.
185. Singh S, Govindarajan R. Presentation and management of congenital myasthenic syndrome with a homozygous Agrin variant (Pro1448Leu). *Clin Neurol Neurosurg*. 2020;199:106277.
186. Xia P, Xie F, Zhou ZJ, Lv W. Novel LG1 mutations in agrin causing congenital myasthenia syndrome. *Intern Med*. 2022;61:887–890.
187. Jacquier A, Risson V, Simonet T, et al. Severe congenital myasthenic syndromes caused by agrin mutations affecting secretion by motoneurons. *Acta Neuropathol*. 2022;144:707–731.
188. Tezuka T, Inoue A, Hoshi T, et al. The MuSK activator agrin has a separate role essential for postnatal maintenance of neuromuscular synapses. *Proc Natl Acad Sci U S A*. 2014;111:16556–16561.
189. Ohkawara B, Shen X, Selcen D, et al. Congenital myasthenic syndrome-associated agrin variants affect clustering of acetylcholine receptors in a domain-specific manner. *JCI Insight*. 2020;5(7):e132023.
190. Nicole S, Shen X, Selcen D, et al. Agrin mutations lead to a congenital myasthenic syndrome with distal muscle weakness and atrophy. *Brain*. 2014;137:2429–2443.
191. Karakaya M, Ceyhan-Birsoy O, Beggs AH, Topaloglu H. A novel missense variant in the AGRN gene; congenital myasthenic syndrome presenting with head drop. *J Clin Neuromuscul Dis*. 2017;18:147–151.
192. Masingue M, Cattaneo O, Wolff N, et al. New mutation in the β1 propeller domain of LRP4 responsible for congenital myasthenic syndrome associated with Cenani-Lenz syndrome. *Sci Rep*. 2023;13:14054.
193. Al Jabry T, Al-Hashmi N, Abdelhadi B, Al-Maawali A. LRP4 site-specific variants in the third β-propeller domain causes congenital myasthenic syndrome type 17. *Eur J Med Genet*. 2024;67:104903.
194. Ohkawara B, Cabrera-Serrano M, Nakata T, et al. LRP4 third β-propeller domain mutations cause novel congenital myasthenia by compromising agrin-mediated MuSK signaling in a position-specific manner. *Hum Mol Genet*. 2014;23:1856–1868.
195. Tsujino A, Maertens C, Ohno K, et al. Myasthenic syndrome caused by mutation of the SCN4A sodium channel. *Proc Natl Acad Sci U S A*. 2003;100:7377–7382.
196. Berghold VM, Koko M, Berutti R, Plecko B. Case report: novel SCN4A variant associated with a severe congenital myasthenic syndrome/myopathy phenotype. *Front Pediatr*. 2022;10:944784.
197. Männikkö R, Wong L, Tester DJ, et al. Dysfunction of NaV1.4, a skeletal muscle voltage-gated sodium channel, in sudden infant death syndrome: a case-control study. *Lancet*. 2018;391:1483–1492.
198. Guergueltcheva V, Müller JS, Dusl M, et al. Congenital myasthenic syndrome with tubular aggregates caused by GFPT1 mutations. *J Neurol*. 2012;259:838–850.
199. Belaya K, Finlayson S, Cossins J, et al. Identification of DPAGT1 as a new gene in which mutations cause a congenital myasthenic syndrome. *Ann N Y Acad Sci*. 2012;1275:29–35.
200. Belaya K, Finlayson S, Slater CR, et al. Mutations in DPAGT1 cause a limb-girdle congenital myasthenic syndrome with tubular aggregates. *Am J Hum Genet*. 2012;91:193–201.
201. Monies DM, Al-Hindi HN, Al-Muhaizea MA, et al. Clinical and pathological heterogeneity of a congenital disorder of glycosylation manifesting as a myasthenic/myopathic syndrome. *Neuromuscul Disord*. 2014;24:353–359.
202. Wu F, Mi W, Fu Y, Struyk A, Cannon SC. Mice with an NaV1.4 sodium channel null allele have latent myasthenia, without susceptibility to periodic paralysis. *Brain*. 2016;139:1688–1699.
203. Nicolau S, Milone M, Liewluck T. Guidelines for genetic testing of muscle and neuromuscular junction disorders. *Muscle Nerve*. 2021;64:255–269.
204. Nicolau S, Milone M. The electrophysiology of presynaptic congenital myasthenic syndromes with and without facilitation: from electrodiagnostic findings to molecular mechanisms. *Front Neurol*. 2019;10:257.
205. Stojkovic T, Masingue M, Turmel H, et al. Diagnostic yield of a practical electrodiagnostic protocol discriminating between different congenital myasthenic syndromes. *Neuromuscul Disord*. 2022;32:870–878.
206. Kosac A, Gavillet E, Whittaker RG. Neurophysiological testing in congenital myasthenic syndromes: a systematic review of published normal data. *Muscle Nerve*. 2013;48:711–715.
207. Elahi B, Laughlin RS, Litchy WJ, Milone M, Liewluck T. Neuromuscular transmission defects in myopathies: rare but worth searching for. *Muscle Nerve*. 2019;59:475–478.
208. Ohno K. Glycosylation defects as an emerging novel cause leading to a limb-girdle type of congenital myasthenic syndromes. *J Neurol Neurosurg Psychiatr*. 2013;84:1064.
209. Chevessier F, Bauché-Godard S, Leroy JP, et al. The origin of tubular aggregates in human myopathies. *J Pathol*. 2005;207:313–323.
210. Luo HY, Zhao L, Mao CY, et al. Novel compound heterozygous GFPT1 mutations in a family with limb-girdle myasthenia with tubular aggregates. *Neuromuscul Disord*. 2019;29:549–553.
211. Huh SY, Kim HS, Jang HJ, Park YE, Kim DS. Limb-girdle myasthenia with tubular aggregates associated with novel GFPT1 mutations. *Muscle Nerve*. 2012;46:600–604.
212. Bauché S, Vellieux G, Sternberg D, et al. Mutations in GFPT1-related congenital myasthenic syndromes are associated with synaptic morphological defects and underlie a tubular aggregate myopathy with synaptopathy. *J Neurol*. 2017;264:1791–1803.
213. Engel AG, Shen XM, Selcen D, Sine SM. Congenital myasthenic syndromes: pathogenesis, diagnosis, and treatment. *Lancet Neurol*. 2015;14(4):420–434.

214. Feresiadou A, Casar-Borota O, Dragomir A, Oldfors CH, Stålberg E, Oldfors A. Tubular aggregates in congenital myasthenic syndrome. *Neuromuscul Disord.* 2018;28:174–175.
215. Ruff RL, Rutecki P. Faster, slower, but never better: mutations of the skeletal muscle acetylcholine receptor. *Neurology.* 2012;79:404–405.
216. Shen XM, Brengman JM, Edvardson S, Sine SM, Engel AG. Highly fatal fast-channel syndrome caused by AChR ε subunit mutation at the agonist binding site. *Neurology.* 2012;79:449–454.
217. Cheung J, Cossins J, Liu W, Belaya K, Beeson D. P42 pathogenic mechanisms of RAPSN mutations in congenital myasthenic syndromes. *Neuromuscul Disord.* 2014;24:S18.
218. Cossins J, Burke G, Maxwell S, et al. Diverse molecular mechanisms involved in AChR deficiency due to rapsyn mutations. *Brain.* 2006;129:2773–2783.
219. Zoltowska K, Webster R, Finlayson S, et al. Mutations in GFPT1 that underlie limb-girdle congenital myasthenic syndrome result in reduced cell-surface expression of muscle AChR. *Hum Mol Genet.* 2013;22:2905–2913.
220. Liewluck T, Selcen D, Engel AG. Beneficial effects of albuterol in congenital endplate acetylcholinesterase deficiency and Dok-7 myasthenia. *Muscle Nerve.* 2011;44:789–794.
221. Vanhaesebrouck AE, Beeson D. The congenital myasthenic syndromes: expanding genetic and phenotypic spectrums and refining treatment strategies. *Curr Opin Neurol.* 2019;32:696–703.
222. Lashley D, Palace J, Jayawant S, Robb S, Beeson D. Ephedrine treatment in congenital myasthenic syndrome due to mutations in DOK7. *Neurology.* 2010;74:1517–1523.
223. Farmakidis C, Pasnoor M, Barohn RJ, Dimachkie MM. Congenital myasthenic syndromes: a clinical and treatment approach. *Curr Treat Options Neurol.* 2018;20:36.
224. Harper CM, Fukodome T, Engel AG. Treatment of slow-channel congenital myasthenic syndrome with fluoxetine. *Neurology.* 2003;60:1710–1713.
225. Rodríguez Cruz PM, Palace J, Ramjattan H, Jayawant S, Robb SA, Beeson D. Salbutamol and ephedrine in the treatment of severe AChR deficiency syndromes. *Neurology.* 2015;85:1043–1047.
226. Verma S, Mazell SN, Shah DA. Amifampridine phosphate in congenital myasthenic syndrome. *Muscle Nerve.* 2016;54:809–810.
227. Arimura S, Okada T, Tezuka T, et al. Neuromuscular disease. DOK7 gene therapy benefits mouse models of diseases characterized by defects in the neuromuscular junction. *Science.* 2014;345:1505–1508.
228. Lin CV, et al. Adeno-associated virus type 9-mediated gene therapy of choline acetyltransferase-deficient mice. *Hum Gene Ther.* 2024;35:123–131.
229. Eguchi T, Tezuka T, Fukudome T, Watanabe Y, Sagara H, Yamanashi Y. Overexpression of Dok-7 in skeletal muscle enhances neuromuscular transmission with structural alterations of neuromuscular junctions: implications in robustness of neuromuscular transmission. *Biochem Biophys Res Commun.* 2020;523:214–219.
230. Rao AK, Sobel J, Chatham-Stephens K, Luquez C. Clinical guidelines for diagnosis and treatment of botulism, 2021. *MMWR Recomm Rep.* 2021;70:1–30.
231. Lúquez C, Edwards L, Griffin C, Sobel J. Foodborne botulism outbreaks in the United States, 2001-2017. *Front Microbiol.* 2021;12:713101.
232. Sobel J. Botulism. *Clin Infect Dis.* 2005;41:1167–1173.
233. Panditrao MV, Dabritz HA, Kazerouni NN, Damus KH, Meissinger JK, Arnon SS. Descriptive epidemiology of infant botulism in California: the first 40 years. *J Pediatr.* 2020;227:247–257.e3.
234. Leclair D, Fung J, Isaac-Renton JL, et al. Foodborne botulism in Canada, 1985-2005. *Emerging Infect Dis.* 2013;19:961–968.
235. Woodruff BA, Griffin PM, McCroskey LM, et al. Clinical and laboratory comparison of botulism from toxin types A, B, and E in the United States, 1975-1988. *J Infect Dis.* 1992;166:1281–1286.
236. Rossetto O, Megighian A, Scorzeto M, Montecucco C. Botulinum neurotoxins. *Toxicon.* 2013;67:31–36.
237. Badell ML, Rimawi BH, Rao AK, Jamieson DJ, Rasmussen S, Meaney-Delman D. Botulism during pregnancy and the postpartum period: a systematic review. *Clin Infect Dis.* 2017;66:S30–S37.
238. Maselli RA, Bakshi N. AAEM case report 16. Botulism American Association of Electrodiagnostic Medicine. *Muscle Nerve.* 2000;23:1137–1144.
239. Cherington M. Clinical spectrum of botulism. *Muscle Nerve.* 1998;21:701–710.
240. Schmidt-Nowara WW, Samet JM, Rosario PA. Early and late pulmonary complications of botulism. *Arch Intern Med.* 1983;143:451–456.
241. Chatham-Stephens K, Fleck-Derderian S, Johnson SD, Sobel J, Rao AK, Meaney-Delman D. Clinical features of foodborne and wound botulism: a systematic review of the literature, 1932-2015. *Clin Infect Dis.* 2017;66:S11–S16.
242. Sobel J. Diagnosis and treatment of botulism: a century later, clinical suspicion remains the cornerstone. *Clin Infect Dis.* 2009;48:1674–1675.
243. Rao AK, Lin NH, Griese SE, Chatham-Stephens K, Badell ML, Sobel J. Clinical criteria to trigger suspicion for Botulism: an evidence-based tool to facilitate timely recognition of suspected cases during sporadic events and outbreaks. *Clin Infect Dis.* 2017;66:S38–S42.
244. Dilena R, Pozzato M, Baselli L, et al. Infant botulism: checklist for timely clinical diagnosis and new possible risk factors originated from a case report and literature review. *Toxins (Basel).* 2021;13(12):860.
245. National Botulism Surveillance | Botulism | CDC. https://www.cdc.gov/botulism/php/national-botulism-surveillance/index.html
246. Rapoport S, Watkins PB. Descending paralysis resulting from occult wound botulism. *Ann Neurol.* 1984;16:359–361.
247. Middaugh N, Edwards L, Chatham-Stephens K, Arguello DF. Wound botulism among persons who inject black tar heroin in New Mexico, 2016. *Front Public Health.* 2021;9:744179.
248. Edwards LD, Gomez I, Wada S, et al. Notes from the Field: wound botulism outbreak among a group of persons who inject drugs – Dallas, Texas, 2020. *MMWR Morb Mortal Wkly Rep.* 2022;71:556–557.
249. Parameswaran L, Rao A, Chastain K, et al. A case of adult intestinal toxemia botulism during prolonged hospitalization in an allogeneic hematopoietic cell transplant recipient. *Clin Infect Dis.* 2017;66:S99–S102.
250. Bai L, Peng X, Liu Y, et al. Clinical analysis of 86 botulism cases caused by cosmetic injection of botulinum toxin (BoNT). *Medicine (Baltimore).* 2018;97:e10659.
251. Arnon SS, Schechter R, Inglesby TV, et al; Working Group on Civilian Biodefense. Botulinum toxin as a biological weapon: medical and public health management. *JAMA.* 2001;285:1059–1070.

252. Sobel J, Rao AK. Making the best of the evidence: toward national clinical guidelines for botulism. *Clin Infect Dis.* 2017;66:S1–S3.
253. Green MA, Heumann MA, Wehr HM, et al. An outbreak of watermelon-borne pesticide toxicity. *Am J Public Health.* 1987;77:1431–1434.
254. Forss N, Ramstad R, Bäcklund T, Lindström M, Kolho E. Difficulties in diagnosing food-borne botulism. *Case Rep Neurol.* 2012;4:113–115.
255. Wakerley BR, Yuki N. Pharyngeal-cervical-brachial variant of Guillain-Barre syndrome. *J Neurol Neurosurg Psychiatr.* 2014;85:339–344.
256. Cherington M. Electrophysiologic methods as an aid in diagnosis of botulism: a review. *Muscle Nerve.* 1982;5:S28–S29.
257. Cornblath DR, Sladky JT, Sumner AJ. Clinical electrophysiology of infantile botulism. *Muscle Nerve.* 1983;6:448–452.
258. Gutmann L, Bodensteiner J, Gutierrez A. Electrodiagnosis of botulism. *J Pediatr.* 1992;121:835.
259. Oh SJ. Botulism: electrophysiological studies. *Ann Neurol.* 1977;1:481–485.
260. Cherington M. Botulism. Ten-year experience. *Arch Neurol.* 1974;30:432–437.
261. Vasa M, Baudendistel TE, Ohikhuare CE, et al. Clinical problem-solving. The eyes have it. *N Engl J Med.* 2012;367:938–943.
262. Mazuet C, Ezan E, Volland H, Popoff MR, Becher F. Toxin detection in patients' sera by mass spectrometry during two outbreaks of type A Botulism in France. *J Clin Microbiol.* 2012;50:4091–4094.
263. Jones RGA, Marks JD. Use of a new functional dual coating (FDC) assay to measure low toxin levels in serum and food samples following an outbreak of human botulism. *J Med Microbiol.* 2013;62:828–835.
264. Devers KG, Nine JS. Autopsy findings in botulinum toxin poisoning. *J Forensic Sci.* 2010;55:1649–1651.
265. Kongsaengdao S, Samintarapanya K, Rusmeechan S, Sithinamsuwan P, Tanprawate S. Electrophysiological diagnosis and patterns of response to treatment of botulism with neuromuscular respiratory failure. *Muscle Nerve.* 2009;40:271–278.
266. Centers for Disease Control and Prevention (CDC). Botulism from drinking prison-made illicit alcohol – Utah 2011. *MMWR Morb Mortal Wkly Rep.* 2012;61:782–784.
267. Simpson L. The life history of a botulinum toxin molecule. *Toxicon.* 2013;68:40–59.
268. Maselli RA, Ellis W, Mandler RN, et al. Cluster of wound botulism in California: clinical, electrophysiologic, and pathologic study. *Muscle Nerve.* 1997;20:1284–1295.
269. Maselli RA, Burnett ME, Tonsgard JH. In vitro microelectrode study of neuromuscular transmission in a case of botulism. *Muscle Nerve.* 1992;15:273–276.
270. O'Horo JC, Harper EP, El Rafei A, et al. Efficacy of antitoxin therapy in treating patients with foodborne botulism: a systematic review and meta-analysis of cases, 1923–2016. *Clin Infect Dis.* 2017;66:S43–S56.
271. Yu PA, Lin NH, Mahon BE, et al. Safety and improved clinical outcomes in patients treated with new equine-derived heptavalent botulinum antitoxin. *Clin Infect Dis.* 2017;66:S57–S64.
272. Garispe A, Cherry S. Infant Botulism. *J Educ Teach Emerg Med.* 2023;8:O33–O60.
273. Friggeri A, Marçon F, Marciniak S, et al. 3,4-Diaminopyridine may improve neuromuscular block during botulism. *Crit Care.* 2013;17:449.
274. Nayak SU, Griffiss JM, McKenzie R, et al. Safety and pharmacokinetics of XOMA 3AB, a novel mixture of three monoclonal antibodies against botulinum toxin A. *Antimicrob Agents Chemother.* 2014;58:5047–5053.
275. Guptill JT, Raja SM, Juel VC, et al. Safety, tolerability, and pharmacokinetics of NTM-1632, a novel mixture of three monoclonal antibodies against botulinum Toxin B. *Antimicrob Agents Chemother.* 2021;65:e0232920.
276. Raja SM, Guptill JT, Juel VC, et al. First-in-Human clinical trial to assess the safety, tolerability and pharmacokinetics of single doses of NTM-1633, a novel mixture of monoclonal antibodies against Botulinum Toxin E. *Antimicrob Agents Chemother.* 2022;66:e0173221.
277. Edlow JA, McGillicuddy DC. Tick paralysis. *Infect Dis Clin North Am.* 2008;22:397–413, vii.
278. Grattan-Smith PJ, Morris JG, Johnston HM, et al. Clinical and neurophysiological features of tick paralysis. *Brain.* 1997;120(Pt 11):1975–1987.
279. Diaz JH. A 60-year meta-analysis of tick paralysis in the United States: a predictable, preventable, and often misdiagnosed poisoning. *J Med Toxicol.* 2010;6:15–21.
280. Cooper BJ, Spence I. Temperature-dependent inhibition of evoked acetylcholine release in tick paralysis. *Nature.* 1976;263:693–695.
281. Emmons P, McLennan H. Failure of acetylcholine release in tick paralysis. *Nature.* 1959;183:474–475.
282. Dworkin MS, Shoemaker PC, Anderson DE. Tick paralysis: 33 human cases in Washington State, 1946-1996. *Clin Infect Dis.* 1999;29:1435–1439.
283. Felz MW, Smith CD, Swift TR. A six-year-old girl with tick paralysis. *N Engl J Med.* 2000;342:90–94.
284. Schaumburg HH, Herskovitz S. The weak child—a cautionary tale. *N Engl J Med.* 2000;342:127–129.
285. Gorman RJ, Snead OC. Tick paralysis in three children. The diversity of neurologic presentations. *Clin Pediatr (Phila).* 1978;17:249–251.
286. Mongan PF. Tick toxicosis in North America. *J Fam Pract.* 1979;8:939–944.
287. Pearn J. Neuromuscular paralysis caused by tick envenomation. *J Neurol Sci.* 1977;34:37–42.
288. Rose I. A review of tick paralysis. *Can Med Assoc J.* 1954;70:175–176.
289. Rose I. Evidence of a neuromuscular block in tick paralysis. *Nature.* 1956;178:95–96.
290. Diaz JH. A comparative meta-analysis of tick paralysis in the United States and Australia. *Clin Toxicol (Phila).* 2015;53:874–883.
291. Pontiff K, Woodward C, McMahon P. Tick paralysis case series: an 11-year institutional case series. *Pediatr Emerg Care.* 2021;37:589–592.
292. Swift TR, Ignacio OJ. Tick paralysis: electrophysiologic studies. *Neurology.* 1975;25:1130–1133.
293. Masina S, Broady KW. Tick paralysis: development of a vaccine. *Int J Parasitol.* 1999;29:535–541.
294. Swift TR. Weakness from magnesium-containing cathartics: electrophysiologic studies. *Muscle Nerve.* 1979;2:295–298.
295. Krishnan AV, Lin CS, Reddel SW, McGrath R, Kiernan MC. Conduction block and impaired axonal function in tick paralysis. *Muscle Nerve.* 2009;40:358–362.
296. Pecina CA. Tick paralysis. *Semin Neurol.* 2012;32:531–532.
297. Cherington M, Synder RD. Tick paralysis. Neurophysiologic studies. *N Engl J Med.* 1968;278:95–97.

298. DeBusk FL, O'Connor S. Tick toxicosis. *Pediatrics*. 1972; 50:328–329.
299. Donat JR, Donat JF. Tick paralysis with persistent weakness and electromyographic abnormalities. *Arch Neurol*. 1981; 38:59–61.
300. Morris HH. Tick paralysis: electrophysiologic measurements. *South Med J*. 1977;70:121–122.
301. Vedanarayanan V, Sorey WH, Subramony SH. Tick paralysis. *Semin Neurol*. 2004;24:181–184.
302. Schmitt N, Bowmer EJ, Gregson JD. Tick paralysis in British Columbia. *Can Med Assoc J*. 1969;100:417–421.
303. Stone BF, Neish AL. Tick-paralysis toxoid: an effective immunizing agent against the toxin of Ixodes holocyclus. *Aust J Exp Biol Med Sci*. 1984;62(Pt 2):189–191.
304. Tabor AE. A review of Australian tick vaccine research. *Vaccines (Basel)*. 2021;9(9):1030.
305. Nakajima T, Ohta S, Morita H, Midorikawa Y, Mimura S, Yanagisawa N. Epidemiological study of sarin poisoning in Matsumoto City, Japan. *J Epidemiol*. 1998;8:33–41.
306. Buckley NA, Eddleston M, Li Y, Bevan M, Robertson J. Oximes for acute organophosphate pesticide poisoning. *Cochrane Database Syst Rev*. 2011;(2):CD005085.
307. Eddleston M, Buckley NA, Eyer P, Dawson AH. Management of acute organophosphorus pesticide poisoning. *Lancet*. 2008;371:597–607.
308. Jokanović M, Prostran M. Pyridinium oximes as cholinesterase reactivators. Structure-activity relationship and efficacy in the treatment of poisoning with organophosphorus compounds. *Curr Med Chem*. 2009;16:2177–2188.
309. Sungur M, Güven M. Intensive care management of organophosphate insecticide poisoning. *Crit Care*. 2001;5:211–215.
310. Besser R, Gutmann L, Dillmann U, Weilemann LS, Hopf HC. End-plate dysfunction in acute organophosphate intoxication. *Neurology*. 1989;39:561–567.
311. Eddleston M, Eyer P, Worek F, et al. Pralidoxime in acute organophosphorus insecticide poisoning—a randomised controlled trial. *PLoS Med*. 2009;6:e1000104.
312. Kularatne SAM, Senanayake N. Venomous snake bites, scorpions, and spiders. *Handb Clin Neurol*. 2014;120:987–1001.
313. Del Brutto OH. Neurological effects of venomous bites and stings: snakes, spiders, and scorpions. *Handb Clin Neurol*. 2013;114:349–368.
314. White J. Bites and stings from venomous animals: a global overview. *Ther Drug Monit*. 2000;22:65–68.
315. Singh G, Pannu HS, Chawla PS, Malhotra S. Neuromuscular transmission failure due to common krait (*Bungarus caeruleus*) envenomation. *Muscle Nerve*. 1999;22:1637–1643.
316. Faiz A, Ghose A, Ahsan F, et al. The greater black krait (*Bungarus niger*), a newly recognized cause of neuro-myotoxic snake bite envenoming in Bangladesh. *Brain*. 2010;133:3181–3193.
317. Bickler PE, Abouyannis M, Bhalla A, Lewin MR. Neuromuscular weakness and paralysis produced by snakebite envenoming: mechanisms and proposed standards for clinical assessment. *Toxins (Basel)*. 2023;15(1):49.
318. Norris RL, Pfalzgraf RR, Laing G. Death following coral snake bite in the United States—first documented case (with ELISA confirmation of envenomation) in over 40 years. *Toxicon*. 2009;53:693–697.
319. Silva A, Hodgson WC, Isbister GK. Antivenom for neuromuscular paralysis resulting from snake envenoming. *Toxins (Basel)*. 2017;9(4):143.
320. Ratanabanangkoon K. Polyvalent snake antivenoms: production strategy and their therapeutic benefits. *Toxins (Basel)*. 2023;15(9):517.
321. Ratanabanangkoon K, Tan KY, Pruksaphon K, et al. A pan-specific antiserum produced by a novel immunization strategy shows a high spectrum of neutralization against neurotoxic snake venoms. *Sci Rep*. 2020;10:11261.
322. Ratanabanangkoon, K. A quest for a universal plasma-derived antivenom against all elapid neurotoxic snake venoms. *Front Immunol*. 2021;12:668328.
323. Pettigrew LC, Glass JP. Neurologic complications of a coral snake bite. *Neurology*. 1985;35:589–592.
324. Poison Control. https://www.poison.org
325. Association of Zoological Parks and Aquariums. https://www.aza.org
326. Clark RF, Wethern-Kestner S, Vance MV, Gerkin R. Clinical presentation and treatment of black widow spider envenomation: a review of 163 cases. *Ann Emerg Med*. 1992;21:782–787.
327. Swift TR. Disorders of neuromuscular transmission other than myasthenia gravis. *Muscle Nerve*. 1981;4:334–353.
328. Golcuk Y, Velibey Y, Gonullu H, Sahin M, Kocabas E. Acute toxic fulminant myocarditis after a black widow spider envenomation: case report and literature review. *Clin Toxicol (Phila)*. 2013;51:191–192.
329. Balhara KS, Stolbach A. Marine envenomations. *Emerg Med Clin North Am*. 2014;32:223–243.
330. Auerbach PS. Marine envenomations. *N Engl J Med*. 1991; 325:486–493.
331. Fuehrer J, Kong EL, Murphy-Lavoie HM. Sea snake toxicity. In: *StatPearls*. StatPearls Publishing; 2024.
332. Kerr LM, Yoshikami D. A venom peptide with a novel presynaptic blocking action. *Nature*. 1984;308:282–284.
333. Sano K, Enomoto K, Maeno T. Effects of synthetic omega-conotoxin, a new type Ca^{2+} antagonist, on frog and mouse neuromuscular transmission. *Eur J Pharmacol*. 1987;141:235–241.
334. Hunter JM. New neuromuscular blocking drugs. *N Engl J Med*. 1995;332:1691–1699.
335. Gooch JL, Moore MH, Ryser DK. Prolonged paralysis after neuromuscular junction blockade: case reports and electrodiagnostic findings. *Arch Phys Med Rehabil*. 1993;74:1007–1011.
336. Howard JF. Adverse drug effects on neuromuscular transmission. *Semin Neurol*. 1990;10:89–102.
337. Atchison WD, Adgate L, Beaman CM. Effects of antibiotics on uptake of calcium into isolated nerve terminals. *J Pharmacol Exp Ther*. 1988;245:394–401.
338. Argov Z, Mastaglia FL. Drug therapy: Disorders of neuromuscular transmission caused by drugs. *N Engl J Med*. 1979;301:409–413.
339. Bever CT, Chang HW, Penn AS, Jaffe IA, Bock E. Penicillamine-induced myasthenia gravis: effects of penicillamine on acetylcholine receptor. *Neurology*. 1982;32:1077–1082.
340. Albers JW, Beals CA, Levine SP. Neuromuscular transmission in rheumatoid arthritis, with and without penicillamine treatment. *Neurology*. 1981;31:1562–1564.
341. Albers JW, Hodach RJ, Kimmel DW, Treacy WL. Penicillamine-associated myasthenia gravis. *Neurology*. 1980;30:1246–1249.
342. Russell AS, Lindstrom JM. Penicillamine-induced myasthenia gravis associated with antibodies to acetylcholine receptor. *Neurology*. 1978;28:847–849.
343. Batocchi AP, Evoli A, Servidei S, Palmisani MT, Apollo F, Tonali P. Myasthenia gravis during interferon alfa therapy. *Neurology*. 1995;45:382–383.

344. Brüggemann W, Herath H, Ferbert A. [Follow-up and immunologic findings in drug-induced myasthenia]. *Med Klin (Munich).* 1996;91:268–271.
345. Fawcett PR, McLachlan SM, Nicholson LV, Argov Z, Mastaglia FL. D-Penicillamine-associated myasthenia gravis: immunological and electrophysiological studies. *Muscle Nerve.* 1982;5:328–334.
346. Liu GT, Bienfang DC. Penicillamine-induced ocular myasthenia gravis in rheumatoid arthritis. *J Clin Neuroophthalmol.* 1990;10:201–205.
347. Masters CL, Dawkins RL, Zilko PJ, Simpson JA, Leedman RJ. Penicillamine-associated myasthenia gravis, antiacetylcholine receptor and antistriational antibodies. *Am J Med.* 1977;63:689–694.
348. Raynauld JP, Lee YS, Kornfeld P, Fries JF. Unilateral ptosis as an initial manifestation of D-penicillamine induced myasthenia gravis. *J Rheumatol.* 1993;20:1592–1593.
349. Vincent A, Newsom-Davis J. Acetylcholine receptor antibody characteristics in myasthenia gravis. II. Patients with penicillamine-induced myasthenia or idiopathic myasthenia of recent onset. *Clin Exp Immunol.* 1982;49:266–272.
350. Vincent A, Newsom-Davis J, Martin V. Anti-acetylcholine receptor antibodies in d-penicillamine-associated myasthenia gravis. *Lancet.* 1978;311:1254.
351. Lensch E, Faust J, Nix WA, Wandel E. Myasthenia gravis after interferon-alpha treatment. *Muscle Nerve.* 1996;19:927–928.
352. Mase G, Zorzon M, Biasutti E, et al. Development of myasthenia gravis during interferon-alpha treatment for anti-HCV positive chronic hepatitis. *J Neurol Neurosurg Psychiatr.* 1996;60:348–349.
353. Pérez A, Perella M, Pastor E, Cano M, Escudero J. Myasthenia gravis induced by alpha-interferon therapy. *Am J Hematol.* 1995;49:365–366.
354. Piccolo G, Franciotta D, Versino M, Alfonsi E, Lombardi M, Poma G. Myasthenia gravis in a patient with chronic active hepatitis C during interferon-alpha treatment. *J Neurol Neurosurg Psychiatr.* 1996;60:348.
355. Streib EW. Adverse effects of magnesium salt cathartics in a patient with the myasthenic syndrome (Lambert-Eaton syndrome). *Ann Neurol.* 1977;2:175–176.
356. Bashuk RG, Krendel DA. Myasthenia gravis presenting as weakness after magnesium administration. *Muscle Nerve.* 1990;13:708–712.

CHAPTER 27

Muscular Dystrophies

Muscular dystrophies are hereditary, progressive muscle diseases in which there is necrosis of muscle tissue and replacement by connective and fatty tissues, which helps to distinguish them from other hereditary myopathies. Before discussing specific types of muscular dystrophies, it is important to understand the relevant muscle proteins that are affected in the various dystrophies. The different forms of muscular dystrophies result from mutations affecting proteins localizable to the sarcolemma, myonuclei, basement membrane and extracellular matrix surrounding muscle fibers, sarcomere, nonstructural enzymes, and proteins and RNA itself that are important in regulating proper transcription and translation.[1-4]

▶ DYSTROPHIN–GLYCOPROTEIN COMPLEX AND RELATED PROTEINS

DYSTROPHIN

The identification and characterization of dystrophin as the abnormal gene product in Duchenne and Becker muscular dystrophies (DMD and BMD) were the major discoveries underlying our current understanding of muscular dystrophies (Fig. 27-1).[1-5] Dystrophin is located on the cytoplasmic face of skeletal and cardiac muscle membrane and constitutes approximately 5% of the sarcolemma cytoskeletal proteins. Dystrophin is a rod-shaped molecule composed of four domains. The amino-terminal domain binds to the cytoskeletal filamentous actin. The second domain bears similarity to spectrin and provides structural integrity to red blood cells. The third domain is a cysteine-rich region, and the fourth domain is the carboxy terminal. The cysteine-rich domain and the first half of the carboxy-terminal domain of dystrophin are important in linking dystrophin to β-dystroglycan and the glycoproteins that span the sarcolemma.

Dystrophin is also present in the brain where it localizes subcellularly to the postsynaptic density, a disc-shaped structure beneath the postsynaptic membrane in chemical synapses. The postsynaptic density may play an important role in synaptic function by stabilizing the synaptic structure, anchoring postsynaptic receptors, and transducing extracellular matrix–cell signals.

DYSTROPHIN-ASSOCIATED PROTEINS/GLYCOPROTEINS

Dystrophin is tightly associated with a large oligomeric complex of sarcolemmal proteins referred to as the dystrophin–glycoprotein complex (Fig. 27-1).[5-7] Mutations in the various genes, which encode for the different proteins of the dystrophin–glycoprotein complex, are now known to be responsible for many forms of muscular dystrophy (Table 27-1). In addition to dystrophin, the dystrophin–glycoprotein complex is composed of an entirely cytoplasmic group of proteins referred to as the syntrophin complex, the dystroglycan complex, and the sarcoglycan complex (Fig. 27-1).

The syntrophin complex binds to the carboxy terminus of dystrophin and is composed of three distinct 59-kD dystrophin-associated proteins (DAPs), which are encoded by separate genes. α-Syntrophin is expressed only in muscle and the gene has been localized to chromosome 20q11.2. β1- and β2-Syntrophin are more widely expressed, and their genes have been localized to chromosomes 8q23–24 and 16q22–23, respectively. Dystrobrevin is encoded on chromosome 2p22–23 and is a cytoplasmic protein, which binds to the syntrophin complex and to the C terminus of dystrophin.

The dystroglycan complex is composed of α- and β-dystroglycan. β-Dystroglycan spans the sarcolemmal membrane and has a cytoplasmic tail that binds to dystrophin, while the extracellular tail binds α-dystroglycan. α-Dystroglycan, which is entirely extracellular, also binds to laminin α2 (merosin), a basal lamina protein. Of note, a gene located on chromosome 3p21 encodes for both the α- and β-dystroglycan. Importantly, α-dystroglycan undergoes N-linked and extensive O-linked glycosylation, which is important for normal binding to merosin and perhaps other extracellular matrix proteins.[8]

The sarcoglycan complex includes four membrane-spanning proteins: (1) α-sarcoglycan (previously known as adhalin), (2) β-sarcoglycan, (3) γ-sarcoglycan, and (4) δ-sarcoglycan. In addition, there is a 25-kD transmembrane protein, sarcospan, which colocalizes with the sarcoglycan complex. The sarcoglycan complex associates with the cysteine-rich domain and/or the first half of the carboxy terminal of dystrophin directly or indirectly via

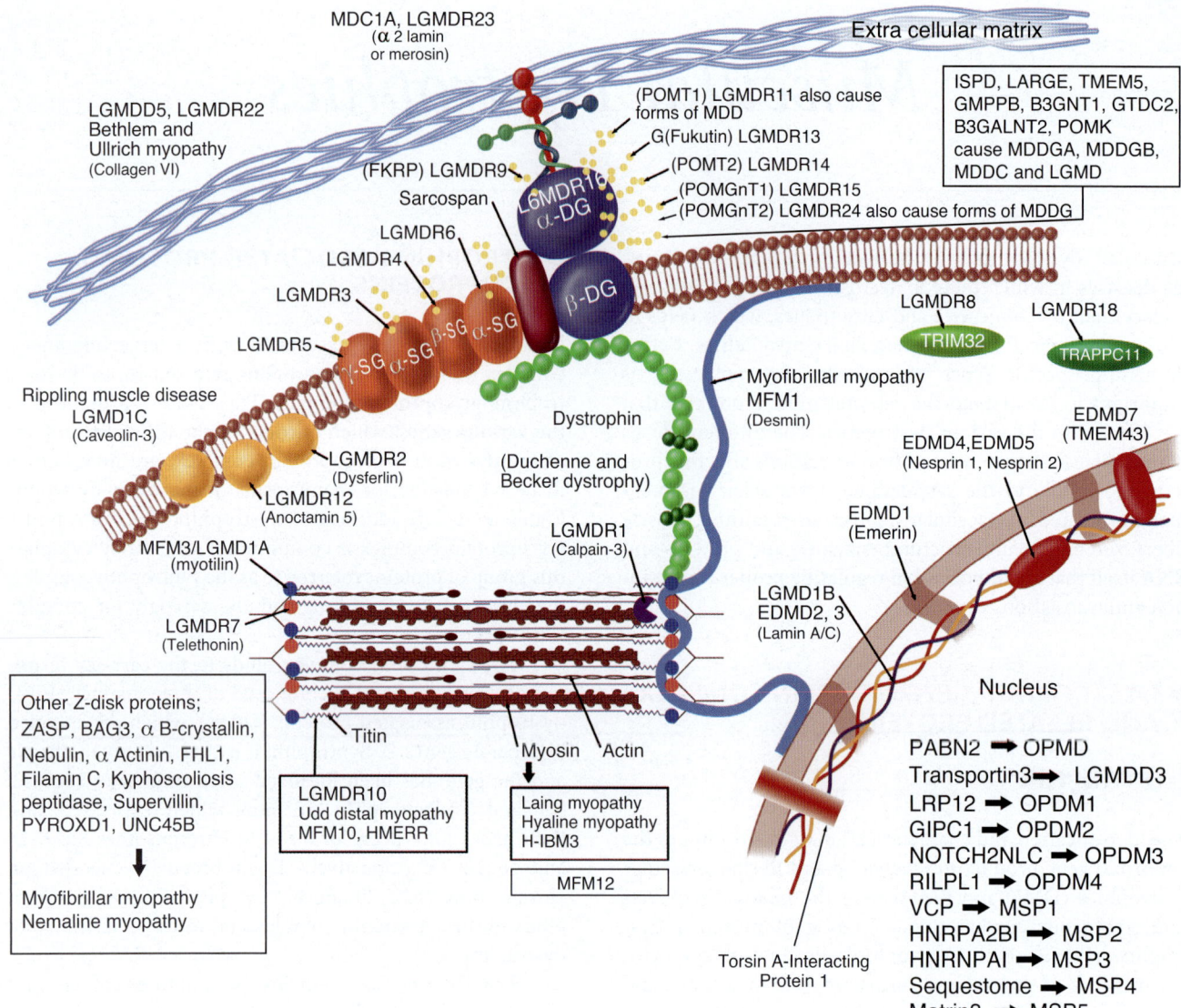

Figure 27-1. Proteins involved in muscular dystrophies. This schematic shows the location of various sarcolemmal, sarcomeric, nuclear, and enzymatic proteins associated with muscular dystrophies. The diseases associated with mutations in the genes responsible for encoding these proteins are shown in boxes. Dystrophin, via its interaction with the dystroglycan complex, connects the actin cytoskeleton to the extracellular matrix. Extracellularly, the sarcoglycan complex interacts with biglycan, which connects this complex to the dystroglycan complex and the extracellular matrix collagen. Various enzymes are important in the glycosylation of the α-dystroglycan and mediate its binding to the extracellular matrix and usually cause a congenital muscular dystrophy with severe brain and eye abnormalities but may cause milder LGMD phenotype. Mutations in genes that encode for sarcomeric and Z-disc proteins cause forms of LGMD and distal myopathies (including myofibrillar myopathy, forms of hereditary inclusion body myopathy) as well as nemaline rod myopathy and other "congenital" myopathies. Mutations affecting nuclear membrane proteins are responsible for most forms of EDMD. Mutations in other nuclear genes cause other forms of dystrophy.

the dystroglycan complex. The exact relationship between the sarcoglycan complex and the dystrophin–dystroglycan complex is still unclear. Mutations in the various sarcoglycan genes are responsible for limb-girdle muscular dystrophies (LGMDs): LGMDR5 (formerly known as LGMD2C), LGMDR3 (formerly known as LGMD2D), LGMDR4 (formerly known as LGMD2E), and LGMDR6 (formerly known as LGMD2F) (Fig. 27-1).

MEROSIN/LAMININ AND ALPHA-DYSTROGLYCAN

The basal lamina surrounding each muscle fiber closely adheres to the sarcolemma and is composed of type I and IV collagen, heparan sulfate, proteoglycan, entactin, fibronectin, and laminin. Laminin is a large, flexible heterotrimer composed of three different but homologous α, β, and γ chains,

▶ TABLE 27-1. MOLECULAR DEFECTS OF MUSCULAR DYSTROPHIES

Disease	Inheritance	Gene	Affected Protein
DYSTROPHINOPATHIES			
Duchenne/Becker	XR	DYS	Dystrophin
LIMB-GIRDLE DYSTROPHIES			
Old/New Nomenclature			
LGMD1A/MFM3	AD	MYOT	Myotilin
LGMD1B/EDMD	AD	LMNA	Lamin A and C
LGMD1C/Rippling muscle disease	AD	CAV3	Caveolin-3
LGMD1D/LMGDD1	AD	DNAJB6	DNAJ heat shock protein family (Hsp40) member B6
LGMD1E/MFM1	AD	DES	Desmin
LGMD1F/LGMDD2	AD	TNPO3	Transportin 3
LGMD1G/LGMDD3	AD	HNRNPDL	Heterogeneous nuclear ribonucleoprotein D like protein
LGMD1H/Discarded due to false linkage			
LGMD1I/LGMDD4	AD	CAPN3	Calpain 3
Bethlem myopathy/LGMDD5	AD	COL6A1/2/3	Collagen type VI alpha
LGMD2A/LGMDR1	AR	CAPN3	Calpain 3
LGMD2B/LGMDR2	AR	DYSF	Dysferlin
LGMD2C/LGMDR5	AR	SGCG	γ-Sarcoglycan
LGMD2D/LGMDR3	AR	SGCA	α-Sarcoglycan
LGMD2E/LGMDR4	AR	SCGB	β-Sarcoglycan
LGMD2F/LGMDR6	AR	SCGD	δ-Sarcoglycan
LGMD2G/LGMDR7	AR	TCAP	Telethonin
LGMD2H/LGMDR8	AR	TRIM32	Tripartite motif-containing 32
LGMD2I/LGMDR9	AR	FKRP	Fukutin-related protein
LGMD2J/LGMDR10	AR	TTN	Titin
LGMD2K/LGMDR11	AR	POMT1	Protein O-mannosyltransferase 1
LGMD2L/LGMDR12	AR	ANO5	Anoctamin-5
LGMD2M/LGMDR13	AR	FKTN	Fukutin
LGMD2N/LGMDR14	AR	POMT2	Protein O-mannosyltransferase 2
LGMD2O/LGMDR15	AR	POMGnT1	Protein O-linked mannose Beta-1,2-N-acetylglucosaminyltranferase-1
LGMD2P/LGMDR16	AR	DAG1	α-Dystroglycan
LGMD2Q/LGMDR17	AR	PLEC1	Plectin-1
LGMD2R/MFM1	AR	DES	Desmin
LGMD2S/LGMDR18	AR	TRAPPC11	Trafficking protein particle complex 11
LMGD2T/LGMDR19	AR	GMPPB	GDP-mannose pyrophosphorylase B
LGMD2U/LGMDR20	AR	CRPPA	CDP-L-ribitol pyrophosphorylase A (also known as ISPD)
LGMD2V/Pompe Disease	AR	GAA	Alpha-glucosidase
LGMD2W/PINCH-2 related myopathy	AR	LIMS2	PINCH-2
LGMD2X/LGMDR25	AR	BVES	Blood vessel endothelial substance
LGMD2Y/TOR1AIP1 related myopathy	AR	TOR1AIP1	Torsin A interacting protein 1 (also know as Lamin-associated protein 1)
LGMD2Z/LGMDR21	AR	POGLUT1	Protein O-glucosyltransferase 1
Ullrich myopathy/LGMDR22	AR	COL6A1/2/3	Collagen VI subunits A1, A2, or A3
Laminin α2-related dystrophy/LGMDR23	AR	LAMA2	Laminin subunit alpha 2
POMGNT2-related dystrophy/LGMDR24	AR	POMGNT2	Protein O-linked mannose beta 1,4-N-acetyl-glucosaminyltransferase 2
NA/LGMDR26	AR	POPDC3	PODC3
NA/LGMDR27	AR	JAG2	Jagged2
CONGENITAL MUSCULAR DYSTROPHIES (MDC)			
MDC1A	AR	LAMA2	Laminin-α$_2$ chain
α$_7$-Integrin-related MDC	AR	ITGA7	α$_7$-Integrin
MDDGA1/MDDGB1/MDDGC1	AR	POMT1	Protein O-mannosyltransferase 1
MDDGA2/MDDGB2/MDDGC2	AR	POMT2	Protein O-mannosyltransferase 12

(continued)

TABLE 27-1. (CONTINUED)

Disease	Inheritance	Gene	Affected Protein
MDDGA3/MDDGB3/ MDDGC3	AR	POMGNT1	Protein O-mannose-β-1,2-N-acetylglucosaminyl transferase
MDDGA4/MDDGB4/ MDDGC4	AR	FKTN	Fukutin
MDDGA5/MDDGB5/ MDDGC5	AR	FKRP	Fukutin-related protein
MDDGA6/MDDGB6/ MDDGC6	AR	LARGE	LARGE
MDDGA7/MDDGB7/ MDDGC7	AR	ISPD	Isoprenoid synthetase domain-containing protein
MDDGA8/MDDGB8/ MDDGC8	AR	POMGNT2	Protein O-mannose beta-1,4-N-acetylglucosaminyltransferase-2
MDDGA9/MDDGB9/ MDDGC9	AR	DAG1	Alpha-dystroglycan
MDDGA10/MDDGB10/ MDDGC10	AR	TMEM5	Transmembrane protein 5
MDDGA11/MDDGB11/ MDDGC11	AR	B3GALNT2	Beta A-1,3-N-acetylgalactosaminyl transferase 2
MDDGA12/MDDGB12/ MDDGC12	AR	POMK	Protein-O-mannose kinase
MDDGA13/MDDGB13/ MDDGC13	AR	B4GAT1	Beta-1,4-glucuronyltransferase 1
MDDGA14/MDDGB14/ MDDGC14	AR	GMPPB	Beta-GDP-mannose pyrophosphorylase
Rigid spine syndrome	AR	SEPN1	Selenoprotein N1
Ullrich/Bethlem	AR/AD	COL6A1, COL6A2, COL6A3	Collagens 6A1, 6A2, and 6A3
DISTAL DYSTROPHIES/MYOPATHIES			
Welander	AD	TIA1	T-cell restricted intracellular antigen
Udd	AD	TTN	Titin
Markesbery-Griggs	AD	LDB3	ZASP
GNE myopathy (Nonaka; h-IBM2)	AR	GNE	UDP-N-acetylglucosamine 2-epimerase/N-acetylmannosamine kinase
Miyoshi 1	AR	DYSF	Dysferlin
Miyoshi 3	AR	ANO5	Anoctamin-5
Laing	AD	MYH7	Myosin heavy chain 7
Williams	AD	FLNC	Filamin C
Distal myopathy with vocal cord and pharyngeal weakness (VCPDM)/MSP5	AD	MTR3	Matrin 3
KLHL9 Myopathy	AD	KLH9	KELCH-like homologue 9
ADSSL Myopathy	AR	ADSSL	Adenylosuccinate synthase
PLIN4 Myopathy	AD	PLIN4	Perilipin-4
FACIOSCAPULOHUMEROL DYSTROPHIES			
FSHD1	AD		Deletion in D4Z4 region with secondary increase in DUX4 expression
FSHD2	AD	SMCHD1	Structural maintenance of chromosomes flexible hinge domain-containing protein 1
FSHD3	AD	LRIF1	Ligand-dependent nuclear receptor interacting factor 1
FSHD4	AD	DNMT3B	DNA methyltransferase 3B
SCAPULOPERONEAL DYSTROPHY	AD	DES	Desmin
	AD	MyHC 7	Myosin heavy chain 7
	XR	FHL1	Four-and-a-half LIM domain 1
EMERY-DREIFUSS MUSCULAR DYSTROPHIES			
EDMD1	XR	EMD	Emerin
EDMD2	AD	LMNA	Lamin A
EDMD3	AR	LMNA	Lamin A
EDMD4	AD	SYNE1	Nesprin-1
EDMD5	AD	SYNE2	Nesprin-2
EDMD6	XR	FHL1	Four-and-one-half LIM1
EDMD7	AD	TMEM5	Transmembrane protein 5

TABLE 27-1. (CONTINUED)

Disease	Inheritance	Gene	Affected Protein
OCULOPHARNGEAL MUSCULAR DYSTROPHY (OPMD)	AD	PABPN1	Poly(A)-binding protein-2
OCULOPHARNGEAL DISTAL MUSCULAR DYSTROPHY (OPDM)			
OPDM1	AD	LRP12	Low-density lipoprotein receptor-related protein 12
OPDM2	AD	GIPC1	GIPC PDZ domain-containing family member 1
OPDM3	AD	NOTCH2NLC	Notch 2 N-terminal like C
OPDM4	AD	RILPL1	Rab interacting lysosomal protein like 1
MYOTONIC DYSTROPHY			
Myotonic dystrophy 1	AD	DMPK	Myotonin protein kinase
Myotonic dystrophy 2	AD	CNBP	Cellular retroviral nucleic acid-binding protein 1
MYOFIBRILLAR MYOPATHIES			
MFM1	AD/AR	DES	Desmin
MFM2	AD	CRYAB	Alpha-B crystallin
MFM3	AD	MYOT	Myotolin
MFM4	AD	LDP3	ZASP
MFM5	AD	FLNC	Filamin C
MFM6	AD	BAG3	Bcl-2–binding protein
MFM7	AD	KY	Kyphoscoliosis peptidase
MFM8	AD	PYROXD1	PYROXD1
MFM9	AD	TTN	Titin
MFM10	AD	SVIL	Supervillin
MFM11	AD	UNC45B	UNC45 myosin chaperone B
MFM12	AD	MYL2	Myosin light chain 2
MULTISYSTEM PROTEINOPATHIES			
MSP1/IBMPFD1	AD	VCP	Valosin-containing protein
MSP2/IBMPFD2	AD	HNRPA2B1	HNRPA2B1
MSP3/IBMPFD3	AD	HNRNPA1	HNRNPA1
MSP4	AD	SQTM1	Sequestome
MSP5	AD	MTR3	Matrin 3

AD, autosomal dominant; AR, autosomal recessive; B3GALNT2, beta-1,4-N-acetlyglucosaminyltransferase; GMPPB, GDP-mannose pyrophosphorylase B; GNE, UDP-N-acetylglucosamine 2-epimerase/N-acetylmannosamine kinase; h-IBM, hereditary inclusion body myopathy; h-IBMPFD, hereditary inclusion body myopathy, Paget disease and frontotemporal dementia; ISPD, isoprenoid synthase domain-containing protein; HNRNPA1, heterogeneous nuclear ribonucleoprotein A1 like 2; HNRPA2B1, heterogeneous nuclear ribonucleoprotein A2/B1; MFM, myofibrillar myopathy; MDDGA1, muscular dystrophy–dystroglycanopathy with brain and eye anomalies (type A); MyHC, myosin heavy chain; POMGnT1, O-mannose-1,2-N-acetylglucosaminyl transferase; POMT1, O-mannosyltransferase; POPDC3, Popeye domain-containing protein 3; PYROXD1, pyridine nucleotide-disulfide oxidoreductase domain-containing protein 1; TIA1, T-cell restricted intracellular antigen; TMEM5, transmembrane protein 5; VCP, valosin-containing protein; ZASP, Z-band alternatively spliced PDZ motif-containing protein.

held together by disulfide bonds. There are five different α chains, three β chains, and two γ chains that have been characterized. The major isoform of laminin heavy chains in muscle is laminin-2, which is composed of α2, β1, and γ1 chains. Muscle also contains laminin-4, composed of α2, β2, and γ1 subunits. Merosin is the collective name for laminins that share a common α2 chain. α-Dystroglycan binds specifically to laminin-2, but not to the other extracellular components (Fig. 27-1). Ligands for the sarcoglycan complex are unknown, but it has been postulated that the complex is directly or indirectly linked to laminin-4.[9] Merosin is also expressed in the endoneurial basement membrane surrounding the myelin sheath of peripheral nerves.[10] Likewise, α-dystroglycan and β-dystroglycan are found in peripheral nerves. Expression of α-dystroglycan and β-dystroglycan is restricted to the outer membrane of Schwann cells and is not present in the inner membrane or on compact myelin.

Proper binding of merosin or laminin α2 requires glycosylation of α-dystroglycan. Impaired glycosylation of α-dystroglycan usually leads to severe congenital muscular dystrophy (MDC) but can be associated with a milder later-onset LGMD. These have been further subdivided into three types based on clinical phenotype: muscular dystrophy-dystroglycanopathy (congenital with brain and eye anomalies), type A (MDDGA); muscular dystrophy-dystroglycanopathy (congenital with or without impaired intellectual development), type B (MDDGB); muscular dystrophy-dystroglycanopathy (limb-girdle), type C (MDDGC).

Transmembrane β-dystroglycan anchors extracellular α-dystroglycan to the outer membrane of Schwann cells and myelin. As in muscle, merosin serves as a ligand in the Schwann cell dystroglycan complex by binding to α-dystroglycan. This complex appears to have a role in peripheral myelinogenesis. Mutations involving the merosin gene not only result in a form of congenital muscular dystrophy, but they also are associated with mild dysmyelination in the central and peripheral nervous systems.

INTEGRINS

Integrins are transmembrane, heterodimeric (α/β) receptors, which play key roles in establishing linkages between the extracellular matrix and the cytoskeleton, as well as in transducing extracellular matrix–cell signals.[11] Integrins are important in cell adhesion, migration, differentiation, proliferation, and cytoskeletal organization. The major integrin expressed throughout the sarcolemma in mature muscle fibers is α7β 1D. Binding of α7β 1D integrin merosin in skeletal muscle appears to be as important as the linkage of α-dystroglycan to merosin in providing structural stability to the sarcolemma (Fig. 27-1). Mutations of the α7 subunit result in abnormal binding of merosin to integrin and cause some forms of MDC.

UTROPHIN (DYSTROPHIN-RELATED PROTEIN)

Utrophin is an autosomal homologue of dystrophin. It is ubiquitously expressed but is localized exclusively at the neuromuscular junction in normal skeletal muscle. Utrophin associates with DAPs, suggesting that the utrophin–glycoprotein complex plays a role in the formation and integrity of the neuromuscular junction. Upregulation of utrophin is evident in the dystrophinopathies, perhaps as a compensatory mechanism.

▶ OTHER SARCOLEMMAL PROTEINS

DYSFERLIN AND ANOCTAMIN-5

Dysferlin is another cytoskeletal protein present in skeletal and cardiac muscles. It is located predominantly on the subsarcolemmal surface of the muscle membrane, but it has a small transmembrane spanning tail (Fig. 27-1). The protein does not appear to be directly connected to the dystrophin–glycoprotein complex. The function of dysferlin is not entirely known. Dysferlin may have a role in membrane fusion and repair by regulating vesicle fusion with the membrane.[12,13] In addition, dysferlin may assist in stabilizing the sarcolemmal membrane or in signal transduction.[14,15] Mutations affecting the dysferlin gene, *DYSF*, result in LGMD2B (now known as LGMDR2) and a form of Miyoshi distal myopathy (MMD1). Interestingly, anoctamin-5 is another sarcolemmal protein that like dysferlin is associated with abnormal repair of the sarcolemma.[16] Mutations in the anoctamin-5 gene, *ANO5*, cause a phenotypically similar limb-girdle muscular dystrophy (LGMDR12, formerly known as LGMD2L) another form of Miyoshi distal myopathy type 3 (MMD3).[17]

CAVEOLAE

Caveolae are 10–100-nm invaginations in the sarcolemma, derived by the oligomerization of approximately 14–16 caveolin-3 monomers that form a scaffolding complex of proteins and lipids (Fig. 27-1).[18,19] Caveolin-3 cofractionates with the dystrophin–glycoprotein complex but is thought to be part of a discrete complex. It does not directly bind to dystrophin or the sarcoglycans but does apparently interact with dysferlin. Caveolin-3 is necessary for the proper formation of T tubules and may assist in organization of signaling complexes, calcium channels (i.e., dihydropyridine and ryanodine receptors), and sodium channels. Mutations in the *CAV3* gene encoding for caveolin-3 are responsible for causing LGMD1C, rippling muscle disease, a form of distal myopathy, and some cases of idiopathic hyper-CK-emia.[20,21] Cavin is another protein that localizes to caveolae that when abnormally expressed leads to a myopathy.

▶ SARCOMERIC PROTEINS

In addition to the above sarcolemmal and related proteins, there are other important proteins that compose and support the sarcomere (Fig. 27-1). The major contractile myofibrillar proteins are the thick and thin filaments. The main component of the thick filaments is a polymer of myosin. A single thick filament is composed of nearly 300 myosin molecules. Each individual myosin molecule, in turn, consists of a single long "tail" attached to two "head" portions that project out from the tail. The head and its projecting part are referred to as a cross-bridge, which has two flexible hinges: one at the head/arm interface and the other at the arm/filament interface. The entire myosin filament is twisted about a central axis, allowing the cross-bridges to extend longitudinally and circumferentially 360 degrees. The head or the myosin heavy chain (MyHC) includes ATP-binding sites that act as an ATPase and also an actin-binding region. The energy liberated by this process is used to maintain the cross-bridge in the extended or "cocked" position. There are three major MyHC isoforms that are expressed in human skeletal muscle (type I, MYH7, expressed in type 1 fibers; IIa, MyH2, expressed in 2A fibers; and IIb, MyH1, expressed in 2B fibers).[22] Mutations in genes that encode for various MyHC isoforms cause various myopathies and cardiomyopathies.

The thin filament is composed of three subcomponents: actin, tropomyosin, and troponin. Polymerized globular or G-actin molecules form two helical strands of filamentous or F-actin. Each G-actin molecule binds one molecule of ADP.

Two chains of tropomyosin molecules wind loosely within the helical structure of the F-actin. The tropomyosin molecules overlie "active sites" on the actin molecules that link with the myosin heads forming the cross-bridges. The third major subcomponent of the thin filament, troponin, consists of three globular proteins: troponin I, T, and C. Troponin I binds strongly to actin, troponin T is attached to tropomyosin, while troponin C has a large affinity for calcium. The troponin complex attaches the tropomyosin molecules to the actin molecules, thereby forming the complete thin filament. The interaction between the myosin cross-bridges and actin filaments causes the muscle fiber to shorten or contract because the above-noted filaments slide past each other.

One end of the actin filaments is firmly anchored to the Z-disc and the other end projects out to between myosin filaments. These Z-discs extend from myofibril to myofibril across the diameter of a muscle fiber. The region of muscle or myofibril between two Z-discs is called a sarcomere. The major protein of the Z-disc is α-actinin. Nebulin is a giant protein, which is attached to α-actinin at the Z-disc and spans the entire length of the thin filament. There are two nebulin molecules for every thin filament. Desmin is an intermediate-size filament that encircles the Z-disc and helps to link the Z-disc to the sarcolemma, myonuclei, and adjacent myofibers. The cytoplasmic heat-shock protein, αB-crystallin, interacts with desmin in the assembly and stabilization of the Z-disc. Syncoilin, together with plectin, may also link desmin filaments to the Z-disc.[23] Furthermore, ZASP (Z-band alternatively spliced PDZ motif-containing protein) binds to α-actinin and assists in cross-linking thin filaments of adjacent sarcomeres.[24]

Other filamentous proteins are also important in providing stability to the sarcomere (Fig. 27-1). The giant protein titin (also known as connectin) is attached to the Z-disc and spans from the M-line to the Z-line of the sarcomere. Titin serves to connect the myosin filaments to the Z-disc. Telethonin is another sarcomeric protein present in skeletal and cardiac muscles. It colocalizes with titin to the Z-discs and along the thick filaments. Telethonin is also linked with myotilin, which in turn interacts with α-actinin and actin. In addition, filamin-c binds actin and is also involved in the formation of the Z-disc. Filamin-c also binds γ- and δ-sarcoglycan at the sarcolemma and may also play a role involved in signaling pathways from the sarcolemma to the myofibril.[25]

The interaction of all these sarcomeric proteins and Z-disc is important in myofibrillogenesis. As will be discussed, mutations affecting the genes encoding for these various sarcomeric proteins are responsible for causing different dystrophies, congenital myopathies, and inherited cardiomyopathies.

The myofibrils are surrounded by intracellular fluid called sarcoplasm. Within the sarcoplasm lies large numbers of mitochondria required for energy and other organelles. Within the sarcoplasm and surrounding the myofibrils there is an intricate series of channels called the sarcoplasmic reticulum. Longitudinal sarcoplasmic reticulum channels terminate along large terminal cisternae at either end of the sarcomere. T tubules closely associate with terminal cisternae. Two terminal cisternae are in close association with one T tubule forming a so-called triad. The T tubule conducts action potentials into the terminal cisternae and the depths of the muscle. The action potentials open voltage-gated L-type calcium channels, called the dihydropyridine receptor, located on the sarcolemmal membrane. The dihydropyridine receptor also serves as a voltage sensor for the calcium release channel, the ryanodine receptor, located on the sarcoplasmic reticulum. Mutations in these genes are responsible for hypokalemic periodic paralysis, malignant hyperthermia, and central core disease. In addition, there is a separate calcium reuptake channel located on the sarcoplasmic reticulum called sarcoplasmic reticulum calcium-ATPase. Mutations in the gene encoding for this protein (SERCA1) lead to Brody disease which is characterized by impaired relaxation of muscles.

▶ NUCLEAR PROTEINS

Emerin is a member of the nuclear lamina-associated protein (LAP) family and is located on the inner nuclear membranes of skeletal, cardiac, and smooth muscle fibers (Fig. 27-1).[26-30] The nuclear lamina is a multimeric matrix composed of a complex of intermediate-sized filaments (lamins A, B, and C), which associates with the nucleoplasmic surface of the inner nuclear membrane. Of note, lamins A and C are produced by alternative splicing of a single gene. Emerin is attached to the inner nuclear membrane through its carboxy-terminal tail, while the remainder of the protein projects into the nucleoplasm. The lamins bind to emerin, specific lamin receptors, and perhaps other LAPs located on the inner nuclear membrane. This complex of proteins is important in the organization and structural integrity of the nuclear membrane. In addition, LAPs, lamin receptors, and the lamins bind to chromatin and promote its attachment to the nuclear membrane. Nesprin-1 and -2 as well as transmembrane protein 43 (TMEM43) are located in the outer and inner nuclear membrane and bind to actin and interact with emerin and the lamins to provide support to the nuclear membrane. Abnormalities in these nuclear envelop proteins apparently disrupt the structure of the nuclear membrane, the organization of interphase chromatin, and perhaps also signal transduction between the nucleus and the sarcoplasm.[29,30] Mutations in the gene that code for emerin are responsible for X-linked Emery–Dreifuss muscular dystrophy (EDMD), while mutations involving the gene that encodes lamin A/C cause autosomal-dominant EDMD2 (and what was previously called LGMD1B) and the autosomal-recessive EDMD3. In addition, mutations in the genes that encode for nesprin-1 and -2 as well as transmembrane protein 43 also cause autosomal-dominant forms of EDMD (i.e., EDMD4, EDMD5, and EDMD7, respectively).

Within the nucleus are important RNA-binding proteins including valosin-containing protein (VCP), heterogeneous nuclear ribonucleoproteins (HNRNPA2B1, HNRNPA1), sequestome 1 (SQSTM1), matrin 3 (MATR3), and T-cell intracellular antigen-1 (TIA1). Mutations in some of their encoding genes cause the so-called multisystem proteinopathy (MSP).[31-39] The clinical spectrum of the MSPs include hereditary inclusion body myopathy (h-IBM), distal myopathy with vocal cord paralysis, amyotrophic lateral sclerosis (ALS), dementia, parkinsonism, and Paget disease of bone (PDB). The gene that encodes for another nuclear protein, poly(A)-binding protein nuclear 1 (PABPN1) is mutated in oculopharyngeal muscular dystrophy (OPMD).

Additionally, myotonic dystrophy type 1 is caused by CTG expansion in the myotonin protein kinase gene (DMPK) gene, while myotonic dystrophy type 2 is caused by CCTG repeat expansions in the cellular retroviral nucleic acid binding protein 1 gene (CNBP) as discussed in greater detail in Chapter 31 (Myotonic Dystrophies). Furthermore, CGG repeat expansions in the 5′ untranslated region (UTR) of LRP12, GIPC1, NOTCH2NLC, and RILPL1 cause oculopharyngeal distal myopathy (OPDM) type 1, 2, 3 and 4, respectively.[40] Possible pathogenic mechanisms of these repeat expansion disorders include loss of function of the protein by interfering normal transcription, RNA-mediated sequestration of RNA-binding proteins and the translation of toxic repeat peptides.

▶ NOTCH SIGNALING PATHWAY PROTEINS

The Notch signaling pathway has recently been appreciated to be very important in maintaining muscle stem cells and regulating the proper development, function, and regeneration of skeletal muscle.[41] Notch receptors are transmembrane proteins with and extracellular and transcellular domain. Binding of Notch receptors to the ligands leads to internalization of the Notch intracellular domain (NICD) into the nucleus where they bind to DNA transcription factors important in regulation of muscle stem cells. In this regard, genes/proteins that are important in the Notch signaling pathway, include TRIM32 (tripartite motif-containing protein 32), JAG2 (jagged 2), MEGF10 (multiple epidermal growth-factor like domains 10), and PAX7 (paired box 7). Mutations in these genes lead to what has been referred to as "satellite cell-opathies."

▶ ENZYMATIC PROTEINS

Calpain-3 is a muscle-specific, calcium-dependent, nonlysosomal, proteolytic enzyme present in muscle. The pathophysiologic mechanism of how mutations involving this enzyme result in a dystrophic process is not completely understood. Calpain-3 exists in both the cytosol and the nuclei of skeletal muscle fibers (Fig. 27-1), where it may be directly involved or may participate in the activation of other enzymes involved in muscle metabolism. Mutations in the calpain-3 gene are responsible for LGMDR1 (formerly known as LGMD2A).

Tripartite motif-containing protein 32, also known as E3-ubiquitine ligase, is encoded by TRIM32. This enzyme may function by tagging proteins (e.g., ubiquitination) for degradation by proteasomes (Fig. 27-1). The protein may also be important in the Notch signaling pathways discussed later. Mutations in TRIM32 cause LGMDR8 (LGMD2H).

Fukutin is a glycosyltransferase, and its deficiency is associated with abnormal glycosylation of α-dystroglycan and results in Fukuyama congenital muscular dystrophy (FCMD) and LGMDR13 (LGMD2M) (Fig. 27-1). Mutations in the fukutin-related protein gene (FKRP) are found in some patients with MDC with normal merosin (MDC1C) and in LGMDR9 (LGMD2I).[42-44] Interestingly, impaired glycosylation of α-dystroglycan is felt to be responsible for other forms of MDC [muscle–eye–brain disease (MEB) and Walker–Warburg syndrome (WWS)].[45] MEB is most commonly caused by mutations in the O-mannose-β-1,2-N-acetylglucosaminyl transferase gene (POMGnT1), which also causes LGMDR15 (LGMD2O). WWS is most commonly caused by mutations in the O-mannosyltransferase gene (POMT1) that also causes LGMDR11 (LGMD2K). Mutations in numerous other genes that encode for enzymes that are important in glycosylation of α-dystroglycan can cause congenital muscular dystrophy or a milder LGMD syndrome (i.e., POMT2, LARGE, ISPD, GTDC2, B3GALNT2, B4GAT1, TMEM5, GMPPB, POMK, DPM1, DPM2, DPM3).[46,47]

Thus, it appears that normal glycosylation of α-dystroglycan is important for muscle function but also for normal development of the central nervous system, which is affected in these forms of MDC. Interestingly, mutations in the gene encoding for α-dystroglycan itself have been found to cause LGMDR16 (LGMD2P). In addition, UDP-N-acetylglucosamine 2-epimerase/N-acetylmannosamine kinase, encoded by GNE, is involved in the posttranslational glycosylation of proteins, and is abnormal in some forms of autosomal-recessive inclusion body myopathy (now known as GNE myopathy and previously also as the Nonaka type of distal myopathy).

▶ MUSCULAR DYSTROPHIES

Muscular dystrophies traditionally have been classified according to their pattern of weakness (e.g., limb-girdle, facioscapulohumeral, and scapuloperoneal), mode of inheritance, and the responsible gene defect (Table 27-1).[1-4,46,47] However, as you will see, there are disparate clinical phenotypes associated with similar genotypes and near identical clinical phenotypes associated with many different genotypes. This is particularly notable for the LGMDs. In addition, with discovery of new genes that were initially reported as being associated with "LGMDs", have been subsequently found to cause distal myopathies, EDMD, or a myofibrillar myopathy (MFM). The advances in genetics have led yet to a recent reclassification of the LGMD by the European Neuromuscular Center (ENMC), which will be discussed in greater detail in the section regarding LGMDs.[1]

▶ THE DYSTROPHINOPATHIES: DUCHENNE AND BECKER

DUCHENNE MUSCULAR DYSTROPHY

Clinical Features

The best known of the muscular dystrophies is DMD.[48–50] DMD is an X-linked recessive disorder, but approximately one-third of patients with DMD are a result of spontaneous mutations. The incidence is roughly 1 per 3,500 male births with a prevalence approaching 1 per 18,000 males.[51]

The natural history of children with DMD (not treated with corticosteroids) is well known.[50,52,53] Most boys appear quite normal at birth and achieve the anticipated milestones of sitting and standing with little or only slight delay. However, some affected boys are hypotonic and weak at birth. Careful inspection of neck flexors in infants and toddlers suspected of having the disease usually reveal some degree of weakness. A wide-base, waddling (Trendelenburg) gait is noted by about 2–6 years of age. The waddling representing a compensatory action for hip abductor weakness. The affected child has difficulty running and jumping. There is a tendency for the child to walk on the toes, related to the center of balance being displaced anteriorly because of axial- and hip-girdle weakness and also from heel cord tightness. Calf hypertrophy may also be appreciated (Fig. 27-2). The progressive leg weakness leads to increasing falls between the ages of 2 and 6 years. Children also have difficulty arising from the floor and employ the characteristic Gower sign to enable them to rise to a standing position. Weakness is characteristically worse proximally and more so in the lower compared to upper limbs. Usually by 8 years of age, affected children have difficulty climbing stairs and need to pull themselves up the stairs using the handrails. Hyperlordosis of the lumbar spine is often noted during standing, a compensatory maneuver for hip extensor weakness. Between 6 and 12 years of age, weakness progresses to the point that the upper-limb and torso muscles are profoundly affected. Ambulation becomes progressively more difficult, and affected children are confined to a wheelchair by 12 years of age. This immobility, in turn, leads to the development of kyphoscoliosis and worsening of contractures. Nowadays as boys with DMD are usually treated with corticosteroids, they can ambulate past the age of 12 years. The biceps brachii, triceps, and quadriceps reflexes diminish and are absent in 50% of children by the age of 10 years. An interesting finding is the persistent ability to obtain an ankle jerk in at least a third of patients, even in end stages of the disease. Contractures about the hip and ankles also significantly impair posture.

Ventilatory function gradually declines and leads to death in most patients by the early 20s. This deterioration may be a consequence not only of ventilatory muscle weakness, but also due to the altered thoracic anatomy related to the kyphoscoliosis. In addition to skeletal muscle, cardiac muscle is also involved. Most patients are asymptomatic early in the course; however, dysrhythmias and congestive heart failure (CHF) can occur late in the disease. Approximately 90% of patients have electrocardiogram (EKG) abnormalities, most commonly sinus tachycardia, tall right precordial R waves, and deep narrow Q waves in the left precordial leads.[54–56] Echocardiogram reveals dilation and/or hypokinesis of ventricular walls. Unfortunately, most patients with DMD die in their late teens or early 20s from ventilatory or cardiac failure. Smooth muscle is also affected, and patients can develop gastroparesis and intestinal pseudo-obstruction.

The central nervous system is also involved in DMD. The average IQ of the affected children is approximately one standard deviation below the normal mean.[57] The mechanism by which the central nervous system is affected is unclear, but, as noted above, dystrophin is expressed at some synapses in the brain.

Laboratory Features

The serum creatine kinase (CK) levels are markedly elevated (50–100 times normal or greater) at birth and peak at around 3 years of age. Subsequently, serum CK levels decline approximately 20% per year as a result of decreasing muscle bulk, although the CK levels never normalize.

Electrodiagnostic testing in dystrophinopathies is of limited value, particularly when there is a family history of the disorder. Diagnosis requires genetic testing for identifiable mutations in the dystrophin gene and, if that is unrewarding, a muscle biopsy utilizing immunostaining and/or immunoblotting techniques. Electrodiagnostic testing may be helpful in sporadic cases and in BMD in which CK levels can be only mildly elevated and the differential diagnosis is much broader. Needle electromyography (EMG) demonstrates increased insertional and spontaneous activity in the form of fibrillation potentials and positive sharp waves. However, as muscle tissue is progressively replaced

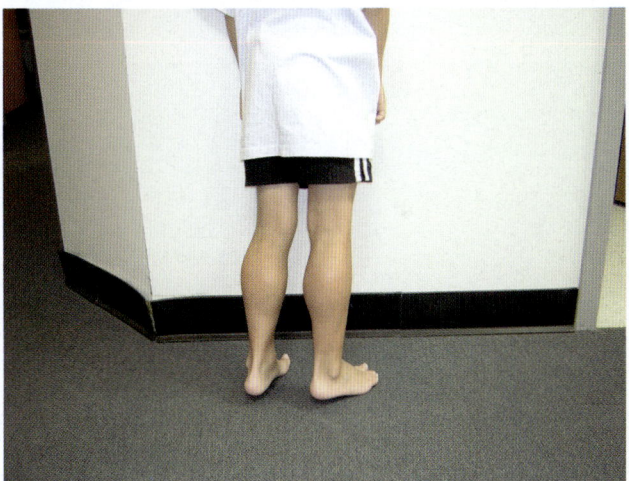

Figure 27-2. Duchenne muscular dystrophy. Enlarged calf muscles (pseudohypertrophy) and tight head cords resulting in toe walk are seen in this affected boy.

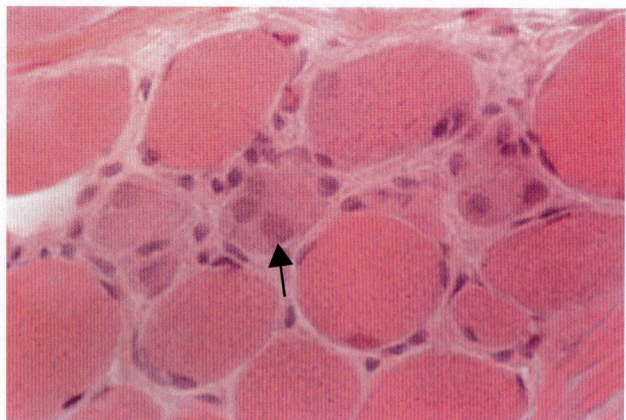

Figure 27-3. Duchenne muscular dystrophy. Muscle biopsy in a patient with DMD demonstrates mild variability in fiber size with small regenerating fibers that have enlarged nuclei (*arrow*). Hematoxylin and eosin (H&E).

with both adipose cells and connective tissue, insertional activity diminishes. The mean amplitudes of nonpolyphasic motor unit action potentials (MUAPs) are reduced, but large amplitude polyphasic potentials can also be seen. Both short- and long-duration MUAPs can be demonstrated in individual muscles, the latter reflecting the chronicity of the myopathic process. An early recruitment pattern of MUAPs is evident at low-force thresholds in weak muscles.

Histopathology

Muscle biopsies reveal scattered necrotic and regenerating muscle fibers, variability in muscle fiber size, increased endomysial and perimysial connective tissue, scattered hypertrophic and hypercontracted fibers in addition to small, rounded, regenerating fibers (Fig. 27-3). Fiber splitting and central nuclei can also be seen but occur less often than in other muscular dystrophies. The process of degeneration and regeneration continues until the limited regenerative capacity of the satellite cells is exceeded, at which time the necrotic muscle tissue is replaced with fat and connective tissue. Endomysial inflammatory cells consisting of cytotoxic T lymphocytes (two-thirds) and macrophages (one-third) are present to a variable degree and phagocytize necrotic fibers.[58]

Immunohistochemistry demonstrates reduced or absent dystrophin on the sarcolemma (Fig. 27-4).[45,50] About 60% of patients with DMD will have some faint staining of the muscle membrane using antibodies directed against the amino terminal or rod domain of dystrophin. However, less than 1% of muscle fibers have sarcolemmal staining with antibodies directed against the carboxy terminal of dystrophin. The few dystrophin-positive muscle fibers are known as revertant fibers. They arise secondary to spontaneous subsequent mutations that restore the "reading frame" and allows transcription of dystrophin, albeit abnormal size and shape. On the other hand, utrophin, which is normally restricted to the neuromuscular junction, is overexpressed in DMD and is present throughout the sarcolemma.

Immunoblot or western blot of muscle tissue assesses both the quantity and the size of the dystrophin present. With use of carboxy-terminal antibodies, the western blot reveals 0%–3% of the normal amount of dystrophin present in muscle tissue, and the size of the remaining dystrophin is usually diminished.[6] With amino-terminal or rod-domain antibodies, approximately 50% of patients with DMD have some detectable truncated dystrophin. Immunohistochemical analysis in dystrophinopathies may also demonstrate a reduction of dystroglycan, dystrobrevin, and all the sarcoglycan proteins, including sarcospan.

BECKER MUSCULAR DYSTROPHY

Clinical Features

BMD represents a milder form of dystrophinopathy. BMD can be distinguished from DMD clinically by its slower rate of progression and by dystrophin analysis.[4,50] The incidence

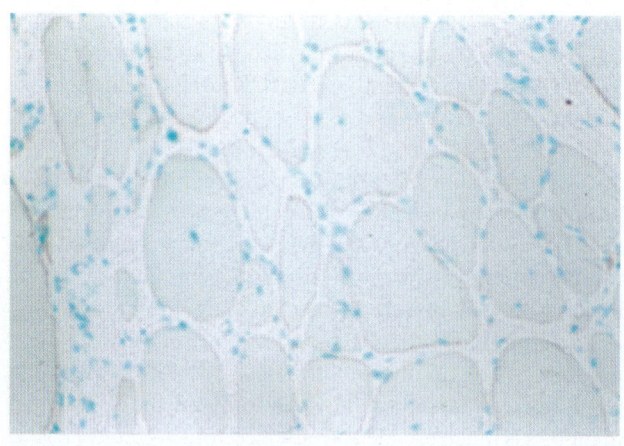

A

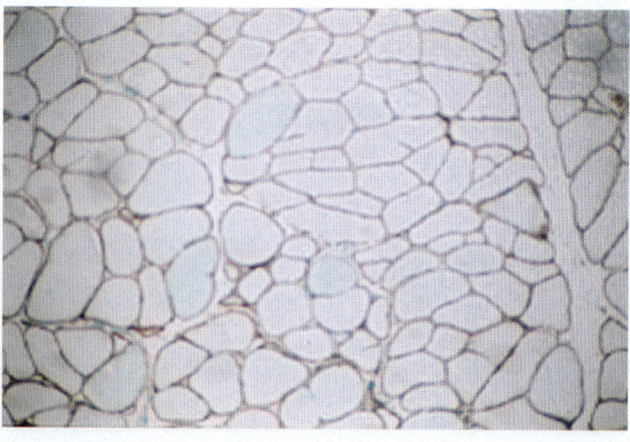

B

Figure 27-4. Immunoperoxidase staining using dystrophin (Dys 2) antibodies demonstrates absence of sarcolemmal staining on muscle fibers in DMD (**A**) and normal staining in a control biopsy (**B**).

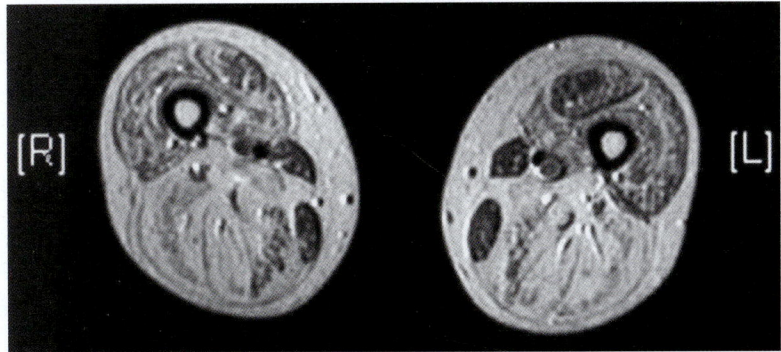

Figure 27-5. Becker muscular dystrophy. Skeletal muscle MRI (T1 weighted) of the thigh in a patient with BMD demonstrates the bright and feathery appearance of fat and connective tissue replacing muscle in the thighs.

of BMD is approximately 5 per 100,000.[51,59] Approximately 10% of cases are the result of spontaneous mutations. Clinical features that help with the diagnosis of possible BMD include (1) a family history compatible with X-linked recessive inheritance, (2) ambulation maintained past the age of 15 years (in the absence of steroid treatment), (3) a limb-girdle pattern of muscle weakness, and (4) calf hypertrophy (pseudohypertrophy).[60] Some patients exhibit preferential involvement of the quadriceps muscle (quadriceps myopathy).[61] BMD patients, unlike DMD, typically have relative sparing of neck flexor strength as a distinctive clinical feature.

A wide spectrum of clinical phenotypes and variability can be seen even within families.[4,62] Most patients develop difficulty in walking; however, by definition, they remain ambulatory past the age of 15 years. Approximately 50% of affected individuals lose the ability to ambulate independently by the fourth decade. Some patients manifesting with isolated myalgias,[63] myoglobinuria,[64] cardiomyopathy,[65,66] and asymptomatic hyper-CK-emia have been demonstrated to have mild forms of dystrophinopathy. Cardiac abnormalities are similar to DMD.[67] Mental abilities have not been investigated as thoroughly as in DMD, but some series have demonstrated a borderline or mildly impaired IQ in patients with BMD.[4,60,62] The life expectancy is reduced, although many patients live well into adulthood.[60]

Laboratory Features

Serum CK levels are elevated, often 20–200 times normal.[4] Patients with only exertional myalgias may have only slightly elevated serum CK levels. EMG is abnormal in weak muscles as discussed in the DMD section. Skeletal muscle magnetic resonance imaging (MRI) scans can demonstrate fatty replacement of affected muscle groups (Fig. 27-5).

Histopathology

The histological features are similar to those observed for DMD but are less severe (Fig. 27-6).[4,68] BMD may be distinguished histologically from DMD with immunostaining, which demonstrates the presence of dystrophin using carboxy-terminal antibodies on muscle membranes in most cases of BMD. In contrast, immunostaining with antibodies directed against the carboxy terminal of dystrophin is usually negative in DMD. However, the degree and intensity of the dystrophin staining are usually not normal in BMD. The staining pattern may be uniformly reduced or can vary between and within fibers. Western blot analysis of muscle tissue typically reveals an abnormal quantity and/or size of the dystrophin protein.[4,6,48,50,69]

OUTLIERS

This older term was used for children who have a clinical phenotype in between that of DMD and BMD. In the pre-steroid era, these children were defined by the ability to ambulate after the age of 12 years but required a wheelchair by the age of 15 years. In early childhood, outliers may be distinguished from children with more severe DMD clinical phenotype by the presence of antigravity neck flexion strength. Children with DMD cannot lift their heads fully against gravity when lying supine (Medical Research Council grade less than 3), unlike outliers and BMD children who typically can. Immunologic studies on muscle tissue usually reveal the presence of some dystrophin, although often reduced in amount and/or size.

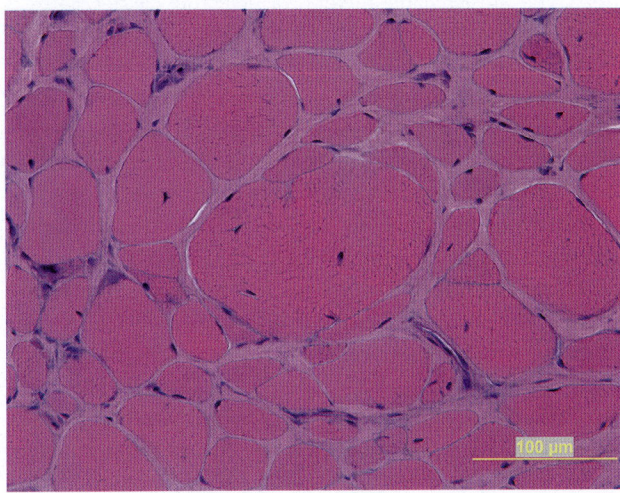

Figure 27-6. Becker muscular dystrophy. Muscle biopsy demonstrates increased endomysial connective tissue, marked variability in muscle fiber size, slightly increased internalized nuclei, and splitting of muscle fibers. Hematoxylin and eosin (H&E).

WOMEN CARRIERS

The daughters of men with BMD (males with DMD are usually infertile) and the mothers of affected children are obligate carriers of the mutated dystrophin gene. Mothers and sisters of isolated patients with DMD or BMD are at risk of being carriers. One of the most important aspects of caring for patients and families with dystrophinopathies is to determine the carrier status of "at-risk" females for the purpose of genetic counseling. There is a 50% chance that males born to women carriers will inherit the disease, and 50% of the daughters born will become carriers themselves. Women carriers are usually asymptomatic, but some develop muscle weakness.[4,60] These cases are usually explained by the Lyon hypothesis: skewed inactivation of the normal X-chromosome and dystrophin gene results in increased transcription of the mutated dystrophin gene. Females with translocations at the chromosomal Xp21 site or Turner syndrome (XO genotype) may also develop dystrophinopathies.

Manifesting carriers typically have a mild limb-girdle phenotype similar to BMD.[4] Prior to the advances in molecular genetics, these women were often diagnosed with LGMD, particularly when there was no family history of DMD or BMD. Rarely, females can develop severe weakness as seen in DMD.

Laboratory and histologic features of manifesting carriers are similar to those discussed for DMD and BMD. Immunostaining for dystrophin demonstrates an absent, decreased, or mosaic pattern of staining in many women carriers (Fig. 27-7); however, staining can be normal.[70–73] Thus, immunostaining and western blot analysis are not very sensitive in identifying carrier status of asymptomatic females.

Serum CK levels are an insensitive measure of carrier status.[74,75] CK levels can be elevated early in life; however, a normal serum CK does not exclude a carrier status. Elevated serum CK levels are identified in less than 50% of obligate carriers. The most reliable method of detecting carrier status is with genetic testing. This analysis is accomplished first by identifying the specific mutation in an affected male relative. The detection of such a mutation makes carrier detection of at-risk female relatives much easier and also allows for subsequent prenatal detection in at-risk fetuses. If a mutation is demonstrated in an affected male relative, at-risk females can be screened for the same mutation. However, it should be noted that the carrier status of a mother of a sporadic DMD case must be interpreted cautiously because of the potential for germline mosaicism.[76] In a germline mosaic, the mutation involves only a percentage of the germ cells (i.e., oocytes) but are not present in the leukocytes in which DNA analysis is performed. In these rare cases, an affected child may have an identifiable mutation on DNA analysis, but the mother could have no demonstrable mutation in the leukocytes but is still capable of having other affected children. The recurrence rate in germline carriers is unknown and dependent on the number of mutated oocytes but has been estimated to be as high as 14%.[76] Prenatal diagnosis can be made with DNA analysis of chorionic villi or amniotic fluid cells when there is an identifiable mutation in the family.

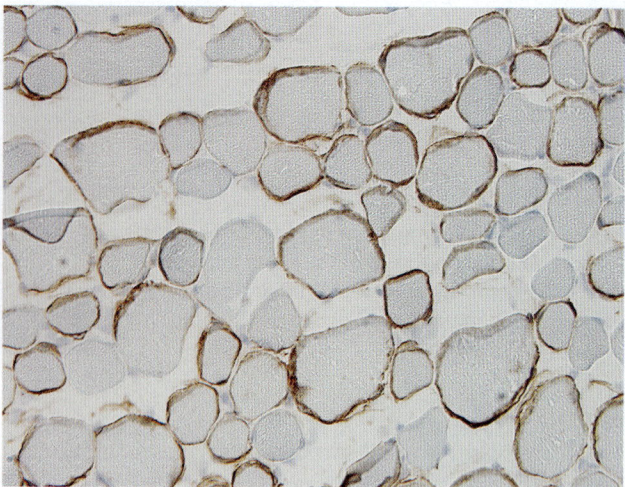

Figure 27-7. Muscle biopsy of a manifesting woman carrier of a dystrophin mutation demonstrates a mosaic pattern of dystrophin expression on the sarcolemma. Immunoperoxidase staining using dystrophin (Dys 2) antibodies.

MOLECULAR GENETICS AND PATHOGENESIS OF THE DYSTROPHINOPATHIES

Dystrophin is a structural protein, which is intimately bound to the sarcolemma and provides structural integrity to the muscle membrane (Fig. 27-1). Abnormal dystrophin quantity or quality results in the muscle losing its ability to maintain its integrity during contraction, leading to membrane tears and subsequent muscle fiber necrosis.

The dystrophin gene, located on chromosome Xp21, is composed of approximately 2.4 Mb of genomic DNA and includes 79 exons, which code for a 14-kb transcript.[5,7] The large size of the gene probably accounts for the high spontaneous mutation rate responsible for one-third of new cases. Large deletions, several kilobases to over 1 million base pairs, can be demonstrated in approximately two-thirds of patients with dystrophinopathy. Approximately 5%–10% of DMD cases are caused by point mutations, resulting in premature stop codons.[77] Duplications are evident in another 5% of cases. Mutations occur primarily in the center (80%) and near the amino terminal (20%) of the gene.[77] Mutations that disrupt the translational reading frame of the gene lead to near total loss of dystrophin and DMD, while in-frame mutations result in the translation of semifunctional dystrophin of abnormal size and/or amount and in outlier or BMD clinical phenotypes.[6] Although there are exceptions to the "reading-frame rule," 92% of phenotypic differences are explained by in-frame and out-of-frame mutations.[77] It appears that the quality or remaining functional capability of the mutated dystrophin protein is more important than the actual quantity. The reduction in the various sarcoglycans, which is also evident in immunohistochemical studies of DMD and BMD, suggests that normal dystrophin is important for the integrity of the sarcoglycan complex.

TREATMENT OF THE DYSTROPHINOPATHIES

Corticosteroids

Prednisone (0.75 mg/kg/day) has been shown to increase strength and function (peaking at 3 months) and slow the rate of deterioration in children with DMD.[48,50,78–83] Steroids also appear to reduce the risk of scoliosis and stabilize pulmonary function. The beneficial effects are noted as early as 10 days and are sustained for at least 3 years. These apparent clinical benefits are accompanied by an increase in muscle mass and decline in the rate of muscle catabolism.[81] The mechanism is not felt to be related to the immunosuppressive action of prednisone on inflammatory infiltrates in the muscle but rather by altering muscle metabolism, particularly protein synthesis and/or breakdown. Lower doses of prednisone (<0.75 mg/kg/day) are not as effective in DMD. There have been no large, double-blinded, placebo-controlled studies assessing the efficacy of steroids in BMD, although small series suggest a possible benefit.[84]

Unfortunately, high-dose prednisone is associated with significant side effects including weight gain, stunted growth, cushingoid appearance, excessive hair growth, irritability, and hyperactivity. In addition, prednisone is also associated with an increased risk of infections, cataract formation, hypertension, glucose intolerance, osteoporosis, and osteonecrosis. Twice-weekly oral prednisone given on a weekend (5 mg/kg/day) appeared to be beneficial compared to historical controls in a small open-label study of 20 boys with DMD.[85] An analog of prednisone, deflazacort is approved for treatment of DMD.[48,50,83,86,87] Small studies have suggested that deflazacort 0.90 mg/kg/day is as effective as prednisone 0.75 mg/kg/day and may be associated with fewer side effects, but the evidence was graded as being very low quality.[88] A recent double-blind, randomized trial compared daily prednisone (0.75 mg/kg) ($n = 65$), daily deflazacort (0.90 mg/kg) ($n = 65$), or intermittent prednisone (0.75 mg/kg for 10 days on and then 10 days off).[89] Both daily prednisone and daily deflazacort were more effective than intermittent prednisone, but there was no significant difference between the two daily corticosteroid regimens. In regard to side effects, weight gain was greater with prednisone, however deflazacort was associated with greater slowing of growth.

Vamorolone was developed as a dissociative corticosteroid that might have similar efficacy but fewer side effects. A recent randomized, double-blind, placebo- and prednisone-controlled 24-week clinical trial compared four groups: placebo; prednisone, 0.75 mg/kg per day; vamorolone, 2 mg/kg per day; and vamorolone, 6 mg/kg per day. Vamorolone was shown to be effective and safe in the treatment of boys with DMD over the 24-week treatment period and maintained in open-label extension trials for 30 months.[90–92] These results led to FDA approval of Vamorolone 6 mg/kg per day (up to a maximum of 300 mg daily for DMD.

Histone Deacetylase Inhibitors

Givinostat is a histone deacetylase (HDAC) inhibitor that was recently approved by the FDA for treatment of DMD ages 6 and older based on the results of a randomized, double-blind, placebo-controlled 18-month phase 3 study that showed statistically significant less decline in the time it took to climb four stairs and also a smaller decline in the North Star Ambulatory Assessment (NSAA) in patients treated givinostat.[93] It is taken orally twice a day in a dosage that is weight dependent. It is recommended that providers assess platelet counts and triglycerides before prescribing givinostat. Patients with a platelet count less than 150×10^9/L should not take givinostat. HDACs regulate muscle gene expression and inhibitors believed to enhance the muscle regeneration and reduce fibrofatty degeneration.[94]

Gene Therapies

Potential strategies for replacing the defective dystrophin protein include somatic gene therapy via myoblast or stem cell transplantation, direct gene replacement using modified viral vectors, and exon-skipping agents to restore the dystrophin gene reading frame.[95–97] Controlled trials of human myoblast transfer in DMD have not resulted in any significant clinical improvement. In our opinion, stem cell therapies are likely not going to be clinically effective. Recent small studies of delandistrogene moxeparvovec, an adeno-associated vector based gene therapy designed to treat DMD with a functionally shortened microdystrophin molecule, resulted in an increase in microdystrophin by Western blot on muscle biopsies and perhaps some clinical improvement.[98,99] This led to accelerated FDA approval for 4 to 5 year old boys with DMD. A larger, randomized trial has been conducted, and although the results have not been published as yet, the sponsor of the study released information that the primary outcome measure was not met.

Most of the recent advances have been with exon-skipping strategies. Antisense oligonucleotides (ASO) designed to induce exon skipping of specific mutations and drugs that allow read-through of nonsense mutations have potential benefit.[50] ASO can be designed to skip over specific exon such that the reading frame might be restored. This could lead to increased expression of dystrophin, albeit at a reduced size. ASO would theoretically be able to correct multiple DMD mutations. For example, skipping of exon 45 might theoretically correct both deletions of exons 46–47 and exons 46–48. It has been estimated that as many as 35% of DMD might theoretically improve by targeting a limited number of exons (44, 45, 51, and 53) and the yield may increase to over 80% with skipping of two exons.[50] Currently, there are four FDA-approved ASO using exon-specific morpholinos: eteplirsen (Exondys51)[100,101] targeting exon 51, golodirsen (Vyondys53)[102,103] targeting exon 53, viltolarsen (Viltepso)[104,105] also targeting exon 53, and casimersen (AmonDys-45)[106,107] targeting exon 45. However, these drugs were approved based on very small studies that demonstrated only very modest increase in dystrophin expression in muscle fibers (0.4%–5%) without definite, clinically meaningful efficacy.

Supportive Therapy

Patients are best managed using a multidisciplinary approach.[4,58–60] Ideally, neuromuscular clinics should involve neurologists, physiatrists, physical therapists, occupational therapists, speech therapists, respiratory therapists, dietitians, cardiologists, pulmonologists, psychologists, and genetic counselors in order to assess all the needs of individual patients. Physical therapy is a key component in the treatment of patients with muscular dystrophy. Because contractures develop early in the disease, particularly of the heel cords, iliotibial bands, and the hips, appropriate stretching exercises must be started early in the disease. Long leg braces may aid ambulation. Rehabilitation issues are discussed in greater detail in Chapter 5.

Cardiac function, including EKG and echocardiogram, should be assessed at diagnosis of DMD or at least by the 6 years of age and then at least once every 2 years until the age of 10 years.[58-60] Afterward, there should be annual cardiac assessments, sooner if cardiac symptoms and signs begin earlier. Holter monitoring should also be considered as arrhythmia may develop before signs of systolic dysfunction. Afterload reduction with angiotensin-converting enzyme inhibitors or angiotensin receptor blockers is considered standard treatment of cardiomyopathy.[58-60] β-Blockers and diuretics are also used to treat heart failure. Likewise, cardiac assessments and treatment are important in management of patients with BMD.[4]

Scoliosis is a universal complication of DMD, particularly once the child is nonambulatory.[58-60] We perform yearly spinal radiographs to assess progression once scoliosis is apparent on clinical examination. Scoliosis results in pain, aesthetic damage, and perhaps ventilatory compromise. Orthopedic consultation should be considered for curves past 20 degrees.[50] We consider spinal fusion in children with 35 degrees scoliosis or more and for those who are in significant discomfort. Ideally, forced vital capacity (FVC) should be greater than 35% to minimize the risk of surgery. Quality of life seems to be improved following spinal stabilization; however, scoliosis surgery does not appear to increase ventilatory function.

DMD, GLYCEROL KINASE DEFICIENCY, AND ADRENAL HYPOPLASIA CONGENITA

DMD and glycerol kinase deficiency (GKD) can occur together as part of a contiguous gene syndrome at chromosome Xp21.[108-110] The gene order for the contiguous loci is Xpter–AHC–GKD–DYS—centromere, and thus patients may also have adrenal hypoplasia congenita (AHC) depending on the extent of the mutation. Microdeletions can span these contiguous genes, producing a clinical phenotype that is different from that seen in patients who have mutations only within the individual DMD, GK, or AHC genes. Most children with combined DMD and GKD exhibit severe psychomotor delay. In addition to muscular weakness, they also often experience episodic nausea, vomiting, and stupor from GKD. Further, mutations involving the DAX1 gene responsible for AHC can result in life-threatening adrenal insufficiency manifested by Addisonian hyperpigmentation of the skin, hypogonadotropic hypogonadism/cryptorchidism, hyperkalemia, hyponatremia, and hypoglycemia. Glycerol kinase is responsible for the first step in glycerol metabolism and is important in glycolysis, gluconeogenesis, and triglyceride metabolism:

$$\text{glycerol} + \text{ATP} \Leftrightarrow \text{glycerol 3-phosphate} + \text{ADP}.$$

GKD results in glyceroluria and hyperglycerolemia. GKD should be considered in a young child with elevated serum triglyceride levels because the standard serum triglyceride test actually measures free glycerol. The neurological side effects of GKD are responsive to a fat-restricted diet and avoidance of prolonged fasting.

AHC is caused by mutations in the dosage-sensitive sex reversal AHC, X-chromosome, gene 1, or *DAX1*. The DAX1 protein is a member of the nuclear hormone receptor superfamily and functions to regulate the transcription of genes involved in the normal development of the adrenal glands. Decreased serum levels of gonadotropins and a subnormal increase in serum cortisol in response to exogenous administration of adrenocorticotropic hormone are found. Treatment of adrenal insufficiency is by replacement of glucocorticoids, mineralocorticoids, and testosterone.

Mutations involving the 3′ (carboxy-terminal) portion of the dystrophin gene usually span into the GK locus. Thus, patients with dystrophinopathies who have three mutations should be evaluated for the contiguous gene syndrome. Most patients have DMD; BMD can also occur. Diagnosis of X-chromosomal microdeletions can be made with Southern blotting, DNA amplification through PCR, or fluorescent in situ hybridization analysis. Further, fluorescent in situ hybridization provides a rapid and accurate evaluation for these microdeletions and can also be used for carrier detection and prenatal diagnosis.

LIMB-GIRDLE MUSCULAR DYSTROPHY

The LGMDs are a heterogeneous group of disorders that clinically resemble the dystrophinopathies, except for the equal occurrence in men and women (Table 27-1).[1-4,111] The prevalence rate of all LGMDs together was recently estimated on meta-analysis to be 1.63 per 100,000 (range 0.56–5.75 per 100,000).[112] The LGMDs are inherited in an autosomal-recessive or autosomal-dominant fashion. Traditionally, the autosomal-dominant LGMDs were classified as type 1 (e.g., LGMD1), while recessive forms were termed type 2 (e.g., LGMD2). Further alphabetical subclassification was applied to these disorders in the order they were discovered in consideration of their distinct genotypes (e.g., LGMD2A, LGMD2B, etc.; see Table 27-1). However, as alluded previously, a new nomenclature was proposed by the ENMC for several reasons.[1] With advances in genetics, we ran into the end of the alphabet for autosomal-recessive LGMDs. Furthermore, with more gene identification, disorders previously classified as an "LGMD" were found to also have been classified as a congenital muscular dystrophy, EDMD, or an MFM. Some "LGMD" designations were applied when only a single family reported. The new nomenclature designates autosomal-dominant and autosomal-recessive LGMDs as LGMDD and LGMDR, respectively, with a numerical number following based on genotype (Table 27-1). An LGMD was further defined as:

> "a genetically inherited condition that primarily affects skeletal muscle leading to progressive, predominantly proximal muscle weakness at presentation caused by a loss of muscle fibres. To be considered a form of limb girdle muscular dystrophy the condition must be described in at least two unrelated families with affected individuals achieving independent walking, must have an elevated serum creatine kinase activity, must demonstrate degenerative changes on muscle imaging over the course of the disease, and have dystrophic changes on muscle histology, ultimately leading to end-stage pathology for the most affected muscles."[1]

As can be seen from Table 27-1, some of the myopathies previously categorized as "LGMD" are no longer designated as such. However, their use is still pervasive in the literature, so we will use both the older and new terminologies in this chapter: Old Classification/New Classification, when applicable, and the associated abnormal protein in parentheses. For the most part, the clinical, laboratory, and histopathological features of the LGMDs are nonspecific, with the few exceptions to be discussed.

Reproduced with permission from Straub V, Murphy A, Udd B. 229th ENMC international workshop: limb girdle muscular dystrophies - nomenclature and reformed classification Naarden, the Netherlands,. *Neuromuscul Disord.* 2018;28:702–710.

▶ AUTOSOMAL-DOMINANT LGMD

LGMD1A/MFM3 (MYOTILIN)

Clinical Features

Gilchrist and colleagues described the original family (144 patients over 7 generations) with this autosomal-dominant inherited LGMD (Table 27-1, Fig. 27-8).[113] Subsequently

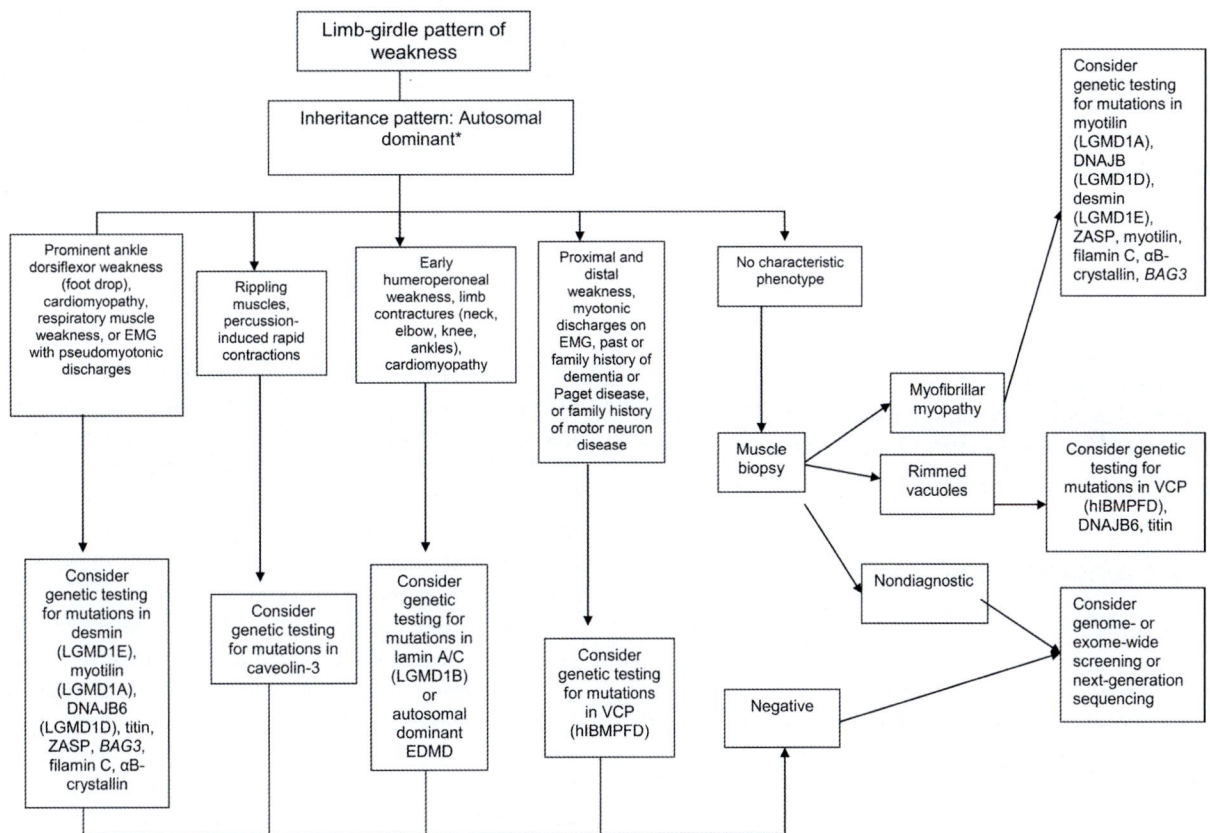

Figure 27-8. Diagnostic approach to patients with a limb-girdle pattern of weakness and suspected muscular dystrophy with an autosomal-dominant inheritance pattern. *Autosomal-dominant, autosomal-recessive, or X-linked inheritance may be responsible in sporadic cases. EDMD, Emery–Dreifuss muscular dystrophy; h-IBMPFD, hereditary inclusion body myopathy with Paget disease and frontotemporal dementia; LGMD, limb-girdle muscular dystrophy; VCP, valosin-containing protein. (Reproduced with permission from Narayanaswami P, Weiss M, Selcen D, et al. Evidence-based guideline summary: diagnosis and treatment of limb-girdle and distal dystrophies: report of the guideline development subcommittee of the American Academy of Neurology and the practice issues review panel of the American Association of Neuromuscular & Electrodiagnostic Medicine. *Neurology.* 2014;83(16):1453–1463.)

there have been many other reports, many under the category of MFM.[1–4,23,114–119] The onset of weakness ranges from the teens to the eighth decade of life. There is often an early predilection for the scapular–humeral–pelvic muscles. However, distal muscles, particularly in the lower extremities, can be weaker than proximal muscles in some patients.[4,23] Patients can also develop an associated cardiomyopathy. Unlike the dystrophinopathies and other LGMDs (e.g., the sarcoglycanopathies), calf hypertrophy is rare. Dysarthria or hypernasal speech occurs in some individuals.[117,118] Because the pattern of weakness can often be predominantly distal and the pathology is of an MFM, the new ENMC criteria no longer classify this myopathy as an LGMD, but rather as MFM3.[1]

Laboratory Features

Serum CK levels are normal or elevated up to nine times normal. Muscle imaging studies have revealed fibrofatty replacement and edema in the medial gastrocnemius, soleus, hip adductors, and biceps femoris with relative sparing of the semitendinosus muscles.[115,116]

Histopathology

Muscle biopsies are notable for the frequent occurrence of rimmed vacuoles and occasional nemaline rod-like inclusions.[4,114] Muscle biopsies can demonstrate features of MFM (see later section regarding MFM) on routine light microscopy, immunohistochemistry, and electron microscopy (EM).[4,23]

Molecular Genetics and Pathogenesis

LGMD1A/MFM3 is caused by autosomal-dominant mutations in the *MYOT* gene that encodes for myotilin located on chromosome 5q22.3–31.3.[4,23,114,119] Spontaneous mutations are common, so the lack of a family history should not exclude the diagnosis. Myotilin is a sarcomeric protein that colocalizes with α-actinin at the Z-disc. Mutations lead to disruption of the Z-disc and sarcomere.

LGMD1B/EDMD2 (LAMIN A/C)

Clinical Features

LGMD1B/EDMD2 can present with weakness in the hip and shoulder girdle or have a predilection for the humeral and peroneal muscles and is often associated with cardiac conduction defects; some affected individuals manifest only with a cardiomyopathy.[4,29,120–123] The cardiomyopathy and associated arrhythmias can result in sudden death and often require pacemaker or intracardiac defibrillator implantation.[4] Some patients require cardiac transplantation because of CHF from dilated cardiomyopathy. This clinical phenotype much more resembles that seen in the more common X-linked EDMD caused by mutation in the gene that encodes for emerin. In this regard LGMD1B and

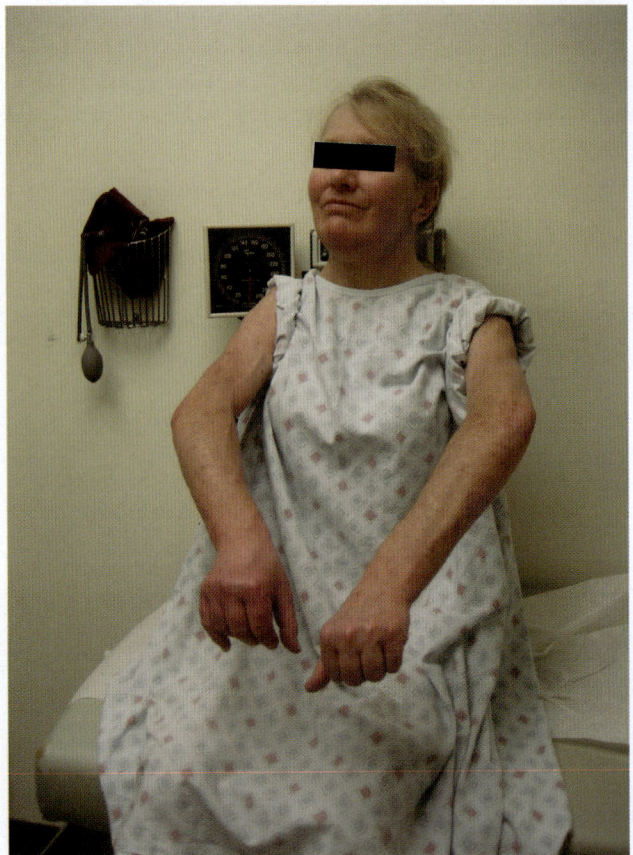

Figure 27-9. A patient with LGMD1B/EDMD2 caused by *LMNA* mutation demonstrated severe early elbow *contractures*.

autosomal-dominant EDMD2 are allelic being caused by mutations in the lamin A/C gene, *LMNA*.[4,29,121]

As mentioned, the pattern of muscle involvement is characterized by proximal arm weakness and atrophy with preferential involvement of humeral muscles, both proximal and distal weakness in the lower extremities, ankle, and elbow contractures (Fig. 27-9), and spinal rigidity (particularly in the neck). However, contractures may not be apparent until late in the disease course or not at all, which is a feature that may help distinguish it from X-linked EDMD caused by mutations in the emerin gene, in which contractures are invariably present early in the disease course.[29,122–126] The LGMD phenotype is associated with proximal leg more than arm weakness, but again often with preferential involvement of humeral muscles. Again, flexion contractures of elbows and Achilles tendons may be seen but can be subtle or not apparent until late in the course. Again, because the pattern of weakness is usually more typical of EDMD, the new ENMC criteria classify this myopathy as EDMD2 as opposed to a LGMD.[1]

Laboratory Features

Serum CK levels may be normal or elevated up to 25 times normal. Skeletal muscle imaging with MRI or CT can show fatty infiltration in the posterior compartment of the thigh and calves.[4,127–130] One imaging study comparing AD-EDMD to LGMDD5, also known as Bethlem or Ullrich myopathy (collagen VI disorders), which have a similar pattern of muscle weakness, found that the quadriceps were relatively spared, and the hamstrings were more severely involved in AD-EDMD.[128]

Histopathology

Muscle biopsies demonstrate variation in fiber size, increased endomysial connective tissue, normal dystrophin, sarcoglycan, and emerin staining. Occasionally, rimmed vacuoles are evident on muscles biopsy.[4,120] Emerin and lamin A/C expressions on the nuclear membrane are typically normal with immunohistochemistry. On EM, myonuclei exhibit the loss of peripheral heterochromatin or its detachment from the nuclear envelop, altered interchromatic texture, and fewer nuclear pores compared to normal.[28]

Molecular Genetics and Pathogenesis

LGMD1B/EDMD2 is caused by mutations in *LMNA* that encodes for lamin A/C.[29,30,121] Of note, Dunnigan type familial partial lipodystrophy, mandibuloacral dysplasia, Hutchinson–Gilford progeria syndrome, restrictive dermopathy, and a form of dominant-intermediate Charcot–Marie–Tooth (CMT) neuropathy are also allelic disorders associated with *LMNA* mutations.[4] Interestingly, phenotypic variability occurs even within family members carrying the same mutation.[4,123] The pathogenic role of lamin A/C is discussed in more detail in the EDMD section.

LGMD1C/RIPPLING MUSCLE DISEASE TYPE 2 (CAVEOLIN-3)

Clinical Features

This myopathy is caused by mutations in the caveolin-3 gene, *CAV3*, and is associated with a heterogeneous phenotype.[4,18–21,131–142] Most are inherited in an autosomal-dominant fashion, though an autosomal-recessive inheritance pattern has also been described.[143] Affected individuals may present in childhood or adult life with proximal weakness or exertional myalgias. Calf hypertrophy may be evident. The rate of progression is variable. Other patients manifest with muscle stiffness, rippling muscle disease, distal weakness (anterior or posterior compartment), asymptomatic hyper-CK-emia, and rarely myoglobinuria.[4,19–21,131,138] Generalized percussion-induced rapid contractions (PIRCs) were apparent in the face, neck, and extremities in all affected patients in one series, while actual rippling muscles are evident in approximately two-thirds.[141] This has led to the classification of this disorder as hereditary rippling muscle disease type 2. Spontaneous mutations are not uncommon, so a lack of a family history does not exclude the diagnosis.[18]

Laboratory Features

Serum CK can be elevated 3- to 30-fold.[4]

Histopathology

Muscle biopsies demonstrate nonspecific myopathic features with normal dystrophin, sarcoglycan, and merosin staining.[4] Reduced caveolin-3 staining may be appreciated along the sarcolemma. EM reveals a decreased density of caveolae on the muscle membrane as well.

Molecular Genetics and Pathogenesis

This myopathy is caused by mutations in the caveolin-3 gene (*CAV3*) located on chromosome 3p25.[4,18,19] Most are autosomal-dominant mutations, but autosomal-recessive mutations have also been reported.[143] Caveolin-3 is located on the sarcolemma ([Fig. 27-1](#)). It cofractionates with the dystrophin–glycoprotein complex but is thought to be part of a discrete complex. Caveolins play a role in the formation of caveolae membranes, where they act as scaffolding proteins to organize and concentrate caveolin-interacting lipids and proteins.[19] Caveolin-3 might also function to facilitate organization of signaling complexes and the sodium channels that contribute to the pathogenesis of rippling muscle disease.

LGMD1D/LGMDD1 (DNAJB6)

Clinical Features

LGMD1D, now called LGMDD1, is a rare dystrophy associated with slowly progressive weakness with a mean age of onset of around 30 years (range 4–69 years).[1–4,144–147] Dysphagia is the most frequent symptom. Affected individuals typically develop proximal muscle weakness in the lower extremities (hamstrings worse than quadriceps) with normal or only mild proximal upper extremity strength.[146] However, the phenotype can be variable and a quarter of patients can manifest more distal lower extremity weakness with preferential involvement of the posterior compartment more than the anterior compartment.[145,147] The median age at loss of ambulation is around 34 years.[147] The largest series of patients (#122) reported mild cardiac and ventilatory muscles abnormalities (minor EKG alterations or FVC slightly below 80% of predicted) occurring in 30% and 38% of patients and at median ages of 46 and 42 years, respectively.[147]

Laboratory Features

Serum CK levels range from normal to 10-fold elevated but are usually 2–3 times the upper limit of normal.

Histopathology

Muscle biopsies reveal muscle fibers with rimmed vacuoles and other features suggestive of MFM.[145,148]

Molecular Genetics and Pathogenesis

The disorder is caused by mutations in the DNAJ (Hsp40) homologue, subfamily B, member gene (*DNAJB6*) located on chromosome 7q36.[145,146]

LGMD1E/MFM1 (DESMIN)

Clinical Features

Myofibrillary myopathy type 1 (MFM1), formerly known as LGMD1E, is an autosomal-dominant disorder caused by mutations in the gene that encodes for desmin (*DES*).[1-4,149-157] It has also been called hereditary inclusion body myopathy type 1 (h-IBM). Additionally, it is allelic with what was previously termed, LGMD2R, which is a desminopathy inherited in an autosomal-recessive fashion. Mutations in *DES* are one of the most common causes of MFM. The age of onset ranges from the first to sixth decades of life.[4] Although patients may have a limb-girdle pattern of weakness, most have more distal involvement with the earliest manifestation being progressive foot drop.[4] Some have proximal equal to distal weakness,[151-153,156] or a scapuloperoneal distribution.[152,155] Dysphagia or dysarthria can also occur.[151,156] Ventilatory muscle weakness[4,154-156] and cardiac involvement are common and may precede skeletal muscle weakness.[4,141-158] Cardiac manifestations include arrhythmia (e.g., atrioventricular conduction block, atrial fibrillation, other tachyarrhythmias, sudden cardiac death) and some patients require pacemaker or cardioverter defibrillator implantation. Dilated cardiomyopathy appears to be more frequent than hypertrophic or restrictive cardiomyopathy. Some patients benefit from cardiac transplantation.[157]

Laboratory Features

Serum CK levels are normal or only moderately elevated (up to five times normal).[4,152-155] EMG is myopathic and often demonstrates increased insertional and spontaneous activity (fibrillation potentials, positive sharp waves). In addition, myotonic, or more appropriately, pseudomyotonic discharges (decrescendo as opposed to crescendo/decrescendo frequency and amplitude of discharges) are seen. Skeletal muscle imaging of the distal leg usually shows involvement of the tibialis anterior and peroneus group more than the posterior compartment (medial gastrocnemius and soleus).[4] In the thighs, the earliest abnormalities may be in the semitendinosus and sartorius.[4]

Histopathology

Muscle biopsies reveal muscle fibers with rimmed vacuoles and other features suggestive of an MFM.

Molecular Genetics and Pathogenesis

The disorder is caused by mutations in the *DES* gene that encodes for desmin, an intermediate filament. In muscle, desmin forms a three-dimensional scaffold extending across the diameter of the myofibril surrounding the Z-discs and linking the entire sarcomere (contractile proteins) to the sarcolemmal membrane, cytoplasmic organelles, and myonuclei.

LGMD1F/LGMDD2 (TRANSPORTIN-3)

Clinical Features

This dystrophy can present in infancy to late adult life with proximal greater than distal weakness and atrophy, legs more than arms.[159-161] Most of the reported patients were from Spain or Italy, but it has been reported in Sweden and Hungary as well. Cardiac and ventilatory muscles appear to be spared.

Laboratory Features

CK level is normal to moderately elevated.

Histopathology

Muscle biopsy can show enlarged myonuclear with central pallor, fibers with rimmed vacuoles, along with and features of MFM.

Molecular Genetics and Pathogenesis

LGMD1F/LGMDD2 is caused by mutation in *TNP03* which encodes for transportin-3, a nuclear import receptor for precursor-mRNA splicing factors.[159-161] Impairment of this important protein may cause muscle destruction by various previous mentioned mechanisms in the section regarding RNA-binding proteins.

LGMD1G/LGMDD3 (HETEROGENEOUS NUCLEAR RIBONUCLEOPROTEIN D LIKE PROTEIN)

Clinical Features

This rare, recently discovered dystrophy is characterized by slowly progressive proximal muscle weakness or distal weakness of the arms and legs.[162-164] Scapular winging is common. Onset is usually in the mid-30s but can occur during the teenage years. Notably, affected individuals may also develop cataracts before the age of 50 years.

Laboratory Features

CK level can be normal or slightly elevated. Skeletal muscle MRI in some patients has revealed particular involvement of adductor magnus and vastus lateralis and medialis in the thigh but preservation of the rectus femoris and the adductor longus muscles.[164]

Histopathology

Muscle biopsies can show muscle fibers with rimmed vacuoles, cytoplasmic bodies, muscle size variability, scattered necrotic and regenerating fibers and endomysial and perimysial fibrosis.[162-164]

Molecular Genetics and Pathogenesis

LGMD1G/LGMDD3 is caused by mutation in *HNRNPDL* which encodes for heterogeneous nuclear ribonucleoprotein D like protein.[162-164] Ribonucleoproteins bind to pre-mRNA and function in splicing and nuclear export. Thus, as discussed previously, RNA-binding proteins when mutated may lead to muscle destruction by several mechanisms.

LGMD1H/LGMDD4 (CALPAIN-3)

Calpainopathy far more commonly arises as an autosomal-recessive condition, LGMD2A/LGMDR1. However, rare individuals have an autosomal-dominant calpainopathy, previously referred to as LGMD1H, but now called LGMDD4.[1,165-167] It is typically associated with a 21-bp, in-frame deletion (c.643_663del21) c.1715G>C p.(Arg572Pro) mutation in the calpain-3 gene, *CAPN3*,[165,166] but has also been associated with a c.1715G>C p.(Arg572Pro) point mutation.[167] Notably, the more common large deletion is missed on most commercially available next-generation sequencing (NGS) panels at this time. The calpain-3 enzyme is a homodimer; evidence suggests that these mutations lead dominant-negative effect on calpain-3: altered calpain-3 polymerizing with normal protein thereby rendering it less active. Affected individuals develop proximal weakness and atrophy in the arms and legs with average age of onset in the mid-30s, although some manifest symptoms in the first or second decade. Back pain and myalgias are common. Serum CK is elevated in most, and muscle biopsies reveal dystrophic changes. Serum CK was elevated in most, but not all, patients, and muscle biopsy, when performed, showed myopathic changes, including increased internal nuclei, variation in fiber size, and occasional fibrosis. Additional features included back pain and myalgia. Overall, the disorder is similar to LGMD2A/LGMDR1 (as discussed greater detail in the next section) but appears less severe.

▶ AUTOSOMAL-RECESSIVE LGMD

LGMD2A/LGMDR1 (CALPAIN-3)

Clinical Features

This LGMD was first described in inhabitants of Reunion Island in the Indian Ocean, but subsequently, the dystrophy has been reported throughout the world (Table 27-1, Fig. 27-10).[1-4,168-174] Epidemiological series report that 18.5%–35% of LGMD are calpainopathies and is the most common form of LGMD in people from eastern Europe, Spain, Italy, the Netherlands, northern England, and Brazil.[2] In this regard, LGMD2A/LGMDR1 is responsible for approximately 28% of LGMD cases in Italy,[149] 26.5% in northern England,[174] and 28% in the Netherlands.[175]

The onset of weakness ranges from early childhood to mid-adult life.[1-4,168-174] There is an early predilection for the pelvic-girdle muscles and posterior thigh (gluteus maximus, thigh adductors, hamstrings, and, to a lesser degree, the gluteus medius and psoas), followed 2–5 years later by periscapular and humeral muscle weakness and atrophy (latissimus dorsi, serratus anterior, rhomboids, pectoralis major, and the biceps brachii). The deltoid and brachioradialis are less severely affected, while the distal leg, supra- and infraspinati, triceps, brachialis, and forearm muscles are relatively spared. Only mild weakness of neck muscles can be detected. Scapular winging is present in most patients. Facial muscles are usually unaffected. Ocular and velopharyngeal muscles are not involved. There is often slight scoliosis from truncal weakness from paraspinal muscle involvement. Abdominal muscles are also affected. Early contractures at the elbows and calves are typically present, such that patients may mimic EDMD. Calf hypertrophy or atrophy may be seen. Muscle stretch reflexes are absent or diminished. Progression is steady, but variable, between and within affected kinships.[4,171] For the most part, the earlier onset of symptoms and signs correlates with a faster evolution of the disease process. Approximately 50% of patients are nonambulatory by the age of 20 years, but some remain ambulatory late in life. Ventilatory function is only moderately affected. Cardiac function is normal, and there is no intellectual impairment. Life expectancy is close to normal.

Laboratory Features

Serum CK levels are usually increased up to 20 times normal early in the disease but decrease close to the normal range later when patients are wheelchair bound. Rarely, there is peripheral eosinophilia evident on blood counts. Skeletal muscle MRI scans demonstrate fat and connective tissue replacing normal muscle fibers. There is a predilection for the posterior thigh and adductors in the upper leg, the soleus and medial gastrocnemius muscles in the lower leg, the serratus anterior in the arms, and the paraspinal muscles (Fig. 27-11).[4,176-178]

Histopathology

Muscle biopsies demonstrate variation in fiber size associated with increased endomysial connective tissue. A lobulated appearance of muscle fibers on NADH staining is a frequent observation; however, this finding is not specific for calpainopathies. Interestingly, there was a report of six unrelated calpainopathy patients presenting as eosinophilic myositis in childhood.[179] We have also found mutations in the calpain-3 gene in adults who were originally misdiagnosed as having

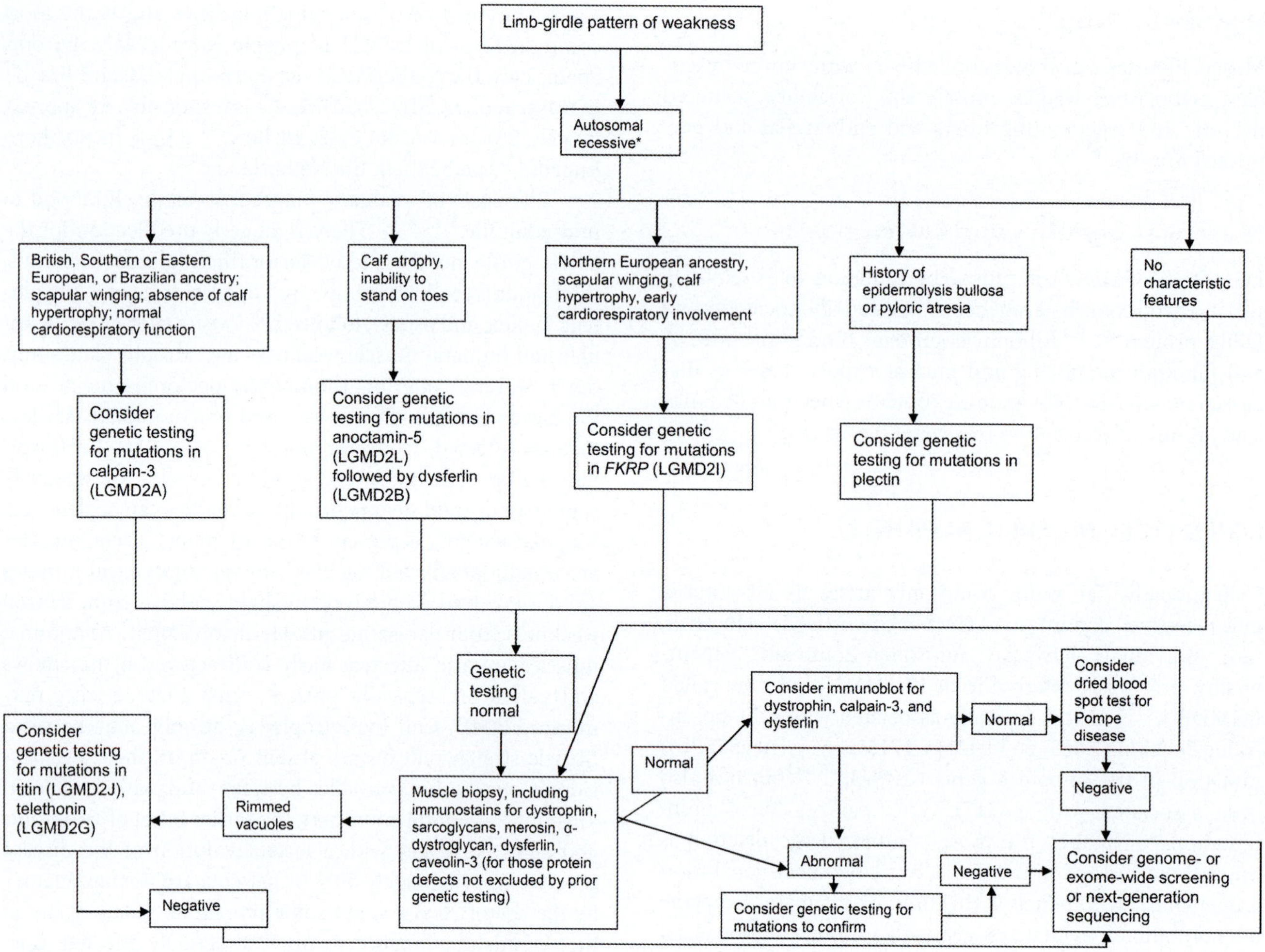

Figure 27-10. Diagnostic approach to patients with a limb-girdle pattern of weakness and suspected muscular dystrophy with an autosomal-recessive inheritance pattern. *Autosomal-dominant, autosomal-recessive, or X-linked inheritance may be responsible in sporadic cases. LGMD, limb-girdle muscular dystrophy. (Reproduced with permission from Narayanaswami P, Weiss M, Selcen D, et al. Evidence-based guideline summary: diagnosis and treatment of limb-girdle and distal dystrophies: report of the guideline development subcommittee of the American Academy of Neurology and the practice issues review panel of the American Association of Neuromuscular & Electrodiagnostic Medicine. *Neurology.* 2014;83(16):1453–1463.)

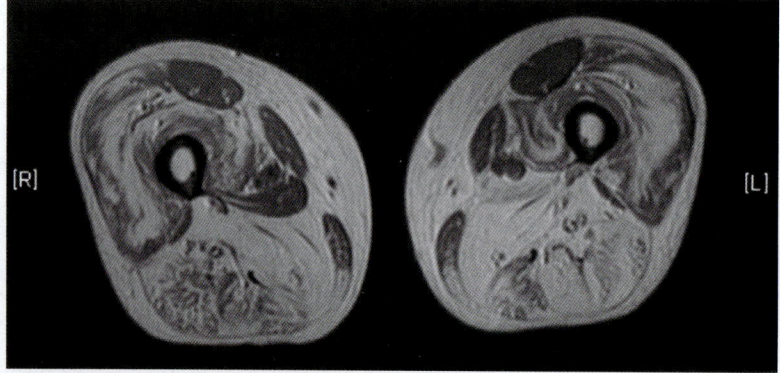

Figure 27-11. LGMD 2A/LGMRR1. Skeletal muscle MRI scan (T1 weighted) of the thigh reveals fat and connective tissue (bright signal) replacing normal muscle fibers with a predilection for the posterior thigh *muscles*.

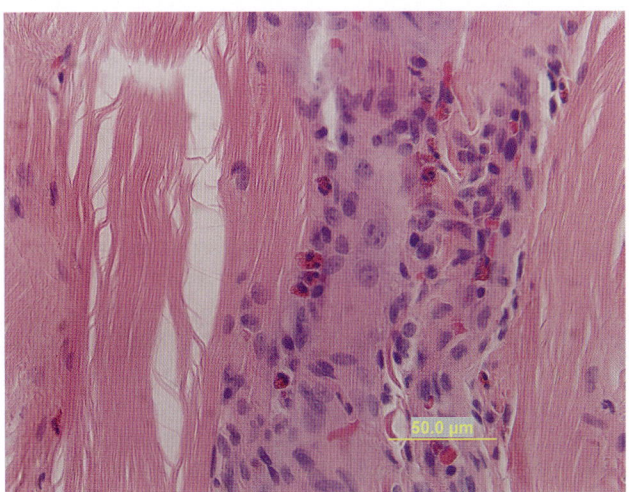

Figure 27-12. LGMD 2A/LGMDR1. Muscle biopsy demonstrates eosinophilic infiltrate that can be mistaken for eosinophilic myositis. Paraffin section, H&E.

eosinophilic myositis that was refractory to immunosuppressive treatment (Fig. 27-12).[180]

As calpain-3 is a cytosolic enzyme, immunostaining cannot be performed for diagnosis. Western blot analysis demonstrates reduced calpain-3 in most biopsies, but in 20% of cases the western blot is normal. The mutation in the gene may not alter the size or amount of calpain-3 but may affect the enzyme activity. Unfortunately, there are no readily available tests to assess enzyme activity. Definite diagnosis requires demonstration of a mutation in calpain-3 gene because secondary deficiency in calpain-3 can be seen in other dystrophies, most notably the dysferlinopathies and titinopathies.

Molecular Genetics and Pathogenesis

LGMD2A/LGMDR1 is caused by mutations in the *CPN3*.[1–4,172,181–185] Over two-thirds of patients with calpainopathy manifest with a BMD-like phenotype, approximately 10% present with severe childhood-onset weakness similar to DMD, while even fewer manifest with a distal myopathy, or have asymptomatic hyper-CK-emia.[4] Prenatal diagnosis is possible through DNA analysis of fetal cells obtained by amniocentesis or chorionic villus sampling.

Calpain-3 is a muscle-specific, calcium-dependent, nonlysosomal, proteolytic enzyme. The mutation leads to an absence or a reduction in this enzyme, but how this results in the dystrophic process is not fully understood. Calpain-3 activates other enzymes involved in muscle metabolism.[182] Lack of calpain-3 might lead to the accumulation of toxic substances in muscle cells. Perhaps, calpain-3 plays a role in gene expression by regulating turnover or activity of transcription factors or their inhibitors.[182]

The reason for the peripheral eosinophilia and the eosinophilic infiltrate noted in biopsies of some affected individuals is not clear. Calpain-3 is highly expressed in T lymphocytes. These cells secrete interleukin-5 and interleukin-3, which are cytokines that are required for the growth and differentiation of eosinophils. Perhaps, the mutation in the gene causes not only LGMD, but also a perturbation of T-cell function leading to eosinophilia.[186]

LGMD2B/LGMDR2 (DYSFERLIN)

Clinical Features

LGMDR2, previously referred to as LGMD2B, usually presents in the late teens or early 20s, although onset as late as the age of 48 years has been reported.[1–4,187–198] The clinical phenotype is quite variable, with some patients having a "limb-girdle" pattern of weakness, others having early involvement of the posterior calf muscles (i.e., Miyoshi myopathy type 1 or MMD1), and still others with anterior tibial weakness or combination of any of the above. Most patients with dysferlinopathies manifest at least initially with atrophy and weakness of the gastrocnemius and soleus muscles, in contrast to many other forms of LGMD which more typically have calf muscle hypertrophy or pseudohypertrophy (Fig. 27-13). Not uncommonly, involvement of the calf muscles is asymmetric. A very uncommon presentation is early involvement of the paraspinal muscles leading to rigid spine syndrome or, on

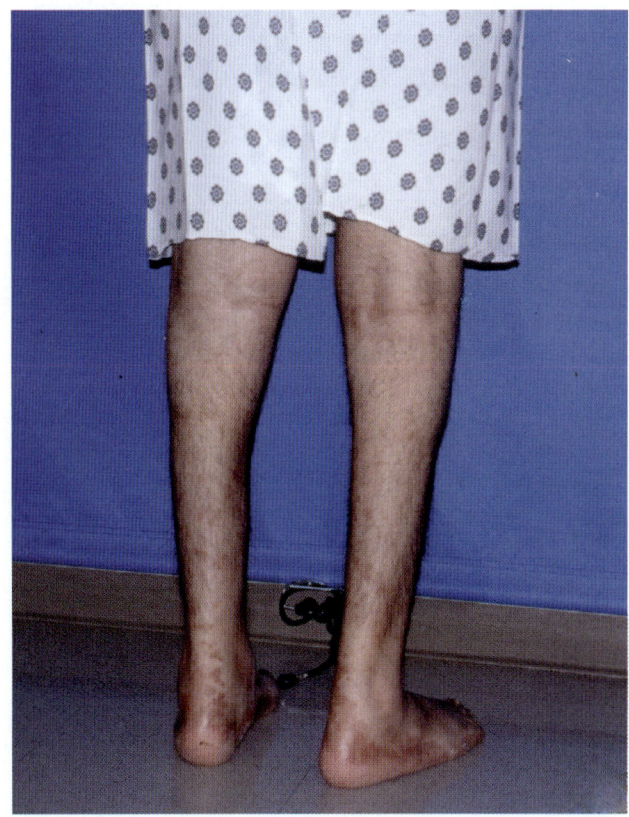

Figure 27-13. LGMD 2B/LGMDR2/Miyoshi myopathy. Note the marked atrophy of the calves in a patient with Miyoshi myopathy caused by dysferlin mutation.

the opposite end of the spectrum, a lax spine with hyperlordosis or kyphosis. A large study comparing the demographic, MRI, functional, and genetic differences between 168 genetically confirmed dysferlinopathy patients with a clinical diagnosis of LGMDR2 or MMD1 examined the spectrum of the two disorders.[198] The authors concluded that these are not phenotypically distinct and therefore should not be split into separate cohorts of LGMDR2 and MMD1 for the purposes of clinical management, enrollment in clinical trials or access to subsequent treatments. LGMD2B/LGMDR2 accounts for approximately 6%–10% of the LGMDs.[4,175]

On examination, patients will have difficulty standing on their tip toes. Over time, the hamstrings and gluteal muscles are affected and then the distal arms. Less commonly, affected individuals manifest with proximal hip-girdle weakness followed by shoulder-girdle weakness. Mild scapular winging may be evident at any stage of the disease. Still other patients have early, prominent involvement of the anterior tibial muscles. In our experience, a good examination will often detect atrophy and weakness of the calf muscles in patients with the "limb-girdle" and the "anterior tibial" phenotypes. A helpful sign in dysferlinopathies is the early loss of the Achilles tendon reflexes. Usually, this is the most preserved reflex in other forms of LGMD but is the first to disappear in the dysferlinopathies. Of note, there is intra- and interfamilial variability in disease progression and pattern of muscle involvement.

Progression is usually slow, although we have seen several patients with a rather abrupt onset and rapid progression to a nonambulatory state. The subacute rapid progression and the prominent inflammatory cell infiltrate seen on muscle biopsy (see Histopathology) can lead to the misdiagnosis of polymyositis.

Laboratory Features

Serum CK levels are usually markedly elevated (usually 35–200 times normal). Because dysferlin is present on white blood cells, western blot analysis on these cells for dysferlin represents a noninvasive method of making the diagnosis.[194] Skeletal muscle imaging has shown the pattern of muscle involvement is similar regardless of whether patients manifest with Miyoshi or limb-girdle phenotype in that there is early involvement of the gastrocnemius and thigh adductors with both presentations.[4,195–198]

Histopathology

Muscle biopsies demonstrate variation in fiber size, scattered necrotic and regenerating fibers, and increased endomysial connective tissue. Immunostaining reveals absent or diminished sarcolemmal staining with dysferlin antibodies. In contrast, there may be increased cytoplasmic staining. The reduced sarcolemmal immunostaining can be secondary and seen in other types of LGMD[199]; therefore, western blot needs to be performed on the muscle or white blood cells to confirm a primary deficiency. Not uncommonly, a prominent mononuclear inflammatory cell infiltrate is evident in the endomysium and surrounding blood vessels, which likely accounts for many cases of dysferlinopathy being misdiagnosed as polymyositis.[200] In contrast to polymyositis, the inflammatory cells do not typically appear to invade nonnecrotic fibers. Another immunohistological feature that is helpful is the deposition of membrane attack complex on the sarcolemma of nonnecrotic muscle fibers (Fig. 27-14A).[201] This is an early finding in dysferlinopathies and other dystrophies with inflammation that is not seen in primary inflammatory myopathies such as polymyositis, dermatomyositis, and inclusion body myositis. Interestingly, amyloid deposition in blood vessel walls, around the sarcolemma, and in the endomysial or perimysial connective tissue may be apparent with Congo red staining (Fig. 27-14B and C).[202] On EM, duplication of the basal lamina, disruption in the sarcolemma, invaginations or papillary exophytic defects of the muscle membrane, and subsarcolemmal vesicles may be appreciated.[201]

Molecular Genetics and Pathogenesis

Mutations within the dysferlin gene are the cause of LGMD2B/LGMDR2, MM1, and some distal myopathies with anterior tibial weakness.[1–4,14,187,203] A study of 407 muscle biopsies from patients with unclassified myopathies (nondystrophinopathy and nonsarcoglycanopathy) demonstrated that 6.5% had abnormal dysferlin by western blot and immunostaining.[185] Dysferlinopathy accounted for 1% of patients with an unknown LGMD and 60% of patients with a distal myopathy. The clinical phenotype of patients with dysferlinopathy broke down as follows: 80% manifested with distal weakness, 8% had LGMD phenotype, and 6% presented with asymptomatic hyper-CK-emia. Dysferlin shares amino acid sequence homology with *Caenorhabditis elegans* spermatogenesis factor FER-1, thus the origin of its name. Dysferlin is located predominantly on the subsarcolemmal surface of the muscle membrane, but it has a small transmembrane spanning tail (Fig. 27-1). It does not appear to have a significant interaction with the dystrophin–glycoprotein complex, and immunostaining for dystrophin, dystroglycans, merosin, and the sarcoglycans is normal. Studies suggest that at least one role of dysferlin is patching defects in skeletal membrane such that mutations in the gene result in defective membrane repair.[13]

SARCOGLYCANOPATHIES (LGMD2C/LGMDR5, LGMD2D/LGMDR3, LGMD2E/LGMFR4, AND LGMD2F/LGMDR6)

Clinical Features

The sarcoglycanopathies account for approximately 10% of LGMD with roughly the following frequencies: α-sarcoglycan 6.6%, β-sarcoglycan 3.1%, γ-sarcoglycan 1.5%, and δ-sarcoglycan <1%.[1–4,204–216] The clinical, laboratory, and histologic features of the sarcoglycanopathies are quite similar

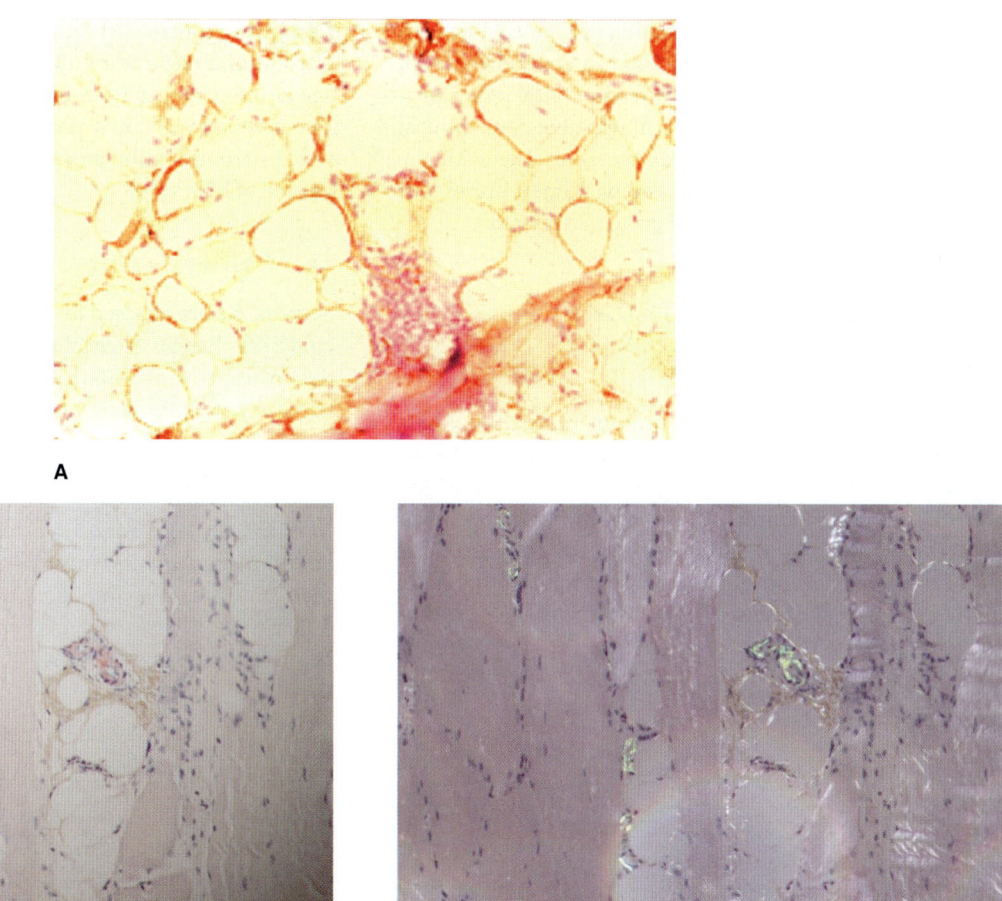

Figure 27-14. Dysferlinopathy. Muscle biopsies often demonstrate endomysial inflammatory cell infiltrate that can lead to misdiagnosis as polymyositis (PM). An early observation is the demonstration of membrane attack complex (MAC) on the sarcolemma of nonnecrotic muscle fibers in dysferlinopathies (also seen in FSHD) that is not appreciated in PM (**A**). Immunoperoxidase with anti-MAC antibodies. Amyloid deposition is apparent in endothelial walls of small vessels in the perimysial and endomysial that appear pink on Congo Red (**B**) and are apple-green birefringent with polarized light (**C**).

to the dystrophinopathies, with some children developing severe weakness resembling DMD, and other patients having a later onset and slower progression similar to BMD. Proximal leg and arm muscles are affected early, and calf pseudohypertrophy can often be appreciated. A recent large study of 396 patients with sarcoglycanopathy from 13 different countries reported patients with LGMDR3 had a later onset and slower progression of the disease, while cardiac involvement was most frequent in LGMDR4.[215] Onset of symptoms before 10 years of age and western blot showing less than 30% sarcoglycan expression were independent risk factors for losing ambulation before 18 years of age, in LGMDR3, LGMDR4, and LGMDR5 patients. Cardiac involvement also occurred in 5 of 23 patients with ultra-rare LGMDR6.[216] In contrast to the dystrophinopathies, there are no significant intellectual impairments. Rare patients manifest with asymptomatic hyper-CK-emia or exercise intolerance.[215]

Laboratory Features

Serum CK levels are markedly elevated. Echocardiogram may reveal evidence of cardiomyopathy.

Histopathology

Muscle biopsies demonstrate normal dystrophin; however, all of the sarcoglycans are usually absent or diminished on the sarcolemma, regardless of the primary sarcoglycan mutation.

Molecular Genetics and Pathogenesis

LGMD2C/LGMDR5, LGMD2D/LGMDR3, LGMD2E/LGMDR5, and LGMD2F/LGMDR6 are caused by mutations in the γ-, α-, β-, and δ-sarcoglycan genes, respectively.[1–4,204–216] The clinical phenotypes appear to correlate with the expression of the sarcoglycans. The proteins of the sarcoglycan complex appear to function as a unit. Mutations involving any of the sarcoglycans result in destabilization of the entire complex and reduced expression of the other proteins. As apparent with the dystrophinopathies, the clinical severity of the sarcoglycanopathies may correlate with the type of mutation (i.e., whether the reading frame is preserved) and subsequent level of functional protein expression.[215]

LGMD2G/LGMDR7 (TELETHONIN)

Clinical Features

This myopathy is associated with prominent early weakness of the quadriceps and anterior tibial muscle groups with an onset between 2 and 15 years of age.[1–4,217–221] Some affected individuals manifest similar to Miyoshi myopathy with calf weakness. However, some have calf hypertrophy. Weakness affects the proximal more than distal muscles in the arms. Progression of weakness varies even within families. Cardiomyopathy can also develop.

Laboratory Features

Serum CKs are elevated 3- to 30-fold.

Histopathology

Besides the usual dystrophic features, many muscle fibers had one or more rimmed vacuoles.[2] Immunohistochemistry and western blot analysis demonstrate a deficiency of telethonin.[217,219] Abnormal features may resemble MFM.

Molecular Genetics and Pathogenesis

LGMD2G/LGMDR7 is caused by mutations in the telethonin gene, *TCAP*, located on chromosome 17q11–12.[1,217,219] Telethonin, also known as titin-cap, is a 19-kD sarcomeric protein that is expressed in skeletal and cardiac muscles where it localizes to the central parts of the Z-disc.[218] It is a ligand for the giant sarcomeric protein, titin, which helps phosphorylate the C-terminal domain of telethonin in early differentiating myocytes. Telethonin may also overlap with myosin as well. It is among the most abundant proteins in muscle. The interaction of telethonin with titin appears to be important in myofibrillogenesis.[218,222]

LGMD2H/LGMDR8 (E3-UBIQUITINE LIGASE OR TRIM 32)

Clinical Features

This genetically distinct LGMD was initially reported in families of Manitoba Hutterite origin but subsequently has been reported elsewhere.[1–4,223–227] Most affected individuals have exercise-induced myalgias and an examination revealing a limb-girdle pattern of weakness with scapular winging, facial weakness, calf hypertrophy, and heel cord contractures. Rarely, prominent distal upper extremity weakness is seen. Cardiac and respiratory muscles seem relatively spared. The age at onset ranges from birth to the seventh decade of life. The myopathy is slowly progressive, and most affected individuals are still ambulatory without assistance in the fourth decade of life.

Laboratory Features

Serum CKs are elevated 5- to 50-fold. There may be nonspecific EKG changes. Skeletal muscle MRI scans reveal preferential involvement of posterior thigh muscles early with eventual involvement of the anterior thigh later in the course.[227]

Histopathology

Muscle biopsies demonstrate typical dystrophic features. In addition, many fibers (mostly type 2) contain small vacuoles that immunostain for sarcoplasmic reticulum-associated ATPase.[224–227] These vacuoles abut T-tubules and appear to be membrane bound on EM.

Molecular Genetics and Pathogenesis

LGMD2H/LGMDR8 and sarcotubular myopathy (discussed in Chapter 28 with Congenital Myopathies) are allelic disorders caused by mutations in the gene, *TRIM32*, that encodes for E3-ubiquitine ligase (also known as tripartite motif-containing 32). This enzyme may function by ubiquitinating proteins that need proteasomal degradation.[226] The mechanism by which this leads to muscle destruction is unclear, but one might speculate on the possible toxic accumulation of "aged" or otherwise abnormal proteins not cleared by proteasomes. Recent studies suggest that TRIM32 is also important in the NOTCH pathway which, as mentioned previously, is of key importance in maintaining muscle stem cells and regulating the proper development, function, and regeneration of skeletal muscle.[41] So, this myopathy may also be considered a satellite cell-opathy.

LGMD2I/LGMDR9 (FKRP)

Clinical Features

LGMD2I/LGMDR9 was initially described in a large consanguineous Tunisian family with 13 affected members.[228] Subsequently, it has been demonstrated worldwide and constitutes 4%–30% of all LGMDs; it is the most common form of LGMD in northern Europe.[2–4,43,175,229–236] One class 1 study found this to be the cause of 19% of LGMDs.[183] The onset can range from infancy (MDC type 1C or MDDGC5) to the fourth decade of life.[2–4,42,43,46,47] The pattern of weakness and course is variable. Some individuals have more hip-girdle involvement, while others are weaker in the proximal arms and neck flexors. Calves are often hypertrophic. Importantly, approximately one-half of patients develop a dilated cardiomyopathy and ventilatory muscle weakness.[4,229,230,236,237] Rare patients present with episodes of myoglobinuria.[234,235]

Laboratory Features

Serum CKs are elevated 10–30 times normal in some younger patients who are affected but may be normal in older individuals. Pulmonary function tests (PFTs) often reveal reduced FVC while echocardiograms demonstrate a dilated cardiomyopathy.[4,232,233,236] MRI of the leg and paraspinal muscles reveal abnormal signal and fatty infiltration, but the findings are not specific.[4,238,239]

Histopathology

Nonspecific dystrophic features are evident on muscle biopsy. Of note, immunohistochemistry demonstrates normal dystrophin and sarcoglycan staining. However, α-dystroglycan and occasionally merosin are reduced or absent with immunostaining (Fig. 27-15).

Molecular Genetics and Pathogenesis

LGMD2I/LMGDR9 is caused by mutations in the gene that encodes for FKRP located on chromosome 19q13.3.[1-4] Mutations in this gene are also responsible for a congenital muscular dystrophy-dystroglycanopathy with or without impaired intellectual development (type B5; MDDGB5) and a severe congenital muscular dystrophy-dystroglycanopathy with brain and eye anomalies (type A5; MDDGA5).[46,47] FKRP is a glycosyltransferase and its deficiency is associated with abnormal glycosylation of α-dystroglycan, which apparently disrupts the dystrophin–glycoprotein complex. Abnormalities in glycosylation of α-dystroglycan are a recurring theme in the MDCs, as this is also causative mechanism in Fukuyama disease, MEB, WWS, and LARGE-related CMD (MDDGA5). There is a correlation between a reduction in α-dystroglycan, causal mutation, and clinical severity.[44]

FKRP localizes in rough endoplasmic reticulum (ER), while fukutin localizes in the *cis*-Golgi compartment (ER).[240] Fukutin and FKRP appear to be involved at different steps in *O*-mannosylglycan synthesis of α-dystroglycan, and FKRP is most likely involved in the initial step in this synthesis. ER retention of mutant FKRP may play a role in the pathogenesis of these dystrophies and potentially explain why the allelic disorder LGMD 2I/LGMDR9 is milder, because the mutated protein is able to reach the Golgi apparatus.[241]

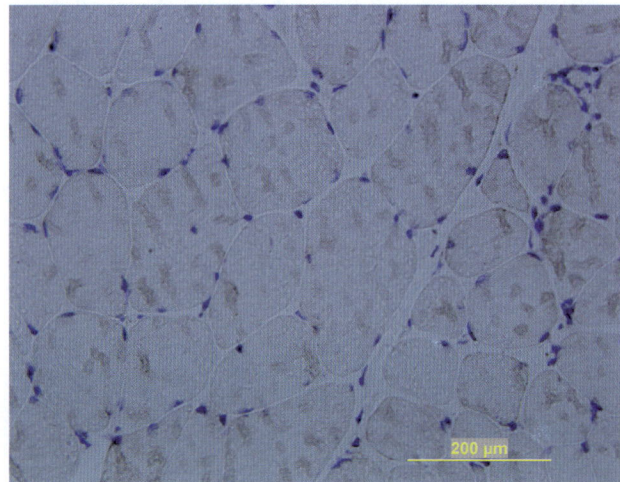

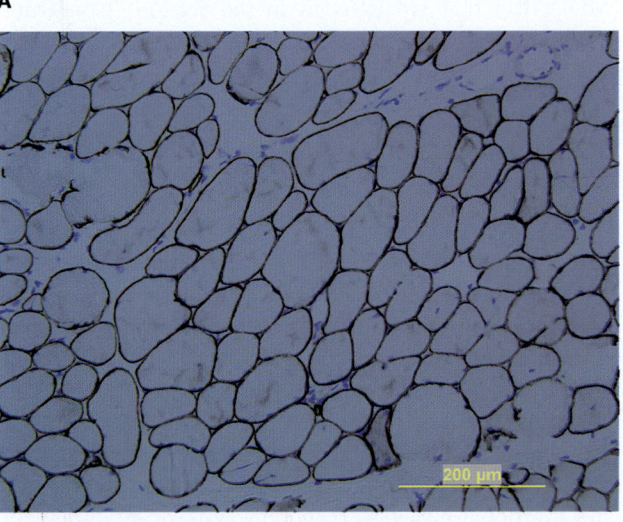

Figure 27-15. LGMD2I/LGMDR9. Muscle biopsies demonstrate reduced or patchy merosin staining (**A**), absent α-dystroglycan staining (**B**), but normal dystrophin staining (**C**) around the sarcolemma. Immunoperoxidase.

TITINOPATHIES

Mutations in the titin gene (*TTN*) are associated with at least three different clinical phenotypes: autosomal-recessive LGMD2J/LGMDR10, autosomal-dominant distal myopathy (Udd type distal myopathy), and autosomal-dominant hereditary myopathy with early respiratory failure (HMERF).[1–4,242–253] The Udd type distal myopathy is the most common phenotype associated with TTN mutations and is discussed in the "Distal Myopathy" section under "Udd type distal myopathy." We will discuss the LGMD2J/LGMDR10 and HMERF phenotypes next.

LGMD2J/LGMDR10 (TITIN)

Clinical Features

LGMD2J/LGMDR10 usually presents in the first three decades of life with proximal leg and arm with milder distal (anterior tibial, gastrocnemius, forearm, and hand) weakness.[1–4,243,244,249] Many affected individuals are wheelchair dependent within 20 years of onset. Scapular winging is uncommon but may be evident.

A somewhat different presentation is that of an early-onset, proximal, and distal weakness leading to delayed motor milestones that is associated with a severe dilated cardiomyopathy.[252] Notably, some affected children exhibit hypertrophy of the thighs and calves along with atrophy of the arms. Spinal rigidity and moderate joint contractures can appear in the first decade. Affected individuals develop CHF and may suffer sudden death from fatal arrhythmias.[252]

Laboratory Features

CK elevation is usually 3–5 times normal. As mentioned, echocardiography may reveal features of a cardiomyopathy, and PFTs can reveal signs of ventilatory muscle weakness. Skeletal muscle MRI has demonstrated fatty replacement of thigh (hamstrings more than quadriceps) and lower leg muscles (anterior more than posterior compartment).[248]

Histopathology

Muscle biopsies revealed dystrophic features, and, unlike the allelic Udd type distal myopathy, rimmed vacuoles are absent or rare.[243,249,253]

Molecular Genetics and Pathogenesis

This LGMD is caused by mutations in *TTN* that encodes the sarcolemmal protein, titin.

HEREDITARY MYOPATHY WITH EARLY RESPIRATORY FAILURE (TITIN)

Clinical Features

HMERF is associated with a clinical phenotype overlaps with that seen in LGMD2J/LGMDR10 and Udd type distal myopathy.[4,250,251,254–256] It is also known as myofibrillary myopathy type 1 (MFM9) given the histopathological abnormalities discussed below. As in Udd type distal myopathy, HMERF is associated with early progressive foot drop and an autosomal-dominant inheritance. However, it tends to affect patients in early adulthood (but can develop in late teens to the eighth decade of life) and may affect the proximal muscles (legs greater than arms), as seen in LGMD2J/LGMDR10. Most patients have prominent calf hypertrophy. As the name of the syndrome implies, HMERF is also associated with severe ventilatory muscle weakness. However, cardiomyopathy is not a common feature.

Laboratory Features

Serum CKs are usually mildly elevated. One study reported that skeletal muscle MRI identified the most commonly affected muscles to be the semitendinosus (20/21 subjects), the peroneus longus (16/21), and the obturator externus (15/21).[250,251,254–256]

Histopathology

Muscle biopsies reveal dystrophic features along with muscle fibers containing rimmed vacuoles and eosinophilic inclusions.[250,251,254–256] Further, light microscopy and EM may reveal extensive myofibrillar degeneration with Z-disc as seen in MFM.

Molecular Genetics and Pathogenesis

HMERF is typically caused by mutations in exon 344 of *TTN* that encodes the fibronectin-3 (FN3) domain in the A-band region of titin.[254]

LGMD2K/LGMDR11 (POMT1)

This LGMD is caused by mutations in the *POMT1* gene which is more commonly associated with severe congenital muscular dystrophy-dystroglycanopathy with brain and eye anomalies (MDDGA1) or congenital muscular dystrophy-dystroglycanopathy with impaired intellectual development (MDDGB1) that is discussed in the section "Congenital Muscular Dystrophy." However, rare patients have a milder, later-onset LGMD phenotype.[1–4]

LGMD2L/LGMDR12 (ANOCTAMIN-5)

Clinical Features

Patients with mutations in *ANO5* that encode for anoctamin-5 can manifested with a limb-girdle pattern of weakness (LGMD2L/LGMDR12) or with distal weakness resembling Miyoshi myopathy (referred to as Miyoshi myopathy type 3 or MM3).[1–4,17,257–265] Similar to what is seen in the dysferlinopathies (i.e., LGMD2B/LGMDR2 and MM1), the clinical phenotypes often overlap in the anoctaminopathies. In addition, some patients have a pseudo-metabolic presentation with exertional myalgias, rhabdomyolysis, or asymptomatic hyper-CK-emia.[258–261] Epidemiological studies suggest that anoctaminopathy is one of the most common adult muscular dystrophies in Northern Europe, with a prevalence of about 20%–26% in unselected undiagnosed cases.[175,262]

Onset of weakness usually ranges from 20 to 55 years with a mean in the mid-30s in both LGMD2L/LGMDR12 and MM3 presentations.[4,17,257–265] As alluded, atrophy and weakness of the calf muscles (gastrocnemius or tibialis anterior) can be seen in combination with proximal muscle involvement. Asymmetric atrophy of the biceps brachii in the arms and quadriceps in the legs appears to be common.

Patients with MM3 manifest with early calf weakness and atrophy that is also often asymmetric.[4,17,257–265] However, some patients initially have calf hypertrophy before the atrophy occurs. The phenotype can merge with LGMD2L/LGMDR12 as some affected individuals develop atrophy or weakness of the quadriceps, biceps brachii, and pectoral muscles.[17,259–261]

Laboratory Features

CK levels are usually moderately elevated, sometimes over 20-fold.[4,17,257–265] Echocardiography, EKG, and PFTs are usually normal.[4,258–261] Skeletal muscle MRI has demonstrated atrophy and fat replacement of the long head of the biceps brachii in the arms and the medial gastrocnemius, soleus, adductor magnus, semimembranosus, biceps femoris long head, tensor fasciae latae, and to a lesser extent the quadriceps in the legs that is often asymmetric.[17,264,265]

Histopathology

Muscle biopsies reveal nonspecific dystrophic features.[258,260] Intramuscular interstitial and perivascular amyloid deposits, as also apparent in dysferlinopathies, are found in approximately 50% of biopsies of patients with anoctaminopathy.[17]

Molecular Genetics and Pathogenesis

LGMD2L/LGMDR12 is caused by mutations in *ANO5* that encode anoctamin-5.[257–262] This protein is located within the ER. The exact function of anoctamin-5 is unclear, but it belongs to a family of proteins found in calcium active chloride channels. Similar to dysferlinopathies, mutations in *ANO5* lead to improper repair of muscle membranes.

LGMD2M/LGMDR13 (FUKUTIN)

LGMD2M/LGMDR13 is caused by mutations in the fukutin gene, *FKTN*, that usually causes severe muscular dystrophy-dystroglycanopathy with brain and eye anomalies (MDDGA4) or a form of congenital muscular dystrophy-dystroglycanopathy without impaired intellectual development (MDDGB4), as discussed in more detail in the section "Congenital Muscular Dystrophy."[46,47] However, mutations may rarely be associated with this more benign LGMD phenotype or MDDGC4.[1–4,266–268]

LGMD2N/LGMDR14 (POMT2)

LGMD2N/LGMDR14 is caused by mutations in the *POMT2* gene that encodes for protein-*O*-mannosyltransferase. Mutations in *POMT2* usually cause MEB disease (MDDGA2 or MDDGB2), as discussed in the section "Congenital Muscular Dystrophy," but rarely can cause a more benign form of LGMD or MDDGC2.[1–4,266,269]

LGMD2O/LGMDR15 (POMGNT1)

Mutations in *POMGnT1* usually cause MDDGA3 or MDDGB3 (discussed in more detail in the section "Congenital Muscular Dystrophy") but have been associated with more benign MDDGC3 or LGMD2O/LGMDR15 that has later onset of weakness and spared cognition.[1–4,46,47,266,267,270]

LGMD2P/LGMDR16 (α-DYSTROGLYCAN)

Clinical Features

LGMD2P/LGMDR16 usually causes MDDGA9 but has been associated with more benign MDDGC9.[271–273]

Laboratory Features

CK levels are markedly elevated.

Histopathology

Muscle biopsies reveal dystrophic features with a reduction of α-dystroglycan on immunohistochemistry.

Molecular Genetics and Pathogenesis

This dystrophy is caused by mutations in the *DAG1* gene that encode for α-dystroglycan. This disorder is in essence a primary α-dystroglycanopathy in which mutations lead to impaired binding to merosin and destabilization of the dystrophin–dystroglycan complex.

LGMD2Q/LGMDR17 (PLECTIN-1)

Clinical Features

LGMD2Q/LGMDR17, also referred to as muscular dystrophy associated with epidermolysis bullosa, is caused by mutations in the gene that encodes for plectin-1.[4,274–286] Interestingly, in this regard, it is also allelic to a form of congenital myasthenia.[274,280,282,283,285] The characteristic clinical feature is the development in infancy or early childhood of epidermolysis bullosa, which manifests as blisters of the skin and mucous membranes, and nail bed abnormalities. Later in life, progressive weakness may ensue. Other patients manifest in early childhood or up to the fourth decade of life with limb-girdle weakness without any skin abnormalities,[4,281] while some affected individuals may have ptosis, ophthalmoplegia, and facial weakness.[4,278,281] Other reported features include dental caries, scarring alopecia, urethral strictures, pyloric atresia, esophageal strictures, respiratory distress, and, rarely, cardiomyopathy.

Laboratory Features

CK levels may be slightly to markedly elevated. EMG demonstrates myopathic features with muscle membrane irritability and repetitive nerve stimulation, at least in cases of congenital myasthenia, have shown decrement and increased jitter on single-fiber EMG. In vitro electrophysiologic studies showed normal quantal release by nerve impulse and small miniature end-plate potentials.[274]

Histopathology

Muscle biopsy may demonstrate type 1 fiber predominance and irregular oxidative staining. One study reported immunohistochemical loss of sarcolemmal staining using the antibody to the rod domain of plectin-1 in type 1 fibers, whereas type 2 fibers retained activity.[282] Plectin-1 deficiency may also be demonstrated on skin biopsy. EM has shown nonspecific myofibrillar disarray and Z-disc streaming. In those with features of congenital myasthenia, the endplates had focal degeneration of the junctional folds, but AChR content was normal.[274]

Molecular Genetics and Pathogenesis

LGMD2Q/LGMDR17 is caused by mutations in *PLEC1* that encodes for plectin-1. Plectin may serve as a scaffolding protein important for the formation of muscle fibers and neuromuscular transmission and also for the structural integrity of skin.[274]

LGMD2R/MFM1 (DESMIN)

This myopathy is no longer classified as an LGMD but rather as a myofibrillar myopathy (MFM1).[1] Patients manifests with progressive proximal muscle weakness and ventilatory failure in early childhood or adulthood. CK levels are mildly elevated. In contrast to most cases of primary desminopathy, it is associated with autosomal-recessive inheritance as opposed to autosomal dominant.[288,289] It is allelic with LGMD1E and is discussed in more detail in the sections regarding LGMD1E and myofibrillar myopathies.

LGMD2S/LGMDR18 (TRAPPC11)

Clinical Features

This LGMD is characterized by an infantile onset of choreiform, athetoid or dystonic movements, seizures, truncal ataxia, and mental intellectual disability.[290-294] Proximal weakness typically develops in childhood along with scoliosis and hip dysplasia. Cataracts, a cardiomyopathy, and liver disease may also be seen.

Laboratory Features

CK is mild to moderately elevated.

Histopathology

Muscle biopsies reveal typical dystrophic features.[290-294] Additionally, there is evidence of hypoglycosylation of alpha-dystroglycan and variably reduced dystrophin-associated complex proteins.[294] On autopsy, the brain from one affected individual revealed cerebellar atrophy, granule cell hypoplasia, Purkinje cell loss, degeneration, and dendrite dystrophy, reduced alpha-dystroglycan expression in Purkinje cells and dentate neurons but an absence of neuronal migration defects.[294]

Molecular Genetics and Pathogenesis

LGMD2S/LGMDR18 is caused by mutations in the gene encoding transport (trafficking) protein particle complex, subunit 11 (*TRAPPC11*), which is important in trafficking proteins between ER and Golgi complex.[290-294] Histopathology also suggests there may be an associated secondary alpha-dystroglycanopathy.

LGMD2T/LGMDR19 (GDP-MANNOSE PYROPHOSPHORYLASE B)

LGMD2T/LGMDR10 is allelic to muscular dystrophy-dystroglycanopathy type C (MDDGC14) and can have onset of proximal weakness in infancy or early childhood.[295-297] Additional signs can include mild intellectual disability or seizures. Serum CK is usually increased. Interestingly, some affected individuals have fatigable weakness and repetitive nerve stimulation can reveal a decrement. So, it is also considered a form of congenital myasthenic syndrome. Muscle biopsies reveal dystrophic features with reduction of alpha-dystroglycan immunostaining. The myopathy is caused by mutations in the gene that encodes for GDP-mannose pyrophosphorylase B, *GMPPB*, which lead to impaired glycosylation of alpha-dystroglycan.

LGMD2U/LGMDR20 (CDP-L-RIBITOL PYROPHOSPHORYLASE A

This is another secondary alpha-dystroglycanopathy LGMD and is allelic to MDDGC7.

The myopathy is characterized by onset of proximal leg greater than arm weakness, tongue and calf hypertrophy, scapular winging, and ventilatory muscle weakness in infancy or childhood. Exertional myalgias and myoglobinuria have occurred.[298-300] Serum CKs are typically elevated 5–7 times normal values. Muscle biopsies showed dystrophic changes with hypoglycosylated alpha-dystroglycan. This dystrophy is caused by mutations in the gene that encodes for CDP-L-ribitol phosphorylase A, *CRPPA*. CDP-L-ribitol phosphorylase A is also known as isoprenoid synthetase domain-containing protein (ISPD) and again is important in glycosylation of alpha-dystroglycan.

LGMD2V/POMPE DISEASE (ALPHA-GLUCOSIDASE)

Some patients classified initially as having a form of LGMD were subsequently linked to mutations in alpha-glucosidase, and so LGMD2V was reclassified as Pompe disease.[1]

LGMD2W/PINCH2-RELATED MYOPATHY (PINCH2)

This rare myopathy was reported in two siblings with progressive, proximal weakness and atrophy of the lower and upper extremities, calf hypertrophy, triangular tongue, and dilated cardiomyopathy with an onset in childhood.[301] Because it has only been reported in one family it is not listed as an "LGMD" in the new ENMC classification but instead is referred to as PINCH2-related myopathy. The PINCH2 protein, also called LIM and senescent cell antigen-lime domains 2, is encoded by *LIMS2*. PINCH2 is a component of a complex that mediates signaling between muscle fibers and the extracellular matrix.

LGMD2X/LGMDR25 (BLOOD VESSEL ENDOTHELIAL SUBSTANCE)

This rare dystrophy is associated with proximal weakness and cardiac arrhythmias beginning in childhood or mid-adult life.[302–305] An EKG can show atrioventricular conduction block and bradycardia that require pacemaker insertion. Serum CK can be normal or elevated, while muscle biopsy shows nonspecific dystrophic features. This myopathy is caused by mutations in the blood vessel endothelial substance gene, *BVES*. The encoded protein is also called Popeye domain-containing protein 1 (POPDC1), and it is a transmembrane protein that appears essential for normal skeletal and cardiac muscle function.

LGMD2Y/TOR1AIP1-RELATED MYOPATHY (TORSIN A INTERACTING PROTEIN 1/ LAMIN-ASSOCIATED PROTEIN 1)

This autosomal-recessive myopathy associated with rigid spine and distal joint contractures (MRRSDC) is not listed as an LGMD in the new classification system.[306–309] Affected individuals manifest with slowly progressive muscle weakness and atrophy with onset in the first or second decades of life. Additional features included rigid spine, joint contractures, restricted pulmonary function, and mild cardiac involvement. Serum CK is increased. Some patients have had evidence of impaired neuromuscular transmission on electrophysiological testing such that they resembled a congenital myasthenic syndrome.[309] Echocardiogram can show diastolic and systolic dysfunction with reduced ejection fraction. Skeletal muscle biopsies show mild dystrophic changes. Notably, electron microscopic studies have revealed nuclear fragmentation and deformation, chromatin clump formation, and naked chromatin resulting from karyoplasmic leakage into the sarcoplasmic compartment. This myopathy is caused by mutations in *TOR1AIP1* that encodes for torsin A interacting protein 1 (also known as lamin-associated protein 1).[306–309] This protein localizes to the inner nuclear membrane where it interacts with both A- and B-type lamins and emerin. In this regard, its pathogenic mechanism may be similar to other nuclear envelopathies that cause EDMD.

LGMD2Z/LGMDR21 (PROTEIN O-GLUCOSYLTRANSFERASE 1)

This rare LGMD was reported in 15 patients from 9 families with onset of weakness at birth to the fifth decade of life.[310] Scapular winging was evident in 11 of the 15 patients and 6 had ventilatory muscle weakness beginning in the fifth decade. Serum CK was normal or mildly elevated. Interestingly, skeletal muscle MRI showed early fatty replacement of internal regions of thigh muscles with sparing of external areas, a so-called "inside-to-outside" pattern of fatty degeneration, which is opposite to the "outside-in" pattern of fatty replacement seen in collagen 6-related disorders (Bethlem and Ullrich myopathies or LGMDR22 discussed in next section). Muscle biopsies reveal a reduction of satellite cells, decreased NOTCH1 intracellular domain expression, and reduced alpha-dystroglycan glycosylation. The disorder is caused by mutations in the protein O-glucosyltransferase 1, *POGLUT1*. This enzyme adds an O-glucose to a specific serine residue of epidermal growth factor-like repeats that are found in Notch extracellular domains. These findings suggest that this is a "satellite cell-opathy"; the pathogenic basis for this myopathy is Notch-dependent loss of muscle satellite cells leading to impaired muscle regeneration.

BETHLEM MYOPATHY/LGMDD5 (COLLAGEN 6 SUBUNITS A1, A2, OR A3)

Clinical Features

Bethlem myopathy/LGMDD5 is usually inherited in an autosomal-dominant fashion and is a mild variant of Ullrich congenital muscular dystrophy (UCMD)/LGMDR22. The clinical features are very similar to EDMD.[311–319] Onset is usually at birth or early childhood. Decreased fetal movements may be noted *in utero*, and neonates may demonstrate generalized hypotonia. Motor milestones are often delayed but are reached. However, weakness may not be evident until early adulthood. Variability in the age of onset and in clinical severity may even be seen within affected family members. There is proximal greater than distal muscle weakness, with the legs being more severely affected than the arms. Extensor muscles are weaker than flexor muscles. There can be mild neck and trunk involvement, but cranial muscles are spared. Muscle strength can be asymmetric. Calf hypertrophy may be seen. As in EDMD, contractures at the elbows and ankles are evident early in the course before any significant weakness manifests. There can be distal joint hyperextensibility. Eventually, contractures develop in the wrists and fingers. These flexor contractures of the wrists and fingers can be best appreciated by asking the patient to abduct their elbows and try to place the palm of their hands and fingers together as if they are praying. Because of the contractors the palm and fingers cannot make full contact (Bethlem sign). Some patients manifest with only proximal hip- and shoulder-girdle weakness without evidence of contractures, thus resembling an LGMD. Muscle stretch reflexes may be normal or reduced. Cardiac function is usually spared in Bethlem myopathy—a feature that might help to distinguish it from EDMD. However, ventilatory muscles appear to be involved in Bethlem myopathy and seem to be related to more severe weakness.

Laboratory Features

Serum CK is normal or mildly elevated. Cardiac studies (e.g., EKG, Holter monitor, and echocardiogram) may be abnormal, as discussed in the previous section. Motor and sensory nerve conduction studies (NCSs) are normal. Insertional and spontaneous activity is usually normal on EMG, although a mixture of small-amplitude, short-duration, polyphasic MUAPs with large-amplitude, long-duration MUAPs can be seen.[314,315]

Skeletal muscle MRI scans may reveal early involvement of the thigh muscles with a fairly specific pattern (Fig. 27-16) in which the preferential involvement of the rectus femoris with focus of fatty replacement in the anterior aspect of the muscle.[317,318] Other muscle fibers have fatty replacement in their periphery with relative sparing of the central regions—an "outside in" pattern of fatty degeneration. This pattern is opposite of what is seen in LGMD2Z/LGMDR21, which was discussed in the preceding section.

Histopathology

Muscle biopsies demonstrate nonspecific myopathic features. There is variability in fiber size, increased splitting, central nuclei, and mild endomysial fibrosis. Lobulated type 1 fibers and moth-eaten fibers may be apparent on NADH-TR stains.

Molecular Genetics and Pathogenesis

Bethlem myopathy/LGMDD5 is most commonly caused by dominant heterozygous mutations of the genes (COL6A1, COL6A2, and COL6A3) encoding for the α1 and α2 subunits of collagen VI located on chromosome 21q and α3 subunit of collagen VI located on 2q37.[314,316] Autosomal-recessive forms of collagen VI mutations typically lead to more severe UCMD discussed in more detail in the section "Congenital Muscular Dystrophy," however, rare causes of autosomal-recessive inherited Bethlem myopathy have also been reported.[319] Collagen VI bridges the extracellular matrix with the sarcolemma. Interestingly, compound heterozygous mutations have been defined in the COL6A2 and COL6A3 genes in the more severe UCMD (see the section "Congenital Muscular Dystrophy"). Collagen VI deficiency in muscle or cultured fibroblasts was complete in severe cases and partial in the milder ones, which suggests a correlation between the degree of collagen VI deficiency and the clinical severity in UCMD.

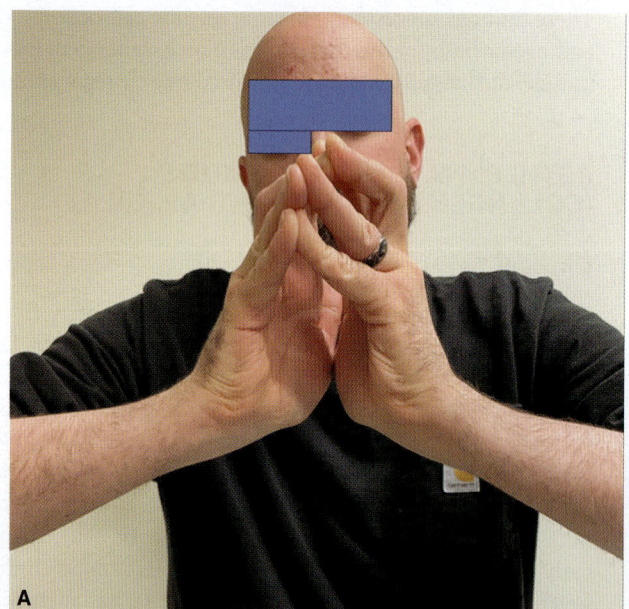
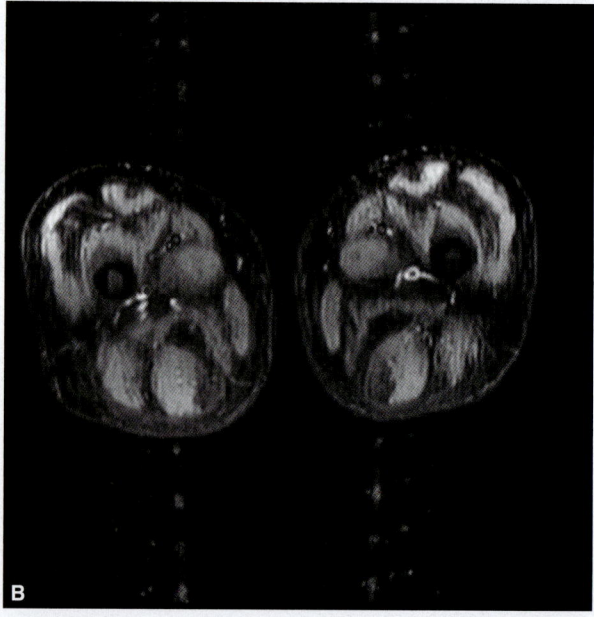

Figure 27-16. Bethlem Myopathy. Because of flexor contractures of wrists and long finger flexors patients are unable to place palms and fingers together as if praying, so-called Bethlem sign (**A**). (Used with the permission from Anthony A. Amato, MD.) Skeletal muscle MRI of the thigh in a patient with Bethlem myopathy reveals moderate involvement of thigh muscles with the "central shadow" within the rectus femoris, atrophy and increased abnormal signal at the periphery of the vastus lateralis, and fatty replacement between the vastus lateralis and the vastus intermedius (**B**).

Treatment

Physical therapy is indicated to prevent progressive contractures that can impair mobility and function.

LAMININ α2-RELATED DYSTROPHY/ LGMDR23 (LAMIN SUBUNIT ALPHA 2)

The laminin α2-related myopathies have clinical spectrum ranging from the congenital muscular dystrophy (MDC1A), to the more benign LGMDR23.[320–325] MDC1A is discussed in section regarding congenital muscular dystrophies. LGMDR23 manifests with slowly progressive proximal and axial muscle weakness, scapular winging, rigidity of the spine, scoliosis, ventilatory muscle weakness, and an increased CK with an age at onset that generally ranges from childhood to mid-adulthood. Reduced cardiac ejection fraction is seen in a few patients. Additional neurologic features, including executive deficits, seizures, and peripheral neuropathy, may also be present. MRI of the brain may show white matter abnormalities, while there can be mild slowing of nerve conduction velocities on neurophysiological testing. Muscle biopsies reveal dystrophic features with partial LAMA2 deficiency. The myopathy is caused by mutations in *LAMA2* which encodes for laminin α2, also known as merosin. Laminin α2 binds to alpha-dystroglycan in the extracellular matrix in muscle in an interaction that is important for proper muscle function. It is also expressed in the central nervous system where it is important for neuronal migration and is also expressed on Schwann cells in peripheral nerves. MDC1A is typically caused by mutations leading to premature termination codons and complete deficiency of laminin α2, while the more benign LGMDR23 is caused by missense mutations that lead to only partial laminin deficiency on muscle biopsies.[323,324]

POMGNT2-RELATED DYSTROPHY/ LGMDR24 (PROTEIN O-LINKED MANNOSE BETA 1,4-*N*-ACETYLGLUCOSAMINYL-TRANSERASE-2)

This rare dystrophy is allelic to MDDGC8 and is associated with congenital or childhood onset of proximal weakness. Some patients have impaired intellectual development.[326] Serum CK is elevated, and muscle biopsy often shows dystrophic features with reduced alpha-dystroglycan immunostaining.

LGMDR26 (POPEYE DOMAIN-CONTAINING PROTEIN 3)

LGMDR26 was reported in five patients from three unrelated consanguineous families of different ethnic origins (Danish, Iranian, and Spanish).[327] Affected individuals presented with slowly proximal weakness with onset in teens to fifth decade. Some patients had calf hypertrophy. CK was markedly elevated. Skeletal muscle MRI showed fatty replacement of the thigh muscles, medial gastrocnemius, and paraspinal muscles. Some patients had calf hypertrophy. Muscle biopsies revealed dystrophic changes and whorled fibers.

LGMDR27 (JAGGED2)

This recently discovered LGMD was reported in 23 patients from 13 unrelated families.[41,328] Onset of muscle weakness occurred from infancy to young adulthood with normal or mildly elevated CKs. Muscle biopsies show typical dystrophic features. Skeletal muscle MRI reveals fatty replacement of internal regions of thigh muscles and tibialis anterior with sparing of external areas, the so-called "inside-to-outside" pattern of fatty degeneration similar to that seen in LGMDR21 (*POGLUT1*-associated muscular dystrophy). Homozygous or compound heterozygous mutations were in *JAG2* that encodes for JAGGED2. Transcriptome analysis of muscle tissue has suggested disease mechanism may be related to Notch pathway dysfunction with misregulation of genes involved in myogenesis, including *PAX7*. Again, this may be considered a satellite cell-opathy.

MEGF10-RELATED MYOPATHY

This is another satellite cell-opathy. Although some have classified this as a congenital myopathy, we discuss this entity in this chapter as onset can be in adult life and the disease mechanism is similar to other disorders such as JAGGED-2 myopathy that is classified as an LGMDR27. The phenotypic spectrum ranges from an early-onset myopathy (birth or infancy), areflexia, respiratory distress, and dysphagia (EMARDD) to onset in the fifth decade of life.[41,329–332] Weakness is often more prominent in the upper extremities and distal muscles. Gastrostomy tubes and invasive ventilation are required to preserve life. Variable features include high-arched palate or cleft palate, contractures of the fingers, and pes equinovarus. CK is normal to mildly elevated. EMG shows myopathic features, while NCSs are normal. Skeletal muscle biopsies may reveal atrophic fibers, increased internalized whorled fibers, cytoplasmic bodies, aggregation of myofibrillar proteins, cores or minicores, and dystrophic features. It is caused by autosomal-recessive mutations in *MEGF10* that encodes for multiple epidermal growth factor 10 which is expressed on muscle satellite cells. It is believed to mediate cell proliferation and differentiation as well as to help regulate muscle development and repair.

DIAGNOSIS AND TREATMENT OF LGMD

Previously, we and others preached a stepwise approach and the use of algorithms developed by the practice guideline

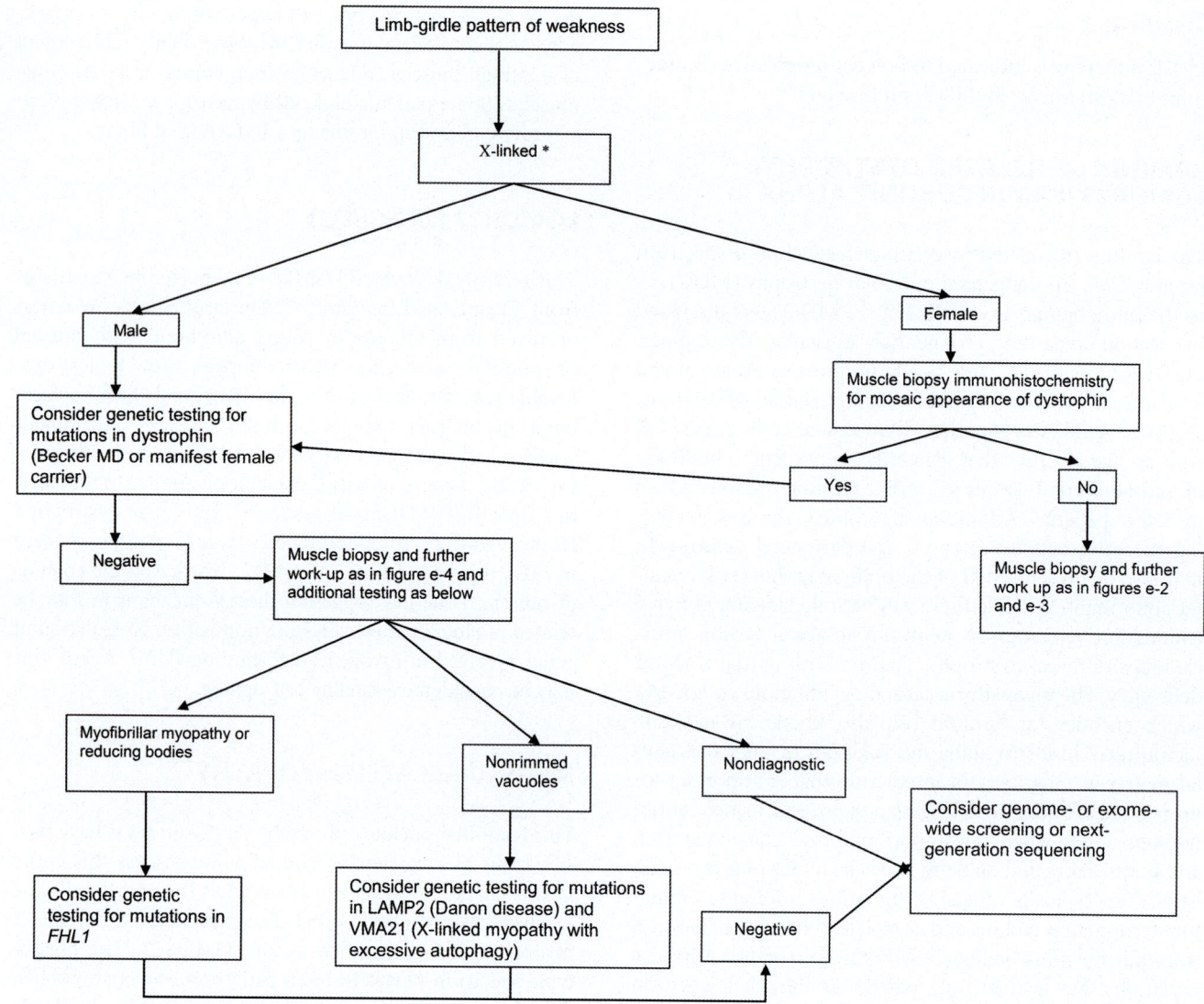

Figure 27-17. Diagnostic approach to patients with a limb-girdle pattern of weakness and suspected muscular dystrophy with an X-linked recessive inheritance pattern. In women, an X-linked disorder may be considered, if there is a familial presentation with men more affected than women. *Autosomal-dominant, autosomal-recessive, or X-linked inheritance may be responsible in sporadic cases. MD, muscular dystrophy. (Reproduced with permission from Narayanaswami P, Weiss M, Selcen D, et al. Evidence-based guideline summary: diagnosis and treatment of limb-girdle and distal dystrophies: report of the guideline development subcommittee of the American Academy of Neurology and the practice issues review panel of the American Association of Neuromuscular & Electrodiagnostic Medicine. *Neurology*. 2014;83(16):1453–1463.)

committee of the American Academy of Neurology (AAN) and American Association of Neuromuscular and Electrodiagnostic Medicine (AANEM) (Figs. 27-8, 27-10, and 27-17).[4,333] However, more recently our diagnostic approach to patients with muscular dystrophy has significantly changed because of the increased availability of NGS panels and their reduced cost. This has made NGS more cost efficient for diagnosis of hereditary myopathies, particularly since the clinical phenotypes (e.g., limb-girdle or distal weakness) are each associated with mutations in many different genes. Importantly though, NGS can miss large deletions, duplications, inversions, and mutations in introns that can affect splicing. Furthermore, many times with sequencing of so many genes, there are often variations of unknown significance (VOUS) found in any number of genes. Therefore, it is important still to know the phenotypes associated with specific hereditary myopathies to see if they match with reported VOUS. Muscle biopsies are also useful to see if the expected histopathological features match with what would be expected if the VOUS were indeed pathogenic.

Treatment is largely supportive.[4] Physical and occupational therapy are important to prevent contractures and improve function. Large therapeutic trials of corticosteroids (similar to those conducted for DMD) have not been performed in patients with LGMD. Gene therapies are just getting started, similar to what was discussed in the section on dystrophinopathies.

CONGENITAL MUSCULAR DYSTROPHY

The congenital muscular dystrophies or MDCs are a heterogeneous group of autosomal-recessive disorders, characterized by the perinatal onset of hypotonia and weakness, dystrophic appearing muscle biopsies, and the exclusion of other recognizable causes of myopathy of the newborn (Table 27-1).[46,47,333–335] The abbreviation assigned by the Human Genome Organization is "MDC" for muscular dystrophy, congenital. The MDCs have been classified in the past according to clinical, ophthalmological, radiological, and pathological features. A more recent classification is based on the location of the defective proteins and purported pathogeneses of the individual dystrophies. The major categories of MDCs include (1) those associated with mutations in genes encoding structural proteins of the basal lamina, extracellular matrix, or sarcolemmal proteins that bind to the basal lamina; (2) those associated with impaired glycosylation of α-dystroglycan; and (3) those associated with selenoprotein 1 mutations. Those with impaired glycosylation of α-dystroglycan have been further subdivided into three types based on clinical phenotype: Muscular dystrophy-dystroglycanopathy (congenital with brain and eye anomalies), type A (MDDGA); muscular dystrophy-dystroglycanopathy (congenital with impaired intellectual development), type B (MDDGB); muscular dystrophy-dystroglycanopathy (limb-girdle), type C (MDDGC).

MDC ASSOCIATED WITH GENETIC DEFECTS OF STRUCTURAL PROTEINS OF THE BASAL LAMINA OR EXTRACELLULAR MATRIX

MDC1A (LAMININ α2/MEROSIN)

Clinical Features

Approximately 30%–40% of patients with MDC have absent or severely decreased laminin α2 (merosin).[237–240] As mentioned previously, MDC1A is allelic to LGMDR23, in which there is partial deficiency of laminin α2, and is associated with a milder clinical phenotype.[336–345] Children with MDC1A usually present at birth with generalized weakness and hypotonia. There is a predilection for neck, shoulder, and hip-girdle muscles. Calf hypertrophy may be appreciated early in the course. Contractures develop, but severe arthrogryposis is rare. Breathing and feeding problems can be present but usually not severe enough to require ventilator support at birth. Some children develop a cardiomyopathy. Limited extraocular movements can be observed in the later stages.

As mentioned, MDC1A is associated with more severe weakness and a much poorer prognosis compared with LGMDR23.[336] Most children with MDC1A never ambulate independently, although rarely children are able to stand and occasionally walk with assistance. Individuals with only partial laminin α2 deficiency have a milder course and can present in childhood with a DMD phenotype or in early adulthood with a phenotype similar to BMD or LGMD.[247,336–338,346]

Most children with MDC1A have normal intelligence despite abnormal white matter changes apparent on MRI. However, there is a high incidence of epilepsy (12%–30%) as well as a few reported cases of occipital dysplasia. Epilepsy can also occur in patients with partial merosin deficiency. Rare patients with MDC1A with epilepsy and occipital agyria also have cognitive impairment.

Laboratory Features

Serum CK levels are markedly elevated, usually over 2,000 IU/L in the merosin-negative infants, while partial merosinopathies are associated with normal or mildly elevated serum CKs. Brain MRI often demonstrates diffuse white matter abnormalities in T2-weighted images suggestive of dysmyelination in most children after the age of 6 months (Fig. 27-18). In addition, occipital polymicrogyria/agyria and hypoplasia of pons and/or cerebellum are evident in rare cases. Patients with partial merosin deficiency may or may not have cerebral hypomyelination on MRI. Visual- and somatosensory-evoked potential may reveal delayed latencies in MDC1A.[347]

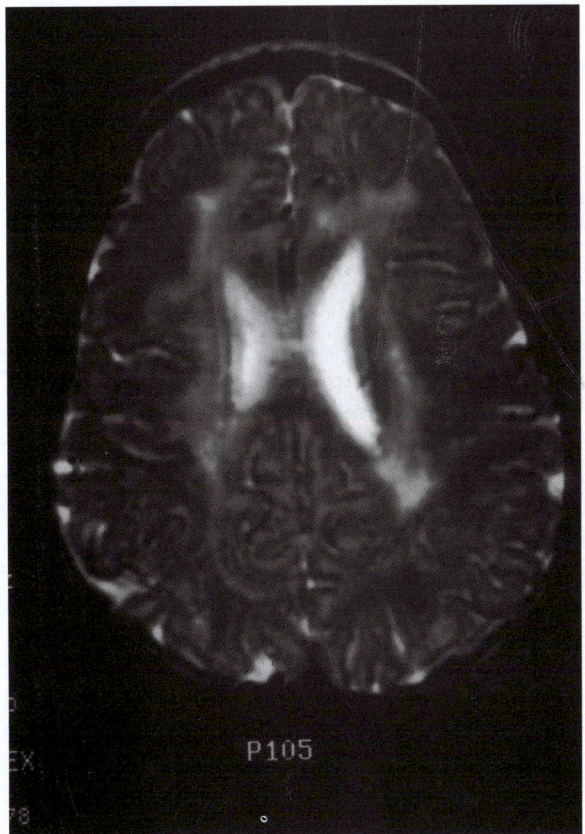

Figure 27-18. Congenital muscular dystrophy. T2-weighted MRI of the brain of an infant with merosin-negative congenital muscular dystrophy reveals increased signal of the subcortical white matter consistent with hypomyelination.

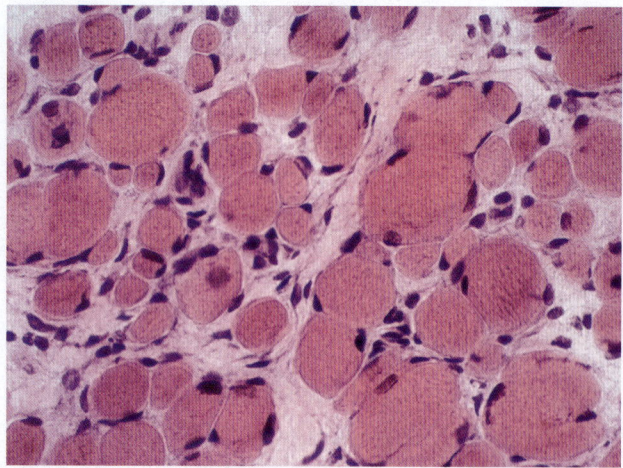

Figure 27-19. Congenital muscular dystrophy. Muscle biopsy demonstrates fiber size variability and increased endomysial and perimysial connective tissue consistent with a dystrophic process. Hematoxylin and eosin (H&E).

Slowing of nerve conduction velocities is also commonly appreciated.[338]

Histopathology

Muscle biopsies demonstrate variation in fiber size with increased endomysial connective tissue (Fig. 27-19) and notably decreased or absent laminin α2.

Molecular Genetics and Pathogenesis

MDC1A is associated with mutations in the gene encoding α2 subchain of merosin or laminin α2, *LAMA2*, on chromosome 6q21–22. The gene codes for a 390-kD protein, which is synthesized as one chain but processed into two fragments. On immunoblot, these two fragments have molecular masses of approximately 80 kD (C terminal) and 300 kD (N terminal).[337,341]

Merosin is also present in the basal lamina of myelinated nerves. Abnormal expression of merosin may interfere with myelinogenesis and may account for the hypomyelination evident in the central and peripheral nervous system. Importantly, merosin is expressed in the skin, and thus MDC1A can be diagnosed on skin biopsies.[341,348] Further, prenatal diagnosis of MDC1A can be made on chorionic villous sampling.[342,349]

Merosin binds to α-dystroglycan and α7β 1D integrin (Fig. 27-1). As with primary dystrophinopathies and sarcoglycanopathies, merosinopathies may result in a disruption of the dystrophin–glycoprotein complex. Mutations in the α2 subchain of merosin result in a markedly diminished expression of α7β 1D integrin, but a normal or only mildly decreased expression of components of the dystroglycan or sarcoglycan complexes on the sarcolemma. Of note, mutations involving the α7 subunit of integrin that binds to merosin also result in a form of MDC.[350]

MEROSIN-POSITIVE CLASSIC MDC

As noted in the previous discussion, merosin-positive forms of classic MDC are clinically more benign than merosin-negative MDC. These merosin-positive MDC cases are genetically heterogeneous. Mutations of the α7 subunit of integrin gene, *ITGA7* been demonstrated in rare patients with merosin-positive MDC.[351] Affected children present with congenital onset of generalized weakness and hypotonia and have delayed motor milestones. Cognitive impairment was evident in one child who had a normal MRI of the brain and EEG. Serum CK is only mildly elevated (less than five times normal). Muscle biopsies reveal only mild variation of fiber size with normal merosin expression on immunohistochemistry.

▶ ULLRICH DISEASE/LGMDR22

Clinical Features

UCMD is associated with weakness at birth or early infancy, contractures of the proximal joints, hyperextensibility of the distal joints, high-arched palate, and protuberant calcanei.[351–354] UCMD is allelic with the more benign Bethlem myopathy (LGMDD5). UCMD is associated with congenital muscle weakness, delayed motor milestones, proximal joint contractures, scoliosis, and marked distal joint hyperextensibility. Intelligence is normal.

Laboratory Features

Serum CK is normal or mildly elevated.

Histopathology

Muscle biopsies reveal variation in muscle fiber size, scattered regenerating and degenerating fibers, and increased endomysial connective tissue. Immunohistochemistry reveals that collagen VI is present in the interstitium but absent from the sarcolemma.[351] EM demonstrates that collagen VI in the interstitium fails to anchor normally to the basal lamina surrounding muscle fibers.

Molecular Genetics and Pathogenesis

Collagen VI is composed of three chains, α1, α2, and α3, and is a ubiquitously expressed extracellular matrix protein. The three chains are encoded by the genes *COL6A1* and *COL6A2* on chromosome 21q22.3 and *COL6A3* on chromosome 2q37. UCMD and the less severe Bethlem myopathy are caused by mutations in these genes.[353] UCMD had been considered a recessive condition caused by homozygous or compound heterozygous mutations in COL6A2 and COL6A3. In contrast, the milder disorder Bethlem myopathy has dominant inheritance and is caused by single mutations in COL6A1, COL6A2, and COL6A3.[353] UCMD is usually inherited in an autosomal-recessive fashion, while Bethlem myopathy is autosomal dominant, but there are mild cases that are autosomal recessively inherited and severe cases that are dominantly inherited.[353] Furthermore, there can be phenotypic variability within affected family members. Collagen VI deficiency in muscle or cultured fibroblasts was complete in severe cases and partial in the milder forms, which suggests a correlation between the degree of collagen VI deficiency and the clinical severity in UCMD.[354]

▶ MDC ASSOCIATED WITH IMPAIRED GLYCOSYLATION OF α-DYSTROGLYCAN: MUSCULAR DYSTROPHY- DYSTROGLYCANOPATHIES

As mentioned previously, this group of CDM is subclassified into: muscular dystrophy-dystroglycanopathy (congenital with brain and eye anomalies), type A (MDDGA); muscular dystrophy-dystroglycanopathy (congenital with impaired intellectual development), type B (MDDGB); muscular dystrophy-dystroglycanopathy (limb-girdle), type C (MDDGC). The primary sequence of α-dystroglycan predicts a molecular mass of 72 kD; however, the mass of α-dystroglycan in the skeletal muscle is 156 kDa. The increase in size is due to posttranslational modification of α-dystroglycan. O-mannosyl and LARGE-dependent glycosylation of α-dystroglycan are apparently important for stable binding of the sarcolemma to merosin in the basement membrane. The α-dystroglycanopathies can be the result of mutations in the α-dystroglycan (DAG1) gene, but also in numerous other genes that are involved in the glycosylation pathway (POMT1, POMT2, POMGNT1, POMGNT2, FKRP, Fukutin, LARGE, ISPD, GTDC2, B3GALNT2, B4GAT1, TMEM5, GMPPB, POMK, and dolichyl-phosphate mannosyltransferase subunit genes—DPM1, DPM2, DPM3).[4,46,47,295,355–375]

The protein O-mannosyltransferase 1 (POMT1) forms a complex with a second protein O-mannosyltransferase (POMT2) to catalyze the first step in O-mannosyl glycosylation. Subsequently, the transfer of N-acetylglucosamine to O-mannose of glycoproteins is catalyzed by O-mannose β-1,2-N-acetylglucosaminyltransferase (POMGNT1). Fukutin, FKRP, LARGE, and other enzymes mentioned above are other secretory enzymes involved in posttranslational glycosylation of α-dystroglycan, although the exact reactions they catalyze are not known. Not only is glycosylation of α-dystroglycan important for proper muscle function, but impaired glycosylation of α-dystroglycan leads to defects in neuronal migration and the abnormalities in the central nervous system.

As previously mentioned, the nomenclature of these disorders has changed in recent years. Muscular dystrophy–dystroglycanopathy with brain and eye anomalies (type A), MDDGA1, previously referred to as the WWS or MEB disease, is genetically heterogeneous and can be caused by mutation in other genes involved in DAG1 glycosylation.

MDDGA1 is caused by mutation in the gene encoding protein O-mannosyltransferase-1 (POMT1); MDDGA2 is caused by mutations in the POMT2 gene; MDDGA3 is caused by mutation in the POMGNT1 gene; MDDGA4 is caused by mutations in the FKTN gene; MDDGA5 is caused by mutations in the FKRP gene; MDDGA6 is caused by mutations in the LARGE gene; MDDGA7 is caused by mutations in the ISPD gene; MDDGA8 is caused by mutations in the POMGNT2 gene; MDDGA9 is caused by mutations in the DAG gene; MDDGA10 is caused by mutations in the TMEM5 gene; MDDGA11 is caused by mutations in the B3GALNT2 gene; MDDGA12 is caused by mutations in the POMK gene; MDDGA13 is caused by mutations in the B4GAT1 gene; and MDDGA14 is caused by mutations in the GMPPB gene.[46,47,295,355–375]

Muscle biopsy findings are indistinguishable from other forms of MDC using routine stains. A striking inflammatory infiltrate is occasionally present, which has led to the erroneous diagnosis of a congenital inflammatory myopathy. Importantly, abnormal glycosylation of α-dystroglycan can be appreciated by reduced immunostaining of the sarcolemmal membrane with antibodies directed against α-dystroglycan and merosin.

▶ FUKUYAMA CONGENITAL MUSCULAR DYSTROPHY

Clinical Features

FCMD was originally described in Japan, where it is the most common form of MDC.[46,47,366–368] The myopathy presents with generalized proximal greater than distal weakness and hypotonia in infants. Mothers of affected children retrospectively recall decreased fetal movements. There is an increased frequency of spontaneous abortions of affected fetuses. Pseudohypertrophy of the calves is recognized in approximately half the children. Muscle stretch reflexes are reduced. Some children are born with arthrogryposis and contractures that are progressive.

In addition to the myopathy, FCMD is associated with severe structural abnormalities of the brain, including microcephaly, cortical dysplasia, lissencephaly, pachygyria, polymicrogyria, and hydrocephalus.[366,367] Intellectual function is markedly compromised. Approximately 50% of children who are affected have seizures. Both physical and mental developments are delayed, with the majority never being able to stand or ambulate independently. Most children die by the age of 10–12 years of age from ventilatory failure.

Laboratory Features

The serum CK level is usually elevated 10–50 times normal values. Electroencephalography is often abnormal, demonstrating epileptiform activity and generalized slowing. MRI and CT scans of the brain reveal structural abnormalities and evidence of hypomyelination.

Molecular Genetics and Pathogenesis

FCMD is most commonly caused by mutations in the fukutin gene, *FKTN* (MDDGA4).[366–368] Fukutin is a secretory enzyme that localizes to the *cis*-Golgi compartment and is thought to have a role in posttranslational glycosylation of α-dystroglycan.[240] In addition to the skeletal muscle involvement, the disruption of normal glycosylation of α-dystroglycan or other proteins leads to defects in neuronal migration and differentiation, which accounts for the many abnormalities seen within the central nervous system. Milder phenotypes associated with *FKTN* mutations are classified as MDDGB4, MDDGC4, or LGMD2M/LGMDR13.

► WALKER–WARBURG SYNDROME

Clinical Features

WWS, or cerebro-ocular dysplasia, is the most severe α-dystroglycanopathy and is associated with a life expectancy of less than 3 years. WWS presents as severe generalized weakness and hypotonia in infancy.[46,47,362–364,367] In addition, the infants are usually born blind secondary to ocular malformations, which include fixed pupils, hypoplasia of the optic nerves, microphthalmia, corneal opacities, cataracts, shallow anterior chambers, ciliary body abnormalities, iridolental synechiae, and retinal dysplasia and detachment. As with FCMD and MEB, WWS is associated with migrational and developmental disturbances of neurons in the brain, which include lissencephaly, polymicrogyria, hydrocephalus, hypomyelination of the subcortical white matter, and hypoplasia of the brainstem and vermis. Seizures are common.

Laboratory Features

Serum CK levels are elevated. Brain MRI scans reveal structural abnormalities, which are alluded to in the above section. Electroencephalography is often abnormal, revealing slowing of the background and epileptiform activity.

Molecular Genetics and Pathogenesis

WWS is caused by mutations in several genes (*POMT1 POMT2, FKRP, FKTN, ISPD, CTDC2, TMEM5, POMGNT1, B3GALNT2, GMPPB, B4GAT1, POMK*).[46,47,362,369,370] Mutations in *POMT1* gene are the most common and account for the 20% of WWS. The clinical phenotype of patients with mutations in the *POMT1* gene is also variable, with rare cases being reported with LGMD and mild cognitive impairment (LGMD2K/LGMDR11).[371]

► MUSCLE–EYE–BRAIN DISEASE

Clinical Features

MEB disease was initially described in Finnish patients but has been subsequently reported in other populations.[363,364,372–374] As in WWS, brain and eye abnormalities accompany the muscle weakness; however, MEB is less severe. Although infants are weak and motor development is slow, most affected children eventually can sit and stand and some ambulate. There are severe cognitive impairments associated with structural abnormalities in the brain, which include pachygyria, polymicrogyria, abnormal midline structures, and hypoplasia of the vermis and pons. MEB is also associated with progressive myopia, glaucoma, and late cataracts.

Laboratory Features

Serum CK levels are elevated. MRI of the brain may demonstrate polymicrogyria, abnormal midline structures, hypoplastic vermis, and pons.[363,372–374]

Molecular Genetics and Pathogenesis

MEB is most commonly caused by mutations in the gene that encodes for O-mannose-β-1,2-N-acetylglucosaminyl transferase (*POMGnT1*) on chromosome 1p32–34 (MDDGA3).[363,364,369] POMGnT1 catalyzes the transfer of N-acetylglucosamine to O-mannose of glycoproteins. Mutations in this gene have also been associated with a milder phenotype, MDDGB3, MDDGC3, or LGMD2O/LGMDR15. Mutations in the *FKRP*, *FKTN*, *ISPD*, and *TMEM5* genes can also cause MEB.

MDC1C/MDDGB5

Clinical Features

MDC1, now referred to as MDDGB5, is caused by mutations in the gene that encodes for FKRP.[44,46,47,375] The FKRP-related myopathies are very common, especially among patients of Northern European and English ancestry, and give rise to the largest phenotypical spectrum of muscular dystrophies so far connected to mutations of a single gene. The age of onset can range from infancy (e.g., congenital) to the fourth decade of life, with a pattern of weakness similar to MDC1A. A phenotype reminiscent of WWS can also be seen in patients with FKRP mutations (MDDGA5) or milder, later-onset disease MDDGC5 or LGMDR9. Early involvement of cardiac and respiratory muscles is common.[229–231]

Laboratory Features

CK levels are always very elevated (10–75× normal). Echocardiogram may reveal features of a dilated cardiomyopathy. PFTs may reveal reduced FVC and inspiratory pressures. MRI of the brain may reveal microcephaly, cerebellar cysts, and hypoplasia of the vermis, and also white matter abnormalities on MRI as in other α-dystroglycanopathies.[375]

Molecular Genetics and Pathogenesis

MDC1C is caused by mutations in *FKRP* that encodes for fukutin related protein (FKRP). FKRP localizes in rough

ER and appears to be involved in one of the initial steps in O-mannosylation of α-dystroglycan.[240] ER retention of mutant FKRP may play a role in the pathogenesis and potentially explain why the allelic disorder LGMD2I/LGMDR9 is milder, because the mutated protein is able to reach the Golgi apparatus.[241] There is a correlation between a reduction in α-dystroglycan and the severity of the clinical phenotype.[44] Patients with MDDGA5 have a profound depletion of α-dystroglycan, those with a Duchenne-like phenotype (MDDGB5) have a moderate reduction in α-dystroglycan, and individuals with the milder form MDDGC5 or LGMD2I/LGMDR9 demonstrate a variable but subtle alteration in α-dystroglycan immunolabeling.

MDC1D/MDDGA6

Clinical Features

MDC1D is now referred to as MDDGA5. This is a very rare dystrophy which, as in other secondary α-dystroglycanopathies, is associated with generalized weakness and global developmental delay.[46,47,355] Motor milestones are delayed, but affected individuals may be able to ambulate. Nystagmus may be evident but no other ocular abnormalities are typically identified.

Laboratory Features

Serum CK is mild to moderately elevated. Mild structural abnormalities have been appreciated on brain MRI.

Molecular Genetics and Pathogenesis

Mutations in the human *LARGE* gene (also is required for glycosylation of α-dystroglycan) is responsible for this rare form of MDC.[46,47,355] This gene encodes for another putative glycosyltransferase.

▶ MDC ASSOCIATED WITH SELENOPROTEIN N1 MUTATIONS

RIGID SPINE SYNDROME

Clinical Features

The rigid spine syndrome or rigid spine muscular dystrophy (RSMD) is a heterogeneous disorder. One subtype, RSMD1, manifests in infancy with hypotonia, proximal weakness, and delayed motor milestones.[376–383] Affected individuals develop progressive limitation of spine mobility often associated with scoliosis and contractures at the knees and elbows. Thus, these patients share many clinical features with EDMD and UCMD/Bethlem myopathy. Of note, some patients previously diagnosed with multi/minicore congenital myopathy have a rigid spine. Respiratory weakness can develop due to stiffness of the rib cage and involvement of the diaphragm. Many patients require noninvasive ventilator support.

Laboratory Features

Serum CK levels are normal to slightly elevated. Conduction defects may be evident on EKG. PFTs reveal a reduced vital capacity in patients old enough to cooperate. EMG demonstrates myopathic appearing MUAPs, while insertional activity is typically normal and abnormal spontaneous activity is sparse.

Histopathology

Muscle biopsies reveal nonspecific myopathic features including variability in fiber size, increased internal nuclei, type 1 fiber predominance, and moth-eaten fibers and lobulated fibers on NADH-TR stains. Some cases are associated with multiple minicores. Cytoplasmic bodies, Mallory bodies, increased desmin expression, and sarcoplasmic and intranuclear tubulofilamentous inclusions may also be present similar to MFM. Endomysial fibrosis is apparent, particularly in axial muscles (i.e., rectus abdominis and paraspinal muscles). Immunostains for dystrophin, sarcoglycans, and the dystroglycans are normal.

Molecular Genetics and Pathogenesis

Some cases of autosomal-recessive RSMD have been linked to mutations in the gene that encodes for selenoprotein N1, *SEPN1*, located on chromosome 1p35–36.[379,382,383] Mutations in this gene have also been shown in some patients with multi/minicore myopathy and MFM. Selenoprotein N1 is an ER glycoprotein. The function of this protein is not known.

▶ DIAGNOSIS AND TREATMENT OF MDC

With the various genes that can cause congenital muscular dystrophy, diagnosis can be daunting, particularly with those more familiar with taking care of adults. Assessment of ocular and brain abnormalities and other features can help point to the right direction of genetic testing, but as per the diagnostic approach of LGMD, the wider availability and reduced cost of NGS panels have made this easier (Fig. 27-20). Treatment of the MDCs is supportive. Corticosteroids have not been associated with any significant benefit even in those cases with associated significant inflammation on muscle biopsy. Antiepileptic medications are necessary for control of seizures. Physical therapy and range-of-motion exercise are important to reduce contractures. Ventilator support, invasive or noninvasive, may be beneficial in patients with ventilatory muscle involvement.

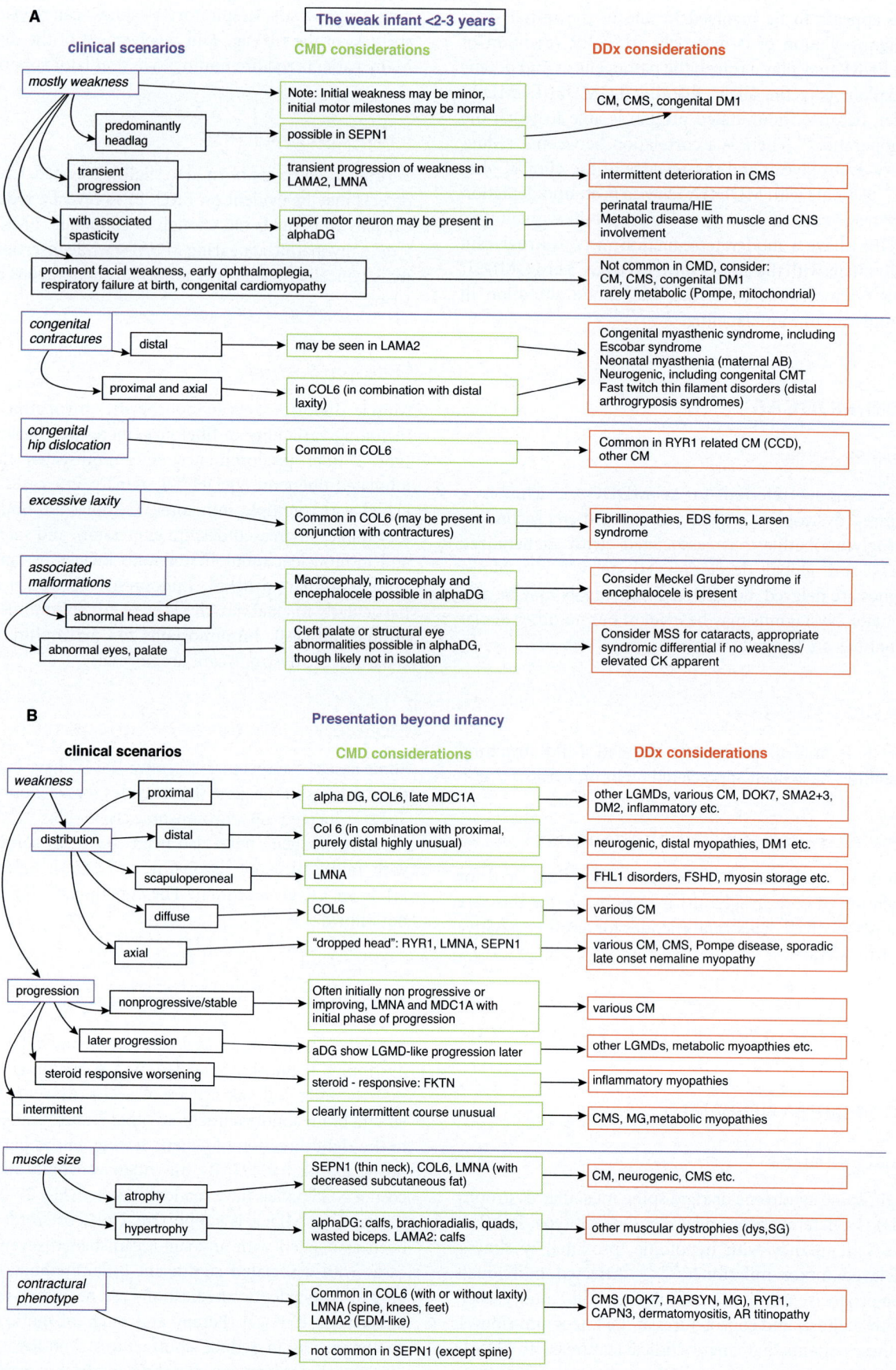

Figure 27-20. Differential diagnostic considerations for various clinical findings in infancy (**A**) and beyond infancy (**B, C**), as well as for various laboratory findings that may be available at the outset of the diagnostic encounter (**D**).

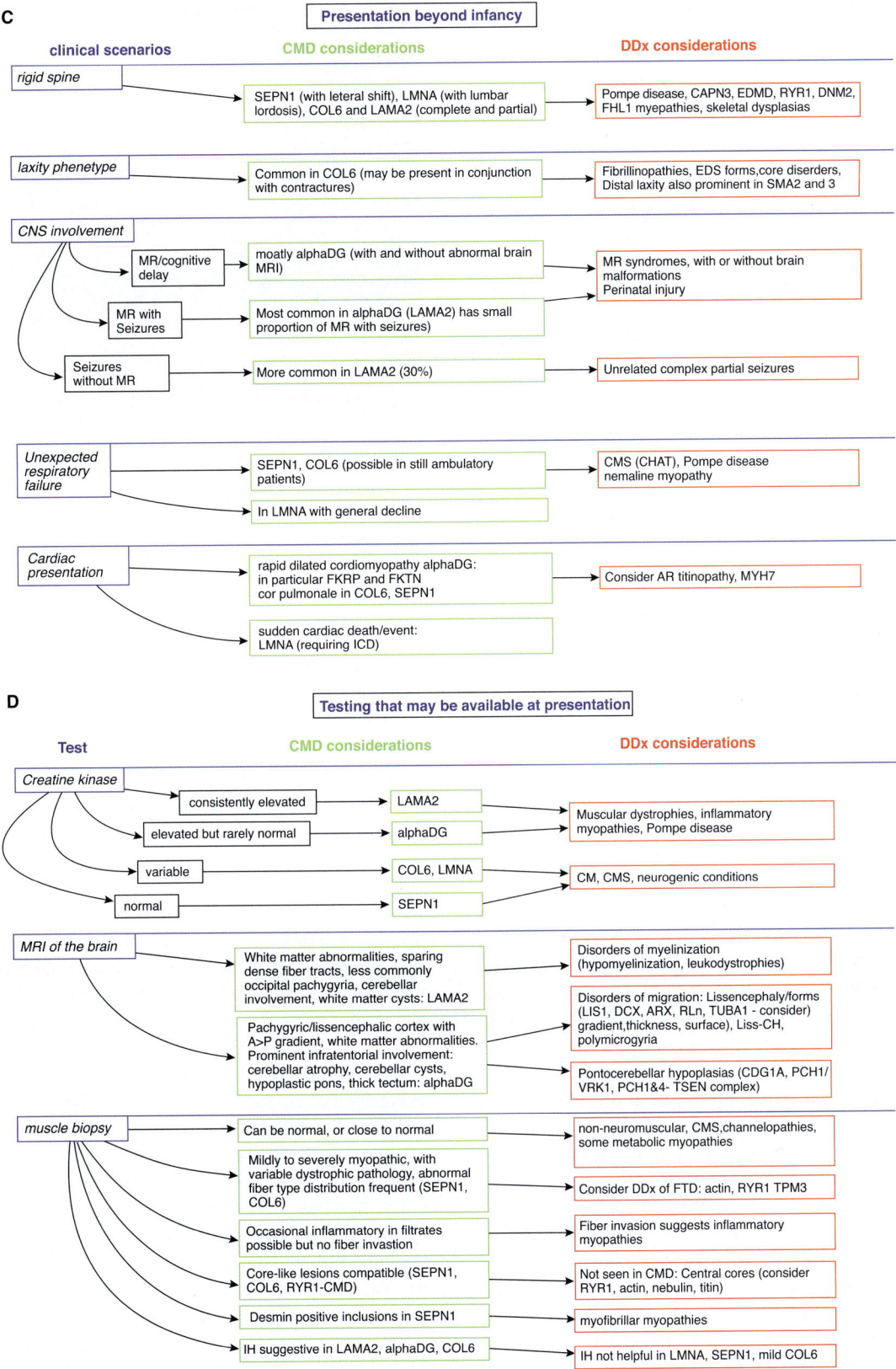

Figure 27-20. (Continued) Note: The most important tools in the clinical differential diagnosis are EMG/NCS to diagnose neurogenic involvement, muscle biopsy, and selective biochemical and genetic testing. The differential diagnostic considerations are not exhaustive but highlight a few of the more relevant conditions to consider with a given clinical picture. To save space we are only using the gene/protein symbols to indicate specific diagnosis. (Reproduced with permission from Bönnemann CG, Wang CH, Quijano-Roy S, et al. Diagnostic approach to the congenital muscular dystrophies. *Neuromuscul Disord*. 2014;24(4):289–311.)

OTHER REGIONAL FORMS OF MUSCULAR DYSTROPHY

FACIOSCAPULOHUMERAL MUSCULAR DYSTROPHY

Clinical Features

Facioscapulohumeral muscular dystrophy (FSHD) is an autosomal-dominant disorder, with an incidence of approximately 4 per million and a prevalence of roughly 50 per million.[384] There is a variable degree of penetrance of clinical findings within families, while around 30% of affected family members are unaware of their deficits. Thus, it is very important to examine family members of patients suspected of having FSHD.

Onset of weakness is usually appreciated between 3 and 44 years, although onset as late as 75 years has been reported.[384–389] As the name suggests, FSHD is characterized by muscle weakness and wasting in a rather specific distribution. The muscles of facial expression, particularly the orbicularis oculi, zygomaticus, and orbicularis oris muscles, are affected early. Patients may be unable to fully close their eyes against resistance and may sleep with incomplete eyelid closure. Affected persons can have a horizontal smile and weak puckering of the lips. Facial weakness may be strikingly asymmetric, mimicking a seventh nerve palsy. The muscles of mastication and the external ocular muscles are typically spared.

The scapula-stabilizer muscles (serratus anterior, rhomboid, middle trapezius, and, to some degree, latissimus dorsi muscles) are also weak and atrophic early in the course. Weakness of these muscles lead to upward and lateral rotation of the shoulder blades with scapular winging and the appearance of a "trapezius hump," which often is mistaken for muscle hypertrophy (Fig. 27-21). Although the deltoids are relatively spared during the early course of the disease, the sternocostal head of the pectoralis major is often atrophic and weak. The clavicles are displaced more horizontally and may angle downward from the sternum to the upper arm. Combined with the internal rotation of the upper arms, the anterior axillary folds, which are normally vertical, become horizontally displaced. There are also significant weakness and atrophy of the biceps brachii and triceps, with relatively normal bulk of the forearm muscles producing the so-called "Popeye arms." Wrist extensors are weaker than wrist flexors. The characteristic facial and upper torso appearance led to the designation of "facioscapulohumeral" muscular dystrophy. Some patients with FSHD manifest only with scapular winging or a limb-girdle pattern of weakness, but without facial weakness, and thus mimic an LGMD.[390] Further, there can be striking asymmetric, and sometimes unilateral, involvement of the facial, scapular stabilizers, or humeral muscles.

The tibialis anterior is usually the earliest lower limb muscle to manifest weakness, and occasionally patients present with foot drop.[388] The gastrocnemius muscles are usually normal, although rarely patients manifest with difficulty walking on their toes.[388] The muscle involvement may progress to the pelvic musculature, producing a hyperlordotic posture and a waddling gait. As in the face and arms, weakness in the legs is often asymmetric. Approximately 20% of patients with FSHD eventually will require wheelchairs.

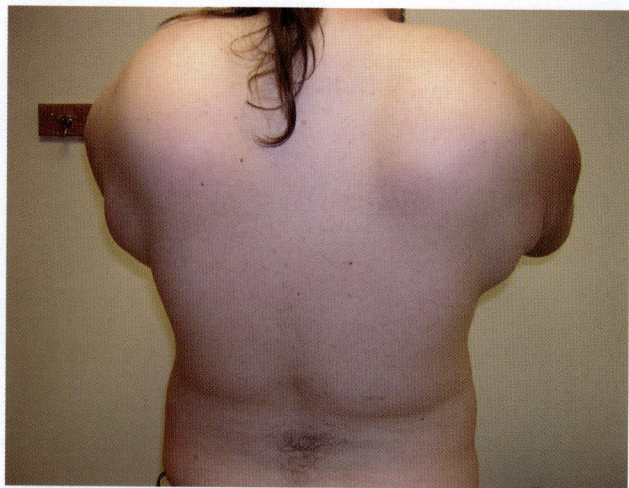

Figure 27-21. Facioscapulohumeral muscular dystrophy (FSHD). Characteristic appearance of a patient diagnosed with FSHD. On attempted forward flexion of the arms at the shoulders the scapulae elevates and laterally deviates off the posterior rib cage under the trapezius musculature, giving the false impression of very muscular individual. Palpation reveals the bone underlying the muscle tissue.

Abdominal muscles may also be involved, producing a positive Beevor sign (the umbilicus may move up or down a few centimeters when the patient is supine and attempts to flex the head because of upper or lower abdominal muscle weakness). Although seldom volunteered, asking a patient if they have to roll on their side to arise from a supine position, may provide insight into possible abdominal wall weakness. Sensation is intact to all modalities, and the reflexes are usually absent or diminished commensurate with the degree of muscle wasting.

Some patients with FSHD appear to experience a late exacerbation of muscle weakness. They may only have mild weakness for years and then suddenly have a marked increase of weakness in the typical distribution over the course of several years. Affected individuals usually have a normal life span; however, severe progressive ventilatory muscle weakness was reported in approximately 1% of patients with FSHD in one large series.[391] Severe extremity weakness, wheelchair dependency, and kyphoscoliosis appear to be risk factors for ventilatory failure. Further, rare patents develop cardiac involvement manifesting as conduction defects, supraventricular, or ventricular arrhythmias that may require pacemaker implantation.[392]

Infantile-onset FSHD is associated with severe weakness presenting in the first 2 years of life. A wheelchair is required to maintain mobility by the time the patient is 9 or 10 years of age. FSHD can also be associated with profound sensorineural hearing loss and retinal telangiectasias (Coats disease). Some infants present with profound facial diplegia mimicking Mobius syndrome.[393]

Laboratory Features

Serum CK levels are normal or moderately elevated. A characteristic finding on skeletal muscle MRI is the involvement of the trapezius and subscapularis muscles with sparing of the iliopsoas along with asymmetric involvement of upper- and lower-limb muscles.[394]

Histopathology

The muscle biopsy demonstrates variation in muscle fiber size with atrophic and hypertrophic fibers, scattered necrotic and regenerating fibers, increased internalized nuclei, lobulated fibers, and increased endomysial connective tissue. Prominent mononuclear inflammatory infiltrate may be appreciated in the endomysium, which can lead to confusion with polymyositis (Fig. 27-22).[395] Immunostaining with antibodies directed against membrane attack complex may demonstrate deposition on the sarcolemma of nonnecrotic muscle fibers.[396]

Molecular Genetics and Pathogenesis

There are at least four genetic distinct causes of FSHD, but the pathogenic mechanisms appear related. Both forms are inherited in an autosomal-dominant fashion, but spontaneous mutations are common, and penetrance is variable in both.

FSHD1 is responsible for 95% of cases and is linked to mutations in the telomeric region of chromosome 4q35 (Fig. 27-23).[384,397–399] An *Eco*RI polymorphism occurs and is variable in size; normally, it is 50–300 kb, but the size is reduced in FSHD1 to 10–30 kb. Within this *Eco*RI polymorphism lies a tandem array of 11–100 *Kpn* I units, each 3.3 kb in size, which is termed D4Z4.[384] Most patients with autosomal-dominant FSHD1 carry one array of 1–10 units. In addition, there is normally an allelic variation of chromosome 4qter, designated 4qA and 4qB, which differ by a few insertion/deletion events in the region distal to D4Z4.[384] The 4qA allele contains a block of beta-satellite DNA directly distal to D4Z4 on 4qA, which is not present on the 4qB allele. Although occurring in similar frequency in the normal population, FSHD1 and the other genetic forms of FSHD are exclusively associated with the 4qA type of allele.

There is an inverse correlation between the size of the D4Z4 repeat unit and the severity of the disease. Patients carrying one to three units are usually severely affected and often represent isolated (de novo mutations) cases, whereas patients carrying 4–10 units typically have an affected parent.[304] Anticipation phenomena may occur in some families, although the size of the mutation appears stable and there can be extreme variability in phenotype even within families.[398] The mutation in FSHD1 is unlike other described genetic disorders, in which anticipation is associated with an increased size of a polymorphic trinucleotide repeat mutation.

Approximately 5% of FSHD patients do not have a deletion affecting D4Z4 repeats. FSHD2 is caused by mutations in the *SMCHD1* gene that encodes the structural maintenance of chromosomes flexible hinge domain-containing 1 protein.[400,401] FSHD3 is caused by a mutations in the ligand-dependent nuclear receptor interacting factor 1 gene, *LRIF1*,[402] and FSHD 4 is due to mutations in *DNMT3B* that encode for DNA methyltransferase 3B (*DNMT3B*).[403] Notably, the D4Z4 region in hypomethylated in all forms of FSHD. Methylation is an epigenic means of reducing transcription. Mutations in *SMCHD1*, *LRIF1*, and *DNMT3B* lead to D4Z4 chromatin relaxation and hypomethylation. Within the D4Z4 repeat lies the *DUX4* gene that is normally not expressed in muscle. Hypomethylation of the D4Z4 region leads to a toxic overexpression of this *DUX4* gene. *DUX4* encodes for double homeobox 4, which itself is a transcription factor controlling the expression of other genes. This in-turn likely leads to the under or overexpression of other genes.

Diagnosis

The diagnosis of FSHD is usually apparent on clinical grounds. Genetic testing is particularly useful for confirmation in patients without family history or unusual clinical phenotypes as well as for genetic counseling. We start off by testing for FSHD1 as it is much more common, and if this is unrevealing, test for other causes of FSHD.

Treatment

Surgery to fix the scapula to the thorax, thereby increasing range of motion, is beneficial in some patients.[404,405]

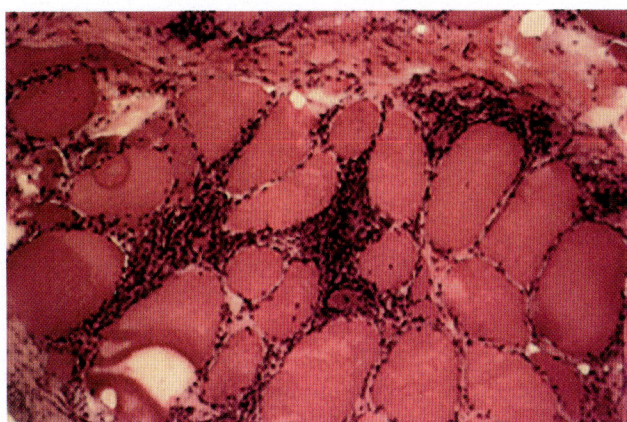

Figure 27-22. Facioscapulohumeral muscular dystrophy. Muscle biopsy demonstrates prominent inflammation (H&E). Physicians need to be aware that such prominent inflammation can be present in muscular dystrophies and can occasionally be misdiagnosed as an inflammatory myopathy (e.g., polymyositis). The inflammatory cells present in the dystrophic muscle usually do not invade nonnecrotic muscle fibers, in contrast to the invasion of nonnecrotic muscle fibers seen in polymyositis and inclusion body myositis.

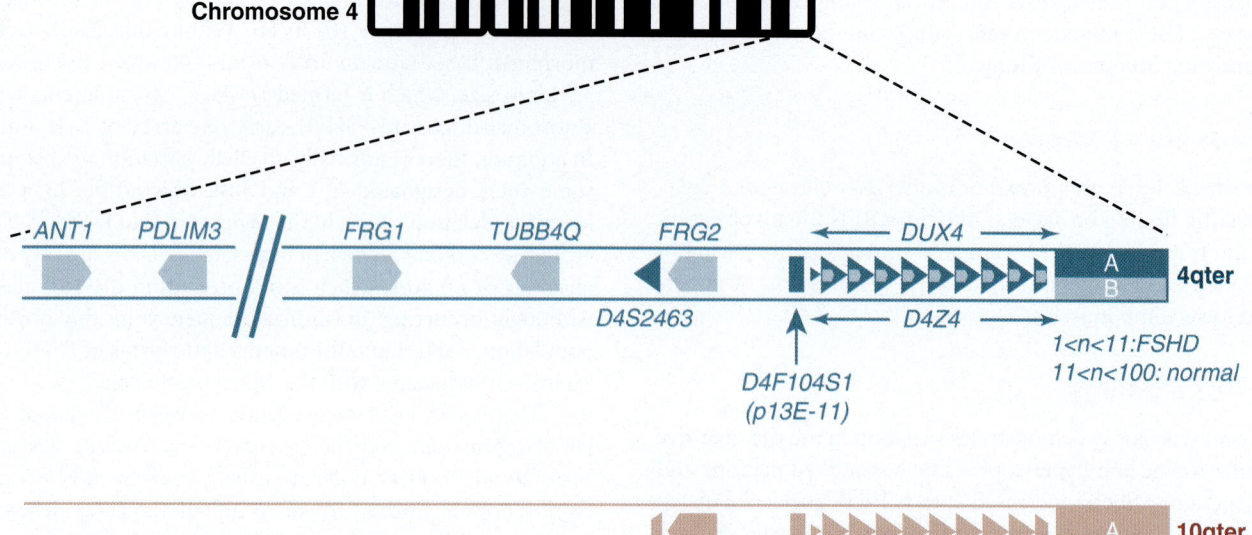

Figure 27-23. Schematic representation of the facioscapulohumeral muscular dystrophy (FSHD) locus. The polymorphic D4Z4 repeat array (*arrowheads*) in the subtelomere of chromosome 4 (blue) can vary between 11 and 100 units in the healthy population. One inversed copy of D4Z4 (D4S2463) is located 37 kb proximally. Just preceding the D4Z4 repeat unit, probe p13E-11 (D4F104S1), used in the DNA diagnosis of FSHD, is situated. Within each unit, a putative open reading frame designated DUX4 (*block arrow*) is located, but expression of this gene has never been established. In a proximal direction, several additional genes have been identified (*block arrows*) including *FRG2*, *TUBB4Q* (a pseudogene), and *FRG1*. At a much larger distance, several other genes have been evaluated for their involvement in FSHD. Most notably, these include *ANT1* and *PDLIM3*. Distal to D4Z4, two allelic variants of 4qter have been identified: 4qA (dark blue) and 4qB (light blue). Both variants are almost equally common in the population and vary by a few insertion and deletion events. FSHD alleles are exclusively linked with the 4qA variant. The subtelomere of chromosome 10q is similarly organized as 4q due to an ancient duplication of the 4q subtelomere. The homology between 4qter and 10qter extends from the telomere to 40 kb proximally to D4Z4 within an incomplete inverted copy of D4Z4. In contrast to 4qter, there is no B variant of the 10q subtelomere. (Reproduced with permission from Tawil R, Van Der Maarel SM. Facioscapulohumeral muscular dystrophy. *Muscle Nerve*. 2006;34(1):1–15.)

However, they need to have sufficient strength of the deltoid muscles in order to benefit from the procedure. Ankle–foot orthotics are useful in patients with foot drop secondary to tibialis anterior weakness.

SCAPULOPERONEAL MUSCULAR DYSTROPHY/MYOPATHY

Clinical Features

Patients with scapuloperoneal muscular dystrophy/myopathy manifest with foot drop followed by scapular weakness within the first two decades of life.[4,406–415] Weakness is often asymmetric, and patients sometimes are misdiagnosed as having a peroneal neuropathy. Furthermore, some with a scapuloperoneal pattern of weakness do indeed suffer from a form of neuropathy or motor neuronopathy.[411] Some patients with myopathic scapuloperoneal syndromes demonstrate preservation or even hypertrophy of the extensor digitorum brevis with the ability to dorsiflex the foot more effectively than the big toe. This feature is not typically seen in neurogenic causes of foot drop that are more usually length-dependant. The hypertrophy may result from attempting to dorsiflex the foot with this muscle. Ankle contractures are prominent features of the disease secondary to the weak anterior compartment muscles. The weak scapular muscles result in an appearance of the shoulder-girdle similar to that seen in FSHD. However, unlike FSHD, the humeral musculature is usually relatively spared. On the other hand, the peroneal muscles are typically more severely affected in scapuloperoneal muscular dystrophy compared to FSHD. Rarely, some patients may manifest mild weakness of the facial muscles, creating a diagnostic confusion with FSHD. However, facial muscle weakness is usually much less prominent than that seen in FSHD. Muscle weakness is slowly progressive.

Laboratory Features

The serum CK levels can be normal or moderately abnormal. The motor and sensory nerve conductions are normal aside from reduced CMAPs in the more severely affected muscles.[4,407–410] Needle EMG may demonstrate sparse fibrillation potentials and myopathic units.

Histopathology

Muscle biopsies reveal nonspecific myopathic features, including fiber size variation with atrophic and hypertrophic fibers, split fibers, necrotic and regenerating fibers, and increased endomysial connective tissue.[409] Some biopsies demonstrate inclusions typical of MFM,[410] hyaline bodies,[414] or nemaline rods.[415]

Molecular Genetics and Pathogenesis

Scapuloperoneal muscular dystrophy/myopathy is genetically heterogeneous. Mutations have been identified in the *DES* encoding for desmin,[152] *FHL1* that encodes four-and-a-half LIM protein,[412] *MYH7* encoding for MyHC 7,[414] and *ACTA1* that encodes alpha-actin.[415] Mutations in *DES* and *FHL1* are also associated with MFM, while mutations in *MYH7* are associated with Laing-type distal myopathy as will be discussed in a later section. Mutations in *FHL1* also cause reducing body myopathy. Mutations in *FHL1*, *MYH7*, and *ACTA1* are discussed in more detail in Chapter 28 regarding Congenital Myopathies.

Treatment

There are no reported studies regarding medical therapy in scapuloperoneal muscular dystrophy. Ankle–foot orthoses are beneficial in patients with ankle dorsiflexor weakness. Surgery to stabilize the scapula may improve arm function in some patients.

EMERY DREIFUSS MUSCULAR DYSTROPHY (EDMD)

There are at least seven subtypes of EDMD that have been associated with mutations in *EMD* (EDMD1), *LMNA* (EDMD2 and EDMD3), *SYNE1* (EDMD4), *SYNE2* (EDMD5), *FHL1*, (EDMD6), *TMEM43* (EDMD7), encoding emerin, lamin A/C, nesprin-1, nesprin-2, FHL1, and LUMA, respectively.[416] Mutations in *EMD* and *FHL* lead to X-linked inheritance while the others can be autosomal dominant (*LMNA*, *SYNE1*, *SYNE2*, *TMEM43*) or autosomal recessive (*LMNA*). As the clinical phenotypes are similar, we will discuss these together.

Clinical Features

EDMD is characterized by (1) early contractures of the Achilles tendons, elbows, and posterior cervical muscles; (2) slowly progressive muscle atrophy and weakness, with a predominantly humeroperoneal distribution in early stages; and (3) cardiomyopathy with conduction defects.[4,416–426] Scapular winging is common. Prominent contractures are evident in early childhood or in the teenage years, with an inability to fully extend the elbows secondary to elbow flexion contractures (Fig. 27-24). Patients may toe walk due to early heel cord contractures. There is reduced mobility of the spine such that EDMD is in the differential diagnosis of the so-called "rigid spine syndrome."[419,426] Patients have

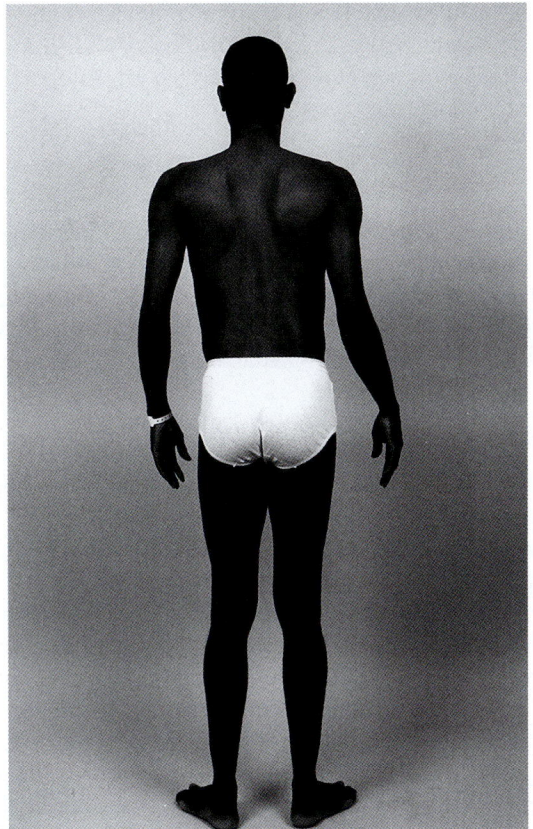

Figure 27-24. Emery–Dreifuss muscular dystrophy (EDMD). Posterior view of a patient with EDMD demonstrates atrophy of the triceps musculature, left more than right, and early contractures of the elbows (patient is unable to straighten the arms down at the side). There is also mild scapular winging.

difficulty flexing their neck and trunk. Importantly, the contractures of the Achilles tendons, elbows, and paraspinal muscles are evident before there is any significant weakness, which helps distinguish EDMD from other types of dystrophies associated with contractures.

Patients with EDMD usually appear normal at birth. Some children develop mild weakness. The characteristic pattern of muscle involvement helps distinguish EDMD from most other forms of dystrophy. There is an early predilection for weakness and atrophy affecting the humeroperoneal muscles (i.e., biceps brachii, triceps, anterior tibial, and peroneal muscles). Pes cavus deformities of the feet are common. Weakness is slowly progressive, and eventually the shoulder- and pelvic-girdle muscles can become involved. Most affected individuals are able to ambulate into the third decade. Unlike many of the LGMDs, which it may be confused with, there is no calf hypertrophy. Muscle stretch reflexes are diminished or absent early in the disease.

Importantly, EDMD is associated with potentially lethal cardiac arrhythmias by the end of the second or beginning of the third decade. Conduction defects range from first-degree A-V block to complete heart block. Syncope and sudden cardiac death can occur. Although women carriers do not manifest muscle weakness or contractures, they may develop a cardiopathy. Affected individuals with *FHL1* mutations (see below) are more apt to develop ventilatory muscle failure.[416,421–424]

Laboratory Features

The serum CK levels may be normal or moderately elevated. EKG frequently reveals sinus bradycardia, prolongation of the PR interval, or more severe degrees of conduction block. Motor and sensory NCSs are typically normal in these patients. EMG reveals myopathic MUAPs.

Histopathology

The muscle biopsy findings can be quite varied, depending on the degree of weakness of the biopsied muscle.[4,416,420,421,425,426] There is usually muscle fiber size variation with type 1 fiber atrophy. There can be a predominance of either type 1 or type 2 muscle fibers. Muscle fiber splitting, increased central nuclei, and endomysial fibrosis may be seen. Immunohistochemistry reveals the absence of emerin as well as abnormal lamin A/C and lamin B2 on the nuclear membrane.[26,27] Ultrastructural studies demonstrate the focal absence of peripheral heterochromatin in areas between the nuclear pores, irregular and uniform thickening of the nuclear lamina, and compaction of heterochromatin in areas of irregular thickening of the nuclear lamina as well as areas where the peripheral heterochromatin does not adhere to the nuclear lamina.[27] Diagnosis can be confirmed by immunostaining muscle or skin tissue for emerin or by immunoblot analysis of leukocytes.

Muscle biopsies in patients with *FHL1* mutations (EDMD6, see below) can be distinguished from those with more common emerin mutations (EDMD1) as the former reveals reducing bodies, cytoplasmic bodies, and sometimes features of MFM.[4,416,421,425,426]

Molecular Genetics and Pathogenesis

EDMD1 (EDMD-X1) is caused by mutations in *EMD* located on chromosome Xq28, which encodes for emerin (Table 27-1).[4,416] EDMD2 is caused by autosomal-dominant mutations in LMNA (previously also known as LGMD1B).[29,30,121,416,427] De novo mutations are responsible for 76% of cases; therefore, mutations in *LMNA* should be considered in all autosomal dominant and sporadic cases of EDMD as well as familial dilated cardiopathy.[29] EDMD3 is rarer and caused by autosomal-recessive mutations in *LMNA*. Interestingly, the clinical phenotypes associated with *LMNA* mutations are quite broad and include "dropped head syndrome," a form of autosomal-recessive axonal CMT neuropathy, an isolated autosomal-dominant dilated cardiomyopathy with conduction defect, and familial partial lipodystrophy.[416] Mutations in EMD and LMNA account for approximately 40% of cases.[416] EDMD4 and EDMD5 are caused by mutations in *SYNE1* and *SYNE2* that encoded for nesprin-1 and nesprin-2, respectively.[416,428] Mutations in *FHL1* that encodes the four-and-a-half LIM1 protein can present with an EDMD phenotype (EDMD6) or as a scapuloperoneal myopathy, an MFM, reducing body myopathy, X-linked myopathy with postural muscle atrophy, rigid spine syndrome, or isolated hypertrophic cardiomyopathy.[4,416,421–426] Autosomal-dominant EDMD is caused by mutations in *TMEM43* that encodes for transmembrane protein 43 or LUMA.[417,429]

Emerin is located on the inner nuclear membranes of skeletal, cardiac, and smooth muscle fibers as well as skin cells.[26–28,416] Its carboxy-terminal tail anchors the protein to the inner nuclear membrane, while the remainder of the protein projects into the nucleoplasm. Emerin is a member of the nuclear LAP family. The nuclear lamina is composed of intermediate-sized filaments (e.g., lamins A, B, and C) associated with the nucleoplasmic surface of the inner nuclear membrane. These lamins bind to various LAPs, including LAP1, LAP2, and lamin B receptor, which are located on the inner nuclear membrane. LAP2, lamin B receptor, and the lamins also bind to chromatin and thereby promote its attachment to the nuclear membrane.[348] Nesprin-1 and -2 (*n*uclear *e*nvelope *sp*ectrin *r*epeat *i*roteins) are spectrin-repeat containing proteins that are anchored in the outer and inner nuclear membranes.[416,428] Nesprin-1 and -2 are transcribed from two genes, *SYNE1* on chromosome 6q24 and *SYNE2* on chromosome 14q23. Nesprin-1 and -2 bind actin and both emerin and lamins A/C, thereby linking the nuclear lamina with the actin cytoskeleton. Transmembrane protein 43 or LUMA is also a nuclear envelope protein that binds emerin and lamin A/C. Mutations in *EMD*, *LMNA*, *SYNE1*, *SYNE2*, *FHL1*, and *TMEM43* lead to disorganization of the nuclear lamina and heterochromatin that is apparent on EM and immunohistochemistry.[416] The myopathies associated with these have also been categorized as nuclear "envelopathies." The pathogenic basis of myopathies caused by FHL1 mutations is unclear.

Diagnostic Approach and Treatment

In patients with clear X-linked inheritance we used to first check for mutations in *EDM*. However, the genes associated with EDMD often come in panels with other muscular dystrophies that are often cheaper and even free. Nonetheless, the algorithm of testing individual genes based on clinical phenotype are still valuable, as discussed in the LGMD section (Figs. 27-8 and 27-25).[4]

We obtain EKGs and echocardiograms on all our patients (as well as on possible female carriers) and longer cardiac monitoring and cardiology consultations on those with abnormalities (e.g., atrioventricular block) or cardiac symptoms. Affected individuals may require pacemakers or intracardiac defibrillators, and some authorities even recommend these prophylactically.[4,416] Those patients with reduced cardiac ejection fraction are treated with angiotensin-converting enzyme inhibitors or angiotensin

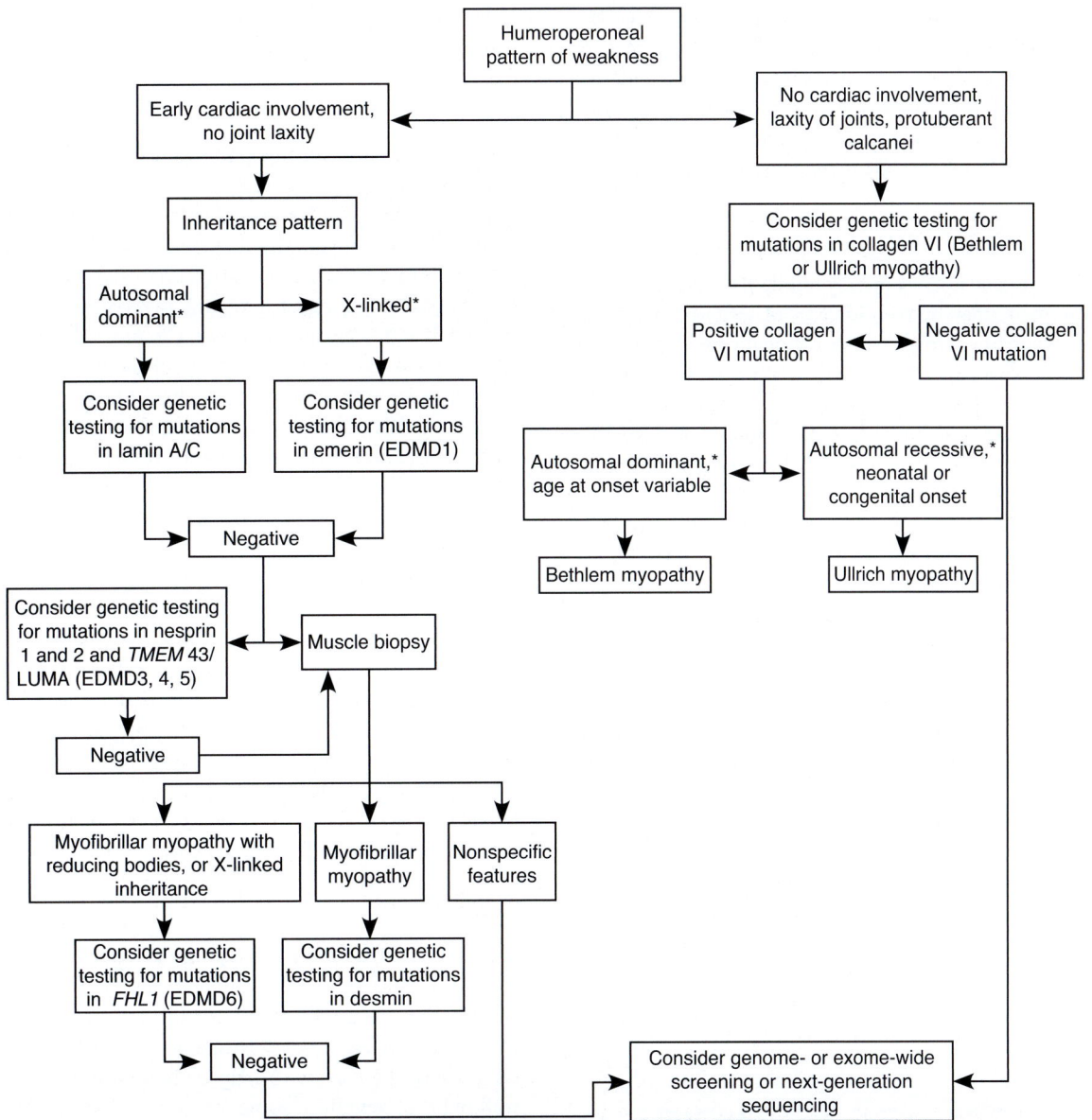

Figure 27-25. Diagnostic approach to patients with a humeroperoneal pattern of weakness and suspected muscular dystrophy (Emery–Dreifuss muscular dystrophy). *Autosomal-dominant, autosomal-recessive, or X-linked inheritance may be responsible in sporadic cases. EDMD, Emery–Dreifuss muscular dystrophy. (Reproduced with permission from Narayanaswami P, Weiss M, Selcen D, et al. Evidence-based guideline summary: diagnosis and treatment of limb-girdle and distal dystrophies: report of the guideline development subcommittee of the American Academy of Neurology and the practice issues review panel of the American Association of Neuromuscular & Electrodiagnostic Medicine. Neurology. 2014;83(16):1453–1463.)

receptor. Some patients benefit from heart transplantation. Physical therapy is aimed at minimizing contractures.

BENT SPINE/DROPPED HEAD SYNDROME

Clinical Features

Neck extensor weakness can be an early and prominent manifestation of several disorders, in particular myasthenia gravis and ALS.[430] However, there are a number of patients with weakness that remains restricted to the cervical and, sometimes, also to the thoracic and paraspinal muscles leading to bent spine syndrome or camptocormia.[430–432] The differential diagnosis is broad (see Chapter 1, Table 1-11). Onset of neck extensor weakness usually begins after 60 years of age, leading to progressive head drop. Involvement of the thoracic paraspinal muscles leads to severe kyphosis or the bent spine posture upon standing (see Chapter 2, Fig. 2-32). When affected individuals patients are supine, their spines straighten, in contrast to patients with fixed contractures of the spine. Weakness may remain clinically isolated to the neck extensors even for several years, although there may be subclinical (radiographic or electromyographic) evidence of disease in the upper thoracic paraspinal muscles. In addition, mild shoulder-girdle weakness may also develop. A family history of bent spine syndrome has been described.[431]

Laboratory Features

Serum CK is usually normal or only mildly elevated. Monoclonal gammopathy may be seen in cases of sporadic late-onset nemaline myopathy, which can occasionally present with a neck extensor myopathy.[433] CT and MRI of the low cervical and upper thoracic spine reveal atrophy and fatty or edematous changes in the paraspinal muscles (see Chapter 2, Fig. 2-32A). Motor and sensory NCSs are normal. EMG reveals fibrillation potentials and positive sharp waves in cervical and thoracic paraspinals.[430,431] Short-duration, small-amplitude MUAPs with early recruitment are seen in the cervical and thoracic paraspinal muscles. EMG of the arms and legs is typically normal.

Histopathology

Muscle biopsies of the cervical paraspinal muscles demonstrate nonspecific myopathic features, including variability in fiber size with atrophic and hypertrophic muscle fibers, increased internalized nuclei, fibers with rimmed vacuoles, fiber splitting, moth-eaten fibers, and increased endomysial connective tissue. Rarely, there is endomysial inflammation. Biopsies of proximal limb muscles may be normal or may demonstrate similar, but less prominent, abnormalities. Ragged red fibers and cytochrome C oxidase (COX)-negative fibers suggestive of mitochondrial dysfunction are not uncommon but may be age related. Cores and minicores may also be appreciated in some cases (Fig. 27-26).[434,435]

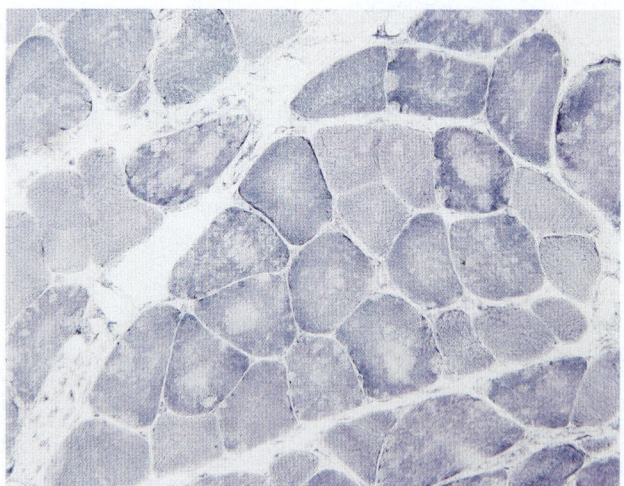

Figure 27-26. Muscle biopsy in patient with bent spine syndrome and ryanodine receptor gene (*RYR1*) mutation demonstrates central cores, multiminicores, and moth-eaten fibers, NADH × 20×.

Late-onset nemaline myopathy also can occasionally present initially as an axial myopathy.[433]

Pathogenesis

Isolated neck extensor myopathy may just represent a "forme fruste" of the bent spine syndrome. The cause of axial myopathy is heterogeneous (see Table 1-11 in Chapter 1). In some cases, the myopathy may be the result of a monophasic inflammatory process restricted to the paraspinal muscles. Sporadic late onset nemaline myopathy (SLONM) can manifest with this pattern (see Chapter 28). We suspect that in most cases this disorder represents a regional form of muscular dystrophy or other hereditary myopathy that predominantly affects the paraspinal muscles. Rarely, dysferlinopathies and FSHD can present with a paraspinal myopathy that can lead to camptocormia. Myotonic dystrophies and late-onset Pompe disease have also been described to manifest initially with head drop or bent spine syndrome. We have seen McArdle disease manifest as bent spine syndrome without any history of exercise intolerance. Several series have reported mutations in *RYR1* (ryanodine receptor), and this has been one of the most common identifiable etiologies that we have encountered.[434,435] *RYR1* mutations are more commonly associated with other phenotypes such as malignant hyperthermia or congenital myopathy with central cores (see Chapter 28 on Congenital Myopathies). Mutations have also been reported in the myosin heavy chain 7 gene, *MHY7*, that more typically leads to Laing type distal myopathy.[436]

Treatment

We refer patients for PT to assist in their gait. Cervical collars (e.g., Headmaster Collar) may help stabilize the head drop. Back braces are usually cumbersome and do not help much in our experience. Use of a rollator walk such that patients can extend their arms to help straighten their backs when walking is of benefit in some.

OCULOPHARYNGEAL MUSCULAR DYSTROPHY

Clinical Features

OPMD is an autosomal-dominant disorder, which usually presents in the fourth to sixth decades of life with increasing ptosis.[437–442] The ptosis is almost always bilateral but can be asymmetric. The extraocular muscles are involved in approximately 50% of patients but are often subtle and double vision is uncommon. The pupils are spared. Approximately one-fourth of patients manifests initially with dysphagia, which is slowly progressive and leads to severe weight loss and aspiration.[438] Facial and masticatory muscles may be slightly weak in some patients. The gag reflex is impaired. Laryngeal involvement can also develop, resulting in dysphonia.

Some patients develop slight weakness of the neck and proximal limbs. Distal muscles weakness may also occur, particularly in the distal oculopharyngeal dystrophy variant (see below). Sensation is normal, but muscle stretch reflexes can be reduced or absent. Life span is not altered.

Laboratory Features

Serum CK levels are normal or only mildly elevated. Swallowing studies demonstrate impaired pharyngeal and esophageal motility. An MRI study on 168 patients with OPMD revealed fatty replacement with a predilection for the most commonly affected muscles, including the tongue, adductor magnus, and soleus muscles.[442] Muscle ultrasound has also been used to demonstrate fatty replacement in affected muscles.[443]

Histopathology

The muscles most severely affected are the extraocular and pharyngeal muscles, although minor abnormalities may be detectable in the limb muscles in advanced cases. Muscle biopsies reveal variation in fiber size, degenerating and regenerating fibers, increased internal nuclei, and an increase in adipose and endomysial connective tissue.[437,438] Rimmed vacuoles similar to those found in inclusion body myositis/myopathy and some of the distal myopathies are often, although not universally, observed. On EM, intranuclear inclusions are evident in up to 9% of muscle nuclei.[443] These tubulofilamentous inclusions have an outer diameter of approximately 8.5 nm and an inner diameter of 3 nm, are up to 0.25 μm in length, and are often arranged in tangles or palisades.[443] In addition, 15–18-nm tubulofilaments may be evident in the cytoplasm, as seen in IBM, h-IBM, and some of the distal myopathies. OPMD can be distinguished from various mitochondrial myopathies, which can also cause ptosis and ophthalmoparesis, by the lack of ragged red fibers. However, there have been a few cases of OPMD with abnormal mitochondrial structure and quantity on EM, although these findings, for the most part, are suspected to be age related. Further, muscle biopsies of pharyngeal muscles (taken at the time of cricopharyngeal myotomy-anecdotal observations) reveal more severe abnormalities along with frequent rimmed vacuoles, ragged red fibers, and nemaline rods. Sural nerve biopsy in a few patients revealed a mild reduction in myelinated and unmyelinated nerve fibers; however, this could be a confounding variable related to the patients' advanced ages.

Molecular Genetics and Pathogenesis

OPMD is caused by expansions of a short GCG repeat within the first exon of PABPN1 located on chromosome 14q11.1 that encodes for poly(A)-binding protein-2 (PABP2) (Table 27-1).[437–440] Normally, there are 10 GCG repeats encoding for a polyalanine tract at the N-terminus of the protein. In OPMD, there is an expansion to 11–18 repeats.[439,440] These expansions are meiotically stable, explaining the lack of anticipation phenomena from one generation to the next. Patients who are homozygous for GCG expansions may manifest at an earlier age and have more severe weakness.

The PABP2 protein is found mostly in dimeric and oligomeric forms with the nuclei (Fig. 27-1).[439,440,444,445] PABP2 is involved in polyadenylation of mRNA and is adjoined to the polyadenylated mRNA complex for transport through the nuclei pores into the cytoplasm. In the cytoplasm, the PABP2 detaches from the mRNA. The mRNA is translated into protein, and the PABP2 is actively transported back into the nuclei. The expansion of the GCG repeats probably results in abnormal folding of the polyalanine domains of PABP2. The misfolded proteins are ubiquitinated but are resistant to nuclear proteasomal degradation. The abnormal PABP2 oligomers then accumulate as the 8.5-nm intranuclear tubulofilamentous inclusions apparent on EM.[444–446] The more severe clinical phenotypes are associated with a large number of myonuclei containing intranuclear inclusions.[445] The aggregation of mutated PAPBN1 may lead to disruption of various nuclear or cytoplasmic processes leading to cell death. Speculated pathogenic mechanisms include: (1) direct toxicity of the intranuclear aggregates; (2) the intranuclear sequestration of essential transcription factors, molecular chaperones, RNA-binding proteins, and RNAs by these intranuclear aggregates; (3) the abnormal PABPN1 protein suppresses the function of wild-type protein.[439,440]

Treatment

Noninvasive therapies include the use of eyelid crutches on glasses or even taping the eyelids, neither of which are commonly popular with patients due to the mechanical irritation of the eyelids they create. Ptosis surgery can also be performed, if patients have sufficient orbicularis oculi strength to allow complete closure of the eyelids postoperatively. There is the risk of corneal abrasions and keratitis if the eyelids cannot close completely. Cricopharyngeal myotomy may be beneficial in patients with dysphagia. Patients with severe dysphagia resulting in aspiration or significant weight loss require a feeding tube.

OCULOPHARYNGEAL DISTAL MYOPATHY

Clinical Features

OPDM is characterized by adult-onset ptosis, external ophthalmoplegia, facial muscle weakness, distal limb muscle weakness and atrophy, and pharyngeal involvement, resulting in dysphagia and dysarthria.[447–457] Occasional patients manifest with only ptosis without pharyngeal or distal weakness.[449]

Laboratory Features

Serum CK levels are normal or only mildly elevated. EMG is myopathic and may show myotonic discharges. Swallowing studies demonstrate impaired pharyngeal and esophageal motility.

Histopathology

Muscle biopsies of affected muscles show dystrophic features with rimmed vacuoles. Intra-myonuclear inclusions that immunostain with anti–phospho-p62/SQSTM1 antibodies are apparent.[452] Intranuclear inclusions are also seen on skin biopsies.[453]

Molecular Genetics and Pathogenesis

OPDM is a genetically heterogeneous autosomal disorder caused by trinucleotide repeat expansions (CTG) in the 5′ UTR regions of *LRP12* (OPDM1), *G1PC1* (OPDM2), *NOTCH2NLC* (OPDM3), and *RILPL1* (OPMD4).[449–452,454–456] The CGG repeat expansion in *NOTCH2NLC* is also the cause of neuronal intranuclear hyaline inclusion disease and other neurodegenerative diseases affecting the brain. Possible pathogenic mechanisms of these repeat expansion disorders include the loss of function of the protein by interfering normal transcription, RNA-mediated sequestration of RNA-binding proteins, and the translation of toxic repeat peptides.

DISTAL MYOPATHY/MUSCULAR DYSTROPHY

Although distal weakness is often presumed to be neuropathic in etiology, a variety of neuromuscular disorders, including myopathies, are associated with distal extremity weakness (Table 27-1, Fig. 27-27).[4,457,458] The distal myopathies are characterized clinically by progressive atrophy and weakness of distal arm or leg muscles and histologically by nonspecific myopathic features on muscle biopsy. We consider many of the distal myopathies to be forms of muscular dystrophy. Advances in the molecular genetics of these disorders support this notion, as some types of distal myopathy have been found to be allelic with specific types of LGMD, as previously discussed. Furthermore, there is a clear overlap of some distal myopathies with some forms of h-IBM and MFM. The distal myopathies can be subdivided based on the clinical features, age of onset, CK levels, muscle histology, and mode of inheritance. At the time of this writing, mutations in 19 genes are known to cause an autosomal-dominant distal myopathy (*ACTN2, CAV3, CRYAB, DNAJB6, DNM2, FLNC, HNRNPA1, HSPB8, KHLH9, LDB3, MATR3, MB, MYOT, PLIN4, TIA1, VCP, NOTCH2NLC, LRP12, GIPS1*), mutations in four genes (*ADSSL, ANO5, DYSF, GNE*) result in an autosomal-recessive distal myopathy; and mutations in five genes can lead to either a dominant or a recessive distal myopathy (*DES, MYH7, NEB, RYR1,* and *TTN*).[457] Many of the myopathies associated with mutations are covered in other sections, but below we cover the more common hereditary distal myopathies.

WELANDER DISTAL MYOPATHY

Clinical Features

Welander originally described the features of this autosomal-dominant myopathy in a report of 249 cases from 72 Scandinavian families.[381] Onset of weakness usually begins in the fifth decade of life, with rare cases beginning before the age of 30 years (mean age of onset 47 years, range 20–77 years). Weakness is usually first noted in the wrist and finger extensors and slowly progresses to involve the distal lower limbs—ankle dorsiflexors more than the plantar flexors.[4,457–462] However, in approximately 10% of cases, weakness is initially appreciated in the legs, or there is simultaneous involvement of the distal arms and legs. Although the extensor muscle groups are more severely affected, the flexor groups are involved in over 40% of cases. Rarely, proximal muscles become weak. Sensation is usually normal. Muscle stretch reflexes are initially preserved, but the brachioradialis and Achilles reflexes diminish or disappear over time.

Laboratory Features

Serum CK levels are usually normal or only minimally abnormal.[2] Motor and sensory NCSs are usually normal for age. Some patients have diminished temperature and vibratory perception quantitative sensory testing.[460–462] Needle EMG demonstrates early recruitment of small-amplitude, short-duration MUAPs.[4,460–462] Quantitative EMG further suggests a myopathic process.[460]

Histopathology

Muscle biopsies demonstrate variability in fiber size, increased central nuclei, split fibers, and increased endomysial connective tissue and adipose cells in longstanding disease.[4,460–464] Furthermore, rimmed vacuoles typical of IBM, h-IBM, and OPMD are seen in scattered muscle fibers. EM also reveals 15–18-nm cytoplasmic and nuclear filaments similar to those observed in IBM, h-IBM, and OPMD. In addition, disruption of myofibrils and accumulation of Z-disc–derived material similar to that found in MFM can also be demonstrated. Nerve biopsies may reveal a moderate reduction of mainly small-diameter, myelinated fibers.[462]

Molecular Genetics and Pathogenesis

Welander myopathy is caused by mutations in the *TIA1* gene that encodes an RNA-binding protein involved in the alternative splicing of specific pre-mRNAs.[465] The TIA1 protein appears to aggregate in granules in muscle biopsy in patients with Welander myopathy. The mutations in *TIA1* may make the transcribed protein more prone to self-aggregation and aggregate with other proteins as well as interfere with normal splicing of mRNA.[465,466] Interestingly, a rare digenic disorder is seen in patients who, while they lack the typical *TIA1* mutation, instead have a polymorphism in the *TIA1* gene along with a mutation in *SQSTM1* that encodes for p62 or sequestome.[467] Mutations in *SQSTM1* typically cause MSP leading to h-IBM, motor neuron disease, frontotemporal dementia (FTD) and PDM, but when combined with this *TIA1* polymorphism only the myopathy occurs.

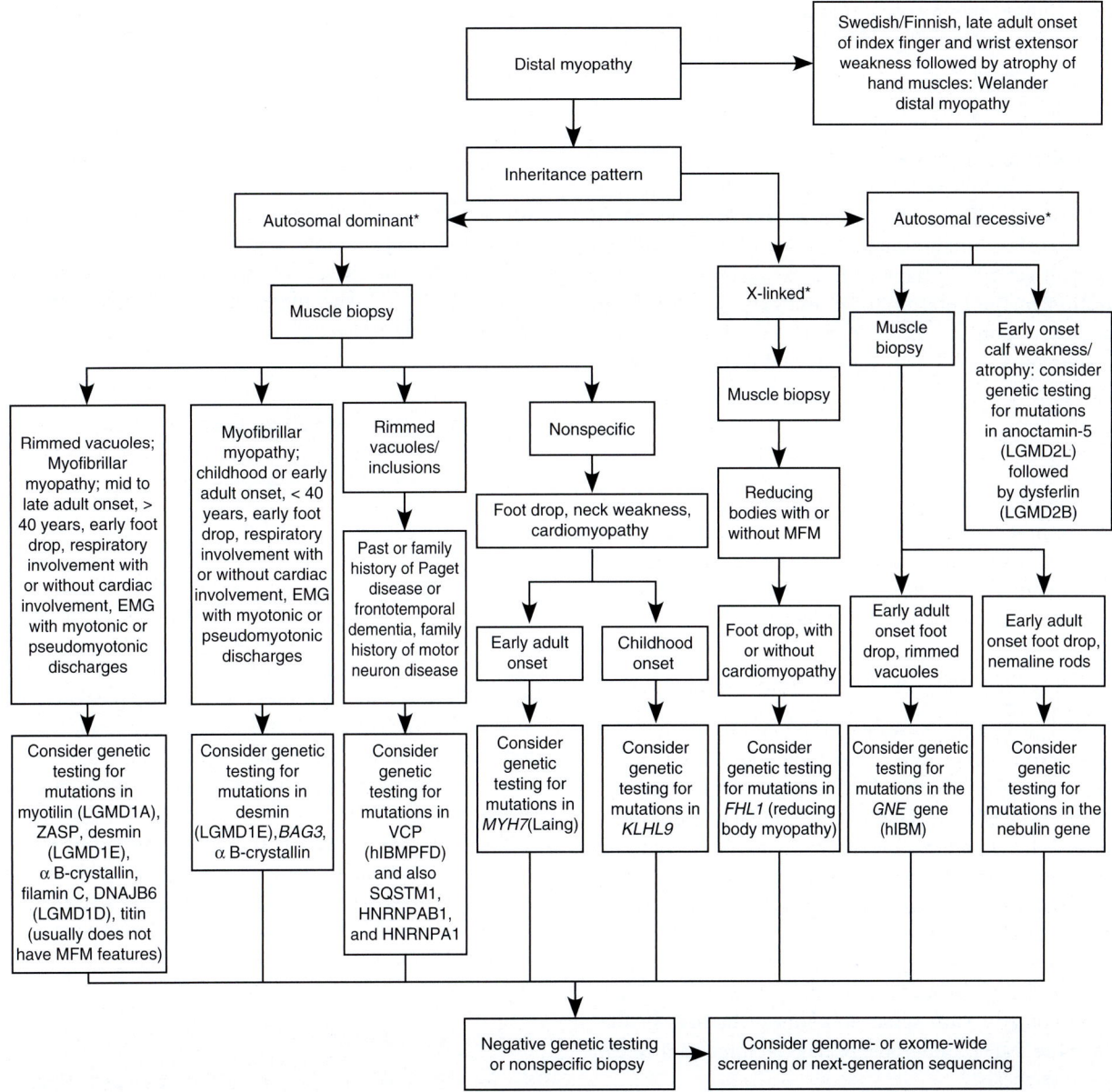

Figure 27-27. Diagnostic approach to patients with a distal pattern of weakness and suspected muscular dystrophy. *Autosomal-dominant, autosomal-recessive, or X-linked inheritance may be responsible in sporadic cases. h-IBM, hereditary inclusion body myopathy; h-IBMPFD, hereditary inclusion body myopathy with Paget disease and frontotemporal dementia. (Reproduced with permission from Narayanaswami P, Weiss M, Selcen D, et al. Evidence-based guideline summary: diagnosis and treatment of limb-girdle and distal dystrophies: report of the guideline development subcommittee of the American Academy of Neurology and the practice issues review panel of the American Association of Neuromuscular & Electrodiagnostic Medicine. *Neurology*. 2014;83(16):1453–1463.)

UDD DISTAL MYOPATHY

Clinical Features

As previously discussed, this autosomal-dominant distal myopathy is associated with mutations in the *TTN*. Udd distal myopathy usually presents after the age of 35 years (usually in the fifth to seventh decades), with weakness of the anterior compartment of the lower legs resulting in unilateral or bilateral foot drop.[4,242–253,457,458] The disorder is slowly progressive, beginning in the toe extensors and gradually involving anterior tibial muscles. Occasionally, the proximal legs and distal upper limbs (predominately the hand intrinsics and wrist extensors) are affected. Rarely, the arms are affected more than the legs, posterior calves are involved with sparing of the anterior tibial muscles, or patients have a limb-girdle distribution of weakness.[242] Facial muscles are usually spared, although bulbar weakness has been reported. Sensation is normal. Achilles tendon reflexes are usually reduced. Unlike other forms of titinopathy, cardiac and ventilatory muscles are usually spared in Udd distal myopathy.

Laboratory Features

Serum CK is normal or only slightly elevated.[4,242–253,457,458] Motor and sensory NCSs are normal. EMG of affected muscles reveals fibrillation potentials and positive sharp waves as well as small-amplitude, brief-duration MUAPs that recruit early.[4,245] Imaging scans of muscle reveal fatty infiltration in the anterior tibial and extensor digitorum longus more than the gastrocnemius muscles; the proximal pelvic muscles, gluteus medius and minimus may be affected later.[243,248]

Histopathology

Muscle biopsies reveal dystrophic features and muscle fibers with rimmed vacuoles.[4,235,457,458] Other features of MFM are usually not seen in titinopathy manifesting with the Udd distal myopathy but may be seen in those with the HMERF presentation, as discussed in the Titinopathy section.

Molecular Genetics and Pathogenesis

Udd distal myopathy is caused by mutations in the *TTN* gene on chromosome 2q31–33 encoding for titin.[4,457,458,468] As previously discussed, the disorder is allelic to autosomal-recessive LGMDJ/LGMDR10 and autosomal-dominant HMERF. Why dominant mutations in the *TTN* typically lead to such different phenotypes and inheritance pattern is not entirely clear. A confounding factor is the variability of clinical phenotype sometimes seen even within families. The giant protein titin (also known as connectin) is attached to the Z-disc and spans from the M- to the Z-line of the sarcomere. Titin serves to connect the myosin filaments to the Z-disc and probably plays an important role in myofibrillogenesis.

MARKESBERY–GRIGGS DISTAL MYOPATHY

Clinical Features

This is another late-onset, autosomal-dominant distal myopathy, typically beginning in the anterior compartment of the legs with onset in third to eighth decades of life.[4,457,458,469,470] Patients can later develop proximal leg and distal arm weakness (wrist and finger extensors). A dilated cardiomyopathy is common.

Laboratory Features

Serum CK is normal or only mildly elevated. Motor and sensory NCSs are usually normal. Serum CK is usually mildly elevated, and EMG reveals features of a myopathy with muscle membrane irritability.

Histopathology

Muscle biopsies demonstrate rimmed vacuoles and features of MFM.

Molecular Genetics and Pathogenesis

Markesbery–Griggs distal myopathy is caused by mutations in LIM domain-binding 3 gene (*LDB3*) that encodes for Z-band alternatively spliced PDZ-motif–containing protein or ZASP.[4,457,458,470] The mutation leads to disruption of actin filaments and the Z-disc.[471]

GNE MYOPATHY (NONAKA DISTAL MYOPATHY OR AUTOSOMAL-RECESSIVE INCLUSION BODY MYOPATHY)

Clinical Features

This autosomal-recessive myopathy was initially reported in Japan,[4,457,458,472–475] but it occurs worldwide and is allelic to autosomal-recessive inclusion body *myopathy* (h-IBM type 1).[4,476–479] The preferred term now is "GNE myopathy." Affected individuals usually develop weakness of the anterior compartment of the distal lower limb, leading to foot drop in the second or third decade of life. The posterior compartment of the legs and distal upper-limb muscles are also affected early, but to a lesser degree. The proximal arm and leg muscles, as well as the neck flexors, become weak over time. The quadriceps may become affected but usually remain relatively spared compared to other muscle groups, as are ocular and bulbar muscles. Sensation is normal. Muscle stretch reflexes can be normal or absent.

Laboratory Features

Serum CK is normal or only mildly elevated. Motor and sensory NCSs are usually normal. EMG reveals positive sharp waves and early recruitment of small-amplitude, brief-duration MUAPs in weak muscles. Skeletal muscle MRI and ultrasound demonstrate muscle atrophy and fatty replacement of affected muscle groups.[402]

Histopathology

Muscle biopsies demonstrate rimmed vacuoles with muscle fibers as well as other nonspecific myopathic features, as described in the other forms of distal myopathy.[4,457,458,472–478] Because of the frequent rimmed vacuoles, the biopsy can be erroneously interpreted as sporadic inclusion body *myositis* (s-IBM). However, inflammation cell infiltrate and major histochemistry antigen 1 expression on muscle fibers are usually absent. EM can demonstrate 15–18-nm intranuclear and cytoplasmic tubulofilaments similar to that found in sporadic IBM.

Molecular Genetics and Pathogenesis

This myopathy is caused by mutations in the *GNE* gene on chromosome 9p1–q1 that encodes for UDP-*N*-acetylglucosamine 2-epimerase/*N*-acetylmannosamine kinase.[4,457,458,477,479,480] This is an enzyme that is important in the production of sialic acid. However, the exact pathogenic mechanism is unclear and may involve reduced production of sialic acid that is located on muscle membranes, impaired posttranslational glycosylation of muscle membrane proteins, or some other mechanism.[477]

MIYOSHI DISTAL MYOPATHY

Miyoshi myopathy is a genetically heterogeneous disorder associated with early adult onset of calf atrophy and weakness with markedly elevated serum CKs. It is caused by mutations in the dysferlin and anoctamin-5 genes and was discussed in greater detail in the sections on LGMD2B/LGMDR2 and LGMD2L/LGMDR12, respectively.

LAING DISTAL MYOPATHY

Clinical Features

Laing and colleagues initially described an Australian family with dominant inheritance (nine affected members over four generations) with weakness beginning in the anterior compartment of the distal lower limbs and neck flexors between the ages of 4 and 25 years.[481] Subsequently, this myopathy has been widely reported.[4,436,482–486] Over time, there is involvement of finger extensors and later, to a lesser extent, the shoulder- and hip-girdle muscles. Finger flexors and hand intrinsic muscles are spared. Scapular winging, scoliosis, pes cavus, ankle contractures, and/or lumbar hyperlordosis are seen in approximately 50% of patients. Hand tremor may occur.

Laboratory Features

Serum CK is normal or slightly elevated.[4,481,484,485] Motor and sensory NCSs are normal. EMG reveals occasional fibrillation potentials and positive sharp waves and small-amplitude, short-duration, polyphasic MUAPs in distal more than proximal muscles.

Histopathology

Muscle biopsies demonstrate nonspecific myopathic features. Rimmed vacuoles are not seen. Large deposits of MyHC in the subsarcolemmal region of type 1 muscle fibers led some authorities to label this as a form of myosin storage myopathy.[22,487–491]

Molecular Genetics and Pathogenesis

Laing distal myopathy is caused by mutations in the slow/beta cardiac MyHC 1 gene, *MYH7*, located on chromosome 14q.[4,488–491] MyHC is the major myosin isoform expressed in type 1 muscle fibers. Of note, mutations have also been identified in the *MYH7* in hyaline body myopathy (discussed in Chapter 28 on Congenital Myopathies). Mutations in *MYH7* are also a common cause of familial hypertrophic and dilated cardiomyopathy, although patients with the cardiomyopathy usually do not have much symptomatic skeletal muscle involvement and vice versa.[19] That said, we have followed patients with Laing myopathy, who also had a severe cardiomyopathy requiring transplantation, so cardiac evaluation in all patients is important. *MYH7* mutations can also lead to bent spine syndrome.[436]

WILLIAMS DISTAL MYOPATHY

Clinical Features

Williams distal myopathy is an autosomal-dominant disorder that manifests as progressive, predominantly lower extremity weakness that can affect proximal or distal muscles either in the arms or legs with an onset in the teens to fifth decade of life.[4,488–495] Some patients develop a cardiomyopathy.

Laboratory Features

Serum CK is usually mildly elevated, and EMG is myopathic. Muscle MRI may demonstrate fatty replacement in posterior compartment of the lower extremities.

Histopathology

Muscle biopsies may demonstrate features of MFM as will be discussed in a later section as well as nemaline rods.

Molecular Genetics and Pathogenesis

William distal myopathy is caused by mutations in the *FLNC* gene that encodes for filamin-C, an actin-binding protein felt to be important in cytoskeletal formation.

▶ OTHER DISTAL MYOPATHIES

DISTAL MYOPATHY WITH NEBULIN MUTATIONS

Mutations in the nebulin gene (*NEB*), although usually associated with nemaline myopathy with a congenital onset, can cause a later-onset distal myopathy with nemaline rods.[496,497] Such affected individuals develop slowly progressive weakness with foot drop along with finger extensor and neck flexor weakness later in childhood or in the teens. CK levels are normal or only slightly elevated. PFTs may reveal a reduced FVC.[496] Fatty degeneration in the anterior compartment of the lower legs may be apparent on skeletal muscle MRI.[496,497] The diagnosis is made by demonstration of nemaline bodies on muscle biopsy in patients with the characteristic phenotype and with confirmatory genetic testing.

DISTAL MYOPATHY WITH KELCH-LIKE HOMOLOGUE 9 (KLHL9) MUTATIONS

Mutations in *KLHL9* that encode for KELCH-like homologue 9 are also associated with progressive foot drop followed by intrinsic hand weakness with onset in the first or second decade of life.[498] Inheritance is autosomal dominant. Weakness is slowly progressive such that affected individuals may retain the ability to walk until late in life. CK levels are normal or mildly elevated. Muscle biopsies reveal nonspecific dystrophic changes without rimmed vacuoles.

ADSSL MYOPATHY

Most patients with this myopathy present with childhood onset of distal extremity and facial weakness that slowly progresses to proximal muscles by early adulthood.[498–504] However, rare patients manifest with predominantly proximal weakness. One patient presented with slowly progressive limb and ventilatory muscle weakness, dysphagia, and Brugada syndrome starting at the age of 56 years; he died of respiratory muscle weakness at the age of 66 years.[504] Serum CK is mildly elevated. Muscle biopsy may reveal rimmed vacuoles or nemaline rods. This autosomal-recessive myopathy is caused by mutations in the *ADSSL* gene that encodes the muscle isozyme of adenylosuccinate synthase, the enzyme catalyzing the initial reaction in the conversion of inosine monophosphate (IMP) to adenosine monophosphate (AMP).[498–504] Notably, mutations in *ADSSL1* are the most common cause of nemaline myopathy in Japan.[503]

PLIN4 MYOPATHY

This rare myopathy is associated with autosomal-dominant adult-onset distal myopathy[505,506] or a proximal myopathy.[507] Serum CK is mildly elevated, and EMG may show myotonic or complex repetitive discharges. Muscle MRI may show severe fatty replacement, with a predilection for the thigh adductors, vastus intermedius, vastus medialis, soleus, and gastrocnemius but relative sparing of the rectus femoris and gracilis. Muscle biopsies show fibers with rimmed vacuoles, lipid droplets, and ubiquitin/p62 protein aggregates. The myopathy is caused by 99 bp repeat expansions in the perilipin-4 gene, *PLIN4*.[506,507] Perilipin-4 is a member of the perilipin family, a group of proteins that coat the surface of lipid droplets. The mechanism on how mutations in the gene lead to myopathy is unclear.

▶ TREATMENT OF THE DISTAL MYOPATHIES

There are no specific medications currently available for distal myopathies. There are drug trials underway, however, for some distal myopathies (e.g., ManNAC in GNE myopathy: NCT04231266).[477] Physical and occupational therapy are the mainstays of treatment. Braces for lower limb weakness and other orthotic devices may be of benefit in improving gait and functional abilities.

▶ MYOFIBRILLAR MYOPATHY

MFM is a clinically and genetically heterogeneous group of disorders, characterized by the pathologic finding of myofibrillar disruption on EM and excessive desmin accumulation in muscle fibers.[4,23,24,149–151,508–517] Because desmin is not the only protein that accumulates, the term "MFM" was suggested to be a more accurate description of the spectrum of the histologic abnormalities.[509,513,517] This myopathy has been reported as desmin storage myopathy, desmin myopathy, familial desminopathy, spheroid body myopathy, cytoplasmic body myopathy, Mallory body myopathy, familial cardiomyopathy with subsarcolemmal vermiform deposits, myopathy with intrasarcoplasmic accumulation of dense granulofilamentous material, and h-IBM with early respiratory failure.[508] In addition, some cases previously diagnosed with other forms of distal myopathy (Markesbery–Griggs distal myopathy) have MFM histopathology.[469] MFM has been classified by some in the past as congenital myopathies, but are probably best considered a form of muscular dystrophy.

Clinical Features

As mentioned, MFM is associated with a wide spectrum of clinical phenotypes.[4,23,24,149–151,508–517] Most affected individuals develop weakness between 25 and 45 years of age, although weakness may be noticeable in infancy or may present later in adulthood. Weakness can be predominantly proximal, distal, or generalized. In addition, some patients have a facioscapulohumeral or scapuloperoneal distribution of weakness. Facial and pharyngeal muscles can also be affected in some individuals. Rigidity of the spine can also be seen.

In addition to skeletal muscle, the heart can also be affected, and cardiac arrhythmias and CHF may be the predominant features of the disease. In severe cardiomyopathies, pacemaker insertion or cardiac transplantation may be required. In addition, severe ventilatory muscle involvement can develop in MFM. Also, smooth muscle involvement may lead to intestinal pseudo-obstructions.

Laboratory Features

Serum CK is normal or usually only slightly increased in MFM.[4] EKGs may demonstrate conduction defects or arrhythmia, while echocardiograms may reveal a dilated or hypertrophic cardiomyopathy. NCSs are usually normal, although low CMAP and SNAP amplitudes and slowing of conduction velocities can be seen. EMG reveals increased insertional and spontaneous activity with fibrillation potentials, positive sharp waves, pseudomyotonic potentials, complex repetitive discharges, and early recruitment of short-duration, small-amplitude, polyphasic MUAPs.[4] Long-duration, large-amplitude MUAPs may also be seen, owing to the chronicity of the disorder.

Histopathology

Muscle biopsies reveal variability in fiber size, increased internalized nuclei, occasionally type 1 fiber predominance, and in some cases, scattered fibers with rimmed vacuoles.[4] In addition, Nakano et al. defined two major types of lesions on light microscopy and EM that characterize MFM: hyaline structures and nonhyaline lesions (Fig. 27-28).[513] The hyaline structures are cytoplasmic granular inclusions, which are typically eosinophilic on H&E and dark blue-green, or occasionally red, on modified Gomori trichrome stains. They do not stain for NADH. On EM, the hyaline lesions resemble

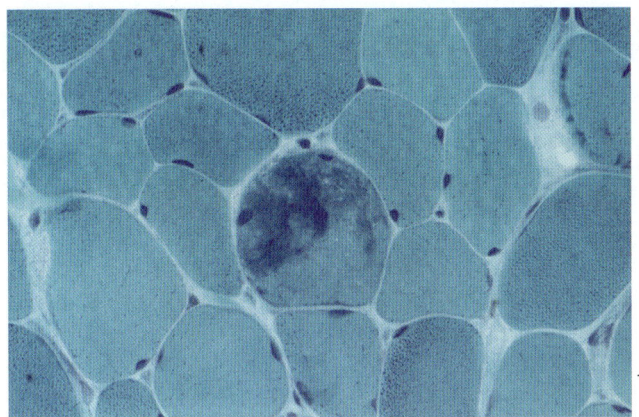

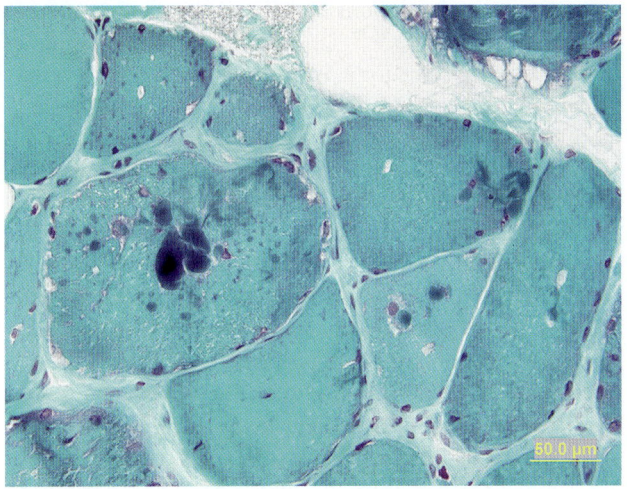

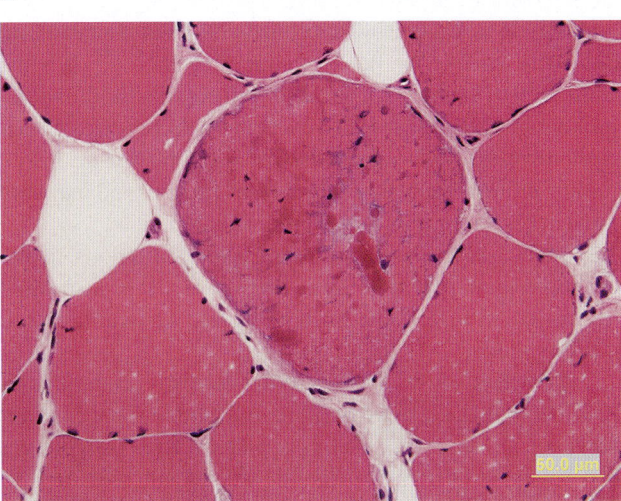

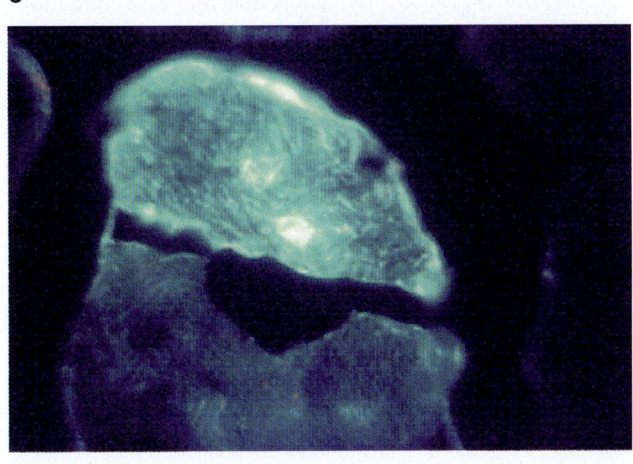

Figure 27-28. Myofibrillar myopathy. Nonhyaline lesions appear as amorphous accumulation of reddish-purple or dark green material (**A**), while the hyaline lesions are denser and can have the appearance of cytoplasmic or spheroid bodies (**B**) on trichrome stain. The hyaline lesions are eosinophilic on H&E but less well seen than on the trichrome stains (**C**). The hyaline and nonhyaline lesions do not stain with NADH-TR (**D**). Immunostaining reveals that the lesions are immunoreactive to desmin (**E**).

cytoplasmic, spheroid, or Mallory bodies. The nonhyaline lesions appear as dark green areas of amorphous material on Gomori trichrome stains. On EM, these nonhyaline lesions correspond to foci of myofibrillar destruction and consist of disrupted myofilaments, Z-disc–derived bodies, dappled dense structures of Z-disc origin, and streaming of the Z-disc.[513,515] In addition, larger-size tubulofilaments (14–20 nm) typical of the inclusion body myopathies may accumulate.

Immunohistochemistry reveals that both the hyaline and the nonhyaline lesions contain desmin and numerous other proteins.[4,25,149–151,508–517] Abnormal accumulation of desmin is not specific for MFM and can be seen in a variety of neuromuscular conditions, including X-linked myotubular myopathy, congenital myotonic dystrophy, spinal muscular atrophy, nemaline rod myopathy, fetal myotubes, IBM, and in regenerating muscle fibers of any etiology. Abnormal accumulation of desmin has been demonstrated in cardiac muscles in MFM patients with cardiomyopathy. Immunohistochemistry also reveals that the nonhyaline lesions react strongly not only for desmin, but also for dystrophin, gelsolin, N terminus of β-amyloid precursor protein, and NCAM in addition to desmin. In addition, the nonhyaline lesions are depleted of actin, α-actinin, myosin, and, less consistently, titin and nebulin. In contrast, the hyaline structures are composed of compacted and degraded remnants of thick and thin filaments that react to actin, α-actinin, and myosin, in addition to dystrophin, gelsolin, filamin-c, and the N terminus of β-amyloid precursor protein; they do not react to NCAM and react variably to desmin. Both types of lesions also react for αB-crystallin, α1 antichymotrypsin, and ubiquitin and can be congophilic. The abnormal muscle fibers also abnormally express several cyclin-dependent kinases (CDC/CDK) in the cytoplasm, including CDC2, CDK2, CDK4, and CDK7.[508,517] Laser capture microdissection and mass spectrometry to evaluate the proteomic profile may be useful in subtyping the aggregates in muscle fibers in patients with MFM.[518]

Nerve and intramuscular nerve biopsies have demonstrated enlarged axons with accumulation of intermediate-sized neurofilaments and formation of axonal spheroids in some patients.[519]

Molecular Genetics and Pathogenesis

MFM is a genetically heterogeneous disorder. The pathogenesis of MFM is likely related to disruption of the Z-disc.[4,23,24,515]

MFM1 is caused by mutations in the desmin gene, *DES*. It was previously classified autosomal-dominant LGMD1E but was reclassified as an MFM because of the histopathology as previously discussed.[4,149–157,515,520,521] Desmin is an intermediate filament protein of skeletal, cardiac, and some smooth muscle cells. This cytoskeletal protein links Z-bands with the sarcolemma and the nucleus. The intermediate filament network is important in the stability of the muscle fiber and during mitosis/regeneration of muscle cells. These abnormal desmin filaments form insoluble aggregates, which prevent the genesis of the normal filamentous network.

MFM2 is caused by autosomal-dominant mutations in the αB-crystallin gene, *CRYAB*.[4,522–525] αB-Crystallin possesses "molecular chaperone" activity and is felt to interact with desmin in the assembly of the intermediate filament network.

MFM3 is caused by mutations in the myotilin gene, *MYOT* and is allelic to LGMD1A as previously discussed.[4,23,114–119] Myotilin is a component of the Z-disc where it interacts with α-actinin, actin, and filamin-c and plays a fundamental role in myofibrillar assembly.

MFM4, also known as Markesbury–Griggs distal myopathy, is caused autosomal-dominant mutations in the *LDP3* gene that encodes for ZASP.[4,24,470] ZASP is expressed in skeletal and cardiac muscles, and it binds to α-actinin, a component of the Z-disc that in turn cross-links thin filaments of adjacent sarcomeres.[24]

MFM5 is caused by mutations in *FLNC* that encodes for filamin-C. It is allelic to Williams distal myopathy, as previously discussed.[4,25,488–495] Filamin-C binds actin and is involved in the formation of the Z-disc. In addition, filamin-c also binds γ- and δ-sarcoglycan at the sarcolemmal membrane and may also play a role in signaling pathways from the sarcolemma to the myofibril.[25]

MFM6 is caused by autosomal-dominant mutations in *BAG3* that encode for Bcl-2–binding protein.[4,522–525] It is the rarest form of MFM. It is associated with proximal and/or distal weakness, hypernasal speech, ventilatory weakness, and dilated cardiomyopathy with onset in the first or second decade. Bcl-2–binding protein interacts with heat shock proteins and may have a role in cellular response to environmental stress.

MFM7 is a caused by homozygous mutations in the kyphoscoliosis peptidase gene, *KY* gene. It is associated with onset in infancy or early childhood of weakness and kyphoscoliosis.[526–528]

MFM8 is caused by autosomal-recessive mutations in *PYROXD1* that encodes pyridine nucleotide-disulfide oxidoreductase domain-containing protein 1, a flavoprotein that catalyzes pyridine-nucleotide–dependent reduction of thiol residues.[529]

MFM9 is caused by autosomal-recessive mutations in *TTN* that encode for titin. It is also known as HMERF (hereditary myopathy with early respiratory failure), which was previously discussed in the section on Titinopathies.

MFM10 is caused by autosomal-recessive mutations in *SVIL* that encode supervillin, which belongs to the villin/gelsolin superfamily of actin-binding proteins.[530]

MFM11 is caused by mutation in the UNC45 myosin chaperone B, *UNC45B*, that is also known as congenital myopathy with eccentric cores.[531,532]

MFM12 is caused by autosomal-recessive mutations in *MYL2* that encode for myosin light chain 2.[533–535]

Mutations in *FHL1*, *SEPN1*, *DNAJB6*, and *TNPO3* can also have MFM-like histopathology as previously discussed, but their associated disorders are not classified as myofibrillar myopathies.

Treatment

There are no proven medications to improve skeletal muscle weakness. Antiarrhythmic and cardiotropic medications are sometimes necessary in patients with cardiopathy. Cardiac transplantation can be lifesaving in patients with severe cardiomyopathy. Patients can benefit from physical and occupational therapy.

HEREDITARY INCLUSION BODY MYOPATHY TYPE 3

Clinical Features

This myopathy usually presents with congenital arthrogryposis and ophthalmoparesis with mild proximal weakness beginning in adulthood. Face and distal extremity weakness may occur. Some patients complain of muscle pain. As muscle biopsies may demonstrate rimmed vacuoles and tubulofilamentous inclusions, this disorder has also been called h-IBM type 3.[4,22,536,537]

Laboratory Features

Serum CK levels are normal or slightly elevated.

Histopathology

Muscle biopsies reveal small and infrequent type 2 fibers, particularly type 2A fibers, focal disorganization of the myofibrils, and rimmed vacuoles, and EM showing 15- to 20-nm tubulofilaments in the sarcoplasm.[2] Lobulated fibers and minicores may be seen.

Molecular Genetics and Pathogenesis

Mutations have been identified in the *MYH2* gene that encodes for MyHCIIa.[4,22,536,537] The MyHCIIa isoform of MyHCs is expressed in type 2A muscle fibers.

MULTISYSTEM PROTEINOPATHIES (MSP)

The MSPs are genetically heterogeneous disorders featured by h-IBM, ALS, parkinsonism, FTD, and PDB.[31,32,39] Most are caused by mutations in genes that encode for RNA-binding proteins or proteins involved in the elimination of other aged proteins. There are at least four types of MSP which are discussed below.

MULTISYSTEM PROTEINOPATHIES 1–4

Clinical Features

MSP1 is also known IBMPFD1, as it is associated with h-IBM, PDB and FTD.[4,538–555] MSP1 is a rare, autosomal-dominant disorder caused by mutations in *VCP* that encodes for VCP. It is characterized by adult onset (range late first to ninth decade, with mean in the 40s) of limb-girdle, distal, or scapuloperoneal weakness. There also appears to be a mild asymmetry and variability in the patterns of muscle weakness. FTD is seen in approximately 30%–50% and has an onset approximately 10 years after weakness (average age 54 years). PDB tends to occur earlier than in the more common sporadic forms of PDB and is seen with variable frequency. The complete triad of h-IBM, PDB, and FTD occurs in only about one-third of cases. In addition, mutations in the same gene cause a form of familial amyotrophic lateral sclerosis (fALS) with or without FTD.[556,557] A dilated cardiomyopathy may be seen in a quarter of patients.[551] Ultimately, the cause of death is through progressive muscle weakness and ventilatory failure. There is significant heterogeneity in clinical phenotype and severity both between and within families.

Laboratory Features

Serum CK levels are normal to slightly elevated. Serum alkaline phosphatase levels can be a screening test but may not be elevated in those without PDB. EMG shows myopathic changes with muscle membrane irritability.

Histopathology

Muscle biopsies reveal fibers with rimmed vacuoles and inclusions that immunostain with ubiquitin, TDP-43, and VCP.[4] Neurogenic features (i.e., fiber type grouping and atrophic, angulated fibers) may also be appreciated, which is notable because *VCP* mutations can also be associated with motor neuron disease.[547,548] EM may show paired helical filaments in muscle and in PDB osteoclasts.

Molecular Genetics and Pathogenesis

MSP1 is caused by mutations in the gene encoding VCP, a member of the AAA-ATPase superfamily.[4,32,538,539] VCP is associated with a variety of cellular activities, including cell-cycle control, membrane fusion, and the ubiquitin–proteasome degradation pathway. VCP normally localizes to nuclei and specifically near nucleoli. Mutations in the VCP gene may disrupt nuclear structure or normal translation of mRNA. In addition, mutations in *HNRPA2B1 (MSP2/IBMPFD2)*, and *HNRNPA1* (MSP3/IBMPFD3) also can cause hIBM, fALS, and PDB; mutations in *SQTM1* (MSP4) are also associated with fALS or hIBM but have not been associated with PDB.[31,558,559]

MULTISYSTEM PROTEINOPATHY 5 (DISTAL MYOPATHY WITH VOCAL CORD PARALYSIS AND PHARYNGEAL WEAKNESS)

Clinical Features

MSP5 is also known as late-onset, autosomal-dominant vocal cord and pharyngeal distal myopathy (VCPDM).[560–563]

Weakness usually begins in the anterior tibial muscles in the fourth to sixth decade. Weakness is asymmetric in some. Vocal cord and pharyngeal involvement develop after the limb weakness manifested. Ventilatory weakness can ensue.

The initial description of a large family in America was that of a vacuolar myopathy.[560,561] Subsequently, some affected individuals developed progressive ventilatory failure resulting in death within 15 years of onset, and examinations showed hyperreflexia of the lower limbs, indicative of upper motor neuron involvement, as well as tongue fasciculations.[562] These clinical findings led to the reclassification of this disorder in this family as a form of slowly progressive familial amyotrophic lateral sclerosis (ALS21) rather than a myopathy.[562] However, other series of families with the same MTR3 mutation report a clearly progressive myopathy without any evidence of lower motor neuron defects by clinical examination, EMG, and histopathology.[563]

Laboratory Features

Serum CK levels are normal to moderately elevated. Motor and sensory NCSs are usually normal but may reveal mild slowing of conduction velocities. EMG may reveal either myopathic or neurogenic features, but the description of these features was limited. Fibrillations and positive sharp waves have been described, but not fasciculation potentials.

Histopathology

Muscle biopsies demonstrated nonspecific myopathic features along with numerous rimmed vacuoles. Spinal cords have shown loss of motor neurons, as well as marked MATR3 immunoreactivity in the nucleus of anterior horn cells with diffuse cytoplasmic staining in many neurons.[562]

Molecular Genetics and Pathogenesis

This disorder is caused by mutations in *MTR3* that encodes for matrin 3.[561–563] Matrin 3 is a component of the nuclear matrix and appears to have roles in DNA replication, transcription, and RNA splicing. This may be similar to other disorders such as seen with mutations affecting similar genes including *VCP*, *SQTM1*, *HNRNPA2B1*, and *HNRNPA1* that can all be associated with forms of familial ALS or h-IBM.

MULTISYSTEM PROTEINOPATHY 6 (H-IBM WITH CENTRAL WHITE MATER DISEASE)

MSP6 has also been known has h-IBM with central white matter disease. It is an autosomal-recessive disorder associated with an infantile onset of progressive, proximal greater than distal weakness, legs worse than arms, and marked cerebral white matter abnormalities on CT and MRI.[37,564] Despite the apparent leukoencephalopathy on radiological imaging, intellectual function was normal in all the cases. Motor NCSs are mildly slow, suggesting dysmyelination of peripheral nerves as well. Mutations have been identified in *ANXA11* that encodes the calcium-dependent phospholipid-binding protein annexin A11.

▶ SUMMARY

With so many different types of muscular dystrophies and the variability of clinical phenotypes associated with specific forms of dystrophy, even within individual families, the evaluation of patients presenting with weakness can be quite daunting. The wider availability and reduced costs of NGS have made it more cost-effective in many instances to order large genetic panels based on clinical phenotype as a first diagnostic step. However, NGS can miss large deletions and duplications, as well as intronic mutations that affect mRNA splicing. Therefore, ordering clinicians need to know the limitations of genetic testing, particularly if one of the myopathies with the above type mutations are highly suspected (e.g., myotonic dystrophy, FSHD, OPMD, OPDM, and many of the MSPs). Furthermore, NGS often showed variations in unclear significance in a number of genes. Therefore, it is still very important to understand the associated clinical phenotype (inheritance pattern, age of onset, pattern of weakness, and associated manifestations—early contractures and cardiac or ventilatory involvement) and histopathological findings associated with pathogenic mutations in the genes that cause the various hereditary myopathies (Figs. 27-8, 27-10, 27-17, 27-20, 27-23, and 27-27).[2,253] Whole genome or exome sequencing, RNA sequencing of muscle biopsies, and proteomic analysis are additional diagnostic tests that may prove useful. Again, accurate clinical assessment will remain a prerequisite to distinguish pathological mutations from the benign polymorphisms that this technology will uncover.

Unfortunately, there are limited medications that have been found clinically beneficial in slowing progression. Still with supportive treatments (physical and occupational therapy, bracing, respiratory, and cardiac), quality of life can be improved in patients. More work needs to be done to further understand the pathogenesis of these disorders and discover targeted and better treatments.

REFERENCES

1. Straub V, Murphy A, Udd B; LGMD workshop study group. 229th ENMC international workshop: limb girdle muscular dystrophies—nomenclature and reformed classification Naarden, the Netherlands, 17–19 March 2017. *Neuromuscul Disord.* 2018;28(8):702–710.
2. Bockhorst J, Wicklund M. Limb girdle muscular dystrophies. *Neurol Clin.* 2020;38(3):493–504.

3. Johnson NE, Statland JM. The limb-girdle muscular dystrophies. *Continuum (Minneap Minn)*. 2022;28(6):1698–1714.
4. Narayanaswami P, Weiss M, Selcen D, et al; Guideline Development Subcommittee of the American Academy of Neurology; Practice Issues Review Panel of the American Association of Neuromuscular & Electrodiagnostic Medicine. Summary of evidence-based guideline: Diagnosis and treatment of limb-girdle and distal muscular dystrophies. *Neurology*. 2014;83(16):1453–1463.
5. Hoffman EP, Brown RH Jr, Kunkel LM. Dystrophin: The protein product of the Duchenne muscular dystrophy locus. *Cell*. 1987;51(6):919–928.
6. Hoffman EP, Fischbeck KH, Brown RH, et al. Characterization of dystrophin in muscle-biopsy specimens from patients with Duchenne's or Becker's muscular dystrophy. *N Engl J Med*. 1988;318(21):1363–1368.
7. Koenig M, Hoffman EP, Bertelson CJ, Monaco AP, Feener C, Kunkel LM. Complete cloning of the Duchenne muscular dystrophy (DMD) cDNA and preliminary genomic organization of the DMD gene in normal and affected individuals. *Cell*. 1987;50(3):509–517.
8. Michele DE, Barresi R, Kanagawa M, et al. Post-translational disruption of dystroglycan–ligand interactions in congenital muscular dystrophies. *Nature*. 2002;418(6896):417–422.
9. Wewer UM, Engvall E. Merosin/laminin-2 and muscular dystrophy. *Neuromuscul Disord*. 1996;6(6):409–418.
10. Matsumura K, Yamada H, Saito F, Sunada Y, Shimizu T. Peripheral nerve involvement in merosin-deficient congenital muscular dystrophy and dy mouse. *Neuromuscul Disord*. 1997;7(1):7–12.
11. Vachon PH, Xu H, Liu L, et al. Integrins (alpha7beta1) in muscle function and survival. Disrupted expression in merosin-deficient congenital muscular dystrophy. *J Clin Invest*. 1997;100(7):1870–1881.
12. Bansal D, Miyake K, Vogel SS, et al. Defective membrane repair in dysferlin-deficient muscular dystrophy. *Nature*. 2003;423(6936):168–172.
13. Cenacchi G, Fanin M, De Giorgi LB, Angelini C. Ultrastructural changes in dysferlinopathy support defective membrane repair mechanism. *J Clin Pathol*. 2005;58(2):190–195.
14. Bashir R, Britton S, Strachan T, et al. A gene related to *Caenorhabditis elegans* spermatogenesis factor fer-1 is mutated in limb-girdle muscular dystrophy type 2B. *Nat Genet*. 1998;20(1):37–42.
15. Matsuda C, Aoki M, Hayashi YK, Ho MF, Arahata K, Brown RH Jr. Dysferlin is a surface membrane-associated protein that is absent in Miyoshi myopathy. *Neurology*. 1999;53(5):1119–1122.
16. Chandra G, Defour A, Mamchoui K, et al. Dysregulated calcium homeostasis prevents plasma membrane repair in anoctamin 5/TMEM16E-deficient patient muscle. *Cell Death Discov*. 2019;5:118.
17. Soontrapa P, Liewluck T. Anoctamin 5 (ANO5) muscle disorders: A narrative review. *Genes (Basel)*. 2022;13(10):1736.
18. Carbone I, Bruno C, Sotgia F, et al. Mutation in the CAV3 gene causes partial caveolin-3 deficiency and hyperCKemia. *Neurology*. 2000;54(6):1373–1376.
19. Minetti C, Sotgia F, Bruno C, et al. Mutations in the caveolin-3 gene cause autosomal dominant limb-girdle muscular dystrophy. *Nat Genet*. 1998;18(4):365–368.
20. Sotgia F, Woodman SE, Bonuccelli G, et al. Phenotypic behavior of caveolin-3 R26Q, a mutant associated with hyperCKemia, distal myopathy, and rippling muscle disease. *Am J Physiol Cell Physiol*. 2003;285(5):C1150–C1160.
21. Woodman SE, Sotgia F, Galbiati F, Minetti C, Lisanti MP. Caveolinopathies: mutations in caveolin-3 cause four distinct autosomal dominant muscle diseases. *Neurology*. 2004;62(4):538–543.
22. Oldfors A, Tajsharghi H, Darin N, Lindberg C. Myopathies associated with myosin heavy chain mutations. *Acta Myol*. 2004;23(2):90–96.
23. Selcen D, Engel AG. Mutations in myotilin cause myofibrillar myopathy. *Neurology*. 2004;62(8):1363–1371.
24. Selcen D, Engel AG. Mutations in ZASP define a novel form of muscular dystrophy in humans. *Ann Neurol*. 2005;57(2):269–276.
25. Vorgerd M, van der Ven PF, Bruchertseifer V, et al. A mutation in the dimerization domain of filamin c causes a novel type of autosomal dominant myofibrillar myopathy. *Am J Hum Genet*. 2005;77(2):297–304.
26. Nagano A, Koga R, Ogawa M, et al. Emerin deficiency at the nuclear membrane in patients with Emery–Dreifuss muscular dystrophy. *Nat Genet*. 1996;12(3):254–259.
27. Ognibene A, Sabatelli P, Petrini S, et al. Nuclear changes in a case of X-linked Emery–Dreifuss muscular dystrophy. *Muscle Nerve*. 1999;22(7):864–869.
28. Sabatelli P, Lattanzi G, Ognibene A, et al. Nuclear alterations in autosomal-dominant Emery–Dreifuss muscular dystrophy. *Muscle Nerve*. 2001;24(6):826–829.
29. Bonne G, Mercuri E, Muchir A, et al. Clinical and molecular genetic spectrum of autosomal dominant Emery-Dreifuss muscular dystrophy due to mutations of the lamin A/C gene. *Ann Neurol*. 2000;48(2):170–180.
30. Felice KJ, Schwartz RC, Brown CA, Leicher CR, Grunnet ML. Autosomal dominant Emery–Dreifuss dystrophy due to mutations in rod domain of the lamin A/C gene. *Neurology*. 2000;55(2):275–280.
31. Chompoopong P, Oskarsson B, Madigan NN, et al. Multisystem proteinopathies (MSPs) and MSP-like disorders: clinical-pathological-molecular spectrum and long-term follow up. *Neurology*. 2023;10(4):632–643.
32. Korb MK, Kimonis VE, Mozaffar T. Multisystem proteinopathy: Where myopathy and motor neuron disease converge. *Muscle Nerve*. 2021;63:442–454.
33. Ghaoui R, Palmio J, Brewer J, et al. Mutations in HSPB8 causing a new phenotype of distal myopathy and motor neuropathy. *Neurology*. 2016;86:391–398.
34. Chompoopong P, Milone M, Niu Z, Cui G, Mer G, Liewluck T. A novel missense HNRNPA1 variant in the PY-NLS domain in a patient with late-onset distal myopathy. *Neuromuscul Disord*. 2022;32:521–526.
35. Kazamel M, Sorenson EJ, McEvoy KM, et al. Clinical spectrum of valosin containing protein (VCP)-opathy. *Muscle Nerve*. 2016;54:94–99.
36. Niu Z, Pontifex CS, Berini S, et al. Myopathy with SQSTM1 and TIA1 variants: clinical and pathological features. *Front Neurol*. 2018;9:147.
37. Leoni TB, González-Salazar C, Rezende TJR, et al. A novel multisystem proteinopathy caused by a missense ANXA11 variant. *Ann Neurol*. 2021;90(2):239–252.
38. Kim HJ, Mohassel P, Donkervoort S, et al. Heterozygous frameshift variants in HNRNPA2B1 cause early-onset oculopharyngeal muscular dystrophy. *Nat Commun*. 2022;13:2306.

39. Benatar M, Wuu J, Fernandez C, et al. Motor neuron involvement in multisystem proteinopathy: implications for ALS. *Neurology*. 2013;80(20):1874–1880.
40. Kumutpongpanich T, Liewluck T. Oculopharyngodistal myopathy: the recent discovery of an old disease. *Muscle Nerve*. 2022;66(6):650–652.
41. Vargas-Franco D, Kalra R, Draper I, Pacak CA, Asakura A, Kang PB. The Notch signaling pathway in skeletal muscle health and disease. *Muscle Nerve*. 2022;66(5):530–544.
42. Brockington M, Blake DJ, Prandini P, et al. Mutations in the fukutin-related protein gene (FKRP) cause a form of congenital muscular dystrophy with secondary laminin alpha2 deficiency and abnormal glycosylation of alpha-dystroglycan. *Am J Hum Genet*. 2001;69(6):1198–1209.
43. Brockington M, Yuva Y, Prandini P, et al. Mutations in the fukutin-related protein gene (FKRP) identify limb girdle muscular dystrophy 2I as a milder allelic variant of congenital muscular dystrophy MDC1C. *Hum Mol Genet*. 2001;10(25):2851–2859.
44. Brown SC, Torelli S, Brockington M, et al. Abnormalities in alpha-dystroglycan expression in MDC1 C and LGMD2I muscular dystrophies. *Am J Pathol*. 2004;164(2):727–737.
45. Beltran-Valero de Bernabe D, Voit T, Longman C, et al. Mutations in the FKRP gene can cause muscle-eye-brain disease and Walker-Warburg syndrome. *J Med Genet*. 2004;41(5):e61.
46. Butterfield RJ. Congenital muscular dystrophy and congenital myopathy. *Continuum (Minneap Minn)*. 2019;25(6):1640–1661.
47. Zambon AA, Muntoni F. Congenital muscular dystrophies: What is new? *Neuromuscul Disord*. 2021;31(10):931–942.
48. Bushby K, Finkel R, Birnkrant DJ, et al. Diagnosis and management of Duchenne muscular dystrophy, part 1: diagnosis, and pharmacological and psychosocial management. *Lancet Neurol*. 2010;9(1):77–93.
49. Bushby K, Finkel R, Birnkrant DJ, et al; DMD Care Considerations Working Group. Diagnosis and management of Duchenne muscular dystrophy, part 2: implementation of multidisciplinary care. *Lancet Neurol*. 2010;9(2):177–189.
50. Flanigan KM. Duchenne and Becker muscular dystrophies. *Neurol Clin*. 2014;32(3):671–688.
51. Emery AE. Population frequencies of inherited neuromuscular diseases—a world survey. *Neuromuscul Disord*. 1991;1(1):19–29.
52. Brooke MH, Fenichel GM, Griggs RC, et al. Duchenne muscular dystrophy: patterns of clinical progression and effects of supportive therapy. *Neurology*. 1989;39(4):475–481.
53. Brooke MH, Griggs RC, Mendell JR, Fenichel GM, Shumate JB. The natural history of Duchenne muscular dystrophy: a caveat for therapeutic trials. *Trans Am Neurol Assoc*. 1981;106:195–199.
54. Farah MG, Evans EB, Vignos PJ Jr. Echocardiographic evaluation of left ventricular function in Duchenne's muscular dystrophy. *Am J Med*. 1980;69(2):248–254.
55. Perloff JK, Roberts WC, de Leon AC Jr, O'Doherty D. The distinctive electrocardiogram of Duchenne's progressive muscular dystrophy. An electrocardiographic-pathologic correlative study. *Am J Med*. 1967;42(2):179–188.
56. Sanyal SK, Johnson WW. Cardiac conduction abnormalities in children with Duchenne's progressive muscular dystrophy: electrocardiographic features and morphologic correlates. *Circulation*. 1982;66(4):853–863.
57. Leibowitz D, Dubowitz V. Intellect and behaviour in Duchenne muscular dystrophy. *Dev Med Child Neurol*. 1981;23(5):577–590.
58. Arahata K, Engel AG. Monoclonal antibody analysis of mononuclear cells in myopathies. I: quantitation of subsets according to diagnosis and sites of accumulation and demonstration and counts of muscle fibers invaded by T cells. *Ann Neurol*. 1984;16(2):193–208.
59. Bushby KM, Thambyayah M, Gardner-Medwin D. Prevalence and incidence of Becker muscular dystrophy. *Lancet*. 1991;337(8748):1022–1024.
60. Bushby KM, Gardner-Medwin D. The clinical, genetic and dystrophin characteristics of Becker muscular dystrophy. I. Natural history. *J Neurol*. 1993;240(2):98–104.
61. Sunohara N, Arahata K, Hoffman EP, et al. Quadriceps myopathy: Forme fruste of Becker muscular dystrophy. *Ann Neurol*. 1990;28(5):634–639.
62. Comi GP, Prelle A, Bresolin N, et al. Clinical variability in Becker muscular dystrophy. Genetic, biochemical and immunohistochemical correlates. *Brain*. 1994;117(Pt 1):1–14.
63. Gospe SM Jr, Lazaro RP, Lava NS, Grootscholten PM, Scott MO, Fischbeck KH. Familial X-linked myalgia and cramps: a nonprogressive myopathy associated with a deletion in the dystrophin gene. *Neurology*. 1989;39(10):1277–1280.
64. Doriguzzi C, Palmucci L, Mongini T, Chiadò-Piat L, Restagno G, Ferrone M. Exercise intolerance and recurrent myoglobinuria as the only expression of Xp21 Becker type muscular dystrophy. *J Neurol*. 1993;240(5):269–271.
65. Muntoni F, Cau M, Ganau A, et al. Brief report: deletion of the dystrophin muscle-promoter region associated with X-linked dilated cardiomyopathy. *N Engl J Med*. 1993;329(13):921–925.
66. Towbin JA, Hejtmancik JF, Brink P, et al. X-linked dilated cardiomyopathy. Molecular genetic evidence of linkage to the Duchenne muscular dystrophy (dystrophin) gene at the Xp21 locus. *Circulation*. 1993;87(6):1854–1865.
67. de Visser M, de Voogt WG, la Rivière GV. The heart in Becker muscular dystrophy, facioscapulohumeral dystrophy, and Bethlem myopathy. *Muscle Nerve*. 1992;15(5):591–596.
68. Kaido M, Arahata K, Hoffman EP, Nonaka I, Sugita H. Muscle histology in Becker muscular dystrophy. *Muscle Nerve*. 1991;14(11):1067–1073.
69. Hoffman EP, Kunkel LM, Angelini C, Clarke A, Johnson M, Harris JB. Improved diagnosis of Becker muscular dystrophy by dystrophin testing. *Neurology*. 1989;39(8):1011–1017.
70. Hoffman EP, Arahata K, Minetti C, Bonilla E, Rowland LP. Dystrophinopathy in isolated cases of myopathy in females. *Neurology*. 1992;42(5):967–975.
71. Arahata K, Ishihara T, Kamakura K, et al. Mosaic expression of dystrophin in symptomatic carriers of Duchenne's muscular dystrophy. *N Engl J Med*. 1989;320(3):138–142.
72. Clerk A, Rodillo E, Heckmatt JZ, Dubowitz V, Strong PN, Sewry CA. Characterisation of dystrophin in carriers of Duchenne muscular dystrophy. *J Neurol Sci*. 1991;102(2):197–205.
73. Minetti C, Chang HW, Medori R, et al. Dystrophin deficiency in young girls with sporadic myopathy and normal karyotype. *Neurology*. 1991;41(8):1288–1292.
74. Hyser CL, Doherty RA, Griggs RC, et al. Carrier assessment for mothers and sisters of isolated Duchenne dystrophy cases: the importance of serum enzyme determinations. *Neurology*. 1987;37(9):1476–1480.
75. Hyser CL, Griggs RC, Mendell JR, et al. Use of serum creatine kinase, pyruvate kinase, and genetic linkage for carrier detection in Duchenne and Becker dystrophy. *Neurology*. 1987;37(1):4–10.

76. Bakker E, Veenema H, Den Dunnen JT, et al. Germinal mosaicism increases the recurrence risk for 'new' Duchenne muscular dystrophy mutations. *J Med Genet.* 1989;26(9):553–559.
77. Prior TW, Bartolo C, Pearl DK, et al. Spectrum of small mutations in the dystrophin coding region. *Am J Hum Genet.* 1995;57(1):22–33.
78. Brooke MH, Fenichel GM, Griggs RC, et al. Clinical investigation of Duchenne muscular dystrophy. Interesting results in a trial of prednisone. *Arch Neurol.* 1987;44(8):812–817.
79. Fenichel GM, Florence JM, Pestronk A, et al. Long-term benefit from prednisone therapy in Duchenne muscular dystrophy. *Neurology.* 1991;41(12):1874–1877.
80. Griggs RC, Moxley RT 3rd, Mendell JR, et al. Prednisone in Duchenne dystrophy. A randomized, controlled trial defining the time course and dose response. Clinical Investigation of Duchenne Dystrophy Group. *Arch Neurol.* 1991;48(4):383–388.
81. Griggs RC, Moxley RT 3rd, Mendell JR, et al. Duchenne dystrophy: randomized, controlled trial of prednisone (18 months) and azathioprine (12 months). *Neurology.* 1993;43(3 Pt 1):520–527.
82. Mendell JR, Moxley RT, Griggs RC, et al. Randomized, double-blind six-month trial of prednisone in Duchenne's muscular dystrophy. *N Engl J Med.* 1989;320(24):1592–1597.
83. Moxley RT 3rd, Ashwal S, Pandya S, et al. Practice parameter: Corticosteroid treatment of Duchenne dystrophy: Report of the Quality Standards Subcommittee of the American Academy of Neurology and the Practice Committee of the Child Neurology Society. *Neurology.* 2005;64(1):13–20.
84. Backman E, Henriksson KG. Low-dose prednisolone treatment in Duchenne and Becker muscular dystrophy. *Neuromuscul Disord.* 1995;5(3):233–241.
85. Connolly AM, Schierbecker J, Renna R, Florence J. High dose weekly oral prednisone improves strength in boys with Duchenne muscular dystrophy. *Neuromuscul Disord.* 2002;12(10):917–925.
86. Angelini C, Pegoraro E, Turella E, Intino MT, Pini A, Costa C. Deflazacort in Duchenne dystrophy: study of long-term effect. *Muscle Nerve.* 1994;17(4):386–391.
87. Bonifati MD, Ruzza G, Bonometto P, et al. A multicenter, double-blind, randomized trial of deflazacort versus prednisone in Duchenne muscular dystrophy. *Muscle Nerve.* 2000;23(9):1344–1347.
88. Matthews E, Brassington R, Kuntzer T, Jichi F, Manzur AY. Corticosteroids for the treatment of Duchenne muscular dystrophy. *Cochrane Database Syst Rev.* 2016;2016(5):CD003725.
89. Guglieri M, Bushby K, McDermott MP, et al. Effect of different corticosteroid dosing regimens on clinical outcomes in boys with Duchenne muscular dystrophy: a randomized clinical trial. *JAMA.* 2022;327(15):1456–1468.
90. Guglieri M, Clemens PR, Perlman SJ, et al. Efficacy and safety of vamorolone vs placebo and prednisone among boys with Duchenne muscular dystrophy: a randomized clinical trial. *JAMA Neurol.* 2022;79(10):1005–1014.
91. Dang UJ, Damsker JM, Guglieri M, et al. Efficacy and safety of vamorolone over 48 weeks in boys with Duchenne muscular dystrophy: a randomized controlled trial. *Neurology.* 2024;102(5):e208112.
92. Mah JK, Clemens PR, Guglieri M, et al. Efficacy and safety of vamorolone in Duchenne muscular dystrophy: a 30-month nonrandomized controlled open-label extension trial. *JAMA Netw Open.* 2022;5(1):e2144178.
93. Mullard A. FDA approves an HDAC inhibitor for Duchenne muscular dystrophy. *Nat Rev Drug Discov.* 2024;23(5):329.
94. Mozzetta C, Sartorelli V, Steinkuhler C, Puri PL. HDAC inhibitors as pharmacological treatment for Duchenne muscular dystrophy: a discovery journey from bench to patients. *Trends Mol Med.* 2024;30(3):278–294.
95. Manini A, Abate E, Nuredini A, Corti S, Comi GP. Adeno-associated virus (AAV)-mediated gene therapy for Duchenne muscular dystrophy: the issue of transgene persistence. *Front Neurol.* 2022;12:814174.
96. Elangkovan N, Dickson G. Gene therapy for Duchenne muscular dystrophy. *J Neuromuscul Dis.* 2021;8(s2):S303–S316.
97. Holm A, Hansen SN, Klitgaard H, Kauppinen S. Clinical advances of RNA therapeutics for treatment of neurological and neuromuscular diseases. *RNA Biol.* 2022;19(1):594–608.
98. Zaidman CM, Proud CM, McDonald CM, et al. Delandistrogene moxeparvovec gene therapy in ambulatory patients (aged ≥4 to <8 years) with Duchenne muscular dystrophy: 1-year interim results from study SRP-9001-103 (ENDEAVOR). *Ann Neurol.* 2023;94(5):955–968.
99. Mendell JR, Sahenk Z, Lehman KJ, et al. Long-term safety and functional outcomes of delandistrogene moxeparvovec gene therapy in patients with Duchenne muscular dystrophy: A phase 1/2a nonrandomized trial. *Muscle Nerve.* 2024;69(1):93–98.
100. Charleston JS, Schnell FJ, Dworzak J, et. Eteplirsen treatment for Duchenne muscular dystrophy: Exon skipping and dystrophin production. *Neurology.* 2018;90(24):e2146–e2154.
101. McDonald CM, Shieh PB, Abdel-Hamid HZ, et al; the Italian DMD Telethon Registry Study Group, Leuven NMRC Registry Investigators, CINRG Duchenne Natural History Investigators, and PROMOVI Trial Clinical Investigators. Open-label evaluation of eteplirsen in patients with Duchenne muscular dystrophy amenable to exon 51 skipping: PROMOVI trial. *J Neuromuscul Dis.* 2021;8(6):989–1001.
102. Frank DE, Schnell FJ, Akana C, et al. Increased dystrophin production with golodirsen in patients with Duchenne muscular dystrophy. *Neurology.* 2020;94(21):e2270–e2282.
103. Servais L, Mercuri E, Straub V, et al. Long-term safety and efficacy data of golodirsen in ambulatory patients with Duchenne muscular dystrophy amenable to exon 53 skipping: a first-in-human, multicenter, two-part, open-label, phase 1/2 trial. *Nucleic Acid Ther.* 2022;32(1):29–39.
104. Clemens PR, Rao VK, Connolly AM, et al. Safety, tolerability, and efficacy of viltolarsen in boys with Duchenne muscular dystrophy amenable to exon 53 skipping: a phase 2 randomized clinical trial. *JAMA Neurol.* 2020;77(8):982–991.
105. Dhillon S. Viltolarsen: First approval. *Drugs.* 2020;80(10):1027–1031.
106. Wagner KR, Kuntz NL, Koenig E, et al. Safety, tolerability, and pharmacokinetics of casimersen in patients with Duchenne muscular dystrophy amenable to exon 45 skipping: a randomized, double-blind, placebo-controlled, dose-titration trial. *Muscle Nerve.* 2021;64(3):285–292.
107. Shirley M. Casimersen: First approval. *Drugs.* 2021;81(7):875–879.
108. Darras BT, Francke U. Myopathy in complex glycerol kinase deficiency patients is due to 3 deletions of the dystrophin gene. *Am J Hum Genet.* 1988;43(2):126–130.

109. Guggenheim MA, McCabe ER, Roig M, et al. Glycerol kinase deficiency with neuromuscular, skeletal, and adrenal abnormalities. *Ann Neurol.* 1980;7(5):441–449.
110. Seltzer WK, Angelini C, Dhariwal G, Ringel SP, McCabe ER. Muscle glycerol kinase in Duchenne dystrophy and glycerol kinase deficiency. *Muscle Nerve.* 1989;12(4):307–313.
111. Liewluck T, Milone M. Untangling the complexity of limb-girdle muscular dystrophies. *Muscle Nerve.* 2018;58(2):167–177.
112. Mah JK, Korngut L, Fiest KM, et al. A systematic review and meta-analysis on the epidemiology of the muscular dystrophies. *Can J Neurol Sci.* 2016;43(1):163–177.
113. Gilchrist JM, Pericak-Vance M, Silverman L, Roses AD. Clinical and genetic investigation in autosomal dominant limb-girdle muscular dystrophy. *Neurology.* 1988;38(1):5–9.
114. Hauser MA, Horrigan SK, Salmikangas P, et al. Myotilin is mutated in limb girdle muscular dystrophy 1A. *Hum Mol Genet.* 2000;9(14):2141–2147.
115. Olivé M, Goldfarb LG, Shatunov A, Fischer D, Ferrer I. Myotilinopathy: refining the clinical and myopathological phenotype. *Brain.* 2005;128:2315–2326.
116. Pénisson-Besnier I, Talvinen K, Dumez C, et al. Myotilinopathy in a family with late onset myopathy. *Neuromuscul Disord.* 2006;16:427–431.
117. Schramm N, Born C, Weckbach S, Reilich P, Walter MC, Reiser MF. Involvement patterns in myotilinopathy and desminopathy detected by a novel neuromuscular whole-body MRI protocol. *Eur Radiol.* 2008;18:2922–2936.
118. Olivé M, Odgerel Z, Martínez A, et al. Clinical and myopathological evaluation of early- and late-onset subtypes of myofibrillar myopathy. *Neuromuscul Disord.* 2011;21:533–542.
119. Reilich P, Krause S, Schramm N, et al. A novel mutation in the myotilin gene (MYOT) causes a severe form of limb girdle muscular dystrophy 1 A (LGMD1 A). *J Neurol.* 2011;258(8):1437–1444.
120. van der Kooi AJ, Ledderhof TM, de Voogt WG, et al. A newly recognized autosomal dominant limb girdle muscular dystrophy with cardiac involvement. *Ann Neurol.* 1996;39(5):636–642.
121. Bonne G, Di Barletta MR, Varnous S, et al. Mutations in the gene encoding lamin A/C cause autosomal dominant Emery–Dreifuss muscular dystrophy. *Nat Genet.* 1999;21(3):285–288.
122. Jimenez-Escrig A, Gobernado I, Garcia-Villanueva M, Sanchez-Herranz A. Autosomal recessive Emery-Dreifuss muscular dystrophy caused by a novel mutation (R225Q) in the lamin A/C gene identified by exome sequencing. *Muscle Nerve.* 2012;45:605–610.
123. Rankin J, Auer-Grumbach M, Bagg W, et al. Extreme phenotypic diversity and nonpenetrance in families with the LMNA gene mutation R644 C. *Am J Med Genet A.* 2008;146A:1530–1542.
124. van der Kooi AJ, Bonne G, Eymard B, et al. Lamin A/C mutations with lipodystrophy, cardiac abnormalities, and muscular dystrophy. *Neurology.* 2002;59:620–623.
125. van der Kooi AJ, van Meegen M, Ledderhof TM, McNally EM, de Visser M, Bolhuis PA. Genetic localization of a newly recognized autosomal dominant limb-girdle muscular dystrophy with cardiac involvement (LGMD1B) to chromosome 1q11–21. *Am J Hum Genet.* 1997;60(4):891–895.
126. Vantyghem M, Pigny P, Maurage CA, et al. Patients with familial partial lipodystrophy of the Dunnigan type due to a LMNA R482-W mutation show muscular and cardiac abnormalities. *J Clin Endocrinol Metab.* 2004;89:5337–5346.
127. Carboni N, Mura M, Marrosu G, et al. Muscle imaging analogies in a cohort of patients with different clinical phenotypes caused by LMNA gene mutations. *Muscle Nerve.* 2010;41:458–463.
128. Deconinck N, Dion E, Ben Yaou R, et al. Differentiating Emery-Dreifuss muscular dystrophy and collagen VI-related myopathies using a specific CT scanner pattern. *Neuromuscul Disord.* 2010;20:517–523.
129. Mercuri E, Counsell S, Allsop J, et al. Selective muscle involvement on magnetic resonance imaging in autosomal dominant Emery-Dreifuss muscular dystrophy. *Neuropediatrics.* 2002;33:10–14.
130. Mercuri E, Clements E, Offiah A, et al. Muscle magnetic resonance imaging involvement in muscular dystrophies with rigidity of the spine. *Ann Neurol.* 2010;67:201–208.
131. Aboumousa A, Hoogendijk J, Charlton R, et al. Caveolinopathy—new mutations and additional symptoms. *Neuromuscul Disord.* 2008;18(7):572–578.
132. González-Pérez P, Gallano P, González-Quereda L, et al. Phenotypic variability in a Spanish family with a Caveolin-3 mutation. *J Neurol Sci.* 2009;276:95–98.
133. Cagliani R, Bresolin N, Prelle A, et al. A CAV3 microdeletion differentially affects skeletal muscle and myocardium. *Neurology.* 2003;61:1513–1519.
134. Catteruccia, M, Sanna T, Santorelli FM, et al. Rippling muscle disease and cardiomyopathy associated with a mutation in the CAV3 gene. *Neuromuscul Disord.* 2009;19:779–783.
135. Dotti MT, Malandrini A, Gambelli S, Salvadori C, De Stefano N, Federico A. A new missense mutation in caveolin-3 gene causes rippling muscle disease. *J Neurol Sci.* 2006;243:61–64.
136. Fischer D, Schroers A, Blümcke I, et al. Consequences of a novel caveolin-3 mutation in a large German family. *Ann Neurol.* 2003;53:233–241.
137. Fulizio L, Nascimbeni AC, Fanin M, et al. Molecular and muscle pathology in a series of caveolinopathy patients. *Hum Mutat.* 2005;25:82–89.
138. Jacobi C, Ruscheweyh R, Vorgerd M, Weber MA, Storch-Hagenlocher B, Meinck HM. Rippling muscle disease: variable phenotype in a family with five afflicted members. *Muscle Nerve.* 2010;41:128–132.
139. Ricker K, Moxley RT, Rohkamm R. Rippling muscle disease. *Arch Neurol.* 1989;46:405–408.
140. Sundblom J, Stålberg E, Osterdahl M, et al. Bedside diagnosis of rippling muscle disease in CAV3 p.A46 T mutation carriers. *Muscle Nerve.* 2010;41:751–757.
141. Vorgerd M, Bolz H, Patzold T, Kubisch C, Malin JP, Mortier W. Phenotypic variability in rippling muscle disease. *Neurology.* 1999;52:1453–1459.
142. Yabe I, Kawashima A, Kikuchi S, et al. Caveolin-3 gene mutation in Japanese with rippling muscle disease. *Acta Neurol Scand.* 2003;108:47–51.
143. Kubisch C, Schoser BG, von During M, et al. Homozygous mutations in caveolin-3 cause a severe form of rippling muscle disease. *Ann Neurol.* 2003;53:512–520.
144. Hackman P, Sandell S, Sarparanta J, et al. Four new Finnish families with LGMD1D; refinement of the clinical phenotype and the linked 7q36 locus. *Neuromuscul Disord.* 2011;21:338–344.
145. Sarparanta J, Jonson PH, Golzio C, et al. Mutations affecting the cytoplasmic functions of the co-chaperone DNAJB6 cause limb-girdle muscular dystrophy. *Nat Genet.* 2012;44:450–455, S1–S2.

146. Harms MB, Sommerville RB, Allred P, et al. Exome sequencing reveals DNAJB6 mutations in dominantly-inherited myopathy. *Ann Neurol.* 2012;71:407–416.
147. Findlay AR, Robinson SE, Poelker S, Seiffert M, Bengoechea R, Weihl CC. LGMDD1 natural history and phenotypic spectrum: implications for clinical trials. *Ann Clin Transl Neurol.* 2023;10(2):181–194.
148. Sandell S, Huovinen S, Palmio J, et al. Diagnostically important muscle pathology in DNAJB6 mutated LGMD1D. *Acta Neuropathol Commun.* 2016;4:9.
149. Goldfarb LG, Park KY, Cervenáková L, et al. Missense mutations in desmin associated with familial cardiac and skeletal myopathy. *Nat Genet.* 1998;19(4):402–403.
150. Dalakas MC, Dagvadorj A, Goudeau B, et al. Progressive skeletal myopathy, a phenotypic variant of desmin myopathy associated with desmin mutations. *Neuromuscul Disord.* 2003;13(3):252–258.
151. Dalakas MC, Park KY, Semino-Mora C, Lee HS, Sivakumar K, Goldfarb LG. Desmin myopathy, a skeletal myopathy with cardiomyopathy caused by mutations in the desmin gene. *N Engl J Med.* 2000;342(11):770–780.
152. Walter MC, Reilich P, Huebner A, et al. Scapuloperoneal syndrome type Kaeser and a wide phenotypic spectrum of adult-onset, dominant myopathies are associated with the desmin mutation R350P. *Brain.* 2007;130:1485–1496.
153. Goudeau B, Rodrigues-Lima F, Fischer D, et al. Variable pathogenic potentials of mutations located in the desmin alpha-helical domain. *Hum Mutat.* 2006;27:906–913.
154. Bär H, Goudeau B, Wälde S, et al. Conspicuous involvement of desmin tail mutations in diverse cardiac and skeletal myopathies. *Hum Mutat.* 2007;28:374–376.
155. Olivé M, Armstrong J, Miralles F, et al. Phenotypic patterns of desminopathy associated with three novel mutations in the desmin gene. *Neuromuscul Disord.* 2007;17:443–450.
156. Greenberg SA, Salajegheh M, Judge DP, et al. Etiology of limb girdle muscular dystrophy 1D/1E determined by laser capture microdissection proteomics. *Ann Neurol.* 2012;71:141–145.
157. Shelly S, Talha N, Pereira NL, Engel AG, Johnson JN, Selcen D. Expanding spectrum of desmin-related myopathy, long-term follow-up, and cardiac transplantation. *Neurology.* 2021;97(11):e1150–e1158.
158. Kubisch C., Ketelsen UP, Goebel I, Omran H. Autosomal recessive rippling muscle disease with homozygous CAV3 mutations. *Ann Neurol.* 2005;57:303–304.
159. Palenzuela L, Andreu AL, Gàmez J, et al. A novel autosomal dominant limb-girdle muscular dystrophy (LGMD 1F) maps to 7q32.1–32.2. *Neurology.* 2003;61(3):404–406.
160. Melià MJ, Kubota A, Ortolano S, et al. Limb-girdle muscular dystrophy 1F is caused by a microdeletion in the transportin 3 gene. *Brain.* 2013;136:1508–1517.
161. Costa R, Rodia MT, Pacilio S, Angelini C, Cenacchi G. LGMD D2 TNPO3-related: from clinical spectrum to pathogenetic mechanism. *Front Neurol.* 2022;13:840683.
162. Vieira NM, Naslavsky MS, Licinio L, et al. A defect in the RNA-processing protein HNRPDL causes limb-girdle muscular dystrophy 1G (LGMD1G). *Hum Mol Genet.* 2014;23:4103–4110.
163. Sun Y, Chen H, Lu Y, et al. Limb girdle muscular dystrophy D3 HNRNPDL related in a Chinese family with distal muscle weakness caused by a mutation in the prion-like domain. *J Neurol.* 2019;266:498–506.
164. Berardo A, Lornage X, Johari M, et al. HNRNPDL-related muscular dystrophy: expanding the clinical, morphological and MRI phenotypes. *J Neurol.* 2019;266(10):2524–2534.
165. Vissing J, Barresi R, Witting N, et al. A heterozygous 21-bp deletion in CAPN3 causes dominantly inherited limb girdle muscular dystrophy. *Brain.* 2016;139:2154–2163.
166. Martinez-Thompson JM, Niu Z, Tracy JA, et al. Autosomal dominant calpainopathy due to heterozygous CAPN3 c.643_663del21. *Muscle Nerve.* 2018;57:679–683.
167. Vissing J, Dahlqvist JR, Roudaut C, et al. A single c.1715G>C calpain 3 gene variant causes dominant calpainopathy with loss of calpain 3 expression and activity. *Hum Mutat.* 2020;41(9):1507–1513.
168. Fardeau M, Eymard B, Mignard C, Tomé FM, Richard I, Beckmann JS. Chromosome 15-linked limb-girdle muscular dystrophy: Clinical phenotypes in Reunion Island and French metropolitan communities. *Neuromuscul Disord.* 1996;6(6):447–453.
169. Fardeau M, Hillaire D, Mignard C, et al. Juvenile limb-girdle muscular dystrophy. Clinical, histopathological and genetic data from a small community living in the Reunion Island. *Brain.* 1996;119(Pt 1):295–308.
170. Kawai H, Akaike M, Kunishige M, et al. Clinical, pathological, and genetic features of limb-girdle muscular dystrophy type 2 A with new calpain 3 gene mutations in seven patients from three Japanese families. *Muscle Nerve.* 1998;21(11):1493–1501.
171. Penisson-Besnier I, Richard I, Dubas F, Beckmann JS, Fardeau M. Pseudometabolic expression and phenotypic variability of calpain deficiency in two siblings. *Muscle Nerve.* 1998;21(8):1078–1080.
172. Spencer MJ, Tidball JG, Anderson LV, et al. Absence of calpain 3 in a form of limb-girdle muscular dystrophy (LGMD2A). *J Neurol Sci.* 1997;146(2):173–178.
173. Guglieri M, Magri F, D'Angelo MG, et al. Clinical, molecular, and protein correlations in a large sample of genetically diagnosed Italian limb girdle muscular dystrophy patients. *Hum Mutat.* 2008;29:258–266.
174. Norwood FL, Harling C, Chinnery PF, Eagle M, Bushby K, Straub V. Prevalence of genetic muscle disease in Northern England: in-depth analysis of a muscle clinic population. *Brain.* 2009;132(Pt 11):3175–3186.
175. Ten Dam L, Frankhuizen WS, Linssen WHJP, et al. Autosomal recessive limb-girdle and Miyoshi muscular dystrophies in the Netherlands: the clinical and molecular spectrum of 244 patients. *Clin Genet.* 2019;96(2):126–133.
176. Mercuri E, Bushby K, Ricci E, et al. Muscle MRI findings in patients with limb girdle muscular dystrophy with calpain 3 deficiency (LGMD2A) and early contractures. *Neuromuscul Disord.* 2005;15:164–171.
177. Barp A, Laforet P, Bello L, et al. European muscle MRI study in limb girdle muscular dystrophy type R1/2A (LGMDR1/LGMD2A). *J Neurol.* 2020;267(1):45–56.
178. Aivazoglou LU, Guimarães JB, Costa MAF, et al. Whole-body MRI in limb girdle muscular dystrophy type R1/2A: correlation with clinical scores. *Muscle Nerve.* 2022;66(4):471–478.
179. Krahn M, Lopez De Munain A, Streichenberger N, et al. CAPN3 mutations in patients with idiopathic eosinophilic myositis. *Ann Neurol.* 2006;59(6):905–911.
180. Amato AA. Adults with eosinophilic myositis and calpain-3 mutations. *Neurology.* 2008;70:730–731.

181. Beckmann JS, Richard I, Broux O, et al. Identification of muscle-specific calpain and beta-sarcoglycan genes in progressive autosomal recessive muscular dystrophies. *Neuromuscul Disord*. 1996;6(6):455–462.
182. Richard I, Broux O, Allamand V, et al. Mutations in the proteolytic enzyme calpain 3 cause limb-girdle muscular dystrophy type 2 A. *Cell*. 1995;81(1):27–40.
183. Richard I, Roudaut C, Saenz A, et al. Calpainopathy-a survey of mutations and polymorphisms. *Am J Hum Genet*. 1999;64(6):1524–1540.
184. Luo SS, Xi JY, Zhu WH, et al. Genetic variability and clinical spectrum of Chinese patients with limb-girdle muscular dystrophy type 2 A. *Muscle Nerve*. 2012;46(5):723–729.
185. Fanin M, Pegoraro E, Matsuda-Asada C, Brown RH Jr, Angelini C. Calpain-3 and dysferlin protein screening in patients with limb-girdle dystrophy and myopathy. *Neurology*. 2001;56(5):660–665.
186. Brown RH Jr, Amato A. Calpainopathy and eosinophilic myositis. *Ann Neurol*. 2006;59(6):875–877.
187. Illa I, Serrano-Munuera C, Gallardo E, et al. Distal anterior compartment myopathy: a dysferlin mutation causing a new muscular dystrophy phenotype. *Ann Neurol*. 2001;49(1):130–134.
188. Illarioshkin SN, Ivanova-Smolenskaya IA, Tanaka H, et al. Clinical and molecular analysis of a large family with three distinct phenotypes of progressive muscular dystrophy. *Brain*. 1996;119(Pt 6):1895–1909.
189. Mahjneh I, Marconi G, Bushby K, Anderson LV, Tolvanen-Mahjneh H, Somer H. Dysferlinopathy (LGMD2B): a 23-year follow-up study of 10 patients homozygous for the same frameshifting dysferlin mutations. *Neuromuscul Disord*. 2001;11(1):20–26.
190. Mahjneh I, Passos-Bueno MR, Zatz M, et al. The phenotype of chromosome 2p-linked limb-girdle muscular dystrophy. *Neuromuscul Disord*. 1996;6(6):483–490.
191. Suzuki N, Aoki M, Takahashi T, et al. Novel dysferlin mutations and characteristic muscle atrophy in late-onset Miyoshi myopathy. *Muscle Nerve*. 2004;29(5):721–723.
192. Takahashi T, Aoki M, Tateyama M, et al. Dysferlin mutations in Japanese Miyoshi myopathy: relationship to phenotype. *Neurology*. 2003;60(11):1799–1804.
193. Vilchez JJ, Gallano P, Gallardo E, et al. Identification of a novel founder mutation in the DYSF gene causing clinical variability in the Spanish population. *Arch Neurol*. 2005;62:1256–1259.
194. Ho M, Gallardo E, McKenna-Yasek D, De Luna N, Illa I, Brown RH Jr. A novel, blood-based diagnostic assay for limb girdle muscular dystrophy 2B and Miyoshi myopathy. *Ann Neurol*. 2002;51(1):129–133.
195. Paradas C, Llauger J, Diaz-Manera J, et al. Redefining dysferlinopathy phenotypes based on clinical findings and muscle imaging studies. *Neurology*. 2010;75:316–323.
196. Kesper K, Kornblum C, Reimann J, Lutterbey G, Schröder R, Wattjes MP. Pattern of skeletal muscle involvement in primary dysferlinopathies: a whole-body 3.0-T magnetic resonance imaging study. *Acta Neurol Scand*. 2009;120:111–118.
197. Brummer D, Walter MC, Palmbach M, et al. Long-term MRI and clinical follow-up of symptomatic and presymptomatic carriers of dysferlin gene mutations. *Acta Myol*. 2005;24:6–16.
198. Moore U, Gordish H, Diaz-Manera J, et al. Miyoshi myopathy and limb girdle muscular dystrophy R2 are the same disease. *Neuromuscul Disord*. 2021;31(4):265–280.
199. Piccolo F, Moore SA, Ford GC, Campbell KP. Intracellular accumulation and reduced sarcolemmal expression of dysferlin in limb-girdle muscular dystrophies. *Ann Neurol*. 2000;48(6):902–912.
200. Gallardo E, Rojas-Garcia R, de Luna N, Pou A, Brown RH Jr, Illa I. Inflammation in dysferlin myopathy: immunohistochemical characterization of 13 patients. *Neurology*. 2001;57(11):2136–2138.
201. Selcen D, Stilling G, Engel AG. The earliest pathologic alterations in dysferlinopathy. *Neurology*. 2001;56(11):1472–1481.
202. Spuler S, Carl M, Zabojszcza J, et al. Dysferlin-deficient muscular dystrophy features amyloidosis. *Ann Neurol*. 2008;63:323–328.
203. Liu J, Aoki M, Illa I, et al. Dysferlin, a novel skeletal muscle gene, is mutated in Miyoshi myopathy and limb girdle muscular dystrophy. *Nat Genet*. 1998;20(1):31–36.
204. Angelini C, Fanin M, Freda MP, Duggan DJ, Siciliano G, Hoffman EP. The clinical spectrum of sarcoglycanopathies. *Neurology*. 1999;52(1):176–179.
205. Duggan DJ, Gorospe JR, Fanin M, Hoffman EP, Angelini C. Mutations in the sarcoglycan genes in patients with myopathy. *N Engl J Med*. 1997;336(9):618–624.
206. Melacini P, Fanin M, Duggan DJ, et al. Heart involvement in muscular dystrophies due to sarcoglycan gene mutations. *Muscle Nerve*. 1999;22(4):473–479.
207. Angelini C, Fanin M, Menegazzo E, Freda MP, Duggan DJ, Hoffman EP. Homozygous alpha-sarcoglycan mutation in two siblings: one asymptomatic and one steroid-responsive mild limb-girdle muscular dystrophy patient. *Muscle Nerve*. 1998;21(6):769–775.
208. Bonnemann CG, Modi R, Noguchi S, et al. Beta-sarcoglycan (A3b) mutations cause autosomal recessive muscular dystrophy with loss of the sarcoglycan complex. *Nat Genet*. 1995;11(3):266–273.
209. Campbell KP. Adhalin gene mutations and autosomal recessive limb-girdle muscular dystrophy. *Ann Neurol*. 1995;38(3):353–354.
210. Duggan DJ, Fanin M, Pegoraro E, Angelini C, Hoffman EP. Alpha-sarcoglycan (adhalin) deficiency: complete deficiency patients are 5% of childhood-onset dystrophin-normal muscular dystrophy and most partial deficiency patients do not have gene mutations. *J Neurol Sci*. 1996;140(1-2):30–39.
211. Duggan DJ, Manchester D, Stears KP, Mathews DJ, Hart C, Hoffman EP. Mutations in the delta-sarcoglycan gene are a rare cause of autosomal recessive limb-girdle muscular dystrophy (LGMD2). *Neurogenetics*. 1997;1(1):49–58.
212. Ljunggren A, Duggan D, McNally E, et al. Primary adhalin deficiency as a cause of muscular dystrophy in patients with normal dystrophin. *Ann Neurol*. 1995;38(3):367–372.
213. McNally EM, Duggan D, Gorospe JR, et al. Mutations that disrupt the carboxyl-terminus of gamma-sarcoglycan cause muscular dystrophy. *Hum Mol Genet*. 1996;5(11):1841–1847.
214. Vainzof M, Souza LS, Gurgel-Giannetti J, Zatz M. Sarcoglycanopathies: an update. *Neuromuscul Disord*. 2021;31(10):1021–1027.
215. Alonso-Pérez J, González-Quereda L, Bello L, et al. New genotype-phenotype correlations in a large European cohort of patients with sarcoglycanopathy. *Brain*. 2020;143(9):2696–2708.
216. Alonso-Pérez J, González-Quereda L, Bruno C, et al. Clinical and genetic spectrum of a large cohort of patients with

δ-sarcoglycan muscular dystrophy. *Brain*. 2022;145(2): 596–606.
217. Moreira ES, Wiltshire TJ, Faulkner G, et al. Limb-girdle muscular dystrophy type 2G is caused by mutations in the gene encoding the sarcomeric protein telethonin. *Nat Genet*. 2000;24(2):163–166.
218. Mues A, van der Ven PF, Young P, Fürst DO, Gautel M. Two immunoglobulin-like domains of the Z-disc portion of titin interact in a conformation-dependent way with telethonin. *FEBS Lett*. 1998;428(1-2):111–114.
219. Chen H, Xu G, Lin F, et al. Clinical and genetic characterization of limb girdle muscular dystrophy R7 telethonin-related patients from three unrelated Chinese families. *Neuromuscul Disord*. 2020;30(2):137–143.
220. Chen Z, Saini M, Koh JS, et al. Unique clinical, radiological and histopathological characteristics of a southeast Asian cohort of patients with limb-girdle muscular dystrophy 2G/LGMD-R7-telethonin-related. *J Neuromuscul Dis*. 2023;10(1):91–106.
221. Huang K, Li QX, Duan HQ, Luo YB, Bi FF, Yang H. Findings of limb-girdle muscular dystrophy R7 telethonin-related patients from a Chinese neuromuscular center. *Neurogenetics*. 2022;23(1):37–44.
222. Mayans O, van der Ven PF, Wilm M, et al. Structural basis for activation of the titin kinase domain during myofibrillogenesis. *Nature*. 1998;395(6705):863–869.
223. Weiler T, Greenberg CR, Zelinski T, et al. A gene for autosomal recessive limb-girdle muscular dystrophy in Manitoba Hutterites maps to chromosome region 9q31-q33: evidence for another limb-girdle muscular dystrophy locus. *Am J Hum Genet*. 1998;63(1):140–147.
224. Schoser BG, Frosk P, Engel AG, Klutzny U, Lochmüller H, Wrogemann K. Commonality of TRIM32 mutation in causing sarcotubular myopathy and LGMD2 H. *Ann Neurol*. 2005; 57(4):591–595.
225. Borg K, Stucka R, Locke M, et al. Intragenic deletion of TRIM32 in compound heterozygotes with sarcotubular myopathy/LGMD2 H. *Hum Mutat*. 2009;30(9):E831–E844.
226. Saccone V, Palmieri M, Passamano L, et al. Mutations that impair interaction properties of TRIM32 associated with limb-girdle muscular dystrophy 2H. *Hum Mutat*. 2008;29: 240–247.
227. Johnson K, De Ridder W, Töpf A, et al. Extending the clinical and mutational spectrum of *TRIM32*-related myopathies in a non-Hutterite population. *J Neurol Neurosurg Psychiatry*. 2019;90(4):490–493.
228. Driss A, Amouri R, Ben Hamida C, et al. A new locus for autosomal recessive limb-girdle muscular dystrophy in a large consanguineous Tunisian family maps to chromosome 19q13.3. *Neuromuscul Disord*. 2000;10(4-5):240–246.
229. Mercuri E, Brockington M, Straub V, et al. Phenotypic spectrum associated with mutations in the fukutin-related protein gene. *Ann Neurol*. 2003;53(4):537–542.
230. Poppe M, Bourke J, Eagle M, et al. Cardiac and respiratory failure in limb-girdle muscular dystrophy 2I. *Ann Neurol*. 2004;56(5):738–741.
231. Poppe M, Cree L, Bourke J, et al. The phenotype of limb-girdle muscular dystrophy type 2I. *Neurology*. 2003;60(8):1246–1251.
232. Boito CA, Melacini P, Vianello A, et al. Clinical and molecular characterization of patients with limb-girdle muscular dystrophy type 2I. *Arch Neurol*. 2005;62:1894–1899.
233. Schwartz M, Hertz JM, Sveen ML, Vissing J. LGMD2I presenting with a characteristic Duchenne or Becker muscular dystrophy phenotype. *Neurology*. 2005;64(9):1635–1637.
234. Lindberg C, Sixt C, Oldfors A. Episodes of exercise-induced dark urine and myalgia in LGMD 2I. *Acta Neurol Scand*. 2012;125(4):285–287.
235. Mathews KD, Stephan CM, Laubenthal K, et al. Myoglobinuria and muscle pain are common in patients with limb-girdle muscular dystrophy 2I. *Neurology*. 2011;76(2):194–195.
236. Müller T, Krasnianski M, Witthaut R, Deschauer M, Zierz S. Dilated cardiomyopathy may be an early sign of the C826 A Fukutin-related protein mutation. *Neuromuscul Disord*. 2005;15(5):372–376.
237. Libell EM, Richardson JA, Lutz KL, et al. Cardiomyopathy in limb girdle muscular dystrophy R9, FKRP related. *Muscle Nerve*. 2020;62(5):626–632.
238. Revsbech KL, Rudolf K, Sheikh AM, et al. Axial muscle involvement in patients with limb girdle muscular dystrophy type R9. *Muscle Nerve*. 2022;65(4):405–414.
239. Palmieri A, Manara R, Bello L, et al. Cognitive profile and MRI findings in limb-girdle muscular dystrophy 2I. *J Neurol*. 2011;258(7):1312–1320.
240. Matsumoto H, Noguchi S, Sugie K. Subcellular localization of fukutin and fukutin-related protein in muscle cells. *J Biochem (Tokyo)*. 2004;135(6):709–712.
241. Esapa CT, McIlhinney RA, Blake DJ. Fukutin-related protein mutations that cause congenital muscular dystrophy result in ER-retention of the mutant protein in cultured cells. *Hum Mol Genet*. 2005;14(2):295–305.
242. Udd B, Vihola A, Sarparanta J, Richard I, Hackman P. Titinopathies and extension of the M-line mutation phenotype beyond distal myopathy and LGMD2J. *Neurology*. 2005;64(4): 636–642.
243. Udd B. Limb-girdle type muscular dystrophy in a large family with distal myopathy: Homozygous manifestation of a dominant gene? *J Med Genet*. 1992;29(6):383–389.
244. Udd B, Rapola J, Nokelainen P, Arikawa E, Somer H. Non-vacuolar myopathy in a large family with both late adult onset distal myopathy and severe proximal muscular dystrophy. *J Neurol Sci*. 1992;113(2):214–221.
245. Udd B, Partanen J, Halonen P, et al. Tibial muscular dystrophy. Late adult-onset distal myopathy in 66 Finnish patients. *Arch Neurol*. 1993;50(6):604–608.
246. Udd B, Haravuori H, Kalimo H, et al. Tibial muscular dystrophy—from clinical description to linkage on chromosome 2q31. *Neuromuscul Disord*. 1998;8(5):327–332.
247. Van den Bergh PY, Bouquiaux O, Verellen C, et al. Tibial muscular dystrophy in a Belgian family. *Ann Neurol*. 2003; 54(2):248–251.
248. Mahjneh I, Lamminen AE, Udd B, et al. Muscle magnetic resonance imaging shows distinct diagnostic patterns in Welander and tibial muscular dystrophy. *Acta Neurol Scand*. 2004;110(2):87–93.
249. Pénisson-Besnier I, Hackman P, Suominen T, et al. Myopathies caused by homozygous titin mutations: limb-girdle muscular dystrophy 2 J and variations of phenotype. *J Neurol Neurosurg Psychiatry*. 2010;81(11):1200–1202.
250. Ohlsson M, Hedberg C, Brådvik B, et al. Hereditary myopathy with early respiratory failure associated with a mutation in A-band titin. *Brain*. 2012;135(Pt 6):1682–1694.

251. Pfeffer G, Elliott HR, Griffin H, et al. Titin mutation segregates with hereditary myopathy with early respiratory failure. *Brain*. 2012;135(Pt 6):1695–1713.
252. Carmignac V, Salih MA, Quijano-Roy S, et al. C-terminal titin deletions cause a novel early-onset myopathy with fatal cardiomyopathy. *Ann Neurol*. 2007;61(4):340–351.
253. Udd B, Kääriänen H, Somer H. Muscular dystrophy with separate clinical phenotypes in a large family. *Muscle Nerve*. 1991;14(11):1050–1058.
254. Palmio J, Leonard-Louis S, Sacconi S, et al. Expanding the importance of HMERF titinopathy: new mutations and clinical aspects. *J Neurol*. 2019;266(3):680–690.
255. Tasca G, Udd B. Hereditary myopathy with early respiratory failure (HMERF): still rare, but common enough. *Neuromuscul Disord*. 2018;28(3):268–276.
256. Lv X, Zhao B, Xu L, et al. Clinical, pathological, and molecular genetic analysis of 7 Chinese patients with hereditary myopathy with early respiratory failure. *Neurol Sci*. 2022;43(5):3371–3380.
257. Hicks D, Sarkozy A, Muelas N, et al. A founder mutation in Anoctamin 5 is a major cause of limb-girdle muscular dystrophy. *Brain*. 2011;134(Pt 1):171–182.
258. Penttilä S, Palmio J, Suominen T, et al. Eight new mutations and the expanding phenotype variability in muscular dystrophy caused by ANO5. *Neurology*. 2012;78(12):897–903.
259. Bolduc V, Marlow G, Boycott KM, et al. Recessive mutations in the putative calcium-activated chloride channel Anoctamin 5 cause proximal LGMD2L and distal MMD3 muscular dystrophies. *Am J Hum Genet*. 2010;86(2):213–221.
260. Mahjneh I, Jaiswal J, Lamminen A, et al. A new distal myopathy with mutation in anoctamin 5. *Neuromuscul Disord*. 2010;20(12):791–795.
261. Schessl J, Kress W, Schoser B. Novel ANO5 mutations causing hyper-CK-emia, limb girdle muscular weakness and Miyoshi type of muscular dystrophy. *Muscle Nerve*. 2012;45(5):740–742.
262. Sarkozy A, Hicks D, Hudson J, et al. ANO5 gene analysis in a large cohort of patients with anoctaminopathy: confirmation of male prevalence and high occurrence of the common exon 5 gene mutation. *Hum Mutat*. 2013;34(8):1111–1118.
263. Vázquez J, Lefeuvre C, Escobar RE, et al. Phenotypic spectrum of myopathies with recessive anoctamin-5 mutations. *J Neuromuscul Dis*. 2020;7(4):443–451.
264. De Wel B, Huysmans L, Peeters R, et al. Prospective natural history study in 24 adult patients with LGMDR12 over 2 years of follow-up: quantitative MRI and clinical outcome measures. *Neurology*. 2022;99(6):e638–e649.
265. Holm-Yildiz S, Witting N, de Stricker Borch J, et al. Muscle biopsy and MRI findings in ANO5-related myopathy. *Muscle Nerve*. 2021;64(6):743–748.
266. Godfrey C, Clement E, Mein R, et al. Refining genotype phenotype correlations in muscular dystrophies with defective glycosylation of dystroglycan. *Brain*. 2007;130(Pt 10):2725–2735.
267. Jimenez-Mallebrera C, Torelli S, Feng L, et al. A comparative study of alpha-dystroglycan glycosylation in dystroglycanopathies suggests that the hypoglycosylation of alpha-dystroglycan does not consistently correlate with clinical severity. *Brain Pathol*. 2009;19(4):596–611.
268. Godfrey C, Escolar D, Brockington M, et al. Fukutin gene mutations in steroid-responsive limb girdle muscular dystrophy. *Ann Neurol*. 2006;60(5):603–610.
269. Biancheri R, Falace A, Tessa A, et al. POMT2 gene mutation in limb-girdle muscular dystrophy with inflammatory changes. *Biochem Biophys Res Commun*. 2007;363(4):1033–1037.
270. Clement EM, Godfrey C, Tan J, et al. Mild POMGnT1 mutations underlie a novel limb-girdle muscular dystrophy variant. *Arch Neurol*. 2008;65(1):137–141.
271. Hara Y, Balci-Hayta B, Yoshida-Moriguchi T, et al. A dystroglycan mutation associated with limb-girdle muscular dystrophy. *N Eng J Med*. 2011;364(10):939–946.
272. Dincer P, Balci B, Yuva Y, et al. A novel form of recessive limb girdle muscular dystrophy with mental retardation and abnormal expression of alpha-dystroglycan. *Neuromusc Disord*. 2003;13:771–778.
273. Dong M, Noguchi S, Endo Y, et al. DAG1 mutations associated with asymptomatic hyperCKemia and hypoglycosylation of alpha-dystroglycan. *Neurology*. 2015;84(3):273–279.
274. Banwell BL, Russel J, Fukudome T, Shen XM, Stilling G, Engel AG. Myopathy, myasthenic syndrome, and epidermolysis bullosa simplex due to plectin deficiency. *J Neuropathol Exp Neurol*. 1999;58(8):832–846.
275. Charlesworth A, Chiaverini C, Chevrant-Breton J, et al. Epidermolysis bullosa simplex with PLEC mutations: new phenotypes and new mutations. *Br J Dermatol*. 2013;168(4):808–814.
276. Chavanas S, Pulkkinen L, Gache Y, et al. A homozygous nonsense mutation in the PLEC1 gene in patients with epidermolysis bullosa simplex with muscular dystrophy. *J Clin Invest*. 1996;98(10):2196–2200.
277. Forrest K, Mellerio JE, Robb S, et al. Congenital muscular dystrophy, myasthenic symptoms and epidermolysis bullosa simplex (EBS) associated with mutations in the PLEC1 gene encoding plectin. *Neuromuscul Disord*. 2010;20(11):709–711.
278. Gache Y, Chavanas S, Lacour JP, et al. Defective expression of plectin/HD1 in epidermolysis bullosa simplex with muscular dystrophy. *J Clin Invest*. 1996;97(10):2289–2298.
279. Pulkkinen L, Smith FJ, Shimizu H, et al. Homozygous deletion mutations in the plectin gene (PLEC1) in patients with epidermolysis bullosa simplex associated with late-onset muscular dystrophy. *Hum Mol Genet*. 1996;5(10):1539–1546.
280. Smith FJ, Eady RA, Leigh IM, et al. Plectin deficiency results in muscular dystrophy with epidermolysis bullosa. *Nat Genet*. 1996;13:450–457.
281. Yiu EM, Klausegger A, Waddell LB, et al. Epidermolysis bullosa with late-onset muscular dystrophy and plectin deficiency. *Muscle Nerve*. 2011;44:135–141.
282. Selcen D, Juel VC, Hobson-Webb LD, et al. Myasthenic syndrome caused by plectinopathy. *Neurology*. 2011;76(4):327–336.
283. Maselli RA, Arredondo J, Cagney O, et al. Congenital myasthenic syndrome associated with epidermolysis bullosa caused by homozygous mutations in PLEC1 and CHRNE. *Clin Genet*. 2011;80(5):444–451.
284. McMillan JR, Akiyama M, Rouan F, et al. Plectin defects in epidermolysis bullosa simplex with muscular dystrophy. *Muscle Nerve*. 2007;35(1):24–35.
285. Fine JD, Stenn J, Johnson L, Wright T, Bock HG, Horiguchi Y. Autosomal recessive epidermolysis bullosa simplex. Generalized phenotypic features suggestive of junctional or dystrophic epidermolysis bullosa, and association with neuromuscular diseases. *Arch Dermatol*. 1989;125:931–938.
286. Bolling MC, Pas HH, de Visser M, et al. PLEC1 mutations underlie adult-onset dilated cardiomyopathy in epidermolysis

bullosa simplex with muscular dystrophy. *J Invest Dermatol.* 2010;130(4):1178–1181.
287. Gundesli H, Talim B, Korkusuz P, et al. Mutation in exon 1f of PLEC, leading to disruption of plectin isoform 1f, causes autosomal-recessive limb girdle muscular dystrophy. *Am J Hum Genet.* 2010;87(6):834–841.
288. Cetin N, Balci-Hayta B, Gundesli H, et al. A novel desmin mutation leading to autosomal recessive limb-girdle muscular dystrophy: distinct histopathological outcomes compared with desminopathies. *J Med Genet.* 2013;50(7):437–443.
289. Henderson M, De Waele L, Hudson J, et al. Recessive desmin-null muscular dystrophy with central nuclei and mitochondrial abnormalities. *Acta Neuropathol.* 2013;125(6):917–919.
290. Bögershausen N, Shahrzad N, Chong JX, et al. Recessive TRAPPC11 mutations cause a disease spectrum of limb girdle muscular dystrophy and myopathy with movement disorder and intellectual disability. *Am J Hum Genet.* 2013;93(1):181–190.
291. Chen Q, Zheng W, Xu H, et al. Digenic variants in the *TTN* and *TRAPPC11* genes co-segregating with a limb-girdle muscular dystrophy in a Han Chinese family. *Front Neurosci.* 2021;15:601757.
292. Fee DB, Harmelink M, Monrad P, Pyzik E. Siblings with mutations in TRAPPC11 presenting with limb-girdle muscular dystrophy 2S. *J Clin Neuromuscul Dis.* 2017;19(1):27–30.
293. Wang X, Wu Y, Cui Y, Wang N, Folkersen L, Wang Y. Novel TRAPPC11 mutations in a Chinese pedigree of limb girdle muscular dystrophy. *Case Rep Genet.* 2018;2018:8090797.
294. Munot P, McCrea N, Torelli S, et al. TRAPPC11-related muscular dystrophy with hypoglycosylation of alpha-dystroglycan in skeletal muscle and brain. *Neuropathol Appl Neurobiol.* 2022;48(2):e12771.
295. Carss KJ, Stevens E, Foley AR, et al. Mutations in GDP-mannose pyrophosphorylase B cause congenital and limb-girdle muscular dystrophies associated with hypoglycosylation of α-dystroglycan. *Am J Hum Genet.* 2013;93(1):29–41.
296. Belaya K, Rodríguez Cruz PM, Liu WW, et al. Mutations in GMPPB cause congenital myasthenic syndrome and bridge myasthenic disorders with dystroglycanopathies. *Brain.* 2015;138(Pt 9):2493–2504.
297. Rodríguez Cruz PM, Belaya K, Basiri K, et al. Clinical features of the myasthenic syndrome arising from mutations in GMPPB. *J Neurol Neurosurg Psychiatry.* 2016;87(8):802–809.
298. Cirak S, Foley AR, Herrmann R, et al. ISPD gene mutations are a common cause of congenital and limb-girdle muscular dystrophies. *Brain.* 2013;136(Pt 1):269–281.
299. Tasca G, Moro F, Aiello C, et al. Limb-girdle muscular dystrophy with α-dystroglycan deficiency and mutations in the ISPD gene. *Neurology.* 2013;80(10):963–965.
300. Song D, Fu X, Ge L, et al. A splice site mutation c.1251G>A of ISPD gene is a common cause of congenital muscular dystrophy in Chinese patients. *Clin Genet.* 2020;97(5):789–790.
301. Chardon JW, Smith AC, Woulfe J, et al. LIMS2 mutations are associated with a novel muscular dystrophy, severe cardiomyopathy and triangular tongues. *Clin Genet.* 2015;88(6):558–564.
302. Schindler RFR, Scotton C, Zhang J, et al. POPDC1-S201F causes muscular dystrophy and arrhythmia by affecting protein trafficking. *J Clin Invest.* 2016;126:239–253.
303. De Ridder W, Nelson I, Asselbergh B, et al. Muscular dystrophy with arrhythmia caused by loss-of-function mutations in BVES. *Neurol Genet.* 2019;5:e321.
304. Indrawati LA, Iida A, Tanaka Y, et al. Two Japanese LGMDR25 patients with a biallelic recurrent nonsense variant of BVES. *Neuromuscul Disord.* 2020;30(8):674–679.
305. Gangfuss A, Hentschel A, Heil L, et al. Proteomic and morphological insights and clinical presentation of two young patients with novel mutations of BVES (POPDC1). *Molec Genet Metab.* 2022;136:226–237.
306. Kayman-Kurekci G, Talim B, Korkusuz P, et al. Mutation in TOR1AIP1 encoding LAP1B in a form of muscular dystrophy: a novel gene related to nuclear envelopathies. *Neuromuscul Disord.* 2014;24(7):624–633.
307. Ghaoui R, Benavides T, Lek M, et al. TOR1AIP1 as a cause of cardiac failure and recessive limb-girdle muscular dystrophy. *Neuromuscul Disord.* 2016;26:500–503.
308. Feng X, Wu J, Xian W, et al. Muscular involvement and tendon contracture in limb-girdle muscular dystrophy 2Y: a mild adult phenotype and literature review. *BMC Musculoskelet Disord.* 2020;21(1):588.
309. Malfatti E, Catchpool T, Nouioua S, et al. A TOR1AIP1 variant segregating with an early onset limb girdle myasthenia-Support for the role of LAP1 in NMJ function and disease. *Neuropathol Appl Neurobiol.* 2022;48(1):e12743.
310. Servián-Morilla E, Cabrera-Serrano M, Johnson K, et al. *POGLUT1* biallelic mutations cause myopathy with reduced satellite cells, α-dystroglycan hypoglycosylation and a distinctive radiological pattern. *Acta Neuropathol.* 2020;139:565–582.
311. Arts WF, Bethlem J, Volkers WS. Further investigations on benign myopathy with autosomal dominant inheritance. *J Neurol.* 1978;217(3):201–206.
312. Bertini E, Pepe G. Collagen type VI and related disorders: Bethlem myopathy and Ullrich scleroatonic muscular dystrophy. *Eur J Paediatr Neurol.* 2002;6(4):193–198.
313. Bethlem J, Wijngaarden GK. Benign myopathy, with autosomal dominant inheritance. A report on three pedigrees. *Brain.* 1976;99(1):91–100.
314. Haq RU, Speer MC, Chu ML, Tandan R. Respiratory muscle involvement in Bethlem myopathy. *Neurology.* 1999;52(1):174–176.
315. Jobsis GJ, Boers JM, Barth PG, de Visser M. Bethlem myopathy: a slowly progressive congenital muscular dystrophy with contractures. *Brain.* 1999;122(Pt 4):649–655.
316. Jobsis GJ, Keizers H, Vreijling JP, et al. Type VI collagen mutations in Bethlem myopathy, an autosomal dominant myopathy with contractures. *Nat Genet.* 1996;14(1):113–115.
317. Mercuri E, Lampe A, Allsop J, et al. Muscle MRI in Ullrich congenital muscular dystrophy and Bethlem myopathy. *Neuromuscul Disord.* 2005;15(4):303–310.
318. ten Dam L, van der Kooi AJ, van Wattingen M, de Haan RJ, de Visser M. Reliability and accuracy of skeletal muscle imaging in limb-girdle muscular dystrophies. *Neurology.* 2012;79(16):2276–2277.
319. Caria F, Cescon M, Gualandi F, et al. Autosomal recessive Bethlem myopathy: a clinical, genetic and functional study. *Neuromuscul Disord.* 2019;29(9):657–663.
320. Chan SHS, Foley R, Phadke R, et al. Limb girdle muscular dystrophy due to LAMA2 mutations: diagnostic difficulties due to associated peripheral neuropathy. *Neuromusc. Disord.* 2014;24:677–683.
321. Gavassini BF, Carboni N, Nielsen JE, et al. Clinical and molecular characterization of limb-girdle muscular dystrophy due to LAMA2 mutations. *Muscle Nerve.* 2011;44:703–709.

322. Lokken N, Born AP, Duno M, Vissing J. LAMA2-related myopathy: frequency among congenital and limb-girdle muscular dystrophies. *Muscle Nerve.* 2015;52:547–553.
323. Magri F, Brusa R, Bello L, et al. Limb girdle muscular dystrophy due to *LAMA2* gene mutations: new mutations expand the clinical spectrum of a still challenging diagnosis. *Acta Myol.* 2020;39(2):67–82.
324. Oliveira J, Gruber A, Cardoso M, et al. LAMA2 gene mutation update: toward a more comprehensive picture of the laminin-alpha-2 variome and its related phenotypes. *Hum Mutat.* 2018;39:1314–1337.
325. Bouman K, Groothuis JT, Doorduin J, et al. *LAMA2*-related muscular dystrophy across the life span: a cross sectional study. *Neurol Genet.* 2023;9(5):e200089.
326. Endo Y, Dong M, Noguchi S, et al. Milder forms of muscular dystrophy associated with POMGNT2 mutations. *Neurol Genet.* 2015;1:e33.
327. Vissing J, Johnson K, Topf A, et al. POPDC3 gene variants associate with a new form of limb girdle muscular dystrophy. *Ann Neurol.* 2019;86:832–843.
328. Coppens S, Barnard A M, Puusepp S, et al. A form of muscular dystrophy associated with pathogenic variants in JAG1. *Am J Hum Genet.* 2021;108: 840–856. Erratum: *Am J Hum Genet.* 2021;108.
329. Logan CV, Lucke B, Pottinger C, et al. Mutations in MEGF10, a regulator of satellite cell myogenesis, cause early onset myopathy, areflexia, respiratory distress and dysphagia (EMARDD). *Nature Genet.* 2011;43:1189–1192.
330. Boyden SE, Mahoney LJ, Kawahara G, et al. Mutations in the satellite cell gene MEGF10 cause a recessive congenital myopathy with minicores. *Neurogenetics.* 2012;13:115–124.
331. Fujii K, Hirano M, Terayama A, et al. Identification of a novel mutation and genotype-phenotype relationship in MEGF10 myopathy. *Neuromuscul Disord.* 2022;32:436–440.
332. Harris E, Marini-Bettolo C, Töpf A, et al. MEGF10 related myopathies: a new case with adult onset disease with prominent respiratory failure and review of reported phenotypes. *Neuromuscul Disord.* 2018;28(1):48–53.
333. Bönnemann CG, Wang CH, Quijano-Roy S, et al. Diagnostic approach to the congenital muscular dystrophies. *Neuromuscul Disord.* 2014;24(4):289–311.
334. Pasrija D, Tadi P. Congenital muscular dystrophy. In: *StatPearls [Internet]*. StatPearls Publishing; 2022.
335. Harmelink M. Differentiating congenital myopathy from congenital muscular dystrophy. *Clin Perinatol.* 2020;47(1):197–209.
336. Prandini P, Berardinelli A, Fanin M, et al. LAMA2 loss-of-function mutation in a girl with a mild congenital muscular dystrophy. *Neurology.* 2004;63(6):1118–1121.
337. Sewry CA, Naom I, D'Alessandro M, et al. Variable clinical phenotype in merosin-deficient congenital muscular dystrophy associated with differential immunolabeling of two fragments of the laminin alpha 2 chain. *Neuromuscul Disord.* 1997;7(3):169–175.
338. Shorer Z, Philpot J, Muntoni F, Sewry C, Dubowitz V. Demyelinating peripheral neuropathy in merosin-deficient congenital muscular dystrophy. *J Child Neurol.* 1995;10(6):472–475.
339. Cohn RD, Herrmann R, Muntoni F, et al. Laminin alpha2 chain-deficient congenital muscular dystrophy: variable epitope expression in severe and mild cases. *Neurology.* 1998;51(1):94–100.
340. Mora M, Moroni I, Uziel G, et al. Mild clinical phenotype in a 12-year-old boy with partial merosin deficiency and central and peripheral nervous system abnormalities. *Neuromuscul Disord.* 1996;6(5):377–381.
341. Morandi L, Di Blasi C, Farina L, et al. Clinical correlations in 16 patients with total or partial laminin alpha2 deficiency characterized using antibodies against 2 fragments of the protein. *Arch Neurol.* 1999;56(2):209–215.
342. Naom I, Sewry C, D'Alessandro M, et al. Prenatal diagnosis in merosin-deficient congenital muscular dystrophy. *Neuromuscul Disord.* 1997;7(3):176–179.
343. Pegoraro E, Marks H, Garcia CA, et al. Laminin alpha2 muscular dystrophy: genotype/phenotype studies of 22 patients. *Neurology.* 1998;51(1):101–110.
344. Tan E, Topaloglu H, Sewry C, et al. Late onset muscular dystrophy with cerebral white matter changes due to partial merosin deficiency. *Neuromuscul Disord.* 1997;7(2):85–89.
345. Bushby K, Anderson LV, Pollitt C, Naom I, Muntoni F, Bindoff L. Abnormal merosin in adults. A new form of late onset muscular dystrophy not linked to chromosome 6 q2. *Brain.* 1998;121(Pt 4):581–588.
346. Philpot J, Cowan F, Pennock J, et al. Merosin-deficient congenital muscular dystrophy: the spectrum of brain involvement on magnetic resonance imaging. *Neuromuscul Disord.* 1999;9(2):81–85.
347. Mercuri E, Pennock J, Goodwin F, et al. Sequential study of central and peripheral nervous system involvement in an infant with merosin-deficient congenital muscular dystrophy. *Neuromuscul Disord.* 1996;6(6):425–429.
348. Sewry CA, D'Alessandro M, Wilson LA, et al. Expression of laminin chains in skin in merosin-deficient congenital muscular dystrophy. *Neuropediatrics.* 1997;28(4):217–222.
349. Guicheney P, Vignier N, Helbling-Leclerc A, et al. Genetics of laminin alpha 2 chain (or merosin) deficient congenital muscular dystrophy: from identification of mutations to prenatal diagnosis. *Neuromuscul Disord.* 1997;7(3):180–186.
350. Hayashi YK, Chou FL, Engvall E, et al. Mutations in the integrin alpha7 gene cause congenital myopathy. *Nat Genet.* 1998;19(1):94–97.
351. Ishikawa H, Sugie K, Murayama K, et al. Ullrich disease due to deficiency of collagen VI in the sarcolemma. *Neurology.* 2004;62(4):620–623.
352. Yonekawa T, Nishino I. Ullrich congenital muscular dystrophy: clinicopathological features, natural history and pathomechanism(s). *J Neurol Neurosurg Psychiatry.* 2015;86(3):280–287.
353. Baker NL, Morgelin M, Peat R, et al. Dominant collagen VI mutations are a common cause of Ullrich congenital muscular dystrophy. *Hum Mol Genet.* 2005;14(2):279–293.
354. Demir E, Ferreiro A, Sabatelli P, et al. Collagen VI status and clinical severity in Ullrich congenital muscular dystrophy: phenotype analysis of 11 families linked to the COL6 loci. *Neuropediatrics.* 2004;35(2):103–112.
355. Meilleur KG, Zukosky K, Medne L, et al. Clinical, pathologic, and mutational spectrum of dystroglycanopathy caused by LARGE mutations. *J Neuropathol Exp Neurol.* 2014;73(5):425–441.
356. Manzani MC, Tambunan DE, Hill RS, et al. Exome sequencing and functional validation in zebrafish identify GTDC2 mutations as a cause of Walker-Warburg syndrome. *Am J Hum Genet.* 2012;91(3):541–547.
357. Buysse K, Riemersma M, Powell G, et al. Missense mutations in [beta]-1,3-N-acetylglucosaminyltransferase 1 (B3GNT1)

358. Stevens E, Carss KJ, Cirak S, et al. Mutations in B3GALNT2 cause congenital muscular dystrophy and hypoglycosylation of [alpha]-dystroglycan. *Am J Hum Genet.* 2013;92(3): 354–365.
357. cause Walker-Warburg syndrome. *Hum Mol Genet.* 2013; 22(9):1746–1754.
359. Hedberg C, Oldfors A, Darin N. B3GALNT2 is a gene associated with congenital muscular dystrophy with brain malformations. *Eur J Hum Genet.* 2014;22(5):707–710.
360. Vuillaumier-Barrot S, Bouchet-Séraphin C, Chelbi M, et al. Identification of mutations in TMEM5 and ISPD as a cause of severe cobblestone lissencephaly. *Am J Hum Genet.* 2012; 91(6):1135–1143.
361. Kim DS, Hayashi YK, Matsumoto H, et al. POMT1 mutation results in defective glycosylation and loss of laminin-binding activity in alpha-DG. *Neurology.* 2004;62(6):1009–1011.
362. Beltran-Valero de Bernabe D, Currier S, Steinbrecher A, et al. Mutations in the O-mannosyltransferase gene POMT1 give rise to the severe neuronal migration disorder Walker–Warburg syndrome. *Am J Hum Genet.* 2002;71(5):1033–1043.
363. Cormand B, Pihko H, Bayés M, et al. Clinical and genetic distinction between Walker–Warburg syndrome and muscle–eye–brain disease. *Neurology.* 2001;56(8):1059–1069.
364. Diesen C, Saarinen A, Pihko H, et al. POMGnT1 mutation and phenotypic spectrum in muscle–eye–brain disease. *J Med Genet.* 2004;41(10):e115.
365. Wewer UM, Durkin ME, Zhang X, et al. Laminin beta 2 chain and adhalin deficiency in the skeletal muscle of Walker–Warburg syndrome (cerebro-ocular dysplasia-muscular dystrophy). *Neurology.* 1995;45(11):2099–2101.
366. Toda T, Kobayashi K, Kondo-Iida E, et al. The Fukuyama congenital muscular dystrophy story. *Neuromuscul Disord.* 2000;10(3):153–159.
367. Toda T, Yoshioka M, Nakahori Y, et al. Genetic identity of Fukuyama-type congenital muscular dystrophy and Walker–Warburg syndrome. *Ann Neurol.* 1995;37(1):99–101.
368. Kobayashi K, Nakahori Y, Miyake M, et al. An ancient retrotransposal insertion causes Fukuyama-type congenital muscular dystrophy. *Nature.* 1998;394(6691):388–392.
369. Yoshida A, Kobayashi K, Manya H, et al. Muscular dystrophy and neuronal migration disorder caused by mutations in a glycosyltransferase, POMGnT1. *Dev Cell.* 2001;1(5):717–724.
370. van Reeuwijk J, Janssen M, van den Elzen C, et al. POMT2 mutations cause alpha-dystroglycan hypoglycosylation and Walker Warburg syndrome. *J Med Genet.* 2005;42(12): 907–912.
371. Balci B, Uyanik G, Dincer P, et al. An autosomal recessive limb girdle muscular dystrophy (LGMD2) with mild mental retardation is allelic to Walker–Warburg syndrome (WWS) caused by a mutation in the POMT1 gene. *Neuromuscul Disord.* 2005;15(4):271–275.
372. Haltia M, Leivo I, Somer H, et al. Muscle–eye–brain disease: a neuropathological study. *Ann Neurol.* 1997;41(2):173–180.
373. Santavuori P, Somer H, Sainio K, et al. Muscle–eye–brain disease (MEB). *Brain Dev.* 1989;11(3):147–153.
374. Santavuori P, Valanne L, Autti T, Haltia M, Pihko H, Sainio K. Muscle–eye–brain disease: clinical features, visual evoked potentials and brain imaging in 20 patients. *Eur J Paediatr Neurol.* 1998;2(1):41–47.
375. Louhichi N, Triki C, Quijano-Roy S, et al. New FKRP mutations causing congenital muscular dystrophy associated with mental retardation and central nervous system abnormalities. Identification of a founder mutation in Tunisian families. *Neurogenetics.* 2004;5(1):27–34.
376. Lotz BP, Stubgen JP. The rigid spine syndrome: a vacuolar variant. *Muscle Nerve.* 1993;16(5):530–536.
377. Mercuri E, Talim B, Moghadaszadeh B, et al. Clinical and imaging findings in six cases of congenital muscular dystrophy with rigid spine syndrome linked to chromosome 1p (RSMD1). *Neuromuscul Disord.* 2002;12(7–8):631–638.
378. Merlini L, Granata C, Ballestrazzi A, Marini ML. Rigid spine syndrome and rigid spine sign in myopathies. *J Child Neurol.* 1989;4(4):274–282.
379. Moghadaszadeh B, Topaloglu H, Merlini L, et al. Genetic heterogeneity of congenital muscular dystrophy with rigid spine syndrome. *Neuromuscul Disord.* 1999;9(6–7):376–382.
380. Reichmann H, Goebel HH, Schneider C, Toyka KV. Familial mixed congenital myopathy with rigid spine phenotype. *Muscle Nerve.* 1997;20(4):411–417.
381. Taylor J, Muntoni F, Robb S, Dubowitz V, Sewry C. Early onset autosomal dominant myopathy with rigidity of the spine: A possible role for laminin beta 1? *Neuromuscul Disord.* 1997;7(4):211–216.
382. Flanigan KM, Kerr L, Bromberg MB, et al. Congenital muscular dystrophy with rigid spine syndrome: a clinical, pathological, radiological, and genetic study. *Ann Neurol.* 2000;47(2):152–161.
383. Ferreiro A, Ceuterick-de Groote C, Marks JJ, et al. Desmin-related myopathy with Mallory body-like inclusions is caused by mutations of the selenoprotein N gene. *Ann Neurol.* 2004; 55(5):676–686.
384. Tawil R, Van Der Maarel SM. Facioscapulohumeral muscular dystrophy. *Muscle Nerve.* 2006;34(1):1–15.
385. Personius KE, Pandya S, King WM, Tawil R, McDermott MP. Facioscapulohumeral dystrophy natural history study: standardization of testing procedures and reliability of measurements. The FSH DY Group. *Phys Ther.* 1994;74(3):253–263.
386. Tawil R, McDermott MP, Mendell JR, Kissel J, Griggs RC. Facioscapulohumeral muscular dystrophy (FSHD): design of natural history study and results of baseline testing. FSH-DY Group. *Neurology.* 1994;44(3 Pt 1):442–446.
387. Tawil R, McDermott MP, Pandya S, et al. A pilot trial of prednisone in facioscapulohumeral muscular dystrophy. FSHDY Group. *Neurology.* 1997;48(1):46–49.
388. van der Kooi AJ, Visser MC, Rosenberg N, et al. Extension of the clinical range of facioscapulohumeral dystrophy: report of six cases. *J Neurol Neurosurg Psychiatry.* 2000;69(1):114–116.
389. Mul K. Facioscapulohumeral muscular dystrophy. *Continuum (Minneap Minn).* 2022;28(6):1735–1751.
390. Felice KJ, North WA, Moore SA, Mathews KD. FSH dystrophy 4q35 deletion in patients presenting with facial-sparing scapular myopathy. *Neurology.* 2000;54(10):1927–1931.
391. Wohlgemuth M, van der Kooi EL, van Kesteren RG, van der Maarel SM, Padberg GW. Ventilatory support in facioscapulohumeral muscular dystrophy. *Neurology.* 2004;63(1):176–178.
392. Laforet P, de Toma C, Eymard B, et al. Cardiac involvement in genetically confirmed facioscapulohumeral muscular dystrophy. *Neurology.* 1998;51(5):1454–1456.
393. Felice KJ, Jones JM, Conway SR. Facioscapulohumeral dystrophy presenting as infantile facial diplegia and late-onset limb-girdle myopathy in members of the same family. *Muscle Nerve.* 2005;32(3):368–372.

394. Monforte M, Bortolani S, Torchia E, et al. Diagnostic magnetic resonance imaging biomarkers for facioscapulohumeral muscular dystrophy identified by machine learning. *J Neurol*. 2022;269(4):2055–2063.
395. Munsat TL, Piper D, Cancilla P, Mednick J. Inflammatory myopathy with facioscapulohumeral distribution. *Neurology*. 1972;22(4):335–347.
396. Spuler S, Engel AG. Unexpected sarcolemmal complement membrane attack complex deposits on nonnecrotic muscle fibers in muscular dystrophies. *Neurology*. 1998;50(1):41–46.
397. Wijmenga C, Hewitt JE, Sandkuijl LA, et al. Chromosome 4q DNA rearrangements associated with facioscapulohumeral muscular dystrophy. *Nat Genet*. 1992;2(1):26–30.
398. Tawil R, Forrester J, Griggs RC, et al. Evidence for anticipation and association of deletion size with severity in facioscapulohumeral muscular dystrophy. The FSH-DY Group. *Ann Neurol*. 1996;39(6):744–748.
399. Himeda CL, Jones PL. The genetics and epigenetics of facioscapulohumeral muscular dystrophy. *Annu Rev Genomics Hum Genet*. 2019;20:265–291.
400. Lemmers RJ, Tawil R, Petek LM, et al. Digenic inheritance of an SMCHD1 mutation and an FSHD-permissive D4Z4 allele causes facioscapulohumeral muscular dystrophy type 2. *Nat Genet*. 2012;44(12):1370–1374.
401. Sacconi S, Lemmers RJ, Balog J, et al. The FSHD2 gene SMCHD1 is a modifier of disease severity in families affected by FSHD1. *Am J Hum Genet*. 2013;93(4):744–751.
402. Hamanaka K, Šikrová D, Mitsuhashi S, et al. Homozygous nonsense variant in *LRIF1* associated with facioscapulohumeral muscular dystrophy. *Neurology*. 2020;94(23):e2441–e2447.
403. van den Boogaard ML, Lemmers RJLF, Balog J, et al. Mutations in DNMT3B modify epigenetic repression of the D4Z4 repeat and the penetrance of facioscapulohumeral dystrophy. *Am J Hum Genet*. 2016;98(5):1020–1029.
404. Andrews CT, Taylor TC, Patterson VH. Scapulothoracic arthrodesis for patients with facioscapulohumeral muscular dystrophy. *Neuromuscul Disord*. 1998;8(8):580–584.
405. Letournel E, Fardeau M, Lytle JO, Serrault M, Gosselin RA. Scapulothoracic arthrodesis for patients who have facioscapulohumeral muscular dystrophy. *J Bone Joint Surg Am*. 1990;72(1):78–84.
406. Chakrabarti A, Pearce JM. Scapuloperoneal syndrome with cardiomyopathy: Report of a family with autosomal dominant inheritance and unusual features. *J Neurol Neurosurg Psychiatry*. 1981;44(12):1146–1152.
407. Kaeser HE. Scapuloperoneal muscular atrophy. *Brain*. 1965;88(2):407–418.
408. Takahashi K, Nakamura H, Nakashima R. Scapuloperoneal dystrophy associated with neurogenic changes. *J Neurol Sci*. 1974;23(4):575–583.
409. Thomas PK, Schott GD, Morgan-Hughes JA. Adult onset scapuloperoneal myopathy. *J Neurol Neurosurg Psychiatry*. 1975;38(10):1008–1015.
410. Wilhelmsen KC, Blake DM, Lynch T, et al. Chromosome 12-linked autosomal dominant scapuloperoneal muscular dystrophy. *Ann Neurol*. 1996;39(4):507–520.
411. Probst A, Ulrich J, Kaeser HE, Heitz P. Scapulo-peroneal muscular atrophy. Full autopsy report. Unusual findings in the anterior horn of the spinal cord. Lipid storage in muscle. *Eur Neurol*. 1977;16(1–6):181–196.
412. Quinzi CM, Vu TH, Min KC, et al. X-linked dominant scapuloperoneal myopathy is due to mutation in the gene encoding four-and-a-half-LIM protein 1. *Am J Hum Genet*. 2008;82:208–213.
413. Thomas PK, Calne DB, Elliott CF. X-linked scapuloperoneal syndrome. *J Neurol Neurosurg Psychiatry*. 1972;35(2):208–215.
414. Pegoraro E, Gavassini BF, Borsato C, et al. MYH7 gene mutation in myosin storage myopathy and scapulo-peroneal myopathy. *Neuromusc Disord*. 2007;17:321–329.
415. Zukosky K, Meilleur K, Traynor BJ, et al. Association of a novel ACTA1 mutation with a dominant progressive scapuloperoneal myopathy in an extended family. *JAMA Neurol*. 2015;72(6):689–698.
416. Heller SA, Shih R, Kalra R, Kang PB. Emery-Dreifuss muscular dystrophy. *Muscle Nerve*. 2020;61(4):436–448.
417. Emery AE, Dreifuss FE. Unusual type of benign x-linked muscular dystrophy. *J Neurol Neurosurg Psychiatry*. 1966;29(4):338–342.
418. Hopkins LC, Jackson JA, Elsas LJ. Emery–Dreifuss humeroperoneal muscular dystrophy: an X-linked myopathy with unusual contractures and bradycardia. *Ann Neurol*. 1981;10(3):230–237.
419. Kubo S, Tsukahara T, Takemitsu M, et al. Presence of emerinopathy in cases of rigid spine syndrome. *Neuromuscul Disord*. 1998;8(7):502–507.
420. Emery AE. Emery–Dreifuss muscular dystrophy—a 40 year retrospective. *Neuromuscul Disord*. 2000;10(4–5):228–232.
421. Schessl J, Columbus A, Hu Y, et al. Familial reducing body myopathy with cytoplasmic bodies and rigid spine revisited: identification of a second LIM domain mutation in FHL1. *Neuropediatrics*. 2010;41(1):43–46.
422. Schoser B, Goebel HH, Janisch I, et al. Consequences of mutations within the C terminus of the FHL1 gene. *Neurology*. 2009;73(7):543–551.
423. Shalaby S, Hayashi YK, Nonaka I, Noguchi S, Nishino I. Novel FHL1 mutations in fatal and benign reducing body myopathy. *Neurology*. 2009;72(4):375–376.
424. Chen DH, Raskind WH, Parson WW, et al. A novel mutation in FHL1 in a family with X-linked scapuloperoneal myopathy: phenotypic spectrum and structural study of FHL1 mutations. *J Neurol Sci*. 2010;296(1–2):22–29.
425. Selcen D, Bromberg MB, Chin SS, Engel AG. Reducing bodies and myofibrillar myopathy features in FHL1 muscular dystrophy. *Neurology*. 2011;77(22):1951–1959.
426. Shalaby S, Hayashi YK, Goto K, et al. Rigid spine syndrome caused by a novel mutation in four-and-a-half LIM domain 1 gene (FHL1). *Neuromuscul Disord*. 2008;18:959–961.
427. Fatkin D, MacRae C, Sasaki T, et al. Missense mutations in the rod domain of the lamin A/C gene as causes of dilated cardiomyopathy and conduction-system disease. *N Engl J Med*. 1999;341(23):1715–1724.
428. Zhang Q, Bethmann C, Worth NF, et al. Nesprin-1 and -2 are involved in the pathogenesis of Emery Dreifuss muscular dystrophy and are critical for nuclear envelope integrity. *Hum Mol Genet*. 2007;16(23):2816–2833.
429. Liang WC, Mitsuhashi H, Keduka E, et al. TMEM43 mutations in Emery-Dreifuss muscular dystrophy-related myopathy. *Ann Neurol*. 2011;69(6):1005–1013.
430. Katz JS, Wolfe GI, Burns DK, et al. Isolated neck extensor myopathy: a common cause of dropped head syndrome. *Neurology*. 1996;46(4):917–921.

431. Serratrice G, Pouget J, Pellissier JF. Bent spine syndrome. *J Neurol Neurosurg Psychiatry.* 1996;60(1):51–54.
432. Suarez GA, Kelly JJ Jr. The dropped head syndrome. *Neurology.* 1992;42(8):1625–1627.
433. Chahin N, Selcen D, Engel AG. Sporadic late onset nemaline myopathy. *Neurology.* 2005;65(8):1158–1164.
434. Duarte S, Oliveira J, Santos R, et al. Dominant and recessive RYR1 mutations in adults with core lesions and mild muscle symptoms. *Muscle Nerve.* 2011;44(1):102–108.
435. Løseth S, Voermans NC, Torbergsen T, et al. A novel late-onset axial myopathy associated with mutations in the skeletal muscle ryanodine receptor (RYR1) gene. *J Neurol.* 2013;260(6):1504–1510.
436. Fiorillo C, Astrea G, Savarese M, et al. MYH7-related myopathies: clinical, histopathological and imaging findings in a cohort of Italian patients. *Orphanet J Rare Dis.* 2016;11(1):91.
437. Brais B, Rouleau GA, Bouchard JP, Fardeau M, Tomé FM. Oculopharyngeal muscular dystrophy. *Semin Neurol.* 1999;19(1):59–66.
438. Hill ME, Creed GA, Bouchard JP, Fardeau M, Tomé FM. Oculopharyngeal muscular dystrophy: phenotypic and genotypic studies in a UK population. *Brain.* 2001;124(Pt 3):522–526.
439. Yamashita S. Recent progress in oculopharyngeal muscular dystrophy. *J Clin Med.* 2021;10(7):1375.
440. Trollet C, Boulinguiez A, Roth F, et al. Oculopharyngeal muscular dystrophy. In: Adam MP, Everman DB, Mirzaa GM, et al., eds. GeneReviews® [Internet]. University of Washington, Seattle; 1993–2022.
441. Kroon RHMJM, Kalf JG, de Swart BJM, et al. Longitudinal assessment of strength, functional capacity, oropharyngeal function, and quality of life in oculopharyngeal muscular dystrophy. *Neurology.* 2021;97(15):e1475–e1483.
442. Alonso-Jimenez A, Kroon R, Alejaldre-Monforte A, et al. Muscle MRI in a large cohort of patients with oculopharyngeal muscular dystrophy. *J Neurol Neurosurg Psychiatry.* 2019;90(5):576–585.
443. Kroon RHMJM, Kalf JG, Meijers RL, et al. Muscle ultrasound is a sensitive biomarker in oculopharyngeal muscular dystrophy. *Muscle Nerve.* 2022;66(4):453–461.
444. Calado A, Tome FM, Brais B, et al. Nuclear inclusions in oculopharyngeal muscular dystrophy consist of poly(A) binding protein 2 aggregates which sequester poly(A) RNA. *Hum Mol Genet.* 2000;9(15):2321–2328.
445. Shanmugam V, Dion P, Rochefort D, Laganière J, Brais B, Rouleau GA. PABP2 polyalanine tract expansion causes intranuclear inclusions in oculopharyngeal muscular dystrophy. *Ann Neurol.* 2000;48(5):798–802.
446. Brais B, Bouchard JP, Xie YG, et al. Short GCG expansions in the PABP2 gene cause oculopharyngeal muscular dystrophy. *Nat Genet.* 1998;18(2):164–167.
447. Fukuhara N, Kumamoto T, Tsubaki T, Mayuzumi T, Nitta H. Oculopharyngeal muscular dystrophy and distal myopathy. Intrafamilial difference in the onset and distribution of muscular involvement. *Acta Neurol Scand.* 1982;65(5):458–467.
448. Amato AA, Jackson CE, Ridings LW, Barohn RJ. Childhood-onset oculopharyngodistal myopathy with chronic intestinal pseudo-obstruction. *Muscle Nerve.* 1995;18(8):842–847.
449. Shimizu T, Ishiura H, Hara M, et al. Expanded clinical spectrum of oculopharyngodistal myopathy type 1. *Muscle Nerve.* 2022;66(6):679–685.
450. Deng J, Yu J, Li P, et al. Expansion of GGC repeat in GIPC1 is associated with oculopharyngodistal myopathy. *Am J Hum Genet.* 2020;106:793–804.
451. Xi J, Wang X, Yue D, et al. 5-Prime UTR CGG repeat expansion in GIPC1 is associated with oculopharyngodistal myopathy. *Brain.* 2021;144:601–614.
452. Ogasawara M, Iida A, Kumutpongpanich T, et al. CGG expansion in NOTCH2NLC is associated with oculopharyngodistal myopathy with neurological manifestations. *Acta Neuropathol Commun.* 2020;8:204.
453. Ogasawara M, Eura N, Nagaoka U, et al. Intranuclear inclusions in skin biopsies are not limited to neuronal intranuclear inclusion disease but can also be seen in oculopharyngodistal myopathy. *Neuropathol Appl Neurobiol.* 2022;48(3):e12787.
454. Yu J, Shan J, Yu M, et al. The CGG repeat expansion in RILPL1 is associated with oculopharyngodistal myopathy type 4. *Am J Hum Genet.* 2022;109(3):533–541.
455. Zeng YH, Yang K, Du GQ, et al. GGC Repeat Expansion of RILPL1 is Associated with Oculopharyngodistal Myopathy. *Ann Neurol.* 2022;92(3):512–526.
456. Huang XR, Tang BS, Jin P, Guo JF. The phenotypes and mechanisms of NOTCH2NLC-related GGC repeat expansion disorders: A Comprehensive Review. *Mol Neurobiol.* 2022;59(1):523–534.
457. Savarese M, Sarparanta J, Vihola A, et al. Panorama of the distal myopathies. *Acta Myol.* 2020;39(4):245–265.
458. Milone M, Liewluck T. The unfolding spectrum of inherited distal myopathies. *Muscle Nerve.* 2019;59(3):283–294.
459. Welander L. Myopathia distalis tarda hereditaria; 249 examined cases in 72 pedigrees. *Acta Med Scand Suppl.* 1951;265:1–124.
460. Borg K, Ahlberg G, Borg J, Edström L. Welander's distal myopathy: clinical, neurophysiological and muscle biopsy observations in young and middle aged adults with early symptoms. *J Neurol Neurosurg Psychiatry.* 1991;54(6):494–498.
461. Lindberg C, Borg K, Edström L, Hedström A, Oldfors A. Inclusion body myositis and Welander distal myopathy: a clinical, neurophysiological and morphological comparison. *J Neurol Sci.* 1991;103(1):76–81.
462. Borg K, Solders G, Borg J, Edström L, Kristensson K. Neurogenic involvement in distal myopathy (Welander). Histochemical and morphological observations on muscle and nerve biopsies. *J Neurol Sci.* 1989;91(1–2):53–70.
463. Borg K, Tome FM, Edström L. Intranuclear and cytoplasmic filamentous inclusions in distal myopathy (Welander). *Acta Neuropathol (Berl).* 1991;82(2):102–106.
464. Edstrom L. Histochemical and histopathological changes in skeletal muscle in late-onset hereditary distal myopathy (Welander). *J Neurol Sci.* 1975;26(2):147–157.
465. Hackman P, Sarparanta J, Lehtinen S, et al. Welander distal myopathy is caused by a mutation in the RNA-binding protein TIA1. *Ann Neurol.* 2013;73(4):500–509.
466. Klar J, Sobol M, Melberg A, et al. Welander distal myopathy caused by an ancient founder mutation in TIA1 associated with perturbed splicing. *Hum Mutat.* 2013;34(4):572–577.
467. Lee Y, Jonson PH, Sarparanta J, et al. TIA1 variant drives myodegeneration in multisystem proteinopathy with SQSTM1 mutations. *J Clin Invest.* 2018;128(3):1164–1177.
468. Hackman P, Vihola A, Haravuori H, et al. Tibial muscular dystrophy is a titinopathy caused by mutations in TTN, the gene encoding the giant skeletal-muscle protein titin. *Am J Hum Genet.* 2002;71(3):492–500.

469. Markesbery WR, Griggs RC, Leach RP, Lapham LW. Late onset hereditary distal myopathy. *Neurology*. 1974;24(2):127–134.
470. Griggs R, Vihola A, Hackman P, et al. Zaspopathy in a large classic late-onset distal myopathy family. *Brain*. 2007;130:1477–1484.
471. Lin X, Ruiz J, Bajraktari I, et al. Z-disc-associated, alternatively spliced, PDZ motif-containing protein (ZASP) mutations in the actin-binding domain cause disruption of skeletal muscle actin filaments in myofibrillar myopathy. *J Biol Chem*. 2014;289(19):13615–13626.
472. Mizusawa H, Kurisaki H, Takatsu M, et al. Rimmed vacuolar distal myopathy: a clinical, electrophysiological, histopathological and computed tomographic study of seven cases. *J Neurol*. 1987;234(3):129–136.
473. Nonaka I, Sunohara N, Ishiura S, Satoyoshi E. Familial distal myopathy with rimmed vacuole and lamellar (myeloid) body formation. *J Neurol Sci*. 1981;51(1):141–155.
474. Nonaka I, Sunohara N, Satoyoshi E, Terasawa K, Yonemoto K. Autosomal recessive distal muscular dystrophy: a comparative study with distal myopathy with rimmed vacuole formation. *Ann Neurol*. 1985;17(1):51–59.
475. Sunohara N, Nonaka I, Kamei N, Satoyoshi E. Distal myopathy with rimmed vacuole formation. A follow-up study. *Brain*. 1989;112(Pt 1):65–83.
476. Argov Z, Eisenberg I, Grabov-Nardini G, et al. Hereditary inclusion body myopathy: The Middle Eastern genetic cluster. *Neurology*. 2003;60(9):1519–1523.
477. Mullen J, Alrasheed K, Mozaffar T. GNE myopathy: history, etiology, and treatment trials. *Front Neurol*. 2022;13:1002310.
478. Sivakumar K, Dalakas MC. The spectrum of familial inclusion body myopathies in 13 families and a description of a quadriceps-sparing phenotype in non-Iranian Jews. *Neurology*. 1996;47(4):977–984.
479. Eisenberg I, Grabov-Nardini G, Hochner H, et al. Mutations spectrum of GNE in hereditary inclusion body myopathy sparing the quadriceps. *Hum Mutat*. 2003;21(1):99.
480. Eisenberg I, Avidan N, Potikha T, et al. The UDP-N-acetylglucosamine 2-epimerase/N-acetylmannosamine kinase gene is mutated in recessive hereditary inclusion body myopathy. *Nat Genet*. 2001;29(1):83–87.
481. Laing NG, Laing BA, Meredith C, et al. Autosomal dominant distal myopathy: linkage to chromosome 14. *Am J Hum Genet*. 1995;56(2):422–427.
482. Mastaglia FL, Phillips BA, Cala LA, et al. Early onset chromosome 14-linked distal myopathy (Laing). *Neuromuscul Disord*. 2002;12:350–357.
483. Meredith C, Herrmann R, Parry C, et al. Mutations in the slow skeletal muscle fiber myosin heavy chain gene (MYH7) cause Laing early-onset distal myopathy (MPD1). *Am J Hum Genet*. 2004;75:703–708.
484. Muelas N, Hackman P, Lugue H, et al. MYH7 gene tail mutation causing myopathic profiles beyond Laing distal myopathy. *Neurology*. 2010;75:732–741.
485. Overeem S, Schelhaas HJ, Blijham PJ, et al. Symptomatic distal myopathy with cardiomyopathy due to a MYH7 mutation. *Neuromuscul Disord*. 2007;17:490–493.
486. Tasca G, Ricci E, Penttilä S, et al. New phenotype and pathology features in MYH7-related distal myopathy. *Neuromuscul Disord*. 2012;22:640–647.
487. Lamont PJ, Udd B, Mastaglia FL, et al. Laing early onset distal myopathy: slow myosin defect with variable abnormalities on muscle biopsy. *J Neurol Neurosurg Psychiatry*. 2006;77(2):208–215.
488. Tajsharghi H, Thornell LE, Lindberg C, Lindvall B, Henriksson KG, Oldfors A. Myosin storage myopathy associated with a heterozygous missense mutation in MYH7. *Ann Neurol*. 2003;54(4):494–500.
489. Tajsharghi H, Oldfors A, Macleod DP, Swash M. Homozygous mutation in MYH7 in myosin storage myopathy and cardiomyopathy. *Neurology*. 2007;68:962.
490. Masuzugawa S, Kuzuhara S, Narita Y, Naito Y, Taniguchi A, Ibi T. Autosomal dominant hyaline body myopathy presenting as scapuloperoneal syndrome: clinical features and muscle pathology. *Neurology*. 1997;48:253–257.
491. Bohlega S, Abu-Amero SN, Wakil SM, et al. Mutation of the slow myosin heavy chain rod domain underlies hyaline body myopathy. *Neurology*. 2004;62:518–521.
492. Williams DR, Reardon K, Roberts L, et al. A new dominant distal myopathy affecting posterior leg and anterior upper limb muscles. *Neurology*. 2005;64:1245–1254.
493. Duff RM, Tay V, Hackman P, et al. Mutations in the N-terminal actin-binding domain of filamin C cause a distal myopathy. *Am J Hum Genet*. 2011;88:729–740.
494. Guergueltcheva V, Peeters K, Baets J, et al. Distal myopathy with upper limb predominance caused by filamin C haploinsufficiency. *Neurology*. 2011;77:2105–2114.
495. Luan X, Hong D, Zhang W, Wang Z, Yuan Y. A novel heterozygous deletion-insertion mutation (2695–2712 del/GTTTGT ins) in exon 18 of the filamin C gene causes filaminopathy in a large Chinese family. *Neuromuscul Disord*. 2010;20:390–396.
496. Wallgren-Pettersson C, Lehtokari VL, Kalimo H, et al. Distal myopathy caused by homozygous missense mutations in the nebulin gene. *Brain*. 2007;130:1465–1476.
497. Lehtokari VL, Pelin K, Herczegfalvi A, et al. Nemaline myopathy caused by mutations in the nebulin gene may present as a distal myopathy. *Neuromuscul Disord*. 2011;21:556–562.
498. Cirak S, von Deimling F, Sachdev S, et al. Kelch-like homologue 9 mutation is associated with an early onset autosomal dominant distal myopathy. *Brain*. 2010;133:2123–2135.
499. Park HJ, Hong YB, Choi YC, et al. ADSSL1 mutation relevant to autosomal recessive adolescent onset distal myopathy. *Ann Neurol*. 2016;79:231–243.
500. Park HJ, Lee JE, Choi GS, et al. Electron microscopy pathology of ADSSL1 myopathy. *J Clin Neurol*. 2017;13:105–106.
501. Park HJ, Shin HY, Kim S, et al. Distal myopathy with ADSSL1 mutations in Korean patients. *Neuromuscul Disord*. 2017;27:465–472.
502. Mroczek M, Durmus H, Bijarnia-Mahay S, et al. Expanding the disease phenotype of ADSSL1-associated myopathy in non-Korean patients. *Neuromuscul Disord*. 2020;30:310–314.
503. Saito Y, Nishikawa A, Iida A, et al. ADSSL1 myopathy is the most common nemaline myopathy in Japan with variable clinical features. *Neurology*. 2020;95(11):e1500–e1511.
504. Motoda A, Takahashi T, Watanabe C, et al. An autopsied case of ADSSL1 myopathy. *Neuromuscul Disord*. 2021;31(11):1220–1225.
505. Di Blasi C, Moghadaszadeh B, Ciano C, et al. Abnormal lysosomal and ubiquitin-proteasome pathways in 19p13.3 distal myopathy. *Ann Neurol*. 2004;56:133–138.
506. Ruggieri A, Naumenko S, Smith MA, et al. Multiomic elucidation of a coding 99-mer repeat-expansion skeletal muscle disease. *Acta Neuropathol*. 2020;140:231–235.
507. Wang Q, Yu M, Zhang W, et al. Subsarcolemmal and cytoplasmic p62 positivity and rimmed vacuoles are distinctive

for PLIN4-myopathy. *Ann Clin Transl Neurol.* 2022;9(11): 1813–1819.
508. Amato AA, Kagan-Hallet K, Jackson CE, et al. The wide spectrum of myofibrillar myopathy suggests a multifactorial etiology and pathogenesis. *Neurology.* 1998;51(6):1646–1655.
509. De Bleecker JL, Engel AG, Ertl BB. Myofibrillar myopathy with abnormal foci of desmin positivity. II. Immunocytochemical analysis reveals accumulation of multiple other proteins. *J Neuropathol Exp Neurol.* 1996;55(5):563–577.
510. Engel AG. Myofibrillar myopathy. *Ann Neurol.* 1999;46(5): 681–683.
511. Goebel HH. Desmin-related neuromuscular disorders. *Muscle Nerve.* 1995;18(11):1306–1320.
512. Goldfarb LG, Vicart P, Goebel HH, Dalakas MC. Desmin myopathy. *Brain.* 2004;127(Pt 4):723–734.
513. Nakano S, Engel AG, Waclawik AJ, Emslie-Smith AM, Busis NA. Myofibrillar myopathy with abnormal foci of desmin positivity. I. Light and electron microscopy analysis of 10 cases. *J Neuropathol Exp Neurol.* 1996;55(5):549–562.
514. Selcen D, Engel AG. Myofibrillar myopathy caused by novel dominant negative alpha B-crystallin mutations. *Ann Neurol.* 2003;54(6):804–810.
515. Selcen D, Ohno K, Engel AG. Myofibrillar myopathy: clinical, morphological and genetic studies in 63 patients. *Brain.* 2004;127(Pt 2):439–451.
516. Vicart P, Caron A, Guicheney P, et al. A missense mutation in the alpha B crystallin chaperone gene causes a desmin-related myopathy. *Nat Genet.* 1998;20(1):92–95.
517. Nakano S, Engel AG, Akiguchi I, Kimura J. Myofibrillar myopathy. III. Abnormal expression of cyclin-dependent kinases and nuclear proteins. *J Neuropathol Exp Neurol.* 1997;56(8):850–856.
518. Liewluck T. A window into the myofibrillar myopathy proteome. *Neurol Genet.* 2021;7(3):e587.
519. Sabatelli M, Bertini E, Ricci E, et al. Peripheral neuropathy with giant axons and cardiomyopathy associated with desmin type intermediate filaments in skeletal muscle. *J Neurol Sci.* 1992;109(1):1–10.
520. Munoz-Marmol AM, Strasser G, Isamat M, et al. A dysfunctional desmin mutation in a patient with severe generalized myopathy. *Proc Natl Acad Sci U S A.* 1998;95(19):11312–11317.
521. Li M, Dalakas MC. Abnormal desmin protein in myofibrillar myopathies caused by desmin gene mutations. *Ann Neurol.* 2001;49(4):532–536.
522. Homma S, Iwasaki M, Shelton GD, Engvall E, Reed JC, Takayama S. BAG3 deficiency results in fulminant myopathy and early lethality. *Am J Path.* 2006;169:761–773.
523. Lee HC, Cherk SW, Chan SK, Wet al. BAG3-related myofibrillar myopathy in a Chinese family. *Clin Genet.* 2012;81: 394–398.
524. Odgerel Z, Sarkozy A, Lee H-S, et al. Inheritance patterns and phenotypic features of myofibrillar myopathy associated with a BAG3 mutation. *Neuromusc Disord.* 2010;20:438–442.
525. Semmler AL, Sacconi S, Bach JE, et al. Unusual multisystemic involvement and a novel BAG3 mutation revealed by NGS screening in a large cohort of myofibrillar myopathies. *Orphanet J Rare Dis.* 2014;9:121.
526. Ebrahimzadeh-Vesal R, Teymoori A, Dourandish AM, Azimi-Nezhad M. Identification of a novel nonsense mutation in kyphoscoliosis peptidase gene in an Iranian patient with myofibrillar myopathy. *Genes Dis.* 2018;5:331–334.
527. Hedberg-Oldfors C, Darin N, Olsson Engman M, et al. A new early-onset neuromuscular disorder associated with kyphoscoliosis peptidase (KY) deficiency. *Europ J Hum Genet.* 2016;24:1771–1777.
528. Straussberg R, Schottmann G. Sadeh M, et al. Kyphoscoliosis peptidase (KY) mutation causes a novel congenital myopathy with core targetoid defects. *Acta Neuropath.* 2016;132: 475–478.
529. O'Grady G L, Best HA, Sztal TE, et al. Variants in the oxidoreductase PYROXD1 cause early-onset myopathy with internalized nuclei and myofibrillar disorganization. *Am J Hum Genet.* 2016;99:1086–1105.
530. Hedberg-Oldfors C, Meyer R, Nolte K, et al. Loss of supervillin causes myopathy with myofibrillar disorganization and autophagic vacuoles. *Brain.* 2020;143:2406–2420.
531. Dafsari HS, Kocaturk NM, Daimaguler H-S, et al. Bi-allelic mutations in uncoordinated mutant number-45 myosin chaperone B are a cause for congenital myopathy. *Acta Neuropath Commun.* 2019;7:211.
532. Donkervoort S, Kutzner CE, Hu Y, et al. Pathogenic variants in the myosin chaperone UNC-45B cause progressive myopathy with eccentric cores. *Am J Hum Genet.* 2020;107:1078–1095.
533. Barth P G, Wanders RJA, Ruitenbeek W, et al. Infantile fibre type disproportion, myofibrillar lysis and cardiomyopathy: a disorder in three unrelated Dutch families. *Neuromusc Disord.* 1998;8:296–304.
534. Manivannan S N, Darouich S, Masmoudi A, et al. Novel frameshift variant in MYL2 reveals molecular differences between dominant and recessive forms of hypertrophic cardiomyopathy. *PLoS Genet.* 2020;16:e1008639.
535. Weterman MAJ, Barth PG, van Spaendonck-Zwarts KY, et al. Recessive MYL2 mutations cause infantile type I muscle fibre disease and cardiomyopathy. *Brain.* 2013;136:282–293.
536. Tajsharghi H, Darin N, Rekabdar E, et al. Mutations and sequence variation in the human myosin heavy chain IIa gene (MYH2). *Eur J Hum Genet.* 2005;13(5):617–622.
537. Martinsson T, Oldfors A, Darin N, et al. Autosomal dominant myopathy: Missense mutation (Glu-706 –>Lys) in the myosin heavy chain IIa gene. *Proc Natl Acad Sci U S A.* 2000;97: 14614–14619.
538. Watts GD, Thorne M, Kovach MJ, Pestronk A, Kimonis VE. Clinical and genetic heterogeneity in chromosome 9p associated hereditary inclusion body myopathy: exclusion of GNE and three other candidate genes. *Neuromuscul Disord.* 2003;13(7-8):559–567.
539. Watts GD, Wymer J, Kovach MJ, et al. Inclusion body myopathy associated with Paget disease of bone and frontotemporal dementia is caused by mutant valosin-containing protein. *Nat Genet.* 2004;36(4):377–381.
540. Watts GD, Thomasova D, Ramdeen SK, et al. Novel VCP mutations in inclusion body myopathy associated with Paget disease of bone and frontotemporal dementia. *Clin Genet.* 2007;72:420–426.
541. Watts GD. Inclusion body myopathy associated with Paget disease of bone and frontotemporal dementia is caused by mutant valosin-containing protein. *Nat Genet.* 2004;36: 377–381.
542. Kimonis VE, Kovach MJ, Waggoner B, et al. Clinical and molecular studies in a unique family with autosomal dominant limb-girdle muscular dystrophy and Paget disease of bone. *Genet Med.* 2000;2:232–241.

543. Kimonis VE, Mehta SG, Fulchiero EC, et al. Clinical studies in familial VCP myopathy associated with Paget disease of bone and frontotemporal dementia. *Am J Med Genet A.* 2008;146A:745–757.
544. Kimonis VE, Watts GD. Autosomal dominant inclusion body myopathy, Paget disease of bone, and frontotemporal dementia. *Alzheimer Dis Assoc Disord.* 2005;19(Suppl 1):S44–S47.
545. Guyant-Maréchal L, Laquierrière A, Duyckaerts C, et al. Valosin-containing protein gene mutations: clinical and neuropathologic features. *Neurology.* 2006;67:644–651.
546. Haubenberger D, Bittner RE, Rauch-Shorny S, et al. Inclusion body myopathy and Paget disease is linked to a novel mutation in the VCP gene. *Neurology.* 2005;65:1304–1305.
547. Miller TD, Jackson AP, Barresi R, et al. Inclusion body myopathy with Paget disease and frontotemporal dementia (IBMPFD): clinical features including sphincter disturbance in a large pedigree. *J Neurol Neurosurg Psychiatry.* 2009;80:583–584.
548. Kim EJ, Park YE, Kim DS, et al. Inclusion body myopathy with Paget disease of bone and frontotemporal dementia linked to VCP p.Arg155Cys in a Korean family. *Arch Neurol.* 2011;68:787–796.
549. Kumar KR, Needham M, Mina K, et al. Two Australian families with inclusion-body myopathy, Paget's disease of bone and frontotemporal dementia: Novel clinical and genetic findings. *Neuromuscul Disord.* 2010;20:330–334.
550. Stojkovic T, Hammouda el H, Richard P, et al. Clinical outcome in 19 French and Spanish patients with valosin-containing protein myopathy associated with Paget's disease of bone and frontotemporal dementia. *Neuromuscul Disord.* 2009;19:316–323.
551. Viassolo V, Previtali SC, Schiatti E, et al. Inclusion body myopathy, Paget's disease of the bone and frontotemporal dementia: Recurrence of the VCP R155 H mutation in an Italian family and implications for genetic counselling. *Clin Genet.* 2008;74:54–60.
552. Waggoner B, Kovach MJ, Winkelman M, et al. Heterogeneity in familial dominant Paget disease of bone and muscular dystrophy. *Am J Med Genet.* 2002;108:187–191.
553. Shi Z, Hayashi YK, Mitsuhashi S, et al. Characterization of the Asian myopathy patients with VCP mutations. *Eur J Neurol.* 2012;19:501–509.
554. van der Zee J, Pirici D, Van Langenhove T, et al. Clinical heterogeneity in 3 unrelated families linked to VCP p.Arg159His. *Neurology.* 2009;73:626–632.
555. Palmio J, Sandell S, Suominen T, et al. Distinct distal myopathy phenotype caused by VCP gene mutation in a Finnish family. *Neuromuscul Disord.* 2011;21:551–555.
556. Johnson JO, Mandrioli J, Benatar M, et al. Exome sequencing reveals VCP mutations as a cause of familial ALS. *Neuron.* 2010;68(5):857–864.
557. González-Pérez P, Cirulli ET, Drory VE, et al. Novel mutation in VCP gene causes atypical amyotrophic lateral sclerosis. *Neurology.* 2012;79(22):2201–2208.
558. Kim HJ, Kim NC, Wang YD, et al. Mutations in prion-like domains in hnRNPA2B1 and hnRNPA1 cause multisystem proteinopathy and ALS. *Nature.* 2013;495:467–473.
559. Bucelli RC, Arhzaouy K, Pestronk A, et al. SQSTM1 splice site mutation in distal myopathy with rimmed vacuoles. *Neurology.* 2015;85(8):665–674.
560. Feit H, Silbergleit A, Schneider LB, et al. Vocal cord and pharyngeal weakness with autosomal dominant distal myopathy: clinical description and gene localization to 5q31. *Am J Hum Genet.* 1998;63(6):1732–1742.
561. Senderek J, Garvey SM, Krieger M, et al. Autosomal-dominant distal myopathy associated with a recurrent missense mutation in the gene encoding the nuclear matrix protein, matrin 3. *Am J Hum Genet.* 2009;84:511–518.
562. Johnson JO, Pioro EP, Boehringer A, et al. Mutations in the Matrin 3 gene cause familial amyotrophic lateral sclerosis. *Nat Neurosci.* 2014;17(5):664–666.
563. Muller TJ, Kraya T, Stoltenburg-Didinger G, et al. Phenotype of the Matrin-3-distal myopathy in 16 German patients. *Ann Neurol.* 2014;76:669–680.
564. Cole AJ, Kuzniecky R, Karpati G, Carpenter S, Andermann E, Andermann F. Familial myopathy with changes resembling inclusion body myositis and periventricular leucoencephalopathy. A new syndrome. *Brain.* 1988;111(Pt 5):1025–1037.

CHAPTER 28

Congenital Myopathies

The term "congenital myopathy" was originally used to describe a group of myopathic disorders presenting preferentially, but not exclusively, at birth and being morphologically distinct from congenital muscular dystrophies (Table 28-1).[1–4] However, disorders that were once considered forms of muscular dystrophy are now known to be allelic to some types of congenital myopathy. For example, congenital muscular dystrophy with rigid spine syndrome, multi/minicore, and some cases of myofibrillar myopathy are caused by selenoprotein N1 mutations; sarcotubular myopathy and limb-girdle muscular dystrophy DR8 (LGMDR8, previously referred to as LGMD2H) are due to mutations in *TRIM32*; reducing body myopathy has been classified as a congenital myopathy, LGMD, scapuloperoneal myopathy, and myofibrillar myopathy. Likewise, some disorders caused by mutations in sarcomeric proteins are classified as forms of LGMD or myofibrillar myopathy (e.g., titinopathies, myotilinopathies, ZASPopathies), while others (e.g., actinomyosin, tropomyosin, α-actin, and troponin) as forms of congenital myopathy (nemaline myopathy). Thus, the nosology of what distinguishes a "congenital myopathy" from a "muscular dystrophy" on clinical and histopathologic grounds is not at all clear, particularly when we consider the advances in genetics. Additionally, with genetics, we are finding heterogeneity of clinical phenotypes associated with mutations in individual genes. For example, *RYR1* mutations are classically associated with central core disease, but may also manifest with malignant hyperthermia, King–Denborough syndrome, late-onset axial myopathy, exertional rhabdomyolysis/myalgia, or asymptomatic hyperCKemia.

Usually, the congenital myopathies present in infancy as generalized hypotonia and weakness. Motor milestones are typically delayed. Affected infants are usually hypotonic and display delayed motor development. Some disorders with mutations in similar genes present later in childhood or even in adulthood. The congenital myopathies were initially considered as nonprogressive, although it is now clear that progressive weakness can occur.

Congenital myopathies can be inherited in an autosomal-dominant, autosomal-recessive, or X-linked pattern. Within families, there can be considerable variation with respect to disease presentation and degree of muscle involvement. The serum creatine kinase (CK) levels can be normal or slightly elevated. The classification of congenital myopathies has been based almost exclusively on clinical presentation and light/electron microscopic structural alterations of the muscle biopsy specimen (Table 28-1).

▶ CENTRAL CORE MYOPATHY

CLINICAL FEATURES

Central core myopathy usually manifests at birth or early childhood as generalized weakness and hypotonia.[1–9] The degree of muscle weakness can vary even within families. Muscle weakness is stable or only slowly progressive. Motor milestones, such as the ability to sit and walk, are delayed. Some affected individuals never achieve independent ambulation, while others have only mild weakness. The proximal muscles, legs more than arms, are preferentially affected, leading to a wide-based hyperlordotic gait. Individuals who are affected may also demonstrate a Gowers sign when arising from the floor. There may be mild facial and neck flexor weakness. Ptosis or extraocular muscle weakness may be evident. Muscle atrophy or hypertrophy is usually not seen in childhood-onset central core disease. Contractures are uncommon. Muscle stretch reflexes are normal or reduced. There are no apparent central nervous system abnormalities. Affected individuals may exhibit mild-to-moderate skeletal deformities including pes planus, pes cavus, kyphoscoliosis, and congenital hip dislocation. Mild ventilatory muscle weakness with reduced forced vital capacity and nocturnal hypoxemia is seen in some patients.

LABORATORY FEATURES

The serum CK levels are normal or slightly elevated. Motor and sensory nerve conduction studies (NCSs) are usually normal. Electromyography (EMG) may reveal fibrillation potentials and positive sharp waves and myopathic appearing motor unit action potentials (MUAPs) that recruit early in weak muscles.[10] Long-duration, polyphasic MUAPs and units with satellite potentials may also be appreciated. Skeletal muscle MRI reveals early involvement of the vasti, sartorius, and adductor magnus in the thigh with relative sparing of the rectus femoris, adductor longus, and hamstrings in the legs and biceps brachii in the arms.[1,9]

HISTOPATHOLOGY

The characteristic histologic features are the structural alterations within the center of muscle fibers, the so-called cores.[1–13] These cores appear only in type 1 muscle fibers and

TABLE 28-1. CONGENITAL MYOPATHIES

Disease	Inheritance	Protein (Gene)	Clinical Features
Central core myopathy	AD (rare AR)	Ryanodine receptor (RYR1)	Onset: infancy or childhood, occasionally adulthood; proximal limbs and mild facial weakness; skeletal anomalies; risk for MH in those with RYR1 mutations
	AR	Muscle slow/β cardiac myosin heavy chain 7 gene (MYH7)	
	AD	α-Actin 1 (ACTA1)	
	AR	Titin (TTN)	
	AD	Coiled–coil domain-containing 78 (CCDC78)	
Multi/minicore myopathy	AR	Selenoprotein N1/(SEPN1)	Onset: infancy or childhood; proximal and facial muscles; rare EOM weak; cardiomyopathy and respiratory weakness; skeletal anomalies; risk for MH in those with RYR1 mutations
	AD/AR	Ryanodine receptor (RYR1)	
	AR	Titin (TTN)	
	AD	Muscle slow/β cardiac myosin heavy chain 7 gene (MYH7) (MYH2)	
	AR	Multiple EGF-like-domains 10 (MEGF10)	
	AR	unc-45 myosin chaperone A (UNC45B)	
Core–rod myopathy[a]	AD/AR	α-Actin 1 (ACTA1)	Onset in infancy or childhood. Phenotypes can resemble those seen with nemaline myopathy
	AR	Nebulin (NEB)	
	AD	Kelch repeat and BTB/(KBTBD13)	
	AR	Thyroid hormone receptor interactor 4 (TRIP4)	
Nemaline rod myopathy[a]	AR	Nebulin (NEB)	*Infantile-onset form*: severe generalized hypotonia/weakness; respiratory weakness; skeletal anomalies; usually fatal in the first year of life
	AD/AR	α-Actin (ACTA1)	
	AD/AR	α-Tropomyosin (TPM3)	
	AD/AR	β-Tropomyosin (TPM2)	*Mild early-onset form*: Most common subtype; onset in infancy or childhood; mild generalized hypotonia and weakness; facial muscles; rare ptosis, EOM weak; dysmorphic facies and skeletal anomalies
	AR	Slow troponin T (TNNT1)	
	AR	Cofilin-2 (CFL2)	
	AD	Kelch repeat and BTB domain-containing 13 (KBTBD13)	
Cap Myopathy[a]	AR	Kelch-like family member 40 and 41 genes (KLHL40 and KLHL41)	*Adult-onset form*: onset in adult life; mild proximal and occasionally distal weakness; no facial or skeletal anomalies
	AR	Leomoidin-3 (LMOD3)	
	AR	Myopalladin (MYPN)	
Zebra body myopathy[a]	AD	β-Tropomyosin (TPM2)	
	AD	α-Tropomyosin (TPM3)	
	AD	α-Actin 1 (ACTA1)	
	AR	Nebulin (NEB)	
	AR	Myopallidin (MYPN)	
	AD	α-Actin 1 (ACTA1)	
Centronuclear/myotubular myopathy	X-linked	Myotubularin (MTM1)	Severe neonatal hypotonia and weakness; respiratory weakness; ptosis and EOM weak; poor prognosis in most
	AD	Dynamin-2 (DYN2)	
	AD/AR	Ryanodine receptor (RYR1)	Onset in late infancy or early childhood of generalized weakness and hypotonia; facial and EOM weakness, ptosis; facial anomalies
	AD/AR	Amphiphysin 2 (BIN2)	
	AR	Titin (TTN)	
	AD	Coiled-coil domain-containing protein 79 (CCDC78)	Onset in late childhood or adulthood of mild proximal and/or distal weakness; ptosis is common; facial and EOM muscles variably involved; no skeletal or facial anomalies; mild sensory abnormalities
	AR	Striated muscle preferentially expressed protein kinase (SPEG)	
	AR	Sterile-alpha motif and leucine zipper-containing kinase (ZAC)	Cases with BIN2 mutations may have severe distal lower extremity weakness
Congenital fiber-type disproportion	AD	α-Tropomyosin (TMP3)	Onset in infancy to adulthood; generalized or proximal weakness; may have facial, respiratory, or asymmetric weakness; skeletal anomalies
	AD	Ryanodine receptor (RYR1)	
	AD/AR	Rarely caused by mutations in ACTA1, SEPN1, MYL2, TPM2, TTN, HACD1, SCN1A, and MHC7	

▶ TABLE 28-1. (CONTINUED)

Disease	Inheritance	Protein (Gene)	Clinical Features
Reducing body myopathy	X-linked AR	Four and a half LIM (*FHL1*) Desmin (*DES*)	Onset in infancy or childhood; generalized nonprogressive weakness; occasional respiratory weakness; skeletal and facial anomalies
Fingerprint body myopathy	AR	One patient was found to have a mutation in *LMOD3*	Infantile onset; slow or nonprogressive proximal weakness
Sarcotubular myopathy (allelic to LGMD R8/LGMD 2H)	AR	Tripartite motif-containing protein 32/(*TRIM 32*)	Onset: infancy or adulthood; slow progressive proximal and/or distal weakness
Trilaminar myopathy	Unknown	Unknown	Infantile onset: generalized weakness; skeletal anomalies
Myosin storage myopathy/hyaline body myopathy/familial myopathy with lysis of myofibrils	AD	Muscle slow/β cardiac myosin heavy chain 7 gene (*MYH7*)	Onset in infancy or adults; limb-girdle, scapuloperoneal, or distal weakness
H-IBM 3/myosin storage myopathy	AD	Myosin heavy chain type IIa (*MYH2*)	Congenital arthrogryposis; ophthalmoparesis; adult onset of mild proximal weakness and myalgias; rimmed vacuoles and inclusions on muscle biopsy (H-IBM type 3)
Tubular aggregate myopathy	AD	Stromal interaction molecule 1 (*STIM1*)	STIM1 and ORAI1 are associated with childhood or early adulthood onset; limb-girdle weakness; immune deficiency; Stormorken syndrome
	AD	Orai1 (*ORAI1*)	
	AD	Calsequestrin (*CASQ1*)	
	AR	UDP-*N*-acetylglucosamine-dolichyl-phosphate *N*-acetylglucosaminephosphotransferase 1 (*DPAGT1*)	*GDPAGT1*, *GFPT1*, and *ALG2* mutations are associated with infantile onset of a myasthenic syndrome with fatigable weakness
	AR	Glutamine-fructose-6-phosphate transaminase 1 (*GFPT1*)	*PGAM* mutations are associated with glycogen storage disease type X
	AR	Alpha-1,3/1,6-mannosyltransferase (*ALG2*)	*SCN4A* mutations are associated with hypokalemic periodic paralysis type 2
	AR	Phosphoglycerate mutase (*PGAM*)	
	AD	Sodium voltage-gated channel, alpha subunit (*SCN4A*)	
Native American Myopathy	AR	SH3 and cysteine-rich domain 3 (*STAC3*)	Congenital onset of trunk and proximal extremity weakness, delayed motor milestones, ptosis, myopathic facies, cleft-plate, feeding difficulties, ptosis, conductive hearing loss, skeletal deformities, and short stature. Increased risk of pulmonary atresia and malignant hyperthermia

AD, autosomal dominant; AR, autosomal recessive; EOM weakness, ophthalmoparesis; MH, malignant hyperthermia.
^aCore–rod myopathy, Cap myopathy, zebra body myopathy are all subtypes nemaline myopathy.

are particularly noticeable on nicotinamide adenine dinucleotide tetrazolium reductase (NADH-TR) stains, where the cores are devoid of stain (Fig. 28-1). The cores can occasionally be eccentric and multiple within a given muscle fiber. The distinction between central core and multi/minicore is that in central core myopathy the "cores" extend along the entire length of the muscle fibers on the longitudinal section. However, in some cases, the distinction between central cores and multi/minicores is not clear, as there can be typical multi/minicores in patients with central core myopathy. Furthermore, repeat biopsies in patients initially diagnosed with minicores may subsequently reveal central cores.[12] In addition, muscle biopsies reveal variation in fiber size, increased internalized nuclei, and often a predominance of type 1 fibers that may be atrophic. Increased endomysial fibrosis and fat may be present,[11] but the other features help distinguish the disorder from muscular dystrophies.

On electron microscopy (EM), the cores may be "structured" or "unstructured" (Fig. 28-2). In structured cores, there is streaming of the Z-band, but the sarcomeres are preserved. In unstructured cores, there is severe myofibrillar disruption and loss of the normal sarcomere organization. In both structured and unstructured cores, mitochondria and glycogen granules are reduced or absent. The cores appear to contain desmin, dystrophin, actin, α-actinin, gelsolin, nebulin, myotilin, β-amyloid precursor protein, NCAM, and various cyclin-dependent kinases based on immunocytochemistry; the cores are also variably congophilic.[13]

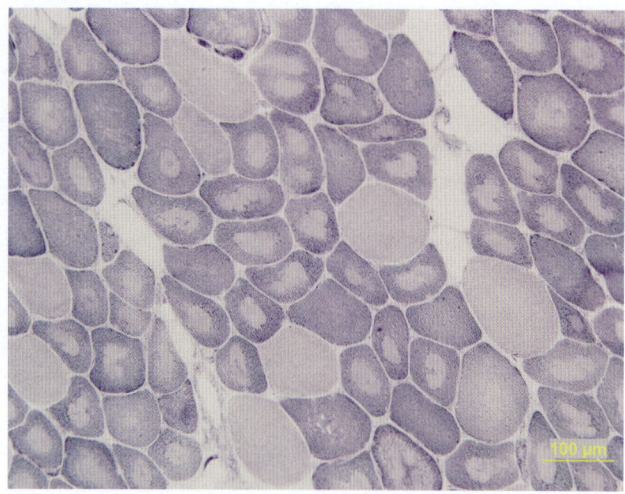 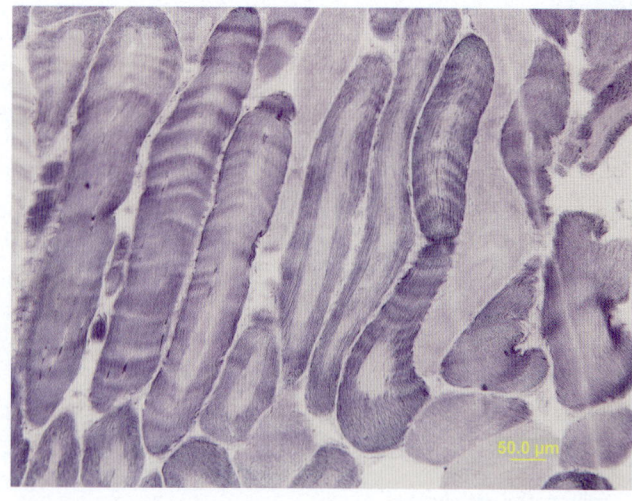

Figure 28-1. Central core myopathy. Nicotinamide adenine dinucleotide tetrazolium reductase (NADH-TR) stain demonstrates areas devoid of oxidated enzyme activity in the center of the fibers or sometimes eccentric regions (**A**) that extend the length of the fiber longitudinally (**B**).

MOLECULAR GENETICS AND PATHOGENESIS

Central core myopathy is an autosomal-dominant disorder caused by mutations in the ryanodine receptor gene (*RYR1*) on chromosome 19q13.1 in most cases.[1–4,14–17] Typically, this involves compound heterozygous mutations, usually a truncating mutation combined with a missense mutation. Rarely, autosomal-recessive inheritance may occur with *RYR1* mutations.[18] Of note, mutations in the *RYR1* are responsible for one form of familial malignant hyperthermia; thus, patients with central core myopathy are at risk of malignant hyperthermia (Table 28-1).[19] Why these "cores" form in the center of the muscle fibers is unknown. The ryanodine receptor is a tetramer

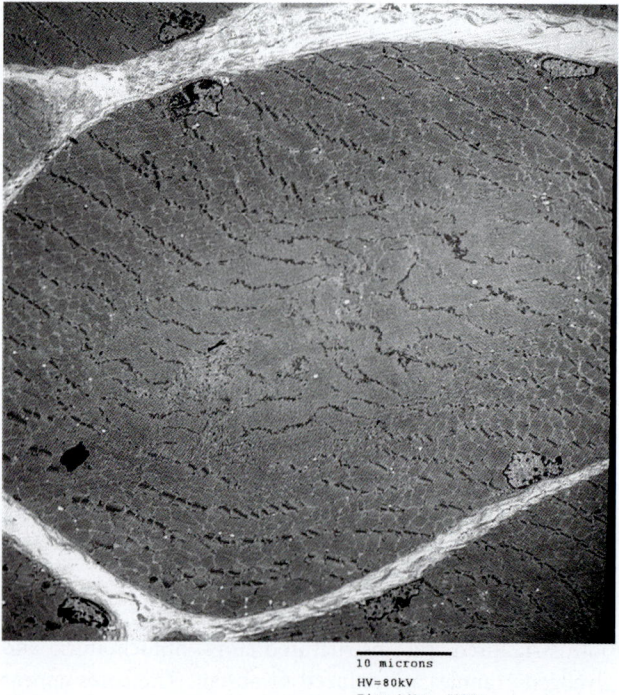 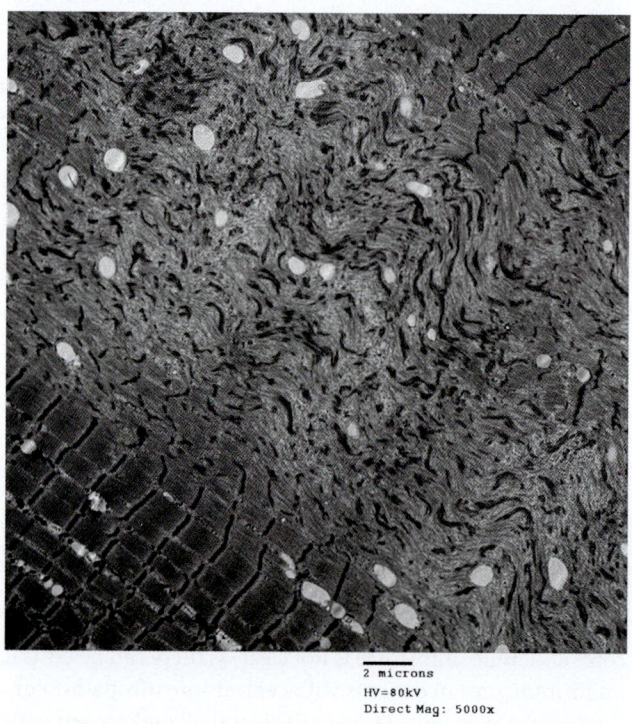

Figure 28-2. Central core myopathy. Electron microscopy reveals areas with poorly aligned sarcomeres and reduced glycogen and mitochondrial in an "unstructured" core (**A**). A core can be seen to extend over a large length of the fibers on a longitudinal section (**B**).

of RYR1 proteins, which bridges the gap between the sarcoplasmic reticulum and the T-tubules in skeletal muscle and forms a calcium-release channel. Thus, the ryanodine receptor likely plays an important role in excitation–contraction coupling.[20] Most of the mutations associated with the classic phenotype are seen in the C-terminal domain that corresponds to the transmembrane domain of the protein. In experimental studies of mutant myotubes, voltage-gated calcium release was reduced by approximately 90%, while caffeine-induced Ca^{2+} release was only marginally reduced in mutant myotubes, indicating the disruption of voltage-sensor activation of calcium release.[21,22]

Mutations in muscle slow/β cardiac myosin heavy chain 7 gene (*MYH7*) have been associated with eccentric cores and multi/minicores.[2–4,23] Mutations in the genes that encode actin 1 (*ACTA1*), titin (*TTN*), coiled–coil domain-containing gene, *CCDC78*, have also been associated with core-like changes on muscle biopsy, while mutations in *NEB* that encodes nebulin and *KBTBD13* encoding Kelch repeat and BTB may cause cores and nemaline rods.[2–4,24,25]

TREATMENT

There is no specific medical treatment available for central core myopathy. Patients may benefit from physical therapy and orthotic devices. Patients with central core disease and their families should be informed of their risk of developing malignant hyperthermia with general anesthesia. Appropriate precautions and avoidance of certain anesthetic agents (e.g., halothane) and neuromuscular-blocking agents (succinylcholine) need to be taken during surgical procedures.

▶ MULTI/MINICORE MYOPATHY

CLINICAL FEATURES

Although it is generally agreed that multi/minicore disease (MmD) constitutes a distinct entity, the morphologic lesions defining it are nonspecific, and the clinical expression of the disease is highly variable.[1–4,23–31] MmD usually presents in infancy or early childhood, but adult-onset cases have been reported as well. Affected infants are usually hypotonic and weak. Motor milestones are delayed, but ambulation is usually achieved. Most patients have generalized muscle weakness and atrophy predominantly affecting axial and proximal extremity muscles. Distal muscles are usually normal or only slightly involved. However, there appears to be a subgroup of MmD that manifests with predominantly distal hand weakness.[28,29] Facial muscle weakness, ptosis, and occasionally ophthalmoparesis can also be seen.

Muscle contractures and multiple skeletal deformities such as kyphoscoliosis, high-arched palate, and club feet are common findings. Weakness is usually stable or only slowly progressive.[29] Neck extensors and trunk muscles may be contracted, leading to rigidity of the spine. Cardiomyopathy and ventilatory muscle involvement can also develop.[30,31] Ventilatory involvement can be disproportionate to the degree of scoliosis.[29] Patients may require intermittent or continuous positive-pressure ventilation.

LABORATORY FEATURES

Serum CK is usually normal or only slightly elevated. Pulmonary function tests often reveal reduced forced vital capacities. Polysomnographic studies may disclose nocturnal oxygen desaturation and short apneic periods. NCSs are normal. EMG usually reveals normal insertional and spontaneous activity, although early recruitment of short-duration, small-amplitude MUAPs may be appreciated.[10]

HISTOPATHOLOGY

Muscle biopsies reveal multiple small regions within muscle fibers of variable size (minicores) formed by disorganization of the myofibrils (Fig. 28-3).[1–4,19,23–31] Minicores are similar to central cores but are much smaller and do not extend the entire length of the muscle fiber as do central cores. In addition, minicores can occur in either type 1 or type 2 muscle fibers. Type 1 fiber predominance and atrophy as well as fiber size variation are also noted. There can be increased endomysial connective tissue as well. EM demonstrates myofibrillar disruption similar to that seen in central cores (Fig. 28-4).

MOLECULAR GENETICS AND PATHOGENESIS

This is a genetically heterogeneous group of disorders.[2–4] The absence of clear dominant transmission in any well-established case and the presence of several consanguineous families

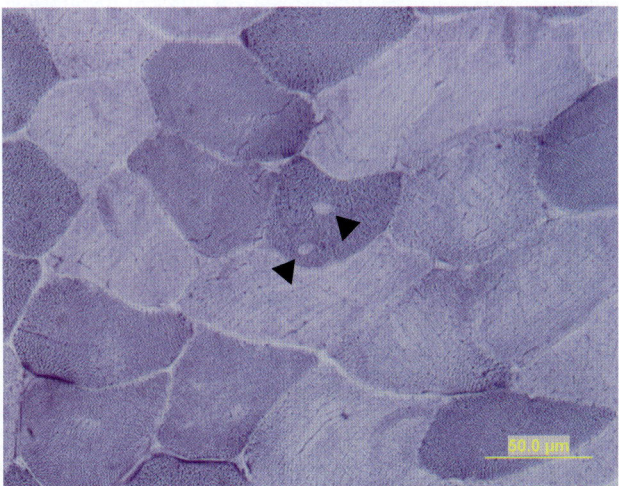

Figure 28-3. Multi/minicore myopathy. NADH stain demonstrates small areas devoid of oxidative enzyme activity (*arrowheads*).

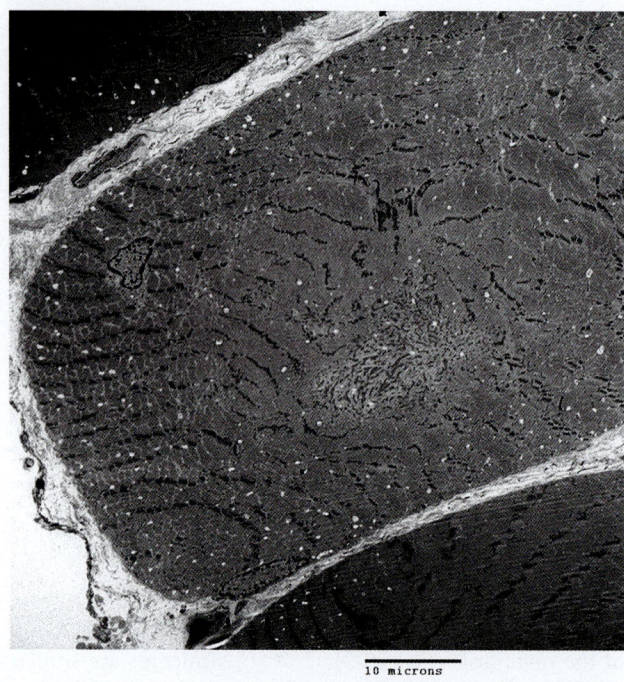

Figure 28-4. Multi/minicore myopathy. Electron microscopy reveals areas of myofibrillar disarray similar to central core myopathy but are much smaller.

strongly suggest that MmD is usually an autosomal-recessive entity or the result of spontaneous mutations.[2–4,29] Interestingly though, some patients with MmD (usually cases associated with external ophthalmoplegia and ptosis) have demonstrable mutations in the *RyR1* gene similar to central core myopathy.[2–4,12,32] Mutations in the selenoprotein N gene (*SEPN1*), which is located on chromosome 1p36, are the most common cause in individuals with classic MmD.[33] Of note, this is the same gene responsible for the congenital muscular dystrophy with rigid spine syndrome and some cases of myofibrillar myopathy.[33] The dystrophic changes and histologic features of myofibrillar myopathy apparent on some muscle biopsies and *SEPN1* mutations identified in some cases of MmD highlight the difficult nosologic boundaries between various types of congenital myopathies and muscular dystrophies. In addition, mutations in the genes that encode for cofilin-2 (*CFL2*), myosin heavy chain 7 (*MYH7*), *MYH2*, titin (*TTN*), multiple EGF-like-domains 10 (*MEGF10*), coiled-coil domain-containing 78 (*CCDC78*), unc-45 myosin chaperone A (*UNC45B*), actinin alpha 2 (*ACTN2*), thyroid hormone receptor interactor 4 (*TRIP4*), and Kelch repeat and BTB (POZ) domain-containing 13 (*KBTBD13*) have been in patients with cores/minicores on muscle biopsy along with possible nemaline rods or central nuclei.[2,34–39]

TREATMENT

No specific medical treatment is available. Patients may be at risk of malignant hyperthermia and should be counseled accordingly (see Central Core Myopathy).[40,41] Early-onset scoliosis is common and may require extensive arthrodesis. Patients may require intermittent or continuous positive-pressure ventilation.

▶ CORE–ROD MYOPATHY

CLINICAL FEATURES

Central core and nemaline rod myopathies are generally considered two genetically and histologically distinct disorders.[2–4,38,39,42–49] However, as noted in the preceding section, there are scattered reports in the literature of the simultaneous occurrence of both cores and rods in the same muscle biopsy. Onset of symptoms is variable (congenital or early adult life) as is severity. The weakness can be proximal, distal, or generalized. Some cases have ptosis and/or skeletal deformities (e.g., contractures, scoliosis).

LABORATORY FEATURES

The serum CK level can be normal or slightly elevated. NCSs are usually normal. Early recruitment of small-amplitude, short-duration MUAPs are appreciated in weak muscles on EMG.

HISTOPATHOLOGY

Muscle biopsies, as implied by the name, can show both cores and rods along with type 1 fiber predominance (Fig. 28-5).

MOLECULAR GENETICS AND PATHOGENESIS

Mutations in the ryanodine receptor gene (*RYR1*) account for most cases, however mutations in the *NEB*, *ACTA1*, *CFL2*, and *KBTBD13* genes have also been associated with muscle biopsies demonstrating both cores and nemaline rods.[2,38,39,42–49]

TREATMENT

No specific medical treatment is available. Those cases with *RYR1* mutations should be counseled regarding the possible risk of malignant hyperthermia.

▶ OTHER PHENOTYPES ASSOCIATED WITH RYR1 MUTATIONS

As previously discussed, the clinical phenotype associated with *RYR1* mutations is large and aside from central core and

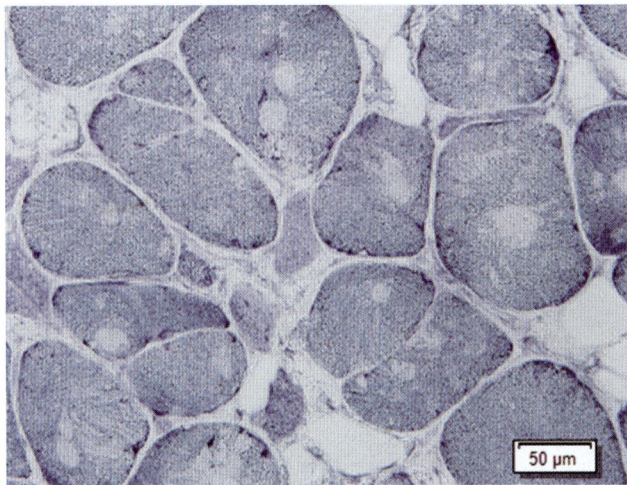
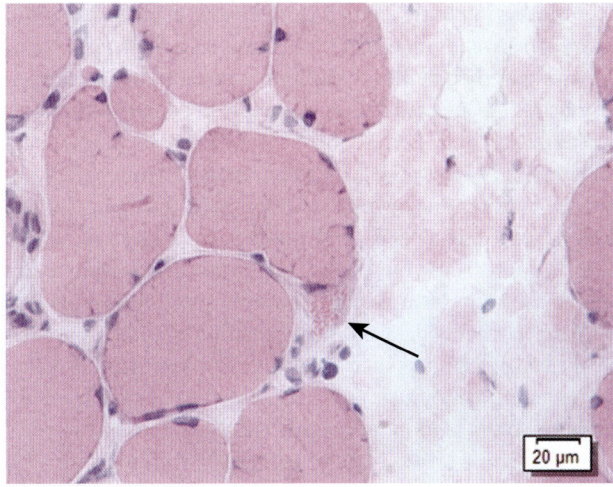
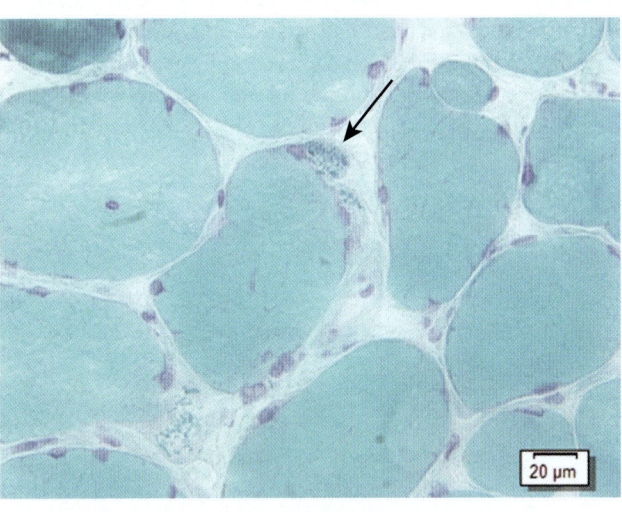

Figure 28-5. Core–rod myopathy in a patient with RYR1 mutation. NADH-TR stain reveals central cores, eccentric cores, and multi/minicores (**A**). H&E stain (**B**) and modified Gomori-trichrome stain (**C**) reveal subsarcolemmal nemaline rods (see *arrows*).

multi/minicore myopathies that usually occur early in life, also cause malignant hyperthermia. In addition, *RYR1* mutations have been identified as a cause of exertional myalgias and rhabdomyolysis in the absence of baseline weakness.[50] King–Denborough syndrome is a rare disorder characterized by a susceptibility to malignant hyperthermia, delayed motor development, short stature, cryptorchidism, skeletal abnormalities, and variable dysmorphic features that in some cases, but not all, have been associated with *RYR1* mutations.[51,52] In addition, mutations in RYR1 are increasing seen in patients with exertional myalgias and rhabdomyolysis.[53,54]

Furthermore, late-onset axial myopathy manifesting as bent spine syndrome (camptocormia), or neck extensor myopathy have been found to have *RYR1* mutations.[55–57] CKs are normal or slightly elevated. EMG may be normal in extremities and demonstrate fibrillation potentials and positive sharp waves only in axial/paraspinal muscles. In our experience, muscle biopsies of extremity muscles that are strong may be unrevealing while biopsy of upper trapezius or paraspinal muscles may demonstrate cores, multi/minicores, or moth-eaten fibers.

▶ NEMALINE MYOPATHY

CLINICAL FEATURES

Nemaline myopathy is clinically and genetically heterogeneous. It can be inherited in an autosomal-dominant or autosomal-recessive fashion. There are three major clinical presentations of nemaline myopathy: (1) a severe infantile form, (2) a static or slowly progressive form, and (3) an adult-onset form.[1–4,58–72]

The severe infantile form is characterized by severe generalized weakness and hypotonia at birth. Muscle stretch and Moro reflexes are usually absent. Affected infants have a weak cry and suck. Because of ventilatory muscle involvement, they often need to be mechanically ventilated. Most children with this severe infantile-onset form of nemaline myopathy die in the first year of life due to ventilatory complications. Arthrogryposis, neonatal ventilatory failure, and failure to achieve early motor milestones are associated with early mortality.[64] Most are inherited in an autosomal-recessive pattern, but autosomal-dominant inheritance also occurs.

More commonly, nemaline myopathy manifests as mild, nonprogressive, or slowly progressive weakness beginning in infancy or early childhood. Both proximal and distal extremity muscles are affected and associated with generalized reduction in muscle bulk. Some patients have a facioscapuloperoneal distribution of weakness. Motor milestones are often delayed, and the children may exhibit a wide-based, waddling, hyperlordotic gait. Slight facial and masticatory muscle weakness may be appreciated, but ptosis and extraocular weakness are not typical. Many have a characteristic dysmorphic narrow face with high-arched palate and micrognathia. In addition, multiple skeletal deformities such as pectus excavatum, kyphoscoliosis, temporal mandibular ankylosis, pes cavus, or club feet are common. Deep tendon reflexes are reduced or absent.

The adult-onset type of nemaline rod myopathy is associated with mild proximal and occasionally distally predominant muscle weakness presenting in adulthood. Some patients have minimal skeletal muscle weakness but manifest with a cardiomyopathy. The adult-onset form is not associated with dysmorphic facial features or skeletal deformities typical of the early-onset forms.

LABORATORY FEATURES

The serum CK level is normal or slightly elevated. NCSs are usually normal. Early recruitment of small-amplitude, short-duration MUAPs are appreciated in weak muscles on EMG. In the severe infantile forms, EMG may demonstrate increased insertional and spontaneous activity in the form of fibrillation potentials and positive sharp waves.[10] Such abnormal spontaneous activity is usually not appreciated in the more benign forms of myopathy.

HISTOPATHOLOGY

Muscle biopsies often reveal type 1 fiber predominance and hypotrophy in the congenital forms but not in the adult-onset form of the disease. On routine histochemistry, the nemaline rods are best appreciated on modified Gomori-trichrome stain, on which the rods appear as small, red or bluish–purple staining bodies in the subsarcolemma and occasionally perinuclear regions (Fig. 28-6). On EM, the

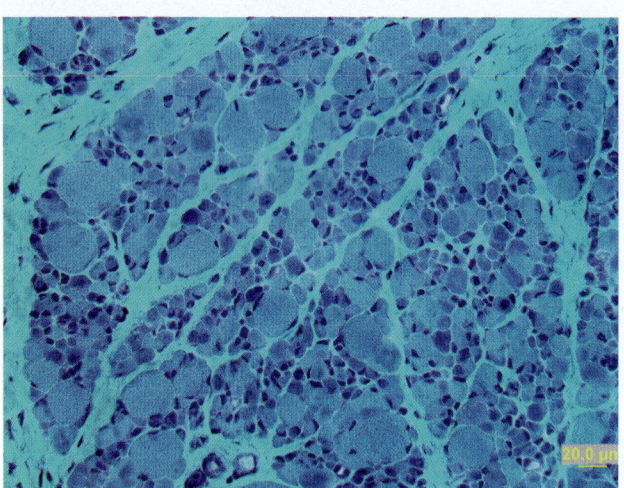

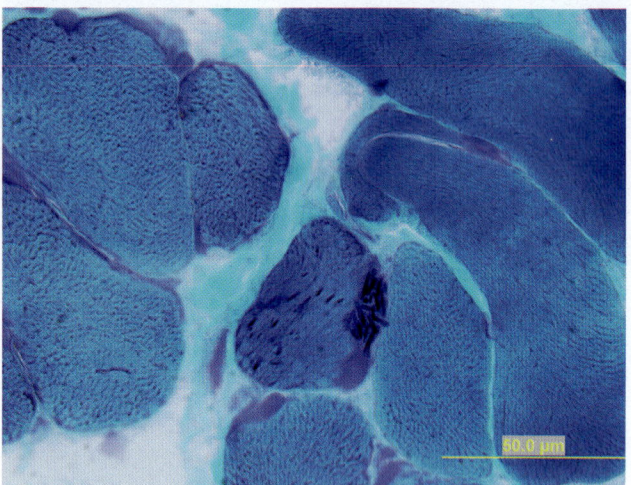

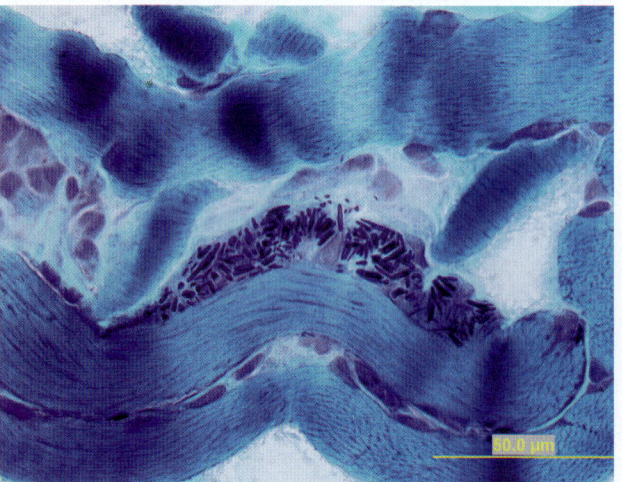

Figure 28-6. Nemaline myopathy. Infantile nemaline myopathy demonstrates many hypotrophic fibers (**A**). In an adult-onset nemaline myopathy, high-power light microscopy reveals subsarcolemmal cluster of bluish-purple staining rods in cross section (**B**) and on longitudinal sections (**C**). Modified Gomori-trichrome stain.

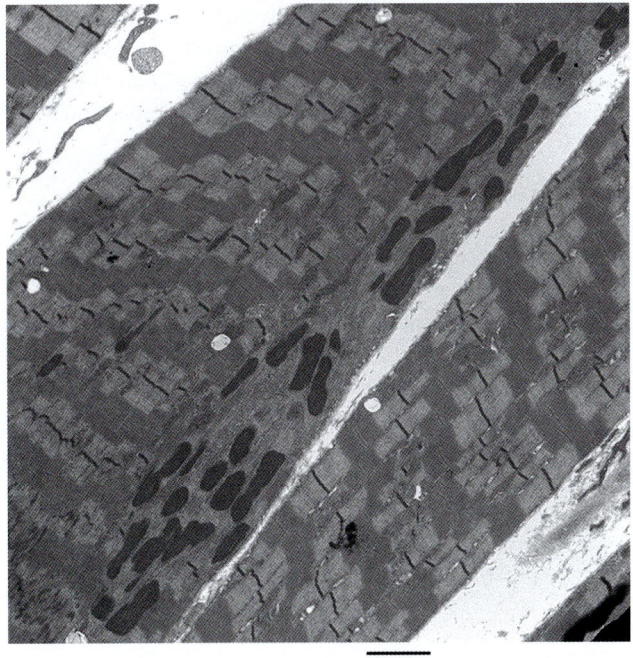

Figure 28-7. Nemaline myopathy. Electron microscopy reveals rods appearing as osmiophilic bodies, which have the same density as the Z discs.

typical "rod bodies" measure 3–6 μm in length and 1–3 μm in diameter, giving the appearance of threads (nemaline: Greek for "thread like"). The nemaline rods have a density similar to the Z-disc (Fig. 28-7). Intranuclear rods may be observed, and early reports suggested that these represent a marker for this severe form of the disease (Fig. 28-8).[69–71] However, intranuclear rods are not demonstrated in all severe infantile cases and can also be found in milder adult-onset cases of nemaline myopathy.[63] Immunohistochemistry reveals that the rods and Z-disc are often strongly immunoreactive for α-actinin.[73] Rods are not specific for congenital nemaline myopathy and have been reported following tenotomy, SLOMN, HIV-associated myopathy, myofibrillar myopathy, inclusion body myositis, and hypothyroidism.

MOLECULAR GENETICS AND PATHOGENESIS

Nemaline rods arise secondary to a derangement of proteins necessary to maintain normal Z-disc structure. The myopathy is genetically heterogeneous, with mutations having been identified in at least 11 genes that encode nebulin (*NEB*), α-tropomyosin (*TPM3*), β-tropomyosin (*TPN2*), troponin T (*TNNT1*), α-actin (*ACTA1*), Cofilin-2/(*CFL2*), Kelch repeat and BTB 13 (*KBTBD13*), Kelch-like family member 40 and 41 (*KLHL40* and *KLHL41*), leomoidin-3 (*LMOD3*), and myopalladin (*MYPN*) (Table 28-1).[1–4,74–93]

Most of the autosomal-recessive cases (around 50%) are caused by mutations in the nebulin gene (*NEB*).[1–4,74–76] The clinical phenotype associated with nebulin mutations can be mild or severe. Mutations in the α-actin gene (*ACTA1*) can cause autosomal-recessive and autosomal-dominant nemaline myopathy.[1–4,60,77–80] *ACTA1* mutations are the second most common cause of nemaline myopathy (15%–30%) but are responsible for about 50% of the severe lethal congenital-onset cases. The severity of the disease ranges from lack of spontaneous movements at birth requiring immediate mechanical ventilation to mild disease compatible with life to adulthood. There are reported cases with adult onset as well.[60] Mutations in the *ACTA1* gene are also responsible for previously reported cases of "congenital myopathy with excess of thin filaments."

Mutations in the α-tropomyosin gene (*TPM3*) can result in autosomal-dominant or autosomal-recessive nemaline myopathy.[2–4,81–83] The severity of cases with *TPM3* mutations vary from severe infantile to late childhood-onset,

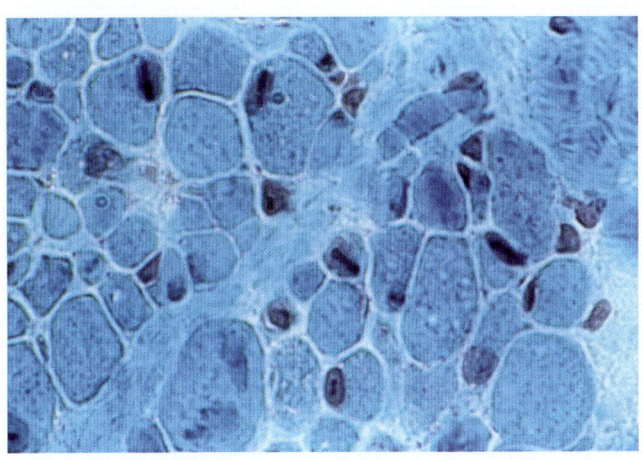
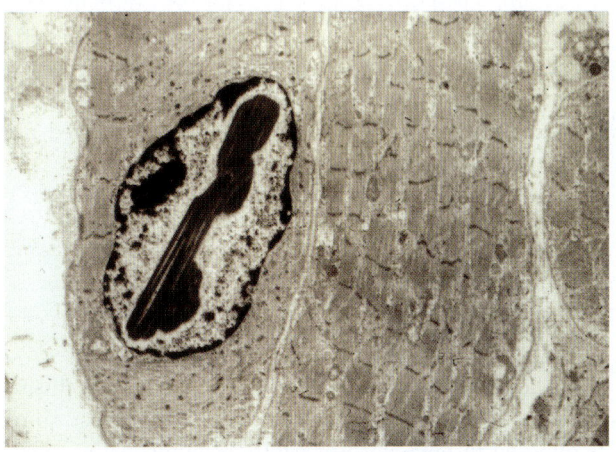

A   **B**

Figure 28-8. Nemaline myopathy. Intranuclear rods are apparent on this modified Gomori-trichrome stain (**A**) and on electron microscopy (**B**).

slowly progressive forms. A useful clue for *TPM3* mutations is when rods are only present in type 1 fibers as *TMP3* is not expressed in type 2 fibers. Mutations in the β-tropomyosin gene (*TPN2*) cause autosomal-dominant rod myopathy that may manifest with neck and distal lower extremity weakness (foot drop) and cardiomyopathy.[84] A severe, rare, infantile form of autosomal-recessive nemaline myopathy found in Amish communities is caused by mutations in the muscle troponin T (*TNNT1*) gene.[85] Mutations in the gene that encodes for the actin-binding protein, coiflin-2 (*CFL2*), have been identified in nemaline myopathy and minicores.[86–88]

A study utilizing whole-exome sequencing found autosomal-recessive mutations in the Kelch-like family member 40 gene (*KLHL40*) in 28 apparently unrelated kindreds of various ethnicities with nemaline myopathy.[89] This accounted for 28% of the tested individuals in the Japanese cohort making *KLHL40* the most common cause of this severe form of nemaline myopathy in this population. Another study using whole-exome sequencing identified recessive small deletions and missense changes mutations in the Kelch-like family member 41 gene (*KLHL41*) in five unrelated individuals.[90] These studies along with cases of core–rod myopathy associated with mutations in Kelch repeat and BTB domain-containing 13 (*KBTBD13*)[49] mutations suggest the importance of BTB-Kelch family members in the maintenance of Z-disc and sarcomeric integrity. Autosomal-recessive mutations in the leomoidin-3 gene, *LMOD3*, and can manifest as a severe congenital myopathy or mild myopathy.[92,93]

As mentioned in the core–rod myopathy section, there are several other genes (*ACTA1*, *NEB*, *KBTBD13*) associated with muscle biopsies showing both nemaline rods with cores. Further, both caps and nemaline rods were found in one patient caused by an autosomal-dominant mutation in the *TPM3* gene (discussed later in the Cap Myopathy section).[91]

TREATMENT

No specific medical treatment is available. Morbidity from respiratory tract infections and feeding difficulties frequently diminish with increasing age; therefore, aggressive early management is warranted in most cases of severe infantile nemaline myopathy. Individuals who are affected may benefit from physical therapy and bracing.

▶ LATE-ONSET NEMALINE MYOPATHY

CLINICAL FEATURES

Sporadic late-onset nemaline myopathy (SLONM) distinct from the congenital, nemaline myopathy and is acquired as opposed to hereditary in nature. The myopathy usually presents after the age of 40 years and can begin as late as the ninth decade with proximal extremity weakness.[94–101] Some patients may present with an axial myopathy isolated head drop or bent spine syndrome from paraspinal muscle weakness. Ventilatory muscle involvement may ensue and be cause of death, particularly in cases associated with a monoclonal gammopathy. In addition, late-onset nemaline rods can sometimes be found in patients with HIV infection.[100,102]

LABORATORY FEATURES

Serum CK is usually normal, but can be slightly elevated and even low. Motor and sensory NCSs are normal. EMG reveals increased insertional and spontaneous activity in the form of positive sharp waves, fibrillation potentials, and early recruitment of short-duration, small-amplitude MUAPs. About 50% of cases are associated with a monoclonal gammopathy (IgG or IgA) of undetermined significance.[94–98] Skeletal muscle MRI demonstrates hyperintensity on both T1-weighted images and T2-weighted short-tau inversion recovery (T2W-STIR) sequences with preferential involvement of paraspinal, gluteus minimus and medius, semimembranosus, and soleus muscles.[101]

HISTOPATHOLOGY

Routine light and electron microscopy demonstrates small nemaline rods, often many trabeculated/lobulated muscle fibers, and occasional inflammatory cell infiltrates (Fig. 28-9). The rods may be very small and appear more like granules than rods, and therefore may be missed on routine light microscopy if the thickness of the sections is greater than 3 μm.[94] However, the rods are almost always appreciated on EM. Immunohistochemistry reveals the rods are usually immunoreactive to anti–α-actinin antibody.[101]

MOLECULAR GENETICS AND PATHOGENESIS

This is an acquired myopathy as opposed to a hereditary disease—no genetic mutations have been found. The relationship between the nemaline myopathy and the monoclonal gammopathy and HIV infection is not clear.

TREATMENT

The response to treatment with various immunotherapies in patients with late-onset nemaline myopathy with a monoclonal gammopathy is generally poor. However, some patients improved at least temporarily to intravenous immunoglobulin or, if they have a monoclonal gammopathy, autologous stem cell transplantation.[96–101]

▶ CAP MYOPATHY

CLINICAL FEATURES

The clinical features of this rare myopathy overlap with those seen in nemaline myopathy given the causal genes are similar.

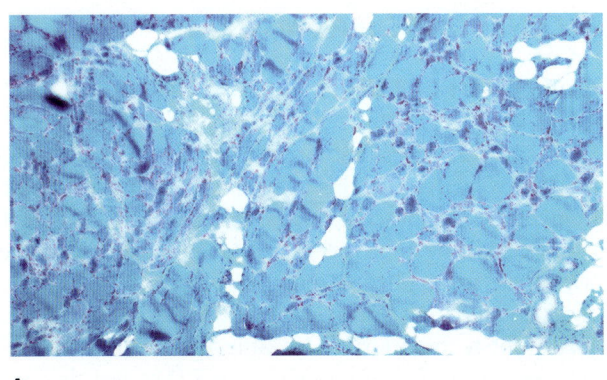
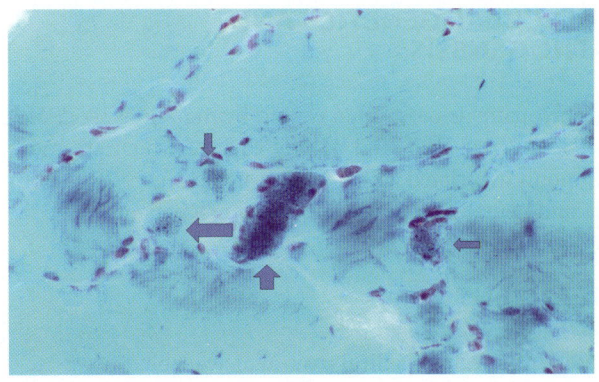
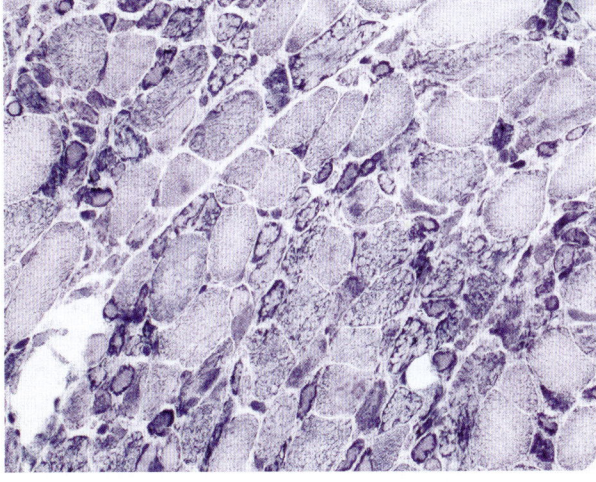
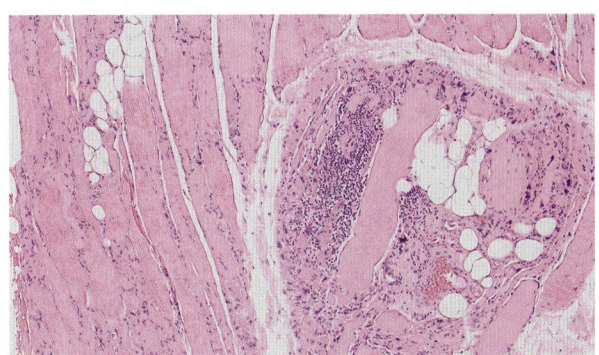
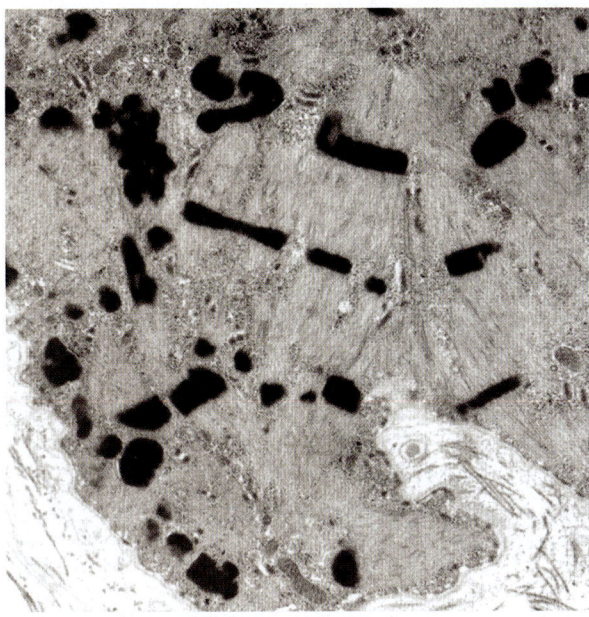

Figure 28-9. Sporadic late onset nemaline myopathy (SLONM). Variability in fiber size and with atrophic fibers with dark-staining, smudginess is appreciated on modified-Gomori trichrome stain (**A**). On higher power, some of these atrophic, smudgy fibers are seen to have very small nemaline rods (**B**). NADH-TR shows many lobulated/trabeculated muscle fibers (**C**). Paraffin stain shows endomyseal inflammatory cell infiltrate (**D**). Electron microscopy shows small nemaline rods/granules (**E**). (Used with the permission from Anthony A. Amato, MD.)

It is usually associated with neonatal onset of generalized muscle weakness and hypotonia associated with skeletal deformities and reduced muscle stretch reflexes.[1,2,103–112] Ventilatory muscles are also frequently affected.

LABORATORY FEATURES

Serum CK is normal. NCSs are normal, while EMG demonstrates myopathic MUAPs.

HISTOPATHOLOGY

Muscle biopsies reveal many muscle fibers that contain a peripheral crescent that reacts strongly to NADH-TR, periodic acid–Schiff (PAS), and phosphorylase, but not to succinic dehydrogenase (SDH) or myofibrillar ATPase. Immunohistochemistry reveals that these "caps" display increased fast-myosin activity, desmin, tropomyosin, and α-actinin.[104] On EM, there is widened Z-bands, disarray of the myofibrils, and lack of thick filaments.

MOLECULAR GENETICS AND PATHOGENESIS

This myopathy is most often caused by mutations in *TPM2*, *TMP3*, *ACTA1*, *NEB*, and *MYPD* each of which are more commonly associated with nemaline myopathy.[1,2,105–110] Both caps and nemaline rods are found in some patients.[91,100]

TREATMENT

There is no specific medical treatment available.

▶ ZEBRA BODY MYOPATHY

CLINICAL FEATURES

Only a few of cases of zebra body myopathy have been reported.[113,114] One child presented with generalized weakness and atrophy from birth.[113] The second report involved a child with severe hypotonia, dysphagia, and asymmetric weakness of the upper limbs.[115] Muscle weakness was stable or only slowly progressive.

LABORATORY FEATURES

Serum CK is two to three times normal. EMG reveals myopathic units without abnormal spontaneous activity.

HISTOPATHOLOGY

Muscle biopsies demonstrate variability in muscle fiber size, increased internal nuclei, and occasional vacuoles. The Z-bodies appear on EM as osmiophilic 270-mm stria, with a periodicity such that these resemble stripes on a zebra.[113,114] The density of the stria is that of Z-discs and measuring up to 2 nm in length. Streaming of the Z-bands and nemaline rods may also be appreciated.

MOLECULAR GENETICS AND PATHOGENESIS

Zebra bodies are associated with mutations in *ACTA1*, so is likely a subtype of nemaline myopathy. However, zebra bodies are not a specific abnormality and can be found in normal individuals at myotendinous junctions, in intrafusal fibers (muscle spindles), extraocular muscles, and cardiac muscles. These may also be found in other pathologic conditions (e.g., myofibrillar myopathy).

TREATMENT

There is no specific medical treatment available.

▶ CENTRONUCLEAR MYOPATHY

CLINICAL FEATURES

Spiro and colleagues first introduced the term "myotubular myopathy" to describe this myopathy, given its resemblance to myotubes on muscle biopsies.[116] However, this myopathy is not caused by an arrest of myotubes and the term "centronuclear myopathy" is more appropriate. At least three clinically different forms of the disease are recognized: (1) a slowly progressive, infantile–early childhood type; (2) a severe X-linked neonatal type; and (3) a late childhood- or adult-onset type.[1–4,116–120] The slowly progressive, infantile–early childhood type is the most common presentation. These cases may be inherited in an autosomal-recessive or autosomal-dominant fashion. Children who are affected are usually the product of a normal pregnancy and delivery. Mild hypotonia and generalized weakness are apparent in infancy or early childhood and motor milestones are typically delayed. Ambulation is usually achieved, but the gait may be wide based and hyperlordotic. As with nemaline myopathy, generalized muscle atrophy, elongated narrow facies, and high-arched palate are often appreciated. Unlike other forms of congenital myopathy, ptosis, and ophthalmoparesis are common in centronuclear myopathy. Muscle stretch reflexes are depressed or absent, but sensation is completely normal. Some children have mental retardation and seizures.

The X-linked recessive myotubular myopathy presents at birth with severe hypotonia and generalized weakness. Affected infants usually require ventilatory support and feeding tubes. Polyhydramnios is a frequent complication of the mother's pregnancy. Ptosis and ophthalmoparesis may not be apparent initially but become more prominent after the newborn period. Arthrogryposis may be evident. X-linked myotubular myopathy is usually fatal in infancy; however, the prognosis is not invariably poor.[119,120] With aggressive medical intervention, the survival rate has increased.[120]

Interestingly, there are several well-described cases of manifesting females with proven X-linked (myotubularin deficiency) centronuclear myopathy.[115,121–124] One large questionnaire study found that roughly 50% of female carries manifested at least mild symptoms.[124] Affected females can present with axial and proximal weakness, bilateral ptosis, and external ophthalmoplegia with onset in childhood or adulthood. The mechanism may be akin to skewed inactivation, as sometimes seen in manifesting female carriers of dystrophin mutations.

A more benign form of centronuclear myopathy can present in late childhood or adulthood. Muscle weakness is usually mild and only slowly progressive. The pattern of muscle weakness is quite variable, with some patients having predominantly proximal weakness, while distal muscles are more affected in others. Facial muscles may be weak, and some have ptosis and ophthalmoparesis. A facioscapulohumeral pattern of weakness has also been described.[125] Unlike infantile- and childhood-onset cases, dysmorphic facial features and skeletal anomalies are not associated with

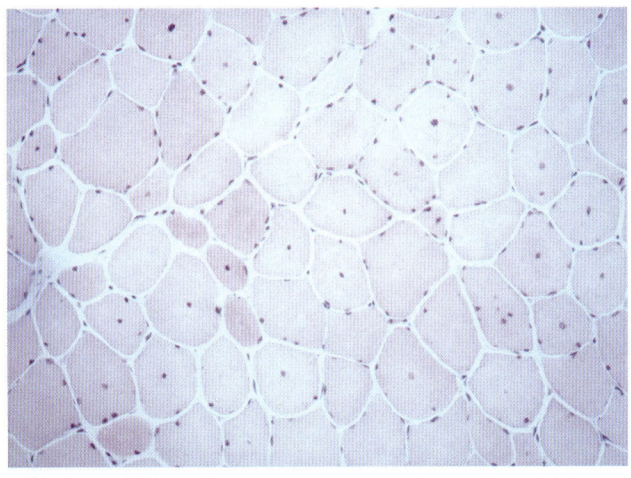
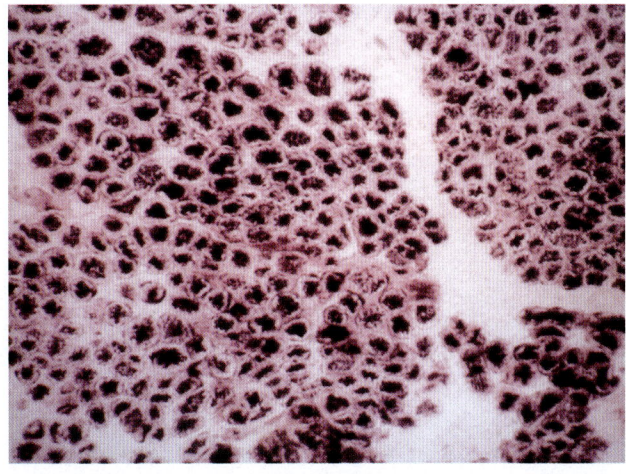

Figure 28-10. Centronuclear myopathy. Increased number of internalized nuclei often in the center of the muscle fiber is appreciated (**A**), hematoxylin and eosin (H&E). Late childhood- and adult-onset cases often have increased nuclei more randomly located throughout the fibers. Central areas appear dark on NADH-TR (**B**).

the adult-onset form of centronuclear myopathy. Some of these cases are felt to be autosomal-dominantly inherited.

LABORATORY FEATURES

Serum CK is normal or slightly elevated. Motor and sensory NCSs are normal. However, EMG is usually very abnormal, particularly in the severe X-linked infantile-onset form, revealing increased insertional and spontaneous activity in the form of positive sharp waves, fibrillation potentials, complex repetitive discharges, and even myotonic discharges.[10] Early recruitment of short-duration, small-amplitude MUAPs are evident in weak muscles. Reduced amplitudes and mild slowing of motor and sensory NCSs have been noted in some individuals with mutations in dynamin-2 gene (discussed in "Pathogenesis" section), which is not surprising, as this is also a cause of dominant intermediate Charcot–Marie–Tooth disease type B (DI-CMTB).

HISTOPATHOLOGY

Muscle biopsies reveal myonuclei in the center of muscle fibers, often forming chains when viewed longitudinally.[1–4,118] The type 1 fibers predominate and appear hypotrophic, while the type 2 fibers are normal in size. In cases associated with *BIN1* mutations, the nuclei often cluster in the center of the fiber rather than forming longitudinal chains. On transverse section, the number of muscle fibers with central nuclei ranges from 25% to 95% (Fig. 28-10A). The central nuclei appear in both fiber types. On ATPase stains, there is a small perinuclear halo devoid of ATPase activity. With oxidative enzyme stains, the center of muscle fibers appears dark (Fig. 28-10B). There can also be a radial arrangement of the intermyofibrillar network, which resembles spokes on a wheel, in cases caused by dynamin-2 (*DYN2*) mutations (Fig. 28-11). Necklace fibers, in which there are rings/loops of oxidative enzyme staining internally within fibers, can be found in late-onset centronuclear myopathy and obligate women carriers with myotubularin 1 (*MTM1*) mutations and in individuals with *DYN2* mutations (see below) (Fig. 28-12).[1–4,120] There can be increased endomysial connective tissue as can be seen in muscular dystrophies. On EM, there are reduced myofibrils and an excess of mitochondria and glycogen granules in the center of muscle fibers that are not occupied by nuclei.

MOLECULAR GENETICS AND PATHOGENESIS

As noted previously, there is genetic heterogeneity in centronuclear myopathy (Table 28-1). The severe X-linked neonatal

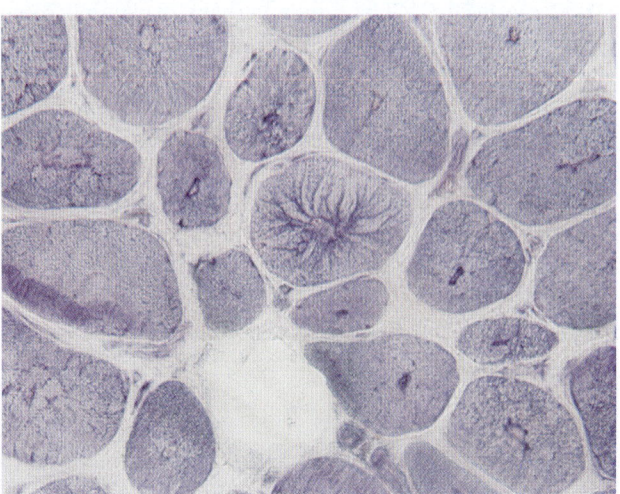

Figure 28-11. Radial spirals. Muscle biopsy in a patient with centronuclear myopathy caused by dynamin-2 (*DYN2*) mutations has radial spirals on NADH-TR. The radial arrangement of the intermyofibrillar network resembles spokes on a wheel.

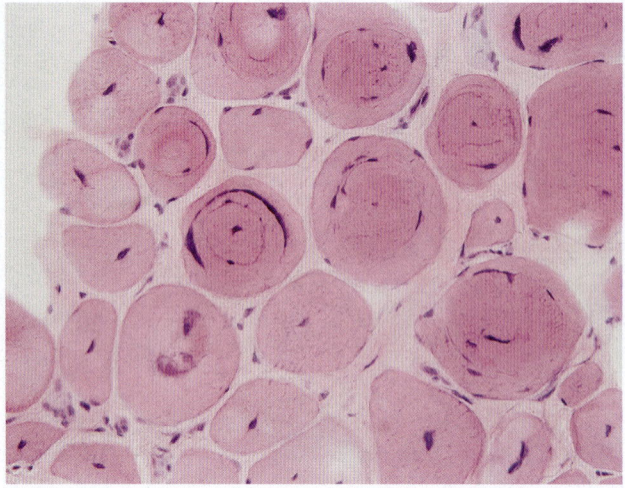 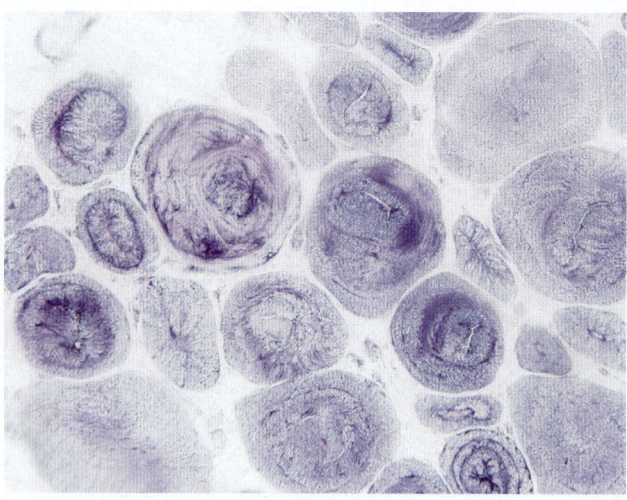

Figure 28-12. Necklace fibers. Muscle biopsy of a patient with centronuclear myopathy caused by dynamin-2 (*DYN2*) mutations has necklace fibers that appear as internal rings/loops within fibers seen here on H&E (**A**) and NADH-TR (**B**) stains.

form is caused by mutations in the myotubularin 1 gene (*MTM1*).[1–4,126,127] Myotubularin is a dual-specificity phosphatase, which plays a role in muscle cell growth and differentiation. Terminal muscle fiber differentiation is dependent on the hypophosphorylation of specific gene-regulating proteins.[128] Myotubularin is thought to dephosphorylate these regulating proteins, and mutations in the myotubularin gene lead to loss of function of this phosphatase activity, resulting in maturational disturbances of muscle.

Some autosomal-dominant cases of late-onset centronuclear myopathy characterized by prominent distal limb weakness and ptosis have been linked to mutations in the *DYN2* gene, which encodes for dynamin-2.[117,129] Mutations in this gene have also been reported in cases of severe neonatal centronuclear myopathy. Of note, mutations in *DYN2* cause DI-CMTB,[130] thus perhaps explaining some of the overlapping features (distal weakness, mild sensory abnormalities) that might be seen. Dynamin-2 belongs to the family of large GTPases and is important in endocytosis, membrane trafficking, actin assembly, and centrosome cohesion.[117]

Rare cases of centronuclear myopathy have been reported associated with *RYR1*, amphiphysin 2 (*BIN2*), titin (*TTN*), coiled-coil domain-containing protein 79 (*CCDC78*), striated muscle preferentially expressed protein kinase (*SPEG*), and sterile-alpha motif and leucine zipper-containing kinase (*ZAC*) mutations.[1,2,131–134]

TREATMENT

Infants with the X-linked form of the disease often require mechanical ventilation and tube feedings to support life. With such aggressive medical intervention, the survival rate has increased.[119]

▶ CONGENITAL FIBER-TYPE DISPROPORTION

CLINICAL FEATURES

Congenital fiber-type disproportion usually manifests as generalized hypotonia and weakness along with a weak cry and suck in infancy.[1–4,135] Motor milestones are delayed, but muscle weakness is usually nonprogressive and functional status improves with age attained. However, there are cases with a progressive and sometimes fatal course secondary to ventilatory muscle insufficiency.[135] Some children who are affected display dysmorphic facial features with a high-arched palate, congenital hip dislocations, kyphoscoliosis, arthrogryposis, and a rigid spine. Muscle stretch reflexes are reduced. Approximately one-third of affected children have some type of central nervous system abnormalities; some of these cases may represent forms of congenital muscular dystrophy with impaired glycosylation of α-dystroglycan (see Chapter 27).

LABORATORY FEATURES

The serum CK is normal or mildly elevated. NCSs are normal. EMG can be normal or can reveal increased insertional and spontaneous activity and early recruitment of myopathic MUAPs.[10]

HISTOPATHOLOGY

Muscle biopsies reveal disproportionate atrophy of type 1 compared to type 2 fibers.[1–4,135] While type 1 fibers are more numerous, they are typically less than 15% the diameter of type 2 fibers, which appear normal in size or slightly hypertrophic (Fig. 28-13). However, type 1 fiber predominance and

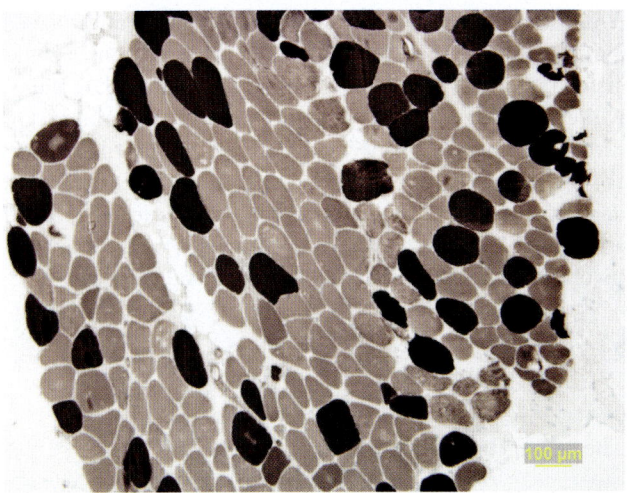

Figure 28-13. Congenital fiber-type disproportion. Type 1 fibers are more numerous but smaller in diameter than the type 2 fibers. However, type 1 fiber predominance and hypotrophy are not specific for this myopathy, and these are also common in other forms of congenital myopathy and congenital muscular dystrophy. ATPase 9.4.

hypotrophy are not specific for this myopathy, and these are also common in centronuclear, central core, nemaline, and fingerprint body myopathy and may also be found in congenital muscular dystrophies, spinal muscular atrophy, and central nervous system disease. With sequential muscle biopsies, nemaline rods or central nuclei may become apparent.[136] No consistent ultrastructural abnormalities have been noted.

MOLECULAR GENETICS AND PATHOGENESIS

Mutations in *TPM3* are the most common cause accounting for 25%–50% of cases and are autosomal dominant in inheritance.[1–4] The second most common cause is mutations in *RYR1* that are inherited in an autosomal-recessive fashion and account for approximately 20% of cases. Mutations in *ACTA1*, *TPM2*, *SEPN1*, *MYL2*, *HACD*, *MYH7*, *TTN*, and *SCN1A* account for most of the remaining cases.[1–4,137–140]

TREATMENT

Supportive measures such as mechanical ventilation and tube feeding may be temporarily required in some patients. Physical therapy and orthotic devices may be beneficial.

▶ SARCOTUBULAR MYOPATHY

CLINICAL FEATURES

Sarcotubular myopathy was initially reported in two Hutterite brothers of a consanguineous marriage.[140] Subsequently, it has been demonstrated that this disorder is allelic to LGMD2H, now referred to as LGMDR8 (see Chapter 27).[141] Patients can present with exertional myalgias or proximal muscle weakness in infancy or adult life. Scapular winging, calf hypertrophy, foot drop, and mild facial weakness may be appreciated. Muscle stretch reflexes are usually diminished.

LABORATORY FEATURES

Serum CK levels have ranged from normal to 20-fold elevated.[140,141] EMG may be normal or may reveal myopathic features.

HISTOPATHOLOGY

Muscle biopsies reveal an increase in internal nuclei, muscle fiber splitting, and many fibers (mostly type 2) with small vacuoles.[140,141] These vacuoles, which abut T-tubules, appear to be membrane bound, and are empty or contain a small amount of amorphous debris on EM. The vacuoles immunostain for sarcoplasmic reticulum-associated ATPase.

MOLECULAR GENETICS AND PATHOGENESIS

Mutations in *TRIM32*, the gene encoding the tripartite motif-containing protein 32, have been demonstrated; thus, this disorder is allelic to LGMDR8.[141] The TRIM 32 protein may be critical for the recognition of other protein(s) targeted to be ubiquitinated by this ligase enzyme.

TREATMENT

There is no specific medical treatment.

▶ FINGERPRINT BODY MYOPATHY

CLINICAL FEATURES

Fingerprint body myopathy is a rare disorder and typically presents as generalized hypotonia, weakness, and muscle atrophy in infancy or early childhood.[142–144] Muscle strength is stable or only slowly deteriorates over time. Muscle stretch reflexes are reduced or absent. Some individuals have a reduced intelligence and febrile seizures. In addition, kyphoscoliosis and pectus excavatum may be evident in some cases.

LABORATORY FEATURES

Serum CKs are normal or slightly elevated. NCSs are normal. EMG may be normal or may demonstrate short-duration, low-amplitude MUAPs without abnormal insertional or spontaneous activity.

HISTOPATHOLOGY

Muscle biopsy reveals type 1 fiber predominance with type 1 fiber hypotrophy and type 2 fiber hypertrophy. On oxidative enzyme stains, there is reduced activity in the subsarcolemma and perinuclear regions in type 1 fibers. EM and phase-contrast microscopy demonstrate a complex lamellar pattern resembling fingerprints that are evident in these areas; these fingerprint bodies appear to be composed of cytoskeletal proteins.[142–144] Fingerprint bodies are nonspecific and have also been noted in myotonic dystrophy, various distal myopathies, nemaline myopathy, dermatomyositis, oculopharyngeal dystrophy, and muscle biopsies from patients with uremia and chronic pulmonary disease.

MOLECULAR GENETICS AND PATHOGENESIS

Most of the cases have been sporadic, although the disease was reported in a pair of male identical twins[142] and in two siblings.[144] Next-generation sequencing panel in one patient with fingerprint bodies and their first biopsy and cytoplasmic bodies along with nemaline rods on a second biopsy were found to have mutations in *LMOD3*, a known rare cause of nemaline myopathy as discussed in the section regarding nemaline myopathy.[145]

TREATMENT

There is no specific medical treatment.

▶ TRILAMINAR MYOPATHY

CLINICAL FEATURES

A single infant with rigidity of its trunk and limbs, decreased spontaneous movements, weak suck and swallowing, and numerous joint contractures has been reported with this disorder.[146] Sensation appeared normal and deep tendon reflexes were intact. By 10 months of age, the infant had some head control, but was still unable to sit. Subsequently, the patient was able to ambulate, albeit with difficulty.

LABORATORY FEATURES

Serum CK was markedly elevated at birth (approximately 40 times normal). EMG and NCSs were normal.

HISTOPATHOLOGY

Muscle biopsy demonstrated variability in fiber size. The unique feature was that approximately 25% of fibers were hypertrophic and had three concentric zones that displayed a differential staining pattern.[146] The inner and outer zones stained intensely with Gomori-trichrome and NADH stains, while the inverse pattern was seen on ATPase staining. On EM, the innermost zone demonstrated myofibrillar disarray and densely packed mitochondria, glycogen granules, and myofilaments. The intermediate zone revealed Z-band streaming. The outer zone was composed of disorganized myofibrils, mitochondria, lipid droplets, and vesicles.

MOLECULAR GENETICS AND PATHOGENESIS

The pathogenesis is unknown.

TREATMENT

No specific medical treatment is available.

▶ MYOSIN STORAGE MYOPATHY/HYALINE BODY MYOPATHY/FAMILIAL MYOPATHY WITH LYSIS OF MYOFIBRILS

CLINICAL FEATURES

Myosin storage/hyaline body myopathy is a rare congenital myopathy, which can present in infancy to as late as the fifth decade of life with limb-girdle or scapuloperoneal pattern of weakness.[1,147–153] Muscle strength is stable or only slowly deteriorates and is nonprogressive. Rare patients have a cardiomyopathy.[152] Muscle stretch reflexes are preserved. Hyaline body myopathy has been reported as occurring sporadically as well as being inherited in an autosomal-dominant or autosomal-recessive fashion. There is variability in the severity of the course even within families.

LABORATORY FEATURES

Serum CK levels can be normal or mildly elevated, while EMG studies may be normal or may reveal an increased number of small-duration, low-amplitude, polyphasic MUAPs. Echocardiography may reveal a dilated cardiomyopathy with reduced ejection fraction.

HISTOPATHOLOGY

Muscle biopsies reveal subsarcolemmal "hyaline" bodies that stain pale green on modified Gomori-trichrome and pale pink on H&E stains (Fig. 28-14).[147–152] The hyaline bodies occur in type 1 fibers, which are hypotrophic. The hyaline bodies do not stain with oxidative enzymes or PAS but demonstrate intense ATPase activity. Angulated neurogenic fibers and fiber-type grouping may also be appreciated.

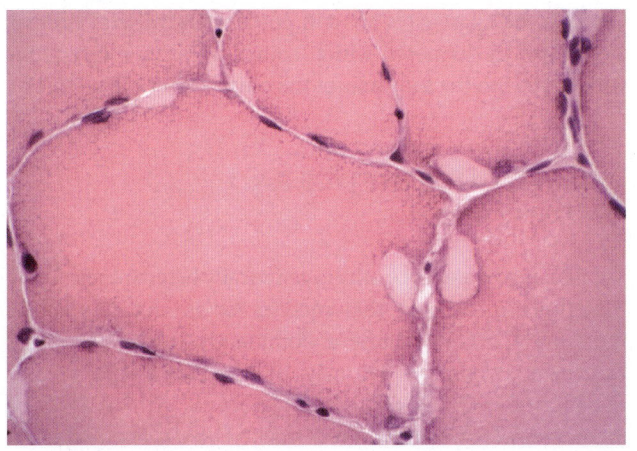

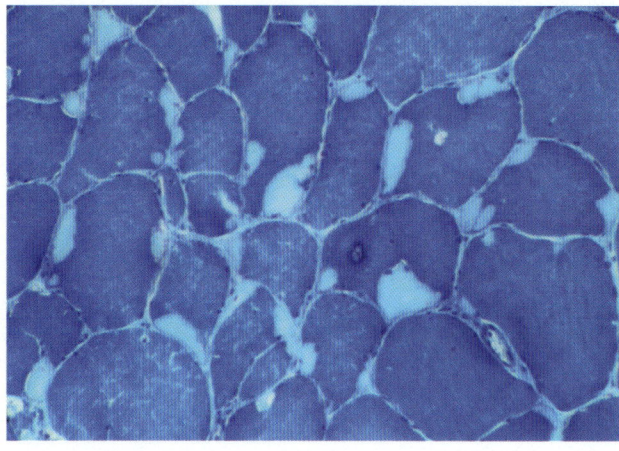

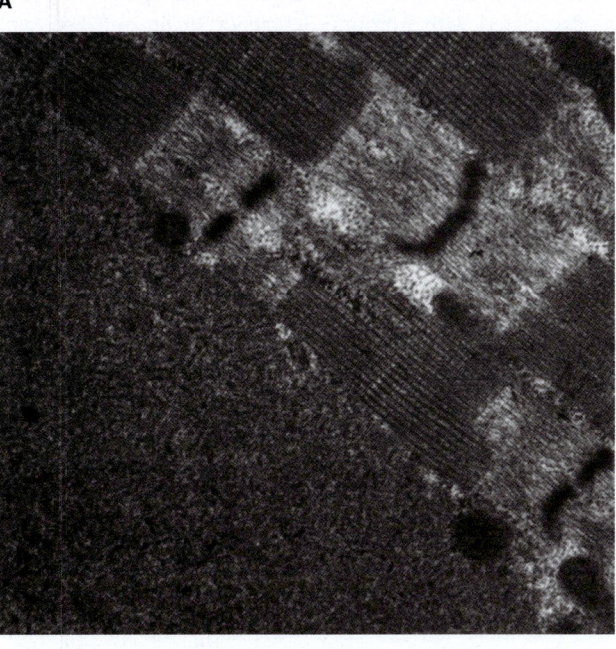

Figure 28-14. Hyaline body myopathy. Subsarcolemmal deposits stain pale pink on H&E (**A**) and pale green on modified trichrome (**B**). Electron microscopy reveals a hyaline body, which appears composed of granular and filamentous debris, adjacent to a normal appearing sarcomere (**C**).

Immunostaining demonstrates strong reactivity for slow myosin heavy chain (MyHC) in some but not all hyaline bodies.[149] The hyaline bodies are nonreactive for αB-crystallin, ubiquitin, tropomyosin, actins, desmin, and components of sarcolemma. On EM, the hyaline bodies appear to be composed of granulofilamentous debris often with fragments of sarcomeres and surrounded by a zone of sarcomeric disorganization.[149]

MOLECULAR GENETICS AND PATHOGENESIS

Missense mutations in the *MYH7* gene that encodes for slow/β-cardiac MyHC cause most cases of autosomal-dominant hyaline body myopathy.[148–153] Mutations in this gene also have been associated with a familial form of cardiomyopathy and Laing-type distal myopathy/dystrophy, and scapuloperoneal myopathy/dystrophy (see Chapter 27). *MYH7* encodes the major myosin isoform seen in type 1 muscle fibers and cardiac muscle. Within this region lies a candidate who exhibits homology to the MyHC. It appears that normal MyHC is essential for the assembly of thick filaments in skeletal muscle.

TREATMENT

There is no specific medical treatment available.

▶ OTHER MYOSIN STORAGE DISORDERS

Another autosomal-dominant myopathy characterized by mild weakness and myalgias with onset in childhood or early adult life has been linked to mutations in the *MYH2* gene, which encodes for MyHC IIa.[154,155] The MyHC IIa isoform of

MyHCs is expressed in type 2 A muscle fibers. Other families present with congenital arthrogryposis, ophthalmoplegia, and mild proximal weakness beginning in adulthood. As muscle biopsies may demonstrate rimmed vacuoles and tubulofilamentous inclusions, this disorder has also been called hereditary inclusion body myopathy type 3 (see Chapter 27).[156,157]

▶ TUBULAR AGGREGATE MYOPATHY

CLINICAL FEATURES

Tubular aggregates are a nonspecific histologic abnormality, which may be found in muscle biopsies of patients with in hypokalemic periodic paralysis type 2 (hypoKPP2, see Chapter 32), some forms of glycogen storage disease [e.g., phosphoglycerate mutase (PGAM) deficiency, see Chapter 29], hyperthyroidism, hypoxia, and some toxic myopathies. In addition, tubular aggregates are also found on muscle biopsy of patients with no symptoms or signs of a myopathy. However, there are several clinical syndromes in which the primary pathologic feature is tubular aggregates on muscle biopsy.[2,158-161] Affected individuals may have slow progressive limb-girdle weakness beginning in childhood or early adulthood. In addition, there are forms of congenital myasthenia with tubular aggregates (see Chapter 26).[159,161] These patients demonstrate fatigable weakness, which improves with anticholinesterase medications. Another clinical subgroup comprises patients with generalized myalgias, which are worse with exertion.[158,161] Muscle tone, bulk, and strength are normal as is the rest of the physical examination. In addition, there is a rare tubular aggregate myopathy associated with Stormorken syndrome (muscle weakness, miosis, thrombocytopenia, hyposplenism, ichthyosis, dyslexia, and short stature).[161]

LABORATORY FEATURES

Serum CK is normal or mildly increased. Routine motor and sensory NCSs are normal. Patients with the myasthenic syndrome demonstrate a decremental response on repetitive stimulation, which improves with pyridostigmine. EMG can be normal or can demonstrate myopathic MUAPs and fibrillation potentials. Patients with the muscle-pain syndrome typically have completely normal electrodiagnostic findings.

HISTOPATHOLOGY

Tubular aggregates stain basophilic on H&E and are red on modified Gomori trichrome (Fig. 28-15A). These react intensely to NADH-TR (Fig. 28-15B), but not to SDH. Tubular aggregates are located in a subsarcolemmal position and are present only in type 2 muscle fibers in the syndromes associated with periodic paralysis and muscle pain but are evident in both fiber types in the limb-girdle syndrome.

On EM, the aggregates are composed of bundles of tubules 60–80 nm in diameter, which course in various directions with respect to the long axis of the muscle fibers (Fig. 28-16).

MOLECULAR GENETICS AND PATHOGENESIS

Tubular aggregate myopathy is genetically heterogeneic.[161-169] Mutations in the gene that encodes for stromal interaction molecule 1, STIM1, cause a dominantly inherited tubular aggregate myopathy that may be associated with immunodeficiency or Stormorken syndrome.[161-163] Mutations in the gene that encodes for Orai-1, ORAI1, also cause an autosomal-dominant tubular aggregate myopathy that can be associated with immune deficiency or Stormorken syndrome.[161,164] Mutations in calsequestrin (CASQ1) also have been associated with tubular aggregates.[161,166,169] STIM1 is a calcium-sensing protein that binds to Orai-1, a calcium-release channel located in the sarcoplasmic reticulum. Calsequestrin 1 is a calcium-binding protein located at terminal cisternae of type 2 muscle fibers, where it serves as the main calcium buffer.[161]

Some forms of congenital myasthenia, which can easily be mistaken for a congenital myopathy, if one does not appreciate fatigability or decrement on repetitive nerve stimulation, are associated with tubular aggregates.[165-167] These include mutations in the genes that encode for UDP-N-acetylglucosamine-dolichyl-phosphate, N-acetylglucosaminephosphotransferase 1 (DPAGT1), glutamine-fructose-6-phosphate transaminase 1 (GFPT1), and alpha-1,3/1,6-mannosyltransferase (ALG2).[161,165-167] Mutations in these genes lead do decreased acetylcholine receptors and the neuromuscular junction but why they lead also to tubular aggregates is unclear.

Mutations in the gene encoding phosphoglycerate mutase (PGAM) lead to glycogen storage disease type X. Mutations in the sodium voltage-gated channel, alpha subunit gene, SCN4A, can result in hypokalemic periodic paralysis type 2 (hypoKPP2). These myopathies are also associated with tubular aggregates on biopsy for unclear reasons.[161]

TREATMENT

Patients with the congenital myasthenic syndrome may benefit from pyridostigmine. Individuals with the muscle pain syndrome may improve with dantrolene or tricyclic antidepressant medications.

▶ REDUCING BODY MYOPATHY

CLINICAL FEATURES

Reducing body myopathy is a rare disorder that has varied clinical presentations.[170-175] It can present in infancy with

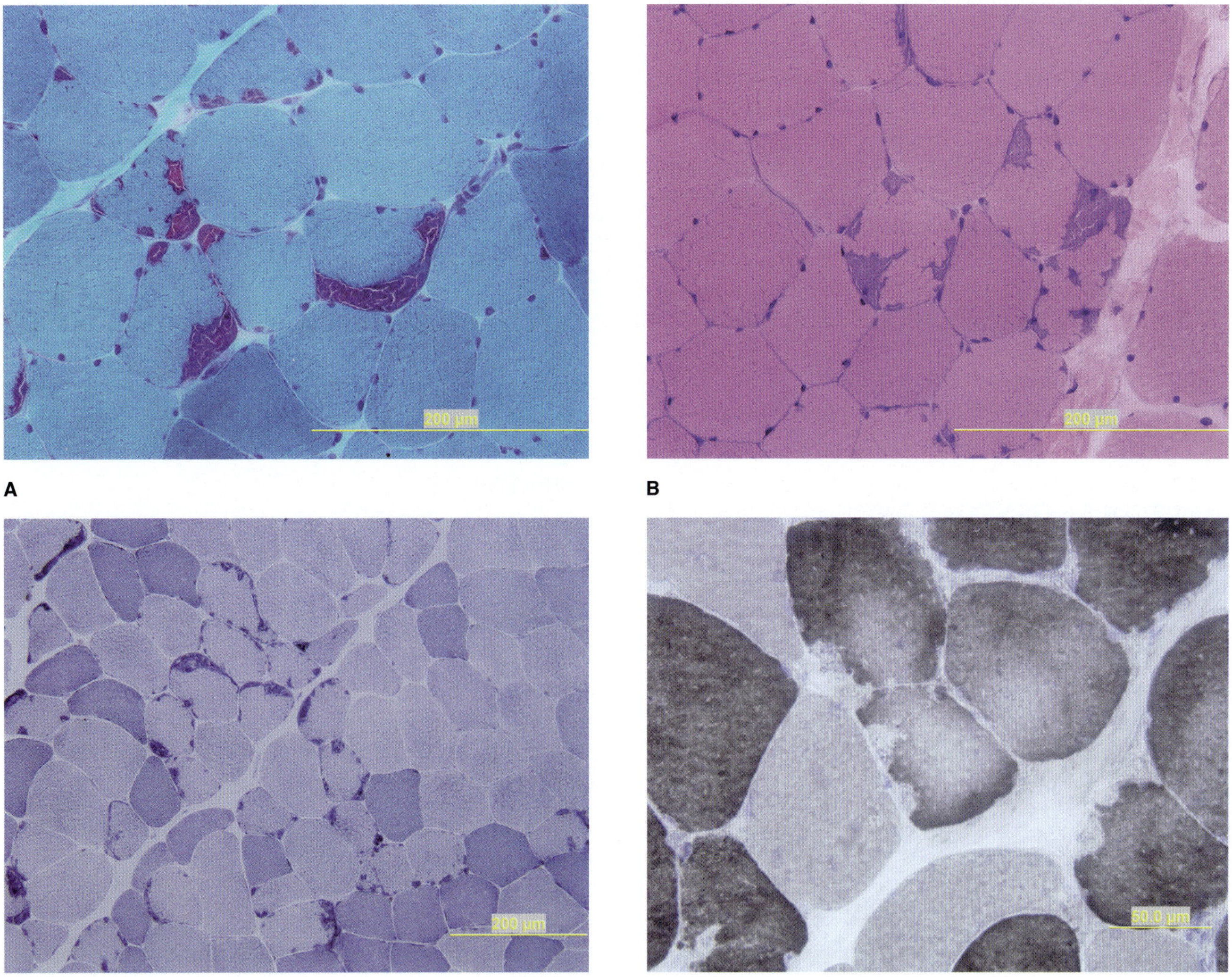

Figure 28-15. Tubular aggregates. Tubular aggregates appear as subsarcolemmal masses of reddish material on modified trichrome (**A**) and are bluish on H&E (**B**). The tubular aggregates occur only in type 2 fibers and appear densely staining on NADH-TR (**C**), but do not stain with ATPase 9.4 (**D**).

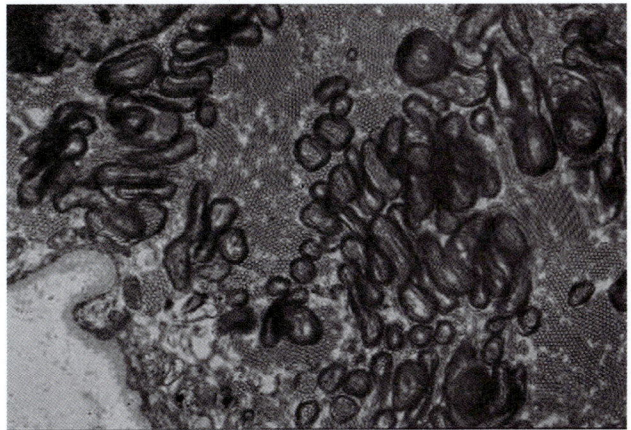

Figure 28-16. Tubular aggregates. On EM, tubular aggregates appear as subsarcolemmal aggregates of long, straight parallel tubules, which are somewhat haphazardly oriented in small bundles.

severe generalized weakness, hypotonia, and joint contractures. Ptosis may be apparent as well. There is an increased mortality due to associated ventilatory muscle weakness. Some affected individuals apparently develop muscle weakness later in childhood or in adulthood. The proximal or distal muscles may be preferentially affected, and involvement can be asymmetric, particularly in the arms. The course can vary from mild stable weakness to progressive deterioration of strength, leading to death. Some affected patients develop contractures of the major joints, scoliosis, and rigidity of the spine.

LABORATORY FEATURES

Serum CK levels are usually normal, although a few patients have demonstrated mild elevations. NCSs are normal. EMG may demonstrate myopathic features.

HISTOPATHOLOGY

The characteristic feature on muscle biopsies is "reducing bodies," named such because of their unique ability to reduce nitroblue tetrazolium when mediated by menadione.[170–175] These reducing bodies stain purple with modified Gomori-trichrome stain and pink on H&E stain and are devoid of oxidative enzyme staining. Immunohistochemistry reveals increased desmin at the periphery of some reducing bodies, but αB-crystallin, α-actinin, titin, and nebulin immunostains are normal. There is usually type 1 fiber predominance as seen in most other congenital myopathies, but the reducing bodies are evident in both fiber types. On EM, the reducing bodies appear to be composed of electron-dense granules and 12–17-nm tubulofilaments.

MOLECULAR GENETICS AND PATHOGENESIS

This rare disorder is usually caused by mutations in the four and a half LIM gene (*FHL1*), located on chromosome Xq26.3 that encodes for four and a half LIM.[175–181] Rare cases of reducing body myopathy have also been reported with mutations in the desmin gene (*DES*).[182] In many ways the histopathology resembles in part what is in myofibrillar myopathy (discussed in Chapter 27).

TREATMENT

No specific treatment is available.

▶ NATIVE AMERICAN MYOPATHY

CLINICAL FEATURES

This rate myopathy was initially described in individuals from the Lumbee Native American tribe,[183–185] but it has since been identified in numerous other populations worldwide.[186–190] It is characterized by infantile onset of trunk and proximal extremity weakness, delayed motor milestones, ptosis, myopathic facies, cleft-plate, feeding difficulties, ptosis, conductive hearing loss, skeletal deformities (e.g., scoliosis, kyphosis or kyphoscoliosis, and contractures), short stature, and an increased risk of malignant hyperthermia. There can be restrictive lung disease due to pulmonary hypoplasia. Intellect is unaffected. There is increased mortality.

LABORATORY FEATURES

Serum CK is usually normal.[186] EMG may show myopathic motor units but there is typically no abnormal muscle membrane irritability.[183–186]

HISTOPATHOLOGY

Muscle biopsies may reveal nonspecific features such as type 1 and type 2 muscle fiber atrophies, increased internalized, and subsarcolemmal mitochondrial proliferation, or increased lipid on EM.[186]

MOLECULAR GENETICS AND PATHOGENESIS

This is an autosomal disorder caused by mutations in *STAC3* that encodes for SH3 and cysteine-rich domain 3. This protein is required for normal excitation-contraction coupling in skeletal muscle.

TREATMENT

There is no specific medical treatment.

▶ MYOFIBRILLAR MYOPATHY

This is a genetically heterogeneous group of disorders, which are now considered to be forms of muscular dystrophy as opposed to congenital myopathies and are discussed in detail in Chapter 27.

▶ SUMMARY

As evident from this chapter, there is significant overlap in what have previously been termed congenital myopathies and congenital and limb-girdle dystrophies. Continued advances in molecular genetics have provided and will likely provide better insight into the classification of these myopathies. Unfortunately, there are no medications yet available to successfully treat these disorders. However, physical and occupational therapy as outlined in Chapter 5 as well as supportive therapy for ventilatory or cardiac muscle involvement can be beneficial.

REFERENCES

1. North KN, Wang CH, Clarke N, et al; International Standard of Care Committee for Congenital Myopathies. Approach to the diagnosis of congenital myopathies. *Neuromuscul Disord.* 2014;24(2):97–116.
2. Claeys KG. Congenital myopathies: an update. *Dev Med Child Neurol.* 2020;62(3):297–302.
3. Butterfield RJ. Congenital muscular dystrophy and congenital myopathy. *Continuum (Minneap Minn).* 2019;25(6):1640–1661.
4. Phadke R. Myopathology of congenital myopathies: bridging the old and the new. *Semin Pediatr Neurol.* 2019;29:55–70.
5. Isaacs H, Heffron JJ, Badenhorst M. Central core disease. A correlated genetic, histochemical, ultramicroscopic, and

biochemical study. *J Neurol Neurosurg Psychiatry*. 1975;38(12): 1177–1186.
6. Magee KR, Shy GM. A new congenital non-progressive myopathy. *Brain*. 1956;79(4):610–621.
7. Quinlivan RM, Muller CR, Davis M, et al. Central core disease: clinical, pathological, and genetic features. *Arch Dis Child*. 2003;88(12):1051–1055.
8. Bharucha-Goebel DX, Santi M, Medne L, et al. Severe congenital RYR1-associated myopathy: the expanding clinicopathologic and genetic spectrum. *Neurology*. 2013;80(17): 1584–1589.
9. Abath Neto O, Moreno CAM, Malfatti E, et al. Common and variable clinical, histological, and imaging findings of recessive RYR1-related centronuclear myopathy patients. *Neuromuscul Disord*. 2017;27(11):975–985.
10. Amato A, Dumitru D. *Hereditary Myopathies*. Hanley & Belfus; 2002.
11. Sewry CA, Müller C, Davis M, et al. The spectrum of pathology in central core disease. *Neuromuscul Disord*. 2002;12(10): 930–938.
12. Ferreiro A, Monnier N, Romero NB, et al. A recessive form of central core disease, transiently presenting as multi-minicore disease, is associated with a homozygous mutation in the ryanodine receptor type 1 gene. *Ann Neurol*. 2002;51(6):750–759.
13. De Bleecker JL, Ertl BB, Engel AG. Patterns of abnormal protein expression in target formations and unstructured cores. *Neuromuscul Disord*. 1996;6(5):339–349.
14. Robinson R, Carpenter D, Shaw MA, Halsall J, Hopkins P. Mutations in RYR1 in malignant hyperthermia and central core disease. *Hum Mutat*. 2006;27:977–989.
15. Wu S, Ibarra MCA, Malicdan MCV, et al. Central core disease is due to RYR1 mutations in more than 90% of patients. *Brain*. 2006;129(Pt 6):1470–1480.
16. Monnier N, Marty I, Faure J, et al. Null mutations causing depletion of the type 1 ryanodine receptor (RYR1) are commonly associated with recessive structural congenital myopathies with cores. *Hum Mutat*. 2008;29:670–678.
17. Monnier N, Laquerrière A, Marret S, et al. First genomic rearrangement of the RYR1 gene associated with an atypical presentation of lethal neonatal hypotonia. *Neuromuscul Disord*. 2009;19:680–684.
18. Zhou H, Brockington M, Jungbluth H, et al. Epigenetic allele silencing unveils recessive RYR1 mutations in core myopathies. *Am J Hum Genet*. 2006;79(5):859–868.
19. Mathews KD, Moore SA. Multiminicore myopathy, central core disease, malignant hyperthermia susceptibility, and RYR1 mutations: one disease with many faces? *Arch Neurol*. 2004;61(1):27–29.
20. Jungbluth H, Treves S, Zorzato F, et al. Congenital myopathies: disorders of excitation-contraction coupling and muscle contraction. *Nat Rev Neurol*. 2018;14(3):151–167.
21. Avila G. Intracellular Ca^{2+} dynamics in malignant hyperthermia and central core disease: established concepts, new cellular mechanisms involved. *Cell Calcium*. 2005;37(2):121–127.
22. Avila G, O'Connell KM, Dirksen RT. The pore region of the skeletal muscle ryanodine receptor is a primary locus for excitation-contraction uncoupling in central core disease. *J Gen Physiol*. 2003;121(4):277–286.
23. Romero NB, Xie T, Malfatti E, et al. Autosomal dominant eccentric core disease caused by a heterozygous mutation in the MYH7 gene. *J Neurol Neurosurg Psychiatry*. 2014;85(10):1149–1152.
24. Kaindl AM, Rüschendorf F, Krause S, et al. Missense mutations of ACTA1 cause dominant congenital myopathy with cores. *J Med Genet*. 2004;41(11):842–848.
25. Majczenko K, Davidson AE, Camelo-Piragua S, et al. Dominant mutation of CCDC78 in a unique congenital myopathy with prominent internal nuclei and atypical cores. *Am J Hum Genet*. 2012;91(2):365–371.
26. Engel AG, Gomez MR, Groover RV. Multicore disease. A recently recognized congenital myopathy associated with multifocal degeneration of muscle fibers. *Mayo Clin Proc*. 1971;46(10):666–681.
27. Ferreiro A, Estournet B, Chateau D, et al. Multi-minicore disease—searching for boundaries: phenotype analysis of 38 cases. *Ann Neurol*. 2000;48(5):745–757.
28. Ferreiro A, Fardeau M. 80th ENMC international workshop on multi-minicore disease: 1st international MmD workshop. 12–13th May, 2000, Soestduinen, The Netherlands. *Neuromuscul Disord*. 2002;12(1):60–68.
29. Jungbluth H, Beggs A, Bönnemann C, et al. 111th ENMC International Workshop on Multi-minicore Disease. 2nd International MmD Workshop, 9–11 November. 2002, Naarden, The Netherlands. *Neuromuscul Disord*. 2004;14(11):754–766.
30. Jungbluth H, Sewry C, Brown SC, et al. Minicore myopathy in children: a clinical and histopathological study of 19 cases. *Neuromuscul Disord*. 2000;10(4–5):264–273.
31. Zeman AZ, Dick DJ, Anderson JR, Watkin SW, Smith IE, Shneerson JM. Multicore myopathy presenting in adulthood with respiratory failure. *Muscle Nerve*. 1997;20(3):367–369.
32. Monnier N, Ferreiro A, Marty I, Labarre-Vila A, Mezin P, Lunardi J. A homozygous splicing mutation causing a depletion of skeletal muscle RYR1 is associated with multi-minicore disease congenital myopathy with ophthalmoplegia. *Hum Mol Genet*. 2003;12(10):1171–1178.
33. Ferreiro A, Quijano-Roy S, Pichereau C, et al. Mutations of the selenoprotein N gene, which is implicated in rigid spine muscular dystrophy, cause the classical phenotype of multiminicore disease: reassessing the nosology of early-onset myopathies. *Am J Hum Genet*. 2002;71(4):739–749.
34. Cullup T, Lamont PJ, Cirak S, et al. Mutations in MYH7 cause multi-minicore disease (MmD) with variable cardiac involvement. *Neuromuscul Disord*. 2012;22(12):1096–1104.
35. Clarke NF, Amburgey K, Teener J, et al. A novel mutation expands the genetic and clinical spectrum of MYH7-related myopathies. *Neuromuscul Disord*. 2013;23(5):432–436.
36. Carmignac V, Salih MAM, Quijano-Roy S, et al. C-terminal titin deletions cause a novel early-onset myopathy with fatal cardiomyopathy. *Ann Neurol*. 2007;61:340–351.
37. Boyden SE, Mahoney LJ, Kawahara G, et al. Mutations in the satellite cell gene MEGF10 cause a recessive congenital myopathy with minicores. *Neurogenetics*. 2012;13(2):115–124.
38. Ogasawara M, Nishino I. A review of core myopathy: central core disease, multiminicore disease, dusty core disease, and core-rod myopathy. *Neuromuscul Disord*. 2021;31: 968–977.
39. Bouman K, Küsters B, De Winter JM, et al. NEM6, KBTBD13-related congenital myopathy: myopathological analysis in 18 Dutch patients reveals ring rods fibers, cores, nuclear clumps, and granulo-filamentous protein material. *J Neuropathol Exp Neurol*. 2021;80(4):366–376.
40. Guis S, Figarella-Branger D, Monnier N, et al. Multiminicore disease in a family susceptible to malignant hyperthermia:

histology, in vitro contracture tests, and genetic characterization. *Arch Neurol.* 2004;61(1):106–113.
41. Koch BM, Bertorini TE, Eng GD, Boehm R. Severe multicore disease associated with reaction to anesthesia. *Arch Neurol.* 1985;42(12):1204–1206.
42. Monnier N, Romero NB, Lerale J, et al. An autosomal dominant congenital myopathy with cores and rods is associated with a neomutation in the RYR1 gene encoding the skeletal muscle ryanodine receptor. *Hum Mol Genet.* 2000;9:2599–2608.
43. Scacheri PC, Hoffman EP, Fratkin JD, et al. A novel ryanodine receptor gene mutation causing both cores and rods in congenital myopathy. *Neurology.* 2000;55(11):1689–1696.
44. Hernandez-Lain A, Husson I, Monnier N, et al. De novo RYR1 heterozygous mutation (I4898 T) causing lethal core-rod myopathy in twins. *EurJ Med Genet.* 2001;54(1):29–33.
45. Pallagi E, Molnár M, Molnár P, Diószeghy P. Central core and nemaline rods in the same patient. *Acta Neuropathol.* 1998;96(2):211–214.
46. Afifi AK, Smith JW, Zellweger H. Congenital nonprogressive myopathy: central core disease and nemaline myopathy in one family. *Neurology.* 1965;15:371–381.
47. Romero NB, Lehtokari V, Quijano-Roy S, et al. Core-rod myopathy caused by mutations in the nebulin gene. *Neurology.* 2009;73(14):1159–1161.
48. Gommans IM, Davis M, Saar K, et al. A locus on chromosome 15q for a dominantly inherited nemaline myopathy with core-like lesions. *Brain.* 2003;126(Pt 7):1545–1551.
49. Sambuughin N, Yau KS, Olivé M, et al. Dominant mutations in KBTBD13, a member of the BTB/Kelch family, cause nemaline myopathy with cores. *Am J Hum Genet.* 2010;87:842–847.
50. Dlamini N, Voermans NC, Lillis S, et al. Mutations in RYR1 are a common cause of exertional myalgia and rhabdomyolysis. *Neuromuscul Disord.* 2013;23(7):540–548.
51. D'Arcy CE, Bjorksten A, Yiu EM, et al. King-Denborough syndrome caused by a novel mutation in the ryanodine receptor gene. *Neurology.* 2008;71(10):776–777.
52. Dowling JJ, Lillis S, Amburgey K, et al. King-Denborough syndrome with and without mutations in the skeletal muscle ryanodine receptor (RYR1) gene. *Neuromuscul Disord.* 2011;21(6):420–427.
53. Iamini N, Voermans NC, Lillis S, et al. Mutations in RYR1 are a common cause of exertional myalgia and rhabdomyolysis. *Neuromuscul Disord.* 2013;23(7):540–548.
54. Knuiman GJ, Küsters B, Eshuis L, et al. The histopathological spectrum of malignant hyperthermia and rhabdomyolysis due to RYR1 mutations. *J Neurol.* 2019;266:876–887.
55. Duarte ST, Oliveira J, Santos R, et al. Dominant and recessive RYR1 mutations in adults with core lesions and mild muscle symptoms. *Muscle Nerve.* 2011;44:102–108.
56. Løseth S, Voermans NC, Torbergsen T, et al. A novel late-onset axial myopathy associated with mutations in the skeletal muscle ryanodine receptor (RYR1) gene. *J Neurol.* 2013;260(6):1504–1510.
57. Jungbluth H, Lillis S, Zhou H, et al. Late-onset axial myopathy with cores due to a novel heterozygous dominant mutation in the skeletal muscle ryanodine receptor (RYR1) gene. *Neuromuscul Disord.* 2009;19(5):344–347.
58. Shy GM, Engel WK, Somers JE, Wanko T. Nemaline myopathy. A new congenital myopathy. *Brain.* 1963;86:793–810.
59. Engel WK, Wanko T, Fenichel GM. Nemaline myopathy; a second case. *Arch Neurol.* 1964;11:22–39.
60. Agrawal PB, Strickland CD, Midgett C, et al. Heterogeneity of nemaline myopathy cases with skeletal muscle alpha-actin gene mutations. *Ann Neurol.* 2004;56(1):86–96.
61. Jungbluth H, Sewry CA, Brown SC, et al. Mild phenotype of nemaline myopathy with sleep hypoventilation due to a mutation in the skeletal muscle alpha-actin (ACTA1) gene. *Neuromuscul Disord.* 2001;11(1):35–40.
62. North KN, Laing NG, Wallgren-Pettersson C. Nemaline myopathy: current concepts. The ENMC International Consortium and Nemaline Myopathy. *J Med Genet.* 1997;34(9):705–713.
63. Ryan MM, Ilkovski B, Strickland CD, et al. Clinical course correlates poorly with muscle pathology in nemaline myopathy. *Neurology.* 2003;60(4):665–673.
64. Ryan MM, Schnell C, Strickland CD, et al. Nemaline myopathy: a clinical study of 143 cases. *Ann Neurol.* 2001;50(3):312–320.
65. Wallgren-Pettersson C. Congenital nemaline myopathy. A clinical follow-up of twelve patients. *J Neurol Sci.* 1989;89(1):1–14.
66. Wallgren-Pettersson C. Nemaline and myotubular myopathies. *Semin Pediatr Neurol.* 2002;9(2):132–144.
67. Wallgren-Pettersson C. Congenital myopathies. *Eur J Paediatr Neurol.* 2005;9(1):27–28.
68. Wallgren-Pettersson C, Laing NG. 138th ENMC Workshop: nemaline myopathy, 20–22 May. 2005, Naarden, The Netherlands. *Neuromuscul Disord.* 2006;16(1):54–60.
69. Barohn RJ, Jackson CE, Kagan-Hallet KS. Neonatal nemaline myopathy with abundant intranuclear rods. *Neuromuscul Disord.* 1994;4(5–6):513–520.
70. Norton P, Ellison P, Sulaiman AR, Harb J. Nemaline myopathy in the neonate. *Neurology.* 1983;33(3):351–356.
71. Rifai Z, Kazee AM, Kamp C, Griggs RC. Intranuclear rods in severe congenital nemaline myopathy. *Neurology.* 1993;43(11):2372–2377.
72. Laitila J, Wallgren-Pettersson C. Recent advances in nemaline myopathy. *Neuromuscul Disord.* 2021;31:955–967.
73. Wallgren-Pettersson C, Jasani B, Newman GR, et al. Alpha-actinin in nemaline bodies in congenital nemaline myopathy: immunological confirmation by light and electron microscopy. *Neuromuscul Disord.* 1995;5(2):93–104.
74. Gurgel-Giannetti J, Reed U, Bang ML, et al. Nebulin expression in patients with nemaline myopathy. *Neuromuscul Disord.* 2001;11(2):154–162.
75. Pelin K, Donner K, Holmberg M, Jungbluth H, Muntoni F, Wallgren-Pettersson C. Nebulin mutations in autosomal recessive nemaline myopathy: an update. *Neuromuscul Disord.* 2002;12(7–8):680–686.
76. Pelin K, Hilpela P, Donner K, et al. Mutations in the nebulin gene associated with autosomal recessive nemaline myopathy. *Proc Natl Acad Sci U S A.* 1999;96(5):2305–2310.
77. Sparrow JC, Nowak KJ, Durling HJ, et al. Muscle disease caused by mutations in the skeletal muscle alpha-actin gene (ACTA1). *Neuromuscul Disord.* 2003;13(7–8):519–531.
78. Marston S, Mirza M, Abdulrazzak H, Sewry C. Functional characterisation of a mutant actin (Met132Val) from a patient with nemaline myopathy. *Neuromuscul Disord.* 2004;14(2):167–174.
79. Nowak KJ, Wattanasirichaigoon D, Goebel HH, et al. Mutations in the skeletal muscle alpha-actin gene in patients with actin myopathy and nemaline myopathy. *Nat Genet.* 1999;23(2):208–212.

80. Wallgren-Pettersson C, Pelin K, Nowak KJ, et al; ENMC International Consortium On Nemaline Myopathy. Genotype phenotype correlations in nemaline myopathy caused by mutations in the genes for nebulin and skeletal muscle alpha-actin. *Neuromuscul Disord.* 2004;14(8–9):461–470.
81. Laing NG, Wilton SD, Akkari PA, et al. A mutation in the alpha tropomyosin gene TPM3 associated with autosomal dominant nemaline myopathy NEM1. *Nat Genet.* 1995;10(2):249.
82. Durling HJ, Reilich P, Müller-Höcker J, et al. De novo missense mutation in a constitutively expressed exon of the slow alpha-tropomyosin gene TPM3 associated with an atypical, sporadic case of nemaline myopathy. *Neuromuscul Disord.* 2002;12(10):947–951.
83. Wattanasirichaigoon D, Swoboda KJ, Takada F, et al. Mutations of the slow muscle alpha-tropomyosin gene, TPM3, are a rare cause of nemaline myopathy. *Neurology.* 2002;59(4):613–617.
84. Donner K, Ollikainen M, Ridanpää M, et al. Mutations in the beta-tropomyosin (TPM2) gene—a rare cause of nemaline myopathy. *Neuromuscul Disord.* 2002;12(2):151–158.
85. Jin JP, Brotto MA, Hossain MM, et al. Truncation by Glu180 nonsense mutation results in complete loss of slow skeletal muscle troponin T in a lethal nemaline myopathy. *J Biol Chem.* 2003;278(28):26159–26165.
86. Agrawal PB, Greenleaf RS, Tomczak KK, et al. Nemaline myopathy with minicores caused by mutation of the CFL2 gene encoding the skeletal muscle actin-binding protein, cofilin-2. *Am J Hum Genet.* 2007;80:162–167.
87. Ockeloen CW, Gilhuis HJ, Pfundt R, et al. Congenital myopathy caused by a novel missense mutation in the CFL2 gene. *Neuromuscul Disord.* 2012;22:632–639.
88. Ong RW, Alsaman A, Selcen D, et al. Novel cofilin-2 (CFL2) four base pair deletion causing nemaline myopathy. *J Neurol Neurosurg Psychiatry.* 2014;85(9):1058–1060.
89. Ravenscroft G, Miyatake S, Lehtokari VL, et al. Mutations in KLHL40 are a frequent cause of severe autosomal-recessive nemaline myopathy. *Am J Hum Genet.* 2013;93(1):6–18.
90. Gupta VA, Ravenscroft G, Shaheen R, et al. Identification of KLHL41 mutations implicates BTB-Kelch-mediated ubiquitination as an alternate pathway to myofibrillar disruption in nemaline myopathy. *Am J Hum Genet.* 2013;93(6):1108–1117.
91. Malfatti E, Schaeffer U, Chapon F, et al. Combined cap disease and nemaline myopathy in the same patient caused by an autosomal dominant mutation in the TPM3 gene. *Neuromuscul Disord.* 2013;23(12):992–997.
92. Schatz UA, Weiss S, Wenninger S, et al. Evidence of mild founder *LMOD3* mutations causing nemaline myopathy 10 in Germany and Austria. *Neurology.* 2018;91:e1690–e1694.
93. Yuen M, Sandaradura SA, Dowling JJ, et al. Leiomodin-3 dysfunction results in thin filament disorganization and nemaline myopathy. *J Clin Invest.* 2014;124:4693–4708.
94. Chahin N, Selcen D, Engel AG. Sporadic late onset nemaline myopathy. *Neurology.* 2005;65(8):1158–1164.
95. Eymard B, Brouet JC, Collin H, Chevallay M, Bussel A, Fardeau M. Late-onset rod myopathy associated with monoclonal gammopathy. *Neuromuscul Disord.* 1993;3(5–6):557–560.
96. Milone M, Katz A, Amato AA, et al. Sporadic late onset nemaline myopathy responsive to IVIg and immunotherapy. *Muscle Nerve.* 2010;41:272–276.
97. Benveniste O, Laforet P, Dubourg O, et al. Stem cell transplantation in a patient with late-onset nemaline myopathy and gammopathy. *Neurology.* 2008;71:531–532.
98. Doppler K, Knop S, Einsele H, Sommer C, Wessig C. Sporadic late onset nemaline myopathy and immunoglobulin deposition disease. *Muscle Nerve.* 2013;48(6):983–988.
99. Naddaf E, Milone M, Kansagra A, Buadi F, Kourelis T. Sporadic late-onset nemaline myopathy: clinical spectrum, survival, and treatment outcomes. *Neurology.* 2019;93:e298–e305.
100. Schnitzler LJ, Schreckenbach T, Nadaj-Pakleza A, et al. Sporadic late-onset nemaline myopathy: clinico-pathological characteristics and review of 76 cases. *Orphanet J Rare Dis.* 2017;12:86.
101. Zhao B, Dai T, Zhao D, et al. Clinicopathologic profiles of sporadic late-onset nemaline myopathy: practical importance of anti-α-actinin immunostaining. *Neurol Neuroimmunol Neuroinflamm.* 2022;9(4):e1184.
102. Dalakas MC, Pezeshkpour GH, Flaherty M. Progressive nemaline (rod) myopathy associated with HIV infection. *N Engl J Med.* 1987;317:1602–1603.
103. Fidziańska A, Badurska B, Ryniewicz B, Dembek I. "Cap disease": new congenital myopathy. *Neurology.* 1981;31(9):1113–1120.
104. Fidziańska A. Cap disease—a failure in the correct muscle fibre formation. *J Neurol Sci.* 2002;201(1–2):27–31.
105. Hung RM, Yoon G, Hawkins CE, Halliday W, Biggar D, Vajsar J. Cap myopathy caused by a mutation of the skeletal alpha-actin gene ACTA1. *Neuromuscul Disord.* 2010;20:238–240.
106. Lehtokari VL, Ceuterick-de Groote C, de Jonghe P, et al. Cap disease caused by heterozygous deletion of the beta-tropomyosin gene TPM2. *Neuromuscul Disord.* 2007;17:433–442.
107. Tajsharghi H, Ohlsson M, Lindberg C, Oldfors A. Congenital myopathy with nemaline rods and cap structures caused by a mutation in the beta-tropomyosin gene (TPM2). *Arch Neurol.* 2007;64:1334–1338.
108. Ohlsson M, Fidziańska A, Tajsharghi H, Oldfors A. TPM3 mutation in one of the original cases of cap disease. *Neurology.* 2009;72:1961–1963.
109. Waddell LB, Kreissl M, Kornberg A, et al. Evidence for a dominant negative disease mechanism in cap myopathy due to TPM3. *Neuromuscul Disord.* 2010;20:464–466.
110. Polavarapu K, Bardhan M, Anjanappa RM, et al. Nemaline rod/cap myopathy due to novel homozygous *MYPN* mutations: the first report from South Asia and comprehensive literature review. *J Clin Neurol.* 2021;17(3):409–418.
111. Schreckenbach T, Schröder JM, Voit T, et al. Novel TPM3 mutation in a family with cap myopathy and review of the literature. *Neuromuscul Disord.* 2014;24:117–124.
112. Schaeffer U, Chapon F, Yang Y, et al. Combined cap disease and nemaline myopathy in the same patient caused by an autosomal dominant mutation in the TPM3 gene. *Neuromuscul Disord.* 2013;23(12):992–997.
113. Lake BD, Wilson J. Zebra body myopathy. Clinical, histochemical and ultrastructural studies. *J Neurol Sci.* 1975;24(4):437–446.
114. Reyes MG, Goldbarg H, Fresco K, Bouffard A. Zebra body myopathy: a second case of ultrastructurally distinct congenital myopathy. *J Child Neurol.* 1987;2(4):307–310.
115. Cocanougher BT, Flynn L, Yun P, et al. Adult *MTM1*-related myopathy carriers: classification based on deep phenotyping. *Neurology.* 2019;93:e1535–e1542.
116. Spiro AJ, Shy GM, Gonatas NK. Myotubular myopathy. Persistence of fetal muscle in an adolescent boy. *Arch Neurol.* 1966;14:1–14.

117. Fischer D, Herasse M, Bitoun M, et al. Characterization of the muscle involvement in dynamin 2-related centronuclear myopathy. *Brain*. 2006;129(Pt 6):1463–1469.
118. Jeannet PY, Bassez G, Eymard B, et al. Clinical and histologic findings in autosomal centronuclear myopathy. *Neurology*. 2004;62(9):1484–1490.
119. McEntagart M, Parsons G, Buj-Bello A, et al. Genotype–phenotype correlations in X-linked myotubular myopathy. *Neuromuscul Disord*. 2002;12(10):939–946.
120. Wallgren-Pettersson C, Clarke A, Samson F, et al. The myotubular myopathies: differential diagnosis of the X linked recessive, autosomal dominant, and autosomal recessive forms and present state of DNA studies. *J Med Genet*. 1995;32(9):673–679.
121. Hammans SR, Robinson DO, Moutou C, et al. A clinical and genetic study of a manifesting heterozygote with X-linked myotubular myopathy. *Neuromuscul Disord*. 2000;10(2):133–137.
122. Jungbluth H, Sewry CA, Buj-Bello A, et al. Early and severe presentation of X-linked myotubular myopathy in a girl with skewed X-inactivation. *Neuromuscul Disord*. 2003;13(1):55–59.
123. Kristiansen M, Knudsen GP, Tanner SM, et al. X-inactivation patterns in carriers of X-linked myotubular myopathy. *Neuromuscul Disord*. 2003;13(6):468–471.
124. Reumers SFI, Braun F, Spillane JE, et al. Spectrum of clinical features in X-linked myotubular myopathy carriers: an international questionnaire study. *Neurology*. 2021;97:e501–e512.
125. Felice KJ, Grunnet ML. Autosomal dominant centronuclear myopathy: report of a new family with clinical features simulating facioscapulohumeral syndrome. *Muscle Nerve*. 1997;20(9):1194–1196.
126. Laporte J, Biancalana V, Tanner SM, et al. MTM1 mutations in X-linked myotubular myopathy. *Hum Mutat*. 2000;15(5):393–409.
127. Laporte J, Guiraud-Chaumeil C, Vincent MC, et al. Mutations in the MTM1 gene implicated in X-linked myotubular myopathy. ENMC International Consortium on Myotubular Myopathy. European Neuro-Muscular Center. *Hum Mol Genet*. 1997;6(9):1505–1511.
128. Cui X, De Vivo I, Slany R, Miyamoto A, Firestein R, Cleary ML. Association of SET domain and myotubularin-related proteins modulates growth control. *Nat Genet*. 1998;18(4):331–337.
129. Bitoun M, Maugenre S, Jeannet PY, et al. Mutations in dynamin 2 cause dominant centronuclear myopathy. *Nat Genet*. 2005;37(11):1207–1209.
130. Zuchner S, Noureddine M, Kennerson M, et al. Mutations in the pleckstrin homology domain of dynamin 2 cause dominant intermediate Charcot–Marie–Tooth disease. *Nat Genet*. 2005;37(3):289–294.
131. Nicot AS, Toussaint A, Tosch V, et al. Mutations in amphiphysin 2 (BIN1) disrupt interaction with dynamin 2 and cause autosomal recessive centronuclear myopathy. *Nat Genet*. 2007;39:1134–1139.
132. Claeys KG, Maisonobe T, Böhm J, et al. Phenotype of a patient with recessive centronuclear myopathy and a novel BIN1 mutation. *Neurology*. 2010;74:519–521.
133. Böhm J, Yiş U, Ortaç R, et al. Case report of intrafamilial variability in autosomal recessive centronuclear myopathy associated to a novel BIN1 stop mutation. *Orphanet J Rare Dis*. 2010;5:35.
134. Ceyhan-Birsoy O, Agrawal PB, Hidalgo C, et al. Recessive truncating titin gene, TTN, mutations presenting as centronuclear myopathy. *Neurology*. 2013;81(14):1205–1214.
135. Cavanagh NP, Lake BD, McMeniman P, et al. Congenital fibre type disproportion myopathy. A histological diagnosis with an uncertain clinical outlook. *Arch Dis Child*. 1979;54(10):735–743.
136. Danon MJ, Giometti CS, Manaligod JR, Swisher C. Sequential muscle biopsy changes in a case of congenital myopathy. *Muscle Nerve*. 1997;20(5):561–569.
137. Laing NG, Clarke NF, Dye DE, et al. Actin mutations are one cause of congenital fibre type disproportion. *Ann Neurol*. 2004;56(5):689–694.
138. Brandis A, Aronica E, Goebel HH. TPM2 mutation. *Neuromuscul Disord*. 2008;18(12):1005.
139. Clarke NF, Kidson W, Quijano-Roy S, et al. SEPN1: associated with congenital fiber-type disproportion and insulin resistance. *Ann Neurol*. 2006;59:546–552.
140. Jerusalem F, Engel AG, Gomez MR. Sarcotubular myopathy. A newly recognized, benign, congenital, familial muscle disease. *Neurology*. 1973;23(9):897–906.
141. Schoser BGH, Frosk P, Engel AG, Klutzny U, Lochmüller H, Wrogemann K. Commonality of TRIM32 mutation in causing sarcotubular myopathy and LGMD2 H. *Ann Neurol*. 2005;57(4):591–595.
142. Curless RG, Payne CM, Brinner FM. Fingerprint body myopathy: a report of twins. *Dev Med Child Neurol*. 1978;20(6):793–798.
143. Engel AG, Angelini C, Gomez MR. Fingerprint body myopathy, a newly recognized congenital muscle disease. *Mayo Clin Proc*. 1972;47(6):377–388.
144. Fardeau M, Tomé FM, Derambure S. Familial fingerprint body myopathy. *Arch Neurol*. 1976;33(10):724–725.
145. Marguet F, Rendu J, Vanhulle C, et al. Association of fingerprint bodies with rods in a case with mutations in the LMOD3 gene. *Neuromuscul Disord*. 2020;30:207–212.
146. Ringel SP, Neville HE, Duster MC, Carroll JE, et al. A new congenital neuromuscular disease with trilaminar muscle fibers. *Neurology*. 1978;28(3):282–289.
147. Barohn RJ, Brumback RA, Mendell JR. Hyaline body myopathy. *Neuromuscul Disord*. 1994;4(3):257–262.
148. Bohlega S, Abu-Amero SN, Wakil SM, et al. Mutation of the slow myosin heavy chain rod domain underlies hyaline body myopathy. *Neurology*. 2004;62(9):1518–1521.
149. Bohlega S, Lach B, Meyer BF, et al. Autosomal dominant hyaline body myopathy: clinical variability and pathologic findings. *Neurology*. 2003;61(11):1519–1523.
150. Laing NG, Ceuterick-de Groote C, Dye DE, et al. Myosin storage myopathy: slow skeletal myosin (MYH7) mutation in two isolated cases. *Neurology*. 2005;64(3):527–529.
151. Masuzugawa S, Kuzuhara S, Narita Y, Naito Y, Taniguchi A, Ibi T. Autosomal dominant hyaline body myopathy presenting as scapuloperoneal syndrome: clinical features and muscle pathology. *Neurology*. 1997;48(1):253–257.
152. Tajsharghi H, Thornell LE, Lindberg C, Lindvall B, Henriksson KG, Oldfors A. Myosin storage myopathy associated with a heterozygous missense mutation in MYH7. *Ann Neurol*. 2003;54(4):494–500.
153. Pegoraro E, Gavassini BF, Borsato C, et al. MYH7 gene mutation in myosin storage myopathy and scapulo-peroneal myopathy. *Neuromuscul Disord*. 2007;17:321–329.
154. Oldfors A, Tajsharghi H, Darin N, Lindberg C. Myopathies associated with myosin heavy chain mutations. *Acta Myol*. 2004;23(2):90–96.

155. Tajsharghi H, Darin N, Rekabdar E, et al. Mutations and sequence variation in the human myosin heavy chain IIa gene (MYH2). *Eur J Hum Genet.* 2005;13(5):617–622.
156. Tajsharghi H, Thornell LE, Darin N, et al. Myosin heavy chain IIa gene mutation E706K is pathogenic and its expression increases with age. *Neurology.* 2002;58:780–786.
157. Martinsson T, Oldfors A, Darin N, et al. Autosomal dominant myopathy: missense mutation (Glu-706 → Lys) in the myosin heavy chain IIa gene. *Proc Natl Acad Sci U S A.* 2000;97(26):14614–14619.
158. Martin JJ, Ceuterick C, Van Goethem G. On a dominantly inherited myopathy with tubular aggregates. *Neuromuscul Disord.* 1997;7(8):512–520.
159. Dobkin BH, Verity MA. Familial neuromuscular disease with type 1 fiber hypoplasia, tubular aggregates, cardiomyopathy, and myasthenic features. *Neurology.* 1978;28(11):1135–1140.
160. Morgan-Hughes JA, Mair WG, Lascelles PT. A disorder of skeletal muscle associated with tubular aggregates. *Brain.* 1970;93(4):873–880.
161. Gang Q, Bettencourt C, Brady S, et al. Genetic defects are common in myopathies with tubular aggregates. *Ann Clin Transl Neurol.* 2022;9:4–15.
162. Böhm J, Chevessier F, Maues De Paula A, et al. Constitutive activation of the calcium sensor STIM1 causes tubular aggregate myopathy. *Am J Hum Genet.* 2013;92:271–278.
163. Hedberg C, Niceta M, Fattori F, et al. Childhood onset tubular aggregate myopathy associated with de novo STIM1 mutations. *J Neurol.* 2014;261(5):870–876.
164. Nesin V, Wiley G, Kousi M, et al. Activating mutations in STIM1 and ORAI1 cause overlapping syndromes of tubular myopathy and congenital miosis. *Proc Natl Acad Sci U S A.* 2014;111(11):4197–4202.
165. Selcen D, Shen XM, Brengman J, et al. DPAGT1 myasthenia and myopathy: genetic, phenotypic, and expression studies. *Neurology.* 2014;82(20):1822–1830.
166. Finlayson S, Palace J, Belaya K, et al. Clinical features of congenital myasthenic syndrome due to mutations in DPAGT1. *J Neurol Neurosurg Psychiatry.* 2013;84(10):1119–1125.
167. Selcen D, Shen XM, Milone M, et al. GFPT1-myasthenia: clinical, structural, and electrophysiologic heterogeneity. *Neurology.* 2013;81(4):370–378.
168. Böhm J, Lornage X, Chevessier F, et al. CASQ1 mutations impair calsequestrin polymerization and cause tubular aggregate myopathy. *Acta Neuropathol.* 2018;135:149–151.
169. Barone V, Del Re V, Gamberucci A, et al. Identification and characterization of three novel mutations in the CASQ1 gene in four patients with tubular aggregate myopathy. *Hum Mutat.* 2017;38:1761–1773.
170. Brooke MH, Neville HE. Reducing body myopathy. *Neurology.* 1972;22(8):829–840.
171. Figarella-Branger D, Putzu GA, Bouvier-Labit C, et al. Adult onset reducing body myopathy. *Neuromuscul Disord.* 1999;9(8):580–586.
172. Nomizu S, Person DA, Saito C, Lockett LJ. A unique case of reducing body myopathy. *Muscle Nerve.* 1992;15(4):463–466.
173. Oh SJ, Meyers GJ, Wilson ER Jr, Alexander CB. A benign form of reducing body myopathy. *Muscle Nerve.* 1983;6(4):278–282.
174. Bertini E, Salviati G, Apollo F, et al. Reducing body myopathy and desmin storage in skeletal muscle: morphological and biochemical findings. *Acta Neuropathol (Berl).* 1994;87(1):106–112.
175. Mota IA, Correia CDC, Fontana PN, Carvalho AAS. Reducing body myopathy – A new pathogenic FHL1 variant and literature review. *Neuromuscul Disord.* 2021;31:847–853.
176. Schessl J, Zou Y, McGrath MJ, et al. Proteomic identification of FHL1 as the protein mutated in human reducing body myopathy. *J Clin Invest.* 2008;118:904–912.
177. Schessl J, Taratuto AL, Sewry C, et al. Clinical, histological and genetic characterization of reducing body myopathy caused by mutations in FHL1. *Brain.* 2009;132:452–464.
178. Schessl J, Columbus A, Hu Y, et al. Familial reducing body myopathy with cytoplasmic bodies and rigid spine revisited: identification of a second LIM domain mutation in FHL1. *Neuropediatrics.* 2010;41:43–46.
179. Shalaby S, Hayashi YK, Nonaka I, Noguchi S, Nishino I. Novel FHL1 mutations in fatal and benign reducing body myopathy. *Neurology.* 2009;72:375–376.
180. Chen DH, Raskind WH, Parson WW, et al. A novel mutation in FHL1 in a family with X-linked scapuloperoneal myopathy: phenotypic spectrum and structural study of FHL1 mutations. *J Neurol Sci.* 2010;296:22–29.
181. Selcen D, Bromberg MB, Chin SS, Engel AG. Reducing bodies and myofibrillar myopathy features in FHL1 muscular dystrophy. *Neurology.* 2011;77:1951–1959.
182. Greenberg SA, Salajegheh M, Judge DP, et al. Etiology of limb girdle muscular dystrophy 1D/1E determined by laser capture microdissection proteomics. *Ann Neurol.* 2012;71:141–145.
183. Stamm DS, Aylsworth AS, Stajich JM, et al. Native American myopathy: congenital myopathy with cleft palate, skeletal anomalies, and susceptibility to malignant hyperthermia. *Am J Med Genet.* 2008;146A:1832–1841.
184. Stamm DS, Powell CM, Stajich JM, et al. Novel congenital myopathy locus identified in Native American Indians at 12q13.13-14.1. *Neurology.* 2008;71:1764–1769.
185. Stewart CR, Kahler SG, Gilchrist JM. Congenital myopathy with cleft palate and increased susceptibility to malignant hyperthermia: King syndrome? *Pediatr Neurol.* 1988;4:371–374.
186. Webb BD, Manoli I, Jabs EW. STAC3 disorder. In: Adam MP, Everman DB, Mirzaa GM, et al., eds. *GeneReviews*® [Internet]. University of Washington, Seattle; 1993–2022.
187. Grzybowski M, Schänzer A, Pepler A, Heller C, Neubauer BA, Hahn A. Novel STAC3 mutations in the first non-Amerindian patient with Native American myopathy. *Neuropediatrics.* 2017;48:451–455.
188. Telegrafi A, Webb BD, Robbins SM, et al. Identification of STAC3 variants in non-Native American families with overlapping features of Carey-Fineman-Ziter syndrome and Moebius syndrome. *Am J Med Genet A.* 2017;173:2763–2771.
189. Murtazina A, Demina N, Chausova P, Shchagina O, Borovikov A, Dadali E. The first Russian patient with native American myopathy. *Genes (Basel).* 2022;13:341.
190. Zaharieva IT, Sarkozy A, Munot P, et al. STAC3 variants cause a congenital myopathy with distinctive dysmorphic features and malignant hyperthermia susceptibility. *Hum Mutat.* 2018;39:1980–1994.

CHAPTER 29

Metabolic Myopathies

The inherited metabolic myopathies are traditionally classified by their underlying biochemical abnormalities as disorders of (1) carbohydrate, (2) lipid, and (3) adenine nucleotide metabolism.[1–3] A fourth possible category includes the mitochondrial disorders. As mitochondrial disorders do not cause defects in a specific biochemical pathway, they are discussed in Chapter 30. The immediate source of energy for muscles comes from the hydrolysis of adenosine triphosphate (ATP). At rest, the major substrate for muscle in terms of ATP production comes from the metabolism of long-chain fatty acids. Therefore, any disorder impairing β-oxidation of long-chain fatty acids in the mitochondria can lead to a myopathy. During exercise, ATP is derived from the metabolism of carbohydrates, fatty acids, and ketones. Early in the course of exercise (e.g., up to 45 minutes), energy is derived mainly from free glucose or glucose made available via glycogenolysis. Subsequently, there is a shift toward the metabolism of fatty acids such that after a few hours 70% of energy is derived from lipid breakdown.

Metabolic myopathies can also be viewed as static or dynamic disorders. The static myopathies are defined by the presence of fixed or progressive weakness. On the other hand, the dynamic myopathies are associated with exercise intolerance (i.e., exertional myalgias, cramps, and myoglobinuria) as the dominant clinical features. Some metabolic defects are associated with both a dynamic and a static myopathy.

▶ DISORDERS OF CARBOHYDRATE METABOLISM

Carbohydrates are stored in liver and muscle as glycogen, a highly branched polymer of glucose. Normal synthesis and breakdown of glycogen is essential to maintain adequate glucose concentration in muscle that can be further metabolized and provide energy in the form of ATP. There are 16+ recognized glycogen storage diseases (GSDs), also called glycogenoses (Table 29-1). This is somewhat a misnomer because some of these glycogenoses do not result in the accumulation of glycogen in tissues.

The glycogenoses predominantly affect liver and muscle. Since there is differential metabolism of carbohydrates in these two tissues, the individual GSDs may produce strictly liver or muscle disease, or some combination of the two. Types I (glucose-6-phosphatase deficiency) and VI (liver phosphorylase deficiency) only cause liver disease and are not further discussed. Types II (lysosomal α-glucosidase deficiency), V (phosphorylase deficiency), VII [phosphofructokinase (PFK) deficiency], X [phosphoglycerate mutase (PGAM) deficiency], and XI (lactate dehydrogenase deficiency) produce almost exclusively muscle disease, while the remaining types produce a varying mixture of muscle disease with systemic disease.

The pathophysiological basis by which the varied enzymatic defects lead to muscle dysfunction remains largely unknown. The inability to metabolize a substrate reduces the ability of muscle cells to form ATP necessary for normal energy production. Furthermore, the enzymatic defects may result in accumulation of metabolites, which may be toxic to muscle.

The exercise forearm test can be helpful diagnosing various disorders of glycolysis. The test can be adequately performed without blood pressure cuff insufflation. In fact, performing this test with the limb ischemic may be hazardous to the patient because it can induce profound muscle damage and myoglobinuria.[4] A butterfly needle is placed in the antecubital fossa and draw baseline lactate and ammonia levels are drawn. The forearm muscles are then exercised by having the patient rapidly and strenuously open and close the hand for 1 minute. Immediately after exercise and then 1, 2, 4, 6, and 10 minutes postexercise, blood samples are again taken and analyzed for lactate and ammonia. The normal response is for lactate and ammonia levels to raise three to four times the baseline levels. If neither the lactate nor the ammonia level increases, the test is inconclusive and implies that the muscles were not sufficiently exercised. A rise in lactate levels, but not ammonia, is seen with myoadenylate deaminase deficiency (MADD). In myophosphorylase, PFK, PGAM, phosphoglycerate kinase (PGK), phosphorylase b kinase (PBK), debranching enzyme, and lactate dehydrogenase deficiencies, the ammonia levels rise appropriately, but the lactic acid does not.

GLYCOGENOSIS TYPE 0 (GLYCOGEN SYNTHASE 1 DEFICIENCY)

Clinical Features

This rare disorder can manifest in children or adults with myalgias, exercise intolerance, and proximal weakness with or without a cardiomyopathy (recurrent attacks of syncope, prolonged QT syndrome, and sudden cardiac death).[1,5–8] However, loss of consciousness was gradual in one patient suggesting metabolic dysfunction within the central nervous system (CNS) as opposed to pure cardiac etiology.[7] Mild proximal weakness may be evident.

► TABLE 29-1. DISORDERS OF CARBOHYDRATE METABOLISM

Disorder	Enzyme Defect	Inheritance	Clinical Features
Type 0	Glycogen synthase 1	Autosomal recessive	Childhood onset weakness, hypertrophic cardiomyopathy
Type I (von Gierke disease)	Glucose-6-phosphate	Autosomal recessive	No neuromuscular signs or symptoms
Type II (Pompe disease)	α-1,4-Glucosidase	Autosomal recessive	Infancy: hypotonia, cardiomyopathy, respiratory failure, generalized weakness Childhood–adult: progressive weakness, respiratory failure
Type III (Cori–Forbes disease)	Debranching enzyme (amylo-1,6-glucosidase)	Autosomal recessive	Infancy: hypotonia, generalized weakness Childhood/adult: proximal or distal weakness, spasticity, learning disability, dementia, incontinence
Type IV (Anderson disease)	Branching enzyme (amylo-1,4–1,6-transglucosidase)	Autosomal recessive	Infancy: hypotonia, generalized weakness Childhood/adult: proximal or distal weakness
Type V (McArdle disease)	Myophosphorylase	Autosomal recessive	Infancy: rare weakness Childhood/adult: exercise intolerance, rare weakness, including axial muscles
Type VI	Liver phosphorylase	Autosomal recessive	No muscle involvement
Type VII (Tarui disease)	Phosphofructokinase	Autosomal recessive	Childhood: exercise intolerance, rare weakness
Type IXB	[a]Phosphorylase b kinase B subunit	Autosomal recessive	Infancy to adult: exercise intolerance, rare weakness
Type IXD	[a]Phosphorylase b kinase A subunit	X-linked	
Type X	Phosphoglycerate mutase	Autosomal recessive	Childhood–adult: exercise intolerance
Type XI	Lactate dehydrogenase	Autosomal recessive	Childhood–adult: exercise intolerance
Type XII	Aldolase A	Autosomal recessive	Infancy–childhood: exercise intolerance and weakness
Type XIII	β-Enolase	Autosomal recessive	Childhood–adult: exercise intolerance
Type XIV	Phosphoglucomutase	Autosomal recessive	Childhood: exercise intolerance and weakness
Type XV	Glycogenin 1	Autosomal recessive	Childhood onset of weakness
Other GSDs	Phosphoglycerate kinase 1	X-linked	Childhood: exercise intolerance, rare weakness, hemolytic anemia, mental retardation, seizures
	Triosephosphate isomerase	Autosomal recessive	Infancy: hypotonia, generalized weakness learning disability

[a]Phosphorylase b kinase deficiency was previously termed GSD VIII. Both phosphorylase b kinase and phosphoglycerate kinase deficiencies have been termed GSD IX in the literature.

Laboratory Features

Exercise forearm test shows failure of lactate elevation and skeletal muscle magnetic resonance imaging (MRI) may reveal fatty degeneration of the gluteal and flexor muscles of the thigh.[7]

Histopathology

Skeletal muscle and cardiac muscle as well as skin fibroblasts have depletion of glycogen, a reduction in glycogen synthetase 1 activity, and abnormal proliferation of mitochondria.[1,5–8] Phosphorylase activity may also be deficient in muscle fibers.

Molecular Genetics and Pathogenesis

Synthesis of glycogen requires glycogen synthase 1 which catalyzes the addition of glucose monomers to the growing glycogen molecule through the formation of α-1,4-glycoside linkages. GSD 0 is caused by mutations in the *GYS1* gene that encodes glycogen synthase 1. Deficiency of this enzyme leads to the depletion of glycogen in skeletal and cardiac muscles.

Treatment

There are no specific medical therapies.

GLYCOGENOSIS TYPE II (POMPE DISEASE; ACID MALTASE DEFICIENCY; α-GLUCOSIDASE DEFICIENCY)

GSD II is an autosomal-recessive disorder caused by a deficiency of lysosomal acid α-glucosidase (Table 29-1, Fig. 29-1). The term "acid maltase deficiency" is a misnomer as humans do not have acid maltase. GSD II, more commonly referred to as Pompe disease and is classified into two forms: a severe infantile form, a juvenile-onset type, and an adult-onset variant.[1,3,9–31] Pompe disease is broadly classified into an

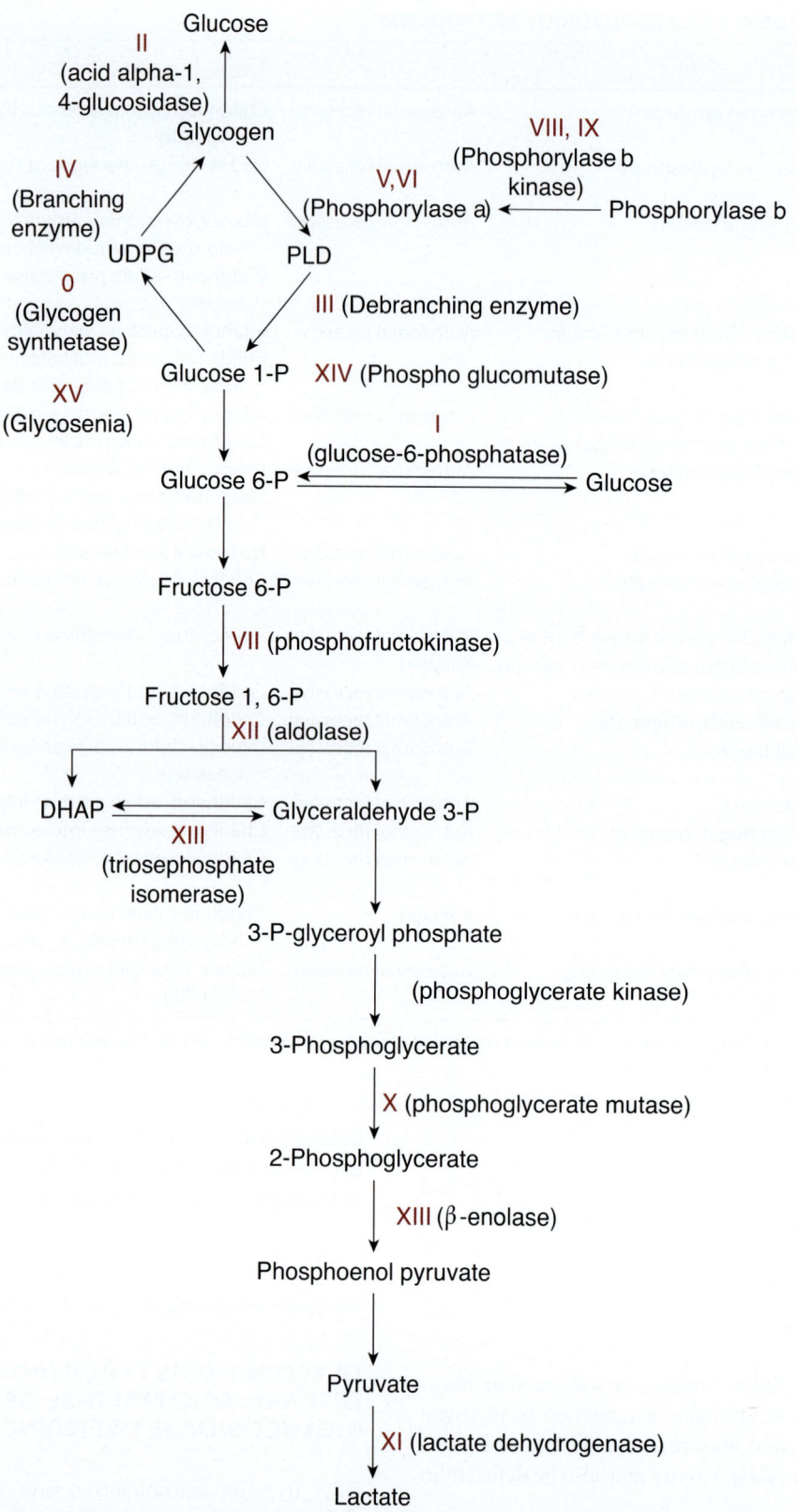

Figure 29-1. Glycolytic pathways. Glycogen metabolism disorders are caused by specific enzyme deficiencies involving each of the pathways illustrated with a Roman numeral. The enzymes corresponding to each numbered glycogen storage disorder are listed in Table 29-1. Diseases I and VI are not included, as these do not involve muscle. (From Amato AA. Sweet success—A treatment for McArdle's disease. *N Engl J Med*. 2003;349:2481–2482. Copyright © 2003, Massachusetts Medical Society. Reprinted with permission from Massachusetts Medical Society.)

infantile form and a late onset form after 1 year of age that can present in childhood, adolescence, or adult. The incidence of infantile Pompe disease ranges from 1 in 31,000 to 1 in 138,000. The incidence of later-onset forms has been purported to be as high as 1 in 53,000, but we think it is far less common in our experience.

Clinical Features

Infantile Pompe disease is characterized by generalized weakness and hypotonia, cardiomegaly, and mild-to-moderate hepatomegaly, with an onset in the first several months of life.[1,3,13,18–20] Infants often have an enlarged tongue (i.e., macroglossia). The weakness and cardiomyopathy are progressive. Feeding difficulties and ventilatory muscle weakness are common. The disease is invariably fatal by 2 years of age secondary to cardioventilatory failure.

The late-onset Pompe disease usually manifests in the first decade of life.[12,16,18,21,31] Motor milestones may be delayed. Weakness is slowly progressive and involves proximal greater than distal muscles in the legs and arms. Children often have hypertrophy of the calf muscles, a waddling gait, and significant lumbar lordosis and demonstrate a Gower maneuver to arise from the floor. Thus, affected children are not uncommonly misdiagnosed with Duchenne or some other form of limb-girdle muscular dystrophy. Rarely, affected children present with rigidity of the spine.[24] Unlike the infantile-onset Pompe disease, cardiomegaly, hepatomegaly, and macroglossia are uncommon. Nevertheless, it is relentlessly progressive, and ventilatory muscles are invariably affected leading to death in the second or third decade of life.

Adult-onset Pompe disease usually manifests in the third or fourth decade (up to the eighth decade, mean 36.5 years).[10,12–14,18,24–27,31] Patients develop generalized proximal greater than distal muscle weakness resembling polymyositis or limb-girdle muscular dystrophy. Some patients have a scapuloperoneal distribution of weakness.[9] Weakness is occasionally asymmetric and may involve the face or tongue.[26] Nearly half of the affected individuals complain of muscle pains, particularly in the thighs. Muscle stretch reflexes may be reduced. Hepatomegaly and cardiomegaly do not typically occur; however, electrocardiographic abnormalities and arrhythmias can be seen. As in the infantile and juvenile forms of the disease, there is a predilection for the involvement of ventilatory muscles. In this regard, 16%–33% of patients present with symptoms related to ventilatory insufficiency (e.g., dyspnea, frequent nocturnal arousals, morning headaches, and excessive daytime sleepiness).[26,31]

Laboratory Features

Serum CK levels are moderately elevated in infantile-onset, but adults may have normal CK levels. α-Glucosidase activity may be assayed in muscle fibers, fibroblasts, leukocytes, lymphocytes, and urine. The reduction of activity generally correlates with the severity of the myopathy. Infantile-onset disease is associated with a severe deficiency of α-glucosidase activity, while the less severe adult-onset form has residual activity, up to 30% in muscle and 53% in lymphocytes.[27] Importantly, false-negative results on leukocyte assay can occur due to contamination with granulocytes or other sources of neutral glucosidase. A dried blood spot analysis of α-glucosidase activity has been used as an initial screening test.[28–31] Of note, activity levels by dried blood spot do not correlate with severity of the myopathy. Confirmatory genetic testing should be performed. In many parts of the world, genetic testing is readily available and free. In these instances, genetic testing should be done when the diagnosis is suspected and dried blood spot can be skipped.

Imaging studies confirm the early and severe involvement of the adductor magnus and semimembranosus in the early stage of the disease and later fatty infiltration of the long head of the biceps femoris, semitendinosus, and the anterior thigh muscles. In advanced phases, selective sparing of sartorius, rectus, femoris, and gracilis muscles, and peripheral portions of the vastus lateralis are also evident.[32,33] Skeletal muscle MRI and CT also reveal early involvement of paravertebral and abdominal trunk muscular.[34,35]

Motor and sensory nerve conduction studies (NCSs) are normal. Electromyography (EMG) reveals increased insertional and spontaneous activity in the form of fibrillation potentials, positive sharp waves, complex repetitive discharges, and even myotonic discharges. In mild forms of the disease, these irritative discharges may be evident only in the paraspinal muscles. Motor unit action potentials (MUAPs) are myopathic in appearance and recruit early.

Electrocardiograms (EKG) may demonstrate nonspecific abnormalities including left-axis deviation, short PR interval, large QRS complexes, inverted T waves, ST depression, and persistent sinus tachycardia in both the severe and mild forms of GSD II.[26] Wolfe–Parkinson–White syndrome occurs in infantile and adult forms of the disease.[3,36,37] Echocardiograms may show hypertrophic cardiomyopathy. Pulmonary function tests show a restrictive defect with decreased forced vital capacity, reduced maximal inspiratory and expiratory pressures, and early fatigue of the diaphragm.[26,31]

Histopathology

Biopsies characteristically demonstrate glycogen-filled vacuoles within muscle fibers (Fig. 29-2).[1,3,9,27,31] These vacuoles are very prominent in the infantile form, but in the childhood and adult forms, these are apparent in only 25%–75% of fibers in clinically affected muscles and may be absent in clinically unaffected muscle groups. Muscle biopsy may show only slight, nonspecific abnormalities in late-onset cases. When present, the vacuoles react strongly to periodic acid–Schiff (PAS), are sensitive to diastase, and stain intensely with acid phosphatase, confirming that the vacuoles are secondary lysosomes filled with glycogen. Glycogen can also be found free in the cytoplasm on electron microscopy (EM). Muscle biopsies also reveal necrotic and regenerating muscle fibers, variation in fiber size and fiber splitting. In later stages, muscle

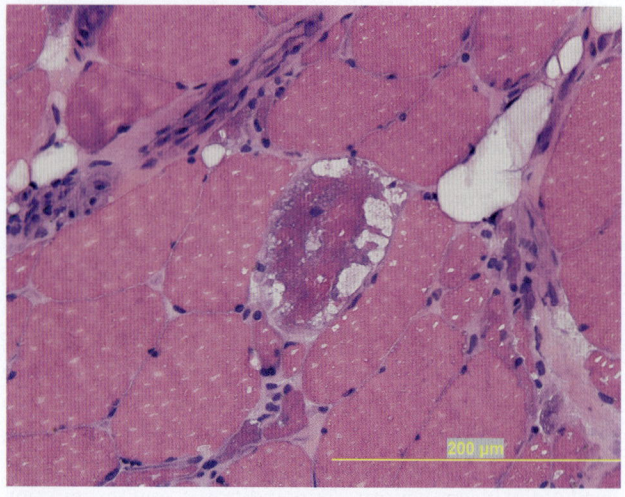
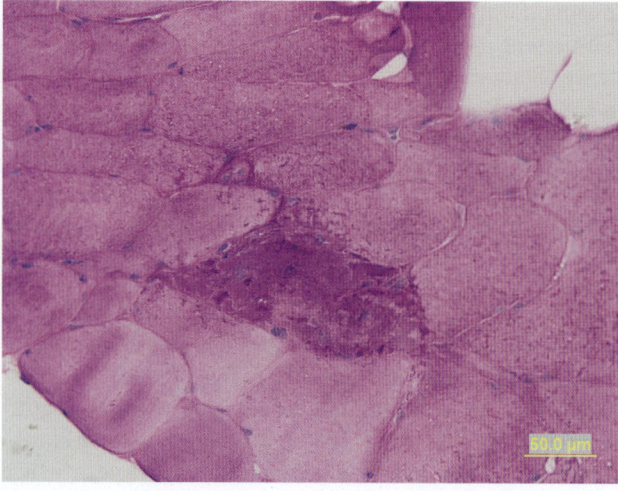
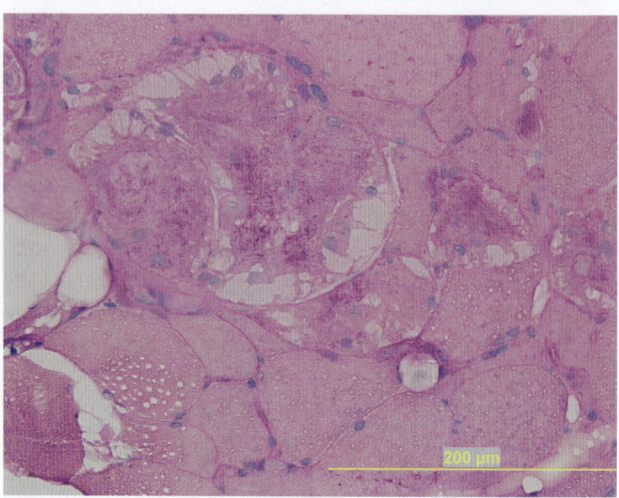

Figure 29-2. Pompe disease. Muscle biopsy in a patient with adult-onset acid maltase deficiency reveals one or more vacuoles within many muscle fibers, hematoxylin and eosin (H&E) (**A**). These vacuoles are filled with glycogen, which stains intensely red on periodic acid–Schiff (PAS) stain (**B**) and are digested by diastase (**C**).

fiber atrophy and increased endomysial connective tissue may be present. Occasionally, fiber-type grouping, and group atrophy may be evident, owing to motor neuron degeneration. In this regard, glycogens accumulate in anterior horn cells and bulbar nuclei as well as Schwann cells accounting for the superimposed neurogenic findings in some patients.[38,39]

Molecular Genetics and Pathogenesis

Missense, nonsense, and frame-shift mutations have been identified in the α-glucosidase gene, *GAA*, located on chromosome 17q21–23 in infantile and late-onset cases.[40,41] Prenatal diagnosis is possible with amniocentesis or chorionic villus sampling.[40–42] Acid α-glucosidase is a lysosomal enzyme, which cleaves 1,4 and 1,6 linkages in glycogen, maltose, and isomaltose. Glycogen within lysosomes is degraded to glucose by α-glucosidase, and the deficiency of the enzyme results in glycogen accumulation. There appears to be an inverse correlation between residual acid α-glucosidase activity and the clinical severity. However, there are cases associated with an adult-onset Pompe disease that have very little residual enzyme activity, so the relationship between disease activity and clinical severity is not 100% accurate. Interestingly, there may be variability in phenotype and severity within families.[19,43]

How acid α-glucosidase leads to muscle fiber dysfunction is not completely understood. The accumulating glycogen that results from the deficiency may displace or replace important cellular organelles. Alternatively, the lysosomes filled with glycogen may rupture, thereby releasing proteases that degrade myofibrils and other important muscle proteins. Muscle catabolism is increased by 31% in Pompe disease compared to normal controls, and mean protein balance is reduced.[17] Furthermore, resting energy expenditure in Pompe disease is increased.[17] Patients do not exhibit exercise intolerance or myoglobinuria because metabolism of nonmembrane-bound glycogen and glucose for energy metabolism is not impaired.

Treatment

In the past, there were no specific treatments for acid maltase deficiency other than supportive therapy for associated cardioventilatory complications. Low carbohydrate and ketogenic diets are ineffective. A small study reported that

4 out of 16 patients treated with high-protein diet demonstrated improvement in muscle and respiratory function.[17]

Enzyme replacement therapy (ERT) with intravenous recombinant α-glucosidase enzyme appears to be safe and beneficial in classic infantile Pompe disease though the results of clinical trials in late-onset Pompe disease have demonstrated only a modest benefit in distance travelled in the 6-minute walk test and in forced vital capacity between the α-glucosidase (alglucosidase alfa) and placebo-treated patients.[44–47] The recommended dose of (alglucosidase alfa) is 20 mg/kg IV every 2 weeks. A newer α-glucosidase ERT, avalglucosidase alfa, was developed to improve uptake into lysosomes via cation-independent-mannose-6-phosphate (M6P) receptors on the cell surface. A recent trial comparing alglucosidase alfa to avalglucosidase alfa in late-onset Pompe disease provided some evidence of clinically meaningful improvement with avalglucosidase alfa therapy over alglucosidase alfa in respiratory function, ambulation, and functional endurance, but it was not statistically superior.[48] Long-term tolerability and sustained efficacy of avalglucosidase alfa were demonstrated in late-onset Pompe disease for up to 6.5 years.[49] The recommended dose of avalglucosidase alfa (20 mg/kg IV for late-onset Pompe patients ≥30 kg or 40 mg/kg for those <30 kg). Cipaglucosidase alfa co-administered with miglustat is another recently FDA approved ERT. Miglastat acts as a stabilizer and prevents loss of enzyme activity during cipaglucosidase alfa infusion. A randomised, double-blind, parallel-group, phase 3 trial of participants with late-onset Pompe disease (18 yrs or older) compared IV cipaglucosidase alfa (20 mg/kg) plus oral miglustat (n = 85) or to IV alglucosidase alfa (20 mg/kg) plus oral placebo (n = 40) once every 2 weeks for 52 weeks demonstrated efficacy of cipaglucosidase and miglustat compared to placebo, but it was not superior to alglucosidase alfa.[50]

As alluded above, not all patients, including infants with classic Pompe disease, respond to ERT. A poor prognostic factor among infants is cross-reactive immunologic material (CRIM) status; CRIM-negative is strongly correlated with a poor outcome.[51,52] Although most CRIM-negative infants initially respond to continuous use of ERT, a resurgence of the natural progression of weakness subsequently ensues. These CRIM-negative infants develop antibodies directed against the infused recombinant α-glucosidase. Presumably, those infants who do not produce even minute amount of α-glucosidase are at increased risk of mounting an antibody response against α-glucosidase, as it is seen to be a foreign protein by the immune system.

GLYCOGENOSIS TYPE III (DEBRANCHING ENZYME DEFICIENCY)

Clinical Features

GSD III, also known as Cori–Forbes disease, accounts for approximately 25% of GSD (Table 29-1, Fig. 29-1).[53–57] GSD III is caused by the deficiency of debranching enzyme. This enzyme has two separate catalytic functions: (1) oligo-1,4-1,4-glucanotransferase activity and (2) α-1,6 glucosidase activity. Both the transferase and the glucosidase activities are vital in breaking down glycogen into glucose, and a deficiency in either or both enzymatic functions lead to myopathy.

There are two principal and two less-common forms of GSD III. In GSD IIIa, debranching enzyme is deficient in both the liver and the muscle. In contrast, enzyme activity is abnormal only in the liver in GSD IIIb, and a myopathy does not occur in this form of the disease. In rare cases, selective loss of only one of the two debranching enzyme activities [glucosidase (type IIIc) or transferase (type IIId)] has also been demonstrated.[58]

Deficiency of the debranching enzyme in muscle leads to weakness in patients with GSD IIIa. Onset of muscle weakness may be appreciated in infancy or childhood, although it usually does not manifest until the third to fourth decades of life.[53–57,59–65] Severe atrophy and weakness of distal extremity muscles, particularly the peroneal and calf muscles, occur in about 50% of patients.[55] Tight heal cords are common, and patients may have the tendency to toe walk. This distal involvement can lead to an initial misdiagnosis of motor neuron disease or a peripheral neuropathy. Some patients do, in fact, have a superimposed mild sensorimotor polyneuropathy. Pseudohypertrophy, particularly of the more proximal muscle groups, may be seen.[62] Generalized muscle weaknesses can also occur. In addition, some patients develop progressive ventilatory muscle weakness with or without extremity weakness. Ventilatory failure can evolve fairly rapidly. Less commonly, some patients develop a cardiomyopathy with or without extremity weakness.[60,66–69] Finally, rare patients manifest with myalgias, cramps, exercise intolerance, or myoglobinuria.[55,61,63,64,70]

Laboratory Features

Deficiency of debranching enzyme can be demonstrated with biochemical assay of muscle, fibroblasts, or lymphocytes. Serum CK levels are usually elevated 2–20 times normal. Exercise forearm testing reveals normal increase in serum ammonia but not in lactate levels. EMG demonstrates abnormalities similar to that described with acid maltase deficiency. Pulmonary function tests show reduced forced vital capacity in patients with ventilatory muscle involvement. Echocardiogram reveals findings suggestive of hypertrophic obstructive cardiomyopathy in most patients with GSD IIIa, while conduction defects and arrhythmias are apparent on EKG.[53,66,69,70]

Histopathology

Muscle biopsies demonstrate a vacuolar myopathy with abnormal accumulation of glycogen in the subsarcolemmal and intermyofibrillar regions of muscle fibers.[59,61,62,71] These vacuoles stain intensely with PAS and are digested by diastase. In contrast to Pompe disease, these vacuoles do not stain with acid phosphatase, suggesting that glycogen does not primarily accumulate in lysosomes. On EM, free pools of glycogen are apparent. Some glycogen appears in lysosomes, but not to the same extent as seen in Pompe disease. Autopsy studies of the heart have revealed fibrosis, moderate-to-severe vacuolization of cardiac myocytes, mild-to-severe glycogen accumulation in the atrioventricular (AV), and glycogen accumulation in smooth muscle cells of intramyocardial arteries associated with smooth muscle hyperplasia and profoundly thickened vascular walls.[72] Abnormal glycogen accumulation can also be found in skin and peripheral nerves.[73–76]

Molecular Genetics and Pathogenesis

The mutations in the debranching enzyme gene, *AGL*, on chromosome 1p21 cause both GSD IIIa and GSD IIIb.[76–79] Prenatal diagnosis is possible.[80] The *AGL* gene is composed of 35 exons spanning 85 kb of genomic DNA. Alternative splicing and differential RNA transcription result in at least six distinct isoforms and underline the differential expression of the debranching enzyme.[81] Tissue-specific expression of different isoforms results from the presence of at least two promoter regions. Of note, mutations within exon 3 mutations appear to be specific for GSD IIIb.[79]

Deficiency of the enzyme leads to the accumulation of glycogen in muscle; the exact mechanism of muscle weakness is not known. Similar amounts of glycogen accumulation in muscle can be demonstrated in patients who do not manifest weakness. Accumulation of glycogen in peripheral nerves may account for some degree of weakness and atrophy, particularly of the distal muscles.

Treatment

Frequent low-carbohydrate meals and maintaining a high-protein intake may prevent fasting hypoglycemia. High-protein nocturnal intragastric feedings led to apparent improvement in exercise tolerance, muscle strength and mass, EMG findings, and growth in one patient,[65] but this observation has not been subsequently confirmed. Supportive therapy is required for patients with congestive heart failure. Liver transplantation has been done on patients with cirrhosis and hepatocellular carcinoma.[81] However, debranching enzyme activity has remained absent in leukocytes after transplantation and is not likely to normalize in muscle.

GLYCOGENOSIS TYPE IV (BRANCHING ENZYME DEFICIENCY)

Clinical Features

GSD IV is rare and caused by the deficiency of the enzyme that helps make the branched glycogen molecule (Table 29-1, Fig. 29-1).[82–99] There are several forms of branching enzyme deficiency. The classic and most common type of GSD IV, also known as Andersen disease, presents in infancy as progressive liver dysfunction with hepatomegaly, splenomegaly, and failure to thrive. Muscular weakness, atrophy, hypotonia, hyporeflexia, and contractures may occur but are overshadowed by the liver disease.[88,93] Most children succumb to severe liver failure by 5 years of age. There is also a benign hepatic form of GSD IV in which the liver disease does not progress.[97] Some patients with GSD IV manifests primarily with muscle weakness, atrophy, and cardiomyopathy in childhood or adult life.[83,91,92] Either proximal or distal muscle groups can be preferentially affected. In addition, a fatal infantile form is associated with congenital onset of severe weakness.[93–96] Finally, there is a variant of branching enzyme deficiency, known as polyglucosan body neuropathy, which usually presents in adults as progressive upper and lower motor neuron loss, sensory nerve involvement, cerebellar ataxia, neurogenic bladder, and dementia.[84,86,98,99] Occasionally, polyglucosan body neuropathy manifests in children.[87] There is a predilection for polyglucosan body neuropathy in the Ashkenazi population.

Laboratory Features

Depending on the subtype of GSD IV, deficiency of branching enzyme may be demonstrated in muscle, peripheral nerve, fibroblasts, or leukocytes.[83,84,89,98,99] In patients with primary neuromuscular involvement, the deficiency may be noted only in muscle.[83] Branching enzyme activity can be normal in the muscle in patients with adult polyglucosan body neuropathy.[84,86] The serum CK may be normal or slightly elevated. EMG reveals myopathic features and muscle membrane instability similar to that observed with GSDs II and III. In patients with polyglucosan body neuropathy, an axonal sensorimotor neuropathy is apparent, while the EMG abnormalities reflect a superimposed polyradiculopathy. EKG can demonstrate progressive conduction defects leading to complete AV block.[91] Echocardiogram may reveal a dilated cardiomyopathy.[91]

Histopathology

Routine light microscopy and EM reveals deposition of varying amounts of finely granular and filamentous polysaccharide (polyglucosan bodies) in the CNS, peripheral nerves (axons and Schwann cells), skin, liver, and cardiac and skeletal muscles.[83,86,87,90–92] These polyglucosan bodies are PAS-positive and diastase resistant, suggesting the accumulation of polysaccharides other than glycogen (Fig. 29-3). They are not specific for this disorder and can be seen occasionally in nerve biopsies from patients with other diseases. This polysaccharide resembles amylopectin in that it has longer than normal peripheral chains and few branch points.

Autopsy studies have demonstrated abnormal polysaccharide material in the liver, heart, skeletal muscle, and in neurons of the brain and the spinal cord. The abnormal polysaccharide material is more abundant in the motor neurons than in other nerve cells and affects all motor neurons of the brainstem and spinal cord.[100]

Molecular Genetics and Pathogenesis

The disease is inherited in an autosomal-recessive manner. Deletions, nonsense, and missense mutations within the glycogen branching enzyme (*GBE1*) gene on chromosome 3p12

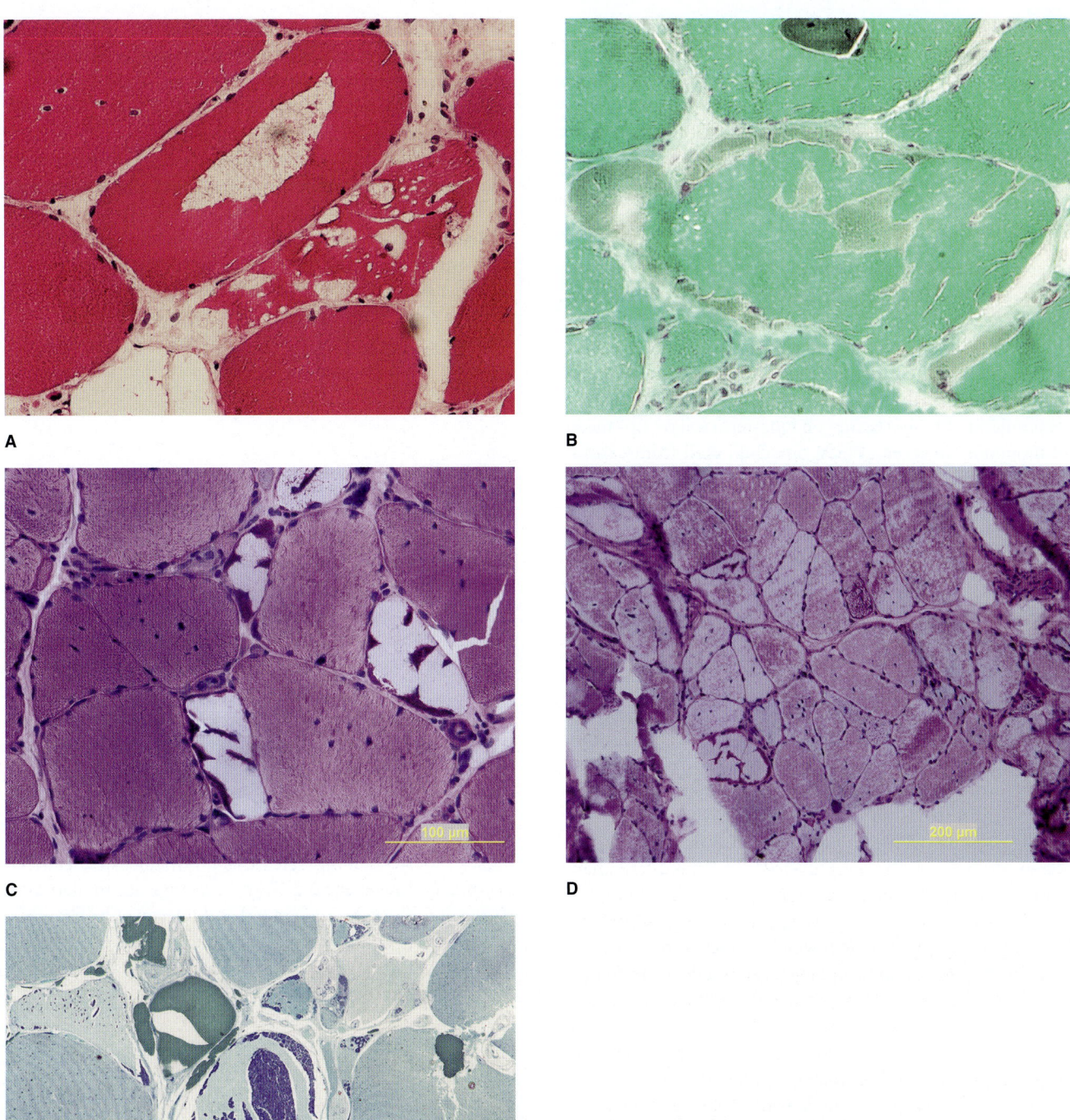

Figure 29-3. Type IV glycogenoses/Anderson disease. Muscle biopsy reveals vacuolated fibers on H&E (**A**) and modified Gomori trichrome (**B**) that appear to contain amorphous debri, which are periodic acid–Schiff (PAS) positive (**C**), and diastase resistant (**D**) suggestive of a filamentous polysaccharide that is not glycogen (i.e., polyglucosan). Semithin plastic sections counterstained with PAS demonstrate increased polysaccharide deposition within muscle fibers (**E**).

have been identified in the severe hepatic, benign hepatic, and the neuromuscular forms of GSD IV, including adult polyglucosan body disease.[82,85,99,100] There are phenotypic variability and differential expression of branching enzyme activity. The mechanism by which the abnormal accumulation of polysaccharide results in muscle damage is not known.

Treatment

Liver transplantation has been performed in some children with GSD IV with beneficial results.[101–103] Apparently, systemic microchimerism occurs after liver allotransplantation and can ameliorate pancellular enzyme deficiencies in this disease. Most of the patients became free of liver, neuromuscular, and cardiac dysfunction, with reduced polysaccharide accumulation in these tissues on long-term follow-up (mean 42 months). However, at least one child died from cardiomyopathy due to massive deposition of polysaccharide in the heart 2½ years after transplantation.[101] No other medical therapies have been demonstrated to be effective.

GLYCOGENOSIS TYPE V (MCARDLE DISEASE; MYOPHOSPHORYLASE DEFICIENCY)

Clinical Features

Glycogenosis type V (myophosphorylase deficiency), more commonly known as McArdle disease, is the most common neuromuscular disorder of carbohydrate metabolism. McArdle disease is an autosomal-recessive disorder that usually presents with exercise intolerance in childhood or young adults (Table 29-1, Fig. 29-1).[104–110] Patients complain of exertional muscle pain and cramps induced by brief, but very intense, activities (e.g., weight-lifting and sprinting), but these can also occur following prolonged low-intensity exercises (e.g., swimming and jogging). If affected individuals ignore these symptoms and continue to exercise at a high level, the muscle pain and cramping can become quite intense and electrically silent contractures may develop. Some patients present with fatigue following exercise without associated cramps or muscle pain. Many patients note a second-wind phenomenon, in which after the onset of mild exertional myalgias or cramps (usually after 10 minutes of exercise), the muscle pain and sense of intolerance may dissipate. Subsequently, the individual may continue with the exercise at the previous or a slightly reduced level.[107] The second-wind phenomenon is the result of mobilization and use of blood-borne glucose.

Not everyone develops myoglobinuria and only about 50% of attacks of myoglobinuria are related to exertion. Myoglobinuria may not occur until the second or third decade, although it has developed in the first decade of life.[105] As many as 10% of attacks may be accompanied by acute renal failure, but this may be high as there probably are subclinical bouts of myoglobinuria that go unreported.[105]

Most patients have normal motor examinations between attacks of muscle cramping. However, fixed proximal weakness develops in as many as one-third of patients, perhaps as a result of recurrent bouts of rhabdomyolysis. Some patients present with progressive proximal muscle atrophy and weakness in late adult life rather than exercise intolerance.[108,111] Weakness may involve the arms more than the legs and can be asymmetric. Scapular winging may be evident. We have seen some patients manifest with camptocormia (bent spine syndrome) from paraspinal muscle involvement that has been recently found to be evident early in the course.[109,112] Finally, a few cases have been reported with congenital weakness, some of which were rapidly progressive, leading to ventilatory failure within the first year of life.[113,114]

Laboratory Features

Serum CK levels are invariably elevated even while patients are asymptomatic. Hyperuricemia was a common finding present in 88 subjects (44.7%) and complicated by gout in 25% of cases in one large series.[108] The exercise forearm test reveals a normal rise in serum ammonia but no significant rise in lactic acid.[115] EMG is usually normal in patients with McArdle disease between attacks of myoglobinuria unless fixed muscle weakness develops. Skeletal muscle MRI scans demonstrate early involvement paraspinal, subscapularis, anterior serratus, erector spinae, and quadratus femoris muscles.[109,112]

Histopathology

Muscle biopsies demonstrate variability in fiber size, scattered necrotic and regenerating fibers, excessive accumulation of glycogen in the subsarcolemmal and intermyofibrillar areas, and absent myophosphorylase staining (Fig. 29-6).[116,117] Biochemical assay for myophosphorylase reveals absent or significantly reduced activity.

Molecular Genetics and Pathogenesis

This disorder is inherited in an autosomal-recessive fashion and is caused by mutations in the *PYGM* gene that encodes myophosphorylase.[114,118,119] This enzyme initiates glycogen breakdown by phosphorylating and lysing α-1,4 glucosyl residues from the outer branches of glycogen, generating glucose-1-phosphate. Mutations result in little detectable protein or enzyme activity. Interestingly, the mutations associated with some of the rare cases of fatal infantile myopathy are the same as evident in the more common clinical presentation of McArdle disease.[114] A pseudodominant pattern of inheritance has been reported and felt to be secondary to heterozygotes that have low levels of residual myophosphorylase.[120] Another mechanism is the mating of a homozygote (or compound heterozygote) with a heterozygote.[120]

Although exercise intolerance and contractures had been postulated to be due to the inability to generate enough ATP, studies have demonstrated that ATP is not depleted during exercise in McArdle disease, Tarui disease, or in the other disorders of glycogenolysis and glycolysis.[121] Exercise is associated with (1) an increase in adenosine diphosphate (ADP); (2) intracellular pH that does not acidify in response to exercise; (3) inorganic phosphate levels in muscle, which are 50% lower than normal muscle tissue; and (4) intracellular calcium concentrations at the onset of contracture, which is more than 10-fold greater than that found in normal control muscle exercised.[122] Perhaps the combination of increased intracellular ADP, reduced inorganic phosphate, and lack of acidification with impaired glycolysis increase the sensitivity of the muscle fiber contractile apparatus to intracellular calcium. Further, the increased intracellular ADP may inhibit ADP dissociation from actin–myosin cross-bridges, thereby increasing the time spent in contraction.

In addition, patients with McArdle disease have reduced concentrations of the sodium–potassium ATPases pump, higher exercise-induced serum potassium concentrations, and a greater increase in heart rate during exercise.[123] Decreased sodium–potassium ATPases may lead to an exercise-induced increase in extracellular potassium because of impaired reuptake of potassium released during muscle contraction. Further, exercise intolerance leads to reduced physical activity, which may result in downregulation of the pump, and the increased ADP may decrease the transport rate of the remaining pumps. The increased concentration of extracellular potassium partially depolarizes the muscle membrane, thereby inactivating sodium channels and reducing membrane excitability.[123] Patients with McArdle disease also develop exaggerated tachycardia with exertion that can limit the exercise capacity of individuals who are affected.[123] It is not known why sodium–potassium pump concentrations in skeletal muscle in patients with McArdle disease are reduced. Reduced physical activity may downregulate the number of sodium–potassium ATPase pumps. Alternatively, myophosphorylase deficiency may reduce the pump concentration by disrupting the normal coupling of muscle glycogenolysis and pump activity.[123]

Treatment

A single-blind, placebo-controlled, crossover study of oral sucrose (75 g) in 12 patients with McArdle disease demonstrated marked improvement in exercise tolerance, supported by the subjects' reduced perceived exertion levels and their diminished maximum heart rates.[107] The limitation of oral sucrose loading is that the beneficial effect is short-lived. Repeated dosing may lead to weight gain, which in and of itself can reduce exercise tolerance. Furthermore, it can cause inhibition of fatty acid use, which also is an important fuel source with prolonged physical activity. Sucrose loading will also not be helpful in situations of unexpected exertional activity and prolonged physical activity or with static exercise (e.g., weight-lifting).

A high-protein diet might help but supplementing the diet with branched-chain amino acid supplementation can actually lower exercise capacity.[124] Creatine monohydrate has been studied but found to be of no significant benefit.[125] Surplus calories may lead to weight gain and subsequent decline in cardiovascular fitness. Some small studies have suggested that vitamin B6 supplementation (50 mg/day) can reduce exercise intolerance and enhance performance.[118] A Cochrane review of clinical trials reported that there was low-quality evidence of improvement in some parameters with creatine, oral sucrose, ramipril, and a carbohydrate rich diet, although none indicated significant, clinical benefit.[106]

We instruct patients to avoid intense isometric exercises (e.g., weight-lifting) and maximum aerobic exercises (e.g., sprinting). However, mild-to-moderate aerobic conditioning may be beneficial, as poor cardiovascular fitness results in a diminished delivery of blood-borne substrates necessary for muscle oxidative metabolism.[107,124] Patients should be instructed on how to moderate their physical activity in order to obtain a "second-wind" response. Any bout of moderate exercise should be preceded by 5–15 minutes of low-level warm-up activity to promote the transition to the second "wind."[124]

GLYCOGENOSIS TYPE VII (PHOSPHOFRUCTOKINASE DEFICIENCY)

Clinical Features

PFK deficiency or Tarui disease is an autosomal-recessive disease, caused by a deficiency in PFK in muscle and erythrocytes (Table 29-1, Fig. 29-1). PFK deficiency is much less common than McArdle disease. The clinical features are very similar to McArdle disease with respect to exercise intolerance, muscle pain, contractures, and relief of discomfort by rest. However, PFK deficiency is not associated with the warm-up phenomena, and there is a lower incidence of myoglobinuria.[126,127] In addition, some patients develop jaundice (due to mild hemolysis) and gouty arthritis due to PFK deficiency in erythrocytes.

The clinical phenotype can vary. Some individuals who are affected manifest with hemolytic anemia without a myopathy. Others present later in adulthood with fixed weakness, which may predominantly affect the proximal or occasionally the scapuloperoneal muscles.[128,129] They may have had only mild exercise intolerance in their younger years but never have a history of cramps or myoglobinuria. In addition, PFK deficiency can present in infancy with severe generalized weakness and cardiomyopathy. Contractures, cortical blindness, and corneal opacifications are evident in some infants, but hemolytic anemia does not occur. Severely affected children may die from cardioventilatory failure in infancy or early childhood.

Laboratory Features

Serum CK is usually elevated, and mild anemia and increased reticulocyte count are often noted.[129] Exercise forearm testing reveals a normal increase in ammonia production but a blunted increase in lactic acid. EMG is usually normal.

Histopathology

Muscle biopsies demonstrate vacuoles and an abnormal accumulation of glycogen.[128] In addition, there is also an abnormal accumulation of polysaccharide, which stains intensely with PAS but is diastase resistant, especially in older patients. Muscle biopsies may reveal only nonspecific myopathic features without evidence of abnormal glycogen accumulation in the infantile form of disease. Definitive diagnosis of Tarui disease can be made by biochemical and histochemical analyses of muscle tissue, which reveal the deficiency of PFK activity and staining.

Molecular Genetics and Pathogenesis

Tarui disease is caused by mutations in the *PFKM* gene which encodes for PFK. PFK catalyzes the ATPase-dependent conversion of fructose 6-phosphate to fructose 1,6-diphosphate. Human PFK comprises three distinct isoenzyme subunits (M—muscle, L—liver, and P—platelet). Skeletal muscles contain only the M isoform, while erythrocytes contain a hybrid of M and L subunits. The gene responsible for the M isoform, PFK-M, was initially mapped to 1q32 but was subsequently reassigned to 12q13. The symptoms reflect inactivation of PFK in muscle and partial inactivation in red blood cells. Different molecular defects may explain the different clinical presentations; however, the biochemical and molecular basis for clinical heterogeneity remains unclear.

As in McArdle disease, there is ADP accumulation in exercised muscle, but whether or not there is also reduction in sodium–potassium pumps in Tarui disease is not known. The normal coupling of muscle glycogenolysis and sodium–potassium pump activity may be disrupted by increased ADP or reduction in pump concentration, as we described in the section on McArdle disease.

Treatment

Unlike in McArdle disease, glucose or fructose administration prior to activity does not help; rather it may be deleterious. Patients with PFK deficiency rely on free fatty acids as a fuel substrate during exercise. Therefore, they experience more exercise intolerance, if given a glucose infusion or they consume high-carbohydrate meals, because glucose reduces the blood levels of free fatty acids.[130] This is just the opposite of the second-wind phenomena and is sometime called the *out-of-wind phenomena*. An aerobic conditioning program similar to those given to patients with McArdle deficiency may improve exercise tolerance.

GLYCOGENOSIS TYPE IX (PHOSPHORYLASE B KINASE DEFICIENCY)

Muscle PBK or phosphorylase kinase (PHK) deficiency was formerly designated GSD VIII but is now more commonly referred to as GSD IX. PHK is a multimeric enzyme composed of four subunits. As will be discussed below, mutations involving PHKA1, encoding subunit α, cause the rare X-linked GSD IXa that is only associated with muscle involvement. Mutations in PHKB, encoding subunit β, cause the more common autosomal-recessive GSD IXb that involves both the liver and muscle. Mutations in other subunits are not associated with muscle involvement.

Clinical Features

PHK deficiency is associated with heterogeneous clinical manifestations.[131–135] It most commonly manifests as exercise intolerance with cramps and myoglobinuria (Table 29-1, Fig. 29-1). However, PHK deficiency can occasionally present in infancy or childhood with mild weakness and a delay in motor milestones. Rarely, a fatal cardiomyopathy can occur in infancy. Approximately 50% of patients develop proximal or distal weakness in adulthood.

Laboratory Features

Serum CK may be normal or mildly elevated. The exercise forearm test may be normal or abnormal. EMG is usually normal. Diagnosis is based on clinical findings, assay of PHK activity in erythrocytes, or liver or muscle tissues (depending upon presentation) and confirmatory findings on molecular genetic testing.

Histopathology

Muscle biopsy may be normal or may demonstrate variability in fiber size, scattered necrotic fibers, and slight subsarcolemmal accumulation of glycogen. Biochemical analysis reveals decreased PHK activity.

Molecular Genetics and Pathogenesis

PHK catalyzes the conversion of inactive myophosphorylase to the active form and converts active glycogen synthetase to an inactive form. As mentioned above, PHK is a multimeric enzyme composed of four different subunits. Mutations in *PHKA1*, encoding subunit α, cause the less-common X-linked GSD IXa that is associated with muscle involvement only, while mutations in *PHKB*, encoding subunit β, cause autosomal-recessive GSD IXb that involves both liver and muscle.[136]

Treatment

There is no specific medical therapy. Patients should be instructed on a mild-to-moderate exercise program and to avoid vigorous activity.

GLYCOGENOSIS TYPE X (PHOSPHOGLYCERATE MUTASE DEFICIENCY)

Clinical Features

PGAM deficiency presents in childhood or early adult life as exercise intolerance, cramps, and recurrent myoglobinuria (Table 29-1, Fig. 29-1).[137,138]

Laboratory Features

Serum CK is mildly elevated. The exercise forearm test is abnormal. EMG is normal.

Histopathology

Muscle biopsies reveal increased glycogen by PAS staining and on EM. Tubular aggregates may be evident in type 2B fibers (Fig. 29-4). Biochemical assay demonstrates normal or only mildly elevated glycogen content and markedly diminished activity of PGAM (<10% of normal).

Molecular Genetics and Pathogenesis

Type X glycogenosis is an autosomal-recessive disorder caused by mutations in the *PGAM2* gene encoded on chromosome 7p13–p12.3. PGAM catalyzes the interconversion of 2- and 3-phosphoglycerate. There are two subunits for PGAM: a muscle-specific subunit (PGAMM) and a non-muscle-specific or brain subunit (PGAMB). Mature muscle contains the homodimer MM form of PGAM, which has diminished enzymatic activity in type X glycogenosis.

Treatment

There is no definitive medical therapy. Dantrolene improved symptoms in one patient with severe cramps and tubular

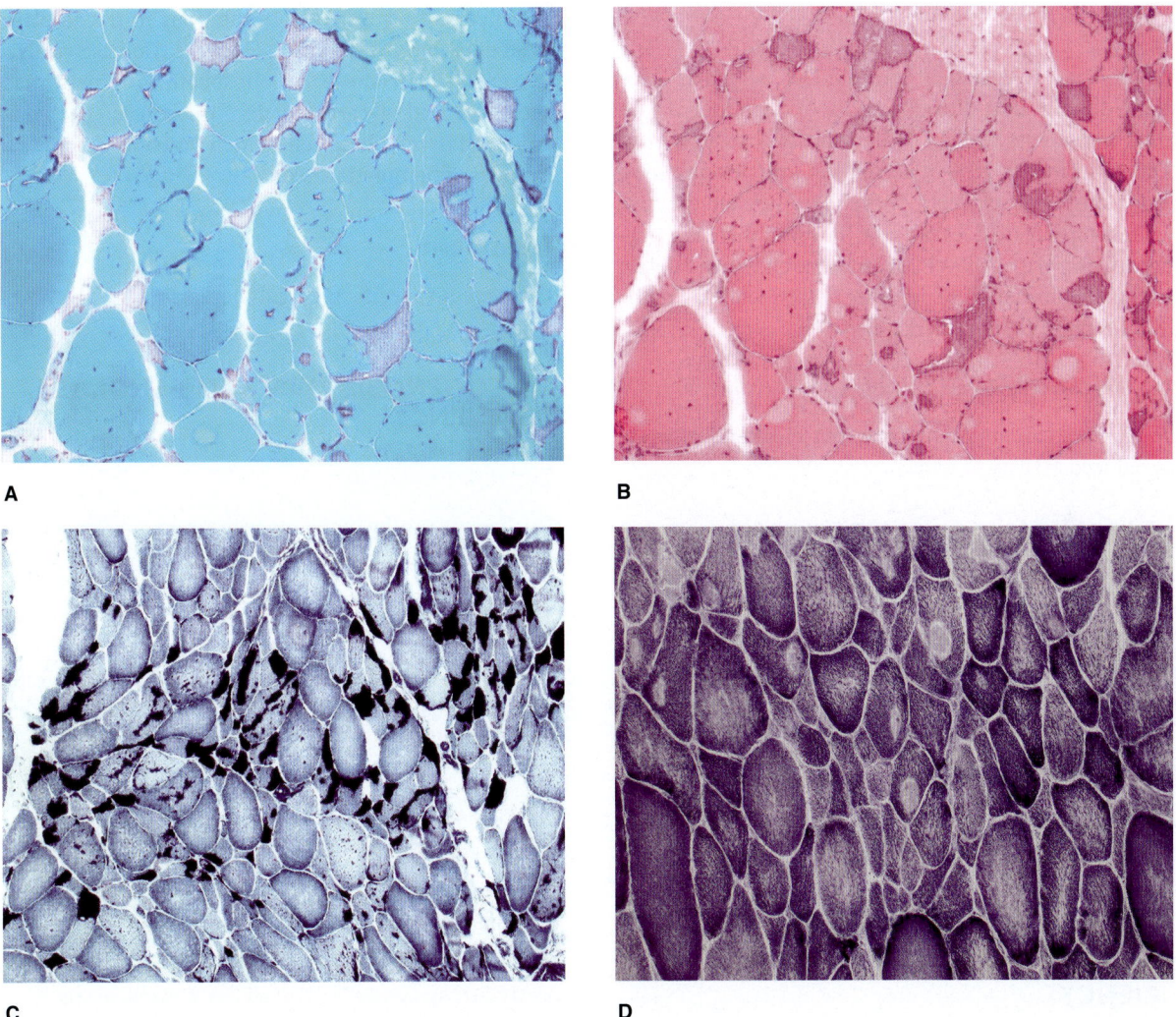

Figure 29-4. Muscle biopsies can reveal scattered fibers with tubular aggregates in patients with phosphoglycerate mutase (PGAM) deficiency. Tubular aggregates appear as subsarcolemmal masses of reddish-purple material on modified trichrome (**A**) and are bluish on H&E (**B**). The tubular aggregates occur only in type 2 fibers and appear densely staining on NADH-TR (**C**), but do not stain with SDH (**D**).

aggregates on muscle biopsy.[137] Nevertheless, dantrolene is not recommended as routine therapy. Patients should be instructed on avoiding strenuous activity and placed on a mild-to-moderate aerobic exercise program.

GLYCOGENOSIS TYPE XI (LACTATE DEHYDROGENASE DEFICIENCY)

Clinical Features

This rare autosomal-recessive disorder manifests as exercise intolerance, myalgia, cramping, and recurrent myoglobinuria (Table 29-1, Fig. 29-1).[139,140] Muscle strength is normal. Patients may also develop a generalized, scaly, erythematous rash, particularly in the summer. Pregnancies may be complicated by uterine stiffness in early stages of delivery and often requires cesarean section. This complication has not been associated with other glycogenoses. Chronic renal failure can develop secondary to recurrent myoglobinuria.

Laboratory Features

Serum CK level is elevated. Serum LDH, which is usually markedly elevated during attacks of rhabdomyolysis, is normal in patients with LDH deficiency. A reduction in the LDH-M isoform (<5% of normal) in muscle and blood can be demonstrated on electrophoretic studies. On exercise forearm testing, lactate does not rise; however, there is a normal increase in pyruvate levels, because the enzymatic defect lies distal to the formation of pyruvate in the metabolic pathway. EMG is typically unremarkable.

Histopathology

Muscle biopsies can appear normal, but biochemical assay reveals reduced activity of LDH.

Molecular Genetics and Pathogenesis

There are five distinct LDH isoenzymes, each comprising tetramers composed of combinations of two different subunits, M and H. Thus far, only mutations involving the muscle M subunits encoded by the *LDH* gene, *LDHA*, on chromosome 11p15.4 have been associated with muscle disease.[139]

Treatment

There is no specific medical therapy. Obstetricians need to be made aware of potential complications of labor in affected pregnant females.

GLYCOGENOSIS TYPE XII (ALDOLASE A DEFICIENCY)

Clinical Features

This rare disorder can manifest in the newborn period or early childhood with rhabdomyolysis and episodes of hemolytic anemia—often following febrile illnesses (Table 29-1, Fig. 29-1).[141–143] Some affected individuals manifest with exercise intolerance and mild proximal weakness. Scapular winging and distal upper extremity weakness have been reported in adults. Learning disabilities and delayed language acquisition may also be evident.

Laboratory Features

Serum CK can be normal or elevated.

Histopathology

Muscle biopsy appeared normal or show nonspecific changes on routine light microscopy, but EM revealed accumulation of lipid. Biochemical analysis revealed markedly reduced aldolase activity.

Molecular Genetics and Pathogenesis

The myopathy is caused by mutations in the aldolase gene located on chromosome 16q22–24.[141] Aldolase catalyzes the conversion of fructose 1,6-phosphate to dihydroxyacetone phosphate and glyceraldehyde 3-phosphate. The enzyme is expressed in red blood cells which probably accounts for the episodes of hemolytic anemia.

Treatment

There are no specific medical therapies.

GLYCOGENOSIS TYPE XIII (β-ENOLASE DEFICIENCY)

Clinical Features

This rare myopathy manifests with severe muscle cramps, postexertional myalgias, myoglobinuria (Table 29-1, Fig. 29-1).[144–147]

Laboratory Features

The serum CK levels were episodically elevated. Either no or an attenuated rise in lactic acid is noted on an exercise forearm test.

Histopathology

Muscle biopsy revealed abnormal accumulation of glycogen in the sarcoplasm. Selective β-enolase deficiency was demonstrated with immunohistochemistry and immunoblotting.

Molecular Genetics and Pathogenesis

Heterozygous and homozygous mutations have been identified within the *ENO3* gene that encodes for β-enolase. β-Enolase catalyzes the step interconverting 2-phosphoglycerate and phosphoenolpyruvate.

Treatment

There are no specific medical therapies.

GLYCOGENOSIS TYPE XIV (PHOSPHOGLUCOMUTASE 1 DEFICIENCY)

Clinical Features

This rare myopathy has also been classified as a congenital disorder of glycosylation, PGM1-CDG (Table 29-1, Fig. 29-1).[148–150] Most cases present in infancy with a multisystem disorder that can include cleft palate, bifid uvula, anal atresia, liver abnormalities, cardiac valve anomalies, and skeletal deformities. However, some patients manifest only with exercise-induced intolerance with episodes of rhabdomyolysis without a second-wind phenomena that can develop in adulthood.

Laboratory Features

CK at rest may be normal. Exercise forearm test reveals a normal elevation of lactate but also an exaggerated rise in ammonia. EMG is myopathic.[150] Serum transferrin glycan isoform analysis by liquid chromatography-mass spectrometry is used as a primary diagnostic screen tool when the disorder is suspected.

Histopathology

Muscle biopsy revealed abnormal accumulation of glycogen in the sarcoplasm.

Molecular Genetics and Pathogenesis

Phosphoglucomutase 1 catalyzes the conversion of glucose-1-phosphate to glucose-6-phosphate. It is caused by mutations in *PGYM1*.

Treatment

D-galactose supplementation was trialed in more than 20 patients who reported improvement in exercise intolerance, fatigability, hypogonadism, rhabdomyolysis and the frequency of hypoglycemia.[150] The dose of D-galactose tried ranged between 0.5 and 3 g/kg/day (maximum dose 50 g/day) and showed no adverse effects in most patients. It is recommended to avoid doses higher than 50 g/day as this may lead to an increase of galactose-1-phosphate and galactitol which could be toxic.

GLYCOGENOSIS TYPE XV (GLYCOGENIN 1 DEFICIENCY)

Clinical Features

This rare myopathy manifests in childhood or adulthood with slowly progressive limb-girdle or scapuloperoneal weakness with or without a cardiomyopathy (ventricular arrhythmia) along with exercise intolerance (Table 29-1, Fig. 29-1).[1,151–154]

Laboratory Features

Serum CKs can be normal or slightly elevated.[151–154] EMG may show increased insertional and spontaneous activity and early recruitment of small myopathic–appearing motor units. EKG may show ventricular arrhythmia, while echocardiogram may show reduced ejection fraction. Cardiac MRI may demonstrate area with late enhancement, and slightly increased left ventricular volume and mass.[151]

Histopathology

Skeletal muscle biopsy may reveal abnormal accumulation of glycogen, polyglucosan bodies, and depletion of glycogenin 1 along with type 1 fiber atrophy and predominance.[151–154]

Molecular Genetics and Pathogenesis

Glycogenin 1 is encoded by *GYG1*. The enzyme catalyzes the formation of short glucose polymers of approximately 10 glucose residues, from uridine diphosphate glucose in an autoglucosylation reaction.[151,152] This enzymatic step is followed by elongation and branching of the polymer, catalyzed by glycogen synthase 1, which as discussed previously is abnormal in GSD type 0.

Treatment

There are no specific medical therapies. Some patients have required cardiac transplantation.

▶ OTHER RELATED DISORDERS

TRIOSEPHOSPHATE ISOMERASE DEFICIENCY

Clinical Features

This rare myopathy is associated with congenital hypotonia and weakness, cardiomyopathy, hemolytic anemia, and CNS involvement (i.e., intellectual disability, epilepsy, dystonia, and dyskinesia) (Table 29-1, Fig. 29-1).[155–158]

Laboratory Features

Serum CKs are normal, but EMG is myopathic.

Histopathology

Muscle biopsy demonstrated increased glycogen on routine light microscopy and EM.

Molecular Genetics and Pathogenesis

Triosephosphate isomerase catalyzes the conversion of dihydroxyacetone phosphate into glyceraldehyde 3-phosphate.

Treatment

There are no specific medical therapies.

PHOSPHOGLYCERATE KINASE DEFICIENCY

Clinical Features

PGK deficiency is an X-linked disorder that commonly presents as hemolytic anemia and CNS disturbances (e.g., intellectual disability and seizures) in boys (Table 29-1, Fig. 29-1). In addition, some patients present with a myopathy.[159–165] The myopathy is characterized by exercise intolerance, cramps, and recurrent myoglobinuria. Slowly progressive proximal weakness has also been described. Presentation with hemolytic anemia, CNS disturbances, and myopathy appears to occur in equal frequencies in patients with PGK deficiency.

Laboratory Features

Serum CK is two to three times normal. Most patients with the myopathy do not have hemolytic anemia, although it has been described.[162] Exercise forearm test fails to show a normal rise in lactate. EMG is usually normal.

Histopathology

Muscle biopsies are typically normal, but mild and diffuse PAS staining may be noted. Abnormal glycogen accumulation is usually apparent by EM. Enzymatic assays reveal reduced PGK enzyme activity.

Molecular Genetics and Pathogenesis

The disorder is caused by mutations in the *PGK1* gene located on chromosome Xq13. PGK catalyzes the transfer of the acyl phosphate group of 1,3-diphosphoglycerate to ADP, with the formation of 3-phosphoglycerate and ATP in the terminal stage of the glycolysis.

Treatment

No specific medical therapy for the myopathy is available.

UBIQUITIN LIGASE (RBCK1) DEFICIENCY

Clinical Features

Ubiquitin ligase deficiency is a rare autosomal-recessive disorder presenting in childhood to late teens with slowly progressive proximal leg weakness.[166,167] Patients with homozygous or compound heterozygous for truncating mutations have developed a rapidly progressive dilated cardiomyopathy with onset in adolescence that required cardiac transplantation. Hepatomegaly with abnormal accumulation of polyglucosan may also occur.

Laboratory Features

Serum CK was normal to six-fold elevated. Echocardiogram may demonstrate features of a dilated cardiomyopathy.

Histopathology

Skeletal and cardiac muscle biopsy fibers are typically devoid of normal glycogen but contain abnormal accumulation of polyglucosan bodies that were PAS-positive that were resistant to diastase. The inclusions are also ubiquitinated and stained for ubiquitin-binding protein sequestosome-1 (p62).[166,167]

Molecular Genetics and Pathogenesis

The disorder is caused by mutations in the *RBCK1* gene that encodes for ubiquitin ligase. *RBCK1* mutations are also known to be associated with recurrent infections and episodes of sepsis and possible autoimmune disorders. The enzyme appears to be involved in myogenesis. It also plays a role in regulating the nuclear factor κB (NFκB) pathways which may explain the recurrent infections and autoimmunity in some patients depending on the site of the mutation.

Treatment

No specific medical therapy for the myopathy is available, though medications treating congestive heart failure and cardiac transplantation have been used to treat the cardiomyopathy.

▶ OTHER VACUOLAR MYOPATHIES

We debated in which chapter to discuss Danon disease and X-linked myopathy with excessive autophagy (XMEA). Danon disease was initially reported as "lysosomal glycogen storage disease with normal acid maltase."[168] Some have termed this GSD IIb. XMEA shares similar histopathological features with Danon disease. As both are in the differential diagnosis of vacuolar myopathies with increased glycogen deposition, we decided to include discussion of these disorders in this chapter.

DANON DISEASE (X-LINKED VACUOLAR CARDIOMYOPATHY AND MYOPATHY)

Clinical Features

Danon and colleagues initially described this rare disorder characterized by the triad of hypertrophic or dilated cardiomyopathy, myopathy, and mental retardation.[169–176] Males are more severely affected than females, but female carriers can also manifest with symptoms.[174,175] Individuals who are affected usually appear normal at birth but develop proximal muscle weakness and a cardiomyopathy in childhood or early adult life. Approximately 70% of males have some degree of mental retardation compared to less than 50% of women.[141,170] Either hypertrophic or dilated cardiomyopathy may occur that can be complicated by arrhythmia and sudden death.[171,174,175] In a review of 82 patients with Danon disease in the literature, the average ages of first symptom, cardiac transplantation, and death were 12.1, 17.9, and 19.0 years in males and 27.9, 33.7, and 34.6 years in females, respectively.[171]

Laboratory Features

Serum CK levels are moderately elevated. Echocardiograms often demonstrate a hypertrophic or dilated cardiomyopathy.[171,175] The most frequent EKG abnormality is Wolff–Parkinson–White syndrome, but AV block, bundle branch blocks, bradycardia, and atrial flutter/fibrillation may also be observed. Cardiac MRI in males shows features of a hypertrophic cardiomyopathy, whereas manifesting females may show either a dilated or hypertrophic cardiomyopathy.[177] Cardiac MRI may be useful in women harboring lysosome-associated membrane protein-2 (LAMP-2) mutations, as it may demonstrate early involvement and guide timely considerations of implantable cardioverter-defibrillator therapy.[175]

NCSs are normal. Increased insertional and spontaneous activity in the form of fibrillation potentials, positive sharp waves, complex repetitive discharges, and myotonic discharges are evident on EMG.[168] There is early recruitment of small-amplitude, short-duration, polyphasic MUAPs.

Histopathology

Muscle biopsies demonstrate variability in fiber size with autophagic vacuoles.[168] Excess free glycogen between disorganized myofibrils and within membrane-bound sacs and vacuoles may be seen on EM. On EM, some of the vacuoles are bound by basal lamina. These histological features are similar to Pompe disease, although α-glucosidase activity is normal in Danon disease. The characteristic feature is the absence of LAMP-2 on immunostaining. Unlike XMEA,[178] which it can resemble, there is no abnormal deposition of membrane attack complex on muscle fibers.

Molecular Genetics and Pathogenesis

Danon disease is caused by mutations in the *LAMP2* gene located on the chromosome Xq24 that encodes for LAMP-2.[169] LAMP-2 is a major lysosomal membrane protein and mutations lead to defects in autophagy.

Treatment

There is no specific medical therapy at this time for the skeletal muscle weakness. Some patients require pacemakers, intracardiac defibrillators, or cardiac transplantation for the cardiomyopathy.[171,174,175,179]

X-LINKED MYOPATHY WITH EXCESSIVE AUTOPHAGY

Clinical Features

XMEA can present in infancy or early adult life with slowly progressive proximal weakness and atrophy.[178,180–185] Respiratory weakness can also ensue. Unlike Danon disease, which it can resemble, individuals with XMEA usually do not develop a cardiomyopathy or intellectual disability. However, a single case resembling XMEA was reported with cardiomyopathy.[182]

Laboratory Features

Serum CK levels may be normal or mildly elevated. Routine motor and sensory NCSs are normal. EMG reveals increased insertional and spontaneous activity with fibrillation potentials, positive sharp waves, complex repetitive discharges, and myotonic discharges.[178,180,181] There is early recruitment of small-amplitude, short-duration, polyphasic MUAPs.

Histopathology

Muscle biopsies reveal muscle fiber size variation and many fibers with autophagic vacuoles (Fig. 29-5A and B).[178,180–183] Unlike Danon disease and Pompe disease, these vacuoles are not PAS-positive. Further, LAMP-2 is present in the vacuoles and within the cytoplasm in XMEA (Fig. 29-5C). Calcium and membrane attack complex (C5b-9) (Fig. 29-5D) deposits along the sarcolemma of abnormal muscle fibers.[178,184] On EM, some of the vacuoles are bound by basal lamina. These are often appreciated in the subsarcolemmal region where they appear to fuse with the cell membrane allowing expression of their contents into the extracellular space. Redundant folds of basal lamina surrounding muscle fibers are also characteristic.

Molecular Genetics and Pathogenesis

The XMEA is caused by mutations in the *VMA21* gene located on chromosome Xq28 that encodes for VMA21.[184,185] Vacuolar ATPases (V-ATPases) are composed of 14 subunits that act as a proton pumps which regulate the levels lysosomes. VMA21 is a chaperone protein that is essential to the assembly of V-ATPase. Defects in VMA21 lead to a rise in lysosomal pH which reduces degradation and blocks autophagy.

Treatment

There is no specific medical therapy for XMEA.

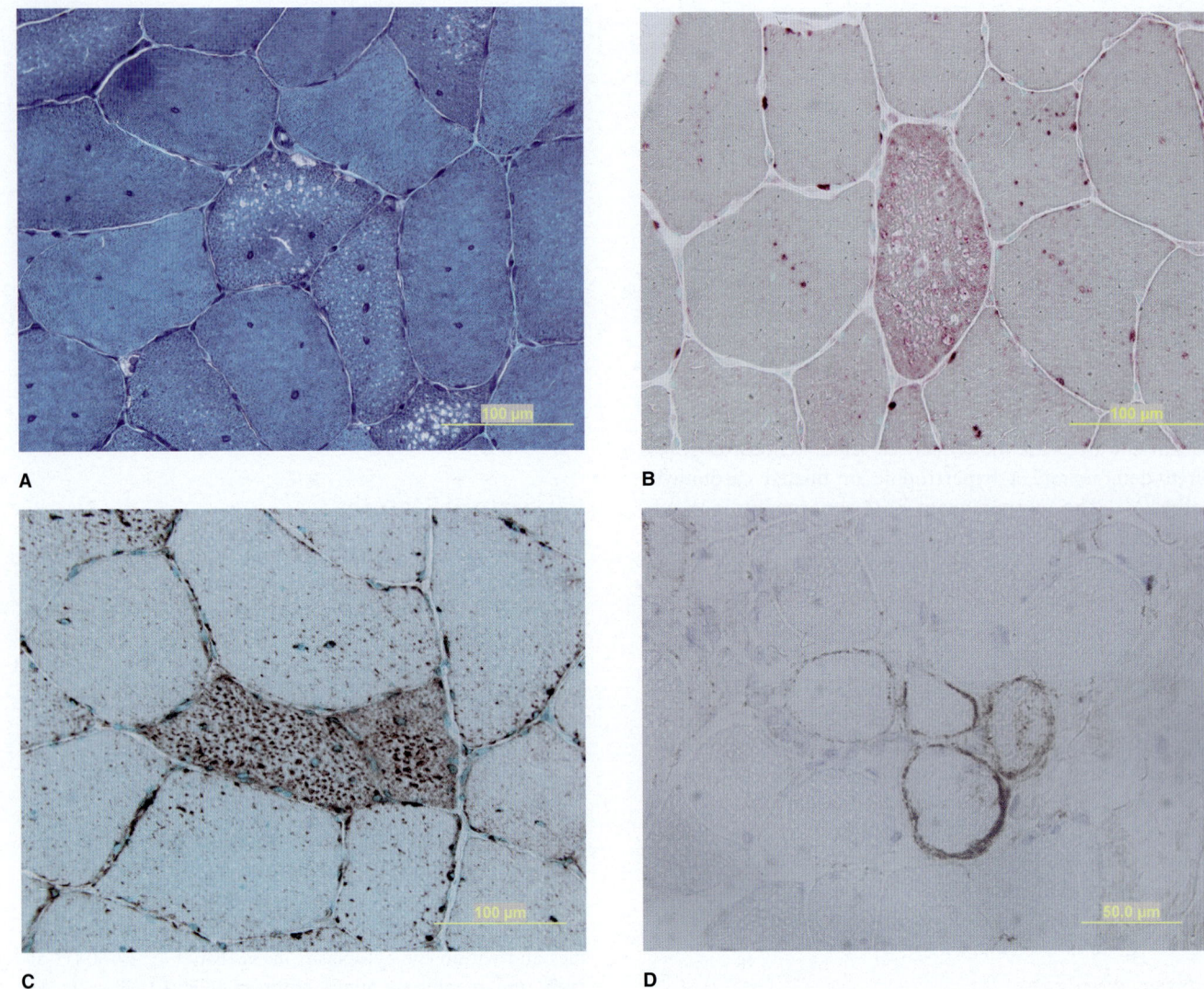

Figure 29-5. X-linked myopathy with excessive autophagia (XMEA). Muscle biopsies reveal fibers with autophagic vacuoles on modified Gomori trichrome (**A**), which stain red with acid phosphatase stain (**B**). Immunoperoxidase stain with antibodies directed against lysosome-associated membrane protein-2 (LAMP-2) demonstrates the presence of LAMP-2 in lysosomes (**C**). Further, immunoperoxidase stain demonstrates membrane attack complex (C5b-9) deposition along the sarcolemma of abnormal muscle fibers (**D**).

► DISORDERS OF PURINE NUCLEOTIDE METABOLISM

Disorders of purine metabolism more commonly cause hyperuricemic syndromes (gout and Lesch–Nyhan syndrome) or immunodeficiency disorders rather than a myopathy. A single disorder of nucleotide metabolism, MADD, has been linked to exercise intolerance and myoglobinuria in the past, but even this association has been questioned.

MYOADENYLATE DEAMINASE DEFICIENCY (MADD)

Clinical Features

Patients with MADD may develop exertional muscle pain and fatigue[186–189] and perhaps myoglobinuria[187] in late adolescence to middle age. However, the relationship between MADD and the exercise intolerance and bouts of myoglobinuria is controversial. The neurological examination is normal. Many individuals with MADD are asymptomatic, and mild exertional muscle pain and fatigue are extremely common symptoms in the general population. MADD has been reported in 1%–2% of muscle biopsies, making it the most common enzyme deficiency in muscle.[188] Additionally, muscle biopsies in patients with other types of neuromuscular disorders such as amyotrophic lateral sclerosis, spinal muscular atrophy, inflammatory myopathies, and various forms of muscular dystrophies have been found to have incidental deficiencies in MAD. Thus, although the frequency of MADD may be increased in muscle biopsies performed for evaluation of exertional myalgias,[186] a cause and effect relationship between the enzymatic deficiency and symptomatic muscle disease has yet to be established.

Laboratory Features

Serum CK is normal or only slightly elevated. The exercise forearm test is abnormal; serum lactate levels rise normally with exercise; however, ammonia levels remain relatively stable. EMG is normal.

Histopathology

The routine muscle biopsy is normal.[186] Specific biochemical assay or histological stain for MADD is essentially the only abnormality noted.

Molecular Genetics and Pathogenesis

MAD catalyzes the removal of an ammonia group from adenosine monophosphate (AMP) to form inosine monophosphate. AMP combines with ATP to form two ADP molecules (2 ADP ↔ ATP + AMP). By catalyzing the conversion of AMP to inosine monophosphate, thereby reducing available AMP, MAD indirectly tilts the above equation in favor of the formation of ATP, maintaining energy supplies. Also, the production of ammonia by MAD buffers the lactic acid formed during exercise. Further, inosine monophosphate stimulates glycolysis by acting on PFK and aids in making fumarate, a substrate integral to the Kreb cycle. Thus, MADD potentially can have wide-reaching metabolic effects in multiple energy production cycles. Reduced phosphocreatine and ADP levels have been demonstrated in MADD patients compared to normal controls.[189] However, a study of sustained, isometric muscle contraction during ischemia in patients with MADD and normal controls found no difference in oxygen use, endurance time, resting, and postexercise lactate and phosphocreatine levels, suggesting a normal exercise capacity.[1,190]

Point mutations have been identified in primary MADD in the gene *AMPD1* (AMP deaminase 1), located on chromosome 1p13–21.[188,191] As noted above, MADD has been associated with a number of neuromuscular disorders. A study in the Dutch population revealed no significant differences in frequencies of the characteristic "mutation" in the MAD gene in patients with exercise intolerance, those with other neuromuscular disorders, and healthy volunteers.[188] It may be that the "mutations" that lead to MADD are no more than harmless polymorphisms.

Treatment

There is no specific medical treatment available.

▶ LIPID METABOLISM DISORDERS

The major source of fuel for muscles at rest and following prolonged or intense physical activity are free fatty acids, particularly long-chain fatty acids. β-Oxidation of free fatty acids occurs within the inner matrix of mitochondria and generates ATP. Fatty acids are divided into short-, medium-, long-, and very–long-chain fatty acids, depending on their size. Short- and medium-chain fatty acids are readily permeable to either the outer or the inner mitochondrial membranes. However, long-chain fatty acids must interact with various carrier proteins and be actively transported across the mitochondrial membranes (Fig. 29-6). First, the long-chain fatty acids combine with coenzyme A (CoA) in a reaction catalyzed by acyl-CoA-synthetase at the outer mitochondrial membrane, creating a long-chain acyl-CoA. Next, the long-chain acyl-CoA must link with carnitine in a reaction reversibly catalyzed by carnitine palmitoyl transferase 1 (CPT1), an enzyme located on the outer face of the outer mitochondrial membrane, in order to cross over the outer membrane. The long-chain acyl–carnitine complex within the intermembrane space is then transported across the inner mitochondrial membrane, in a reaction catalyzed by carnitine palmitoyl transferase 2 (CPT2) located on the inner surface of the inner membrane. This liberates carnitine from the long-chain acyl-CoA. The carnitine is then transported in the opposite direction, in a reaction catalyzed by carnitine/acylcarnitine translocase. The long-chain acyl-CoA, now within the mitochondrial matrix, can be metabolized by β-oxidation into ATP.

β-Oxidation of the fatty acids within the mitochondria proceeds through repeated cycles consisting of four sequential enzymatic reactions (Fig. 29-7). First, flavin-dependent, length-specific acyl-CoA dehydrogenases [note that there are short-, medium-, long-, and very–long-chain acyl-CoA dehydrogenases (SCADs, MCADs, LCADs, and VLCADs)] convert the acyl-CoA substrates into enoyl-CoAs and reduce flavin adenine dinucleotide (FAD). Second, length-specific enoyl-CoA hydratase catalyzes the formation of 3-hydroxyacyl-CoA derivatives. Third, length-specific, NAD-dependent 3-hydroxyacyl-CoA dehydrogenases (HADs) catalyze the formation of 3-ketoacyl-CoA esters by a second dehydrogenation reaction. In the fourth and final step, length-dependent 3-ketothiolase catalyzes the conversion of the 3-ketoacyl-CoA ester to acetyl-CoA and fatty acyl-CoA, which are now two carbon atoms shorter than the acyl-CoA that entered the initial first step. This sequential cycle of four enzymatic reactions is then repeated.

Electrons transferred to $FADH_2$ and NADH are then transferred to the respiratory chain, which is composed of five multimeric protein complexes embedded in the inner mitochondrial membrane. FADH delivers its electrons to coenzyme Q via two flavoproteins: electron-transferring flavoprotein (ETF) and ETF-coenzyme Q oxidoreductase (ETF-QO). NADH delivers its electrons to complex I of the respiratory chain. The electrons are then transported down an energy gradient from one complex to another, generating a proton motive force, which is necessary to produce ATP.

Defects in the transport of long-chain fatty acids and lipid metabolism affect multiple organs, including muscle. Two major muscle manifestations are (1) progressive muscle weakness and hypotonia (e.g., as seen in carnitine transporter and carnitine/acylcarnitine defects) and (2) acute, recurrent rhabdomyolysis (e.g., as seen in deficiencies

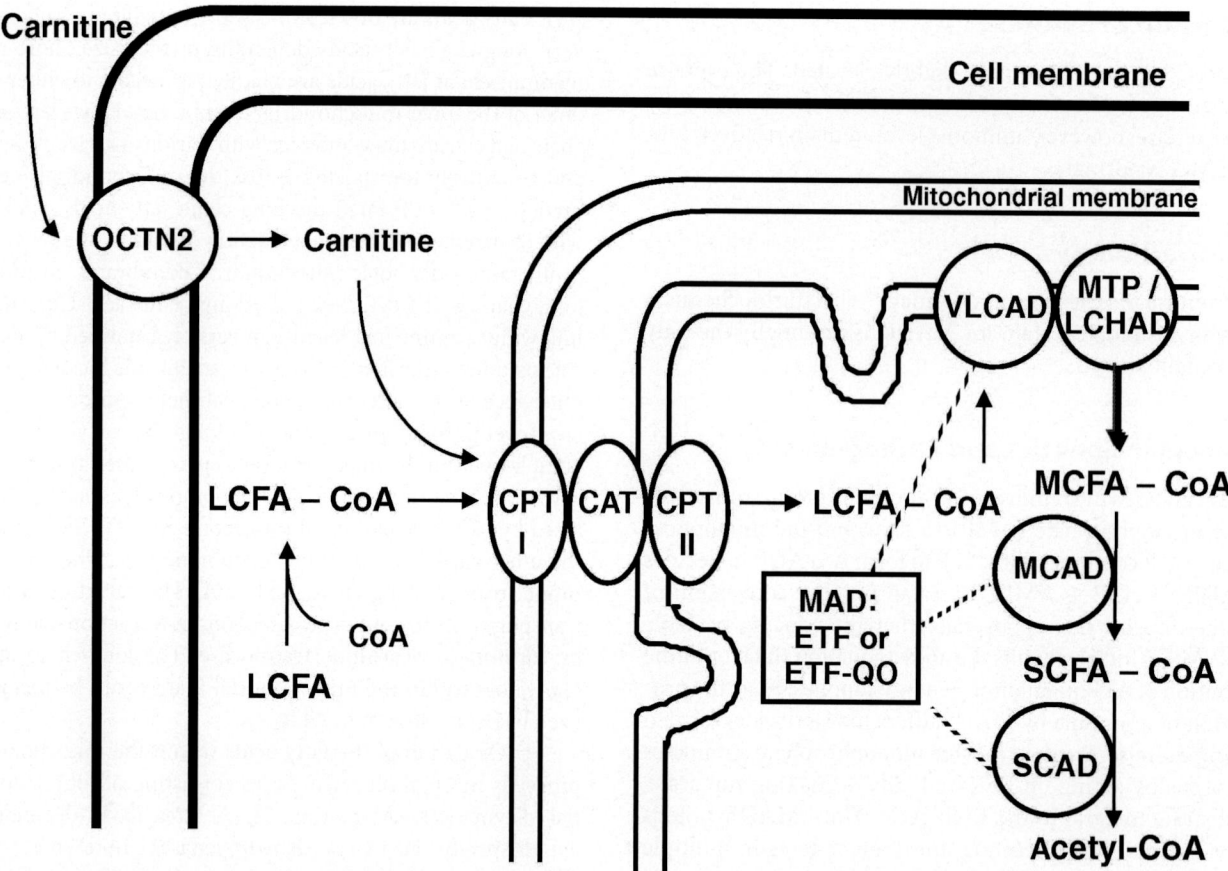

Figure 29-6. Simplified scheme of mitochondrial fatty acid oxidation. CAT, carnitine acylcarnitine translocase; CPT I, carnitine palmitoyl transferase I; CPT II, carnitine palmitoyl transferase II; LCFA, long-chain fatty acid; LCHAD, long-chain 3-hydroxyacyl-CoA dehydrogenase; MAD, multiple acyl-CoA dehydrogenase; MCAD, medium-chain acyl-CoA dehydrogenase; MCFA, medium-chain fatty acid; MTP, mitochondrial trifunctional protein; OCTN2, plasma membrane sodium-dependent carnitine transporter; SCAD, short-chain acyl-CoA dehydrogenase; SCFA, short-chain fatty acid; VLCAD, very-long-chain acyl-CoA dehydrogenase. (Reproduced with permission from Laforet P, Vianey-Sabab C. Disorders of muscle lipid metabolism: diagnostic and therapeutic changes. *Neuromuscul Disord.* 2010;20(11):693–700.)

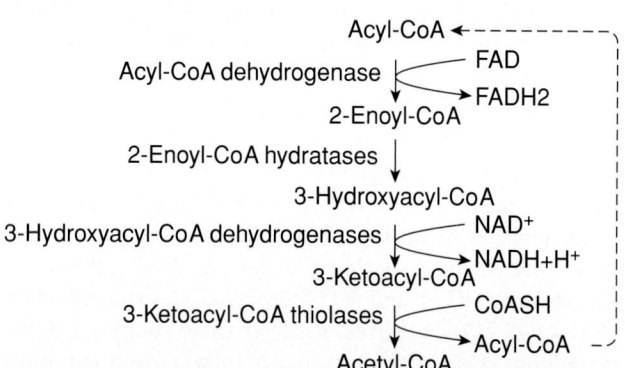

Figure 29-7. β-Oxidation of fatty acids pathway. There are four steps involved in the complete oxidation of fatty acids. The main defects in this pathway affecting muscle involve deficiencies of the acyl-CoA dehydrogenases. The details of each reaction are given in the text. (Reproduced with permission from Walsh RJ. Metabolic Myopathies. *Continuum.* 2006; 12(3):76–120.)

of CPT2, VLCAD, and trifunctional protein). Some defects result in both fixed weakness and recurrent bouts of rhabdomyolysis (e.g., VLCAD and trifunctional protein deficiencies).

Diagnostic workup depends on the clinical presentation.[160-163] In patients with fixed progressive weakness, other more common disorders as muscular dystrophy or congenital myopathy are typically suspected. The diagnosis of a lipid storage disease is often only suspected after a biopsy is performed and it shows a vacuolar myopathy with abnormal lipid accumulation (Fig. 29-8). The next step is to assess total and free carnitine levels and serum acylcarnitine. Typically, the carnitine and acylcarnitine levels are markedly reduced in primary carnitine deficiency. In the acyl-CoA dehydrogenases deficiencies including multi–acyl-CoA dehydrogenase deficiency (MADD), specific patterns are seen on the acylcarnitine and urine organic acid profiles. If the carnitine levels, acylcarnitine profile, and the urine for organic acids are not remarkable, then one needs to consider a form of neutral lipid storage disease. In such cases, there is increase in triglycerides (TGs) in the tissues

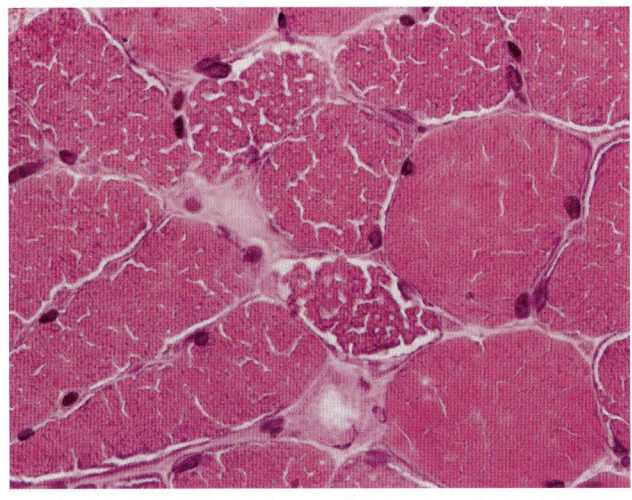
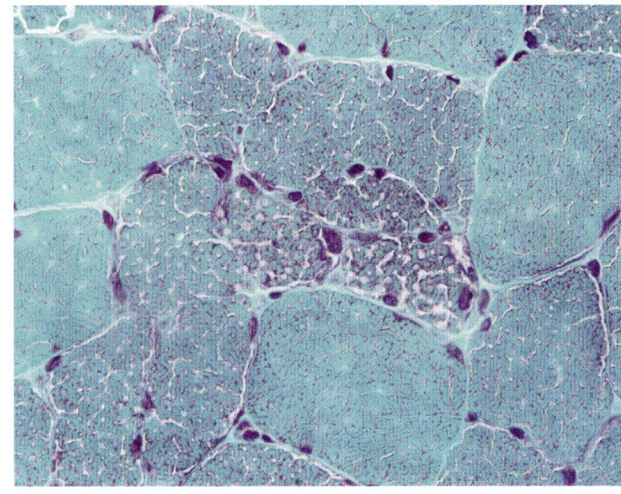
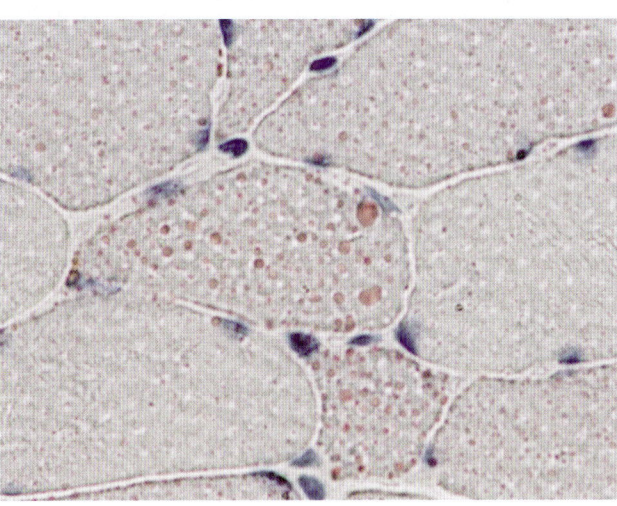

Figure 29-8. Multi-acyl-CoA dehydrogenase deficiency (MADD). Muscle biopsy demonstrates vacuoles within muscle fibers on H&E (**A**) and modified Gomori trichrome (**B**) that are filled by lipid deposition within fibers on oil red O stain (**C**).

(not fatty acids). A blood smear may show the accumulation of TG droplets, the so-called Jordan anomaly (Fig. 29-9).

Lipid storage disorders should also be suspected in cases of recurrent myoglobinuria following prolonged physical exertion—the time when fatty acid metabolism is needed for ATP production. Also, cases of myoglobinuria following a febrile illness or fasting should lead to consideration of a lipid storage disease. We usually start the workup with an exercise forearm test, which should be normal. Serum for acylcarnitine profile and urine for organic acid analysis are sent, and if abnormal may give a clue as to the exact enzyme defect and subsequent targeted genetic testing. The most common cause of recurrent myoglobinuria (when one is found) is CPT2 deficiency. Therefore, if the above tests are not revealing, the next step is to do genetic testing for the most common mutations associated with CPT2 deficiency. If this is normal, then we usually proceed with a muscle biopsy or skin biopsy for fibroblasts and send specimens for analysis of various lipid enzymes. In children with recurrent episodes of myoglobinuria in the setting of febrile illness, who have

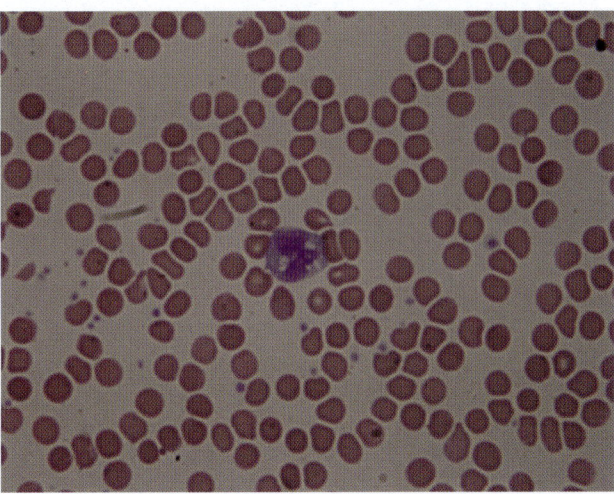

Figure 29-9. Jordan anomaly. Blood smear demonstrates clear lipid droplets (triglyceride) within a polymorphonuclear cell in a case of neutral lipid storage disorder.

normal serum acylcarnitine profile and urine organic acids, one needs to also consider lipin deficiency.

Please see the below discussion of specific lipid storage diseases for further details.

CARNITINE TRANSPORTER DEFICIENCY (PRIMARY CARNITINE DEFICIENCY)

Clinical Features

Primary systemic carnitine deficiency is a clinically heterogeneous disorder.[192–210] Some patients with primary carnitine deficiency develop symptoms and signs resembling Reye syndrome in early childhood with acute attacks of vomiting, altered mental status, hypoglycemia, and hepatomegaly.[193,195,202,204,205] These children may become weak, but the systemic manifestations tend to overshadow the myopathy. More commonly, individuals who are affected present with a hypertrophic or dilated cardiomyopathy and progressive proximal muscle weakness, and atrophy in childhood or early adult life.[197,198,206–210] Rhabdomyolysis and respiratory weakness can occur.[211] Infantile onset has also been described. A few cases have worsened significantly during pregnancy or in the postpartum period.[210]

Secondary carnitine deficiency may result from a variety of disorders, including respiratory chain defects, organic aciduria, endocrinopathies, dystrophies, and renal and liver failure, malnutrition, and as a toxic effect of certain medications.[199,212] It is not known if the secondary deficiency of carnitine can in and of itself causes a myopathy.

Laboratory Features

Plasma and tissue (including muscle) carnitine levels are markedly diminished in primary carnitine deficiency, while the levels are only moderately reduced (25%–50% normal) in secondary forms of carnitine deficiency.[192–195,199,206,213] Serum acylcarnitine levels are also reduced. Serum CK levels are normal in approximately 50% of patients with the myopathic form of the disease but can be elevated to as much as 15 times normal. In primary systemic carnitine deficiency, liver enzymes are also elevated. Fasting individuals with carnitine deficiency may develop hypoglycemia, acidosis, and elevated CK levels and liver function tests. However, ketones are not elevated in the urine during fasting.

EMG may reveal increased insertional activity with positive sharp waves, fibrillation potentials, and complex repetitive discharges. Early recruitment of short-duration, small-amplitude, and polyphasic MUAPs can be observed. An echocardiogram can demonstrate a dilated or hypertrophic cardiomyopathy.

Histopathology

Muscle biopsies reveal variability in muscle fiber size and abnormal accumulation of lipid in the subsarcolemma and intermyofibrillar regions (Fig. 29-10). Type 1 fibers are preferentially affected, as would be expected, given that oxidative metabolism primarily occurs in these fibers. EM also demonstrates increased lipid (Fig. 29-11). Muscle carnitine levels are dramatically decreased (<2%–4% of normal) in patients with primary carnitine deficiency (this may serve to distinguish from patients with secondary deficiency).

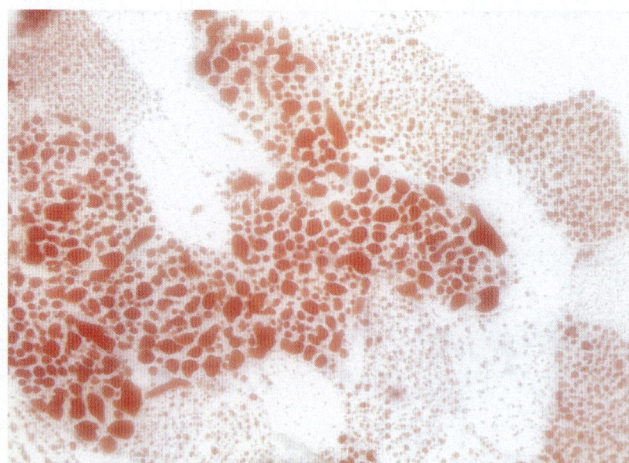

Figure 29-10. Carnitine deficiency. Muscle biopsy demonstrates increased lipid droplets within muscle fibers (*Oil red O*).

Molecular Genetics and Pathogenesis

Primary carnitine deficiency is caused by mutations in the gene encoding for the sodium-dependent carnitine transporter protein, *OCTN2* (also called *SLC22A5*) located on chromosome 5q33.1.[214] Carnitine is supplied to tissues by diet and endogenous synthesis. Intracellular carnitine levels are maintained at 20–50 times the extracellular concentration by this active transport system (Fig. 29-6). The deficiency of carnitine impairs the transport of long-chain fatty acids into the inner mitochondrial matrix, thus severely affecting energy production from these fatty acids.

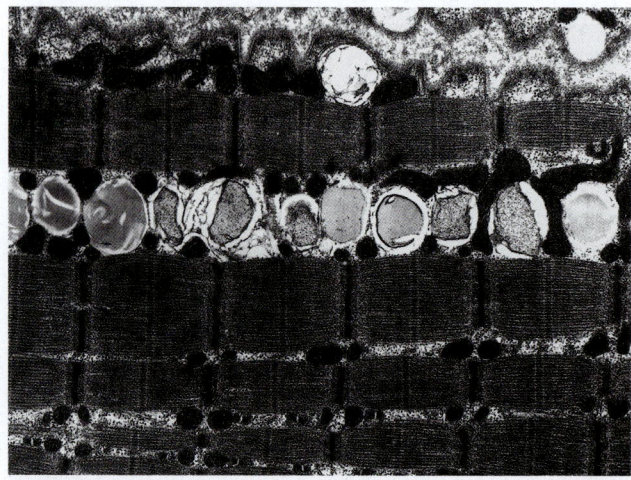

Figure 29-11. Electron microscopy reveals increased endomysial lipid droplets.

Treatment

Oral L-carnitine (100–200 mg/kg/day) benefits some, but not all patients, with carnitine deficiency.[192–194,200,206,211,215–217] There can be a dramatic clinical response to oral L-carnitine in patients with severe cardiomyopathy and muscle weakness.[206] However, only modest increases in muscle carnitine levels have been demonstrated, even in those who improved in muscle strength.[206] Perhaps, intracellular (muscle) concentration of carnitine only needs to be more than 2%–4% of normal to allow for normal lipid metabolism.

CARNITINE PALMITOYL TRANSFERASE 2 DEFICIENCY

Clinical Features

Carnitine palmitoyl transferase 2 (CPT2) deficiency is inherited in an autosomal-recessive manner and typically presents in the second or third decade of life with muscular pain and myoglobinuria following intense or prolonged exertion.[192–194,218–221] Prolonged fasting and infection are other precipitating factors. The neuromuscular examination is usually normal between bouts of rhabdomyolysis. Rarely CPT2 deficiency can manifest as a severe and fatal cardiomyopathy in infancy or early childhood.

Laboratory Features

Serum CK levels are usually normal, except when the patient performs intense physical activities or fasts. Exercise forearm test is normal, which can also help distinguish CPT2 deficiency from the glycogen storage disorders which can also cause exercise-induced rhabdomyolysis. Muscle and serum carnitine levels are normal. EMG is usually unremarkable, although myopathic units may be seen. EKG is also normal.

Histopathology

There is usually no gross abnormality noted on light microscopic examination of muscle tissue. However, an increase in the lipid content of muscle may be apparent on EM.

Molecular Genetics and Pathogenesis

This disorder is caused by mutations in the *CPT2* gene located on chromosome 1p32.[220] The resultant deficiency of CPT2 impairs the transport of acylcarnitine across the inner mitochondrial membrane (Fig. 29-6). Thus, the generation of ATP from fatty acid metabolism is diminished. Interestingly, CPT1 deficiency does not usually cause a myopathy.

Treatment

A high-protein, low-fat diet with frequent meals should be advised. Avoidance of prolonged strenuous activity, cold temperatures, and fasting may prevent episodes of rhabdomyolysis. During febrile illness, patients should be instructed to increase their intake of complex carbohydrates and again avoid fasting.

VERY LONG-CHAIN ACYL-CoA DEHYDROGENASE (VLCAD) DEFICIENCY

Clinical Features

VLCAD deficiency is a clinically heterogeneous disorder with three major phenotypes.[222–231] The disorder most commonly manifests in childhood with an early onset of hypertrophic cardiomyopathy, recurrent episodes of hypoketotic hypoglycemia and dicarboxylic aciduria, and a high mortality rate (50%–75%). There is a milder form characterized by episodes of hypoketotic hypoglycemia and dicarboxylic aciduria, minimal if any cardiac involvement, and low mortality. In addition, VLCAD deficiency can rarely present similar to CPT deficiency, with exercise-induced myoglobinuria beginning in early childhood to early adulthood.

Laboratory Features

Serum CK is elevated with myoglobinuria as expected. Between attacks, the CK may be normal. There can be a secondary deficiency of carnitine, in particular with muscle. There is an increase in plasma concentration of tetradecanoic acid ($C_{14:1}$) with normal levels of myristic acid ($C_{14:1}$), consistent with a defect in β-oxidation of long-chain fatty acids.[227,230] Reduced VLCAD activity can be demonstrated in cultured fibroblasts and lymphocytes.[230] EMG may reveal myopathic-appearing MUAPs.

Histopathology

Muscle biopsies may demonstrate abnormal accumulation of lipid.

Molecular Genetics and Pathogenesis

This myopathy is caused by mutations in the *ACADVL*, which is located on chromosome 17p11.2–p13.1 that encodes for VLCAD.[222,223,229,230] Patients with this enzyme deficiency have impaired ability to metabolize very–long-chain fatty acids (Fig. 29-6). Some of the previously described cases of long-chain acyl-CoA deficiency probably in fact had very–long-chain CoA deficiency.[229]

Treatment

A low-fat/high-carbohydrate diet in which long-chain fatty acids are partially replaced by medium-chain TGs may be effective in preventing attacks of hypoketotic hypoglycemia, dicarboxylic aciduria, and myoglobinuria in some,[226,231] but not all patients.[227] Affected individuals should be instructed to avoid fasting.

LONG-CHAIN ACYL-CoA DEHYDROGENASE (LCAD) DEFICIENCY

Clinical Features

LCAD usually presents in infancy with failure to thrive, hepatomegaly, cardiomegaly, nonketotic hypoglycemia, and an encephalopathy resembling Reye syndrome.[232–234] Individuals who are affected may develop exercise intolerance with attacks of rhabdomyolysis and proximal weakness.

Laboratory Features

Serum CK is elevated during attacks of muscle pain and cramps. Total and free carnitine levels are reduced in the plasma, liver, and muscle, but long-chain acylcarnitine esters are increased. Diagnosis is suggested by demonstrating decreased LCAD activity in cultured fibroblasts.[232]

Histopathology

Muscle biopsies reportedly demonstrate abnormal accumulation of lipid.

Molecular Genetics and Pathogenesis

LCAD is caused by mutations in the *ACADL* gene located on 2q34–q35. However, as previously noted, some reported cases of LCAD deficiency were in fact patients with VLCAD deficiency.[229] LCAD acts on fatty acyl-CoA derivatives whose acyl residues contain more than 12 carbon atoms. Patients with LCAD deficiency have an impaired ability to metabolize long-chain fatty acids.

Treatment

Intravenous glucose has led to relief of the myalgias and lowering of the serum CK levels in some patients.[232] Carnitine can improve the cardiomyopathy but does not affect skeletal muscle strength.[232]

MEDIAN-CHAIN ACYL-CoA DEHYDROGENASE (MCAD) DEFICIENCY

Clinical Features

MCAD is the most common form of acyl-CoA deficiency, but unlike defects in long-chain fatty acid metabolism, this deficiency is only rarely associated with cardiac or skeletal muscle involvement.[235–239] However, rare episodes of rhabdomyolysis and acute encephalopathy have been reported in infancy and late in life.[235,238,240,241]

Laboratory Features

MCAD activity is diminished to <10% in muscle, fibroblasts, lymphocytes, and liver.[235,236,240] A secondary deficiency of carnitine may be evident in the plasma, liver, and muscle. Dicarboxylic, adipic, and sebacic acids are increased in the urine.

Histopathology

Muscle biopsy is notable only for excess lipid.

Molecular Genetics and Pathogenesis

The disorder is caused by mutations within the *ACADM* gene located on chromosome 1p31 that encodes for MCAD. MCAD acts on fatty acyl-CoA derivatives whose acyl residues contain 4–14 carbon atoms.

Treatment

Carnitine may improve the hepatomegaly and urinary organic acid profile and prevent attacks of rhabdomyolysis and encephalopathy, although there is some concern that carnitine supplementation is ineffective and possibly dangerous.[239] Fasting should be avoided.

SHORT-CHAIN ACYL-CoA DEHYDROGENASE (SCAD) DEFICIENCY

Clinical Features

Patients with SCAD deficiency may manifest with a wide range of features, including dysmorphic facial features, feeding difficulties, failure to thrive, metabolic acidosis, ketotic hypoglycemia, lethargy, developmental delay, seizures, hypotonia, dystonia, and myopathy.[237,242–248] In regard to the myopathy, it presents as exercise intolerance, myalgias, or progressive proximal weakness, which may be present in infancy or may develop in early to mid-adulthood. Facial weakness, ptosis, progressive external ophthalmoplegia, respiratory weakness, and cardiomyopathy have also been described.[243] Some infants present with failure to thrive and nonketotic hypoglycemia.

Laboratory Features

Serum CK and carnitine levels are usually normal. Serum acylcarnitine profile reveals increased butyrylcarnitine (C4) concentration.[245,246] There is increased urinary excretion of short-chain metabolites ethylmalonate and methylsuccinate.

Histopathology

The few reports of muscle biopsies have demonstrated excess lipid. Muscle carnitine levels may be secondarily reduced. SCAD deficiency can be demonstrated in muscle tissue. Multicore myopathy has also been reported in the setting of SCAD.[243]

Molecular Genetics and Pathogenesis

Genetic defects have been localized to the *ACADS* located at 12q22–qter, which encodes for SCAD.[248,249] SCAD acts on fatty acyl-CoA derivatives whose acyl residues contain four to six carbon atoms.

Treatment

No specific medical therapy has been shown to be beneficial, including carnitine supplementation.

MITOCHONDRIAL TRIFUNCTIONAL PROTEIN DEFICIENCY/HYDROXYACYL-CoA DEHYDROGENASE DEFICIENCY

Clinical Features

Mitochondrial trifunctional protein (MTP) is a complex of eight subunits, that includes long-chain hydroxyacyl-CoA dehydrogenase (HAD). MTP/long-chain HAD deficiency is clinically heterogeneous. It can present in infancy or early childhood with Reye-like syndrome, nausea, vomiting, seizures, hypoketotic hypoglycemia, respiratory failure, and cardiomyopathy.[250–258] Mortality is high (approximately 50%) due to the cardiomyopathy. Progressive weakness and recurrent episodes of myoglobinuria become more prevalent later in childhood. Some individuals who are affected develop a progressive sensorimotor polyneuropathy, sensory ganglionopathy, and pigmentary retinopathy.[255,258] Mothers of an affected fetus can develop distinctive complications of pregnancy: hemolysis, elevated liver enzymes, low platelets (HELLP) and acute fatty liver of pregnancy (AFLP).[253]

Laboratory Features

Serum CK and lactate levels may be elevated. Urinary organic acids reveal dicarboxylic aciduria and 3-hydroxydicarboxylic aciduria. Acylcarnitine profile demonstrates increased long chains. An assay of cultured fibroblasts can demonstrate the deficiency of long-chain HAD deficiency or genetic testing can be done to confirm the diagnosis. NCS may reveal features suggestive of an axonal sensorimotor neuropathy, while myopathic MUAPs are apparent on EMG in weak muscles.

Histopathology

Muscle biopsies reveal an abnormal accumulation of lipids, although this increase is not as prominent as that observed in other disorders of β-oxidation. A nerve biopsy in one patient demonstrated marked loss of myelinated nerve fibers and axonal degeneration.

Molecular Genetics and Pathogenesis

The disorder is inherited in an autosomal-recessive pattern and is caused by mutations in the *HADHB* gene located on chromosome 2p23 that encodes for long-chain HAD. Long-chain HAD catalyzes the third step in β-oxidation: the conversion of 3-hydroxyacyl-CoA derivatives to 3-ketoacyl-CoA derivatives. Deficiency of the enzyme leads to impairment in metabolism of long-chain fatty acids (Fig. 29-5).

Treatment

Patients may benefit from a high-carbohydrate, low-fat protein diet with or without supplementation with medium-chain TGs, riboflavin, and L-carnitine supplementation.[250,257] Patients should avoid fasting.

MULTI–ACYL-CoA DEHYDROGENASE DEFICIENCY (MADD)

Clinical Features

MADD, also known as glutaric aciduria type II, usually manifests with progressive proximal weakness and atrophy associated with episodes of confusion, ataxia, tremor, nausea, vomiting, hypoketotic hypoglycemia, lethargy, and hepatomegaly in infancy or early childhood.[192–194,259–269] Some patients present with recurrent episodes of exercise-induced myoglobinuria later in childhood or adult life similar to CPT2 deficiency or with proximal or distal weakness.[262,263]

Laboratory Features

NCSs demonstrate an axonal sensory neuropathy, while the EMG may reveal myopathic-appearing MUAPs. Serum acylcarnitine analysis usually reveals increased concentrations of all chain lengths, but mainly medium- and long-chain acylcarnitines. The plasma-free carnitine level is usually decreased but can sometimes be normal. Urine organic acid demonstrates C5–C10 dicarboxylic aciduria and acylglycine derivatives. Reduced ETF-QO activity can be demonstrated in cultured fibroblasts.[261] Genetic testing is available to confirm a mutation.

Histopathology

Muscle biopsies reveal vacuoles with abnormal accumulation of lipid (Fig. 29-8).

Molecular Genetics and Pathogenesis

The disorder can result from deficiency of any of three subunits of the enzyme complex: the alpha or β subunits of ETF (ETFA or ETFB) and ETF dehydrogenase (ETF-QO). These genes map as follows: ETFA to 15q23–q25, ETFB to 19q13.3, and ETF-QO to 4q32–qter. ETF transfers electrons from reduced forms of acyl-CoA dehydrogenase to the respiratory chain via ETF-QO. ETF-QO transfers electrons from ETF to ubiquinone (Fig. 29-5). Defects in these enzymes result in the inability to oxidize the reduced forms of various dehydrogenases including VLCAD, LCAD, MCAD, and SCAD.

Treatment

Fasting should be avoided. Carnitine supplementation does not appear to help, although both low-fat diets[260,268] and riboflavin[261,264-267] have been reported to provide significant benefit.

NEUTRAL LIPID STORAGE DISEASE

Clinical Features

Neutral lipid storage disease is characterized by systemic accumulation of TGs in the cytoplasm and includes two distinct diseases: (1) neutral lipid storage disease with myopathy (NLSDM), (2) neutral lipid storage disease with ichthyosis (NLSDI) also called Chanarin–Dorfman syndrome (Fig. 29-12).[192-194,270-274] Patients with NLSDM may present with generalized weakness, distal myopathy, or cardiomyopathy. Patients with NLSDI present with similar weakness along with ichthyosis.

Laboratory Features

Serum CK is usually mildly elevated. EMG is myopathic and can show muscle membrane irritability. Plasma carnitine profile reveals normal or mildly reduced total and free carnitine. Plasma acylcarnitine profile and serum/urine organic acids are normal. Peripheral blood smear reveal lipid-containing vacuoles in leukocytes (Jordan anomaly) (Fig. 29-9).

Histopathology

Muscle biopsies reveal excess lipid.

Molecular Genetics and Pathogenesis

NLSDM is caused by mutations in the *PNPLA2* gene that encodes adipose triglyceride lipase (ATGL), which is also referred to as patatin-like phospholipase domain–containing protein 2 (PNPLA2).[272,273] This protein catalyzes the initial step in TG hydrolysis. NLSDI is due to defects in the gene that encodes the co-activator of ATGL, comparative gene identification-58 (CGI-58), which is also known as abhydrolase domain–containing 5 (ABHD5).[274] Mutations in these genes lead to accumulation of TGs in muscle.

Treatment

There is no specific medical therapy.

PHOSPHATIDIC ACID PHOSPHATASE (LIPIN) DEFICIENCY

Clinical Features

Phosphatidic acid phosphatase (lipin) deficiency is another recently recognized disorder associated with TG metabolism. It usually manifests in children with recurrent bouts of myoglobinuria in the setting of febrile illness, but it has also been associated with exertional myalgias and has been reported in adults.[275-280] Clinical examination is otherwise unremarkable.

Laboratory Features

Serum CK is elevated. Total and free carnitine, plasma acylcarnitine profile, and urine organic acid levels are normal.

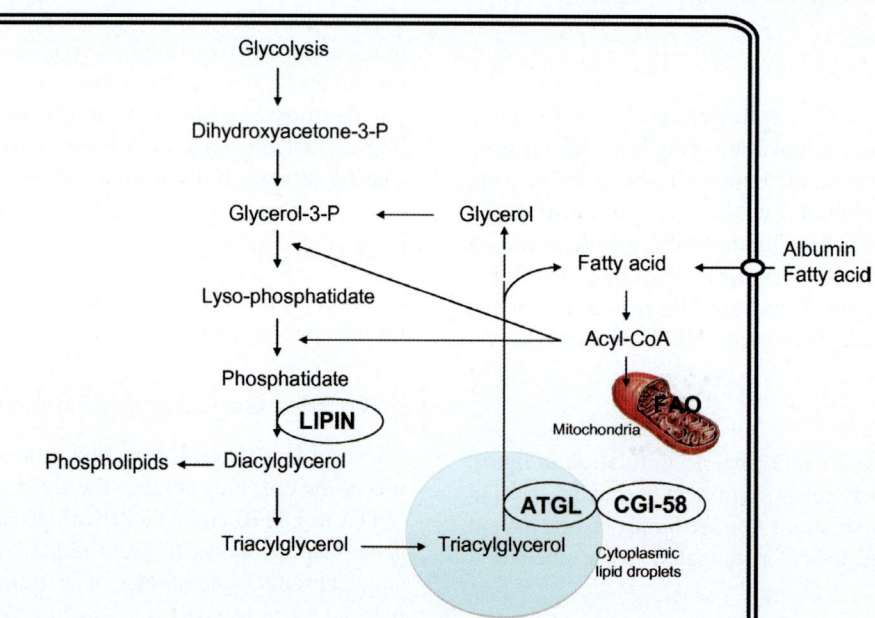

Figure 29-12. Simplified scheme of lipid metabolism. ATGL, adipose triglyceride lipase; CGI-58, activator of ATGL; FAO, fatty acid oxidation; LIPIN, phosphatidic acid phosphatase. (Reproduced with permission from Laforet P, Vianey-Sabab C. Disorders of muscle lipid metabolism: diagnostic and therapeutic changes. *Neuromuscul Disord*. 2010;20(11):693–700.)

Histopathology

Muscle biopsies may reveal excess lipid or can be normal.

Molecular Genetics and Pathogenesis

Phosphatidic acid phosphatase (lipin) deficiency is caused by mutations in the *LPN1* gene. Phosphatidic acid phosphatase is important in TG synthetase and catalyzes the conversion of phosphatidate to diacylglycerol (Fig. 29-12).

Treatment

There is no specific medical therapy.

▶ SUMMARY

Evaluating patients with possible metabolic myopathies can be quite daunting. A basic understanding of carbohydrate and lipid metabolism and effects of exercise as provided in this chapter is necessary. We hope that clinicians will find our approach to these patients helpful.

REFERENCES

1. Tarnopolsky MA. Myopathies related to glycogen metabolism disorders. *Neurotherapeutics*. 2018;15:915–927.
2. Cohen BH. Mitochondrial and metabolic myopathies. *Continuum (Minneap Minn)*. 2019;25:1732–1766.
3. DiMauro S, Miranda AF, Sakoda S, et al. Metabolic myopathies. *Am J Med Genet*. 1986;25(4):635–651.
4. Meinck HM, Goebel HH, Rumpf KW, Kaiser H, Neumann P. The forearm ischaemic work test—hazardous to McArdle's patients? *J Neurol Neurosurg Psychiatry*. 1982;45:1144–1146.
5. Kollberg G, Tulinius M, Gilljam T, et al. Cardiomyopathy and exercise intolerance in muscle glycogen storage disease 0. *N Engl J Med*. 2007;357(15):1507–1514.
6. Cameron JM, Levandovskiy V, MacKay N, et al. Identification of a novel mutation in GYS1 (muscle-specific glycogen synthase) resulting in sudden cardiac death, that is diagnosable from skin fibroblasts. *Mol Genet Metab*. 2009;98(4):378–382.
7. Sukigara S, Liang WC, Komaki H, et al. Muscle glycogen storage disease 0 presenting recurrent syncope with weakness and myalgia. *Neuromuscul Disord*. 2012;22(2):162–165.
8. Musumeci O, Pugliese A, Oteri R, et al. A new phenotype of muscle glycogen synthase deficiency (GSD0B) characterized by an adult onset myopathy without cardiomyopathy. *Neuromuscul Disord*. 2022;32(7):582–589.
9. Barohn RJ, McVey AL, DiMauro S. Adult acid maltase deficiency. *Muscle Nerve*. 1993;16:672–676.
10. Engel AG. Acid maltase deficiency in adults: studies in four cases of a syndrome which may mimic muscular dystrophy or other myopathies. *Brain*. 1970;93:599–616.
11. Hogan GR, Gutmann L, Schmidt R, Gilbert E. Pompe's disease. *Neurology*. 1969;19:894–900.
12. Hudgson P, Gardner-Medwin D, Worsfold M, Pennington RJ, Walton JN. Adult myopathy from glycogen storage disease due to acid maltase deficiency. *Brain*. 1968;91:435–460.
13. Karpati G, Carpenter S, Engel AG, et al. The syndrome of systemic carnitine deficiency: clinical, morphologic, biochemical, and pathophysiologic features. *Neurology*. 1975;25(1):16–24.
14. Rosen EC, Engel AG. Acid maltase deficiency in adults presenting as respiratory failure. *Am J Med*. 1978;64:485–491.
15. Roth JC, Williams HE. The muscular variant of Pompe's disease. *J Pediatr*. 1967;71:567–573.
16. Smith J, Zellweger H, Afifi AK. Muscular form of glycogenosis, type II (Pompe). *Neurology*. 1967;17:537–549.
17. Bodamer OA, Leonard JV, Halliday D. Dietary treatment in late-onset acid maltase deficiency. *Eur J Pediatr*. 1997;156(suppl 1):S39–S42.
18. Engel AG, Gomez MR, Seybold ME, Lambert EH. The spectrum and diagnosis of acid maltase deficiency. *Neurology*. 1975;23:95–106.
19. Loonen MC, Busch HF, Koster JF, et al. Family with different clinical forms of acid maltase deficiency (glycogenosis type II): biochemical and genetic studies. *Neurology*. 1981;31(10):1209–1216.
20. Pompe JC. Over idiopatsche hypertrophie van net hart. *Ned Tijdschr Geneeskd*. 1932;76:304–312.
21. Smith HL, Amick LD, Sidbury JB. Type II glycogenosis: report of a case with four-year survival and absence of acid maltase associated with abnormal glycogen. *Am J Dis Child*. 1966;111:475–481.
22. Swaiman KF, Kennedy WR, Sauls HS. Late infantile acid maltase deficiency. *Arch Neurol*. 1968;18:642–648.
23. Zellweger H, Brown BI, McCormick WF, Tu J. A mild form of muscular glycogenosis in two brothers with alpha-1,4-glucosidase deficiency. *Ann Pediatr (Paris)*. 1965;205:413–437.
24. Fadic R, Waclawik AJ, Brooks BR, Lotz BP. The rigid spine syndrome due to acid maltase deficiency. *Muscle Nerve*. 1997;20:364–366.
25. Engel AG, Dale AJ. Autophagic glycogenosis of late onset with mitochondrial abnormalities: light and electron microscopic observations. *Mayo Clin Proc*. 1968;43:233–279.
26. Felice KJ, Alesssi AG, Grunnet ML. Clinical variability in adult-onset acid maltase deficiency: report of affected sibs and review of the literature. *Medicine*. 1995;74:131–135.
27. Wokke JH, Ausems MG, van den Boogaard MJ, et al. Genotype–phenotype correlation in adult-onset acid maltase deficiency. *Ann Neurol*. 1995;38(3):450–454.
28. Umapathysivam K, Hopwood JJ, Meikle PJ. Determination of acid alpha-glucosidase activity in blood spots as a diagnostic test for Pompe disease. *Clin Chem*. 2001;47:1378–1383.
29. Kallwass H, Carr C, Gerrein J, et al. Rapid diagnosis of late-onset Pompe disease by fluorometric assay of alpha-glucosidase activities in dried blood spots. *Mol Genet Metab*. 2007;90(4):449–452.
30. Vissing J, Lukacs Z, Straub V. Diagnosis of Pompe disease: muscle biopsy vs blood-based assays. *JAMA Neurol*. 2013;70:923–927.
31. American Association of Neuromuscular & Electrodiagnostic Medicine. Diagnostic criteria for late-onset (childhood and adult) Pompe disease. *Muscle Nerve*. 2009;40:149–160.
32. de Jager AE, van der Vliet TM, van der Ree TC, Oosterink BJ, Loonen MC. Muscle computer tomography in adult-onset acid maltase deficiency. *Muscle Nerve*. 1998;21:398–400.
33. Pichiecchio A, Uggetti C, Ravaglia S, et al. Muscle MRI in adult-onset acid maltase deficiency. *Neuromuscul Disord*. 2004;14:51–55.

34. Alejaldre A, Díaz-Manera J, Ravaglia S, et al. Trunk muscle involvement in late-onset Pompe disease: study of thirty patients. *Neuromuscul Disord.* 2012;22(suppl 2):S148–S154.
35. Díaz-Manera J, Walter G, Straub V. Skeletal muscle magnetic resonance imaging in Pompe disease. *Muscle Nerve.* 2021;63:640–650.
36. Buckley BH, Hutchins GM. Pompe's disease presenting as hypertrophic myocardiopathy with Wolfe–Parkinson–White syndrome. *Am Heart J.* 1978;96:246–252.
37. Francesconi M, Auff E, Ursin C, Sluga E. WPW-syndrome kombiniert mit AV-block 2 bei einer adulten form einer glycogenose type II. *Wien Klin Wochenschr.* 1982;94:401–404.
38. Gambetti PL, DiMauro S, Baker L. Nervous system in Pompe's disease. *J Neuropathol Exp Neurol.* 1971;30:412–430.
39. Mancall EL, Aponte GE, Berry RG. Pompe's disease (diffuse glycogenosis) with neuronal storage. *J Neuropathol Exp Neurol.* 1965;24:85–96.
40. Raben N, Nichols RC, Boerkoel C, Plotz P. Genetic defects in patients with glycogenosis type II (acid maltase deficiency). *Muscle Nerve.* 1995;(suppl 3):S70–S74.
41. Reuser AJ, Kroos MA, Hermans MM, et al. Glycogenosis type II (acid maltase deficiency). *Muscle Nerve.* 1995;(suppl 3):S61–S69.
42. Kleijer WJ, van der Kraan M, Kroos MA, et al. Prenatal diagnosis of glycogen storage disease type II: enzyme assay or mutation analysis? *Pediatr Res.* 1995;38:103–106.
43. Kroos MA, Van der Kraan M, Van Diggelen OP, Klejer WJ, Reuser AJ. Two extremes of the clinical spectrum of glycogen storage disease type II in one family: a matter of genotype. *Hum Mutat.* 1997;9:17–22.
44. Kishnani PS, Corzo D, Nicolino M, et al. Recombinant human acid [alpha]-glucosidase: major clinical benefits in infantile-onset Pompe disease. *Neurology.* 2007;68:99–109.
45. van der Ploeg AT, Clemens P, Corzo D, et al. A randomized study of alglucosidase alfa in late-onset Pompe's disease. *N Engl J Med.* 2010;362(15):1396–1406.
46. Toscano A, Schoser B. Enzyme replacement therapy in late-onset Pompe disease: a systematic literature review. *J Neurol.* 2013;260:951–959.
47. Cupler EJ, Berger KI, Leshner RT, et al; AANEM Consensus Committee on Late-onset Pompe Disease. Consensus treatment recommendations for late-onset Pompe disease. *Muscle Nerve.* 2012;45:319–333.
48. Diaz-Manera J, Kishnani PS, Kushlaf H, et al; COMET Investigator Group. Safety and efficacy of avalglucosidase alfa versus alglucosidase alfa in patients with late-onset Pompe disease (COMET): a phase 3, randomised, multicentre trial. *Lancet Neurol.* 2021;20(12):1012–1026. Erratum in: *Lancet Neurol.* 2022;21(4):e4.
49. Dimachkie MM, Barohn RJ, Byrne B, et al; NEO-EXT investigators. Long-term safety and efficacy of avalglucosidase alfa in patients with late-onset pompe disease. *Neurology.* 2022:99(5):e536–e548.
50. Schoser B, et al; PROPEL Study Group. Safety and efficacy of cipaglucosidase alfa plus miglustat versus alglucosidase alfa plus placebo in late-onset Pompe disease (PROPEL): an international, randomised, double-blind, parallel-group, phase 3 trial. *Lancet Neurol.* 2021;20(12):1027–1037.
51. Kishnani PS, Goldenberg PC, DeArmey SL, et al. Cross-reactive immunologic material status affects treatment outcomes in Pompe disease infants. *Mol Genet Metab.* 2010;99:26–33.
52. Banugaria SG, Prater SN, Ng YK, et al. The impact of antibodies on clinical outcomes in diseases treated with therapeutic protein: lessons learned from infantile Pompe disease. *Genet Med.* 2011;13:729–736.
53. Brunberg JA, McCormick WF, Schochet SS. Type III glycogenosis: an adult with diffuse weakness and muscle wasting. *Arch Neurol.* 1971;25:171–178.
54. Coleman RA, Winter HS, Wolf B, Gilchrist JM, Chen YT. Glycogen storage disease type III (glycogen debranching enzyme deficiency): correlation of biochemical defects with myopathy and cardiomyopathy. *Ann Intern Med.* 1992;116:896–900.
55. Cornelio G, Bresolin N, Singer PA, DiMauro S, Rowland LP. Clinical varieties of neuromuscular disease in debrancher deficiency. *Arch Neurol.* 1984;41:1027–1032.
56. Moses SW, Gadoth N, Bashan N, Ben-David E, Slonim A, Wanderman KL. Neuromuscular involvement in glycogen storage disease type III. *Acta Paediatr Scand.* 1986;75:289–296.
57. Decostre V, Laforêt P, De Antonio M, et al. Long term longitudinal study of muscle function in patients with glycogen storage disease type IIIa. *Mol Genet Metab.* 2017;122(3):108–116.
58. Ding JH, de Barsy T, Brown BI, Coleman RA, Chen YT. Immunoblot analyses of glycogen debranching enzyme in different subtypes of glycogen storage disease type III. *J Pediatr.* 1990;116(1):95–100.
59. DiMauro S, Hartwig GB, Hays A, et al. Debrancher deficiency: neuromuscular disorder in 5 adults. *Ann Neurol.* 1979;5:422–436.
60. Fukuda T, Sugie H, Ioto M, Tsurui S, Sugie Y, Igarashim Y. Nine cases of debrancher deficiency (glycogen storage disease type III) presenting with muscle weakness—study in clinicobiochemical analysis [Japanese]. *Rinsho Shika Clin Neurol.* 1996;36:540–543.
61. Hattori Y, Nohara C, Hirasawa E, Mori H, Imai H, Mizuno Y. A 21-year-old man with distal dominant progressive muscle atrophy (clinical conference) [Japanese]. *No To Shinei—Brain Nerve.* 1995;47(5):509–518.
62. Marbini A, Gemignani F, Saccardi F, Rimoldi M. Debrancher deficiency neuromuscular disorder with pseudohypertrophy in two brothers. *J Neurol.* 1989;236:418–420.
63. Murase T, Ikeda H, Muro T, Nakao K, Sugita H. Myopathy with type III glycogenosis. *J Neurol Sci.* 1973;20:287–295.
64. Ozand P, Tokatli M, Amiri S. Biochemical investigation of an unusual case of glycogenosis. *J Pediatr.* 1967;71:225–232.
65. Slonim AE, Weisberg C, Benke P, Evans OB, Burr IM. Reversal of debrancher deficiency myopathy by the use of high-protein nutrition. *Ann Neurol.* 1982;11:420–422.
66. Cuspidi C, Sampieri L, Pelizzoli S, et al. Obstructive hypertrophic cardiomyopathy in type III glycogen storage disease. *Acta Cardiol.* 1997;52:117–123.
67. Kiechl S, Kohlendorfer U, Thaler C, et al. Different clinical aspects of debrancher deficiency myopathy. *J Neurosurg Psychiatry.* 1999;67(3):364–368.
68. Miller CG, Alleyne GA, Brooks SE. Gross cardiac involvement in glycogen storage disease type III. *Br Heart J.* 1972;34:862–864.
69. Tada H, Kurita T, Ohe T, et al. Glycogen storage disease type III associated with ventricular tachycardia. *Am Heart J.* 1995;130:911–912.
70. Preisler N, Pradel A, Husu E, et al. Exercise intolerance in glycogen storage disease type III: weakness or energy deficiency? *Mol Genet Metab.* 2013;109:14–20.
71. Laforêt P, Inoue M, Goillot E, et al. Deep morphological analysis of muscle biopsies from type III glycogenesis (GSDIII), debranching enzyme deficiency, revealed stereotyped

71. vacuolar myopathy and autophagy impairment. *Acta Neuropathol Commun.* 2019;7:167.
72. Austin SL, Proia AD, Spencer-Manzon MJ, Butany J, Wechsler SB, Kishnani PS. Cardiac pathology in glycogen storage disease type III. *JIMD Rep.* 2012;6:65–72.
73. Powell HC, Haas R, Hall CL, Wolff JA, Nyhan W, Brown BI. Peripheral nerve in type III glycogenosis: selective involvement of unmyelinated fiber Schwann cells. *Muscle Nerve.* 1985;8:667–671.
74. Sancho S, Navarro C, Fernández JM, et al. Skin biopsy findings in glycogenosis III: clinical, biochemical, and electrophysiological correlations. *Ann Neurol.* 1990;27(5): 480–486.
75. Ugawa Y, Inoue K, Takemura T, Iwamasa T. Accumulation of glycogen in sural nerve axons in adult-onset type III glycogenosis. *Ann Neurol.* 1986;19:294–296.
76. Okubo M, Horinishi A, Nakumura N, et al. A novel point mutation in an acceptor splice site of intron 32 (IVS32 A-12->G) but no exon 3 mutations in the glycogen debranching enzyme gene in a homozygous patient with glycogen storage disease type IIIb. *Hum Genet.* 1998;102(1):1–5.
77. Pavari R, Shen J, Hershkowitz E, Chen YT, Moses SW. Two new mutations in the 3 coding region of the glycogen debranching enzyme in a glycogen storage disease type IIIa Ashkenazi Jewish patient. *J Inherit Metab Dis.* 1998;21:141–148.
78. Shen J, Bao Y, Chen YT. A nonsense mutation due to a single base insertion in the 3′-coding region of glycogen debranching enzyme gene associated with a severe phenotype in a patient with glycogen storage disease type IIIa. *Hum Mutat.* 1997;9:37–40.
79. Shen J, Bao Y, Liu HM, Lee P, Leonard JV, Chen YT. Mutations in exon 3 of the glycogen debranching enzyme gene are associated with glycogen storage disease type III that is differentially expressed in liver and muscle. *J Clin Invest.* 1996;98: 352–357.
80. Shen J, Liu HM, McConkie-Rosell A, Chen YT. Prenatal diagnosis and carrier detection for glycogen storage disease type III using polymorphic DNA markers. *Prenat Diagn.* 1998;18:61–64.
81. Haagsma EB, Smit GP, Niezen-Koning KE, Gouw AS, Meerman L, Slooff MJ. Type IIIb glycogen storage disease associated with end-stage cirrhosis and hepatocellular carcinoma. The liver transplant group. *Hepatology.* 1997;25:537–540.
82. Bao Y, Kishnani P, Wu JY, Chen YT. Hepatic and neuromuscular forms of glycogen storage disease IV caused by mutations in the same glycogen-branching enzyme gene. *J Clin Invest.* 1996;97:941–948.
83. Bornemann A, Besser R, Shin YS, Goebel HH. A mild adult myopathic variant of type IV glycogenosis. *Neuromuscul Disord.* 1996;6:95–99.
84. Bruno C, Servidei S, Shanske S, et al. Glycogen branching enzyme deficiency in adult polyglucosan body disease. *Ann Neurol.* 1993;33:88–93.
85. Bruno C, van Diggelen OP, Cassandrini D, et al. Clinical and genetic heterogeneity of branching enzyme deficiency (glycogenosis type IV). *Neurology.* 2004;63(6):1053–1058.
86. Cafferty MS, Lovelace RE, Hays AP, Servidei S, DiMauro S, Rowland LP. Polyglucosan body disease. *Muscle Nerve.* 1991;14:102–107.
87. Felice KJ, Grunnet ML, Rao KR, Wolfson LI. Childhood-onset spinocerebellar syndrome associated with massive polyglucosan body deposition. *Acta Neurol Scand.* 1997;95:60–64.
88. Fernandes J, Huijing F. Branching enzyme-deficiency glycogenosis: studies in therapy. *Arch Dis Child.* 1968;43:347–352.
89. Fishbein WN, Armbrustmacher VW, Griffin JL. Myoadenylate deaminase deficiency: a new disease of muscle. *Science.* 1978;200:545–548.
90. McMaster KR, Powers JM, Hennigar GR Jr, et al. Nervous system involvement in type IV glycogenosis. *Arch Neurol.* 1979;103:105–111.
91. Nase S, Kunse KP, Sigmund M, Schoeder JM, Shin Y, Hanrath P. A new variant of type IV glycogenosis with primary cardiac manifestation and complete branching enzyme deficiency. In vivo detection by heart muscle biopsy. *Eur Heart J.* 1995;16:1695–1704.
92. Servidei S, Riepe RE, Langston C, et al. Severe cardiopathy in branching enzyme deficiency. *J Pediatr.* 1987;111:51–56.
93. Zellweger H, Mueller S, Ionasescu V, Schochet SS, McCormick WF. Glycogenosis IV: a new cause of infantile hypotonia. *J Pediatr.* 1972;80:842–844.
94. Taratuto AL, Akman HO, Saccoliti M, et al. Branching enzyme deficiency/glycogenosis storage disease type IV presenting as a severe congenital hypotonia: muscle biopsy and autopsy findings, biochemical and molecular genetic studies. *Neuromuscul Disord.* 2010;20:783–790.
95. Li SC, Hwu WL, Lin JL, et al. Association of the congenital neuromuscular form of glycogen storage disease type IV with a large deletion and recurrent frameshift mutation. *J Child Neurol.* 2012;27:204–208.
96. Escobar LF, Wagner S, Tucker M, Wareham J. Neonatal presentation of lethal neuromuscular glycogen storage disease type IV. *J Perinatol.* 2012;32:810–813.
97. McConkie-Rosell A, Wislon C, Picolli DA, et al. Clinical and laboratory findings in four patients with the non-progressive hepatic form of type IV glycogen storage disease. *J Inherit Metab Dis.* 1996;29:51–58.
98. Lossos A, Meiner Z, Barash V, et al. Adult polyglucosan body disease in Ashkenazi Jewish patients carrying the Tyr329 ser mutation in the glucogen-branching enzyme gene. *Ann Neurol.* 1998;44:867–872.
99. Ziemssen F, Sinderm E, Schroder JM, et al. Novel missense mutations in the glycogen-branching enzyme gene in adult polyglucosan body disease. *Ann Neurol.* 2000;47: 536–540.
100. Tay SK, Akman HO, Wendy K, et al. Fatal infantile neuromuscular presentation of glycogen storage disease type IV. *Neuromuscul Disord.* 2004;14(4):253–260.
101. Rosenthal P, Podesta L, Grier R, et al. Failure of liver transplantation to diminish cardiac deposits of amylopectin and leukocyte inclusions in type IV glycogen storage disease. *Liver Transpl Surg.* 1995;1:373–376.
102. Selby R, Starzl TE, Yunis E, Brown BI, Kendall RS, Tzakis A. Liver transplantation for type IV glycogen storage disease. *N Engl J Med.* 1991;324:39–42.
103. Starzl TE, Demetris AJ, Trucco M, et al. Chimerism after liver transplantation for type IV glycogen storage disease and type 1 Gaucher's disease. *N Engl J Med.* 1993;328:745–749.
104. McArdle B. Myopathy due to a defect in muscle glycogen breakdown. *Clin Sci.* 1951;10:13–35.
105. Quinlivan R, Buckley J, James M, et al. McArdle disease: a clinical review. *J Neurol Neurosurg Psychiatry.* 2010;81(11):1182–1188.
106. Quinlivan R, Martinuzzi A, Schoser B. Pharmacological and nutritional treatment for McArdle disease (glycogen

storage disease type V). *Cochrane Database Syst Rev.* 2010;(12):CD003458.
107. Vissing J, Haller RG. The effect of oral sucrose on exercise tolerance in patients with McArdle's disease. *N Engl J Med.* 2003;349:2503–2509.
108. Pizzamiglio C, Mahroo OA, Khan KN, Patasin M, Quinlivan R. Phenotype and genotype of 197 British patients with McArdle disease: an observational single-centre study. *J Inherit Metab Dis.* 2021;44:1409–1418.
109. Álvarez-Velasco R, Nuñez-Peralta CA, Alonso-Pérez J, et al. High prevalence of paraspinal muscle involvement in adults with McArdle disease. *Muscle Nerve.* 2022;65:568–573.
110. Tobaly D, Laforêt P, Stojkovic T, et al. Whole-body muscle MRI in McArdle disease. *Neuromuscul Disord.* 2022;32:5–14.
111. Wolfe GI, Baker NS, Haller RG, Burns DK, Barohn RJ. McArdle's disease presenting with asymmetric, late-onset arm weakness. *Muscle Nerve.* 2000;23:641–645.
112. Løkken N, Revsbech KL, Jacobsen LN, et al. Muscle MRI in McArdle disease: a European multicenter observational study. *Neurology.* 2022;99(15):e1664–e1675.
113. DiMauro S, Hartlage PL. Fatal infantile form of muscle phosphorylase deficiency. *Neurology.* 1978;28:1124–1129.
114. Tsujino S, Shanske S, DiMauro S. Molecular genetic heterogeneity of myophosphorylase deficiency (McArdle's disease). *N Engl J Med.* 1993;329:241–245.
115. Kazemi-Esfarjani P, Skomorowska E, Jensen TD, Haller RG, Vissing J. A nonischemic forearm exercise test for McArdle disease. *Ann Neurol.* 2002;52:153–159.
116. Brandt NJ, Buchthal F, Ebbesen F, Kamieniecka Z, Krarup C. Post-tetanic mechanical tension and evoked action potentials in McArdle's disease. *J Neurol Neurosurg Psychiatry.* 1977;40:920–925.
117. Gruener R, McArdle B, Ryman BE, Weller RO. Contracture of phosphorylase deficient muscle. *J Neurol Neurosurg Psychiatry.* 1968;31:268–283.
118. Beynon RJ, Bartham C, Hopkins P, et al. McArdle's disease: molecular genetics and metabolic consequences of the phenotype. *Muscle Nerve.* 1995;3:S18–S22.
119. Fernandez R, Navarro C, Andreu AL, et al. A novel missense mutation (W797R) in the myophosphorylase gene in Spanish patients with McArdle's disease. *Arch Neurol.* 2000;57:217–219.
120. Manfredi G, Silvestri G, Servidei S, et al. Manifesting heterozygotes in McArdle's disease: clinical, morphological, and biochemical studies in a family. *J Neurol Sci.* 1992;115:91–94.
121. Ruff RL. Why do patients with McArdle's disease have decreased exercise capacity? *Neurology.* 1998;50:6–7.
122. Ruff RL. Elevated intracellular Ca^{2+} and myofibrillar Ca^{2+} sensitivity cause iodoacetate-induced muscle contractures. *J Appl Physiol.* 1996;81:1230–1239.
123. Haller RG, Clausen T, Vissing J. Reduced levels of skeletal muscle Na+K+-ATPase in McArdle disease. *Neurology.* 1998;50:37–40.
124. Haller RG. Treatment of McArdle disease. *Arch Neurol.* 2000;57:923–924.
125. Vorgerd M, Zange J, Kley R, et al. Effect of high-dose creatine therapy on symptoms of exercise intolerance in McArdle disease: double-blind, placebo-controlled crossover study. *Arch Neurol.* 2002;59(1):97–101.
126. Haller RG, Vissing J. No spontaneous second wind in muscle phosphofructokinase deficiency. *Neurology.* 2004;62(1):82–86.
127. Musumeci O, Bruno C, Mongini T, et al. Clinical features and new molecular findings in muscle phosphofructokinase deficiency (GSD type VII). *Neuromuscul Disord.* 2012;22:325–330.
128. Malfatti E, Birouk N, Romero NB, et al. Juvenile-onset permanent weakness in muscle phosphofructokinase deficiency. *J Neurol Sci.* 2012;316:173–177.
129. Hays AP, Hallett M, Delfs J, et al. Muscle phosphofructokinase deficiency: abnormal polysaccharide in a case of late-onset myopathy. *Neurology.* 1981;31(9):1077–1086.
130. Haller RG, Lewis SF. Glucose-induced exertional fatigue in muscle phosphofructokinase deficiency. *N Engl J Med.* 1991;324:364–369.
131. Abarbanel JM, Bashan N, Potashnik R, Osimani A, Moses SW, Herishanu Y. Adult muscle phosphorylase "b" kinase deficiency. *Neurology.* 1986;36:560–562.
132. Clemens PR, Yamamoto M, Engel AG. Adult phosphorylase b kinase deficiency. *Ann Neurol.* 1990;28:529–538.
133. Van den Berg IE, Berger R. Phosphorylase b kinase deficiency in man: a review. *J Inherit Metab Dis.* 1990;13:442–451.
134. Wilkinson DA, Tonin P, Shanske S, Lombes A, Carlson GM, DiMauro S. Clinical and biochemical features of 10 adult patients with muscle phosphorylase kinase deficiency. *Neurology.* 1994;44:461–466.
135. Kishnani PS, Goldstein J, Austin SL, et al; ACMG Work Group on Diagnosis and Management of Glycogen Storage Diseases Type VI and IX. Diagnosis and management of glycogen storage diseases type VI and IX: a clinical practice resource of the American College of Medical Genetics and Genomics (ACMG). *Genet Med.* 2019;21(4):772–789.
136. Burwinkel B, Maichele AJ, Aagenaes O, et al. Autosomal glycogenosis of liver and muscle due to phosphorylase kinase deficiency is caused by mutations in the phosphorylase kinase beta subunit (PHKB). *Hum Mol Genet.* 1997;6:1109–1115.
137. Vissing J, Schmalbruch H, Haller RG, Clausen T. Muscle phosphoglycerate mutase deficiency with tubular aggregates: effect of dantrolene. *Ann Neurol.* 1999;46:274–277.
138. Naini A, Toscano A, Musumeci O, Vissing J, Akman HO, DiMauro S. Muscle phosphoglycerate mutase deficiency revisited. *Arch Neurol.* 2009;66(3):394–398.
139. Kanno T, Maekawa M. Lactate dehydrogenase M-subunit deficiencies: clinical features, metabolic background, and genetic heterogeneities. *Muscle Nerve.* 1995;(suppl 3):S54–S60.
140. Yue D, Zhu W, Zhao C. Exertional myalgia, contractures and annular erythema in a patient with muscle lactate dehydrogenase (LDH) deficiency. *Neuromuscul Disord.* 2018;28:59.
141. Kreuder J, Borkhardt A, Repp R, et al. Inherited metabolic myopathy and hemolysis due to a mutation in aldolase A. *N Engl J Med.* 1996;334:1100–1104.
142. Yao DC, Tolan DR, Murray MF, et al. Hemolytic anemia and severe rhabdomyolysis caused by compound heterozygous mutations of the gene for erythrocyte/muscle isozyme of aldolase, ALDOA(Arg303X/Cys338Tyr). *Blood.* 2004;103:2401–2403.
143. Papadopoulos C, Svingou M, Kekou K, et al. Aldolase a deficiency: report of new cases and literature review. *Mol Genet Metab Rep.* 2021;27:100730.
144. Comi GP, Fortunato F, Lucchiari S, et al. Beta-enolase deficiency, a new metabolic myopathy of distal glycolysis. *Ann Neurol.* 2001;50:202–207.
145. Musumeci O, Brady S, Rodolico C, et al. Recurrent rhabdomyolysis due to muscle beta-enolase deficiency: very rare or underestimated? *J Neurol.* 2014;261:2424–2428.

146. Wigley R, Scalco RS, Gardiner AR, et al. The need for biochemical testing in beta-enolase deficiency in the genomic era. *JIMD Rep.* 2019;50:40–43.
147. Buch AE, Musumeci O, Wigley R, et al. Energy metabolism during exercise in patients with β-enolase deficiency (GSDXIII). *JIMD Rep.* 2021;61:60–66.
148. Stojkovic T, Vissing J, Petit F, et al. Muscle glycogenosis due to phosphoglucomutase 1 deficiency. *N Engl J Med.* 2009; 361:425–427.
149. Preisler N, Laforêt P, Echaniz-Laguna A, et al. Fat and carbohydrate metabolism during exercise in phosphoglucomutase type 1 deficiency. *J Clin Endocrinol Metab.* 2013;98:E1235-E1240.
150. Altassan R, Radenkovic S, Edmondson AC, et al. International consensus guidelines for phosphoglucomutase 1 deficiency (PGM1-CDG): diagnosis, follow-up, and management. *J Inherit Metab Dis.* 2021;44:148–163.
151. Moslemi AR, Lindberg C, Nilsson J, Tajsharghi H, Andersson B, Oldfors A. Glycogenin-1 deficiency and inactivated priming of glycogen synthesis. *N Engl J Med.* 2010;362:1203–1210.
152. Malfatti E, Nilsson J, Hedberg-Oldfors C, et al. A new muscle glycogen storage disease associated with glycogenin-1 deficiency. *Ann Neurology.* 2014;76:891–898.
153. Akman HO, Aykit Y, Amuk OC, et al. Late-onset polyglucosan body myopathy in five patients with a homozygous mutation in GYG1. *Neuromuscul Disord.* 2016;26:16–20.
154. Ben Yaou R, Hubert A, Nelson I, et al. Clinical heterogeneity and phenotype/genotype findings in 5 families with GYG1 deficiency. *Neurol Genet.* 2017;3:e208.
155. Bardosi A, Eber SW, Hendrys M, Pelrun A. Myopathy with altered mitochondria due to a triosephosphate isomerase (TPI) deficiency. *Acta Neuropathol (Berl).* 1990;79:387–394.
156. Schneider AS, Valentine WN, Hattori M, Heins HL Jr. Hereditary hemolytic anemia with triosephosphate isomerase deficiency. *NEJM.* 1965;272:229–235.
157. Linarello RE, Shetty AK, Thomas T, Warrier RP. Triosephosphate isomerase deficiency in a child with congenital hemolytic anemia and severe hypotonia. *Pediatr Hematol Oncol.* 1998;15:553–556.
158. Harris C, Nelson B, Farber D, et al. Child Neurology: Triosephosphate isomerase deficiency. *Neurology.* 2020;95(24): e3448–e3451.
159. Fujii H, Kanno H, Hirono A, Shiomura T, Miwa S. A single amino acid substitution (157 Gly to Val) in a phosphoglycerate kinase variant (PGK Shizuoka) associated with chronic hemolysis and myoglobinuria. *Blood.* 1992;79:1582–1585.
160. Sugie H, Sugie Y, Nishida M, et al. Recurrent myoglobinuria in a child with mental retardation: phosphoglycerate kinase deficiency. *J Child Neurol.* 1989;4:95–99.
161. Tonin P, Shanske S, Miranda AF, et al. Phosphoglycerate kinase deficiency: biochemical and molecular genetic studies in a new myopathic variant (PGK Alberta). *Neurology.* 1993;43:387–391.
162. Tsujino S, Tonin P, Shanske S, et al. A splice junction mutation in a new myopathic variant of phosphoglycerate kinase deficiency (PGK North Carolina). *Ann Neurol.* 1994;35(3):349–353.
163. Echaniz-Laguna A, Nadjar Y, Béhin A, et al. Phosphoglycerate kinase deficiency: a nationwide multicenter retrospective study. *J Inherit Metab Dis.* 2019;42:803–808.
164. Coppens S, Koralkova P, Aeby A, et al. Recurrent episodes of myoglobinuria, mental retardation and seizures but no hemolysis in two brothers with phosphoglycerate kinase deficiency. *Neuromuscul Disord.* 2016;26:207–210.
165. Baba K, Fukuda T, Furuta M, et al. A Case of a mild clinical phenotype with myopathic and hemolytic forms of phosphoglycerate kinase deficiency (PGK Osaka): a case report and literature review. *Intern Med.* 2022;61(23):3589–3594.
166. Nilsson J, Schoser B, Laforet P, et al. Polyglucosan body myopathy caused by defective ubiquitin ligase RBCK1. *Ann Neurol.* 2013;74(6):914–919.
167. Thomsen C, Malfatti E, Jovanovic A, et al. Proteomic characterisation of polyglucosan bodies in skeletal muscle in RBCK1 deficiency. *Neuropathol Appl Neurobiol.* 2022;48:e12761.
168. Danon MJ, Oh SJ, DiMauro S, et al. Lysosomal glycogen storage disease with normal acid maltase. *Neurology.* 1981;31(1):51–57.
169. Nishino I, Fu J, Tanji K, et al. Primary LAMP-2 deficiency causes X-linked vacuolar cardiomyopathy and myopathy (Danon disease). *Nature.* 2000;406:906–910.
170. Sugie K, Yamatoto A, Murayama K, et al. Clinicopathological features of genetically confirmed Danon disease. *Neurology.* 2002;58(12):1773–1778.
171. Boucek D, Jirikowic J, Taylor M. Natural history of Danon disease. *Genet Med.* 2011;13:563–568.
172. Stevens-Lapsley JE, Kramer LR, Balter JE, Jirikowic J, Boucek D, Taylor M. Functional performance and muscle strength phenotypes in men and women with Danon disease. *Muscle Nerve.* 2010;42:908–914.
173. Kim H, Cho A, Lim BC, et al. A 13-year-old girl with proximal weakness and hypertrophic cardiomyopathy with Danon disease. *Muscle Nerve.* 2010;41:879–882.
174. Cheng Z, Fang Q. Danon disease: focusing on heart. *J Hum Genet.* 2012;57:407–410.
175. Miani D, Taylor M, Mestroni L, et al. Sudden death associated with Danon disease in women. *Am J Cardiol.* 2012;109(3):406–411.
176. Cenacchi G, Papa V, Pegoraro V, Marozzo R, Fanin M, Angelini C. Review: Danon disease: review of natural history and recent advances. *Neuropathol Appl Neurobiol.* 2020;46:303–322.
177. Hanneman K. Cardiac MRI in Danon disease: sex-specific differences and characteristic imaging findings. *Radiology.* 2021;299:311–312.
178. Yamamoto A, Morisawa Y, Verloes A, et al. Infantile lysosomal glycogen storage disease with normal acid maltase is genetically distinct from Danon disease (X-linked vacuolar cardiomyopathy and myopathy). *Neurology.* 2001;57:903–905.
179. Hong KN, Battikha C, John S, et al. Cardiac transplantation in Danon disease. *J Card Fail.* 2022;28:664–669.
180. Kalimo H, Savonataus ML, Lang H, et al. X-linked myopathy with excessive autophagia: a new hereditary muscle disease. *Ann Neurol.* 1988;23:258–265.
181. Villanova M, Louboutin JP, Chateau D, et al. X-linked vacuolated myopathy: complement membrane attack complex on surface of injured muscle fibers. *Ann Neurol.* 1995;37:637–645.
182. Kaneda D, Sugie K, Yamatoto A, et al. A novel form of autophagic vacuolar myopathy with late-onset and multiorgan involvement. *Neurology.* 2003;61:128–131.
183. Saraste A, Koskenvuo JW, Airaksinen J, et al. No cardiomyopathy in X-linked myopathy with excessive autophagy. *Neuromuscul Disord.* 2015;25:485–487.
184. Ramachandran N, Munteanu I, Wang P, et al. VMA21 deficiency prevents vacuolar ATPase assembly and causes

autophagic vacuolar myopathy. *Acta Neuropathol.* 2013;125(3): 439–457.
185. Ruggieri A, Ramachandran N, Wang P, et al. Non-coding VMA21 deletions cause X-linked myopathy with excessive autophagy. *Neuromuscul Disord.* 2015;25:207–211.
186. Kelemen J, Rice DR, Bradley WG, Munsat TL, DiMauro S, Hogan EL. Familial myoadenylate deaminase deficiency and exertional myalgia. *Neurology.* 1982;32:857–863.
187. Tonin P, Lewis P, Servidei S, DiMauro S. Metabolic causes of myoglobinuria. *Ann Neurol.* 1990;27:181–185.
188. Verzijl HT, van Engelen BG, Luyten JA, et al. Genetic characteristics of myoadenylate deaminase deficiency. *Ann Neurol.* 1998;44:140–143.
189. Sabina RL, Swain JL, Olanow W, et al. Myoadenylate deaminase deficiency: functional and metabolic abnormalities associated with disruption of purine nucleotide cycle. *J Clin Invest.* 1984;73(3):720–730.
190. Vissing J, Lewis SF, Galbo H, Haller RG. Effect of deficient muscular glycogenolysis on extramuscular fuel production in exercise. *J Appl Physiol.* 1992;72:1773–1779.
191. Sabina RL, Fishbein WN, Pezeshkpour G, Clarke PR, Holmes EW. Molecular analysis of the myoadenylate deaminase deficiencies. *Neurology.* 1992;42:170–179.
192. Liang WC, Nishino I. Lipid storage myopathy. *Curr Neurol Neurosci Rep.* 2011;11:97–103.
193. Laforet P, Vianey-Sabab C. Disorders of muscle lipid metabolism: diagnostic and therapeutic changes. *Neuromuscular Dis.* 2010;20:693–700.
194. Ohkuma A, Noguchi S, Sugie H, et al. Clinical and genetic analysis of lipid storage myopathies. *Muscle Nerve.* 2009;39:333–342.
195. Di Donato S, Rimoldi M, Bertagnolio B, Uziel G, Wiesmann UN. A biochemical approach to lipid storage myopathies. *Biochem Exp Biol.* 1977;13(1):85–91.
196. Chapoy PF, Angelini C, Brown WJ, Stiff JE, Shug AL, Cederbaum SD. Systemic carnitine deficiency: a treatable inherited lipid storage disease presenting as Reye's syndrome. *N Engl J Med.* 1980;303:1389–1394.
197. Cornelio F, Di Donato S, Testa D, et al. Carnitine deficient myopathy and cardiomyopathy with fatal outcome. *Ital J Neurol Sci.* 1980;1(2):95–100.
198. Cornelio G, Di Donato S, Peluchetti D, et al. Fatal cases of lipid storage myopathy with carnitine deficiency. *J Neurol Neurosurg Psychiatry.* 1977;40:170–178.
199. Di Donato S. Primary and secondary carnitine deficiency in man. *Ital J Biochem.* 1984;33(4):285A–291A.
200. Di Donato S, Pelucchetti D, Rimoldi M, Mora M, Garavaglia B, Finocchiaro G. Systemic carnitine deficiency: clinical, biochemical, and morphological cure with L-carnitine. *Neurology.* 1984;34(2):157–162.
201. DiMauro S, Trevisan C, Hays A. Disorders of lipid metabolism in muscle. *Muscle Nerve.* 1980;3(5):369–388.
202. Engel AG, Banker BQ, Eiben RM. Carnitine deficiency: clinical, morphological, and biochemical observations in a fatal case. *J Neurol Neurosurg Psychiatry.* 1977;40:313–322.
203. Garavaglia B, Uziel G, Dworsak F, Carrar F, DiDonato S. Primary carnitine deficiency: heterozygote and intrafamilial phenotypic variation. *Neurology.* 1991;41:1691–1693.
204. Karpati G, Carpenter S, Eisen A, Aubé M, DiMauro S. The adult form of acid maltase (a-1,4-glucosidase) deficiency. *Ann Neurol.* 1977;1:276–280.
205. Morand P, Despert F, Carrier N, et al. Myopathie lipidique avec cardiomyopathie severe par deficit generalise en carnitine. *Arch Mal Coeur Vaiss.* 1979;5:536–544.
206. Stanley CA, DeLeeuw S, Coates PM, et al. Chronic cardiomyopathy and weakness or acute coma in children with a defect in carnitine uptake. *Ann Neurol.* 1991;30:709–716.
207. Bautista J, Rafel E, Martinez A, et al. Familial hypertrophic cardiomyopathy and muscle carnitine deficiency. *Muscle Nerve.* 1990;13:192–194.
208. Hart ZH, Chang CH, DiMauro S, Farooki Q, Ayyar R. Muscle carnitine deficiency and fatal cardiomyopathy. *Neurology.* 1978;28:147–151.
209. Markesbery WR, McQuillen MP, Procopis PG, Harrison AR, Engel AG. Muscle carnitine deficiency. *Arch Neurol.* 1974;31:320–324.
210. Angelini C, Govoni E, Bragaglia MM, Vergani L. Carnitine deficiency: acute postpartum crisis. *Ann Neurol.* 1978;4:558–562.
211. Prockop LD, Engel WK, Shug AL. Nearly fatal muscle carnitine deficiency with full recovery after replacement therapy. *Neurology.* 1983;33:1629–1631.
212. Engel AG, Rebouche CJ, Wilson DM, Glasgow AM, Romshe CA, Cruse RP. Primary systemic carnitine deficiency. II. Renal handling of carnitine. *Neurology.* 1981;31(7):819–825.
213. Treem WR, Stanley CA, Finegold DN, Hale DE, Coates PM. Primary carnitine deficiency due to a failure of carnitine transport in kidney, muscle, and fibroblasts. *N Engl J Med.* 1988;319(20):1331–1336.
214. Nezu JI, Tamai I, Oku A, et al. Primary systemic carnitine deficiency is caused by mutations in a gene encoding a sodium-dependent carnitine transporter. *Nat Genet.* 1999;21:91–94.
215. Angelini C, Lucke S, Cantarutti F. Carnitine deficiency of skeletal muscle: report of a treated case. *Neurology.* 1976;26:633–637.
216. Snyder TM, Little BW, Roman-Campos G, McQuillen JB. Successful treatment of familial idiopathic lipid storage myopathy with L-carnitine and modified lipid diet. *Neurology.* 1982;32:1106–1115.
217. Tripp ME, Katcher ML, Peters HA, et al. Systemic carnitine deficiency presenting as familial endocardial fibroelastosis: a treatable cardiomyopathy. *N Engl J Med.* 1981;305:385–390.
218. Angelini C, Trevisan C, Isaya G, Pegolo G, Vergani L. Clinical varieties of carnitine and carnitine palmitoyltransferase deficiency. *Clin Biochem.* 1987;20(1):1–7.
219. Demaugre F, Bonnefont JP, Mitchell G, et al. Hepatic and muscular presentations of carnitine palmitoyl transferase deficiency: two distinct entities. *Pediatr Res.* 1988;24(3):308–311.
220. Taroni F, Verderio E, Dworzak F, Willems PJ, Cavadini P, Di Donato S. Identification of a common mutation in the carnitine palmitoyltransferase II gene in familial recurrent myoglobinuria patients. *Nat Genet.* 1993;4:314–320.
221. Trevisan CP, Isaya G, Angelini C. Exercise-induced recurrent myoglobinuria: defective activity of inner carnitine palmitoyltransferase in muscle mitochondria of two patients. *Neurology.* 1987;37(7):1184–1188.
222. Andresen BS, Bross P, Vianey-Saban C, et al. Cloning and characterization of human very-long-chain acyl-CoA dehydrogenase cDNA, chromosomal assignment of the gene and identification in four patients of nine different mutations within the VLCAD gene. *Hum Mol Genet.* 1996;5(4):461–472. Erratum in: *Hum Mol Genet.* 1996;5(9):1390.
223. Aoyama T, Souri M, Ueno I, et al. Cloning of human very-long-chain acyl coenzyme A dehydrogenase and molecular

characterization of its deficiency in two patients. *Am J Hum Genet.* 1995;57:273–283.
224. Brown-Harrison MC, Nada MA, Sprecher H, et al. Very long chain acyl-CoA dehydrogenase deficiency: successful treatment of acute cardiomyopathy. *Biochem Mol Med.* 1996;58(1): 59–65.
225. Merinero B, Cerdra-Perez C, Garcia MJ, Vianey-Saban C, Duran M, Ugarte M. Mitochondrial very-long-chain acyl-CoA dehydrogenase deficiency with a mild course. *J Inherit Metab Dis.* 1996;19:173–176.
226. Minetti C, Garavaglia B, Bado M, et al. Very-long-chain acyl-coenzyme A dehydrogenase deficiency in a child with recurrent myoglobinuria. *Neuromuscul Disord.* 1998;8:3–6.
227. Smelt AH, Poorthuis BJ, Onkenhout W, et al. Very long chain acyl-coenzyme A dehydrogenase deficiency with adult onset. *Ann Neurol.* 1998;43(4):540–544.
228. Taroni F, Uziel G. Fatty-acid mitochondrial β-oxidation and hypoglycemia in children. *Curr Opin Neurol.* 1996;9:477–485.
229. Yamaguchi S, Indo Y, Coates PM, Hashimoto T, Tanaka K. Identification of a very-long-chain acyl-CoA dehydrogenase deficiency in three patients previously diagnosed with long-chain acyl-CoA dehydrogenase deficiency. *Pediatr Res.* 1993;34:111–113.
230. Laforêt P, Acquaviva-Bourdain C, Rigal O, et al. Diagnostic assessment and long-term follow-up of 13 patients with Very Long-Chain Acyl-Coenzyme A dehydrogenase (VLCAD) deficiency. *Neuromuscul Disord.* 2009;19:324–329.
231. Ogilvie I, Porfarzam M, Jackson S, Stockdale C, Bartlett K, Turnbull DM. Very long-chain acyl coenzyme A dehydrogenase deficiency presenting with exercise-induced myoglobinuria. *Neurology.* 1994;44(3 Pt 1):467–473.
232. Hale DE, Batshaw ML, Coates PM, et al. Long-chain acyl coenzyme A dehydrogenase deficiency: an inherited cause of nonketotic hypoglycemia. *Pediatr Res.* 1985;19:666–671.
233. Parini R, Garavaglia B, Saudubray JM, et al. Clinical diagnosis of long-chain acyl-coenzyme A-dehydrogenase deficiency: use of stress and fat-loading tests. *J Pediatr.* 1991;119(1 Pt 1): 77–80.
234. Tein I, Vajsar J, MacMillan L, Sherwood WG. Long-chain L-3-hydroxyacyl-coenzyme A dehydrogenase deficiency neuropathy: response to cod liver oil. *Neurology.* 1999;52(3):640–643.
235. Zierz S, Engel AG, Romshe CA. Assay of acyl-CoA dehydrogenases in muscle and liver and identification of four new cases of medium-chain acyl-CoA dehydrogenase deficiency associated with systemic carnitine deficiency. *Adv Neurol.* 1988;48:231–237.
236. Coates PM, Hale DE, Stanley CA, Corkey BE, Cortner JA. Genetic deficiency of medium-chain acyl coenzyme A dehydrogenase: studies in cultured skin fibroblasts and peripheral mononuclear leukocytes. *Pediatr Res.* 1985;19(7):671–676.
237. Di Donato S, Gellera C. Short-chain and medium-chain acyl-CoA dehydrogenases are lowered in riboflavin-responsive lipid myopathies with multiple acyl-CoA dehydrogenase deficiency. *Prog Clin Biol Res.* 1990;321:325–332.
238. Ding JH, Roe CR, Iafolla AK, Chen YT. Medium-chain acyl-coenzyme A dehydrogenase deficiency and sudden infant death [letter]. *N Engl J Med.* 1991;325:61–62.
239. Treem WR, Stanley CA, Goodman SI. Medium-chain acyl-CoA dehydrogenase deficiency: metabolic effects and therapeutic efficacy of long-term carnitine supplementation. *J Inherit Metab Dis.* 1989;12:112–119.
240. Ruitenbeek W, Poels PJ, Turnbull DM, et al. Rhabdomyolysis and acute encephalopathy in late onset medium chain acyl-CoA dehydrogenase deficiency. *J Neurol Neurosurg Psychiatry.* 1995;58:209–214.
241. Zierz S, Engel AG, Romsche CA. Assay for acyl-CoA dehydrogenase in muscle and liver and identification of four cases of medium-chain acyl-CoA dehydrogenase deficiency associated with carnitine deficiency. In: Di Donato S, DiMauro S, Mamoli A, Rowland LP, eds. *Molecular Genetics of Neurological and Neuromuscular Diseases: Advances in Neurology*, Vol. 48. Raven Press; 1988:231–237.
242. Coates PM, Hale DE, Fiocchario G, Tanaka K, Winter SC. Genetic deficiency of short-chain acyl-coenzyme A dehydrogenase in cultured fibroblasts from a patient with muscle carnitine deficiency and severe muscle weakness. *J Clin Invest.* 1988;81:171–175.
243. Tein I, Haslam RH, Rhead WJ, Bennett MJ, Becker LE, Vockley J. Short-chain acyl-CoA dehydrogenase deficiency. A cause of ophthalmoplegia and multicore myopathy. *Neurology.* 1999;52:366–372.
244. Turnbull DM, Bartlett K, Stevens DL, et al. Short-chain acyl-CoA dehydrogenase deficiency associated with a lipid storage myopathy and secondary carnitine deficiency. *N Engl J Med.* 1984;311:1232–1236.
245. van Maldegem BT, Duran M, Wanders RJ, et al. Clinical, biochemical, and genetic heterogeneity in short-chain acyl-coenzyme A dehydrogenase deficiency. *JAMA.* 2006; 296(8):943–952.
246. van Maldegem BT, Wanders JA, Wijburg FA. Clinical aspects of short-chain acyl-CoA dehydrogenase deficiency. *J Inherit Metab Dis.* 2010;33:507–511.
247. Baerlocher KE, Steinmann B, Aguzzi A, Krähenbühl S, Roe CR, Vianey-Saban C. Short-chain acyl-CoA dehydrogenase deficiency in a 16-year-old girl with severe muscle wasting and scoliosis. *J Inherit Metab Dis.* 1997;20(3):427–431.
248. Corydon MJ, Andresen BS, Bross P, et al. Structural organization of the human short-chain acyl-CoA dehydrogenase gene. *Mamm Genome.* 1997;8:922–926.
249. Naito E, Indo Y, Tanaka K. Short chain acyl-coenzyme A dehydrogenase (SCAD) deficiency: immunochemical demonstration of molecular heterogeneity due to variant SCAD with differing stability. *J Clin Invest.* 1989;84:1671–1674.
250. Jackson S, Baartlett K, Land J, et al. Long-chain 3-hydroxyacyl-CoA dehydrogenase deficiency. *Pediatr Res.* 1991;29:406–411.
251. Rocchiccioli F, Wanders RJ, Augburg P, et al. Deficiency of long-chain 3-hydroxyacyl-CoA dehydrogenase: a cause of lethal myopathy and cardiomyopathy in early childhood. *Pediatr Res.* 1990;28:657–662.
252. Thiel C, Baudach S, Schnackenberg U, Vreken P, Wanders RJ. Long-chain 3-hydroxyacyl-CoA dehydrogenase deficiency: neonatal manifestation at the first day of life presenting with tachypnoea. *J Inherit Metab Dis.* 1999;22:839–840.
253. Tyni T, Pihko H. Long-chain 3-hydroxyacyl-CoA dehydrogenase deficiency. *Acta Pediatr.* 1999;88:237–245.
254. Wanders RJ, IJlst L, van Gennip AH, et al. Long-chain 3-hydroxyacyl-CoA dehydrogenase deficiency: identification of a new inborn error of mitochondrial fatty acid beta-oxidation. *J Inherit Metab Dis.* 1990;13(3):311–314.
255. Bertini E, Dionisi-Vici C, Garavaglia B, et al. Peripheral sensory-motor neuropathy, pigmentary retinopathy, and fatal

255. ... cardiomyopathy in long-chain 3-hydroxyacyl-CoA dehydrogenase deficiency. *Eur J Pediatr.* 1992;151(2):121–126.
256. Wanders RJ, Vreken P, den Boer ME, Wijburg FA, van Gennip AH, IJlst L. Disorders of mitochondrial fatty acyl-CoA beta-oxidation. *J Inherit Metab Dis.* 1999;22:442–487.
257. Korenke GC, Wanders RJ, Hanefeld F. Striking improvement of muscle strength under creatine therapy in a patient with long-chain 3-hydroxyacyl-CoA dehydrogenase deficiency. *J Inherit Metab Dis.* 2003;26(1):67–68.
258. Nadjar Y, Souvannanorath S, Maisonobe T, et al. Sensory neuronopathy as a major clinical feature of mitochondrial trifunctional protein deficiency in adults. *Rev Neurol (Paris).* 2020;176:380–386.
259. Di Donato S, Frerman FE, Rimoldi M, Rinaldo P, Taroni F, Wiesmann UN. Systemic carnitine deficiency due to lack of electron transfer flavoprotein: ubiquinone oxidoreductase. *Neurology.* 1986;36(7):957–963.
260. Dusheiko G, Kew MC, Joffe BI, Lewin JR, Mantagos S, Tanaka K. Recurrent hypoglycemia associated with glutaric aciduria type II in an adult. *N Engl J Med.* 1979;301:1405–1409.
261. Gregersen N, Wintzensen H, Christensen SK, Christensen MF, Brandt NJ, Rasmussen K. C(6)-C(10)-dicarboxylic aciduria: investigations of a patient with riboflavin responsive multiple acyl-CoA dehydrogenation defects. *Pediatr Res.* 1982;16:861–868.
262. Izumi R, Suzuki N, Nagata M, et al. A case of late onset riboflavin-responsive multiple acyl-CoA dehydrogenase deficiency manifesting as recurrent rhabdomyolysis and acute renal failure. *Intern Med.* 2011;50:2663–2668.
263. Pollard LM, Williams NR, Espinoza L, et al. Diagnosis, treatment, and long-term outcomes of late-onset (type III) multiple acyl-CoA dehydrogenase deficiency. *J Child Neurol.* 2010;25:954–960.
264. Liang WC, Ohkuma A, Hayashi YK, et al. ETFDH mutations, CoQ10 levels, and respiratory chain activities in patients with riboflavin-responsive multiple acyl-CoA dehydrogenase deficiency. *Neuromuscul Disord.* 2009;19:212–216.
265. Olsen RK, Olpin SE, Andresen BS, et al. ETFDH mutations as a major cause of riboflavin-responsive multiple acyl-CoA dehydrogenation deficiency. *Brain.* 2007;130:2045–2054.
266. Wen B, Dai T, Li W, et al. Riboflavin-responsive lipid-storage myopathy caused by ETFDH gene mutations. *J Neurol Neurosurg Psychiatry.* 2010;81:231–236.
267. Maillart E, Acquaviva-Bourdain C, Rigal O, et al. Multiple acyl-CoA dehydrogenase deficiency (MADD): a curable cause of genetic muscular lipidosis. *Rev Neurol.* 2010;166:289–294.
268. Mongini T, Doriguzzi C, Palmucci L, et al. Lipid storage myopathy in multiple acyl-CoA dehydrogenase deficiency: an adult case. *Eur Neurol.* 1992;32(3):170–176.
269. Wen B, Tang S, Lv X, et al. Clinical, pathological and genetic features and follow-up of 110 patients with late-onset MADD: a single-center retrospective study. *Hum Mol Genet.* 2022;31:1115–1129.
270. Dorfman ML, Hershko C, Eisenberg S, Sagher F. Ichthyosiform dermatosis with systemic lipidosis. *Arch Dermatol.* 1974;110:261–266.
271. Chanarin I, Patel A, Slavin G, Wills EJ, Andrews TM, Stewart G. Neutral-lipid storage disease: a new disorder of lipid metabolism. *Br Med J.* 1975;1:553–555.
272. Ohkuma A, Nonaka I, Malicdan MC, et al. Distal lipid storage myopathy due to PNPLA2 mutation. *Neuromuscul Disord.* 2008;18:671–674.
273. Fischer J, Lefevre C, Morava E, et al. The gene encoding adipose triglyceride lipase (PNPLA2) is mutated in neutral lipid storage disease with myopathy. *Nat Genet.* 2007;39:28–30.
274. Lefevre C, Jobard F, Caux F, et al. Mutations in CGI-58, the gene encoding a new protein of the esterase/lipase/thioesterase subfamily, in Chanarin-Dorfman syndrome. *Am J Hum Genet.* 2001;69:1002–1012.
275. Zeharia A, Shaag A, Houtkooper RH, et al. Mutations in LPIN1 cause recurrent acute myoglobinuria in childhood. *Am J Hum Genet.* 2008;83(4):489–494.
276. Michot C, Hubert L, Brivet M, et al. LPIN1 gene mutations: a major cause of severe rhabdomyolysis in early childhood. *Hum Mutat.* 2010;31:E1564–E73244.
277. Michot C, Hubert L, Romero NB, et al. Study of LPIN1, LPIN2 and LPIN3 in rhabdomyolysis and exercise-induced myalgia. *J Inherit Metab Dis.* 2012;35:1119–1128.
278. Indika NLR, Vidanapathirana DM, Jasinge E, Waduge R, Shyamali NLA, Perera PPR. Lipin-1 deficiency-associated recurrent rhabdomyolysis and exercise-induced myalgia persisting into adulthood: a case report and review of literature. *Case Rep Med.* 2020;2020:7904190.
279. Che R, Wang C, Zheng B, et al. A rare case of pediatric recurrent rhabdomyolysis with compound heterogenous variants in the LPIN1. *BMC Pediatr.* 2020;20(1):218.
280. Minton T, Forrester N, Baba SA, Urankar K, Brady S. A rare case of adult onset LPIN1 associated rhabdomyolysis. *Neuromuscul Disord.* 2020;30:241–245.

CHAPTER 30

Mitochondrial Disorders

Mitochondrial myopathies and neuropathies or neuromyopathies refer to a heterogeneous group of disorders caused by dysfunction of mitochondria.[1-13] Mitochondrial disorders can be classified according to the associated biochemical, genetic defects, or clinical phenotype (Tables 30-1 to 30-3). One difficulty in classifying patients by any particular scheme is the clinical-phenotypic heterogeneity associated with specific mitochondrial mutations and the genetic heterogeneity in well-defined clinical phenotypes that are seen with mitochondrial disorders.

The mitochondria are responsible for converting fuels (carbohydrates, lipids, and proteins) into energy for the cells. Fatty acids are metabolized into molecules of acetyl-CoA within the mitochondria. Amino acids are converted to pyruvate in the mitochondria. Carbohydrates are metabolized to pyruvate in the cytoplasm and then transported into the mitochondria. Pyruvate from either source is converted into acetyl-CoA. Acetyl-CoA, then enters into the Krebs cycle from which electrons are generated. Electrons derived from the Krebs cycle are shuttled to the respiratory chain and processed through complexes I–V to generate ATP molecules. Thus, mitochondrial disorders can be classified according to the metabolic defect present (1) transport, (2) substrate utilization, (3) Krebs cycle, (4) oxidation/phosphorylation coupling, and (5) respiratory chain (Table 30-1).

Some of the biochemical abnormalities seen in various mitochondrial disorders are nonspecific and the result of primary "upstream" defects in metabolic pathways. For example, cytochrome oxidase (COX) deficiency is seen in many types of mitochondrial myopathy and does not imply that the primary mutation lies in one of the genes encoding for subunits of COX. The rapid advances of molecular genetics may provide a better classification scheme. The mitochondrial disorders may be classified by their genetic defect (1) mitochondrial DNA (mtDNA), (2) nuclear DNA (nDNA) mutations directly or indirectly affecting the mitochondrial respiratory chain complex, or (3) nDNA mutations that are involved in mtDNA maintenance or mitochondrial dynamics (Table 30-2; Fig. 30-1).[1,4-9] Notably though, there is significant phenotypic variability even in patients with the same genetic mutation. Therefore, a combined classification scheme is currently favored because of phenotypical variability and problems inherent in current genotyping capabilities (Table 30-3). Prior to discussing specific disorders, we will review a few basic principles regarding the mitochondrial genome and different inheritance patterns of mitochondrial disorders.

► COMPOSITION OF MITOCHONDRIAL DNA AND PROTEINS

The mitochondrial genome comprises 16.5-kb circular double-stranded DNA. It is composed of a 1.1-kb D-loop that is involved in the regulation of transcription and replication of the molecule, and is the only region not directly involved in the synthesis of respiratory chain polypeptides. Contiguous mitochondrial genes overlap in some areas and transcription is polycistronic such that mitochondrial genes are transcribed as two large RNAs. These are subsequently cleaved into 13 respective messenger RNAs (mRNA), 2 ribosomal RNAs (rRNA) encoding 12S and 16S rRNA, and 22 transfer RNAs (tRNA) that provide the necessary RNA components for intramitochondrial protein synthesis. Interestingly, the genetic code for translation of human mitochondrial genes differs from the standard code which governs the translation of human nuclear genes. The 13 mRNAs are translated into 13 polypeptides that are subunits of the respiratory chain complexes. These include ND1 through ND6 and ND4L that encode seven subunits of respiratory chain complex I, CYT b encodes the only mtDNA-encoded respiratory chain complex III subunit, CO I to CO III encode for three of respiratory chain complex IV (cytochrome c oxidase, or COX) subunits, and ATPase6 and ATPase8 encode for two subunits of respiratory chain complex V.[1]

Note that any mutation in a mitochondrial tRNA gene can impair the proper translation of the 13 mitochondrial mRNAs. Importantly, the 13 proteins encoded by the mitochondrial genome account for less than 5% of all mitochondrial proteins. The majority of mitochondrial proteins (>1,400) are encoded by the nuclear genome that are translated in the cytoplasm and subsequently are transported into the mitochondria. Furthermore, the nucleus appears to regulate replication of the mitochondrial genome.

The respiratory chain comprises five multienzyme complexes (complexes I–V) (Fig. 30-2). Complex I (NADH-CoQ reductase) contains 45 subunits, 7 encoded by mtDNA; complex II [succinate dehydrogenase (SDH) CoQ reductase] comprises 4 subunits, each encoded by nuclear genes; complex III (CoQH$_2$-cytochrome c reductase) comprises 11 polypeptide units, one of which is encoded by mtDNA; complex IV (COX) has 13 subunits, 3 encoded by mtDNA; and complex V (ATPase synthetase) comprises 19 subunits, 2 encoded by mtDNA (Table 30-4).

▸ TABLE 30-1. CLASSIFICATION OF THE MITOCHONDRIAL MYOPATHIES BY METABOLIC FUNCTION AFFECTED

Metabolic Function	Defects
Substrate transport	Carnitine palmitoyltransferase (CPT)
	Primary systemic/muscle carnitine deficiency
	Secondary carnitine deficiency
	Combined carnitine and CPT deficiency
Substrate utilization	Pyruvate decarboxylase deficiency
	Pyruvate dehydrogenase deficiency
	Pyruvate carboxylase deficiency
	Fatty acid β-oxidation defects
Kreb cycle	Fumarase
	α-Ketoglutarate dehydrogenase deficiency
	Dihydrolipoyl dehydrogenase
Oxidation/phosphorylation coupling	Luft syndrome: Loose coupling with hypermetabolism
Respiratory chain	Complex I
	Complex II
	Complex III
	Complex IV
	Complex V
	Combinations of I–V

Reproduced with permission from Walsh RJ. Metabolic Myopathies. *Continuum.* 2006;12(3):76–120.

▸ GENETICS OF MITOCHONDRIAL DISORDERS

A population-based study in Northern England found that 6.57 per 100,000 adults have a mitochondrial disease and 12.48 per 100,000 of children and adults are at risk for developing a mitochondrial disorder on the basis of identifiable mtDNA mutations.[14] Because this study included only disorders caused by mtDNA mutations and not nDNA mutations affecting mitochondria, the prevalence of mitochondrial disorders is certainly higher. A study in adults that included pathogenic mutations of both the mitochondrial and nuclear genomes found a prevalence of around 1 in 4,300, making mitochondrial cytopathies among the commonest adult forms of inherited neurological disorders.[15]

Remember that during fertilization, all the mitochondria are contributed by the mother. Hundreds of mitochondria are present in most cells in the body and every mitochondrion has several copies of mtDNA. Mutations involving mtDNA are more common and more likely to manifest clinically than mutations in nuclear genes because of the lack of introns and decreased DNA repair mechanisms in the mitochondrial genome. mtDNA mutations are randomly distributed in subsequent generations of somatic cells during mitosis and germ

▸ TABLE 30-2. CLASSIFICATION OF MITOCHONDRIAL DISORDERS BY GENETIC MUTATIONS

I. Mitochondrial DNA mutations
   A. Large-scale deletions
      1. Kearns–Sayre syndrome
      2. PEO
   B. Mutations in mtDNA protein–coding genes
      1. ATP6 is associated with Leigh syndrome and NARP
      2. Cytochrome b is associated with exercise intolerance and recurrent myoglobinuria
      3. Cytochrome c oxidase is associated with fatal and benign infantile myopathies, Leigh syndrome, MELAS, recurrent rhabdomyolysis
   C. Mutations in mitochondrial tRNA and rRNA genes
      1. MERRF is usually associated with mutations in tRNALys gene. MERRF has also been associated with mutations in tRNALeu and tRNASer
      2. MELAS is usually associated with mutations in tRNALeu gene. MELAS also occurs with mutations in tRNAVal, tRNACys, ND5 of complex 1, and in cytochrome b
II. Nuclear gene mutations
   A. Nuclear mutations associated with mtDNA maintenance and replication (multiple mtDNA deletions and mtDNA depletion)
      1. Thymidine phosphorylase gene (*TYMP*) is associated with autosomal recessive MNGIE
      2. Adenine nucleotide translocator 1 (*ANT1*) is associated with autosomal dominant PEO
      3. Twinkle (*C10orf2*) is associated with autosomal dominant PEO and SANDO
      4. Polymerase gamma (*POLG1* and *POLG2*) is associated with autosomal recessive and dominant PEO, SANDO, MIRAS
      5. Ribonucleotidase reductase (*RRM2B*) is associated with MNGIE and PEO
      6. Thymidine kinase 2 (*TK2*) is associated with severe myopathy
      7. DNA replication helicase/nuclease 2 (*DNA2*) is associated with PEO
      8. Deoxyguanosine kinase (*DGUOK*) is associated with PEO, recurrent rhabdomyolysis, and mtDNA depletion myopathy
      9. Paraplegin (*SGP7*) is usually associated with hereditary spastic paraplegia but can be associated with PEO and spasticity
   B. Nuclear mutations associated with abnormal mitochondrial fusion/fission
      1. Mitofusin 2 (*MFN2*) associated with CMT2A
      2. Ganglioside-induced differentiation associated-protein 1 (*GDAP1*) associated with CMT2K and CMT4A
      3. Optic atrophy 1 (*OPA1*) associated with optic atrophy 1 syndrome/CMT with optic atrophy
      4. Mitochondrial inner protein 17 (*MPV17*) associated with Navajo neurohepatopathy and PEO
   C. Nuclear DNA mutations directly affecting components of mitochondrial respiratory chain
      1. Leigh syndrome may be caused by mutations in SURF1 and several different subunits of Complexes I, II, IV of the respiratory chain encoded by nuclear genes
      2. NARP caused by mutations in *MTATP6*
      3. SDH mutations can be associated with exercise intolerance

MELAS, mitochondrial encephalopathy, lactic acidosis; MIRAS; mitochondria recessive ataxic syndrome; MNGIE, myo-neuro-gastrointestinal encephalopathy; mtDNA, mitochondrial DNA; PEO, progressive external ophthalmoplegia; NARP, neuropathy ataxia and retinitis pigmentosa; SANDO, sensory ataxic neuropathy, dysarthria/dysphagia, ophthalmoplegia; SDH, succinate dehydrogenase.

▶ TABLE 30-3. CLASSIFICATION OF MITOCHONDRIAL MYOPATHIES BY CLINICAL FEATURES AND GENOTYPE

Disease	Mode of Inheritance	Mitochondrial DNA Mutation	Gene Location
Kearns–Sayre syndrome	Sporadic	Single large mtDNA mutation	Large area of mt genome
PEO	Sporadic	Single large mtDNA mutation	Large area of mt genome
PEO	Maternal	Point mutations of mtDNA	tRNA^{Leu}, tRNA^{Ile}, tRNA^{Asn}
PEOA	Autosomal dominant	Multiple mtDNA deletions	*POLG1, C10orf2* (twinkle); less common: *ANT1, POLG2, TK2, OPA1, DGOUK, RRM2B*
PEOB	Autosomal recessive	Multiple mtDNA deletions	*POLG1*; less common: *TK2, DGOUK, RRM2B, MPV17, DNA2, SGP7*
ARCO	Autosomal recessive	Multiple mtDNA deletions	Unknown nuclear gene
MERRF	Maternal	Point mutations of mtDNA	tRNA^{Lys}, tRNA^{Leu}, tRNA^{His}, tRNA^{Phe}, tRNA^{Ser}, *MTND5*
MERRF	Autosomal recessive	Multiple mtDNA deletions	*POLG1*
MELAS	Maternal	Point mutations of mtDNA	tRNA^{Leu}, tRNA^{Val}, tRNA^{Lys}, tRNA^{Phe}, tRNA^{Ser}, *ND5, ND4, ND1, MTCYB*
MNGIE	Autosomal recessive	Multiple mtDNA deletions	*TYPM, POLG1, RRM2B*
MNGIE	Maternal	Point mutations of mtDNA	tRNA^{Lys}
Leigh syndrome	Maternal	Point mutations of mtDNA	*MTND3, MTND5, MTND6, MTCO3, MTATP6,* tRNA^{Val}, tRNA^{Lys}, tRNA^{Trp}, tRNA^{Leu}
Leigh syndrome	Autosomal recessive	None	*NDUFV1, NDUFS1, NDUFS3, NDUFS4, NDUFS7, NDUFS8, SDHA BCS1L, COX10, COX15, SCO2, SURF1, LRPPRC*
Leigh syndrome	X-linked	None	*PDHA1*
Leigh syndrome	Sporadic	Single large mtDNA mutation	Large area of mt genome
Recurrent myoglobinuria	Sporadic or autosomal recessive	Mutations and microdeletions of mtDNA	*MTCO1, 2, and 3, MTCYB, ND4*
Recurrent myoglobinuria	Maternal	Point mutations of mtDNA	tRNA^{Phe}
MLASA	Autosomal recessive	None	*PUS1*
SANDO	Autosomal recessive	Multiple mtDNA deletions	*POLG1, C10orf2*
SANDO	Autosomal dominant	Multiple mtDNA deletions	*C10orf2*
Navajo neurohepatopathy	Autosomal recessive	None	*MPV17*
Optic atrophy 1	Autosomal recessive	None	*OPA1*

PEO, progressive external ophthalmoplegia; ARCO, autosomal recessive cardiopathy and ophthalmoplegia; MELAS, mitochondrial encephalopathy, lactic acidosis, and strokes; MERRF, myoclonic epilepsy and ragged red fibers; MNGIE, myo-neuro-gastrointestinal encephalopathy; MLASA, mitochondrial myopathy and sideroblastic anemia; mtDNA, mitochondrial DNA; SANDO, sensory ataxic neuropathy, dysarthria/dysphagia, ophthalmoplegia.

cells during meiosis. Therefore, some cells will have few or no mutant genomes (normal homoplasmy), some will have a mixture of mutant and normal or wild-type mtDNA (heteroplasmy), and some will have predominantly mutant genomes (mutant homoplasmy). Phenotypic expression depends on the relative proportion of mutant and wild-type mitochondria within each cell within a given organ system. When the number of mitochondria bearing sufficient mutated mtDNA exceed a certain threshold, mitochondrial function becomes impaired, and patients manifest clinical symptoms and signs of disease (threshold affect).

During mitosis and meiosis, the proportion of mutant mitochondria in daughter cells can shift, thus changing the genotype and possibly the phenotype (mitotic/meiotic segregation). In addition, mutant mitochondria may utilize the mitochondrial-encoded mRNAs and tRNAs from neighboring normal mitochondria in a process called complementation. Thus, there can be some degree of normal translation of mtDNA-encoded proteins even in mitochondria harboring large DNA deletions.

Different organs have differing susceptibility for mitochondrial abnormalities depending on their energy requirements. Because the central nervous system (CNS) is in constant demand for energy, small decreases in energy production can lead to severe abnormalities. In contrast, skeletal muscle has low-energy demands at rest, but these demands drastically increase with exercise. This is the basis for exercise-intolerance in many patients with mitochondrial myopathies.

Primary mutations of mtDNA can only be inherited from the mother. Unlike X-linked disorders that are also passed on only from the mother, males and females are equally affected in inherited mitochondrial diseases, while males are generally more severely affected with an X-linked inheritance pattern. Further, based on the degree of mitochondrial segregation and heteroplasmy, all the children of an affected mother may be affected to a variable degree, which is different from autosomal dominant and recessive inheritance patterns.

Mitochondrial disorders are not strictly inherited from an affected mother. Because over 95% of mitochondrial

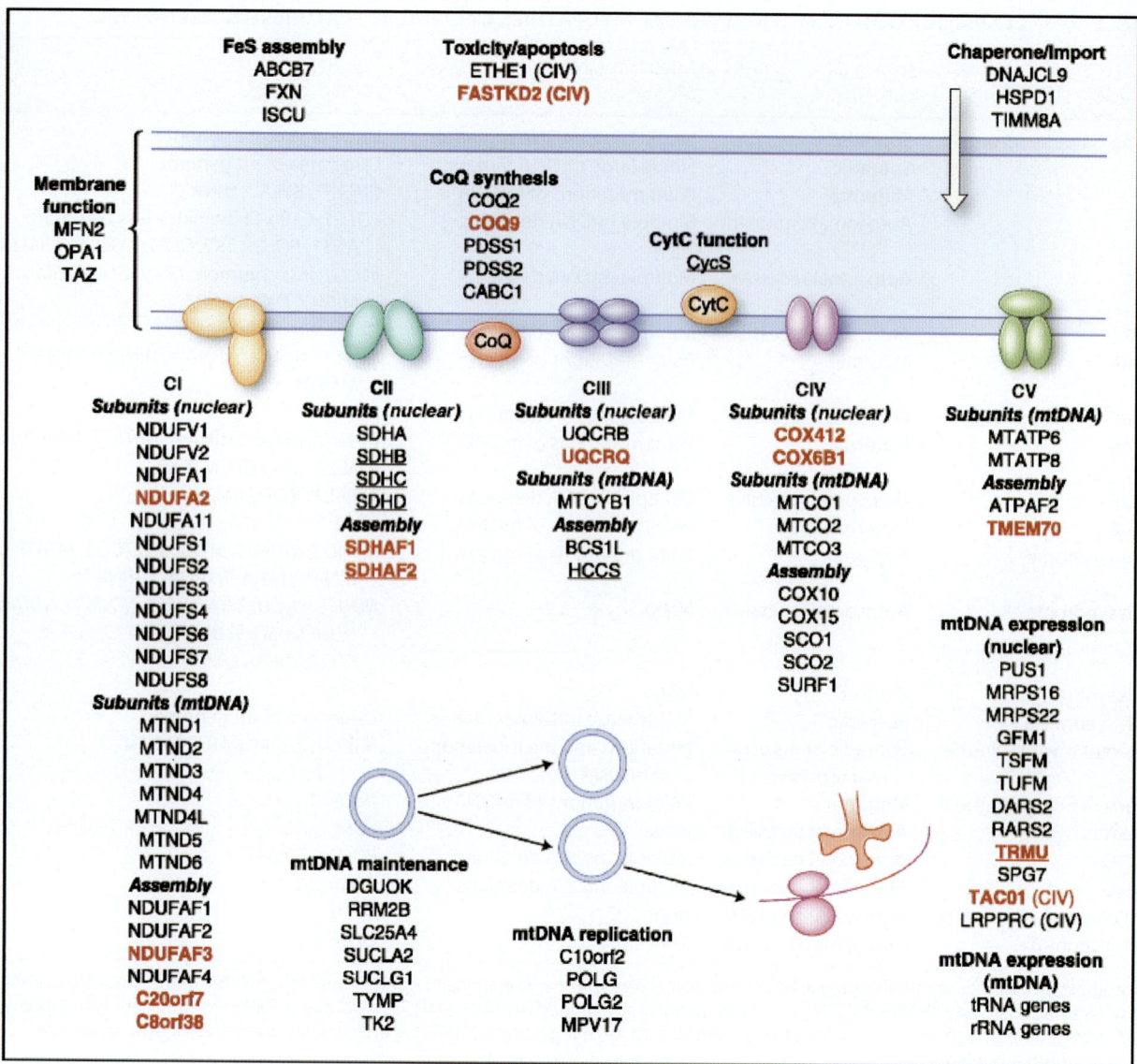

Figure 30-1. Genes associated with mitochondrial disease. Mutations have been identified in genes encoding CI, CII, CIII, CIV, and CV subunits and assembly factors; genes involved in mitochondrial DNA (mtDNA) maintenance (via nucleotide metabolism), mtDNA replication, and mtDNA expression; genes affecting the electron carriers, coenzyme Q (CoQ) and cytochrome c (CytC); genes affecting FeS assembly; and genes involved in protein import, toxicity/apoptosis, and membrane function. Recently identified genes described in this review are highlighted in red. Genes affecting oxidative phosphorylation for which mutations are not reported to cause neuropathology are underlined. rRNA, ribosomal RNA; tRNA, transfer RNA. Currently, most cases of mitochondrial encephalopathy are untreatable, other than by relieving certain symptoms. Therefore, there is a great need to better understand the genetics of mitochondrial disease, which will enable prenatal diagnoses and will deliver the deeper understanding of mitochondrial function needed for the development of effective therapies. Recent advances in sequencing technology indicate that we may be on the cusp of a revolution in the way genetic diseases, such as mitochondrial encephalopathy, are diagnosed. (Reproduced with permission from Tucker EJ, Compton AG, Thorburn DR. Recent advances in the genetics of mitochondrial encephalopathies. *Curr Neurol Neurosci Rep.* 2010;10(4):277–285.)

proteins are encoded from nuclear genes, mitochondrial disorders can be inherited in an autosomal dominant [e.g., some forms of progressive external ophthalmoplegia (PEO)], autosomal recessive [e.g., mitochondrial neurogastrointestinal encephalomyopathy (MNGIE) syndrome], and even X-linked (e.g., some forms of Leigh syndrome) fashion. In addition, the presence of mutations involving mtDNA does not imply a maternal/mitochondrial inheritance pattern. In this regard, Kearns–Sayre syndrome (KSS) is associated with large mtDNA deletions but is sporadic in nature. In addition, as noted earlier there appears to be some nuclear control over the replication and/or maintenance mitochondrial genome. Thus, mutations in some nuclear genes result in syndromes associated with depletion or multiple deletions of mtDNA. These disorders can

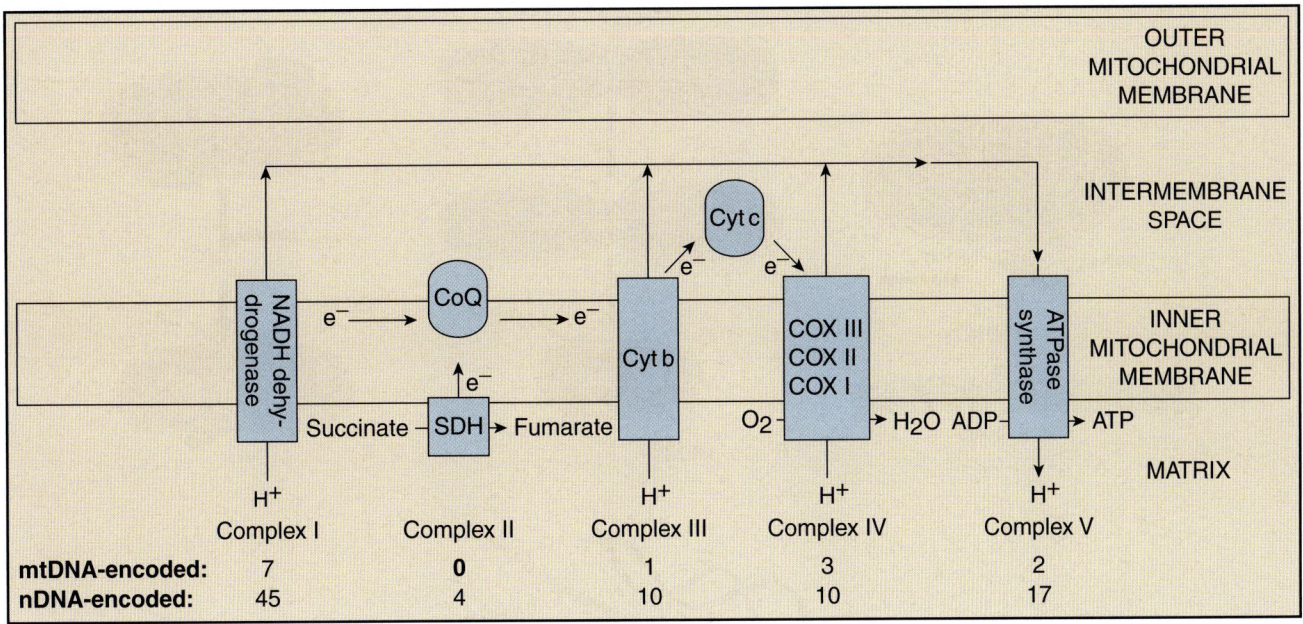

Figure 30-2. Schematic view of the respiratory chain. This diagram shows the number of subunits encoded by mitochondrial DNA (mtDNA) and nuclear DNA (nDNA) for each complex. All of the subunits for complex II are encoded by nDNA. Electrons (e−) flow down the respiratory chain and protons (H+) are pumped from the matrix to the intermembranous space through complexes I, III, and IV, then back into the matrix through complex V (ATPase synthase). Cytochrome c (Cyt c) and coenzyme Q (CoQ) are electron carriers. This process generates adenosine triphosphate (ATP). (Reproduced with permission from Walsh RJ. Metabolic myopathies. *Continuum*. 2006;12(3):76–120.)

demonstrate autosomal recessive or dominant inheritance patterns and are caused by defects in enzymes required for mtDNA replication and for maintaining the proper balance within mitochondria of deoxynucleoside triphosphates (dNTPs) that serve as the building blocks for mtDNA (Figs. 30-1 and 30-3). Replication of mtDNA requires the catalytic subunit of polymerase (encoded by the *POLG1* gene), the accessory subunit (encoded by *POLG2*), and the replicative helicases, twinkle (encoded by *PEO1*), and DNA replication helicase/nuclease 2 (encoded by *DNA2*). Mutations in these genes result in mtDNA depletion and/or multiple mtDNA deletions that are found in various mitochondrial disorders [e.g., PEO, MNGIE, sensory ataxia neuropathy dysarthria/dysphagia ophthalmoplegia (SANDO)], which are discussed later.[1-9] A delicate balance of the four dNTPs (dATP, dGTP, dCTP, and dTTP) is also necessary for mtDNA replication. Several nuclear-encoded enzymes are key in preserving this balance (i.e., *TK2, DGUOK SUCLA2, SUCLG1, RRM2B, TYMP,* and *MPV17*). Mutations in these genes also lead to mtDNA depletion and cause various mitochondrial disorders (e.g., mitochondrial depletion myopathy, MNGIE, Navajo neurohepatopathy).[1-9] Furthermore, some nuclear genes are responsible for normal mitochondrial dynamics (Figs. 30-1 and 30-3). For example, fusion of mitochondria is dependent on nuclear-encoded profusion GTPases that are located in the mitochondrial membranes and mitofusin 1 and 2 (MFN1 and MFN2).[1-9]

There can be significant genetic heterogeneity even within well-defined clinical syndromes. For example, PEO can be associated with multiple mtDNA deletions, point mutations in various mitochondrial tRNA genes, or have no mtDNA mutations. In addition, specific mutations of mitochondrial-encoded genes can manifest with heterogeneous clinical phenotypes. For example, point mutations in the mitochondrial tRNA^{Leu} can result in mitochondrial myopathy lactic acidosis and strokes (MELAS), PEO, an encephalomyopathy, or a generalized myopathy with exercise intolerance. Variability in clinical phenotype can also be apparent within families with identical mtDNA mutations. The vast clinical and genetic heterogeneity of the various mitochondrial disorders can be explained by the different segregation patterns of mutant mitochondria, the degree of mutant heteroplasmy, tissue-specific thresholds, and the severity of the biochemical impairment related to the specific mutations.

▶ **TABLE 30-4. COMPOSITION AND GENETIC CONTROL OF THE MITOCHONDRIAL RESPIRATORY CHAIN**

Complex	Respiratory Chain	
	Total Number Polypeptides	mtDNA Encoded
I	45	7
II	4	0
III	11	1
IV	13	3
V	19	2

Modified with permission from Zeviani M, Bonilla E, DeVivo DC, DiMauro S. Mitochondrial diseases. *Neurol Clin*. 1989;7:123–156.

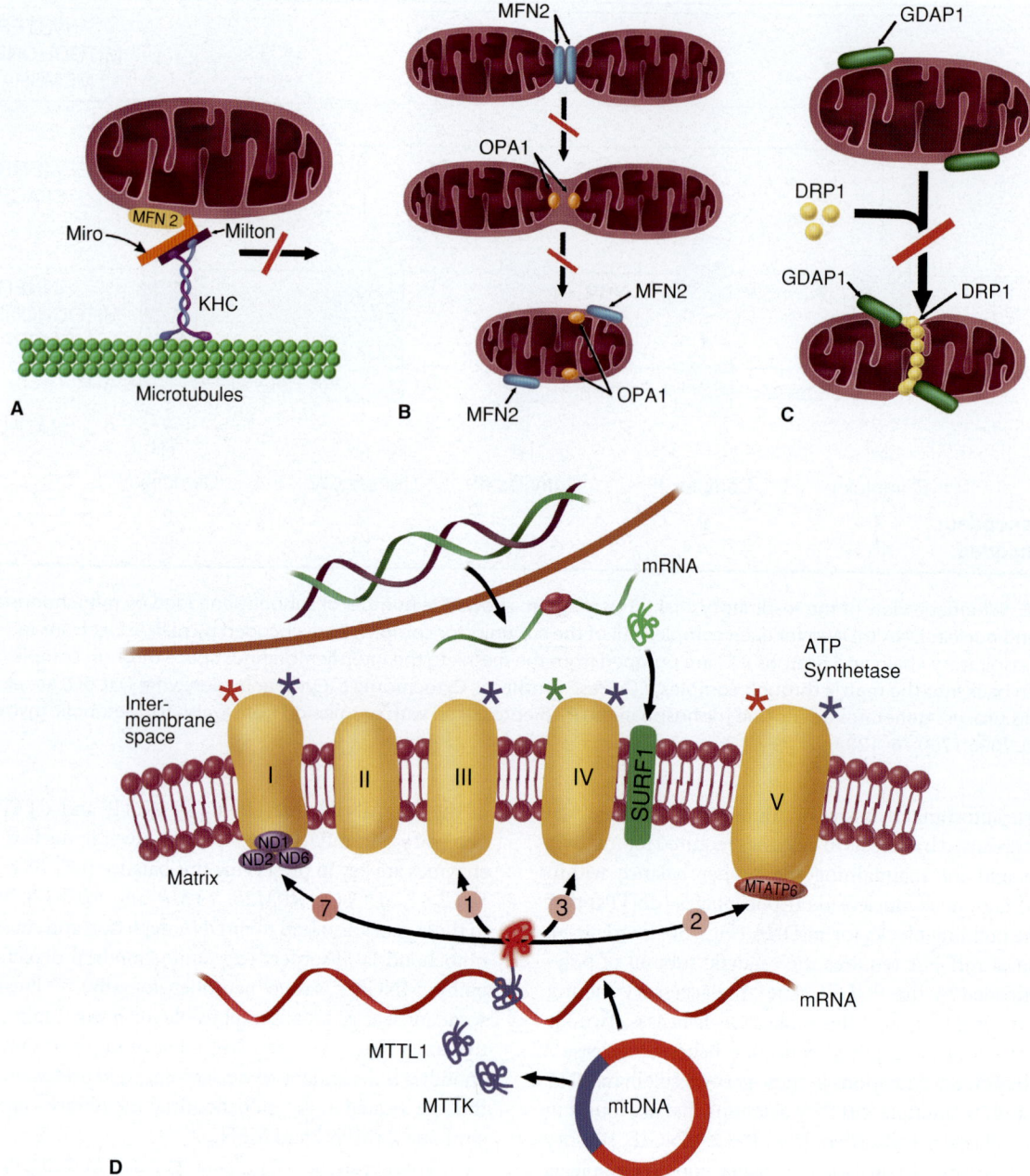

Figure 30-3. Overview of mechanisms underlying the main mitochondrial peripheral neuropathies. (**A**) *MFN2* is located in the outer mitochondrial membrane and interacts with Miro and Milton proteins, which belong to the molecular complex that links mitochondria to kinesin (KHC) motors. (**B**) *MFN2* participates in bringing the outer membranes of two mitochondria into close proximity. Thus, *MFN2* mutations can lead to defects in mitochondrial motility along the cytoskeletal microtubular tracks, and to dysfunction in fusion of the outer mitochondrial membranes of opposing mitochondria. Similarly, mutations involving OPA1, which is located in the inner mitochondrial membrane, lead to dysfunction in the fusion process of the inner mitochondrial membrane. **C:** Loss-of-function mutations affecting GDAP1, located in the outer mitochondrial membrane, can lead to dysfunction in the mitochondrial fission process, since GDAP1 might be a positive effector of assembly of the fission mediator DRP1. Dysfunction is shown by red oblique bars. **D:** Dysfunctions in the respiratory chain can be due to the following: direct mutations in mitochondrial protein-coding genes (*red segment* of circular mtDNA) *ND1*, *ND4*, and *ND6*, which encode for subunits of complex I (NADH dehydrogenase), and *MTATP6*, which encodes for a subunit of complex V (ATP-synthase); mutations in mitochondrial tRNA-coding genes (*light blue segment*) *MTTL1* and *MTTK*, which lead to dysfunction in transcription of mitochondrial protein-coding genes; or direct mutations in the nuclear gene *SURF1* (in *green*), which encodes an ancillary protein involved in complex IV (cytochrome c oxidase) assembly. Dysfunction in the corresponding respiratory chain complexes are shown by *red*, *light blue*, and *green asterisks*, respectively. Encircled numbers show the number of subunits encoded by mtDNA.

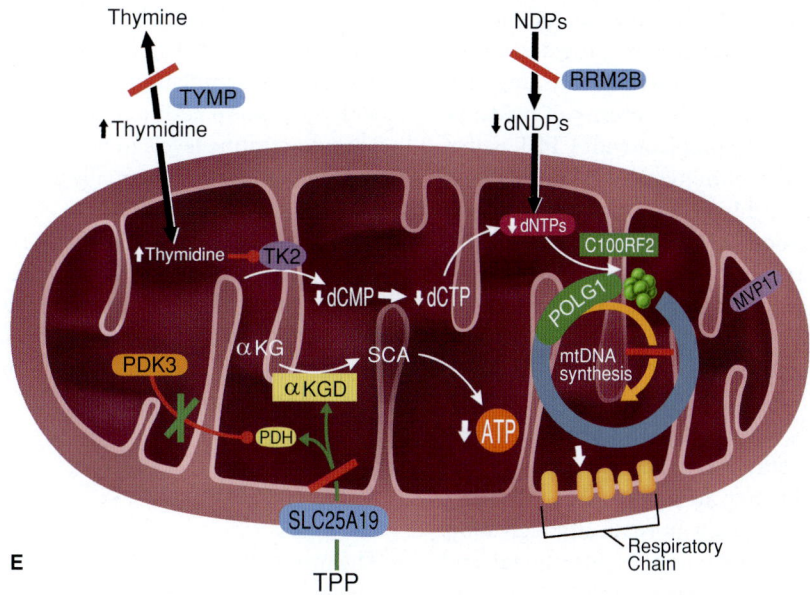

Figure 30-3. *(Continued)* **E:** Dysfunctions of the respiratory chain can also occur as a result of changes in mtDNA synthesis (*red oblique bar*), which lead to mtDNA depletion or multiple mtDNA deletions. mtDNA synthesis might be disturbed by the following: mutations in nuclear genes encoding components of the mitochondrial replisome—that is, polymerase gamma *POLG* and the helicase *C10orf2* genes; loss-of-function mutations (*red oblique bar*) in genes involved in the synthesis of nucleotides—that is, *RRM2B* and *TYMP*—which lead to nucleotide depletion (*red lines* show inhibition); or mutations in *MPV17*, a nuclear gene encoding an inner mitochondrial membrane protein of unknown function. Finally, mitochondrial peripheral neuropathies might result from changes in intermediary metabolism that eventually leads to decreased ATP synthesis. Mutations in *SLC25A19* inhibit the passage of TPP from the cytosol to the mitochondrial matrix, thus leading to lactate accumulation and an increase in αKG (an intermediate of the Krebs cycle), since TPP is an essential cofactor of PDH and αKGD (*green lines* show stimulation); similarly, a gain-of-function mutation (*green tick mark*) in *PDK3* might lock PDH in an inactive state, limiting glucose oxidation and favoring a switch toward anaerobic lactate production. mtDNA, mitochondrial DNA; NDPs, nucleoside diphosphates; dNDPs, deoxynucleoside diphosphates; dCTD, deoxycytidine; dCMP, deoxycytosine monophosphate; dCTP, deoxycytosine triphosphate; α-KG, α-ketoglutarate; α-KGD, α-ketoglutarate dehydrogenase; SCA, succinyl-CoA; TPP, thiamine pyrophosphate; PDH, pyruvate dehydrogenase.

► LABORATORY FEATURES

Serum creatine kinase (CK), lactic acid, and pyruvate levels can be normal or elevated. In addition, lactic acid levels may also be elevated in cerebrospinal fluid (CSF). Some mitochondrial disorders (e.g., mtDNA depletion) can be associated with renal tubular defects characterized by glycosuria, proteinuria, and aminoaciduria. Serum levels of fibroblast growth factor 21 (FGF-21) and growth and differentiation factor 15 (GDF-15) have recently been found to be useful in the diagnostic evaluation of mitochondrial disease, particular those with associated with myopathy. GDF-15 is a member of the transforming growth factor beta superfamily, while FGF-21 is a hormone-like cytokine secreted in response to starvation and leads to mobilization of lipid stores and production of ketone bodies.[16] Some studies have found GDF-15 levels to be a more sensitive marker,[16–18] while others demonstrate that FGF-21 levels are more sensitive.[19,20]

Cardiopulmonary exercise testing (CPET) has been used to evaluate for possible metabolic myopathies, including mitochondrial disorders.[21,22] Low levels of workload lead to an excessive rise in pulse rate and oxygen consumption. The degree of exercise intolerance correlates directly with the severity of impaired muscle oxidative phosphorylation as indicated by the peak capacity for muscle oxygen extraction and mitochondrial mutation load.[23,24] The diagnostic value of a constant workload protocol may be superior to an incremental cycle test, but the test is less sensitive for mitochondrial myopathies than simple testing of resting lactate and muscle morphology.[25] A forearm exercise test can be performed where bicycle ergometry testing is not available.[26] The patient is instructed to open and close their hand (about once every 2 seconds at 40% of maximal voluntary contraction for 3 minutes). A butterfly needle can be placed in the antecubital fossa and venous oxygen and lactate levels can be measured at baseline and each minute during and immediately following exercise. Patients with mitochondrial myopathies and exercise intolerance often demonstrate excessive and prolonged lactate production and paradoxically increased venous oxygen saturation.[26] The range of elevated venous PO_2 during forearm exercise in mitochondrial myopathy patients (32–82 mm Hg) correlates closely with the severity of oxidative impairment appreciated during cycle exercise.[27] Thus, the measurement of venous PO_2 during aerobic forearm exercise provides an easily performed screening test that sensitively detects impaired oxygen use and accurately assesses the severity of oxidative impairment in patients with the problem with CPET is that abnormalities are not specific for mitochondrial myopathies. People who are deconditioned (e.g., unfit, sedentary), those with chronic fatigue syndrome, and fibromyalgia often have abnormal reduced have reduced oxygen extraction, higher heart rate, and lactate rises that overlap with those who have a mitochondrial disorder.[21,28,29]

Nerve conduction studies (NCSs) may be normal or abnormal. Some mitochondrial disorders are associated with a myopathy and/or a neuropathy. The neuropathy can be an axonal [i.e., neuropathy ataxia and retinitis pigmentosa (NARP)] or demyelinating in nature (e.g., MNGIE). Electromyography (EMG) is usually normal, although some myopathies are associated with increased insertional and spontaneous activity as well as early recruitment of small motor unit action potentials (MUAPs), while neurogenic disorders may be associated with decreased recruitment and large MUAPs. Conduction defects may be apparent on electrocardiograms (EKG).

Magnetic resonance imaging (MRI) and CT of the brain as well as electroencephalography (EEG) are typically abnormal in patients with a mitochondrial encephalomyopathy. Brain CT may show basal ganglia calcification and/or diffuse atrophy. MRI may show focal atrophy of the cortex or cerebellum, or high signal change on T2-weighted images, particularly in the basal ganglia, thalamus, and occipital cortex.[1]

MRI of skeletal muscle can reveal morphologic changes that resemble muscular dystrophies.[30] Magnetic resonance spectroscopy (MRS) with ^{31}P and ^{1}H compounds permits the analysis of ATP, creatine phosphate, inorganic phosphate, and pH in muscle and brain.[31,32] In mitochondrial disorders, there is a rapid fall in levels of creatine phosphate and an abnormal accumulation of inorganic phosphates in tissues with exercise. In addition, there is a delay in the recovery of phosphocreatine levels to normal after exercise. These techniques may also be potentially valuable in evaluating efficacy of various treatments.[33]

If a mitochondrial disorder is suspected from the clinical history and laboratory results, a muscle biopsy may be useful to confirm the diagnosis. Mutational analysis may be done on white blood cells. However, in certain syndromes, this is not as sensitive in finding mitochondrial mutations as in muscle tissue, particularly in those with large mtDNA deletions.

▶ HISTOPATHOLOGY

The histopathological abnormalities in nerve biopsies of the various mitochondrial disorders are nonspecific and generally not helpful. However, muscle biopsies are often useful in diagnosing a mitochondrial disorder, particularly if there is significant muscle involvement. The characteristic histological features are the presence of ragged red fibers on the modified Gomori trichrome stain, but abnormalities are also evident on H&E and other stains (Fig. 30-4). Oxidative enzyme stains nicotinamide adenine dinucleotide dehydrogenase (NADH), SDH, and COX are invaluable. The aggregated mitochondria intensely react to NADH and SDH stains forming ragged blue fibers. Some patients with mitochondrial myopathies (in particular disorders not associated with mitochondrial tRNA mutations) may have no ragged red fibers and normal NADH and SDH staining. COX stain (directed against one of the subunits encoded by mtDNA) appears to be the most sensitive stain and can demonstrate

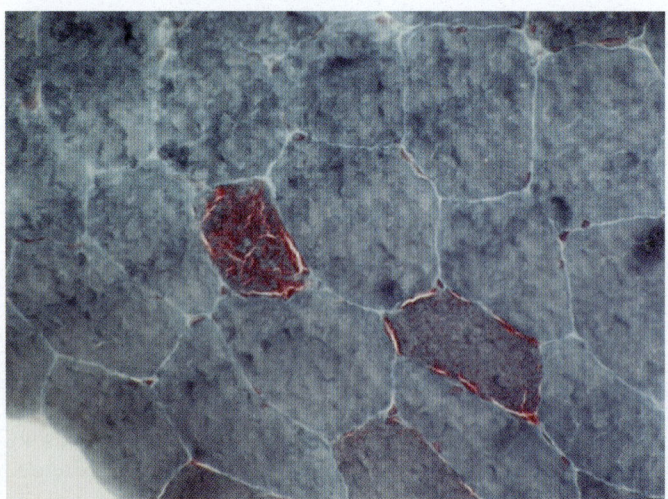

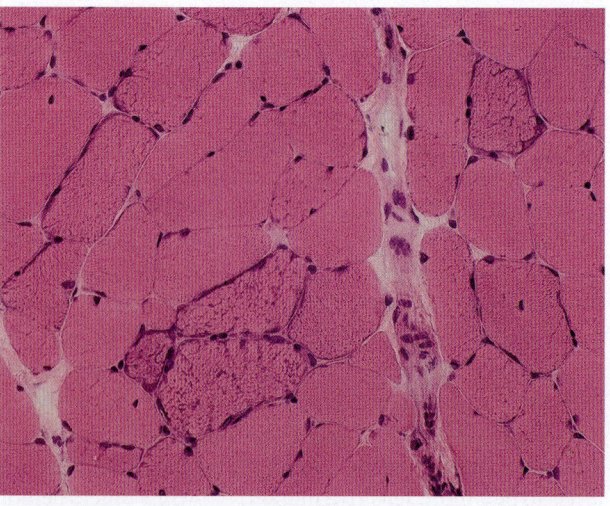

Figure 30-4. Muscle biopsy demonstrates ragged red fibers resulting from the accumulation of abnormal mitochondrial below the sarcolemma of muscle fibers on modified Gomori trichrome stain (**A**). The abnormal accumulation is also evident on H&E (**B**) and appears as "ragged blue fibers" on NADH staining (**C**).

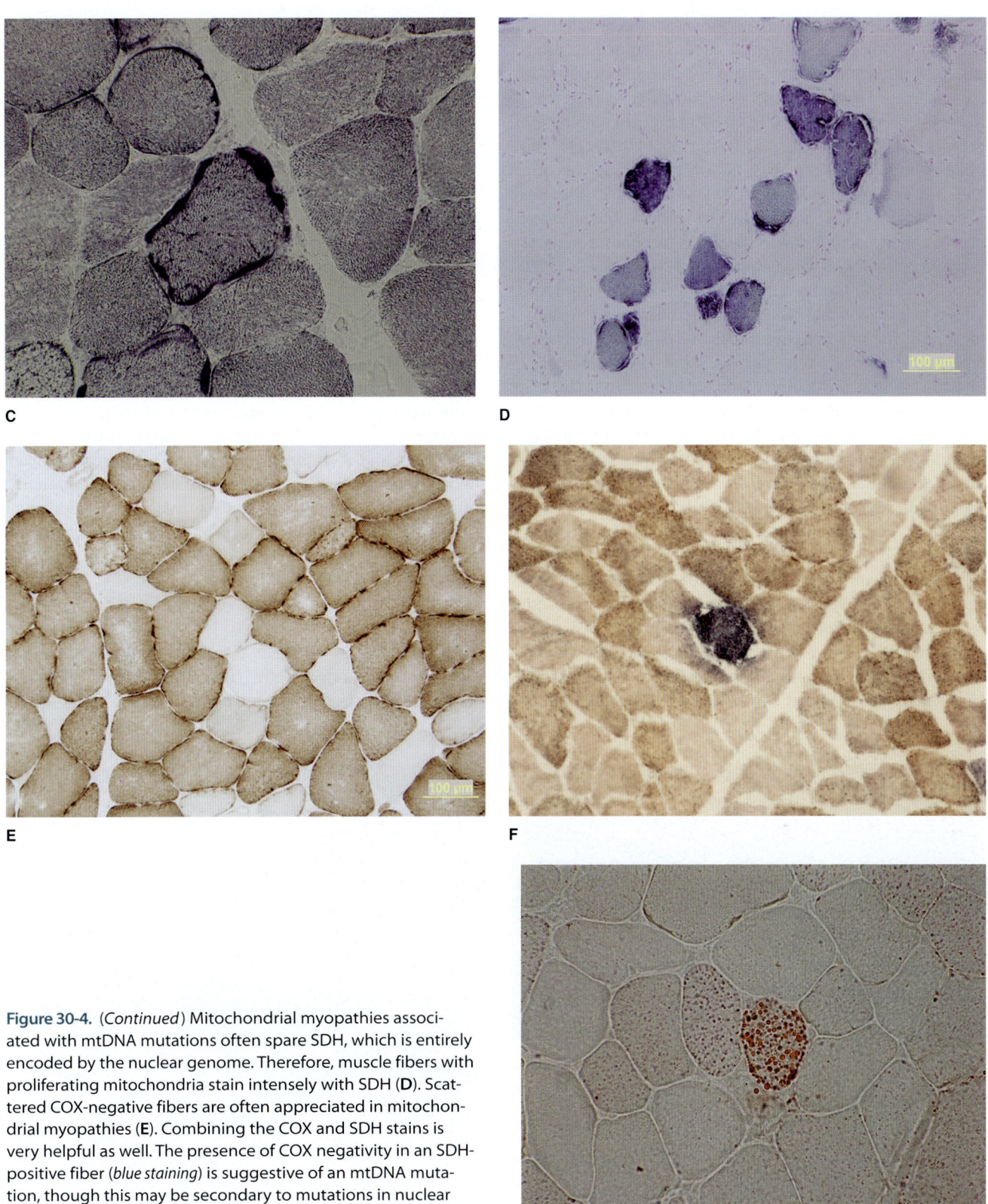

Figure 30-4. (Continued) Mitochondrial myopathies associated with mtDNA mutations often spare SDH, which is entirely encoded by the nuclear genome. Therefore, muscle fibers with proliferating mitochondria stain intensely with SDH (D). Scattered COX-negative fibers are often appreciated in mitochondrial myopathies (E). Combining the COX and SDH stains is very helpful as well. The presence of COX negativity in an SDH-positive fiber (*blue staining*) is suggestive of an mtDNA mutation, though this may be secondary to mutations in nuclear genes regulating mtDNA (F). Because mitochondria are vital in metabolism of fatty acids, there is often accumulation of fat droplets in the "ragged red fibers" on Oil Red O stain (G).

scattered muscle fibers with reduced or absent stain. In addition, COX can highlight the subsarcolemmal accumulations of mitochondria. Reduced COX staining can be seen in both ragged red and otherwise normal-appearing muscle fibers. The variability of COX staining in combination with intense SDH staining is characteristic of disorders with mtDNA mutations. Remember, the SDH component of complex II is entirely encoded by nDNA, while 3 of 13 subunits of complex IV (COX) are encoded by mtDNA. Mutations of mtDNA often lead to a proliferation of mitochondria, perhaps in a compensatory response. Because SDH is entirely encoded by nDNA, its transcription is generally increased in disorders caused by mtDNA mutations. The variability of COX staining reflects the heteroplasmic population of mutant and wild-type mitochondria. COX staining is not always abnormal in mitochondrial myopathies. Some patients with MELAS, point mutations in either ND genes or cytochrome b, or multiple mtDNA deletions (e.g., due to *POLG1* and other nDNA mutations) can have normal muscle histochemistry, including COX staining.[12] An increased number of lipid droplets are also often evident, particularly within ragged red fibers.

Ultrastructural alterations in mitochondria are usually apparent on EM. These abnormalities include an increased number of normal-appearing mitochondria, enlarged mitochondria with abnormal cristae, and mitochondria with paracrystalline inclusions (Fig. 30-5). The paracrystalline inclusions are accumulations of dimeric mitochondrial creatine kinase (mtCK). This enzyme exists in both a dimeric and octamer form, but the increased radical generation in patients with mitochondrial disorders favors the production and crystallization of dimeric mtCK.[34]

▶ BIOCHEMICAL ANALYSIS OF MITOCHONDRIAL FUNCTION

Mitochondrial enzyme activities can be assayed in muscle biopsy specimens. This can be useful when the routine muscle histochemistry is unrevealing, but the diagnosis of a mitochondrial myopathy is still suspected because of the clinical phenotype. It has also been used in the past to target genes for mutation screening, though advances in genetic testing has drastically reduced the need for enzyme activity analysis. There is no standard method for performing mitochondrial metabolic analysis. Some centers prefer to assay only fresh muscle biopsy specimens (this is necessary for measurement of substrate oxidation). Rates of flux, substrate oxidation, and ATP production can be measured by polarography or using ^{14}C-labeled substrates. More commonly, measurement of enzyme activity of each of the individual respiratory complexes is performed on frozen muscle tissue.

▶ MOLECULAR GENETIC ANALYSIS

Mutation analysis of mtDNA and nuclear genes traditionally has been guided by the clinical phenotype, laboratory features, histochemistry, and biochemistry (Fig. 30-6).[1-13]

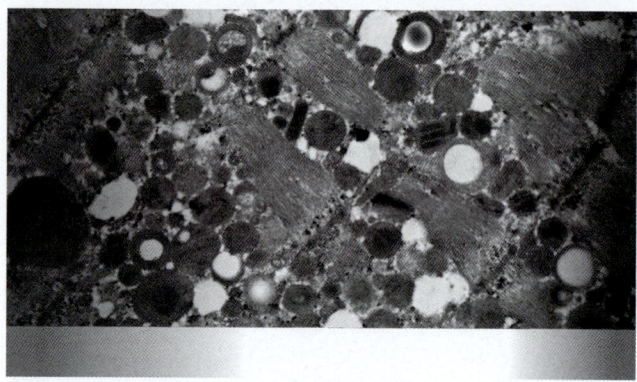

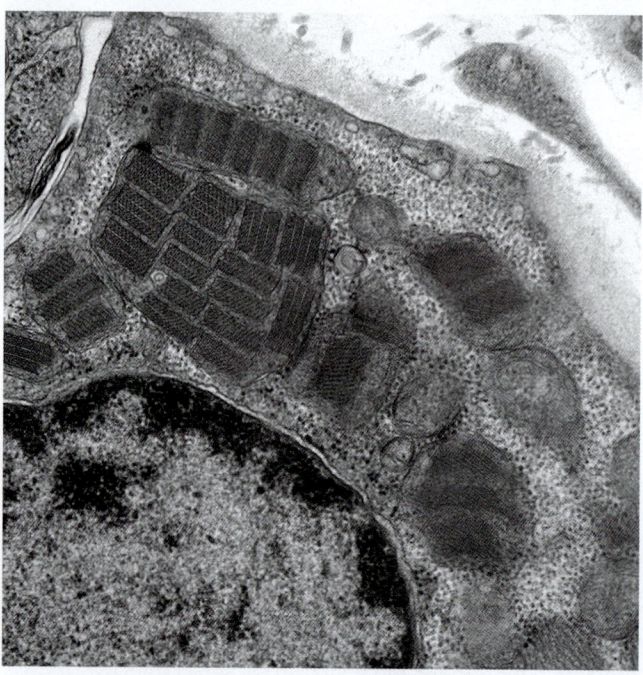

Figure 30-5. Electron microscopy. EM reveals increased numbers of mitochondria below the sarcolemma and intermixed throughout the sarcoplasm of abnormal size and shape (some quite large) along with abnormal paracrystalline inclusions cristae replacing the normal morphology of the cristae (**A**). The abnormal cristae can resemble racetracks or as here a parking lot (**B**).

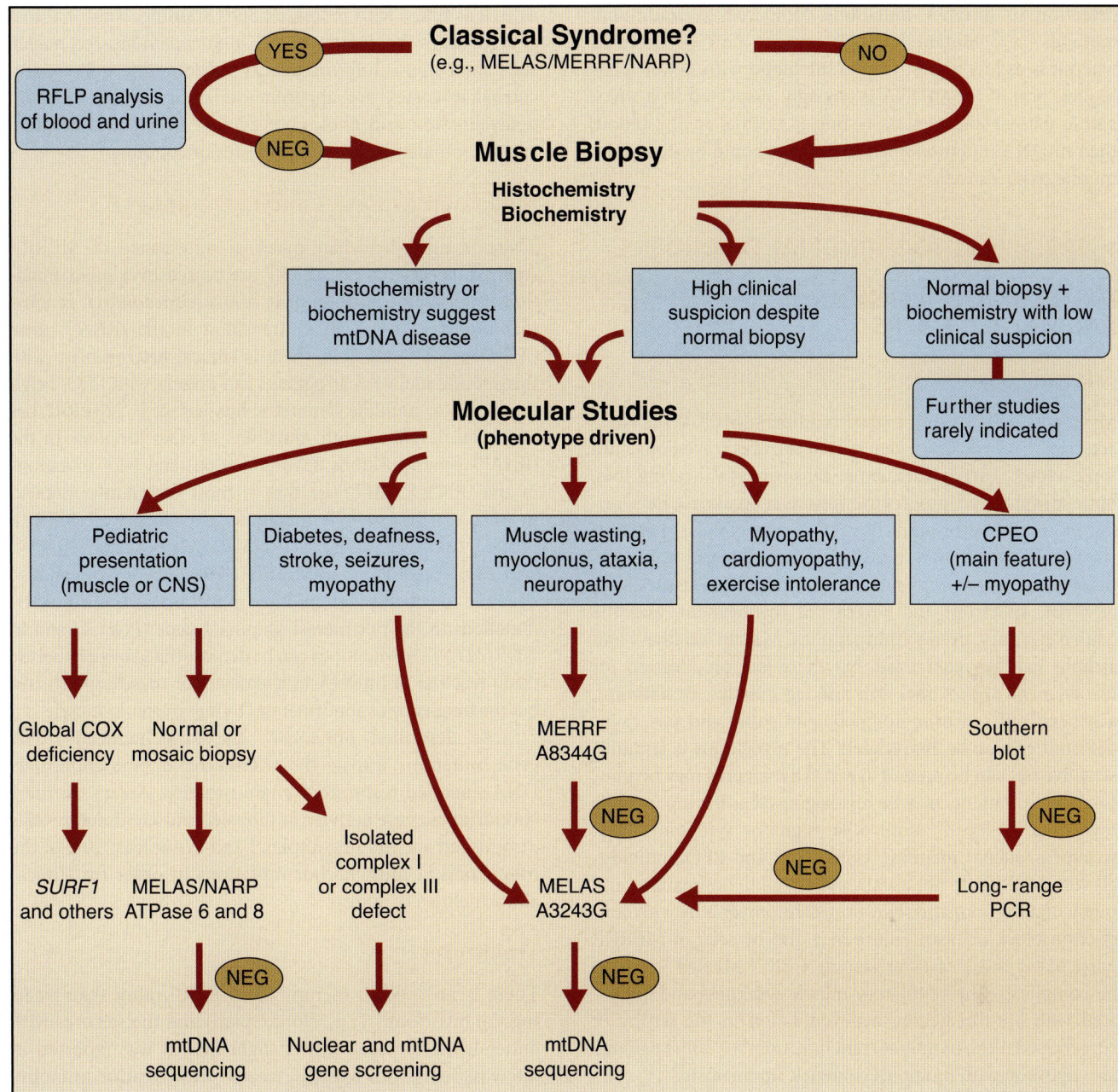

Figure 30-6. Flowchart illustrating traditional routes of investigation in cases of suspected mitochondrial muscle disease. This has largely been replaced by recent advances in genetic testing allowing less expensive testing of nuclear and mitochondrial DNA and ability to greater detect mutant homoplasmy. (Reproduced with permission from Taylor RW, Schaefer AM, Baron MJ, et al. The diagnosis of mitochondrial muscle disease. *Neuromuscul Disord.* 2004;14(4):237–245.)

In patients with classic clinical syndromes (e.g., MERRF, MELAS), one can proceed directly toward mutation screening for the most common mutations associated with these disorders. As will be discussed, however, there is wide genetic heterogeneity even within well-defined clinical phenotypes. If a pathogenic mutation is not found in white blood cells, then genetic testing can be performed on other tissues (e.g., muscle or epithelial cells in saliva or urine). Genetic testing of epithelial cells in urine is valuable in cases of MELAS as the mutant homoplasmy is greater in these cells that white blood cells in this disorder. Traditionally, screening for mutations has been done based on clinical phenotype aided by histochemical features and biochemical analysis. However, recent advances in molecular genetics have allowed for less expensive and extensive screening of mtDNA and nDNA by next-generation sequencing (NGS) and other techniques. NGS-based method with combined sequencing of the complete mtDNA and nuclear genes (either a panel of known genes that cause mitochondrial disease or whole genome sequencing) which enables a more sensitive heteroplasmy detection of mtDNA mutations compared to traditional methods.[1,25–38] Mutant homoplasmy can now be detected when it is as low as 5%–10% in the blood with newer techniques. Still, if an mtDNA is strongly suspected in a myopathic patient and genetic testing is normal in the blood, then mtDNA mutation analysis testing should be done on a muscle tissue as well.

► SPECIFIC MITOCHONDRIAL DISORDERS

MYOCLONIC EPILEPSY AND RAGGED RED FIBERS

Clinical Features

Myoclonic epilepsy and ragged red fibers (MERRF) is characterized by myoclonus, generalized seizures (myoclonic and tonic–clonic), ataxia, dementia, sensorineural hearing loss, optic atrophy, and progressive muscular weakness developing in childhood or adult life.[1–6,39–48] The clinical spectrum is variable, which may reflect the percentage of abnormal mitochondria that segregate into the respective tissues. Age of onset, spectrum and severity of involvement, and the course can vary, even within families. Muscle weakness and atrophy can be generalized, but there is a predilection for involvement of proximal arm and leg muscles. In addition, a generalized sensorimotor polyneuropathy and pes cavus deformities may be appreciated. The myoclonus is stimulus sensitive but can be present at rest. The seizures may be photosensitive. Patients may be misdiagnosed as having juvenile myoclonic epilepsy,[49] until other signs or symptoms (e.g., weakness, ataxia) manifest. Unlike KSS and PEO, individuals with MERRF do not usually ptosis, ophthalmoparesis, and pigmentary retinopathy. However, cardiomyopathy with conduction block or heart failure may also be seen in MERRF, particularly those cases presenting early.[45] MERRF can also be complicated by ventilatory muscle weakness and associated with life-threatening hypoventilation in the setting of surgery, sedation, or intercurrent infection.[45,50] Some patients also manifest with multiple symmetric lipomatosis.[51,52]

Laboratory Features

Serum CK can be normal or mildly elevated. Serum lactate can be normal or elevated as well. Generalized slowing of the background activity and bursts of spikes and slow waves may be apparent on EEG. MRI or CT scan of the brain often reveals cerebral and cerebellar atrophy. NCSs may demonstrate reduced decreased amplitudes of sensory nerve action potentials consistent with a superimposed axonopathy in some patients.[40,53,54] EMG is usually normal, although early recruitment of small MUAPs might be evident in weak muscles.

Histopathology

Muscle histopathology is abnormal as noted previously. Many ragged red fibers and COX-negative fibers are evident as well as fibers with increased SDH staining. Neuronal loss and gliosis of the dentate nuclei, globus pallidus, red nuclei, substantia nigra, inferior olivary nuclei, optic nerves, and cerebellar cortex are apparent on autopsy.[41] In addition, demyelination and gliosis are evident in the corticospinal and spinothalamic tracts, and posterior columns.

Molecular Genetics and Pathogenesis

There is non-Mendelian maternal inheritance of MERRF. Approximately 80% of MERRF are caused by a point mutation at nucleotide position 8344 of the mitochondrial genome that results in an A to G transition in the tRNA^{Lys} gene (*MTTK*).[1,47,55–57] Of note, there is clinical heterogeneity with this specific mutation as patients can present with PEO, Leigh syndrome, or multiple symmetric lipomatosis.[41,52] MERRF has also been described with mutations at other locations in the tRNA^{Lys} gene (positions 8356 and 8366) and with mutations in the tRNA^{Leu} (*MTTL1*) that is most commonly mutated in MELAS. Other tRNA mutations associated with MERRF include tRNA^{His} (*MTTH*), tRNA^{Phe} (*MTTF*), and tRNA^{Ser} (*MTTS1*). In addition, an MERRF clinical phenotype can also be found in patients with multiple mtDNA deletions caused by mutations in the polymerase gamma 1 gene (*POLG1*) and in ND5 (*MTND5*). Mutations can be demonstrated by polymerase chain reaction of mtDNA in leukocytes or muscle specimens, but the frequency of abnormal mtDNA is greater in muscle.

As described previously, the mitochondrial tRNA gene mutations impair the translation of mitochondrial-DNA–encoded respiratory chain proteins. Assays of mitochondrial enzyme activity in biopsied muscle tissue reveals diminished activity of complex I and IV. At least 90% of the mitochondria must harbor mutations in order for clinical abnormalities to appear.[51]

Treatment

There is no specific therapy for MERRF other than treating the myoclonus (e.g., clonazepam) and the seizures with antiepileptic medications. A slight benefit was reported in a few patients with MERRF treated with creatine monohydrate (5–10 g/day).[58,59] Special care must be taken as patients with mitochondrial myopathies can develop marked alveolar hypoventilation in response to sedating medications and anesthetic agents.[3,60]

MITOCHONDRIAL MYOPATHY LACTIC ACIDOSIS AND STROKES

Clinical Features

MELAS is characterized by muscle weakness, high lactate levels in the serum or CSF, and stroke-like episodes.[1–6,60–66] Onset occurs in the first year of life in fewer than 10% with 60%–80% developing symptoms and signs of the illness by the age of 15 years.[61,64] Rarely, MELAS can present as late as the eighth decade.[62] Most affected individuals have recurrent stroke-like episodes manifesting as migraine-type headaches with nausea and vomiting, hemiparesis, hemianopsia, or cortical blindness. These stroke-like attacks may be provoked by exercise or intercurrent infection. Progressive dementia may ensue. Most patients exhibit proximal muscle weakness and complain of easy fatigue and myalgias with exercise.

As with other mitochondrial disorders, many patients with MELAS are short-statured. Some affected individuals develop myoclonus, seizures, or ataxia and thus overlap clinically with MERRF. Ptosis, ophthalmoparesis, pigmentary retinopathy, and/or cardiomyopathy occur in less than 10% of patients. Some individuals with the most common 3243 mutation in the *MTTL1* gene manifest with only diabetes mellitus and/or deafness.

Laboratory Features

Serum CK can be normal or elevated. Lactate levels are elevated in the serum and CSF in the majority of patients. EEG may demonstrate epileptiform activity. NCSs are normal, but EMG may reveal early recruitment of myopathic-appearing MUAPs.

MRI scans of the brain reveal cortical atrophy and increased signal on T(2), FLAIR, and DWI imaging in the cerebral cortex, basal ganglia, and thalamus (Fig. 30-7). The apparent diffusion coefficient (ADC) of the lesions may be increased or decreased.[66] MRS of acute cortical lesions reveal severely elevated lactate levels and reduced concentrations of *N*-acetylaspartyl compounds, glutamate, and myo-inositol.[32] In addition, MRS of skeletal muscle may demonstrate a reduced phosphocreatine level, elevated concentrations of inorganic phosphate and free adenosine 5′-diphosphate, and an abnormally low phosphorylation potential.[32]

Histopathology

Muscle biopsies are indistinguishable from other mitochondrial myopathies as described previously. There are many ragged red fibers that have variable COX staining, ranging from increased reactivity to absent staining. This variability in COX staining is more prominent than that seen in MERRF. The COX-negative fibers intensely stain with SDH. Arterioles are also strongly SDH-reactive, and an increased number of mitochondria are evident in the muscular walls of small blood vessels. Mitochondrial enzyme analysis of muscle tissue may reveal reduced activities of complexes I, III, IV, and V.

Molecular Genetics and Pathogenesis

MELAS is inherited maternally in a non-Mendelian pattern. Over 70% of cases are caused by an mtDNA mutation, an A to G substitution, at nucleotide position 3243 in the gene (*MTTL1*) encoding for tRNA^{Leu}.[1,3,61] There is genetic heterogeneity of MELAS as mutations have also been identified at positions 3252, 3260, 3271, 3291 in the tRNA^{Leu} gene as well as in the genes for tRNA^{Val} (*MTTV*), tRNA^{Lys} (*MTTK*), tRNA^{Phe} (*MTTF*), tRNA^{Ser} (*MTTS1*), the dehydrogenase-ubiquinone oxidoreductase (ND) subunits of complex I: ND1 (*MTND1*), ND4 (*MTND4*), ND5 (*MTND5*), and cytochrome b of complex III (*MTCYB*).[67] In addition, there is phenotypic heterogeneity even within different family members who carry the common 3243 mutation within the tRNA^{Leu} gene. Abnormal mitochondria in cerebral blood vessels or the neurons both may be responsible for the stroke-like episodes secondary to impaired energy production in metabolically active regions of the brain.

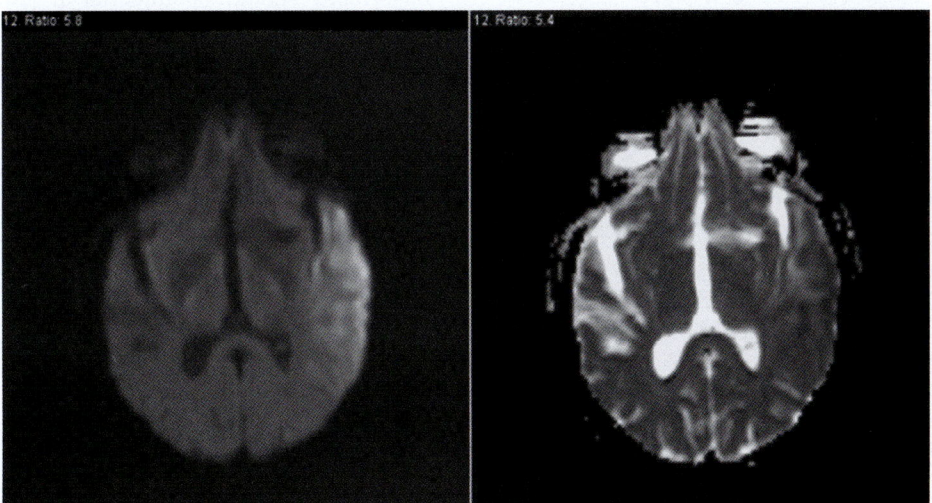

Figure 30-7. MRI in MELAS. The MRI brain imaging, during a stroke-like episode in a 61-year-old patient with genetically proven MELAS, shows a DWI high-intensity lesion in the left temporal lobe in the first image and absence of corresponding hypointensity on the corresponding ADC image. (Reproduced with permission from Walsh RJ. Metabolic myopathies. *Continuum.* 2006;12(3):76–120. Figure 3-11, p. 106.)

Treatment

No specific medical therapy is available other than treatment for seizures and myoclonus. Coenzyme Q does not appear to be of any significant benefit. A small study reported some improvement with dichloroacetate (DCA),[68] but a double-blind, placebo-controlled, randomized, 3-year crossover trial of DCA (25 mg/kg/day) in 30 patients demonstrated no efficacy with peripheral nerve toxicity.[69] Creatine monohydrate (5–10 g/day) modestly improved strength in a few patients with MELAS,[58,59,70] but again, blinded controlled studies are lacking. L-Arginine is often recommended, but a recent meta-analysis of 37 articles that included 91 patients (0 randomized controlled trials; 3 open-label; 1 retrospective cohort; 33 case reports/case series) concluded that the available evidence is of poor methodologic quality and concluded oral L-arginine confers no demonstrable clinical benefit in either the acute or prophylactic treatment of MELAS.[71]

KEARNS–SAYRE SYNDROME

Clinical Features

KSS is characterized by the clinical triad of PEO, pigmentary retinopathy, and cardiomyopathy with onset usually before the age of 20 years.[1–6,72–78] Other clinical features include short stature, proximal muscle weakness, sensorineural hearing loss, dementia, ataxia, depressed ventilatory drive, and multiple endocrinopathies (e.g., diabetes mellitus, hypothyroidism, hypoparathyroidism, delayed secondary sexual characteristics). Affected individuals are very sensitive to sedatives and anesthetic agents can provoke ventilatory failure.[79,80]

Laboratory Features

Serum CK level is typically normal; however, lactate and pyruvate levels may be elevated. CSF protein is usually increased. The EKG often reveals conduction defects. NCSs are usually normal, although diminished amplitudes suggestive of an axonal sensory or sensorimotor polyneuropathy may be seen. EMG usually demonstrates normal insertional and spontaneous activity but may reveal early recruitment of small polyphasic MUAPs in weak muscles.

Histopathology

Muscle biopsies demonstrate ragged red fibers; however, unlike MERRF and MELAS, there is little variability of COX staining with most of the ragged red fibers lacking COX reactivity.[81] The number of ragged red fibers and COX-negative fibers correlates with the percentage of mitochondria harboring large deletions. Autopsy may reveal spongy degeneration of the cerebral white matter.

Molecular Genetics and Pathogenesis

Single large mtDNA deletions (ranging from 1.3 to 8.8 kb) can be demonstrated in most patients with KSS.[1,74,76,78,81] As many as 43% of patients have a characteristic 4.9-kb deletion, suggesting there may be "hot spots" in the mitochondrial genome for these large deletions. One is more likely to find mtDNA mutations in muscle tissue than in peripheral white blood cells with the percentage of affected mitochondrial genomes in muscle biopsies ranging from 20% to 90%.[76] These large deletions most likely arise during oogenesis.[5] Mitochondrial disorders with single large deletions need to be differentiated from disorders with multiple deletions (see later). The large deletions usually involve several tRNA genes, thus impairing the adequate translation of mtDNA-encoded proteins. The single deletion mutations are usually sporadic in nature, although rare cases with familial occurrences have been reported.[74]

The clinical phenotype of individuals harboring single large mtDNA is again heterogeneous. Some patients develop migraines and stroke-like episodes with or without PEO, some have PEO with or without limb weakness, retinopathy, or deafness, others have an encephalopathy without PEO (including Leigh syndrome), while rare patients manifest only with diabetes mellitus, deafness, or Pearson syndrome.

Treatment

Some patients with KSS treated with creatine supplementation (0.08–0.35 g/kg body weight/day) have improved exercise capacity measured with bicycle ergometry.[70] Patients with cardiac conduction defects may require pacemaker insertion. Ptosis may be treated with eyelid surgery provided there is sufficient facial strength to allow full eye closure. Tarsorraphy should be undertaken judiciously, however, as there is risk for corneal injury due to exposure/trauma if the eyelids cannot completely close, and risk of ptosis recurrence. Patients and their physicians need to be made aware of the extreme sensitivity to CNS depressants and potential for decreased respiratory drive.[3,79,80]

PROGRESSIVE EXTERNAL OPHTHALMOPLEGIA

Clinical Features

Patients with PEO have ptosis and ophthalmoparesis (Fig. 30-8) with or without extremity weakness, but they lack pigmentary retinopathy, cardiac conduction defects, or other systemic manifestations (e.g., endocrinopathies).[1–6,74–84]

Some cases that are sporadic in nature and associated with single large deletions of mtDNA probably represent a partial clinical expression of KSS. There are autosomal dominant and recessive forms as well as maternally (mitochondrial) inherited forms of PEO.

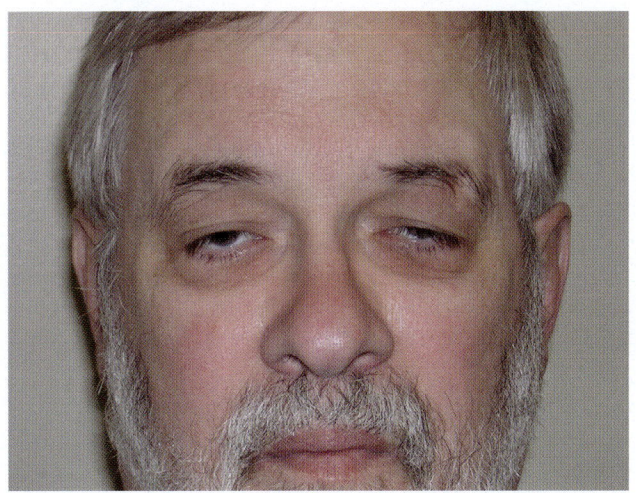

Figure 30-8. Progressive external ophthalmoplegia. A patient has ptosis and inability to move the eyes.

Laboratory Features

Serum CK, serum lactate, and CSF lactate can be normal or elevated. CSF protein may be increased. In contrast to classic KSS, the EKG does not demonstrate cardiac conduction defects. NCSs are normal. EMG is also usually normal, although myopathic MUAPs may be found in weak extremity muscles.

Histopathology

Muscle pathology is indistinguishable from KSS.

Molecular Genetics and Pathogenesis

Approximately 40%–70% of patients with PEO have single large mtDNA deletions similar to KSS.[1,74–84] Such cases are generally sporadic in nature and PEO is not passed on to subsequent generations. Point mutations have been identified within various mitochondrial tRNAs (Leu, Ile, Asn, Trp) genes in several kinships with maternal inheritance of PEO.[64]

Autosomal dominant PEO is usually associated with multiple mtDNA deletions and is genetically heterogeneous (Table 30-2).[1,74–77,81–84]

Several genes have been identified in autosomal dominant PEO (PEOA): PEOA1 due to mutations in the polymerase gamma 1 gene (POLG1); PEOA2 is caused by mutations in the ANT1 gene that encodes for adenine nucleotide translocator (ANT); and PEOA3 caused by mutation in the twinkle gene (C10orf2). ANT is the most abundant mitochondrial protein and is responsible for transporting adenosine triphosphate across the inner mitochondrial membrane, while twinkle and POLG are involved in mtDNA replication. Less common, PEO has been associated with mutations in POLG2, TK2, OPA1, DGOUK, and RRM2B.

Autosomal recessive progressive external ophthalmoplegia (PEOB) is also most commonly caused by mutations in the POLG1 gene. Mutations in this gene also have been implicated in Alper syndrome, which causes a clinical triad of psychomotor retardation, intractable epilepsy, and liver failure in infants and young children. Less common mutations have been identified in the TK2, DGOUK, RRM2B, MPV17, DNA2, and SPG7 genes.[1,4–7,85–87]

Treatment

Surgery to correct ptosis may help. As with other mitochondrial disorders, individuals with PEO can develop hypoventilation in the setting of infection and in response to sedatives or anesthetic agents.[3,79,80]

AUTOSOMAL RECESSIVE CARDIOMYOPATHY AND OPHTHALMOPLEGIA (ARCO)

Clinical Features

Only a few patients have been reported with this rare syndrome characterized by childhood-onset PEO, facial and proximal limb weakness, and severe cardiomyopathy.[88,89] Affected individuals frequently complained of chest pain, dyspnea, and palpitations secondary to severe dilated cardiomyopathy and some require heart transplantation. The severe cardiomyopathy and autosomal recessive inheritance pattern help to distinguish this myopathy from autosomal dominant and maternally inherited PEO. The reported patients had no evidence of pigmentary retinopathy, hearing loss, ataxia, or peripheral neuropathy, although deep tendon reflexes were reduced.

Laboratory Features

Serum CK levels are mildly elevated. Serum lactate can be normal at rest but increases excessively during exercise. The EKG reveals cardiac conduction defects, while echocardiogram usually demonstrates dilated ventricles and a reduced ejection fraction. NCSs are normal, but EMG may reveal myopathic-appearing MUAPs.

Histopathology

Muscle biopsies reveal ragged red fibers which are strongly reactive to SDH but COX-negative.[88,89] However, there are also many COX-negative fibers which do not co-localize to ragged red and SDH-positive fibers. Biochemical assay has demonstrated decreased activity of respiratory chain enzymes containing mtDNA-encoded subunits, sparing the entirely nuclear-encoded SDH and citrate synthetase.

Molecular Genetics

Multiple mtDNA deletions may be found and the genetic defect is suspected to lie in nuclear genes involved in regulating the mitochondrial genome.

Treatment

Many patients will die from severe cardiomyopathy within the first two decades of life unless they receive cardiac transplantation.

MITOCHONDRIAL DNA DEPLETION MYOPATHY

Clinical Features

The mtDNA depletion syndromes (MDSs) are a heterogeneous group of autosomal recessive disorders characterized by decreased mtDNA copy number in affected tissues (Table 30-2).[1–10,90–115] The MDSs are associated with a severe myopathy that usually presents in infancy or early childhood, but milder cases manifesting in adult life have been reported. There is a predilection for proximal muscle involvement but ptosis and ophthalmoplegia are also common. Some also have a superimposed polyneuropathy. Muscle stretch reflexes are diminished or absent. In addition, some affected individuals can develop a cardiomyopathy, De Toni–Fanconi–Debré syndrome (a renal tubular defect), seizures, or liver failure. When the onset is in infancy, the muscle weakness is typically severe and progressive leading to feeding difficulties, respiratory failure, and death usually within the first year of life. Some forms of PEO (previously discussed) and MNGIE, mitochondria recessive ataxic syndrome (MIRAS), optic atrophy 1 (OA1), and Navajo neurohepatopathy (discussed in subsequent sections) are other mitochondrial disorders associated with MDS.

Laboratory Features

Serum CK can be normal or elevated as can serum lactate levels. The associated renal tubular defect results in glycosuria, proteinuria, and aminoaciduria. Cerebral atrophy and patchy areas of hypomyelination of subcortical white matter may be apparent on MRI scans.[97] Unlike most other mitochondrial myopathies, EMG may demonstrate numerous fibrillation potentials and positive sharp waves in those myopathies with mtDNA depletion. Motor units can have a mixed myopathic and neuropathic appearance. NCSs can be normal or reveal features of an axonal or demyelinating sensorimotor neuropathy.

Histopathology

Muscle biopsies demonstrate many COX-negative fibers, although ragged red fibers may not be apparent.[91,97] EM shows enlarged mitochondria, some with concentric or whorled cristae, dense bodies, or paracrystalline inclusions. Biochemical assay of COX activity in skeletal muscle tissue of affected patients is greatly diminished or absent.

Molecular Genetics and Pathogenesis

MDS is associated with mutations in nuclear genes that control and maintain mtDNA.[1–10] At least half the cases are sporadic in nature, but some are inherited in an autosomal recessive fashion. A depletion of mtDNA was first reported by Moraes et al. in 1991[98] and subsequently confirmed by others.[91,94–115] The quantity of mtDNA indirectly correlates with the clinical severity of the disorder. As much as a 99% reduction in mtDNA is present in the fatal infantile myopathy form of the disease, while the more benign myopathy has been demonstrated to have lesser depletions (36%–88%) of mtDNA. Mitochondrial depletion myopathy is usually caused by mutations in the gene that encodes for thymidine kinase 2 (*TK2*),[94,103–114] but rare cases are caused by mutations in the deoxyguanosine kinase gene (*DGOUK*).[85,114,115]

Mitochondrial depletion can be seen by mutations in other genes that are associated with other clinical syndromes: thymidine phosphorylase (*TYMP*), *POLG1* and *2*, twinkle (*C10orf2*), mitochondrial inner membrane protein 17 (*MPV17*), ribonucleotide reductase (*RRM2B*), optic atrophy 1 (*OPA1*), succinate-CoA ligase alpha subunit (*SUCLG1*), and succinate-CoA ligase ADP-forming, beta subunit (*SUCLA2*).[1] Disorders associated with mutations in these genes are discussed in other sections.

Treatment

No specific medical therapy has been demonstrated to be effective. Patients and their physicians need to be made aware of the extreme sensitivity to CNS depressants and potential for decreased respiratory drive.[3]

MITOCHONDRIAL NEUROGASTROINTESTINAL ENCEPHALOMYOPATHY

Clinical Features

MNGIE, also referred to as POLIP syndrome (*P*olyneuropathy, *O*phthalmoplegia, *L*eukoencephalopathy, and *I*ntestinal *P*seudo-obstruction) is an autosomal recessive mitochondrial disorder.[1–10,73,116–121] As the acronyms imply, the disorder is associated with a sensorimotor polyneuropathy, leukoencephalopathy on MRI of the brain, ragged red fibers on muscle biopsy, and chronic intestinal pseudo-obstruction. The disorder usually manifests before the age of 20 years (mean 13.9 years, range 2.5–32 years).[122] The course is progressive with severe disability or death by the third or fourth decade of life. The earliest symptoms are often caused by gastrointestinal dysmotility (i.e., dyspepsia, bloating, eructation, cramps, intolerance of large meals, and episodic nausea, vomiting, and diarrhea). Affected individuals gradually develop distal greater than proximal muscle weakness and atrophy, a stocking–glove distribution of sensory loss, and reduced muscle stretch reflexes throughout. Most patients have ptosis and extraocular muscle weakness. Despite the leukoencephalopathy apparent on MRI and on autopsies, most affected patients have little in the way of CNS symptoms or signs. However, rare patients have mental retardation. Other clinical features include pigmentary retinopathy, sensorineural hearing loss, facial weakness, hoarseness, or dysarthria.

Laboratory Features

Serum CK can be normal or mildly elevated. Lactate, pyruvate, and CSF protein levels are typically elevated. Thymidine phosphorylase activity is decreased in leukocytes and platelets, thymidine levels are increased in the plasma, and deoxyuridine is increased in serum and plasma in those cases caused by mutation in the *TYMP* gene that encodes for thymidine phosphorylase.

Leukoencephalopathy of the cerebral and cerebellar white matter is apparent on MRI scans. Radiological studies also demonstrate dilatation and dysmotility of the esophagus, stomach, and small intestine. EKG has shown conduction defects in some patients, although they remained asymptomatic from a cardiac standpoint. Motor and sensory nerve conduction velocities may be slow to within the demyelinating range, while F-wave latencies are usually markedly prolonged.[118,122,123] Other cases are more suggestive of a primary axonopathy with reduced SNAP and CMAP amplitudes. EMG may reveal fibrillation potentials and positive sharp waves.[122] Recruitment of MUAPs can be decreased, suggestive of denervation in distal muscles. However, quantitative EMG of proximal muscles may reveal small duration MUAPs suggesting a superimposed myopathic process. The generalized weakness coupled with the demyelinating polyneuropathy can lead to misdiagnosis as chronic inflammatory demyelinating polyneuropathy.[123]

Histopathology

Muscle biopsies may demonstrate ragged red fibers, ragged blue fibers with NADH and SDH staining, and COX-negative fibers.[122] Neurogenic atrophy may be apparent biopsies of distal muscles. Nerve biopsies have shown loss of myelinated nerve fibers, demyelination/remyelination, and rare onion-bulb formation, in addition to features of axonal degeneration. Abnormal mitochondria with paracrystalline inclusions occur in both muscle fibers and Schwann cells. Diminished COX and other respiratory complex activities can be demonstrated on enzymatic assays of muscle tissue.[122]

Autopsies have revealed widespread endoneurial fibrosis and demyelination in the peripheral nervous system and poorly defined white matter changes in the cerebral and cerebellar white matter.[118] Cranial nerves and spinal roots are less severely involved. Neurons of the brainstem and spinal cord appeared relatively intact. Interestingly, a loss of neurons and fibrotic changes of the autonomic ganglia and of the celiac and myenteric plexuses has been noted, which likely explains the associated gastrointestinal dysmotility.[118]

Molecular Genetics and Pathogenesis

Multiple mtDNA deletions similar to those found in some cases of autosomal dominant PEO have been demonstrated in some patients with autosomal recessive MNGIE.[1–10,117,124,125] Some cases of MNGIE are caused by mutations in the thymidine phosphorylase (*TYPM* or *ECGG1*) gene located on chromosome 22q13.32-qter.[1,117,125,126] Thymidine phosphorylase converts thymidine to 2-deoxy D-ribose 1-phosphate and may regulate thymidine availability for DNA synthesis. Interestingly, thymidine phosphorylase is not normally expressed in muscle tissue, so how it leads to multiple mtDNA deletions is unclear. It may lead to a reduction in the nucleotide pool within the mitochondria. Rare cases of MNGIE have been shown to be caused by mutations in *POLG1*, *RRM2B*, and the tRNA^{Lys} (*MTTK*) gene.[10,127–129] Neuropathy is demyelinating in patients carrying *TYPM* or *RRM2B* mutations, whereas patients with *POLG1* mutations mainly have axonal electrodiagnostic (EDX) features.[10]

Treatment

No specific proven medical therapy is available. Again, patients and their physicians need to be made aware of the extreme sensitivity to CNS depressants and potential for decreased respiratory drive.[3] Some studies have reported that hemodialysis peritoneal dialysis, and platelet infusion can temporarily improve of the biochemical imbalance in in MNGIE patients, but this does not necessarily translate into clinical improvement, and there are practical limitations and safety concerns with these treatments.[119] Allogeneic hematopoietic stem cell transplantation (HSCT) can restore thymidine phosphorylase enzyme function in patients with MNGIE and small series have reported improvement in clinical manifestations in some patients.[120,121] However, there are significant short- and long-term risks associated with HSC (e.g., infection, graft-vs.-host disease, secondary malignancies). Allogeneic HSCT should be considered for selected patients with an optimal donor. PEG tube or parenteral feedings for nutritional support are required in the majority of cases. Ankle foot orthotics may be beneficial in patients with foot drop.

SENSORY ATAXIA NEUROPATHY DYSARTHRIA/DYSPHAGIA OPHTHALMOPLEGIA

Clinical Features

SANDO (sensory ataxic neuropathy, dysarthria, ophthalmoplegia) is a disorder that may occur sporadically or in either a dominantly or recessively inherited fashion.[8–10,130–134] The onset of sensory ataxia is typically in early adulthood. Not all patients have each element of the SANDO syndrome. In addition to the phenotypic features described in the acronym, cerebellar ataxia, facial weakness, mild proximal weakness, exercise intolerance, Parkinsonism, myoclonus epilepsy, and hepatic failure have been described.[130,132]

Laboratory Features

NCSs may reveal amplitude reduction and/or slowing of sensory SNAPs.[8–10,130–134]

Histopathology

Muscle biopsies may reveal ragged red and COX-negative muscle fibers. Sural nerve biopsy is not routinely performed but has revealed loss of large and small myelinated fibers and demonstrated onion-bulb formations.[8,9] Autopsy studies have shown axonal and dorsal column degeneration, suggesting involvement of dorsal root ganglia.[10]

Molecular Genetics and Pathogenesis

SANDO is usually autosomal recessively inherited and caused by mutations in *POLG1* that results in multiple mtDNA deletions and mtDNA depletion as mentioned previously.[131,133,134] SANDO can also result from mutations in *C10orf2*, which encodes twinkle helicase that also is involved in mtDNA replication.[135] Mutations in this gene can cause an autosomal dominant or recessive syndrome.

Treatment

No specific medical therapy is available.

MITOCHONDRIA RECESSIVE ATAXIC SYNDROME

MIRAS is very similar to SANDO and typically presents as a juvenile- or adult-onset ataxic neuropathy. Associated phenotypic features may include CPEO, dysarthria, seizures, nystagmus, cognitive impairment, involuntary movements, and psychiatric symptoms.[135-140] Like SANDO, it is usually caused by mutations in *POLG1*.

NEUROPATHY ATAXIA AND RETINITIS PIGMENTOSA

Clinical Features

NARP is associated with a childhood- or adult-onset axonal neuropathy, cerebellar ataxia, and retinitis pigmentosa. There may be proximal or distal weakness as well as pes cavus on examination.[8-10,141-144]

Laboratory Features

NCSs reveal features suggestive of an axonal sensory neuropathy.

Histopathology

Muscle biopsy does not generally reveal ragged red or COX-negative fibers as the causal gene (see below) is involved only in the last step of ATP production. Nerve biopsy reveals loss of myelinated nerve fibers.[8,9]

Molecular Genetics and Pathogenesis

NARP is caused by mutations in mitochondrial-encoded ATPase 6 (*MTATP6*), which is also a cause of Leigh syndrome.

Treatment

No specific medical therapy is available.

NAVAJO NEUROHEPATOPATHY

Clinical Features

This manifests in infancy or early childhood with failure to thrive, diarrhea, vomiting, and signs of liver failure, including recurrent metabolic acidosis. In addition, infants have generalized hypotonia and weakness. Other neurological signs included microcephaly, seizures, ataxia, and dystonia. Those individuals who survive typically develop a severe sensorimotor polyneuropathy.[8,9,145-148] Loss of sensation leads to acromutilation and corneal ulcerations.

Laboratory Features

Serum transaminases and bilirubin are elevated while albumin is low. There may be evidence of a coagulopathy. Aminoaciduria is evident on urine screen. MRI scans reveal abnormal signal intensity in cortex and subcortical white matter as well as the dentate nuclei and cerebellar white matter.[8,9] NCSs reveal slowing of conduction velocities suggestive of a demyelinating sensorimotor polyneuropathy.[8-10,145,146]

Histopathology

Nerve biopsies have demonstrated loss of myelinated and unmyelinated nerve fibers.[145,148]

Molecular Genetics and Pathogenesis

This is caused by homozygous mutations (Arg50Trp) in the mitochondrial inner membrane protein gene (*MPV17*).[145,146]

Treatment

No specific medical therapy is available.

OPTIC ATROPHY 1 (OA1) SYNDROME

Clinical Features

OA1 usually manifests with progressive optic atrophy and is inherited in an autosomal dominant pattern.[10,149-152] It is allelic to what has also been called HMSN VI (CMT with optic atrophy). Approximately 20% of affective individuals develop neurological abnormalities, such as PEO, peripheral neuropathy, proximal myopathy, and hearing loss. The neuropathy is usually mild, and mostly sensory, but mild distal muscle atrophy and weakness along with pes cavus may be seen. Some patients have a sensory or cerebellar ataxia.

Laboratory Features

NCSs are most suggestive of an axonal sensory greater than motor polyneuropathy.[150,153]

Histopathology

Muscle biopsy often shows multiple mtDNA deletions and sometimes depletion, ragged red fibers, and COX-negative fibers. Literature on nerve biopsy findings is lacking.

Molecular Genetics and Pathogenesis

This is caused my mutations in the *OPA1* gene, encoding a dynamin-related GTPase, which is important in mitochondrial fusion, fission, and cristae organization.[8,9,152,153]

Treatment

There is no specific medical treatment for OPA1.

LEIGH SYNDROME

Clinical Features

Leigh syndrome, or subacute necrotizing encephalomyopathy, usually presents in infancy or early childhood, but can rarely develop in adult life.[1–3,151,154] Affected individuals can manifest with recurrent vomiting, psychomotor retardation, hypotonia, generalized weakness and atrophy, ptosis, ophthalmoplegia, poor suck, respiratory failure, nystagmus, optic atrophy, hearing loss, involuntary movements, seizures, spasticity, ataxia, and peripheral neuropathy. The rate of progression varies, but the disorder is generally fatal.

Laboratory Features

Serum and CSF lactate levels are elevated as can be the lactate:pyruvate ratio. The syndrome is biochemically heterogeneous. Defects in activity of the pyruvate dehydrogenase (PDH), pyruvate decarboxylase (PDC), COX, and complex I have been described in some patients with Leigh syndrome. MRI demonstrates symmetric lesions in the thalamus, brainstem, cerebellum, and spinal cord reflecting the underlying pathology.

Histopathology

Muscle biopsy can demonstrate reduced or absent COX staining (mitochondrial- and nuclear-encoded COX subunits) of muscle fibers, although ragged red fibers are usually not seen. Unlike fatal infantile myopathy, COX staining is also deficient in muscle spindles and in the smooth muscle of intramuscular blood vessels. Autopsy studies of the brain and spinal cord demonstrate symmetric cystic necrosis, spongiform changes, demyelination, and vascular proliferation in the thalamus, basal ganglia, brainstem, cerebellar white matter, dentate nuclei, and posterior columns.

Molecular Genetics and Pathogenesis

Leigh syndrome is genetically heterogeneous. Mutations have been identified in both nuclear- and mitochondrial-encoded genes. These genes are all involved in energy metabolism, including the generation of ATP, components of the PDH complex and mitochondrial respiratory chain complexes I, II, III, IV, and V, which are involved in oxidative phosphorylation.

Complex I comprises at least 45 subunits, of which 7 are encoded by the mitochondrial genome (ND1–6, ND4 L) and the others are encoded by nuclear genes. Multiple complex I genes have been implicated in Leigh syndrome including mitochondrial-encoded *MTND3*, *MTND5*, and *MTND6*, and nuclear-encoded *NDUFV1*, *NDUFS1*, *NDUFS3*, *NDUFS4*, *NDUFS7*, and *NDUFS8* genes.[155,156]

From complex II, a mutation has been found in the nDNA gene flavoprotein subunit A (*SDHA*).[157] In complex III, a mutation has been found in the nDNA gene BCS1 L, which is involved in the assembly of complex III.

Complex IV mutated genes include mitochondrial-encoded cytochrome c oxidase subunit 3 (*MTCO3*) and nuclear-encoded cytochrome c oxidase assembly proteins 10 (*COX10*) and 15 (*COX15*). Two other nuclear-encoded genes with mutations are: (1) synthesis of cytochrome c oxidase 2 (*SCO2*), and (2) surfeit 1 (*SURF1*). Surfeit1 is involved in the assembly of complex IV.[158] Mutations have been found in a complex V gene, the mitochondrial-encoded ATPase 6 (*MTATP6*).[159] Of note, mutations in this gene are also responsible for the mitochondrial disorder termed NARP (neuropathy, ataxia, and retinitis pigmentosa) as previously discussed. When the proportion of mutated mtDNA is high (>90%), Leigh syndrome occurs; but NARP develops when the burden of mtDNA mutations is lower.

Mutations in multiple genes encoding mitochondrial tRNA proteins have also been identified in patients with maternally inherited Leigh syndrome: TRNA^{Val} (*MTTV*), tRNA^{Lys} (*MTTK*), tRNA^{Trp} (*MTTW*), and tRNA^{Leu} (*MTTL1*).[154,160] Single large deletions of mtDNA have also been demonstrated.[161]

Leigh syndrome may also be caused by mutations in components of the PDH complex. The gene *DLD* encodes for dihydrolipoamide dehydrogenase, which is a component not only of the PDH complex, but also of the alpha-ketoglutarate dehydrogenase complex, and the branched-chain alpha-keto acid dehydrogenase complex. Compound heterozygous mutations in *DLD* have been implicated in Leigh syndrome. X-linked Leigh syndrome is caused by mutation in the gene encoding the E1-alpha subunit of the PDH complex (*PDHA1*).[162–164]

The French–Canadian (or Saguenay–Lac-Saint-Jean) type of Leigh syndrome with COX deficiency (LSFC) is caused by mutation in the leucine-rich PPR motif-containing protein gene (*LRPPRC*). This gene encodes for an mRNA-binding protein involved in the processing and trafficking of mtDNA-encoded transcripts, but how this causes COX deficiency is not yet clear.

FOCAL MITOCHONDRIAL DEPLETION

Clinical Features

This disorder has been described in only a few patients.[165,166] A sister and brother presented in the second decade of life with exertional muscle pain and fatigue, myoglobinuria, and mild proximal weakness.[165] Their father of this pair was asymptomatic but had an elevated serum CK. Congenital weakness, hypotonia, delayed motor milestones, and mental retardation have also been reported.[166]

Laboratory Features

Serum CK levels are mild to moderately elevated and serum lactate levels are normal. A decreased selenium level has been described in one patient.[166] NCSs are normal, but EMG may reveal myopathic MUAPs.

Histopathology

The most striking histologic feature, for which this disorder is named, is focal depletion of mitochondria in the center of the sarcoplasm in type 2 muscle fibers. At the periphery of muscle fibers, the mitochondria are enlarged. Scattered degenerating and regenerating fibers can be appreciated.

Molecular Genetics and Pathogenesis

This myopathy is presumably autosomal dominant. No molecular or quantitative defects of mtDNA have been reported in patients with this syndrome. Similar histological findings have been demonstrated in patients with myopathy felt to be related to selenium deficiency.[167]

Treatment

There is no specific medical therapy. A trial of selenium replacement should be considered in patients who are deficient in selenium.

MITOCHONDRIAL MYOPATHIES ASSOCIATED WITH EXERCISE INTOLERANCE/RECURRENT MYOGLOBINURIA

Clinical Features

Some patients with mitochondrial myopathy manifest only with exercise-induced myalgias beginning in infancy or early adulthood.[4–6,168–179] They are typically short-statured and have generalized reduction in muscle bulk. Muscle strength may be normal or there can be mild proximal weakness. Recurrent episodes of myoglobinuria can also occur and be provoked by exercise and alcohol intake. However, provocative factors often are not present. We have seen patients with progressive deafness as well.

Laboratory Features

Serum lactate and pyruvate may be normal or slightly at rest but become significantly elevated with aerobic exercise. Serum CK can be normal or mildly elevated between episodes of myoglobinuria. EMG and NCSs are typically normal.

Histopathology

Muscle biopsies may reveal scattered ragged red fibers, increased SDH and NADH stains (ragged blue fibers), as well as COX-negative fibers. However, COX stain can be normal, particularly in patients with mutations in *MTCO1*, *MTCO2*, *MTCO3*, *ND4*, and *MTCYB* (see below). Decreased COX activity has been found on enzyme analysis of muscle tissue in some,[168] but not all cases.[169] Abnormal mitochondria with paracrystalline inclusions can be detected on EM.

Molecular Genetics and Pathogenesis

This is a genetically heterogeneous group of disorders. Multiple mtDNA deletions, point mutations in tRNA^{Phe}, and gene encoding for subunits of COX (*MTCO1*, *MTCO2*, *MTCO3*) have been reported.[15,93,94,172] Other cases of exercise intolerance and recurrent myoglobinuria have be ascribed to mutations in the mtDNA genes encoding for tRNA^{Gly143} subunit 4 of NADH dehydrogenase (*ND4*),[174] and cytochrome b (*MTCYB*).[175,176] Mutations in *ND4*, may also produce Leber hereditary optic neuropathy[177] or Wolfram syndrome.[178] In addition, mutations in the gene encoding the iron-sulfur cluster assembly protein (*ISCU*) have been associated with exercise intolerance and myoglobinuria and muscle biopsies demonstrating SDH deficiency and accumulation of iron in muscle fibers.[179]

Treatment

There is no specific medical therapy other than treatment of myoglobinuria and avoidance of strenuous activity and alcohol.

Charcot–Marie–Tooth Disease

There are at least three proteins involved in mitochondrial dynamics that cause forms of CMT: CMT2 A caused by mutations in the mitofusin 2 gene (*MFN2*). CMT2K and CMT4A are associated with mutations in ganglioside-induced differentiation associated-protein 1 (*GDAP1*), and OPA1 mutations are associated with CMT associated with optic atrophy as previously discussed (Fig. 30-3).[8,9] CMT caused by mutations involving MFN2 and GDAP1 are discussed in more detail in Chapter 11 (Charcot–Marie–Tooth Disease and Related Disorders). MFN and GDAP1 are involved in the fusion and fission of mitochondria which are essential in controlling the shape, size, number, and transport of mitochondria within cells. Dynamin-like GTPases located in the outer membrane (e.g., MFN2) and inner membrane (e.g., OPA1) control mitochondrial fusion. MFN2 helps tether mitochondria during fusion, while OPA1 is important for fusion of the inner membrane and formation of cristae. GDAP1, located in the outer membrane, is important in mitochondrial fission.

► SUMMARY

There is a wide range of phenotypic and genotypic variability in patients with mitochondrial disorders. Due to high-energy requirements, many of these disorders are associated with disorders of peripheral nerve and/or muscle. This phenotypic and genotypic heterogeneity has made definitive diagnosis (i.e., identifying specific genetic mutation) more difficult and expensive, though advances in genetic testing have markedly facilitated diagnosis. Although there is a greater understanding regarding the molecular pathogenesis of the different forms of mitochondrial disorders, these advances have not as yet led to easy diagnosis in many cases or effective medical treatments, other than supportive measures. There is a high morbidity and mortality that is independently predicted by braining involvement, cardiac conduction defects, and concurrent diabetes mellitus.[180]

REFERENCES

1. Chinnery PF. Primary mitochondrial disorders overview. In: Adam MP, Mirzaa GM, Pagon RA, et al., eds. *GeneReviews® [Internet]*. University of Washington, Seattle; 1993–2022.
2. Olimpio C, Tiet MY, Horvath R. Primary mitochondrial myopathies in childhood. *Neuromuscul Disord.* 2021;31:978–987.
3. Parikh S, Goldstein A, Koenig MK, et al. Diagnosis and management of mitochondrial disease: a consensus statement from the Mitochondrial Medicine Society. *Genet Med.* 2015;17(9):689–701.
4. DiMauro S, Schon EA, Carelli V, Hirano M. The clinical maze of mitochondrial neurology. *Nat Rev Neurol.* 2013;9(8):429–444.
5. Milone M, Wong L-J. Diagnosis of mitochondrial myopathies. *Mol Genet Metab.* 2013;110(1–2):35–41.
6. Pfeffer G, Chinnery PF. Diagnosis and treatment of mitochondrial myopathies. *Ann Med.* 2013;45(1):4–16.
7. Tucker EJ, Compton AG, Thorburn DR. Recent advances in the genetics of mitochondrial encephalopathies. *Curr Neurol Neurosci Rep.* 2010;10(4):277–285.
8. Finsterer J, Ahting U. Mitochondrial depletion syndromes in children and adults. *Can J Neurol Sci.* 2013;40(5):635–644.
9. Finsterer J. Inherited mitochondrial neuropathies. *J Neurol Sci.* 2011;304(1–2):9–16.
10. Pareyson D, Piscosquito G, Moroni I, Salsano E, Zeviani M. Peripheral neuropathy in mitochondrial disorders. *Lancet Neurol.* 2013;12(10):1011–1024.
11. Schmiedel J, Jackson S, Schäfer J, Reichmann H. Mitochondrial cytopathies. *J Neurol.* 2003;250(3):267–277.
12. Taylor RW, Schaefer AM, Baron MJ, McFarland R, Turnbull DM. The diagnosis of mitochondrial muscle disease. *Neuromuscul Disord.* 2004;14:237–245.
13. Vu TH, Hirano M, DiMauro S. Mitochondrial diseases. *Neurol Clin.* 2002;20(3):809–839, vii-viii.
14. Chinnery PF, Johnson MA, Wardell TM, et al. The epidemiology of pathogenic mitochondrial DNA mutations. *Ann Neurol.* 2000;48(2):188–193.
15. Gorman GS, Schaefer AM, Ng Y, et al. Prevalence of nuclear and mitochondrial DNA mutations related to adult mitochondrial disease. *Ann Neurol.* 2015;77(5):753–759.
16. Varhaug KN, Hikmat O, Nakkestad HL, Vedeler CA, Bindoff LA. Serum biomarkers in primary mitochondrial disorders. *Brain Commun.* 2021;3:fcaa222.
17. Yatsuga S, Fujita Y, Ishii A, et al. Growth differentiation factor 15 as a useful biomarker for mitochondrial disorders. *Ann Neurol.* 2015;78(5):814–823.
18. Davis RL, Liang C, Sue CM. A comparison of current serum biomarkers as diagnostic indicators of mitochondrial diseases. *Neurology.* 2016;86:2010–2015.
19. Riley LG, Nafisinia M, Menezes MJ, et al. FGF21 outperforms GDF15 as a diagnostic biomarker of mitochondrial disease in children. *Mol Genet Metab.* 2022;135(1):63–71.
20. Lehtonen JM, Forsström S, Bottani E, et al. FGF21 is a biomarker for mitochondrial translation and mtDNA maintenance disorders. *Neurology.* 2016;87(22):2290–2299.
21. Riley MS, Nicholls DP, Cooper CB. Cardiopulmonary exercise testing and metabolic myopathies. *Ann Am Thorac Soc.* 2017;14(Supplement_1):S129–S139.
22. Bhatia R, Cohen BH, L McNinch N. A novel exercise testing algorithm to diagnose mitochondrial myopathy. *Muscle Nerve.* 2021;63:715–723.
23. Jeppesen TD, Schwartz M, Olsen DB, Vissing J. Oxidative capacity correlates with muscle mutation load in mitochondrial myopathy. *Ann Neurol.* 2003;54(1):86–92.
24. Taivassalo T, Jensen TD, Kennaway N, DiMauro S, Vissing J, Haller RG. The spectrum of exercise tolerance in mitochondrial myopathies: a study of 40 patients. *Brain.* 2003;126:413–423.
25. Jeppesen TD, Olsen D, Vissing J. Cycle ergometry is not a sensitive diagnostic test for mitochondrial myopathy. *J Neurol.* 2003;250(3):293–299.
26. Jensen TD, Kazemi-Esfarjani P, Skomorowska E, Vissing J. A forearm exercise screening test for mitochondrial myopathy. *Neurology.* 2002;58(10):1533–1538.
27. Taivassalo T, Abbott A, Wyrick P, Haller RG. Venous oxygen levels during aerobic forearm exercise: an index of impaired oxidative metabolism in mitochondrial myopathy. *Ann Neurol.* 2002;51(1):38–44.
28. Riley MS, O'Brien CJ, McCluskey DR, Bell NP, Nicholls DP. Aerobic work capacity in patients with chronic fatigue syndrome. *BMJ.* 1990;301:953–956.
29. Joseph P, Arevalo C, Oliveira RKF, et al. Insights from invasive cardiopulmonary exercise testing of patients with myal-

gic encephalomyelitis/chronic fatigue syndrome. *Chest.* 2021; 160:642–651.
30. Olsen DB, Langkilde AR, Ørngreen MC, Rostrup E, Schwartz M, Vissing J. Muscle structural changes in mitochondrial myopathy relate to genotype. *J Neurol.* 2003;250(11):1328–1334.
31. Laforet P, Wary C, Duteil S, et al. Exploration of exercise intolerance by 31P NMR spectroscopy of calf muscles coupled with MRI and ergometry. *Rev Neurol.* 2003;159(1):56–67.
32. Moller HE, Wiedermann D, Kurlemann G, Hilbich T, Schuierer G. Application of NMR spectroscopy to monitoring MELAS treatment: a case report. *Muscle Nerve.* 2002;25(4):593–600.
33. Bendahan D, Mattei JP, Kozak-Ribbens G, Cozzone PJ. Non invasive investigation of muscle diseases using 31P magnetic resonance spectroscopy: potential in clinical applications. *Rev Neurol.* 2002;158(5 pt 1):527–540.
34. Tarnopolsky MA, Simon DK, Roy BD, et al. Attenuation of free radical production and paracrystalline inclusions by creatine supplementation in a patient with a novel cytochrome *b* mutation. *Muscle Nerve.* 2004;29(4):537–547.
35. Nicolau S, Milone M, Liewluck T. Guidelines for genetic testing of muscle and neuromuscular junction disorders. *Muscle Nerve.* 2021;64:255–269.
36. Kerr M, Hume S, Omar F, et al. MITO-FIND: a study in 390 patients to determine a diagnostic strategy for mitochondrial disease. *Mol Genet Metab.* 2020;131(1-2):66–82.
37. Wagner M, Berutti R, Lorenz-Depiereux B, et al. Mitochondrial DNA mutation analysis from exome sequencing—A more holistic approach in diagnostics of suspected mitochondrial disease. *J Inherit Metab Dis.* 2019;42(5):909–917.
38. Abicht A, Scharf F, Kleinle S, et al. Mitochondrial and nuclear disease panel (Mito-aND-Panel): combined sequencing of mitochondrial and nuclear DNA by a cost-effective and sensitive NGS-based method. *Mol Genet Genomic Med.* 2018;6(6):1188–1198.
39. Blumenthal DT, Shanske S, Schochet SS, et al. Myoclonus epilepsy with ragged red fibers and multiple mtDNA deletions. *Neurology.* 1998;50(2):524–525.
40. Fang W, Huang CC, Chu NS, et al. Myoclonic epilepsy with ragged-red fibers (MERRF) syndrome: report of a Chinese family with mitochondrial DNA point mutation in the tRNA^{Lys} gene. *Muscle Nerve.* 1994;17(1):52–57.
41. Fukuhara N. Clinicopathological features of MERRF. *Muscle Nerve.* 1995;(suppl 3):S90–S94.
42. Fukuhara N. MERRF: a clinicopathological study. Relationships between myoclonus epilepsy and mitochondrial myopathies. *Rev Neurol.* 1991;147:476–479.
43. Fukuhara N, Tokiguchi S, Shirakawa K, Tsubaki T. Myoclonus epilepsy associated with ragged-red fibers (mitochondrial abnormalities): disease entity or a syndrome? Light- and electron-microscopic studies of two cases and review of literature. *J Neurol Sci.* 1980;47:117–133.
44. Lombes A, Mendell JR, Nakase H, et al. Myoclonic epilepsy and ragged red fibers with cytochrome oxidase deficiency: neuropathology, biochemistry, and molecular genetics. *Ann Neurol.* 1989;26(1):20–33.
45. Ozawa M, Goto Y, Sakuta R, Tanno Y, Tsuji S, Nonaka I. The 8,344 mutation in mitochondrial DNA: a comparison between the proportion of mutant DNA and clinical pathologic findings. *Neuromuscul Disord.* 1995;5:483–488.
46. Rosing HS, Hopkins LC, Wallace DC, Epstein CM, Weidenheim K. Maternally inherited mitochondrial myopathy and myoclonic epilepsy. *Ann Neurol.* 1985;17:228–237.
47. Silvestri G, Ciafoni E, Santorelli FM, et al. Clinical features associated with the A→G transition at nucleotide 8344 of mtDNA ("MERRF mutation"). *Neurology.* 1993;43(6):1200–1206.
48. Tsairis P, Engel WK, Kark P. Familial myoclonic epilepsy syndrome associated with skeletal muscle mitochondrial abnormalities [abstract]. *Neurology.* 1973;23:408.
49. Greenberg DA, Durner M, Keddache M, et al. Reproducibility and complications in gene searches: linkage on chromosome 6, heterogeneity, association, and maternal inheritance in juvenile myoclonic epilepsy. *Am J Hum Genet.* 2000;66:508–516.
50. Bryne E, Dennet X, Trounce I. Burdon J. Mitochondrial myoneuropathy with respiratory failure and myoclonic epilepsy. A case report with biochemical studies. *J Neurol Sci.* 1985;71:273–281.
51. Larsson NG, Tulinius MH, Holme E, Oldfors A. Pathogenetic aspects of the A8344G mutation of mitochondrial DNA associated with MERRF syndrome and multiple symmetric lipomas. *Muscle Nerve.* 1995;(suppl 3):S102–S106.
52. Muñoz-Málaga A, Bautista J, Salazar JA, et al. Lipomatosis, proximal myopathy, and the mitochondrial 8344 mutation. A lipid storage myopathy? *Muscle Nerve.* 2000;23:538–542.
53. Mizusawa H, Watanabe M, Kanazawa I, et al. Familial mitochondrial myopathy associated with peripheral neuropathy: partial deficiencies of complex I and complex IV. *J Neurol Sci.* 1988;86:171–184.
54. Pezeshkpour G, Krarup C, Buchthal F, DiMauro S, Bresolin N, McBurney J. Peripheral neuropathy in mitochondrial disease. *J Neurol Sci.* 1987;77:285–304.
55. Hammans SR, Sweeny MG, Brockington M, et al. The mitochondrial DNA transfer RNA^{Lys} A → G$^{(8344)}$ mutation and the syndrome of myoclonic epilepsy with ragged red fibres (MERRF). Relationship of the clinical phenotype to proportion of mutant mitochondrial DNA. *Brain.* 1993;116:617–632.
56. Shoffner JM, Lott MT, Lezza AMS, Seibel P, Ballinger SW, Wallace DC. Myoclonic epilepsy and ragged-red fiber disease (MERRF) is associated with a mitochondrial DNA tRNA^{Lys} mutation. *Cell.* 1990;61:931–937.
57. Yoneda M, Miyatake T, Attardi G. Heteroplasmic mitochondrial tRNA^{Lys} mutation and its complementation in MERRF patient-derived mitochondrial transformants. *Muscle Nerve Suppl.* 1995;(suppl 3):S95–S101.
58. Tarnopolsky M, Martin J. Creatine monohydrate increases strength in patients with neuromuscular disease. *Neurology.* 1999;52:854–857.
59. Tarnopolsky MA, Roy BD, MacDonald JR. A randomized, controlled trial of creatine monohydrate in patients with mitochondrial cytopathies. *Muscle Nerve.* 1997;20:1502–1509.
60. Feit H, Kirkpatrick J, VanWoert MH, Pandian G. Myoclonus, ataxia, and hypoventilation: response to L-5-hydroxytrptophan. *Neurology.* 1983;33:109–112.
61. Ciafaloni E, Ricci E, Shanske S, et al. MELAS: clinical features, biochemistry, and molecular genetics. *Ann Neurol.* 1992;31:391–398.
62. Crimmins D, Morris JGL, Walker GL, et al. Mitochondrial encephalomyopathy: variable clinical expression within a single kindred. *J Neurol Neurosurg Psychiatry.* 1993;56:900–905.
63. Goto YI. Clinical features of MELAS and mitochondrial DNA mutations. *Muscle Nerve.* 1995;3:S107–S112.
64. Goto Y, Horai S, Matsuoka T, et al. Mitochondrial myopathy, encephalopathy, lactic acidosis and stroke-like episodes

64. (MELAS): correlative study of the clinical features and mitochondrial DNA mutation. *Neurology*. 1992;42:545–550.
65. Pavlakis SG, Phillips PC, DiMauro S, De Vivo DC, Rowland LP. Mitochondrial myopathy, encephalopathy, lactic acidosis, and stroke-like episode: a distinctive clinical syndrome. *Ann Neurol*. 1984;16:481–488.
66. Iizuka T, Sakai F, Kan S, Suzuki N. Slowly progressive spread of the stroke-like lesions in MELAS. *Neurology*. 2003;61(9): 1238–1244.
67. Servidei S. Mitochondrial encephalomyopathies: gene mutation. *Neuromuscul Disord*. 2000;10:10–15.
68. Saitoh S, Momoi MY, Yamagata T, Mori Y, Imai M. Effects of dichloroacetate in three patients with MELAS. *Neurology*. 1998;50:531–534.
69. Kaufmann P, Engelstad K, Wei Y, et al. Dichloroacetate causes toxic neuropathy in MELAS: a randomized, controlled clinical trial. *Neurology*. 2006;66(3):324–330.
70. Komura K, Hobbiebrunken E, Wilichowski EK, Hanefeld FA. Effectiveness of creatine monohydrate in mitochondrial encephalomyopathies. *Pediatr Neurol*. 2003;28(1):53–58.
71. Stefanetti RJ, Ng YS, Errington L, Blain AP, McFarland R, Gorman GS. L-Arginine in mitochondrial encephalopathy, lactic acidosis, and stroke-like episodes: a systematic review. *Neurology*. 2022;98:e2318–e2328.
72. Berenberg RA, Pellock JM, DiMauro S, et al. Lumping or splitting? "Ophthalmoplegia-plus" or Kearns-Sayre syndrome? *Ann Neurol*. 1977;1:37–54.
73. DiMauro S, Bonilla E, Lombes A, Shanske S, Minneti C, Moraes CT. Mitochondrial encephalomyopathies. *Neurol Clin*. 1990;8:483–506.
74. Holt IJ, Harding AE, Cooper JM, et al. Mitochondrial myopathies: clinical and biochemical features of 30 patients with major deletions of muscle mitochondrial DNA. *Ann Neurol*. 1989;26:699–708.
75. Laforêt P, Lombès A, Eymard B, et al. Chronic progressive external ophthalmoplegia with ragged-red fibers: clinical, morphological, and genetic investigations in 43 patients. *Neuromuscul Disord*. 1995;5:399–413.
76. Moraes CT, DiMauro S, Zeviani M, et al. Mitochondrial deletions in progressive external ophthalmoplegia and Kearns-Sayre syndrome. *N Engl J Med*. 1989;320:1293–1299.
77. Rowland LP. Progressive external ophthalmoplegia and ocular myopathies. In: Rowland LP, DiMauro S, eds. *Handbook of Clinical Neurology*. Vol 18(62). Elsevier Science Publishers BV; 1992:287–329.
78. Zeviani M, Moraes CT, DiMauro S, et al. Deletions of mitochondrial DNA in Kearns-Sayre syndrome. *Neurology*. 1988;38:1339–1346.
79. Barohn RJ, Clanton T, Sahenk Z, Mendell JR. Recurrent respiratory insufficiency and depressed ventilatory drive complicating mitochondrial myopathies. *Neurology*. 1990;40:103–106.
80. Carroll JE, Zwillich C, Weil JV, Brooke MH. Depressed ventilatory response in oculocraniosomatic neuromuscular disease. *Neurology*. 1976;26:140–146.
81. Goto Y, Koga S, Horai S, Nonaka I. Chronic progressive external ophthalmoplegia: a correlative study of mitochondrial DNA deletions and their phenotypic expression in muscle biopsies. *J Neurol Sci*. 1990;100:63–69.
82. Orsucci D, Angelini C, Bertini E, et al. Revisiting mitochondrial ocular myopathies: a study from the Italian Network. *J Neurol*. 2017;264:1777–1784.
83. Orsucci D, Caldarazzo Ienco E, Rossi A, Siciliano G, Mancuso M. Mitochondrial syndromes revisited. *J Clin Med*. 2021;10:1249.
84. Gutiérrez-Gutiérrez G, San Millán-Tejado B, Muelas N, et al. Clinical, pathological and genetic spectrum in 89 cases of mitochondrial progressive external ophthalmoplegia. *J Med Genet*. 2020;57:643–646.
85. Ronchi D, Garone C, Bordoni A. Next-generation sequencing reveals *DGUOK* mutations in adult patients with mitochondrial DNA multiple deletions. *Brain*. 2012:135:3404–3415.
86. Ronchi D, Di Fonzo A, Lin W, et al. Mutations in DNA2 link progressive myopathy to mitochondrial DNA instability. *Am J Hum Genet*. 2013;92:293–300.
87. Pfeffer G, Gorman GS, Griffin H, et al. Mutations in the SPG7 gene cause chronic progressive external ophthalmoplegia through disordered mitochondrial DNA maintenance. *Brain*. 2014;137:1323–1336.
88. Bohlega S, Tanji K, Santorelli FM, Hirano M, al-Jishi A, DiMauro S. Multiple mitochondrial DNA deletions associated with autosomal recessive ophthalmoplegia and severe cardiomyopathy. *Neurology*. 1996;46:1329–1334.
89. Carrozzo R, Hirano M, Fromenty B, et al. Multiple mtDNA deletions in autosomal dominant and recessive diseases suggests distinct pathogeneses. *Neurology*. 1998;50:99–106.
90. Minchum PE, Dormer RL, Hughs IA, et al. Fatal infantile myopathy due to cytochrome c oxidase deficiency. *J Neurol Sci*. 1983;60:453–463.
91. Tritschler H-J, Andreetta F, Moraes CT, et al. Mitochondrial myopathy of childhood associated with depletion of mitochondrial DNA. *Neurology*. 1992;42:209–217.
92. Tritschler HJ, Bonilla E, Lombes A, et al. Differential diagnosis of fatal and benign cytochrome c oxidase deficient myopathies of infancy: an immunohistochemical approach. *Neurology*. 1991;41:300–305.
93. Zeviani M, Peterson P, Servidei S, Bonilla E, DiMauro S. Benign reversible muscle cytochrome c oxidase deficiency: a second case. *Neurology*. 1987;37:64–67.
94. Mancuso M, Filosto M, Bonilla E, et al. Mitochondrial myopathy of childhood associated with mitochondrial DNA depletion and a homozygous mutation (T77M) in the TK2 gene. *Arch Neurol*. 2003;60(7):1007–1009.
95. Mancuso M, Filosto M, Stevens JC, et al. Mitochondrial myopathy and complex III deficiency in a patient with a new stop-codon mutation (G339X) in the cytochrome b gene. *J Neurol Sci*. 2003;209(1–2):61–63.
96. Campos Y, Martin MA, García-Silva T, et al. Clinical heterogeneity associated with mitochondrial DNA depletion in muscle. *Neuromuscul Disord*. 1998;8:568–573.
97. Vu TH, Sciacco M, Tanji K, et al. Clinical manifestations of mitochondrial DNA depletion. *Neurology*. 1998;50:1783–1790.
98. Moraes CT, Shanske S, Tritschler HJ, et al. Mitochondrial DNA depletion with variable tissue specificity: a novel genetic abnormality in mitochondrial diseases. *Am J Hum Genet*. 1991;48:492–501.
99. Durham SE, Bonilla E, Samuels DC, DiMauro S, Chinnery PF. Mitochondrial DNA copy number threshold in mtDNA depletion myopathy. *Neurology*. 2005;65:453–455.
100. Figarella-Branger D, Pelssier JF, Scheiner C, Wernert F, Desnuelle C. Defects of the mitochondrial respiratory chain complexes in three pediatric cases with hypotonia and cardiac involvement. *J Neurol Sci*. 1992;108:105–113.

101. Mazziotta MR, Ricci E, Bertini E, et al. Fatal infantile liver failure associated with mitochondrial DNA depletion. *J Pediatr.* 1992;121:896–901.
102. Telerman-Toppet N, Biarent D, Bouton JM, et al. Fatal cytochrome c oxidase-deficient myopathy of infancy associated with mtDNA depletion. Differential involvement of skeletal muscle and cultured fibroblasts. *J Inherit Metab Dis.* 1992;15:323–326.
103. Saada A, Ben-Shalom E, Zyslin R, Miller C, Mandel H, Elpeleg O. Mitochondrial deoxyribonucleoside triphosphate pools in thymidine kinase 2 deficiency. *Biochem Biophys Res Commun.* 2003;310(3):963–966.
104. Saada A, Shaag A, Elpeleg O. MtDNA depletion myopathy: elucidation of the tissue specificity in the mitochondrial thymidine kinase (TK2) deficiency. *Mol Genet Metab.* 2003;79(1):1–5.
105. Saada A, Shaag A, Mandel H, Nevo Y, Eriksson S, Elpeleg O. Mutation mitochondrial thymidine kinase in mitochondrial DNA depletion myopathy. *Nat Genet.* 2001;29:342–344.
106. Vila MR, Segovia-Silvestre T, Gamez J, et al. Reversion of mtDNA depletion in a patient with TK2 deficiency. *Neurology.* 2003;60(7):1203–1205.
107. Chanprasert S, Wang J, Weng SW, et al. Molecular and clinical characterization of the myopathic form of mitochondrial DNA depletion syndrome caused by mutations in the thymidine kinase (TK2) gene. *Mol Genet Metab.* 2013;110(1–2):153–161.
108. Paradas C, Gutiérrez Ríos P, Rivas E, Carbonell P, Hirano M, DiMauro S. TK2 mutation presenting as indolent myopathy. *Neurology.* 2013;80(5):504–506.
109. Béhin A, Jardel C, Claeys KG, et al. Adult cases of mitochondrial DNA depletion due to TK2 defect: an expanding spectrum. *Neurology.* 2012;78(9):644–648.
110. Lesko N, Naess K, Wibom R, et al. Two novel mutations in thymidine kinase-2 cause early onset fatal encephalomyopathy and severe mtDNA depletion. *Neuromuscul Disord.* 2010;20(3):198–203.
111. Collins J, Bove KE, Dimmock D, Morehart P, Wong LJ, Wong B. Progressive myofiber loss with extensive fibro-fatty replacement in a child with mitochondrial DNA depletion syndrome and novel thymidine kinase 2 gene mutations. *Neuromuscul Disord.* 2009;19(11):784–787.
112. Blakely E, He L, Gardner JL, et al. Novel mutations in the TK2 gene associated with fatal mitochondrial DNA depletion myopathy. *Neuromuscul Disord.* 2008;18(7):557–560.
113. Oskoui M, Davidzon G, Pascual J, et al. Clinical spectrum of mitochondrial DNA depletion due to mutations in the thymidine kinase 2 gene. *Arch Neurol.* 2006;63(8):1122–1126.
114. Wang L, Limongelli A, Vila MR, Carrara F, Zeviani M, Eriksson S. Molecular insight into mitochondrial DNA depletion syndrome in two patients with novel mutations in the deoxyguanosine kinase and thymidine kinase 2 genes. *Mol Genet Metab.* 2005;84(1):75–82.
115. Buchaklian AH, Helbling D, Ware SM, Dimmock DP. Recessive deoxyguanosine kinase deficiency causes juvenile onset mitochondrial myopathy. *Mol Genet Metab.* 2012;107(1–2):92–94.
116. Bardosi A, Creutzfeldt W, DiMauro S, et al. Myo-neuro-, gastrointestinal encephalopathy (MNGIE syndrome) due to partial deficiency of cytochrome-c-oxidase. A new mitochondrial multisystem disorder. *Acta Neuropathol (Berl).* 1987;74:248–258.
117. Nishino I, Spinazzola A, Papadimitriou A, et al. Mitochondrial neurogastrointestinal encephalomyopathy: an autosomal recessive disorder due to thymidine phosphorylase mutations. *Ann Neurol.* 2000;47:729–800.
118. Simon LT, Horoupian DS, Dorfman LJ, et al. Polyneuropathy, ophthalmoplegia, leukoencephalopathy, and intestinal pseudo-obstruction: POLIP syndrome. *Ann Neurol.* 1990;28:349–360.
119. Hirano M, Carelli V, De Giorgio R, et al. Mitochondrial neurogastrointestinal encephalomyopathy (MNGIE): position paper on diagnosis, prognosis, and treatment by the MNGIE International Network. *J Inherit Metab Dis.* 2021;44:376–387.
120. Zaidman I, Elhasid R, Gefen A, et al. Hematopoietic stem cell transplantation for mitochondrial neurogastrointestinal encephalopathy: a single-center experience underscoring the multiple factors involved in the prognosis. *Pediatr Blood Cancer.* 2021;68:e28926.
121. Halter JP, Michael W, Schüpbach M, et al. Allogeneic haematopoietic stem cell transplantation for mitochondrial neurogastrointestinal encephalomyopathy. *Brain.* 2015;138(Pt 10):2847–2858.
122. Hirano M, Silvestri G, Blake DM, et al. Mitochondrial neurogastrointestinal encephalomyopathy (MNGIE): clinical, biochemical, and genetic features of an autosomal recessive mitochondrial disorder. *Neurology.* 1994;44:721–727.
123. Bedlack RS, Vu T, Hammans S, et al. MNGIE neuropathy: five cases mimicking chronic inflammatory demyelinating polyneuropathy. *Muscle Nerve.* 2004;29(3):364–368.
124. Servidei S, Zeviani M, Manfredi G, et al. Dominantly inherited mitochondrial myopathy with multiple deletions of mitochondrial DNA: clinical, morphologic, and biochemical studies. *Neurology.* 1991;41:1053–1059.
125. Nishino I, Spinazzola A, Hirano M. Thymidine phosphorylase gene mutations in MNGIE, a human mitochondrial disorder. *Science.* 1999;283:689–692.
126. Hirano M, Garcia-de-Yebenes J, Jones AC, et al. Mitochondrial neurogastrointestinal encephalomyopathy syndrome maps to chromosome 22q13.32-qter. *Am J Hum Genet.* 1998;63:526–533.
127. Van Goethem G, Schwartz M, Löfgren A, Dermaut B, Van Broeckhoven C, Vissing J. Novel POLG mutations in progressive external ophthalmoplegia mimicking mitochondrial neurogastrointestinal encephalomyopathy. *Eur J Hum Genet.* 2003;11:547–549.
128. Tang S, Dimberg EL, Milone M, Wong LJ. Mitochondrial neurogastrointestinal encephalomyopathy (MNGIE)-like phenotype: an expanded clinical spectrum of POLG1 mutations. *J Neurol.* 2012;259:862–868.
129. Shaibani A, Shchelochkov OA, Zhang S, et al. Mitochondrial neurogastrointestinal encephalopathy due to mutations in RRM2B. *Arch Neurol.* 2009;66:1028–1032.
130. Fadic R, Russell JA, Russell JA, Lehar M, Kuncl RW, Johns DR. Sensory ataxic neuropathy as the presenting feature of a novel mitochondrial disease. *Neurology.* 1997;49:239–245.
131. Mancuso M, Filosto M, Bellan M, et al. POLG mutations causing ophthalmoplegia, sensorimotor polyneuropathy, ataxic and deafness. *Neurology.* 2004;62:316–318.
132. van Domburg PH, Gabreëls-Festen AA, ter Laak H, et al. Mitochondrial cytopathy presenting as hereditary sensory neuropathy with progressive external ophthalmoplegia, ataxia and fatal myoclonic epileptic status. *Brain.* 1996;119:997–1010.

133. Milone M, Brunetti-Pierri N, Tang L-Y, et al. Sensory ataxic neuropathy with ophthalmoparesis caused by POLG mutations. *Neuromuscul Disord.* 2008;18;626–632.
134. Wong LJ, Naviaux RK, Brunetti-Pierri N, et al. Molecular and clinical genetics of mitochondrial diseases due to POLG mutations. *Hum Mutat.* 2008;29(9):E150–E172.
135. Hakonen AH, Heiskanen S, Juvonen V, et al. Mitochondrial DNA polymerase W748 S mutation: a common cause of autosomal recessive ataxia with ancient European origin. *Am J Hum Genet.* 2005;77:430–441.
136. Wintgerthun S, Ferrari G, He L, et al. Autosomal recessive mitochondrial ataxic syndrome due to mitochondrial polymerase gamma mutations. *Neurology.* 2005;64:1204–1208.
137. Rantamaki MT, Soini HK, Finnila SM, Majamaa K, Udd B. Adult-onset ataxia and polyneuropathy caused by mitochondrial 8993T->C mutation. *Ann Neurol.* 2005;58:337–340.
138. Van Goethem G, Luoma P, Rantamäki M, et al. POLG mutations in neurodegenerative disorders with ataxia but no muscle involvement. *Neurology.* 2004;63:1251–1257.
139. Luoma PT, Luo N, Löscher WN, et al. Functional defects due to spacer-region mutations of human mitochondrial DNA polymerase in a family with an ataxia-myopathy syndrome. *Hum Mol Genet.* 2005;14:1907–1920.
140. Tzoulis C, Engelsen BA, Telstad W, et al. The spectrum of clinical disease caused by the A467 T and W748 S POLG mutations: a study of 26 cases. *Brain.* 2006;129:1685–1692.
141. Holt IJ, Harding AE, Petty RK, Morgan-Hughes JA. A new mitochondrial disease associated with mitochondrial DNA heteroplasmy. *Am J Hum Genet.* 1990;46:428–433.
142. Santorelli FM, Tanji K, Shanske S, DiMauro S. Heterogeneous clinical presentation of the mtDNA NARP/T8993G mutation. *Neurology.* 1997;49:270–273.
143. Childs AM, Hutchin T, Pysden K, et al. Variable phenotype including Leigh syndrome with a 9185T>C mutation in the MTATP6 gene. *Neuropediatrics.* 2007;38:313–316.
144. Gelfand JM, Duncan JL, Racine CA, et al. Heterogeneous patterns of tissue injury in NARP syndrome. *J Neurol.* 2011;258:440–448.
145. Karadimas CL, Vu TH, Holve SA, et al. Navajo neurohepatopathy is caused by a mutation in the MPV17 gene. *Am J Hum Genet.* 2006;79:544–548.
146. Spinazzola A, Viscomi C, Fernandez-Vizarra E, et al. MPV17 encodes an inner mitochondrial membrane protein and is mutated in infantile hepatic mitochondrial DNA depletion. *Nat Genet.* 2006;38:570–575.
147. Lawlor MW, Holve S, Stubbs EB Jr. Assessment of serum-mediated neurotoxicity in Navajo neuropathy. *Electromyogr Clin Neurophysiol.* 2000;40:211–214.
148. Appenzeller O, Kornfeld M, Snyder R. Acromutilating, paralyzing neuropathy with corneal ulceration in Navajo children. *Arch Neurol.* 1976;33:733–738.
149. Yu-Wai-Man P, Griffiths PG, Gorman GS, et al. Multi-system neurological disease is common in patients with OPA1 mutations. *Brain.* 2010;133:771–786.
150. Amati-Bonneau P, Valentino ML, Reynier P, et al. OPA1 mutations induce mitochondrial DNA instability and optic atrophy 'plus' phenotypes. *Brain.* 2008;131:338–351.
151. Hudson G, Amati-Bonneau P, Blakely EL, et al. Mutation of OPA1 causes dominant optic atrophy with external ophthalmoplegia, ataxia, deafness and multiple mitochondrial DNA deletions: a novel disorder of mtDNA maintenance. *Brain.* 2008;131:329–337.
152. Liguori M, La Russa A, Manna I, et al. A phenotypic variation of dominant optic atrophy and deafness (ADOAD) due to a novel OPA1 mutation. *J Neurol.* 2008;255:127–129.
153. Voo I, Allf BE, Udar N, Silva-Garcia R, Vance J, Small KW. Hereditary motor and sensory neuropathy type VI with optic atrophy. *Am J Ophthalmol.* 2003;136:670–677.
154. Chalmers RM, Lamont PJ, Nelson I, et al. A mitochondrial DNA tRNA^{Val} point mutation associated with adult-onset Leigh syndrome. *Neurology.* 1997;49:589–592.
155. Loeffen J, Smeitink J, Triepels R, et al. The first nuclear-encoded complex 1 mutation in a patient with Leigh syndrome. *Am J Hum Genet.* 1998;63:1598–1604.
156. Triepels RH, Vanden Heuven L, Loeffen JL, et al. Leigh syndrome associated with a mutation in the NDUFS7 (PSST) nuclear encoded subunit of complex I. *Ann Neurol.* 1999;45:787–790.
157. Bougeron T, Roustin P, Chretien D, et al. Mutation of a nuclear succinate dehydrogenase gene results in mitochondrial respiratory chain deficiency. *Nat Genet.* 1995;11:144–149.
158. Ahu Z, Yao J, Johns T, et al. SURF1, encoding a factor involved in the biogenesis of cytochrome c oxidase, is mutated in Leigh syndrome. *Nat Genet.* 1998;20:337–343.
159. Shoffner JM, Fernhoff PM, Krawiecki NS, et al. Subacute necrotizing encephalopathy: oxidative phosphorylation defects and the ATPase 6 point mutation. *Neurology.* 1992;42:2168–2174.
160. Sweeney MG, Hammans SR, Duchen LW, et al. Mitochondrial DNA mutation underlying Leigh's syndrome: clinical, pathological, biochemical, and genetic studies of a patient presenting with progressive myoclonic epilepsy. *J Neurol Sci.* 1994;121:57–65.
161. Yamamoto M, Clemens PR, Engel AG. Mitochondrial DNA deletions in mitochondrial cytopathies: observations in 19 patients. *Neurology.* 1991;41:1822–1828.
162. DeVivo D. Complexities of the pyruvate dehydrogenase complex. *Neurology.* 1998;51:1247–1249.
163. Lissens W, Desguerre I, Benelli C, et al. Pyruvate dehydrogenase deficiency in a female due to a 4 base pair deletion in exon 10 of the E1 alpha gene. *Hum Mol Genet.* 1995;4:307–308.
164. Matthews PM, Marchington DR, Squire M, Land J, Brown RM, Brown GK. Molecular genetic characterization of an X-linked form of Leigh's syndrome. *Ann Neurol.* 1993;33:652–655.
165. Genge A, Karpati G, Arnold D, Shoubridge EA, Carpenter S. Familial myopathy with conspicuous depletion of mitochondria in muscle fibers: a morphologically distinct disease. *Neuromuscul Disord.* 1995;5:139–144.
166. Nishino I, Kobayshi O, Goto Y, et al. A new distinct muscular dystrophy with mitochondrial structural abnormalities. *Muscle Nerve.* 1998;21:40–47.
167. Osaki Y, Nishino I, Murakami N, et al. Mitochondrial abnormalities in selenium-deficient myopathy. *Muscle Nerve.* 1998;21:637–639.
168. Saunier P, Chretien D, Wood C, et al. Cytochrome c oxidase deficiency presenting as recurrent neonatal myoglobinuria. *Neuromuscul Disord.* 1995;5:285–289.
169. Ohno K, Tanaka M, Sahashi K, et al. Mitochondrial DNA deletions in inherited recurrent myoglobinuria. *Ann Neurol.* 1991;29:364–369.
170. Chinnery PF, Johnson MA, Taylor RW, Durward WF, Turnbull DM. A novel mitochondrial tRNA isoleucine gene mutation causing chronic progressive external ophthalmoplegia. *Neurology.* 1997;49:1166–1168.

171. Moslemi AR, Lindberg C, Toft J, Holme E, Kollberg G, Oldfors A. A novel mutation in the mitochondrial tRNA(Phe) gene associated with mitochondrial myopathy. *Neuromuscul Disord.* 2004;14:46–50.
172. Keightley JA, Hoffbuhr KC, Burton MD, et al. A microdeletion in cytochrome c oxidase (COX) subunit III associated with COX deficiency and recurrent myoglobinuria. *Nat Genet.* 1996;12(4):410–416.
173. Nishigaki Y, Bonilla E, Shanske S, Gaskin DA, DiMauro S, Hirano M. Exercise-induced muscle "burning," fatigue, and hyper-CKemia: mtDNA T10010C mutation in tRNA^{Gly}. *Neurology.* 2002;8(8):1282–1285.
174. Andreu AL, Tanji K, Bruno C, et al. Exercise intolerance due to a nonsense mutation in the mtDNA ND4 gene. *Ann Neurol.* 1999;45:820–823.
175. Andreu AL, Bruno C, Dunne TC, et al. A nonsense mutation (G15059 A) in the cytochrome *b* gene in a patient with exercise intolerance and myoglobinuria. *Ann Neurol.* 1999;45:127–130.
176. Andreu AL, Bruno C, Shanske S, et al. Missense mutation in the mtDNA cytochrome *b* gene in a patient with myopathy. *Neurology.* 1998;51:1444–1447.
177. Wallace DC, Singh G, Lott MT, et al. Mitochondrial DNA mutation associated with Leber's hereditary optic neuropathy. *Science.* 1988;242:1427–1430.
178. Pilz D, Quarrell OW, Jones EW. Mitochondrial mutation commonly associated with Leber's hereditary optic neuropathy observed in a patient with Wolfram syndrome (DIDMOAD). *J Med Genet.* 1994;31:328–330.
179. Kollberg G, Melberg A, Holme E, Oldfors A. Transient restoration of succinate dehydrogenase activity after rhabdomyolysis in iron-sulphur cluster deficiency myopathy. *Neuromuscul Disord.* 2011;21:115–120.
180. Papadopoulos C, Wahbi K, Behin A, et al. Incidence and predictors of total mortality in 267 adults presenting with mitochondrial diseases. *J Inherit Metab Dis.* 2020;43:459–466.

CHAPTER 31

Myotonic Dystrophies

Myotonic dystrophy is the most common myotonic disorder (Table 31-1). There are two genetically distinct forms of myotonic dystrophy: dystrophica myotonia type 1 (DM1) and dystrophica myotonia type 2 (DM2), the latter of which is also known as proximal myotonic myopathy (PROMM).

▶ MYOTONIC DYSTROPHY (DM1)

CLINICAL FEATURES

DM1 in an autosomal dominant manner with estimated prevalence ranging from 5 to 20 per 100,000,[1-4] but a recent cross-sectional cohort study of deidentified dried blood spots from the newborn screening program in the state of New York showed the prevalence was closer to 47.6 per 100,000 or 1 in every 2,100 births.[5] DM1 can present at any age, including infancy. Limb weakness begins distally in the extremities and can progress slowly to affect proximal muscles. Wrist flexors are often weaker than wrist extensors. Finger flexors can also be weak.[6] The neck flexors, including the sternocleidomastoids, are also affected early. Atrophy and weakness of temporalis and other facial muscles, as well as the jaw muscles giving rise to the characteristic "hatchet face" appearance (Fig. 31-1). Ptosis is often evident though extraocular movements are unaffected. Some patients develop dysarthria and dysphagia due to pharyngeal and lingual muscles involvement.

Many patients do not complain or are not aware of their myotonia, although it is usually readily apparent on examination, particularly in the hands. Delayed relaxation of the fingers is seen following a forceful hand grip (action myotonia). The myotonia is lessened with repeated muscle contractions, a so-called warm-up phenomenon. Percussion of muscle groups, in particular of the thenar eminence or finger extensors also gives rise to delayed relaxation (percussion myotonia). Muscle reflexes are diminished, but sensory testing is normal.[7] Adult patients with DM1 may have a mild reduction in cognitive abilities, while severe cognitive impairment is associated with congenital myotonic dystrophy.[8,9]

Congenital myotonic dystrophy is much more severe than adult-onset DM1. Affected infants are invariably born to mothers with myotonic dystrophy.[10,11] It is important to examine mothers of floppy infants, as they may not even be aware that they have the disorder. Pregnancy may be complicated by polyhydramnios and diminished fetal movements. Infants with congenital myotonic dystrophy have severe generalized weakness and hypotonia and may also have arthrogryposis. Clinical myotonia is not apparent in the neonatal period and may not be noticeable until about 5 years of age. However, myotonic discharges can be appreciated on electromyography (EMG) before the appearance of clinical myotonia. Many infants require ventilatory assistance due to ventilatory insufficiency. The mortality rate in infancy is approximately 25%. Severe psychomotor abnormalities affect 75% of surviving children. Most will have some degree of cognitive impairment. Life expectancy is reduced in DM1 patients, particularly those with early onset of the disease and significant proximal, in addition to distal, weakness.[12,13]

ASSOCIATED MANIFESTATIONS

DM1 is a systemic disorder affecting the gastrointestinal tract, the uterus, ventilatory muscles, cardiac muscle, the lens, and the endocrine system.[14-16] In addition to dysphagia, reduced gastrointestinal motility can lead to chronic pseudo-obstruction.[17,18] Alveolar hypoventilation can arise from involvement of the diaphragm and intercostal muscles.[19,20] It is more severe in congenital myotonic dystrophy and may lead to ventilatory failure, but this certainly occurs in later-onset cases as well.[11] Reduction in forced vital capacity correlates with the severity of overall weakness, size of the mutation (see Pathogenesis) and duration of disease.[19] Many patients develop symptoms suggestive of sleep apnea: frequent nocturnal arousals, excessive daytime hypersomnolence, and morning headaches.[21] Decreased central drive likely contributes to hypoventilation.[21-23] Pulmonary hypertension can develop and may lead to cor pulmonale.

Cardiac abnormalities are common with approximately 90% of patients having conduction defects on electrocardiograms (EKGs), while 10% have atrial fibrillation.[24-26] Sudden cardiac death secondary to arrhythmia is well documented. Importantly, the size of the mutation (discussed in Pathogenesis section) and the severity of the skeletal muscle weakness do not correlate with the occurrence of cardiac conduction abnormalities or sudden death.[26] It seems that risk of sudden death increases with duration of disease and age, and that risk is higher in male patients.[26]

Neurobehavioral abnormalities are common in patients with DM1.[27,28] Neuropsychological testing demonstrates elements of obsessive–compulsive, passive–aggressive, dependent, and avoidant personality traits in many patients. Apathy and depression are also frequent. Cognitive impairment,

▶ **TABLE 31-1. MYOTONIC DISORDERS**

Myotonic dystrophy type 1
Myotonic dystrophy type 2/proximal myotonic myopathy
Myotonia congenita (autosomal dominant and recessive)
Paramyotonia congenita
Potassium-aggravated myotonia
Hyperkalemic periodic paralysis
Chondrodystrophic myotonia (Schwartz–Jampel syndrome)
Drug-induced
    Cholesterol-lowering agents (statin medications, fibrates)
    Cyclosporine
    Chloroquine

particularly in memory and spatial orientation, may be demonstrated. The neuropsychological deficits appear to correlate with brain single photon emission computed tomography, which shows frontal and parieto-occipital hypoperfusion.[28]

Other systemic manifestations include posterior subscapular cataracts, frontal balding, testicular atrophy and impotence in men, and a high rate of fetal loss and complications of pregnancy in women. An increase in fetal insulin receptor-A relative to adult insulin receptor can result in insulin resistance predisposing to diabetes.[16,29] There is also an increased risk for hyperlipidemia, nonalcoholic fatty liver disease, osteoporosis and malignant thyroid nodules, bone fractures, miscarriage, preterm delivery, and failed labor during delivery.

Epidemiological studies have reported an increased risk of cancer in patients with DM1.[30–34] In a study of Swedish and Danish populations, the risk of malignancy was double that of the general population.[30] Specifically, they observed an increased risk of endometrial, ovarian, colon, and brain cancer. In a study from the Mayo Clinic, there was an increased risk of thyroid cancer and choroidal melanoma, as well as perhaps testicular and prostate cancer.[31] However, they found no increased risk of endometrial, ovarian, breast, colorectal, lung, renal, bladder, or brain cancers. Pilomatricoma, a benign hair matrix cells-derived calcifying skin tumor, which manifests as small firm papules/nodules, is the most common cutaneous tumor in DM1, but do not appear to be increased in DM1.[32,35]

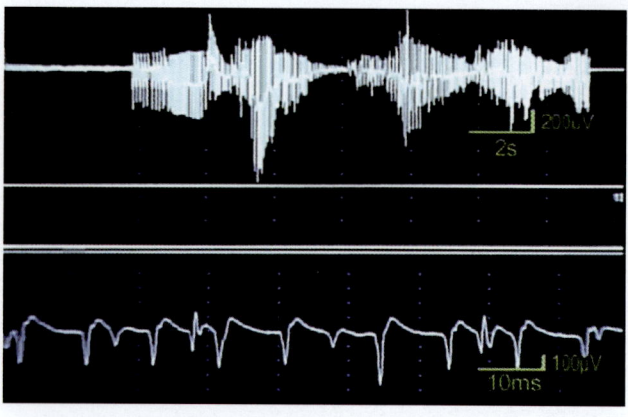

Figure 31-2. Myotonic dystrophy. Electromyography reveals myotonic discharges which wax and wane in frequency and amplitude.

LABORATORY FEATURES

Serum creatine kinase (CK) may be normal or mildly increased. Motor and sensory nerve conduction studies (NCSs) are usually normal. EMG demonstrates myotonic discharges (Fig. 31-2). It is important to sample multiple muscles as myotonic discharges are not necessarily appreciated in every muscle studied.[36] Facial and intrinsic hand muscles are the most commonly affected. In congenital myotonic dystrophy, electrical myotonia may be observed as early as 5 days to 3 weeks following birth and increases with age.[37,38] Fibrillation potentials, positive sharp waves, and myopathic motor unit action potentials (MUAPs) may also be seen but they can be obscured by the myotonic discharges. As mentioned, EKG and pulmonary function tests (PFTs) can be abnormal.

Skeletal muscle imaging is not routinely performed but may have a role as a biomarker in clinical trials. Magnetic resonance imaging (MRI) scans have revealed fatty replacement of the tongue, sternocleidomastoid, paraspinals, gluteus minimus, distal quadriceps, and gastrocnemius medialis on T1 images.[39] Interestingly, hyperintensity on short tau inversion recovery (STIR) sequences precedes fat replacement. Abnormalities on MRI are evident even in patients with mild disease correlate with clinical severity and disease duration.

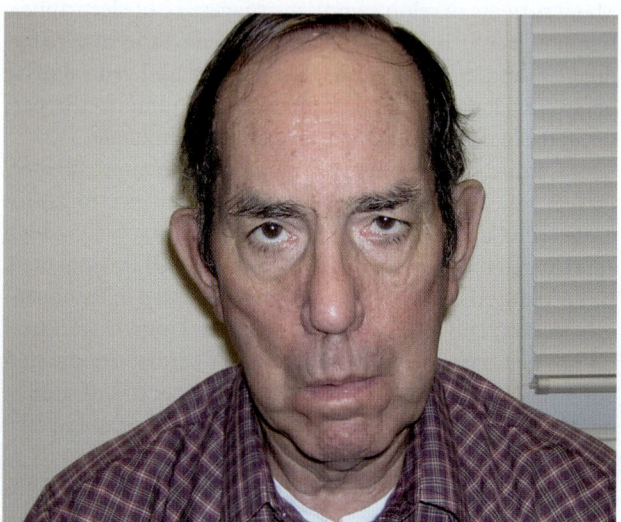

Figure 31-1. Myotonic dystrophy type 1. Note the typical myotonic facies of a DM 1 patient with frontal balding and temporal jaw, and facial muscle atrophy, and weakness.

HISTOPATHOLOGY

Muscle biopsies demonstrate an increased number of internalized nuclei in the muscle fibers (Fig. 31-3). Type 1 predominance and atrophy are very common. In addition, hypertrophic

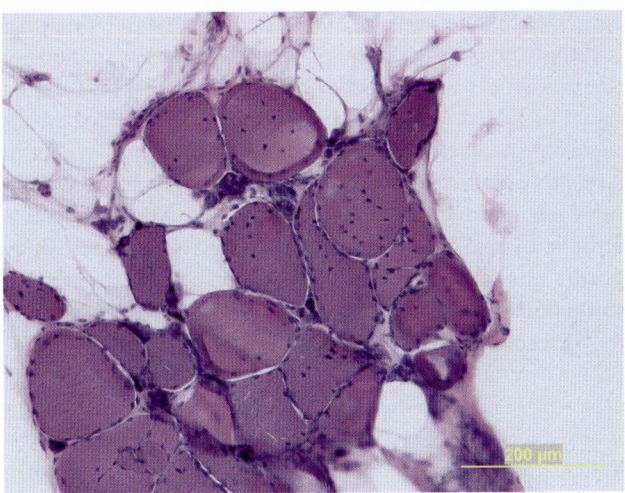

Figure 31-3. Myotonic dystrophy type 1. Muscle biopsies reveal adipose tissue and remaining muscle fibers with numerous internalized nuclei and atrophic fibers with pyknotic nuclear clumps.

type 2 fibers, ring fibers, small angulated fibers, atrophic fibers with pyknotic nuclear clumps, and sarcoplasmic masses are also frequently observed. In contrast to other muscular dystrophies, necrotic fibers and increased connective tissue are less conspicuous. Autopsy studies of the brain demonstrate neurofibrillary degeneration with abnormal tau expression.[40]

MOLECULAR GENETICS AND PATHOGENESIS

DM1 is caused by an expansion of unstable polymorphic cytosine–thymine–guanine (CTG) trinucleotide repeats in the 3′ untranslated region of the dystrophia myotonica protein kinase gene (*DMPK*), that is located on chromosome 19q13.2.[14,41-49] This CTG repeat is copied in the gene up to 27 times in the normal population, but 50 to more than 4,000 copies are found in DM1 patients. Individuals with CTG repeat numbers between 38 and 50 are considered to have a "pre-mutation" allele and may remain asymptomatic throughout their lives. The severity of the myopathy directly correlates with the size of the CTG repeat, which is unstable. The mutation size usually expands from one generation to the next, which accounts for the anticipation phenomena (i.e., the earlier presentation and/or more severe disease in each generation). More marked expansion of the CTG repeat usually occurs in children of mothers with DM1 with CTG repeat size usually over 750.

It is not the abnormal expression of myotonin protein kinase itself that is responsible for the disorder. Rather, DM1 seems to be a consequence of nuclear retention of mutant mRNA containing expanded CTG repeats, rather than a specific lack or gain of function of the *DMPK* protein. Indeed, the myopathy and other systemic features appear to be due to a toxic gain of function of the mutant mRNA.[49,50]

The transcribed mRNA with expanded CTG (DM1) accumulates as abnormal focal collections in the nucleus that cannot be transported to the cytoplasm, where RNA translation into protein takes place.[49-54] Aggregates of mutated mRNA are directly toxic to cells by sequestering RNA-binding proteins (such as muscleblind proteins), which in turn, lead to abnormal splicing of pre-mRNA from various target genes (e.g., chloride ion channel [CIC-1], insulin receptor, tau protein, cardiac troponin, ryanodine receptor, and sarcoplasmic/endoplasmic reticulum Ca^{2+}-ATPase).[49,51-59] Therefore, there is abnormal translation of the RNAs into functional proteins, and this explains the multiple organ/systemic manifestations of DM1. Other studies have shown that mutant RNA binds and sequesters transcription factors with up to 90% depletion of selected transcription factors from active chromatin.[60] This leads to reduced expression of a variety of genes, including the CIC-1, which is also mutated in myotonia congenita and is the likely origin of the myotonic discharges that occur in both disorders.

TREATMENT

There are no medical therapies that clearly improve muscle strength, though various gene therapies are being developed and studied. Patients are usually not so bothered by the myotonia to warrant treatment. Further, some drugs that may improve myotonia, such as quinine, procainamide, and tocainide can also potentiate cardiac arrhythmias and should be avoided. A study of mexiletine did show that it was helpful in reducing myotonia.[61] In patients with bothersome myotonia, we initiate treatment with mexiletine 150 mg daily and gradually increase as tolerated and as necessary to control the symptoms, up to a maximum of 300 mg three times daily. We assess baseline EKG and with each increment of dosage. In addition, aerobic training is safe and may improve fitness effectively in patients with myotonic dystrophy.[62]

We obtain yearly EKGs to monitor for evidence of conduction defects/arrhythmias.[15,63] If abnormalities are detected, we obtain a cardiology consultation and prolonged cardiac monitoring and echocardiogram as these patients may require antiarrhythmic medication or insertion of a pacemaker or intracardiac defibrillator insertion.[15,63] PFTs are routinely performed. Patients with DM1 are at risk for pulmonary and cardiac complications from general anesthesia and neuromuscular-blocking medications.[64-67] These agents should be used with extreme caution.

We order overnight polysomnography in patients with symptoms and signs of sleep apnea. Patients with significant hypoventilation or sleep apnea may benefit from noninvasive ventilatory assistance with bilevel positive airway pressure (BiPAP). Modafinil 200–400 mg per day is also effective in reducing the excessive daytime somnolence that is commonly associated with DM1.[68-70] Because of increased risk of endocrinopathies consensus guidelines recommend checking fasting blood glucose or HbA1c, if diabetes is suspected, as well as thyroid-stimulating hormone and circulating thyroid hormone (TSH and free T4) level and at least every 3 years; more frequently if indicated. Additional serum lipid levels are assessed at baseline and every 3 years.[15] Some patients require excision of their cataracts. Occasionally for bothersome ptosis, we refer patients for blepharoplasty. However, it is important to discuss with patients the associated risk of inadvertent exposure keratitis. Physical and occupational therapy are important. Orthotic devices such as ankle braces are indicated in patients with foot drop to assist their gait.

Genetic counseling is of utmost importance. Patients need to know that the risk of passing the disease on to their children is 50% with each pregnancy. Further, the disease severity is generally worse from one generation to the next, particularly when the mother has DM1. Prenatal diagnosis is possible via amniocentesis or chorionic villus sampling.

▶ MYOTONIC DYSTROPHY TYPE 2 OR PROXIMAL MYOTONIC MYOPATHY

CLINICAL FEATURES

Myotonic dystrophy type 2 (DM2) is a multisystem, autosomal dominant disorder that resembles DM1 with myotonia, weakness, cataracts, testicular failure, glucose intolerance, hypogammaglobulinemia, and cardiac conduction defects.[2-4,14,29,54,71-82] The prevalence of DM1 was found to be 1 in 1,830 persons in an epidemiological study carried out in Finland.[83] In a study of 234 individuals with DM2, 90% had electrical myotonia, 82% weakness, 61% cataracts, 23% diabetes, and 19% cardiac involvement.[71] Most patients with DM2 become symptomatic between the ages of 20 and 60 years, although onset can occur in childhood. The initial symptoms are usually intermittent stiffness and pain of the thigh muscles in one or both legs. Myotonia may be evident in proximal and distal extremity muscles, as well as facial muscles, however, it is variable and not always present. Myotonia can initially manifest or worsen during pregnancy.[84,85] There is an associated "warm-up" phenomenon with decreased myotonia following repeated muscle contractions. The clinical myotonia does not exacerbate with cold temperature, although a few affected individuals have described worsening of symptoms with warm temperatures.[86]

Pain is prevalent in around 75% of patients.[81] The pain is often described as episodic and disabling, with burning, tearing, or jabbing qualities. This pain typically affects the thighs, shoulders, and upper arms and is not necessarily related to the myotonic stiffness of the muscles. They may complain of peculiar chest pains as well, leading to cardiac evaluations to rule out coronary artery disease.

Slowly progressive proximal and distal weakness develops in the majority of patients. The characteristic pattern of muscle weakness involves the neck flexors, elbow extensors, thumb and deep finger flexors, and hip flexors and extensors in the legs. In general, the proximal muscle is often affected earlier than one sees in DM1, thus the name "proximal myotonic myopathy." Some patients describe fluctuations of their weakness with episodes of increased weakness lasting hours or weeks.[76] During these periods of increased weakness, repeated activity can lead to transient improvement in strength. Significant loss of muscle bulk is not apparent early, however, approximately 9% of patients develop considerable atrophy of proximal muscles late in life.[71] Calf hypertrophy occurs in some patients, which can be asymmetric. Rarely, myoglobinuria can occur as a complication of DM2.

Symptoms and severity can vary within families. Studies have demonstrated an earlier onset of symptoms among offspring of affected individuals, suggesting that anticipation is also a feature of DM2.[71,76,78] However, in contrast to DM1, anticipation in DM2 is much milder and a congenital form has never been described.[71,78]

ASSOCIATED MANIFESTATIONS

Cataracts that are indistinguishable from those seen in DM1 are common in DM2.[14,71] These cataracts usually appear before the age of 50 years and have even developed in patients in their late childhood. Cardiac abnormalities may also develop.[14,71,87] Syncope, near-syncopal spells, or symptomatic tachycardia occur in 8%, cardiac conduction defects in 20%, and a potentially life-threatening cardiomyopathy occur in as many as 7% of individuals who are affected.[71] Unlike DM1, most series have not reported an increased incidence of alveolar hypoventilation in patients with DM2, however, some patients develop sleep apnea and excessive daytime somnolence.[21]

Also, in contrast to DM1, cognitive impairment is not a prominent feature. However, white matter abnormalities may be appreciated on MRI of the brain.[17] In addition, some affected individuals have stroke-like symptoms, seizures, parkinsonian features, and hypersomnia. Further, neuropsychological testing reveals lower scores on tests of frontal lobe function compared to normal along with avoidant personality traits; brain single-photon emission and computed tomography can show frontal and parieto-occipital hypoperfusion similar to DM1.[20] Frontal balding has been reported in as many as 20%–50% of men aged 21–34 years. There is an increased risk of endocrinopathies with testicular atrophy, diabetes, and thyroid dysfunction, as well as hyperlipidemia as in DM1.[16,81,82] Additionally, there is an increased risk of cancer.[30-33]

LABORATORY FEATURES

Serum CK levels are often mildly elevated. Low testosterone levels may be seen in as many as 29% of affected males and insulin insensitivity in 75% of patients.[71] A high gamma-glutamyl transpeptidase (GGT) was demonstrated in 64%, low IgG in 65%, and low IgM in 11%.[71] Abnormalities are common in EKG as previously described.

Motor and sensory NCSs are normal. EMG reveals myotonic discharges even in patients without clinical myotonia, although these discharges can be difficult to detect in some patients. Despite the prominent proximal muscle involvement clinically, electrical myotonia is often more easily detected in distal muscles.

HISTOPATHOLOGY

Muscle biopsy reveals nonspecific myopathic features including a mild-to-moderate increase in internalized nuclei, variability of fiber size with atrophy of type 2 fibers, small angular fibers, and atrophic fibers with pyknotic nuclear clumps.[71,88,89] In contrast to that seen in DM1, selective type 1 fiber atrophy, sarcoplasmic masses, and ringed fibers are not usually appreciated on DM2 muscle biopsies. Autopsy studies demonstrate neurofibrillary degeneration with abnormal tau expression as in DM1.[40]

MOLECULAR GENETICS AND PATHOGENESIS

DM2 and PROMM are allelic disorders caused by CCTG repeat expansions in intron 1 of the *CNBP* (cellular nucleic acid-binding protein), previously known as *ZNF9* (zinc finger protein 9), located on chromosome 3.[49,54,71,81] The smallest mutations in *CNBP* range from 55 to 75 CCTG repeats while the largest are about 11,000 repeats in size. The transcribed mRNA with expanded CCTG repeats accumulates as abnormal focal collections in the nucleus similar to expanded CTG repeats seen in DM1.[49,51–54] As with DM1, the aggregates of mutated mRNA appear to exert their toxic effect on cells by sequestering RNA-binding proteins that leads to abnormal splicing of pre-mRNA from various target genes (e.g., ClC-1, insulin receptor, tau protein, cardiac troponin).[49,51–53,56,59] The subsequent abnormal translation of the RNAs into functional proteins explains the multiple organ/systemic manifestations of both DM1 and DM2.

TREATMENT

There is no specific treatment for DM2. There is insufficient information regarding the efficacy of various antimyotonia agents, but mexiletine or carbamazepine, or phenytoin can be tried if the myotonia or muscle pain is bothersome to the patient.[81,82,90] Cataracts may need surgical excision. It seems prudent to carefully monitor patients during surgery and the postoperative period.

As with DM1, we obtain yearly EKGs to monitor for evidence of conduction defects/arrhythmias.[82] If abnormalities are detected, we obtain a cardiology consultation and prolonged cardiac monitoring and echocardiogram. We obtain baseline PFTs and repeat if patients develop dyspnea or signs of sleep apnea. In addition, we order overnight polysomnography in patients with symptoms and signs of sleep apnea. Patients with significant hypoventilation or sleep apnea may benefit from noninvasive ventilatory assistance with BiPAP. Modafinil 200–400 mg per day may be effective in reducing the excessive daytime somnolence. As discussed in DM1 section, because of increased risk of endocrinopathies consensus guidelines recommend checking fasting blood glucose or HbA1c, if diabetes is suspected, as well as thyroid-stimulating hormone and circulating thyroid hormone (TSH and free T4) level and at least every 3 years; more frequently if indicated. Additional serum lipid levels are assessed at baseline and every 3 years.[82] Genetic counseling is again very important.

▶ SUMMARY

DM1 and DM2 are multisystemic disorders caused by expanded repeats in the noncoding regions of the *DMPK* and *CNBP* genes, respectively. The novel pathogenic consequence of these mutations is not due to a loss of function created by loss of *DMPK* and *CNBP* protein products, but rather a toxic effect on the cells by the accumulation of abnormal mRNA. The mutant mRNA sequesters necessary RNA-binding proteins, and this results in abnormal splicing of pre-mRNA from various target genes (e.g., ClC-1, insulin receptor, tau protein, cardiac troponin), thus explaining the multisystemic manifestations of DM1 and DM2.

REFERENCES

1. Emery AE. Population frequencies of inherited neuromuscular diseases—a world survey. *Neuromuscul Disord*. 1991;1(1):19–29.
2. Machuca-Tzili L, Brook D, Hilton-Jones D. Clinical and molecular aspects of the myotonic dystrophies: a review. *Muscle Nerve*. 2005;32(1):1–18.
3. Tramonte JJ, Burns TM. Myotonic dystrophy. *Arch Neurol*. 2005;62(8):1316–1319.
4. van Engelen BG, Eymard B, Wilcox D. 123rd ENMC International Workshop: management and therapy in myotonic dystrophy, 6–8 February 2004, Naarden, The Netherlands. *Neuromuscul Disord*. 2005;15(5):389–394.
5. Johnson NE, Butterfield RJ, Mayne K, et al. Population-based prevalence of myotonic dystrophy type 1 using genetic analysis of statewide blood screening program. *Neurology*. 2021;96(7):e1045–e1053.
6. Nicolau S, Liewluck T, Milone M. Myopathies with finger flexor weakness: not only inclusion-body myositis. *Muscle Nerve*. 2020;62(4):445–454.
7. Messina C, Tonali P, Scoppetta C. The lack of deep reflexes in myotonic dystrophy. *J Neurol Sci*. 1976;30(2-3):303–311.
8. Bird TD, Follett C, Griep E. Cognitive and personality function in myotonic dystrophy. *J Neurol Neurosurg Psychiatry*. 1983;46(11):971–980.
9. Portwood MM, Wicks JJ, Lieberman JS, Duveneck MJ. Intellectual and cognitive function in adults with myotonic muscular dystrophy. *Arch Phys Med Rehabil*. 1986;67(5):299–303.
10. Hageman AT, Gabreels FJ, Liem KD, Renkawek K, Boon JM. Congenital myotonic dystrophy; a report on thirteen cases and a review of the literature. *J Neurol Sci*. 1993;115(1):95–101.

11. Reardon W, Newcombe R, Fenton I, Sibert J, Harper PS. The natural history of congenital myotonic dystrophy: mortality and long term clinical aspects. *Arch Dis Child*. 1993;68(2):177–181.
12. de Die-Smulders CE, Howeler CJ, Thijs C, et al. Age and causes of death in adult-onset myotonic dystrophy. *Brain*. 1998;121(Pt 8):1557–1563.
13. Mathieu J, Allard P, Potvin L, Prevost C, Begin P. A 10-year study of mortality in a cohort of patients with myotonic dystrophy. *Neurology*. 1999;52(8):1658–1662.
14. Meola G. Clinical and genetic heterogeneity in myotonic dystrophies. *Muscle Nerve*. 2000;23(12):1789–1799.
15. Ashizawa T, Gagnon C, Groh WJ, et al. Consensus-based care recommendations for adults with myotonic dystrophy type 1. *Neurol Clin Pract*. 2018;8(6):507–520.
16. Winters SJ. Endocrine dysfunction in patients with myotonic dystrophy. *J Clin Endocrinol Metab*. 2021;106(10):2819–2827.
17. Hund E, Jansen O, Koch MC, et al. Proximal myotonic myopathy with MRI white matter abnormalities of the brain. *Neurology*. 1997;48(1):33–37.
18. Nowak TV, Anuras S, Brown BP, Ionasescu V, Green JB. Small intestine motility in myotonic dystrophy patients. *Gastroenterology*. 1984;86(5 pt 1):808–813.
19. Hartog L, Zhao J, Reynolds J, et al. Factors influencing the severity and progression of respiratory muscle dysfunction in myotonic dystrophy type 1. *Front Neurol*. 2021;12:658532.
20. Hawkins AM, Hawkins CL, Abdul Razak K, Khoo TK, Tran K, Jackson RV. Respiratory dysfunction in myotonic dystrophy type 1: a systematic review. *Neuromuscul Disord*. 2019;29(3):198–212.
21. Subramony SH, Wymer JP, Pinto BS, Wang ET. Sleep disorders in myotonic dystrophies. *Muscle Nerve*. 2020;62(3);309–320.
22. Begin R, Bureau MA, Lupien L, Lemieux B. Control and modulation of respiration in Steinert's myotonic dystrophy. *Am Rev Respir Dis*. 1980;121(2):281–289.
23. Hansotia P, Frens D. Hypersomnia associated with alveolar hypoventilation in myotonic dystrophy. *Neurology*. 1981;31(10):1336–1337.
24. Motta J, Guilleminault C, Billingham M, Barry W, Mason J. Cardiac abnormalities in myotonic dystrophy. Electrophysiologic and histologic studies. *Am J Med*. 1979;67(3):467–473.
25. Russo V, Papa AA, Lioncino M, et al. Prevalence of atrial fibrillation in myotonic dystrophy type 1: a systematic review. *Neuromuscul Disord*. 2021;31(4):281–290.
26. Sabovic M, Medica I, Logar N, Mandic E, Zidar J, Peterlin B. Relation of CTG expansion and clinical variables to electrocardiogram conduction abnormalities and sudden death in patients with myotonic dystrophy. *Neuromuscul Disord*. 2003;13(10):822–826.
27. Delaporte C. Personality patterns in patients with myotonic dystrophy. *Arch Neurol*. 1998;55(5):635–640.
28. Meola G, Sansone V, Perani D, et al. Executive dysfunction and avoidant personality trait in myotonic dystrophy type 1 (DM-1) and in proximal myotonic myopathy (PROMM/DM-2). *Neuromuscul Disord*. 2003;13(10):813–821.
29. Moxley RT 3rd, Griggs RC, Goldblatt D, VanGelder V, Herr BE, Thiel R. Decreased insulin sensitivity of forearm muscle in myotonic dystrophy. *J Clin Invest*. 1978;62(4):857–867.
30. Gadalla SM, Lund M, Pfeiffer RM, et al. Cancer risk among patients with myotonic muscular dystrophy. *JAMA*. 2011;306(22):2480–2486.
31. Win AK, Perattur PG, Pulido JS, Pulido CM, Lindor NM. Increased cancer risks in myotonic dystrophy. *Mayo Clin Proc*. 2012;87(2):130–135.
32. D'Ambrosio ES, Chuang K, David WS, Amato AA, Gonzalez-Perez P. Frequency and type of cancers in myotonic dystrophy: a retrospective cross-sectional study. *Muscle Nerve*. 2023;68(2):142–148.
33. Abbott D, Johnson NE, Cannon-Albright LA. A population-based survey of risk for cancer in individuals diagnosed with myotonic dystrophy. *Muscle Nerve*. 2016;54(4):783–785.
34. Alsaggaf R, St George DMM, Zhan M, et al. Benign tumors in myotonic dystrophy type I target disease-related cancer sites. *Ann Clin Transl Neurol*. 2019;6(8):1510–1518.
35. Kong HE, Pollack BP. Cutaneous findings in myotonic dystrophy. *JAAD Int*. 2022;7:7–12.
36. Streib EW, Sun SF. Distribution of electrical myotonia in myotonic muscular dystrophy. *Ann Neurol*. 1983;14(1):80–82.
37. Dodge PR, Gamstrop I, Byers RK, Russell P. Myotonic dystrophy in infancy and childhood. *Pediatrics*. 1965;35:3–19.
38. Swift TR, Ignacio OJ, Dyken PR. Neonatal dystrophia myotonica. Electrophysiologic studies. *Am J Dis Child*. 1975;129(6):734–737.
39. Garibaldi M, Nicoletti T, Bucci E, et al. Muscle magnetic resonance imaging in myotonic dystrophy type 1 (DM1): refining muscle involvement and implications for clinical trials. *Eur J Neurol*. 2022;29(3):843–854.
40. Maurage CA, Udd B, Ruchoux MM, et al. Similar brain tau pathology in DM2/PROMM and DM1/Steinert disease. *Neurology*. 2005;65(10):1636–1638.
41. Brook JD, McCurrach ME, Harley HG, et al. Molecular basis of myotonic dystrophy: expansion of a trinucleotide (CTG) repeat at the 3′ end of a transcript encoding a protein kinase family member. *Cell*. 1992;68(4):799–808.
42. Fischbeck KH. The mechanism of myotonic dystrophy. *Ann Neurol*. 1994;35(3):255–256.
43. Fu YH, Friedman DL, Richards S, et al. Decreased expression of myotonin-protein kinase messenger RNA and protein in adult form of myotonic dystrophy. *Science*. 1993;260(5105):235–238.
44. Fu YH, Pizzuti A, Fenwick RG Jr, et al. An unstable triplet repeat in a gene related to myotonic muscular dystrophy. *Science*. 1992;255(5049):1256–1258.
45. Harper PS, Harley HG, Reardon W, Shaw DJ. Anticipation in myotonic dystrophy: new light on an old problem. *Am J Hum Genet*. 1992;51(1):10–16.
46. Mahadevan M, Tsilfidis C, Sabourin L, et al. Myotonic dystrophy mutation: an unstable CTG repeat in the 3′ untranslated region of the gene. *Science*. 1992;255(5049):1253–1255.
47. Ptacek LJ, Johnson KJ, Griggs RC. Genetics and physiology of the myotonic muscle disorders. *N Engl J Med*. 1993;328(7):482–489.
48. Shelbourne P, Davies J, Buxton J, et al. Direct diagnosis of myotonic dystrophy with a disease-specific DNA marker. *N Engl J Med*. 1993;328(7):471–475.
49. Soltanzadeh P. Myotonic dystrophies: a genetic overview. *Genes (Basel)*. 2022;13(2):367.
50. Tian B, White RJ, Xia T, et al. Expanded CUG repeat RNAs form hairpins that activate the double-stranded RNA-dependent protein kinase PKR. *RNA*. 2000;6(1):79–87.
51. Mankodi A, Takahashi MP, Jiang H, et al. Expanded CUG repeats trigger aberrant splicing of ClC-1 chloride channel pre-mRNA and hyperexcitability of skeletal muscle in myotonic dystrophy. *Mol Cell*. 2002;10(1):35–44.

52. Mankodi A, Teng-Umnauay P, Krym M, Henderson D, Swanson M, Thornton CA. Ribonuclear inclusions in skeletal muscle in myotonic dystrophy types 1 and 2. *Ann Neurol.* 2003; 54(6):760–768.
53. Mankodi A, Thornton CA. Myotonic syndromes. *Curr Opin Neurol.* 2002;15(5):545–552.
54. Udd B, Meola G, Krahe R, et al. Myotonic dystrophy type 2 (DM2) and related disorders report of the 180th ENMC workshop including guidelines on diagnostics and management 3–5 December 2010, Naarden, The Netherlands. *Neuromuscul Disord.* 2011;21(6):443–450.
55. Berg J, Jiang H, Thornton CA, Cannon SC. Truncated ClC-1 mRNA in myotonic dystrophy exerts a dominant-negative effect on the Cl current. *Neurology.* 2004;63(12):2371–2375.
56. Day JW, Ranum LP. RNA pathogenesis of the myotonic dystrophies. *Neuromuscul Disord.* 2005;15(1):5–16.
57. Kimura T, Nakamori M, Lueck JD, et al. Altered mRNA splicing of the skeletal muscle ryanodine receptor and sarcoplasmic/endoplasmic reticulum Ca^{2+}-ATPase in myotonic dystrophy type 1. *Hum Mol Genet.* 2005;14(15):2189–2200.
58. Pascual M, Vicente M, Monferrer L, Artero R. The Muscleblind family of proteins: an emerging class of regulators of developmentally programmed alternative splicing. *Differentiation.* 2006;74(2-3):65–80.
59. Kanadia RN, Johnstone KA, Mankodi A, et al. A muscleblind knockout model for myotonic dystrophy. *Science.* 2003;302(5652):1978–1980.
60. Ebralidze A, Wang Y, Petkova V, Ebralidse K, Junghans RP. RNA leaching of transcription factors disrupts transcription in myotonic dystrophy. *Science.* 2004;303(5656):383–387.
61. Logigian EL, Martens WB, Moxley RT 4th, et al. Mexiletine is an effective antimyotonia treatment in myotonic dystrophy type 1. *Neurology.* 2010;74(18):1441–1448.
62. Orngreen MC, Olsen DB, Vissing J. Aerobic training in patients with myotonic dystrophy type 1. *Ann Neurol.* 2005;57(5):754–757.
63. McNally EM, Mann DL, Pinto Y, et al. Clinical care recommendations for cardiologists treating adults with myotonic dystrophy. *J Am Heart Assoc.* 2020;9(4):e014006.
64. Aldridge LM. Anesthetic problems in myotonic dystrophy. A case report and review of the Aberdeen experience comprising 48 general anaesthetics in a further 16 patients. *Br J Anaesth.* 1985;57(11):1119–1130.
65. Brahams D. Postoperative monitoring in patients with muscular dystrophy. *Lancet.* 1989;2(8670):1053–1054.
66. Harper PS. Postoperative complications in myotonic dystrophy. *Lancet.* 1989;2(8674):1269.
67. Mathieu J, Allard P, Gobeil G, Girard M, De Braekeleer M, Begin P. Anesthetic and surgical complications in 219 cases of myotonic dystrophy. *Neurology.* 1997;49(6):1646–1650.
68. Damian MS, Gerlach A, Schmidt F, Lehman E, Reichmann H. Modafinil for excessive daytime sleepiness in myotonic dystrophy. *Neurology.* 2001;56(6):794–796.
69. MacDonald JR, Hill JD, Tarnopolsky MA. Modafinil reduces excessive somnolence and enhances mood in patients with myotonic dystrophy. *Neurology.* 2002;59(12):1876–1880.
70. Talbot K, Stradling J, Crosby J, Hilton-Jones D. Reduction in excess daytime sleepiness by modafinil in patients with myotonic dystrophy. *Neuromuscul Disord.* 2003;13(5):357–364.
71. Day JW, Ricker K, Jacobsen JF, et al. Myotonic dystrophy type 2: molecular, diagnostic, and clinical spectrum. *Neurology.* 2003;60(4):657–664.
72. Meola G, Sansone V, Radice S, Skradski S, Ptacek L. A family with an unusual myotonic and myopathic phenotype and no CTG expansion (proximal myotonic myopathic syndrome): a challenge for future molecular studies. *Neuromuscul Disord.* 1996;6(3):143–150.
73. Moxley RT 3rd. Proximal myotonic myopathy: mini-review of a recently delineated clinical disorder. *Neuromuscul Disord.* 1996; 6(2):87–93.
74. Ricker K, Grimm T, Koch MC, et al. Linkage of proximal myotonic myopathy to chromosome 3q. *Neurology.* 1999;52(1): 170–171.
75. Ricker K, Koch MC, Lehmann-Horn F, et al. Proximal myotonic myopathy: a new dominant disorder with myotonia, muscle weakness, and cataracts. *Neurology.* 1994;44(8): 1448–1452.
76. Ricker K, Koch MC, Lehmann-Horn F, et al. Proximal myotonic myopathy. Clinical features of a multisystemic disorder similar to myotonic dystrophy. *Arch Neurol.* 1995;52(1):25–31.
77. Ricker K, Moxley RT 3rd, Heine R, Lehmann-Horn F. Myotonia fluctuans. A third type of muscle sodium channel disease. *Arch Neurol.* 1994;51(11):1095–1102.
78. Schneider C, Ziegler A, Ricker K, et al. Proximal myotonic myopathy: evidence for anticipation in families with linkage to chromosome 3q. *Neurology.* 2000;55(3):383–388.
79. Thornton CA, Ashizawa T. Getting a grip on the myotonic dystrophies. *Neurology.* 1999;52(1):12–13.
80. Thornton CA, Griggs RC, Moxley RT 3rd. Myotonic dystrophy with no trinucleotide repeat expansion. *Ann Neurol.* 1994;35(3):269–272.
81. Meola G. Myotonic dystrophy type 2: the 2020 update. *Acta Myol.* 2020;39(4):222–234.
82. Schoser B, Montagnese F, Bassez G, et al; Myotonic Dystrophy Foundation. Consensus-based care recommendations for adults with myotonic dystrophy type 2. *Neurol Clin Pract.* 2019;9(4):343–353.
83. Suominen T, Bachinski LL, Auvinen S, et al. Population frequency of myotonic dystrophy: higher than expected frequency of myotonic dystrophy type 2 (DM2) mutation in Finland. *Eur J Hum Genet.* 2011;19(7):776–782.
84. Newman B, Meola G, O'Donovan DG, Schapira AH, Kingston H. Proximal myotonic myopathy (PROMM) presenting as myotonia during pregnancy. *Neuromuscul Disord.* 1999;9(3): 144–149.
85. Rudnik-Schoneborn S, Schneider-Gold C, Raabe U, Kress W, Zerres K, Schoser BG. Outcome and effect of pregnancy in myotonic dystrophy type 2. *Neurology.* 2006;66(4): 579–580.
86. Sander HW, Tavoulareas GP, Chokroverty S. Heat-sensitive myotonia in proximal myotonic myopathy. *Neurology.* 1996; 47(4):956–962.
87. Schoser BG, Ricker K, Schneider-Gold C, et al. Sudden cardiac death in myotonic dystrophy type 2. *Neurology.* 2004;63(12): 2402–2404.
88. Schoser BG, Schneider-Gold C, Kress W, et al. Muscle pathology in 57 patients with myotonic dystrophy type 2. *Muscle Nerve.* 2004;29(2):275–281.
89. Vihola A, Bassez G, Meola G, et al. Histopathological differences of myotonic dystrophy type 1 (DM1) and PROMM/DM2. *Neurology.* 2003;60(11):1854–1857.
90. Moxley RT 3rd. Carrell-Krusen Symposium Invited Lecture-1997. Myotonic disorders in childhood: diagnosis and treatment. *J Child Neurol.* 1997;12(2):116–129.

CHAPTER 32

Nondystrophic Myotonias and Periodic Paralysis

In this chapter, we describe the pathophysiology, clinical presentation, laboratory findings, and treatment of the nondystrophic myotonias and periodic paralyses (Table 32-1). There are several inherited myopathic disorders associated with clinical or electrical myotonia in which muscle is not dystrophic.[1-9] These disorders are caused by mutations in various ion channels and are thus referred to here as muscle channelopathies. Mutations in the chloride channel cause myotonia congenita (MC). The sodium channelopathies include potassium-sensitive (hyperkalemic) periodic paralysis (HyperKPP), paramyotonia congenita (PMC), potassium-aggravated myotonia (PAM) (e.g., myotonia fluctuans, myotonia permanens, and acetazolamide-responsive myotonia), and familial hypokalemic periodic paralysis type 2 (HypoKPP2). HyperKPP and PMC are usually associated with episodes of transient generalized or focal weakness. Hypokalemic periodic paralysis type 1 (HypoKPP1) is not associated with myotonia clinically or electrophysiologically and is caused by mutations of muscle dihydropyridine (DHP) receptor (a type of calcium channel). Andersen–Tawil syndrome (ATS) is another rare form of hereditary periodic paralysis of which some forms are usually caused by mutations in a *KCNJ2* gene that encodes for the inwardly rectifying potassium channel (Kir2.1). The estimated prevalence for the different forms of periodic paralyses are 1 per 100,000 for HypoPP, 1 per 200,000 for HyperPP, and 1 per 1,000,000 for ATS.[9]

Electrophysiological studies, in particular the short- and long-exercise tests (SETs and LETs), also described in Chapter 2, can be useful in distinguishing subtypes of muscle channelopathy and thus deserve special comment (Tables 32-1 and 32-2).[1-14] The SET is performed by having the patient isometrically exercise a muscle [e.g., abductor digiti minimi (ADM)] for 10 seconds, followed by measurement of compound muscle action potential (CMAP) amplitudes immediately after exercise and every 10 seconds thereafter up to 60 seconds. Fournier et al. modified the test by having the SET repeated twice more with a rest period of 60 seconds between trials. In addition, the SET should be done at room temperature and then with cooling of the muscle. In normal individuals, immediately after short exercise, there is a mild increase in the CMAP amplitudes compared to baseline (mean 4%–5%, range −28% to +27%) with the amplitudes returning to baseline within 10 seconds.[11,12] If the SET is performed after cooling the limb (e.g., with an ice pack), the CMAP amplitudes decrease (−25% to −65%), but the durations of the CMAPs increase.

The LET is performed by having the patient isometrically exercise a muscle (e.g., ADM) for 5 minutes (with 3–4 seconds of rest every 30–45 seconds), while CMAP amplitudes are recorded every minute during the exercise period, immediately after cessation of exercise, then every minute for 5 minutes, and finally every 5 minutes for 40–45 minutes. In normal people, CMAP amplitudes only slightly decrease after the exercise period (range −16 to +5%), and the amplitudes then return to normal within the next 30–60 seconds and remain so during the next 40–50 minutes.[11,12] In a study of 45 patients with genetically confirmed HypoKPP or HyperKPP, significant decrement was present in 71% of patients and the sensitivity was highest in 8/8 (100%) with frequent (daily or weekly) attacks, evident in 15/21 (71%) with up to monthly attacks, but present in only 9/15 (56%) with less frequent attacks. So, a negative study in patients with frequent attack of periodic paralysis makes a hereditary form of periodic paralysis very unlikely, but a negative test in a patient with rare attacks of weakness does not exclude the disorder.[14]

Changes in CMAP amplitudes with the SET separate muscle channelopathies into five patterns (Table 32-2; Fig. 32-1).[11] The first three patterns help distinguish the nondystrophic myotonias, particularly when performed at room temperature and then in cold, while patterns IV and V are useful in diagnosing periodic paralysis in combination with the LET.[11,12]

▶ CHLORIDE CHANNELOPATHIES

MYOTONIA CONGENITA

Clinical Features

The autosomal-dominant form of MC, or Thomsen disease, often presents in the first few years of life.[1-4,7,8,15-21] Affected infants may have difficulty opening their eyes after crying. Stiffness in the legs upon arising and taking the first few steps may lead to tripping and falling. As patients become older, their muscle stiffness may become more noticeable in the arms. Myotonia of muscles of mastication may result in difficulties in chewing and swallowing. As with most forms of myotonia, the stiffness in the muscles eases with repeated contractions, the so-called warm-up phenomena. Thus,

TABLE 32-1. NONDYSTROPHIC MYOTONIAS AND HEREDITARY PERIODIC PARALYSIS

Disorder	Inheritance	Gene (Location)	Clinical or EMG Myotonia	Short-Exercise Test	Long-Exercise Test	Fournier Electrophysiologic Pattern
Myotonia congenita (MC) Thomsen disease Becker disease	AD AR	CLCN-1 (7q35)	Yes	±PEMPs; transient decrease in CMAP amplitudes after the first trial in AR-MC but less common with AD MC; reduction in amplitudes is less in the second and third trials. No change with cold in AR-MC, but reduction in amplitudes occurs after the first trial in AD-MC that improves with subsequent trials	Slight or no decrease in amplitudes immediately after exercise with no change over time	Pattern II
Hyperkalemic periodic paralysis (HyperKPP)	AD	SCN4A (17q13.1–13.3)	Maybe	No PEMPs; Increase in amplitudes after the first trial with further increase after the second and third trials	Transient increase in amplitudes immediately after exercise with subsequent gradual decrease in amplitudes over a prolonged period of time (as much as 40 minutes or more)	Pattern IV
Paramyotonia congenita (PMC)	AD	SCN4A (17q13.1–13.3)	Yes	PEMPs are common; amplitudes may increase or decrease with the initial trial but gradually decline after the second and third trials (most common with T1313M mutations—other forms of PMC usually have normal SET); reduction in amplitudes is more prominent in cold. PMC with Q270 m mutation may have normal SET at rest but has decrement with cooling	Decrease in amplitudes during and following exercise that may persist for hours	Pattern I
Potassium-aggravated myotonias Myotonia permanens Myotonia fluctuans Acetazolamide-responsive MC	AD	SCN4A (17q13.1–13.3)	Yes	No PEMPs; usually no change even with cooling	No change	Pattern III
Hypokalemic periodic paralysis type 1 (HypoKPP1)	AD	CACNA1S (1q31–32)	No	No PEMPs; usually no change even with cooling	Slight increase or no immediate change with exercise but gradually decline of amplitudes over time is seen in most	Pattern V
Hypokalemic periodic paralysis type 2 (HypoKPP2)	AD	SCN4A (17q13.1–13.3)	No	No PEMPs; usually no change even with cooling	A slight increase in amplitudes may be seen during and immediately after exercise followed by a delayed reduction in amplitudes after 10–20 minutes	Pattern V
Andersen–Tawil syndrome (ATS)	AD	KCNJ2 (17q23.1–q24.2)	No	Unknown	A decrement in CMAP area and to a lesser extent the amplitude may be appreciated	
Schwartz–Jampel syndrome	AR	HSPG2 (1p34.1–36.1)	Yes	Unknown	Unknown	

AD, autosomal dominant; AR, autosomal recessive; CMAP, compound muscle action potential; PEMPs, postexercise myotonic potentials on the motor conduction studies.

▶ TABLE 32-2. ELECTRODIAGNOSTIC PATTERNS[10]

Patterns	SET	LET
I	Postexercise amplitude decrement that worsens with each trial	Postexercise amplitude decrement that does not return to baseline over 40 minutes
II	Postexercise amplitude decrement that improves with each trial	No postexercise amplitude change or small transient decrement
III	No postexercise amplitude change	No postexercise amplitude change
IV	Postexercise amplitude increment that increases with each trial	Transient postexercise amplitude increment followed by late continuous decrement over 40 minutes
V	No postexercise amplitude change	Late continuous postexercise amplitude decrement over 40 minutes

Stunnenberg BC, LoRusso S, Arnold WD, et al. Guidelines on clinical presentation and management of nondystrophic myotonias. *Muscle Nerve*. 2020;62:430–444.

although an affected individual may have initial stiffness in their legs when they begin to walk, within a short time ambulation becomes easier. After rest, the same stereotypical pattern of stiffness returns on initiation of physical activity. The myotonia can worsen with cold similar to that seen in PMC.[18] The severity of the myotonia can fluctuate and is variable even within affected family members. The stiffness may worsen during pregnancy. Of note, people with MC usually do not typically complain of muscle pain with their stiffness. In contrast to the myotonic dystrophies, there are no systemic disorders (e.g., cataracts, endocrinopathies, cardiopathy, ventilatory muscle weakness) associated with MC

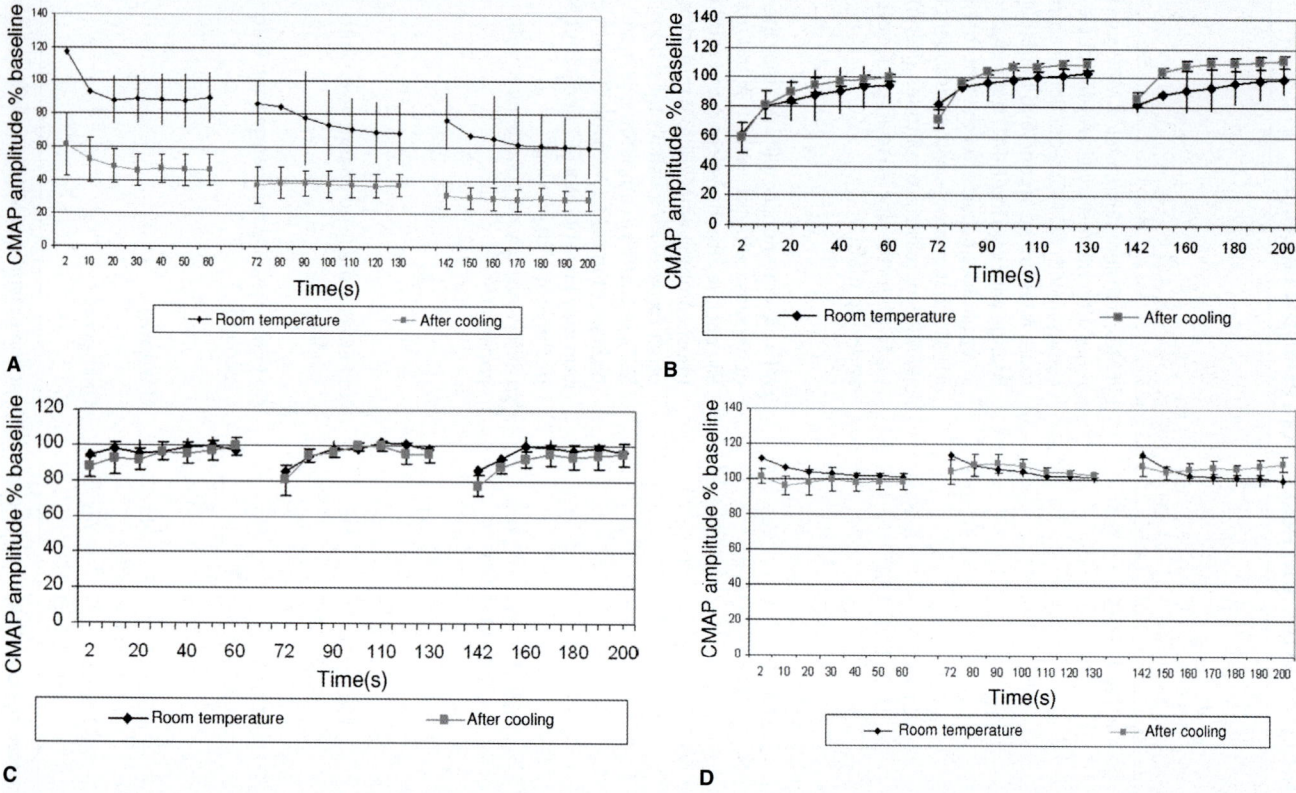

Figure 32-1. Short-exercise test (SET) and Fournier Patterns in the nondystrophic myotonias. (**A**) Fournier Pattern I. Paramyotonia congenita (PMC) associated with T1313M *SCN4A* mutation. The SET is associated with a decrease in compound muscle action potential (CMAP) amplitudes that worsens with repeated trials of short exercise at room temperature. The SET with cooling shows even greater decrement of CMAP amplitude. PMC associated with (**B**) Fournier Pattern II. Autosomal-recessive myotonia congenita. The SET is associated with a decrease in CMAP amplitudes immediately after exercise that returns to baseline after 20–40 seconds. The reduction in the CMAP amplitudes decreases with repeated trials of short exercise. (**C**) Autosomal-dominant myotonia congenita. The SET at room temperature often shows no decrement, but with cooling there is reversion to Fournier Pattern II with decrement that improves with repeated activity. (**D**) Fournier Pattern III. The SET at room temperature and after cooling is normal as seen in most cases of potassium-associated myotonia (PAM), PMC that are not associated with T1313M mutation, and in the myotonic dystrophies. (Reproduced with permission from Matthews E, Fialho D, Tan SV, et al. CINCH Investigators. The non-dystrophic myotonias: molecular pathogenesis, diagnosis and treatment. *Brain*. 2010;133(Pt 1):9–22.)

or increased mortality. However, some individuals present later in life with stiffness and proximal weakness and resemble myotonic dystrophy type 2 (DM2) or proximal myotonic myopathy (PROMM).[4,18] There may be an increased risk of malignant hyperthermia (MH) with anesthetic agents.

On examination, affected individuals usually appear extremely muscular (e.g., Herculean). Muscle strength is usually normal, but some patients develop mild proximal weakness. Action myotonia can be elicited by having the patient make a strong grip and then try to relax their fingers, or by having patients forcefully close their eyes and then try to open them. One sees delayed relaxation, which improves with repeated activity due to the warm-up phenomena discussed above. In addition, myotonia can be demonstrated by percussing a muscle (e.g., the thenar eminence) with a reflex hammer (percussion myotonia).

Becker described the features of the autosomal-recessive form of MC which bears his name. The clinical features of the autosomal-recessive and dominant forms of MC are similar, but there are some differences.[1–4,7,8,15,16,19,20] The autosomal-recessive or Becker type of MC usually presents between 4 and 12 years of age, somewhat later than that seen in the autosomal-dominant form, however, the severity of weakness is typically worse.[1,2,18] Transient muscle weakness, particularly in the distal arms, may occur following a severe bout of myotonia. On examination, muscle bulk is usually increased. Mild fixed weakness is apparent in proximal muscles of the arms and legs as well as in the neck. Systemic complications are not seen, though there is an increased risk of MH.

Laboratory Features

Skeletal muscle MRI is usually not that helpful as it may[22] or may not[23] demonstrate signal abnormalities, which if present are nonspecific. Serum creatine kinase (CK) is normal or only slightly elevated. Routine motor and sensory nerve conduction studies (NCSs) are normal. On repetitive nerve stimulation, a decrement may be appreciated when a prolonged train of stimuli are delivered at 10 Hz or more. In such cases, the CMAP amplitudes may decrease to 65% of normal and even large degrees of decrement can occur with stimulation at higher rates.[6,24]

The SET is associated with a decrease in CMAP amplitude immediately after exercise that returns to baseline after 20–40 seconds, in 48%–80% of individuals with MC (Fig. 32-1B).[2,4,10,12] The reduction in the CMAP amplitude decreases with repeated trials of short exercise, corresponding to the clinical warm-up phenomena. Fournier et al.[10] called this Pattern II (Table 32-2). A greater than 40% decrement of SET is specific for MC.[4,12] More accurately though, it is the autosomal-recessive cases that usually have the reduction in CMAP amplitudes, while the autosomal-dominant cases typically are not associated with significant change in amplitude.[3,11,12] Performing the SET in cooled limb patients with autosomal-dominant MC may result in a drop in amplitude that improves with repeated short exercise (e.g., a conversion from normal to Pattern II with cold). In contrast, there is usually no significant difference in the results of the short exercise performed at room temperature; in comparison to cold in individuals with autosomal-recessive MC (they remain with Pattern II).[4,11] Overall, Fournier Pattern II is seen in over 60% of autosomal-recessive MC, but less than 30% of autosomal-dominant MC.[4,11] In addition, postexercise repetitive discharges or myotonic potentials (PEMPs) are seen in about one-third of MC patients after short exercise.[10] These PEMPs disappear within 10–30 seconds after exercise. The LET is usually normal, but 10%–30% of patients with MC (usually AR-MC) have an initial transient decrement greater than normal (Fig. 32-2).[10,12,25]

On needle electromyography (EMG), myotonic discharges are evident at rest and during volitional activity. Cooling a limb does not lead to exacerbation of the clinical or electrical myotonia or development of weakness, unlike that seen in PMC.[26] It may be difficult to appreciate motor unit action potential (MUAP) as the myotonic discharges obscure the voluntary MUAPs, but morphology and recruitment are usually normal. However, short duration, small amplitude MUAPs may occasionally be appreciated in weak muscles. Single-fiber EMG reveals normal fiber density but slightly increased jitter.

Molecular Genetics and Pathogenesis

Both the autosomal-dominant form (Thomsen) and recessive form (Becker) of MC are caused by mutations in the muscle chloride channel gene (*CLCN1*) on chromosome 7q35 (Fig. 32-3).[1,5,27–29] Of note, there is a so-called painful variant of MC that resembles the Thomsen and Becker forms, except patients with this disorder more frequently complain of myalgias. This painful variant of MC is usually caused by mutations in the muscle sodium channel gene, *SCN4A* (discussed later). Structurally, the chloride ion channel is a homotetramer with each subunit encoded by the *CLCN1* gene.[28] The function of the chloride ion channel is to maintain the high resting membrane conductance in muscle fibers.[30] Mutations of the *CLCN1* gene are associated with reduced chloride conductance. Because chloride ions are responsible for 70% of the skeletal muscle resting membrane potential, reduced chloride conductance leads to a decrease in the rate of muscle membrane repolarization. Thus, sodium channels are able to recover from inactivation faster. As a result of the muscle membrane being in a state of depolarization, recurrent firings of action potentials or myotonic discharges occur.[30]

Treatment

Many individuals with MC do not require medical treatment. However, when the myotonia is severe and impairs function, treatment with antiarrhythmic or antiepileptic medications (e.g., mexiletine, phenytoin, carbamazepine) that interfere with the muscle sodium channel can be beneficial. In this regard, a randomized, placebo-controlled trial demonstrated that mexiletine (200 mg three times daily) reduced muscle stiffness.[30] We have also found mexiletine diminishing the transient exacerbations of weakness that can accompany

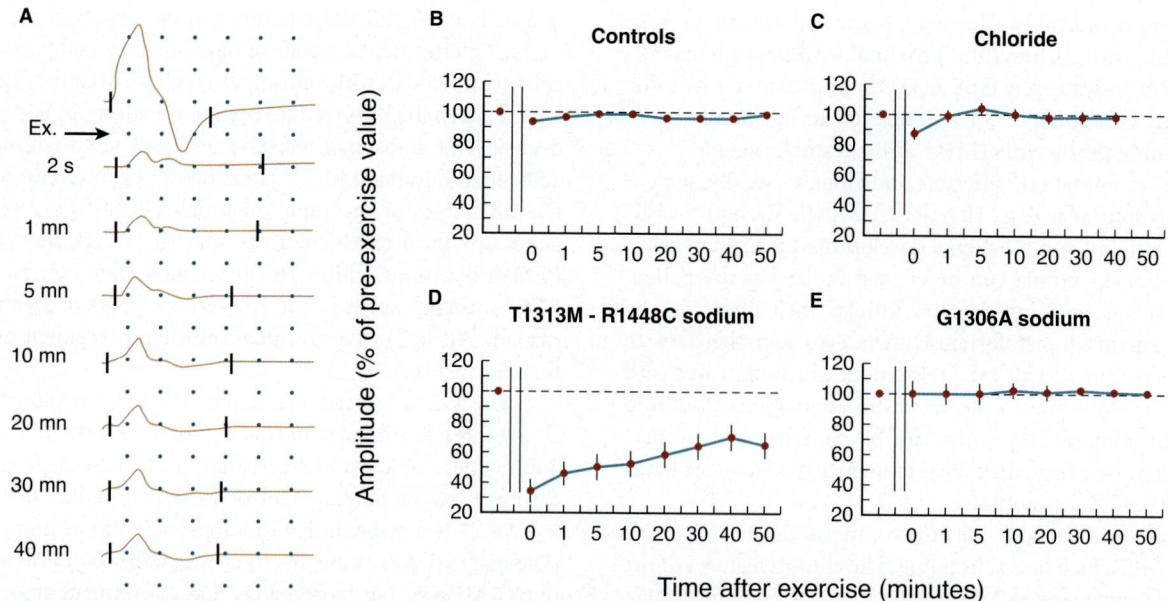

Figure 32-2. Long-exercise test in myotonic syndromes. (**A**) Immediate and persistent decrease of compound muscle action potential (CMAP) amplitude (−85%) after long exercise in a paramyotonia congenita (PMC) patient with the T1313M sodium channel mutation. Pre-exercise *(top trace)* and postexercise recordings *(bottom trace)* at various times following the trial (Ex.) as indicated to the left of the tracings. Scale between two dots: 5 ms, 5 mV. Changes in CMAP amplitude of the abductor digiti minimi (ADM) muscle after long exercise *(double bars)* in 41 unaffected controls (**B**), 6 myotonia congenita (MC) patients with chloride channel mutations (**C**), 16 PMC patients with T1313M or R1448C sodium channel mutations (**D**), and 2 patients with G1306A sodium channel mutations (**E**). The amplitude of the CMAP, expressed as a percentage of its pre-exercise value, is plotted against the time elapsed after the exercise trial *(symbols* and *vertical bars)*. Means ± standard errors of the means. (Reproduced with permission from Fournier E., Arzel M, Sternberg D, et al. Electromyography guides toward subgroups of mutations in muscle channelopathies. *Ann Neurol.* 2004;56(5):650–661.)

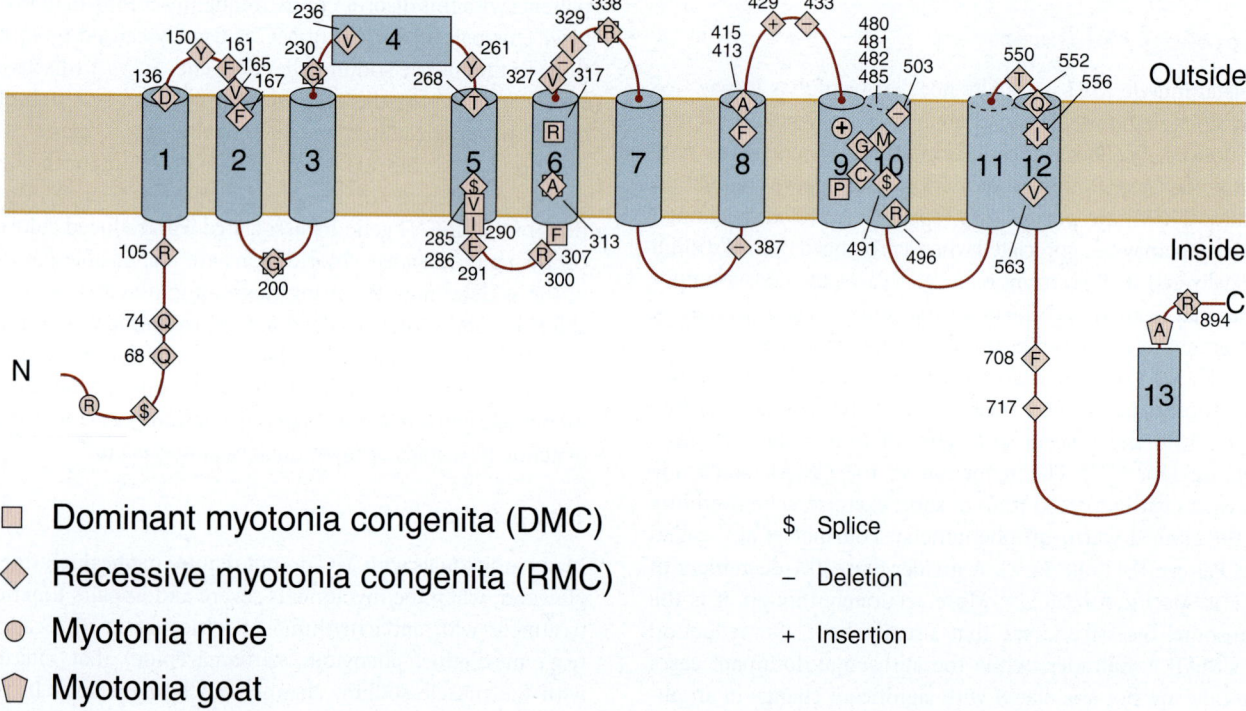

Figure 32-3. The chloride channel monomer, ClC-1, is functional as homodimeric channel complex. Different symbols used for known mutations leading to dominant Thomsen-type myotonia, recessive Becker-type myotonia, recessive myotonic mice, and dominant myotonic goat are explained on *bottom left*. Conventional one-letter abbreviations were used for replaced amino acids located at positions given by respective numbers of human protein. (Reproduced with permission from Lehmann-Horn F, Jurkat-Rott K. Voltage-gated ion channels and hereditary disease. *Physiol Rev.* 1999;79(4):1317–1372.)

the myotonia. Prior to starting mexiletine, we obtain a baseline electrocardiogram (EKG) as the drug can prolong the QT interval. If the EKG reveals a significant abnormality, we obtain a cardiology consultation before beginning mexiletine. Lightheadedness, diarrhea, and dyspepsia are dose-limiting side effects of mexiletine. Dantrolene, which blocks the release of calcium from the sarcoplasmic reticulum, may reduce myotonia as well, but is usually avoided because of side effects.

SODIUM CHANNELOPATHIES

The sodium channelopathies include HyperKPP, PMC, the PAMs (e.g., myotonia fluctuans, myotonia permanens, and acetazolamide responsive myotonia)[1–9,31–47] and familial HypoKPP2.[9,34,36–39] They are myopathies that share some similar clinical and laboratory features but have differences (Table 32-1). These disorders are inherited in an autosomal-dominant fashion. They are all caused by missense mutations in the pore-forming subunit of the voltage-gated skeletal-muscle sodium channel Nav1.4 (encoded by the SCN4A gene that is located on chromosome 17q23–25) (Fig. 32-4).[1,5,31,33–47] For the most part, each missense mutation in SCN4A is consistently associated with one of the four allelic sodium channel disorders, suggesting the presence of separate classes of functional defects. However, some variability exists, and the distinction is often blurred between PMC and Hyper-KPP, even in affected members of the same family.

POTASSIUM-SENSITIVE OR HYPERKALEMIC PERIODIC PARALYSIS (ADYNAMIA EPISODICA HEREDITARIA)

Clinical Features

Potassium-sensitive periodic paralysis or hyperkalemic periodic paralysis (HyperKPP) is an autosomal-dominant

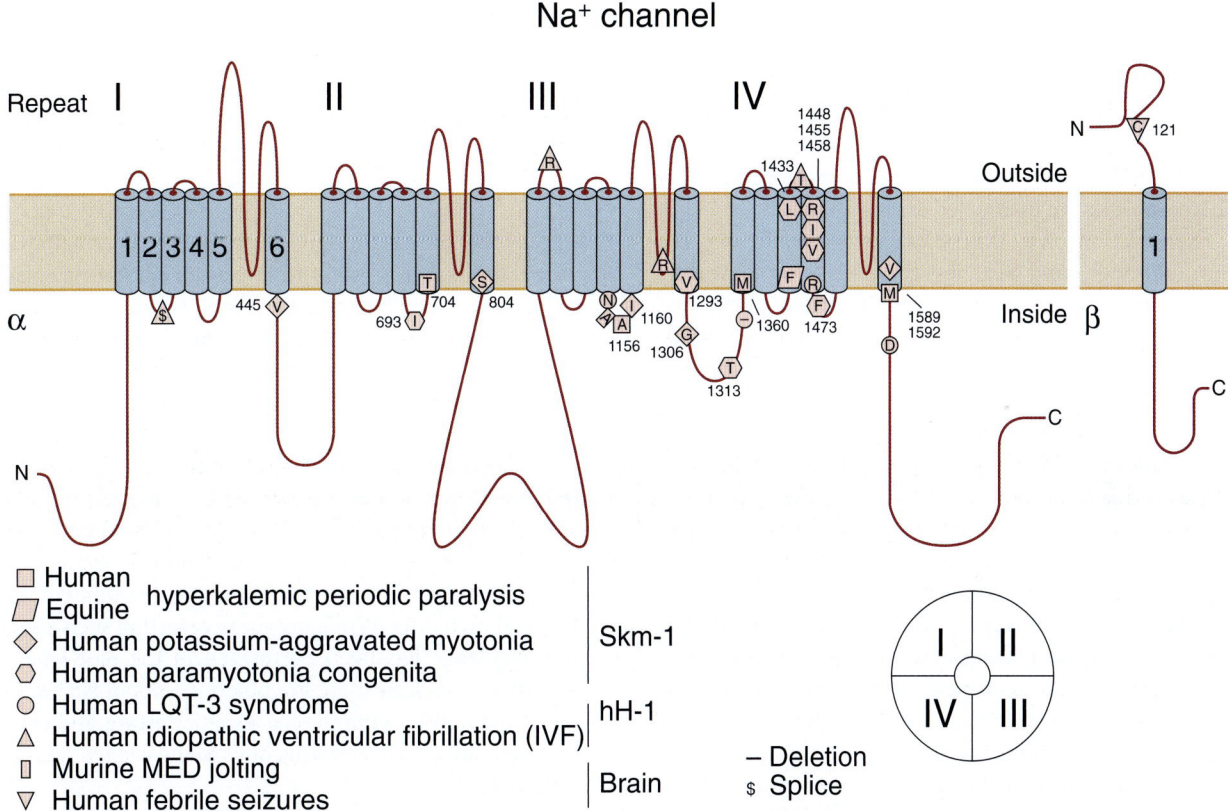

Figure 32-4. Subunits of voltage-gated sodium channel. α-Subunit consists of four highly homologous domains (repeats I–IV) containing two transmembrane segments each (S1–S6). S5–S6 loops form ion-selective pores, and S4 segments contain positively charged residues conferring voltage dependence to the protein. Repeats are connected by intracellular loops; one of them, III–IV linker, contains supposed inactivation particle of channel. β1 and β2 are auxiliary subunits. When inserted in membrane, four repeats of protein fold to generate a central pore as schematically indicated on *bottom right*. Mutations have been described for α-subunits of various species and tissues: human and equine adult skeletal muscle (Skm-1), human heart (hH-1), and murine brain. So far, only one mutation has been reported for a sodium channel subunit, that is, one of human brain. Conventional one-letter abbreviations are used for replaced amino acids whose positions are given by respective numbers of human skeletal muscle channel. Different symbols used for point mutations indicate resulting diseases as explained at *bottom left*. (Reproduced with permission from Lehmann-Horn F, Jurkat-Rott K. Voltage-gated ion channels and hereditary diseases. *Physiol Rev*. 1999;79(4): 1317–1372.)

disorder with a high degree of penetrance.[9,17,33,39–41,48–58] A large study in England revealed the prevalence to be 0.17 per 100,000.[5] HyperKPP manifests in three forms: (1) without myotonia, (2) with clinical or electrical myotonia, or (3) associated with paramyotonia. The course of the attacks of weakness is similar in each form, except that cooling triggers weakness in those with paramyotonia. Clinical myotonia is often mild, and can be elicited in the face (e.g., eyelids), tongue, forearm (e.g., finger extensors), and the thenar eminence with percussion or activity. The myotonia eases with repetitive activity, except in individuals with paramyotonia who exhibit paradoxical myotonia in which muscle stiffness is induced or worsened by exercise and cold temperature.

Approximately 50% of affected individuals become initially symptomatic with attacks of weakness in the first decade of life. These attacks usually develop in the morning, although can occur at any time, and are often precipitated by rest following exercise, intake of potassium rich food, fasting, pregnancy, exposure to cold, and even by emotional stress. The weakness can be mild or severe, with the latter more commonly occurring after strenuous physical activity. People may note paresthesia and achiness in the muscles prior to the development of weakness. The thigh and calf muscles are often affected, and weakness may progress to other muscle groups. However, the weakness can also be focal. In contrast to HypoKPP, generalized flaccid paralysis is uncommon. Rarely, the bulbar and ventilatory muscles are affected. The sphincter muscles are unaffected during attacks.

The duration of weakness attacks is usually less than 2 hours, although mild weakness can persist for a few days. The frequency of attacks is highly variable, ranging from several times a day to less than once a year. The attacks of weakness in HyperPP tend to be shorter in duration but more frequent that those occurring in HypoKPP. In addition, there is great variation of attack severity and frequency within and between families. The frequency of paretic attacks often decreases with age. Sustained mild exercise after a period of strenuous activity may postpone or prevent weakness from developing in the exercising muscles, while resting muscle groups become weak. Following a bout of weakness, it is not uncommon for pain to be experienced in the affected muscles up to several days. During attacks, the reflexes are diminished or absent, while sensation remains normal. Between the attacks, sensation and muscle stretch reflexes are normal and lid lag or eyelid myotonia may be the only clinical signs present. As many as 80% affected individuals develop fixed or slowly progressive weakness, independent of the episodic attacks, usually involving the more proximal muscles.[9]

Laboratory Features

Skeletal muscle MRI scans may reveal nonspecific signal abnormalities in thigh and calf muscles.[22] Serum CK levels are usually mildly elevated. In between the attacks, serum potassium levels are within normal limits. Increase in serum potassium levels (usually to 5–6 mEq/L) are associated with

TABLE 32-3. ETIOLOGIES OF SECONDARY HYPOKALEMIC AND HYPERKALEMIC PARALYSES

Hypokalemic paralysis
  Thyrotoxic periodic paralysis
  Renal tubular acidosis
  Gitelman syndrome
  Villous adenoma
  Bartter syndrome
  Hyperaldosteronism
  Chronic or excessive use of diuretics, corticosteroids, licorice
  Amphotericin B toxicity
  Alcoholism
  Toluene toxicity
  Barium poisoning
Hyperkalemic paralysis
  Addison disease
  Hypoaldosteronism (hyporeninemic)
  Isolated aldosterone deficiency
  Excessive potassium supplementation
  Potassium-sparing diuretics (e.g., spironolactone, triamterene)
  Chronic renal failure
  Rhabdomyolysis

Reproduced with permission from Amato AA, Dumitru D. Hereditary myopathies. In: Dumitru D, Amato AA, Swartz MJ, eds. *Electrodiagnostic Medicine*. 2nd ed. Hanley & Belfus, Inc.; 2002.

attacks of weakness, though serum levels may remain within normal limits. Serum sodium levels can fall during episodes of weakness. During attacks, there is increased urinary excretion of potassium that can actually result in transient hypokalemia at the end of an attack. On EKG, the hyperkalemia can result in increased amplitudes of the precordial T waves.

Secondary causes of hyperkalemia can cause generalized weakness and must be excluded particularly in individuals with no family history (Table 32-3). Usually, the serum potassium levels are greater than 7 mEq/L. Patients with secondary causes of hyperkalemic do not exhibit clinical or electrical myotonia. While provocative testing such as potassium challenge has been performed in the past when the diagnosis is unclear, there are obvious risks of such testing. The availability of commercial genetic testing and features on electrophysiological testing obviate the need for such provocative testing.

Routine motor and sensory NCSs are normal between attacks of weakness.[49,50,57–59] However, during an attack of weakness, the CMAP amplitudes may be reduced in affected muscles. As previously mentioned, the SET and LET can be useful in distinguishing subtypes of channelopathies.[9–14] With the SET test, some patients with HyperKPP, depending on the exact mutation (e.g., T704M), have abnormal increased CMAP amplitudes that persist for a longer period of time than normal individuals.[10,12] Further, repetition of short exercise amplifies the increase in CMAP amplitudes. With the LET,

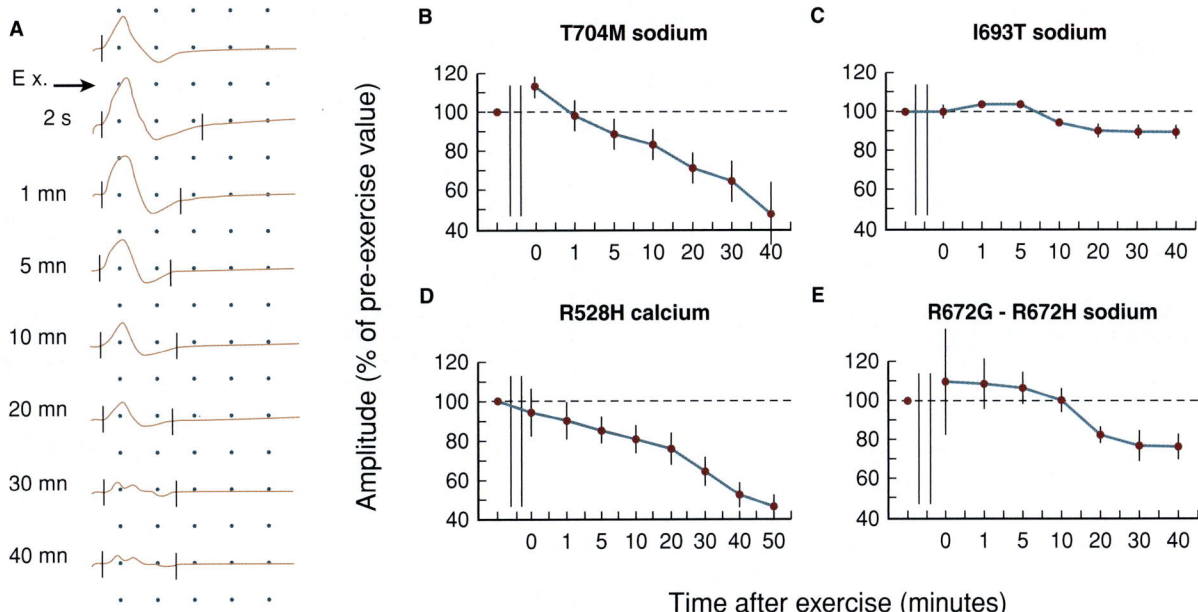

Figure 32-5. Long-exercise test in periodic paralyses. (**A**) Early increase (+38%) and delayed decrease (−74%) of compound muscle action potential (CMAP) amplitude after long exercise in HyperKPP patient with the T704M sodium channel mutation. Pre-exercise *(top trace)* and postexercise recordings *(bottom trace)* at different times following the trial (Ex.) as indicated left of the traces. Scale between two dots: 5 ms, 5 mV. Changes in CMAP amplitude of the abductor digiti minimi (ADM) muscle after long exercise *(double bars)* in 6 HyperKPP patients with T704M sodium channel mutations (**B**), 6 Myotonia-HyperKPP patients with the I693T mutation of the sodium channel (**C**), 13 HypoKPP1 patients with the R528H calcium channel mutation (**D**), and 2 HypoKPP2 patients with R672G or R672G sodium channel mutations (**E**). The amplitude of the CMAP, expressed as a percentage of its pre-exercise value, is plotted against the time elapsed after the exercise trial *(symbols* and *vertical bars)*. Means ± standard errors of the means. (Reproduced with permission from Fournier E, Arzel M, Sternberg D, et al. Electromyography guides toward subgroups of mutations in muscle channelopathies. *Ann Neurol.* 2004;56(5):650–661.)

during the exercise period and immediately afterwards, there is an initial increase in CMAP amplitudes from baseline that is followed by a progressive decline in the amplitudes over the next 40–50 minutes. Brief exercise (e.g., 10 seconds) during this paretic phase may induce an increment in the CMAP amplitudes (Fig. 32-5).[10] This constellation of findings on SET and LET is termed Fournier Pattern IV.

Needle EMG reveals variable findings. Myotonic discharges are found in 50%–75% of affected individuals, though clinical myotonia is apparent in less than 20%.[10,59] In patients with clinical myotonia, examination of the muscle between attacks of weakness reveals an increase in insertional activity, in the form of fibrillation potentials and positive sharp waves, in addition to myotonic discharges. These abnormal discharges reflect the hyperexcitability or instability of the muscle membrane and are not due to denervation. Reducing the limb temperature may exacerbate the runs of myotonic discharges. Analysis of MUAP parameters may reveal a slight increase in small amplitude, short duration, and polyphasic potentials. In people with HyperKPP without clinical myotonia, the insertional and spontaneous activity is normal between attacks of weakness. During an attack of weakness, the MUAPs decrease in duration and amplitude, and may disappear altogether in plegic muscles.

Histopathology

Muscle biopsies in patients with HyperKPP may reveal non-rimmed vacuoles.[17,60,61]

Molecular Genetics and Pathogenesis

Potassium-sensitive periodic paralysis is caused by mutations in the α-subunit of the voltage-dependent sodium channel gene (*SCN4A*) (Fig. 32-4).[5,9,18,41,43,62–64]

Treatment

Attack frequency may be reduced with a low-potassium, high-carbohydrate diet and avoidance of fasting, strenuous activity, and cold. Mild, short-lasting attacks of weakness usually do not require treatment. Sometimes a simple ingestion of simple carbohydrates (e.g., fruit juices, glucose-containing candies) decreases the serum potassium level by increasing insulin secretion and may improve strength. Beta-adrenergic agonists (e.g., metaproterenol, albuterol, and salbutamol) also may increase strength but one needs to take care in regard to associated cardiac arrhythmias. Beta-adrenergic medications may have their effect through the sodium–potassium pump. Only in severe attacks of weakness is treatment with intravenous glucose, insulin, or calcium carbonate warranted. Prophylactic use of acetazolamide (125–1,000 mg per day), chlorothiazide (250–1,000 mg per day), or dichlorphenamide (50–150 mg per day) are beneficial in reducing the frequency of attacks and perhaps the myotonia.[9,21,32,39,65,66] Mexiletine may be useful in managing myotonia when it is bothersome.

PARAMYOTONIA CONGENITA (EULENBURG DISEASE)

Clinical Features

PMC is an autosomal-dominant disorder with high penetrance that is allelic to potassium-sensitive periodic paralysis, which probably explains why many patients have clinical features of both disorders (paralysis periodica paramyotonia).[1–4,7,8,17,32,33,55,67–71] The name derives from the "para"-doxical reaction to exercise. In contrast to the warm-up phenomena observed in other myotonic syndromes, repeated exercise worsens the muscle stiffness in patients with PMC. Paramyotonia, particularly of the eyelids, is typically evident in most affected individuals. Myotonia is also exacerbated by exercise or cold exposure. A cold-induced attack of weakness can last for several hours even after return to a warm environment. Weakness can also be induced in some cases by potassium intake. Further attacks of weakness can be focal or generalized attacks of weakness.

Symptoms and signs of PMC usually manifest within the first decade of life. During a crying spell, infants may be noted to have difficulty opening their eyes secondary to the "exercise"-induced myotonia of the orbicularis oculi muscles. While percussion myotonia may be demonstrated, it is usually not prominent. Some people complain of mild muscle pain, but myalgias are usually not as prominent as that seen in patients with DM2/PROMM which PMC can resemble. In addition, fixed or progressive weakness of proximal or distal muscles can develop over time.

Laboratory Features

Serum CK levels are usually mildly to moderately elevated. Serum potassium levels may be normal or elevated in some patients during an attack of paralysis. Skeletal muscle MRI scans may reveal nonspecific signal abnormalities.[22]

Routine sensory and motor NCSs are normal between attacks of weakness.[67] Prolonged repetitive stimulation at rates exceeding 5 Hz or repetitive stimulation following a minute or more of exercise can induce a decrement in the CMAP in some patients.[24,67] The SET may demonstrate several distinctive abnormalities (Tables 32-1 and 32-2).[4,10–12] Immediately after 10 seconds of exercise, repetitive after-discharges may be seen on recorded CMAPs evoked by a single supramaximal stimulus (PEMPs) (Fig. 32-6). Subsequent

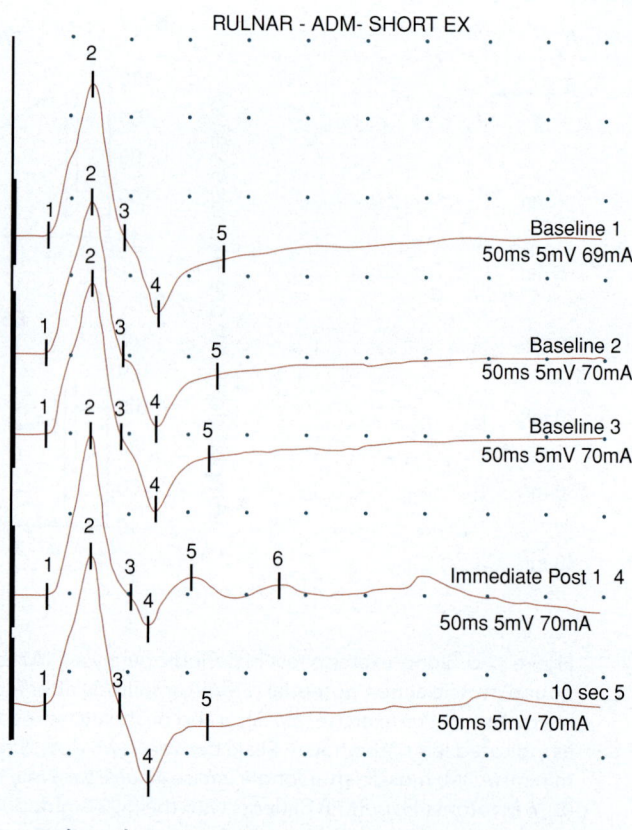

Figure 32-6. Postexercise myotonic potentials (PEMPs). PEMPs are seen following short-exercise test (SET) in a patient with paramyotonia congenita. The top three tracings are baseline compound muscle action potentials (CMAPs). Following short exercise of 10 seconds, the fourth trace from the top demonstrates PEMPs following the CMAP (labeled as 5 and 6 with tracer). The fifth CMAP 10 seconds no longer demonstrates any PEMPs.

stimuli are associated with reduction of these PEMPs. Also, there is decrement in the amplitudes of the main CMAP waveforms compared to baseline with repeated stimuli following the short exercise in some patients. We repeat the SET with a 10-second break in between epochs to increase the yield of finding abnormalities. Upon repetition of the short exercise, even in those patients who do not show any CMAP decline after the first trial, one may see marked reduction of CMAP amplitudes by the third trial (Fig. 32-1A). In some patients, there is also a gradual decrease in PEMPs. This so-called Fournier Pattern I is seen in approximately 90% of patients with PMC caused by a T1313M mutation in the *SCN4A* gene (Tables 32-1 and 32-2).[4,10,12] Fournier et al. reported patients with R1448C also had Pattern I, but other series reported no decrement on SET in individuals with this mutation.[4,10,12] This pattern is for the most part distinct from that seen in MC and DM2, which PMC may clinical resemble. Individuals with PMC mutations caused by Q270K mutations in the *SCN4A* gene may have SET that resemble those seen in MC (Fournier Pattern II).[11] To further increase the yield, the SET should be repeated after the extremity has been cooled.[4,11,12] Cooling may bring out further abnormalities (even more marked reduction in amplitudes that worsen with repetition of short exercises than seen when the SET is performed at room temperature). Upon cooling, the SET in patients with Q270M mutations may convert to Fournier Pattern I that is more typical of PMC. With the LET, the CMAP amplitudes are markedly reduced during and following the exercise compared to baseline.[4,10,12,26,67] The amplitudes remain reduced for prolonged periods, sometimes exceeding an hour.

EMG reveals normal MUAPs though they are often difficult to appreciate with the background of diffuse myotonic discharges.[4,10,69–72] In patients with PMC and periodic paralysis, local cooling of the muscle results in dense fibrillation potentials and the gradual reduction in MUAP activity. As the muscle becomes flaccid, the myotonic discharges abate, and complete electrical silence is observed. In contrast, in patients with pure PMC without periodic paralysis, local cooling of the muscle results in increased myotonic discharges, but MUAP morphology and recruitment as well as muscle strength remain normal. Single-fiber EMG reveals a slight increase in jitter and fiber density.[70]

Histopathology

Muscle biopsies can reveal nonspecific myopathic features and mild fiber size variation with a mixture of normal, atrophic and hypertrophic fibers.[71] Intracytoplasmic vacuoles may be appreciated, particularly in those individuals with superimposed periodic paralysis. Electron microscopy (EM) may show myofibrillar disarray and tubular aggregates.

Molecular Genetics and Pathogenesis

PMC with and without episodes of periodic paralysis are caused by mutations in *SCN4A* (Fig. 32-4).[1,5,7,8,42,44,65]

Treatment

A randomized, placebo-controlled trial of mexiletine (200 mg by mouth three times daily) was helpful in reducing muscle stiffness.[73] Cold-induced decrements of baseline CMAP amplitudes following exercise or repetitive stimulation may also improve with mexiletine.[74]

POTASSIUM-AGGRAVATED MYOTONIAS (MYOTONIA FLUCTUANS, MYOTONIA PERMANENS, AND ACETAZOLAMIDE-RESPONSIVE MYOTONIA)

The PAMs are also caused by mutations in the muscle sodium channel gene and are allelic to HyperKPP and PMC (Table 32-1).[1,4,7,8,10–12] Individuals with these disorders have myotonia without episodes of weakness. The electrophysiology of these disorders is more variable. Most of the time, SET is normal (Fig. 32-1D), but Fournier Patterns I and II may be seen. In those with normal SET at room temperature, cooling may result in reduced CMAP amplitudes that worsen with repeated short exercises similar to what is seen in PMC (conversion to Fournier Pattern I).[11] The LET in patients with PAM is usually normal. A randomized, placebo-controlled trial of mexiletine (200 mg three times daily) was helpful in reducing muscle stiffness in a study of nondystrophic myotonias that included PAM.[73]

MYOTONIA FLUCTUANS

Clinical Features

Myotonia fluctuans is characterized by (1) fluctuating myotonia of varying severity, (2) increased myotonia of delayed onset (several minutes) following exercise, (3) paramyotonia of eyelids, (4) warm-up phenomena of myotonia in the limbs, (5) no episodes of weakness nor weakness following potassium loading, exercise, or cold, and (6) increased myotonia with potassium but not with exposure to cold.[33,46,47,75] The fluctuating severity of the myotonia is unlike that seen in MC, PMC, and HyperKPP associated with myotonia. The severity of the myotonia can range from absolutely no stiffness to severe myotonia affecting the extraocular muscles, the muscles of mastication and swallowing, and the extremities. Myotonia fluctuans is also dissimilar from other myotonic disorders in that exercise induces myotonia, which is delayed in onset. The stiffness is not worse in the cold.

Laboratory Features

Serum CK levels are usually slightly elevated. The SET may be normal or shows mild reduction in amplitude that improves with repeated stimulation (i.e., Fournier Pattern II); similar to what is seen in MC without change in response to cooling.[10,11] The LET is normal.

Histopathology

Muscle biopsies may be normal or show increased internalized nuclei and fiber size variability.[43] Subsarcolemmal vacuoles may be appreciated on EM.[46]

Molecular Genetics and Pathogenesis

Myotonia fluctuans is caused by mutations in *SCN4A*.[18,46,47]

Treatment

Mexiletine[73] and avoidance of high-potassium foods may be helpful.

MYOTONIA PERMANENS

Clinical Features

Myotonia permanens is associated with constant muscle stiffness that is aggravated by potassium and following activity.[31,32,56,76,77] Affected people may develop dyspnea, acidosis, and hypoxia related to severe myotonia affecting ventilatory muscles. Neither episodic weakness nor exacerbation of myotonia with cold is seen.

Laboratory Features

Serum CK levels are normal or only mildly elevated.

Histopathology

Biopsy results have not been well described.

Molecular Genetics and Pathogenesis

Myotonia permanens is usually caused by G1306A mutations in *SCN4A*.[31,76,77]

Treatment

Mexiletine may be beneficial.[73]

ACETAZOLAMIDE-RESPONSIVE MYOTONIA

Clinical Features

Individuals with this disorder complain of painful muscle stiffness that begins in childhood but worsens with age into early adulthood.[18,35,78] The myotonia is most severe in the face and hands and is aggravated by potassium, fasting, and to a lesser extent by exercise. Muscle stiffness and pain may be eased by ingestion of high carbohydrate meals. Action and percussion myotonia are appreciated. Paradoxical myotonia may be found in the eyelids. Strength is normal.

Laboratory Features

Serum CK is usually mildly elevated. The SET may be normal or show mild reduction in amplitude that improves with repetitive activity (i.e., Fournier Pattern II) that is similar to what is seen in MC. There is no change with cooling.[10,11]

Histopathology

Muscle biopsies have been performed in only a few patients and have been normal or revealed generalized muscle fiber hypertrophy.

Molecular Genetics and Pathogenesis

Acetazolamide-responsive myotonia is also caused by mutations in *SCN4A*.[18,35,78]

Treatment

Acetazolamide may help diminish muscle stiffness and pain. We initiate treatment with acetazolamide 125 mg per day and titrated as tolerated to 250 mg three times daily. Mexiletine may also be helpful.

FAMILIAL HYPOKALEMIC PERIODIC PARALYSIS TYPE 2

Clinical Features

Most cases of familial HypoKPP are caused by mutations in the skeletal muscle voltage-gated calcium channel α-1 subunit (*CACNA1S*) gene (HypoKPP1).[5,9,17,38,39] However, a less common form is associated with mutations in the *SCN4A* gene, so-called HypoKPP2.[5,9,17,36–39] HypoKPP2 is clinically similar to HypoKPP1, though in a large retrospective series of molecularly defined HypoKPP1 and HypoKPP2 cases, the age of onset was earlier (average 10 years) and the duration of episodes longer (average 20 hours) in HypoKPP1 compared with HypoKPP2 (16 years of age and 1 hour of duration, respectively).[38] However, a study by a different group demonstrated a slightly older onset of symptoms in some cases of HypoKPP1 depending on the site of the mutation compared to HypoKPP2.[17] Greater than 70% of HypoKPP1 patients developed fixed proximal weakness compared with none of the HypoKPP2 patients.[38] Also, in regard to treatment, acetazolamide, which can be helpful in HypoKPP1, can occasionally exacerbate attacks of weakness in HypoKPP2.[38]

Laboratory Features

Serum potassium is reduced during the attacks. Serum CK may be normal or elevated. On the LET, a decrease of CMAP amplitudes is seen approximately 10–20 minutes after cessation of exercise (Table 32-1).[10] However, this decrement is less than what is typically observed in patients with a HyperKPP. EMG between attacks of muscle paralysis is usually normal and in particular, there are no myotonic discharges.[10,37,38]

Histopathology

While muscle biopsies in HypoKPP1 often demonstrate non-rimmed vacuoles within muscle fibers, biopsies in HypoKPP2 often reveal muscle fibers with tubular aggregates.[33,34]

Treatment

Some individuals with HypoKPP2 have a reduction of attacks with acetazolamide, but much fewer improve than in those with HypoKPP1.[40] More importantly, some patients with HypoKPP2 experience an exacerbation of weakness with acetazolamide rather than improvement.[38–40] Therefore, initiation of a trial of acetazolamide or dichlorphenamide should be done cautiously in a patient with HypoKPP2 or HypoKPP in whom the genotype is unknown.

MOLECULAR GENETICS AND PATHOGENESIS/PATHOPHYSIOLOGY OF THE SODIUM CHANNELOPATHIES

The voltage-gated muscle sodium channel is a heterodimer composed of subunits that are encoded on chromosomes 17q23–25 and 19q13.1, respectively.[1,18,39] Point mutations in the subunit gene, *SCN4A*, are responsible for HyperKPP, PMC, and the various PAMs as previously discussed. No disorders are known to be caused by mutations in the β-subunit. The subunit has four homologous domains (I–IV) each containing six hydrophobic segments (S1–S6) that transverse the sarcolemmal membrane (Fig. 32-4).[1,18,30,33] An extracellular loop dips within the plasma membrane between S5 and S6 of each domain and participates in the formation of the pore. The S4 helix contains a repeating motif of positively charged amino acids at every third position suggesting that this region serves as the voltage sensor.[33] The S4 segment appears to be critical for inactivation of the open channel, while the S3 segment is important in the recovery of inactivated channels.[56] The interaction between the S3 and S4 segments is important for transition to and from inactivation states (Fig. 32-7).

Numerous different point mutations in *SCN4A* have been reported and most are located in regions of the α-subunit critical for fast inactivation. Most of these

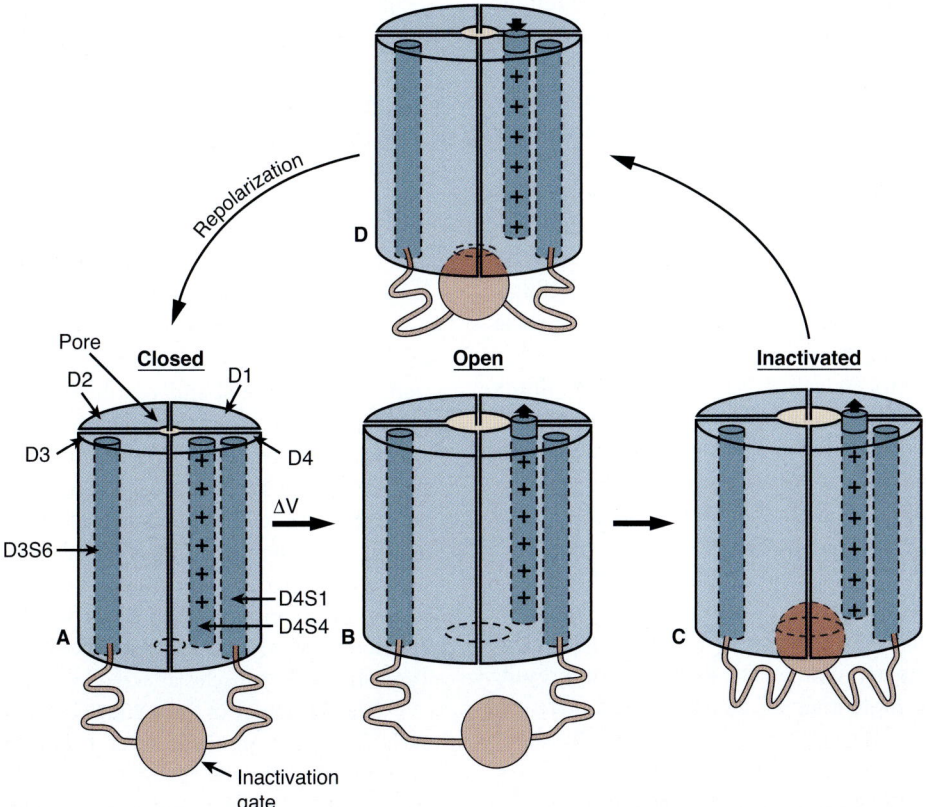

Figure 32-7. Cation channel model. Voltage-gated sodium and calcium channels are believed to have similar structures and physiology. These cation channels have four domains (D1–D4) each containing six transmembrane segments. This model shows the four domains (D1–D4, *blue*) of the cation channel arranged around the ion pore (*blue*) in the membrane. The S4 segments of cation channels contain a repeating motif of positively charged (+) amino acids (arginine or lysine) at every third position separated by two neutral amino acids. In the closed state (**A**), the pore (*blue*) is closed, and the inactivation gate (*brown*) is open. In response to depolarization, the S4 segments (*darker blue*) shown here move slightly under the influence of electrostatic forces. The S4 segment of domain 4 is the site of two of the recognized mutations in patients with paramyotonia congenita. Depolarization leads to a conformational shift that results in the pore (*blue*) opening (**B**). Channel closing is thought to result from a "ball-valve" mechanism where the cytoplasmic loop (*brown*) between domains D3 and D4 falls into the ion pore, thus blocking it (**C**). In this model, repolarization would then result in the protein assuming its closed conformation (**D**) and release of the inactivation gate. The channel is now in the closed state (**A**) and is ready to open in response to the next depolarization. (Reproduced with permission from Ptacek LJ. The familial periodic paralyses and nondystrophic myotonias. *Am J Med*. 1998;105(1):58–70.)

missense mutations are associated with gain-of-function defects, which are either disrupted inactivation or enhanced activation. The notable exception is the mutations associated with HypoKPP2, which are all clustered in the voltage-sensor region of the second repeat (D2S4) and diminish activity by enhancing inactivation. The fast inactivation limits the number of sodium channels available for activation, which in turn leads to a refractory period, until there is repolarization of the muscle membrane.[1,9,31,56,62,79] The gain-of-function mutations associated with PMC and PAM typically slow the rate of inactivation three- to fivefold, resulting in a longer duration of the action potentials and increased availability of Na+ channels (i.e., fraction not inactivated) at the end of each action potential that augment the membrane excitability and resulting myotonic discharges. In addition to slow inactivation, many PMC mutations also disrupt the final extent of inactivation. The steady inward Na current generated through the small fraction of mutant channels that have failed to inactivate, depolarizes the membrane to a new stable resting potential of approximately −50 mV. This results in inactivation of the wild-type and most of the mutant Na channels, resulting in a system that is refractory from generating an action potential, leading to a paralytic attack.[31,62,79] In these individuals, increased extracellular potassium results in further depolarization of the muscle membrane, thus leading to muscle fiber inexcitability.

In contrast, a process called "slow inactivation" limits the availability of sodium channels on a time scale of seconds to minutes, which can also affect muscle membrane excitability. Rare patients with SCN4A mutations manifesting as HyperKPP and myotonia have impaired slow inactivation, as opposed to defective fast inactivation.[80]

Patch clamp studies of intercostal muscles of patients with PMC demonstrate normal resting membrane potentials at 37°C, but cooling to 27°C leads to depolarization of the muscle membrane to approximately −40 mV.[62,79] As a result, spontaneous action potentials are generated secondary to the approximation of the resting membrane and threshold potentials that correlate with the cold-induced myotonia. Subsequently, the muscle membrane may remain in a depolarized state for a prolonged period of time such that it is no longer capable of generating further action potentials, and therefore, the muscles become weak.[31,62,79]

In HyperKPP, mutant sodium channels are associated with large persistent currents that further increase, when extracellular potassium levels are elevated.[31,62,79] Increased extracellular potassium leads to depolarization of the muscle membrane and increased late openings of the noninactivated sodium channels.[56] The continued sodium influx sustains the depolarization of the membrane, which in turn leads to inactivation of normal sodium channels and subsequent muscle fiber inexcitability.

In HypoKPP2, mutations in gating-charge–carrying argentine residues in an S4 segment induce a hyperpolarization-activated cationic leak through the voltage sensor of the skeletal muscle sodium channel.[81,82] A sustained proton leak may contribute to instability of ion conductance indirectly, by interfering with intracellular pH homeostasis.[82]

▶ CALCIUM CHANNELOPATHIES

PRIMARY HYPOKALEMIC PERIODIC PARALYSIS TYPE 1 (HYPOKPP1)

Clinical Features

HypoKPP1 is an autosomal-dominant disorder with reduced penetrance in women (a male to female ratio of 3 or 4 to 1) and an overall prevalence of 0.13 to 1/100,000.[5,9,18,39] Onset of episodic weakness usually occurs in the first two decades of life. Individuals with HypoKPP1 do not have clinical or electrophysiological myotonia or paramyotonia which may be useful in distinguishing from the HyperKPP and PMC.

Attacks of weakness may be precipitated by strenuous physical activity followed by rest or sleep, high carbohydrates and sodium meals, alcohol consumption, emotional stress, concurrent viral illness, lack of sleep, and/or menstruation. Specific medications (e.g., beta agonists, corticosteroids, and insulin) are also triggers for attacks. Episodes of weakness can occur at any time of day, although most occur in the morning.

The severity of an attack can range from mild focal weakness of an isolated muscle group to severe generalized paralysis. Facial and ventilatory muscles as well as the sphincter muscles are typically spared or only minimally affected. Nevertheless, ventilatory muscle involvement and cardiac arrhythmia secondary to hypokalemia have occurred.[83] When weakness is profound, the muscle is electrically unexcitable. Reflexes are absent when muscles are severely affected. Severe muscle weakness usually lasts for several hours to more than a day, though many individuals note a residual weakness for several days following an attack. Typically, those muscles affected last are the first to recover.

The frequency of these attacks of weakness is also highly variable—they can occur several times a week to less than once a year. After the age of 30 years the frequencies of the attacks often diminish, and some individuals become free of attacks in their 40s or 50s. On the other hand, many patients develop permanent fixed or slowly progressive weakness over time.[17,39,84,85] Proximal muscles, especially in the legs, are more prone to developing fixed weakness.

Often an attack of periodic weakness is heralded by a sensation of heaviness or aching in the low back, thighs, and calves which spreads to involve other muscle groups, primarily those in the proximal upper limbs. Mild exercise during this prodrome may stave off the full-blown attack of weakness; however, this is not always successful.

Laboratory Features

Serum potassium levels are usually below 3.0 mEq/L during an attack of weakness, though between attacks the serum potassium is normal. The EKG may demonstrate bradycardia, flattened T waves, prolonged PR and QT intervals, and notably U waves secondary to the hypokalemia. Serum CK levels are usually mildly elevated and increase during attacks of weakness. Provocative testing using intravenous glucose load, and sometimes insulin, was used in the past to lower the serum potassium to assist in diagnosis but is no longer performed.

Sensory and motor NCSs are normal between attacks of weakness.[84–86] However, surface recordings have revealed reduced muscle fiber conduction velocity between paralytic attacks.[87] During paralytic attacks, sensory studies remain normal, but the CMAP amplitudes are reduced secondary to muscle membrane inexcitability. Repetitive stimulation of mildly affected muscles demonstrates preservation of CMAP amplitudes to some degree, supporting the clinical impression that mild exercise can stave off an attack.

In contrast to individuals with HyperKPP, there are minimal changes in CMAP amplitudes immediately after the exercise phase of the SETs/LETs in those with HypoKPP (Table 32-1).[10,12] However, with the LET, there is usually a delayed decline in CMAP amplitudes (−51 ± 10%). The reduction in amplitudes is usually less in those with HypoKPP2 compared to HypoKPP1.[10]

EMG between attacks of muscle paralysis is usually normal.[86] However, EMG early in an attack of weakness reveals a slight increase in insertional and spontaneous potentials (e.g., fibrillation potentials and positive sharp waves), which are a reflection of the hyperirritable muscle membranes and not indicative of denervation. As the paralytic attack progresses, there is a decrease in the amplitude and duration of voluntary MUAPs as well as an overall decrease in the number of MUAPs contributing to the interference pattern. When the paralytic attack is maximal, there is marked reduction or complete absence of insertional activity, and there are minimal, if any, voluntary MUAPs. In patients who develop persistent muscle weakness, small amplitude, short duration, polyphasic MUAPs that recruit early may be appreciated in weak muscles along with rare fibrillation potentials and positive sharp waves.

Between attacks, single-fiber EMG shows normal jitter along with a slight increase in fiber density. The latter is likely the result of a mild myopathic process with muscle fiber splitting which can be appreciated on histopathology. During an attack, the reduction in muscle membrane excitability results in a dropout of single muscle fibers and a decrease in fiber density, compared to both normal and interattack values for the patients. This is accompanied by a slight increase in jitter with occasional blocking of potentials.[88]

Muscle MRI reveals abnormal replacement of muscle by fat in most patients, even those without fixed weakness.[85] Such fatty replacement is most commonly appreciated in the paraspinal muscles, psoas, iliacus, the posterior muscles of the thigh and gastrocnemius, and soleus of the calf.

Histopathology

Muscle biopsies may reveal intracellular vacuoles, tubular aggregates, and dilation of the sarcoplasmic reticulum

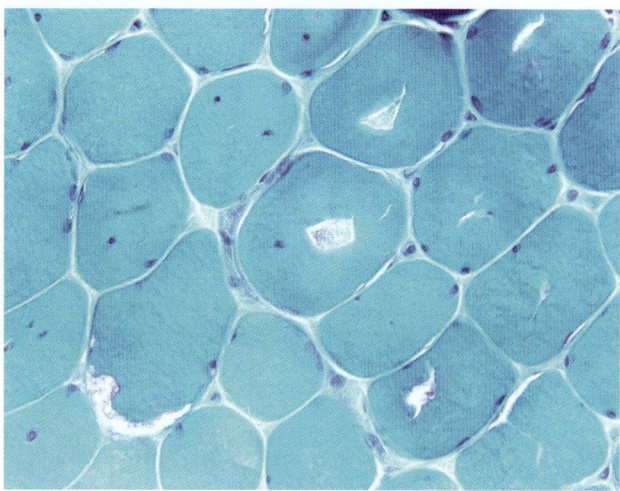

Figure 32-8. Muscle biopsy in a patient with HypoKPP reveals muscle fibers with vacuoles. Modified Gomori trichrome stain.

(Fig. 32-8).[17,38,61] HypoKPP1 is more likely to be associated with vacuoles on biopsy, while tubular aggregates are more common in HypoKPP2.[17,38] Muscle fiber size variation, split fibers, hypertrophic, and some atrophic fibers can also be present. Rarely, necrotic and degenerating muscle fibers are noted.

Molecular Genetics and Pathogenesis

Approximately 70% of cases of familial HypoKPP1 are caused by mutations in the α-subunits of skeletal muscle L-type calcium channel gene, *CACNA1S*, located on chromosome 1q31–3245.[5,9,18,36,83] In 10% of affected individuals (HypoKPP2), the mutations are present in the α-subunits of skeletal muscle sodium channel gene, *SCN4A*, and no identifiable mutation is found in the remaining 20% of patients. For both HypoKPP1 and HypoKPP2, the mutations occur in highly conserved arginine residues in the voltage-sensing segments of the calcium channel.[18,36] In addition, rare cases of HypoKPP have been associated with mutations in another potassium channel gene, *KCNE3*.[89] Further, Gitelman syndrome, caused by mutations affecting the thiazide-sensitive sodium chloride co-transporter, may also cause hypokalemic paralysis.[90]

The voltage-gated calcium channel (Cav1.1), also known as the DHP receptor, is composed of five subunits (α1, α2, β, δ, and γ). The α1-subunit is composed of four domains, each containing six transmembrane segments (S1–S6), and links to the ryanodine receptor (Fig. 32-9).[41] This receptor that functions not only as a calcium ion channel for the transverse tubules of skeletal muscle, but also as a voltage sensor for excitation–contraction coupling (Fig. 32-10).[30] The other subunits of the calcium channel regulate the function of the α1-subunit.[41] The S4 segment of the α1-subunit confers the voltage-sensing properties to the channel, and is the site for most of the mutations identified in patients with HypoKPP1.

The mechanism for the induced attacks of weakness in HypoKPP1 is not completely understood.[18,83,91–93] Myofibers

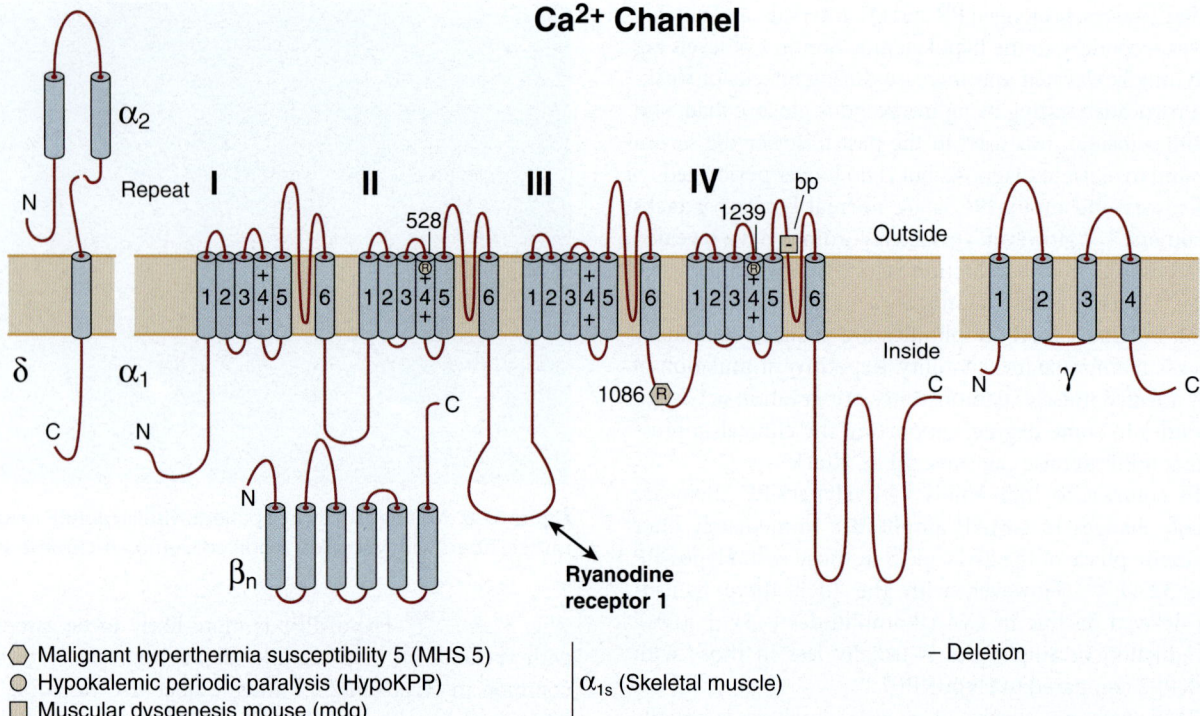

Figure 32-9. Subunits of voltage-gated calcium channel. α-Subunit resembles that of sodium channel; however, function of various parts, for example, III–IV linker, may not be the same. α_2/δ, $\beta_1–\beta_4$, and γ are auxiliary subunits. Mutations shown here, α_{1S}-subunit of skeletal muscle L-type calcium channel (= dihydropyridine receptor), have been described for humans (HypoKPP, MHS 5) and mice (mdg). Conventional one-letter abbreviations are used for replaced amino acids whose positions are given by respective numbers of α_{1S}-subunit. Symbols used for point mutations indicate resulting diseases as explained at bottom left. (Reproduced with permission from Lehmann-Horn F, Jurkat-Rott K. Voltage-gated ion channels and hereditary disease. Physiol Rev. 1999;79:1317–1372.)

are depolarized and inexcitable during an attack. In vitro, muscle fibers from patients with HypoKPP1 exposed to low K-solutions paradoxically depolarize. However, the source of the depolarizing current has remained elusive. The available data suggest a loss-of-function defect with reduced ionic current density. A study on fibers biopsied from a patient with an R528H calcium channel mutation detected a reduction in ATP-sensitive K current, more easily tying it to the depolarization seen with hypokalemia and suggesting a secondary channelopathy resulting from altered calcium homeostasis. It has also been posited that reduced calcium influx through the T-tubule may be the cause of impaired excitation–contraction coupling.

The DHP receptor functions as a calcium channel as well as a voltage sensor for excitation–contraction coupling. Electrophysiological recordings of myotubes expressing mutant calcium channels reveal diminished calcium current and a negative shift of the steady-state inactivation current.[83] Decreased calcium influx through the T-tubule may impair excitation–contraction coupling. Furthermore, the kinetics of the sodium channel also appears to be influenced by mutations involving *CACNA1S*. The sodium conductance is increased in the resting state leading depolarization of the resting membrane potential from about −80 mV to around −50 mV. In this partially depolarized state, the number of sodium channels available to activate is likely reduced, thus, creating an inexcitable membrane and clinical weakness.

Treatment

The primary mode of therapy is reducing exposure to known triggers (e.g., avoiding ingestion of high-carbohydrate meals, extremely strenuous exercise). Acetazolamide (125–1,500 mg/day) and potassium salts (0.25–0.5 mEq/kg) are often prescribed prophylactically in order to prevent hypokalemia and reduce attacks of weakness. However, a large retrospective study found that only approximately 50% of genotyped patients with HypoKPP1 responded to acetazolamide and even fewer with HypoKPP2.[40] Importantly, acetazolamide may actually induce attacks of weakness in individuals with HypoKPP2 caused by *SCNA4* mutations.[17,39,40] Dichlorphenamide (50–150 mg/day) also may be effective in reducing attack frequency and severity in HypoKPP1 but would be very cautious in using to treat HypoKPP2 as per use of acetazolamide.[21,65,66] Triamterene (25–100 mg/day) or spironolactone (25–100 mg/day) may be used in an attempt to prevent attacks and perhaps to improve interattack weakness when acetazolamide is not effective. Acute attacks of weakness

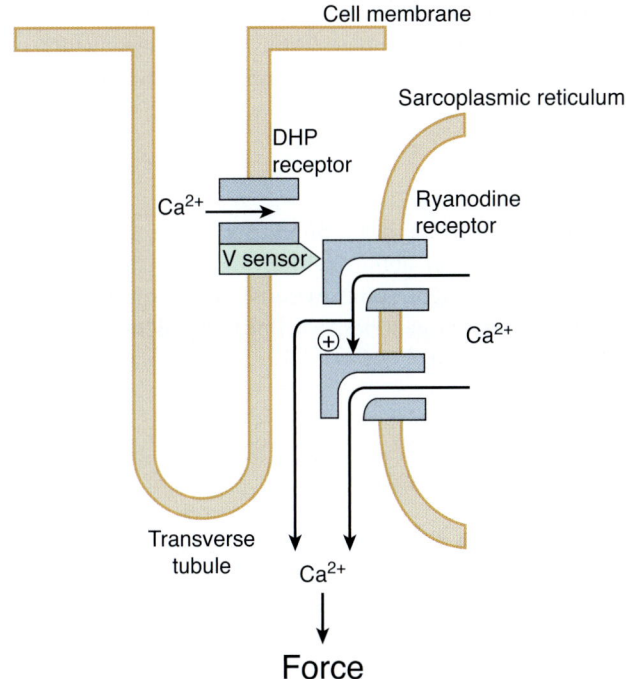

Figure 32-10. Triadic junction between a transverse tubule and sarcoplasmic reticulum: position of two calcium channels of skeletal muscle, L-type calcium channel, also called dihydropyridine (DHP) receptor, and calcium release channel, also called ryanodine receptor. Coupling between the two channels is not fully elucidated. Mutations in respective genes cause hypokalemic periodic paralysis, malignant hyperthermia, or central core disease. (Reproduced with permission from Lehmann-Horn F, Jurkat-Rott K. Voltage gated ion channels and hereditary disease. *Physiol Rev.* 1999;79:1317–1372.)

can be treated with oral potassium salts (0.25 mEq/kg body weight) every 30 minutes until strength improves.

In severe attacks and if the patient's condition precludes oral potassium, intravenous potassium (KCL bolus 0.05–0.1 mEq/kg body weight or 20–40 mEq/L of KCL in 5% mannitol) may be administered. Cardiac monitoring is essential throughout treatment. HypoKPP1 may be allelic with MH, so it is not surprising that MH without periodic paralysis has been described with mutation in *CACNA1S*. Hence, all HypoKPP patients undergoing surgery should be monitored for MH-like reactions (rigidity and marked elevation in CK). However, postoperative paralysis in this group of patients is more likely related to the stress of surgery.

SECONDARY HYPOKALEMIC PARALYSIS

Secondary HypoKPP needs to be excluded, particularly if there is no family history or in those with onset after the third decade of life (Table 32-3). Urinary or gastrointestinal dumping of potassium may precipitate attacks of weakness and cause a necrotizing myopathy. Muscle strength improves with correction of the hypokalemia.

THYROTOXIC PERIODIC PARALYSIS

Thyrotoxic periodic paralysis (TPP) resembles HypoKPP, except that there is typically no family history.[94] TPP is more common in Asian adults, but it occurs worldwide. Interestingly, although hyperthyroidism is more common in women, the majority of cases of TPP occur in men. Affected individuals can also develop progressive muscle weakness secondary to hyperthyroidism itself. The attacks of weakness dissipate with treatment and correction of the dysthyroid state but can recur with redevelopment of hyperthyroidism. Acetazolamide does not appear to have any significant benefit. However, β-blockers may be effective in reducing the frequency and severity of the paralytic attacks in thyrotoxic patients. Mutations in the *KCNJ18* gene that encodes an inwardly rectifying potassium (Kir) channel, Kir2.6, has been reported in about 33% of patients in the United States, France, and Brazil with TPP.[86,87] In addition, genome-wide screening of Asians with TPP found linkage to possible genetic mutation in *KCNJ2* which encodes for the Kir2.1 potassium channel.[95–98]

▶ OTHER FORMS OF PERIODIC PARALYSIS

ANDERSEN–TAWIL SYNDROME (ANDERSEN SYNDROME OR KLEIN–LISAK–ANDERSEN SYNDROME)

Clinical Features

ATS is a rare ion channel disorder characterized by the clinical triad of periodic paralysis, ventricular arrhythmias associated with long QT, and skeletal developmental anomalies.[9,39,99–107] A diagnosis of ATS can be made when an individual exhibits two of these three cardinal features. Only about 60% of affected individuals manifest the complete triad, while approximately 80% express two of the three cardinal features. Inheritance is autosomal-dominant although de novo mutations are frequent, and phenotypic expression is extremely variable. A large study found the prevalence in England to be approximately 0.08 per 100,000.[5]

The neuromuscular manifestations of ATS consist of episodic weakness that may arise spontaneously or be triggered by rest following exertion. The attacks of paralysis usually begin in the first or second decade of life and may be associated with elevated, normal, or most commonly decreased serum potassium levels. The attacks vary in duration (hours to days), severity, and frequency ranging from a single lifetime event to daily bouts of weakness. Permanent proximal weakness often develops over time. A recent large study reported fixed weakness in 25% of patients and 13.5% required a wheelchair or other assistive devices to aid in ambulation.[99] Patients with ATS do not show evidence of myotonia or paramyotonia.

Cardiac manifestations include potentially life-threatening arrhythmias, including bidirectional ventricular tachycardia (VT), polymorphic VT, and *torsades de pointes*.

The cardiac arrhythmias may be asymptomatic or manifest as palpitations, syncope, or even cardiac arrest necessitating defibrillator implantation. No specific triggers have been associated with the ventricular arrhythmias of ATS. One of the most common EKG findings is a long QT interval, which is recognized as an integral feature of ATS and may serve as a trigger for fatal ventricular arrhythmias. Thus, ATS must be considered in all individuals presenting with episodic weakness and/or a long QT syndrome.

Developmental anomalies associated with ATS include clinodactyly, hypertelorism, low set ears, mandibular hypoplasia, syndactyly, and scoliosis. Other features less commonly associated are short stature, a broad nose and forehead, cleft or high-arched palate, short digits, vaginal atresia, brachydactyly, cardiac valve abnormalities, and hypoplastic kidneys. Neurocognitive abnormalities characterized by deficits in executive function and abstract reasoning may also be seen.

Laboratory Features

Serum CK can be normal or only slightly elevated. Serum potassium levels may be normal, elevated or decreased during attacks of weakness. Skeletal muscle MRI often reveals fatty infiltration.[99] A prolonged QT interval is present in 80% of patients, while some have even more ominous ventricular tachyarrhythmias as previously discussed. Routine motor and sensory NCSs are normal. The LET may reveal a decrement in the CMAP area and to a lesser extent the amplitude,[12,100] but a large recent series did not find LET to be very reliable in ATS.[99] EMG is usually normal as well between attacks of weakness. Myotonic discharges are not seen.

Histopathology

Tubular aggregates, similar to those observed in other forms of periodic paralysis, may be appreciated on muscle biopsies.[99]

Molecular Genetics and Pathogenesis

Approximately two-thirds of ATS patients have missense mutations or small deletions in the *KCNJ2* gene (ATS1).[5,9,99,101,103,106,107] This gene encodes for the inwardly rectifying potassium channel (Kir2.1) and is predominantly expressed in heart, skeletal muscle, and brain. This mutation leads to impairment of muscle membrane and perhaps neuronal depolarization and repolarization, but its role in the associated skeletal developmental anomalies is not well understood. Kir2.1 channels help stabilize resting membrane potentials. The majority of *KCNJ2* mutations result in the failure of appropriate conduction, and many alter the binding of phosphatidylinositol bisphosphate, an important regulator of Kir2.1 channel function. It is postulated that reduced Kir2.1 channel function in skeletal muscle may result in sustained membrane depolarization, failure of action potential propagation, and flaccid paralysis. It may also prolong the most terminal phase of repolarization in the heart and lead to delayed after-depolarizations. Approximately 20% of patients with an ATS phenotype have no mutation of *KCJN2* (ATS2).

Treatment

It is important to be aware of and recognize the potential cardiac conduction abnormalities. Malignant arrhythmias may be treated with antiarrhythmic agents or pacemaker insertion. In one large series, two-thirds of patients improved with acetazolamide.[99]

▶ OTHER SKELETAL MUSCLE CHANNELOPATHIES

OTHER POTASSIUM CHANNELOPATHIES

A few kindreds with periodic paralysis have been found to have mutations in another potassium channel gene, *KCNE3*.[89] Attacks of weakness have been associated with low serum potassium levels in some but not other cases.

OTHER CALCIUM CHANNELOPATHIES

Some cases of central core disease and MH are caused by mutations in the ryanodine receptor gene, *RYR1*. The ryanodine receptor is responsible for the release of calcium from the sarcoplasmic reticulum. Central core disease is discussed in Chapter 28 regarding Congenital Myopathies. Notably, rare patients with *RYR1* mutations may manifest late-onset periodic paralysis and muscle pain with or without fixed weakness.[108,109] Malignant hyperthermia is in Chapter 35 regarding Toxic Myopathies. Mutations in the stromal interaction molecule 1 gene (*STIM1*) and the ORA1 calcium release-activated calcium modulator 1 gene (*ORA1*) are causes of hereditary tubular aggregate myopathy (TAM). This myopathy manifests with progressive weakness or myalgias, hyperCKemia, and an increased risk of MH. Because TAM is also discuss this myopathy in Chapter 28 regarding on Congenital Myopathies. Brody disease is caused by mutations in SERCA1 gene, *ATP2A1*, which encodes the fast-twitch skeletal muscle sarcoplasmic reticulum calcium ATPase and is discussed below as it clinical resembles and can be mistake for a myotonic disorder.

BRODY DISEASE

Clinical Features

This rare disorder is characterized by impaired skeletal muscle relaxation following exercise.[110-113] Affected individuals complain of exercise-induced cramping and stiffness in the arms and legs. Recurrent myoglobinuria is an uncommon complication. Having the patient repeatedly open and close their fists or do several deep knee bends may induce delayed muscle relaxation that can be painful. Some patients also have impaired relaxation of the eyelids after forced eyelid closure. The muscle stiffness resembles paramyotonia as the stiffness worsens with activity. However, there is no percussion myotonia. Some people have mild proximal weakness on examination. Patients may be at risk for MH.[110]

Laboratory Features

Serum CK levels are normal or only slightly elevated.[110–113] Potassium levels are normal. Unlike the dynamic glycogen storage disorders, which it may mimic due to the exercise-induced cramps, an exercise forearm test reveals a normal rise in lactic acid and ammonia in Brody disease. NCSs and EMG are normal.[110–113] Importantly, muscles exhibiting impaired relaxation are electrically silent, unlike what is observed in the myotonic disorders.

Histopathology

Muscle biopsies demonstrate type 2 muscle fiber atrophy and increased internalized nuclei.[11] Sarcoplasmic/endoplasmic reticulum Ca^{2+} ATPase (SERCA1) immunohistochemistry and enzyme activity are reduced, while western blot analysis can show decreased or absence of the SERCA1 protein.[110] On EM, swollen mitochondria with crystalline inclusions are rarely noted. As with MH, skeletal muscle fibers are extremely sensitive to caffeine.

Molecular Genetics and Pathogenesis

Brody disease is an autosomal-recessive disorder caused by mutations in the *ATP2A1* gene located on chromosome 16p12.2–12.2.[110–113] This gene encodes for SERCA1, a calcium channel present on the sarcoplasmic reticulum of type 2 muscle fibers. These mutations cause a decreased rate of ATP-dependent calcium transport across the channel. Normally, upon depolarization of the T tubules, calcium ions are released from the lateral cisterns of the sarcoplasmic reticulum into the sarcoplasm. Relaxation requires the calcium concentration in the sarcoplasm to return to baseline, which is accomplished by calcium-ATPase located in the sarcoplasmic reticulum membrane. This enzyme pumps calcium back into the sarcoplasmic reticulum, but the activity is reduced in Brody disease. This results in an increased intracellular calcium and impaired relaxation following phasic (fast-twitch) activity. Not all patients with Brody disease have been found to have mutations in the *ATP2A1* gene, thus, the disorder is genetically heterogeneous.[111]

Treatment

Response to treatment with dantrolene, various calcium channel blockers (e.g., verapamil), and mexiletine have been variable.[110,112]

SCHWARTZ–JAMPEL SYNDROME (CHONDRODYSTROPHIC MYOTONIA)

Clinical Features

Schwartz–Jampel syndrome (SJS) is an autosomal-recessive disorder associated with developmental skeletal abnormalities and myotonia.[113–123] Affected children often have dysmorphic facies with micrognathia, narrowed palpebral fissures, and low set ears. In addition, over time kyphoscoliosis, bowing of the diaphyses, irregular epiphyses, reduced stature, and pectus carinatum become apparent. Infants may have a decreased suck and a weak high-pitched cry. As seen in MC, facial muscles may distort during or following a crying spell due to myotonia. Muscles often appear hypertrophied, and movement is slow due to stiffness related to the myotonia. Developmental motor milestones may be delayed.

Laboratory Features

Serum CK levels can be normal or mildly elevated. Routine motor and sensory NCSs are usually normal. Needle EMG may reveal complex repetitive,[123] myokymic,[121] pseudomyotonic (decrescendo runs of waning positive sharp waves), or myotonic discharges.[115–120,124]

Histopathology

Muscle biopsies reveal variation in fiber size with hypertrophic and atrophic fibers along with scattered degeneration and regenerating fibers.[123] Replacement of muscle fibers by fatty and connective tissue may be seen over time.

Molecular Genetics and Pathogenesis

SJS results from mutations in the *HSPG2* gene located on chromosome 1p34–36.1, which encodes perlecan, the major heparan sulfate proteoglycan component of basement membranes.[125–128] Analyses of *HSPG2* messenger RNA (mRNA) and perlecan immunostaining on patients' cells revealed a hypomorphic effect of the studied mutations.[128] Truncating mutations result in instability of *HSPG2* mRNA through nonsense mRNA-mediated decay, whereas missense mutations involving cysteine residues lead to intracellular retention of perlecan. How mutations in the *HSPG2* lead to myotonia is unclear but may indirectly affect the kinetics of the skeletal muscle sodium channel. Synchronous opening of sodium channels following a stimulus to the muscle membrane following repolarization of the membrane and delayed sodium channel activation have been demonstrated.

Treatment

Procainamide or mexiletine may be beneficial in reducing the muscle stiffness associated with SJS.

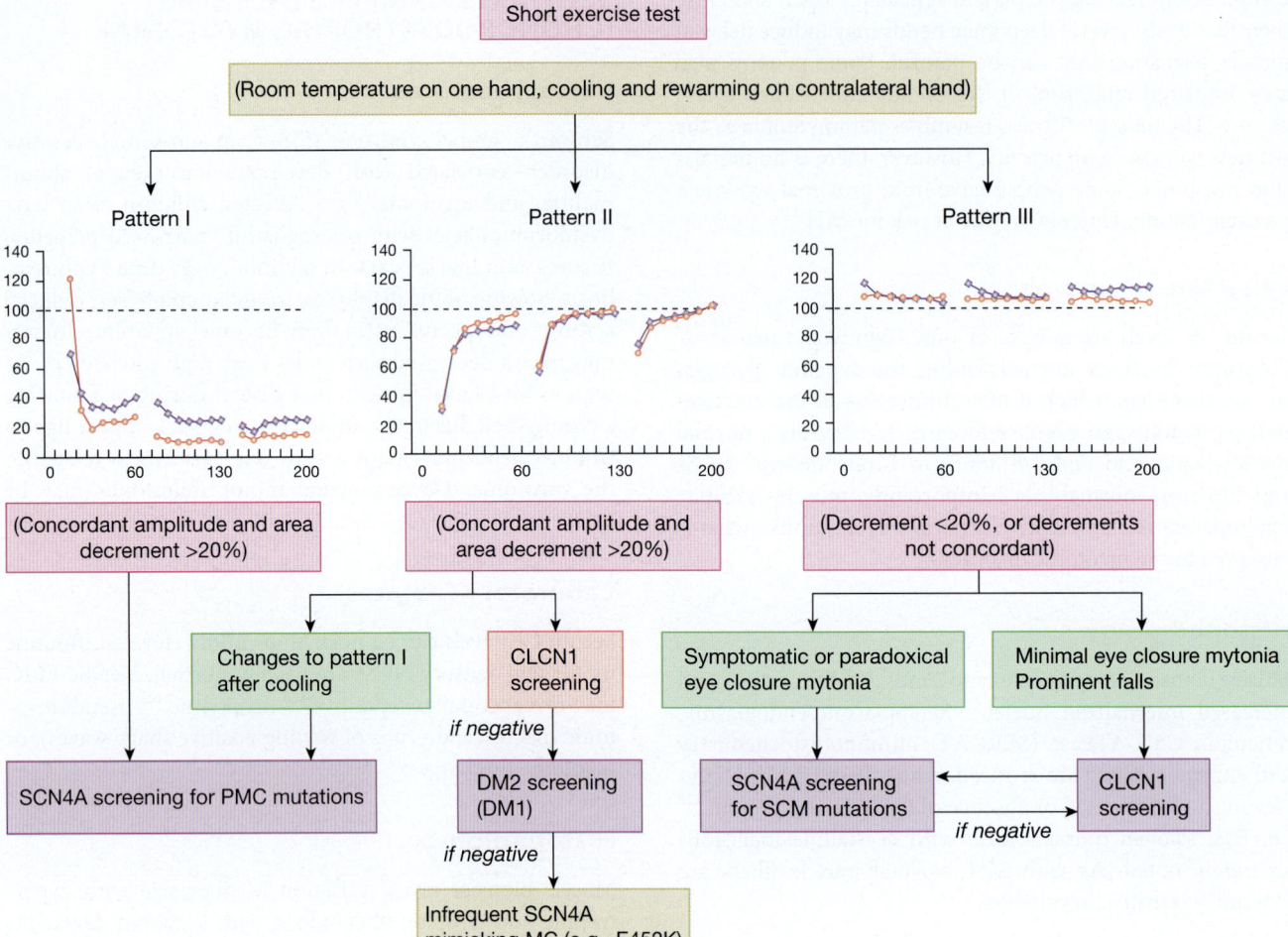

Figure 32-11. Suggested algorithm when using electrophysiological exercise tests for guiding genetic testing in patients with suspected nondystrophic myotonia. DM1, myotonic dystrophy type 1; DM2, myotonic dystrophy type 1 or proximal myotonic myopathy; MC, myotonia congenita; PMC, paramyotonia congenita; SCM, sodium channel myotonia. (Reproduced with permission from Tan SV, Matthews E, Barber M, et al. Refined exercise testing can aid DNA-based diagnosis in muscle channelopathies. *Ann Neurol.* 2011;69(2):328–340.)

▶ SUMMARY

Mutations affecting different muscle ion channels (sodium, calcium, chloride, and potassium) are associated with a variety of neuromuscular manifestations including clinical and electrical myotonia, periodic and sometimes progressive weakness, and occasionally skeletal deformities as seen in ATS. The overlapping features in these disorders can make them difficult to diagnose. The combination of a good clinical history (including family history), neuromuscular exam, and electrophysiological studies (EMG combined with SET performed at room temperature and with the extremity cooled) can be very helpful in guiding which genetic tests may be more useful in order to confirm the diagnosis for nondystrophic myotonias (Fig. 32-11). The LET can be helpful in diagnosing a hereditary periodic paralysis. Attacks of periodic paralysis may be reduced in some patients with acetazolamide, but this may make others worse (i.e., HypoKPP2).

Mexiletine appears to be beneficial in alleviating bothersome myotonia in some patients.

REFERENCES

1. Matthews E, Fialho D, Tan SV, et al; CINCH Investigators. The non-dystrophic myotonias: molecular pathogenesis, diagnosis and treatment. *Brain.* 2010;133(Pt 1):9–22.
2. Trip J, Drost G, Ginjaar HB, et al. Redefining the clinical phenotypes of non-dystrophic myotonic syndromes. *J Neurol Neurosurg Psychiatry.* 2009;80(6):647–652.
3. Heatwole CR, Statland JM, Logigian EL. The diagnosis and treatment of myotonic disorders. *Muscle Nerve.* 2013;47(5):632–648.
4. Trivedi JR, Bundy B, Statland J, et al; CINCH Consortium. Non-dystrophic myotonia: prospective study of objective and patient reported outcomes. *Brain.* 2013;136(Pt 7):2189–2200.
5. Horga A, Raja Rayan DL, Matthews E, et al. Prevalence study of genetically defined skeletal muscle channelopathies in England. *Neurology.* 2013;80(16):1472–1475.

6. Streib EW, Sun SF, Yarkowsky T. Transient paresis in myotonic syndromes: a simplified electrophysiologic approach. *Muscle Nerve*. 1982;5:719–723.
7. Stunnenberg BC, LoRusso S, Arnold WD, et al. Guidelines on clinical presentation and management of nondystrophic myotonias. *Muscle Nerve*. 2020;62(4):430–444.
8. Vereb N, Montagnese F, Gläser D, Schoser B. Non-dystrophic myotonias: clinical and mutation spectrum of 70 German patients. *J Neurol*. 2021;268(5):1708–1720.
9. Statland JM, Fontaine B, Hanna MG, et al. Review of the diagnosis and treatment of periodic paralysis. *Muscle Nerve*. 2018;57(4):522–530.
10. Fournier E, Arzel M, Sternberg D, et al. Electromyography guides toward subgroups of mutations in muscle channelopathies. *Ann Neurol*. 2004;56(5):650–661.
11. Fournier E, Viala K, Gervais H, et al. Cold extends electromyography distinction between ion channel mutations causing myotonia. *Ann Neurol*. 2006;60(3):356–365.
12. Tan SV, Matthews E, Barber M, et al. Refined exercise testing can aid DNA-based diagnosis in muscle channelopathies. *Ann Neurol*. 2011;69(2):328–340.
13. Simmons DB, Lanning J, Cleland JC, et al. Long exercise test in periodic paralysis: a Bayesian analysis. *Muscle Nerve*. 2019;59(1):47–54.
14. Ribeiro A, Suetterlin KJ, Skorupinska I, et al. The long exercise test as a functional marker of periodic paralysis. *Muscle Nerve*. 2022;65(5):581–585.
15. Colding-Jorgensen E. Phenotypic variability in myotonia congenita. *Muscle Nerve*. 2005;32(1):19–34.
16. Kuhn E, Fiehn W, Seiler D, Schroder JM. The autosomal recessive (Becker) form of myotonia congenita. *Muscle Nerve*. 1979;2(2):109–117.
17. Miller TM, Dias da Silva MR, Miller HA, et al. Correlating phenotype and genotype in the periodic paralyses. *Neurology*. 2004;63(9):1647–1655.
18. Ptacek LJ. The familial periodic paralyses and nondystrophic myotonias. *Am J Med*. 1998;105(1):58–70.
19. Sanders DB. Myotonia congenita with painful muscle contractions. *Arch Neurol*. 1976;33(8):580–582.
20. Sun SF, Streib EW. Autosomal recessive generalized myotonia. *Muscle Nerve*. 1983;6(2):143–148.
21. Tawil R, McDermott MP, Brown R, Jr, et al. Randomized trials of dichlorphenamide in the periodic paralyses. Working group on periodic paralysis. *Ann Neurol*. 2000;47(1):46–53.
22. Morrow JM, Matthews E, Raja Rayan DL, et al. Muscle MRI reveals distinct abnormalities in genetically proven nondystrophic myotonias. *Neuromuscul Disord*. 2013;23(8):637–646.
23. Kornblum C, Lutterbey GG, Czermin B, et al. Whole-body high-field MRI shows no skeletal muscle degeneration in young patients with recessive myotonia congenita. *Acta Neurol Scand*. 2010;121(2):131–135.
24. Aminoff MJ, Layzer RB, Satya-Murti S, Faden AI. The declining electrical response of muscle to repetitive nerve stimulation in myotonia. *Neurology*. 1977;27(9):812–816.
25. Streib EW. AAEE minimonograph #27: differential diagnosis of myotonic syndromes. *Muscle Nerve*. 1987;10(7):603–615.
26. Subramony SH, Malhotra CP, Mishra SK. Distinguishing paramyotonia congenita and myotonia congenita by electromyography. *Muscle Nerve*. 1983;6(5):374–379.
27. George AL Jr, Crackover MA, Abdalla JA, Hudson JA, Ebers GC. Molecular basis of Thomsen's disease (autosomal dominant myotonia congenital). *Nat Genet*. 1993;3(4):305–310.
28. Lorenz C, Meyer-Kleine C, Steinmeyer K, Koch MC, Jentsch TJ. Genomic organization of the human muscle chloride channel CIC-1 and analysis of novel mutations leading to Becker-type myotonia. *Hum Mol Genet*. 1994;3(6):941–946.
29. Wu FF, Ryan A, Devaney J, et al. Novel CLCN1 mutations with unique clinical and electrophysiological consequences. *Brain*. 2002;125(Pt 11):2392–2407.
30. Hoffman EP, Lehman-Horn F, Rudel R. Overexcited or inactive: ion channels in muscle disease. *Cell*. 1995;80(5):681–686.
31. Cannon SC. From mutation to myotonia in sodium channel disorders. *Neuromuscul Disord*. 1997;7(4):241–249.
32. Moxley RT 3rd. Carrell-Krusen symposium invited lecture-1997. Myotonic disorders in childhood: diagnosis and treatment. *J Child Neurol*. 1997;12(2):116–129.
33. Ptacek LJ, Johnson KJ, Griggs RC. Genetics and physiology of the myotonic muscle disorders. *N Engl J Med*. 1993;328(7):482–489.
34. Bulman DE, Scoggan KA, van Oene MD, et al. A novel sodium channel mutation in a family with hypokalemic periodic paralysis. *Neurology*. 1999;53(9):1932–1936.
35. Ptáček LJ, Tawil R, Griggs RC, et al. Sodium channel mutations in acetazolamide-responsive myotonia congenita, paramyotonia congenita, and hyperkalemic periodic paralysis. *Neurology*. 1994;44(8):1500–1503.
36. Jurkat-Rott K, Mitrovic N, Hang C, et al. Voltage-sensor sodium channel mutations cause hypokalemic periodic paralysis type 2 by enhanced inactivation and reduced current. *Proc Natl Acad Sci USA*. 2000;97(17):9549–9554.
37. Ptáček LJ, Tawil R, Griggs RC, et al. Dihydropyridine receptor mutations cause hypokalemic periodic paralysis. *Cell*. 1994;77(6):863–868.
38. Sternberg D, Maisonobe T, Jurkatt-Rott K, et al. Hypokalaemic periodic paralysis type 2 caused by mutations at codon 672 in the muscle sodium channel gene SCN4A. *Brain*. 2001;124(Pt 6):1091–1099.
39. Venance SL, Cannon SC, Fialho D, et al; CINCH investigators. The primary periodic paralyses: diagnosis, pathogenesis and treatment. *Brain*. 2006;129(Pt 1):8–17.
40. Matthews E, Portaro S, Ke Q, et al. Acetazolamide efficacy in hypokalemic periodic paralysis and the predictive role of genotype. *Neurology*. 2011;77(22):1960–1964.
41. Lehmann-Horn F, Jurkat-Rott K. Voltage-gated ion channels and hereditary diseases. *Physiol Rev*. 1999;79(4):1317–1372.
42. Ptacek LJ, George AL Jr, Barchi RL, et al. Mutations in an S4 segment of the adult skeletal muscle sodium channel cause paramyotonia congenita. *Neurology*. 1992;8(5):891–897.
43. Ptacek LJ, Tawil R, Griggs RC, Storvick D, Leppert M. Linkage of atypical myotonia congenita to a sodium channel locus. *Neurology*. 1992;42(2):431–433.
44. Ptacek LJ, Gouw L, Kwienciński H, et al. Sodium channel mutations in paramyotonia congenita and hyperkalemic periodic paralysis. *Ann Neurol*. 1993;33(3):300–307.
45. Ricker K, Camacho LM, Grafe P, Lehmann-Horn F, Rudel R. Adynamia episodica hereditaria: what causes the weakness? *Muscle Nerve*. 1989;12(11):883–891.
46. Ricker K, Lehmann-Horn F, Moxley RT 3rd. Myotonia fluctuans. *Arch Neurol*. 1990;47(3):268–272.

47. Ricker K, Moxley RT 3rd, Heine R, Lehmann-Horne F. Myotonia fluctuans. A third type of muscle sodium channel disease. *Arch Neurol.* 1994;51(11):1095–1102.
48. Subramony SH, Wee AS. Exercise and rest in hyperkalemic periodic paralysis. *Neurology.* 1986;36(2):173–177.
49. Bradley WG. Adynamia episodica hereditaria. Clinical, pathological and electrophysiological studies in an affected family. *Brain.* 1969;92(2):345–378.
50. Brooks JE. Hyperkalemic periodic paralysis. Intracellular electromyographic studies. *Arch Neurol.* 1969;20(1):13–18.
51. Bradley WG, Taylor R, Rice DR, Hausmanowa Petruzewicz I, Adelman LS, Jenkinson M. Progressive myopathy in hyperkalemic periodic paralysis. *Arch Neurol.* 1990;47(9):1013–1017.
52. Carson MJ, Pearson CM. Familial hyperkalemic periodic paralysis with myotonic features. *J Pediatr.* 1964;64:853–865.
53. Gamstorp I. [Adynamia episodica hereditaria.] *Acta Paediatr Suppl (Upps).* 1956;45(Suppl 108):1–126.
54. McArdle B. Adynamia episodica hereditaria and its treatment. *Brain.* 1962;85:121–148.
55. Rüdel R, Ricker K, Lehman-Horn F. Genotype-phenotype correlations in human skeletal muscle sodium channel diseases. *Arch Neurol.* 1993;50(11):1241–1248.
56. Rüdel R, Lehmann-Horn F. Workshop report. Paramyotonia, potassium-aggravated myotonias, and periodic paralyses. *Neuromuscul Disord.* 1997;7(2):127–132.
57. Hoskins B, Vroom FQ, Jarrell MA. Hyperkalemic periodic paralysis. Effects of potassium, exercise, glucose, and acetazolamide on blood chemistry. *Arch Neurol.* 1975;32(8):519–523.
58. Layzer RB, Lovelace RE, Rowland LP. Hyperkalemic periodic paralysis. *Arch Neurol.* 1967;16(5):445–472.
59. Amato AA, Dumitru D. Hereditary myopathies. In: Dumitru D, Amato AA, Swartz MJ, eds. *Electrodiagnostic Medicine.* 2nd ed. Hanley & Belfus, Inc.; 2002:1265–1370.
60. Meyers KR, Gilden DH, Rinaldi CF, Hansen JL. Periodic muscle weakness, normokalemia, and tubular aggregates. *Neurology.* 1972;22(3):269–279.
61. Tomé FMS, Borg K. Periodic paralysis and electrolyte disorders. In: Mastaglia FL, Walton JN, eds. *Skeletal Muscle Pathology.* Churchill Livingstone; 1992:343–366.
62. Lehmann-Horn F, Kuther G, Ricker K, Grafe P, Ballanyi K, Rudel R. Adynamia episodica hereditaria with myotonia: a noninactivating sodium current and the effect of extracellular pH. *Muscle Nerve.* 1987;10(4):363–374.
63. Lehmann-Horn F, Iaizzo PA, Hatt H, Franke C. Altered gating and conductance of Na+ channels in hyperkalemic periodic paralysis. *Pflugers Arch.* 1991;418(3):297–299.
64. Ptácek LJ, George AL Jr, Griggs RC, et al. Identification of a mutation in the gene causing hyperkalemic periodic paralysis. *Cell.* 1991;67(5):1021–1027.
65. Sansone VA, Burge J, McDermott MP, et al. Randomized, placebo-controlled trials of dichlorphenamide in periodic paralysis. *Neurology.* 2016;86(15):1408–1416.
66. Sansone VA, Johnson NE, Hanna MG, et al. Long-term efficacy and safety of dichlorphenamide for treatment of primary periodic paralysis. *Muscle Nerve.* 2021;64(3):342–346.
67. Streib EW, Sun SF, Hanson M. Paramyotonia congenita: clinical and electrophysiologic studies. *Electromyogr Clin Neurophysiol.* 1983;23(4):315–325.
68. Streib EW. Paramyotonia congenita. *Semin Neurol.* 1991;11(3):249–257.
69. Lajoie WJ. Paramyotonia congenita, clinical features and electromyographic findings. *Arch Phys Med Rehabil.* 1961;42:507–512.
70. Lundberg PO, Stalberg E, Thiele B. Paralysis periodica paramyotonia. A clinical and neurophysiological study. *J Neurol Sci.* 1974;21(3):309–321.
71. Thrush DC, Morris CJ, Salmon MV. Paramyotonia congenita: a clinical, histochemical and pathological study. *Brain.* 1972;95(3):537–552.
72. Jackson CE, Barohn RJ, Ptacek LJ. Paramyotonia congenita: abnormal short exercise test, and improvement after mexiletine therapy. *Muscle Nerve.* 1994;17(7):763–768.
73. Statland JM, Bundy BN, Wang Y, et al; Consortium for clinical investigation of neurologic channelopathies. Mexiletine for symptoms and signs of myotonia in nondystrophic myotonia: a randomized controlled trial. *JAMA.* 2012;308(13):1357–1365.
74. Streib EW. Paramyotonia congenita: successful treatment with tocainide. Clinical and electrophysiologic findings in seven patients. *Muscle Nerve.* 1987;10(2):155–162.
75. Lennox G, Purves A, Marsden D. Myotonia fluctuans. *Arch Neurol.* 1992;49(10):1010–1011.
76. Colding-Jorgensen E, Duno M, Vissing J. Autosomal dominant monosymptomatic myotonia permanens. *Neurology.* 2006;67(1):153–155.
77. Avila-Smirnow D, Vargas Leal CP, Beytía Reyes MLA, et al. Non-dystrophic myotonia Chilean cohort with predominance of the SCN4A Gly1306Glu variant. *Neuromuscul Disord.* 2020;30(7):554–561.
78. Trudell RG, Kaiser KK, Griggs RC. Acetazolamide-responsive myotonia congenita. *Neurology.* 1987;37(3):488–491.
79. Lehmann-Horn F, Rudel R, Dengler R, Lorkovic H, Haass A, Ricker K. Membrane defects in paramyotonia congenita with and without in a warm environment. *Muscle Nerve.* 1981;4(5):396–406.
80. Haywood LJ, Sandoval GM, Cannon SC. Defective slow inactivation of sodium channels contributes to familial periodic paralysis. *Neurology.* 1999;52(7):1447–1453.
81. Sokolov S, Scheuer T, Catterall WA. Gating pore current in an inherited ion channelopathy. *Nature.* 2007;446(7131):76–78.
82. Struyk AF, Cannon SC. A Na+ channel mutation linked to hypokalemic periodic paralysis exposes a proton-selective gating pore. *J Gen Physiol.* 2007;130(1):11–20.
83. Lapie P, Lory P, Fontaine B. Hypokalemic periodic paralysis: an autosomal dominant muscle disorder caused by mutations in a voltage-gated calcium channel. *Neuromusc Disord.* 1997;7(4):234–240.
84. Links TP, Zwarts MJ, Wilmink JT, Molenaar WM, Oosterhuis HJ. Permanent muscle weakness in familial hypokalemic periodic paralysis. Clinical, radiological and pathological aspects. *Brain.* 1990;113(Pt 6):1873–1889.
85. Holm-Yildiz S, Witting N, Dahlqvist J, et al. Permanent muscle weakness in hypokalemic periodic paralysis. *Neurology.* 2020;95(4):e342–e352.
86. Gordon AM, Green JR, Lagunoff D. Studies on a patient with hypokalemic familial periodic paralysis. *Am J Med.* 1970;48(2):185–195.

87. Links TP, Smit AJ, Molenaar WM, Zwarts MJ, Oosterhuis HJ. Familial hypokalemic periodic paralysis. Clinical, diagnostic, and therapeutic aspects. *J Neurol Sci*. 1994;122(1):33–43.
88. De Grandis D, Fiaschi A, Tomelleri G, Orrico D. Hypokalemic periodic paralysis: a single fiber electromyographic study. *J Neurol Sci*. 1978;37(1-2):107–112.
89. Abbot GW, Butler MH, Bendahhou S, Dalakas MC, Ptacek LJ, Goldstein SA. MiRP2 forms potassium channels in skeletal muscle with Kv3.4 and is associated with periodic paralysis. *Cell*. 2001:104(2):217–231.
90. Ng HY, Lin SH, Hsu CY, Tsai YZ, Chen HC, Lee CT. Hypokalemic paralysis due to Gitelman syndrome: a family study. *Neurology*. 2006;67(6):1080–1082.
91. Grafe P, Quasthoff S, Strupp M, Lehmann-Horn F. Enhancement of K+ conductance improves in vitro the contraction force of skeletal muscle in hypokalemic periodic paralysis. *Muscle Nerve*. 1990;13(5):451–457.
92. Hofmann WW, Smith RA. Hypokalemic periodic paralysis studies in vitro. *Brain*. 1970;93(3):445–474.
93. Rudel R, Lehmann-Horn F, Ricker K, Kuther G. Hypokalemic periodic paralysis: in vitro investigation of muscle fiber membrane parameters. *Muscle Nerve*. 1984;7(2):110–120.
94. Falhammar H, Thorén M, Calissendorff J. Thyrotoxic periodic paralysis: clinical and molecular aspects. *Endocrine*. 2013;43(2):274–284.
95. Ryan DP, da Silva MR, Soong TW, et al. Mutations in potassium channel Kir2.6 cause susceptibility to thyrotoxic hypokalemic periodic paralysis. *Cell*. 2010;140(1):88–98.
96. Jongjaroenprasert W, Phusantisampan T, Mahasirimongkol S, et al. A genome-wide association study identifies novel susceptibility genetic variation for thyrotoxic hypokalemic periodic paralysis. *J Hum Genet*. 2012;57(5):301–304.
97. Cheung CL, Lau KS, Ho AY, et al. Genome-wide association study identifies a susceptibility locus for thyrotoxic periodic paralysis at 17q24.3. *Nat Genet*. 2012;44(9):1026–1029.
98. Wang X, Chow CC, Yao X, et al. The predisposition to thyrotoxic periodic paralysis (TPP) is due to a genetic variant in the inward-rectifying potassium channel, KCNJ2. *Clin Endocrinol*. 2014;80(5):770–771.
99. Vivekanandam V, Männikkö R, Skorupinska I, et al. Andersen–Tawil syndrome: deep phenotyping reveals significant cardiac and neuromuscular morbidity. *Brain*. 2022;145(6):2108–2120.
100. Song J, Luo S, Cheng X, et al. Clinical features and long exercise test in Chinese patients with Andersen-Tawil syndrome. *Muscle Nerve*. 2016;54(6):1059–1063.
101. Davies NP, Imbrici P, Fialho D, et al. Andersen–Tawil syndrome: new potassium channel mutations and possible phenotypic variation. *Neurology*. 2005;65(7):1083–1089.
102. Klein R, Ganelin R, Marks JF. J Periodic paralysis with cardiac arrhythmia. *J Pediatr*. 1963;62:371–385.
103. Ma D, Tang XD, Rogers TB, Welling PA. An Andersen–Tawil syndrome mutation in Kir2.1 (V302M) alters the G-loop cytoplasmic K+ conduction pathway. *J Biol Chem*. 2007;282(8):5781–5789.
104. Salajegheh MK, Amato AA. Channelopathies: Paroxysmal paralysis. In: Squire LR, Albright TD, Bloom FE, eds. *New Encyclopedia of Neuroscience*. 2009;496–507.
105. Tawil R, Ptacek LJ, Pavlkis SG, et al. Andersen's syndrome: potassium-sensitive periodic paralysis, ventricular ectopy, and dysmorphic features. *Ann Neurol*. 1994;35(3):326–330.
106. Tan SV, Z'graggen WJ, Boërio D, et al. Membrane dysfunction in Andersen–Tawil syndrome assessed by velocity recovery cycles. *Muscle Nerve*. 2012;46(2):193–203.
107. Plaster NM, Tawil R, Trisani-Firouzi M, et al. Mutations in Kir2.1 cause the developmental and episodic electrical phenotypes of Andersen's syndrome. *Cell*. 2001;105(4):511–519.
108. Zhou H, Lillis S, Loy RE, et al. Multi-minicore disease and atypical periodic paralysis associated with novel mutations in the skeletal muscle ryanodine receptor (RYR1) gene. *Neuromuscul Disord*. 2010;20(3):166–173.
109. Matthews E, Neuwirth C, Jaffer F, et al. Atypical periodic paralysis and myalgia: a novel *RYR1* phenotype. *Neurology*. 2018;90(5):e412–e418.
110. Molenaar JP, Verhoeven JI, Rodenburg RJ, et al. Clinical, morphological and genetic characterization of Brody disease: an international study of 40 patients. *Brain*. 2020;143(2):452–466.
111. Voermans NC, Laan AE, Oosterhof A, et al. Brody syndrome: a clinically heterogeneous entity distinct from Brody disease: a review of literature and a cross-sectional clinical study in 17 patients. *Neuromuscul Disord*. 2012;22(11):944–954.
112. Benders AA, Veerkamp JH, Oosterhof A, et al. Ca^{2+} homeostasis in Brody's disease. A study in skeletal muscle and cultured muscle cells and the effects of dantrolene and verapamil. *J Clin Invest*. 1994;94(2):741–748.
113. Odermatt A, Taschner PE, Khanna VK, et al. Mutations in the gene-encoding SERCA1, the fast-twitch skeletal muscle sarcoplasmic reticulum Ca^{2+} ATPase, are associated with Brody disease. *Nat Genet*. 1996;14(2):191–194.
114. Pavone L, Mollica F, Grasso A, Cao A, Gullotta F. Schwartz-Jampel syndrome in two daughters of first cousins. *J Neurol Neurosurg Psychiatry*. 1978;41(2):161–169.
115. Aberfeld DC, Namba T, Vye MV, Grob D. Chondrodystrophic myotonia: report of two cases. Myotonia, dwarfism, diffuse bone disease, and unusual ocular and facial abnormalities. *Arch Neurol*. 1970;22(5):455–462.
116. Brown SB, Carcia-Mullin R, Murai Y. The Schwartz-Jampel syndrome (myotonic chondrodystrophy) in the adult. *Neurology*. 1975;25:365–366.
117. Cadilhac J, Baldet P, Greze J, Duday H. EMG studies of two family cases of the Schwartz and Jampel syndrome (osteochondro-muscular dystrophy with myotonia). *Electromyogr Clin Neurophysiol*. 1975;15(1):5–12.
118. Cao A, Cianchetti C, Calisti L, de Virgiliis S, Ferreli A, Tangheroni W. Schwartz-Jampel syndrome. Clinical, electrophysiological and histopathological study of a severe variant. *J Neurol Sci*. 1978;35(2-3):175–187.
119. Fowler WM Jr, Layzer RB, Taylor RG, et al. The Schwartz-Jampel syndrome. Its clinical, physiological, and histological expressions. *J Neurol Sci*. 1974;22(1):127–146.
120. Huttenlocher PR, Landwirth J, Hanson V, Gallagher BB, Bensch K. Osteo-chondro-muscular dystrophy. A disorder manifested by multiple skeletal deformities, myotonia, and dystrophic changes in muscle. *Pediatrics*. 1969;44(6):945–958.
121. Pascuzzi RM, Gratianne R, Azzarelli B, Kincaid JC. Schwartz-Jampel syndrome with dominant inheritance. *Muscle Nerve*. 1990;13(12):1152–1163.

122. Pascuzzi RM. Schwartz-Jampel syndrome. *Semin Neurol.* 1991;11(3):267-273.
123. Spanns F, Theunissen P, Reekers AD, Smit L, Veldman H. Schwartz-Jampel syndrome: I. Clinical, electromyographic and histologic studies. *Muscle Nerve.* 1990;13(6):516-527.
124. Taylor RG, Layzer RB, Davis HS, Fowler WM Jr. Continuous muscle fiber activity in the Schwartz-Jampel syndrome. *Electroencephalogr Clin Neurophysiol.* 1972;33(5):497-509.
125. Arikawa-Hirasawa E, Le AH, Nishino I, et al. Structural and functional mutations of the perlecan gene cause Schwartz-Jampel syndrome, with myotonic myopathy and chondrodysplasia. *Am J Hum Genet.* 2002;70(5):1368-1375.
126. Nicole S, Davoine CS, Topaloglu H, et al. Perlecan, the major proteoglycan of basement membranes, is altered in patients with Schwartz-Jampel syndrome (chondrodystrophic myotonia). *Nat Genet.* 2000;26(4):480-483.
127. Stum M, Davoine CS, Fontaine B, Nicole S. Schwartz-Jampel syndrome and perlecan deficiency. *Acta Myol.* 2005;24(2):89-92.
128. Stum M, Davoine CS, Vicart S, et al. Spectrum of HSPG2 (Perlecan) mutations in patients with Schwartz-Jampel syndrome. *Hum Mutat.* 2006;27(11):1082-1091.

CHAPTER 33

Inflammatory Myopathies

There are five major categories of idiopathic inflammatory myopathy (IIM): dermatomyositis (DM), polymyositis (PM), antisynthetase syndrome (ASyS), immune-mediated necrotizing myopathy (IMNM), and inclusion body myositis (IBM), which are clinically, histologically, and pathogenically distinct (Tables 33-1 to 33-4).[1–13] However, the category of PM is increasingly diminishing as most cases are now known to be IBM, ASyS, and IMNM.[14–19] The IIMs may occur in isolation or in association with cancer, various connective tissue diseases (overlap syndromes), and autoantibodies. Other less common myositides (i.e., granulomatous and myositis associated with infections) will also be discussed in this chapter. It is important to emphasize that not all myopathies with inflammation are classified as "inflammatory myopathies." In this regard, various muscular dystrophies (e.g., congenital, facioscapulohumeral, and dysferlinopathies) may be associated with profound inflammation and are not uncommonly misdiagnosed as PM.

There are a few reports of IMNM occurring in parents, children, and siblings of affected patients, suggesting a genetic predisposition to developing these disorders, possibly secondary to inherited human leukocyte antigen (HLA) haplotypes.[20–25] There are hereditary forms of inclusion body myopathy, but with rare exceptions, the muscle biopsies in these cases lack inflammation, and the clinical phenotype (i.e., age of onset and pattern of weakness) is different from sporadic IBM.

The annual incidence of the DM and "PM" has ranged between 0.1 and 4 per 100,000 person-years,[4,6,23–27] with recent studies suggesting the incidence may up to 16 per 100,000 in some populations[32] with prevalence in the range of 14 to 32 per 100,000.[6,28–32] However, defining the actual incidence and prevalence of the individual myositides has been limited by the different diagnostic criteria employed in various epidemiological studies. Most published papers regarding epidemiology and treatment of DM and PM have used the outdated Bohan and Peter criteria.[33–35] PM will be over diagnosed with Bohan and Peter criteria. These criteria were fine in 1975, but these criteria do not require a muscle biopsy and the only feature that distinguishes PM from DM is the presence of a rash in DM. Further, the biopsy abnormalities as listed are nonspecific (except for perifascicular atrophy—a finding specific for DM, but not seen in PM) and do not help in distinguishing PM from DM or for that matter any myopathy with necrosis, including muscular dystrophies. Importantly, the Bohan and Peter histological criteria do not take into account the advances in autoantibodies (e.g., antisynthetase antibodies), histopathology, and the distinct diagnoses of ASyS, IBM, and IMNM. This can have implications regarding treatment strategies and prognosis as we will discuss.[1,6,7,36]

Criteria for diagnosis of the various inflammatory myopathies need to take into account the advances in understanding of the pathogeneses of these disorders. We emphasize that DM is not simply PM with a rash (or the converse: PM is not DM without a rash). Furthermore, IBM is not PM with inclusions (or the converse: IBM is not PM with inclusions). For this reason, revised criteria for the various IIM have been devised to take into account the recent advancements in the field, including histopathological features and presence of autoantibodies (Tables 33-2 to 33-4).[1,6,14–17,37–39] With the caveats noted above, we will begin our discussion of the individual inflammatory myopathies.

▶ DERMATOMYOSITIS

CLINICAL FEATURES

DM can present at any age, including infancy. Like most other autoimmune disorders, there is an increased incidence of DM in women compared to men. Although the pathogenesis of childhood and adult DM is presumably similar, there are important differences in some of the clinical features and associated disorders.[1,2,4,6,40–44] Weakness can develop rather acutely (over days or several weeks), or insidiously (over months). Proximal leg and arm muscles as well as neck flexors are usually the earliest and most severely affected muscle groups. Thus, the earliest patient complaints are often difficulty lifting their arms over their heads, climbing steps, and arising from chairs. Distal muscles are also involved. Children are more likely to present with an insidious onset of muscle weakness and myalgias that are often preceded by fatigue, low-grade fevers, and a rash. Dysphagia occurs in approximately 30% of patients with DM probably due to involvement of oropharyngeal and esophageal muscles. Speech, chewing, and swallowing difficulties can arise secondary to involvement of the masseter muscle. We have even seen speech difficulties as a result of involvement of the pharyngeal, laryngeal, and the tongue muscles. Sensation is normal, and muscle stretch reflexes are preserved unless a severe degree of weakness has developed.

DM is usually diagnosed earlier than other forms of myositis because of the characteristic rash, which typically accompanies or precedes the onset of muscle weakness.

▶ TABLE 33-1. INFLAMMATORY MYOPATHIES: CLINICAL AND LABORATORY FEATURES

Disorder	Sex	Age of Onset	Rash	Pattern of Weakness	Laboratory Features	Muscle Biopsy	Cellular Infiltrate	Response to IS Therapy	Common Associated Conditions
DM	F > M	Childhood and adult	Yes	Proximal > distal	Normal or increased CK (up to 50× normal or higher); various MSAs (anti-MDA5, anti-TIF1, anti-Mi-2, anti-NXP2, anti-SAE)	Perimysial and perivascular inflammation; IFN-1 regulated proteins (MHC-1, MxA), MAC deposition on capillaries	CD4+ Dendritic cells; B cells; macrophages	Yes	Myocarditis, ILD, malignancy, vasculitis, other CTDs
PM	F > M	Adult	No	Proximal > distal	Increased CK (up to 50× normal or higher)	Endomysial and perivascular inflammation; ubiquitous expression of MHC-1	CD8+ T cells; macrophages; plasma cells	Yes	Myocarditis, ILD, other CTDs
NM	M = F	Children and adults	No	Proximal > distal	Elevated CK (>10× normal or higher); anti-HMGCR or anti-SRP antibodies	Necrotic muscle fibers; minimal inflammatory infiltrate	Macrophages in necrotic fibers undergoing phagocytosis	Yes	Malignancy, CTD, HMGCR antibody cases can be triggered by statin use
ASyS	F > M	Children and adults	Sometimes	Proximal > distal	Elevated CK (>10× normal or higher); antisynthetase antibodies	Perimysial and perivascular inflammation; perimysial fragmentation with alkaline phosphatase staining; perimysial muscle damage with necrosis	CD4+ Dendritic cells; B cells; macrophages	Yes	Nonerosive arthritis, ILD, Raynaud phenomenon, mechanic hands, and fever
IBM	M > F	Older adults (>50 years)	No	Proximal and distal; predilection for: finger/wrist flexors, knee extensors	Normal or mildly increased CK (usually <10× normal); anti-cN-1A antibodies; large granular lymphocytes on flow cytometry and reduced CD4/CD8 ratio with increased CD8 count	Endomysial and perivascular inflammation; CD57+ CD8+ expressing KLRG1; ubiquitous expression of MHC-1; rimmed vacuoles; p62, LC3, TDP-43 aggregates; EM: 15–18 nm tubulofilaments; ragged red and COX negative fibers	CD8+ T cells; macrophages; plasma cells; myeloid dendritic cells; large granular lymphocytes	None or minimal	Granular lymphocytic leukemia/ lymphocytosis, sarcoidosis, SICCA or Sjögren syndrome

CK, creatine kinase; cN-1A, cytosolic 5′-nucleotidase 1A; CTDs, connective tissue diseases; COX, cytochrome oxidase; DM, dermatomyositis; F, female; IBM, inclusion body myositis; IFN-1, type 1 interferon; ILD, interstitial lung disease; IS, immunosuppressive; KLRG1, killer cell lectin-like receptor G1; M, male; MAC, membrane attack complex; MDA5, melanoma differentiation antigen; MHC-1, major histocompatibility antigen 1; NXP2, nuclear matrix protein 2; NM, necrotizing myopathy; PM, polymyositis; anti-SAE, anti–small ubiquitin-like modifier activating enzyme; anti–TIF1-γ, anti-transcription intermediary factor 1-γ.

▶ **TABLE 33-2. DIAGNOSTIC CRITERIA FOR POLYMYOSITIS, DERMATOMYOSITIS, IMMUNE-MEDIATED NECROTIZING MYOPATHY, AND NONSPECIFIC/UNSPECIFIED MYOSITIS**

I. *Polymyositis (PM)*
  1. Clinical features
     a. Inclusion criteria
        i. Onset usually over 18 years (post puberty)
        ii. Subacute or insidious onset
        iii. Pattern of weakness: symmetric proximal > distal weakness
     b. Exclusion criteria
        i. Clinical features of IBM (see Griggs et al.: asymmetric weakness, wrist/finger flexors same or worse than deltoids; knee extensors and/or ankle dorsiflexors same or worse than hip flexors)
        ii. Ocular weakness, isolated dysarthria, neck extensor > neck flexor weakness
     c. Exposure to myotoxic drugs, active endocrinopathy (hyperthyroid or hypothyroid and hyperparathyroid), amyloidosis, family history of muscular dystrophy or proximal motor neuropathies (e.g., SMA)
  2. Serum creatine kinase level must be elevated
  3. Other laboratory criteria (one of three): EMG criteria, skeletal muscle MRI, or presence of myositis-specific antibodies
     a. Electromyography:
        i. Inclusion criteria
           • Increased insertional and spontaneous activity in the form of fibrillation potentials, positive sharp waves, or complex repetitive discharges
           • Morphometric analysis reveals the presence of short-duration, small-amplitude, polyphasic MUAPs
        ii. Exclusion criteria
           • Prominent myotonic discharges that would suggest proximal myotonic dystrophy or other channelopathy
           • Morphometric analysis reveals predominantly long-duration, large-amplitude MUAPs
           • Decreased recruitment pattern of MUAPs
     b. Skeletal muscle MRI shows diffuse or patchy increased signal (edema) within muscle tissue on STIR images
     c. Myositis-specific antibodies are detected in the serum
  4. Muscle biopsy
     a. Definite PM requires endomysial inflammatory cell infiltrate (T cells) surrounding and invading nonnecrotic muscle fibers
     b. Probable PM
        i. Endomysial CD8+ T cells surrounding and but no definite invasions of nonnecrotic muscle fibers or
        ii. Ubiquitous MHC-1 expression
        iii. Also requires exclusion of "necrotizing myopathies" and dystrophies with immunopathology/electron microscopy and clinical history/examination
     c. Exclusion criteria
        i. Rimmed vacuoles, ragged red fibers, cytochrome oxidase-negative fibers that would suggest IBM
        ii. Perifascicular atrophy, deposition of MAC on small blood vessels, reduced capillary density, tubuloreticular inclusions in endothelial cells, or pipestem capillaries that would suggest dermatomyositis (DM) or another type of humorally mediated microangiopathy
        iii. Dystrophic features or MAC deposition on nonnecrotic muscle fibers that would suggest a muscular dystrophy
  A. Definite PM
     1. All clinical criteria
     2. Elevated serum CK
     3. Muscle biopsy with features of histological features of definite PM
  B. Probable PM
     1. All clinical criteria
     2. Elevated serum CK
     3. Other laboratory criteria (one of three)
     4. Muscle biopsy with features of histological features of probable PM

II. *Dermatomyositis (DM)*
  1. Clinical features
     a. Inclusion criteria
        i. Onset in childhood (juvenile DM) or adulthood (adult DM)
        ii. Subacute or insidious onset
        iii. Pattern of weakness: symmetric proximal legs > arms, neck flexors > neck extensors
        iv. Rash suggestive of DM: heliotrope, Gottron papules/sign, V-sign, shawl sign, holster sign
     b. Exclusion criteria
        i. Ocular weakness, isolated dysarthria, neck extensor > neck flexor weakness
        ii. Exclusion of other causes of weakness (see PM clinical exclusion criteria)

(continued)

► TABLE 33-2. (CONTINUED)

   2. Muscle biopsy:
      a. Definite DM requires perifascicular atrophy
      b. Probable DM requires:
         Myxovirus resistance 1 protein (or other type 1–interferon-regulated proteins) deposition on small blood vessels or muscle fibers
         Or
         MAC deposition on small blood vessels
         Or
         Reduced capillary density
         Or
         Tubuloreticular inclusions in endothelial walls on EM
         Or
         MHC-1 expression of perifascicular fibers
         Or
         Perivascular, perimysial inflammatory cell infiltrate (this is a nonspecific abnormality in and of itself)
   A. Definite DM
      1. All clinical criteria
      2. Muscle biopsy demonstrates perifascicular atrophy
   B. Probable DM
      1. All clinical criteria
      2. Muscle biopsy fulfills probable DM histological criteria or elevated serum CK or other laboratory criteria (one of three: EMG, MRI, or MSA)
   C. Amyopathic DM
      1. Rash typical of DM: heliotrope, Gottron papules/sign, V-sign, shawl sign, and holster sign
      2. Skin biopsy demonstrates a reduced capillary density, deposition of MAC on small blood vessels along the dermal–epidermal junction, and variable keratinocyte decoration for MAC
      3. No subjective or objective muscle weakness
      4. Normal serum CK
      5. Normal EMG
   D. Possible DM sine dermatitis
      1. Clinical criteria but classic DM rash is absent
      2. Muscle biopsy demonstrates:
         Perifascicular atrophy
         Or
         MxA deposition on small blood vessels or muscle fibers
         Or
         MAC deposition on small blood vessels
         Or
         Reduced capillary density
         Or
         Tubuloreticular inclusions in endothelial walls on EM
         Or
         MHC-1 expression of perifascicular fibers
      3. Elevated CK plus other laboratory criteria (one of three: EMG, MRI, or MSA)
III. *Nonspecific/unspecified myositis*
   1. Clinical features
      a. Inclusion criteria
         i. Onset in childhood or adulthood
         ii. Subacute or insidious onset
         iii. Pattern of weakness: symmetric proximal > distal weakness
      b. Exclusion criteria: Rash typical of DM; PM clinical exclusion criteria
   2. Muscle biopsy
      a. Perivascular, perimysial inflammatory cell infiltrate but there is no perifascicular atrophy, perifascicular MHC-1 expression, MAC deposition on small blood vessels, reduced capillary density, or tubuloreticular inclusions on EM
         Or
      b. Scattered endomysial CD8+ T cells infiltrate but that does not clearly surround or invade muscle fibers
         And
      c. Requires exclusion of "necrotizing myopathies," dystrophies, and "possible IBM" with immunopathology/electron microscopy and clinical history/examination
   3. Serum creatine kinase (CK) level is elevated
   4. Other laboratory criteria (one of three): EMG criteria, skeletal muscle MRI, or presence of myositis-specific antibodies

▶ **TABLE 33-2. (CONTINUED)**

IV. *Immune-mediated necrotizing myopathy*
1. Clinical features
    a. Inclusion criteria
        i. Onset usually over 18 years (post puberty)
        ii. Subacute or insidious onset
        iii. Pattern of weakness: symmetric proximal > distal weakness
    b. Exclusion criteria: Rash typical of DM; PM clinical exclusion criteria
2. Muscle biopsy
    a. The predominant abnormal histological feature of the muscle biopsy is the presence of many necrotic muscle fibers
    b. Inflammatory cells are sparse or only slightly perivascular; perimysial infiltrate is evident
    c. MAC deposition on small blood vessels may be seen
    d. Tubuloreticular inclusions in endothelial cells are uncommon or not evident
    e. Pipestem capillaries may be evident on EM
    f. No evidence of mononuclear inflammatory cells invading nonnecrotic muscle fibers
    g. No perifascicular atrophy
3. Serum CK level must be elevated
4. Other laboratory criteria (one of three): EMG criteria, skeletal muscle MRI, or presence of myositis-specific antibodies

IBM, inclusion body myositis; MRI, magnetic resonance imaging; DM, dermatomyositis; MUAP, motor unit action potential; MHC-1, major histocompatibility-1; MAC, membrane attack complex; CK, creatine kinase; EM, electron microscopy; MSA, myositis-specific antibody; MxA, myxovirus resistance 1 protein.

Reproduced with permission from Hoogendijk JE, Amato AA, Lecky BR, et al. 119th ENMC international workshop: trial design in adult idiopathic inflammatory myopathies, with the exception of inclusion body myositis, 10–12 October 2003, Naarden, The Netherlands. *Neuromuscul Disord.* 2004;14(5):337–345.

However, the rash can develop years after the onset of weakness, which could lead to an erroneous diagnosis of PM. Some patients have the characteristic rash but never develop weakness (the so-called amyopathic DM or DM *sine* myositis).[43,44] Rare patients do not have an appreciable rash at the time they present with weakness. We have seen some patients with histopathological features characteristic of DM who have developed the rash months or years after onset of weakness or not at all (adermatopathic DM or DM *sine* dermatitis). These patients would be erroneously classified as PM using Bohan and Peter criteria.

The classical skin manifestations include a purplish discoloration of the eyelids (heliotrope rash) often associated with periorbital edema and a papular, erythematous

▶ **TABLE 33-3. EUROPEAN NEUROMUSCULAR CENTER 2011 WORKSHOP CRITERIA FOR INCLUSION BODY MYOSITIS**

Clinical and Laboratory Features	Classification	Pathological Features
Duration >12 months Age at onset >45 years Knee extension weakness ≥ hip flexion weakness And/Or Finger flexion weakness > shoulder abduction weakness CK no greater than 15× ULN	Clinicopathologically defined IBM	All of the following: Endomysial inflammatory infiltrate Rimmed vacuoles Protein accumulation[a] or 15–18 nm filaments
Duration >12 months Age at onset >45 years Knee extension weakness ≥ hip flexion weakness And Finger flexion weakness > shoulder abduction weakness CK no greater than 15× ULN	Clinically defined IBM	One or more, but not all, of: Endomysial inflammatory infiltrate Upregulation of MHC class I Rimmed vacuoles Protein accumulation[a] or 15–18 nm filaments
Duration >12 months Age at onset >45 years Knee extension weakness ≥ hip flexion weakness Or Finger flexion weakness > shoulder abduction weakness CK no greater than 15× ULN	Probable IBM	One or more, but not all, of: Endomysial inflammatory infiltrate Upregulation of MHC class I Rimmed vacuoles Protein accumulation[a] or 15–18 nm filaments

[a]Demonstration of amyloid or other protein accumulation by established methods (e.g., for amyloid Congo red, crystal violet, thioflavin T/S, for other proteins p62, SMI-31, TDP-43).

Reproduced with permission from Rose MR, ENMC IBM Working Group. 188th ENMC International Workshop: Inclusion Body Myositis, 2–4 December 2011, Naarden, The Netherlands. *Neuromuscul Disord.* 2013;23(12):1044–1055.

▶ **TABLE 33-4. EUROPEAN NEUROMUSCULAR CENTER 2023 WORKSHOP CRITERIA FOR INCLUSION BODY MYOSITIS**[13]

ENMC Diagnosis of IBM is confirmed when there is:

1. Common presentation (age of onset > 45 years, progression over 12 months, and CK < 15 × upper limited of normal associated with pattern of weakness involving finger flexor <u>AND</u> knee extensor weakness that is often asymmetric and also often accompanied by dysphagia) <u>AND</u> a muscle biopsy demonstrating endomysial inflammation surround non-necrotic muscle fibers (with or without invasion), OR
2. Common presentation (as above) and a muscle biopsy demonstrating endomysial inflammation surround non-necrotic muscle fibers (with or without invasion), and <u>at least one supportive</u> investigation finding(s) (rimmed vacuoles or cytoplasmic protein aggregates, mitochondrial abnormalities, anti-cN1a antibodies, typical pattern of muscle involvement on MRI or ultrasound imaging), OR
3. Uncommon presentation (e.g., axial weakness, proximal limb weakness only, foot drop, facial diplegia, isolated dysphagia) and a muscle biopsy demonstrating endomysial inflammation surround non-necrotic muscle fibers (with or without invasion), and <u>at least two</u> supportive investigation finding(s) as noted above

rash over the knuckles (Gottron papules) (Fig. 33-1). In addition, an erythematous, macular, sun-sensitive rash may appear on the face, neck, and anterior chest (V-sign), shoulders and upper back (shawl sign), hips (holster sign), and extensor surfaces of elbows, knuckles, knees, and malleoli (Gottron sign). The nail beds often have dilated capillary loops occasionally with thrombi or hemorrhage. The skin lesions can be subtle at times and difficult to appreciate in individuals who are darker skinned—another common reason for misdiagnosing patients with PM rather than DM.

Subcutaneous calcifications occur in 30%–70% of children, but in our experience, these are less common in adults (Fig. 33-2).[45,46] These lesions tend to develop over pressure points (buttocks, knees, and elbows) and can be complicated by ulceration of the overlying skin. Once the calcinosis appears, treatment is very difficult. Colchicine, probenecid, warfarin, and phosphate buffers have been tried with limited success. Surgery may be performed, but the lesions may recur or worsen.

ASSOCIATED MANIFESTATIONS

Cardiac

Conduction defects, arrhythmias, ventricular, and septal wall motion abnormalities, and reduced ejection fractions may be seen on electrocardiograms, echocardiography, and radionucleotide scintigraphy.[41,42,47–51] Nevertheless, most patients do not develop any cardiac symptoms. However, pericarditis, myocarditis, and congestive heart failure can occasionally develop secondary to involvement of cardiac muscle and may be lethal.

Pulmonary

Older epidemiological studies report interstitial lung disease (ILD) complicating approximately 10–20% of patients with DM, although many of these cases would likely be classified as ASyS nowadays.[41,42,52–59] Nonetheless, ILD can be seen in DM, particularly in patients with anti-MDA5 (melanoma differentiation antigen 5) antibodies. Rarely, patients develop bronchiolitis obliterans with organizing pneumonia. ILD manifests clinically as dyspnea and nonproductive cough. It can begin abruptly or insidiously and even precede the development of the characteristic rash and muscle weakness. Chest radiographs reveal a diffuse reticulonodular pattern with a predilection for involvement at the lung bases. A diffuse alveolar pattern or ground-glass appearance is seen in the more fulminant cases.[52] A restrictive defect with reduced forced vital capacity and decreased diffusion capacity are evident on pulmonary function tests. A less common pulmonary complication is ventilatory muscle weakness, but it does occur. Furthermore, aspiration pneumonia can be a complication of oropharyngeal and esophageal weakness.

Gastrointestinal

Involvement of the skeletal and smooth muscles of the gastrointestinal tract can lead to dysphagia, aspiration, and delayed gastric emptying. Vasculopathy affecting the gastrointestinal tract is a serious complication that appears to be much more common in juvenile DM compared to adult DM. The vasculopathy can result in mucosal ulceration, perforation, and life-threatening hemorrhage.

Joints

Arthralgias of large and small joints with or without arthritis are common. Joint and muscle pain often eases when the limbs are flexed, and this can lead to the formation of flexion contractures across the major joints. This emphasizes the importance of early physical therapy and range-of-motion exercises to prevent contractures from developing. Flexion contractures at the ankles leading to toe walking are a common early finding in childhood DM.

Vasculopathy

A vasculopathy affects the skin, muscle, and gastrointestinal system. Ulcerations and gangrene of digits can be seen, particularly in anti-MDA5 cases. Rarely, massive muscle infarction can lead to myoglobinuria and acute renal tubular necrosis.

Malignancy

There is an increased incidence of cancer ranging from 6% to 45% in DM.[34,35,41,42,59,60] More recent epidemiological studies suggest the risk is closer to 12% within the first 2–3 years in adults. Among patients with cancer-associated DM the risk is highest in patients with anti–TIF1-γ antibodies and to a

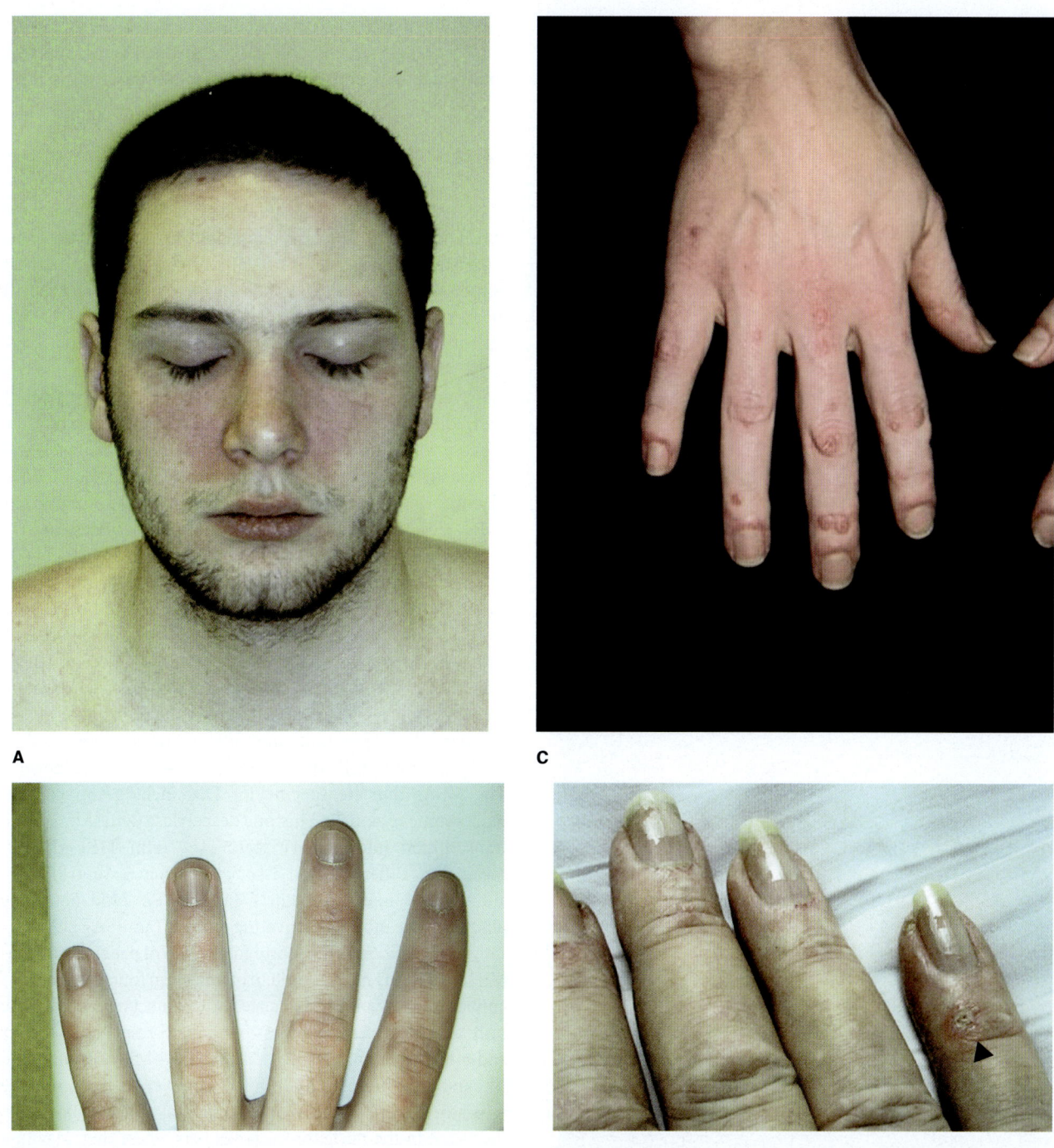

Figure 33-1. Dermatomyositis. Moderate erythematous rash is appreciated along the hairline of the scalp, the malar region of the face, and the eyelids—later the heliotrope rash (**A**). Macular erythematous rash is seen over the extensor surface of the knuckles (Gottron sign) (**B**). Gottron papules are the papular lesions seen here on the knuckles (**C**). Dilated capillary loops are evident in the nail bed changes as well as a small ulceration involving the distal aspect of the little finger (**D**).

lesser extent in those with anti-NXP and anti-SAE antibodies (see Laboratory section below).[61] The association with cancer has not been demonstrated in juvenile DM and the increased risk is predominantly seen in adults over the age of 40 years. Although women are more likely to develop DM than men, the risk of malignancy is equal in both sexes. Most malignancies are identified within 2 years of the presentation of the myositis. The clinical severity of rash or muscle weakness does not appear to correlate with the presence or absence of a neoplasm. Treatment of the underlying malignancy sometimes results in improvement of muscle strength.

We perform a comprehensive history and annual physical examination with breast and pelvic examinations for women and testicular and prostate examinations for men to

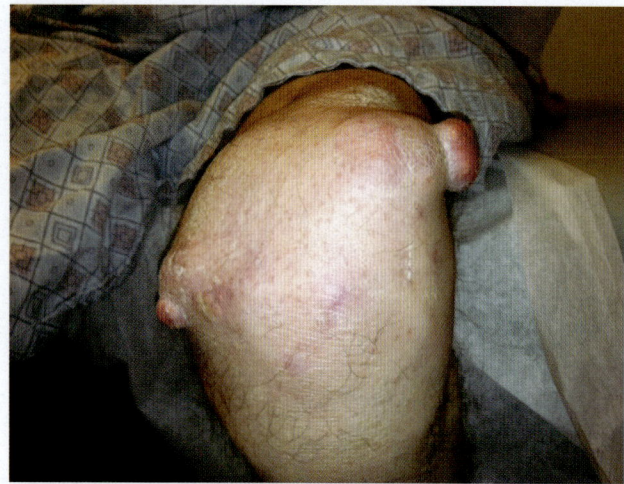

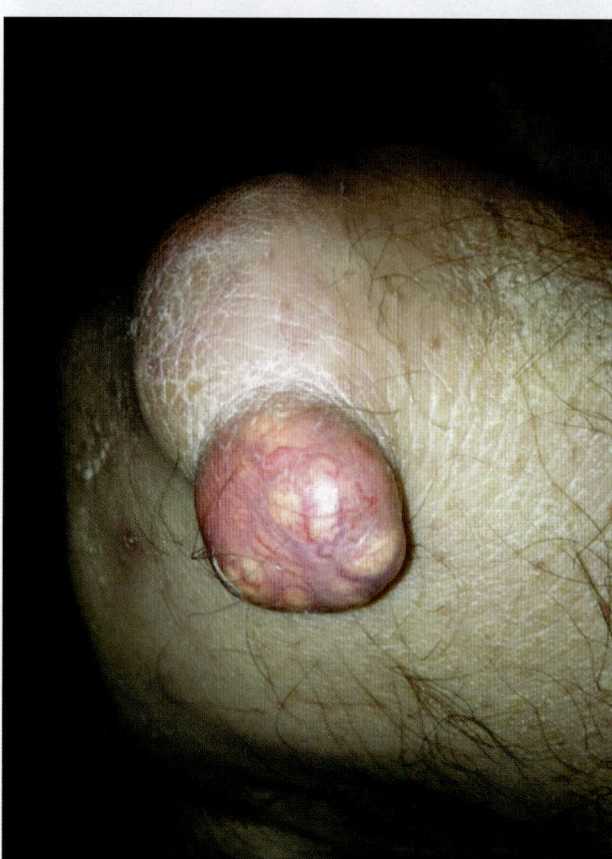

Figure 33-2. Calcinosis. This adult patient, who had under treated juvenile dermatomyositis as a child, has severe calcinosis on the medial and lateral aspects of the left knee (**A**); lateral lesion is seen at higher magnification (**B**).

search for an underlying malignancy. In addition, we obtain a complete blood count (CBC), routine blood chemistries, urinalysis, and stool specimens for occult blood. We order computerized tomographic (CT) scans of the chest, abdomen, and pelvis (PET/CT for patients with anti–TIF1-γ antibodies, see below), and mammography. Colonoscopy should be done on all patients over the age of 50 years or in those who have attributable gastrointestinal symptoms (e.g., abdominal pain, constipation, or blood in the stool).

LABORATORY FEATURES

Necrosis of muscle fibers usually leads to increased serum creatine kinase (CK), aldolase, myoglobin, lactate dehydrogenase, aspartate aminotransferase (AST), and alanine aminotransferase (ALT) levels. Serum CK is the most sensitive and specific marker for muscle damage and is elevated in at least 90% of patients with DM.[34,41,42] However, serum CK levels do not correlate with the severity of weakness. The CK level can be normal even in individuals who are markedly weak, particularly in childhood DM, in patients with slow, insidious disease, and in those with little residual muscle mass. In approximately 10% of cases with a normal CK, the aldolase level is elevated.[62–64] Erythrocyte sedimentation rate (ESR) is usually normal or only mildly elevated and is not a reliable indicator of disease severity.

Antinuclear antibodies (ANAs) are detected in 24%–60% of patients with DM.[41,57,58] These antibodies are much more common in patients with overlap syndromes (to be discussed later). Some patients have the so-called "myositis-specific antibodies" (MSAs; Table 33-5).[1,6,57,58,65–90] Recent studies have shown that these myositis autoantibodies accumulate in the same subcellular compartment as the autoantigen inside myofibers.[91,92] These autoantibodies may not only be diagnostic and prognostic biomarkers but may also be pathogenic. The MSAs that are specific for DM include anti–complex nucleosome remodeling histone deacetylase (anti–Mi-2), anti–transcription intermediary factor 1-γ (anti–TIF1-γ), anti–melanoma differentiation-associated gene 5 (anti-MDA5), anti–nuclear matrix protein 2 (anti-NXP2), and anti–small ubiquitin-like modifier activating enzyme (anti-SAE).[6,57,58,67–74]

Mi-2 antibodies are found in 15–20% of patients with DM. Mi-2 is a 240-kD nuclear protein of unknown function. The Mi-2 antibodies are typically associated with an acute onset, a florid rash, and prominent weakness but a good response to therapy and a favorable prognosis.[6,57,58,67–71,74] Anti-Mi2 autoantibodies recognize the nuclear Mi2/NuRD complex, a transcriptional repressor. Recent studies demonstrate that these antibodies are deposited in the nuclei of the myofibers where they may bind to this complex and inhibit its function.[91,92] Antibodies directed against melanoma differentiation-association protein 5 (anti-MDA5), also known as anti–CADM-140 antibodies, are found in 10–20% of DM patients and up to 65% of patients with clinically amyopathic DM with palmar rash and papules along with severe skin ulcerations from ischemia, and rapidly progressive ILD.[75–80] Anti-MDA5 antibody levels closely correlate with the severity of skin ulcerations, ILD, and disease prognosis.

Autoantibodies targeting transcriptional intermediary factor 1-γ (TIF1-γ), also known p155 antibodies, are found in adult cancer-associated DM with an 89% specificity and 70% sensitivity.[72,81–85,87] Particular vigilance for cancer is needed in DM patients with TIF1-γ antibodies. Patients with antibodies often have severe skin involvement and milder myositis.

▶ TABLE 33-5. AUTOANTIBODIES ASSOCIATED WITH INFLAMMATORY MYOPATHIES

Antisynthetase Autoantibodies	Autoantigen	Clinical Features
Anti–Jo-1	Histidyl t-RNA synthetase	PM, DM + ILD, Raynaud, arthritis, mechanic hands
Anti–PL-7	Threonyl t-RNA synthetase	PM, DM + ILD. Raynaud, arthritis, mechanic hands
Anti–PL-12	Alanyl t-RNA synthetase	ILD > PM, DM
Anti-EJ	Glycyl t-RNA synthetase	PM > DM + ILD. Raynaud, arthritis, mechanic hands
Anti-OJ	Isoleucyl t-RNA synthetase	ILD + PM/DM, Raynaud, arthritis, mechanic hands
Anti-KS	Asparaginyl t-RNA synthetase	ILD > PM, DM, Raynaud, arthritis, mechanic hands
Anti-Zo	Phenylalanyl t-RNA synthetase	ILD + PM, DM, Raynaud, arthritis, mechanic hands
Anti-Ha	Tyrosyl t-RNA synthetase	ILD + PM, DM, Raynaud, arthritis, mechanic hands
Dermatomyositis Autoantibodies		
Anti–Mi-2	Chromatin remodeling enzyme	Severe skin disease, treatment responsive
Anti–MDA5	Melanoma differentiation-associated gene 5	ILD, palmar lesions, rash > myopathy
Anti–TIF1 γ	Transcriptional intermediary factor 1 γ	Cancer-associated dermatomyositis
Anti-NXP2	Nuclear matrix protein	Severe muscle weakness
Anti-SAE	Small ubiquitin-like modifier-activating enzyme	Rapidly progressive, ILD, rash > myopathy
IMNM Autoantibodies		
Anti-SRP	Signal recognition particle	Severe, treatment-resistant, myopathy, cardiac involvement
Anti-HMGCR	HMGCR	Severe myopathy that continues despite stopping statin
Inclusion Body Myositis Autoantibody		
Anti-cN1A/anti-Mup44	Cytosolic 5′-nucleotidase	Inclusion body myositis

PM, polymyositis; DM, dermatomyositis; ILD, interstitial lung disease; HMGCR, HMG-CoA reductase; cN1A, cytosolic 5′-nucleotidase.
Reproduced with permission from Ciafaloni E, Chinnery P, Griggs R. *Evaluation and Treatment of Myopathies*. 2nd ed. Oxford University Press; 2014.

Antibodies directed against nuclear matrix protein NXP2 (also known as MORC3) have been found in as many as 17% of patients with DM and are also associated calcinosis, subcutaneous edema, distal weakness, and cancer.[86,88,89]

Anti-SAE antibodies have been reported in 1.5–8% of DM with a frequency of cancer in 14–57%.[90,93] Most patients manifest with a skin rash alone and CK if often normal, but aldolase elevated in around a third of patients. In contrast to, ILD can also be seen in anti-SAE DM, but unlike anti-MDA5 amyopathic DM the ILD is usually mild.[93]

Magnetic resonance imaging (MRI) can provide information on the pattern of muscle involvement by looking at the cross-sectional area of axial and limb muscles.[94–99] MRI may demonstrate signal abnormalities in affected muscles secondary to inflammation and edema or replacement by fibrotic tissue. However, the changes on MRI are not usually specific for myositis. Some have advocated MRI as a method to guide which muscle to biopsy.[97] However, we have found that MRI usually adds little to a good clinical examination and electromyography (EMG) in defining the pattern of muscle involvement and determining the muscle for biopsy.

ELECTROPHYSIOLOGICAL FEATURES

The characteristic EMG abnormalities observed in patients with myositis include (1) increased insertional and spontaneous activity with fibrillation potentials, positive sharp waves, and occasionally pseudomyotonic discharges (e.g., decrescendo waves of positive waves that do not wax or wane in frequency and amplitude) or complex repetitive discharges; (2) small-duration, low-amplitude, polyphasic motor unit action potentials (MUAPs); and (3) MUAPs that recruit early but at normal frequencies.[100] Recruitment may also be decreased (fast firing MUAPs) in advanced disease, if there is marked loss of muscle fibers. Decreased insertional activity may be seen in chronic disease secondary to fibrosis. In addition, long-duration, polyphasic MUAPs may also be evident later in longstanding disease due to muscle fiber splitting and regeneration rather than a superimposed neurogenic process.

The degree of abnormal spontaneous EMG activity reflects the ongoing disease activity. EMG can be used to assist determining which muscle to biopsy in patients with only mild weakness. In addition, EMG may also be useful in the assessment of previously responsive patients with myositis who become weaker by differentiating an increase in disease activity from weakness secondary to type 2 muscle fiber atrophy from disuse or chronic steroid administration. Abnormal insertional and spontaneous activity is expected in active myositis, while isolated type 2 muscle fiber atrophy is not associated with such abnormal activity on EMG. Along these lines, it is our opinion that a multifocal or diffuse pattern of abnormal insertional and spontaneous activity without obvious changes in MUAP morphology or recruitment is much more likely to represent an acute myopathy, like DM, than a neurogenic disorder.

HISTOPATHOLOGY

The pathological process is multifocal, and the frequency and severity of histological abnormalities can vary within the muscle biopsy specimens. The pathognomonic histological feature is perifascicular atrophy (Fig. 33-3A), although this is a late finding and in our experience is found in <50% of adult-onset cases (it is somewhat more frequent in juvenile-onset DM). The perifascicular area contains small regenerating and degenerating fibers. Oxidative enzyme stains highlight the microvacuolation within these fibers. Combined COX/SDH stain may demonstrate COX-negative/SDH-positive staining perifascicular muscle fibers (Fig. 33-3B). Scattered necrotic fibers and much less frequently, wedge-shaped microinfarcts may be evident. Even though DM is an IIM, inflammatory cell infiltrates are not evident with routine histochemistry in some patients. The inflammatory infiltrate is composed primarily of macrophages, B cells, and CD4+ cells in the perivascular and perimysial regions around blood vessels (perivascular).[39,101] These CD4+ cells are mainly plasmacytoid dendritic cells (PDCs) and not T-helper cells as they are often CD3 negative.[102] Importantly, in contrast to PM, ASyS, IMNM, and IBM (discussed later), invasion of nonnecrotic fibers is not prominent. Immunohistochemistry (IHC) staining demonstrates that muscle fibers express MHC-1 antigen, STAT1, and various interferon-α/β inducible proteins, including myxovirus resistance 1 (MxA) and ISG15 on the sarcolemma, particularly in the perifascicular regions (Fig. 33-4), and can be seen even before the development of perifascicular atrophy.[102–106] However, there is no overexpression of interferon-gamma inducible proteins on muscle fibers.

DM is associated with a reduction in the capillary density (number of capillaries per area of muscle) and compensatory dilation of the remaining small vessels.[107] One of the earliest demonstrable histological abnormalities in DM is deposition of the C5b-9 complement membrane attack complex (MAC) around small blood vessels (Fig. 33-5).[107–109] Deposition of MAC precedes inflammatory cell infiltration and other structural abnormalities (e.g., perifascicular atrophy) in the muscle on light microscopy and is relatively specific for DM.[107] Other complement components (C3 and C9) and immunoglobulins (IgM and less often IgG) are also deposited on or around the walls of intramuscular blood vessels.[110] These observations have led to the hypothesis that DM is caused by deposition of immunoglobulins on capillaries, subsequent activation of complement, and MAC-induced necrosis of the vessels, which then lead to ischemic damage of muscle. However, as discussed in section "Pathogenesis," this hypothesis is purely speculative, and DM is currently felt to be a type 1 interferonopathy. In addition to expression of MxA on muscle fibers, MxA also is expressed on capillaries in DM (Fig. 33-4).

Electron microscopy (EM) reveals small intramuscular blood vessels (arterioles and capillaries) with endothelial hyperplasia, microvacuoles, and tubuloreticular cytoplasmic inclusions.[111,112] Notably, tubuloreticular inclusions in endothelial and other cells have long been found to be induced by type 1 intereferons.[113]

A few studies have been conducted comparing histopathological abnormalities between various subtypes of DM based on MSAs. A large study from Japan reported anti–TIF1-γ was associated with vacuolated/punched out perifascicular muscle fibers and more likely expression of MHC-1; anti–Mi-2 with prominent muscle fiber damage (perifascicular necrosis and atrophy, inflammatory cell infiltration, increased perimysial alkaline phosphatase activity, and sarcolemmal MAC deposition; anti-MDA5 with scattered/diffuse staining pattern of MxA staining with less muscle fiber damage and inflammatory cell infiltrate; anti-NXP2 with more evidence of microinfarction); and anti-SAE and seronegative DM with HLA-DR expression.[114] A North American study also found that anti–Mi-2 cases had more inflammatory cell infiltrate; anti–TIF1-γ was associated with more

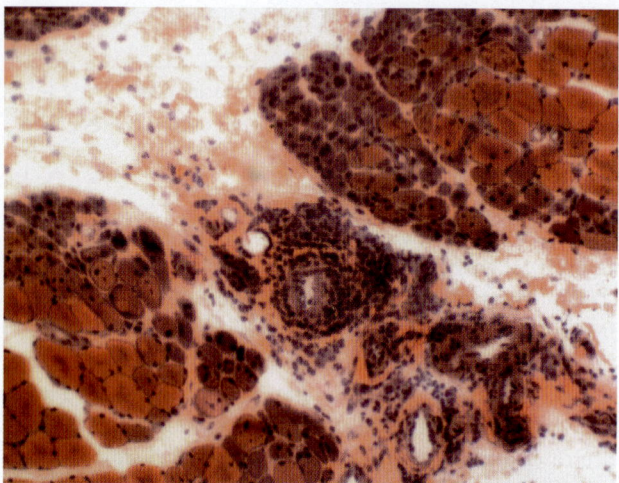

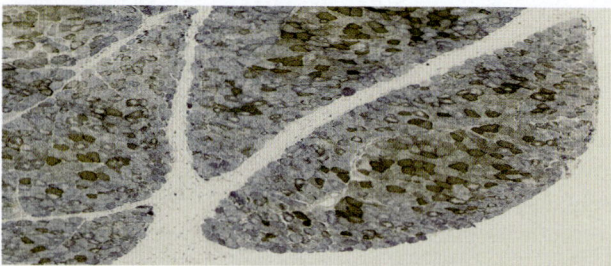

Figure 33-3. Dermatomyositis. Muscle biopsy demonstrates classic perifascicular atrophy of muscle fibers and perivascular inflammation within the perimysium (**A**), hematoxylin and eosin (H&E). Combined cytochrome oxidase/succinic dehydrogenase (COX/SDH) stain demonstrates COX-negative/SDH-positive staining of perifascicular muscle fibers (**B**).

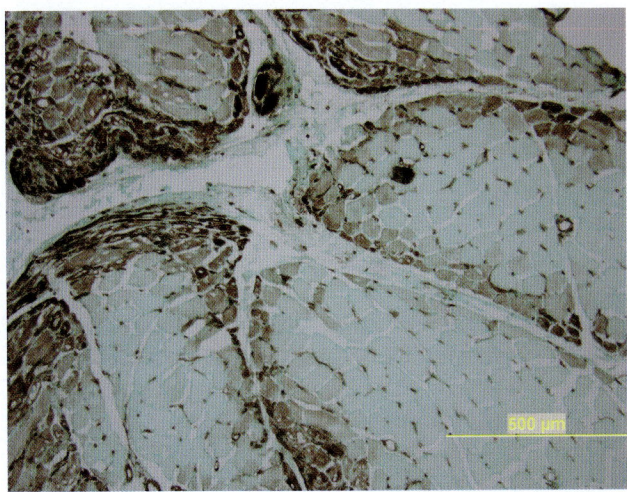

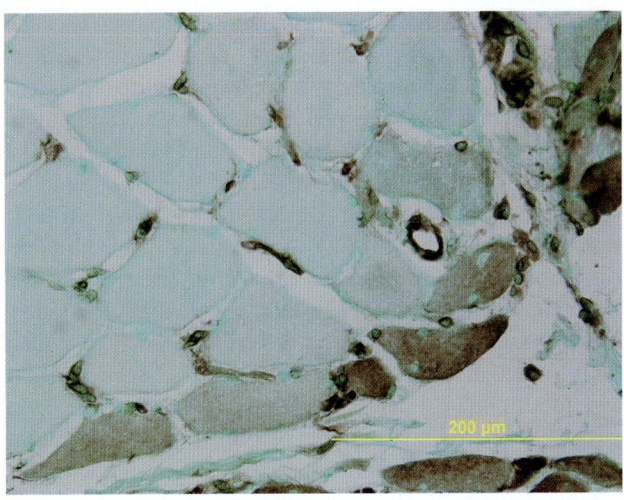

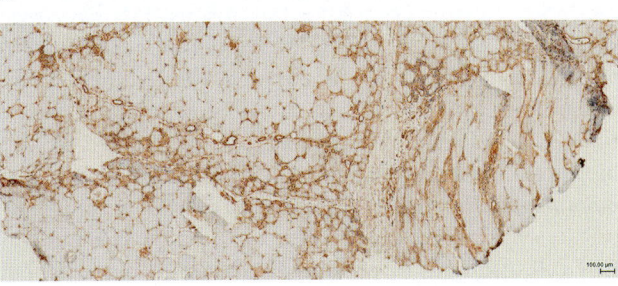

Figure 33-4. Dermatomyositis. Immunoperoxidase stain reveals the expression of the interferon-α/β-inducible myxovirus resistance 1 (MxA) protein on perifascicular muscle fibers (**A**) as well as small arterioles and capillaries (**B**). There is also increased expression of major histocompatibility antigen 1 (MHC1) on the perifascicular muscle fibers (**C**). Note that MHC1 is not normally expressed on muscle fibers but is normally expressed on blood vessels.

mitochondrial abnormalities (perifascicular COX negative fibers); and anti-NXP2 had less inflammatory cell infiltrate.[115]

PATHOGENESIS

Previously, DM was felt to be caused by a complement mediated microangiopathy, but recent research suggests that this is not the case.[116] The prevailing hypothesis now is that DM is a type 1 interferonopathy.[102–106,117,118] Although the presence of MAC is well established, its frequency is not, and this is important with regard to the possibility of varied mechanisms of disease and distinct subtypes of DM. Its presence on blood vessels could be due to complement activation by either the classical antibody-mediated or alternative pathways. Even classical pathway activation, which is antibody dependent, can still be relatively antigen nonspecific; some IgM antibodies are highly polyclonal, binding with low avidity to many self-antigens. The specificity of MAC presence is also in question, as it is present in abnormal vascular tissue (e.g., atherosclerotic coronary arteries). It may be that the microvasculature is damaged by some other mechanism (e.g., interferon or other cytokine-related toxicity), and the deposition of immunoglobulins and complement on the damaged vascular tissue might be a secondary phenomenon. That some individuals have developed DM with hereditary complement deficiencies argues against primary destruction of capillaries by complement and MAC.[119,120]

The microangiopathy has been postulated to cause ischemic damage and occasionally infarction of muscle fibers. It has been suggested that the perifascicular atrophy is the result of hypoperfusion to the watershed region of muscle fascicles. However, it has never been demonstrated that the perifascicular region is indeed the watershed area in muscle fibers and that perifascicular fibers are more prone to ischemic damage.[121] Perifascicular atrophy and endomysial capillary MAC deposition were found, in one study, to be inversely

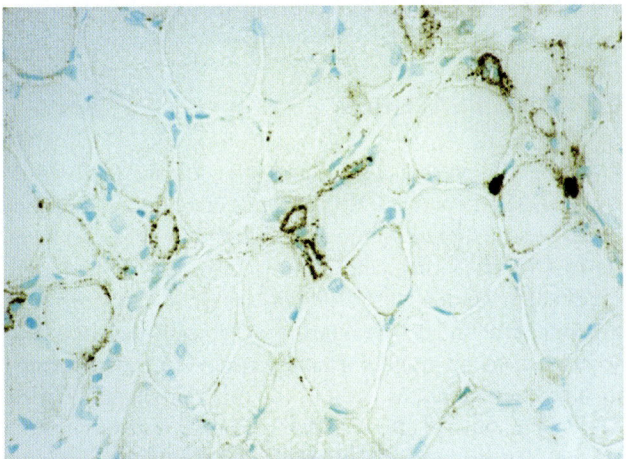

Figure 33-5. Dermatomyositis. Immunoperoxidase stain demonstrates deposition of membrane attack complex (MAC) around small blood vessels and capillaries.

correlated,[108] and another study found no correlation between perifascicular atrophy and capillary depletion.[107] Furthermore, perifascicular atrophy has not been reported in vasculitis, a condition with known muscle ischemia and infarction, nor has perifascicular atrophy been found in experimental models of skeletal muscle ischemia.[121] In another model of ischemic myopathy, resulting from micro arterial embolization with particles 20–80 m in diameter, the pathological changes were located centrally within fascicles and the perifascicular regions were instead preferentially spared.[122] Finally, perifascicular atrophy is not evident in ischemic muscle in animal models when muscle is rendered ischemic from vasculitis or other small vessel injury.

Gene microarray studies of biopsied muscle tissue demonstrate an increased expression of genes induced by type 1 interferons.[102,123,124] Although this is not specific, it is compatible with the hypothesis of a viral infection triggering the autoimmune attack as interferons have a well-defined role in antiviral innate immunity. However, there are other possibilities. Type 1 interferons (i.e., interferon-α and interferon-β) are synthesized by PDCs in response to a serum factor(s) containing immune complexes of antibody, double-stranded DNA, or RNA viruses. Abundant PDCs are evident in the muscle biopsies of patients with DM.[102] PDCs are CD4+ and comprise a large component of the inflammatory cell infiltrate in DM. These CD4+ cells were originally thought to be CD4+ T-helper cells, but it was subsequently demonstrated that most are CD3−. Therefore, these CD4+ cells are predominantly PDCs and not lymphocytes. Increased expression of the type 1 interferon inducible protein MxA is evident on blood vessels and muscle fibers (with a predilection for the perifascicular fibers). Interestingly, one postulated function of MxA is to form tubuloreticular inclusions around RNA viruses. These inclusions have the same morphology as the tubuloreticular inclusions seen on EM in blood vessels in DM. Using immunoelectron microscopy, MxA was demonstrated within inclusions in vessels in DM muscle biopsies.[102] As previously mentioned, tubular reticular inclusions can be induced in endothelial cells when exposed to type 1 interferon. Interestingly, increased expression of type 1 interferon regulated genes are also evident in the peripheral blood and on skin biopsies of patients with active DM, like what has been described in systemic lupus erythematosus (SLE). Further, expression levels in the blood appear to correlate with disease activity. A recent study reported a toxic autocrine effect of type 1 interferon on muscle stem cells that was blocked by interferon-1 inhibition.[118,124] Given the recent advances in the field, we suspect that dysregulated interferon-β production plays a major role in the pathogenesis of DM and could be directly toxic to the small blood vessels and muscle fibers themselves.

PROGNOSIS

In the absence of malignancy, prognosis is generally favorable in patients with DM. Poor prognostic features are increased age, associated ILD, cardiac disease, and late or previous inadequate treatment with 5-year survival rates ranging from 70% to 93%.[42,67,125,126]

▶ POLYMYOSITIS

PM, as reported in the literature, is a heterogeneous group of disorders rather than a distinct entity. A major source of debate among clinicians who primarily take care of patients with PM (e.g., neurologists and rheumatologists) is the criteria for diagnosing PM. The most commonly employed criteria were developed by Bohan and Peter in 1975,[33,34] but these do not take into account advancements in our understanding of the immunopathogenesis of the various inflammatory myopathies or even the existence of IBM, IMNM, and ASyS. Revised criteria for the various IIMs have been proposed (Tables 33-2 and 33-3). For definitive histopathological diagnosis of PM, some have advocated the requirement of seeing CD8+ T cells invading *nonnecrotic* muscle fibers that express MHC-1 antigen.[4,5,37,39,101] Even so, this biopsy feature is not diagnostic for PM, as most cases that demonstrate this finding are in fact IBM. More frequently on biopsy we appreciate perivascular/perimysial inflammatory cell infiltrates or endomysial inflammatory cells, but no actual invasion on nonnecrotic muscle fibers.[12,38] Such perivascular, perimysial inflammation is common, particularly in patients with DM, ASyS, overlap syndromes with myositis, IBM and, occasionally, in dystrophies.

For the various reasons listed above, it is impossible to extract from the literature the true incidence and prognosis of PM or its subtypes and the associated laboratory abnormalities, medical conditions [e.g., connective tissue disorder (CTD), ILD, myocarditis, and cancer]. We need prospective studies using contemporary clinical, laboratory, and histopathological criteria for PM to address these issues. Nevertheless, we will summarize the available literature regarding "PM."

CLINICAL FEATURES

PM generally presents in patients over the age of 20 years. Unlike DM, idiopathic PM in absence of an underlying connective tissue disease is rare in childhood in our experience. As in DM and other autoimmune disorders, PM is more prevalent in women.[23–35,41,42] Patients present with symmetric proximal arm and leg weakness that typically develops over several weeks or months. Distal muscles may also become involved but are not as weak as the more proximal muscles. Muscle pain and tenderness are frequently noted, but these are not the primary symptoms—weakness is the primary complaint. Old series have reported as many as one-third of patients complaining of swallowing difficulties, though many of these cases may have been unrecognized IBM. Mild facial weakness occasionally may be demonstrated on examination. Sensation is normal and muscle stretch reflexes are usually preserved.

ASSOCIATED MANIFESTATIONS

The cardiac and pulmonary complications of PM are reportedly similar to that described in the DM section. Myositis with secondary congestive heart failure or conduction abnormalities occur in up to one-third of patients, but again histopathological confirmation of definite PM using more up-to-date criteria is lacking in most of these studies.[41,42,47–51] ILD has been reported to occur in at least 10% of patient with PM, but most have had antisynthetase antibodies.[41,52–55,57,58,69] So, it is really unclear if or how many patients with "PM" develop myocarditis or ILD. Likewise, polyarthritis has been reported in as many as 45% of patients with PM at the time of diagnosis, but this is a common sign as well in patients with ASyS.[42] The risk of malignancy with PM seems to be lower than that seen in DM but is slightly higher than expected in the general population.[35,42,60]

LABORATORY FEATURES

Serum CK level is elevated fivefold or more in most PM cases.[34,35,41,42] Unlike DM and IBM (to be discussed later) in which the CK can be normal, the serum CK should be elevated in active PM. Serum CK can be useful in monitoring response to therapy, but only in conjunction with the physical examination, as the CK level does not necessarily correlate with the degree of weakness. ESR is normal in most patients and does not correlate with disease activity or severity. Positive ANAs are reportedly present in 16–40% of patients with PM.[34,41,42,57]

MRI may demonstrate T2 signal abnormalities in affected muscles secondary to inflammation and edema or T1 abnormalities as a result of replacement by fibrotic tissue (Fig. 33-6).[94–97]

ELECTROPHYSIOLOGICAL FEATURES

EMG is usually abnormal in PM with increased insertional and spontaneous activity, small polyphasic MUAPs, and early recruitment.[100] These abnormal features do not distinguish PM from other inflammatory myopathies or myopathies with muscle membrane instability.

HISTOPATHOLOGY

The histological features of PM are distinct from DM. The predominant histological features in PM are variability in fiber size, scattered necrotic and regenerating fibers, and inflammatory cell infiltrates. However, as mentioned previously, the specific characteristics of this inflammatory cell infiltrate have been the subject of recent debate. Small studies of PM reported that muscle biopsies demonstrate CD8+ T cells and macrophages invading nonnecrotic muscle fibers expressing MHC-1 antigen (Fig. 33-7).[39,101] Subsequently, some have suggested that this histopathological feature is required for the diagnosis of definite PM.[5,37] However, other authorities argue that invasion of nonnecrotic muscle fibers is not necessary and perivascular, perimysial, or endomysial inflammation without actual invasion of nonnecrotic muscle fibers can suffice for the diagnosis of PM in the proper

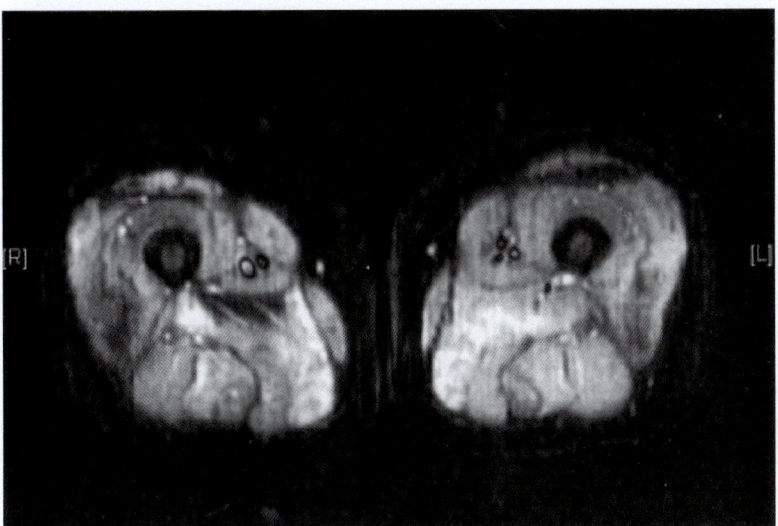

Figure 33-6. Polymyositis. Skeletal muscle MRI (STIR image) reveals patchy areas of increased signal consistent with edema/inflammation in the semitendinosus and semimembranosus in the posterior thigh and to a lesser extent in the quadriceps muscles on both legs.

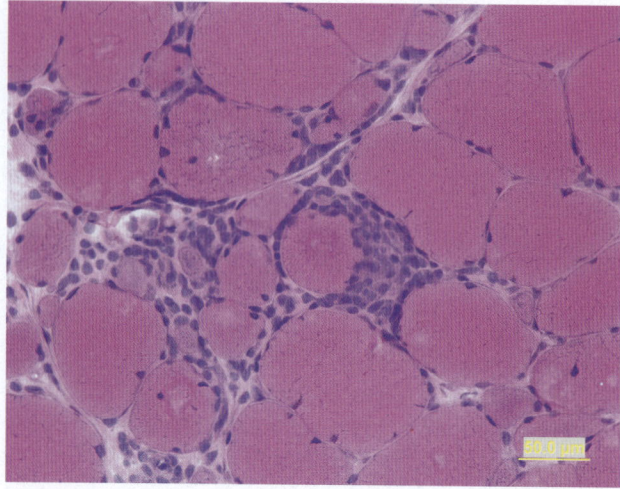

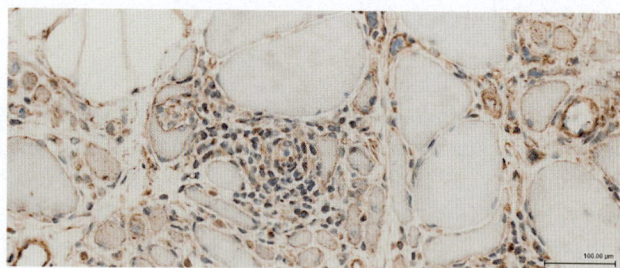

Figure 33-7. Polymyositis. Muscle biopsy demonstrates endomysial mononuclear inflammatory cell infiltrate surrounding and invading nonnecrotic muscle fibers, H&E (**A**). Immunoperoxidase stain demonstrates perivascular and endomysial inflammatory cells surrounding and appearing to invade nonnecrotic muscle fibers expressing major histocompatibility antigen type 1 (MHC1) on the sarcolemma (**B**).

clinical context.[66,127] Importantly, invasion of nonnecrotic muscle fibers is not diagnostic for PM and most patients with this histopathological feature have IBM as will be discussed later.

The endomysial inflammatory cells consist primarily of activated CD8+ (cytotoxic), *alpha, and beta* T cells and macrophages.[39,101,129] Rare cases of PM with CD4- and CD8-*gamma/delta* T-cell infiltrates have been reported.[130–132] The T-cell receptors of endomysial T cells have an oligoclonal pattern of gene rearrangements and a restricted motif in the CD3R region, suggesting that the immune response is antigen specific.[133,134] Further, there are many myeloid dendritic cells in the endomysium that appear to surround nonnecrotic muscle fibers and may serve to present antigens to cytotoxic T cells. Although B cells are rare, plasma cells are common in the endomysium and likely account for the increased expression of immunoglobulin genes on microarray experiments.[135] There is also evidence of oligoclonal pattern of gene rearrangements in plasma cells in PM muscle biopsies. MAC, complement, or immunoglobulins are not deposited on the microvasculature in PM as the may be seen in DM.

PATHOGENESIS

PM is believed to be the result of an HLA-restricted, antigen-specific, cell-mediated immune response directed against muscle fibers. The trigger of this autoimmune attack is not known, but viral infections have been speculated. However, there is no conclusive evidence supporting this hypothesis.[136] MHC-1 molecules on the surface of cells usually express endogenous self-peptides rather than viral particles. Neither viral proteins nor DNA have been identified in muscle fibers. Thus, the autoimmune response may be directed against endogenous self-antigens rather than processed viral antigens. Nonetheless, a viral infection could indirectly trigger an immune response secondary to antigenic mimicry with muscle proteins, altering the expression of proteins on the surface of muscle fibers such that these become antigenic, or by the loss of physiological self-tolerance. Myositis may complicate human immunodeficiency virus (HIV) and human T-lymphocyte virus-1 (HTLV-1) infections (discussed in a subsequent section in this chapter). In these cases, the myositis appears to be the result of such indirect triggering of the immune response against muscle fibers.

The cytotoxic T cells appear to destroy muscle fibers via the perforin pathway. These autoinvasive T cells contain perforin granules oriented next to the sarcolemma of muscle fibers.[137] Upon release of these granules by exocytosis, pore formations are induced on the sarcolemma, leading to osmolysis of muscle fibers.

DIFFERENTIAL DIAGNOSIS

A diagnosis of PM relies on a thorough search to exclude other causes of weakness (Table 33-6). A detailed clinical examination of an appreciation of the pattern of weakness can help differentiate IBM and muscular dystrophies with inflammation from PM. MSAs should be sought to exclude other inflammatory myopathies. Serum CK should be elevated in PM, while it is normal in patients with "fibromyalgia" and polymyalgia rheumatica (PMR) and can be normal in IBM. Skeletal muscle MRI is often interpreted as showing "myositis." However, these increased signal abnormalities are not specific and can be seen in dystrophies, rhabdomyolysis from toxic medications (e.g., statins) metabolic myopathy, and muscle infarcts from various causes (e.g., vasculitis and diabetic vasculopathy). The specific pattern of muscle involvement and extensive fatty replacement in the absence of edematous changes on MRI scans would be helpful, suggesting a dystrophy as opposed to PM. EMG can be useful, as the presence of diffuse myotonic discharges should lead to the consideration of proximal myotonic myopathy or late-onset Pompe disease—conditions that we have seen misdiagnosed as PM.

Importantly, the diagnosis of PM requires a muscle biopsy and the lack of MSAs associated with DM, ASyS, IMNM, and IBM. It is important to look for histopathological features that would suggest IBM (e.g., rimmed vacuoles,

▶ **TABLE 33-6. DISORDERS THAT CAN RESEMBLE POLYMYOSITIS**

Inclusion body myositis
Dermatomyositis *sine* dermatitis
Necrotizing myopathy
Antisynthetase syndrome
Inflammatory myopathy associated with infections (e.g., HIV, HTLV-1, and hepatitis B and C)
Muscular dystrophies (e.g., facioscapulohumeral, congenital, dysferlinopathies, and other limb-girdle dystrophies) and late-onset congenital myopathies
Proximal myotonic myopathy (myotonic dystrophy type 2)
Amyloid myopathy (light chain or familial)
Metabolic and mitochondrial myopathies
Endocrine myopathies (e.g., hypothyroidism, hyperparathyroidism, and diabetic muscle infarction)
Drug-induced myopathies (e.g., cholesterol lowering agents, cyclosporine, chloroquine, amiodarone, colchicine, and D-penicillamine)
Juvenile or adult-onset spinal muscular atrophy (including Kennedy disease)
Polymyalgia rheumatica

HIV, human immunodeficiency virus; HTLV-1, human T-lymphocyte virus-1.
Reproduced with permission from Amato AA, Griggs RC. Unicorns, dragons, polymyositis, and other mythological beasts. *Neurology*. 2003;61(3):288–289.

inclusions, ragged red fibers, etc.). However, the absence of these findings does not exclude the diagnosis of IBM. Muscle biopsy is essential to look for features that might suggest a dystrophy, metabolic myopathy, or IMNM.

PROGNOSIS

Most patients with PM improve with immunotherapies but usually require life-long treatment.[41,67,125] Some retrospective studies suggest that PM does not respond to immunosuppressive agents as well as DM. However, interpretation of the results of these retrospective series is difficult, as the diagnosis of PM was usually made based on the Bohan and Peter criteria rather than on more up-to-date criteria based on strict clinical and histological criteria.

▶ **ANTISYNTHETASE SYNDROME**

CLINICAL FEATURES

The sine qua non of ASyS is the presence of an autoantibody to one of several aminoacyl transfer RNA synthetases (antisynthetase, anti-ARS), included anti–Jo-1 (histidyl), anti–PL-7 (threonyl), anti–PL-12 (alanyl), anti-EJ (glycyl), anti-OJ (isoleucyl), anti-KS (asparaginyl), anti-Ha (tyrosyl), and anti-Zo (phenylalanyl) antibodies.[6,14–16,36,56–58,138,139,140] ASyS is characterized by the presence of myositis, nonerosive arthritis, ILD, Raynaud phenomenon, mechanic hands, and fever associated with antibodies against aminoacyl-tRNA synthetase as noted above. Some patients have no myositis, but just ILD or other clinical features, so one can argue that these antibodies are not necessarily specific for myositis. Some studies have shown an increased severity of ILD in black patients and patients with anti–PL-7 and anti–PL-12 autoantibodies.[140] Notably, some patients can have an erythematous rash and muscle biopsies share histopathological features of DM, which likely accounts for many of these patients being classified as having DM. It has been suggested that the AS is associated with only a moderate response to treatment and a poor long-term prognosis though prognosis has not been studied in a prospective fashion.[67–69]

LABORATORY FEATURES

All patients have an antisynthetase antibodies the most common of which Jo-1 antibodies (directed against histidyl t-RNA synthetase). Jo-1 are demonstrated in as many as 20% of patients with IIM and over 7% of all cases of ASyS.[6,67–69] The other antisynthetases are much less common. As previously mentioned in the dermatomyositis section, these myositis autoantibodies may accumulate in the same subcellular compartment as the autoantigen inside myofibers and be directly pathogenic.[92] Serum CK level is elevated. MRI may demonstrate T2 signal abnormalities in affected muscles secondary to inflammation and edema or T1 abnormalities as a result of replacement by fibrotic tissue.

HISTOPATHOLOGY

Most studies of muscle histopathology have been on anti–Jo-1 cases as other antisynthetase antibodies are much less common, although some comparison studies exist.[139] Muscle biopsies demonstrate a predilection for inflammatory cell infiltrate in the perimysium and around blood vessels, perimysial fragmentation and staining with alkaline phosphatase, and similar to DM, there is perifascicular muscle fiber damage (Fig. 33-8). However, in ASyS there is more perifascicular muscle fiber necrosis that typically seen in DM in which perifascicular atrophy is more prominent.[138] HLA-DR, MHC-1, and MAC are often expressed on the sarcolemma of perifascicular of muscle fibers.[139] In contrast to DM, there much less likelihood of expression of MxA on muscle fibers or capillaries.[139,141]

PATHOGENESIS

The presence of HLA-DR expression on muscle fibers and absence of MxA expression suggests that the type II interferon pathway is involved in the pathogenesis of ASyS and not the type 1 interferon pathway as seen in DM.[139] Much more work needs to be done on unraveling the specific cause(s) and possible differences between those with different antibodies.

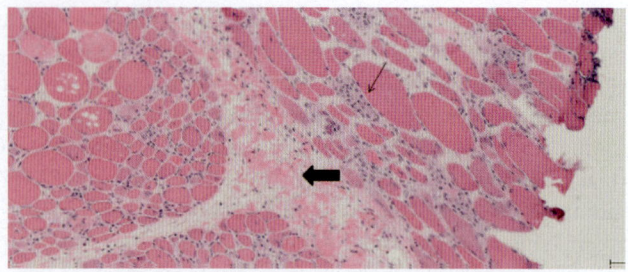
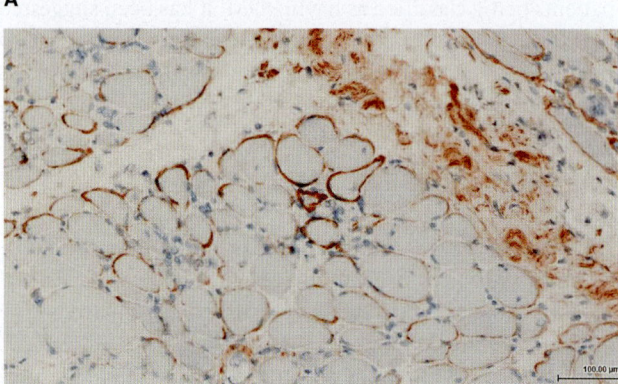
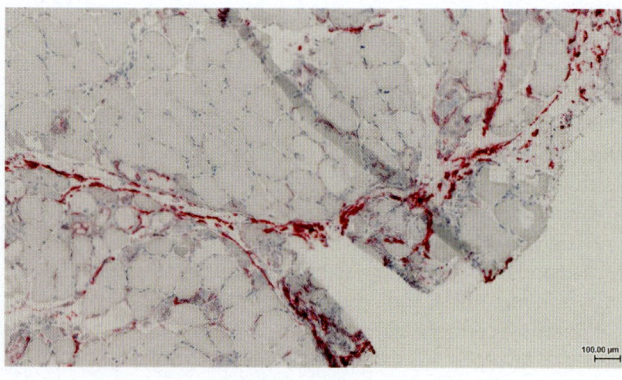

Figure 33-8. Antisynthetase syndrome (anti–Jo-1). Perifascicular/perimysial muscle fiber atrophy and necrosis (*thin arrow*) associated with perimysial connective tissue is edematous and fragmented in appearance (*thick arrow*) (**A**), H&E stain. The perimysial connective tissue intensely stains red with alkaline phosphatase stain (**B**). Immunostaining demonstrates deposition of membrane attack complex (MAC) deposits on the sarcolemma of nonnecrotic perifascicular muscle fibers (**C**).

▶ INCLUSION BODY MYOSITIS

CLINICAL FEATURES

IBM is characterized clinically by the insidious onset of slowly progressive proximal and distal weakness, which generally develops after the age of 40 years (and usually after 50 years) (Tables 33-1, 33-3, and 33-4).[1–4,10,13,142–149] IBM is the most common myopathy (apart from sarcopenia of aging) in patients over the age of 50 years. An increase in the diagnosis of IBM is likely based on improved awareness of the clinically pattern of muscle involvement, improved diagnostic tools (antibody detection and imaging), and identification of specific histopathological features.[150] A recent epidemiological study from Sweden reported a prevalence of 320 per 100,000 (190 per 100,000 women and 450 per 100,000 men) with an incidence of 25 per 100,000 per year.[151] Another study from the Mayo Clinic found the prevalence of IBM to be 18.20 per 100,000 people in adults over 50 years of age to be in Olmsted County, Minnesota, USA.[152] The slow progressive nature of the myopathy probably accounts in part for the delay in diagnosis that averages 5–7 years after the onset of symptoms. Men are much more commonly affected than women, in contrast to the female predominance seen in DM and PM.

The clinical hallmark of IBM is early weakness and atrophy of the quadriceps, flexor forearm muscles (i.e., wrist and finger flexors) (Fig. 33-9), and ankle dorsiflexors.[1–4,10,143–145] In a large retrospective series comparing various criteria for IBM, 97% of patients had finger flexors weaker that shoulder abductors by manual muscle strength testing, though quadriceps were weaker than hip flexors in less than 50%.[149] With manual muscle testing, the MRC grades of the finger and wrist flexors (in particular the deep finger flexors such as the flexor pollicis longus) are usually lower than those of the shoulder abductors, and the muscle scores of the knee extensors and ankle dorsiflexors may be the same or lower than those of the hip flexors in patients with IBM.[3,146–149] In contrast, the proximal muscles (shoulder abductors and hip flexors) are usually weaker than distal muscle groups by manual muscle testing grades in DM, PM, ASyS, and IMNM. In addition, muscle involvement in IBM is often asymmetric, in contrast to the symmetrical involvement in other inflammatory myopathies. The asymmetric involvement of muscle, not uncommonly, leads to the misdiagnosis of amyotrophic lateral sclerosis (ALS). However, the muscle groups affected early are different in IBM compared to ALS. Again, in IBM, there is an atrophy of the flexor forearm compartment, but the hand intrinsics (thenar and hypothenar eminence) are spared, in contrast to ALS in which atrophy in the upper limbs usually is first seen in the hand intrinsics. The presence of slowly progressive, asymmetric, quadriceps and wrist/finger flexor weakness, and atrophy in a patient over 50 years of age strongly suggests the diagnosis of IBM even in the absence of histological confirmation.[3,146–149] Although slowly progressive, IBM is very debilitating. Longitudinal studies have reported that 37% of patients used a wheelchair after 14 years,[145] while others have reported 47% of IBM patients being completely confined to a wheelchair after only 12 years.[144]

Swallowing difficulties develop in up to 60% of patients due to esophageal and pharyngeal muscle involvement. This can lead to weight loss or aspiration. In severe cases, cricopharyngeal myotomy may be beneficial.[143,149,153,154] We have

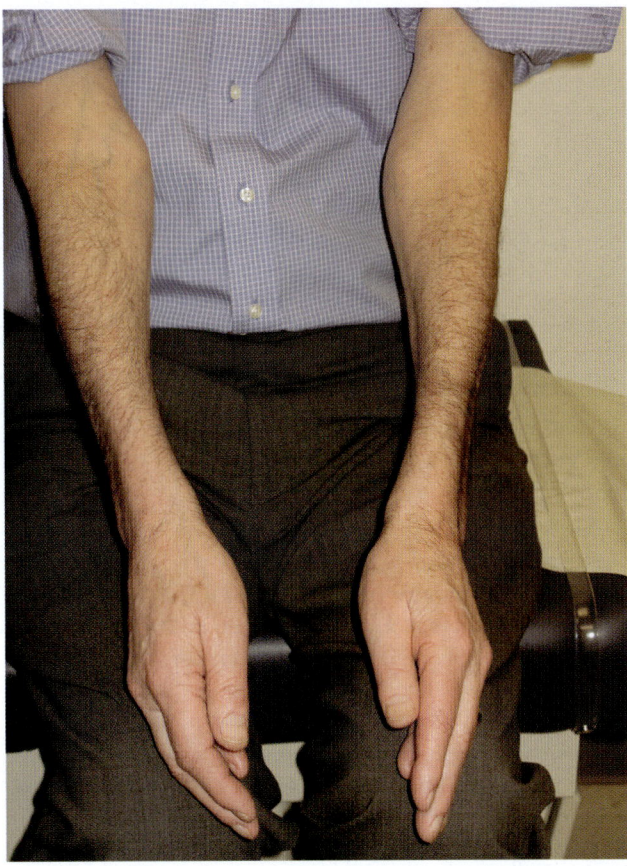 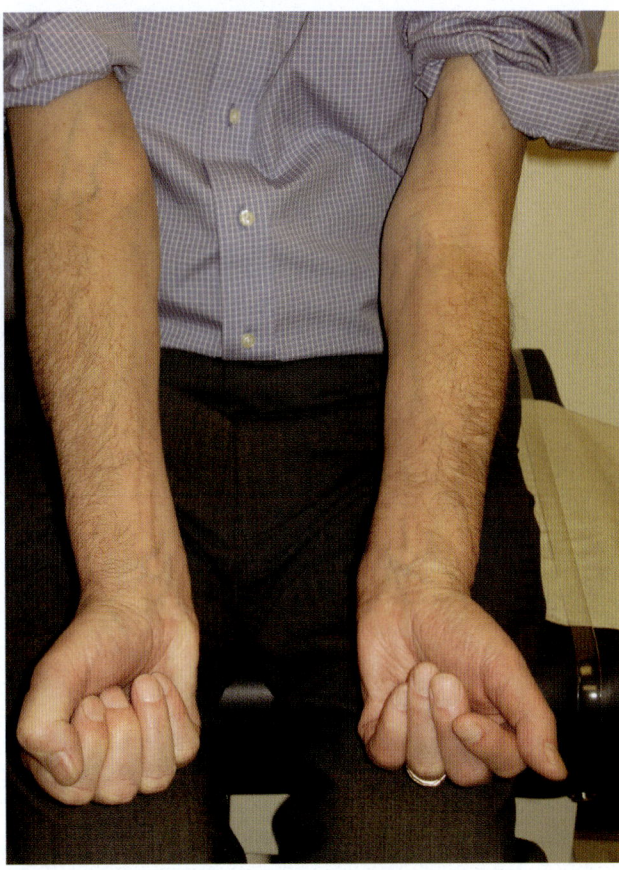

Figure 33-9. Inclusion body myositis. The clinical hallmark of IBM is early, and often asymmetric, atrophy flexor forearm muscles (**A**). This patient was asked to make a grip (flex the fingers) and one can see the asymmetrical weakness flexing the fingers of the left hand, particularly the deep finger flexors and flexor pollicis longus (**B**). (Reproduced with permission from Amato AA, Barohn RJ. Inclusion body myositis: old and new concepts. *J Neurol Neurosurg Psychiatry.* 2009;80(11):1186–1193. Figure 1.)

followed several patients in whom dysphagia was the presenting feature of the disease. Only after following patients for several years did they develop weakness in the extremities that are more characteristic of IBM. Mild facial weakness is evident in one-third of cases.[3,143] Rare patients may have severe facial diplegia.[1,155] In keeping with other inflammatory myopathies, neck flexor weakness is the rule, but some patients manifest with atypical features such as with head drop or bent spine syndrome/camptocormia owing to severe paraspinal muscle involvement.[156,157] Most patients have no sensory symptoms, but as many as 30% have evidence of a generalized sensory peripheral neuropathy on clinical examination and electrophysiological testing.[3] Muscle stretch reflexes are normal or slightly decreased. In particular, the patellar reflexes are lost early.

ASSOCIATED MANIFESTATIONS

IBM is not associated with myocarditis, lung disease, or an increased risk of malignancy. However, as many as 20% of patients with IBM have underlying autoimmune disorders such as Sjögren syndrome, SLE, scleroderma, sarcoidosis, variable immunoglobulin deficiency, or thrombocytopenia.[2,4,151,158]

LABORATORY FEATURES

Serum CK is normal or only mildly elevated (usually less than 10-fold above normal).[3,10,13,143] Positive ANAs and a monoclonal gammopathy of unclear significance are found in approximately 20% of patients with IBM. Antibodies directed against cytosolic 5′-nucleotidase 1 A (cN1A) have been detected in as many as two-thirds of IBM patients, whereas this antibody is very uncommon in other neuromuscular disorders.[159,160] Therefore, cN1A antibody testing may well be useful as a screening test to complement the clinical examination and muscle biopsy, particularly when not all the characteristic features of IBM are present clinically or on muscle biopsy. There is a significant incidence of the HLA-DR3 phenotype (*0301/0302) in IBM.[161] Skeletal muscle imaging (MRI, ultrasound, PET/CT) demonstrate atrophy, fibrofatty replacement, and signal abnormalities in affected muscle groups (Fig. 33-10).[94,162] Video-swallow

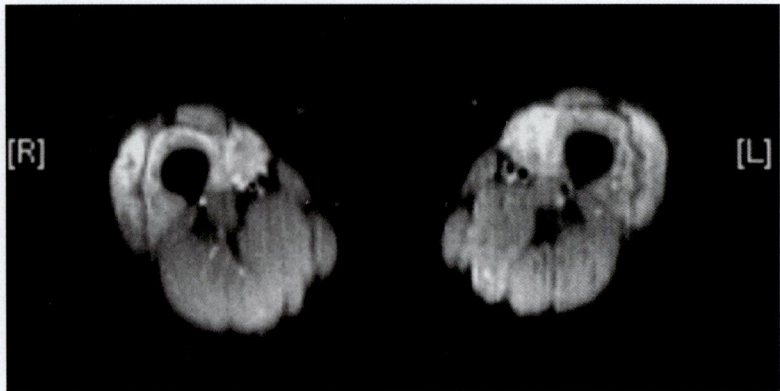

Figure 33-10. Inclusion body myositis. Skeletal muscle MRI (STIR images) reveals patchy areas of increased signal in the vastus lateralis and vastus medialis with relative sparing of the rectus femoris in both thighs.

studies in individuals with dysphagia often demonstrate prominence of the cricopharyngeal muscle (Fig. 33-11).[163]

ELECTROPHYSIOLOGICAL STUDIES

Nerve conduction studies (NCSs) reveal evidence of a mild axonal sensory neuropathy in up to 30% of patients.[3,100] EMG demonstrates increased spontaneous and insertional activity, small polyphasic MUAPs, and early recruitment.[100,143] In addition, large polyphasic MUAPs can also be demonstrated in one-third of patients, which has led to the misinterpretation of a neurogenic process and misdiagnosis in some patients as having ALS.[143,164] However, large polyphasic MUAPs can also be seen in myopathies and probably reflects the chronicity of the disease process rather than a neurogenic etiology.

HISTOPATHOLOGY

Muscle biopsy characteristically reveals endomysial inflammation, small groups of atrophic fibers, eosinophilic cytoplasmic inclusions, and muscle fibers with one or more rimmed vacuoles lined with granular material (Fig. 33-12).[3,8,143,165–174] Amyloid deposition in vacuolated muscle fibers and to a lesser extent within nuclei can be demonstrated on Congo-red staining using polarized light or fluorescence techniques (Fig. 33-13).[165,166] The number of vacuolated and amyloid-positive fibers may increase with time in individual patients.[167] An increased number of ragged red fibers and COX-negative fibers are also evident in patients with IBM compared to patients with DM and PM and age-matched controls (Fig. 33-12).[168] The myonuclei also appear strikingly abnormal. Some are enlarged, contain eosinophilic inclusions, or are located within the vacuoles and appear to be exploding into the vacuoles themselves.

IHC may reveal inclusions react to antibodies directed against p62 (Fig. 33-13), B amyloid, C- and N-terminal epitopes of B-amyloid precursor protein, neurofilament heavy chain, prion protein, apolipoprotein E, 1-antichymotrypsin, and ubiquitin within muscle fibers.[10,148,175] In addition, IHC demonstrates that rimmed vacuoles are lined with the nuclear membrane proteins lamin A/C and emerin, as well as other nuclear proteins (histone H1, histone 2AX, DNA-PK, Hu70, and Hu80).[7,176] An accumulation of mislocalized nucleic acid–binding proteins [including TDP-43, a predominantly nuclear heterogeneous nuclear ribonucleoprotein (hnRNP) that undergoes nucleocytoplasmic shuttling and associates with translation machinery in the cytoplasm] has also identified in IBM nuclear sarcoplasm.[177–179] Studies have shown that both LC3 and p62 are sensitive markers of IBM.[180] In contrast, TDP-43 immunopositivity was highly specific for IBM, but the sensitivity of this test was lower, with definitive staining present in just 67% of IBM cases in one series.[1,180]

On EM, 15–21-nm cytoplasmic and intranuclear tubulofilaments are found in vacuolated muscle fibers, although a minimum of three vacuolated fibers often needs to be scrutinized to confirm their presence (Fig. 33-14).[143] Vacuolated fibers also contain cytoplasmic clusters of 6–10-nm amyloid-like fibrils. Because of sampling error, repeat muscle biopsies may be required to demonstrate the rimmed vacuoles and abnormal tubulofilaments or amyloid accumulation, to

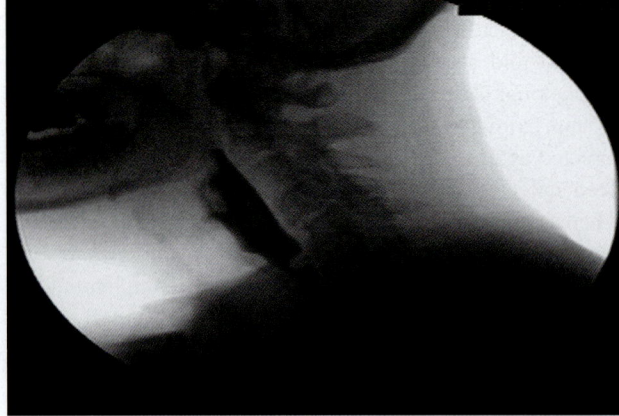

Figure 33-11. Video-swallow studies in an IBM patient with dysphagia demonstrate prominence of the cricopharyngeal muscle that narrows the esophagus.

histologically confirm the diagnosis of "definite" IBM.[3] This sampling error likely accounts for many cases of IBM being misdiagnosed as PM.

In IBM, there is endomysial inflammatory cell infiltrate composed of macrophages and CD8+ cytotoxic/suppressor T lymphocytes, which surround and invade nonnecrotic fibers.[10,101] In addition, there are many myeloid dendritic cells in the endomysium that appear to surround nonnecrotic muscle fibers and may serve to present antigens to cytotoxic T cells. MHC class 1 antigens are expressed on necrotic and nonnecrotic muscle fibers (Fig. 33-12C).[129] The T-cell receptor repertoire of the inflammatory cells has an oligoclonal pattern of gene rearrangement, although there is heterogeneity in the CDR3 domain.[134,169] These findings suggest that the T-cell response is not directed against a muscle-specific antigen, although a superantigen could trigger the response. Persistent clonal restriction of T-cell receptors in infiltrating lymphocytes has been demonstrated on repeat muscle biopsies in some individual patients, suggesting that there is a continuous antigen-driven attack against the muscle fibers.[170] Plasma cells are also quite prominent in the endomysium.[135]

Recent studies have identified highly differentiated CD57+CD8+ T-cell effector memory and terminally differentiated effector cells in IBM muscle invading T cells and in the blood; these cells express killer cell lectin-like receptor G1 (KLRG1).[171] KLRG1 expression in these highly differentiated T cells patients with IBM is confined to the effector memory reexpressing CD45RA cells (TemRA) and Tem cellular compartments. This highly differentiated T-cell population is known to be relatively resistant to apoptosis and control with various forms of immunotherapy, including corticosteroids.[172,173] Importantly, there is minimal KLRG1 expression on IBM patient blood regulator T cells (Tregs) that are important in suppressing undesired autoimmunity. As such, immunotherapy targeting highly differentiated T cells by targeting KLRG1 is a rationale therapeutic approach and such a large randomized, placebo-controlled trial is on-going.

PATHOGENESIS

The pathogenesis of IBM is unknown. There has been debate if IBM is a primary IIM or a primary degenerative myopathy with a secondary inflammatory response (such as seen in a variety of muscular dystrophies). The clonally restricted inflammatory cell infiltrate is suggestive of an autoimmune disorder mediated by cytotoxic T cells. As mentioned in the previous section, there terminally differentiated effector T cells in IBM muscle invading T cells and in the blood expressing KLRG1. This is the strongest evidence of a primary autoimmune condition in addition to the common occurrence of anti-NT5C1A antibodies. The frequency of muscle fibers invaded by inflammatory cells is usually greater than necrotic or amyloidogenic fibers, suggesting that the inflammatory response plays a more important role than the accumulation

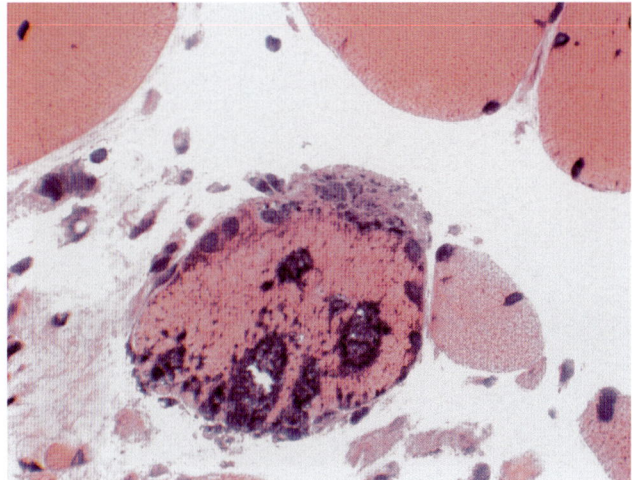

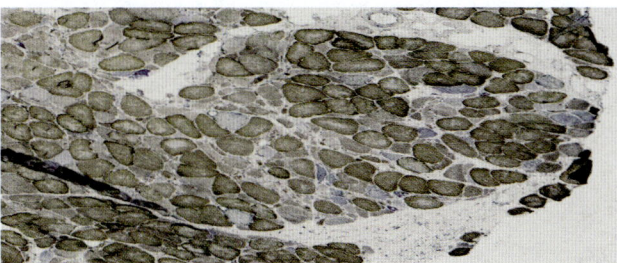

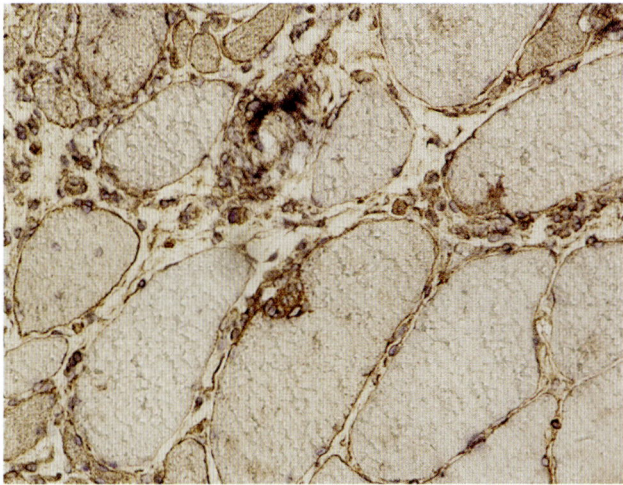

Figure 33-12. Inclusion body myositis. Muscle biopsy reveals muscle fiber with rimmed vacuoles, H&E (**A**). There is also an increased number of cytochrome oxidase negative fibers as seen here on a combined cytochrome oxidase/succinic dehydrogenase stain in which the COX-negative fibers stain more blue (**B**). Endomysial inflammatory cells appear to surround and invade nonnecrotic muscle fibers that express major histocompatibility antigen type 1 or MHC1 on the sarcolemma (**C**).

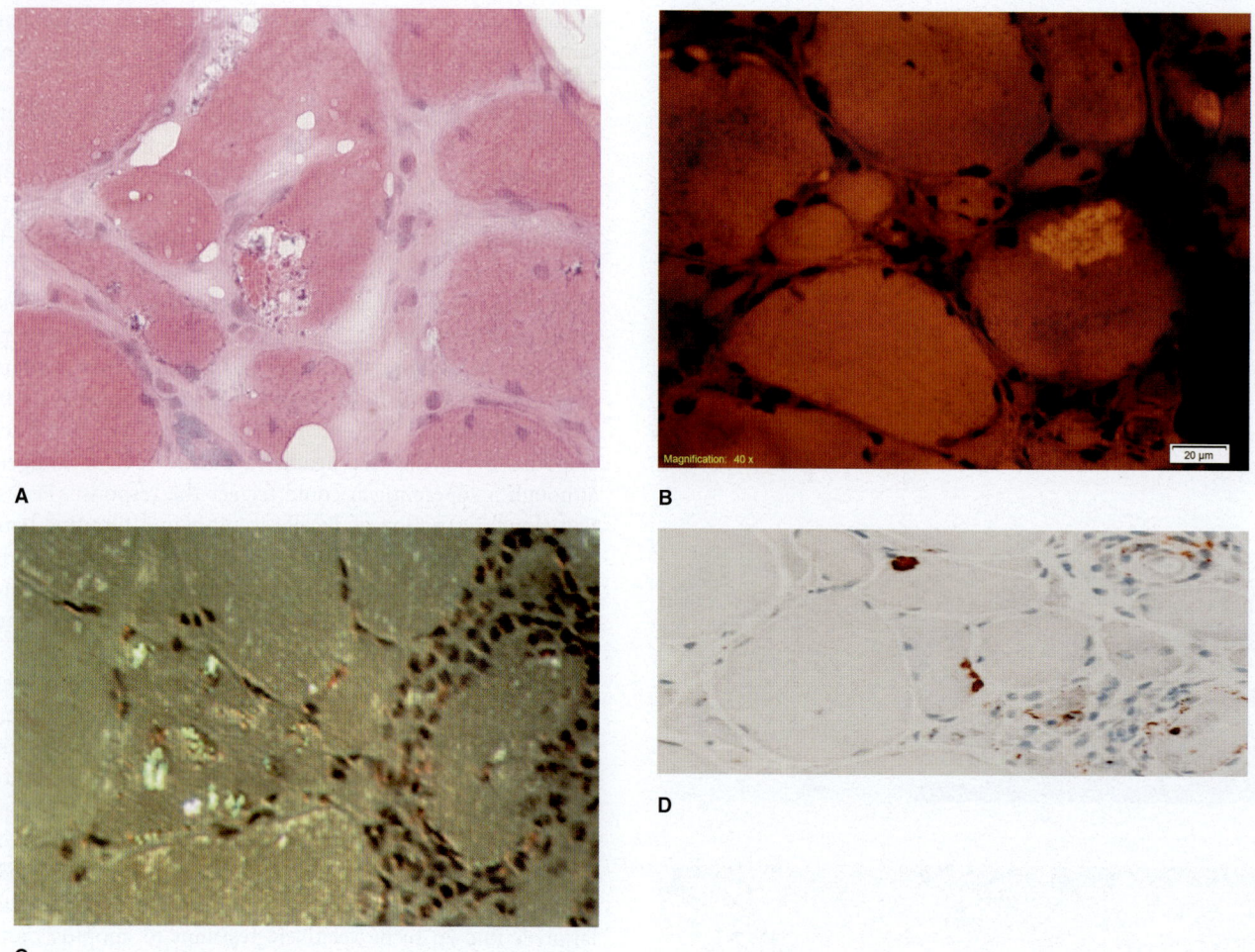

Figure 33-13. Inclusion body myositis. The vacuolated muscle fibers may contain intracytoplasmic (**A**) eosinophilic inclusions (H&E stain), that can appear intensely red on Congo-red stain under rhodamine immunofluorescence (Texas-red filter) (**B**), and as small apple-green birefringent deposits with Congo-red stain under polarized light (**C**) as well as p62 (**D**).

of vacuoles or amyloidogenic filaments in the pathogenesis of IBM.[174] The autoinvasive T cells in IBM release perforin granules; pores form on the muscle membrane, resulting in osmolysis. RNA expression studies demonstrate an increase in immunoglobulin-related genes.[123] This may be explained by the prominent plasma cell infiltration in the endomysium. However, the pathogenic role, if any, of these plasma cells and immunoglobulins is unclear. No abnormal deposition of immunoglobulins or complement has been demonstrated on nonnecrotic muscle fibers or the vasculature in IBM.

The lack of significant clinical response with various immunosuppressive agents has lent support to the argument raised against IBM being a primary autoimmune disorder. We treated eight patients with IBM for 6–24 months with immunosuppressive medications.[167] None of the patients improved in strength or function despite lower serum CK levels and reduced inflammation on the posttreatment muscle biopsies. Interestingly, the amounts of vacuolated muscle fibers and fibers with amyloid deposition were increased in the follow-up biopsies. IBM could be a degenerative disorder of muscle. Although "Alzheimer-characteristic proteins" accumulate in vacuolated muscle fibers by IHC,[10,175] similar degrees of increased mRNA of these proteins are also seen in muscle biopsies of patients with PM and DM.[123] Thus, the increased expression of these proteins in IBM is not likely secondary to increased transcription of mRNA but involves a more distal mechanism. Perhaps, one or more of these proteins become modified post translation, causing misfiling and impaired elimination by the proteasomes.[175]

Ragged red fibers and mitochondrial DNA mutations are more frequent in patients with IBM than in the other inflammatory myopathies and in age-matched controls but are thought to be secondary abnormalities.[10,168,181] Vacuolated muscle fibers express increased nitro tyrosine and both the inducible and the nuclear forms of nitric oxide syntheses, suggesting that nitric oxide–induced oxidative stress (NOS) may play a role in muscle fiber destruction in IBM.[182] Of note, B-crystalline, a member of the heat-shock protein family, is also overexpressed in both normal and abnormal muscle fibers, indicating that the pathological stress is acting upstream from the development of rimmed vacuoles and the accumulation of Alzheimer-like proteins, NOS expression, and mitochondrial mutations.[183]

As mentioned, the myonuclei are very abnormal in IBM. Filamentous inclusions are evident within some myonuclei,

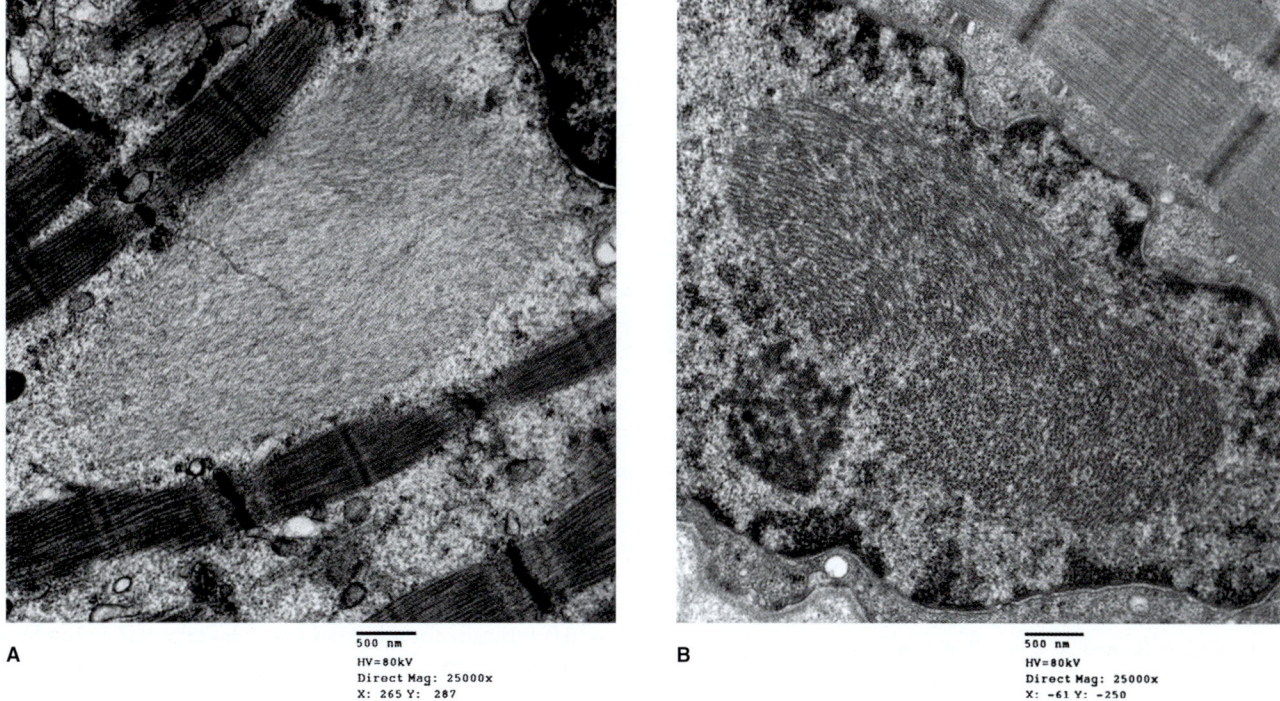

Figure 33-14. Inclusion body myositis. Electron microscopy demonstrates 15–21-nm tubulofilamentous inclusions in the cytoplasm (**A**) and nucleus (**B**). (Courtesy of Dr. Steven A. Greenberg.)

rimmed vacuoles immunostain with antibodies directed against various nuclear membrane proteins as well as nucleic acid–binding proteins (including TDP-43 and hnRNP), and furthermore nucleic acid–binding proteins seem to be extruded out of the nuclei and accumulate as deposits in the sarcoplasm. These features suggest that abnormalities in RNA processing play a role in the pathology of this disease, as has been suggested in some of the hereditary neurodegenerative disorders of the central nervous system (e.g., some forms of familial ALS and frontotemporal dementia) and in some forms of hereditary inclusion body myopathy (see Chapter 27). TDP-43 is an RNA-binding protein that is important for normal splicing of messenger RNA. In this regard, a recent study demonstrated the loss of TDP-43–mediated splicing repression and the abnormal inclusion of cryptic exons in IBM skeletal muscle biopsies.[184] Detection of such cryptic exons had an 84% sensitivity and 99% specificity for IBM diagnosis compared to other inflammatory myopathies that served as disease controls. Most cryptic exons lead to nonsense-mediated-decay of the mRNA so protein is not translated. However, some missplicing events result in proteins that contain "cryptic peptides". Such proteins may have impaired function. Furthermore, autoantibodies may also be generated against such cryptic peptides that serve as neoantigens. This could tie in the degenerative process with secondary inflammation.

A viral etiology has been speculated to be involved in the pathogenesis of IBM but has never been proven. Chronic persistent mumps was previously hypothesized based on immunostaining of inclusions by antimumps antibodies[185] but was subsequently rejected after in situ hybridization and polymerase chain reaction (PCR) studies failed to confirm mumps infection.[186,187] Interestingly, patients with retroviral infections (HIV and HTLV-1) and postpolio syndrome can have histological abnormalities on muscle biopsy similar to IBM.[188,189]

DIFFERENTIAL DIAGNOSIS

Most of the patients that we have seen with IBM were previously diagnosed as having PM or ALS. It is important to remember that because of sampling error, histopathological confirmation of IBM is not always possible. The presence of slowly progressive, asymmetric quadriceps and wrist/finger flexor weakness and atrophy in a patient over 50 years of age strongly suggests the diagnosis of IBM even in the absence of histological confirmation. That said, there are occasional patients with IBM that manifest initially with only hip girdle weakness such that they mimic PM.

As alluded above, the asymmetric muscle atrophy and distal weakness unfortunately may lead to the misdiagnosis of ALS. However, the muscle groups affected early are different in IBM compared to ALS. Again in IBM, there is atrophy of the flexor forearm compartment but the hand intrinsics (thenar and hypothenar eminence) are spared, in contrast to ALS in which atrophy in the arms usually is first seen in the hand intrinsics.

Rimmed vacuoles, amyloid/TDP-43/SMI-31/p62 deposition, and tubulofilamentous inclusions are not usually seen in other forms of IIM but can be observed in patients with various forms of hereditary inclusion body *myopathy* (h-IBM discussed in Chapter 27). The age of onset is usually in early adult life and the pattern of weakness differs (preferential involvement of the tibialis anterior muscles) in patients with autosomal-recessive h-IBM. Autosomal-dominant h-IBM is less common, and the clinical phenotype is more variable but usually predominantly affects the shoulder and hip girdle. One form of autosomal-dominant h-IBMs caused by mutations in the valosin-containing protein gene is associated with Paget disease and frontotemporal dementia.[190] Rimmed vacuoles are also commonly seen in other types of muscular dystrophy, including limb-girdle muscular oculopharyngeal dystrophy, some distal myopathies/dystrophies, hereditary inclusion body myopathy (multisystem proteinopathies), and the myofibrillar myopathies. However, there is a lack of inflammatory cells invading nonnecrotic muscle fibers in these myopathies. A large retrospective study of 371 IBM patients comparing various proposed diagnostic criteria for IBM found that finger flexion weakness, rimmed vacuoles, and invasion of nonnecrotic muscle fibers used in combination were highly performing features. Demonstration of (1) finger flexor or quadriceps weakness, and (2) endomysial inflammation, and (3) either invasion of nonnecrotic muscle fibers or rimmed vacuoles had 90% sensitivity and 96% specificity.[149]

PROGNOSIS

Life expectancy is reduced in IBM, most often related to aspiration pneumonia due to dysphagia.[151,152] The myopathy is slowly progressive, and unfortunately it is not responsive to immunosuppressive or immunomodulating therapies. As mentioned above many patients require a scooter or wheelchair within 10–15 years of onset of symptoms.[143–145,151,152]

▶ IMMUNE-MEDIATED NECROTIZING MYOPATHY

CLINICAL FEATURES

Despite the paucity of inflammatory cells, IMNM is best categorized as an IIM due to its suspected autoimmune nature.[1,6,12,38,128,191–207] IMNM makes up approximately 20% of inflammatory myopathies. Patients present with proximal weakness, which may begin acutely or more insidiously. Some patients complain of myalgias. Patients may have an underlying connective tissue disease [usually scleroderma or mixed connective tissue disease (MCTD)], cancer (paraneoplastic necrotizing myopathy), or the cause may be idiopathic. The most common associated malignancies are gastrointestinal tract adenocarcinomas and small and nonsmall cell carcinomas of the lung. Muscular dystrophies, metabolic myopathies, and toxic myopathies (e.g., statin myotoxicity) need to be excluded. Regarding this, we have seen many necrotizing myopathies that developed in the setting of a patient taking a statin medication but continued to progress for 6 or more months after discontinuation of the statin.[197] These patients only improved once they were treated with immunosuppressive therapy and often relapsed when these medications were tapered. Thus, we feel that statin medications may rarely induce an autoimmune necrotizing myopathy, besides the more typical toxic myopathy that may also be necrotizing in appearance. Patients with necrotizing myopathies generally improve with immunotherapies but, in our experience, they are more difficult to treat than patients with DM, ASyS, or PM.

LABORATORY FEATURES

Serum CK is usually markedly elevated. Positive ANAs suggestive of an underlying CTD may be found. Studies have demonstrated that patients with statin-associated IMNM, particularly if over 50 years of age, often have autoantibodies directed, interestingly enough, against 3-hydroxy-3-methyl-glutaryl coenzyme A (HMG-CoA) reductase.[196–207] The levels may correlate with serum CK and strength of patients.[178] Importantly, these antibodies can also be detected in adults never exposed to statin medications and well as children; they may initially be erroneously diagnosed with limb-girdle muscular dystrophy. Notably also, anti-HMGCR antibodies are not typically found in patients who take statins but have no symptoms or in those who have myopathic symptoms/signs that reverse upon discontinuation of statins.[201] Approximately, 70% of patients with IMNM have anti-HMGCR antibodies.[203–207] Approximately, 10% of anti-signal recognition particle (anti-SRP antibodies) which are associated with severe weakness, dilated cardiomyopathy, and poor responsiveness to standard immunosuppression.[6,12,128,191–202]

EMG demonstrates increased insertional and spontaneous activity, myopathic MUAPs, and early recruitment similar to the other described inflammatory myopathies.

HISTOPATHOLOGY

The most prominent features on muscle biopsy are scattered necrotic muscle fibers (Fig. 33-15A).[1,6,12,191–207] By Bohan and Peter criteria, patients with necrotizing myopathy could be diagnosed as PM. Nevertheless, the pathogenic basis appears to be quite distinct from PM and, in other reported cases, more closely resembles a microangiopathy. The so-called pipestem capillaries may be evident on routine histochemistry and EM.[192] Deposition of MAC on small blood vessels and depletion of capillaries can be seen, although not as prominent as that noted in DM. There is usually expression of MAC and MHC1 on the sarcolemma of nonnecrotic fibers (Fig. 33-15B and C). There is no perifascicular atrophy, perivascular inflammation is sparse, and tubuloreticular inclusions in endothelium are not commonly seen on EM.

PATHOGENESIS

The pathogenesis of the autoimmune necrotizing myopathies is unknown. The deposition of MAC on small arterioles and capillaries with thickened endothelial walls and on the sarcolemma has suggested that in some cases complement-mediated damage may be playing a role, however a randomized,

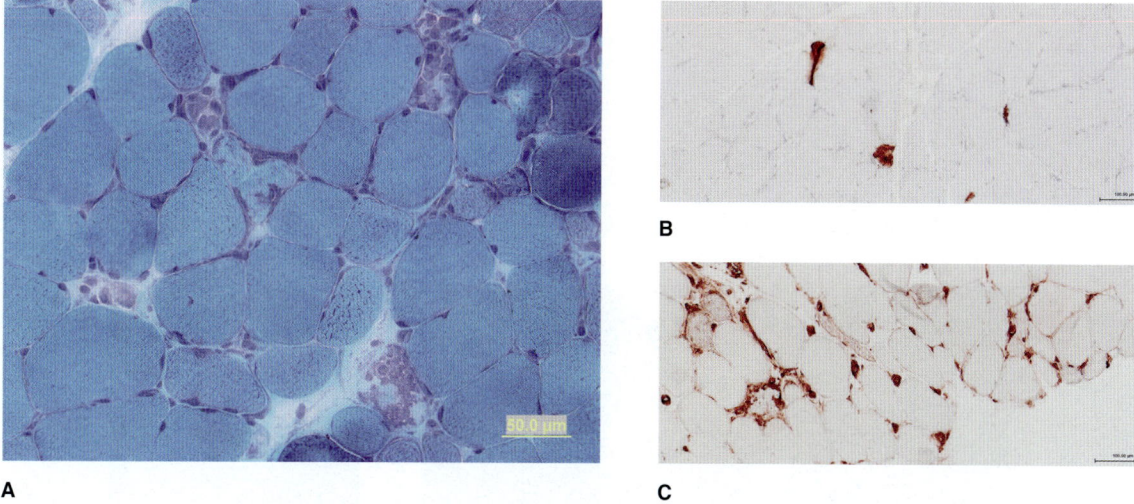

Figure 33-15. Immune-mediated necrotizing myositis. Muscle biopsy reveals scattered necrotic fibers, some in the process of undergoing phagocytosis (**A**). Unlike polymyositis, there is scant, if any, inflammatory cell infiltrate, except in fibers undergoing phagocytosis. Immunohistochemistry may reveal deposition of membrane attack complex (MAC) on small vessels (**B**) and of major histocompatibility antigen 1 (MHC1) on the sarcolemma of non-necrotic muscle fibers (**C**). MAC deposits may also be appreciated on the sarcolemma of nonnecrotic fibers and diffusely in necrotic fibers. Note that blood vessels normally stain for MHC1.

placebo-controlled trial of a complement inhibitor in anti-HMGCR and anti-SRP myositis failed to demonstrate improvement in CK levels or clinical signs of efficacy.[371] A recent study found a cytoplasmic pattern of immunoglobulin deposition in muscle biopsies in patients with anti-HMGCR and anti-SRP myositis again suggesting that perhaps the associated autoantibodies may be pathogenic and not just diagnostic biomarkers.[92] Interesting, recently a rare autosomal recessive limb girdle muscular dystrophy has been reported in patients with pathogenic mutations in the gene that encodes HMGCR.[208,209] Perhaps, these antibodies directly interfere with the function of the receptor in muscle tissue leading to muscle damage.

TREATMENT

In our experience as many as 70% of patients with anti-HMGCR myositis can be managed with intravenous immunoglobulin (IVIG) monotherapy. Anti-SRP and seronegative IMNM are more difficult to treat. As such, we typically always start treatment with corticosteroids plus a second-line immunosuppressive agent (e.g., methotrexate). Furthermore, it is not uncommon that we need to add IVIG or rituximab.

▶ OVERLAP SYNDROMES

The term "overlap syndrome" is applied when non-IBM myositis is associated with other well-defined CTDs such as scleroderma, MCTD, Sjögren syndrome, SLE, or rheumatoid arthritis.[2,4,5,12] In our experience[123] and others,[12,38] the muscle biopsies in patients with overlap syndrome are associated with nonspecific (e.g., perivascular, perimysial and endomysial inflammatory cell infiltrates without invasion of nonnecrotic muscle fibers). The prognoses in these patients are related in part to the underlying CTD. Retrospective series of patients that suggest that myositis associated with overlap syndromes is more responsive to immunosuppressive treatment than isolated DM and PM, but again prospective studies are lacking.[11,41,56,67,125]

SCLERODERMA

Weakness is common in scleroderma. Most patients have normal serum CKs and EMG, while muscle biopsies demonstrate only mild variability in fiber size with atrophy of type 2 muscle fibers and perimysial fibrosis. However, 5%–17% of patients with scleroderma have myositis which can occur in either of its two major forms—progressive systemic sclerosis or CREST (Calcinosis, Raynaud phenomena, Esophageal dysmotility, Sclerodactyly, Telangiectasia) syndrome (Fig. 33-16).[42,211–214] Patients with scleroderma myositis may have mildly increased serum CK levels and irritable and myopathic EMGs. Detailed descriptions of the immunohistopathology on muscle biopsies are lacking, and therefore it is difficult to ascertain if these have features of DM or PM.

Most patients with CREST syndrome have anticentromere antibodies, while anti–Scl-70 antibodies are common in patients with progressive systemic sclerosis. Some patients with scleroderma myositis have anti–PM-Scl antibodies.[58,215] Of note, anti-PM/Scl autoantibodies recognize key components of the nuclear RNA exosome complex. Muscle biopsies of patients with anti-PM/Scl antibodies have demonstrated immunoglobulin deposition within nucleoli of myonuclei and increased expression of genes that are normally degraded by the nuclear RNA exosome complex.[91] Anti–PM/Scl-positive myositis patients have a unique pattern of weakness with arm abductors weaker than hip flexors and increased risk of ILD.[216]

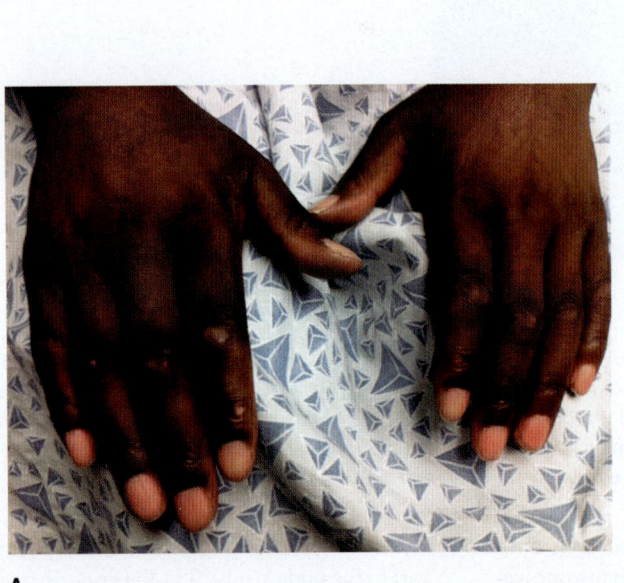
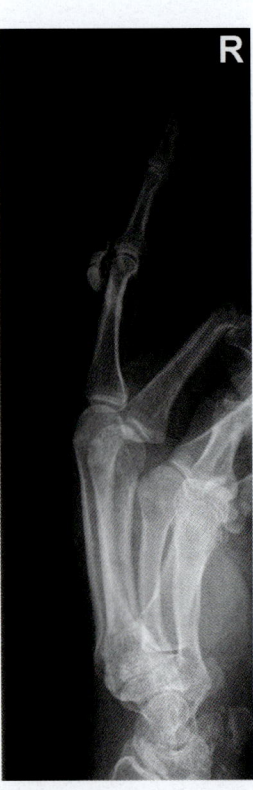

Figure 33-16. Scleroderma-associated myositis. Sclerodactyly is appreciated along with discoloration of the skin on some of the knuckles (**A**). An x-ray reviews calcinosis involving a finger (**B**).

SJÖGREN SYNDROME

Sjögren syndrome is characterized by dryness of the eyes and mouth (sicca syndrome) and other mucosal membranes. Fatigue, subjective weakness, and myalgias are common in Sjögren syndrome, but true myositis is rare. Muscle weakness is usually due to disuse atrophy secondary to arthritis and pain. Nonetheless, myositis with proximal weakness can occur with Sjögren syndrome.[42,217–219] About 90% of patients have ANAs directed against ribonucleoproteins, specifically SS-A (Ro) and less commonly SS-B (La) antibodies. Of note, there is an association of IBM with Sjögren syndrome and sicca syndrome as well as an increased prevalence of anti-NT5C1A antibodies. One needs to be careful in differentiation Sjögren syndrome with overlap myositis with IBM.[220–222] Recognizing the pattern of weakness and histopathology are helpful in this regard.

SYSTEMIC LUPUS ERYTHEMATOSUS

SLE is an autoimmune disorder affecting multiple organ systems. As with other CTDs, weakness is not unusual in SLE but is most often the result of disuse atrophy. Nevertheless, myositis can occur with SLE.[42,102,222,223]

Most patients with SLE have positive ANA titers that are directed against native DNA (highly specific for SLE) and ribonuclear proteins (RNPs). The anti-RNP antibodies are present in less than half of patients with SLE and include anti-SS-A and anti-SS–B (also present in Sjögren syndrome), anti-U1 RNP (also present in MCTD), and anti-Sm (specific for SLE).

Of note, gene expression studies in peripheral blood of patients with SLE demonstrated an upregulation of type 1 interferon-inducible genes, like what is seen in gene expression studies of muscle biopsies in DM.[102] In this regard, MxA is highly expressed in both SLE blood and DM muscle. Both disorders are also associated with tubular reticular inclusions in endothelial cells on EM. Thus, DM and SLE likely share a similar pathogenic basis with abnormalities involving the innate immune system and overexpression of type 1 interferons.

RHEUMATOID ARTHRITIS

The most common etiology of weakness in RA is type 2 muscle fiber atrophy from chronic steroids or disuse secondary to arthritis, but myositis can infrequently occur.[42]

MIXED CONNECTIVE TISSUE DISEASE

Patients with MCTD have clinical features of scleroderma, SLE, rheumatoid arthritis, and myositis.[42,102,211,224] High titers of anti–U1-ribonucleoprotein (U1 RNP) antibodies are common in MCTD but are nonspecific, as these can also be detected in SLE.

ANTI-KU ASSOCIATED MYOSITIS

Anti-Ku autoantibodies are a myositis-associated antibody that can be found in patients with SLE, Sjögren syndrome, RA, and MCTD.[225] Muscle weakness is presenting feature in approximately 38% of patients and develops in over 81% with these antibodies in some large studies. It is frequently also associated with ILD.

▶ OTHER IDIOPATHIC INFLAMMATORY MYOPATHIES

EOSINOPHILIC MYOPATHY

Clinical Features

Eosinophilic myopathy may occur as part of the hypereosinophilic syndrome (HES) and has been subclassified into focal eosinophilic myositis, eosinophilic PM, and eosinophilic perimyositis.[226–235] The diagnostic criteria for a HES are (1) persistent eosinophilia of 1,500 eosinophils/mm^3 for at least 6 months, (2) no evidence of parasitic or other recognized causes of eosinophilia, and (3) signs and symptoms of organ system involvement related to infiltration of eosinophils. Patients with focal eosinophilic myositis and eosinophilic PM present with focal or generalized muscle weakness with or without myalgias and skin changes, while those with perimyositis typically have myalgias without significant weakness. Patients may have other systemic manifestations of HES, including encephalopathy, peripheral neuropathy, myocarditis/pericarditis (manifesting as CHF or arrhythmia), pulmonary (i.e., fibrosis, pleuritis, and asthma), renal and gastrointestinal involvement, and skin changes (i.e., petechial rash, splinter hemorrhages of the nail beds, livedo reticularis, and Raynaud phenomena). The constellation of clinical and laboratory features suggests that eosinophilic PM, HES, and eosinophilic granulomatosis with polyangiitis (EGPA), also known as Churg–Strauss syndrome, may fall into the spectrum of the same or similar disease process.

Laboratory Features

Serum CK is usually elevated in focal eosinophilic myositis and eosinophilic PM but is often normal in eosinophilic perimyositis.[226–235] Hypereosinophilia is generally present. Hypergammaglobulinemia, anemia, and rheumatoid factor may also be seen. ESR is elevated in <50%. Serum ANA is usually negative. EKG may demonstrate cardiac arrhythmia, and chest x-rays may reveal pulmonary infiltrates. Increased insertional and spontaneous activity (i.e., fibrillation potentials and positive sharp waves) with early recruitment of small polyphasic MUAPs are observed on EMG. In addition, there may be evidence of superimposed multiple mononeuropathies, which may also be evident on EMG/NCSs.

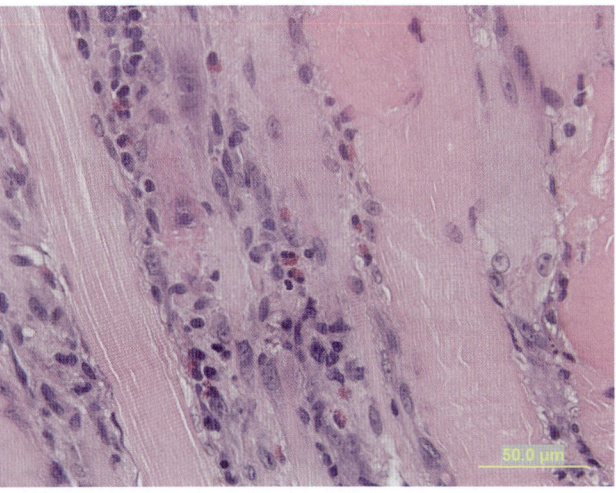

Figure 33-17. Eosinophilic myositis. Muscle biopsy demonstrates necrotic fibers and endomysial inflammatory cell infiltrate that includes many eosinophils. Paraffin-embedded tissue with H&E stain.

Histopathology

Muscle biopsies in patients with focal eosinophilic myositis and eosinophilic PM reveal an endomysial inflammatory cell infiltrate, often but not invariably, including eosinophils.[226–235] Inflammatory cells may appear to surround and invade muscle fibers (Fig. 33-17). Nodular granulomas may also be seen. In patients with eosinophilic perimyositis, muscle biopsies reveal an inflammatory cell infiltrate (eosinophils are not a constant feature) restricted to the fascia and superficial perimysium.

Pathogenesis

The etiology of HES and the eosinophilic myopathies is unknown. Eosinophilia may be the result of a perverse effect on T-cell clones.[234,235] T lymphocytes secrete interleukin-5 and interleukin-3, cytokines that are required for the growth and differentiation of eosinophils.[182] Eosinophils, in turn, damage muscle fibers by their release of the eosinophilic major basic protein, which causes lysis of the membranes of target cells.[231]

Of note, a couple of series have reported children and adults incorrectly diagnosed as having eosinophilic myositis who had mutations in the calpain-3 gene.[236] Thus, these patients had LGMDR1 (LGMD2A).

Differential Diagnosis

The differential diagnosis of myopathies associated with eosinophilia includes parasitic infection, vasculitides (e.g., EGPA), nonhematological and hematological malignancies (T-cell lymphomas and aplastic anemia), toxic oil and L-tryptophan–induced eosinophilic-myalgia syndrome, idiopathic eosinophilic fasciitis (Shulman syndrome), HES, and eosinophilic myopathy as well as LGMDR1. Peripheral blood eosinophil count is elevated in each condition.

Prognosis and Treatment

A poor prognosis for long-term survival with fewer than 20% of patients surviving 3 years was suggested in early reports, but these series of patients may have been biased by the inclusion of autopsied cases. Response to corticosteroids is variable, but some patients do respond. Most patients require the addition of second-line cytotoxic agents (see section "Treatment"). Bone marrow transplantation may be required for refractory cases. Certainly, in childhood cases and refractory adult cases, patients should be screened for mutations in the calpain-3 gene to make sure that they do not have this form of muscular dystrophy.

DIFFUSE FASCIITIS WITH EOSINOPHILIA

Clinical Features

Diffuse fasciitis with eosinophilia or Shulman syndrome is characterized by diffuse fasciitis and peripheral eosinophilia.[237,238] Men are affected more commonly than women in a 2:1 ratio. Most patients are between 30 and 60 years of age; however, children can be affected. Patients complain of myalgias, muscle tenderness, arthralgias, and low-grade fever. On examination, proximal muscles may be weak, although the motor examination is often limited due to decreased effort because of the pain. Joint contractures may develop in the hands, elbows, and knees and, less commonly, at the shoulders and hips secondary to immobilization due to severe pain. Dermatological assessment reveals thickening of the skin with edema and dimpling (the so-called "peau d'orange") in the extremities and occasionally in the trunk. Unlike HES with eosinophilic PM, the heart, lungs, kidneys, and other visceral organs are usually not involved. However, there do appear to be a disproportionate number of hematological complications including aplastic anemia, idiopathic thrombocytopenia, leukemia, lymphoma, and other lymphoproliferative disorders.

Laboratory Features

Over two-thirds have peripheral eosinophilia >7%, while hypergammaglobulinemia and elevated ESR are evident in at least one-third of patients.[237,238] ANAs are detected in about 25% of patients. Serum CK is usually normal. EMG may demonstrate myopathic MUAPs and muscle membrane instability in the superficial subfascial layers. Skeletal muscle MRI reveals increased signal in the fascia overlying the muscle fibers (Fig. 33-18).

Histopathology

A full-thickness biopsy extending from the skin to muscle reveals that the fascia is thickened and contains many lymphocytes, macrophages, plasma cells, and eosinophils (Fig. 33-19).[237,238] Immunoglobulin and C3 deposition in the fascia have also been reported in some patients. The inflammatory infiltrate may invade the adjacent subcutaneous tissues, perimysium, and endomysium. In addition, scattered necrotic fibers and perifascicular atrophy may be seen.

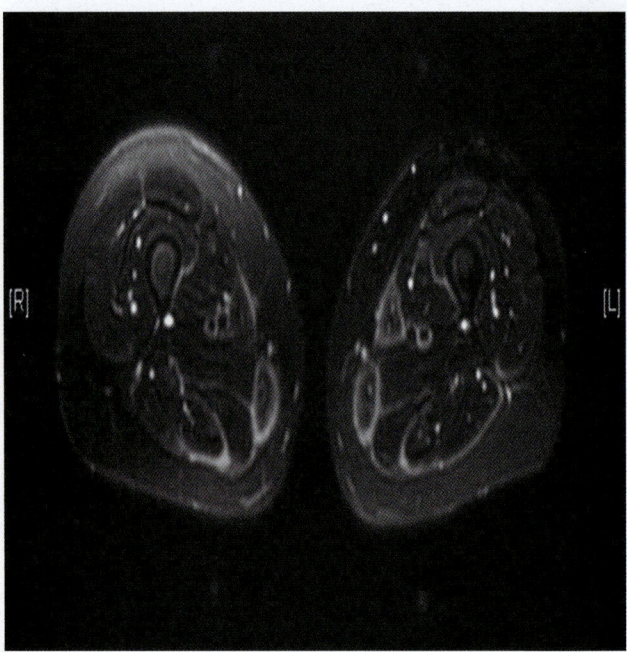

Figure 33-18. Skeletal muscle MRI (T-2 with fat saturation) of the thigh in a patient with fasciitis demonstrates increased signal in fascia surrounding individual large muscle groups, particularly in the posterior compartment.

Pathogenesis

The etiology of diffuse fasciitis with eosinophilia is not known but likely has an autoimmune basis. The clinical and histological features overlap with the eosinophilic myalgia syndrome[239] and toxic oil syndromes,[240] which are caused by the ingestion of tryptophan and denatured rapeseed, respectively. This suggests the possibility of a toxin-induced fasciitis; however, most patients with eosinophilic fasciitis report no known toxic exposures.

Prognosis and Treatment

Corticosteroid treatment usually leads to a rapid improvement. Spontaneous remission may have also been reported. Relapses occur in a minority of patients. The prognosis is not as favorable in cases with hematological complications.

GRANULOMATOUS AND GIANT CELL MYOSITIS

Clinical Features

Granulomatous or giant cell myositis may occur in patients who also have myasthenia gravis (MG) and/or thymoma,[241–250] in patients with IBM, or independently. Regarding MG and thymoma, the myositis may develop before or after the myasthenia thymoma diagnoses, and the thymoma can be benign

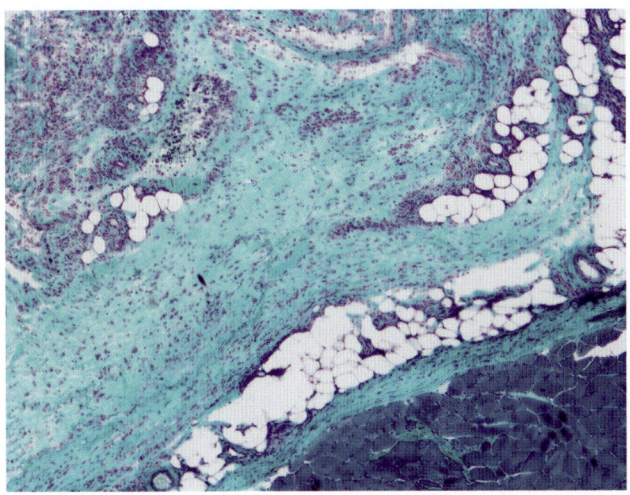 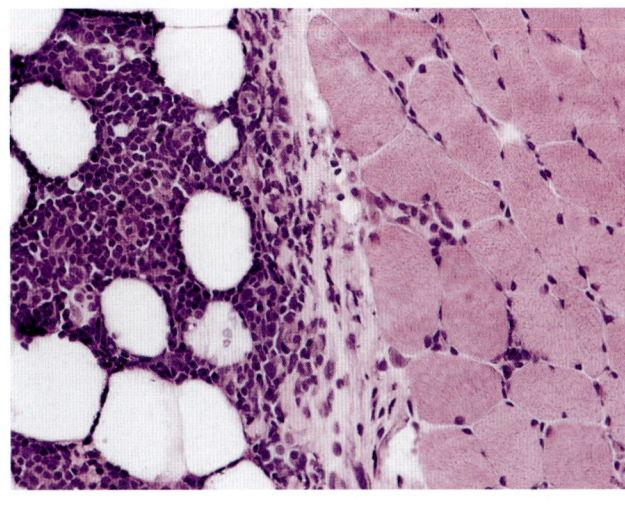

Figure 33-19. Muscle and fascia biopsy reveals inflammatory cell infiltrate including eosinophils in the fascia with sparing of the underlying muscle at low power (**A**, modified Gomori trichrome) and at higher power (**B**, H&E).

or malignant. In addition to proximal weakness, patients with concomitant MG also often have diplopia, ptosis, and bulbar dysfunction. Importantly, there is also an association with a severe and sometimes deadly granulomatous myocarditis.

Nearly 50% of patients with granulomatous myositis have clinical and histological features identical to IBM; these patients do not respond to immunotherapy.[246] Those patients without signs of IBM may respond to immunotherapy, thus highlighting the importance of looking for features of IBM in patients with granulomatous myositis.

Laboratory Features

Serum CK is usually elevated. Myasthenic patients may also have acetylcholine receptor and striated muscle antibodies.

EMG demonstrates myopathic MUAPs and muscle membrane instability. In patients with MG, repetitive nerve stimulation may reveal an abnormal decrement. Chest CT should be ordered to look for a thymoma. Echocardiogram can reveal reduced ejection fraction and ventricular wall motion abnormalities, and EKG may demonstrate conduction block or arrhythmia in patients with myocarditis.

Histopathology

Skeletal and often cardiac muscle biopsies reveal granulomatous inflammation and multinucleated giant cells (Fig. 33-20). Those with IBM also have histopathological features discussed in the section in this chapter regarding IBM.[246–250]

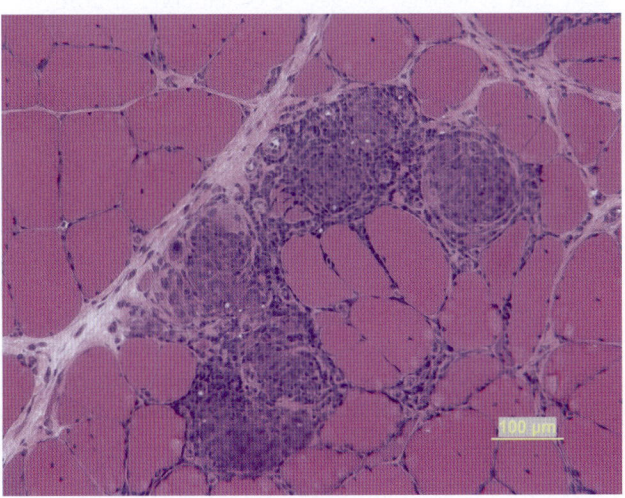 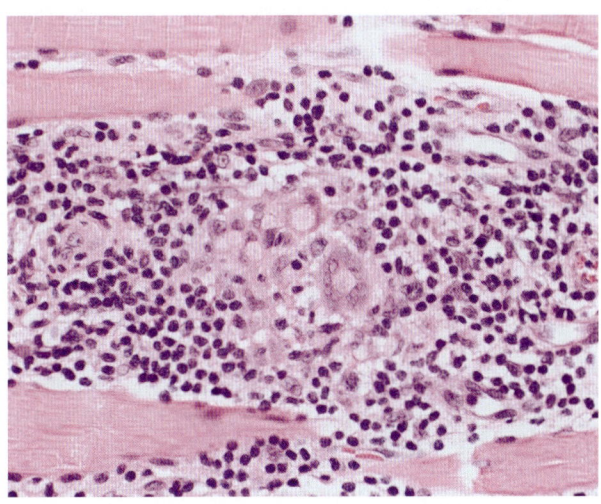

Figure 33-20. Granulomatous myositis. Muscle biopsy reveals granuloma formation in the endomysium (**A**) and a multinucleated giant cell (**B**), H&E.

Pathogenesis

The etiology of this disorder is unknown, but the granulomatous inflammation and giant cell formation suggest a disorder of cell-mediated immunity. However, occurrence of MG in some supports the fact that aberrant humorally mediated immunity may play a role as well. The frequent association of IBM with granulomatous myositis suggests a shared immunopathogenesis (see section on IBM).[247]

Prognosis and Treatment

Some patients improve with immunotherapy, but those with IBM typically do not.

SARCOID MYOPATHY

Clinical Features

Incidental granulomas can be seen in muscle biopsies of patients with sarcoidosis even when they lack symptoms or signs of a myopathy.[242–252] The granulomas may even be palpated within the muscle. Weakness can be mainly proximal or distal. Some patients develop focal myalgias, tenderness, and atrophy. Many patients have clinical and histological features of IBM as mentioned in the proceeding section regarding granulomatous myositis.[244–250] Signs and symptoms of a superimposed neuropathy due to sarcoidosis can also be seen.

Sarcoidosis is more prevalent in black people than white people and in women more than in men. Although uncommon, it can occur in children. Most patients present with pulmonary symptoms and lymphadenopathy. Erythema nodosum and arthralgias are also early features.

Laboratory Features

Serum CK is usually normal or only mildly elevated.[243,251,252] Serum angiotensin-converting enzyme levels can be normal or elevated. Patients are frequently anergic to antigen skin testing. Chest films may demonstrate hilar lymphadenopathy and parenchymal involvement of the lungs. EMG can be normal or show myopathic features. Mixed myopathic and neurogenic MUAPs may be found in patients with a chronic myopathy or with a superimposed neuropathy.

Histopathology

Muscle biopsy reveals noncaseating granulomas consisting of clusters of epithelioid cells, lymphocytes, and giant cells usually around blood vessels in the perimysium and in the endomysium.[243,251,252] As discussed with in the granulomatous myositis section, some patients also have histopathological features of IBM.

Pathogenesis

The exact pathogenic mechanism of sarcoidosis is unknown but likely involves abnormal cell-mediated immunity, given the presence of granulomas and the T-cell anergy in vitro and in vivo. There may be a shared immunopathogenesis with IBM.[247]

Prognosis and Treatment

Treatment of sarcoidosis is usually focused on other systemic manifestations, as the myositis is typically asymptomatic. Corticosteroids are usually effective in treating the myositis, although methotrexate, cyclosporine, or TNF-alpha blockade is occasionally required. In refractory patients, one should consider IBM and perform a repeat biopsy, as we have seen several cases of patients with both sarcoidosis and histologically confirmed IBM. In such cases, the granulomas may have been incidental with the weakness actually due to IBM.

GIANT CELL ARTERITIS

Clinical Features

Giant cell arteritis is a medium and large vessel vasculitis typically affecting women more commonly that men who are older than 50 years of age.[253–255] Patients can present shoulder hip pain like PMR as well as headache, jaw claudication, fevers, weight loss, vision loss, or stroke. Strength examination can be difficult owing to give-way weakness due to pain, although some patients may exhibit mild weakness. Tenderness of the scalp can be found due to temporal arteritis.

Laboratory Features

Most patients have an elevated ESR and C-reactive protein (CRP) in over 90% of patients, however they can be normal.[253–255] In patients with headache and scalp tenderness an ultrasound of temporal artery may reveal a hypoechoic "halo sign" that is strongly suggestive of temporal arteritis.[253–255] Other imaging modalities such as MRA and PET/CT are also highly sensitive in picking up inflamed large vessels throughout the body (Fig. 33-21).[253–255] Serum CK levels are usually normal, but we have seen rare cases in which the CK is actually below normal.

Histopathology

Temporal artery biopsy has been the gold standard for tissue diagnosis, but demonstration of arteritis is not necessary for diagnosis when the clinical, laboratory, and imaging features are strongly suggestive. Muscle biopsies are generally not needed or done for diagnosis but can reveal vasculitis in medium size vessels.

Pathogenesis

The immunohistological findings reveal a cell-mediated attack directed against medium and large size blood vessels.

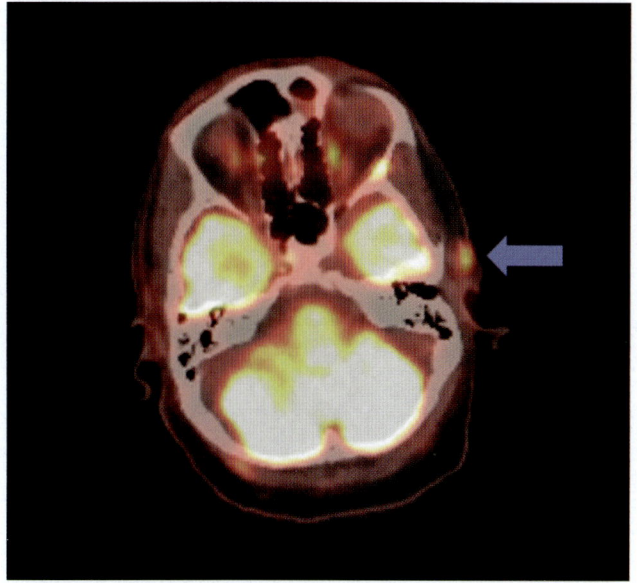
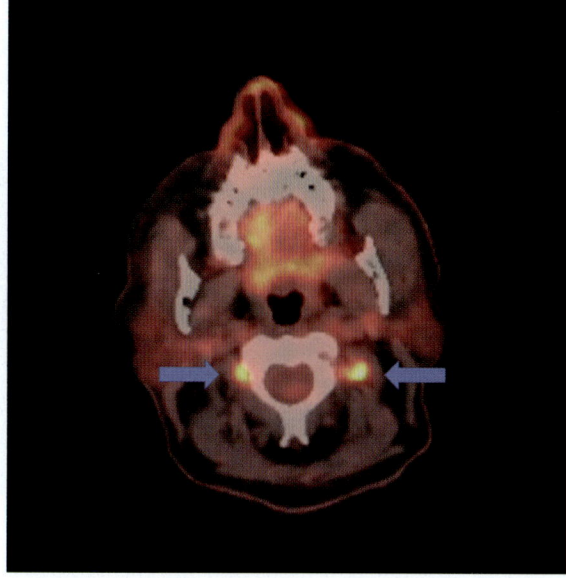

Figure 33-21. Giant cell arteritis. PET/CT scan reveals increased avidity in the temporal arteries (**A**), vertebral arteries (**B**), and iliac arteries (**C**), see arrows.

Prognosis and Treatment

Most patients respond to high-dose corticosteroids that is gradually tapered over several months. However, many patients relapse or have side effects.[253–255] Recently, tocilizumab, an interleukin-6 receptor alpha inhibitor, received weekly or every other week, combined with a 26-week prednisone taper was found to be superior to either 26-week or 52-week prednisone tapering plus placebo with regard to sustained glucocorticoid-free remission in patients with giant cell arteritis.[256]

MYOSITIS/MYASTHENIA/THYMOMA OVERLAP SYNDROMES

A very rare overlap syndrome is associated with thymoma and/or MG with an IIM. Large retrospective series have reported myositis occurring in approximately 1% of patients with MG.[257,258] At least two types of IIM have been reported. In one, giant cell myositis is often associated with myocarditis and occasionally complicated by aplastic anemia.[259–266] Most of these cases have been associated with antiacetylcholine receptor–associated MG, antistriational and antititin antibodies, giant cells in skeletal muscle with or without granulomas, and sometimes myocardial muscles. Rare cases also had aplastic anemia. Some patients improve with thymectomy and immunotherapy but those with aplastic anemia may need allogeneic stem cell transplantation. Another rare type of myositis associated with MG and thymoma is eosinophilic myositis (Fig. 33-22).[267–272] There is also often eosinophilia in the blood stream and increased level of interleukin-5. Additionally, there can be myocarditis. Patients often improve with immunotherapy.

CHECK-POINT INHIBITOR-ASSOCIATED MYOSITIS/MYASTHENIA

Another interesting autoimmune syndrome worth mentioning here is skeletal muscle myositis, myocarditis, and MG that occur as a complication of check-point inhibition uses to treat certain malignancies. We discuss this more in Chapter 35 (Toxic Myopathies).

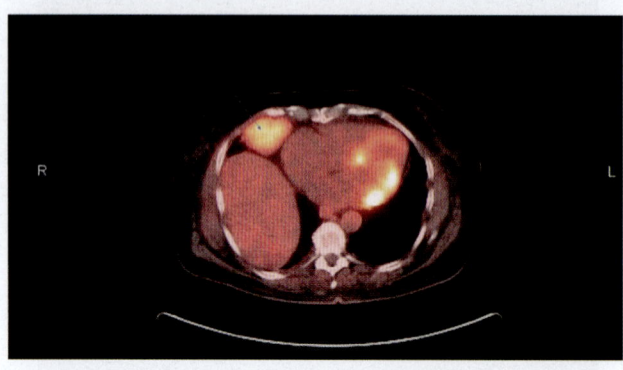
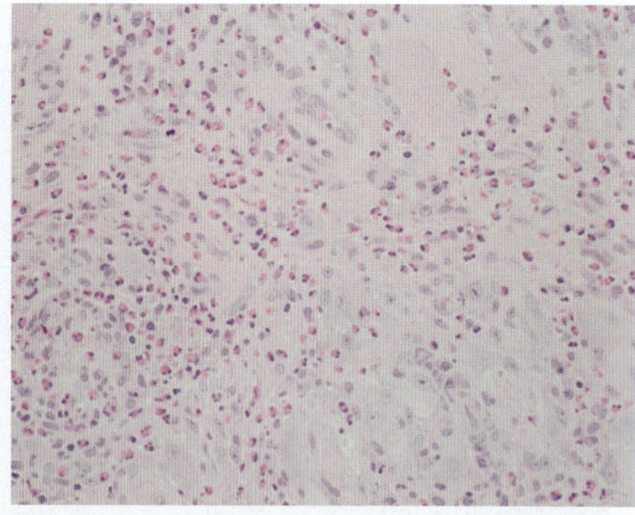

Figure 33-22. Eosinophilic myositis with myasthenia gravis and thymoma overlap. A thymoma is evidence in the mediastinum abutting the heart on PET/CT of chest (**A**). Muscle biopsy demonstrates marked endomysial inflammatory cell infiltrate with abundant eosinophils (**B**).

BEHCET DISEASE

Clinical Features

Behcet disease is a multisystemic disorder characterized by recurrent mucocutaneous and ocular lesions (e.g., oral and genital ulcers, hypopyon, and iritis), erythema nodosum, thrombophlebitis, colitis, meningoencephalitis, and peripheral neuropathy. Onset can occur in childhood or late adult life. In addition, patients may develop focal or generalized myalgias with or without weakness due to myositis.[273–277] The lower extremities, particularly the calves, are primarily affected. Myocarditis may occur.

Laboratory Features

Serum CK levels are normal or mildly elevated. Usually there is leukocytosis, elevated ESR, and increased CRP levels. Approximately 50% of patients are HLA-B5 positive.

Histopathology

Muscle biopsy may reveal macrophages along with CD4+ and CD8+ lymphocytes and neutrophils surrounding and invading nonnecrotic muscles and widespread expression of MHC-1 antigen on muscle fibers like PM.[277] In addition, deposits of complement factor C3 and immunoglobulins have been demonstrated in blood vessel walls as seen in DM.[277]

Pathogenesis

The immunohistological findings reveal a cell-mediated attack directed against muscle fibers, but the enhanced neutrophil migration and immune complex deposition on blood vessels support a leukocytoclastic vasculitis or vasculopathy in the pathogenesis of the disease.

Prognosis and Treatment

The myositis is responsive to immunosuppressive therapy.

FOCAL MYOSITIS

Clinical Features

Focal myositis is a rare disorder, which usually manifests as a solitary, painful, and rapidly expanding skeletal muscle mass.[278–282] It can develop at any age. The most common site of involvement is the leg, but focal myositis can also occur in the upper extremities, abdomen, head, and neck. Focal myositis may be mistaken for a malignant soft tissue tumor (i.e., sarcoma). Rarely, focal myositis generalizes.[280] The disorder needs to be distinguished from focal muscle infarction (most commonly seen in diabetes), sarcoidosis, Behcet syndrome, vasculitis, soft tissue tumors, and focal infections such as pyomyositis (bacterial infection of muscle seen in immunosuppressed patients). The lesions may resolve spontaneously or with corticosteroid treatment.

Laboratory Features

Serum CK and ESR are usually normal. MRI and CT imaging demonstrate edema within the affected muscle groups (Fig. 33-23).[278,281,282]

Histopathology

Muscle biopsies reveal CD4+ and CD8+ T lymphocytes and macrophages in the endomysium along with necrosis and

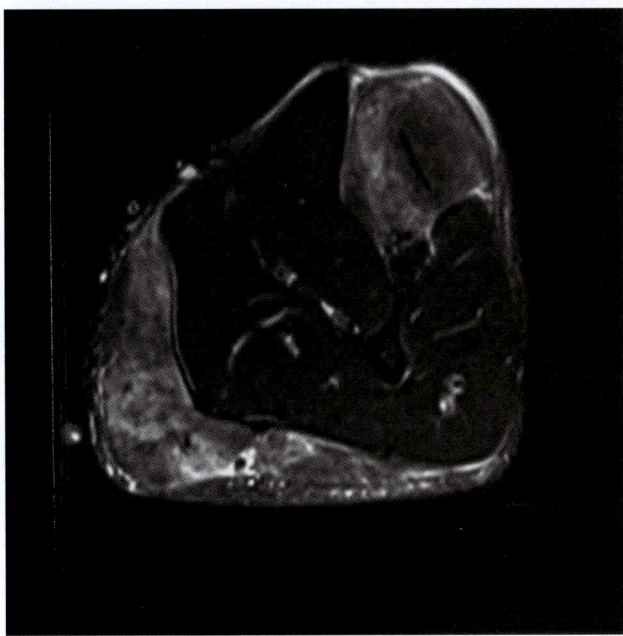

Figure 33-23. Focal myositis. Skeletal muscle MRI (STIR) reveals increased signal in the tibialis anterior and medial gastrocnemius muscles in a patient with focal myositis.

phagocytosis of muscle fibers.[278] In addition, fiber size variability, split fibers, increased centronuclei, and endomysial fibrosis are seen. One report noted that MHC class 1 antigens were not expressed on muscle fibers.[278]

Pathogenesis

The etiology is unknown.

▶ MYOSITIS ASSOCIATED WITH INFECTIONS

VIRAL INFECTIONS

Human Immunodeficiency Virus

Clinical Features

Patients with HIV infection may develop an IIM (Table 33-7).[283] This complication is more common in adults compared to children with HIV infection. IIM usually develops in patients with AIDS but can occur in the early stages of HIV infection. Patients may present with subacute or chronic, progressive, symmetrical proximal weakness, and myalgias. Occasionally, patients with HIV who have a clinical phenotype and muscle biopsies diagnostic of IBM.[284–286] Patients may have concurrent HIV-related neuropathy and may complain also of sensory loss and painful paresthesia. Rhabdomyolysis has also been reported as a rare complication of HIV infection usually but not always in association with antiretroviral therapies and/or statin medications.[287–290] HIV-related myositis needs to be distinguished from zidovudine (AZT) myotoxicity,

▶ **TABLE 33-7. INFLAMMATORY MYOPATHY ASSOCIATED WITH INFECTIONS**

Viral
  Human immunodeficiency virus (HIV)
  Human T-leukemia virus 1 (HTLV-1)
  Influenza types A, B, and C (rare)
  COVID-19
  Hepatitis B and C
  Less common: adenovirus, coxsackie virus, echovirus, parainfluenza virus, Epstein–Barr virus, arbovirus, respiratory syncytial virus, and cytomegalovirus herpes simplex

Bacterial
  Staphylococcus aureus
  Streptococci
  Escherichia coli
  Yersinia
  Legionella
  Leptospirosis
  Lyme disease

Fungal
  Candida
  Cryptococcus
  Sporotrichosis
  Actinomycosis
  Histoplasmosis

Parasites
  Protozoans
    Toxoplasmosis
    Sarcocystis
    Trypanosomiasis
  Cestodes (tapeworms)
    Cysticercosis
    Hydatidosis
    Coenurosis
    Sparganosis
  Nematodes (unsegmented roundworms)
    Trichinosis
    Visceral/cutaneous larva migrans
    Dracunculiasis

HIV-wasting syndrome, and other neuromuscular diseases that can complicate HIV infection (e.g., HIV-related myositis is usually associated with higher CK and more abnormal insertional and spontaneous activity on EMG).[290–294]

Laboratory Features

Serum CK is mildly elevated in most patients. EMG demonstrates muscle membrane instability (i.e., fibrillation potentials, PSWs, and complex repetitive discharges) and early recruitment of small myopathic-appearing MUAPs.

Histopathology

Muscle biopsies reveal perimysial and endomysial inflammation consisting mainly of CD8+ cytotoxic T cells and macrophages, which surround and invade nonnecrotic muscle fibers.[207] Perivascular inflammation is common, but actual necrotizing vasculitis is not seen. Occasional ragged red fibers, nemaline rods, and cytoplasmic bodies are found.[294] Some biopsies reveal features characteristic of IBM.[164,284–286]

Pathogenesis
HIV has been detected by PCR in muscle biopsy specimens; however, the virus is evident by ultrastructural studies only in inflammatory cells.[295] The myositis is not a direct effect of infection of muscle by HIV. Rather, the HIV infection triggers a T-cell–mediated and MHC-1–restricted immune response against unknown antigen(s) on muscle fibers.

Prognosis and Treatment
There are no large uncontrolled studies assessing the efficacy of various treatment options in HIV-related myositis. A trial of antiretroviral medications may be of benefit, if these are not already prescribed. Corticosteroids may be effective in those patients who do not have IBM, but need to be used with caution, given the risk of further immunosuppression in the patient who is already immunocompromised.

Human T-Cell Leukemia Virus Type 1
Clinical Features
HTLV-1 infection can cause adult T-cell leukemia and tropical spastic paraparesis (TSP).[286,296–298] In addition, a myositis may occur in patients who are infected with or without leukemia or TSP. Patients can develop progressive proximal muscle weakness and myalgias like HIV-related myositis. In a patient with TSP, concurrent myositis should be suspected, if the patient has concurrent proximal upper extremity and neck weakness in addition to leg weakness and spasticity. As with HIV, some patients have clinical features and histopathology that are diagnostic of IBM.[286]

Laboratory Features
Serum CK is usually elevated. EMG demonstrates typical myopathic features. In addition, an upper motor neuron pattern of recruitment can be seen in patients who also have TSP (i.e., inadequate activation of MUAPs resulting in a reduced interference pattern without rapidly firing MUAPs).

Histopathology
Muscle biopsy findings are similar to that observed in idiopathic PM and HIV myositis.[286,296–298] As mentioned, patients with HIV-associated IBM have histopathological features characteristic of IBM.[286]

Pathogenesis
As with HIV-related myositis, HTLV-1 can be demonstrated within some inflammatory cells, but not in the muscle fibers themselves. A T-cell–mediated and MHC-1–restricted cytotoxic process similar to HIV is suspected.

Prognosis and Treatment
Although there are only a small number of patients reported who were treated with immunosuppressive agents, non-IBM myositis cases may improve with corticosteroid treatment. In contrast, the myelopathy is relatively refractory to immunosuppression.

Influenza Viruses
Clinical Features
Influenza A, B, and rarely C are associated with upper respiratory infection. As most of us have experienced the common cold or flu and know that, myalgias are common when fever and other constitutional symptoms of influenza infection appear. The myalgias are usually an indirect effect of influenza infection, probably related to the systemic release of cytokines. Nevertheless, active myositis can develop, and the associated clinical syndromes appear different in children and adults.[299–303]

In children, the myositis manifests as severe pain, swelling, and tenderness of the calves when the upper respiratory infection symptoms begin to reside.[299,300,303] Because of the severe muscle pain, affected children may prefer to walk on the toes or crawl and limit their movements. Importantly, prolonged inactivity can lead to muscle contractures. The severe pain limits adequate assessment of muscle strength. Most cases are self-limited, with symptoms lasting less than a week. Myoglobinuria can complicate associated influenza infection, particularly if there is an underlying metabolic defect such as carnitine palmitoyl transferase deficiency.[304]

Influenza virus myositis tends to be more severe in adults.[2,301,302] Generalized or proximal weakness develops in half the adult patients with myositis. Myoglobinuria is more common in adults and can be complicated by renal failure. Patients complain of generalized muscle pain, but this a less prominent symptom than seen in children.

Laboratory Features
CK is usually elevated in patients with acute myositis, while it is typically normal in uncomplicated influenza infection. EMG may show the typical features of an active necrotizing myopathy.

Histopathology
In children, biopsies have revealed scattered necrotic and regenerating muscle fibers with interstitial mononuclear and polymorphonuclear inflammatory cells.[299] EM has not demonstrated any viral-like particles in the muscle biopsies. Viral cultures are only rarely positive.[305]

In adults, the muscle biopsies have demonstrated scattered necrotic and regenerating fibers; however, mononuclear inflammatory cell infiltration is scant. Rare muscle fibers containing viral particles within membrane-bound vacuoles near the sarcolemma have been seen on EM.[306] In addition, intranuclear inclusions consisting of 7–9 nm parallel filaments were present in fibers that did not contain viral particles.[306]

Pathogenesis
It is not known why only rare patients with influenza infection develop myositis. It is possible that the muscle destruction is

a direct effect of the viral infection or alternatively an indirect effect secondary to altering the immune system.

Prognosis and Treatment

The disorder is usually self-limiting, although rare patients have been reported with recurrences associated with infection of different influenza types.[303] Treatment is supportive with bed rest and hydration to avoid renal failure from myoglobinuria. Acetaminophen and nonsteroidal anti-inflammatory drugs (NSAIDs) can be used to treat myalgias and fever.

Severe Acute Respiratory Syndrome Coronavirus 2

Severe acute respiratory syndrome coronavirus 2 (SARS-CoV-2) is the cause of coronavirus disease 2019 (COVID-19). Myalgia and fatigue have been reported in 11%–70% of large series of patients admitted for COVID-19.[307-313] Serum CK has been elevated in 9%–33%, and rhabdomyolysis is estimated to occur in 0.2%–16.9%.[307,308,312-315] Most patients who develop weakness when hospitalized likely have a component of critical illness myopathy. In an autopsy series of 35 patients who died following COVID-19 infection, we reported type 2 atrophy in 32 patients, necrotizing myopathy in 9, and myositis (defined by inflammatory cell infiltrates) in 7, and MxA expression on capillaries in 9.[316] Major histocompatibility complex-1 (MHC-1) expression was observed in all cases of necrotizing myopathy and myositis and in 8 other patients (24 of 35 in total). Another large autopsy series published the saw week found similar findings with endomysial inflammatory cells, including natural killer cells, MHC-I expression on the sarcolemma in 23 of 42 specimens and upregulation of MHC-II antigens in 7 of 42 specimens from patients, but neither were found in any of the controls.[317]

In addition, there are scattered rare reports of patients who developed myositis, some with clinical features (weakness and rash), laboratory features, and histopathological features of a DM-like myopathy or overlap myositis complicating their COVID-19 infection.[318-334] Interestingly, various MSAs (e.g., MDA5, Mi-2, NXP1, SAE) and myositis-associated antibodies (e.g., ANA, anti-Ku) were reported in some of these patients. In these cases, the myositis was not self-limited and required immunotherapy. It is not clear at this time if the myositis was coincidental or if COVID-19 triggered the myositis, though there is no evidence that these cases were the result of direct infection of muscle fibers by SARS-CoV-2. Type 1 interferon is crucial for an effective antiviral response, but we suspect that dysregulated expression could lead to collateral damage in skeletal muscle and capillaries similar to DM. Interferon-gamma and other cytokines probably also contribute muscle damage.[307,316,318]

Other Viral-Related Myositis

Acute viral myositis can also occur in other viral infections including coxsackie virus, parainfluenza, mumps, measles, adenovirus, herpes simplex, cytomegalovirus, hepatitis B and C, Epstein–Barr virus, respiratory syncytial virus, echovirus, and possibly arboviruses. Diagnosis requires acute and convalescent titers (3 or 4 weeks after infection) titers being measured in the serum. The blood, stool, urine, and throat can be cultured to isolate the virus. As in influenza, the myositis associated with these other viruses is usually self-limited and requires only supportive therapy and treatment of myoglobinuria to prevent renal failure.

BACTERIAL INFECTIONS

Clinical Features

The term "pyomyositis" is used to describe focal or multifocal abscesses associated with bacterial infection of the muscle. Pyomyositis is more common in the tropics but has been increasing in frequency in developed countries secondary to HIV infection[335,336] and intravenous drug abuse.[337] Patients present with focal muscle pain, tenderness, and fever. The most common sites of the abscesses are the quadriceps, glutei, and deltoids.[338] If not treated early, the patients can become septic.

Laboratory Features

Serum CK may be normal or elevated. Neutrophilic pleocytosis and elevated ESRs are the rule. Initially, blood cultures may show no growth or organisms until the patient becomes septic.[339] Ultrasound, CT, and MRI of skeletal muscle can be useful in localizing pyogenic abscesses for fine-needle aspiration and diagnosis.[339,340]

Histopathology

Muscle biopsy reveals necrotic tissue containing neutrophils, macrophages, lymphocytes, and occasionally eosinophils.[335,337,338,340] Bacterial infection may be difficult to visualize on light microscopy, but the organisms can be cultured from the drained abscesses.

Pathogenesis

Staphylococcus aureus, streptococci, *Escherichia coli*, *Yersinia*, and *Legionella* are the most common organisms responsible for pyomyositis.[338-340] Pyomyositis usually arises as an extension of the infection from adjacent tissues or via hematological spread of the organisms. Infection of the muscle does not usually develop in the absence of primary infection elsewhere.

Prognosis and Treatment

Early in the course of the illness, microabscesses may respond to appropriate antibiotics. More severe infections require incision and drainage of the abscesses in addition to antibiotics. Despite aggressive treatment, mortality rates range from 1% to 10% in cases complicated by sepsis.[338]

MYOSITIS ASSOCIATED WITH LYME DISEASE

Clinical Features

Lyme disease is often associated with the central nervous system and peripheral nerve manifestations. Rarely, myositis can complicate Lyme disease.[341–346] Rhabdomyolysis may complicate severe myositis.[343] Patients with myositis usually present with focal or generalized weakness and myalgias and may have concomitant manifestations such as rash, arthritis, myocarditis, or more typical neurologic syndromes (e.g., cranial neuropathy, radiculopathy) associated with Lyme disease.

Laboratory Features

Serum CK levels are normal or only slightly increased in most patients; very high levels are rare. Lyme antibody testing may be positive.

Electrophysiological Features

EMG demonstrates myopathic findings often with concomitant polyradiculoneuropathy.[343,345]

Histopathology

Muscle biopsies of suspected Lyme-associated myositis have demonstrated focal nodular infiltrates, perimysial inflammation, and necrotic muscle fibers. Diffuse mononuclear infiltration and invasion of nonnecrotic muscle fibers are usually not seen. Interstitial lymphohistiocytic infiltrates with plasma cells are found predominantly in the vicinity of small endomysial vessels. Immunohistology shows infiltrates that mainly consist of CD4+ T lymphocytes and macrophages and fewer CD8+ T and B cells. Occasionally, the organisms can be seen with silver stains. We have seen a case with perifascicular atrophy characteristic of DM.

Pathogenesis

The histopathological features are suggestive of a vasculopathy.

Prognosis and Treatment

Corticosteroids can help with the myalgias, but the infection needs to be treated with appropriate antibiotics to ultimately improve muscle strength and function.

FUNGAL MYOSITIS

Fungal infection of the muscles is uncommon unless the patient is immunosuppressed. *Candida* is the most common fungal organism and almost always occurs in the setting of diffuse candidiasis.[347,348] Patients manifest with diffuse myalgias, tenderness, weakness, fever, and a papular erythematous rash. However, the myositis is often overshadowed by other systemic involvement. Muscle biopsy demonstrates infiltration of the muscle by hyphal and yeast forms of the organism, inflammation, and hemorrhagic necrosis. Myositis has also been reported complicating actinomycosis, histoplasmosis, sporotrichosis, and cryptococcal infection.[349,350]

PARASITIC INFECTIONS

Trichinosis

Clinical Features

Trichinosis is caused by the nematode *Trichinella spiralis* and is the most common parasitic disease of skeletal muscle. Two to twelve days following ingestion of inadequately cooked meat (usually pork), larvae disseminate through the blood stream and invade muscle tissue. The most frequent muscles involved in order of frequency are the diaphragm, extraocular, tongue, laryngeal, jaw, intercostal, trunk, and limbs.[351,352] Patients complain of generalized muscle pain and weakness, fever, abdominal pain, and diarrhea. In addition, periorbital edema, ptosis, subconjunctival hemorrhage, and an erythematous urticarial or petechial rash are often evident. Myalgias and weakness peak in the third week of the infection but can last for several months. Occasionally, the parasite invades the heart muscle leading to myocarditis and the central nervous system causing meningoencephalitis.

Laboratory Features

Most patients have eosinophilic leukocytosis and elevated serum CK. Serum antibodies against *T. spiralis* can be demonstrated 3–4 weeks after infection.[351]

Histopathology

Muscle biopsies reveal prominent infiltration of the muscle by eosinophils and polymorphonuclear leukocytes in the early stage of infection.[351,352] In chronic stages of infection, mononuclear inflammatory cells become more prevalent. Larvae, cysts, focal calcification of the cysts, fibrosis, and granulomas may be observed (Fig. 33-24).

Pathogenesis

Following ingestion of meat infected with encysted larvae, gastric juices liberate the larvae that infect the gut. Maturation of the parasite occurs in the gut. Subsequently, second-generation larvae disseminate into the bloodstream and lymphatics to invade muscle and provoke the inflammatory response.

Prognosis and Treatment

The treatment of choice for the larvae and adult nematode is thiabendazole, but efficacy has not been established against

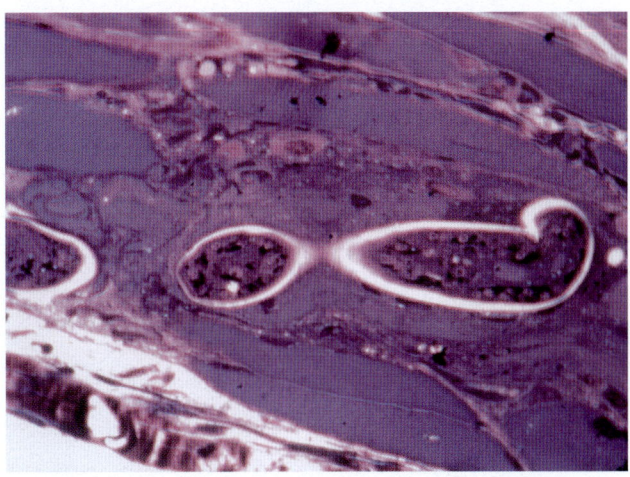

Figure 33-24. Trichinosis. Muscle biopsy demonstrates the parasite cut multiple times. Toluidine blue.

the encysted larvae. Mebendazole may be effective against both circulating and encysted larvae. A 2-week course of prednisone is recommended because a Herxheimer-like reaction may develop as the larvae degenerate. Most patients respond quickly to treatment.

Cysticercosis

Clinical Features
Cysticercosis is caused by the tape worm—*Taenia solium*. Infection of skeletal muscles is manifested by myalgias; tenderness; pseudohypertrophy of infected muscles, especially the tongue and calves, and mild weakness.[353,354] Involvement of the central nervous system may cause focal neurologic deficits, encephalopathy, and seizures.

Laboratory Features
Serum CK and peripheral eosinophil counts are usually increased.

Histopathology
Muscle biopsies reveal eosinophils, plasma cells, macrophages, lymphocytes, and occasionally giant cells along with larvae surrounded by fibrotic changes.[353,354] The encysted larvae eventually calcify.

Pathogenesis
Infection results from ingestion of undercooked meat, mainly pork, which contains the larva form of *T. solium*. The tape worms mature in the small intestine and release ova. Ingestion of food or water contaminated by these ova results in hematogenous spread and infection of the muscle.

Prognosis and Treatment
Praziquantel reduces the size and number of cysts in the central nervous system, but efficacy in myositis has not been established. Niclosamide and paromomycin are the drugs of choice for removing the adult tapeworm. Concomitant administration of corticosteroids is helpful in decreasing the inflammatory reaction directed against degenerating parasites.

Toxoplasmosis

Clinical Features
Toxoplasmosis is caused by the protozoa *Toxoplasma gondii* and manifests as fever, lymphadenopathy, meningoencephalitis, hepatosplenomegaly, uveitis, pneumonia, myocarditis, and/or rash. It is more common in patients who are immunosuppressed. Myositis is uncommon but can occur in isolation or associated with systemic symptoms and presents as fever, myalgias, and weakness.[355–357]

Laboratory Features
Serum CK is usually elevated. The diagnosis of toxoplasmosis can be confirmed with serologic studies (i.e., Sabin–Feldman dye, complement fixation, indirect hemagglutination, and indirect fluorescent antibody). EMG reveals typical features of an IIM.

Histopathology
Muscle biopsies reveal lymphocytes, macrophages, and occasionally giant cells in the endomysium and perimysium. Cysts containing the bradyzoite stage of *T. gondii* are more commonly identified in muscle than the free tachyzoite form.

Pathogenesis
The most common mode of infection is by ingestion of food contaminated by oocysts or ingestion of cysts containing bradyzoites in undercooked food. The organism usually matures to the tachyzoite form and invades the bloodstream and lymphatics and disseminates to other tissues. Systemic disease is most common in patients who are immunosuppressed.

Prognosis and Treatment
The combination of pyrimethamine and sulfadiazine or trisulfapyrimidines are treatments of choice. Combination therapy is effective against the trophozoites but not against encysted protozoa.

▶ TREATMENT OF INFLAMMATORY MYOPATHIES

There are many published retrospective studies and small case reports regarding the use of various immunosuppressive and immunomodulating therapies in different types of IIM (Table 33-8; also see Chapter 4). Unfortunately, most of these older studies are difficult to interpret because they group adult and childhood DM together with PM, ASyS, IBM, and IMNM. Many of these reports were retrospective and unblinded and lacked placebo controls. Further,

▶ TABLE 33-8. IMMUNOTHERAPY FOR INFLAMMATORY MYOPATHIES

Therapy	Route	Dose	Side Effects	Monitor
Prednisone	Oral	0.75–1.5 mg/kg per day to start	Hypertension, fluid and weight gain, hyperglycemia, hypokalemia, cataracts, gastric irritation, osteoporosis, infection, aseptic femoral necrosis	Weight, blood pressure, serum glucose/potassium, cataract formation
Methylprednisolone	Intravenous	1 g in 100 mL/normal saline over 1–2 hours, daily or every other day for 3–6 doses	Arrhythmia, flushing, dysgeusia, anxiety, insomnia, fluid and weight gain, hyperglycemia, hypokalemia, infection	Heart rate, blood pressure, serum glucose/potassium
Azathioprine	Oral	2–3 mg/kg/day; single or two divided doses	Flu-like illness, hepatotoxicity, pancreatitis, leukopenia, macrocytosis, neoplasia, infection, teratogenicity	Blood count, liver enzymes
Methotrexate	Oral	7.5–20 mg weekly, single or divided doses; one day a week dosing	Hepatotoxicity, pulmonary fibrosis, infection, neoplasia, infertility, leukopenia, alopecia, gastric irritation, stomatitis, teratogenicity	Liver enzymes, blood count
	Subcutaneously	20–50 mg weekly; one day a week dosing	Same as oral.	Same as p.o.
Cyclophosphamide	Oral intravenous	1.5–2 mg/kg/day; single a.m. dose 0.5–1.0 g/m^2 per month × 6–12 months	Bone marrow suppression, infertility, hemorrhagic cystitis, alopecia, infections, neoplasia, teratogenicity	Blood count, urinalysis
Cyclosporine	Oral	4–6 mg/kg/day, split into two daily doses	Nephrotoxicity, hypertension, infection, hepatotoxicity, hirsutism, tremor, gum hyperplasia, teratogenicity	Blood pressure, creatinine/BUN, liver enzymes, cyclosporine levels,
Tacrolimus	Oral	0.1–0.2 mg/kg/day in two divided doses	Nephrotoxicity, hypertension, infection, hepatotoxicity, hirsutism, tremor, gum hyperplasia, teratogenicity	Blood pressure, creatinine/BUN, liver enzymes, tacrolimus levels
Mycophenolate mofetil	Oral	Adults (1 g BID to 1.5 g BID), Children (600 mg/m^2/dose BID) (no more than 1 g/day in patients with renal failure)	Bone marrow suppression, hypertension, tremor, diarrhea, nausea, vomiting, headache, sinusitis, confusion, amblyopia, cough, teratogenicity, infection, neoplasia	Blood count
Intravenous immunoglobulin	Intravenous	2 g/kg over 2–5 days; then 1 g/kg every 4–8 weeks as needed	Hypotension, arrhythmia, diaphoresis, flushing, nephrotoxicity, headache, aseptic meningitis, anaphylaxis, stroke	Heart rate, blood pressure, creatinine/BUN
Rituximab	Intravenous	A loading course is typically 750 mg/m^2 (up to 1 g) and repeated in 2 weeks or 375 mg/m^2 weekly Maintenance courses are then repeated usually every 6–18 months	Infusion reactions (as per IVIG), infection, progressive multifocal leukoencephalopathy, hepatitis B reactivation	Some check B-cell count prior to subsequent courses (but this may not be warranted)

in several reports, patients with subjective improvement or lower serum CK levels were defined as positive responses rather than the more important objective improvement in muscle strength and function. There have been only a few published prospective, double-blinded, placebo-controlled trials in the treatment of PM,[358,359] DM,[359–361,364] IBM,[362–370] and IMNM.[371] Nevertheless, there has been a trend in recent years to perform more rigorous studies. Despite the paucity of prospective, double-blinded, placebo-controlled trials demonstrating efficacy of the studied treatment, it is clear to experienced clinicians that various modes of immunotherapy are helpful in DM, ASyS, PM, and IMNM in improving muscle strength and function. In contrast, IBM is generally refractory to immunosuppressive therapy.

CORTICOSTEROIDS

Prednisone is our first-line treatment of choice for DM, PM, ASyS, and IMNM.[1,2,6,8] In patients with severe weakness, we often initiate treatment with a short course of intravenous methylprednisolone (1 g daily for 3 days) prior to starting oral agents. High-dose prednisone appears to reduce morbidity and improve muscle strength and function.[42,67,125,126] Retrospective series report that 58%–100% of patients with DM at least partially improve, while 30%–66% respond completely with prednisone.[3,67] Over 80% of patients with "PM" at least partially improve, but only 10%–33% completely respond to prednisone.[3,67] Likely, many of these "responsive PM" would be classified today as having ASyS or IMNM, while the poorly responsive cases included IBM. Noticeable clinical improvement begins within 3–6 months of starting prednisone in most patients with non-IBM myositis.[3,42] In our experience, ASyS and non-HMGCR IMNM (e.g., anti-SRP and seronegative cases) are more difficult to treat than DM, often requires more than just prednisone alone, and usually takes longer to see a beneficial effect. When no response is noted after an adequate trial of high-dose prednisone, other alternative diagnoses (e.g., IBM or an inflammatory muscular dystrophy) and repeat muscle biopsy should be considered.

Most authorities have found minimal, if any, clinically significant improvement in strength of function with prednisone or other second-line agents in patients with IBM.[3,4,143–145,167,372] However, a few retrospective, unblinded studies reported mild or transient improvement with prednisone.[67,373] A partial response to prednisone was noted in 40%–58% of patients with IBM, although none had complete return of strength. Careful review of these retrospective, unblinded studies shows that the investigators considered *subjective* improvement or lower serum CK levels with treatment a "positive" response. No demonstration of objective improvement in muscle strength was evident. One large retrospective series reported that IBM patients treated with immunotherapy fared worse than those who were not treated.[145]

In patients with DM, PM, ASyS, non-anti-HMGCR necrotizing myositis (e.g., anti-SRP and seronegative) and other idiopathic inflammatory myosities other than IBM (i.e., sarcoidosis), we initiate treatment with single-dose prednisone (0.75–1.5 mg/kg up to 100 mg) every morning (the most common dose used in adults is 60 mg daily).[1,2,4,6,7,374–376] Some studies have suggested that treating patients with alternate steroids or intermittent pulses of intravenous corticosteroids may be equally efficacious and associated with fewer side effects than daily steroids.[376,377] So, one can treat patients with daily prednisone for about 2 weeks and then switch to alternate day prednisone (e.g., 100 mg every other day). Some patients do not tolerate alternate day dosing, or it is challenging in the setting of diabetes in trying to control blood sugar with this regimen, so daily dosing is necessary. We typically follow patients initially at every 2–4 weeks. We maintain the high-dose prednisone until patients are back to normal strength or until improvement in strength has reached a plateau (usually 4–6 months). Subsequently, we slowly taper the prednisone by 5–10 mg every 2–4 weeks. Once the dose is reduced to 10 mg every day or 20 mg every other day, we usually taper prednisone by 2.5–5 mg every 2–4 weeks. Although most patients improve, the response may not be complete, and most will require at least a small dose of prednisone or a second-line agent to have a sustained remission.

We monitor the serum CK levels; however, adjustments of prednisone and other immunosuppressive agents should be based on the objective clinical examination and not the CK levels or the patients' subjective response. Serum CKs can be elevated in patients with no objective weakness or can be normal or only mildly elevated in patients with active disease. An increasing serum CK can herald a relapse, but without objective clinical deterioration, we usually do not increase the dose of the immunosuppressive agent. However, we may hold the dose or the slow the taper. A maintenance dose of prednisone may be required to sustain the clinical response. We try to get patients to 10 mg daily (20 mg every other day) or less of prednisone.

Relapse of the myositis needs to be distinguished from steroid myopathy. This quandary may occur in patients who initially improved but then start developing progressive muscle weakness following long-term corticosteroid treatment because it can cause type 2 muscle fiber atrophy. Features that would suggest a "steroid myopathy" as opposed to relapse of myositis would be a normal serum CK, other clinical features of steroid excess such as ecchymoses and "moon facies," and absence of muscle membrane irritability on EMG. In contrast, patients who become weaker during prednisone taper, have increasing serum CK levels, and abnormal spontaneous activity on EMG are more likely experiencing a flare of the myositis.

CONCURRENT MANAGEMENT

We obtain a chest x-ray and, in at-risk individuals, testing for tuberculosis (TB) prior to initiating immunosuppressive medications. Patients with prior history of TB or a positive testing may need to be treated prophylactically with isoniazid. If patients have ILD and are to be placed on prednisone plus another immunosuppressive agent, we also start an antibiotic (e.g., Bactrim) for pneumocystis prophylaxis.

We measure bone density with dual-energy x-ray absorptiometry at baseline and yearly while patients are receiving corticosteroids. A bone density score of less than 2.5 standard deviations below normal is considered positive for osteoporosis. Calcium supplementation (1 g/day) and vitamin D (400–800 IU/day) are started for prophylaxis against steroid-induced osteoporosis. Postmenopausal women are also started on a bisphosphonate for prevention and treatment of osteoporosis. We prescribe alendronate 35 mg/week (or another bisphosphonate) as prophylaxis against steroid-induced osteoporosis or 70 mg/week in those with osteoporosis. Because the long-term side effects of bisphosphonates are not known, particularly in men and young premenopausal women, we prophylactically treat (alendronate 35 mg/week) these individuals, only if the dual-energy x-ray absorptiometry scan demonstrates a density between 1 and 2.5 standard deviations below normal at baseline or if significant bone loss occurs on follow-up scans. If bone densities are in the osteoporosis range, we treat with alendronate 70 mg/week. Alendronate can cause severe esophagitis, and absorption is impaired if taken with meals. Therefore, patients must be instructed to remain upright and not to eat for at least 30 minutes following the dose of alendronate in the morning.

Antihistamine-H_2 blockers are not routinely started, unless the patient develops gastrointestinal discomfort or has a history of peptic ulcer disease. We instruct patients to start a low-sodium, low-carbohydrate, high-protein diet to prevent excessive weight gain. Physical therapy and an aerobic exercise program are helpful in fending off side effects of prednisone (e.g., weight gain) and preventing contractures and calcinosis that may result from immobility. Blood pressure is measured at each visit as accelerated hypertension and renal failure may occur, particularly in patients with scleroderma or MCTD. In addition, periodic eye examinations for cataracts and glaucoma should be performed. We periodically check fasting blood glucose and serum potassium levels, while they are on high doses of prednisone. Potassium supplementation may be required, if the patient becomes hypokalemic.

INTRAVENOUS IMMUNOGLOBULIN

IVIG has become increasingly popular in the treatment of refractory myositis. Small, uncontrolled studies have reported beneficial response in DM, ASyS, IMNM, and PM.[368,378–381] A prospective, double-blinded, placebo-controlled study of IVIG in 15 patients with DM demonstrated significant clinical improvement with IVIG.[361] A recent study demonstrated efficacy of intravenous immunoglobulin (IVIG) as a first-line treatment in DM.[364] The study utilized the American College of Rheumatology/European League Against Rheumatism criteria for minimal, moderate, and major clinical response in adult DM and PM.[381] Thus, and argument can be made for using IVIG as a first-line treatment of DM.[382] We and others have also found IVIG can be quite effective as a monotherapy in anti-HMGCR myositis, and it is our treatment of choice in this disorder.[205,210]

Mild improvement in muscle strength was reported in three of four patients with IBM treated with IVIG.[380] However, we were unable to document any significant clinical improvement in nine patients with IBM treated with IVIG.[372] Subsequently several prospective, double-blinded, placebo-controlled studies of IVIG in IBM have revealed no significant improvement.[364,365]

We initiate IVIG (2 g/kg) slowly over 2–5 days and repeat infusions at monthly intervals for at least 3 months. Subsequently, we try to decrease or spread out the dose: 2 g/kg every 2 months or 1 g/kg/month. Treatment needs to be individualized. Patients should also have renal function checked beforehand, especially those with diabetes mellitus, because of a risk of IVIG-induced renal failure. Flu-like symptoms—headaches, myalgias, fever, chills, nausea, and vomiting—are common and occur in as many as half the patients. Rash, aseptic meningitis, and stroke can also occur.

SECOND-LINE THERAPIES

These agents are used primarily in patients poorly responsive to prednisone or who relapse during prednisone taper as well as for their potential steroid-sparing effect (Table 33-8). There is equipoise regarding when to start second-line agents (e.g., methotrexate, azathioprine, mycophenolate). The clinician must review with the patient the increased risks of immunosuppression versus possible benefits (e.g., faster improvement, steroid-sparing effect and/or avoidance of the morbidities associated with long-term steroid use). We usually start a second-line agent along with corticosteroids in patients with severe weakness or other organ system involvement (e.g., myocarditis, ILD), those with increased risk of steroid complications (e.g., diabetics, patients with osteoporosis, or postmenopausal women), and patients, who we know from experience have difficult to treat myositis (e.g., IMNM). A second-line agent should also be strongly considered in patients who fail to significantly improve after 2–4 months of treatment or if there is an exacerbation during taper of prednisone. In patients who relapse during the taper, we double the dose of prednisone (no more than 60 mg/day). Once a patient has regained their strength, we resume the prednisone taper at a slower rate. We instruct patients taking immunosuppressant medications to use sunscreen and be vigilant because of the increased risk of cancer, in particular of the skin.

METHOTREXATE

Retrospective studies report that as many as 71%–88% of patients with DM and "PM," including those refractory to prednisone, improve at least partially with the addition of methotrexate.[67,383–388] In addition, a recent randomized trial comparing prednisone versus prednisone plus cyclosporine versus prednisone plus methotrexate showed the addition of methotrexate was better.[389] Methotrexate appears to reduce morbidity in refractory childhood DM,[220] but its side-effect profile has limited its use in children. Methotrexate was not shown to be beneficial in a randomized, placebo-controlled trial in IBM patients.[362]

Methotrexate is administered only 1 day a week. We usually begin methotrexate orally at 5.0 mg/week. The dose is gradually increased by 2.5 mg each week up to 20 mg/week given in three divided doses 12 hours apart. The dose should be reduced and used cautiously in patients with renal insufficiency. If there is no improvement after 1 month of 20 mg/week of oral methotrexate, we switch to weekly parenteral (usually subcutaneous) methotrexate and increase the dose by 5 mg every week up to 60 mg/week. The major side effects of methotrexate are alopecia, stomatitis, ILD, teratogenicity, oncogenicity, risk of infection, and pulmonary fibrosis, along with bone marrow, renal, and liver toxicity. Doses over 50 mg/week require leucovorin rescue, although we rarely use such high doses. However, all patients are concomitantly treated with folate.

Because methotrexate can cause pulmonary fibrosis, we generally avoid using it in myositis patients with ILD and are wary of its use in those with antisynthetase antibodies. We obtain baseline and periodic pulmonary function tests including forced vital capacity and diffusion capacity and repeat these periodically on patients treated with methotrexate. We monitor CBC and liver function tests (LFTs)—AST, ALT, bilirubin, and gamma-glutamyl transpeptidase (GGT) every 2 weeks until the patient is on a stable dose of methotrexate, then every 1–3 months. It is important to check the GGT, as it is the most reliable indicator of hepatic dysfunction, because the AST and ALT can be elevated from muscle involvement.

AZATHIOPRINE

Retrospective studies indicate that azathioprine is an effective therapy in DM and "PM."[42,67] In one study, the addition of azathioprine was associated with improvement in 64% of patients with DM and "PM," although a complete response occurred in only 11%.[67] Not surprisingly, patients who previously responded to prednisone were more likely than patients who are prednisone-refractory to improve with the addition of azathioprine. A prospective, double-blinded study comparing azathioprine (2 mg/kg) in combination with prednisone to placebo plus prednisone found no significant difference in objective improvement at 3 months.[358] However, in the open-label follow-up period, patients on the combination of azathioprine and prednisone did better than those on prednisone alone and required lower doses of prednisone.[390] Azathioprine appears to be effective in some cases of childhood DM but is generally avoided, given its oncogenic potential with long-term use.

Prior to beginning azathioprine, patients can be screened for thiopurine methyltransferase (TPMT) deficiency. Patients who are heterozygous for a mutation in TPMT may be able to tolerate azathioprine at lower dosages, but those who are homozygous for TPMT mutations should not receive the drug as they cannot metabolize it and may have severe bone marrow toxicity. In those patients without TPMT mutations, we initiate azathioprine at a dose of 50 mg/day in adults and increase the dose by 50 mg every 2 weeks up to 2–3 mg/kg/day. Approximately 12% of patients develop a systemic reaction characterized by fever, abdominal pain, nausea, vomiting, and anorexia that requires discontinuation of the drug.[383] This systemic reaction generally occurs within the first few weeks of therapy and resolves within a few days of discontinuing the medication. Recurrence of the systemic reaction usually follows restarting azathioprine. Other major side effects of azathioprine are bone marrow suppression, hepatic toxicity, pancreatitis, teratogenicity, oncogenicity, and increased risk of infection. Allopurinol should be avoided, because combination with azathioprine increases the risk of bone marrow and liver toxicity. A major drawback of azathioprine is that it may take 6–18 months to be effective.

CBCs and LFTs need to be followed closely. If the white blood count (WBC) falls below 3,000/mm^3, we decrease the dose. Azathioprine is held if the WBC declines to 2,500/mm^3 or the absolute neutrophil count falls to 1,000/mm^3. Leukopenia can develop as early as 1 week or as late as 2 years after initiating azathioprine. The leukopenia usually reverses within 1 month, and it is possible to then rechallenge the patient with azathioprine without recurrence of the severe leukopenia.[383] In addition, we discontinue azathioprine if the LFTs increase more than twice the baseline values. Liver toxicity generally develops within the first several months of treatment and can take several months to resolve. Patients can occasionally be successfully rechallenged with azathioprine after LFTs return to baseline without recurrence of hepatic dysfunction.[383]

MYCOPHENOLATE MOFETIL

Mycophenolate mofetil inhibits the proliferation of T and B lymphocytes by blocking purine synthesis in only lymphocytes. Mycophenolate has been used in patients who require transplant to prevent rejection and has recently been tried in a few patients with myositis with reported benefit. The starting dose is 1.0 g twice daily and can be increased to 3 g daily in divided doses if necessary. Mycophenolate is renally excreted; therefore, the dose should be decreased (no more than 1 g/day total dose) in patients with renal insufficiency. A benefit of mycophenolate compared to other immunosuppressive agents is the lack of renal or liver toxicity. Mycophenolate appears to be beneficial in some patients; however, we have seen several severe infections as a complication.[391–394] The most frequent side effect is diarrhea. Less common side effects include abdominal discomfort, nausea, peripheral edema, fever, and leukopenia.

RITUXIMAB

Rituximab is a monoclonal antibody directed against CD20+ B cells, which it depletes for 6 months or more. A number of small series have suggested that rituximab may be effective in DM, PM, ASyS, and IMNM.[395–405] A large prospective, double-blinded, NIH trial found no benefit, but there were significant flaws in the study design.[359] A subset of patients do likely respond,[406] and it has been our experience that rituximab can be beneficial in patients with refractory DM, PM, ASyS, and IMNM. We use it in patients who are refractory to prednisone and at least one of the other second-line agents discussed above. The typical dosage is 750 mg/m^2 (up to 1 g) IV and then repeat the infusion in 2 weeks. Alternatively, patients can be treated with a 4-week course (375 mg/m^2 weekly × 4 weeks). A course of rituximab as above is usually repeated every 6–18 months depending on how well they are doing. There is a very small risk of progressive multifocal leukoencephalopathy, which is discussed with patients before prescribing. Patients should also be assessed for hepatitis B infection as treatment with rituximab can lead to reactivation of this virus.

CYCLOPHOSPHAMIDE

Some reports note improvement in individual patients with oral and intravenous cyclophosphamide.[42,407–411] However, other reports have found increased morbidity with intravenous cyclophosphamide without significant benefit.[412,413] Cyclophosphamide has been advocated for use in myositis associated with ILD or vasculitis, but clinical studies are lacking. Given the controversy regarding the efficacy and the toxicity profile of cyclophosphamide, we reserve it for patients who are refractory to prednisone, methotrexate, azathioprine, mycophenolate, IVIG, and rituximab. When used, we usually pulse patients with cyclophosphamide at 0.5–1 g intravenously/m^2 per month for 6–12 months. Cyclophosphamide can be given orally at a dose of 1.0–2.0 mg/kg/day, but there may be a greater risk of hemorrhagic cystitis. The major side effects include gastrointestinal upset, bone marrow toxicity, alopecia, hemorrhagic cystitis, teratogenicity, sterilization, increased risk of infection and secondary malignancy. Hydration with intravenous fluids prior to intravenous treatment, maintaining a high fluid intake (oral or intravenous therapy), and treatment with mesne are important precautions to help avoid hemorrhagic cystitis. Urinalysis and CBCs are monitored closely (every 1–2 weeks at the onset of therapy and then at least monthly). The dose of cyclophosphamide should be decreased if the WBC decreases below 4,000/mm^3. Cyclophosphamide is held if the WBC declines below 3,000/mm^3, the absolute neutrophil count falls below 1,000/mm^3, or there is evidence of hematuria. It can be restarted at a lower dose once the leukopenia has resolved, but we do not restart the medication in patients with hematuria.

CHLORAMBUCIL

Chlorambucil is uncommonly used because of the significant side effects, which include bone marrow suppression, increased risk of cancer, infection, hepatotoxicity, Stevens–Johnson syndrome, and gastrointestinal disturbance. However, there are a few reports of chlorambucil being used to treat PM and DM.[384,414,415] CBCs and LFTs need to be monitored closely in patients treated with chlorambucil.

CYCLOSPORINE AND TACROLIMUS

Cyclosporine (2.5–10 mg/kg/day) may be effective in some patients with DM and "PM," including childhood DM.[416–424] Improvement in strength may be seen within 2–6 weeks, and it may also serve as a steroid-sparing agent. However, the cost and potential side effects have limited its use in most patients with myositis. A recent randomized trial comparing prednisone versus prednisone plus cyclosporine versus prednisone plus methotrexate showed the addition of methotrexate was better.[389] Tacrolimus has also been reported to help patients with refractory myositis.[324] Side effects of cyclosporine and tacrolimus are renal toxicity, hypertension, electrolyte imbalance, gastrointestinal upset, hypertrichosis, gingival hyperplasia, oncogenicity, tremor, and risk of infection.

We start cyclosporine at a dose of 3.0–4.0 mg/kg/day in two divided doses and gradually increase to 6.0 mg/kg/day as necessary. The cyclosporine dose should initially be titrated to maintain trough serum cyclosporine levels of 50–200 ng/mL. Blood pressure, electrolytes and renal function, and trough cyclosporine levels need to be monitored closely.

Tacrolimus is started at a dose of 0.1 mg/kg and increased up to 0.2 mg/kg (in two divided doses daily). Dosing is titrated to maintain a trough level of 5–15 mg/mL. Blood pressure, electrolytes, and renal function need to be monitored closely and doses adjusted should renal insufficiency develop. With both of these agents, patients should be given a list of drugs to avoid that may increase the risk of renal toxicity.

INFLIXIMAB AND ETANERCEPT

These agents block TNF-alpha and are effective treatments in rheumatoid arthritis and other autoimmune disorders. A few small reports suggest that these medications may be effective in PM and DM.[260,425–431] However, others small reports have found no benefit, and some individuals worsening.[432–435] Therefore, we save TNF-alpha blockers as a last resort in refractory patients.

TOCILIZUMAB

There have been several small reports of tocilizumab, an interleukin-6 blocker, being effective in DM.[436–440] However, a recent trial of 36 patients with DM or PM randomized 1:1 to receive tocilizumab (8 mg/kg intravenously) or placebo every 4 weeks for 24 weeks demonstrated no signs of efficacy.[441]

PLASMAPHERESIS AND LEUKAPHERESIS

Uncontrolled series have reported improvement in DM, PM, and IBM with plasmapheresis or leukapheresis.[442–444] However, a controlled trial of 36 patients with DM and PM comparing plasmapheresis with leukapheresis and with sham apheresis demonstrated no improvement with either plasmapheresis or leukapheresis over the sham apheresis.[445]

TOTAL BODY IRRADIATION

There are a few case reports of refractory cases of DM and PM improving following total body irradiation.[446–448] Others have not found total body irradiation to be effective in PM.[449] Total body irradiation is ineffective in IBM and may aggravate the disease.[450]

THYMECTOMY

Thymectomy has been performed on a small number of patients with PM and DM with improvement.[451]

EMERGING TREATMENTS

The Janus kinase/signal transducer and activator of transcription (JAK/STAT) signaling pathway is felt to be an import regulator of type 1 interferons. As mentioned earlier, DM is felt to be a type 1 interferonopathy. JAK inhibitors (i.e., ruxolitinib, baricitinib, tofacitinib) have been reported in case reports and small series to be beneficial in DM[452–457] and large, randomized trials are underway and being planned (ClinicalTrials.gov Identifiers: NCT04966884: NCT04972760; NCT05361109; NCT05524311). A study of a monoclonal antibody directly inhibiting type 1 interferon pathway looked promising in phase 2 trial (NCT03181893) and a phase 3 trial is underway in DM.

Efgartigimod is a neonatal Fc receptor (FCRN) antagonist that is effective and approved for treatment of MG (discussed in Chapter 25 regarding Myasthenia Gravis). FCRN binds to IgG antibodies and protects them from lysosomal degradation by recycling them back into the circulation. Inhibition of FCRN thus increased elimination of autoantibodies. Given the frequent occurrence of autoantibodies in patients with DM, ASyS, and IMNM (anti-HMGCR, anti-SRP) and that these autoantibodies may be pathogenic, a phase two-thirds trial is underway.

As discussed in the section regarding IBM, there is invasion of muscle fibers by well-differentiated cytotoxic T cells that express KLRG1. An intriguing potential therapy is a monoclonal antibody targeting these KLRG1+ T cells and such a trial is underway in IBM (NCT04659031).

▶ SUMMARY

DM, ASyS, PM, NM, and IBM are clinically, histologically, and pathogenically distinct categories of idiopathic IIM. Features of DM, ASyS, PM, and IMNM can overlap with those of other autoimmune connective tissue diseases. Other types of IIM are much less common but are clinically and histologically distinguishable. DM is an immune-mediated microangiopathy, perhaps due to over expression of type 1 interferons (interferon-beta) that may be directly toxic to muscle fibers as well. The pathogenesis of ASyS, IMNM, IBM, and remaining cases of "PM" are less clear. DM, ASyS, PM, IMNM are responsive to immunotherapy, in contrast to IBM, which is generally refractory to therapy. More prospective, double-blinded, placebo-controlled trials are necessary to determine prognostic features for treatment responsiveness and the best treatment options for the different disorders.

REFERENCES

1. McGrath EM, Doughty CT, Amato AA. Autoimmune myopathies: an update on classification and treatment modalities. *Neurotherapeutics* 2018;15:976–994.
2. Amato AA, Barohn RJ. Idiopathic inflammatory myopathies. *Neurol Clin.* 1997;15(3):615–648.
3. Amato AA, Gronseth GS, Jackson CE, et al. Inclusion body myositis: clinical and pathological boundaries. *Ann Neurol.* 1996;40:581–586.
4. Dalakas MC. Polymyositis, dermatomyositis and inclusion-body myositis. *N Engl J Med.* 1991;325(21):1487–1498.
5. Hoogendijk JE, Amato AA, Lecky BR, et al. 119th ENMC international workshop: trial design in adult idiopathic inflammatory myopathies, with the exception of inclusion body myositis, 10–12 October 2003, Naarden, the Netherlands. *Neuromuscul Disord.* 2004;14(5):337–345.
6. Mammen A, Amato AA. Inflammatory myopathies. In: Griggs RC, Tawil R, eds. *Evaluation and Treatment of Myopathies.* 2nd ed. F.A. Davis Company; 2014.
7. Amato AA, Greenberg SA. Inflammatory myopathies. *Continuum (Minneap Minn).* 2013;19(6 Muscle Disease):1615–1633.
8. Amato AA, Barohn RJ. Evaluation and treatment of inflammatory myopathies. *J Neurol Neurosurg Psychiatry.* 2009;80(10):1060–1068.
9. Amato AA, Barohn RJ. Inclusion body myositis: old and new concepts. *J Neurol Neurosurg Psychiatry.* 2009;80(11): 1186–1193.
10. Griggs RC, Askanas V, DiMauro S, et al. Inclusion body myositis and myopathies. *Ann Neurol.* 1995;38(5):705–713.
11. Pestronk A. Acquired immune and inflammatory myopathies: pathologic classification. *Curr Opin Rheumatol.* 2011; 23(6):595–604.
12. Fernandez C, Bardin N, De Paula AM, et al. Correlation of clinicoserologic and pathologic classifications of inflammatory myopathies: study of 178 cases and guidelines for diagnosis. *Medicine.* 2013;92(1):15–24.
13. Lilleker JB, Naddaf E, Saris CGJ, Schmidt J, de Visser M, Weihl CC; 272nd ENMC workshop participants. 272nd ENMC international workshop: 10 Years of progress—revision of the ENMC 2013 diagnostic criteria for inclusion body myositis and clinical trial readiness. 16–18 June 2023, Hoofddorp, The Netherlands. *Neuromuscul Disord.* 2024;37:36–51.
14. Lundberg IE, Tjärnlund A, Bottai M, et al; International Myositis Classification Criteria Project consortium, The Euro-

myositis register and The Juvenile Dermatomyositis Cohort Biomarker Study and Repository (JDRG) (UK and Ireland). 2017 European League Against Rheumatism/American College of Rheumatology classification criteria for adult and juvenile idiopathic inflammatory myopathies and their major subgroups. *Ann Rheum Dis.* 2017;76(12):1955–1964.
15. Selva-O'Callaghan A, Pinal-Fernandez I, Trallero-Araguás E, Milisenda JS, Grau-Junyent JM, Mammen AL. Classification and management of adult inflammatory myopathies. *Lancet Neurol* 2018;17:816–828.
16. Mariampillai K, Granger B, Amelin D, et al. Development of a new classification system for idiopathic inflammatory myopathies based on clinical manifestations and myositis-specific autoantibodies. *JAMA Neurol.* 2018;75(12):1528–1537.
17. Casal-Dominguez M, Pinal-Fernandez I, Pak K, et al. Performance of the 2017 European Alliance of Associations for Rheumatology/American College of Rheumatology classification criteria for idiopathic inflammatory myopathies in patients with myositis-specific autoantibodies. *Arthritis Rheumatol.* 2022;74(3):508–517.
18. Tanboon J, Uruha A, Stenzel W, Nishino I. Where are we moving in the classification of idiopathic inflammatory myopathies? *Curr Opin Neurol.* 2020;33:590–603.
19. Banker BQ. Dermatomyostis of childhood, ultrastructural alterations of muscle and intramuscular blood vessels. *J Neuropathol Exp Neurol.* 1975;34(1):46–75.
20. Harati Y, Niakan E, Bergman EW. Childhood dermatomyositis in monozygotic twins. *Neurology.* 1986;36(5):721–723.
21. Lewkonia RM, Buxton PH. Myositis in father and daughter. *J Neurol Neurosurg Psychiatry.* 1973;36(5):820–825.
22. Amato AA, Shebert RT. Inclusion body myositis in twins. *Neurology.* 1998;51:598–600.
23. Medsger TA Jr, Dawson WN Jr, Masi AT. The epidemiology of polymyositis. *Am J Med.* 1970;48(6):715–723.
24. Vargas-Leguas H, Selva-O'Callaghan A, Campins-Marti M, et al. Polymyositis-dermatomyositis: incidence in Spain (1997–2004). *Med Clin (Barc).* 2007;129(19):721–724.
25. Gaubitz M. Epidemiology of connective tissue disorders. *Rheumatology (Oxford).* 2006;45(suppl 3):iii3–iii4.
26. Prieto S, Grau JM. The geoepidemiology of autoimmune muscle disease. *Autoimmun Rev.* 2010;9(5):A330–A334.
27. Hengstman GJ, van Venrooij WJ, Vencovsky J, Moutsopoulos HM, van Engelen BG. The relative prevalence of dermatomyositis and polymyositis in Europe exhibits a latitudinal gradient. *Ann Rheum Dis.* 2000;59(2):141–142.
28. Smoyer Tomic KE, Amato AA, Fernandes AW. Incidence and prevalence of idiopathic inflammatory myopathies among commercially insured, Medicare supplemental insured, and Medicaid enrolled populations: an administrative claims analysis. *BMC Musculoskelet Disord.* 2012;13(1):103.
29. Bernatsky S, Joseph L, Pineau CA, et al. Estimating the prevalence of polymyositis and dermatomyositis from administrative data: age, sex and regional differences. *Ann Rheum Dis.* 2009;68(7):1192–1196.
30. Ohta A, Nagai M, Nishina M, Tomimitsu H, Kohsaka H. Prevalence and incidence of polymyositis and dermatomyositis in Japan. *Mod Rheumatol.* 2014;24(3):477–480.
31. Furst DE, Amato AA, Iorga ŞR, Gajria K, Fernandes AW. Epidemiology of adult idiopathic inflammatory myopathies in a U.S. managed care plan. *Muscle Nerve.* 2012;45:676–683.
32. Essouma M, Noubiap JJ, Singwe-Ngandeu M, Hachulla E. Epidemiology of idiopathic inflammatory myopathies in Africa: a contemporary systematic review. *J Clin Rheumatol.* 2022;28(2):e552–e562.
33. Bohan A, Peter JB. Polymyositis and dermatomyositis (first of two parts). *N Engl J Med.* 1975;292(7):344–347.
34. Bohan A, Peter JB. Polymyositis and dermatomyositis (second of two parts). *N Engl J Med.* 1975;292(8):403–407.
35. Bohan A, Peter JB, Bowman RL, Pearson CM. Computer-assisted analysis of 153 patients with polymyositis and dermatomyositis. *Medicine (Baltimore).* 1977;56(4):255–286.
36. Lundberg IE, Fujimoto M, Vencovsky J, Aggarwal R, Holmqvist M, Christopher-Stine L, Mammen AL, Miller FW. Idiopathic inflammatory myopathies. *Nat Rev Dis Primers.* 2021;7(1):86.
37. Dalakas MC, Hohlfeld R. Polymyositis and dermatomyositis. *Lancet.* 2003;362(9388):971–982.
38. van der Meulen MF, Bronner IM, Hoogendijk JE, et al. Polymyositis: an over diagnosed entity. *Neurology.* 2003;61(3):316–321.
39. Arahata K, Engel AG. Monoclonal antibody analysis of mononuclear cells in myopathies. I: quantitation of subsets according to diagnosis and sites of accumulation and demonstration and counts of muscle fibers invaded by T cells. *Ann Neurol.* 1984;16(2):193–208.
40. Bruguier A, Texier P, Clement MC, Dulac O, Ponsot G, Arthuis M. Pediatric dermatomyositis. Apropos of 28 cases. *Arch Fr Pediatr.* 1984;41(1):9–14.
41. Hochberg MC, Feldman D, Stevens MB. Adult onset polymyositis/dermatomyositis: an analysis of clinical and laboratory features and survival in 76 patients with a review of the literature. *Semin Arthritis Rheum.* 1986;15(3):168–178.
42. Tymms KE, Webb J. Dermatopolymyositis and other connective tissue diseases: a review of 105 cases. *J Rheumatol.* 1985;12(6):1140–1148.
43. Sontheimer RD. Cutaneous features of classic dermatomyositis and amyopathic dermatomyositis. *Curr Opin Rheumatol.* 1999;11(6):475–482.
44. Euwer RL, Sontheimer RD. Amyopathic dermatomyositis: a review. *J Invest Dermatol.* 1993;100(1):124S–127S.
45. Cohen MG, Nash P, Webb J. Calcification is rare in adult-onset dermatopolymyositis. *Clin Rheumatol.* 1986;5(4):512–516.
46. Pachman LM. Juvenile dermatomyositis: immunogenetics, pathophysiology, and disease expression. *Rheum Dis Clin North Am.* 2002;28(3):579–602, vii.
47. Askari AD. Inflammatory disorders of muscle. Cardiac abnormalities. *Clin Rheum Dis.* 1984;10(1):131–149.
48. Denbow CE, Lie JT, Tancredi RG, Bunch TW. Cardiac involvement in polymyositis: a clinicopathologic study of 20 autopsied patients. *Arthritis Rheum.* 1979;22(10):1088–1092.
49. Gottdiener JS, Sherber HS, Hawley RJ, Engel WK. Cardiac manifestations in polymyositis. *Am J Cardiol.* 1978;41(7):1141–1149.
50. Haupt HM, Hutchins GM. The heart and cardiac conduction system in polymyositis-dermatomyositis: a clinicopathologic study of 16 autopsied patients. *Am J Cardiol.* 1982;50(5):998–1006.
51. Strongwater SL, Annesley T, Schnitzer TJ. Myocardial involvement in polymyositis. *J Rheumatol.* 1983;10(3):459–463.
52. Dickey BF, Myers AR. Pulmonary disease in polymyositis/dermatomyositis. *Semin Arthritis Rheum.* 1984;14(1):60–76.

53. Frazier AR, Miller RD. Interstitial pneumonitis in association with polymyositis and dermatomyositis. *Chest*. 1974;65(4):403–407.
54. Park S, Nyhan WL. Fatal pulmonary involvement in dermatomyositis. *Am J Dis Child*. 1975;129(6):723–726.
55. Schwarz MI, Matthay RA, Sahn SA, Stanford RE, Marmorstein BL, Scheinhorn DJ. Interstitial lung disease in polymyositis and dermatomyositis: analysis of six cases and review of the literature. *Medicine (Baltimore)*. 1976;55(1):89–104.
56. Hochberg MC, Feldman D, Stevens MB, Arnett FC, Reichlin M. Antibody to Jo-1 in polymyositis/dermatomyositis: association with interstitial pulmonary disease. *J Rheumatol*. 1984;11(5):663–665.
57. Love LA, Leff RL, Fraser DD, et al. A new approach to the classification of idiopathic inflammatory myopathy: myositis specific autoantibodies define useful homogeneous patient groups. *Medicine (Baltimore)*. 1991;70(6):360–374.
58. Targoff IN, Miller FW, Medsger TA Jr, Oddis CV. Classification criteria for the idiopathic inflammatory myopathies. *Curr Opin Rheumatol*. 1997;9(6):527–535.
59. Callen JP. Relationship of cancer to inflammatory muscle diseases. Dermatomyositis, polymyositis, and inclusion body myositis. *Rheum Dis Clin North Am*. 1994;20(4):943–953.
60. Sigurgeirsson B, Lindelof B, Edhag O, Allander E. Risk of cancer in patients with dermatomyositis or polymyositis. A population-based study. *N Engl J Med*. 1992;326(6):363–367.
61. Leatham H, Schadt C, Chisolm S, et al. Evidence supports blind screening for internal malignancy in dermatomyositis: data from 2 large US dermatology cohorts. *Medicine (Baltimore)*. 2018;97:e9639.
62. Carter JD, Kanik KS, Vasey FB, Valeriano-Marcet J. Dermatomyositis with normal creatine kinase and elevated aldolase levels. *J Rheumatol*. 2001;28(10):2366–2367.
63. Nozaki K, Pestronk A. High aldolase with normal creatine kinase in serum predicts a myopathy with perimysial pathology. *J Neurol Neurosurg Psychiatry*. 2009;80(8):904–908.
64. Casciola-Rosen L, Hall JC, Mammen AL, Christopher-Stine L, Rosen A. Isolated elevation of aldolase in the serum of myositis patients: a potential biomarker of damaged early regenerating muscle cells. *Clin Exp Rheumatol*. 2012;30(4):548–553.
65. Hengstman GJ, Brouwer R, Egberts WTM, et al. Clinical and serological characteristics of 125 Dutch myositis patients. Myositis specific autoantibodies aid in the differential diagnosis of the idiopathic inflammatory myopathies. *J Neurol*. 2002;249(1):69–75.
66. Hengstman GJ, van Engelen BG. Polymyositis, invasion of non-necrotic muscle fibres, and the art of repetition. *BMJ*. 2004;329(7480):1464–1467.
67. Joffe MM, Love LA, Leff RL, et al. Drug therapy of the idiopathic inflammatory myopathies: predictors of response to prednisone, azathioprine, and methotrexate and a comparison of their efficacy. *Am J Med*. 1993;94(4):379–387.
68. Miller FW. Myositis-specific autoantibodies. Touchstones for understanding the inflammatory myopathies. *JAMA*. 1993;270(15):1846–1849.
69. Plotz PH, Rider LG, Targoff IN, Raben N, O'Hanlon TP, Miller FW. NIH conference. Myositis: immunologic contributions to understanding cause, pathogenesis, and therapy. *Ann Intern Med*. 1995;122(9):715–724.
70. Mammen AL, Allenbach Y, Stenzel W, Benveniste O; ENMC 239th Workshop Study Group. 239th ENMC International Workshop: classification of dermatomyositis, Amsterdam, the Netherlands, 14–16 December 2018. *Neuromuscul Disord*. 2020;30:70–92.
71. Tanboon J, Inoue M., Hirakawa S, et al. Pathologic features of anti-Mi-2 dermatomyositis. *Neurology*. 2021;96(3):e448–e459.
72. Hida A, Yamashita T, Hosono Y, et al. Anti-TIF1-γ antibody and cancer-associated myositis: a clinicohistopathologic study. *Neurology*. 2016;87:299–308.
73. Inoue M, Tanboon J, Hirakawa S, et al. Association of dermatomyositis sine dermatitis and with anti-nuclear matrix protein 2 autoantibodies. *JAMA Neurol* 2020;77:872–877.
74. Pinal-Fernandez I, Mecoli CA, Casal-Dominguez M, et al. More prominent muscle involvement in patients with dermatomyositis with anti-Mi2 autoantibodies. *Neurology*. 2019;93:e1768–e1777.
75. Sato S, Hirakata M, Kuwana M, et al. Autoantibodies to a 140-kd polypeptide, CADM-140, in Japanese patients with clinically amyopathic dermatomyositis. *Arthritis Rheum*. 2005;52(5):1571–1576.
76. Sato S, Hoshino K, Satoh T, et al. RNA helicase encoded by melanoma differentiation-associated gene 5 is a major autoantigen in patients with clinically amyopathic dermatomyositis: association with rapidly progressive interstitial lung disease. *Arthritis Rheum*. 2009;60(7):2193–2200.
77. Nakashima R, Imura Y, Kobayashi S, et al. The RIG-I-like receptor IFIH1/MDA5 is a dermatomyositis-specific autoantigen identified by the anti-CADM-140 antibody. *Rheumatology (Oxford)*. 2010;49(3):433–440.
78. Fiorentino D, Chung L, Zwerner J, Rosen A, Casciola-Rosen L. The mucocutaneous and systemic phenotype of dermatomyositis patients with antibodies to MDA5 (CADM-140): a retrospective study. *J Am Acad Dermatol*. 2011;65(1):25–34.
79. Chaisson NF, Paik J, Orbai AM, et al. A novel dermato-pulmonary syndrome associated with MDA-5 antibodies: report of 2 cases and review of the literature. *Medicine (Baltimore)*. 2012;91(4):220–228.
80. Cao H, Pan M, Kang Y, et al. Clinical manifestations of dermatomyositis and clinically amyopathic dermatomyositis patients with positive expression of anti-melanoma differentiation-associated gene 5 antibody. *Arthritis Care Res (Hoboken)*. 2012;64(10):1602–1610.
81. Targoff IN, Mamyrova G, Trieu EP, et al. A novel autoantibody to a 155-kd protein is associated with dermatomyositis. *Arthritis Rheum*. 2006;54(11):3682–3689.
82. Kaji K, Fujimoto M, Hasegawa M, et al. Identification of a novel autoantibody reactive with 155 and 140 kDa nuclear proteins in patients with dermatomyositis: an association with malignancy. *Rheumatology (Oxford)*. 2007;46(1):25–28.
83. Trallero-Araguas E, Rodrigo-Pendas JA, Selva-O'Callaghan A, et al. Usefulness of anti-p155 autoantibody for diagnosing cancer-associated dermatomyositis: a systematic review and meta-analysis. *Arthritis Rheum*. 2012;64(2):523–532.
84. Ghirardello A, Bassi N, Palma L, et al. Autoantibodies in polymyositis and dermatomyositis. *Curr Rheumatol Rep*. 2013;15(6):335.
85. Casciola-Rosen L, Mammen AL. Myositis autoantibodies. *Curr Opin Rheumatol*. 2012;24(6):602–608.
86. Fiorentino DF, Chung LS, Christopher-Stine L, et al. Most patients with cancer-associated dermatomyositis have antibodies to nuclear matrix protein NXP-2 or transcription intermediary factor 1γ. *Arthritis Rheum*. 2013;65(11):2954–2962.

87. Kotobuki Y, Tonomura K, Fujimoto M. Transcriptional intermediary factor 1 (TIF1) and anti-TIF1γ antibody-positive dermatomyositis. *Immunol Med*. 2021;44(1):23–29.
88. Albayda J, Pinal-Fernandez I, Huang W, et al. Antinuclear matrix protein 2 autoantibodies and edema, muscle disease, and malignancy risk in dermatomyositis patients. *Arthritis Care Res*. 2017;69(11):1771–1776.
89. Gunawardena H, Wedderburn LR, Chinoy H, et al. Autoantibodies to a 140-kd protein in juvenile dermatomyositis are associated with calcinosis. *Arthritis Rheum* 2009;60:1807–1814.
90. Muro Y, Sugiura K, Nara M, Sakamoto I, Suzuki N, Akiyama M. High incidence of cancer in anti-small ubiquitin-like modifier activating enzyme antibody-positive dermatomyositis. *Rheumatology*. 2015;54(9):1745–1747.
91. Pinal-Fernandez I, Milisenda JC, Pak K, et al. Transcriptional derepression of CHD4/NuRD-regulated genes in the muscle of patients with dermatomyositis and anti-Mi2 autoantibodies. *Ann Rheum Dis*. 2023.
92. Pinal-Fernandez I, Muñoz-Braceras S, Casal-Dominguez M, et al. Pathogenic autoantibody internalization in myositis. medRxiv [Preprint]. 2024 Jan 17:2024.01.15.24301339
93. Albayda J, Mecoli C, Casciola-Rosen L, et al. A North American Cohort of anti-SAE dermatomyositis: clinical phenotype, testing, and review of cases. *ACR Open Rheumatol*. 2021;3(5):287–294.
94. Fraser DD, Frank JA, Dalakas MC. Inflammatory myopathies: MR imaging and spectroscopy. *Radiology*. 1991;179(2):341–342; discussion 343–344.
95. Hernandez RJ, Sullivan DB, Chenevert TL, Keim DR. MR imaging in children with dermatomyositis: musculoskeletal findings and correlation with clinical and laboratory findings. *AJR Am J Roentgenol*. 1993;161(2):359–366.
96. Mastaglia FL, Laing NG. Investigation of muscle disease. *J Neurol Neurosurg Psychiatry*. 1996;60(3):256–274.
97. Pitt AM, Fleckenstein JL, Greenlee RG Jr, Burns DK, Bryan WW, Haller R. MRI-guided biopsy in inflammatory myopathy: initial results. *Magn Reson Imaging*. 1993;11(8):1093–1099.
98. Del Grande F, Carrino JA, Del Grande M, Mammen AL, Christopher Stine L. Magnetic resonance imaging of inflammatory myopathies. *Top Magn Reson Imaging*. 2011;22(2):39–43.
99. Albayda J, Demonceau G, Carlier PG. Muscle imaging in myositis: MRI, US, and PET. *Best Pract Res Clin Rheumatol*. 2022;36(2):101765.
100. Amato A, Dumitru D. *Acquired Myopathies*. Hanley & Belfus; 2002.
101. Engel AG, Arahata K. Monoclonal antibody analysis of mononuclear cells in myopathies. II: phenotypes of autoinvasive cells in polymyositis and inclusion body myositis. *Ann Neurol*. 1984;16(2):209–215.
102. Greenberg SA, Pinkus JL, Pinkus GS, et al. Interferon-alpha/beta-mediated innate immune mechanisms in dermatomyositis. *Ann Neurol*. 2005;57(5):664–678.
103. Salajegheh M, Kong SW, Pinkus JL, et al. Interferon-stimulated gene 15 (ISG15) conjugates proteins in dermatomyositis muscle with perifascicular atrophy. *Ann Neurol*. 2010;67:53–63.
104. Pinal-Fernandez I, Casal-Dominguez M, Derfoul A, et al. Identification of distinctive interferon gene signatures in different types of myositis. *Neurology*. 2019;93:e1193–e1204.
105. Uruha A, Nishikawa A, Tsuburaya RS, et al. Sarcoplasmic MxA expression: a valuable marker of dermatomyositis. *Neurology*. 2017;88(5):493–500.
106. Uruha A, Goebel HH, Stenzel W. Updates on the Immunopathology in Idiopathic Inflammatory Myopathies. *Curr Rheumatol Rep*. 2021;23(7):56.
107. Emslie-Smith AM, Engel AG. Microvascular changes in early and advanced dermatomyositis: a quantitative study. *Ann Neurol*. 1990;27(4):343–356.
108. Kissel JT, Halterman RK, Rammohan KW, Mendell JR. The relationship of complement-mediated microvasculopathy to the histologic features and clinical duration of disease in dermatomyositis. *Arch Neurol*. 1991;48(1):26–30.
109. Kissel JT, Mendell JR, Rammohan KW. Microvascular deposition of complement membrane attack complex in dermatomyositis. *N Engl J Med*. 1986;314(6):329–334.
110. Whitaker JN, Engel WK. Vascular deposits of immunoglobulin and complement in idiopathic inflammatory myopathy. *N Engl J Med*. 1972;286(7):333–338.
111. De Visser M, Emslie-Smith AM, Engel AG. Early ultrastructural alterations in adult dermatomyositis. Capillary abnormalities precede other structural changes in muscle. *J Neurol Sci*. 1989;94(1–3):181–192.
112. Grimley PM, Kang YH, Frederick W, et al. Interferon-related leukocyte inclusions in acquired immune deficiency syndrome: localization in T cells. *Am J Clin Pathol*. 1984;81(2):147–155.
113. Tanboon J, Inoue M, Saito Y, et al Dermatomyositis: Muscle Pathology According to Antibody Subtypes. *Neurology*. 2022;98(7):e739–e749.
114. Pinal-Fernandez I, Casciola-Rosen LA, Christopher-Stine L, Corse AM, Mammen AL. The prevalence of individual histopathologic features varies according to autoantibody status in muscle biopsies from patients with dermatomyositis. *J Rheumatol*. 2015;42:1448–1454.
115. Greenberg SA, Amato AA. Uncertainties in the pathogenesis of adult dermatomyositis. *Curr Opin Neurol*. 2004;17(3):359–364.
116. Ladislau L, Suárez-Calve, X, Toquet S, et al. JAK inhibitor improves type I interferon induced damage: proof of concept in dermatomyositis. *Brain*. 2018;141(6):1609–1621.
117. Pinal-Fernandez I, Greenberg SA. Type I Interferons in Dermatomyositis Myoblasts: Toxic Effect and a Potential Autocrine Loop. *Neurology*. 2022;98(21):869–870.
118. Ichikawa E, Furuta J, Kawachi Y, Imakado S, Otsuka F. Hereditary complement (C9) deficiency associated with dermatomyositis. *Br J Dermatol*. 2001;144(5):1080–1083.
119. Leddy JP, Griggs RC, Klemperer MR, Frank MM. Hereditary complement (C2) deficiency with dermatomyositis. *Am J Med*. 1975;58(1):83–91.
120. Karpati G, Carpenter S, Melmed C, Eisen AA. Experimental ischemic myopathy. *J Neurol Sci*. 1974;23(1):129–161.
121. Hathaway PW, Engel WK, Zellweger H. Experimental myopathy after microarterial embolization; comparison with childhood x-linked pseudohypertrophic muscular dystrophy. *Arch Neurol*. 1970;22(4):365–378.
122. Greenberg SA, Sanoudou D, Haslett JN, et al. Molecular profiles of inflammatory myopathies. *Neurology*. 2002;59(8):1170–1182.
123. Gallay L, Fermon C, Lessard L, et al. Involvement of type I interferon signaling in muscle stem cell proliferation during dermatomyositis. *Neurology*. 2022;98(21):e2108–e2119.

124. Hochberg MC, Lopez-Acuna D, Gittelsohn AM. Mortality from polymyositis and dermatomyositis in the United States, 1968–1978. *Arthritis Rheum.* 1983;26(12):1465–1471.
125. Murabayashi K, Saito E, Okada S, Ogawa T, Kinoshita M. Prognosis of life in polymyositis/dermatomyositis. *Ryumachi.* 1991;31(4):391–397.
126. Hengstman GJ, van Engelen BG. Polymyositis: an over-diagnosed entity. *Neurology.* 2004;63(2):402–403; author reply 403.
127. Miller T, Al-Lozi MT, Lopate G, Pestronk A. Myopathy with antibodies to the signal recognition particle: clinical and pathological features. *J Neurol Neurosurg Psychiatry.* 2002;73(4):420–428.
128. Mozaffar T, Pestronk A. Myopathy with anti-Jo-1 antibodies: pathology in perimysium and neighbouring muscle fibres. *J Neurol Neurosurg Psychiatry.* 2000;68(4):472–478.
129. Emslie-Smith AM, Arahata K, Engel AG. Major histocompatibility complex class I antigen expression, immunolocalization of interferon subtypes, and T cell-mediated cytotoxicity in myopathies. *Hum Pathol.* 1989;20(3):224–231.
130. Mor F. Polymyositis mediated by lymphocytes expressing the gamma/delta receptor. *N Engl J Med.* 1991;325(8):587–588.
131. Hohlfeld R, Engel AG, Ii K, Harper MC. Polymyositis mediated by T lymphocytes that express the gamma/delta receptor. *N Engl J Med.* 1991;324(13):877–881.
132. O'Hanlon TP, Messersmith WA, Dalakas MC, Plotz PH, Miller FW. Gamma delta T cell receptor gene expression by muscle-infiltrating lymphocytes in the idiopathic inflammatory myopathies. *Clin Exp Immunol.* 1995;100(3):519–528.
133. Hofbauer M, Wiesener S, Babbe H, et al. Clonal tracking of autoaggressive T cells in polymyositis by combining laser microdissection, single-cell PCR, and CDR3-spectratype analysis. *Proc Natl Acad Sci USA.* 2003;100(7):4090–4095.
134. Mantegazza R, Andreetta F, Bernasconi P, et al. Analysis of T cell receptor repertoire of muscle-infiltrating T lymphocytes in polymyositis. Restricted V alpha/beta rearrangements may indicate antigen-driven selection. *J Clin Invest.* 1993;91(6):2880–2886.
135. Greenberg SA, Bradshaw EM, Pinkus JL, et al. Plasma cells in muscle in inclusion body myositis and polymyositis. *Neurology.* 2005;65(11):1782–1787.
136. Leff RL, Love LA, Miller FW, et al. Viruses in idiopathic inflamma-tory myopathies: absence of candidate viral genomes in muscle. *Lancet.* 1992;339(8803):1192–1195.
137. Goebels N, Michaelis D, Engelhardt M, et al. Differential expression of perforin in muscle-infiltrating T cells in polymyositis and dermatomyositis. *J Clin Invest.* 1996;97(12):2905–2910.
138. Amato AA, Griggs RC. Unicorns, dragons, polymyositis, and other mythological beasts. *Neurology.* 2003;61(3):288–289.
139. Tanboon J, Inoue M, Hirakawa S, et al. Muscle pathology of antisynthetase syndrome according to antibody subtypes. *MedRxiv.* 2023;33(4):e13155.
140. Pinal-Fernandez I, Casal-Dominguez M, Huapaya JA, et al. A longitudinal cohort study of the anti-synthetase syndrome: increased severity of interstitial lung disease in black patients and patients with anti-PL7 and anti-PL12 autoantibodies. *Rheumatology (Oxford).* 2017;56:999–1007.
141. Inoue M, Tanboon J, Okubo M, et al. Absence of sarcoplasmic myxovirus resistance protein A (MxA) expression in antisynthetase syndrome in a cohort of 194 cases. *Neuropathol Appl Neurobiol.* 2019;45:523–524.
142. Yunis EJ, Samaha FJ. Inclusion body myositis. *Lab Invest.* 1971;25(3):240–248.
143. Lotz BP, Engel AG, Nishino H, Stevens JC, Litchy WJ. Inclusion body myositis. Observations in 40 patients. *Brain.* 1989;112(pt 3):727–747.
144. Cox FM, Titulaer MJ, Sont JK, Wintzen AR, Verschuuren JJ, Badrising UA. A 12-year follow-up in sporadic inclusion body myositis: an end stage with major disabilities. *Brain.* 2011;134(pt 11):3167–3175.
145. Benveniste O, Guiguet M, Freebody J, et al. Long-term observational study of sporadic inclusion body myositis. *Brain.* 2011;134(pt 11):3176–3184.
146. Brady S, Squier W, Hilton-Jones D. Clinical assessment determines the diagnosis of inclusion body myositis independently of pathological features. *J Neurol Neurosurg Psychiatry.* 2013;84(11):1240–1246.
147. Chahin N, Engel AG. Correlation of muscle biopsy, clinical course, and outcome in PM and sporadic IBM. *Neurology.* 2008;70(6):418–424.
148. Rose MR, ENMC IBM Working Group. 188th ENMC international workshop: inclusion body myositis, 2–4 December 2011, Naarden, The Netherlands. *Neuromuscul Disord.* 2013;23:1044–1055.
149. Lloyd TE, Mammen AL, Amato AA, Weiss MD, Needham M, Greenberg SA. Evaluation and construction of diagnostic criteria for inclusion body myositis. *Neurology.* 2014;83(5):426–433.
150. Greenberg SA. Counting people with inclusion body myositis. *Neurology.* 2021;96(21):977–979.
151. Lindgren U, Pullerits R, Lindberg C, Oldfors A. Epidemiology, survival, and clinical characteristics of inclusion body myositis. *Ann Neurol.* 2022;92(2):201–212.
152. Shelly S, Mielke MM, Mandrekar J, et al. Epidemiology and natural history of inclusion body myositis: a 40-year population-based study. *Neurology.* 2021;96(21):e2653–e2661.
153. Darrow DH, Hoffman HT, Barnes GJ, Wiley CA. Management of dysphagia in inclusion body myositis. *Arch Otolaryngol Head Neck Surg.* 1992;118(3):313–317.
154. Verma A, Bradley WG, Adesina AM, Sofferman R, Pendlebury WW. Inclusion body myositis with cricopharyngeus muscle involvement and severe dysphagia. *Muscle Nerve.* 1991;14(5):470–473.
155. Ghosh PS, Laughlin RS, Engel AG. Inclusion-body myositis presenting with facial diplegia. *Muscle Nerve.* 2014;49(2):287–289.
156. Ma H, McEvoy KM, Milone M. Sporadic inclusion body myositis presenting with severe camptocormia. *J Clin Neurosci.* 2013;20(11):1628–1629.
157. Goodman BP, Liewluck T, Crum BA, Spinner RJ. Camptocormia due to inclusion body myositis. *J Clin Neuromuscul Dis.* 2012;14(2):78–81.
158. Danon MJ, Perurena OH, Ronan S, Manaligod JR. Inclusion body myositis associated with systemic sarcoidosis. *Can J Neurol Sci.* 1986;13(4):334–336.
159. Pluk H, van Hoeve BJ, van Dooren SH, et al. Autoantibodies to cytosolic 5′-nucleotidase 1 A in inclusion body myositis. *Ann Neurol.* 2013;73(3):397–407.
160. Larman HB, Salajegheh M, Nazareno R, et al. Cytosolic 5′-nucleotidase 1 A autoimmunity in sporadic inclusion body myositis. *Ann Neurol.* 2013;73(3):408–418.
161. Garlepp MJ, Laing B, Zilko PJ, Ollier W, Mastaglia FL. HLA associations with inclusion body myositis. *Clin Exp Immunol.* 1994;98(1):40–45.

162. Sekul EA, Chow C, Dalakas MC. Magnetic resonance imaging of the forearm as a diagnostic aid in patients with sporadic inclusion body myositis. *Neurology.* 1997;48(4):863–866.
163. Taira K, Yamamoto T, Mori-Yoshimura M, et al. Cricopharyngeal bar on videofluoroscopy: high specificity for inclusion body myositis. *J Neurol.* 2021;268(3):1016–1024.
164. Joy JL, Oh SJ, Baysal AI. Electrophysiological spectrum of inclusion body myositis. *Muscle Nerve.* 1990;13(10):949–951.
165. Askanas V, Engel WK, Alvarez RB. Enhanced detection of Congo-red-positive amyloid deposits in muscle fibers of inclusion body myositis and brain of Alzheimer's disease using fluorescence technique. *Neurology.* 1993;43(6):1265–1267.
166. Mendell JR, Sahenk Z, Gales T, Paul L. Amyloid filaments in inclusion body myositis. Novel findings provide insight into nature of filaments. *Arch Neurol.* 1991;48(12):1229–1234.
167. Barohn RJ, Amato AA, Sahenk Z, Kissel JT, Mendell JR. Inclusion body myositis: explanation for poor response to immunosuppressive therapy. *Neurology.* 1995;45(7):1302–1304.
168. Rifai Z, Welle S, Kamp C, Thornton CA. Ragged red fibers in normal aging and inflammatory myopathy. *Ann Neurol.* 1995;37(1):24–29.
169. O'Hanlon TP, Dalakas MC, Plotz PH, Miller FW. The alpha beta T-cell receptor repertoire in inclusion body myositis: diverse patterns of gene expression by muscle-infiltrating lymphocytes. *J Autoimmun.* 1994;7(3):321–333.
170. Amemiya K, Granger RP, Dalakas MC. Clonal restriction of T-cell receptor expression by infiltrating lymphocytes in inclusion body myositis persists over time. Studies in repeated muscle biopsies. *Brain.* 2000;123(pt 10):2030–2039.
171. Greenberg SA, Pinkus JL, Amato AA, Kristensen T, Dorfman DM. Association of inclusion body myositis with T cell large granular lymphocytic leukaemia. *Brain.* 2016;139(Pt 5):1348–1360.
172. Greenberg SA, Pinkus JL, Kong SW, Baecher-Allan C, Amato AA, Dorfman DM. Highly differentiated cytotoxic T cells in inclusion body myositis. *Brain.* 2019;142(9):2590–2604.
173. Goyal NA, Coulis G, Duarte J, et al. Immunophenotyping of inclusion body myositis blood T and NK cells. *Neurology.* 2022;98(13):e1374–e1383.
174. Pruitt JN 2nd, Showalter CJ, Engel AG. Sporadic inclusion body myositis: counts of different types of abnormal fibers. *Ann Neurol.* 1996;39(1):139–143.
175. Askanas V, Engel WK. Proposed pathogenetic cascade of inclusion-body myositis: importance of amyloid-beta, misfolded proteins, predisposing genes, and aging. *Curr Opin Rheumatol.* 2003;15(6):737–744.
176. Greenberg SA, Pinkus JL, Amato AA. Nuclear membrane proteins are present within rimmed vacuoles in inclusion-body myositis. *Muscle Nerve.* 2006;34:406–416.
177. Salajegheh M, Pinkus JL, Taylor JP, et al. Sarcoplasmic redistribution of nuclear TDP-43 in inclusion body myositis. *Muscle Nerve.* 2009;40(1):19–31.
178. Olive M, Janue A, Moreno D, Gamez J, Torrejon-Escribano B, Ferrer I. TAR DNA-binding protein 43 accumulation in protein aggregate myopathies. *J Neuropathol Exp Neurol.* 2009;68(3):262–273.
179. Kusters B, van Hoeve BJ, Schelhaas HJ, Ter Laak H, van Engelen BG, Lammens M. TDP-43 accumulation is common in myopathies with rimmed vacuoles. *Acta Neuropathol.* 2009;117(2):209–211.
180. Hiniker A, Daniels BH, Lee HS, Margeta M. Comparative utility of LC3, p62 and TDP-43 immunohistochemistry in differentiation of inclusion body myositis from polymyositis and related inflammatory myopathies. *Acta Neuropathol Commun.* 2013;1(1):1–14.
181. Oldfors A, Larsson NG, Lindberg C, Holme E. Mitochondrial DNA deletions in inclusion body myositis. *Brain.* 1993;116(pt 2):325–336.
182. Yang CC, Alvarez RB, Engel WK, Askanas V. Increase of nitric oxide synthases and nitrotyrosine in inclusion-body myositis. *Neuroreport.* 1996;8(1):153–158.
183. Banwell BL, Engel AG. AlphaB-crystallin immunolocalization yields new insights into inclusion body myositis. *Neurology.* 2000;54(5):1033–1041.
184. Britson KA, Ling JP, Braunstein KE, et al. Loss of TDP-43 function and rimmed vacuoles persist after T cell depletion in a xenograft model of sporadic inclusion body myositis. *Sci Transl Med.* 2022;14(628):eabi9196.
185. Chou SM. Inclusion body myositis: a chronic persistent mumps myositis? *Hum Pathol.* 1986;17(8):765–777.
186. Kallajoki M, Hyypia T, Halonen P, Orvell C, Rima BK, Kalimo H. Inclusion body myositis and paramyxoviruses. *Hum Pathol.* 1991;22(1):29–32.
187. Nishino H, Engel AG, Rima BK. Inclusion body myositis: the mumps virus hypothesis. *Ann Neurol.* 1989;25(3):260–264.
188. Cupler EJ, Leon-Monzon M, Miller J, Semino-Mora C, Anderson TL, Dalakas MC. Inclusion body myositis in HIV-1 and HTLV-1 infected patients. *Brain.* 1996;119(pt 6):1887–1893.
189. Semino-Mora C, Dalakas MC. Rimmed vacuoles with beta-amyloid and ubiquitinated filamentous deposits in the muscles of patients with long-standing denervation (postpoliomyelitis muscular atrophy): similarities with inclusion body myositis. *Hum Pathol.* 1998;29(10):1128–1133.
190. Watts GD, Wymer J, Kovach MJ, et al. Inclusion body myopathy associated with Paget disease of bone and frontotemporal dementia is caused by mutant valosin-containing protein. *Nat Genet.* 2004;36(4):377–381.
191. Bronner IM, Hoogendijk JE, Wintzen AR, et al. Necrotising myopathy, an unusual presentation of a steroid-responsive myopathy. *J Neurol.* 2003;250(4):480–485.
192. Emslie-Smith AM, Engel AG. Necrotizing myopathy with pipestem capillaries, microvascular deposition of the complement membrane attack complex (MAC), and minimal cellular infiltration. *Neurology.* 1991;41(6):936–939.
193. Levin MI, Mozaffar T, Al-Lozi MT, Pestronk A. Paraneoplastic necrotizing myopathy: clinical and pathological features. *Neurology.* 1998;50(3):764–767.
194. Vosskamper M, Korf B, Franke F, Schachenmayr W. Paraneoplastic necrotizing myopathy: a rare disorder to be differentiated from polymyositis. *J Neurol.* 1989;236(8):489–490.
195. Hengstman GJ, ter Laak HJ, Vree Egberts WT, et al. Anti-signal recognition particle autoantibodies: marker of a necrotising myopathy. *Ann Rheum Dis.* 2006;65(12):1635–1638.
196. Needham M, Fabian V, Knezevic W, Panegyres P, Zilko P, Mastaglia FL. Progressive myopathy with up-regulation of MHC-I associated with statin therapy. *Neuromuscul Disord.* 2007;17(2):194–200.
197. Grable-Esposito P, Katzberg HD, Greenberg SA, Srinivasan J, Katz J, Amato AA. Immune-mediated necrotizing myopathy associated with statins. *Muscle Nerve.* 2010;41(2):185–190.

198. Mammen AL, Amato AA. Statin myopathy: a review of recent progress. *Curr Opin Rheumatol.* 2010;22(6):644–650.
199. Christopher-Stine L, Casciola-Rosen LA, Hong G, Chung T, Corse AM, Mammen AL. A novel autoantibody recognizing 200-kd and 100-kd proteins is associated with an immune-mediated necrotizing myopathy. *Arthritis Rheum.* 2010;62:2757–2766.
200. Mammen AL, Chung T, Christopher-Stine L, et al. Autoantibodies against 3-hydroxy-3-methylglutaryl-coenzyme A reductase in patients with statin-associated autoimmune myopathy. *Arthritis Rheum.* 2011;63(3):713–721.
201. Mammen AL, Pak K, Williams EK, et al. Rarity of anti-3-hydroxy-3-methylglutaryl-coenzyme A reductase antibodies in statin users, including those with self-limited musculoskeletal side effects. *Arthritis Care Res (Hoboken).* 2012;64(2):269–272.
202. Werner J, Christopher-Stine L, Ghazarian SR, et al. Antibody levels correlate with creatine kinase levels and strength in anti-HMG-CoA reductase-associated autoimmune myopathy. *Arthritis Rheum.* 2012;64(12):4087–4093.
203. Allenbach Y, Mammen AL, Benveniste O, Stenzel W; Immune-Mediated Necrotizing Myopathies Working Group. 224th ENMC International Workshop: Clinico-sero-pathological classification of immune-mediated necrotizing myopathies Zandvoort, The Netherlands, 14–16 October 2016. *Neuromuscul Disord.* 2018;28(1):87–99.
204. Mohassel P, Mammen AL. Anti-HMGCR Myopathy. *J Neuromuscul Dis.* 2018;5(1):11–20.
205. Allenbach Y, Benveniste O, Stenzel W, Boyer O. Immune-mediated necrotizing myopathy: clinical features and pathogenesis. *Nat Rev Rheumatol.* 2020;16(12):689–701.
206. Watanabe Y, Uruha A, Suzuki S, et al. Clinical features and prognosis in anti-SRP and anti-HMGCR necrotising myopathy. *J Neurol Neurosurg Psychiatry.* 2016;87(10):1038–1044.
207. Nicolau S, Milone M, Tracy JA, Mills JR, Triplett JD, Liewluck T. Immune-mediated necrotizing myopathy: unusual presentations of a treatable disease. *Muscle Nerve.* 2021;64(6):733–739.
208. Morales-Rosado JA, Schwab TL, Macklin-Mantia SK, et al. Bi-allelic variants in HMGCR cause an autosomal-recessive progressive limb-girdle muscular dystrophy. *Am J Hum Genet.* 2023;110(6):989–997.
209. Yogev Y, Shorer Z, Koifman A, et al. Limb girdle muscular disease caused by HMGCR mutation and statin myopathy treatable with mevalonolactone. *Proc Natl Acad Sci USA.* 2023;120(7):e2217831120.
210. Mammen AL, Tiniakou E. Intravenous Immune Globulin for Statin-Triggered Autoimmune Myopathy. *N Engl J Med.* 2015;373(17):1680–1682.
211. Greenberg SA, Amato AA. Inflammatory myopathy associated with mixed connective tissue disease and scleroderma renal crisis. *Muscle Nerve.* 2001;24(11):1562–1566.
212. Follansbee WP, Zerbe TR, Medsger TA Jr. Cardiac and skeletal muscle disease in systemic sclerosis (scleroderma): a high risk association. *Am Heart J.* 1993;125(1):194–203.
213. Marguerie C, Bunn CC, Copier J, et al. The clinical and immunogenetic features of patients with autoantibodies to the nucleolar antigen PM-Scl. *Medicine (Baltimore).* 1992;71(6):327–336.
214. Ringel RA, Brick JE, Brick JF, Gutmann L, Riggs JE. Muscle involvement in the scleroderma syndromes. *Arch Intern Med.* 1990;150(12):2550–2552.
215. Brouwer R, Vree Egberts WT, Hengstman GJ, et al. Autoantibodies directed to novel components of the PM/Scl complex, the human exosome. *Arthritis Res.* 2002;4(2):134–138.
216. De Lorenzo R, Pinal-Fernandez I, Huang W, et al. Muscular and extramuscular clinical features of patients with anti-PM/Scl autoantibodies. *Neurology.* 2018;90:e2068–e2076.
217. Denko CW, Old JW. Myopathy in the Sicca syndrome (Sjogren's syndrome). *Am J Clin Pathol.* 1969;51(5):631–637.
218. Ponge T, Mussini JM, Ponge A, et al. Primary Gougerot–Sjogren syndrome with necrotizing polymyositis: favorable effect of hydroxychloroquine. *Rev Neurol (Paris).* 1987;143(2):147–148.
219. Ringel SP, Forstot JZ, Tan EM, Wehling C, Griggs RC, Butcher D. Sjogren's syndrome and polymyositis or dermatomyositis. *Arch Neurol.* 1982;39(3):157–163.
220. Chung SH, Bent EI, Weiss MD, Gardner GC. Sporadic inclusion body myositis and primary Sjogren's syndrome: an overlooked diagnosis. *Clin Rheumatol.* 2021;40(10):4089–4094.
221. Naddaf E, Shelly S, Mandrekar J, et al. Survival and associated comorbidities in inclusion body myositis. *Rheumatology (Oxford).* 2022;61(5):2016–2024.
222. Levy D, Nespola B, Giannini M, et al. Significance of Sjögren's syndrome and anti-cN1A antibody in myositis patients. *Rheumatology (Oxford).* 2022;61(2):756–763.
223. Tiniakou E, Goldman D, Corse A, Mammen A, Petri MA. Clinical and histopathological features of myositis in systemic lupus erythematosus. *Lupus Sci Med.* 2022;9(1):e000635.
224. Sharp GC, Irvin WS, Tan EM, Gould RG, Holman HR. Mixed connective tissue disease—an apparently distinct rheumatic disease syndrome associated with a specific antibody to an extractable nuclear antigen (ENA). *Am J Med.* 1972;52(2):148–159.
225. Casal-Dominguez M, Pinal-Fernandez I, Derfoul A, et al. The phenotype of myositis patients with anti-Ku autoantibodies. *Semin Arthritis Rheum.* 2021;51:728–734.
226. Fermon C, Authier FJ, Gallay L. Idiopathic eosinophilic myositis: a systematic literature review. *Neuromuscul Disord.* 2022 Feb;32(2):116–124.
227. Fermon C, Lessard LER, Fenouil T, et al. Revisiting idiopathic eosinophilic myositis: toward a clinical-pathological continuum from the muscle to the fascia and skin. *Rheumatology (Oxford).* 2023;62(6):2220–2229.
228. Kobayashi Y, Fujimoto T, Shiiki H, Kitaoka K, Murata K, Dohi K. Focal eosinophilic myositis. *Clin Rheumatol.* 2001;20(5):369–371.
229. Layzer RB, Shearn MA, Satya-Murti S. Eosinophilic polymyositis. *Ann Neurol.* 1977;1(1):65–71.
230. Moore PM, Harley JB, Fauci AS. Neurologic dysfunction in the idiopathic hypereosinophilic syndrome. *Ann Intern Med.* 1985;102(1):109–114.
231. Murata K, Sugie K, Takamure M, Fujimoto T, Ueno S. Eosinophilic major basic protein and interleukin-5 in eosinophilic myositis. *Eur J Neurol.* 2003;10(1):35–38.
232. Serratrice G, Pellissier JF, Cros D, Gastaut JL, Brindisi G. Relapsing eosinophilic perimyositis. *J Rheumatol.* 1980;7(2):199–205.
233. Serratrice G, Pellissier JF, Roux H, Quilichini P. Fasciitis, perimyositis, myositis, polymyositis, and eosinophilia. *Muscle Nerve.* 1990;13(5):385–395.
234. Dunand M, Lobrinus JA, Spertini O, Kuntzer T. Eosinophilic perimyositis as the presenting feature of a monoclonal T-cell expansion. *Muscle Nerve.* 2005;31(5):646–651.

235. Simon HU, Plotz SG, Simon D, Dummer R, Blaser K. Clinical and immunological features of patients with interleukin-5-producing T cell clones and eosinophilia. *Int Arch Allergy Immunol.* 2001;124(1–3):242–245.
236. Amato AA. Adults with eosinophilic myositis and calpain-3 mutations. *Neurology.* 2008;70(9):730–731.
237. Lakhanpal S, Ginsburg WW, Michet CJ, Doyle JA, Moore SB. Eosinophilic fasciitis: clinical spectrum and therapeutic response in 52 cases. *Semin Arthritis Rheum.* 1988;17(4):221–231.
238. Shulman LE. Diffuse fasciitis with eosinophilia: a new syndrome? *Trans Assoc Am Physicians.* 1975;88:70–86.
239. Hertzman PA, Blevins WL, Mayer J, Greenfield B, Ting M, Gleich GJ. Association of the eosinophilia-myalgia syndrome with the ingestion of tryptophan. *N Engl J Med.* 1990;322(13):869–873.
240. Kilbourne EM, Rigau-Perez JG, Heath CW Jr, et al. Clinical epidemiology of toxic-oil syndrome. Manifestations of a new illness. *N Engl J Med.* 1983;309(23):1408–1414.
241. Namba T, Brunner NG, Grob D. Idiopathic giant cell polymyositis. Report of a case and review of the syndrome. *Arch Neurol.* 1974;31(1):27–30.
242. Pascuzzi RM, Roos KL, Phillips LH 2nd. Granulomatous inflammatory myopathy associated with myasthenia gravis. A case report and review of the literature. *Arch Neurol.* 1986;43(6):621–623.
243. Mozaffar T, Lopate G, Pestronk A. Clinical correlates of granulomas in muscle. *J Neurol.* 1998;245(8):519–524.
244. Scangarello FA, Angel-Buitrago L, Lang-Orsini M, et al. Giant cell myositis associated with concurrent myasthenia gravis: a case-based review of the literature. *Clin Rheumatol.* 2021;40(9):3841–3851.
245. Jin J, Isfort MC, Ascherman DP, Lacomis D. Granulomatous myositis associated with acetylcholine receptor antibodies Without Clinical Myasthenia. *J Clin Neuromuscul Dis.* 2021;23(1):49–52.
246. Dieudonné Y, Allenbach Y, Benveniste O, et al. Granulomatosis-associated myositis: high prevalence of sporadic inclusion body myositis. *Neurology.* 2020;94:e910–e920.
247. Nelke C, Kleefeld F, Preusse C, Ruck T, Stenzel W. Inclusion body myositis and associated diseases: an argument for shared immune pathologies. *Acta Neuropathol Commun.* 2022;10(1):84.
248. Danon MJ, Perurena OH, Ronan S, Manaligod JR. Inclusion body myositis associated with systemic sarcoidosis. *Can J Neurol Sci J Can Sci Neurol.* 1986;13:334–336.
249. Sanmaneechai O, Swenson A, Gerke AK, Moore SA, Shy ME. Inclusion body myositis and sarcoid myopathy: coincidental occurrence or associated diseases. *Neuromuscul Disord.* 2015;25(4):297–300.
250. Alhammad RM, Liewluck T. Myopathies featuring non-caseating granulomas: Sarcoidosis, inclusion body myositis and an unfolding overlap. *Neuromuscul Disord.* 2019;29(1):39–47.
251. Silverstein A, Siltzbach LE. Muscle involvement in sarcoidosis. Asymptomatic, myositis, and myopathy. *Arch Neurol.* 1969;21(3):235–241.
252. Stjernberg N, Cajander S, Truedsson H, Uddenfeldt P. Muscle involvement in sarcoidosis. *Acta Med Scand.* 1981;209(3):213–216.
253. Younger DS. Giant cell arteritis. *Neurol Clin.* 2019;37(2):335–344.
254. Buttgereit F, Matteson EL, Dejaco C. Polymyalgia rheumatica and giant cell arteritis. *JAMA.* 2020;324(10):993–994.
255. Serling-Boyd N, Stone JH. Recent advances in the diagnosis and management of giant cell arteritis. *Curr Opin Rheumatol.* 2020;32(3):201–207.
256. Stone JH, Tuckwell K, Dimonaco S, et al. Trial of tocilizumab in giant-cell arteritis. *N Engl J Med.* 2017;377(4):317–328.
257. Suzuki S, Motomura M, Maruta T, et al. Autoimmune targets of heart and skeletal muscles in myasthenia gravis. *Arch Neurol.* 2009;66(11):1334–1338.
258. Uchio N, Taira K, Ikenaga C, et al. Inflammatory myopathy with myasthenia gravis. *Neurol – Neuroimmunol Neuroinflam.* 2019;6(2):e535.
259. Bernard C, Frih H, Pasquet F, et al. Thymoma associated with autoimmune diseases: 85 cases and literature review. *Autoimmun Rev.* 2016;15(1):82–92.
260. Scangarello FA, Angel-Buitrago L, Lang-Orsini M, et al. Giant cell myositis associated with concurrent myasthenia gravis: a case-based review of the literature. *Clinical Rheumatology.* 2021;40(9):3841–3851.
261. Burke JS, Medline NM, Katz A. Giant cell myocarditis and myositis. Associated with thymoma and myasthenia gravis. *Arch Pathol.* 1969;88(4):359–366.
262. Bourgeois-Droin C, Sauvanet A, Lemarchand F, De Roquancourt A, Cottenot F, Brocheriou C. Thymoma associated with myasthenia, erythroblastopenia, myositis and giant cell myocarditis. One case (author's transl). *Nouv Press Med.* 1981;10(25):2097–2098, 2103–2104.
263. Pascuzzi RM, Roos KL, Philips 2nd LH. Granulomatous inflammatory myopathy associated with myasthenia gravis. *Arch Neurol.* 1986;43(6):621–623.
264. Kon T, Mori F, Tanji K, Miki Y, Kimura T, Wakabayashi K. Giant cell polymyositis and myocarditis associated with myasthenia gravis and thymoma. *Neuropathology.* 2013;33(3):281–287.
265. Illac C, Boudat AM, Larrieu JM, Delisle MB. Giant cell myositis and myasthenia gravis: a case report. *Ann Pathol.* 2013;33(1):53–56.
266. Grbelja LD, Vrhovac R, Ulamec M. Myasthenia gravis associated with thymoma and aplastic anemia: case report. *Acta Clinica Croatica.* 2017;56(4):817–820.
267. Avni I, Sharabi Y, Sadeh M, Buchman AS. Eosinophilia, myositis, and myasthenia gravis associated with a thymoma. *Muscle Nerve.* 2006;34(2):242–245.
268. Ikeda Y, Tanaka M, Mizushima K, Okamoto K. A case of eosinophilic polymyositis complicated by myasthenia gravis. *Muscle Nerve.* 1998;21(10):1356–1358.
269. Ishida Y, Hayashi M, Higaki A, et al. Hypereosinophilic syndrome with generalized myasthenia gravis. *J Pediatr.* 1996;128(3):369–372.
270. Inoue M, Kojima Y, Shinde A, et al. Concurrence of myasthenia gravis, polymyositis, thyroiditis and eosinophilia in a patient with type B1 thymoma. *Rinsho Shinkeigaku.* 2007;47(7):423–428.
271. Fitzmaurice RJ, Gardner DL. Thymoma with bone marrow eosinophilia. *J R Soc Med.* 1990;83(4):270–271.
272. Sumi M, Nunoda K, Mizutani T, et al. Hypereosinophilia in a patient with invasive thymoma with clonal T-lymphocyte expansion expressing CD4, CD8, and CD25 antigens. *Int J Hematol.* 2006;83(3):243–246.
273. Afifi AK, Frayha RA, Bahuth NB, Tekian A. The myopathology of Behcet's disease—a histochemical, light-, and electron-microscopic study. *J Neurol Sci.* 1980;48(3):333–342.

274. Di Giacomo V, Carmenini G, Meloni F, Valesini G. Myositis in Behcet's disease. *Arthritis Rheum*. 1982;25(8):1025.
275. Finucane P, Doyle CT, Ferriss JB, Molloy M, Murnaghan D. Behcet's syndrome with myositis and glomerulonephritis. *Br J Rheumatol*. 1985;24(4):372–375.
276. Lingenfelser T, Duerk H, Stevens A, Grossmann T, Knorr M, Saal JG. Generalized myositis in Behcet disease: treatment with cyclosporine. *Ann Intern Med*. 1992;116(8):651–653.
277. Worthmann F, Bruns J, Türker T, Gosztonyi G. Muscular involvement in Behcet's disease: case report and review of the literature. *Neuromuscul Disord*. 1996;6(4):247–253.
278. Caldwell CJ, Swash M, Van der Walt JD, Geddes JF. Focal myositis: a clinico-pathological study. *Neuromuscul Disord*. 1995;5(4):317–321.
279. Colding-Jorgensen E, Laursen H, Lauritzen M. Focal myositis of the thigh: report of two cases. *Acta Neurol Scand*. 1993;88(4):289–292.
280. Heffner RR Jr, Barron SA. Polymyositis beginning as a focal process. *Arch Neurol*. 1981;38(7):439–442.
281. Moreno-Lugris C, Gonzalez-Gay MA, Sanchez-Andrade A, et al. Magnetic resonance imaging: a useful technique in the diagnosis and follow up of focal myositis. *Ann Rheum Dis*. 1996;55(11):856.
282. Moskovic E, Fisher C, Westbury G, Parsons C. Focal myositis, a benign inflammatory pseudotumour: CT appearances. *Br J Radiol*. 1991;64(762):489–493.
283. Illa I, Nath A, Dalakas M. Immunocytochemical and virological characteristics of HIV-associated inflammatory myopathies: similarities with seronegative polymyositis. *Ann Neurol*. 1991;29(5):474–481.
284. Lloyd TE, Pinal-Fernandez I, Michelle EH, et al. Overlapping features of polymyositis and inclusion body myositis in HIV-infected patients. *Neurology*. 2017;88:1454–1460.
285. Dalakas MC, Rakocevic G, Shatunov A, Goldfarb L, Raju R, Salajegheh M. Inclusion body myositis with human immunodeficiency virus infection: four cases with clonal expansion of viral-specific T cells. *Ann Neurol*. 2007;61:466–475.
286. Cupler EJ, Leon-Monzon M, Miller J, Semino-Mora C, Anderson TL, Dalakas MC. Inclusion body myositis in HIV-1 and HTLV-1 infected patients. *Brain*. 1996;119:1887–1893.
287. Callens S, De Roo A, Colebunders R. Fanconi-like syndrome and rhabdomyolysis in a person with HIV infection on highly active antiretroviral treatment including tenofovir. *J Infect*. 2003;47(3):262–263.
288. Mahe A, Bruet A, Chabin E, Fendler JP. Acute rhabdomyolysis coincident with primary HIV-1 infection. *Lancet*. 1989;2(8677):1454–1455.
289. McDonagh CA, Holman RP. Primary human immunodeficiency virus type 1 infection in a patient with acute rhabdomyolysis. *South Med J*. 2003;96(10):1027–1030.
290. Rastegar D, Claiborne C, Fleisher A, Matsumoto A. A patient with primary human immunodeficiency virus infection who presented with acute rhabdomyolysis. *Clin Infect Dis*. 2001;32(3):502–504.
291. Arnaudo E, Dalakas M, Shanske S, Moraes CT, DiMauro S, Schon EA. Depletion of muscle mitochondrial DNA in AIDS patients with zidovudine-induced myopathy. *Lancet*. 1991;337(8740):508–510.
292. Cupler EJ, Danon MJ, Jay C, Hench K, Ropka M, Dalakas MC. Early features of zidovudine-associated myopathy: histopathological findings and clinical correlations. *Acta Neuropathol (Berl)*. 1995;90(1):1–6.
293. Dalakas M. HIV or zidovudine myopathy? *Neurology*. 1994;44(2):360–361; author reply 362–364.
294. Dalakas MC, Pezeshkpour GH, Flaherty M. Progressive nemaline (rod) myopathy associated with HIV infection. *N Engl J Med*. 1987;317(25):1602–1603.
295. Pezeshkpour G, Illa I, Dalakas MC. Ultrastructural characteristics and DNA immunocytochemistry in human immunodeficiency virus and zidovudine-associated myopathies. *Hum Pathol*. 1991;22(12):1281–1288.
296. Caldwell CJ, Barrett WY, Breuer J, Farmer SF, Swash M. HTLV-1 polymyositis. *Neuromuscul Disord*. 1996;6(3):151–154.
297. Evans BK, Gore I, Harrell LE, Arnold T, Oh SJ. HTLV-I-associated myelopathy and polymyositis in a US native. *Neurology*. 1989;39(12):1572–1575.
298. Morgan OS, Rodgers-Johnson P, Mora C, Char G. HTLV-1 and polymyositis in Jamaica. *Lancet*. 1989;2(8673):1184–1187.
299. Mejlszenkier JD, Safran AP, Healy JJ, Embree L, Ouellette EM. The myositis of influenza. *Arch Neurol*. 1973;29(6):441–443.
300. Middleton PJ, Alexander RM, Szymanski MT. Severe myositis during recovery from influenza. *Lancet*. 1970;2(7672):533–535.
301. Minow RA, Gorbach S, Johnson BL Jr, Dornfeld L. Myoglobinuria associated with influenza A infection. *Ann Intern Med*. 1974;80(3):359–361.
302. Morgensen JL. Myoglobinuria and renal failure associated with influenza. *Ann Intern Med*. 1974;80(3):362–363.
303. Ruff RL, Secrist D. Viral studies in benign acute childhood myositis. *Arch Neurol*. 1982;39(5):261–263.
304. Christenson JC, San Joaquin VH. Influenza-associated rhabdomyolysis in a child. *Pediatr Infect Dis J*. 1990;9(1):60–61.
305. Farrell MK, Partin JC, Bove KE. Epidemic influenza myopathy in Cincinnati in 1977. *J Pediatr*. 1980;96(3 pt 2):545–551.
306. Gamboa ET, Eastwood AB, Hays AP, Maxwell J, Penn AS. Isolation of influenza virus from muscle in myoglobinuric polymyositis. *Neurology*. 1979;29(10):1323–1335.
307. Suh J, Amato AA. Neuromuscular complications of coronavirus disease-19. *Curr Opin Neurol*. 2021;34(5):669–674.
308. Chen N, Zhou M, Dong X, et al. Epidemiological and clinical characteristics of 99 cases of 2019 novel coronavirus pneumonia in Wuhan, China: a descriptive study. *Lancet*. 2020;395:507–513.
309. Li LQ, Huang T, Wang YQ, et al. COVID-19 patients' clinical characteristics, discharge rate, and fatality rate of meta-analysis. *J Med Virol*. 2020;92:577–583.
310. Borges do Nascimento IJ, Cacic N, Abdulazeem HM, et al. Novel coronavirus infection (COVID-19) in humans: a scoping review and meta-analysis. *J Clin Med*. 2020;9:941.
311. Wang D, Hu B, Hu C, et al. Clinical characteristics of 138 hospitalized patients with 2019 novel coronavirus-infected pneumonia in Wuhan, China. *JAMA*. 2020; 323: 1061–1069.
312. Mao L, Jin H, Wang M, et al. Neurologic manifestations of hospitalized patients with coronavirus disease 2019 in Wuhan, China. *JAMA Neurol*. 2020;77:683–690.
313. Guan WJ, Ni ZY, Hu Y, et al. Clinical characteristics of coronavirus disease 2019 in China. *N Engl J Med*. 2020;382: 1708–1720.
314. Geng Y, Ma Q, Du YS, et al. Rhabdomyolysis is associated with in-hospital mortality in patients with COVID-19. *Shock (Augusta, Ga)*. 2021;56(3):360–367.
315. Haroun MW, Dieiev V, Kang J, et al. Rhabdomyolysis in COVID-19 patients: a retrospective observational study. *Cureus*. 2021;13:e12552.

316. Suh J, Mukerji SS, Collens SI, et al. Skeletal muscle and peripheral nerve histopathology in COVID-19. *Neurology*. 2021;97:e849–e858.
317. Aschman T, Schneider J, Greuel S, et al. Association between SARS-CoV-2 infection and immune-mediated myopathy in patients who have died. *JAMA Neurol*. 2021;78:948–960.
318. Manzano GS, Woods JK, Amato AA. Covid-19-associated myopathy caused by type I interferonopathy. *N Engl J Med*. 2020;383:2389–2390.
319. Zhang H, Charmchi Z, Seidman RJ, Anzika Y, Velayudhan V, Perk J. COVID-19-associated myositis with severe proximal and bulbar weakness. *Muscle Nerve*. 2020;62:E57–e60.
320. Tanboon J, Nishino I. COVID-19-associated myositis may be dermatomyositis. *Muscle Nerve*. 2021;63:E9–e10.
321. Okada Y, Izumi R, Hosaka T, et al. Anti-NXP2 antibody-positive dermatomyositis developed after COVID-19 manifesting as type I interferonopathy. *Rheumatology*. 2022;61:e90–e92.
322. Shi Z, de Vries HJ, Vlaar APJ, et al. Diaphragm Pathology in critically Ill patients with COVID-19 and postmortem findings from 3 medical centers. *JAMA Internal Medicine*. 2021;181:122–124.
323. Hooper JE, Uner M, Priemer DS, Rosenberg A, Chen L. Muscle biopsy findings in a case of SARS-CoV-2-associated muscle injury. *J Neuropathol Exp Neurol*. 2021;80:377–378.
324. Dodig D, Tarnopolsky MA, Margeta M, Gordon K, Fritzler MJ, Lu J. COVID-19-associated critical illness myopathy with direct viral effects. *Ann Neurol*. 2022;91:568–574.
325. Gokhale Y, Patankar A, Holla U, et al. Dermatomyositis during COVID-19 pandemic (a case series): is there a cause effect relationship? *J Assoc Physicians India*. 2020;68(11):20–24.
326. Saud A, Naveen R, Aggarwal R, Gupta L. COVID-19 and myositis: What we know so far. *Curr Rheumatol Rep*. 2021;23(8):63.
327. Movahedi N, Ziaee V. COVID-19 and myositis; true dermatomyositis or prolonged post viral myositis? *Pediatr Rheumatol Online J*. 2021;19(1):86.
328. Okada Y, Izumi R, Hosaka T, et al. Anti-NXP2 antibody-positive dermatomyositis developed after COVID-19 manifesting as type I interferonopathy. *Rheumatology (Oxford)*. 2022;61(4):e90–e92.
329. Kogami M, Suzuki S, Nanjo Y, Ikeda K, Tamura N, Sasaki S, et al. Complication of coronavirus disease 2019 during remission induction therapy against anti-MDA5 antibody-positive dermatomyositis. *Rheumatol Adv Pract*. 2020;4:rkaa068.
330. Cao M, Zhang S, Chu D, et al. COVID-19 or clinical amyopathic dermatomyositis associated rapidly progressive interstitial lung disease? A case report. *BMC Pulm Med*. 2020;20:304.
331. Borges NH, Godoy TM, Kahlow BS. Onset of dermatomyositis in close association with COVID-19 – a first case reported. *Rheumatol (Oxford)*. 2021;60:SI96.
332. Quintana-Ortega C, Remesal A, Ruiz de Valbuena M, et al. Fatal outcome of anti-MDA5 juvenile dermatomyositis in a paediatric COVID-19 patient: a case report. *Mod Rheumatol Case Rep*. 2021;5:101–107.
333. Ho BVK, Seger EW, Kollmann K, Rajpara A. Dermatomyositis in a COVID-19 positive patient. *JAAD Case Rep*. 2021;13:97–99.
334. Liquidano-Perez E, García-Romero MT, Yamazaki-Nakashimada M, et al. Juvenile dermatomyositis triggered by SARS-CoV-2. *Pediatr Neurol*. 2021;121:26–27.
335. Antony SJ, Kernodle DS. Nontropical pyomyositis in patients with AIDS. *J Natl Med Assoc*. 1996;88(9):565–569.
336. Rodgers WB, Yodlowski ML, Mintzer CM. Pyomyositis in patients who have the human immunodeficiency virus. Case report and review of the literature. *J Bone Joint Surg Am*. 1993;75(4):588–592.
337. Hsueh PR, Hsiue TR, Hsieh WC. Pyomyositis in intravenous drug abusers: report of a unique case and review of the literature. *Clin Infect Dis*. 1996;22(5):858–860.
338. Chiedozi LC. Pyomyositis. Review of 205 cases in 112 patients. *Am J Surg*. 1979;137(2):255–259.
339. Akman I, Ostrov B, Varma BK, Keenan G. Pyomyositis: report of three patients and review of the literature. *Clin Pediatr (Phila)*. 1996;35(8):397–401.
340. O'Neill DS, Baquis G, Moral L. Infectious myositis. A tropical disease steals out of its zone. *Postgrad Med*. 1996;100(2):193–194, 199–200.
341. Atlas E, Novak SN, Duray PH, Steere AC. Lyme myositis: muscle invasion by *Borrelia burgdorferi*. *Ann Intern Med*. 1988;109(3):245–246.
342. Horowitz HW, Sanghera K, Goldberg N, et al. Dermatomyositis associated with Lyme disease: case report and review of Lyme myositis. *Clin Infect Dis*. 1994;18(2):166–171.
343. Jeandel C, Perret C, Blain H, Jouanny P, Penin F, Laurain MC. Rhabdomyolysis with acute renal failure due to *Borrelia burgdorferi*. *J Intern Med*. 1994;235(2):191–192.
344. Muller-Felber W, Reimers CD, de Koning J, Fischer P, Pilz A, Pongratz DE. Myositis in Lyme borreliosis: an immunohistochemical study of seven patients. *J Neurol Sci*. 1993;118(2):207–212.
345. Reimers CD, de Koning J, Neubert U, et al. *Borrelia burgdorferi* myositis: report of eight patients. *J Neurol*. 1993;240(5):278–283.
346. Schmutzhard E, Willeit J, Gerstenbrand F. Meningopolyneuritis Bannwarth with focal nodular myositis. A new aspect in Lyme borreliosis. *Klin Wochenschr*. 1986;64(22):1204–1208.
347. Arena FP, Perlin M, Brahman H, Weiser B, Armstrong D. Fever, rash, and myalgias of disseminated candidiasis during antifungal therapy. *Arch Intern Med*. 1981;141(9):1233.
348. Jarowski CI, Fialk MA, Murray HW, et al. Fever, rash, and muscle tenderness. A distinctive clinical presentation of disseminated candidiasis. *Arch Intern Med*. 1978;138(4):544–546.
349. Halverson PB, Lahiri S, Wojno WC, Sulaiman AR. Sporotrichal arthritis presenting as granulomatous myositis. *Arthritis Rheum*. 1985;28(12):1425–1429.
350. Wrzolek MA, Sher JH, Kozlowski PB, Rao C. Skeletal muscle pathology in AIDS: an autopsy study. *Muscle Nerve*. 1990;13(6):508–515.
351. Davis MJ, Cilo M, Plaitakis A, Yahr MD. Trichinosis: severe myopathic involvement with recovery. *Neurology*. 1976;26(1):37–40.
352. Gross B, Ochoa J. Trichinosis: clinical report and histochemistry of muscle. *Muscle Nerve*. 1979;2(5):394–398.
353. Jacob JC, Mathew NT. Pseudohypertrophic myopathy in cysticercosis. *Neurology*. 1968;18(8):767–771.
354. Sawhney BB, Chopra JS, Banerji AK, Wahi PL. Pseudohypertrophic myopathy in cysticerosis. *Neurology*. 1976;26(3):270–272.
355. Gherardi R, Baudrimont M, Lionnet F, et al. Skeletal muscle toxoplasmosis in patients with acquired immunodeficiency syndrome: a clinical and pathological study. *Ann Neurol*. 1992;32(4):535–542.
356. Pollock JL. Toxoplasmosis appearing to be dermatomyositis. *Arch Dermatol*. 1979;115(6):736–737.

357. Rowland LP, Greer M. Toxoplasmic polymyositis. *Neurology.* 1961;11:367–370.
358. Bunch TW, Worthington JW, Combs JJ, Ilstrup DM, Engel AG. Azathioprine with prednisone for polymyositis. A controlled, clinical trial. *Ann Intern Med.* 1980;92(3):365–369.
359. Oddis CV, Reed AM, Aggarwal R, et al. Rituximab in the treatment of refractory adult and juvenile dermatomyositis and adult polymyositis: a randomized, placebo-phase trial. *Arthritis Rheum.* 2013;65:314–324.
360. Muscle Study Group. A randomized, pilot trial of etanercept in dermatomyositis. *Ann Neurol.* 2011;70(3):427–436.
361. Dalakas MC, Illa I, Dambrosia JM, et al. A controlled trial of high-dose intravenous immune globulin infusions as treatment for dermatomyositis. *N Engl J Med.* 1993;329(27): 1993–2000.
362. Badrising UA, Maat-Schieman ML, Ferrari MD, et al. Comparison of weakness progression in inclusion body myositis during treatment with methotrexate or placebo. *Ann Neurol.* 2002;51(3):369–372.
363. Dalakas MC, Koffman B, Fujii M, Spector S, Shivkumar K, Cupler E. A controlled study of intravenous immunoglobulin combined with prednisone in the treatment of IBM. *Neurology.* 2001;56(3):323–327.
364. Aggarwal R, Charles-Schoeman C, Schessl J, et al; ProDERM Trial Group. Trial of Intravenous Immune Globulin in Dermatomyositis. *N Engl J Med.* 2022;387(14):1264–1278.
365. Dalakas MC, Sonies B, Dambrosia J, Sekul E, Cupler E, Sivakumar K. Treatment of inclusion-body myositis with IVIG: a double-blind, placebo-controlled study. *Neurology.* 1997;48(3):712–716.
366. Muscle Study Group. A randomized trial of ßINF1 a (Avonex) in patients with inclusion body myositis (IBM). *Neurology.* 2001;57:1566–1570.
367. Muscle Study Group. Randomized pilot trial of high dose ßINF1 a in patients with inclusion body myositis. *Neurology.* 2004;63:718–720.
368. Gordon PA, Winer JB, Hoogendijk JE, Choy EH. Immunosuppressant and immunomodulatory treatment for dermatomyositis and polymyositis. *Cochrane Database Syst Rev.* 2012;8:CD003643.
369. Hanna MG, Badrising UA, Benveniste O, et al; RESILIENT Study Group. Safety and efficacy of intravenous bimagrumab in inclusion body myositis (RESILIENT): a randomised, double-blind, placebo-controlled phase 2b trial. *Lancet Neurol.* 2019;18(9):833–844.
370. Amato AA, Hanna MG, Machado PM, et al; RESILIENT Study Extension Group. Efficacy and Safety of Bimagrumab in Sporadic Inclusion Body Myositis: Long-term Extension of RESILIENT. *Neurology.* 2021;96(12):e1595–e1607.
371. Mammen A, Amato AA, DiMachie M, et al. Zilucoplan in immune-mediated necrotizing myopathy: a phase 2, randomised, double-blind, placebo-controlled, multicentre trial. *Lancet Rheumatol.* 2023;5(2):e67–e76
372. Amato AA, Barohn RJ, Jackson CE, Pappert EJ, Sahenk Z, Kissel JT. Inclusion body myositis: treatment with intravenous immunoglobulin. *Neurology.* 1994;44(8):1516–1518.
373. Leff RL, Miller FW, Hicks J, Fraser DD, Plotz PH. The treatment of inclusion body myositis: a retrospective review and a randomized, prospective trial of immunosuppressive therapy. *Medicine (Baltimore).* 1993;72(4):225–235.
374. Oddis CV. Idiopathic inflammatory myopathies: a treatment update. *Curr Rheumatol Rep.* 2003;5(6):431–436.
375. Uchino M, Araki S, Yoshida O, Uekawa K, Nagata J. High single-dose alternate-day corticosteroid regimens in treatment of polymyositis. *J Neurol.* 1985;232(3):175–178.
376. Uchino M, Yamashita S, Uchino K, et al. Long-term outcome of polymyositis treated with high single-dose alternate-day prednisolone therapy. *Eur Neurol.* 2012;68(2):117–121.
377. van de Vlekkert J, Hoogendijk JE, de Haan RJ, et al. Oral dexamethasone pulse therapy versus daily prednisolone in sub-acute onset myositis, a randomised clinical trial. *Neuromuscul Disord.* 2010;20(6):382–389.
378. Wang DX, Shu XM, Tian XL, et al. Intravenous immunoglobulin therapy in adult patients with polymyositis/dermatomyositis: a systematic literature review. *Clin Rheumatol.* 2012;31(5):801–806.
379. Patwa HS, Chaudhry V, Katzberg H, Rae-Grant AD, So YT. Evidence-based guideline: intravenous immunoglobulin in the treatment of neuromuscular disorders: report of the Therapeutics and Technology Assessment Subcommittee of the American Academy of Neurology. *Neurology.* 2012;78(13):1009–1015.
380. Soueidan SA, Dalakas MC. Treatment of inclusion-body myositis with high-dose intravenous immunoglobulin. *Neurology.* 1993;43(5):876–879.
381. Aggarwal R, Rider LG, Ruperto N, et al. 2016 American College of Rheumatology/European League Against Rheumatism Criteria for Minimal, Moderate, and Major Clinical Response in Adult Dermatomyositis and Polymyositis: An International Myositis Assessment and Clinical Studies Group/Paediatric Rheumatology International Trials Organisation Collaborative Initiative. *Arthr Rheum.* 2017;69:898–910.
382. Amato AA. Intravenous Immune Globulin Therapy in Dermatomyositis. *N Engl J Med.* 2022;387(14):1320–1321.
383. Kissel JT, Levy RJ, Mendell JR, Griggs RC. Azathioprine toxicity in neuro-muscular disease. *Neurology.* 1986;36(1):35–39.
384. Cagnoli M, Marchesoni A, Tosi S. Combined steroid, methotrexate and chlorambucil therapy for steroid-resistant dermatomyositis. *Clin Exp Rheumatol.* 1991;9(6):658–659.
385. Giannini M, Callen JP. Treatment of dermatomyositis with methotrexate and prednisone. *Arch Dermatol.* 1979; 115(10):1251–1252.
386. Metzger AL, Bohan A, Goldberg LS, Bluestone R, Pearson CM. Polymyositis and dermatomyositis: combined methotrexate and corticosteroid therapy. *Ann Intern Med.* 1974;81(2):182–189.
387. Sokoloff MC, Goldberg LS, Pearson CM. Treatment of corticosteroid-resistant polymyositis with methotrexate. *Lancet.* 1971;1(7688):14–16.
388. Miller LC, Sisson BA, Tucker LB, DeNardo BA, Schaller JG. Methotrexate treatment of recalcitrant childhood dermatomyositis. *Arthritis Rheum.* 1992;35(10):1143–1149.
389. Ruperto N, Pistorio A, Oliveira S, et al; Paediatric Rheumatology International Trials Organisation (PRINTO). Prednisone versus prednisone plus ciclosporin versus prednisone plus methotrexate in new-onset juvenile dermatomyositis: a randomised trial. *Lancet.* 2016;387(10019):671–678.
390. Bunch TW. Prednisone and azathioprine for polymyositis: long-term followup. *Arthritis Rheum.* 1981;24(1):45–48.
391. Rowin J, Amato AA, Deisher N, Cursio J, Meriggioli MN. Mycophenolate mofetil in dermatomyositis: is it safe? *Neurology.* 2006;66(8):1245–1247.

392. Schneider C, Gold R, Schafers M, Toyka K. Mycophenolate mofetil in the therapy of polymyositis associated with a polyautoimmune syndrome. *Muscle Nerve.* 2002;25(2):286–288.
393. Majithia V, Harisdangkul V. Mycophenolate mofetil (Cellcept): an alternative therapy for autoimmune inflammatory myopathy. *Rheumatology.* 2005;44(3):386–389.
394. Tausche AK, Meurer M. Mycophenolate mofetil for dermatomyositis. *Dermatology.* 2001;202:341–343.
395. Levine TD. Rituximab in the treatment of dermatomyositis: an open-label pilot study. *Arthritis Rheum.* 2005;52(2):601–607.
396. Mok CC, Ho LY, To CH. Rituximab for refractory polymyositis: an open-label prospective study. *J Rheumatol* 2007;34(9):1864–1868.
397. Valiyil R, Casciola-Rosen L, Hong G, Mammen A, Christopher-Stine L. Rituximab therapy for myopathy associated with anti-signal recognition particle antibodies: a case series. *Arthritis Care Res (Hoboken).* 2010;62(9):1328–1334.
398. Mahler EA, Blom M, Voermans NC, van Engelen BG, van Riel PL, Vonk MC. Rituximab treatment in patients with refractory inflammatory myopathies. *Rheumatology.* 2011;50(12):2206–2213.
399. Fasano S, Gordon P, Hajji R, Loyo E, Isenberg DA. Rituximab in the treatment of inflammatory myopathies: a review. *Rheumatology (Oxford).* 2017;56(1):26–36.
400. Leclair V, Galindo-Feria AS, Dastmalchi M, Holmqvist M, Lundberg IE. Efficacy and safety of rituximab in antisynthetase antibody positive and negative subjects with idiopathic inflammatory myopathy: a registry-based study. *Rheumatology (Oxford).* 2019;58:1214–1220.
401. Allenbach Y, Guiguet M, Rigolet A, et al. Efficacy of rituximab in refractory inflammatory myopathies associated with anti-synthetase auto-antibodies: an open-label, phase II trial. *PLoS One.* 2015;10:e0133702.
402. Zhang W, Prince HM, Reardon K. Statin-induced anti-HMGCR antibody-related immune-mediated necrotising myositis achieving complete remission with rituximab. *BMJ Case Rep.* 2019;12:e232406.
403. Landon-Cardinal O, Allenbach Y, Soulages A, et al. Rituximab in the treatment of refractory anti-HMGCR immune-mediated necrotizing myopathy. *J Rheumatol.* 2019;46:623–627.
404. He C, Li W, Xie Q, Yin G. Rituximab in the Treatment of Interstitial Lung Diseases Related to Anti-Melanoma Differentiation-Associated Gene 5 Dermatomyositis: A Systematic Review. *Front Immunol.* 2022;12:820163.
405. Janardana R, Amin SN, Rajasekhar L, et al. Low dose rituximab is efficacious in refractory idiopathic inflammatory myopathies. *Rheumatology (Oxford).* 2023;62(3):1243–1247.
406. Aggarwal R, Bandos A, Reed AM, et al. Predictors of clinical improvement in rituximab-treated refractory adult and juvenile dermatomyositis and adult polymyositis. *Arthritis Rheum.* 2013;66(3):740–749.
407. Bombardieri S, Hughes GR, Neri R, Del Bravo P, Del Bono L. Cyclophosphamide in severe polymyositis. *Lancet.* 1989;1(8647):1138–1139.
408. Haga HJ, D'Cruz D, Asherson R, Hughes GR. Short term effects of intravenous pulses of cyclophosphamide in the treatment of connective tissue disease crisis. *Ann Rheum Dis.* 1992;51(7):885–888.
409. Kono DH, Klashman DJ, Gilbert RC. Successful IV pulse cyclophosphamide in refractory PM in 3 patients with SLE. *J Rheumatol.* 1990;17(7):982–983.
410. Leroy JP, Drosos AA, Yiannopoulos DI, Youinou P, Moutsopoulos HM. Intravenous pulse cyclophosphamide therapy in myositis and Sjogren's syndrome. *Arthritis Rheum.* 1990;33(10):1579–1581.
411. Niakan E, Pitner SE, Whitaker JN, Bertorini TE. Immunosuppressive agents in corticosteroid-refractory childhood dermatomyositis. *Neurology.* 1980;30(3):286–291.
412. Cronin ME, Miller FW, Hicks JE, Dalakas M, Plotz PH. The failure of intravenous cyclophosphamide therapy in refractory idiopathic inflammatory myopathy. *J Rheumatol.* 1989;16(9):1225–1228.
413. Fries JF, Sharp GC, McDevitt HO, Holman HR. Cyclophosphamide therapy in systemic lupus erythematosus and polymyositis. *Arthritis Rheum.* 1973;16(2):154–162.
414. Sinoway PA, Callen JP. Chlorambucil. An effective corticosteroid-sparing agent for patients with recalcitrant dermatomyositis. *Arthritis Rheum.* 1993;36(3):319–324.
415. Wallace DJ, Metzger AL, White KK. Combination immunosuppressive treatment of steroid-resistant dermatomyositis/polymyositis. *Arthritis Rheum.* 1985;28(5):590–592.
416. Borleffs JC. Cyclosporine as monotherapy for polymyositis? *Transplant Proc.* 1988;20(3 suppl 4):333–334.
417. Correia O, Polonia J, Nunes JP, Resende C, Delgado L. Severe acute form of adult dermatomyositis treated with cyclosporine. *Int J Dermatol.* 1992;31(7):517–519.
418. Girardin E, Dayer JM, Paunier L. Cyclosporine for juvenile dermatomyositis. *J Pediatr.* 1988;112(1):165–166.
419. Heckmatt J, Hasson N, Saunders C, et al. Cyclosporin in juvenile dermatomyositis. *Lancet.* 1989;1(8646):1063–1066.
420. Jones DW, Snaith ML, Isenberg DA. Cyclosporine treatment for intractable polymyositis. *Arthritis Rheum.* 1987;30(8):959–960.
421. Lueck CJ, Trend P, Swash M. Cyclosporin in the management of polymyositis and dermatomyositis. *J Neurol Neurosurg Psychiatry.* 1991;54(11):1007–1008.
422. Mehregan DR, Su WP. Cyclosporine treatment for dermatomyositis/polymyositis. *Cutis.* 1993;51(1):59–61.
423. Pistoia V, Buoncompagni A, Scribanis R, et al. Cyclosporin A in the treatment of juvenile chronic arthritis and childhood polymyositis-dermatomyositis. Results of a preliminary study. *Clin Exp Rheumatol.* 1993;11(2):203–208.
424. Oddis CV, Sciurba FC, Elmagd KA, Starzl TE. Tacrolimus in refractory polymyositis with interstitial lung disease. *Lancet.* 1999;353(9166):1762–1763.
425. Hengstman GJ, van den Hoogen FH, Barrera P, et al. Successful treatment of dermatomyositis and polymyositis with anti-tumor-necrosis-factor-alpha: preliminary observations. *Eur Neurol.* 2003;50(1):10–15.
426. Hengstman GJD, van den Hoogen FHJ, van Engelen BGM. Treatment of dermatomyositis and polymyositis with anti-tumor necrosis factor-alpha: long-term follow-up. *Eur Neurol.* 2004;52(1):61–63.
427. Efthimiou P, Schwartzman S, Kagen LJ. Possible role for tumour necrosis factor inhibitors in the treatment of resistant dermatomyositis and polymyositis: a retrospective study of eight patients. *Ann Rheum Dis.* 2006;65(9):1233–1236.
428. Riley P, McCann LJ, Maillard SM, Woo P, Murray KJ, Pilkington CA. Effectiveness of infliximab in the treatment of refractory juvenile dermatomyositis with calcinosis. *Rheumatology (Oxford).* 2008;47(6):877–880.
429. Korkmaz C, Temiz G, Cetinbas F, Büyükkidan B. Successful treatment of alveolar hypoventilation due to dermatomyositis

with anti-tumour necrosis factor-alpha. *Rheumatology (Oxford)*. 2004;43(7):937–938.
430. Labioche I, Liozon E, Weschler B, Loustaud-Ratti V, Soria P, Vidal E. Refractory polymyositis responding to infliximab: extended follow-up. *Rheumatology (Oxford)*. 2004;43(4):531–532.
431. Sprott H, Glatzel M, Michel BA. Treatment of myositis with etanercept (Enbrel), a recombinant human soluble fusion protein of TNF-alpha type II receptor and IgG1. *Rheumatology (Oxford)*. 2004;43(4):524–526.
432. Dastmalchi M, Grundtman C, Alexanderson H, et al. A high incidence of disease flares in an open pilot study of infliximab in patients with refractory inflammatory myopathies. *Ann Rheum Dis*. 2008;67(12):1670–1677.
433. Hengstman GJ, De Bleecker JL, Feist E, et al. Open-label trial of anti-TNF-alpha in dermato- and polymyositis treated concomitantly with methotrexate. *Eur Neurol*. 2008;59:159–163.
434. Klein R, Rosenbach M, Kim EJ, Kim B, Werth VP, Dunham J. Tumor necrosis factor inhibitor-associated dermatomyositis. *Arch Dermatol*. 2010;146:780–784.
435. Iannone F, Scioscia C, Falappone PC, Covelli M, Lapadula G. Use of etanercept in the treatment of dermatomyositis: a case series. *J Rheumatol*. 2006;33(9):1802–1804.
436. Zhang X, Zhou S, Wu C, et al. Tocilizumab for refractory rapidly progressive interstitial lung disease related to anti-MDA5-positive dermatomyositis. *Rheumatology (Oxford)*. 2021;60:e227–e228.
437. Murphy SM, Lilleker JB, Helliwell P, Chinoy H. The successful use of tocilizumab as third-line biologic therapy in a case of refractory anti-synthetase syndrome. *Rheumatology (Oxford)*. 2016;55:2277–2278.
438. Kondo M, Murakawa Y, Matsumura T, et al. A case of overlap syndrome successfully treated with tocilizumab: a hopeful treatment strategy for refractory dermatomyositis? *Rheumatology (Oxford)*. 2014;53:1907–1908.
439. Narazaki M, Hagihara K, Shima Y, Ogata A, Kishimoto T, Tanaka T. Therapeutic effect of tocilizumab on two patients with polymyositis. *Rheumatology (Oxford)*. 2011;50:1344–1346.
440. Li S, Li W, Jiang W, et al. The efficacy of tocilizumab in the treatment of patients with refractory immune-mediated necrotizing myopathies: an open-label pilot study. *Front Pharmacol*. 2021;12:635654.
441. Oddis CV, Rockette HE, Zhu L, et al. Randomized trial of tocilizumab in the treatment of refractory adult polymyositis and dermatomyositis. *ACR Open Rheumatol*. 2022;4(11):983–990.
442. Brewer EJ Jr, Giannini EH, Rossen RD, Patten B, Barkley E. Plasma exchange therapy of a childhood onset dermatomyositis patient. *Arthritis Rheum*. 1980;23(4):509–513.
443. Dau PC. Plasmapheresis in idiopathic inflammatory myopathy. Experience with 35 patients. *Arch Neurol*. 1981;38(9):544–552.
444. Herson S, Cherin P, Coutellier A. The association of plasma exchange synchronized with intravenous gamma globulin therapy in severe intractable polymyositis. *J Rheumatol*. 1992;19(5):828–829.
445. Miller FW, Leitman SF, Cronin ME, et al. Controlled trial of plasma exchange and leukopheresis in polymyositis and dermatomyositis. *N Engl J Med*. 1992;326(21):1380–1384.
446. Hubbard WN, Walport MJ, Halnan KE, Beaney RP, Hughes GR. Remission from polymyositis after total body irradiation. *Br Med J (Clin Res Ed)*. 1982;284(6333):1915–1916.
447. Kelly JJ, Madoc-Jones H, Adelman LS, Andres PL, Munsat TL. Response to total body irradiation in dermatomyositis. *Muscle Nerve*. 1988;11(2):120–123.
448. Morgan SH, Bernstein RM, Coppen J, Halnan KE, Hughes GR. Total body irradiation and the course of polymyositis. *Arthritis Rheum*. 1985;28(7):831–835.
449. Cherin P, Herson S, Coutellier A, Bletry O, Piette JC. Failure of total body irradiation in polymyositis: report of three cases. *Br J Rheumatol*. 1992;31(4):282–283.
450. Kelly JJ Jr, Madoc-Jones H, Adelman LS, Andres PL, Munsat TL. Total body irradiation not effective in inclusion body myositis. *Neurology*. 1986;36(9):1264–1266.
451. Cumming WJ. Thymectomy in refractory dermatomyositis. *Muscle Nerve*. 1989;12(5):424.
452. Kim H, Dill S, O'Brien M, et al. Janus kinase (JAK) inhibition with baricitinib in refractory juvenile dermatomyositis. *Ann Rheum Dis*. 2021;80(3):406–408.
453. Fischer K, Aringer M, Steininger J, et al. Improvement of cutaneous inflammation and panniculitis in patients with dermatomyositis by the Janus kinase inhibitor baricitinib. *Br J Dermatol*. 2022;187(3):432–435.
454. Le Voyer T, Gitiaux C, Authier FJ, et al. JAK inhibitors are effective in a subset of patients with juvenile dermatomyositis: a monocentric retrospective study. *Rheumatology (Oxford)*. 2021;60(12):5801–5808.
455. Paik JJ, Casciola-Rosen L, Shin JY, et al. Study of tofacitinib in refractory dermatomyositis: an open-label pilot study of ten patients. *Arthritis Rheumatol*. 2021;73(5):858–865.
456. Hornung T, Janzen V, Heidgen F-J, Wolf D, Bieber T, Wenzel J. Remission of recalcitrant dermatomyositis treated with ruxolitinib. *N Engl J Med*. 2014;371:2537–2538.
457. Ladislau L, Suárez-Calvet X, Toquet S, et al. JAK inhibitor improves type I interferon induced damage: proof of concept in dermatomyositis. *Brain*. 2018;141:1609–1621.

CHAPTER 34

Myopathies Associated With Systemic Disease

Myopathies occur in the setting of a variety of systemic diseases. Previous chapters have discussed inflammatory myopathies that can occur in the setting of connective tissue diseases (e.g., systemic lupus erythematosus, mixed connective tissue disease, Sjögren syndrome, and rheumatoid arthritis) and systemic infections (e.g., HIV, COVID-19). Myopathies occurring as complications of medications (toxic myopathies) are also dealt with elsewhere in the book. In this chapter, we will focus on myopathies related to endocrine disturbances, electrolyte imbalance, nutritional deficiency, and amyloidosis. We will also discuss some other less well-defined syndromes such as fibromyalgia.

▶ ENDOCRINE MYOPATHIES

Myopathies can complicate various endocrinopathies.[1–4] In this section, we review myopathies associated with thyroid, parathyroid, adrenal, pituitary, and pancreatic disorders.

THYROID DISORDERS

Both hyperthyroidism and hypothyroidism can be associated with myopathy.[1–17] In addition, polyneuropathy and neuromuscular junction disorders can occur with dysthyroid states and these need to be differentiated from one another.

THYROTOXIC MYOPATHY

Clinical Features

The mean age of onset of thyrotoxicosis is in the fifth decade. The severity of the myopathy does not necessarily correlate with the severity of the thyrotoxicosis. Muscle symptoms usually appear several months after the onset of other clinical symptoms associated with mild hyperthyroidism. Interestingly, thyrotoxicosis is more common in females; however, thyrotoxic myopathy occurs more commonly in men. Anywhere from 61% to 82% of patients with thyrotoxicosis have some degree of detectable weakness on examination, but only about 5% of patients with thyrotoxicosis present with muscle weakness as their chief complaint.[1–7]

Thyrotoxic myopathy is characterized by proximal muscle weakness and atrophy.[1–9] Some affected individuals have severe shoulder-girdle atrophy and scapular winging.[4] Distal extremity weakness can be the predominant feature in approximately 20% of patients.[6] Myalgias and fatigue are common. Some patients develop dysphagia, dysphonia, and respiratory distress due to involvement of bulbar, esophageal–pharyngeal muscles, and ventilatory muscles.[10,11] Weakness of extraocular muscles and proptosis occur in the setting of Graves disease. Rarely, rhabdomyolysis with myoglobinuria can develop in severe thyrotoxicosis.[12]

Muscle stretch tendon reflexes are often brisk. In addition, fasciculations and myokymia are occasionally seen which probably reflects thyrotoxicosis-induced irritability of anterior horn cells or peripheral nerves.[13–15] Peripheral neuropathy in hyperthyroidism is quite rare, but a demyelinating polyneuropathy has been reported.[13] Other manifestations of hyperthyroidism include nervousness, anxiety, psychosis, tremor, increased perspiration, heat intolerance, palpitations, insomnia, diarrhea, increased appetite, and weight loss. Common signs include goiter, tachycardia, atrial fibrillation, widened pulse pressure, as well as warm, thin, and moist skin.

Myasthenia gravis can develop in association with Graves disease. It can be a challenge distinguishing which neuromuscular symptoms are related to Graves disease or to myasthenia gravis. Muscle weakness associated with hyperthyroidism does not fluctuate or significantly improve with anticholinesterase medications.

Thyrotoxicosis is also associated with an unusual form of hypokalemic periodic paralysis. Thyrotoxic periodic paralysis (TPP) may occur sporadically, although a dominantly inherited mutation in a potassium channel has been identified in some patients. TPP has been commonly reported in Asians, but it is not restricted to this population. The attacks of weakness are similar in onset, frequency, duration, and pattern to familial hypokalemic periodic paralysis (Chapter 32). The one distinguishing feature is that familial hypokalemic periodic paralysis typically has its onset within the first three decades of life, while the onset of TPP usually develops later in adult life. Also, TPP is also more common in males. Serum potassium levels tend to be low during the attacks of weakness, but levels can be normal. Muscle strength returns with treatment and normalization of thyroid function. β-Adrenergic blocking agents also improve the myopathy.

Laboratory Features

Serum creatine kinase (CK) levels are usually normal in hyperthyroidism and can even be on the low side. Thyroid-stimulating hormone (TSH) level is low in primary hyperthyroidism, while the thyroxine (T4) level and, occasionally, only the triiodothyronine (T3) level are elevated. In TPP serum potassium levels also are usually decreased. Routine motor and sensory nerve conduction studies (NCSs) are normal.[14,18] Electromyography (EMG) is usually normal, although fasciculation potentials and motor unit action potential (MUAP) multiplets may be evident due to motor nerve hyperactivity.

Histopathology

Routine muscle biopsies are usually unremarkable, however, mild fatty infiltration, muscle fiber atrophy (types 1 and 2), variability in muscle fiber size, scattered isolated necrotic fibers, decreased glycogen, and increased internal nuclei can be noted.[14,16–18] Nonspecific ultrastructural findings on electron microscopy (EM) may be seen including Z-band streaming, focal swelling of the T tubules, elongated mitochondria, decreased mitochondria, and subsarcolemmal glycogen deposition.[19]

In patients with TPP, muscle biopsies can reveal changes similar to that seen in familial hypokalemic periodic paralysis: vacuoles may be appreciated, on routine light microscopy, while subsarcolemmal blebs filled with glycogen and dilated terminal cisternae of the sarcoplasmic reticulum might be apparent on EM.

Pathogenesis

The thyroid gland produces T4 that is converted to the more active T3 hormone in the periphery. These thyroid hormones are largely bound to plasma proteins. Free thyroid hormones bind to cytoplasmic receptors on target cells and are internalized into the nucleus, where they regulate the transcription of specific genes. Type 1 muscle fibers have a greater density of these thyroid receptors than do type 2 fibers.[20]

The pathogenic basis of thyrotoxic myopathy is unknown but is thought to be due to enhanced muscle catabolism. There is an increase in the basal metabolic rate with enhanced mitochondrial consumption of oxygen, pyruvate, and malate.[20] Glucose uptake and glycolysis are stimulated in muscle independent of insulin.[21] This can lead to an insulin-resistant state with fasting hyperglycemia and glucose intolerance and subsequent depletion of glycogen and reduced ATP production. Insulin resistance also may interfere with insulin's anabolic effect on amino acid and protein metabolism.[22] There is an inadequate level of protein synthesis to meet the demands of accelerated breakdown, which in turn, may be driven by increased lysosomal protease activity.[23,24]

A mutation in the *KCNJ18* gene that encodes an inwardly rectifying potassium channel, Kir2.6, has been discovered in some TPP patients.[25] Mutations were present in up to 33% of the unrelated TPP patients from the United States, Brazil, and France, but in only one of 83 patients from Hong Kong and 0 of 31 Thai patients. Thus, TPP is genetically heterogeneous. The demonstrated mutations appear to lead to muscle membrane inexcitability. In addition, thyroid hormones increase potassium efflux from muscle, which can lead to an increase in the number and activity of sodium-potassium ATPase pumps.[26] This, in turn, results in partial depolarization of the muscle membrane, rendering it less excitable. Depolarization-induced sodium-channel inactivation[6] and impaired propagation of the action potential across altered T tubules further renders the muscle membrane less excitable.[27]

Treatment

Muscle strength improves gradually over several months with treatment of the hyperthyroidism.[2] Beta-blockers (e.g., propranolol) can prevent and lessen the attacks of TPP. Unlike the familial form of hypokalemic periodic paralysis, acetazolamide is ineffective in preventing attacks of weakness associated with thyrotoxicosis.

Extraocular muscle weakness associated with Graves disease can persist for months or years after treatment. Artificial tears and ophthalmic ointments may be beneficial in preventing drying of the cornea and exposure keratitis that can result from severe lid retraction. Corticosteroids and other immunotherapies have been beneficial in some patients but may be associated with significant side effects.[28] Teprotumumab is a monoclonal antibody that inhibits the insulin-like growth factor 1 receptor (IGF-1R) and was recently approved for the treatment of thyroid eye disease (TED) based on results of clinical trials.[29,30] IGF-1R is overexpressed on orbital fibroblasts as well as B and T cell's in Grave's disease and plays a central role in TED.

HYPOTHYROID MYOPATHY

Clinical Features

Approximately one-third of individuals with hypothyroidism develop proximal arm and leg weakness along with myalgias, cramps, and generalized fatigue.[1–4,9,31] Rare patients develop muscle hypertrophy; rhabdomyolysis may occur. Further, ventilatory muscles may be affected in severe cases.[32]

Delayed relaxation of the muscle stretch reflexes may be demonstrated, particularly at the ankle. This finding is best appreciated by having the patient kneel on a chair or bench while striking the Achilles tendon. Myoedema refers to painless and electrically silent mounding of muscle tissue when firmly percussed and is observed in approximately one-third of affected individuals.[33] Myasthenia gravis can also occur in association with hypothyroidism.[34]

Laboratory Features

The serum CK levels are elevated as much as 10–100 times of normal. A TSH level should be checked in any patient with idiopathic hyper-CK-emia. In primary hypothyroidism, serum T4 and T3 levels are low, while TSH levels are elevated. Motor and sensory NCSs are usually normal unless the patient has a concomitant polyneuropathy. Needle EMG is also usually normal, although short-duration, low-amplitude polyphasic MUAPs may be appreciated in severely affected muscles.[35–39]

Histopathology

Muscle biopsy abnormalities are nonspecific and may include variability in muscle fiber size with atrophy of type 2 and occasionally type 1 fibers, hypertrophic muscle fibers, rare necrotic fibers, increased internalized nuclei, ring fibers, glycogen accumulation, vacuoles, and increased connective tissue.[17,40,41] Mitochondrial swellings and inclusions, myofibrillar disarray with central core-like changes, autophagic vacuoles, glycogen accumulation, excess lipid, dilated sarcoplasmic reticulum, and T-tubule proliferation may be appreciated on EM.[40]

Pathogenesis

Hypothyroidism leads to reduced anaerobic and mitochondrial aerobic metabolism of carbohydrates and fatty acids decreasing ATP production.[42,43] Hypothyroidism also impairs adrenergic function and produces a concomitant insulin-resistant state. Protein synthesis and catabolism are reduced.

Treatment

The myopathy improves with treatment of hypothyroidism. However, some degree of weakness can persist even 1 year after return to a euthyroid state.

PARATHYROID DISORDERS

Myopathies are common in disorders of calcium and phosphate homeostasis. The regulation of calcium and phosphate levels requires a complex interaction of intestinal, renal, hepatic, endocrine, skin, and skeletal functions. Vitamin D regulates calcium absorption in the intestines. There are several forms of vitamin D: (1) vitamin D3 or cholecalciferol, which is derived from the skin; (2) vitamin D2 or ergocalciferol, which is dietary and absorbed through the intestines; and (3) 25-hydroxy-vitamin D, which is made in the liver and converted to the more potent metabolite 1,25-dihydroxy-vitamin D in the kidneys. Parathyroid hormone (PTH) assists in the regulation of serum calcium levels by promoting bone resorption, increasing renal calcium absorption and phosphate excretion, and enhancing 1,25-vitamin D conversion. Diet, intestinal absorption, and renal excretion contribute to serum phosphate levels. Increased PTH leads to increased levels of 1,25-dihydroxy-vitamin D, hypercalcemia, and hypophosphatemia. Persistently elevated PTH results in resorption of minerals within bone and replacement by fibrous tissue, a condition termed "osteitis fibrosa" or "osteitis fibrosa cystica" in severe forms.

HYPERPARATHYROIDISM AND OSTEOMALACIA

Clinical Features

Muscle weakness is very common in osteomalacia, which is caused by vitamin D deficiency and secondary hyperparathyroidism in adults, and occurs in as many as 72% of affected patients.[44] Weakness develops, however, in only 2%–10% of patients with isolated hyperparathyroidism.[44,45] The earlier diagnosis and treatment of hyperparathyroidism and osteomalacia have led to fewer and less severe neuromuscular complications than appreciated in the past.[44–49]

The myopathy associated with primary hyperparathyroidism or osteomalacia is characterized by symmetric proximal weakness and atrophy, which are worse in the lower extremities. Concomitant bone pain is common due to associated microfractures. Involvement of the neck extensor muscles can lead to the so-called "dropped head syndrome." There are rare reports of hoarseness, dysphagia, ventilatory involvement, and spasticity,[45,50–52] although the majority of these cases were likely patients with amyotrophic lateral sclerosis and coincidental hyperparathyroidism.[52]

Muscle stretch reflexes are often brisk, but plantar responses are flexor. As many as 50% of patients complain of cramps and paresthesia. In addition, in 29%–57% of patients there is stocking-glove loss of pain or vibratory sensation and decreased muscle stretch reflexes suggestive of an associated peripheral neuropathy.[45] Finally, hypercalcemia can be associated with neurobehavioral abnormalities (memory loss, poor concentration, personality changes, inappropriate behavior including catatonia, anxiety, and hallucinations).

Secondary hyperparathyroidism and muscle weakness can develop in patients with chronic renal failure.[53] Multifocal muscle infarcts and myoglobinuria due to calcification of the arteries (calciphylaxis) can develop in this setting.[54–56] Calciphylaxis can also occur in patients with renal failure without overt hyperparathyroidism.[57]

Laboratory Features

Serum CK levels are usually normal in primary and secondary hyperparathyroidism and osteomalacia. CK may be slightly elevated in patients with muscle infarcts due to calciphylaxis.[56] In primary hyperparathyroidism, serum calcium levels are usually elevated, and serum phosphate levels are low, while urinary excretion of calcium is low, and excretion of phosphate is high. In patients with concurrent hypoalbuminemia, serum calcium levels may be normal, so it is imperative to measure the ionized calcium levels which are typically elevated. Increased urinary excretion of cyclic adenosine monophosphate in the presence of hypercalcemia is also seen in hyperparathyroidism. Serum PTH levels and 1,25-dihydroxy-vitamin D levels are elevated in primary hyperparathyroidism. In contrast, 1,25-dihydroxy-vitamin D levels are low in secondary hyperparathyroidism due to renal failure. Noninvasive imaging techniques, such as ultrasound, thallium/technetium scintigraphy, computed tomography, and magnetic resonance imaging (MRI), may be useful in localizing abnormal parathyroid glands.[58]

Serum calcium level is low or normal, serum phosphate is variably low, and 25-OH-vitamin D levels are also usually low in patients with osteomalacia. 1,25-OH-vitamin D levels may be normal, however, as the body attempts to convert remaining vitamin D to this more potent form. Serum PTH levels are elevated in an attempt to normalize serum calcium levels that are reduced in response to vitamin D deficiency. Urinary excretion of calcium is low in an attempt to preserve serum calcium levels (except in cases secondary to renal tubular acidosis), while excretion of phosphate is high in response to secondary hyperthyroidism. In addition, serum alkaline phosphatase levels are elevated in 80%–90% of cases of osteomalacia, again due to the body's attempt to normalize serum calcium by increasing bone resorption.[58] Skeletal survey reveals decreased bone density along with loss of trabeculae, blurring of trabecular margins, variably thinned cortices, and microfractures that are most evident in the pelvis and proximal femur.[46] EMG and NCSs are normal unless the patients have a neuropathy related to their renal failure.

Histopathology

Muscle biopsies usually demonstrate nonspecific myopathic features with atrophy predominantly of type 2 fibers, but occasionally also of type 1 fibers. Muscle biopsies may reveal multifocal infarcts and calcium deposition primarily within vessel walls in patients with calciphylaxis.[56]

Pathogenesis

Primary hyperparathyroidism can be caused by parathyroid adenomas or hyperplasia as well as pituitary adenomas. Secondary hyperparathyroidism usually occurs in the setting of chronic renal failure which results in the reduction of 1,25-dihydroxy-vitamin D conversion or in malabsorption of vitamin D in disorders such as celiac disease. Vitamin D deficiency leads to diminished intestinal absorption of calcium and decreased renal phosphate clearance, which promotes secondary hyperparathyroidism and osteomalacia. In addition to acquired forms, there are hereditary forms of primary hyperparathyroidism[59] and of vitamin D deficiency and osteomalacia.[46]

The mechanism(s) of weakness in hyperparathyroidism and osteomalacia are not known. PTH stimulates proteolysis in muscle[60] and impairs energy production, transfer, and utilization.[4,61] In addition, PTH may reduce the sensitivity of contractile myofibrillar proteins to calcium and activate a cytoplasmic protease, thus impairing the bioenergetics of muscle. Calcium and phosphate levels do not correlate well with the severity of muscle weakness.[44,45,62] Some studies suggest that an increase PTH might upregulate the ubiquitin–proteosome proteolytic system therapy leading to increased degradation of muscle proteins.[63] Vitamin D also has a direct effect on muscle by increasing muscle adenosine triphosphatase concentration, accelerating amino acid incorporation into muscle proteins,[64] and enhancing the uptake of calcium by the sarcoplasmic reticulum and mitochondria.[65,66]

Treatment

Hyperparathyroidism is diagnosed earlier than in the past because of routine screening of serum calcium levels. Thus, affected individuals are frequently asymptomatic or only mildly affected when they are diagnosed. Medical therapies and surgery are very effective for improvement of muscle weakness when detected within a few months.[45,58,67]

The treatment of choice of symptomatic patients with primary hyperparathyroidism is parathyroidectomy.[58] If a patient has a parathyroid adenoma, the affected gland is removed, while additional glands may be biopsied. Individuals with hyperplasia of all four glands generally have subtotal (three and a half glands) parathyroidectomies. Those who are asymptomatic or have significant perioperative risk may be managed medically.[67] Secondary hyperparathyroidism improves with vitamin D and calcium replacement or renal transplantation, if it is due to end-stage renal failure.[68] Occasionally, subtotal parathyroidectomy may need to be performed in patients with secondary hyperparathyroidism. Likewise, the myopathy associated with osteomalacia responds well to vitamin D and calcium replacement and to treatment of the underlying responsible condition.[44,46–48,69–71]

HYPERPARATHYROIDISM AND MOTOR NEURON DISEASE

Some authors have suggested that hyperparathyroidism can cause a neuromuscular syndrome that mimics amyotrophic lateral sclerosis and that patients may improve following resection of parathyroid adenomas.[45] However, we suspect most of these patients who improved with parathyroidectomy did not have a motor neuron disorder, but rather, hyperparathyroid-related myopathy.[52] In our experience, hyperparathyroidism in patients, who meet clinical and electrophysiologic criteria for amyotrophic lateral sclerosis, is rare and coincidental. These patients do not improve with parathyroidectomy.[52]

HYPOPARATHYROIDISM

Clinical Features

Hypoparathyroidism does not typically cause a myopathy, although a few patients do develop mild proximal weakness.[72–74] In addition, painless myoglobinuria without objective weakness or tetany has been reported.[75] On the other hand, paresthesia and tetany can develop in hypoparathyroidism secondary to hypocalcemia. The examiner may be able to demonstrate Chvostek sign (ipsilateral facial contraction upon tapping the facial nerve at the external auditory meatus) and Trousseau sign (thumb adduction, metacarpophalangeal joint flexion, and interphalangeal joint extension) in these hypocalcemic patients.

Laboratory Features

Serum CK may be normal or mildly elevated in patients.[76,77] Hypoparathyroidism is associated with low serum PTH and calcium levels and high serum phosphate levels. Motor and sensory NCSs are normal. Needle EMG may reveal normal insertional activity. Fasciculation potentials result from motor nerve hyperexcitability induced by the hypocalcemia.[78–80] Multiplets (clusters of MUAPs activated with voluntary effort with interdischarge intervals between 2 and 20 ms) are another manifestation of nerve hyperexcitability and is the most characteristic electrodiagnostic abnormality seen in hypoparathyroidism or tetany. Otherwise, MUAP morphology and recruitment are normal.

Histopathology

Muscle biopsies may be normal or demonstrate mild variability in fiber size and increased internalized nuclei that reflect previous muscle damage caused by episodes of tetany.[17] Decreased glycogen phosphorylase activity of muscle biopsy specimens has also been described.[3]

Pathogenesis

Hypoparathyroidism is seen in a number of conditions including osteomalacia, complications of surgery, hypomagnesemia or hypermagnesemia, irradiation, drugs, sepsis, infiltrative diseases of the parathyroid, and autoimmune, hereditary, or developmental disorders of the parathyroid glands.[81] Decreased PTH leads to reduced synthesis of 1,25-dihydroxyvitamin D, hypocalcemia, and hyperphosphatemia.

The pathogenic mechanism of muscle weakness associated with hypoparathyroidism is poorly understood. Decreased serum calcium concentration causes a shift in the resting membrane potential closer to threshold.[75,82–84] Therefore, less current is required to elicit an action potential, which can lead to tetany. Elevated serum CK and mild histologic abnormalities on muscle biopsy are generally considered secondary to muscle damage from tetany.

Treatment

Muscle weakness improves following correction of the hypocalcemia and hyperphosphatemia with vitamin D and calcium administration.[74]

ADRENAL DISORDERS

The adrenal gland comprises three major regions: (1) zona fasciculata, (2) zona glomerulosa, and (3) zona reticularis. The zona fasciculata produces and secretes glucocorticoids, which when produced in excess by an adrenal tumor can cause a myopathy. Mineralocorticoids such as aldosterone are generated by the zona glomerulosa, and when produced in excess can cause hypokalemia which in turn leads to muscle weakness. The zona reticularis generates androgens but excess or deficiency of these hormones does not result in a muscle weakness. In contrast, these so-called anabolic steroids may increase muscle strength and mass. In the following section, we discuss myopathies associated with glucocorticoid excess or deficiency.

STEROID MYOPATHY

Steroid myopathy is the most common endocrine-related myopathy. An excess of glucocorticoids may arise directly from adrenal tumors, indirectly from pituitary tumors, or from iatrogenic sources (corticosteroid medications).

Clinical Features

Approximately 50%–80% of patients with Cushing disease develop some degree of proximal weakness prior to treatment.[85] Distal extremity, oculobulbar, and facial muscles are spared. Patients classically have an increase in truncal adipose tissue, a rounded facial appearance, and thin, frequently ecchymotic, and hyperpigmented skin (i.e., the so-called Cushingoid appearance).

The incidence of iatrogenic steroid myopathy is not at all clear. Women appear to be more at risk for developing a steroid myopathy than men, approximately 2:1 but the reasons are unclear. An increased risk of the myopathy is seen with prednisone doses of 30 mg/day or more (or equivalent doses of other corticosteroids). Fluorinated corticosteroids have a greater propensity for producing muscle weakness than the nonfluorinated compounds (e.g., risk for myopathy: triamcinolone > betamethasone > dexamethasone).[86] Alternate day therapy may reduce the risk of corticosteroid-induced weakness, but this has never been proven in a clinical study. Weakness can develop within several weeks of starting high doses of corticosteroids but more typically develops after chronic administration. In addition, an acute onset of severe generalized weakness can occur in patients receiving high dosages of intravenous corticosteroids (e.g., 1 g of methylprednisolone/day for multiple consecutive days) with or without concomitant administration of neuromuscular blocking agents (see section on Acute Quadriplegic Myopathy/Critical Illness Myopathy in Chapter 35).

Laboratory Features

Serum CK is normal. Serum potassium can be low, and sodium may be elevated. Motor and sensory NCSs and EMG are normal.

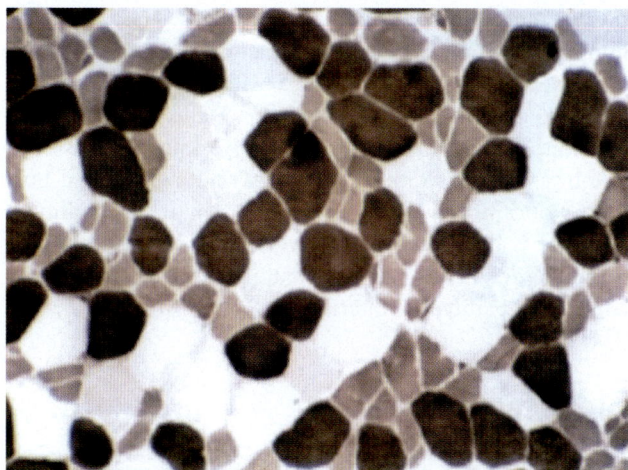

Figure 34-1. Steroid myopathy. Atrophy of type 2B fibers, which are intermediate staining, are appreciated on ATPase 4.5.

Histopathology

Muscle biopsy characteristically reveals preferential atrophy of type 2B fibers (Fig. 34-1).[17,87] Milder degrees of atrophy and increased lipid deposition of type 1 muscle may be seen as well.

Pathogenesis

Corticosteroids bind to receptors on target cells and are subsequently internalized into the nuclei, where they regulate the transcription of specific genes. It is not precisely known how corticosteroids lead to muscle dysfunction. Corticosteroids may result in diminished protein synthesis, increased protein degradation, altered carbohydrate metabolism, impaired mitochondrial function, or decreased sarcolemmal membrane excitability (i.e., in the setting of acute quadriplegic myopathy). In addition, hypokalemia associated with excess corticosteroid can also cause muscle weakness.

Treatment

In cases of adrenal tumors, treatment is surgical when possible. In patients with iatrogenic steroid myopathy, treatment requires reduction in the corticosteroid dose, switching to an alternate day regimen, and encouraging exercise to prevent concomitant disuse atrophy. Experimental studies suggest that insulin-like growth factor-1 may have a prophylactic effect on preventing steroid myopathy.[88] Increasing the dietary protein content of the diet is a suggested treatment of unproven benefit.

A common dilemma that physicians face is renewed or exacerbated weakness in a patient receiving corticosteroids for treatment of an immune-mediated neuromuscular disorder (e.g., inflammatory myopathy, inflammatory neuropathies, or myasthenia gravis).[87,88] Following an initial improvement in their strength with corticosteroid treatment, some patients later experience a subsequent decline in muscle function. The question then arises: Is this a relapse/exacerbation of the disease or a steroid myopathy? Several clinical and laboratory features may be helpful in these situations. Patients with steroid myopathy usually have other manifestations of steroid excess, such as a Cushingoid appearance. If the weakness developed while the patient was tapering the corticosteroids, a relapse of the underlying disease process should be considered. In contrast, if weakness occurred while the patient was on a chronic high dose of steroids, a steroid myopathy is then perhaps more likely. In the case of an inflammatory myopathy, an increasing serum CK would point to an exacerbation of the myositis.[89] An EMG can be useful in that it is usually normal in steroid myopathy, while abnormal insertion and spontaneous activity along with early recruitment of myopathic MUAPs would be expected in exacerbation of inflammatory myopathy. Abnormally increased signal on STIR images of skeletal muscle MRI scans would also favor active myositis. Likewise, in myasthenia gravis flare, one might expect to find fluctuation of clinical deficits on examination (ptosis and ophthalmoplegia are not seen in steroid myopathy) and an increase in decrement with repetitive stimulation tests, or increased jitter and blocking on single fiber EMG. Steroid myopathy typically affects the proximal muscles of the lower extremities first in a symmetric fashion, which can also help to distinguish it from aggravation of other steroid responsive autoimmune neuromuscular disorders that may not follow this pattern of weakness (e.g., chronic inflammatory demyelinating polyneuropathy, oculobulbar myasthenia). However, sometimes it is impossible to state with certainty whether the new weakness is related to a relapse of the underlying disease or secondary to the corticosteroid treatment. In such cases, the best approach is to taper the corticosteroid medication and closely observe the patient. If improvement in strength follows, one can assume the patient had a steroid myopathy. If the patient deteriorates, the worsening weakness is more likely related to the underlying autoimmune neuromuscular disorder, and they may require increased doses of corticosteroids or other forms of immunotherapy.

ADRENAL INSUFFICIENCY

Adrenal insufficiency can result from adrenal or pituitary dysfunction and may be associated with subjective weakness (asthenia) and fatigue.[1–4] Objective weakness is usually the result of electrolyte disturbances (e.g., hyperkalemia) or concurrent endocrinopathies. Serum CK levels, EMG, and muscle biopsies are usually normal. Symptoms improve with proper replacement of adrenal hormones.

▶ PITUITARY DISORDERS

ACROMEGALY

Clinical Features

Patients with acromegaly may develop slowly progressive proximal arm and leg weakness without muscle atrophy.[3,90,91] If anything, muscle hypertrophy is appreciated. Acromegaly can cause bony overgrowth leading to nerve root or spinal cord compression. In addition, there is a predisposition for developing multiple entrapment neuropathies such as carpal and cubital tunnel syndromes. Degenerative joint changes can produce pain that limits activity which may result in disuse muscle atrophy as well.

Laboratory Features

Serum CK levels can be normal or mildly elevated. Motor and sensory NCSs can be normal or demonstrate features of a mononeuropathy (i.e., carpal tunnel syndrome).[91–93] Short-duration and low-amplitude MUAPs may be detected on EMG of proximal muscles of the arms and legs owing to the myopathy.[90] In addition, the EMG can reveal neurogenic features of involved muscle groups, if a patient has a mononeuropathy or radiculopathy related to their acromegaly.

HISTOPATHOLOGY

Muscle biopsies reveal variation in muscle fiber size with hypertrophy and atrophy of all fiber types.[94] Hypertrophy of satellite cells is often appreciated. In addition, rare necrotic fibers may be seen. Myofibrillar loss and abnormal glycogen accumulation may be found on EM.

Pathogenesis

The development and severity of muscle weakness correlate with the duration of acromegaly rather than the levels of serum growth hormone.[90,95] Growth hormone increases protein synthesis within muscle fibers and may lead to muscle fiber hypertrophy.[96,97] However, the pathogenic basis for the muscle weakness that develops despite increased muscle bulk is not known. Studies have demonstrated that the respiratory quotient of resting forearms muscles of patients with acromegaly is lower than normal (0.68 vs. 0.76).[98] Administration of growth hormone increases fatty acid oxidation and decreases glucose utilization.[99] It appears that growth hormone causes muscle to preferentially metabolize lipid as opposed to carbohydrates and this could alter dynamic muscle activity and fatigue. In addition, growth hormone may reduce myofibrillar ATPase activity.[100] In addition, muscle membranes are slightly depolarized compared to normal resting activity which would make them less excitable.

Treatment

Surgical resection of the pituitary adenoma with subsequent reduction of the growth hormone levels leads to improved muscle strength.[90]

PANHYPOPITUITARISM

Pituitary failure in adults commonly leads to muscle weakness and fatigue, probably due to secondary deficiencies of thyroid and glucocorticoid hormones.[101] The myopathy improves with replacement of these hormones. Prepubertal panhypopituitarism is associated with dwarfism and lack of sexual and muscular development. Deficiency of growth hormone may contribute to muscle weakness in this condition, as administration of only thyroid and adrenal hormones does not result in improved strength unless growth hormone is also replaced.[102] However, it is less clear if growth hormone deficiency can contribute to muscle weakness in adults with panhypopituitarism.

DIABETES MELLITUS

Neuromuscular complications of diabetes are usually referable to peripheral neuropathies (see Chapter 21). The only myopathic disorder clearly associated with diabetes is muscle infarction.

DIABETIC MUSCLE INFARCTION

Clinical Features

Diabetic muscle infarction, also known as diabetic myonecrosis, usually occurs in the setting of poorly controlled diabetes. Most patients have other evidence of end-organ damage (retinopathy, nephropathy, neuropathy).[103–110] Patients most commonly present with acute pain and swelling in one thigh. Occasionally, the calf is affected and rarely an upper extremity. A tender mass may be palpated in the quadriceps (most often the vastus lateralis), biceps femoris, or thigh adductors, and occasionally in the gastrocnemius muscle.

Laboratory Features

Serum CK levels may be normal or elevated. Hemoglobin A1C level and erythrocyte sedimentation rate (ESR) are elevated in the majority of patients. MRI or CT of the leg demonstrates signal abnormalities in areas of infarcted muscle (Fig. 34-2). EMG demonstrates fibrillation potentials and positive sharp waves as well as small, polyphasic MUAPs with early recruitment in the involved muscles.[104]

Histopathology

The focal swelling and MRI changes (see below) often lead to a misdiagnosis of a sarcoma or focal myositis. Muscle biopsy should be avoided, if possible, because of the risk of subsequent hemorrhage into the tissue.[57] When performed, muscle biopsies demonstrate large areas of necrosis, edema, hemorrhage, and inflammatory infiltrate consistent with muscle infarction (Fig. 34-3). This infarcted area is later replaced by connective and adipose tissue. Thickening of the basement membranes, hyperplasia of the media, and lumens

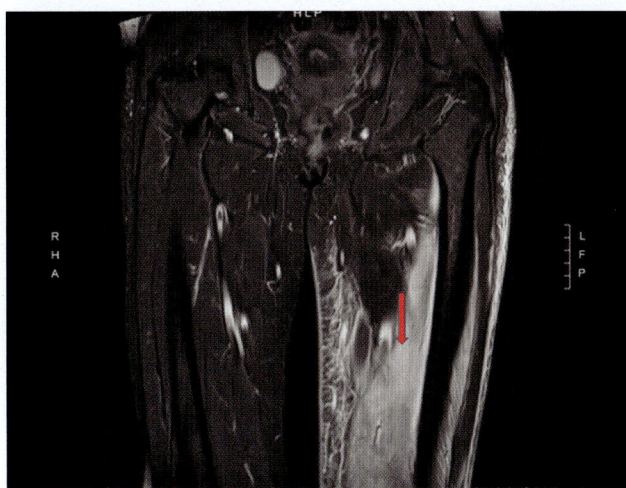

Figure 34-2. Diabetic muscle infarct. MRI (STIR) of the medial thigh reveals bright signal in area of infarct (arrow).

occluded by fibrin, calcium, and lipid of small- and medium-sized blood vessels may be appreciated.[57]

Pathogenesis

Ischemic damage and secondary hemorrhagic infarction result from long-standing, diabetic vasculopathy.

Treatment

The muscle pain and swelling resolve after several weeks, although symptoms may recur in the contralateral leg. Treatment consists of immobilization and pain control. Sometimes we give a short course of prednisone to help with the pain by reducing edema and release of cytokines. However, one must closely monitor the serum glucose levels in such cases.

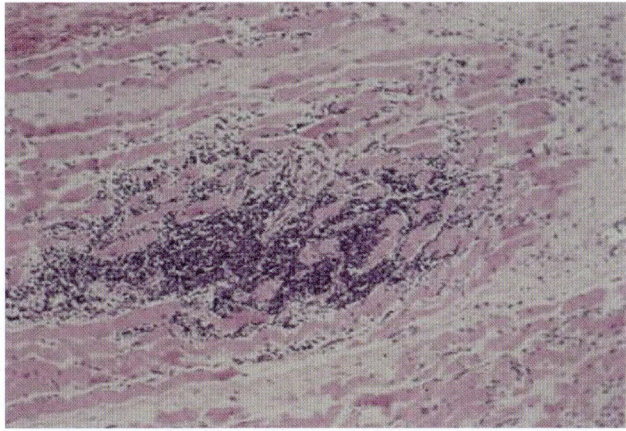

Figure 34-3. Diabetic muscle infarct. Quadriceps muscle biopsy reveals widespread necrosis and endomysial inflammatory cell infiltrate. Paraffin section, stained with hematoxylin and eosin.

▶ MYOPATHIES ASSOCIATED WITH ELECTROLYTE IMBALANCE

DISORDERS OF POTASSIUM (HYPOKALEMIA)

Clinical Features

Hypokalemia is the most common electrolyte abnormality that causes muscle weakness.[111] Clinical, laboratory, and electrophysiological features are similar to familial hypokalemic periodic paralysis (see Chapter 32). Patients must be evaluated for other etiologies of hypokalemia (Table 34-1) before assuming a diagnosis of familial hypokalemic periodic paralysis. Patients usually present with acute to subacute symmetric proximal or generalized weakness, although asymmetric muscle weakness can be seen. The presentation can be mistaken for Guillain–Barré syndrome. Weakness is often accompanied by complaints of myalgias and cramps. A severe complication of hypokalemia is rhabdomyolysis with myoglobinuria and secondary renal failure.

Laboratory Features

Usually, the potassium levels are less than 2.5 mEq/L before any muscle breakdown and weakness occur. Serum CK levels are usually elevated in patients with hypokalemic myopathy. NCSs are normal. EMG of weak muscles may demonstrate fibrillation potentials and positive sharp waves as well as early recruitment of small-duration, low-amplitude MUAPs. The EKG may demonstrate bradycardia, flattened T waves, prolonged PR and QT intervals, and notable U waves.

▶ TABLE 34-1. ETIOLOGIES OF SECONDARY HYPOKALEMIC AND HYPERKALEMIC PARALYSES

Hypokalemic Paralysis
Thyrotoxic periodic paralysis
Renal tubular acidosis
Villous adenoma
Bartter syndrome
Hyperaldosteronism
Chronic or excessive use of diuretics, corticosteroids, licorice
Amphotericin B toxicity
Alcoholism
Toluene toxicity
Barium poisoning

Hyperkalemic Paralysis
Addison disease
Hypoaldosteronism (hyporeninemic)
Isolated aldosterone deficiency
Excessive potassium supplementation
Potassium-sparing diuretics (e.g., spironolactone, triamterene)
Chronic renal failure
Rhabdomyolysis

Histopathology

Biopsies of very weak muscles may demonstrate vacuoles and scattered necrotic fibers.

Pathogenesis

The mechanism of muscle fiber destruction and weakness is not fully known. Reduced extracellular potassium concentration may render the muscle membrane less excitable. Hypokalemia may also diminish blood flow and suppress the synthesis and storage of glycogen in muscles.

Treatment

Muscle strength returns with correction of the hypokalemia. The patients need a medical workup to elucidate the underlying cause of the hypokalemia.

HYPERKALEMIA

Clinical Features

Hyperkalemia can also cause generalized muscle weakness. In addition, there is evidence of increased neuronal or muscle membrane excitability as manifested by the presence of Chvostek sign or myotonic lid lag. There are a number of causes of hyperkalemia that must be excluded before concluding a patient has familial hyperkalemic periodic paralysis (Table 34-1).

Laboratory Features

Most patients with severe generalized weakness have serum potassium levels greater than 7 mEq/L. Renal insufficiency and acidosis may accompany the hyperkalemia but serum CK levels are usually normal. EKG may demonstrate tall, peaked T waves.

Routine NCSs are normal. EMG may demonstrate early recruitment of small "myopathic" MUAPs, but fibrillation potentials and positive sharp waves are atypical. Unlike, familial hyperkalemic (potassium-sensitive) periodic paralysis, myotonic discharges are never seen in the acquired forms of hyperkalemic myopathy.

Histopathology

Muscle biopsies are typically normal.

Pathogenesis

Hyperkalemia causes a prolonged depolarization of the muscle membrane that in turn inactivates the sodium channel, inactivation reduces the excitability of the muscle membrane.

Treatment

Muscle strength returns with correction of hyperkalemia. The underlying cause of the hyperkalemia must be elucidated and treated.

DISORDERS OF CALCIUM

The muscle symptoms of hypercalcemia and hypocalcemia were discussed in the section regarding parathyroid myopathies. Hypercalcemia in the absence of parathormone excess usually manifests with primarily central nervous system rather than neuromuscular symptoms.

DISORDERS OF PHOSPHATE

Hypophosphatemia

Hypophosphatemia can occur in diabetic ketoacidosis, acute alcohol intoxication, hyperalimentation with phosphate-poor preparations, severe diarrhea, and in patients taking phosphate-binding antacids. Serum phosphate levels less than 0.4 mM/L may lead to generalized muscle weakness potentially severe enough to produce ventilatory failure, rhabdomyolysis, and myoglobinuria.[112] Some patients develop paresthesia and diminished muscle stretch reflexes. Severe hypophosphatemia is another potential Guillain–Barré syndrome mimic. In the authors' experience of a single case, the electrophysiologic signature was that of a sensorimotor axonopathy with muscle biopsy demonstrating type 2 fiber atrophy. Symptoms resolve with correction of the serum phosphate levels.

DISORDERS OF MAGNESIUM

Hypermagnesemia most often occur secondary to overusage of magnesium-containing laxatives, particularly if the patient has renal insufficiency.[113] It can also develop during treatment of eclampsia with magnesium sulfate. Severe generalized and ventilatory muscle weakness may ensue but resolves with correction of the serum magnesium levels.

Muscle and nerve hyperexcitability, as characterized by Chvostek and Trousseau signs as well as tetany, may be seen in hypomagnesemia. However, hypocalcemia and other electrolyte disturbances typically accompany hypomagnesemia, and therefore, it is difficult to attribute the neuromuscular abnormality solely to the low serum magnesium levels.

▶ MYOPATHIES ASSOCIATED WITH MALIGNANCY

Patients with malignancies frequently develop generalized weakness, although most do not represent a true paraneoplastic syndrome. Muscle weakness in patients with cancer are much more likely related to impaired nutrition, increased catabolic state induced by the tumor, disuse atrophy, and perhaps toxic effects of chemotherapeutic agents. There are a few well-defined paraneoplastic syndromes, including sensory neuronopathies or sensorimotor neuropathies (e.g., anti-Hu syndrome as discussed in Chapter 19) and Lambert–Eaton syndrome (see Chapter 26), resulting in generalized weakness. Inflammatory and necrotizing myopathies can occur in the setting of cancer (as discussed in more detail in Chapter 33). Rarely, patients with malignancy can have spread of the tumor into a region of muscle.[114,115] Any muscle group can be invaded by resulting in pain, swelling, and weakness in the local region. EMG of the affected muscles may reveal membrane instability and MUAPs with short duration and low amplitudes. Muscle biopsy can demonstrate evidence of tumor emboli.

▶ OTHER MYOPATHIES SECONDARY TO SYSTEMIC DISEASE

AMYLOID MYOPATHY

Clinical Features

Amyloid myopathy usually occurs in the setting of primary amyloidosis (light-chain amyloidosis, AL) and is less frequent with familial amyloidosis.[116–134] Amyloid myopathy does not typically occur in secondary amyloidosis (AA), however we have seen it in rare cases of senile amyloidosis.

With primary and familial amyloidosis, cardiac muscles, peripheral nerves, skin, kidneys, and other organs can also be affected in addition to skeletal muscle. In fact, most patients present with non–muscle-related symptoms. Approximately 20% of patients have a coexistent generalized peripheral neuropathy; mononeuropathies such as carpal tunnel syndrome and ulnar neuropathy also occur. Amyloid myopathy is more common in men and usually manifests with an insidious onset of progressive proximal weakness and myalgia, although distal muscles can also be affected.[121,123,130] The distal muscle weakness may be in part related to a superimposed amyloid neuropathy. Hypertrophy of involved muscle groups can be appreciated; the tongue is often involved with notable macroglossia. However, other patients develop atrophic muscles; again, this could be related to the associated neuropathy. Rare patients have been reported presenting with neck extensor weakness (dropped head syndrome).[126] Ventilatory failure can occur due to involvement of the diaphragm muscle and phrenic nerves. Muscle induration, stiffness, and pain are also variably present.

Laboratory Features

Serum CK is usually normal but can be elevated.[121,130] AL is associated with monoclonal light chain immunoglobulins (λ greater than κ) in the serum or urine.[130–135] Renal insufficiency and proteinuria result from amyloid deposition in the kidneys.

NCSs are abnormal in patients with coexistent peripheral neuropathy. They often reveal reduced motor and sensory amplitudes and mild slowing of conduction velocities.[118,120–122,130] Superimposed carpal tunnel syndrome is a

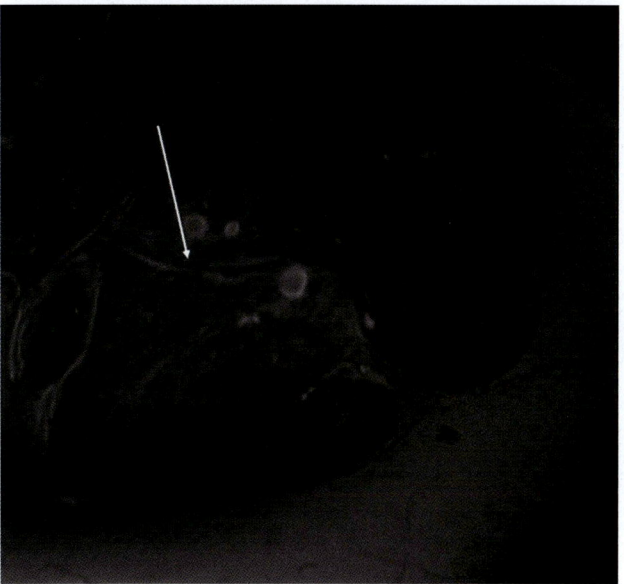

Figure 34-4. Amyloid myopathy. MRI of the thigh demonstrates extensive edema in multiple muscle groups but most notably in the posterior compartment. There is also prominent interfascial edema (*arrow*). There is no focal muscle atrophy. There is no reticulation of the subcutaneous fat. (Reproduced With permission from Budhu J, Holroyd K, Balaban D, et al. Clinical Reasoning: A 63-year-old-woman presenting with bilateral leg pain. *Neurology* 2021; 96(7):343–348. Figure 1.)

common finding. EMG reveals muscle membrane irritability with frequent fibrillation potentials and positive sharp waves, particularly in the paraspinal and proximal extremity muscles.[116,118–123,127,130] Complex repetitive discharges and myotonic discharges may also be appreciated. Early recruitment of short-duration, low-amplitude, polyphasic MUAPs is present in weak proximal muscles. In addition, patients with superimposed amyloid neuropathy often have decreased recruitment of long-duration, large-amplitude potential MUAPs in distal muscles.

MRI scans may reveal hypointense reticulum in the subcutaneous fat with or without increased T2 and STIR signal in affected extremities suggestive of edema (Fig. 34-4).[127–130] Furthermore, MRI may show decreased T1 signaling in the bone marrow, suggesting hematologic malignancies.[128]

Histopathology

Muscle biopsies demonstrate variability in fiber size with an admixture of hypertrophic and atrophic fibers.[121,130] Scattered necrotic and regenerating fibers and increased internalized nuclei may be seen. Group atrophy related to denervation may be appreciated. Amyloid deposition can be visualized using Congo-red stained section with polarized light or rhodamine fluorescence (Fig. 34-5).[121,130–135] On polarized light, amyloid deposits appear apple green in color and with rhodamine fluorescence it appears bright red. After employing this technique in the routine evaluation of all

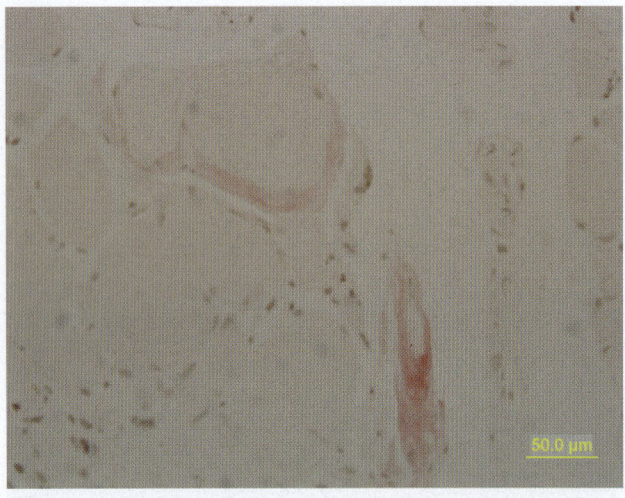
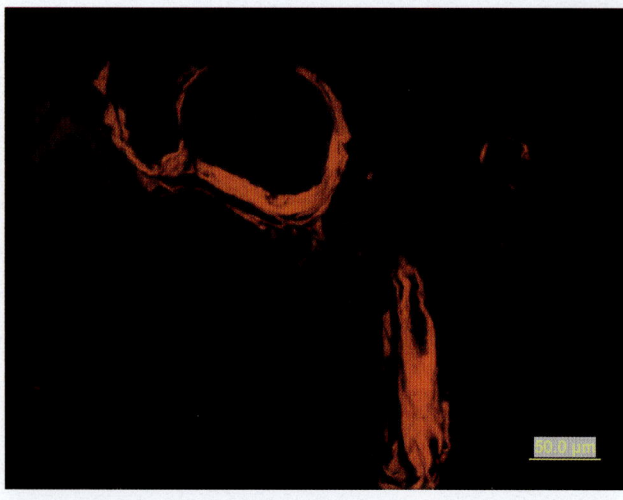

Figure 34-5. Amyloid myopathy. Amyloid deposition is appreciated surrounding blood vessels and occasionally encasing individual muscle fibers on Congo red staining. The deposits are pink on routine light microscopy (A) and bright red using rhodamine optics (B).

muscle specimens, the Mayo Clinic demonstrated a 10-fold increase in the diagnosis of amyloid myopathy, suggesting it is probably an underdiagnosed entity.[121]

The amyloid deposits are best appreciated surrounding small arterioles and venules. In addition, muscle fibers are also partially or completely encased by amyloid deposits. In AL amyloidosis, immunohistochemical studies reveal that the amyloid deposits are composed of λ or κ light chains (Fig. 34-6).[121,130] Immunohistochemistry employing antibodies directed against gelsolin and transthyretin are useful in excluding or diagnosing familial amyloidosis. Mass spectroscopy can also be utilized to identify the subtype of the amyloid deposits.[135] Membrane attack complex may colocalize with amyloid deposition. ApoE was deposited in all patients regardless of the type to systemic amyloidosis in one large series of patients.[121] EM confirms the deposition of short, nonbranching 10-nm amyloid filaments around small blood vessel and muscle fibers.

Pathogenesis

The exact mechanism by which amyloid deposition causes muscle fiber damage is not known. Ischemic damage may arise due to deposition of amyloid in blood vessel walls. Encasement of muscle fibers by the amyloid may interfere with the transport of oxygen, nutrients, and wastes into and out of muscle fibers. There may also be mechanical interference of muscle contraction secondary to amyloid infiltration. Alternatively, the amyloid may interfere with electrical conduction along the sarcolemma.

Treatment

The prognosis of AL amyloidosis is generally poor with a mean life expectancy from time of diagnosis of 21.7 months.[125] However, some patients respond to chemotherapy and autologous stem bone marrow transplantation. Antisense oligonucleotides and small interfering RNA drugs have been beneficial in cases of familial amyloid polyneuropathy (see Chapter 12), but it is not clear if it improves those rare cases of amyloid myopathy.

CRITICAL ILLNESS MYOPATHY/ACUTE QUADRIPLEGIC MYOPATHY

This entity is usually associated with high-dose steroids with or without nondepolarizing neuromuscular agents and is discussed in detail in Chapter 35 regarding Toxic Myopathies.

▶ ILL-DEFINED DISORDERS

POLYMYALGIA RHEUMATICA

Clinical Features

Polymyalgia rheumatica usually occurs in patients over the age of 50 years (peak incidence of 70–79 years).[136–140] The prevalence is approximately of 1 case for every 133 people older than 50 years.[138] There is a female predilection for the development of polymyalgia rheumatica. Patients usually complain of an insidious or acute onset of diffuse nonarticular pain and stiffness, particularly in the morning, beginning about the neck and shoulder region. Other body regions may be affected. A low-grade fever, anorexia, and malaise may accompany the myalgias. Affected individuals may complain of feeling weak or fatigued but on manual muscle testing, their strength should be normal. Approximately 16% of patients develop giant cell arteritis which can be complicated by acute vision loss.[136] Temporal artery biopsy should be performed on all such patients with headaches or visual disturbances to look for evidence in giant-cell arteritis.

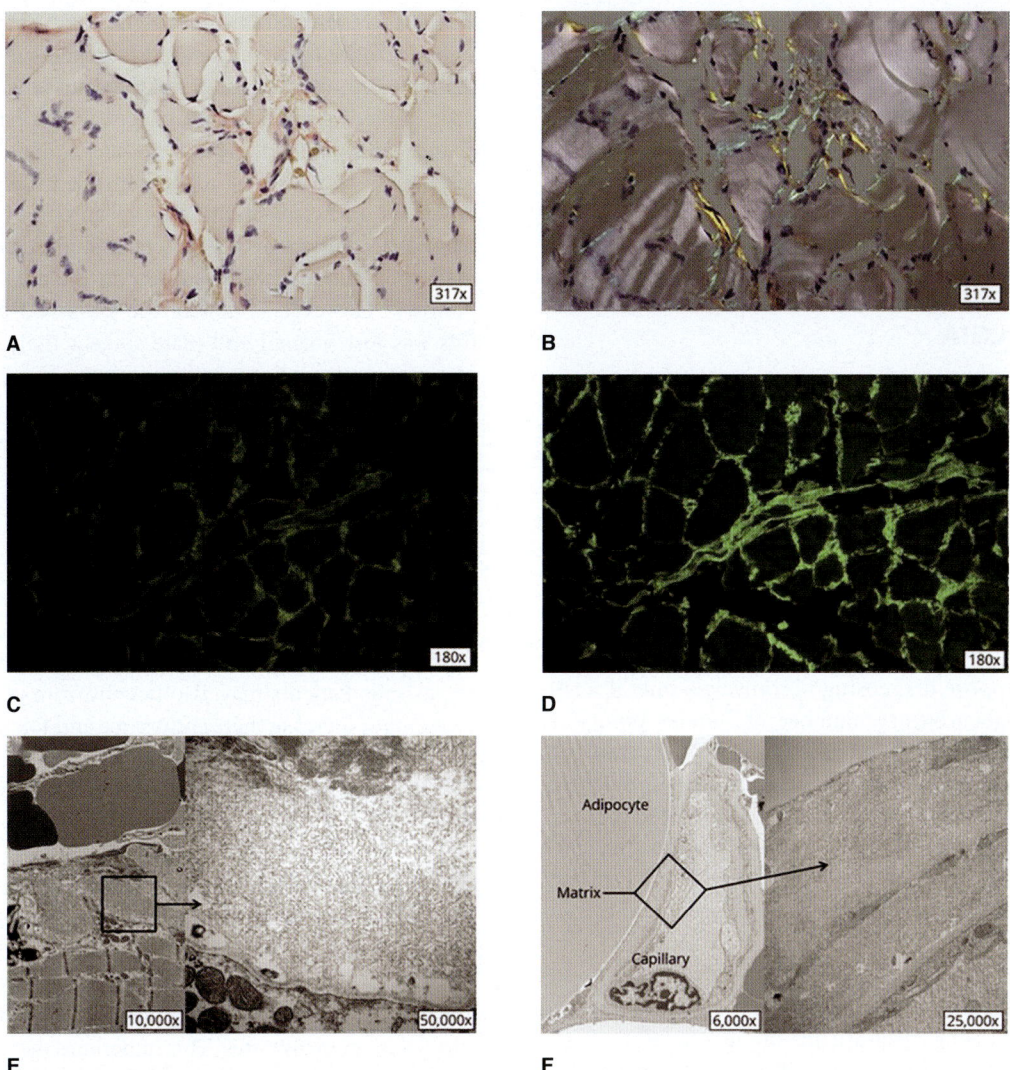

Figure 34-6. Amyloid myopathy. Congo red staining without polarized light demonstrates reddish staining material in the endomysium surrounding muscle fibers and small blood vessels (**A**) that reveals greenish birefringence under polarized light, confirming amyloid deposition (**B**) seen with amyloid deposition. Immunofluorescence staining for kappa light chains shows normal background staining (**C**), while immunostaining strongly reactive for lambda light chains is supportive of the diagnosis of AL amyloid composed of lambda light chain (**D**). Electron microscopy demonstrates fibrillary amyloid deposits surrounding muscle fibers (**E**) as well as perivascular amyloid deposition in the subcutaneous tissue (**F**). (Reproduced With permission from Budhu J, Holroyd K, Balaban D, et al. Clinical Reasoning: A 63-year-old-woman presenting with bilateral leg pain. *Neurology.* 2021; 96(7):343–348. Figure 2.)

Laboratory Features

The diagnosis requires an elevated ESR (over of 40 mm/h) or C-reactive protein level (>6 mg/dl). Serum CK should be normal. Likewise, EMG and NCSs should be normal.

Histopathology

The muscle biopsies should be normal, but mild nonspecific findings (e.g., type 2 fiber atrophy, fiber size variation, and moth-eaten fibers) have been reported.[137] Also note, there is no evidence of significant inflammation in the muscle or overlying fascia.

Pathogenesis

The exact pathogenic basis for polymyalgia rheumatica is unclear. The elevated ESR and CRP, combined with excellent response to corticosteroids suggest an immunologic mechanism. Some cases are clearly associated with arteritis/vasculitis, but it is not usually related to a true myositis or fasciitis.

Treatment

The administration of corticosteroids, usually at low dose (e.g, prednisone 15 mg daily), results in considerable symptom relief within a few days. Dose can be slowly increased in 5 mg increments every 5 days as needed. Once symptoms are under control the prednisone can be decreased by 2.5 mg every two to four weeks.

FIBROMYALGIA

Fibromyalgia and myofascial pain syndrome (MPS), and the fatigue that often accompany them, are commonly diagnosed disorders that are controversial in regard to their nature.[141-149] Fibromyalgia is often dominated by subjective complaints of generalized muscle pain in addition to other somatic complaints including headaches, fatigue, and abdominal cramps. In this regard, it shares many features with the somatoform disorders and "chronic fatigue syndrome."[135,150]

There is no "gold standard" for diagnosing fibromyalgia. Some propose diagnosing fibromyalgia only if a sufficient, although arbitrary, number of "tender points" at specific locations on the body are found.[145] Unfortunately, the study by which these criteria were based was scientifically flawed.[141,142] The investigators predetermined that tender points were necessary for the diagnosis and they each received training in how to identify such tender points. Patients diagnosed with fibromyalgia based on the presence of tender points were then evaluated by other investigators to confirm their presence. That these tender points were reproducible (good interobserver reliability), served as a validation of the diagnosis for the investigators. Sceptics criticized the study for confirming the established bias of the investigators.[141,142,146] Detecting tender points is dependent on the patient's subjective input and is in no way a truly objective marker. The neurological examination including muscle strength testing and laboratory evaluation is otherwise normal in fibromyalgia. Likewise, serum CK, NCSs, and EMG (even of in the areas of tender points) are normal. Finally, there is no difference in the frequency of abnormal muscle histopathology compared to control populations. That said, many patients have reduced epidermal nerve fiber density (IENFD) on skin biopsy.[151,152] Though some have suggested that this proves that fibromyalgia is a small fiber neuropathy, this is of great debate. One study utilizing laser-evoked brain potentials (LEPs) to physiologically assess thermonociception function showed no difference between fibromyalgia patients and healthy controls.[153] Another study showed no correlation of evoked amplitudes and topography of LEPs with IENFD.[154] The cause and effect relationship of fibromyalgia and IENFD is not clear. Conceivably, the reduction of IENFD might be from central desensitization.[155] Perhaps, plasticity within the nervous system leads to reduction in small nerve fibers in response to the chronic pain.

MPS is similar to fibromyalgia, but the pain is described as being more focal as opposed to generalized.[141,142] Rather than tender points, advocates of the disorder suggest patients have "trigger points." These trigger points have been associated with "taut bands," "nodules," and "local twitch responses." However, blinded, controlled studies have demonstrated a low sensitivity and specificity of this so-called diagnostic marker of MPS.[147] One study described abnormal "spontaneous EMG" activity in the area of the trigger points.[148] However, review of the published figures suggest this was just normal end plate spike activity. The majority of electromyographers, including ourselves, have not been able to verify the presence of any abnormalities in MPS.[141,142] As with fibromyalgia, the clinical examination, serum CK, EMG, and NCSs, and muscle biopsies are normal.

Regardless of the organicity of the pain related to fibromyalgia or MPS, the patients' symptoms are often quite distressing and disabling to them. We often recommend treatment with tricyclic antidepressant medications, pregabalin, or gabapentin, as we do with other chronic pain syndromes, in addition to maintenance of as normal a lifestyle as possible. Patients may also benefit from physical therapy program to increase their endurance and tolerance.

▶ SUMMARY

Many systemic disorders can be associated with a myopathy. The myopathy may be a direct effect of the systemic process or may be toxic, related to drugs used to treat the underlying condition. The regenerative capability of muscle allows for improvement in strength with effective treatment of the underlying cause in many cases. This underlines the importance of a detailed evaluation in patients referred for possible myopathy.

REFERENCES

1. Rodolico C, Bonanno C, Pugliese A, Nicocia G, Benvenga S, Toscano A. Endocrine myopathies: clinical and histopathological features of the major forms. *Acta Myol*. 2020;39: 130–135.
2. Katzberg HD, Kassardjian CD. Toxic and endocrine myopathies. *Continuum (Minneap Minn)*. 2016;22(6, Muscle and Neuromuscular Junction Disorders):1815–1828.
3. Kaminski HJ, Ruff RL. Endocrine myopathies (hyper- and hypofunction of adrenal, thyroid, pituitary, and parathyroid glands and iatrogenic corticosteroid myopathy). In: Engel AG, Franzini-Armstrong C, eds. *Myology*. 2nd ed. McGraw-Hill; 1994:1726–1753.
4. Kissel JT, Mendell JR. The endocrine myopathies. In Rowland LP, DiMauro S, Vinken PJ, Bruyn GW, Klawans HL, eds. *Handbook of Clinical Neurology*, Vol 18(62). Elsevier Science Publishers BV; 1992:527–551.
5. Sindoni A, Rodolico C, Pappalardo MA, Portaro S, Benvenga S. Hypothyroid myopathy: a peculiar clinical presentation of thyroid failure. Review of the literature. *Rev Endocr Metab Disord*. 2016;17:499–519.

6. Puvanendran K, Cheah JS, Naganathan N, Wong PK. Thyrotoxic myopathy: a clinical and quantitative analytic electromyographic study. *J Neurol Sci.* 1979;42:441–451.
7. Sataysohi E, Murakami K, Kowa H, Kinishita M, Nishiyama Y. Periodic paralysis in hyperthyroidism. *Neurology.* 1963;13:746–752.
8. Ruff RL, Weissmann J. Endocrine myopathies. *Neurol Clin.* 1988;6:575–592.
9. Ludin HP, Spiess H, Koenig MP. Neuromuscular dysfunction associated with thyrotoxicosis. *Eur Neurol.* 1969;2:269–278.
10. McElvaney GN, Wilcox PG, Fairborn MS, et al. Respiratory muscle weakness and dyspnea in thyrotoxic patients. *Am Rev Respir Dis.* 1990;141(5 pt 1):1221–1227.
11. Mier A, Brophy C, Wass JA, Besser GM, Green M. Reversible muscle weakness in hyperthyroidism. *Am Rev Respir Dis.* 1989;139:529–533.
12. Bennet WR, Huston DP. Rhabdomyolysis in thyroid storm. *Am J Med.* 1984;77:733–735.
13. Feibel JH, Campa JF. Thyrotoxic neuropathy (Basedow's paraplegia). *J Neurol Neurosurg Psychiatry.* 1976;39:491–497.
14. Havard CW, Campbell ED, Ross HB, Spence AW. Electromyographic and histologic findings in the muscles of patients with thyrotoxicosis. *Q J Med.* 1963;32:145–163.
15. McCommas AJ, Sica RE, McNabb AR, Goldberg WM, Upton AR. Evidence for reversible motoneurone dysfunction in thyrotoxicosis. *J Neurol Neurosurg Psychiatry.* 1974;37:548–558.
16. Engel AG. Neuromuscular manifestations of Grave's disease. *Mayo Clin Proc.* 1972;47:919–925.
17. Hudgson P, Kendall-Taylor P. Endocrine myopathies. In: Mastaglia FL, Walton JN, eds. *Skeletal Muscle Pathology.* Churchill Livingstone; 1992:493–509.
18. Waldstein SS, Bronsky D, Shrifter HB, Oester YT. The electromyogram in myxedema. *AMA Arch Intern Med.* 1958;101:97–102.
19. Engel AG. Electron microscopic observations in thyrotoxic and corticosteroid-induced myopathies. *Mayo Clin Proc.* 1966;41:785–796.
20. Janssen JW, Delange-Berkout IW, Van Hardeveld C, Kassenaar AA. The disappearance of l-thyroxine and triiodothyronine from plasma, red and white skeletal muscle after administration of one subcutaneous dose of l-thyroxin to hyperthyroid and euthyroid rats. *Acta Endocrinol (Copenh).* 1981;97:226–230.
21. Celsing F, Blomstrand E, Melichna J, et al. Effect of hyperthyroidism in fibre-type composition, fibre area, glycogen content, and enzyme activity in human muscle protein activity in human skeletal muscle. *Clin Physiol.* 1986;6:171–181.
22. Dubaniewicz A, Kaciuba-Uscilko H, Nazar K, Budohoski L. Sensitivity of the soleus to insulin in resting and exercising with experimental hypo- and hyperthyroidism. *Biochem J.* 1989;263:243–247.
23. Brown JG, Millward DJ. The influence of thyroid status on skeletal muscle protein metabolism. *Biochem Soc Trans.* 1980;8:366–367.
24. Morrison WL, Gibson JN, Jung RT, Rennie MJ. Skeletal muscle and whole body protein turnover in thyroid disease. *Eur J Clin Invest.* 1988;18:62–68.
25. Ryan DP, da Silva MRD, Soong TW, et al. Mutations in potassium channel Kir2.6 cause susceptibility to thyrotoxic hypokalemic periodic paralysis. *Cell.* 2010;140:88–98.
26. Everts ME, Dørup I, Flyvberg A, Marshall SM, Jørgensen KD. Na(+)-K(+) pump in rat muscle: effects of hypophysectomy, growth hormone, and thyroid hormone. *Am J Physiol.* 1990;259(2 pt 1):E278–E283.
27. Dulhunty AF, Gage PW, Lamb GD. Differential effects of thyroid hormone on T-tubules and terminal cisternae in rat muscles: an electrophysiological and morphometric analysis. *J Muscle Res Cell Motil.* 1986;7:225–236.
28. Prummel MF, Mourits MP, Berout A, et al. Prednisone and cyclosporine in the treatment of severe Graves' ophthalmopathy. *N Engl J Med.* 1989;321:1353–1359.
29. Douglas RS, Kahaly GJ, Patel A, et al. Teprotumumab for the treatment of active thyroid eye disease. *N Engl J Med.* 2020;382(4):341–352.
30. Douglas RS, Kahaly GJ, Ugradar S, et al. Teprotumumab efficacy, safety, and durability in longer-duration thyroid eye disease and re-treatment: OPTIC-X study. *Ophthalmology.* 2022;129(4):438–449.
31. Salick AI, Colachis SC Jr, Pearson CM. Myxedema myopathy: clinical, electrodiagnostic, and pathologic findings in advanced case. *Arch Phys Med Rehabil.* 1968;49:230–237.
32. Martinez FJ, Bermudez-Gomez M, Celli BR. Hypothyroidism. A reversible cause of diaphragmatic dysfunction. *Chest.* 1989;96:1059–1063.
33. Salick AI, Pearson CM. Electrical silence of myoedema. *Neurology.* 1967;17(9):899–901.
34. Takamori M, Gutman L, Crosby TW, Martin JD. Myasthenic syndromes in hypothyroidism. Electrophysiological study of neuromuscular transmission and muscle contraction in two patients. *Arch Neurol.* 1972;26:326–335.
35. Afifi AK, Najjar SS, Mire-Salam J, Bergman RA. The myopathology of the Kocher-Debré-Sémélaigne syndrome. Electromyography, light- and electron-microscopic study. *J Neurol Sci.* 1974;22:445–470.
36. Astrom KE, Kugelberg E, Muller R. Hypothyroid myopathy. *Arch Neurol.* 1961;5:472–482.
37. Emser W, Schimrigk K. Myxedema myopathy: a case report. *Eur Neurol.* 1977;16:286–291.
38. Klein I, Parker M, Shebert R, Ayyar DR, Levey GS. Hypothyroidism presenting as muscle stiffness and pseudohypertrophy: Hoffman's syndrome. *Am J Med.* 1981;70:891–894.
39. Norris FH Jr, Panner BJ. Hypothyroid myopathy. Clinical, electromyographical, and ultrastructural observations. *Arch Neurol.* 1966;14:574–589.
40. Evans RM, Watanabe I, Singer PA. Central changes in hypothyroid myopathy: a case report. *Muscle Nerve.* 1990;13:952–956.
41. Laycock MA, Pascuzzi RM. The neuromuscular effects of hypothyroidism. *Semin Neurol.* 1991;11:288–294.
42. Ho KL. Basophilic bodies of skeletal muscle in hypothyroidism: enzyme histochemical and ultrastructural studies. *Hum Pathol.* 1989;20:1119–1124.
43. Schwartz HL, Oppenheimer JH. Physiologic and biochemical actions of thyroid hormone. *Pharmacol Ther B.* 1978;3:349–376.
44. Smith R, Stern G. Muscular weakness in osteomalacia and hyperparathyroidism. *J Neurol Sci.* 1969;8:511–520.
45. Patten BM, Bilezikian JP, Mallette LE, Prince A, Engel WK, Aurbach GD. Neuromuscular disease in primary hyperparathyroidism. *Ann Intern Med.* 1974;80:182–193.
46. Goldring SR, Krane SM, Avioli LV. Disorders of calcification: Osteomalacia and rickets. In: De Groot, ed. *Endocrinology.* 3rd ed. WB Saunders; 1994:1204–1227.
47. Mallette LE, Patten BM, Engel WK. Neuromuscular disease in secondary hyperparathyroidism. *Ann Intern Med.* 1975;82:474–483.

48. Smith R, Stern G. Myopathy, osteomalacia and hyperparathyroidism. *Brain*. 1967;90:593–602.
49. Vicale CT. Diagnostic features of a muscular syndrome resulting from hyperparathyroidism, osteomalacia, owing to renal tubular acidosis, and perhaps to related disorders of calcium metabolism. *Trans Am Neurol Assoc*. 1949;74:143–147.
50. Berenbaum F, Rajzbaum G, Bonnchon P, Amor B. Une hyperparathyroide revelee une chute de la tete. *Rev Rhum Mal Osteoartic*. 1993;60:467–469.
51. Gentric A, Pennec YL. Fatal primary hyperparathyroidism with myopathy involving respiratory muscles. *J Am Geriatr Soc*. 1994;42:1306.
52. Jackson CE, Amato AA, Bryan WW, Wolfe GI, Sakhee K, Barohn RJ. Primary hyperparathyroidism and ALS: is there a relation? *Neurology*. 1998;50:1795–1799.
53. Floyd M, Ayyar DR, Barwick DD, Hudson P, Weightman D. Myopathy in chronic renal failure. *Q J Med*. 1974;53:509–524.
54. Richardson JA, Herron G, Reitz R, Layzer R. Ischemic ulcerations of the skin and necrosis of muscle in azotemic hyperparathyroidism. *Ann Intern Med*. 1969;71:129–138.
55. Randall DP, Fisher MA, Thomas C. Rhabdomyolysis as the presenting manifestation of calciphylaxis. *Muscle Nerve*. 2000;23:289–293.
56. De Luca GC, Eggers SD. A rare complication of azotemic hyperparathyroidism: ischemic calcific myopathy. *Neurology*. 2010;75:1942.
57. Banker BQ, Chester CS. Infarction of thigh muscle in the diabetic patient. *Neurology*. 1973;23:667–677.
58. Norton JA, Sugg SL. Surgical management of hyperparathyroidism. In: De Groot, ed. *Endocrinology*. 3rd ed. WB Saunders; 1994:1106–1122.
59. Habener J, Arnold A, Potts JT. Hyperparathyroidism. In: De Groot, ed. *Endocrinology*. 3rd ed. WB Saunders; 1994:1044–1060.
60. Garber AJ. Effects of parathyroid hormone on skeletal muscle protein and amino acid metabolism in the rat. *J Clin Invest*. 1983;71:1806–1821.
61. Baczynski R, Massry SG, Magott M, El-Belbessi S, Kohan R, Brautbar N. Effect of parathyroid hormone on energy metabolism of skeletal muscle. *Kidney Int*. 1985;28:722–727.
62. Frame B, Heinze EG Jr, Block MA, Manson GA. Myopathy in primary hyperparathyroidism. Observations in three patients. *Ann Intern Med*. 1968;68:1022–1027.
63. Romagnoli C, Brandi ML. Muscle physiopathology in parathyroid hormone disorders. *Front Med (Lausanne)*. 2021;8:764346.
64. Birge SG, Haddad JG. 25-hydroxycholecalciferol stimulation of muscle metabolism. *J Clin Invest*. 1975;56:1100–1107.
65. Curry OB, Basten JF, Francis MJ, Smith R. Calcium up-take by the sarcoplasmic reticulum of muscle from vitamin D deficiency in rabbits. *Nature*. 1974;249:83–84.
66. Pointon JJ, Francis MJO, Smith R. Effect of vitamin D deficiency on sarcoplasmic reticulum and troponin C concentration of rabbit skeletal muscle. *Clin Sci (Lond)*. 1979;57: 257–263.
67. Nussbaum SR, Neer RM, Potts JT Jr. Medical management of hyperparathyroidism and hypercalcemia. In: De Groot, ed. *Endocrinology*. 3rd ed. WB Saunders; 1994:1094–1105.
68. Probhala A, Garg R, Dandona P. Severe myopathy associated with vitamin D deficiency in western New York. *Arch Intern Med*. 2000;160(8):1119–1203.
69. Russell JA. Osteomalacic myopathy. *Muscle Nerve*. 1994;17(6):578–580.
70. Irani PF. Electromyography in nutritional osteomalacic myopathy. *J Neurol Neurosurg Psychiatry*. 1976;39:686–693.
71. Schott GD, Wills MR. Myopathy in hypophosphataemic osteomalacia presenting in adult life. *J Neurol Neurosurg Psychiatry*. 1975;38:297–304.
72. Kruse K, Scheunemann W, Baier W, Schaub J. Hypocalcemic myopathy in idiopathic hypoparathyroidism. *Eur J Pediatr*. 1982;138:280–282.
73. Snowdon JA, Macfie AC, Pearce JB. Hypocalcemic myopathy and parathyroid psychosis. *J Neurol Neurosurg Psychiatry*. 1976;38:48–52.
74. Yamaguchi H, Okamoto K, Shooji M, Morimatsu M, Hirai S. Muscle histology of hypocalcemic myopathy in hypoparathyroidism. *J Neurol Neurosurg Psychiatry*. 1987;50:817–818.
75. Akmal M. Rhabdomyolysis in a patient with hypocalcemia due to hypoparathyroidism. *Am J Nephrol*. 1993;13:61–63.
76. Hower J, Struck H, Tackman W, Stolecke H. CPK activity in hypoparathyroidism. *N Engl J Med*. 1972;287:1098.
77. Shane E, McClane KA, Olarte MR, Bilezikian JP. Hypoparathyroidism and elevated serum enzymes. *Neurology*. 1980;30:192–195.
78. Kugelberg E. Neurologic mechanism for certain phenomena in tetany. *Arch Neurol Psychiatry*. 1946;56:507–521.
79. Kugelberg E. Activation of human nerves by ischemia; Trousseau's phenomenon in tetany. *Arch Neurol Psychiatry*. 1948;60:140–164.
80. Kugelberg E. Activation of human nerves by hyperventilation and hypocalcemia. *Arch Neurol Psychiatry*. 1948;60:153–164.
81. Fitzpatrick LA, Arnold A. Hypoparathyroidism. In: De Groot, ed. *Endocrinology*. 3rd ed. WB Saunders; 1994:1123–1135.
82. Brink F. The role of calcium ion in neural processes. *Pharmacol Rev*. 1954;6:243–298.
83. Frankenhaeuser B. The effect of calcium on the myelinated nerve fiber. *J Physiol*. 1957;137:245–260.
84. Frankenhaeuser B, Hodgkin AL. The action of calcium on the electric properties of squid axons. *J Physiol*. 1957;137:218–244.
85. Muller R, Kugelberg E. Myopathy in Cushing's syndrome. *J Neurol Neurosurg Psychiatry*. 1959;22:314–319.
86. Faludi G, Gotlieb J, Meyers J. Factors influencing the development of steroid-induced myopathy. *Ann N Y Acad Sci*. 1966;138:62–72.
87. Pleasure DE, Walsh GO, Engel WK. Atrophy of skeletal muscle in patients with Cushing's syndrome. *Arch Neurol*. 1970;22: 118–125.
88. Kanda F, Takatani K, Okuda S, Matsushi T, Chihara K. Preventive effects of insulin-like growth factor-1 on steroid-induced muscle atrophy. *Muscle Nerve*. 1999;22:213–217.
89. Askari A, Vignos PJ Jr, Moskowitz RW. Steroid myopathy in connective tissue disease. *Am J Med*. 1976;61:485–492.
90. Pickett JB, Layzer RB, Levin SR, Scheider V, Campbell MJ, Sumner AJ. Neuromuscular complications of acromegaly. *Neurology*. 1975;25:638–645.
91. Lundberg PO, Osterman PO, Stalberg E. Neuromuscular signs and symptoms in acromegaly. In: Canal N, Scarlato G, Walton JN, eds. *Muscle Diseases: Proceedings of an International Congress. Milan 19–21st May 1969*. Excerpta Medica; 1970: 531–534.
92. Low PA, McLeod JG, Turtle JR, Donnelly P, Wright RG. Peripheral neuropathy in acromegaly. *Brain*. 1974;97:139–152.
93. Stewart BM. The hypertrophic neuropathy of acromegaly. *Arch Neurol*. 1966;14:107–110.

94. Mastaglia FL, Barwick DD, Hall R. Myopathy in acromegaly. *Lancet.* 1970;2:907–909.
95. Naglespasen M, Trickey R, Davies MJ, Jenkins JS. Muscle changes in acromegaly. *Br Med J.* 1976;2:914–915.
96. Bigland B, Jehring B. Muscle performance in rats, normal and treated with growth hormone. *J Physiol.* 1952;116:129–136.
97. Prysor-Jones RA, Jenkins JS. Effect of excessive secretion of growth hormone ion tissues of the rat, with particular reference to the heart and skeletal muscle. *J Endocrinol.* 1980;85:75–82.
98. Rabinowitz D, Zierler KL. Differentiation of active from inactive acromegaly by studies of forearm metabolism and response to intra-arterial insulin. *Bull Johns Hopkins Hosp.* 1963;113:211–224.
99. Winckler B, Steele R, Altszuller N, Debodo RC. Effect of growth hormone on free fatty acid metabolism. *Am J Physiol.* 1964;206:174–178.
100. Florini JR, Ewton DZ. Skeletal muscle fiber types and myosin ATPase activity do not change with age or growth hormone administration. *J Gerontol.* 1989;44:B110–B117.
101. Brasel JA, Wright JC, Wilkins L, Blizzard RM. An evaluation of seventy-five patients with hypopituitarism. *Am J Med.* 1965;38:484–498.
102. Raben MS. Growth hormone. 2. Clinical use of growth hormone. *N Engl J Med.* 1962;266:82–86.
103. Anglada M, Vidaller A, Bolao F, Ferrer I, Olivé M. Diabetic muscular infarction. *Muscle Nerve.* 2000;23:825–826.
104. Barohn RJ, Kissel JT. Case-of-the-month: painful thigh mass in a young woman: diabetic thigh infarction. *Muscle Nerve.* 1992;15:850–855.
105. Bjornskowve EK, Carry MR, Katz FH, Lefkowitz J, Ringel SP. Diabetic muscle infarction: a new perspective on pathogenesis and management. *Neuromuscul Disord.* 1995;5(1):39–45.
106. Bodner RA, Younger DS, Rosoklija G. Diabetic muscle infarction. *Muscle Nerve.* 1994;17:949–950.
107. Chester CS, Banker BQ. Focal infarctions of muscle in diabetics. *Diabetic Care.* 1986;9:623–630.
108. Umpierrez GE, Stiles RG, Kleinbart J, Krendel DA, Watts NB. Diabetic muscle infarction. *Am J Med.* 1996;101:245–250.
109. Huang BK, Monu JU, Doumanian J. Diabetic myopathy: MRI patterns and current trends. *AJR Am J Roentgenol.* 2010;195:198–204.
110. Joshi R, Reen B, Sheehan H. Upper extremity diabetic muscle infarction in three patients with end-stage renal disease: a case series and review. *J Clin Rheumatol.* 2009;15:81–84.
111. Comi G, Testa D, Cornelio F, Comola M, Canal M. Potassium depletion myopathy: a clinical and morphological study of six cases. *Muscle Nerve.* 1985;8:17–21.
112. Knochel JP. The clinical status of hypophosphatemia: an update. *N Engl J Med.* 1985;313:447–449.
113. Mordes JP, Wacker WE. Excess magnesium. *Pharmacol Rev.* 1977;29:273–300.
114. Doshi R, Fowler T. Proximal myopathy due to discrete carcinomatous metastases in muscle. *J Neurol Neurosurg Psychiatry.* 1983;46:358–360.
115. Heffner RR Jr. Myopathy of embolic origin in patients with carcinoma. *Neurology.* 1971;21:840–846.
116. Jennekens FG, Wokke JH. Proximal weakness of the extremities as a main feature of amyloid myopathy. *J Neurol Neurosurg Psychiatry.* 1987;50:1353–1358.
117. Nardkarni N, Freimer M. Mendell JR. Amyloidosis causing a progressive myopathy. *Muscle Nerve.* 1995;18:1016–1018.
118. Ringel SP, Claman HN. Amyloid-associated muscle pseudohypertrophy. *Arch Neurol.* 1982;39:413–417.
119. Roke ME, Brown WF, Boughner D, Ang LC, Rice GP. Myopathy in primary systemic amyloidosis. *Can J Neurol Sci.* 1988;15:314–316.
120. Rubin DI, Hermann RC. Electrophysiologic findings in amyloid myopathy. *Muscle Nerve.* 1999;22:355–359.
121. Spuler S, Emslie-Smith A, Engel AG. Amyloid myopathy: an underdiagnosed entity. *Ann Neurol.* 1998;43:719–728.
122. Whitaker JN, Hashimoto K, Quinones M. Skeletal muscle pseudohypertrophy in primary amyloidosis. *Neurology.* 1977;27:47–54.
123. Smetstad C, Monstad P, Lindboe CF, Mygalns A. Amyloid myopathy present with distal atrophic weakness. *Muscle Nerve.* 2004;29:605–609.
124. Bruni J, Bilbao JM, Prtzker PH. Myopathy associated with amyloid angiopathy. *Can J Neurol Sci.* 1977;4:77–80.
125. Yamada M, Tsukagoshi H, Hatakeyama S. Skeletal muscle amyloid deposition in AL- (primary or myeloma-associated), AA- (secondary), and prealbumin-type amyloidosis. *J Neurol Sci.* 1988;85:223–232.
126. Chuquilin M, Al-Lozi M. Primary amyloidosis presenting as "dropped head syndrome." *Muscle Nerve.* 2011;43:905–909.
127. Chapin JE, Kornfeld M, Harris A. Amyloid myopathy: characteristic features of a still underdiagnosed disease. *Muscle Nerve.* 2005;31(2):266–272.
128. Hull KM, Griffith L, Kuncl RW, Wigley FM. A deceptive case of amyloid myopathy: clinical and magnetic resonance imaging features. *Arthritis Rheum.* 2001;8:1954–1958.
129. Mandl LA, Folkerth RD, Pick MA, Weinblatt ME, Gravallese EM. Amyloid myopathy masquerading as polymyositis. *J Rheumatol.* 2000;27:949–952.
130. Budhu J, Holroyd K, Balaban D, et al. Clinical reasoning: a 63-year-old-woman presenting with bilateral leg pain. *Neurology.* 2021;96(7):343–348.
131. Chawla J. Stepwise approach to myopathy in systemic disease. *Front Neurol.* 2011;2:49.
132. Muchtar E, Derudas D, Mauermann M, et al. Systemic immunoglobulin light chain amyloidosis–associated myopathy: presentation, diagnostic pitfalls, and outcome. *Mayo Clin Proc.* 2016;91:1354–1361.
133. Liewluck T, Milone M. Characterization of isolated amyloid myopathy. *Eur J Neurol.* 2017;24:1437–1445.
134. Accardi F, Papa V, Capozzi AR, et al. A rare case of systemic AL amyloidosis with muscle involvement: a misleading diagnosis. *Case Rep Hematol.* 2018;2018:9840405.
135. Muchtar E, Gertz MA, Kyle RA, et al. A modern primer on light chain amyloidosis in 592 patients with mass spectrometry–verified typing. *Mayo Clin Proc.* 2019;94:472–483.
136. Chuang TY, Hunder GG, Ilstrup DM, Kurland LT. Polymyalgia rheumatica: a 10-year epidemiologic and clinical study. *Ann Intern Med.* 1982;97:672–680.
137. Coomes EN. The rate of recovery of reversible myopathies and the effects of anabolic agents in steroid myopathy. *Neurology.* 1965;18:523–530.
138. Salvarani C, Cantini F, Boiardi L, Hunder GG. Polymyalgia rheumatica and giant-cell arteritis. *N Engl J Med.* 2002;347(4):261–271.

139. Buttgereit F, Dejaco C, Matteson EL, Dasgupta B. Polymyalgia rheumatica and giant cell artritis: a systematic review. *JAMA.* 2016;315:2442–2458.
140. Mahmood SB, Nelson E, Padniewski J, Nasr R. Polymyalgia rheumatica: an updated review. *Cleve Clin J Med.* 2020;87:549–556.
141. Bohr T. Problems with myofascial pain syndrome and fibromyalgia syndrome. *Neurology.* 1996;46:593–597.
142. Bohr TW. Fibromyalgia syndrome and myofascial pain syndrome: Do they exist? *Neurol Clin.* 1995;13:365–384.
143. Goldenberg DL. Fibromyalgia, chronic fatigue syndrome, and myofascial pain syndrome. *Curr Opin Rheumatol.* 1993;5:199–208.
144. Komaroff AL, Goldenberg D. The chronic fatigue syndrome: definition, current studies, and lessons for fibromyalgia research. *J Rheumatol Suppl.* 1989;19:23–27.
145. Wolfe F, Smythe HA, Yunus MB, et al. The American College of Rheumatology 1990 criteria for the classification of fibromyalgia. Report of the Multicenter Criteria Committee. *Arthritis Rheum.* 1990;33(2):160–172.
146. Cohen ML, Quinter JL. Fibromyalgia syndrome, a problem of tautology. *Lancet.* 1993;342:906–909.
147. Wolfe F, Simons DG, Fricton J, et al. The fibromyalgia and myofascial pain syndromes: a preliminary study of tender points and trigger points in persons with fibromyalgia, myofascial pain syndrome and no disease. *J Rheumatol.* 1992;19(6):944–951.
148. Hubbard D, Berkoff G. Myofascial trigger points show spontaneous needle EMG activity. *Spine (Phila Pa 1976).* 1993;18:1803–1807.
149. Alciati A, Nucera V, Masala IF, et al. One year in review 2021: fibromyalgia. *Clin Exp Rheumatol.* 2021;39 Suppl 130(3):3–12.
150. Metzler JP, Fleckenstein JL, White CL III, Haller RG, Frenkel EP, Greenlee RG Jr. MRI evaluation of amyloid myopathy. *Skeletal Radiol.* 1992;21:463–465.
151. Sarzi-Puttini P, Giorgi V, Atzeni F, et al. Fibromyalgia position paper. *Clin Exp Rheumatol.* 2021;39 Suppl 130(3):186–193.
152. Kosmidis ML, Koutsogeorgopoulou L, Alexopoulos H, et al. Reduction of Intraepidermal Nerve Fiber Density (IENFD) in the skin biopsies of patients with fibromyalgia: a controlled study. *J Neurol Sci.* 2014;347:143–147.
153. Van Assche DCR, Plaghiki L, Masquelier E, Hatem SM. Fibromyalgia syndrome—a laser-evoked potentials study unsupportive of small nerve fibre involvement. *Eur J Pain.* 2020;24:448–456.
154. Vecchio E, Quitadamo SG, Ricci K, et al. Laser evoked potentials in fibromyalgia with peripheral small fiber involvement. *Clin Neurophysiol.* 2022;135:96.
155. de Tommaso M, Vecchio E, Nolano M. The puzzle of fibromyalgia between central sensitization syndrome and small fiber neuropathy: a narrative review on neurophysiological and morphological evidence. *Neurol Sci.* 2022;43:1667–1684.

CHAPTER 35

Toxic Myopathies

Many drugs can cause a myopathy.[1-10] The pathophysiological mechanisms are diverse and, in many instances, unclear. Medications can have either a direct or an indirect adverse effect on muscle. The direct effect can be focal, as might occur secondary to a drug being injected into tissue, or more commonly generalized. Indirect toxic effects may result from the agent creating an electrolyte imbalance or inducing an immunological reaction. Muscle fibers may undergo necrosis as a result of the drug directly disrupting the sarcolemma, nuclear or mitochondria function, or that of other organelles. Additionally, some drugs trigger and autoimmune myositis. In this chapter, we classify the toxic myopathies according to their presumed pathogenic mechanisms (Table 35-1).

▶ NECROTIZING MYOPATHIES

A number of drugs can cause a generalized necrotizing myopathy. Affected individuals may complain of myalgias or weakness, or they might just have asymptomatic elevations of their serum creatine kinase (CK) levels. Severe necrotizing myopathy may be complicated by myoglobinuria and renal failure. The degree of serum CK elevation is proportionate to the amount of muscle damaged.

CHOLESTEROL-LOWERING DRUGS

Cholesterol-lowering medications including 3-hydroxy-3-methyl-glutaryl-coenzyme A (3-HMG-CoA) reductase inhibitors,[11-19] fibric acid derivatives,[16,20-30] niacin,[31,32] and ezetimibe[33-36] may cause a toxic myopathy. Most patients just have mild elevations in serum CK without any symptoms. Others have myalgias and less frequently weakness. Myoglobinuria is a rare event but can be complicated by death. With discontinuation of the offending agent, the myalgias, weakness, and elevated serum CK levels tend to completely resolve, but it may take several days to months. However, rarely these agents may trigger an immune-mediated inflammatory myopathy, usually necrotizing, that requires treatment with immunosuppressive medications.

HMG-CoA REDUCTASE INHIBITORS (STATINS)

Clinical Features

Statin agents inhibit 3-HMG-CoA reductase, the rate controlling enzyme in cholesterol synthesis (Fig. 35-1). Adverse side effects including asymptomatic hyperCKemia, myalgias, proximal weakness, and, less commonly, myoglobinuria occur with all of the major HMG-CoA reductase inhibitors: lovastatin,[13,16,18,19,32,37,38] simvastatin,[12,14,15,38,39] provastatin,[17,38] atorvastatin,[11,38,40] fluvastatin,[38] and cerivastatin.[38,41,42] The nomenclature regarding statin-induced toxic myopathies in the published literature is unfortunately quite unsatisfactory, listing "myalgias," "myositis," and "myopathy" as three independent types of muscle disorders caused by statin use, when these three subtypes may just reflect the spectrum of severity of the myopathy.[43-45]

Reviews discussing statin myopathies cite a 2%–7% incidence of myalgias, 0.1%–1.0% incidence of weakness or elevated CK, and myoglobinuria developing in <0.5% of patients.[1,43,46-49] The National Heart Lung and Blood Institute advisory panel estimated the incidence of severe myopathy to be approximately 0.08% for lovastatin, simvastatin, and pravastatin.[44] The risk of toxic myopathy increases with the concomitant use of fibric acids,[18,19,27,31,32,40] niacin,[31,32] cyclosporine,[18,19] ezetimibe,[33-36] triazole antibiotics,[50] rapamycin,[51] and sirolimus[48] as well as in the presence of renal insufficiency or hepatobiliary dysfunction. In this regard, 5% of patients taking both lovastatin and gemfibrozil developed a severe myopathy,[27] while a severe myopathy complicated as many as 30% of patients receiving both lovastatin and cyclosporine.[13,18,19]

Most patients with a statin myopathy improve within a few weeks of stopping the agent. One dilemma we face is if patients who exhibited symptoms or signs of statin-intolerance might be rechallenged once the muscle symptoms have resolved. In one study of 51 patients, who previously experienced myalgias or elevated transaminase levels on a variety of different statins, 37 (72.5%) were able to tolerate every other day rosuvastatin.[52]

Although the term "myositis" has been used to denote cases associated with markedly elevated serum CK levels, histopathological confirmation is lacking in most cases. "Myositis" denotes an infection or an autoimmune attack on muscle. Rare cases of dermatomyositis have been described in association with statin use.[17,53-60] There is increasing appreciation of an immune-mediated necrotizing myopathy (anti-HMGCR myositis) that appears to be triggered statin use, but it can occur in absence of statin use (discussed in greater detail in Chapter 33).[49,61-64] In anti-HMGCR myositis weakness continues to progress and CKs remain elevated despite discontinuation of the statin, and only improve if the patients are treated with immunotherapy. Furthermore, disease activity often flares if the immunosuppressive medications are discontinued.

▶ TABLE 35-1. TOXIC MYOPATHIES

Pathogenic Classification	Drug	Clinical Features	Laboratory Features	Histopathology
Necrotizing myopathy	Cholesterol-lowering agents Cyclosporine Labetalol Propofol Alcohol	Acute or insidious onset Proximal weakness Myalgias	Elevated serum CK EMG: fibrillation potentials (fibs), positive sharp waves (PSWs), myotonic discharges (statins, cyclosporine), myopathic MUAPs	Many necrotic muscle fibers No evidence of endomysial inflammatory cell infiltrate invading nonnecrotic muscle fibers
Amphiphilic	Chloroquine Hydroxychloroquine Amiodarone	Acute or insidious onset Proximal and distal weakness Myalgias Sensorimotor neuropathy Hypothyroid (amiodarone)	Elevated serum CK EMG: fibs, PSWs, myotonia (chloroquine), myopathic MUAPs NCS: axonal sensorimotor neuropathy	Autophagic vacuoles and inclusions are apparent in some muscle fibers and in Schwann cells
Antimicrotubular	Colchicine Vincristine	Acute or insidious onset Proximal and distal weakness Myalgias Sensorimotor neuropathy	Normal or elevated CK EMG: fibs, PSWs, myotonic discharges (colchicine), myopathic MUAPs NCS: axonal sensorimotor neuropathy	Autophagic vacuoles and inclusions are evident in some muscle fibers Nerve biopsies demonstrate axonal degeneration
Mitochondrial myopathy	Zidovudine Other HIV and hepatitis B antiretrovirals	Acute or insidious onset Proximal weakness Myalgias Rhabdomyolysis Painful sensory neuropathy	Normal or elevated CK EMG: normal or myopathic NCS: axonal sensory neuropathy/neuronopathy	Muscle biopsies reveal ragged red fibers, COX-negative fibers May also see inflammatory cell infiltrates, cytoplasmic bodies, nemaline rods
Inflammatory myopathy	Statins (anti-HMGCR myositis) Immune checkpoint inhibitors Tyrosine-kinase inhibitors Vascular endothelial growth factor inhibitors L-tryptophan D-penicillamine Cimetidine Phenytoin Alpha-interferons Tumor necrosis alpha blockers	Acute or insidious onset Proximal weakness Myalgias	Elevated serum CK EMG: fibs, PSWs, myopathic MUAPs	Perivascular, perimysial, or endomysial inflammatory cell infiltrates, necrotic and regenerating muscle fibers
Hypokalemic myopathy	Diuretics Laxatives Amphotericin Toluene abuse Licorice Corticosteroids Alcohol abuse	Acute proximal or generalized weakness Myalgias	Serum CK may be elevated Low serum potassium	May see scattered necrotic fibers and vacuoles
Critical illness myopathy	Corticosteroids Nondepolarizing neuromuscular blocking agents	Acute generalized weakness including respiratory muscles	Serum CK can be normal or elevated NCS: low-amplitude CMAPs with relatively normal SNAPs EMG: fibs, PSWs, myopathic MUAPs or no voluntary MUAPs	Atrophy of muscle fibers, scattered necrotic fibers; absence of myosin thick filaments

▶ TABLE 35-1. (CONTINUED)

Pathogenic Classification	Drug	Clinical Features	Laboratory Features	Histopathology
Unknown	Omeprazole	Acute or insidious onset Proximal weakness Myalgias Sensorimotor neuropathy	Normal or slightly elevated serum CK EMG: myopathic MUAPs NCS: axonal sensorimotor neuropathy	Type II muscle fiber atrophy may be seen
	Isotretinoin	Acute or insidious onset Proximal weakness Myalgias	Normal or elevated CK	Atrophy of fibers
	Finasteride and other 5-α-reductase inhibitors	Proximal weakness and atrophy	Serum CK is normal EMG: myopathic MUAPs	Variability in fiber size, type II fiber atrophy, increased internalized nuclei
	Emetine	Acute or insidious onset Proximal weakness Myalgias	Serum CKs mild to moderately elevated	Myofibrillar myopathy

Laboratory Features

Asymptomatic elevation of serum CK is common in patients taking statin medications. Marked elevations of CK occur in patients with severe weakness and myoglobinuria. Routine motor and sensory nerve conduction studies (NCSs) are normal. Fibrillation potentials, positive sharp waves, and myotonic discharges with early recruitment of small-duration motor unit action potentials (MUAPs) are apparent in weak muscles.[65] Electromyography (EMG) in patients with asymptomatic serum CK elevations is often normal.

Interestingly, autoantibodies directed against HMG-CoA reductase occur in cases of statin-associated immune-mediated necrotizing myopathies.[61,62] These antibodies are not usually seen in patients who just take statin medications or those that have the more typical statin myotoxicity that resolves upon discontinuation of the offending medication.

Histopathology

Muscle biopsies reveal muscle fiber necrosis with phagocytosis and small regenerating fibers in patients with elevated serum CKs and weakness or myalgias (Fig. 35-2). Lipid-filled vacuoles within myofibers and cytochrome oxidase–negative myofibers may be appreciated, but these are not consistent findings.[66] Patients with anti-HMGCR myositis often have increased expression of major histocompatibility antigen 1 (MHC1) and membrane attack complex (MAC) deposition on the sarcolemma of scattered, nonnecrotic muscle fibers.[61–64]

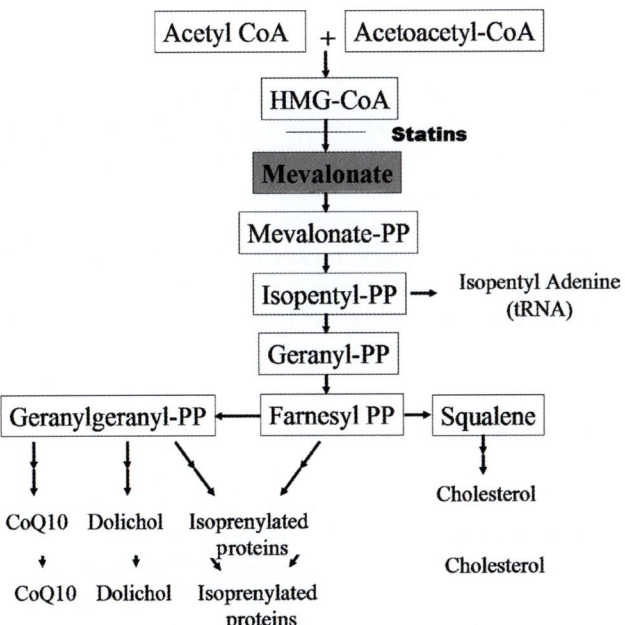

Figure 35-1. Hydroxy-3-methyl-glutaryl-coenzyme A pathway. (Reproduced with permission from Greenberg SA, Amato AA. Statin myopathies. *Continuum.* 2006;12(3):169–184.)

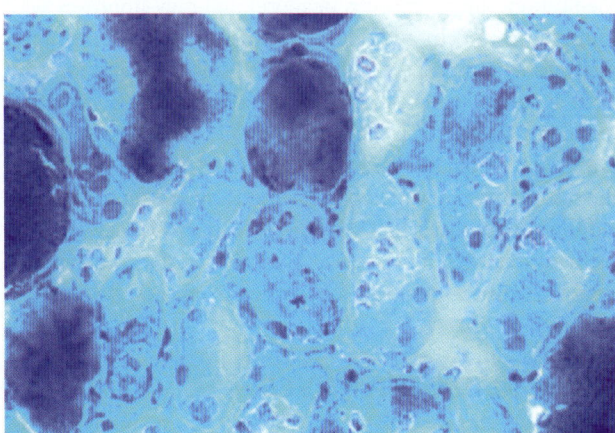

Figure 35-2. Statin myopathy (toxic rhabdomyolysis). Muscle biopsy demonstrates many, clustered necrotic muscle fibers. Modified Gomori trichrome.

Pathogenesis

The pathogenesis of the myopathy secondary to HMG-CoA reductase inhibitors is unclear, as several pathways may potentially be interrupted downstream (Fig. 35-1).[1,49,67] Mevalonate is the immediate product of HMG-CoA reductase metabolism. Subsequently, mevalonate is metabolized to farnesol, which is converted to either squalene or geranylgeraniol. Squalene is the first metabolite committed to the synthesis of cholesterol. In contrast, geranylgeraniol is important in the biosynthesis of coenzyme Q_{10} (a mitochondrial enzyme important in the production of adenosine triphosphate), dolichol (important in glycoprotein synthesis), and isopentylamine (a component of tRNA), and in the activation of regulatory proteins (G-proteins). It is possible that statins could diminish cholesterol within muscle membranes, thereby predisposing the muscle fibers to rhabdomyolysis. However, the depletion of metabolites of geranylgeraniol, and not the inhibition of cholesterol synthesis, may be the primary cause of myotoxicity. In this regard, HMG-CoA reductase inhibitors decrease the levels of coenzyme Q, which could impair energy production.

A couple genome-wide association study conducted in patients with suspected statin-induced toxic myopathy revealed a strong association of myopathy with a single nucleotide polymorphism (SNP), rs4363657, located within the *SLCO1B1* gene on chromosome 12.[68] This gene encodes a protein that regulates the hepatic uptake of statins. Of note, more than 60% statin myopathy patients carried this SNP. No SNPs in any other region were clearly associated with myopathy, including those genes associated with metabolic myopathies.

There are several reports of patients treated with statins who developed dermatomyositis[55–57,59,60] or polymyositis.[17,53,54,58] The most common myositis that we and others have seen in patients on a statin medication is a necrotizing myopathy (anti-HMGCR myositis - see Chapter 33).[61–64] Unlike polymyositis, muscle biopsies in these cases many necrotic fibers without much in the way of endomysial inflammation, except around and within the necrotic fibers. In many instances, the myositis does not improve following discontinuation of the statin medication (after 6 months or more) and only improves with immunotherapy. In addition, the myopathy may worsen after discontinuation of the immunosuppressant agent and improve once again upon reinstituting immunotherapy. In addition, as noted previously, there are autoantibodies directed against the HMG-CoA reductase and deposition of MAC and MHC-1 on the sarcolemma of scattered nonnecrotic muscle fibers.[61,62] This led to the hypothesis that anti-HMGCR myositis may be complement mediated, but a recent clinical trial of a complement-inhibitor failed to demonstrate any sign of efficacy.

FIBRIC ACID DERIVATIVES

Clinical Features

Clofibrate and gemfibrozil are branched-chain fatty acid esters, which are used to treat hyperlipidemia. These fibric acid derivatives can cause a myopathy that typically presents within 2 or 3 months after starting the drug.[16,20–30,40] However, the toxic myopathy may develop up to 2 years following initiation of treatment. Affected individuals complain of generalized weakness, myalgias, and cramps. Myoglobinuria is also a rare complication. Patients with renal insufficiency, those taking both clofibrate and gemfibrozil, and especially also those receiving an HMG-CoA inhibitor, are particularly at increased risk of developing myotoxicity.

Laboratory Features

Elevated serum CK levels are usually noted. Motor and sensory NCSs are normal.[22,24,28] Needle EMG may demonstrate fibrillation potentials, positive sharp waves, complex repetitive discharges, myotonic discharges, and short-duration, small-amplitude polyphasic MUAPs in affected muscle groups.[20,21,25,29,69]

Histopathology

Muscle biopsies demonstrate scattered necrotic muscle fibers. In animal models, clofibrate is also known to result in noninflammatory necrosis of muscle tissue with fiber size variation and groups of small atrophic muscle fibers.[70]

Pathogenesis

The pathogenic mechanism of the myopathy associated with fibric acid derivatives is not known. These medications might somehow destabilize the lipophilic muscle membrane leading to muscle fiber degeneration.[27]

NIACIN

Rarely, niacin use is complicated by myalgias and cramps.[31] Serum CK levels can be elevated as much as 10-fold. The symptoms improve and CK levels normalize after discontinuation of niacin. Electrodiagnostic studies and muscle biopsies have not been reported in detail. In most cases, rhabdomyolysis occurred in patients who were also taking a statin agent.[31] Of note, niacin can inhibit HMG-CoA reductase; therefore, the pathogenic mechanism of the myopathy is likely similar to that of the statins.

EZETIMIBE

Ezetimibe selectively inhibits the absorption of intestinal cholesterol. There are a few reports of ezetimibe-induced myopathy.[33,36,71] Similar to other cholesterol-lowering agents, patients may develop hyperCKemia with or without myalgias or weakness. Most cases occur in patients who are already on a statin agent, but some occur with ezetimibe monotherapy. The toxic myopathy usually resolves within a few weeks after the medication is discontinued.

USE OF CHOLESTEROL-LOWERING AGENTS IN PATIENTS WITH KNOWN MYOPATHIES

A common question posed to neuromuscular specialists is if patients with known myopathies (e.g., muscular dystrophy, metabolic myopathies, polymyositis) can be treated with cholesterol-lowering agents to control their hypercholesterolemia. There is very little evidence that there is increased risk of statin-induced myotoxicity in patients with an underlying myopathy, aside from anti-HMGCR myositis. Furthermore, there is no strong evidence that statin medications (or other lipid-lowering agents) can exacerbate any underlying myopathy. Given the well-known benefits of statins in patients at risk for cardiovascular disease and lack of any strong evidence of increased risk of these medications in patients with underlying myopathy, we again see no contraindication to their use in most patients. We do tend to follow them closer and periodically check their CK levels.

CYCLOSPORINE AND TACROLIMUS

Clinical Features

The immunophilins (i.e., cyclosporine and tacrolimus) are commonly used as immunosuppressive agents, especially in patients requiring transplantation.[72] Rarely, generalized myalgias and proximal muscle weakness develop within months after starting these medications.[72–77] Myoglobinuria can also occur, particularly in patients receiving cyclosporine or tacrolimus concurrent with cholesterol-lowering agents or colchicine.[18,19,78–81] Tacrolimus has also been associated with hypertrophic cardiomyopathy and congestive heart failure.[82] Myalgias, muscle strength, and cardiac function improve with reduction or discontinuation of the offending cyclophilin.

Laboratory Features

Serum CK is usually elevated. NCSs are normal. EMG often reveals increased muscle membrane instability with fibrillation potentials, positive sharp waves, and myotonic potentials.[74] Early recruitment of small-amplitude, short-duration MUAPs may be demonstrated in weak muscle groups.

Histopathology

Muscle biopsies demonstrate necrosis, vacuoles, and type 2 muscle fiber atrophy.

Pathogenesis

The pathogenic basis of immunophilin-induced myopathy and cardiomyopathy is not known. Perhaps, the agents destabilize the lipophilic muscle membrane leading to muscle fiber degeneration, similar to the cholesterol-lowering agents. In this regard, cyclosporine itself has a cholesterol-lowering effect. This may explain the increased risk of myopathy in patients receiving cyclosporine and the more classic lipid-lowering agents (e.g., fibric acid derivatives and statins).

LABETALOL

Clinical Features

There are a few reports of necrotizing myopathy associated with the use of the antihypertensive agent, labetalol.[83,84] Patients can develop acute or insidious onset of proximal weakness or myalgias, which resolve following discontinuation of the medication.

Laboratory Features

Serum CK can be markedly elevated. EMG may demonstrate increased insertional and spontaneous activity with fibrillation potentials and positive sharp waves. Short-duration, small-amplitude, polyphasic MUAPs, which recruit early, are evident.

Histopathology

Routine light microscopy can be normal[83] or can reveal necrotic and regenerating fibers.[84] Electron microscopy (EM) revealed subsarcolemmal vacuoles in one case.[83]

Pathogenesis

The pathogenic etiology for the muscle necrosis seen is not known.

PROPOFOL

Clinical Features

Propofol is an anesthetic agent that is frequently used for sedating patients who are mechanically ventilated and sometimes for the treatment of status epilepticus. Myoglobinuria, metabolic acidosis, hypoxia, and myocardial arrest are rare adverse events associated with the use of propofol.[85–88] Propofol does not appear to be associated with malignant hyperthermia. The myopathy in these individuals could be explained by the high-dose corticosteroids rather than the use of propofol. It remains to be determined if propofol is an independent risk factor for the development of acute quadriplegic myopathy (AQM). There may be an increased risk in patients with underlying mitochondrial disorder.[88]

Laboratory Features

Serum CK levels are markedly elevated. Electrophysiological studies have not been performed or were not reported in the cases associated with rhabdomyolysis in children. The adult patients with AQM have low-amplitude compound muscle action potentials (CMAPs), profuse fibrillation potentials, positive sharp waves, and early recruitment of short-duration, small-amplitude polyphasic MUAPs.

Histopathology

Muscle biopsies reveal necrosis of skeletal and cardiac muscles.[85–87] Patients with AQM, may have prominent necrosis and loss of thick filaments.[88]

Pathogenesis

The mechanism for muscle destruction is unknown though some animal studies suggest that propofol disrupts the respiratory chain enzymes within mitochondria.

Treatment

Propofol should be discontinued, and supportive therapy instituted for myoglobinuria, metabolic acidosis, hyperkalemia, and renal failure.

AMPHIPHILIC DRUG MYOPATHY (DRUG-INDUCED AUTOPHAGIC LYSOSOMAL MYOPATHY)

Amphiphilic drugs contain separate hydrophobic and hydrophilic regions, which allow the drugs to interact with the anionic phospholipids of cell membranes and organelles. In addition to a myopathy, these agents can also cause a toxic neuropathy that is even more severe than the direct toxicity on muscle.

CHLOROQUINE

Clinical Features

Chloroquine, a quinoline derivative, is used to treat malaria, sarcoidosis, systemic lupus erythematosus (SLE), and other connective tissue diseases.[1,2,89–93] Some patients develop slowly progressive, painless, proximal weakness and atrophy, which affect the legs more than the arms. A cardiomyopathy can also occur. Sensation is often reduced as are muscle stretch reflexes, particularly at the ankles, secondary to a concomitant neuropathy. This "neuromyopathy" usually does not occur unless patients take 500 mg a day for a year or more but has been reported with doses as low as 200 mg/day. The neuromyopathy improves after chloroquine discontinuation.

Laboratory Features

Serum CK levels are usually elevated. Motor and sensory NCSs reveal mild-to-moderate reduction in the amplitudes with slightly slow velocities in patients with a superimposed neuropathy.[90,92] Individuals with only the myopathy usually have normal motor and sensory studies.[89] Increased insertional activity in the form of positive sharp waves, fibrillation potentials, and myotonic discharges are seen primarily, but not exclusively, in the proximal limb muscles.[89,90,92] Early recruitment of small-amplitude, short-duration polyphasic MUAPs are appreciated in weak proximal muscles. Neurogenic appearing units and reduced recruitment may be seen in distal muscles that are more affected by the toxic neuropathy.

Histopathology

Autophagic vacuoles are evident in as many as 50% of skeletal and cardiac muscle fibers (Fig. 35-3).[1,2,89–93] Type 1 fibers appear to be preferentially affected. The vacuoles stain positive for acid phosphatase, suggesting lysosomal origin. On EM, the vacuoles are noted to contain concentric lamellar myeloid debris and curvilinear structures. Autophagic vacuoles are also evident in nerve biopsies.

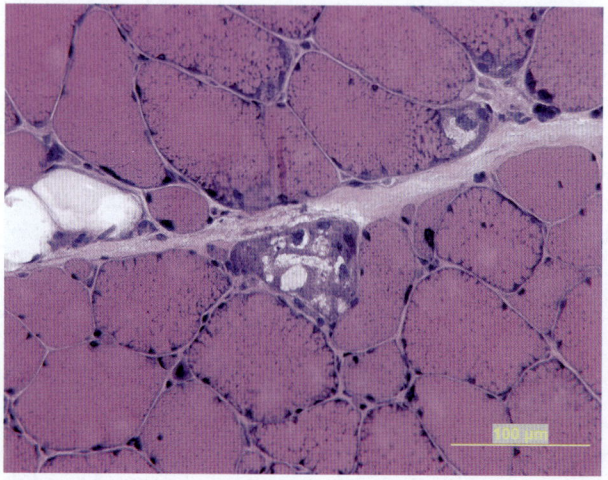
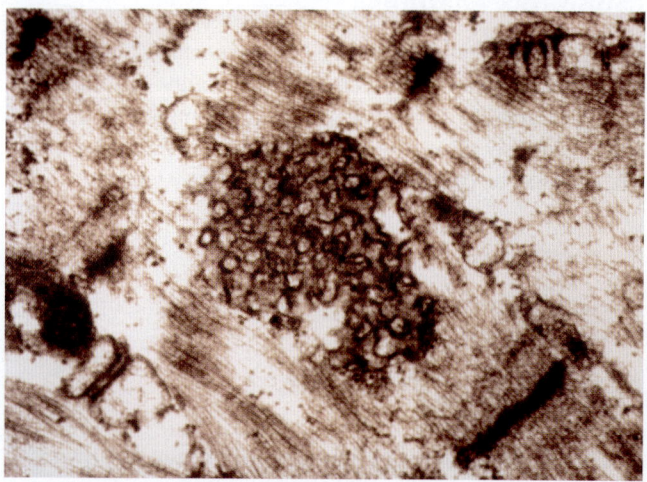

Figure 35-3. Chloroquine myopathy. Chloroquine can cause a vacuolar myopathy (**A**), hematoxylin and eosin (H&E). Electron microscopy reveals a bundle of dilated tubules (**B**). (Reproduced with permission from Wasay M, Wolfe GI, Herrold JM, Burns DK, Barohn RJ. Chloroquine myopathy and neuropathy with elevated CSF protein. *Neurology.* 1998;51(4):1226–1227. Figure 2.)

Pathogenesis

Chloroquine is believed to interact with lipid membranes, forming drug–lipid complexes that are resistant to digestion by lysosomal enzymes. This results in the formation of the autophagic vacuoles filled with myeloid debris.

HYDROXYCHLOROQUINE

Hydroxychloroquine is structurally similar to chloroquine and can cause a neuromyopathy.[1,2,89–93] The myopathy is usually not as severe as seen in chloroquine. Vacuoles are less appreciated on routine light microscopy, but EM still usually demonstrates the abnormal accumulation of myeloid and curvilinear bodies.

AMIODARONE

Clinical Features

Amiodarone is an antiarrhythmic medication that can also cause a neuromyopathy.[94–97] The neuromyopathy is characterized by severe proximal and distal weakness along with distal sensory loss and reduced muscle stretch reflexes. The legs are more affected than the arms. Some patients develop tremor or ataxia. Amiodarone can also cause hypothyroidism, which may also contribute to proximal weakness. Patients with renal insufficiency are predisposed to developing the toxic neuromyopathy. Muscle strength gradually improves following discontinuation of amiodarone.

Laboratory Features

Serum CK levels are elevated. Motor and sensory NCSs reveal reduced amplitudes and slow conduction velocities, particularly in the lower extremities.[96,97] EMG demonstrates fibrillation potentials and positive sharp waves in proximal and distal muscles. In proximal muscles, MUAPs are typically polyphasic, short in duration, small in amplitude, and recruit early. Distal muscles are more likely to have large-amplitude, long-duration polyphasic MUAPs with decreased recruitment.

Histopathology

Muscle biopsies demonstrate scattered fibers with autophagic vacuoles. In addition, neurogenic atrophy can also be appreciated, particularly in distal muscles. EM reveals myofibrillar disorganization and autophagic vacuoles filled with myeloid debris. Myeloid inclusions are also apparent on nerve biopsies. These lipid membrane inclusions may be evident in muscle and nerve biopsies as long as 2 years following discontinuation of amiodarone.

Pathogenesis

The pathogenesis is presumably similar to other amphiphilic medications (e.g., chloroquine).

▶ ANTIMICROTUBULAR MYOPATHIES

COLCHICINE

Clinical Features

Colchicine is commonly prescribed for individuals with gout. Colchicine can also cause a generalized toxic neuromyopathy. It is weakly amphiphilic, but its toxic effect is believed to arise secondary to its binding with tubulin and prevention of tubulin's polymerization into microtubular structures.[1,2] The neuromyopathy usually develops after chronic administration, but it can also develop secondary to acute intoxication.[98–100] Chronic renal failure and age over 50 years are risk factors for the development of neuromyopathy. Patients usually manifest with progressive proximal muscle weakness over several months. Clinical myotonia has been described.[101] A superimposed toxic neuropathy leads to distal sensory loss as well as diminished reflexes. The neuromyopathy weakness typically resolves within 4–6 months after discontinuing the colchicine.

Laboratory Features

Serum CK level is elevated up to 50-fold in symptomatic patients.[1,2,98–100] Serum CK may also be mildly elevated in asymptomatic patients taking colchicine. NCSs reveal reduced amplitudes, slightly prolonged latencies, and mildly slow conduction velocities of motor and sensory nerves in the arms and legs.[98–100,102] Needle EMG demonstrates positive sharp waves, fibrillation potentials, and complex repetitive discharges, which are detected with ease in all muscle regions. Myotonic discharges may also be seen.[101] The myopathic MUAP abnormalities can be masked in the distal limb muscles secondary to the superimposed peripheral neuropathy.

Histopathology

Muscle biopsy demonstrates acid phosphatase–positive autophagic vacuoles containing membranous debris (Fig. 35-4). In addition, nerve biopsies can reveal evidence suggestive of a mild axonal neuropathy.

Pathogenesis

The abnormal assembly of microtubules most likely disrupts intracellular movement or localization of lysosomes, leading to the accumulation of autophagic vacuoles.[1,2]

VINCRISTINE

Clinical Features

Vincristine is a chemotherapeutic agent, which disrupts gene transcription and also promotes the polymerization

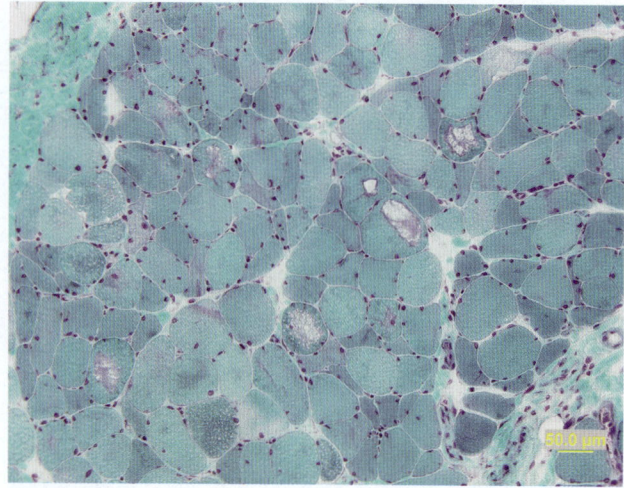 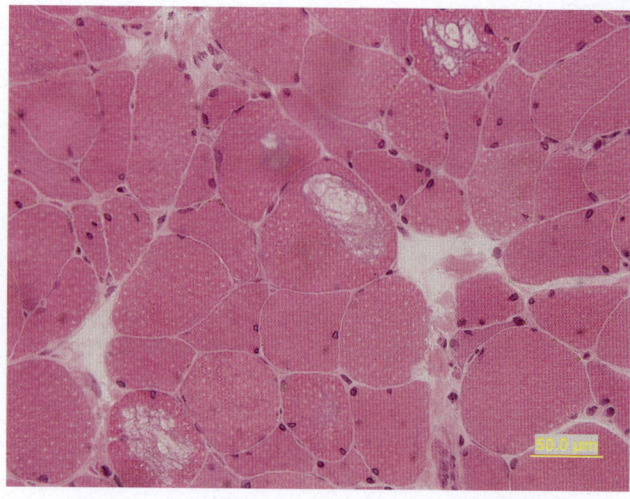

Figure 35-4. Colchicine myopathy. Colchicine can cause a vacuolar myopathy as evident on modified Gomori trichrome stain (**A**) and hematoxylin and eosin stain (**B**).

of tubulin into microtubules. The dose limiting side effect of vincristine is a toxic axonal sensorimotor polyneuropathy that is associated with distal muscle weakness and sensory loss. Proximal muscle weakness and myalgias are less common.[103]

Laboratory Features

Serum CK levels have not been reported in patients suspected of having a superimposed myopathy. NCSs demonstrate markedly reduced amplitudes of sensory nerve action potentials (SNAPs) and CMAPs, while the distal latencies are slightly prolonged, and conduction velocities are mildly slow.[103] Needle EMG demonstrates positive sharp waves, fibrillation potentials, and neurogenic appearing MUAPs in the distally located muscles of the upper and lower extremities.

Histopathology

Biopsies of distal muscles demonstrate evidence of neurogenic atrophy and, occasionally, the accumulation of lipofuscin granules. Proximal muscle biopsies reveal scattered necrotic fibers.[103] On EM, there is prominent myofibrillar disarray and subsarcolemmal accumulation of osmiophilic material. In addition, some myonuclei contain membrane-bound inclusions. Autophagic vacuoles with pseudomembranous debris have been noted in research animals[104,105] but have not been appreciated in humans.[103]

Pathogenesis

The pathogenic basis of the neuromyopathy is presumably similar to that of colchicine.

▶ DRUG-INDUCED MITOCHONDRIAL MYOPATHY

ZIDOVUDINE (AZIDOTHYMIDINE)

Clinical Features

Patients with azidothymidine (AZT) myopathy usually present with an insidious onset of progressive proximal muscle weakness and myalgias.[106–116] However, these clinical features do not help in distinguishing AZT myopathy from other HIV-related myopathies. Other myopathies related to HIV infection are heterogeneous and include inflammatory myopathy (inclusion body myositis is probably the most common form), microvasculitis, noninflammatory necrotizing myopathy, and type 2 muscle fiber atrophy secondary to disuse or wasting due to their chronic debilitated state.[107,110–112,114–124] Furthermore, weakness in an HIV-infected patient can also be secondary to peripheral neuropathy (e.g., chronic inflammatory demyelinating polyneuropathy) or myasthenia gravis. Clinically, AZT myopathy and the other myopathic disorders associated with HIV infection are indistinguishable, compounding the diagnostic difficulty. Regardless of etiology of the myopathy, patients manifest with progressive proximal muscle weakness and myalgias. In addition, muscle weakness may be multifactorial.

Laboratory Features

Serum CK levels are normal or only mildly elevated in AZT myopathy. However, similar elevations are evident in other forms of HIV-related myopathy. An elevated serum CK (e.g., greater than five times the upper limited of normal) is more suggestive of an HIV-associated myositis. Motor and sensory NCSs are normal unless there is a concomitant peripheral neuropathy. Needle EMG may demonstrate positive sharp waves and fibrillation potentials and early recruitment of

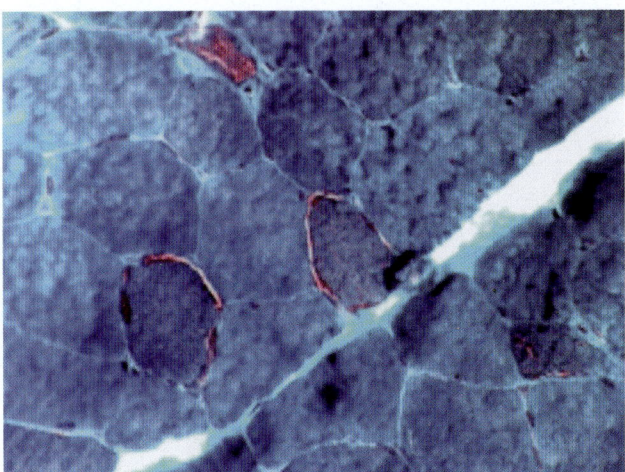

Figure 35-5. Azidothymidine myopathy. Ragged red fibers suggestive of abnormal mitochondria are evident on modified Gomori trichrome stain.

short-duration, small-amplitude polyphasic MUAPs.[114,119,122,125] In addition, small polyphasic MUAPs with early recruitment but no abnormal spontaneous activity was reported in patients with AIDS, along with ultrastructural mitochondrial abnormalities but no inflammation or nemaline rods on biopsy.[112]

Histopathology

Muscle biopsies are remarkable for the presence of ragged red fibers, suggesting mitochondrial abnormalities in AZT myopathy (Fig. 35-5). The number of ragged red fibers correlates with the cumulative dose of AZT.[110,111] In addition, necrotic fibers, cytoplasmic bodies, nemaline rods, and fibers with microvacuolation may be seen in addition to ragged red fibers.[107,110,111] In contrast to HIV-associated inflammatory myopathy, significant endomysial inflammation with or without invasion of nonnecrotic fibers should not be present in cases of pure AZT myopathy. EM can reveal structural abnormalities of the mitochondria.

Pathogenesis

AZT acts as a false substitute for the viral reverse transcriptase, thereby inhibiting its enzymatic activity and replication of the HIV virus. However, AZT also inhibits the activity of mitochondrial DNA polymerase, which probably accounts for the mitochondrial abnormalities. When treated with AZT, patients with HIV have a decrease in quantity of mitochondrial DNA and decline in respiratory chain enzymatic activity, compared to untreated infected patients.[121,126] The histological and molecular abnormalities on repeated muscle biopsies resolve coinciding with clinical improvement following discontinuation of AZT.[127] Although, AZT is responsible for at least some of the mitochondrial abnormalities evident on muscle biopsy, the contribution of these mitochondrial abnormalities to the muscle weakness remains controversial.

Treatment

In the past, anywhere from 18% to 100% of patients with "AZT" myopathy improved following discontinuation of the medication.[107,110,112,114,116,119,120,128] AZT is not used as much anymore as other antiviral agents are typical used nowadays in the treatment of HIV (see below).

OTHER ANTIVIRAL AGENTS

The risk of mitochondrial myopathy with other nucleoside reverse transcriptase inhibitors (e.g., lamivudine), zalcitabine, didanosine used to treat HIV is probably less than that of AZT.[128–130] In addition, nucleoside analogs (lamivudine, adefovir, and clevudine) used to treat hepatitis B infection by reducing virus replication also inhibit mitochondrial DNA replication leading to mitochondrial DNA depletion and mitochondrial myopathy.[131,132] The AIDS Clinical Trial group randomized 2,467 patients to receive one of four single or combination regimens with AZT, didanosine, zalcitabine, and their respective placebo.[123] Approximately 10% of patients had myalgias prior to treatment and 7% developed myalgia during treatment. There was no significant difference between treatment arms and the rate of myalgia or muscle weakness in any group. Five patients (0.5%) had elevated serum CK (>4× normal) prior to treatment, and 52 (5%) developed increased CK during treatment. Serum CK levels were significantly higher in the AZT-zalcitabine group, but this did not correlate with symptoms of myopathy. Unfortunately, there was no comment on muscle biopsies, and thus it is unclear if the myopathies were secondary to mitochondrial toxicity or myositis.

The main treatment of HIV infection currently is with highly active antiretroviral therapy (HAART) consisting of a combination of nucleoside reverse transcriptase inhibitors and protease inhibitors.[128] Rare cases of rhabdomyolysis and myoglobinuria occur in patients taking other HAART medications including tenofovir[133] and ritonavir.[134] A review of 563 patients between 1995 and 1998 demonstrated a prevalence of "HIV-associated myopathy" in 1.5% of patients treated with HAART.[128] It was not clearly stated how the myopathy was defined (e.g., clinical symptoms or signs, elevated serum CK, EMG, or biopsy). Further, it is unclear if the myopathy was felt to be due to mitochondrial toxicity, myositis, or wasting syndrome.

▶ DRUG-INDUCED INFLAMMATORY MYOPATHIES

CHOLESTEROL-LOWERING AGENTS

As discussed in the Necrotizing Myopathies section, an immune-mediated necrotizing myopathy, anti-HMGCR myositis, can occur in patients taking statin medications (see Chapter 33).[1,2,131,132] Anti-HMGCR myositis does improve with the discontinuation of the cholesterol-lowering agent. Rather, patients need to be treated with immunotherapy. Intravenous immunoglobulin can be effective as a monotherapy in many patients.

CHECK-POINT INHIBITORS

Clinical Features

Immune checkpoint inhibitors (ICIs) are increasingly used to treat cancer in order to increase the body's natural immune response to cancer cells by blocking receptors and ligands that inhibit such an attack on cells. The ICIs include monoclonal IgG antibodies directed against programmed cell death-1 (PD1: nivolumab and pembrolizumab), programmed cell death ligand-1 (PDL1: atezolizumab, avelumab, and durvalumab), and the cytotoxic T-lymphocyte–associated antigen 4 (CTLA4: ipilimumab) with many more in development. Important side effects of ICI are autoimmune attack against normal tissues. Neurologic immune-related adverse events (n-irAEs) are rare occurring in approximately 1% of treated patients.[2,135–153] Notably, peripheral nervous system complications (i.e., myositis, myasthenia, Guillain–Barré syndrome and other forms of neuritis) are three times more frequent than reports of central nervous system disorders (encephalitis, hypophysitis). The average time to patients manifesting symptoms is about a month after starting ICI, usually after the second course.

Myositis represents about one-third of neuromuscular complications. Patients may present with asymptomatic hyperCKemia to severe generalized weakness. Notably, unlike other inflammatory myopathies, there is an overlap with myasthenia gravis such that 40%–50% of patients present with ocular or bulbar symptoms with or without axial or proximal extremity muscle involvement. Importantly, life-threatening myocarditis manifesting as malignant arrhythmias or congestive heart failure is also a common comorbidity. Ventilatory muscle involvement can also occur.

Laboratory Features

Serum CK levels can be normal or elevated.[2,135–153] Aldolase may be elevated in rare cases in which the CK is normal. High-sensitivity cardiac troponin levels are elevated in patients with myocarditis but are not specific as they can be elevated in patients with just skeletal muscle involvement. Cardiac MRI and echocardiogram as well as electrocardiograms should be ordered on all patients because of the high mortality and sudden cardiac death that is associated with myocarditis. EMG revealed irritability and early recruitment of small myopathic MUAPs. Antiacetylcholine receptor antibodies, repetitive nerve stimulation, and single-fiber EMG may be normal or abnormal even in patients with severe oculobulbar involvement typical of myasthenia. MRI of muscles can demonstrate muscle edema suggestive of inflammation and may have a predilection for orbital, bulbar, an paraspinal muscles (Fig. 35-6).

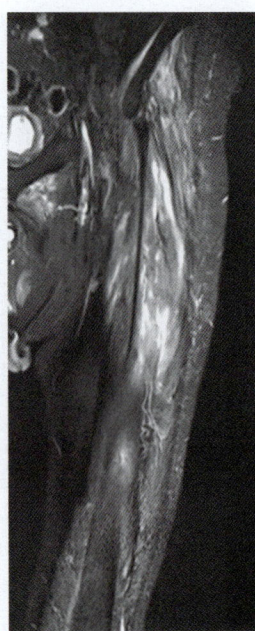

Figure 35-6. Immune checkpoint inhibitor myopathy. Magnetic resonance imaging (STIR) of left thigh reveals increased signal (bright) suggestive of myositis.

Histopathology

Muscle biopsies show perivascular, perimysial, and endomysial infiltrates along with necrotic and regenerating fibers (Fig. 35-7). Some series have noted that necrotic muscle fibers appear clustered as opposed to being scattered diffusely.[137]

Pathogenesis

As discussed above the ICIs unleash the immune system to target cancer cells but this can be complicated by an attack against normal "self-antigens" in various tissues.

Treatment

Most patients at least partially respond to discontinuing the ICI and a short course of immunotherapy (e.g., corticosteroids, other second-line immunosuppressive agents, or intravenous immunoglobulin). In patients with severe weakness or myocarditis we are aggressive in our treatment and usually pulse patients with solumedrol 1 g IV for 5 days and IVIG (2 g/kg over 5 days) before putting them on prednisone 0.75 to 1 mg/kg orally a day. We try to taper prednisone over 6 weeks, as this is usually a monophasic myositis.

L-TRYPTOPHAN/EOSINOPHILIA–MYALGIA SYNDROME

Clinical Features

Eosinophilia–myalgia syndrome was described in the late 1980s and early 1990s and was found to be caused by a contaminant used in the production of L-tryptophan.[154–160]

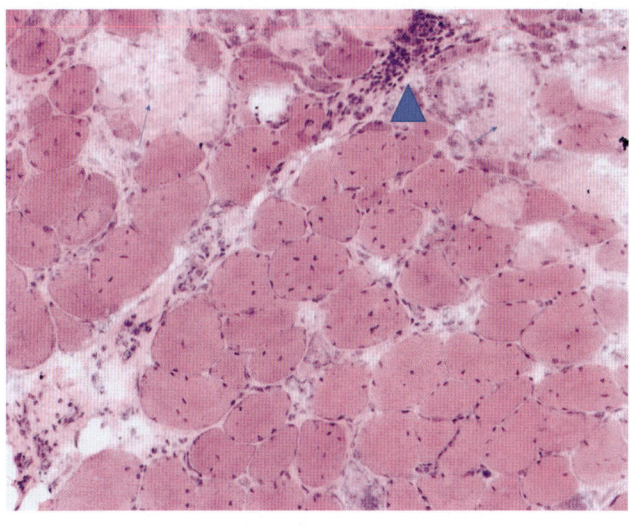
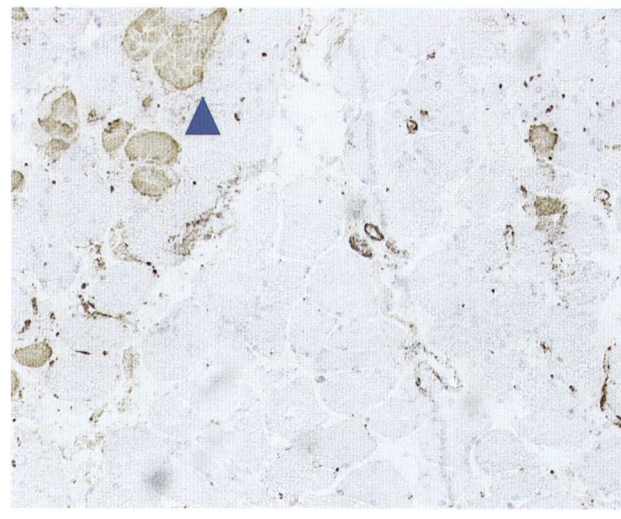

Figure 35-7. Immune checkpoint inhibitor myopathy. Muscle biopsy of thigh reveals perivascular inflammation (*blue arrowhead*), clusters of necrotic muscle fibers (*blue arrows*), and many fibers with increased internalized nuclei on H&E stain (**A**). Immunoperoxidase stain shows membrane attack complex deposition diffusely in sarcoplasm of necrotic fibers (see brownish staining fibers, *blue arrowhead*) (**B**).

The clinical, laboratory, electrophysiological, and histopathological features were similar to that seen in diffuse fasciitis with eosinophilia (Shulman syndrome).[161] Patients developed a subacute onset of generalized muscle pain and tenderness with variable degrees of weakness. Onset could have been within a few weeks or after several years of starting tryptophan. Numbness, paresthesias, arthralgias, lymphadenopathy, dyspnea, abdominal pain, mucocutaneous ulcers, and an erythematous rash were also common. Some patients developed a severe generalized sensorimotor polyneuropathy mimicking Guillain–Barré syndrome[159,162] or multiple mononeuropathies suggestive of a vasculitis.[163]

Laboratory Features

Serum CK levels are normal or elevated. Autoantibodies are absent and ESR is usually normal. The absolute eosinophil count is usually elevated ($>1 \times 10^9$ cells/L). Decreased amplitudes of CMAPs and SNAPs with normal or mildly reduced conduction velocities are evident in patients with a polyneuropathy.[159,164] A few patients with severe Guillain–Barré syndrome had electrophysiological studies showing multifocal conduction block and slowing of conduction velocities.[162] Needle EMG revealed muscle membrane instability in the form of fibrillation potentials, positive sharp waves, and complex repetitive discharges.[157,159,162] Small and large polyphasic MUAPs with early recruitment are seen as a result of the chronic myopathy.[157,159] Large polyphasic MUAPs with decreased recruitment are seen in patients with severe neuropathy.[159] The electrophysiological abnormalities improve with discontinuation of tryptophan.

Histopathology

Muscle biopsies demonstrated diffuse or perivascular inflammatory infiltrate in the fascia, perimysium, and, to a lesser extent, in the endomysium.[159] The majority of inflammatory cells are CD8+ T cells and macrophages, while eosinophils and B cells comprised <3% of the infiltrating cells. Unlike dermatomyositis, there is no deposition of MAC on small blood vessels. Nerve biopsies show predominately perivascular inflammatory infiltrates, mainly mononuclear, with occasional eosinophils in the epineurium, endoneurium, and/or perineurium with axonal degeneration.[157,159,162,164,165]

Pathogenesis

The disorder was caused by a contaminant(s) in the manufacture of tryptophan. Two trace adulterants were identified as the possible toxins: 3-phenylaminoalanine and 1,1′-ethylidenebis tryptophan.[166] The mechanism by which this contaminant resulted in the disorder is unknown, but the eosinophilia and eosinophilic infiltrate in tissues suggest some form of allergic reaction.

Treatment

Discontinuation of L-tryptophan and treatment with high-dose corticosteroids were usually effective in the prior epidemic. Some patients experienced relapses upon withdrawal of steroids.

TOXIC OIL SYNDROME

The toxic oil syndrome occurred as a single epidemic in Spain and has not recurred since 1981. It was quite similar to the eosinophilia–myalgia syndrome associated with tryptophan.[167] The disorder was linked to the ingestion of illegally marked, denatured rapeseed oil as a cooking substitute for olive oil. Interestingly, the toxic contaminant in the rapeseed oil, 3-phenylamino-1, 2-propanediol, is chemically similar to 3-phenylaminoalanine, the presumed adulterant in tryptophan causing the eosinophilia–myalgia syndrome.[166]

D-PENICILLAMINE

D-Penicillamine is rarely used nowadays to treat Wilson disease, rheumatoid arthritis (RA), and other connective tissue disorders. Approximately 0.2%–1.4% of patients treated with D-penicillamine developed an inflammatory myopathy.[168–171] It has also been associated with myasthenia. Discontinuation of the drug results in resolution of the symptoms. The medication may be restarted at a lower dosage without recurrence of the inflammatory myopathy.

CIMETIDINE

Rare cases of inflammatory myopathy have been reported with cimetidine, a histamine H_2 receptor antagonist.[172] One patient developed generalized weakness and myalgias associated with CK elevations up to 40,000 U/L and interstitial nephritis. The muscle biopsy revealed perivascular inflammation, predominantly consisting of CD8+ lymphocytes. No deposition of immunoglobulin or complement on small blood vessels was noted, nor did the patients have a cutaneous rash to suggest dermatomyositis. However, cases of cutaneous vasculitis have been described with cimetidine use.[173]

PROCAINAMIDE

Proximal muscle weakness and myalgias rarely occur with procainamide usage.[174,175] Serum CK levels are elevated, and EMG has been reported as being consistent with a "patchy" myopathy. Muscle biopsies demonstrate perivascular inflammation and rare necrotic muscle fibers. The pathogenesis may be related to lupus-like vasculitis, which can occur in patients treated with procainamide. The myopathy resolves following withdrawal of procainamide.

PHENYTOIN

Myalgias and weakness may develop in patients treated with phenytoin due to hypersensitivity reactions.[176–181] Serum CK levels can be elevated, and muscle biopsies show scattered necrotic and regenerating muscle fibers. EMG can reveal abnormal insertional and spontaneous activity in the form of fibrillation potentials and positive sharp waves. Small-amplitude, short-duration, polyphasic MUAPs, which recruit early may be observed. The myopathy improves with discontinuation of the phenytoin and a short course of corticosteroids.

ALPHA-INTERFERON

Alpha-interferon is used in the treatment of viral hepatitis and certain malignancies (e.g., chronic myelogenous leukemia and melanoma). A rare side effect of alpha-interferon is the occurrence of autoimmune disorders including myasthenia gravis and myositis.[182–184] Further, as discussed in Chapter 33, the overproduction of type 1 interferons, such as alpha-interferon, have been implicated in the pathogenesis of dermatomyositis.

TUMOR NECROSIS FACTOR-ALPHA BLOCKERS

Tumor necrosis factor alpha (TNF-α) blockers are used to treat RA, ankylosing spondylitis, and psoriatic arthritis. Side effects of TNF-α blockers include induction of other autoimmune disorders such as SLE and autoimmune neuropathies. Some patients with myositis patients treated with various TNF-α blockers improve, while others worsen.[185] In addition, there are reports of patients with previous history of myositis, who develop an inflammatory myopathy while being treated with a TNF-α blocker.[186,187]

TYROSINE KINASE INHIBITORS

Tyrosine kinase inhibitors are used to treat a number of cancers and several including imatinib, sorafenib, sunitinib, erlotinib, and osimertinib have been associated with myalgias, weakness, hyperCKemia, and rarely myocarditis.[188–193] We reported a patient with CML who developed polymyositis while taking imatinib.[188] CML28 antibodies were detected in the patient's serum. CML28 is identical to hRrp46p, a component of the human exosome, a multiprotein complex involved in processing of RNA. Antibodies directed against hRrp46p and other components of the human exosome (e.g., PM-Scl 100 and PMScl 75) have been noted in patients with polymyositis (see Chapter 33). The patient's strength and serum CK normalized with discontinuation of the imatinib and a course of corticosteroids.

Tyrosine kinases are involved in signal transduction, cell growth, and differentiation. The mechanism by which tyrosine kinase inhibitors therapy could cause myopathy is unclear. These inhibitors may interact with other medications via effects on the cytochrome P450–dependent metabolism, uridine diphosphate glucuronosyltransferase, and transporter proteins thereby increasing myotoxicity of some medicines (e.g., statins).[2] Perhaps, the rapid apoptosis of malignant cells and subsequent release tumor antigens may have cross-reactivity with muscle antigens and generate an autoimmune response.

VASCULAR ENDOTHELIAL GROWTH FACTOR INHIBITORS

Bevacizumab is used to treat certain tumors. It is a monoclonal antibody that binds and blocks circulating vascular endothelial growth factor. There are rare reports of rhabdomyolysis and myositis with its use.[94,194] The pathogenic mechanism is not clear.

MYOPATHIES SECONDARY TO IMPAIRED PROTEIN SYNTHESIS OR INCREASED CATABOLISM

CORTICOSTEROID MYOPATHY

Clinical Features

Corticosteroid myopathy manifests as proximal muscle weakness and atrophy affecting the legs more than the arms.[1,2,195–202] The distal extremities, oculobulbar, and facial muscles are normal as are sensation and muscle stretch reflexes. Most patients exhibit a Cushingoid appearance with facial edema and increased truncal adipose tissue. Prednisone at doses of 30 mg/day or more (or equivalent doses of other corticosteroids) is associated with an increased risk of myopathy.[199] Any synthetic glucocorticoid can cause the myopathy, but those that are fluorinated (triamcinolone > betamethasone > dexamethasone) are more likely to result in muscle weakness than nonflourinated compounds.[202] Women appear to be more at risk than men (approximately 2:1) of developing a steroid myopathy. Alternate-day dosing may reduce the risk of corticosteroid-induced weakness.

Muscle weakness can develop within several weeks following the administration of corticosteroids; however, it more commonly occurs as a complication of chronic administration of oral high–dose corticosteroids. Acute onset of severe generalized weakness can occur in patients receiving high dosages of intravenous corticosteroids with or without concomitant administration of neuromuscular blocking agents or sepsis (see section regarding Acute Quadriplegic Myopathy).

Laboratory Features

Serum CK is normal. Serum potassium can be low as a result of glucocorticoid excess and can cause some degree of weakness. Motor and sensory nerve conductions are normal in steroid myopathy.[203] Repetitive stimulation studies should not demonstrate a significant decrement or increment. Needle EMG is normal as well. The paucity of abnormalities is understandable, as corticosteroids preferentially affect type 2 muscle fibers. The first recruited motor units are comprised of type 1 muscle fibers. Because these are not affected as severely as type 2 fibers, there is little in the way of electrophysiological abnormality to observe.

Histopathology

Muscle biopsies reveal atrophy of type 2 fibers, especially the fast-twitch, glycolytic-type 2B fibers (Fig. 35-8).[198,199,204,205] There may also be a lesser degree of atrophy of type 1 muscle fibers.

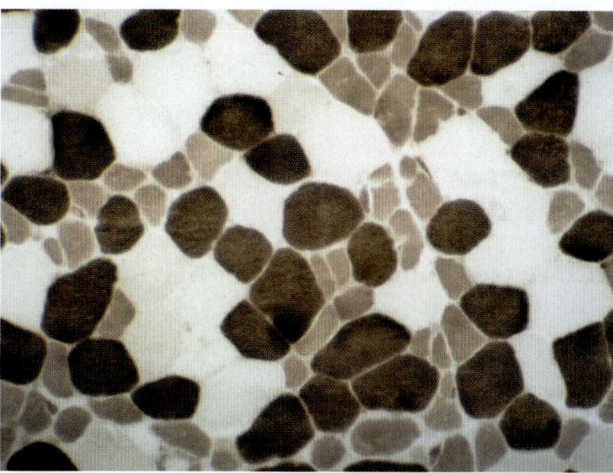

Figure 35-8. Steroid myopathy. Selective atrophy of the intermediately staining type 2B fibers is evident. ATPase pH 4.5.

Pathogenesis

Corticosteroids bind to receptors on target cells and are subsequently internalized into the nuclei, where these regulate the transcription of specific genes. How corticosteroids cause a myopathy is not known, but could be the result of decreased protein synthesis, increased protein degradation, alterations in carbohydrate metabolism, mitochondrial alterations, or reduced sarcolemmal excitability.[1,2,198,199]

Treatment

Reduction in the dose, tapering to an alternate-day regimen, or switching to a nonflourinated steroid along with a low carbohydrate diet and exercise to prevent concomitant disuse atrophy are major modes of therapy.[198,199]

Of particular concern is to distinguish steroid myopathy from an exacerbation of underlying immune-mediated neuromuscular disorder (e.g., inflammatory myopathy, myasthenia gravis, and chronic inflammatory demyelinating polyneuropathy) in a patient being treated with corticosteroids.[1,199,202,204] If the weakness occurs while the patient is tapering the corticosteroid, relapse of the underlying disease process would be most likely. In contrast, if weakness developed while the patient was on chronic high doses of steroids, a steroid myopathy should be considered. In the case of an inflammatory myopathy, an increasing serum CK, EMG with prominent increase in insertional and spontaneous activity, and skeletal muscle MRI showing edema (suspected inflammation) would point to an exacerbation of the myositis. In some cases, it is impossible to state with certainty whether the new weakness is related to a relapse of the underlying disease or secondary to the corticosteroid treatment. In such cases, we taper the corticosteroid medication and closely observe the patient. If muscle strength improves presumably, the patient had a steroid myopathy. If patient's strength declines, then more likely the weakness is caused by an exacerbation of the underlying autoimmune disease and requires increased doses of corticosteroids or other immunosuppressive medication.

TOXIC MYOPATHIES WITH MULTIFACTORIAL OR UNKNOWN PATHOGENIC MECHANISMS

ACUTE QUADRIPLEGIC MYOPATHY/ CRITICAL ILLNESS MYOPATHY

Patients in the ICU may develop generalized weakness due to critical illness polyneuropathy,[206,207] prolonged neuromuscular blockage,[208,209] or secondary to a myopathic process. The myopathic disorder has been termed AQM, acute illness myopathy, critical illness myopathy, and myopathy associated with thick filament (myosin loss).[1,2,210–223] It can be difficult to differentiate AQM from critical illness neuropathy or prolonged neuromuscular blockade, and patients can potentially have a combination of the above. Some series of ICU weakness report critical illness neuropathy to be more frequent than AQM,[224,224] but most, including the authors, have found the myopathy to be much more prevalent.[217,220,225] In the largest series involving 88 patients who developed weakness while in an ICU, AQM was three times as common as critical illness neuropathy (42% vs. 13%); prolonged neuromuscular blockade occurred in only one patient who also had AQM.[217]

Clinical Features

The first reported case of AQM was a 24-year-old woman with status asthmaticus who developed severe generalized weakness following treatment with high doses of intravenous corticosteroids and neuromuscular blockade.[22] Subsequently, there have been numerous reports of AQM usually developing in patients who received high-dose intravenous corticosteroids and/or nondepolarizing neuromuscular blockers.[209–212,215–231] The myopathy can also develop in patients with sepsis or multiorgan failure who never received either corticosteroids or nondepolarizing neuromuscular blocking agents.[213,214,222] Recent organ transplantation appears to be an increased risk factor for the development of AQM, perhaps related to high doses of intravenous corticosteroids used for prevention of rejection and neuromuscular blocking agents in the perioperative period. Because of their immunosuppressed state, patients undergoing transplantation are also prone to infection and sepsis, which also predisposes to AQM.

The incidence of AQM is uncertain because there have been only a few prospective series published on the subject.[226,229] In a study of 25 consecutive patients requiring mechanical ventilation for severe asthma, myopathy developed in 9/25 (36%) and elevated serum CK levels in 19/22 (86%) of patients tested.[229] The patients were treated with dexamethasone 10 mg every 8 hours or hydrocortisone 250 mg every 6 hours; 22 of the 25 patients also received vecuronium. Mechanical ventilation lasted an average of 3.1 ± 3.1 days in patients without myopathy and 12.9 ± 6.6 days in those with myopathy. In a prospective study of 100 consecutive adult patients undergoing liver transplantation, 7 patients developed AQM.[226] Patients were treated with nondepolarizing neuromuscular blocking agents and high-dose steroids in the perioperative period. Three of six patients tested had elevated serum CK levels, as high as 10 times the upper limit of normal by the 25th postoperative day. Four patients had muscle biopsies demonstrating necrosis and selected loss of myosin (see below). Three patients later died from sepsis and multiorgan failure. The remaining patients slowly regained strength and the ability to ambulate over 1–3 months.

Patients with AQM usually exhibit severe generalized weakness of the trunk, extremities, and respiratory muscles which can rarely involve the extraocular muscles.[209,228] The myopathy is usually initially recognized by the inability to wean the patient from the ventilator. Sensory examination is usually normal, but this of course can be difficult to determine in an intubated patient with altered mental status. Muscle reflexes are decreased or absent. The mortality is high, approximately 30% in one large series, secondary to multiple organ failure and sepsis rather than the myopathy.[217] The morbidity and mortality in AQM and critical illness neuropathy appear to be similar.[217] In patients who survive, muscle strength recovers slowly over several months.

Laboratory Features

Serum CK levels can be normal but are moderately elevated in about 50% of patients. NCSs reveal marked CMAP amplitude reduction with normal distal latencies and conduction velocities. In contrast, SNAP amplitudes should be normal or mildly reduced (>80% of the lower limit of normal) in comparison. Markedly reduced amplitudes of SNAPs should lead to the consideration of critical illness neuropathy. However, the SNAPs may be affected, if the patient has a baseline (unrelated poly neuropathy), and many of these patients have illnesses that are associated with poly neuropathy (diabetes mellitus and renal or liver failure). SNAPs in the lower extremities may be obscured by edema as well. Thus, reduced SNAP amplitudes in and of itself do not exclude AQM.

Direct muscle stimulation may help to distinguish AQM from critical illness neuropathy, but these studies are fraught with the possibility of technical error.[220,221,230] Direct muscle stimulation bypasses the distal motor nerve and neuromuscular junction. In critical illness neuropathy or prolonged neuromuscular blockade, the muscle membranes should retain their excitability, and direct muscle stimulation CMAP (dmCMAP) should be near normal despite a low or absent nerve stimulation-evoked CMAP (neCMAP). In contrast, if the muscle membrane excitability is reduced as seen in AQM, both the neCMAP and the dmCMAP should be very low. Theoretically, the ratio of neCMAP to dmCMAP should be close to 1:1 in a myopathy and should approach zero in

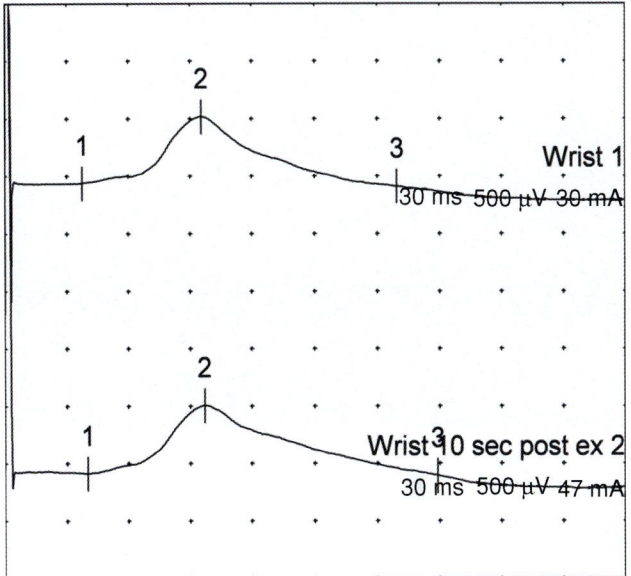

Figure 35-9. Synchronous dispersion causing a reduced amplitude and a long tail of the negative phase of the CMAP resulting in a prolonged duration of the ulnar CMAP (15 ms) from a patient with critical illness myopathy.

a neuropathy or neuromuscular junction disorder. In this regard, absent or reduced amplitudes of the dmCMAP with neCMAP/dmCMAP ratios >0.9 were demonstrated in 11 patients with AQM, while neCMAP/dmCMAP ratios were 0.5 or less in patients with severe neuropathy.[220,221] Significant slowing of muscle-fiber conduction velocity (MFCV) and muscle-fiber conduction block during the acute phase of AQM can be demonstrated. This correlates with prolonged CMAP durations, clinical severity, and course (Fig. 35-9).[231]

EMG usually demonstrates prominent fibrillation potentials and positive sharp waves, however such abnormal spontaneous activity is not always evident. Early recruitment of short-duration, small-amplitude, polyphasic MUAPs may be seen if the patient has sufficient strength to generate any MUAPs. Patients with severe weakness may be unable to volitionally recruit any MUAP. The inability to quantitate MUAP morphology and recruitment can make it difficult to distinguish AQM from critical illness neuropathy in patients who may have incidentally abnormal sensory conduction studies. Sequential EMG studies in AQM have reported profuse spontaneous activity and inability to actively recruit MUAPs early, followed by the appearance of small polyphasic MUAPs with early recruitment during the recovery period.[227]

Histopathology

Muscle biopsies reveal a wide spectrum of histological abnormalities. Type 2 muscle fiber atrophy with or without type 1 fiber atrophy is common.[210,211,214,215,222,223,228] Scattered necrotic and regenerating muscle fibers may be seen (Fig. 35-10A).[210,217,219,222,226,228] Focal or diffuse loss of reactivity for myosin ATPase activity in type 1 fibers more than type 2 fibers, corresponding to the loss of thick filaments (myosin) apparent on EM, is typically observed (Fig. 35-10B and C).[210,212,213,215–217,222,226] Other structural proteins (actin, titin, and nebulin) are relatively spared.[222]

Pathogenesis

The variable laboratory, histological, and electrophysiological features suggest that the pathogenesis is multifactorial. Some biopsies demonstrate widespread necrosis, which certainly can account for the muscle weakness observed in patients. The mechanism of muscle fiber necrosis is not known, and, importantly, not all patients have this feature on biopsy. Myosin is selectively lost in some but not all patients. Calcium-activated proteases (calpains) may be responsible for proteolysis of myosin.[222] Perhaps, glucocorticoids, nondepolarizing neuromuscular agents, or the milieu of critical illness induces the expression of calpains. In addition, the enhanced expression of cytokines during sepsis may, in turn, lead to a catabolic state in muscle with breakdown of proteins, glycogen, and lipid.

The reduced muscle membrane excitability may be the result of a combination of several factors: (1) partial depolarization of the resting membrane potential, (2) reduced muscle membrane resistance, and (3) decreased sodium currents.[220,221,230–232] Denervation and neuromuscular blockade normally decrease the resting membrane muscle potential, increase membrane resistance secondary to decreased chloride conductance, and increase the number of sodium channels on the muscle membrane. In denervated rats treated with corticosteroids, the resting membrane potential does not significantly decrease but muscle membrane resistance decreases (rather than increase) as a result of increased chloride conductance. The reduced membrane resistance decreases the depolarization caused by the opening of sodium channels. In addition, there is diminished sodium current secondary to a reduction in the number of sodium channels, decreased sodium channel conductance, or impaired voltage-dependent gating.

Treatment

Supportive care and treating underlying systemic abnormalities (e.g., antibiotics in sepsis and dialysis in renal failure) are the only modes of therapy. Corticosteroids or nondepolarizing neuromuscular blockers should be discontinued if possible. Patients require extensive physical and occupational therapies to prevent contractures and help regain muscle strength and functional abilities.

FINASTERIDE

Finasteride is used to treat benign prostatic hypertrophy and male pattern baldness. It is a 4-azasteroid that inhibits

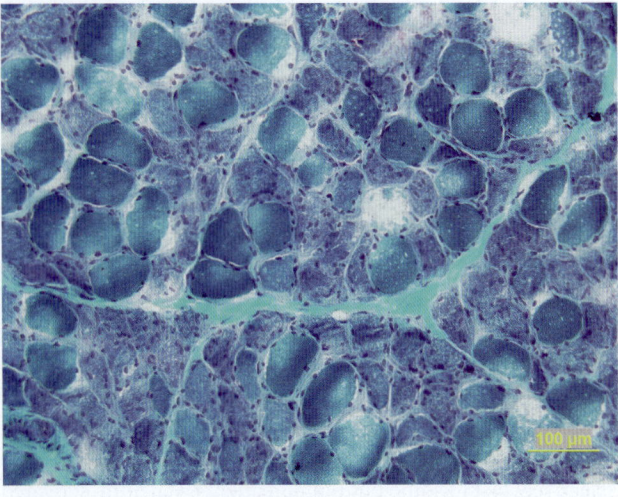

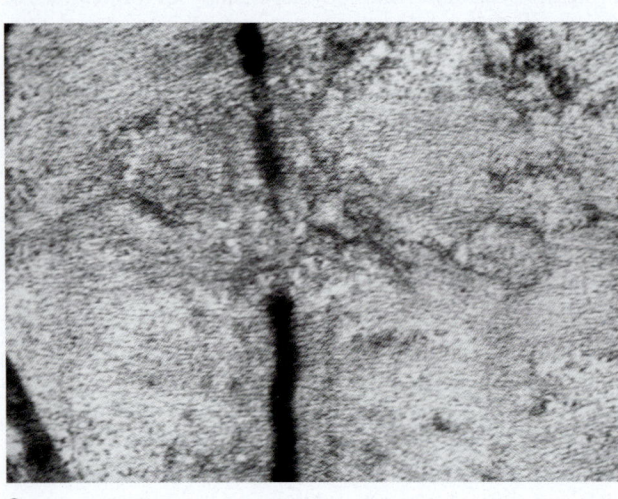

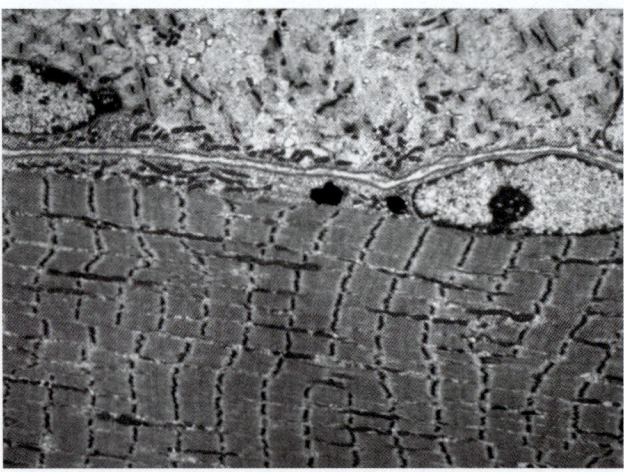

Figure 35-10. Critical illness/acute quadriplegic myopathy. Muscle biopsy demonstrates marked degeneration and atrophy of muscle fibers on modified Gomori trichrome (**A**). Electron microscopy demonstrates a muscle fiber with a preserved sarcomeres adjacent to a degenerating muscle fiber just above it (**B**). Higher-power view on EM reveals the preserved Z-disc and thin filaments but the loss of the myosin thick filaments (**C**).

5α-reductase, and thus blocks dihydrotestosterone production, and androgen action in the prostate and skin. There are rare reports of reversible myalgia, weakness, and hyperCKemia with use of finasteride and other 5α-reductase inhibitors.[233–236] There is limited information on electrophysiology and muscle biopsies, though some have shown variability in fiber size, type 2 muscle fiber atrophy, and increased internalized nuclei. The pathophysiological mechanism for the myopathy is not known. Discontinuation of finasteride is associated with resolution of clinical abnormalities and normalization of CK.

OMEPRAZOLE

Clinical Features

Omeprazole inhibits the H^+/K^+ ATPase enzyme system (the proton pump) at the secretory surface of the gastric parietal cell and is used for the treatment of gastric and duodenal ulcers and reflux. Rare cases of neuromyopathy have been reported with the use of omeprazole.[237,238] Patients develop proximal weakness and myalgias along with paresthesias and a length-dependent loss sensory loss, predominantly in the legs. Muscle reflexes are diminished or absent.

Laboratory Features

Serum CK levels are normal or mildly elevated. NCSs may be normal or reveal an axonal sensorimotor polyneuropathy.[237] EMG can be normal or show small polyphasic MUAPs.

Histopathology

Only a few muscle biopsies have been done and have shown only type 2 muscle fiber atrophy.

Pathogenesis

The pathogenic mechanism for the neuromyopathy is unknown.

Treatment

Muscle strength and sensation improve and serum CK levels normalize following discontinuation of omeprazole. Symptoms may recur if omeprazole is restarted.

ISOTRETINOIN

Clinical Features

Isotretinoin (Accutane) is used for the treatment of severe acne. Exercise-induced myalgias, rhabdomyolysis, and proximal weakness can occur.[239–242]

Laboratory Features

Serum CK levels can be normal or elevated 100-fold.[239–242] Decreased serum carnitine levels may be seen. EMG can demonstrate small polyphasic MUAPs.

Histopathology

Muscle biopsy in a single reported patient demonstrated only atrophy of muscle fibers.

Pathogenesis

The basis for the myopathy is not clear. The diminished carnitine levels and response to L-carnitine in some patients suggest that perturbation of lipid metabolism may be contributory.

Treatment

The myalgias, weakness, and CK elevations improve with discontinuation of isotretinoin.

EMETINE (IPECAC)

Clinical Features

Emetine hydrochloride is an emetic agent that has been abused, particularly in patients with anorexia nervosa and bulimia. A severe proximal myopathy and cardiomyopathy can occur with overuse of emetine (500–600 mg/day for over 10 days).[243–245] Patients also complain of muscle pain, tenderness, and stiffness. Muscle stretch reflexes are usually diminished, but the sensory examination is completely normal. The myopathy is reversible following discontinuation of the medication.

Laboratory Features

The serum CK levels may be mildly to moderately elevated. Sensory and motor NCSs are normal.[243–245] Needle EMG examination can be normal although, positive sharp waves and fibrillation potentials are usually apparent. There is early recruitment of small-amplitude, short-duration MUAPs.

Histopathology

Muscle biopsies reveal scattered necrotic fibers, small atrophic and regenerating fibers as well as many fibers containing cytoplasmic bodies. Oxidative enzyme stains demonstrate targetoid or moth-eaten structures. On EM, there is evidence of myofibrillar degeneration in addition to compacted myofibrillar debris (cytoplasmic bodies). The histological appearance of light microscopy and EM is similar to myofibrillar myopathy (see Chapter 27).[246]

Pathogenesis

The exact pathogenic basis for the disorder is not known, but it is postulated that emetine might inhibit the synthesis of important muscle proteins.

Treatment

The myopathy resolves following discontinued use of emetine.

DRUG-INDUCED HYPOKALEMIC MYOPATHY

Hypokalemia can be a complication of a variety of medications (e.g., diuretics, laxatives, mineralocorticoids, amphotericin, and lithium). Further, excessive eating of licorice may have an aldosterone-like effect and cause hypokalemia. Hypokalemic myopathy has also been associated with alcohol abuse and inhalation of toluene. The clinical, laboratory, histopathological, and electrophysiological features of hypokalemic myopathy are similar, regardless of the etiology of the hypokalemia. Affected individuals develop acute or subacute generalized weakness that can resemble Guillain–Barré syndrome. Weakness usually does not occur unless the serum potassium levels are less than 2 mEq/L. The serum CK levels are elevated. EMGs can be normal or demonstrate mild irritability in the form of fibrillation potentials and positive sharp waves in severely weakened muscles. Muscle biopsies are not typically performed as the diagnosis is apparent with the appropriate laboratory testing. However, muscle biopsies may demonstrate scattered necrotic and regenerating muscle fibers as well as vacuoles that arise from T tubules. The weakness improves with correction of the hypokalemia.

▶ MYOPATHIES ASSOCIATED WITH ANESTHETIC AGENTS AND CENTRALLY ACTING MEDICATIONS

MALIGNANT HYPERTHERMIA

Clinical Features

Malignant hyperthermia is a genetically heterogeneous group of disorders characterized by severe muscle rigidity, myoglobinuria, fever, tachycardia, cyanosis, and cardiac arrhythmias precipitated by depolarizing muscle relaxants (e.g., succinylcholine) and inhalational anesthetic agents (e.g., halothane).[247–249] The incidence of malignant hyperthermia ranges from 0.5% to 0.0005%.[247] At least 50% of patients may have had previous anesthesia without any problems. The signs of malignant hyperthermia usually appear during surgery but can develop in the postoperative period. Rarely, attacks of malignant hyperthermia have been triggered by exercise, ingestion of caffeine, and stress.

Laboratory Features

Serum CK can be normal or mildly elevated between attacks in patients susceptible to malignant hyperthermia. During attacks of malignant hyperthermia, serum CK levels are markedly elevated and myoglobinuria can develop. Hyperkalemia is also usually present. Metabolic and respiratory acidosis is evident with lactic acidosis, hypoxia, and hypercarbia. NCSs and EMG are usually normal in the interictal periods. However, EMG performed shortly after an attack of malignant hyperthermia may demonstrate increased spontaneous activity and, perhaps, small polyphasic MUAPs that recruit early.

The in vitro muscle contracture test can be performed to assess the susceptibility of malignant hyperthermia in individuals who may be at risk (i.e., family members with history of malignant hyperthermia).[247] However, the test is not routinely available and false-positive and false-negative tests occur. Varying concentrations of halothane and caffeine are applied to strips of muscle that are stimulated at 0.1–0.2 Hz for 1–5 seconds, while tension is measured by a stain gauge. In patients susceptible to malignant hyperthermia, much lower concentrations of caffeine and halothane produce muscle contractions than are required to produce a similar in normal muscle tissue.

Histopathology

Muscle biopsies demonstrate nonspecific myopathic features including fiber size variability, increased internal nuclei, moth-eaten fibers, and necrotic fibers after an attack of malignant hyperthermia.

Pathogenesis and Molecular Genetics

Malignant hyperthermia susceptibility is genetically very heterogeneous, as families have been linked to different chromosomes and genes.[250] Mutations in the ryanodine receptor gene, *RYR1*, account for around 85% of cases (MHS1).[250] Mutations in RYR1 are also responsible for central core myopathy (see Chapter 28). The ryanodine receptor bridges the gap between the sarcoplasmic reticulum and the T tubule. Mutations in the ryanodine receptor may result in a functional alteration of the associated calcium channel such that there is an excessive release of calcium into the cytoplasm upon activation. The next most common cause of MHS is mutations in *CACNA1S*, the gene that encodes the alpha-1S subunit of the voltage-dependent L-type calcium channel, also known as the dihydropyridine calcium channel.[250] Notably, this calcium channel is physically coupled with the ryanodine receptor. Mutations in the *STAC3* also can cause MHS. The STAC3 protein interacts with both the ryanodine receptor and dihydropyridine calcium channel.[250] Mutations in the STAC3 gene also cause what has been called Native American myopathy.[251] In addition, patients with muscular dystrophies, myotonic dystrophies, mitochondrial myopathies, and other channelopathies are susceptible to developing malignant hyperthermia.[252]

Thus, it appears that malignant hyperthermia can occur in various myopathic disorders, affecting the structural proteins of the muscle membrane or ion channels. Malignant hyperthermia appears to arise secondary to excessive calcium release by the sarcoplasmic reticulum calcium channels. Increased intracytoplasmic calcium leads to excessive muscle contraction, increased use of oxygen and ATP, and overproduction of heat. Why various anesthetic agents and depolarizing muscle relaxants trigger this exaggerated release of calcium from the sarcoplasmic reticulum in predisposed individuals is not known.

Treatment

Individuals at risk of malignant hyperthermia should not be given known triggering anesthetic agents if possible. Malignant hyperthermia is a medical emergency, requiring several therapeutic steps.[237] The anesthetic agent must be discontinued, while 100% oxygen is delivered. Dantrolene 2–3 mg/kg every 5 minutes for a total of 10 mg/kg should be administered. The stomach, bladder, and lower gastrointestinal tract are lavaged with iced saline solution, and cooling blankets are applied. Acidosis and hyperkalemia are treated with sodium bicarbonate, hyperventilation, dextrose, insulin, and occasionally calcium chloride. Urinary output must be maintained with hydration, furosemide, or mannitol. The patient must be monitored and treated for cardiac arrhythmias.

► MYOPATHIES SECONDARY TO DRUGS OF ABUSE

ALCOHOLIC MYOPATHY

Chronic alcohol abuse is more often attributed to causing neuropathy than myopathy. However, several forms of a toxic myopathy due to alcohol have been described: (1) acute necrotizing myopathy, (2) acute hypokalemic myopathy, (3) chronic alcoholic myopathy, (4) asymptomatic alcoholic myopathy, and (5) alcoholic cardiomyopathy.[253–257]

An acute necrotizing myopathy manifests as acute muscle pain, tenderness to palpation, cramping, swelling, and weakness following or during a recent particularly intense binge. The severity of the myopathy is highly variable. Severe cases can be associated with myoglobinuria and acute renal failure. The muscle cramps resolve over the course of several days, while the remainder of symptoms may last several weeks. Serum CK levels are markedly elevated during these attacks. Muscle biopsies reveal widespread muscle fiber necrosis and occasionally fibers with tubular aggregates. Disorganization of the sarcomeres and degeneration of mitochondria may be appreciated on EM. Patents require appropriate supportive medical care and nutritional supplementation as many are malnourished.

Alcohol abuse can lead to acute hypokalemia, which can cause generalized weakness. Muscle weakness evolves over the time period of 1 or 2 days. Serum potassium is very low, <2 mEq/L, and the CK levels are elevated. Muscle biopsy performed in the acute time frame may reveal vacuoles with the muscle fibers. The myopathy resolves with correction of the serum potassium.

Some alcoholics develop the insidious onset of primarily proximal limb-girdle weakness, especially of the lower limbs, which has been attributed to a chronic alcoholic myopathy. Muscle biopsy may reveal scattered muscle fiber atrophy, necrosis, and regeneration. Whether the muscle weakness is caused by a toxic influence of alcohol on muscle, a toxic peripheral neuropathy, or malnutrition is unclear.

An asymptomatic alcoholic myopathy has been suggested in some patients on the basis of an elevated serum CK levels found coincidentally. There is no complaint of weakness, and the physical examination does not reveal striking evidence of a myopathic disorder. Histological findings are not available for this class of patients, and the true nature of this presumed form of alcoholic myopathy is questionable. The elevated serum CK may be related to subclinical necrotizing myopathy, hypokalemia, or muscle trauma.

Laboratory Features

Serum CK levels may be normal or slightly elevated and potassium levels may be reduced or normal. Reduced amplitudes of the sensory and, occasionally, motor nerve conductions studies may be seen, if patients have a concomitant alcoholic neuropathy. Needle EMG may reveal positive sharp waves, fibrillation potentials, and early recruitment of short-duration, low-amplitude MUAPs firing at high rates with minimal force production in weak muscles in patients with a necrotizing alcoholic myopathy.[253–257]

Pathogenesis

The pathogenic basis for the various forms of alcoholic myopathies is not known. The metabolism of alcohol may lead to the accumulation of toxic metabolites (e.g., acetaldehyde) or free radicals that may be toxic to lipid membranes.

▶ MYOPATHIES SECONDARY TO ILLICIT DRUGS

Illicit drugs including opioids (e.g., heroin, meperidine, cocaine, pentazocine, piritramide, amphetamines, etc.) may be myotoxic.[258–261] Muscle injury can be related to direct muscle trauma (e.g., needle injury), rhabdomyolysis secondary to pressure and ischemic necrosis related to prolonged loss of consciousness, ischemia due to vasoconstriction, rhabdomyolysis caused by generalized status epilepticus, or the direct toxic effects of the drugs (or adulterants) on muscle tissue. Serum CK levels should be markedly elevated, and muscle biopsies reveal widespread necrosis in such cases.

Inhalation of volatile agents (e.g., toluene) can also cause generalized muscle weakness and, occasionally, myoglobinuria. Toluene causes distal renal tubular acidosis with associated severe hypokalemia, hypophosphatemia, and mild hypocalcemia. Muscle strength returns after correction of the electrolyte abnormalities and abstinence from further exposure.

▶ SUMMARY

Various drugs can cause muscle damage and from a variety of different mechanisms. It is imperative to take a good medical history including current and previous medication history (as well as history of illicit drug use and alcohol abuse), as stopping the offending agent usually leads to improvement of the myopathy. However, continued use can be associated with significant morbidity and even death (e.g., from myoglobinuria). The most common toxic myopathy is associated with statin use in keeping with how frequently these medications are prescribed. That said, most individuals treated with statin medications and other medications known to cause toxic myopathy have no complications.

REFERENCES

1. Doughty CT, Amato AA. Toxic myopathies. *Continuum (Minneap Minn)*. 2019;25:1712–1731.
2. Mastaglia FL. The changing spectrum of drug-induced myopathies. *Acta Myol*. 20201;39:283–288.
3. Amato AA, Dumitru D. Acquired myopathies. In: Dumitru D, Amato AA, Zwarts MJ, eds. *Electrodiagnostic Medicine*. 2nd ed. Hanley & Belfus; 2002:1371–1432.
4. Argov Z, Mastaglia FL. Drug-induced neuromuscular disorders in man. In: Walton JN, ed. *Disorders of Voluntary Muscle*. 5th ed. Churchill-Livingstone; 1988:981–1014.
5. Baker PC. Drug-induced and toxic myopathies. *Semin Neurol*. 1983;3:265–273.
6. Griggs RC, Mendell JR, Miller RG. Myopathies of systemic disease. In: *Evaluation and Treatment of Myopathies*. FA Davis; 1995:355–385.
7. Kuncl RW, Wiggins WW. Toxic myopathies. *Neurol Clin*. 1988;6:593–619.
8. Mastaglia FL. Toxic myopathies. In: Rowland LP, DiMauro S, eds. *Handbook of Clinical Neurology*. Vol 18, No. 62: Myopathies. Elsevier Science Publishers BV; 1992:595–622.
9. Victor M, Sieb JP. Myopathies due to drugs, toxins, and nutritional deficiency. In: Engel AG, Franzini-Armstrong C, eds. *Myology*. 2nd ed. McGraw-Hill; 1994:1697–1725.
10. Mastaglia FL. Iatrogenic myopathies. *Curr Opin Neurol*. 2010; 23:445–449.

11. Bakker-Arema RG, Best J, Fayyad R, et al. A brief review paper on the efficacy and safety of atorvastatin in early clinical trials. *Atherosclerosis*. 1997;131:17–23.
12. Berland Y, Coponat H, Durand C, Baz M, Laugier R, Musso JL. Rhabdomyolysis and simvastatin use. *Nephron*. 1991;57:365–366.
13. Corpier C, Jones P, Suki W, et al. Rhabdomyolysis and renal injury with lovastatin use. *JAMA*. 1988;260:239–241.
14. Davidson MH, Stein EA, Dujoven CA, et al. The efficacy and six week tolerability of simvastatin 80 and 160 mg/day. *Am J Cardiol*. 1997;79:38–42.
15. Deslypere J, Vermuelen A. Rhabdomyolysis and simvastatin. *Ann Intern Med*. 1991;114:342.
16. Marais GE, Larson KK. Rhabdomyolysis and acute renal failure induced by combination lovastatin and gemfibrozil therapy. *Ann Intern Med*. 1990;112:228–230.
17. Schalke BB, Schmidt B, Toyka K, Hartung HP. Pravastatin-associated inflammatory myopathy. *N Engl J Med*. 1992;327:649–650.
18. Tobert J. Efficacy and long-term adverse effect pattern of lovastatin. *Am J Cardiol*. 1988;62:28J–33J.
19. East C, Alivizatos PA, Grundy SM, Jones PH, Farmer JA. Rhabdomyolysis in patients receiving lovastatin after cardiac transplantation. *N Engl J Med*. 1988;318:48.
20. Abourizk N, Khalil BA, Bahuth N, Afifi AK. Clofibrate induced muscular syndrome. *J Neurol Sci*. 1979;42:1–9.
21. Denizot M, Fabre J, Pometa D, Wildi E. Clofibrate, nephrotic syndrome, and histological changes in muscle. *Lancet*. 1973;1:1326.
22. Gabriel R, Pearce JM. Clofibrate induced myopathy and neuropathy. *Lancet*. 1976;2:906.
23. Kwiecinski H. Myotonia induced with clofibrate in rats. *J Neurol*. 1978;219:107–116.
24. Langer T, Levy RI. Acute muscular syndrome associated with administration of clofibrate. *N Engl J Med*. 1968;279:856–858.
25. London F, Gross KF, Ringel SP. Cholesterol-lowering agent myopathy (CLAM). *Neurology*. 1991;41:1159–1160.
26. Magarian GJ, Lucas LM. Gemfibrozil-induced myopathy. *Arch Intern Med*. 1991;151:1873–1874.
27. Pierce LR, Wysowski DK, Gross TP. Myopathy and rhabdomyolysis associated with lovastatin-gemfibrozil combination therapy. *JAMA*. 1990;264:71–75.
28. Pierides AM, Alvarez-Ude F, Kerr DN. Clofibrate induced muscle damage in patients with chronic renal failure. *Lancet*. 1975;2:1279–1282.
29. Rush P, Baron M, Kapusta M. Clofibrate myopathy: a case report and a review of the literature. *Semin Arthritis Rheum*. 1986;15:226–229.
30. Shepherd J. Fibrates and statins in the treatment of hyperlipidemia: an appraisal of their efficacy and safety. *Eur Heart J*. 1995;16:5–13.
31. Litin SC, Andersone CF. Nicotinic acid-associated myopathy: a report of three cases. *Am J Med*. 1989;86:481–483.
32. Reaven P, Witzum J. Lovastatin, nicotinic acid and rhabdomyolysis [letter]. *Ann Intern Med*. 1988;109:597–598.
33. Fux R, Morike K, Gundel UF, Hartmann R, Gleiter CH. Ezetimibe and statin-associated myopathy. *Ann Intern Med*. 2004;140(8):671–672.
34. Havranek JM, Wolfsen AR, Warnke GA, Phillips PS. Monotherapy with ezetimibe causing myopathy. *Am J Med*. 2006;119(3):285–286.
35. Simard C, Poirier P. Ezetimibe-associated myopathy in monotherapy and in combination with a 3-hydroxy-3-methylglutaryl coenzyme A reductase inhibitor. *Can J Cardiol*. 2006;22(2):141–144.
36. Perez-Calvo J, Civeira-Murillo F, Cabello A. Worsening myopathy associated with ezetimibe in a patient with McArdle disease. *QJM*. 2005;98(6):461–462.
37. Dujovne CA, Chremos AN, Pool JL, et al. Expanded Clinical Evaluation of Lovastatin (EXCEL) study results. IV. Additional perspectives on the tolerability of lovastatin. *Am J Med*. 1991;91(suppl 1B):25–30.
38. Jones P, Kafonek S, Laurora I, Hunningshake D. Comparative dose efficacy study of atorvastatin versus simvastatin, provastatin, lovastatin, and fluvastatin in patients with hypercholesterolemia (the CURVES Study). *Am J Cardiol*. 1998;81:582–587.
39. Galper JB. Increase incidence of myositis in patients treated with high dose simvastatin. *Am J Cardiol*. 1998;81:259.
40. Duell PB, Connor WE, Illingsworth DR. Rhabdomyolysis after taking atorvastatin with gemfibrozil. *Am J Cardiol*. 1998;81:368–369.
41. Furberg CD, Pitt B. Commentary: withdrawal of cervistatin from the world market. *Curr Control Trials Cardiovasc Med*. 2001;2:205–207.
42. von Keutz E, Schluter G. Preclinical safety evaluation of cerivastation, a novel HMG-CoA reductase inhibitor. *Am J Cardiol*. 1998;82(4B):11J–17J.
43. Hamilton-Craig I. Statin-associated myopathy. *Med J Aust*. 2001;175:486–489.
44. Pasternak RC, Smith SC, Bairey-Merz CN, Grundy S, Cleeman J, Lenfant C. ACC/AHA/NHLBI clinical advisory on the use and safety of statins. *J Am Coll Cardiol*. 2002;40:556–572.
45. Ucar M, Mjorndal T, Dahlqvist R. HMG-CoA reductase inhibitors and myotoxicity. *Drug Saf*. 2000;22:441–457.
46. Hodel C. Myopathy and rhabdomyolysis with lipid-lowering drugs. *Toxicol Lett*. 2002;128:159–168.
47. Thompson PD, Clarkson P, Karas RH. Statin-associated myopathy. *JAMA*. 2003;289:1681–1690.
48. dos Santos AG, Guardia AC, Pereira TS, et al. Rhabdomyolysis as a clinical manifestation of association with ciprofibrate, sirolimus, cyclosporine, and pegylated interferon-α in liver-transplanted patients: A case report and literature review. *Transplant Proc*. 2014;46:1887–1888.
49. Mammen AL, Amato AA. Statin myopathy: a review of recent progress. *Curr Opin Rheumatol*. 2010;22:644–650.
50. Shanmugam VK, Matsumoto C, Pien E, et al. Voriconazole associated myositis. *J Clin Rheumatol*. 2009;15:350–353.
51. Basic-Jukic N, Kes P, Bubic-Filipi L, Vranjican Z. Rhabdomyolysis and acute kidney injury secondary to concomitant use of fluvastatin and rapamycin in a renal transplant recipient. *Nephrol Dial Transplant*. 2010;25:2036.
52. Backes JM, Venero CV, Gibson CA, et al. Effectiveness and tolerability of every-other-day rosuvastatin dosing in patients with prior statin intolerance. *Ann Pharmacother*. 2008;42:341–346.
53. Fauchais AL, Iba Ba J, Maurage P, et al. Polymyositis induced or associated with lipid-lowering drugs: five cases. *Rev Med Interne*. 2004;25(4):294–298.
54. Giordano N, Senesi M, Mattii G, Battisti E, Villanova M, Gennari C. Polymyositis associated with simvastatin. *Lancet*. 1997;349(9065):1600–1601.

55. Hill C, Zeitz C, Kirkham B. Dermatomyositis with lung involvement in a patient treated with simvastatin. *Aust N Z J Med*. 1995;25(6):745–746.
56. Khattak FH, Morris IM, Branford WA. Simvastatin-associated dermatomyositis. *Br J Rheumatol*. 1994;33(2):199.
57. Noel B, Cerottini JP, Panizzon RG. Atorvastatin-induced dermatomyositis. *Am J Med*. 2001;110(8):670–671.
58. Riesco-Eizaguirre G, Arpa-Gutierrez FJ, Gutierrez M, Toribio E. Severe polymyositis with simvastatin use. *Rev Neurol*. 2003;37(10):934–936.
59. Rodriguez-Garcia JL, Serrano Commino M. Lovastatin-associated dermatomyositis. *Postgrad Med J*. 1996;72(853):694.
60. Vasconcelos OM, Campbell WW. Dermatomyositis-like syndrome and HMG-CoA reductase inhibitor (statin) in-take. *Muscle Nerve*. 2004;30(6):803–807.
61. Christopher-Stine L, Casciola Rosen L, Hong G, Chung T, Corse AM, Mammen AL. A novel autoantibody recognizing 200 and 100 kDa proteins is associated with an immune mediated necrotizing myopathy. *Arthritis Rheum*. 2010;62:2757–2766.
62. Mammen AL, Chung T, Christopher-Stine L, et al. Autoantibodies against 3-hydroxy-3-methylglutaryl-coenzyme A reductase in patients with statin-associated autoimmune myopathy. *Arthritis Rheum*. 2011;63:713–721.
63. Needham M, Fabian V, Knezevic W, Panegyres P, Zilko P, Mastaglia FL. Progressive myopathy with up-regulation of MHC-I associated with statin therapy. *Neuromuscul Disord*. 2007;17(2):194–200.
64. Grable-Esposito P, Katzberg HD, Greenberg SA, Srinivasan J, Katz J, Amato AA. Immune-mediated necrotizing myopathy associated with statins. *Muscle Nerve*. 2010;41:185–190.
65. Meriggioli MN, Barboi A, Rowin J, Cochran EJ. HMGCoA reductase inhibitor myopathy: clinical, electrophysiologic, and pathologic data in five patients. *J Clin Neuromuscul Dis*. 2001;2:129–134.
66. Phillips PS, Haas RH, Bannykh S, et al. Statin-associated myopathy with normal creatine kinase levels. *Ann Intern Med*. 2002;137:581–585.
67. Greenberg SA, Amato AA. Statin myopathies. *Continuum*. 2006;12:169–184.
68. SEARCH Collaborative Group; Link E, Parish S, Armitage J, et al. SLCO1B1 variants and statin-induced myopathy: a genomewide study. *N Engl J Med*. 2008;359:789–799.
69. Kra SJ. Muscle syndrome with clofibrate usage. *Conn Med*. 1974;38:348–349.
70. Afifi AK, Hajj SS, Tekian A, et al. Clofibrate-induced myotoxicity in rats. *Eur Neurol*. 1984;23:182–197.
71. Slim H, Thompson PD. Ezetimibe-related myopathy: a systematic review. *J Clin Lipidol*. 2008;2:328–234.
72. Amato AA, Barohn RJ. Neurological complications of transplantations. In: Harati Y, Rolack LA, eds. *Practical Neuroimmunology*. Butterworth-Heineman; 1997:341–375.
73. Arellano F, Krup P. Muscular disorders associated with cyclosporine [letter]. *Lancet*. 1991;337:915.
74. Costigan DA. Acquired myotonia, weakness and vacuolar myopathy secondary to cyclosporine [abstract]. *Muscle Nerve*. 1989;12:761.
75. Goy JJ, Stauffer JC, Deruaz JP, et al. Myopathy as a possible side effect cyclosporine. *Lancet*. 1989;1:1446–1449.
76. Grezard O, Lebranchu Y, Birmele B, Sharobeem R, Nivet H, Bagros P. Cyclosporine-induced muscular toxicity. *Lancet*. 1990;1:177.
77. Noppen D, Verlkeriers B, Dierckx R, Bruyland M, Vanhaelst L. Cyclosporine and myopathy. *Ann Intern Med*. 1987;107:945–946.
78. Hibi S, Hisawa A, Tamai M, et al. Severe rhabdomyolysis with tacrolimus [letter]. *Lancet*. 1995;346:702.
79. Norman D, Illingworth DR, Munson J, Hosenpud J. Myolysis and acute renal failure in heart transplant recipient receiving lovastatin. *N Engl J Med*. 1988;318:46–47.
80. Rieger EH, Halasz NA, Wahlstrom HE. Colchicine neuromyopathy after renal transplantation. *Transplantation*. 1990;49:1196–1198.
81. Volin L, Jarventie G, Ruut U. Fatal rhabdomyolysis as a complication of bone marrow transplantation. *Bone Marrow Transplant*. 1990;6:59–60.
82. Atkinson P, Joubert G, Barron A, et al. Hypertrophic cardiomyopathy with tacrolimus in paediatric transplant patient. *Lancet*. 1995;345:894–896.
83. Teicher A, Rosenthal T, Kissen E, Sarova I. Labetalol-induced toxic myopathy. *Br Med J*. 1981;282:1824–1825.
84. Willis JK, Tilton AH, Harkin JC, Boineau FG. Reversible myopathy due to labatolol. *Pediatr Neurol*. 1990;6:275–276.
85. Hanna JP, Ramundo ML. Rhabdomyolysis and hypoxia associated with prolonged propofol infusion in children. *Neurology*. 1988;50:301–303.
86. Parke TJ, Steven JE, Rice AS, et al. Metabolic acidosis and myocardial failure after propofol infusion in children: five case reports. *Br Med J*. 1992;305:613–616.
87. Strickland RA, Murray MJ. Fatal metabolic acidosis in pediatric patient receiving and infusion of propofol in the intensive care unit: is there a relationship? *Crit Care Med*. 1995;23:405–409.
88. Shimizu J, Tabata T, Tsujita Y, et al. Propofol infusion syndrome complicated with mitochondrial myopathy, encephalopathy, lactic acidosis, and stroke-like episodes: a case report. *Acute Med Surg*. 2019;7:e473.
89. Eadie MJ, Ferrier TM. Chloroquine myopathy. *J Neurol Neurosurg Psychiatry*. 1966;29:331–337.
90. Estes ML, Ewing-Wilson D, Chou SM, et al. Chloroquine neuromyotoxicity. Clinical and pathological perspective. *Am J Med*. 1987;82:447–455.
91. Alderson K, Griffin JW, Cornblath DR, Levine JH, Kuncl RW, Griffin LSC. Neuromuscular complications of amiodarone therapy. *Neurology*. 1987;37(suppl):355.
92. Mastaglia FL, Papadimitriou JM, Dawkins RL, Beveridge B. Vacuolar myopathy associated with chloroquine, lupus erythematosus and thymoma. *J Neurol Sci*. 1977;34:315–328.
93. Naddaf E, Paul P, AbouEzzeddine OF. Chloroquine and hydroxychloroquine myopathy: clinical spectrum and treatment outcomes. *Front Neurol*. 2021;11:616075.
94. Costa-Jussa FR, Jacobs JM. The pathology of amiodarone neurotoxicity. I. Experimental changes with reference to changes in other tissues. *Brain*. 1985;108:735–752.
95. Jacobs JM, Costa-Jussa FR. The pathology of amiodarone neurotoxicity. II. Peripheral neuropathy in man. *Brain*. 1985;108:753–769.
96. Meier C, Kauer B, Muller U, Ludin HP. Neuromyopathy during amiodarone treatment: a case report. *J Neurol*. 1979;220:231–239.
97. Roth R, Itabashi H, Louie J, Anderson T, Narahara KA. Amiodarone toxicity: myopathy and neuropathy. *Am Heart J*. 1990;119:1223–1225.

98. Kuncl RW, Duncan G, Watson D, Alderson K, Rogawski MA, Peper M. Colchicine myopathy and neuropathy. *N Engl J Med.* 1987;316:1562–1568.
99. Kuncl RW, Cornblath DR, Avila O, Duncan G. Electrodiagnosis of human colchicine myoneuropathy. *Muscle Nerve.* 1989;12:360–364.
100. Riggs JE, Schochet SS, Gutmann L, Crosby TW, DiBartolomeo AG. Chronic colchicine neuropathy and myopathy. *Arch Neurol.* 1986;43:521–523.
101. Rutkove SB, De Girolami U, Preston DC, et al. Myotonia in colchicine myoneuropathy. *Muscle Nerve.* 1996;19:870–875.
102. Kontos HA. Myopathy associated with chronic colchicine toxicity. *N Engl J Med.* 1962;266:38–39.
103. Bradley WG, Lassman LP, Pearce GW, Walton JN. The neuromyopathy of vincristine in man: clinical, electrophysiological and pathological studies. *J Neurol Sci.* 1970;10:107–131.
104. Anderson P, Song S, Slotwiner P. The fine structure of spheromembranous degeneration of skeletal muscle induced by vincristine. *J Neuropathol Exp Neurol.* 1967;26:15–24.
105. Slotwiner P, Song S, Andersone P. Spheromembranous degeneration of muscle induced by vincristine. *Arch Neurol.* 1966;15:172–176.
106. Dalakas M. HIV or zidovudine myopathy? [letter]. *Neurology.* 1994;44:360–361.
107. Dalakas MC, Illa I, Pezeshkpour GH, Laukaitis JP, Cohen B, Griffin JL. Mitochondrial myopathy caused by long-term zidovudine therapy. *N Engl J Med.* 1990;322:1098–1105.
108. Gherardi R, Chariot P. HIV or zidovudine myopathy [letter]? *Neurology.* 1994;44:361–362.
109. Grau JM, Casademont J. HIV or zidovudine myopathy? [letter]. *Neurology.* 1994;44:361.
110. Grau JM, Masanes F, Pedreo E, Casdemont J, FernandezSola J, Urbano-Marquez A. Human immunodeficiency virus type 1 infection and myopathy: clinical relevance of zidovidine therapy. *Ann Neurol.* 1993;34:206–211.
111. Mhiri C, Baudrimont M, Bonne G, et al. Zidovudine myopathy: a distinctive disorder associated with mitochondrial dysfunction. *Ann Neurol.* 1991;29:606–614.
112. Peters BS, Winer J, Landon DN, Stoffer A, Pinching AJ. Mitochondrial myopathy associated with chronic zidovudine therapy in AIDS. *Q J Med.* 1993;86:5–15.
113. Richman DD, Fischl MA, Grieco HM, et al. The toxicity of azidothymidine (AZT) in the treatment of patients with AIDS and AIDS-related complex. *N Engl J Med.* 1987;317:192–197.
114. Simpson DM, Bender AN. Human immunodeficiency virus-associated myopathy: analysis of 11 patients. *Ann Neurol.* 1988;24:79–84.
115. Simpson DM, Bender AN, Farraye J, Mendelson SG, Wolfe DE. Human immunodeficiency virus wasting syndrome represents a treatable myopathy. *Neurology.* 1990;40:535–538.
116. Simpson DM, Slasor P, Dafni U, Berger J, Fischl MA, Hall C. Analysis of myopathy in a placebo-controlled zidovudine trial. *Muscle Nerve.* 1997;20:382–385.
117. Bailey RO, Turok DI, Jaufmann BP, Singh JK. Myositis and acquired immunodeficiency syndrome. *Hum Pathol.* 1987;18:749–751.
118. Bessen LJ, Green JB, Louie E, Seitzman P, Weinberg H. Severe polymyositis-like syndrome associated with zidovudine therapy of AIDS and ARC. *N Engl J Med.* 1988;318:708.
119. Chalmers AC, Greco CM, Miller RG. Prognosis in AZT myopathy. *Neurology.* 1991;41:1181–1184.
120. Manji H, Harrison MJ, Round JM, et al. Muscle disease, HIV and zidovudine: the spectrum of muscle disease in HIV-infected individuals treated with zidovudine. *J Neurol.* 1993;240:479–488.
121. Reyes MG, Casanova J, Varricchio F, Sequeira W, Fresco K. Zidovudine myopathy. *Neurology.* 1992;42:1252.
122. Simpson DM, Citak KA, Godfrey E, Godbold J, Wolfe D. Myopathies associated with human immunodeficiency virus and zidovudine: can their effects be distinguished? *Neurology.* 1993;43:971–976.
123. Simpson DA, Katzenstein DA, Hughes MD, et al. Neuromuscular function in HIV infection: analysis of a placebo-controlled combination antiviral trial. AIDS Clinical Group 175/801 Study Team. *AIDS.* 1998;12:2425–2432.
124. Till M, McDonnel KB. Myopathy with human immunodeficiency virus type 1 (HIV) infection. HIV-1 or zidovudine? *Ann Intern Med.* 1990;113:492–494.
125. Panegyres PK, Papadimitriou JM, Hollingsworth PN, Armstrong JA, Kakulas BA. Vesicular changes in the myopathies of AIDS. Ultrastructural observations and their relationship to zidovudine treatment. *J Neurol Neurosurg Psychiatry.* 1990;53:649–655.
126. Arnaudo E, Dalakas M, Shanske S, Moraes CT, DiMauro S, Schon EN. Depletion of mitochondrial DNA in AIDS patients with zidovudine-induced myopathy. *Lancet.* 1991;1:508–510.
127. Masanes F, Barrientos A, Cebrian M, et al. Clinical, histological, and molecular reversibility of zidovudine myopathy. *J Neurol Sci.* 1998;159:225–228.
128. Maschke M, Kastrup O, Esser S, Ross B, Hengge U, Hufnagel A. Incidence and prevalence of neurological disorders associated with HIV since the introduction of highly active antiretroviral therapy (HAART). *J Neurol Sci.* 2000;69:376–380.
129. Benbrik E, Chariot P, Boanvaud S, et al. Cellular and mitochondrial toxicity of zidovudine (AZT), didanosione (ddI), and zacitabine (ddC) on cultured human muscle cells. *J Neurol Sci.* 1997;149:19–25.
130. Pedrol E, Masanes F, Fernandez-Sola J, et al. Lack of myotoxicity with didanosine (dI). Clinical and experimental studies. *J Neurol Sci.* 1996;138:42–48.
131. Fujii T, Takase KI, Honda H, et al. Toxic myopathy with multiple deletions in mitochondrial DNA associated with long-term use of oral anti-viral drugs for hepatitis B: A case study. *Neuropathology.* 2019;39:162–167.
132. Seok JI, Lee DK, Lee CH, et al. Long-term therapy with clevudine for chronic hepatitis B can be associated with myopathy characterized by depletion of mitochondrial DNA. *Hepatology.* 2009;49:2080–2086.
133. Callens S, De Roo A. Fanconi-like syndrome and rhabdomyolysis in a person with HIV infection on highly active antiretroviral treatment occluding tenofovir [letter]. *J Infect Dis.* 2003;47:262–263.
134. Mah Ming JB, Gill MJ. Drug-induced rhabdomyolysis after concomitant use of clarithermycine, atorvastatin, lopinivir/ritanovir in a patient with HIV. *AIDS Patient Care STDS.* 2003;17:207–210.
135. Khan E, Shrestha AK, Elkhooly M, et al. CNS and PNS manifestation in immune checkpoint inhibitors: a systematic review. *J Neurol Sci.* 2022;432:120089.
136. Marini A, Bernardini A, Gigli GL, et al. Neurologic adverse events of immune checkpoint inhibitors: a systematic review. *Neurology.* 2021;96:754–766.

137. Shelly S, Triplett JD, Pinto MV, et al. Immune checkpoint inhibitor-associated myopathy: a clinicoseropathologically distinct myopathy. *Brain Commun*. 2020;2(2):fcaa181.
138. Anquetil C, Salem J-E, Lebrun-Vignes B, et al. Immune checkpoint inhibitor-associated myositis: expanding the spectrum of cardiac complications of the immunotherapy revolution. *Circulation*. 2018;138:743–745.
139. Bilen MA, Subudhi SK, Gao J, et al. Acute rhabdomyolysis with severe polymyositis following ipilimumab-nivolumab treatment in a cancer patient with elevated anti-striated muscle antibody. *J Immunother Cancer*. 2016;4:36.
140. Bitton K, Michot J-M, Barreau E, et al. Prevalence and clinical patterns of ocular complications associated with anti-PD-1/PD-L1 anticancer immunotherapy. *Am J Ophthalmol*. 2019;202:109–117.
141. Brahmer JR, Lacchetti C, Schneider BJ, Atkins MB, Brassil KJ, Caterino JM; in oration with the National Comprehensive Cancer Network, et al; Management of immune-related adverse events in patients treated with immune checkpoint inhibitor therapy: American Society of Clinical Oncology Clinical Practice Guideline. *J Clin Oncol*. 2018;36:1714–1768.
142. Delyon J, Brunet-Possenti F, Leonard-Louis S, et al. Immune checkpoint inhibitor rechallenge in patients with immune-related myositis. *Ann Rheum Dis*. 2019;78:e129.
143. Kao JC, Liao B, Markovic SN, et al. Neurological complications associated with anti-programmed death 1 (PD-1) antibodies. *JAMA Neurol*. 2017;74:1216–1222.
144. Kao JC, Brickshawana A, Liewluck T. Neuromuscular complications of programmed cell death-1 (PD-1) inhibitors. *Curr Neurol Neurosci Rep*. 2018;18: 63.
145. Liewluck T, Kao JC, Mauermann ML. PD-1 inhibitor-associated myopathies: emerging immune-mediated myopathies. *J Immunother*. 2018;41:208–211.
146. Robbins NM, Mozaffar T, Mammen AL, et al. Reader response: pearls & oysters: pembrolizumab-induced myasthenia gravis. *Neurology*. 2019;93:183–184.
147. Seki M, Uruha A, Ohnuki Y, et al. Inflammatory myopathy associated with PD-1 inhibitors. *J Autoimmun*. 2019;100: 105–113.
148. Suzuki S, Ishikawa N, Konoeda F, et al. Nivolumab-related myasthenia gravis with myositis and myocarditis in Japan. *Neurology*. 2017;89:1127–1134.
149. Touat M, Maisonobe T, Knauss S, et al. Immune checkpoint inhibitor-related myositis and myocarditis in patients with cancer. *Neurology*. 2018;91:e985–e994.
150. Vogrig A, Muñiz-Castrillo S, Farina A, Honnorat J, Joubert B. How to diagnose and manage neurological toxicities of immune checkpoint inhibitors: an update. *J Neurol*. 2022; 269:1701–1714.
151. Puwanant A, Isfort M, Lacomis D, et al. Clinical spectrum of neuromuscular complications after immune checkpoint inhibition. *Neuromuscul Dis*. 2019;29:127–133.
152. Garcia-Santibanez R, Khoury M, Harrison TB. Immune-related neuromuscular complications of check-point inhibitors. *Curr Treat Options Neurol*. 2020;22:27.
153. Garibaldi M, Calabro F, Merlonghi G, et al. Immune checkpoint inhibitors related ocular myositis. *Neuromuscul Dis*. 2020;30:420–423.
154. Belongia EA, Hedberg CW, Gleich GJ, et al. An investigation of the case of the eosinophilia myalgia syndrome associated with tryptophan use. *N Engl J Med*. 1990;323:357–365.
155. Donofrio PD, Stanton C, Miller VS, et al. Demyelinating polyneuropathy in eosinophilia-myalgia syndrome. *Muscle Nerve*. 1992;15:796–805.
156. Hertzman PA, Blevins WL, Mayer J, Greenfield B, Ting M, Gleich GJ. Association of the eosinophilia-myalgia syndrome with the ingestion of tryptophan. *N Engl J Med*. 1990;322: 869–873.
157. Sagman DL, Melamed JC. L-Tryptophan induced eosinophilia-myalgia syndrome and myopathy. *Neurology*. 1990; 40:1629–1630.
158. Sakimoto K. The cause of the eosinophilia-myalgia syndrome associated with tryptophan use. *N Engl J Med*. 1990;323:992.
159. Smith BE, Dyck PJ. Peripheral neuropathy in the eosinophilic-myalgia syndrome associated with L-tryptophan ingestion. *Neurology*. 1990;40:1035–1040.
160. Tanhehco JL, Wiechers DO, Golbus J, Neely SE. Eosinophilia-myalgia syndrome: myopathic electrodiagnostic characteristics. *Muscle Nerve*. 1992;15:561–567.
161. Shulman LE. Diffuse fasciitis with eosinophilia: a new syndrome? *Trans Assoc Am Physicians*. 1975;88:70–86.
162. Heiman-Patterseon TD, Bird SJ, Parry GJ, et al. Peripheral neuropathy associated with eosinophilia-myalgia syndrome. *Ann Neurol*. 1990;28:522–528.
163. Quane KA, Keating KE, Manning BM, et al. Detection of a common mutation in the ryanodine receptor gene in malignant hyperthermia: implication for diagnosis and heterogenetic studies. *Hum Mol Genet*. 1994;3:471–476.
164. Selwa JF, Feldman EL, Blaivas M. Mononeuropathy multiplex in tryptophan-associated eosinophilic-myalgia syndrome. *Neurology*. 1990;40:1632–1633.
165. Turi GK, Solitaire GB, James N, Dicker R. Eosinophiliamyalgia syndrome (L-tryptophan-associated neuromyopathy). *Neurology*. 1990;40:1793–1796.
166. Mayeno AN, Belongia EA, Lin F, Lundy SK, Gleich GJ. 3-(Phenylamino) alanine—a novel aniline-derived aminoacid associated with the eosinophilic-myalgia syndrome: a link to the toxic oil syndrome. *Mayo Clin Proc*. 1992;67:1134.
167. Kilbourne EM, Rigau-Perez JG, Heath CW, et al. Clinical epidemiology of toxic-oil syndrome. *N Engl J Med*. 1983;309: 1408–1414.
168. Dawkins RL, Zilko PJ, Carrano J, Garlepp MJ, McDonald BL. Immunobiology of D-penicillamine. *J Rheumatol*. 1981;8(suppl):56–61.
169. Hall JT, Fallahi S, Koopman WJ. Penicillamine-induced myositis: observations and unique features in two patients and review of the literature. *Am J Med*. 1984;77:719.
170. Takahashi K, Ogita T, Okudaira H, Yoshinoya S, Yoshizawa H, Miyamoto T. D-penicillamine induced polymyositis in patients with rheumatoid arthritis. *Arthritis Rheum*. 1986;29:560–564.
171. Taneja V, Mehra N, Singh YN, Kumar A, Malaviya A, Singh RR. HLA-D region genes and susceptibility to D-penicillamine-induced polymyositis. *Arthritis Rheum*. 1990;33:1445–1447.
172. Watson AJ, Dalbow MH, Stachura I, et al. Immunologic studies in cimetidine-induced nephropathy and polymyositis. *N Engl J Med*. 1983;308:142–145.
173. Mitchell CG, Magnussen AR, Weiler JM. Cimetidine-induced cutaneous vasculitis. *Am J Med*. 1983;75:875.
174. Lewis CA, Boheimer N, Rose P, Jackson G. Myopathy after short term administration of procainamide. *Br Med J*. 1986; 292:593–597.

175. Fontiveros ES, Cumming WJ, Hudgson P. Procainamide-induced myositis. *J Neurol Sci.* 1980;45:143–147.
176. Harney J, Glasberg MR. Myopathy and hypersensitivity to phenytoin. *Neurology.* 1983;33:790–791.
177. Kim H, Jo S, Park KW, Han S, Lee S. A case of phenytoin-induced rhabdomyolysis in status epilepticus. *J Epilepsy Res.* 2016;6:36–38.
178. Michael JR, Mitch WE. Reversible renal failure and myositis caused by phenytoin hypersensitivity. *JAMA.* 1976;236:2773–2775.
179. Santos-Calle FJ, Borras-Blasco J, Navarro-Ruiz A, Plaza Macias I. Unsuspected rhabdomyolysis associated with phenytoin. *Int J Clin Pharmacol Ther.* 2005;43:436–440.
180. Olaniran, K, Keshishyan, S, Assallum, H. Phenytoin-induced rhabdomyolysis. *J Case Reports Med.* 2015;4:1–3.
181. MacIsaac R, Brust T. Painful proximal weakness and hyper-CKemia related to intravenous loading of phenytoin. *Can J Neurol Sci.* 2018;45:709–711.
182. Cirigliano G, Della RA, Tavoni A, Tavoni A, Vicava P, Bombardieri S. Polymyositis occurring during alpha-interferon treatment for malignant melanoma: a case report and review of the literature. *Rheumatol Int.* 1999;19:65–67.
183. Dietrich L, Bridges AJ, Albertini MR. DM after interferon alpha treatment. *Med Oncol.* 2000;17:64–69.
184. Hengstman GJ, Vogels OJ, ter Laak HJ, de Witte T, van Engelen BG. Myositis during ling-term interferon-alpha treatment. *Neurology.* 2000;54:2186.
185. The Muscle Study Group. A randomized, pilot trial of etanercept in dermatomyositis. *Ann Neurol.* 2011;70(3):427–436.
186. Klein R, Rosenbach M, Kim EJ, Kim B, Werth VP, Dunham J. Tumor necrosis factor inhibitor-associated dermatomyositis. *Arch Dermatol.* 2010;146:780–784.
187. Ishikawa Y, Yukawa N, Ohmura K, et al. Etanercept-induced anti-Jo-1-antibody-positive polymyositis in a patient with rheumatoid arthritis: a case report and review of the literature. *Clin Rheumatol.* 2010;29:563–566.
188. Srinivasan J, Wu C, Amato AA. Inflammatory myopathy associated with imitinab therapy. *J Clin Neuromuscul Dis.* 2004;5:119–121.
189. Asawaeer M, Barton D, Radio S, Chatzizisis YS. Tyrosine kinase inhibitor-induced acute myocarditis, myositis, and cardiogenic shock. *Methodist Debakey Cardiovasc J.* 2018;14:e5–e6.
190. Stump SE, Whang YE, Crona DJ. Cabozantinib-induced serum creatine kinase elevation and musculoskeletal complaints. *Invest New Drugs.* 2018;36:1143–1146.
191. Parafianowicz P, Krishan R, Beutler BD, Islam RX, Singh T. Myositis—A common but underreported adverse effect of osimertinib: case series and review of the literature. *Cancer Treat Res Commun.* 2020;25:100254.
192. Crowley F, Fitzgerald BG, Bhardwaj AS, Siraj I, Smith C. Life-threatening myositis in a patient with *EGFR*-mutated NSCLC on osimertinib: case report. *JTO Clin Res Rep.* 2021;3:100260.
193. Sakellaropoulou A, Theofilos D, Bisirtzoglo D, et al. A rare adverse effect while treating lung adenocarcinoma. *Pneumon.* 2015;28:262–265. www.pneumon.org/assets/files/789/file612_97.pdf.
194. Ruggeri M, Cecere FL, Moscetti L, et al. Severe rhabdomyolysis during sunitinib treatment of metastatic renal cell carcinoma. A report of two cases. *Ann Oncol.* 2010;21:1926-1927.
195. Coomes EN. The rate of recovery of reversible myopathies and the effects of anabolic agents in steroid myopathy. *Neurology.* 1965;18:523–530.
196. Engel AG. Metabolic and endocrine myopathies. In: Walton JN, ed. *Disorders of Voluntary Muscle.* 5th ed. Churchill-Livingstone; 1988:811–868.
197. Golding DN, Murray SM, Pearce GW, Thompson M. Corticosteroid myopathy. *Ann Phys Med.* 1962;6:171–177.
198. Kaminski HJ, Ruff RL. Endocrine myopathies (hyper- and hypofunction of adrenal, thyroid, pituitary, and parathyroid glands and iatrogenic corticosteroid myopathy). In: Engel AG, Franzini-Armstrong C, eds. *Myology.* 2nd ed. McGraw-Hill; 1994:1726–1753.
199. Kissel JT, Mendell JR. The endocrine myopathies. In: Rowland LP, DiMauro S, eds. *Handbook of Clinical Neurology.* Vol 18. No. 62: *Myopathies.* Elsevier Science Publishers BV; 1992:527–551.
200. Muller R, Kugelberg E. Myopathy in Cushing's syndrome. *J Neurol Neurosurg Psychiatry.* 1959;22:314–319.
201. Williams RS. Triamcinolone myopathy. *Lancet.* 1959;516:698–700.
202. Faludi G, Gotlieb J, Meyers J. Factors influencing the development of steroid-induced myopathy. *Ann NY Acad Sci.* 1967;138:61–72.
203. Buchthal F. Electrophysiological abnormalities in metabolic myopathies and neuropathies. *Acta Neurol Scand.* 1970;46(suppl 43):129–176.
204. Hudgson P, Kendall-Taylor P. Endocrine myopathies. In: Mastaglia FL, Walton JN, eds. *Skeletal Muscle Pathology.* Churchill Livingstone; 1992:493–509.
205. Pleasure DE, Walsh GO, Engel WK. Atrophy of skeletal muscle in patients with Cushing's syndrome. *Arch Neurol.* 1970;22:118–125.
206. Bolton CF, Gilbert JJ, Hahn AF, Sibbald WJ. Polyneuropathy in critically ill patients. *J Neurol Neurosurg Psychiatry.* 1984;47:1223–1231.
207. Zochodne DW, Bolton CF, Wells GF, et al. Critical illness polyneuropathy. A complication of sepsis and multiorgan failure. *Brain.* 1987;110:819–842.
208. Gooch JL. AAEM case report #29: prolonged paralysis after neuromuscular blockade. *Muscle Nerve.* 1995;18:937–942.
209. McFarlane IA, Rosenthal FD. Severe myopathy after status asthmaticus. *Lancet.* 1977;2:615.
210. Rodriguez B, Larsson L, Z'Graggen WJ. Critical illness myopathy: diagnostic approach and resulting therapeutic implications. *Curr Treat Options Neurol.* 2022 Mar 28:1–10.
211. Al-Lozi MT, Pestronk A, Yee WC, Flaris N, Cooper J. Rapidly evolving myopathy with myosin-deficient fibers. *Ann Neurol.* 1994;35:273–279.
212. Danon MJ, Carpenter S. Myopathy with thick filament (myosin) loss following prolonged paralysis with vecuronium during steroid treatment. *Muscle Nerve.* 1991;14:1131–1139.
213. Deconinck N, Van Parijs V, Beckers-Bleukx G, Van den Bergh P. Critical illness myopathy unrelated to corticosteroids or neuromuscular blocking agents. *Neuromuscul Disord.* 1998;8:186–192.
214. Gutmann L, Blumenthal D, Schochet SS. Acute type II myofiber atrophy in critical illness. *Neurology.* 1996;46:819–821.

215. Hirano M, Ott BR, Rapps EC, et al. Acute quadriplegic myopathy: a complication of treatment with steroids, nondepolarizing blocking agents, or both. *Neurology.* 1992;42:2082–2087.
216. Lacomis D, Giuliani MJ, Van Cott A, Kramer DJ. Acute myopathy of the intensive care: clinical, electromyographic, and pathological aspects. *Ann Neurol.* 1996;40:645–654.
217. Lacomis D, Petrella JT, Giuliani MJ. Causes of neuromuscular weakness in the intensive care unit: a study of ninety-two patients. *Muscle Nerve.* 1998;21:610–617.
218. Lacomis D, Smith TW, Chad DA. Acute myopathy and neuropathy in status asthmaticus: case report and literature review. *Muscle Nerve.* 1993;16:84–90.
219. Ramsay DA, Zochodne DW, Robertson DM, Nag S, Ludwin SK. A syndrome of acute severe muscle necrosis in intensive care unit patients. *J Neuropathol Exp Neurol.* 1993;52:387–398.
220. Rich MM, Bird SJ, Raps EC, McClaskey LF, Teener JW. Direct muscle stimulation in acute quadriplegic myopathy. *Muscle Nerve.* 1997;20:665–673.
221. Rich MM, Teener JW, Raps EC, Schotland DL, Bird SJ. Muscle is electrically inexcitable in acute quadriplegic myopathy. *Neurology.* 1996;46:731–736.
222. Showalter CJ, Engel AG. Acute quadriplegic myopathy: analysis of myosin isoforms and evidence for calpain-mediated proteolysis. *Muscle Nerve.* 1997;20:316–322.
223. Sitwell LD, Weishenker BG, Monipetit V, Reid D. Complete ophthalmoplegia as a complication of acute corticosteroid- and pancuronium-associated myopathy. *Neurology.* 1991;41:921–922.
224. Op de Coul AA, Lambregts PC, Koeman J, van Puyenbroek MJ, Ter Laak HJ, Gabreels-Festen AA. Neuromuscular complications in patients given Pavulon (pancuronium bromide) during artificial ventilation. *Clin Neurol Neurosurg.* 1985;87:17–22.
225. Latronico N, Fenzi F, Recupero D, et al. Critical illness myopathy and neuropathy. *Lancet.* 1996;347:1579–1582.
226. Campellone JV, Lacomis D, Kramer DJ, Van Cott AC, Giuliani MJ. Acute myopathy after liver transplantation. *Neurology.* 1998;50:46–53.
227. Road J, Mackie G, Jiang TX, Stewart H, Eisen A. Reversible paralysis with status asthmaticus, steroids, and pancuronium: clinical electrophysiological correlates. *Muscle Nerve.* 1997;20:1587–1590.
228. Zochodne DW, Ramsey DA, Saly V, Shelley S, Moffatt S. Acute necrotizing myopathy of the intensive care: electrophysiological studies. *Muscle Nerve.* 1994;17:285–292.
229. Douglass JA, Tuxen DV, Horne M, et al. Myopathy in severe asthma. *Am Rev Respir Dis.* 1992;146:517–519.
230. Rich MM, Pinter MJ, Kraner SD, Barchi RL. Loss of electrical excitability in an animal model of acute quadriplegic myopathy. *Ann Neurol.* 1998;43:171–179.
231. Allen DC, Arunachalam R, Mills KR. Critical illness myopathy: further evidence from muscle-fiber excitability studies of an acquired channelopathy. *Muscle Nerve.* 2008;37:14–22.
232. Ruff RL. Why do ICU patients become paralyzed? *Ann Neurol.* 1998;43:154–155.
233. Haan J, Hollander JM, van Duinin SG, Sacena PR, Wintzen AR. Reversible severe myopathy during treatment with finasteride. *Muscle Nerve.* 1997;20:502–504.
234. Al-Harbi TM, Kagan J; Tarnopolsky MA. Finasteride-induced myalgia and HyperCKemia. *J Clin Neuromuscul Dis.* 2008;10:76–78.
235. Ryu HJ, Kwon DY. Reversible myopathy and ophthalmoparesis after low-dose finasteride administration for androgenic alopecia. *Dermatol Surg.* 2014;40:595–597.
236. Welk B, McArthur E, Ordon M, Dirk J, Dixon S, Garg AX. Risk of rhabdomyolysis from 5-α reductase inhibitors. *Pharmacoepidemiol Drug Saf.* 2018;27:351–355.
237. Faucheux JM, Tourneize P, Viguier A, Arne-Bes MC, Larrue M, Geraud G. Neuromyopathy secondary to omeprazole treatment. *Muscle Nerve.* 1998;21:261–262.
238. Colmenares EW, Pappas AL. Proton pump inhibitors: risk for myopathy? *Ann Pharmacother.* 2017;51:66–71.
239. Sarifakioglu E, Onur O, Kart H, Yilmaz AE. Acute myopathy and acne fulminans triggered by isotretinoin therapy. *Eur J Dermatol.* 2011;21(5):794–795.
240. Chroni E, Monastirli A, Tsambaos D. Neuromuscular adverse effects associated with systemic retinoid dermatotherapy: monitoring and treatment algorithm for clinicians. *Drug Saf.* 2010;33:25–34.
241. Kaymak Y. Creatine phosphokinase values during isotretinoin treatment for acne. *Int J Dermatol.* 2008;47:398–401.
242. Marson JW, Baldwin HE. The creatine kinase conundrum: a reappraisal of the association of isotretinoin, creatine kinase, and rhabdomyolysis. *Int J Dermatol.* 2020;59:279–283.
243. Bennett HS, Spiro AJ, Pollack MA, Zucker P. Ipecac-induced myopathy simulating dermatomyositis. *Neurology.* 1982;32:91–94.
244. Mateer JE, Farrell BJ, Chou SS, Gutmann L. Reversible ipecac myopathy. *Arch Neurol.* 1985;42:188–190.
245. Palmer EP, Guay AT. Reversible myopathy secondary to abuse of ipecac in patients with major eating disorders. *N Engl J Med.* 1985;313:1457–1459.
246. Amato AA, Kagan-Hallet K, Jackson CE, et al. The wide spectrum of myofibrillar myopathy suggests a multifactorial etiology and pathogenesis. *Neurology.* 1998;51:1646–1655.
247. Bertorini TE. Myoglobinuria, malignant hyperthermia, neuroleptic malignant syndrome and serotonin syndrome. *Neurol Clin.* 1997;15:649–671.
248. Nelson TE, Flewellen EH. Current concepts: the malignant hyperthermia syndrome. *N Engl J Med.* 1983;309:416–418.
249. MacLennan DH, Phillips MS. Malignant hyperthermia. *Science.* 1992;256:789–794.
250. Beebe D, Puram VV, Gajic S, Thyagarajan B, Belani KG. Genetics of malignant hyperthermia: a brief update. *J Anaesthesiol Clin Pharmacol.* 2020;36:552–555.
251. Horstick EJ, Linsley JW, Dowling JJ, et al. Stac3 is a component of the excitation-contraction coupling machinery and mutated in Native American myopathy. *Nat Commun.* 2013;4:1952.
252. Sethna NF, Rockoff MA, Worthen HM, Rosnow JM. Anesthesia-related complications of children with Duchenne muscular dystrophy. *Anesthesiology.* 1988;68:462–465.
253. Ekbom K, Hed R, Kirstein L, Astrom KE. Muscular affections in chronic alcoholism. *Arch Neurol.* 1964;10:449–458.
254. Mayer RF, Garcia-Mullin R, Eckholdt JW. Acute alcoholic myopathy. *Neurology.* 1968;18:275.
255. Oh SJ. Chronic alcoholic myopathy: an entity difficult to diagnose. *South Med J.* 1972;65:449–452.

256. Perkoff GT, Dioso MM, Bleisch V, Klinkerfuss G. A spectrum of myopathy associated with alcoholism. I. Clinical and laboratory features. *Ann Intern Med*. 1967;67:481–492.
257. Rubenstein AE, Wainapel SF. Acute hypokalemic myopathy in alcoholism: a clinical entity. *Arch Neurol*. 1977;34:553–555.
258. Cogen FC, Rigg G, Simmons JL, Domino EF. Phencyclidine-associated acute rhabdomyolysis. *Ann Intern Med*. 1978;88:210–212.
259. Richter RW, Challenor YB, Pearson J, Kagen LJ, Hamilton LL, Ramsey WH. Acute myoglobinuria associated with heroin addiction. *J Am Med Assoc*. 1971;216:1172–1176.
260. Richter RW, Pearson J, Bruun B, Challenor YB, Brust JC, Baden MM. Neurological complications of heroin addiction. *Bull N Y Acad Med*. 1973;49:1–21.
261. Van den Bergh PY, Guettat L, Vande Berg BC, Martine JJ. Focal myopathy associated with chronic intramuscular injection of piritramide. *Muscle Nerve*. 1997;20(12):1598–1600.

CHAPTER 36

Neuromuscular Mimics

Sabrina Paganoni and Erik Ensrud

We define "neuromuscular mimic" as any musculoskeletal condition that presents with pain and apparent weakness and can mimic a neuromuscular etiology such as radiculopathy or entrapment neuropathy. "Limb pain" is a common reason for referral to the clinic and EMG laboratory and the identification of the underlying pain generator is often challenging. For example, in two series of patients referred for electrodiagnostic testing for suspected cervical or lumbosacral radiculopathy, the prevalence of musculoskeletal disorders was 42% and 32%, respectively.[1,2] Thus, musculoskeletal disorders are common in patients suspected of having a radiculopathy. They can mimic radiculopathy or coexist with it in many individuals.[1,2] Importantly, neuromuscular mimics can often be diagnosed quickly at the bedside and are eminently treatable. Their prompt recognition may avoid unnecessary and expensive diagnostic procedures and result in more efficient clinical practice. It is common for physicians from many specialties to be unfamiliar with recognizing these conditions.[3]

In this chapter, we will describe some of the most common mimics of radiculopathy and neuropathy in the upper and lower limbs (Table 36-1). We will not perform an exhaustive review of these pathologies. Rather, this chapter will serve as an entry point for physicians with minimal musculoskeletal training with the goal of providing them with time-efficient and resource-efficient tools to screen for these common conditions in their busy daily practice.

A few key "pearls" are worth remembering when performing a musculoskeletal examination. First, it is important to check the bilateral limbs for side-to-side comparison, starting from the noninvolved side first, whenever possible. If the test maneuver elicits pain, one needs to ask the patient whether the elicited pain is the same that they have been experiencing. This is important in order to avoid overcalling pathology as musculoskeletal examination maneuvers can trigger some discomfort even in healthy individuals, particularly if palpation and provocative tests are performed too vigorously. Finally, when assessing whether the maneuver reproduces the patient's chief complaint, it is very helpful to look for the "wince sign," with the patient blinking and grimacing as the pain is reproduced. Referral to musculoskeletal specialists may be helpful when a "neuromuscular mimic" is suspected based on the screening examination maneuvers described in this chapter.

▶ TOP MIMICS IN THE UPPER LIMBS

SUPRASPINATUS TENDINOPATHY

Supraspinatus tendinopathy is a common cause of shoulder pain and can mimic C5/6/7 radiculopathy.

Symptoms

The rotator cuff consists of four muscles that are responsible for securing the arm into the glenohumeral (shoulder) joint. These muscles are the supraspinatus, infraspinatus, teres minor, and subscapularis. The tendon most commonly injured within the rotator cuff is the supraspinatus.[4] Risk factors include older age, repetitive overhead activity, whether work- or sport-related, anatomic variants, instability of the glenohumeral joint, and periscapular muscle weakness and imbalance.[5-7] The latter are common in people with underlying neurologic diseases.

Patients complain of shoulder pain that is aggravated by arm movement, especially overhead. Painful daily activities may include putting on a shirt or brushing hair. The pain may be localized to the deltoid area but may also radiate upward toward the neck or distally down the arm, thus mimicking cervical radiculopathy, most often in a C5–C7 distribution. Often, patients have difficulty sleeping on the side of the affected shoulder due to pain.

Diagnosis

Shoulder examination includes inspection, range of motion (ROM), strength testing, palpation, and special tests.[8] With long-standing rotator cuff tendinopathy, inspection may reveal atrophy of the supra- and infraspinatus muscles. ROM above 90 degrees of abduction, either actively or passively, is often painful. Active ROM may be limited by pain, but passive ROM is preserved. There may be tenderness to palpation over the affected muscles or focal subacromial tenderness at the posterolateral border of the acromion. Pain may also be elicited by one of the many special tests that are available to examine the shoulder.[8,9] A simple and sensitive screening test for supraspinatus tendinopathy is the Hawkins test (Fig. 36-1). Reduced passive ROM and weakness with resisted abduction and/or external rotation suggest the presence of adhesive capsulitis and rotator cuff tear, respectively.

► TABLE 36-1. **NEUROMUSCULAR MIMICS**

Upper Limb Mimics
  Supraspinatus tendinopathy
  Biceps tendinopathy
  Lateral epicondylitis
  De Quervain syndrome
  Carpometacarpal (CMC) joint osteoarthritis

Lower Limb Mimics
  Hip joint osteoarthritis
  Greater trochanteric bursitis
  Pes anserine bursitis
  Plantar fasciitis

Musculoskeletal ultrasound and magnetic resonance imaging (MRI) can be considered if further investigation and confirmation of the etiology are desired.[10]

Treatment

Conservative treatment for supraspinatus tendinopathy includes rest, activity modification, ice, nonsteroidal anti-inflammatory drugs (NSAIDs), and physical therapy. Physical therapy is directed to preserving ROM while restoring proper muscle activation and strength balance among the muscles of the rotator cuff.[11,12] A subacromial steroid injection may reduce pain and enable earlier participation in ROM exercises and rehabilitation.[13] Referral to orthopedics, physiatry, or rheumatology for further diagnostic and

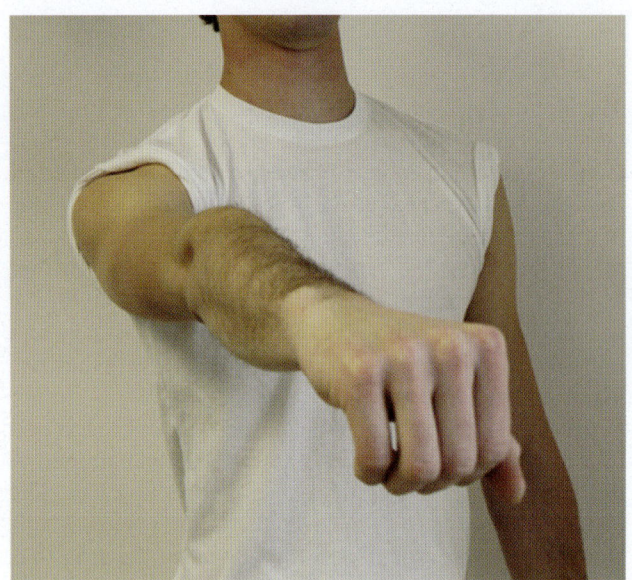

A

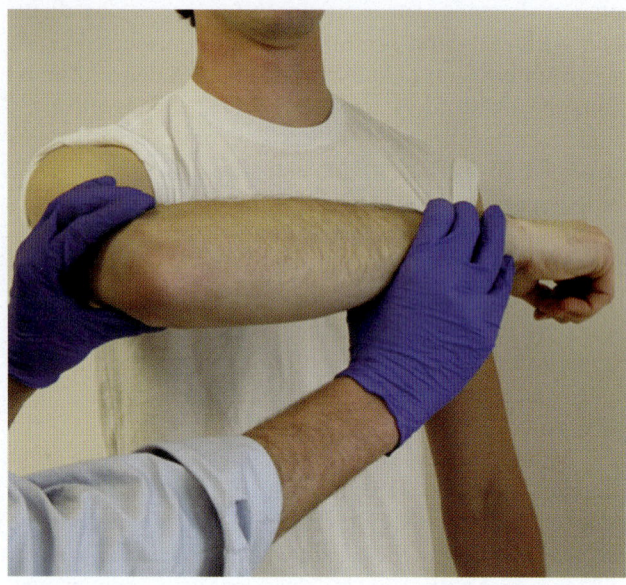

B

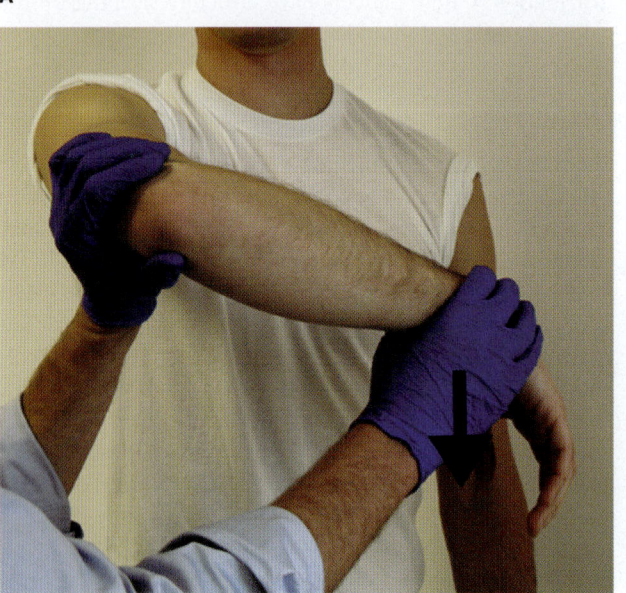

C

Figure 36-1. **Hawkins test.** Correct positioning is important to perform the test. The patient forward flexes the arm to 90 degrees (**A**) and the examiner flexes the elbow to 90 degrees (**B**). The examiner then forcibly internally rotates the shoulder (**C**). The maneuver drives the greater tuberosity of the humerus farther under the coracoacromial ligament. Pain with this maneuver is considered positive for impingement of the supraspinatus tendon under the acromion.

therapeutic management is warranted if there is no response to several weeks of conservative management or if additional pathology is suspected.

BICEPS TENDINOPATHY

Biceps tendinopathy is a common cause of anterior shoulder pain and can mimic C5/C6 cervical radiculopathy.

Symptoms

The tendon of the long head of the biceps, with its synovial lining, lies within the bicipital groove which is located in the anterior upper humerus and is bordered laterally by the greater tuberosity and medially by the lesser tuberosity. The bicipital groove is easily palpable in the anterior upper arm when the arm is externally rotated (Fig. 36-2). Tendinopathy occurs where the tendon passes through the bicipital groove and over the head of the humerus, just like a rope through a pulley. The underlying pathology may involve inflammation of the tendon and tendon sheath (tendonitis, tenosynovitis) and/or chronic overuse injury and degeneration (tendinosis).[14]

Affected individuals complain of a deep, throbbing ache in the anterior shoulder. Tenderness is usually localized to the bicipital groove but may radiate to the deltoid region or downward to the anterolateral arm, making it difficult to distinguish from upper cervical radicular pain. The pain often worsens at night, especially if sleeping on the affected side, and may increase with lifting, pulling, or repetitive overhead reaching. The risk of developing biceps tendinopathy increases with age and is higher in people who routinely perform activities that require repetitive overhead movements. Importantly, biceps tendinopathy often coexists with other pathologies of the shoulder, including rotator cuff tendinopathy and tears, as well as intra-articular injuries such as a labral tear.[15,16]

Diagnosis

Clinical diagnosis includes assessing for Yergason test, which is tenderness identified by palpation of the long head of the biceps tendon in the bicipital groove while internally and externally rotating the humerus (Fig. 36-2).[17] Another helpful test is the Speed test.[18] For the Speed test, the patient is asked to flex the arm (lift upward) against resistance from the examiner with the elbow extended and the forearm fully supinated (Fig. 36-3). The test is considered positive when pain is localized to the bicipital groove, implying biceps tendonitis and/or tenosynovitis. Of note, the Speed test may be positive with other shoulder degenerative pathologies.

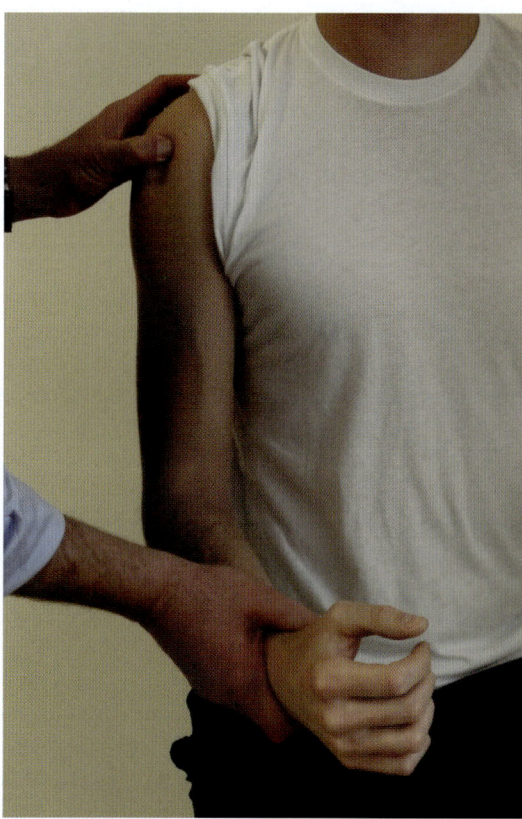

Figure 36-2. Yergason test. The long head of the biceps tendon is palpated for tenderness in the bicipital groove, between the greater and lesser tuberosities of the humeral head. Localization of the bicipital groove is aided by internally and externally rotating the shoulder with the elbow flexed at 90 degrees while feeling for the tuberosities.

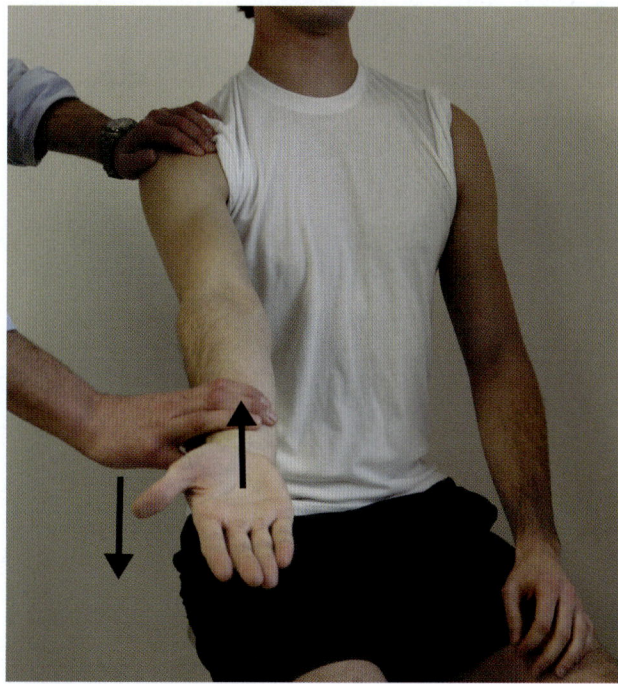

Figure 36-3. Speed test. The patient is asked to flex the shoulder against resistance from the examiner while the elbow is extended and the forearm is supinated. The test is positive for biceps tendon pathology when pain is localized to the bicipital groove.

Ultrasound[19] and/or MRI[20] are not needed for the diagnosis of biceps tendinopathy, but may be considered in patients who are suspected of having additional concurrent shoulder pathologies or are refractory to treatment.

Treatment

Conservative treatment is appropriate for most patients with biceps tendinopathy.[21,22] Treatment includes rest and activity modification to allow the tendon to heal. Oral or topical NSAIDs and modalities, such as ice therapy, help reduce pain and inflammation. The superficial location of the biceps tendon as it runs through the bicipital groove makes it particularly amenable to ice massage. Patients can be instructed to ice the tender area by directly applying ice to the skin using gentle stroking motions ("ice massage"). The paper cup method is a comfortable, convenient, and inexpensive method of performing ice massage. Water is frozen in a paper cup and ice is exposed by tearing the top rim of paper (Fig. 36-4). Ice is then applied to the affected area multiple times a day until the area is numb, which usually occurs within 5 minutes.

If symptoms do not improve with use of rest, activity modification, NSAIDs, and ice therapy, referral to a musculoskeletal medicine expert (from physiatry, sports medicine, or orthopedic surgery) may be considered. Physical therapy is used to improve muscle strength and tendon stability. An ultrasound-guided injection of steroid in the biceps tendon sheath is an option for both diagnostic and therapeutic purposes.[23,24] Ultrasound guidance is needed to avoid injecting the tendon with resulting risk of rupture. Surgical intervention is used only in selected patients and includes tenotomy and tenodesis.[20,25]

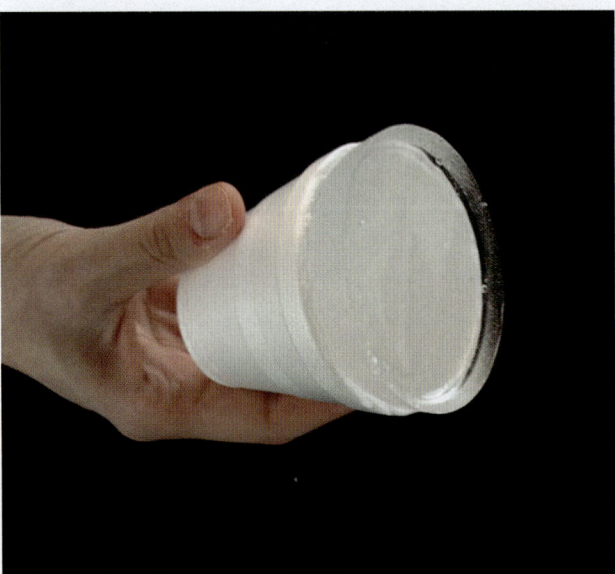

Figure 36-4. Frozen paper cup for ice therapy. A paper cup is filled with water and placed in a freezer. When the water is frozen, the top of the cup can be peeled away to expose the ice. Ice massage is then performed by placing the cup over the injury in a circular pattern allowing the ice to melt away.

LATERAL EPICONDYLITIS

Lateral epicondylitis (colloquially known as "tennis elbow") is a common tendinopathy that presents as lateral elbow pain. Pain may radiate distally along the forearm, mimicking C6 cervical radiculopathy or ulnar neuropathy.

Symptoms

The lateral epicondyle of the humerus is located lateral to the olecranon process and is the origin of the wrist and finger extensors. Overuse and poor mechanics can lead to an overload of the extensor tendons.[26,27] The underlying pathology is not inflammatory, but rather degenerative and consists of tendon microtearing.[28] Pathology most often involves the extensor carpi radialis brevis, approximately 1–2 cm distal to the attachment to the lateral epicondyle, but can affect the other extensors as well.

In most cases, the pain begins shortly after a period of overuse and slowly worsens over weeks and months. There is usually no specific injury associated with the start of symptoms. The point of maximal pain and tenderness is typically located just distal to the lateral epicondyle over the extensor tendon mass. However, pain can extend into the distal forearm mimicking C6 radiculopathy. Pain is exacerbated by arm use, especially repetitive wrist extension and pronation/supination activities. There may be perceived weakness in grip strength. Lateral epicondylitis is most often associated with tennis and other racquet sports. Poor technique including improper backhand, string tension, and grip size are contributing factors.[29] However, any activity that places excessive repetitive stress on the lateral forearm musculature can cause this condition.[30,31]

Diagnosis

Clinical diagnosis includes assessing for tenderness by palpation over the lateral epicondyle and 1–2 cm distal to it over the common extensor tendon, which usually represents the point of maximal tenderness in lateral epicondylitis. The provocative maneuver or "tennis elbow test" consists of resisted radial wrist extension with the forearm in pronation (Fig. 36-5). The examiner stabilizes the elbow with a thumb over the lateral epicondyle. The test is positive if pain is elicited when the patient makes a fist and extends the wrist against resistance by the examiner. The pain is usually worse with the elbow in extension than with the elbow in flexion. Imaging is generally not needed to diagnose this condition, but a plain x-ray of the elbow may be considered to rule out intra-articular pathology and/or loose body fragments. In addition, an x-ray may reveal calcification over the lateral epicondyle. Ultrasound and MRI may be considered if there is no response to conservative treatment.

Treatment

Despite the prevalence of lateral epicondylitis and the availability of different treatment options, only few high-quality

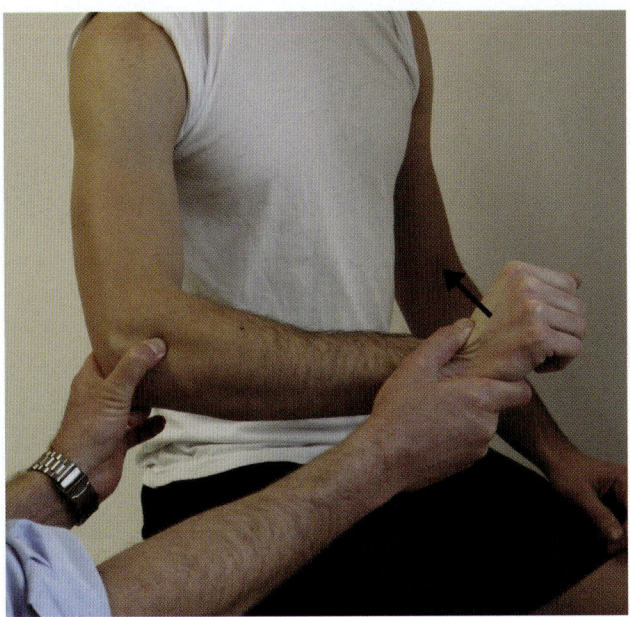

Figure 36-5. Tennis elbow test. The examiner stabilizes the elbow while palpating along the lateral epicondyle. With the elbow pronated and a closed fist, the patient extends the wrist against the examiner's resistance. The point of maximal tenderness is generally located one fingerbreadth distal to the lateral epicondyle over the extensor tendon mass. The pain is usually worse with the elbow in extension than with the elbow in flexion.

clinical trials are available to support evidence-based management algorithms for this condition. Activity modification is an important first step in management and includes correcting training or technique errors such as grip size of the tennis racket when appropriate. Initial conservative management also includes pain control by using a short course of topical or oral NSAIDs[32] and ice massage (as described above). Wrist extensor stretching (Fig. 36-6)[33] and bracing[34] are often helpful. Bracing consists of using a counterforce elbow strap. Elbow or "tennis straps" are placed on the forearm a few centimeters distal to the elbow joint, are easy to use and inexpensive.

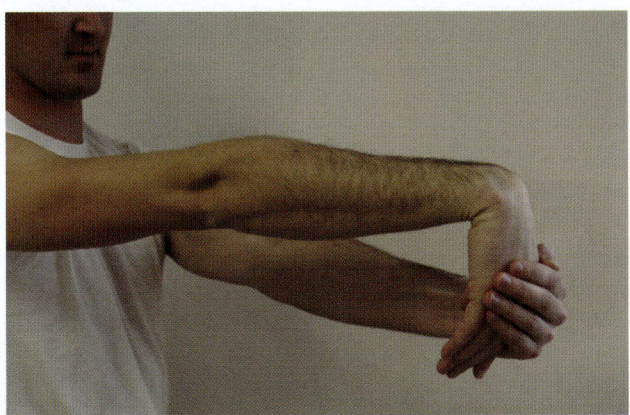

Figure 36-6. Wrist extensor stretch.

Counterforce bracing may reduce tendon and muscle strain at the origin of the forearm extensor muscles, thus relieving pain during activities. Physical therapy has been found to be effective in lateral epicondylitis.[35,36] Therapy includes progressive isometric and eccentric strengthening and incorporates stretching and modalities as needed. Eccentric exercise occurs when muscles contract while lengthening. Application of this technique for lateral epicondylitis involves contracting the wrist extensors against the resistance of an exercise band.[37,38] Steroid injections have also been used to treat "tennis elbow."[39] Their use, however, is controversial.[40] Trials have found that corticosteroid injections improve short-term outcomes in lateral epicondylitis, but do not prevent recurrence and may actually lead to worse long-term outcomes.[36,41,42]

DE QUERVAIN SYNDROME

De Quervain syndrome is a common cause of wrist pain and can mimic carpal tunnel syndrome, C6 cervical radiculopathy, and superficial radial sensory neuropathy.

Symptoms

De Quervain syndrome is the most common tenosynovitis of the wrist. It results from inflammation of the fluid-filled sheath (synovium) that surrounds the tendons of the abductor pollicis longus (APL) and extensor pollicis brevis (EPB) in the first dorsal compartment of the wrist. These tendons run over the dorsal aspect of the radial styloid process.

The exact causes of De Quervain syndrome are unclear, but they probably include shear and repetitive microtrauma. Postures where the thumb is held in abduction and extension are considered predisposing factors,[43,44] although evidence regarding a possible relation with certain occupations is controversial. A systematic review of potential risk factors did not find evidence of an association with specific occupation-related activities.[45] Women are affected more than men[46] and the syndrome commonly occurs during and after pregnancy, due to hormonal changes and possibly lifting the newborn repetitively in a cradled position thus putting stress on the wrist and thumb. Because of the latter postulated risk factor, De Quervain syndrome is also known as "mother's wrist."

Patients with this condition present with insidious onset of pain over the dorsal radial aspect of the wrist which may be accompanied by swelling. The pain may radiate distally into the thumb or proximally along the radial aspect of the forearm. Symptoms are exacerbated by grasping or ulnar deviation of the wrist.

Diagnosis

De Quervain syndrome can be easily diagnosed on physical examination. Patients usually have tenderness to palpation over the dorsal radial wrist. Finkelstein test is pathognomonic for the condition (Fig. 36-7). To perform the test, the patient

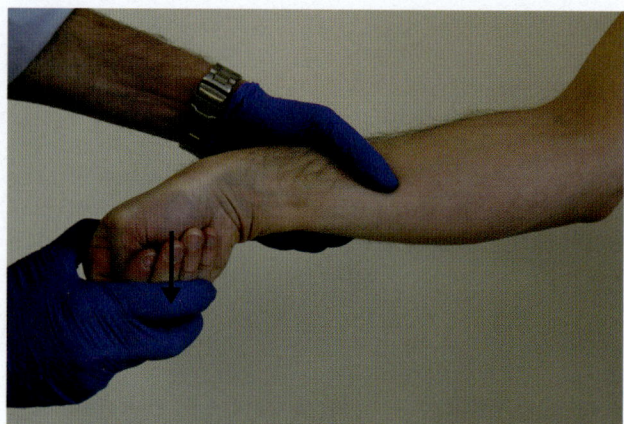

Figure 36-7. Finkelstein test. The patient is asked to make a fist over the thumb. The examiner ulnarly deviates the wrist. A positive test is indicated by exquisite pain in the region of the radial styloid.

is first asked to wrap the fingers around the thumb. To avoid having tight finger flexor tendons splint and immobilize the wrist, it is helpful to ask the patient to wrap the fingers around the thumb lightly, as if the thumb were an egg. The examiner then deviates the wrist in an ulnar direction. A positive test occurs when the patient experiences sharp and intense pain over the radial styloid process, exactly where the tendon sheath takes its course. De Quervain tenosynovitis is a clinical diagnosis and imaging is not needed.

Treatment

Conservative treatment includes rest, ice, anti-inflammatory medications (oral or topical), steroid injections, and a thumb spica splint. The splint is worn during the day, but the patient should remove it several times a day to perform gentle ROM exercises to prevent the complications of prolonged immobilization. Iontophoresis can help with inflammation and pain control. Steroid injections are highly effective in providing pain relief and have a favorable side effect profile.[47] They work best when used in conjunction with a thumb spica splint.[48] Ultrasound guidance for steroid injection is recommended to localize the site of injection more precisely.[49] Surgery is rarely indicated and carries a small risk of injury to the superficial radial nerve.[50]

CARPOMETACARPAL JOINT OSTEOARTHRITIS

Carpometacarpal (CMC) joint osteoarthritis (OA) (colloquially known as "thumb arthritis") is a common cause of hand pain and can mimic carpal tunnel syndrome.

Symptoms

The CMC joint of the thumb connects the trapezium to the first metacarpal bone and plays a key role in the normal

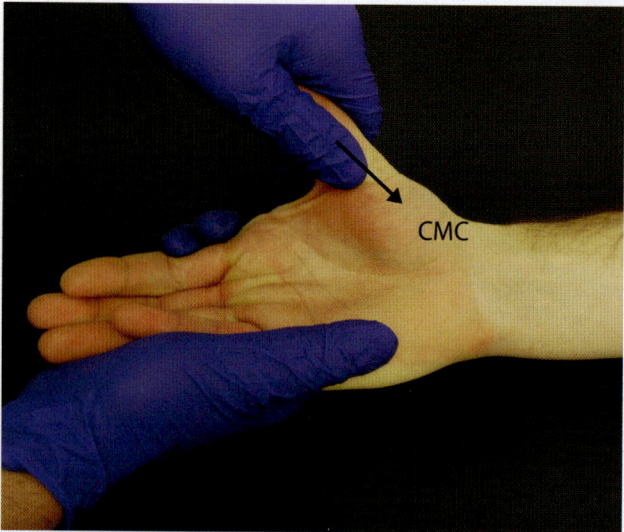

Figure 36-8. Thumb osteoarthritis. The location of the first CMC joint at the base of the thumb is demonstrated in the figure. The grind test is performed by gripping the metacarpal bone of the thumb, loading it with axial forces to push it against the carpal bone (trapezium), and rotating it in circular motion.

functioning of the thumb (Fig. 36-8). Degenerative changes in this joint result in "thumb arthritis" which can cause severe hand pain, swelling, decreased ROM, and reduced grip strength.[51] Pain and swelling occur at the base of the thumb. The discomfort is exacerbated by activities that involve using the thumb to apply force or grasping an object. Thumb arthritis can make it difficult to perform simple household tasks, such as opening jars, pulling a zipper, and turning doorknobs.[52] Patients may complain of reduced grip strength.[52]

The condition is more common in postmenopausal women.[53] Risk factors include genetic predisposition,[54] history of prior trauma to the joint, occupations involving repetitive thumb use,[55] history of rheumatoid arthritis or articular hypermobility,[56] and the presence of OA in other joints.[57,58]

Diagnosis

Thumb OA can be easily diagnosed by using the grind test (Fig. 36-8).[59] The examiner holds the wrist in one hand and grasps the first metacarpal bone in the other hand. Axial pressure toward the wrist is applied while rotating the metacarpal bone in a wide circular arc, resulting in compression of the CMC joint. The test is considered positive if the patient reports pain at the base of the thumb. In a positive test, the examiner will also note a grinding or catch sensation while rotating the metacarpal bone in the circular arc. In addition, the CMC joint may appear enlarged from osteoarthritic hypertrophy. Radiographic evaluation has higher sensitivity than the grind test, but the presence of radiographic OA only has a modest association with clinical symptoms such as hand pain and disability.[60]

Treatment

Treatment for thumb arthritis includes both nonsurgical and surgical options. Activity modification can be tried first to reduce the activities that most exacerbate pain. As an example, one can use pens with a bigger grip, change doorknobs to latches, and use jar openers. Splints can be effective in early stages and can be used at night and/or during the day depending on the patient's job and needs. Different splints are available to support the thumb, place the joint in a resting position, and decrease pain.[61-63] No one splint is superior to the other. Customized braces may provide a better fit and have been associated with improved outcomes but are more expensive.[62] Oral acetaminophen and NSAIDs can be used to manage pain. If a combination of splinting and oral medications is not effective, an intra-articular steroid injection can reduce inflammation and provide pain relief for a few months.[64,65] In severe cases, surgical treatment may be needed and includes different procedures that are tailored to the extent of arthritic involvement.[66] Surgery may include ligament reconstruction and tendon interposition (LRTI), metacarpal osteotomy, trapeziectomy, arthrodesis (joint fusion), and arthroplasty[67] (joint replacement). Recovery after surgery includes 6 weeks of bracing and about 3 months of hand therapy to work on ROM and flexibility of the thumb.[68] Most patients regain their strength and return to normal activities at the 6-month time point.

▶ TOP MIMICS IN THE LOWER LIMBS

HIP JOINT OSTEOARTHRITIS

Hip OA is a common[69] cause of hip, groin, and thigh pain and can mimic L2/3/4 radiculopathy.

Symptoms

The characteristic symptoms of hip OA include anterior hip and groin pain that is exacerbated by weight bearing/physical activity and improves with rest. These characteristics help differentiate hip OA from greater trochanteric bursitis which presents with lateral hip pain aggravated by direct pressure. The pain of hip OA can radiate down the thigh and may also involve the groin area, knee region, and buttock area. Patients may complain of difficulty walking and leg "stiffness." The pain can either be stabbing and sharp or it can be a dull ache. While the causes of hip OA are not completely known, risk factors include increasing age, genetic predisposition, prior hip injury or developmental deformities, heavy manual labor, participation in weight-bearing sports, and being overweight.[70-73]

Diagnosis

The key clinical finding suggestive of hip OA on examination is the ability to reproduce the patient's pain when ranging the femur into full internal rotation (Fig. 36-9).[74] Furthermore, with hip OA, internal rotation is generally limited more than external rotation. The reason underlying these findings is that sharp forceful internal rotation of the femur compresses the femoral acetabular joint space, approximating the bony acetabulum and femoral head, which is uncomfortable when the articular cartilage is degenerated. External rotation is generally better tolerated. Patients may also develop an antalgic gait because they tend to spend a shorter time weight bearing on the affected side due to pain. Diagnosis can be confirmed by weight-bearing anteroposterior (AP) pelvis x-ray to assess the articular width of the hip joints. Joint space narrowing, sclerosis of the joint space margins, and periarticular osteophyte formation are consistent with OA.[75] An ultrasound-guided intra-articular anesthetic and/or steroid injection can be a valuable diagnostic tool when there are questions about the location of the pain generator.[76,77]

Treatment

Treatment of hip OA starts with education about joint protection, weight loss (if appropriate), use of modalities for pain reduction, physical therapy[78,79] to preserve strength and ROM, and use of mobility aids as needed.[80,81] A cane held on the nonaffected side helps to off load the affected hip resulting in improved pain and gait mechanics. Pharmacologic treatment includes acetaminophen, NSAIDs, and ultrasound-guided intra-articular steroid injections.[82] Surgical intervention (either hip resurfacing or replacement) followed by rehabilitation may ultimately be needed to ensure optimal pain control and function in advanced cases.[81]

GREATER TROCHANTERIC BURSITIS

Greater trochanteric bursitis causes lateral hip/thigh pain and can mimic L3/L4/L5 radiculopathy.[83]

Symptoms

Greater trochanteric bursitis presents as tenderness to palpation over the greater trochanter, in the lateral hip and thigh.[84,85] Some prefer the term "greater trochanteric pain syndrome," which may be more accurate because the etiology of this condition is not fully understood. The pain generator may be related to an inflammation of the trochanteric bursa located on the outer side of the femur. However, contributing pain generators may include the gluteus medius and gluteus minimus muscles, their attachments into the greater trochanter of the femur and the femoral shaft, and overlying tissue such as the iliotibial (IT) band.[86-89] All of these structures are associated with the greater trochanter and may be affected by abnormal lower limb biomechanics and disturbances in gait, which are common occurrences in people with underlying neurologic diseases.[83,90-92] Gait abnormalities affect the biomechanics around the greater trochanter and lead to altered pressure on the bursae and friction in the

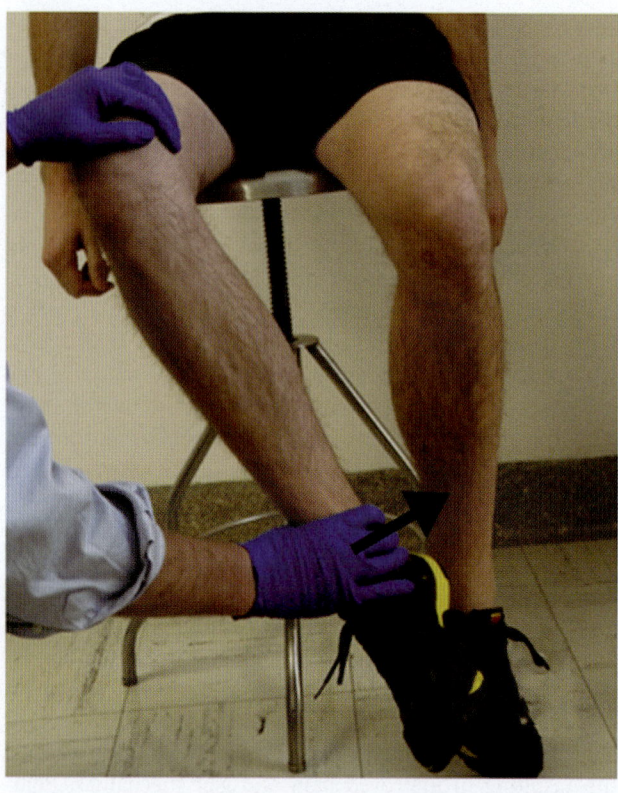 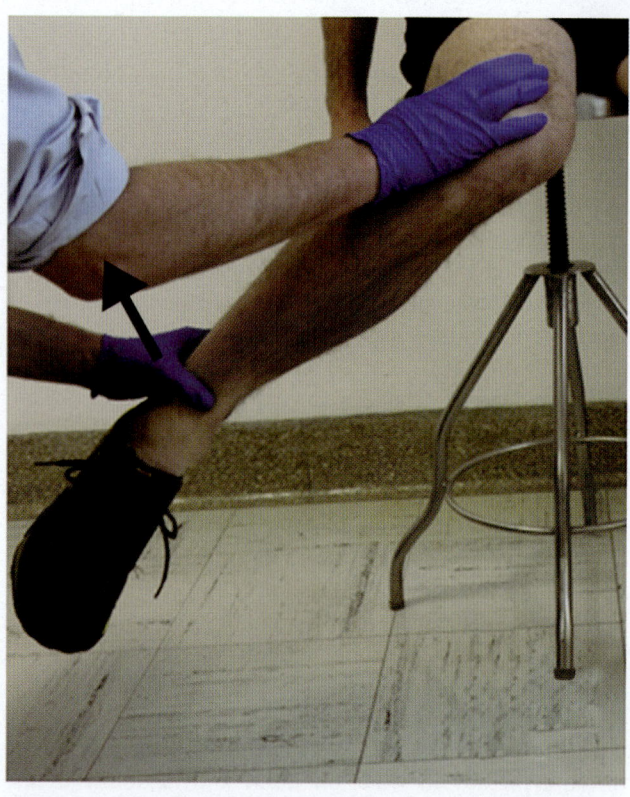

Figure 36-9. **Hip internal and external rotation.** Hip external rotation (**A**) is not typically associated with pain in hip osteoarthritis, whereas hip internal rotation (**B**) does reproduce the patient's pain. Hip ROM can be tested in a sitting position, as demonstrated here, or with the patient lying down on the examination table.

tendons and other soft tissue structures, which ultimately result in local pain and tenderness.[90]

Patients typically complain of lateral hip pain that may radiate into the buttock and outer thigh into the knee. Patients may rub their thigh when describing the pain. The pain is characteristically exacerbated by direct pressure to the point that patients may describe intolerance to sleeping on the affected side. Pain can also be aggravated by walking, especially climbing stairs, and can be disabling with a negative impact on quality of life.[93]

Diagnosis

The diagnosis is based on history and clinical findings of exquisite pain on direct palpation of the region of the greater trochanter.[94] Palpation can be performed in the lateral decubitus position with the affected side placed upward. The trochanteric process is the most prominent portion of the femur. Side-to-side comparison can be easily accomplished by palpating the outer thighs and hips with the patient in a seated position facing the examiner (Fig. 36-10). The examiner palpates along the lateral femurs from distal to proximal until reaching the greater trochanters (Fig. 36-10). Note that palpation of the lateral thigh can elicit some discomfort in people with tight IT bands. However, when trochanteric bursitis is present, direct palpation will elicit prominent sharp pain that reproduces the patient's pain.

Pain relief with local anesthetic and/or steroid injection corroborates the diagnosis and provides excellent pain relief.[95,96] Plain radiographs of the hip can be performed to exclude structural abnormalities, while ultrasound and MRI can be considered in refractory cases.[87]

Treatment

NSAIDs and ice therapy help relieve pain and reduce the inflammation. Ice therapy to the lateral hip every 4–6 hours can be accomplished by ice massage with a paper cup (Fig. 36-4) or by using flexible frozen gels or a bag of frozen peas against the hip to cover a larger area. Typically, uncomplicated greater trochanteric pain syndrome responds very well to local injections of an anesthetic and/or steroid.[91,95,96] The pain may actually worsen for 1 or 2 days immediately following the procedure before improving. Injection aftercare is critical to the success of the injection. The patient should rest, avoid direct pressure and repetitive bending, and use NSAIDs and ice as needed for pain relief. To help prevent recurrence, predisposing factors should be addressed as much as possible. Physical therapy can be helpful to stretch the back and IT band and strengthening the hip muscles can relieve tension in the hip and reduce friction. Daily stretches

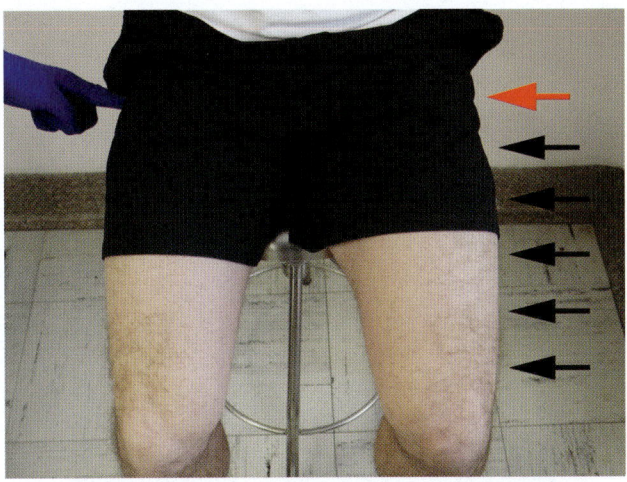

Figure 36-10. **Greater trochanter palpation.** To localize the greater trochanter, the examiner palpates the lateral thigh starting distally (*arrows*) and moving proximally until the greater trochanter of the femur is identified (as indicated by the examiner in the picture). Palpating the greater trochanter will elicit pain in patients with greater trochanteric bursitis. Performing the maneuver in sitting, as demonstrated here, allows a quick side-to-side comparison. Note that palpation of the lateral thigh can elicit some discomfort in people with tight iliotibial bands. However, when greater trochanteric bursitis is present, there will be additional, sharp pain localized to the greater trochanter. The maneuver can also be performed with the patient lying down on the examination table and the affected leg placed upward. Lying down on the side of the affected leg produces exquisite pain in patients with greater trochanteric bursitis.

should be incorporated into an individualized home exercise program (HEP) for best results. Stretches are most effective and best tolerated after the steroid injection of the bursae has been performed.

PES ANSERINE BURSITIS

Bursitis is a common cause of lower extremity pain. Pes anserine bursitis presents as medial knee and leg pain and can mimic L4 lumbar radiculopathy.

Symptoms

The pes anserinus ("goose's foot") is the insertion of the conjoined tendons of three muscles (semitendinosus, sartorius, and gracilis) onto the anteromedial surface of the proximal tibia. It lies superficial to the superficial fibers of the medial collateral ligament (MCL) of the knee. Inflammation of the anserine bursa that lies just under the tendons near their insertion is termed pes anserine bursitis.[97]

Pes anserine bursitis should be suspected when pain occurs in the medial knee region over the upper tibia.[98] Pain is exacerbated by repetitive knee flexion such as when ascending stairs and climbing. Sports that involve side-to-side cutting activity (e.g., tennis and soccer) as well as underlying knee medial compartment OA and obesity may predispose to bursitis. Muscle imbalances involving the hip adductors, hip flexors, and hamstrings may cause an abnormal pull at the insertion point of the three tendons resulting in pes anserine bursitis.[99,100]

Diagnosis

The diagnosis of pes anserine bursitis is made clinically by direct palpation of the bursa, which elicits localized tenderness (Fig. 36-11). The entire tibial plateau needs to be palpated to differentiate between the localized tenderness of anserine bursitis and medial joint line tenderness from an intra-articular injury. In addition, there may be more extensive tenderness along the medial femoral epicondyle to the medial tibia which is present with MCL injury. Imaging is usually not indicated unless there is suspicion for stress fracture or intra-articular pathology such as meniscal injury or knee OA.

Treatment

In the acute phase, treatment includes rest, ice massage (as described above), and a short course of topical or oral NSAIDs to reduce the pain and swelling in the bursa. Activity modification to "rest" the bursa include avoiding direct

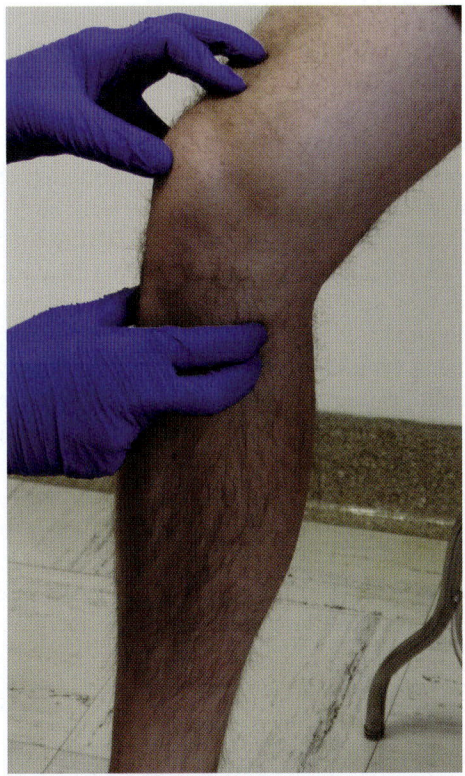

Figure 36-11. **Pes anserine bursa.** The figure depicts the location of the anserine bursa in the medial leg.

pressure (which can be accomplished at night by using a pillow between the knees) as well as activities such as squatting, repetitive knee bending, and crossing the legs.[101] A corticosteroid injection into the bursa can be used both as a diagnostic and therapeutic tool and often provides quick relief.[102] A rehabilitation program is needed to treat any underlying cause of anterior to posterior and medial to lateral muscle imbalance. Therapy focuses on maximizing flexibility, strength, and endurance of the muscles whose tendons form the pes anserinus as well as addressing any muscle imbalances of the entire kinetic chain. Core control should be maximized to allow for proper hamstring and hip adductor and flexion function. Running shoes and inserts need to be appropriate for each individual's biomechanical characteristics. Surgery (bursectomy) is rarely needed.

PLANTAR FASCIITIS

Plantar fasciitis is a common cause of plantar foot pain. It can occur on both sides and mimic the pain associated with distal sensory polyneuropathy. It can also present unilaterally mimicking S1 radiculopathy.

Symptoms

The plantar fascia is a band of thick connective tissue that originates on the calcaneus (or heel bone) and fans out on the sole of the foot to connect it to the base of the toes and support the arch of the foot. It is also related to the Achilles tendon, with connecting fibers between the two from the distal aspect of the Achilles tendon to the origin of the plantar fascia at the calcaneal tubercle.[103] Poor foot biomechanics can cause increased tension on the fascia and pain. This can occur in patients with pes planus, pes cavus, increased subtalar pronation, limited ankle dorsiflexion, decreased intrinsic foot muscle strength, and tight heel cords, all conditions that place stress on the plantar fascia.[104,105] Therefore, plantar fasciitis can coexist with many underlying neuromuscular conditions that are associated with foot deformity and weakness. Obesity, pregnancy, and prolonged standing are additional risk factors.[104,106]

Patients typically describe the worst pain as occurring with weight bearing after getting out of bed in the morning or after a period of inactivity. Pain can be gnawing, stabbing, or burning. History of pain when taking the first steps in the morning helps differentiate this condition from the pain experienced by patients with sensory polyneuropathy whose foot pain is characteristically worse at night when off their feet. In some patients, the pain may radiate to the dorsolateral foot due to the patient offloading the pressure on the heel and walking on the outside of the foot creating an overuse condition to the lateral foot and ankle.

Diagnosis

The history and clinical examination are the mainstay of diagnosis. On physical examination there is tenderness to palpation

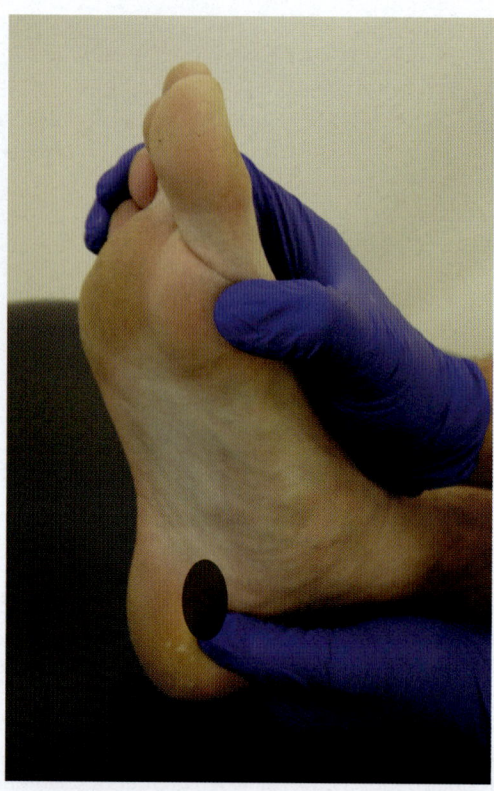

Figure 36-12. Medial calcaneus palpation. This maneuver reveals the area of maximal tenderness in plantar fasciitis at the site of the plantar fascia insertion on the heel bone (*shaded area*).

on the medial plantar aspect of the heel bone (Fig. 36-12). This area corresponds to the site of the plantar fascia insertion on the calcaneus. Palpation of the medial slip of the plantar fascia may also reveal tightness and discomfort (Fig. 36-13), but the area of maximal tenderness corresponds to the medial tubercle of the calcaneus (Fig. 36-12). Discomfort in the proximal plantar fascia can also be elicited by passive ankle and toe dorsiflexion. Diagnostic imaging is rarely needed for the initial diagnosis. Ultrasound and MRI are reserved for cases that do not respond to treatment or to exclude other heel pathology.[107,108] Plain x-rays of the foot can reveal a calcaneal heel spur in many individuals.[108] The heel spur, however, is not pathognomonic of plantar fasciitis and is not the cause of pain in this condition. Rather, the heel spur is thought to represent a byproduct of the chronic pulling of the fascia off the calcaneus and exists in many patients without symptoms of plantar fasciitis.

Treatment

Plantar fasciitis is a self-limiting condition that usually improves within 1 year regardless of treatment. Conservative treatment usually starts with patient-directed therapies. If these are not effective within a few weeks to a few months, management is advanced to include physician-prescribed interventions.

Initial patient-directed modalities include rest, activity modification, ice massage, oral analgesics (acetaminophen or

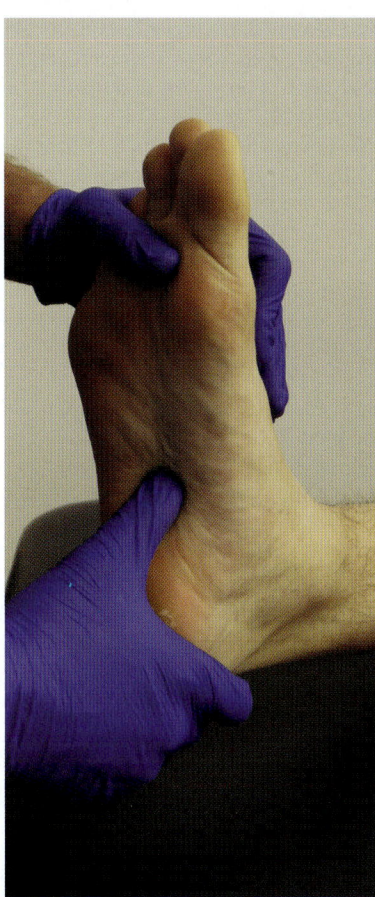

Figure 36-13. Plantar fascia palpation. Palpating the plantar fascia in the arch of the foot can elicit pain in people with plantar fasciitis.

NSAIDs), and stretching.[109,110] Ice massage is performed by having the patient roll the arch of the foot over a frozen soda can or plastic bottle until numb. Treatment can be repeated multiple times a day. Stretching is performed both in bed before getting up in the morning and several times during the day. Before getting up, the patient is asked to stretch the Achilles tendon by dorsiflexing the foot and holding on to it for at least 30 seconds. This exercise is repeated 10 times and can be modified by including a large towel if limited flexibility prevents the patient from reaching the foot. While seated, the patient is also asked to stretch the plantar fascia by dorsiflexing the toes, holding the metatarsophalangeals and stretching the fascia in the arch region. During the day, the patient may stretch by leaning against a wall and performing wall leans, alternating between knee bent and knee extended while the heel is on the ground. Again, each stretch is held for a minimum of 30 seconds and repeated several times. Intrinsic foot and calf strengthening exercises can help as well.

If pain persists, physician-prescribed treatments should be considered. These include shoe inserts, night splinting, physical therapy, and corticosteroid injections. Shoe inserts are commonly recommended for people with plantar fasciitis to aid in limiting overpronation of the foot and to unload the tensile forces on the plantar fascia. These include heel cups, prefabricated longitudinal arch supports, and custom-made full-length shoe insoles.[111-113] Night splints can be used to prevent foot plantar flexion during sleep by keeping the foot and ankle in a neutral 90-degree position. Night splints have been shown to improve plantar fasciitis pain,[113] but poor compliance because of sleep disturbance and foot discomfort has limited their long-term use. Multiple physical therapy modalities may be used, often in combination. Deep myofascial massage and iontophoresis can be performed by a physical therapist. In iontophoresis, electrical pulses are used to cause absorption of topical medications into the soft tissues beneath the skin. A small study found iontophoresis of acetic acid or dexamethasone to be helpful in plantar fasciitis.[114] Corticosteroid injections have been found to be effective in the treatment of plantar fasciitis and may be part of the initial approach in patients who desire an expedited return to normal activity.[115,116] Risks associated with corticosteroid injection include fat pad atrophy and plantar fascia rupture. In recent years, platelet-rich plasma injections have been proposed as an alternative treatment for plantar fasciitis and are currently being tested in clinical trials to determine their efficacy.[117,118] Patients with recalcitrant plantar fasciitis can consider extracorporeal shock wave therapy (ESWT) or, as a last resort, plantar fasciotomy. ESWT is thought to promote neovascularization and induce tissue repair. The technique is commonly used as it is noninvasive and has a good side effect profile although clinical trials have resulted in conflicting evidence.[119-123]

▶ SUMMARY

Musculoskeletal disorders are a common cause of limb pain and are likely to be encountered in daily practice, whether in the neuromuscular clinic or in the EMG laboratory. Musculoskeletal problems can "mimic" radiculopathy or entrapment neuropathy, thus posing a diagnostic challenge. In addition, musculoskeletal pain can complicate chronic neuromuscular diseases such as motor neuron disease and muscular dystrophy. Importantly, many common musculoskeletal problems can be diagnosed quickly at the bedside and are eminently treatable. Therefore, their prompt recognition has the potential to improve clinical flow and patient outcomes.

▶ ACKNOWLEDGMENTS

We would like to thank Farah Hameed, MD for helpful comments and suggestions, and Andrew Sandefer, DO for technical assistance during the initial drafting of this chapter.

REFERENCES

1. Cannon DE, Dillingham TR, Miao H, Andary MT, Pezzin LE. Musculoskeletal disorders in referrals for suspected cervical radiculopathy. *Arch Phys Med Rehabil*. 2007;88:1256–1259.

2. Cannon DE, Dillingham TR, Miao H, Andary MT, Pezzin LE. Musculoskeletal disorders in referrals for suspected lumbosacral radiculopathy. *Am J Phys Med Rehabil*. 2007;86:957–961.
3. Stockard AR1, Allen TW. Competence levels in musculoskeletal medicine: comparison of osteopathic and allopathic medical graduates. *J Am Osteopath Assoc*. 2006;106(6):350–355.
4. Fu FH, Harner CD, Klein AH. Shoulder impingement syndrome. A critical review. *Clin Orthop Relat Res*. 1991;269:162–173.
5. Yi Y, Shim JS, Kim K, et al. Prevalence of the rotator cuff tear increases with weakness in hemiplegic shoulder. *Ann Rehabil Med*. 2013;37:471–478.
6. Gumina S, Carbone S, Campagna V, Candela V, Sacchetti FM, Giannicola G. The impact of aging on rotator cuff tear size. *Musculoskelet Surg*. 2013;97(suppl 1):69–72.
7. Bodin J, Ha C, Petit Le Manac'h A, et al. Risk factors for incidence of rotator cuff syndrome in a large working population. *Scand J Work Environ Health*. 2012;38:436–446.
8. Jain NB, Wilcox RB 3rd, Katz JN, Higgins LD. Clinical examination of the rotator cuff. *PM R*. 2013;5:45–56.
9. Hegedus EJ, Goode AP, Cook CE, et al. Which physical examination tests provide clinicians with the most value when examining the shoulder? Update of a systematic review with meta-analysis of individual tests. *Br J Sports Med*. 2012;46:964–978.
10. Teefey SA, Rubin DA, Middleton WD, Hildebolt CF, Leibold RA, Yamaguchi K. Detection and quantification of rotator cuff tears. Comparison of ultrasonographic, magnetic resonance imaging, and arthroscopic findings in seventy-one consecutive cases. *J Bone Joint Surg Am*. 2004;86-A:708–716.
11. Green S, Buchbinder R, Hetrick S. Physiotherapy interventions for shoulder pain. *Cochrane Database Syst Rev*. 2003;(2):CD004258.
12. Gebremariam L, Hay EM, van der Sande R, Rinkel WD, Koes BW, Huisstede BM. Subacromial impingement syndrome—effectiveness of physiotherapy and manual therapy. *Br J Sports Med*. 2014;48(16):1202–1208.
13. Dogu B, Yucel SD, Sag SY, Bankaoglu M, Kuran B. Blind or ultrasound-guided corticosteroid injections and short-term response in subacromial impingement syndrome: a randomized, double-blind, prospective study. *Am J Phys Med Rehabil*. 2012;91:658–665.
14. Mazzocca AD, McCarthy MB, Ledgard FA, et al. Histomorphologic changes of the long head of the biceps tendon in common shoulder pathologies. *Arthroscopy*. 2013;29:972–981.
15. Beall DP, Williamson EE, Ly JQ, et al. Association of biceps tendon tears with rotator cuff abnormalities: degree of correlation with tears of the anterior and superior portions of the rotator cuff. *AJR Am J Roentgenol*. 2003;180:633–639.
16. Murthi AM, Vosburgh CL, Neviaser TJ. The incidence of pathologic changes of the long head of the biceps tendon. *J Shoulder Elbow Surg*. 2000;9:382–385.
17. Gazzillo GP, Finnoff JT, Hall MM, Sayeed YA, Smith J. Accuracy of palpating the long head of the biceps tendon: an ultrasonographic study. *PM R*. 2011;3:1035–1040.
18. Bennett WF. Specificity of the Speed's test: arthroscopic technique for evaluating the biceps tendon at the level of the bicipital groove. *Arthroscopy*. 1998;14:789–796.
19. Chen HS, Lin SH, Hsu YH, Chen SC, Kang JH. A comparison of physical examinations with musculoskeletal ultrasound in the diagnosis of biceps long head tendinitis. *Ultrasound Med Biol*. 2011;37:1392–1398.
20. Schaeffeler C, Waldt S, Holzapfel K, et al. Lesions of the biceps pulley: diagnostic accuracy of MR arthrography of the shoulder and evaluation of previously described and new diagnostic signs. *Radiology*. 2012;264:504–513.
21. Longo UG, Loppini M, Marineo G, Khan WS, Maffulli N, Denaro V. Tendinopathy of the tendon of the long head of the biceps. *Sports Med Arthrosc*. 2011;19:321–332.
22. Snyder GM, Mair SD, Lattermann C. Tendinopathy of the long head of the biceps. *Med Sport Sci*. 2012;57:76–89.
23. Zhang J, Ebraheim N, Lause GE. Ultrasound-guided injection for the biceps brachii tendinitis: results and experience. *Ultrasound Med Biol*. 2011;37:729–733.
24. Hashiuchi T, Sakurai G, Morimoto M, Komei T, Takakura Y, Tanaka Y. Accuracy of the biceps tendon sheath injection: ultrasound-guided or unguided injection? A randomized controlled trial. *J Shoulder Elbow Surg*. 2011;20:1069–1073.
25. Galasso O, Gasparini G, De Benedetto M, Familiari F, Castricini R. Tenotomy versus tenodesis in the treatment of the long head of biceps brachii tendon lesions. *BMC Musculoskelet Disord*. 2012;13:205.
26. Chourasia AO, Buhr KA, Rabago DP, et al. Relationships between biomechanics, tendon pathology, and function in individuals with lateral epicondylosis. *J Orthop Sports Phys Ther*. 2013;43:368–378.
27. Lucado AM, Kolber MJ, Cheng MS, Echternach JL Sr. Upper extremity strength characteristics in female recreational tennis players with and without lateral epicondylalgia. *J Orthop Sports Phys Ther*. 2012;42:1025–1031.
28. Regan W, Wold LE, Coonrad R, Morrey BF. Microscopic histopathology of chronic refractory lateral epicondylitis. *Am J Sports Med*. 1992;20:746–749.
29. Abrams GD, Renstrom PA, Safran MR. Epidemiology of musculoskeletal injury in the tennis player. *Br J Sports Med*. 2012;46:492–498.
30. Titchener AG, Fakis A, Tambe AA, Smith C, Hubbard RB, Clark DI. Risk factors in lateral epicondylitis (tennis elbow): a case-control study. *J Hand Surg Eur*. 2013;38:159–164.
31. Shiri R, Viikari-Juntura E, Varonen H, Heliovaara M. Prevalence and determinants of lateral and medial epicondylitis: a population study. *Am J Epidemiol*. 2006;164:1065–1074.
32. Pattanittum P, Turner T, Green S, Buchbinder R. Non-steroidal anti-inflammatory drugs (NSAIDs) for treating lateral elbow pain in adults. *Cochrane Database Syst Rev*. 2013;5:CD003686.
33. Sölveborn SA. Radial epicondylalgia ('tennis elbow'): treatment with stretching or forearm band. A prospective study with long-term follow-up including range-of-motion measurements. *Scand J Med Sci Sports*. 1997;7:229–237.
34. Sadeghi-Demneh E, Jafarian F. The immediate effects of orthoses on pain in people with lateral epicondylalgia. *Pain Res Treat*. 2013;2013:353597.
35. Nilsson P, Baigi A, Swärd L, Möller M, Månsson J. Lateral epicondylalgia: a structured programme better than corticosteroids and NSAID. *Scand J Occup Ther*. 2012;19(5):404–410.
36. Olaussen M, Holmedal O, Lindbaek M, Brage S, Solvang H. Treating lateral epicondylitis with corticosteroid injections or non-electrotherapeutical physiotherapy: a systematic review. *BMJ Open*. 2013;3:e003564.
37. Svernlov B, Adolfsson L. Non-operative treatment regime including eccentric training for lateral humeral epicondylalgia. *Scand J Med Sci Sports*. 2001;11:328–334.

38. Martinez-Silvestrini JA, Newcomer KL, Gay RE, Schaefer MP, Kortebein P, Arendt KW. Chronic lateral epicondylitis: comparative effectiveness of a home exercise program including stretching alone versus stretching supplemented with eccentric or concentric strengthening. *J Hand Ther.* 2005;18(4): 411–419, quiz 420.
39. Titchener AG, Booker SJ, Bhamber NS, Tambe AA, Clark DI. Corticosteroid and platelet-rich plasma injection therapy in tennis elbow (lateral epicondylalgia): a survey of current UK specialist practice and a call for clinical guidelines. *Br J Sports Med.* 2013.
40. Krogh TP, Bartels EM, Ellingsen T, et al. Comparative effectiveness of injection therapies in lateral epicondylitis: a systematic review and network meta-analysis of randomized controlled trials. *Am J Sports Med.* 2013;41:1435–1446.
41. Coombes BK, Bisset L, Brooks P, Khan A, Vicenzino B. Effect of corticosteroid injection, physiotherapy, or both on clinical outcomes in patients with unilateral lateral epicondylalgia: a randomized controlled trial. *JAMA.* 2013;309:461–469.
42. Krogh TP, Fredberg U, Stengaard-Pedersen K, Christensen R, Jensen P, Ellingsen T. Treatment of lateral epicondylitis with platelet-rich plasma, glucocorticoid, or saline: a randomized, double-blind, placebo-controlled trial. *Am J Sports Med.* 2013; 41:625–635.
43. Armstrong TJ, Fine LJ, Goldstein SA, Lifshitz YR, Silverstein BA. Ergonomics considerations in hand and wrist tendinitis. *J Hand Surg Am.* 1987;12:830–837.
44. Luopajarvi T, Kuorinka I, Virolainen M, Holmberg M. Prevalence of tenosynovitis and other injuries of the upper extremities in repetitive work. *Scand J Work Environ Health.* 1979; 5(suppl 3):48–55.
45. Stahl S, Vida D, Meisner C, et al. Systematic review and meta-analysis on the work-related cause of de Quervain tenosynovitis: a critical appraisal of its recognition as an occupational disease. *Plast Reconstr Surg.* 2013;132(6):1479–1491.
46. Hartwell SW Jr, Larsen RD, Posch JL. Tenosynovitis in women in industry. *Cleve Clin Q.* 1964;31:115–118.
47. Ashraf MO, Devadoss VG. Systematic review and meta-analysis on steroid injection therapy for de Quervain's tenosynovitis in adults. *Eur J Orthop Surg Traumatol.* 2014;24(2): 149–157.
48. Mardani-Kivi M, Karimi Mobarakeh M, Bahrami F, Hashemi-Motlagh K, Saheb-Ekhtiari K, Akhoondzadeh N. Corticosteroid injection with or without thumb spica cast for de Quervain tenosynovitis. *J Hand Surg Am.* 2014;39:37–41.
49. McDermott JD, Ilyas AM, Nazarian LN, Leinberry CF. Ultrasound-guided injections for de Quervain's tenosynovitis. *Clin Orthop Relat Res.* 2012;470:1925–1931.
50. Kang HJ, Koh IH, Jang JW, Choi YR. Endoscopic versus open release in patients with de Quervain's tenosynovitis: a randomised trial. *Bone Joint J.* 2013;95-B:947–951.
51. Gehrmann SV, Tang J, Li ZM, Goitz RJ, Windolf J, Kaufmann RA. Motion deficit of the thumb in CMC joint arthritis. *J Hand Surg Am.* 2010;35:1449–1453.
52. Zhang Y, Niu J, Kelly-Hayes M, Chaisson CE, Aliabadi P, Felson DT. Prevalence of symptomatic hand osteoarthritis and its impact on functional status among the elderly: The Framingham Study. *Am J Epidemiol.* 2002;156:1021–1027.
53. Wilder FV, Barrett JP, Farina EJ. Joint-specific prevalence of osteoarthritis of the hand. *Osteoarthritis Cartilage.* 2006; 14:953–957.
54. Jonsson H, Manolescu I, Stefansson SE, et al. The inheritance of hand osteoarthritis in Iceland. *Arthritis Rheum.* 2003;48:391–395.
55. Fontana L, Neel S, Claise JM, Ughetto S, Catilina P. Osteoarthritis of the thumb carpometacarpal joint in women and occupational risk factors: a case-control study. *J Hand Surg Am.* 2007;32:459–465.
56. Jonsson H, Valtysdottir ST, Kjartansson O, Brekkan A. Hypermobility associated with osteoarthritis of the thumb base: a clinical and radiological subset of hand osteoarthritis. *Ann Rheum Dis.* 1996;55:540–543.
57. Kessler S, Stove J, Puhl W, Sturmer T. First carpometacarpal and interphalangeal osteoarthritis of the hand in patients with advanced hip or knee OA. Are there differences in the aetiology? *Clin Rheumatol.* 2003;22:409–413.
58. Chaisson CE, Zhang Y, McAlindon TE, et al. Radiographic hand osteoarthritis: incidence, patterns, and influence of pre-existing disease in a population based sample. *J Rheumatol.* 1997;24:1337–1343.
59. Merritt MM, Roddey TS, Costello C, Olson S. Diagnostic value of clinical grind test for carpometacarpal osteoarthritis of the thumb. *J Hand Ther.* 2010;23:261–267; quiz 268.
60. Dahaghin S, Bierma-Zeinstra SM, Ginai AZ, Pols HA, Hazes JM, Koes BW. Prevalence and pattern of radiographic hand osteoarthritis and association with pain and disability (the Rotterdam study). *Ann Rheum Dis.* 2005;64:682–687.
61. Sillem H, Backman CL, Miller WC, Li LC. Comparison of two carpometacarpal stabilizing splints for individuals with thumb osteoarthritis. *J Hand Ther.* 2011;24(3):216–225; quiz 126; discussion 227–230.
62. Bani MA, Arazpour M, Kashani RV, Mousavi ME, Hutchins SW. Comparison of custom-made and prefabricated neoprene splinting in patients with the first carpometacarpal joint osteoarthritis. *Disabil Rehabil Assist Technol.* 2013;8:232–237.
63. Egan MY, Brousseau L. Splinting for osteoarthritis of the carpometacarpal joint: a review of the evidence. *Am J Occup Ther.* 2007;61:70–78.
64. Maarse W, Watts AC, Bain GI. Medium-term outcome following intra-articular corticosteroid injection in first CMC joint arthritis using fluoroscopy. *Hand Surg.* 2009;14:99–104.
65. Joshi R. Intraarticular corticosteroid injection for first carpometacarpal osteoarthritis. *J Rheumatol.* 2005;32:1305–1306.
66. Hentz VR. Surgical treatment of trapeziometacarpal joint arthritis: a historical perspective. *Clin Orthop Relat Res.* 2014; 472(4):1184–1189.
67. Badia A, Sambandam SN. Total joint arthroplasty in the treatment of advanced stages of thumb carpometacarpal joint osteoarthritis. *J Hand Surg Am.* 2006;31:1605–1614.
68. Ataker Y, Gudemez E, Ece SC, Canbulat N, Gulgonen A. Rehabilitation protocol after suspension arthroplasty of thumb carpometacarpal joint osteoarthritis. *J Hand Ther.* 2012;25(4): 374–382; quiz 383.
69. Nho SJ, Kymes SM, Callaghan JJ, Felson DT. The burden of hip osteoarthritis in the United States: epidemiologic and economic considerations. *J Am Acad Orthop Surg.* 2013;21 (suppl 1):S1–S6.
70. Evangelou E, Kerkhof HJ, Styrkarsdottir U, et al. A meta-analysis of genome-wide association studies identifies novel variants associated with osteoarthritis of the hip. *Ann Rheum Dis.* 2014;73(12):2130–2136.
71. Richmond SA, Fukuchi RK, Ezzat A, Schneider K, Schneider G, Emery CA. Are joint injury, sport activity, physical activity,

72. Prieto-Alhambra D, Judge A, Javaid MK, Cooper C, Diez-Perez A, Arden NK. Incidence and risk factors for clinically diagnosed knee, hip and hand osteoarthritis: influences of age, gender and osteoarthritis affecting other joints. *Ann Rheum Dis.* 2014;73(9):1659–1664.
73. Franklin J, Ingvarsson T, Englund M, Lohmander S. Association between occupation and knee and hip replacement due to osteoarthritis: a case-control study. *Arthritis Res Ther.* 2010;12:R102.
74. Chong T, Don DW, Kao MC, Wong D, Mitra R. The value of physical examination in the diagnosis of hip osteoarthritis. *J Back Musculoskelet Rehabil.* 2013;26:397–400.
75. Xu L, Hayashi D, Guermazi A, et al. The diagnostic performance of radiography for detection of osteoarthritis-associated features compared with MRI in hip joints with chronic pain. *Skeletal Radiol.* 2013;42:1421–1428.
76. Yoong P, Guirguis R, Darrah R, Wijeratna M, Porteous MJ. Evaluation of ultrasound-guided diagnostic local anaesthetic hip joint injection for osteoarthritis. *Skeletal Radiol.* 2012;41:981–985.
77. Deshmukh AJ, Thakur RR, Goyal A, Klein DA, Ranawat AS, Rodriguez JA. Accuracy of diagnostic injection in differentiating source of atypical hip pain. *J Arthroplasty.* 2010;25:129–133.
78. Svege I, Nordsletten L, Fernandes L, Risberg MA. Exercise therapy may postpone total hip replacement surgery in patients with hip osteoarthritis: a long-term follow-up of a randomised trial. *Ann Rheum Dis.* 2015;74(1):164–169.
79. Jensen C, Roos EM, Kjaersgaard-Andersen P, Overgaard S. The effect of education and supervised exercise vs. education alone on the time to total hip replacement in patients with severe hip osteoarthritis. A randomized clinical trial protocol. *BMC Musculoskelet Disord.* 2013;14:21.
80. Zhang W, Moskowitz RW, Nuki G, et al. OARSI recommendations for the management of hip and knee osteoarthritis, Part II: OARSI evidence-based, expert consensus guidelines. *Osteoarthritis Cartilage.* 2008;16:137–162.
81. Hochberg MC, Altman RD, April KT, et al. American College of Rheumatology. 2012 recommendations for the use of non-pharmacologic and pharmacologic therapies in osteoarthritis of the hand, hip, and knee. *Arthritis Care Res (Hoboken).* 2012;64:465–474.
82. Lambert RG, Hutchings EJ, Grace MG, Jhangri GS, Conner-Spady B, Maksymowych WP. Steroid injection for osteoarthritis of the hip: a randomized, double-blind, placebo-controlled trial. *Arthritis Rheum.* 2007;56:2278–2287.
83. Swezey RL. Pseudo-radiculopathy in subacute trochanteric bursitis of the subgluteus maximus bursa. *Arch Phys Med Rehabil.* 1976;57:387–390.
84. Schapira D, Nahir M, Scharf Y. Trochanteric bursitis: a common clinical problem. *Arch Phys Med Rehabil.* 1986;67:815–817.
85. Shbeeb MI, Matteson EL. Trochanteric bursitis (greater trochanter pain syndrome). *Mayo Clin Proc.* 1996;71:565–569.
86. Bird PA, Oakley SP, Shnier R, Kirkham BW. Prospective evaluation of magnetic resonance imaging and physical examination findings in patients with greater trochanteric pain syndrome. *Arthritis Rheum.* 2001;44:2138–2145.
87. Blankenbaker DG, Ullrick SR, Davis KW, De Smet AA, Haaland B, Fine JP. Correlation of MRI findings with clinical findings of trochanteric pain syndrome. *Skeletal Radiol.* 2008;37:903–909.
88. Fearon AM, Scarvell JM, Cook JL, Smith PN. Does ultrasound correlate with surgical or histologic findings in greater trochanteric pain syndrome? A pilot study. *Clin Orthop Relat Res.* 2010;468:1838–1844.
89. Long SS, Surrey DE, Nazarian LN. Sonography of greater trochanteric pain syndrome and the rarity of primary bursitis. *AJR Am J Roentgenol.* 2013;201:1083–1086.
90. Segal NA, Felson DT, Torner JC, et al; Multicenter Osteoarthritis Study Group. Greater trochanteric pain syndrome: epidemiology and associated factors. *Arch Phys Med Rehabil.* 2007;88:988–992.
91. Sayegh F, Potoupnis M, Kapetanos G. Greater trochanter bursitis pain syndrome in females with chronic low back pain and sciatica. *Acta Orthop Belg.* 2004;70:423–428.
92. Sloan RL. Greater trochanteric pain syndrome, another cause of hip or thigh pain in multiple sclerosis. *Pract Neurol.* 2009;9:163–165.
93. Fearon AM, Cook JL, Scarvell JM, Neeman T, Cormick W, Smith PN. Greater trochanteric pain syndrome negatively affects work, physical activity and quality of life: a case control study. *J Arthroplasty.* 2014;29(2):383–386.
94. Karpinski MR, Piggott H. Greater trochanteric pain syndrome. A report of 15 cases. *J Bone Joint Surg Br.* 1985;67:762–763.
95. McEvoy JR, Lee KS, Blankenbaker DG, del Rio AM, Keene JS. Ultrasound-guided corticosteroid injections for treatment of greater trochanteric pain syndrome: greater trochanter bursa versus subgluteus medius bursa. *AJR Am J Roentgenol.* 2013;201:W313–W317.
96. Brinks A, van Rijn RM, Willemsen SP, et al. Corticosteroid injections for greater trochanteric pain syndrome: a randomized controlled trial in primary care. *Ann Fam Med.* 2011;9:226–234.
97. Forbes JR, Helms CA, Janzen DL. Acute pes anserine bursitis: MR imaging. *Radiology.* 1995;194:525–527.
98. Rennie WJ, Saifuddin A. Pes anserine bursitis: incidence in symptomatic knees and clinical presentation. *Skeletal Radiol.* 2005;34:395–398.
99. Alvarez-Nemegyei J. Risk factors for pes anserinus tendinitis/bursitis syndrome: a case control study. *J Clin Rheumatol.* 2007;13:63–65.
100. Devan MR, Pescatello LS, Faghri P, Anderson J. A prospective study of overuse knee injuries among female athletes with muscle imbalances and structural abnormalities. *J Athl Train.* 2004;39:263–267.
101. Butcher JD, Salzman KL, Lillegard WA. Lower extremity bursitis. *Am Fam Physician.* 1996;53:2317–2324.
102. Cardone DA, Tallia AF. Diagnostic and therapeutic injection of the hip and knee. *Am Fam Physician.* 2003;67:2147–2152.
103. Stecco C, Corradin M, Macchi V, et al. Plantar fascia anatomy and its relationship with Achilles tendon and paratenon. *J Anat.* 2013;223:665–676.
104. Riddle DL, Pulisic M, Pidcoe P, Johnson RE. Risk factors for Plantar fasciitis: a matched case-control study. *J Bone Joint Surg Am.* 2003;85-A:872–877.
105. Bolivar YA, Munuera PV, Padillo JP. Relationship between tightness of the posterior muscles of the lower limb and plantar fasciitis. *Foot Ankle Int.* 2013;34:42–48.

106. Werner RA, Gell N, Hartigan A, Wiggerman N, Keyserling WM. Risk factors for plantar fasciitis among assembly plant workers. *PM R*. 2010;2:110–116; quiz 1 p following 167.
107. Karabay N, Toros T, Hurel C. Ultrasonographic evaluation in plantar fasciitis. *J Foot Ankle Surg*. 2007;46:442–446.
108. McMillan AM, Landorf KB, Barrett JT, Menz HB, Bird AR. Diagnostic imaging for chronic plantar heel pain: a systematic review and meta-analysis. *J Foot Ankle Res*. 2009;2:32.
109. Donley BG, Moore T, Sferra J, Gozdanovic J, Smith R. The efficacy of oral nonsteroidal anti-inflammatory medication (NSAID) in the treatment of plantar fasciitis: a randomized, prospective, placebo-controlled study. *Foot Ankle Int*. 2007;28:20–23.
110. Digiovanni BF, Nawoczenski DA, Malay DP, et al. Plantar fascia-specific stretching exercise improves outcomes in patients with chronic plantar fasciitis. A prospective clinical trial with two-year follow-up. *J Bone Joint Surg Am*. 2006;88:1775–1781.
111. Lee SY, McKeon P, Hertel J. Does the use of orthoses improve self-reported pain and function measures in patients with plantar fasciitis? A meta-analysis. *Phys Ther Sport*. 2009;10:12–18.
112. Hawke F, Burns J, Radford JA, du Toit V. Custom-made foot orthoses for the treatment of foot pain. *Cochrane Database Syst Rev*. 2008;3:CD006801.
113. Roos E, Engstrom M, Soderberg B. Foot orthoses for the treatment of plantar fasciitis. *Foot Ankle Int*. 2006;27:606–611.
114. Osborne HR, Allison GT. Treatment of plantar fasciitis by LowDye taping and iontophoresis: short term results of a double blinded, randomised, placebo controlled clinical trial of dexamethasone and acetic acid. *Br J Sports Med*. 2006;40:545–549; discussion 549.
115. McMillan AM, Landorf KB, Gilheany MF, Bird AR, Morrow AD, Menz HB. Ultrasound guided corticosteroid injection for plantar fasciitis: randomised controlled trial. *BMJ*. 2012;344:e3260.
116. Schulhofer SD. Short-term benefits of ultrasound-guided corticosteroid injection in plantar fasciitis. *Clin J Sport Med*. 2013;23:83–84.
117. Kim E, Lee JH. Autologous platelet-rich plasma versus dextrose prolotherapy for the treatment of chronic recalcitrant plantar fasciitis. *PM R*. 2014;6(2):152–158.
118. Peerbooms JC, van Laar W, Faber F, Schuller HM, van der Hoeven H, Gosens T. Use of platelet rich plasma to treat plantar fasciitis: design of a multi centre randomized controlled trial. *BMC Musculoskelet Disord*. 2010;11:69.
119. Buchbinder R, Ptasznik R, Gordon J, Buchanan J, Prabaharan V, Forbes A. Ultrasound-guided extracorporeal shock wave therapy for plantar fasciitis: a randomized controlled trial. *JAMA*. 2002;288:1364–1372.
120. Kudo P, Dainty K, Clarfield M, Coughlin L, Lavoie P, Lebrun C. Randomized, placebo-controlled, double-blind clinical trial evaluating the treatment of plantar fasciitis with an extracoporeal shockwave therapy (ESWT) device: A North American confirmatory study. *J Orthop Res*. 2006;24:115–123.
121. Dizon JN, Gonzalez-Suarez C, Zamora MT, Gambito ED. Effectiveness of extracorporeal shock wave therapy in chronic plantar fasciitis: a meta-analysis. *Am J Phys Med Rehabil*. 2013;92:606–620.
122. Speed C. A systematic review of shockwave therapies in soft tissue conditions: focusing on the evidence. *Br J Sports Med*. 2014;48(21):1538–1542.
123. Rhim HC, Kwon J, Park J, Borg-Stein J, Tenforde AS. A systematic review of systematic reviews on the epidemiology, evaluation, and treatment of plantar fasciitis. *Life (Basel)*. 2021;11(12):1287.

INDEX

Note: Page number followed by *f* and *t* indicates figure and table respectively.

A

AAC devices, 159
Abdominal wall innervation, 568
Abductor pollicis brevis, 523
Abductor pollicis longus, 523
Abetalipoproteinemia, 306–307
    clinical features of, 306–307
    histopathology of, 307
    laboratory features of, 307
    molecular genetics of, 307
    pathogenesis of, 307
    treatment of, 307, 434
Abscesses
    spinal, 533
    spinal dural, 587
    spinal epidural, 220*t*
Acanthocytosis, vitamin E and, 434
Accessibility issues, management of, 186*t*
Accessory nerve conduction, 26
Acetazolamide, 874, 878–879
Acetazolamide-responsive myotonia, 873, 874
Acetylcholine receptors (AChRs)
    antibodies to, 58, 64–65, 67–68, 240
        in Lambert-Eaton myasthenic syndrome, 665
        in myasthenia gravis, 607, 609–610
    antinicotinic, 240
    in congenital myasthenic syndromes, 673–674
    deficiency of, 672
    function of, 58
    kinetic abnormalities, 673–674
    in Lambert-Eaton myasthenic syndrome, 660
    mutations in, 668, 678
    response to therapy, 115
    senescent, 609
    testing for, 175
    turnover of, 609
Acetylcholine (ACh) release, 33
Acetylcholinesterase (AChE)
    deficiency, 672, 678
    mutations in, 668
Acetylcholinesterase inhibitors (AChEIs), 607, 621, 633–634
Acid maltase deficiency, 799–803
Acid phosphatase stains, 87, 89*f*
Acquired neuromyotonia, 239
Acrocyanosis in PPMA, 225
Acrodermatitis chronica atrophicans, 416
Acromegaly
    myopathies and, 945–946
    neuropathies associated with, 499
Acrylamide, toxic neuropathies and
    clinical features of, 479–480, 479*t*
    diagnostic testing for, 479*t*
    histopathology of, 480
    laboratory features of, 480
    mechanism of, 479*t*
    pathogenesis of, 480
ACTA1 mutations, 743
Actin 1 *(ACTA1)* mutations, 777
Actin filaments, 91, 707
α-Actin *(ACTA1)* mutations, 781–782, 784
Actinin alpha 2 *(ACTN2)* mutations, 778
Activities of daily living (ADLs)
    adaptive equipment for, 146–150
    bathing, 148–149, 148*f*
    dressing, 148, 148*f*
    driving, 149
    leisure activities, 149
    management of, 186*t*
    meal preparation, 147–148
    myasthenia gravis severity and, 631–632, 631*t*
    position transfers, 149
    proximal lower limb weakness and, 152
    self-feeding, 147–148
    toileting, 148–149
Acupuncture for spasticity, 155
Acute autonomic neuropathy, 65
Acute brachial plexitis. *See* Immune-mediated brachial plexus neuropathies (IBPN)
Acute flaccid paralysis, 221–222
Acute flaccid paralysis (AFP)
    differential diagnoses, 220–221, 220*t*
    poliomyelitis and, 219
    viral agents causing, 221*t*
Acute inflammatory demyelinating polyneuropathy (AIDP)
    antiganglioside antibodies associated with, 329*f*
    clinical features of, 327–328, 327*t*
    differential diagnoses of, 330
    electrodiagnosis of, 328–330
    histopathology of, 331*f*
    HIV-related, 419–420
    laboratory features of, 328
    pathogenesis of, 331
Acute lower extremity monoplegia, 591
Acute motor and sensory axonal neuropathy (AMSAN), 335–336. *See also* Inflammatory demyelinating polyradiculoneuropathy (AIDP)
    clinical features of, 335–336
    histopathology of, 336
    laboratory features of, 336
    pathogenesis of, 336
Acute motor axonal neuropathy (AMAN). *See also* Inflammatory demyelinating polyradiculoneuropathy (AIDP)
    antiganglioside antibodies associated with, 329*f*
    autoantibodies linked to, 67
    clinical features of, 334
    electrodiagnostic features of, 329–330
    histopathology of, 331, 335, 335*f*
    laboratory features of, 334–335
    pathogenesis of, 331, 335
    treatment of, 335
Acute quadriplegic myopathy (AQM), 970–971
    clinical features of, 970
    histopathology of, 971, 972*f*
    laboratory features of, 970–971
    pathogenesis of, 971
    treatment of, 971
Acute small fiber sensory neuropathies
    clinical features of, 337
    histopathology of, 338
    laboratory features of, 337
    pathogenesis of, 338
    treatment of, 338
Acyclovir, 422
Acyl-dehydrogenase deficiency, 64
Adalimumab, toxic neuropathies and, 477
Adaptive equipment, 143–150
Adaptive sports, 138–139, 138*f*
Adenoleukodystrophy, 177
Adenosine triphosphatase (ATPase) stains
    myofibrillar, 87*f*
    pH ranges of, 87*f*
    targetoid fibers on, 94
    use of, 93
Adernomyeloneuropathy, 197–198
Adrenal disorders, myopathies and, 944–945
Adrenal hypoplasia congenita (AHC), 714
Adrenal insufficiency
    cramps and, 236
    myopathies and, 945
Adrenergic dysfunction, detection of, 59
Adrenoleukodystrophy (ALD), 300–302
    clinical features of, 300–301
    differential diagnosis of, 197–298
    histopathology of, 302*f*
    laboratory features of, 301
    molecular genetics of, 302
    pathogenesis of, 302
    treatment of, 302
Adrenomyeloneuropathy (AMN), 300–302
ADSSL myopathy, 752
Adult polyglucosan body disease (APBD), 311–313
    clinical features of, 311, 311*f*
    histopathology of, 311–313, 312*f*, 313*f*
    laboratory features of, 311
Adulthood causes of weakness in, 4*t*

Adult-onset limb-girdle muscular dystrophy, 70. *See also* Limb girdle muscular dystrophies (LGMDs)
Adynamia episodica hereditaria, 869–872
Aerobic exercises
　benefits of, 134–137, 134t
　guidelines, 139
Afterdischarges, 30f
Agalsidase alfa, 300
Age/aging
　cramps and, 233
　muscle fiber size and, 93
　myasthenia gravis and, 614
Agrin antibodies, 67
Agrin deficiency, 672f, 674–675, 678
AIDP. *See* Acute inflammatory demyelinating polyneuropathy (AIDP)
Albuterol, oral, 678
Alcian blue
　for amyloid disposition, 89
　amyloid stained by, 103f
　for nerve biopsies, 101
Alcock canal, 576
Alcohol abuse
　myopathies related to, 974–975
　neuropathies related to, 435–436
　peripheral neuropathy related to, 485–486
Aldolase A deficiency, 810
Alendronate, 923–924
ALG2 deficiency, 670t–671t, 671
Alkalosis, tetany and, 245
Alopecia, Satoyoshi syndrome and, 246
Alpha-dystroglycan staining, 89
Alpha-glucosidase, Pompe disease and, 729
Alpha-interferon-related myopathies, 968
Alpha-tocopherol. *See* Vitamin E
ALS. *See* Amyotrophic lateral sclerosis (ALS)
ALS Cognitive Behavioral Screen (ALS CBS), 174
ALS-functional rating scale (ALSFRS-R), 184
ALS-Parkinson-Dementia complex, 168
Amblyomma americanum, 684
Amblyomma maculatum, 684
Amifampridine phosphate, 643, 667
Aminopyridines, 667
Amiodarone
　myopathies related to, 963
　toxic neuropathies and
　　clinical features of, 474t, 477
　　diagnostic testing for, 474t
　　laboratory features of, 477
　　nerve histopathology in, 474t, 477
Amitriptyline, 238t, 495t
Amoxicillin for Lyme disease, 417
Amphetamines, myopathies related to, 975
Amphilic drug myopathy, myopathies related to, 962–963
Amphiphilic myopathies, drugs related to, 958t
Amphiphysin 2 *(BIN2)* mutations, 786
Amphiphysin antibodies, 65, 240, 249, 441
Amphiphysin protein, 249–250
Amygdalar complex, 442f
Amyloid disposition
　endoneurium, 107–108
　staining for, 89, 90f
Amyloid myopathy
　clinical features of, 949

　histopathology of, 949–950, 949f, 950f, 951f
　laboratory features of, 949
　prognosis, 950f
Amyloidosis, 949
　amyloid disposition in, 107–108
　nerve biopsies for, 98–99
　primary
　　clinical features of, 449
　　histopathology of, 450
　　laboratory features of, 449–450
　　pathogenesis of, 450–451
　　treatment of, 451
　signs of, 98–99
Amyotrophic lateral sclerosis (ALS)
　age of onset, 168
　ALSFRS-R scale, 184
　alsin, 182
　ancillary testing in suspected, 174t
　bulbar symptoms in, 11
　bulbar-onset, 172
　characteristics of, 166
　clinical features of, 170–174
　clinical guidelines for, 184–185
　CMAP amplitude in, 41
　course of, 16
　decision-making in support of, 185
　differential diagnosis of, 226
　EMG studies in, 177
　executive function in, 173
　exercise studies in, 135–136
　familial, 168, 178
　FDA-approved medications for, 183t
　genes associated with, 168, 169t, 172
　Gold Coast Criteria for, 167, 167t
　histopathology of, 179–180
　juvenile-onset, 182
　laboratory features of, 177–179
　life expectancy with, 169, 170
　management of, 182–187
　Mills variant, 172
　motor unit numbers in, 41–42
　mutations related to, 708
　nerve conduction studies in, 177
　neuromyotonic discharges in, 240t
　pain in, 155
　pathogenesis of, 180–182
　in polio victims, 226
　presentation of, 170
　progression of, 56
　revised EEC for, 167t
　risk factors for, 168
　second opinion requests in, 177
　spinal cord histopathology, 181f
　sporadic, 166, 168, 174
　support services in, 185
　symptom management in, 186t
Amyotrophy, diabetic, 496–497
Anal sphincter innervation, 576
Anaphylaxis, IVIgs and, 123
ANCA-associated vasculitis, 391
Andersen disease, 804–806, 805f
Andersen syndrome, 879–880
Andersen-Tawil syndrome (ATS), 879–880
Anesthesia for biopsies, 84, 100
ANG mutations, 182
Angiofollicular lymph node hyperplasia, 451
Angiotrophic large-cell lymphomas, 444

Anhidrosis, detection of, 15
Ankle-foot-orthoses (AFOs), 141–143, 142f, 143f, 153
Annulus fibrosis, 565, 566
Anoctamin-5, 706
Anoctamin-5 *(ANO5)* mutations, 726–727
Anterior horn cells, 517
Anterior interosseous neuropathy (AIN), 548, 550, 550t
Anti-Ro/La antibodies, 64
Anti-AChR antibody-positive myasthenia, 124
Antibody-drug conjugates, toxic neuropathies and, 457t, 461
Anticoagulation agents, electromyography safety and, 25
Anticonvulsants for neuropathic pain, 591
Anti-cytoxic T-lymphocyte-associated antigen 4 (anti-CTLA-4), 461
Antidromic technique, 28
Antigliadin, 402
Anti-Hu. *See* Antineuronal nuclear antibody type 1 (ANA-1, anti-Hu)
Anti-Ku associated myositis, 911
Antimicrotubular myopathies, 958t, 963–964
Antineuronal nuclear antibody type 1 (ANA-1, antiHu), 65, 441–442, 511
Antinuclear antibodies (ANAs), 64, 397, 895t
Antinuclear neuronal type 4 antibodies, 240
Anti-programmed cell death-1 receptor (anti-PD1), 461
Anti-programmed death-ligand 1 (anti-PDL1), 461
Antisaccade testing, 173
Antisynthetase syndrome (ASyS)
　clinical features of, 901
　histopathology of, 901, 902f
　laboratory features of, 901
　pathogenesis of, 901
　rituximab for, 124
　use of steroids for, 118
Anti-TG6 antibodies, 402
Antiviral agents, myopathies related to, 965
ANXA11 mutations, 756
Aortic occlusion, 591
Apolipoprotein A1-related amyloidosis, 316
Apraxias
　type 1, 307
Arachnoid membrane, 105
Arachnoiditis, polyradiculopathies and, 588
Arcade de Fröhse, 523
Argyll Robertson pupils, 417
Arm
　medial cutaneous nerve, 522
ARSA gene, 297
Arsenic, toxic neuropathies and
　clinical features of, 484–485
　detection of, 483t
　histopathology of, 485
　laboratory features of, 483t, 484–485
　pathogenesis of, 485
　treatment of, 485
Arthralgias in PPMA, 225
Arthropod venom, 689
Arylsulfatase A (ARSA), 297
Asparagine-related glycosylation (ALG), 676
Asparagine-related glycosylation 2 (ALG2) deficiency, 676

Asparagine-related glycosylation 14 (ALG14) deficiency, 670t–671t, 671, 676
Aspen Vista Collar, 140, 140f
Assistive devices for HSP, 200
Asthenia. See Weakness
Ataxia with oculomotor apraxia (AOA)
　type 1, 307
　type 2, 307–308
Ataxias
　hereditary, 305–310
　progressive, 434
　vitamin E deficiency and, 434
Ataxia-telangiectasia, 308–309
Atezolizumab, 461
Atlastin gene, 198
Atorvastatin, myopathy and, 957–960
Atovaquone, 115–116
Atropine
　for organophosphate toxicity, 688
　for tetanus, 245
Atypical mycobacteria, polyradiculopathies and, 587
Augmentative and alternative communication (AAC), 132, 159
Autoimmune autonomic neuropathy
　clinical features of, 338
　histopathology of, 338
　laboratory features of, 338
　pathogenesis of, 338
　treatment of, 338–339
Autoimmune regulator (AIRE) expression, 611
Autonomic function
　bedside screening tests of, 15
　indications for, 62
Autonomic nervous system (ANS)
　impaired function of, 10
　pharmacology of, 58
　testing, 58–62
Autonomic neuropathies
　diabetic, 493–494
　HIV-related, 421
　malignancies and, 440
　paraneoplastic, 443
　Sjögren syndrome and, 397
Autosomal recessive cardiomyopathy and ophthalmoplegia (ARCO), 845–846
Avelumab, 461
Axial weakness
　in myasthenia gravis, 619–620
　neck muscle weakness and, 9t
　rehabilitation approach for, 150–151
Axilla roll slings, 141
Axillary crutches, 144f
Axillary nerve
　anatomy of, 522–523, 545
　nerve conduction studies using, 27
Axillary neuropathies
　conditions associated with, 545, 545t
Axonal degeneration, 106–108. See also Wallerian degeneration
Axonal sensorimotor polyneuropathies
　alcohol use and, 435–436
　　histopathology of, 436
　　pathogenesis of, 436
　　treatment of, 436
Axonopathies, G ratios in, 106

Axonotmesis, 524
Axons
　breakdown products, 107
　damage to, 107
　degeneration of, 93–94
　enlarged, 107
　loss of, 51
　　pathology localization in, 53
　severance of, 51
Azathioprine
　adverse effects of, 119
　for chronic inflammatory demyelinating polyneuropathy, 357t, 358
　dosage, 119
　dosage of, 113t
　drug interactions with, 120
　for inflammatory myopathies, 922t, 925
　management considerations for, 119–120
　mechanism of action, 119
　monitoring of, 113t, 120
　for multifocal motor neuropathy, 367
　for myasthenia gravis, 641–642
　side effects of, 113t
　uses, 119
Azidothymidine (AZT), 964–965, 965f

B

B3GALNT2 mutations, 735
B4GAT1 mutations, 735
Babinski sign
　in ALS, 171
　cervical radiculopathies and, 533
　UMN pathology and, 14
Back pain, causes of, 565–566
Backpack palsy, 540
Baclofen
　for cramps, 211, 238t
　for HSP management, 199t, 200
　intrathecal
　　for HSP management, 200
　　for spasticity, 155
　for Isaacs syndrome, 242
　for Morvan syndrome, 242
　for stiff person syndrome, 250
　for tetanus, 245
Balance, impaired causes of, 10
Balance exercises, 134t
Balance training, 137–138
Bariatric surgery, deficiencies after
　histopathology of, 434
　neuropathies and, 434
　pathogenesis of, 434
Basement membrane, 91
Bassen-Kornzweig disease, 306–307. See Abetalipoproteinemia
Bathing, 147f
Bathroom safety, 186t
Batoclimab
　function of, 638
　trials of, 639t
B-cell directed therapies
　for myasthenia gravis, 639–641, 640t
　side effects of, 640
BCG vaccinations, 116
BCL2 mutations, 176
Bcl-2-binding protein *(BAG3)* mutations, 754
Becker muscular dystrophy

carriers of, 712, 712f
clinical features of, 710–711
diagnosis of, 711
dystrophin in, 702
dystrophin staining in, 89
histopathology of, 711, 711f, 712f
laboratory features of, 711
muscle in, 711f
outliers, 711
Bed mobility
　adaptive equipment for, 149
　management of, 186t
Behçet syndrome, 388, 916
　clinical features of, 916
　histopathology of, 916
　laboratory features of, 916
　pathogenesis of, 916
　prognosis, 916
Benadryl for cramps, 238t
Benign focal amyotrophies (BFAs), 211–213
　clinical features of, 211–212
　differential diagnosis of, 212
　electrodiagnosis of, 213
　histopathology of, 213
　laboratory features of, 212–213
　management of, 213
　pathophysiology of, 213
Bent spine syndrome, 745–746, 779
Benzodiazepines
　for HSP management, 199t
　for stiff person syndrome, 250
　for tetanus, 245
Beradinelli-Seip congenital lipodystrophy 2 (BSCL2) mutations, 176
Beriberi. See Thiamine deficiency
Beta-adrenergic agonists, 871–872
B2-microglobulin, hemodialysis and, 403
Beta-blockers
　caution in use of, 626t
　in myasthenia gravis, 626t
　for thyrotoxic myopathy, 941
Betamethasone, 969
Bethanechol, 338
Bethlem myopathy, 730–731, 730f
Bevacizumab, myopathies related to, 968–969
Biceps tendinopathy
　diagnosis of, 985–986
　symptoms of, 985
　treatment of, 986, 986f
Bickerstaff encephalitis syndrome, 336
Bing-Neel syndrome, 453
Biopsies of nerves, 98–108
Bisphosphonates, 923–924
Black widow spiders, 689
Blinking, repetitive, 14
Blood sugar testing, 62
Blood testing
　cost effectiveness of, 62
　for peripheral neuropathy, 62–64
Blood vessel endothelial substance *(BVES)* mutations, 729
Blood-nerve barriers, 105
Bobath slings, 141
Bodian stain, 101
Bone density screening, 923

Borrelia burgdorferi. See also Lyme disease
  Lyme disease and, 416
  neuropathies and, 412*f*
Bortezomib (Velcade), 457*t*, 460
Botulinum toxin
  contraindication for, 626*t*
  for cramps, 238*t*
  denaturation of, 681
  foodborne, 679, 681
  for HSP management, 199*t*, 200
  in myasthenia gravis, 625
  response to, 625
  for spasticity, 155
  for stiff person syndrome, 250
  terrorism and, 681
Botulism, 679–684
  clinical features of, 679–681
  cranial nerve involvement in, 19
  diagnosis of, 220*t*, 680, 681–682
  differential diagnoses, 681–682
  features of, 220*t*, 221
  fibrillation potentials in, 56
  "hidden," 681
  histopathology of, 683
  iatrogenic, 681
  infantile, 679–681, 683–684
  laboratory features of, 682–683
  mechanisms of, 680
  morbidity of, 680
  pathogenesis of, 683
  treatment of, 683–684
  wound, 681
Botulism immune globulin (BIG), 683–684
Bouin's fluid, 84
Boxsero for myasthenia gravis, 637
Braces (orthoses), 140–143, 140*f*
Brachial amyotrophic diplegia (BAD), 172
Brachial plexopathies, 446–447
  classification of, 533–535
  surgical treatment of, 542
Brachial plexus
  anatomy of, 518–521, 519*f*, 528*f*, 529*f*
  disorders of, 535–542
  injuries to, 535*t*
  neoplasms of, 541*f*
  neoplastic invasion of, 447
Brachial plexus neuritis
  features of, 17
Bracing, rehabilitation using, 154–155
Brain-computer interfaces (BCIs), 159
Brentuzimab vedotin, toxic neuropathies and, 457*t*, 461
Brody disease, 880–881
  electrical silence and, 234
  features of, 234
  SRCA1 mutations and, 707
Brown widow spiders, 689
Brown-Vialetto-Van Laere syndrome
  features of, 204*t*
Brown-Vialetto-Van Laere (BVVLS) syndrome, 209
Brunina body in ALS, 179
Bruns-Garland syndrome, 496–497, 590. See also Diabetic lumbosacral radiculoplexus neuropathy
Bulbar syndromes, evaluation of, 11

Bulbar weakness, 156
Bulbospinal muscular atrophy (SBMA), 209
  clinical features of, 209
Bupivacaine for tetanus, 245
Burners/stingers, 540

C

C5 radiculopathies, 531
C6 radiculopathies, 531–532
C7 radiculopathies, 532
C8/T1 radiculopathies, 532
Cafe-au-lait patches, 13
Calcinosis in dermatomyositis, 894*f*
Calciphylaxis, 942
Calcium
  ACh release and, 666
  for cramps, 236, 238*t*
  serum levels of, 943
  for tetany, 246
Calcium channel α-1 subunit, 877
Calcium channel α-1 subunit *(CACNA1S)* mutations, 874, 877
N-type calcium channel antigen antibody, 65
Calcium channelopathies, 876–879
Calcium channels, 879*f*
Calcium supplementation, 923, 943
Calf-spasms, Satoyoshi syndrome and, 246
Calpain-3, function of, 708
Calpain-3 *(CAPN3)* mutation, 719, 721
Calsequestrin *(CASQ1)* mutations, 790
Camptocormia
  in myasthenia gravis, 617
  neck muscle weakness and, 9*t*
  rehabilitation approach for, 150
Campylobacter jejuni, 334
  gangliosides on surface of, 355
  Guillain-Barré syndrome and, 326
  multifocal motor neuropathy and, 367
Cancers. See also Malignancies
  immunotherapies and, 117–118
Candida infections, myositis and, 920
Canes, 143–145
Cannabinoids for HSP management, 199*t*
CANVAS, 308
CAP myopathy, 782–784
Capsaicin
  for HVZ infections, 422
  for painful sensory neuronopathies, 495*t*, 510*t*
  for urinary urgency
    in HSP, 200
Carbamate poisoning, 686–688
  diagnosis of, 687
  features of, 686–687
  laboratory features of, 687
  treatment of, 687–688
Carbamazepine
  for cramps, 211, 238*t*, 239
  for HVZ infections, 422
  for hyperekplexia, 251
  for Isaacs syndrome, 242
  for Morvan syndrome, 242
  for neuropathic pain, 591
  for painful sensory neuronopathies, 510*t*
  for Satoyoshi syndrome, 247

Carbohydrate metabolism disorders, 798–811, 799*t*
Carbon disulfide, toxic neuropathies and
  clinical features of, 479*t*
  diagnostic testing for, 479*t*
  laboratory features of, 479*t*, 480
  mechanism of, 479*t*
  pathogenesis of, 480
Carbon fiber dorsiflexion assist orthoses, 142*f*
Carbon fiber posterior leaf spring ankle-foot orthoses, 142*f*
Carboplatin, neuropathies secondary to
  clinical features of, 455
  histopathology of, 455
  laboratory features of, 455
  pathogenesis of, 455
Cardiac medications, toxic neuropathies and, 477
Cardiomyopathies
  AChR mutations in, 673
  in Duchenne muscular dystrophy, 714
Cardiovagal dysfunction, detection of, 59
Caregivers, lifting assistance for, 149
Carfilzomib, toxic neuropathies and, 457*t*, 460
Carnitine deficiencies, 64, 818–819, 818*f*
  L-carnitine supplementation in, 819
Carnitine palmitoyl transferase 2 (CPT2) deficiency, 819
Carnitine transporter deficiency, 818–819
Carpal spasm, tetany and, 245
Carpal tunnel syndrome (CTS), 552*t*
  acromegaly and, 499
  hypothyroidism and, 499–500
  renal failure and, 403
  symptoms of, 17
Carpometacarpal joint osteoarthritis, 988–989
  diagnosis of, 988
  symptoms of, 988
  treatment of, 989
Caspr-I antibody, 362
Casting, serial, 155
Castleman disease, 451, 452
Cataracts, 924
Cauda equina syndrome, 584
Caveolae-associated protein 4 (cavin-4) autoantibodies, 234
Caveolin staining, 89
Caveolin-3, function of, 706
Caveolin-3 gene *(CAV3)* mutation, 234, 717
Cavus deformity in HSP, 196*f*
CDP-L-ribitol phosphorylase A *(CRPPA)* mutations, 729
Ceftriaxone for Lyme disease, 417
Celiac disease
  clinical features of, 402
  histopathology of, 402
  identification of, 69
  laboratory features of, 402
  pathogenesis of, 402
  treatment of, 402
Cellular nucleic acid-binding protein *(CNBP)* mutations, 861
Cemiplimab, 461
Central and peripheral demyelination (CCPD), 362

Central core myopathy
   clinical features of, 773
   histopathology of, 773, 776, 776f
   laboratory features of, 773
   molecular genetics of, 776–777
   pathogenesis of, 776–777
Centronuclear myopathy
   clinical features of, 784–785
   histopathology of, 785, 785f, 786f
   laboratory features of, 785
   molecular genetics of, 785–786
   pathogenesis of, 785–786
Cephalosporins for tetanus, 245
Cerebellar ataxia, malignancies and, 440
Cerebellar ataxia, neuropathy and vestibular areflexia syndrome (CANVAS), 308, 509
Cerebellar dysfunction, malignancies and, 440
Cerebral palsy, diagnosis of, 198
Cerebrospinal fluid (CSF)
   analysis of, 69
   oligoclonal bands in, 249
   in poliomyelitis, 221
   testing in peripheral neuropathy, 62
Cerebrospinal fluid (CSF) barrier, 105
Cerebrotendinous xanthomatosis, 305
Cerivastatiin, myopathy and, 957–960
Certolizumab, toxic neuropathies and, 477
Ceruloplasmin, serum levels of, 177
Cervical canal stenosis, spastic paresis in, 197
Cervical collars, 170f
Cervical orthoses, 140, 140f
Cervical radiculopathies, 527–531
   C5, 527
   multiple, 532
Cervical spine, MRI of, 530f
Cervical spondylotic myelopathy, 176
Cervical vertebrae, anatomy of, 517–518
Cervical-medullary junction degeneration, 198
CFS, histopathology of, 236
Charcot-Marie-Tooth disease (CMT), 850–851
   classification of, 257t–258t, 259f
   exercise studies in, 136
   features of, 10, 12
   gait analysis in, 153
   genes involved in, 257t–258t
   genetic testing in, 70
   inheritance of, 256, 257t–258t
   neuromyotonic discharges in, 240, 240t
   orthotic devices for, 153
   sacral nerve roots in, 585, 586f
   subtypes of, 256
   type 1, 256–263
      clinical features of, 256, 257–259, 261f
      description of, 256
      histopathology of, 261, 262f
      laboratory features of, 259–261, 267
      molecular genetics of, 261
   type 1A (CMT-De-AD-PMP22), 261–263
   type 1B (CMT-De-AD-MPZ), 262f, 263
   type 1C (CMT-De-AD-LITAF), 262f
   type 1D (CMT-De-AD-ERG2), 263
   type 1E (CMT-De-AD-PMP22), 263
   type 1F (CMT-De-AD-NEFL), 263
   type 1G (CMT-De-AD-PMP22), 263
   type 2
      description of, 256
      histopathology of, 267–268
      laboratory features of, 267–268
      molecular genetics of, 268–269
      pathogenesis of, 268–269
   type 2A1, 268
   type 2A2, 268
   type 2A2 (CMT-Ax-AD-MFN2), 268
   type 2B1 (CMT-Ax-AR-LMN), 266, 268
   type 2B2 (CMT-Ax-AR-PNPK), 266, 268
   type 2C (CMT-Ax-AD-TRPV), 266, 268
   type 2D (CMT-Ax-AD-GARS1), 266, 268
   type 2E (CMT-Ax-AD-NEFL), 266, 268
   type 2EE (CMT-Ax-AD-MPV17), 266, 268
   type 2F (CMT-Ax-AR-HSPB1), 266, 268
   type 2I (CMT-Ax-AD-MPZ), 266, 268
   type 2J (CMT-Ax-AD-MPZ), 266, 268
   type 2K (CMT-Ax-AD-GADP1), 266
   type 2K (CMT-Ax-AD-GDAP1), 268–269
   type 2L (CMT-Ax-AD-HSPB8), 266, 269
   type 2M (CMT-Ax-IN-AD-DNM2), 266
   type 2M (CMT-Ax-In-AD-DNM2), 269
   type 2N (CMT-Ax-AD-AARS), 266, 269
   type 2O (CMT-Ax-AD-DYNC1H1), 266, 269
   type 2P (CMT-Ax-AD-LRSAM), 267, 269
   type 2P (CMT-Ax-AD-LRSAM1), 267
   type 2Q (CMT-Ax-AD-DHTKD1), 267, 269
   type 2R (CMT-Ax-AR-TRIM2), 267, 269
   type 2S (CMT-Ax-AR-IGHMBP2), 267, 269
   type 2T (CMT-Ax-AD-MME), 267, 269
   type 2U (CMT-Ax-AD-MARS1), 267, 269
   type 2V (CMT-Ax-AD-NAGLU), 267, 269
   type 2W (CMT-Ax-AD-HARS1), 267, 268–269
   type 2X (CMT-Ax-AR-SPB11), 267
   type 2X (CMT-Ax-AR-SPG11), 269
   type 2Y (CMT-Ax-AD-VCP), 267, 269
   type 2Z (CMT-Ax-AD-MORC2), 267
   type 3
      clinical features of, 270–271
      description of, 256
      histopathology of, 271
      laboratory features of, 271
      molecular genetics of, 271
      pathogenesis of, 271
   type 4, 256
   type 4 (CMT-De-AR-GENE), 272
   type 4A (CMT-De-AR-GDAP1), 271
   type 4B, 271–274
   type 4B1 (CMT-De-AR-MTMR2), 271
   type 4B2 (CMT-De-AR-SBF2), 272
   type 4B3 (CMT-De-AR-SBF1), 272
   type 4C (CMT-De-AR-SG3TC2), 272, 273
   type 4D (CMT-De-AR-NDRG1), 272
   type 4E, 273
   type 4E (CMT-Di-AR-ERG2), 272
   type 4F (CMT-De-AR-PRX), 272, 273
   type 4G (CMT-De-AR-HK1), 272, 273–274
   type 4H (CMT-De-AR-FDG4), 272, 273–274
   type 4J (CMT-De-AR-FIG4), 272, 274
   type 4K (CMT-De-AR-SIRF1), 274
   type CMTRC (CMT-In-AR-PLEKHG5), 270
   type CMTRIB (CMT-In-AR-KARS1), 270
   type DIB (CMT-In-AD-DNM2), 270
   type DIC (CMT-In-AD-YARS1), 270
   type DIE (CMT-In-AD-IFN2), 270
   type DIF (CMT-In-AD-GNB4), 270
   type DIG (CMT-De-AD-NEFL), 270
   type X4 (CMT-Ax-XLR-AIFM1), 275
   type X5 (CMT-Ax-XLR-PRPS1), 275
   type X6 (CMT-In-XLD-PDK3), 275
   X-linked (CMT-In-XLD-GJB1), 274
Check-point inhibitor-associated myasthenia, 915
Check-point inhibitor-associated myositis, 915
Chelation therapy, 482
Chemotherapy, neuropathies secondary to, 455–463
Chicken pox, neuropathies and, 421–422
Chimeric autoantibody receptor (CCART) cell therapy, 642, 643t
Chin tuck technique, 157
Chlorambucil, 926
Chloramphenicol, 405
Chloride channel (CLCN1) mutations, 869
Chloride channels, myotonia congenita and, 28, 36–37
Chloroquine
   caution in use of, 626t
   in myasthenia gravis, 626t
   myopathies related to, 962–963, 962f
   toxic neuropathies and, 473t, 475–476
Cholestanolosis, 305
Cholesterol-lowering drugs
   inflammatory myopathies and, 965–966
   myopathies and, 961
   toxic myopathies and, 957
Choline acetyltransferase (ChAT)
   in congenital myasthenic syndromes, 672
   deficiency, 672, 678
Choline transporter 1 (CHT1) mutations, 672
Cholinergic dysautonomia
   features of, 19
   testing for, 175
Cholinergic receptor nicotinic alpha 1 subunit (CHRNA1) gene, 612
Cholinergic receptor nicotinic beta 1 subunit (CHRNB1) gene, 612
Chondrodystrophic myotonia, 881
Chorioretinitis, WNV and, 223
Chromosome 9 open reading frame (C9ORF72) mutation, 168, 181, 182
Chronic acquired demyelinating polyneuropathies
   diagnostic algorithm for, 348f
Chronic ataxia neuropathy with disialosyl antibodies (CANDA), 454
Chronic ataxic neuropathy, ophthalmoplegia, IgM paraprotein, cold agglutinins and disialosyl antibodies (CANOMAD), 454
Chronic demyelinating neuropathies, 64, 106f
Chronic immune sensory polyradiculopathy (CISP)
   clinical features of, 368
   histopathology of, 368, 370f
   laboratory features of, 368, 369f
   treatment of, 368

Chronic inflammatory demyelinating
    polyneuropathy (CIDP), 67
  assessment for, 64, 115
  azathioprine for, 119
  clinical features of, 349–350
  corticosteroids for, 118
  cyclophosphamide for, 122
  diagnosis of, 350–352
  diagnostic algorithm for, 348f
  diagnostic criteria, 353t
  differential diagnosis of, 328, 330, 350–352, 590
  disease associations in, 351t
  distal, 346
  electrodiagnostic features of, 352
  features of, 347t
  focal, 346
  histopathologic features of, 104f, 354, 355f
  HIV-related
    clinical features of, 419–420
    laboratory features of, 420
    treatment of, 420
  IVIGs for, 122
  laboratory features of, 352, 354
  mimics for, 351t
  motor, 346
  multifocal, 346
  neuroimaging features of, 352, 354
  neuromyotonic discharges in, 240, 240t
  pathogenesis of, 354–356
  phenotypes of, 346
  plasma exchange for, 125
  rituximab for, 123–124
  SCIg for, 123
  sensory, 346
  treatment of, 356–358, 357t
Chronic inflammatory sensory
    polyradiculopathy (CISP), 346
  CIDP and, 346
  diagnostic algorithm for, 348f
  features of, 347t
  treatment of, 357t
Chronic liver disease, neuropathies associated
    with, 404
Chronic renal failure, hyperparathyroidism
    and, 942
Churg-Strauss syndrome (CSS), 108f, 387–388
Chvostek sign, 239, 245, 948
Cimetidine, myopathies related to, 968
Cisapride, 338
Cisplatin, toxic neuropathies and
  clinical features of, 455, 456t
  histopathology of, 455
  laboratory features of, 455
  mechanism of, 456t
  nerve histopathology of, 456t
  pathogenesis of, 455
Clindamycin for tetanus, 245
Clobazam for hyperekplexia, 251
Clofazimine for leprosy, 413, 416
Clofibrate, myopathies related to, 960
Clonazepam for hyperekplexia, 251
Clonidine for tetanus, 245
Clonus, sustained
  in ALS, 171
  cervical radiculopathies and, 533
Clostridium tetani
  culturing of, 243–244
  exotoxins of, 244
  spores of, 244
  tetanus and, 244
Clumsiness, weakness and, 14
Cobalamin
  deficiency of, 431–432
  function of, 432
Cobra (*Naja* sp.) venom, 688
Cocaine, myopathies related to, 975
Cockayne syndrome, 309
Cogan eyelid twitch sign, 11–12, 619t
Coiflin-2 (*CFL2*) mutations, 778, 782
Coiled-coil domain-containing (*CCDC78*)
    mutation, 777, 778, 786
Colchicine, 477
  for amyloidosis, 451
  drug interactions with, 433
  myopathies related to, 963, 964f
  toxic neuropathies and, 477
    clinical features of, 474t
    diagnostic testing for, 474t
    nerve histopathology in, 474t
Collagen 6 (*COL6*) mutations, 730–731, 734–735
Collagen Q, MuSK and, 611
Collapsing response-mediator protein-5
    (CRMP-5) antibody, 65, 67, 441
COLQ gene, 673
Common fibular nerve, anatomy of, 574
Common fibular neuropathy, 598–599
Common peroneal nerve, conduction studies
    using, 26
Communication issues, management of, 186t
Compartment syndromes, monomelic
    polyneuropathy and, 600
Complement system
  inhibitors of, 636–638, 636t
  role in myasthenia gravis, 610–611
Complex repetitive discharges, 43f, 44
Compound motor action potentials
    (CMAPs)
  aftercharges, 27–28
  cecline between responses, 33
  demyelination and, 50
  orthodromic response, 31
  parameters for, 26–28
  pathology localization and, 53
  short segmental stimulation in, 28f
  temperature considerations in, 23, 24f
  waveform changes, 50
Compression gloves, 152
Compression neuropathies, 384t
Compression stockings, 155–156
Computed tomography (CT) scans
  efficacy of, 71
  lumbosacral spine, 578
Conduction block
  demyelination and, 50
  focal demyelination and
    ulnar neuropathy and, 28f
  timing of studies of, 26
Conduction slowing
  axon loss and, 51
  demyelination and, 51
Conduction velocity, 30
Cone snail venom, 690
Congenital fiber-type disproportion, 786–787, 787f
Congenital hypomyelinating neuropathy. See
    Charcot-Marie-Tooth disease (CMT),
    type 3
Congenital indifference to pain. See Hereditary
    sensory and autonomic neuropathies
    (HSANs), type 5
Congenital insensitivity to pain with
    anhidrosis. See Hereditary sensory and
    autonomic neuropathies (HSANs),
    type 4
Congenital muscular dystrophies (MDCs)
  affected proteins, 703t–704t
  alpha-dystroglycan staining for, 89
  causes of, 733
  classification of, 733
  diagnosis of, 737, 738f–739f
  dystroglycanopathies, 735
  genetic testing in, 70
  MDC1C/MDDGB5, 736–737
  MDC1D/MDDGA6, 737
  MDCA
    clinical features of, 733
    histopathology of, 734, 734f
    laboratory features of, 733, 733f
    molecular genetics of, 734
    pathogenesis of, 734
  merosin staining for, 89
  merosin-positive, 734
  selenoprotein N1-associated, 737
  treatment of, 737
Congenital myasthenic syndromes (CMSs)
  clinical features of, 668, 669t, 671–677
  diagnosis of, 670t–671t, 676–677
    neonatal period, 676
  differential diagnosis of, 676–677
  electrophysical features of, 669t
  histopathology of, 677
  pathogenesis of, 677–678
  postsynaptic, 673
  protein deficiencies, 669t
  response to AChE inhibitors, 669t
  treatment of, 669t, 678
Congenital myopathies, 773–797
  central cores in, 94
  clinical features of, 774t–775t
  inheritance of, 774t–775t
  type 1 fibers in, 87
Congenital myotonic dystrophy, 857
Congo red stain
  for amyloid disposition, 89, 90f
  amyloid stained by, 103f
  for nerve biopsies, 101
Connectin. See Titin
Connective tissue diseases, neuropathies
    associated with, 397–400
Constipation, management of, 186t
Contactin-1 (CNTN1) antibodies, 67
Contactin-associated protein like-2 (CASPR2)
    antibodies, 240, 242
Contactin-associated protein-1 (Caspr1), 67
Contractures
  hip, 152
  joint, 12t
  knee, 152
  management of, 186t

muscle, 12
  neuromuscular diseases and, 154–155
  surgical management of, 155
Conus medullaris syndrome, 586
Coordination, impaired, 171
Copper deficiency
  in ALS, 177
  clinical features of, 435
  histopathology of, 435
  laboratory features of, 435
  pathogenesis of, 435
  presentation of, 198
  treatment of, 435
Core-rod myopathy, 778, 779f
Cori-Forbes disease, 803–804
Coronavirus disease 2019. *See* Severe acute respiratory syndrome coronavirus 2 (SARS-CoV-2)
Corticobulbar tract, pseudobulbar palsy and, 6
Corticospinal tracts
  degeneration of, 198
  motor function and, 14
Corticosteroid myopathy, 969–970
Corticosteroids
  adverse effects of, 118
  caution in use of, 626t
  for chronic immune sensory polyradiculopathy, 368
  for chronic inflammatory demyelinating polyneuropathy, 356
  for HIV-related mononeuropathies, 421
  for inflammatory myopathies, 112, 923
  for Lambert-Eaton myasthenic syndrome, 667
  for leprosy, 416
  management considerations for, 118–119
  mechanism of action, 118, 969f
  for myasthenia gravis, 112, 626t
  for neurolymhomatosis, 445–446
  for nodopathies, 365
  for paranodopathies, 365
  for polymyalgia rheumatica, 951
  for radioplexus neuropathies, 591
  risk of infectious diseases and, 115
  for Satoyoshi syndrome, 247
  steroid myopathy and, 944–945
  strongyloidiasis infection and, 117
  uses of, 118
  for vasculitis, 391
Corynebacterium diphtheriae, 412f, 418
COVID-19, postinfectious LRPN, 590
COVID-19 vaccines, 117, 648
Coxsackievirus A16, 221, 221t
Cramp discharges, 235
Cramp potentials, disorders associated with, 45
Cramp-fasciculation syndrome (CFS)
  clinical features of, 233–234
  diagnosis of, 234–235
  histopathology of, 236
  laboratory features of, 235–236
  pathogenesis of, 236–237
  treatment of, 237–239, 238t
Cramps. *See* Muscle cramps
  management of, 211
Cranial nerves
  motor examination of, 11
  sensory function and, 7

Creatine kinase (CK)
  serum levels of
    in dystrophinopathies, 709–710
    myopathies and, 64
    in RHB/MGU, 20–21
Creatinine for cramps, 236, 238t
Cresyl violet, 89, 101
Cricopharyngeal myotomy, 158
Critical illness mononeuropathy (CIM), 405–406
Critical illness myopathy (CIM), 970–971, 971f
  drugs related to, 958t
  sarcomeres in, 92f
Critical illness polyneuropathy (CIP), 405–406
  clinical features of, 405
  histopathology of, 405–406
  laboratory features of, 405
  pathogenesis of, 406
  treatment of, 406
CRMP-5 antibodies, 240
Crohn disease (CD), neuropathies associated with, 402–403
Crow-Fukase syndrome, 451
Crutches, 144, 144f
Crystallin, 707
αβ-Crystallin *(CRYAB)* mutations, 754
Cuprophane membranes for dialysis, 403
Curtain's sign, 618, 619t
Cushing disease, 944–945
Cutaneous nerves
  dermatomal representation of, 520f
Cutaneous nerves, leprosy and, 411
Cyanocobalamin deficiency, 74f
Cyclophosphamide
  adverse effects of, 122
  for chronic inflammatory demyelinating polyneuropathy, 357t, 359
  contraindications for, 646–647
  dosage of, 122
  for HIV-related mononeuropathies, 421
  for inflammatory myopathies, 922t, 926
  management of, 122
  mechanism of action for, 122
  for neuromuscular disorders
    dosage, 113t
    monitoring of, 113t
    side effects of, 113t
  for radioplexus neuropathies, 591
  uses of, 122
  for vasculitis, 391
Cyclosporine
  adverse effects of, 121
  for chronic inflammatory demyelinating polyneuropathy, 357t, 358
  dosage of, 121
  for inflammatory myopathies, 922t, 926
  management of, 121
  mechanism of action, 121
  for multifocal motor neuropathy, 367
  myopathies related to, 961
  statin myopathy and, 957
  uses for, 121
Cystic fibrosis, vitamin E deficiency and, 434
Cysticercosis, myositis associated with, 921
Cytomegalovirus (CMV)
  Guillain-Barré syndrome and, 326
  neuropathies and, 412f, 421

  polyradiculopathies and, 230, 587
  polyradiculopathies secondary to, 420
Cytosine arabinoside (ARA-C)
  toxic neuropathies and, 457t
Cytosine arabinoside (ARA-C) toxicity, 457t
Cytotoxic T-lymphocyte-associated protein 4 (CTLA-4), 611

D

DADS. *See* Distal acquired demyelinating sensory neuropathy (DADS)
Danon disease, 812–813
Dantrolene
  for Brody disease, 881
  for HSP management, 199t, 200
  for stiff person syndrome, 250
Dapsone
  for leprosy, 413
  for pneumocystic pneumonia, 115–116
  toxic neuropathies and
    clinical features of, 473t
    diagnostic testing for, 473t
    mechanism of, 475
    nerve histopathology in, 473t, 475
Darifenacin for urinary urgency, 200
Davidenkow disease, 215
  clinical features of, 215
  differential diagnosis of, 215
  electrodiagnosis of, 215
  histopathology of, 215
  management of, 215
  pathogenesis of, 215
DAX1 gene, 714
DCTN1 mutations, 176
De Quervain tenosynovitis, 987–988
  diagnosis of, 987–988
  pain in, 155
  symptoms of, 987
  treatment of, 987–988
Decrement, definition of, 624
Deep breathing
  heart rate response to, 60f
  pulse variation and, 15
Deep tendon reflexes
  in ALS, 171
  diminished, 16
  hyperactive, 14
  in myasthenia gravis, 19
  in stiff-person syndrome, 248
Deferoxamine, caution in use of in, 626t
Defibrillators, conduction considerations with, 25
Deflazacort for Duchenne muscular dystrophy, 713
Déjérine-Sottas disease. *See* Charcot-Marie-Tooth disease (CMT), type 3
Demyelination
  conduction slowing and, 51
  focal
    conduction block with, 28f
    pathology localization an d, 53
  forms of, 51
  MRI of, 73
  nerve injury and, 106–108
Denervation
  muscle fibers and, 93–94, 94f
  reinnervation and, 96

Dengue virus, 221, 221t
Dental care in myasthenia gravis, 648
Deoxyguanosine kinase *(DGOUK)* mutations, 846
Depression, management of, 186t
Dermacentor andersoni (wood tick), 684
Dermacentor variabilis (dog tick), 684, 684f
Dermatomes
　clinical map, 580f
　cutaneous nerves, 520f
　description of, 517
Dermatomyositis (DM)
　associated conditions, 888t, 892–894
　autoantibodies in, 894–895, 895t
　clinical features of, 887, 888t, 891–892, 893f, 894f
　diagnosis of, 109
　diagnostic criteria for, 889t–891t
　electrophysiological features of, 895–896
　exercise studies in, 137
　histopathologic features of, 97, 888t
　histopathology of, 896–897, 896f, 897f
　laboratory features of, 888t, 894–895
　pathogenesis of, 897–898
　prognosis in, 898
　tacrolimus for, 122
　tofacitinib for, 125
　treatment of, 888t
　use of steroids for, 118
Desmin, 707
Desmin *(DES)* mutations, 718, 728, 743, 754–755, 792
Dexamethasone, 969
Dextromethorphan, 495t
Diabetes mellitus
　meralgia paresthetica and, 596–597
　microvasculitis associated with, 389
　myopathies and, 946–947
　neuropathies related to, 491–498
Diabetic amyotrophy, 496–497. *See also* Diabetic lumbosacral radiculoplexus neuropathy; Diabetic lumbosacral radiculoplexus neuropathy (DLRPN)
Diabetic autonomic neuropathies
　clinical features of, 493–494
　histopathology of, 494–495
　laboratory features of, 494
　mechanisms of, 494f
　pathogenesis of, 495
　treatment of, 495
Diabetic cachexia, 590
Diabetic femoral neuropathy, 590. *See also* Diabetic lumbosacral radiculoplexus neuropathy
Diabetic ketoacidosis, 948
Diabetic lumbosacral radiculoplexopathy, 496–497, 497f
Diabetic lumbosacral radiculoplexus neuropathy (DLRPN), 589–591
Diabetic multiple mononeuropathies, 498
Diabetic muscle infarctions, 946–947, 947f
Diabetic myonecrosis, 946–947
Diabetic neuropathic cachexia (DNC)
　clinical features of, 495
　histopathology of, 495
　laboratory features of, 495
　treatment of, 495

Diabetic neuropathy
　clinical features of, 491
　diagnosis of, 63
　incidence of, 491
Diabetic patients, thermal testing of, 57
Diabetic polyradiculopathy, 496
　asymmetric, painful, 496–497
　symmetric, painless, 497–498
　　clinical features of, 497
　　histopathology of, 497
　　laboratory features of, 497
　　pathogenesis of, 497
　　treatment of, 497–498
Diabetic radiculoplexopathy
　features of, 17
　plasma exchange for, 125
Diagnoses, symptom development and, 2
3,4-Diaminopyridine (3,4-DAP), 667
Diaphragm
　weakness of, 9–10
Diastase, PAS stains with, 87
Diatase, PAS stains with, 88f
Diazepam
　for hyperekplexia, 251
　for stiff person syndrome, 250
Dichlorphenamide for hypoKPP1, 878–879
Didanosine
　myopathies related to, 965
　toxic neuropathies and, 476
Diffuse fasciitis with eosinophilia, 912, 912f
Digits
　extension of, 13
　weakness of, 7
Dihydropyridine receptors, 707, 879f
Diphtheritic neuropathy, 418
　clinical features of, 418
　histopathology of, 418
　laboratory features of, 418
　pathogenesis of, 418
　treatment of, 418
Diplopia
　extraocular muscles and, 7
　myasthenia gravis and, 616–617
Disc herniation, lumbar, 581f
Disorders of neuromuscular transmission (DNMT), 660–700
　antibody testing for, 67–68
　electrodiagnostic approach to, 34–35
　fibrillation potentials in, 44
　other than autoimmune mg, 661t
　temperature considerations in, 23
Distal acquired demyelinating sensory neuropathy (DADS), 66
　CIDP and, 346
　clinical features of, 360
　cyclophosphamide for, 122
　diagnostic algorithm for, 348f
　electrodiagnostic features of, 360–361
　features of, 347t
　histopathology of, 361
　IgM monoclonal gammopathy and, 361
　laboratory features of, 361, 453
　pathogenesis of, 361
　treatment of, 357t, 361
　use of steroids in, 118
Distal dystrophies, affected proteins, 704t
Distal myopathies, treatment of, 752

Distal myopathy with vocal cord paralysis, 708
Distal myopathy/muscular dystrophy, 748, 749f
Distal spinal muscular atrophy (dSMA), 213–214
　classification of, 214
　clinical features of, 214
　differential diagnosis of, 214
　electrodiagnosis of, 214
　histopathology of, 214–215
　laboratory features of, 214
　management of, 215
　pathogenesis of, 215
Distal symmetric sensory polyneuropathy (DSPN)
　clinical features of, 491
　definition of, 55
　diabetes and, 491–493
　HIV-related
　　clinical features of, 419
　　histopathology of, 419
　　laboratory features of, 419
　　pathogenesis of, 419
　　treatment of, 419
　laboratory features of, 491–492
　nerve histopathology in, 492–493, 492f, 493f
　pathogenesis of, 493
　treatment of, 493
Disulfiram
　toxic neuropathies and, 478
　　clinical features of, 474t
　　diagnostic testing for, 474t
　　nerve histopathology in, 474t
Disuse myopathy, type 2B fibers in, 87
DNA repair disorders, 308–310
DNMT3B mutations, 741
Docetaxel (Taxotere)
　toxic neuropathies and, 456t, 458–459
Dok-7 deficiency, 670t–671t, 671
　in congenital myasthenic syndromes, 672, 678
　presentation of, 673
Dolichy-phosphate N-acetylglucosamine-phosphotransferase 1 (DPAGT1) deficiency, 675–676
Dopa-responsive dystonia, 176
Dorsal cutaneous ulnar nerve, conduction studies, 28
Dorsal nerve of the penis, 576
Dorsal root ganglionopathies, 442f
　causes of, 55
　etiologies of, 16
　features of, 16
Dorsal root ganglions (DRGs), 517
Dorsal roots, spinal nerve, 517
Dorsal scapular nerve
　anatomy of, 521, 522
　damage to, 542–543
Dostarlimab, 461
Doxycycline for Lyme disease, 417
DPAGT1 deficiency, 670t–671t, 671
Dressing, adaptive equipment for, 148f
Driving, adaptive equipment for, 149
Drooling, 157
Dropped head syndrome, 745–746
Drug-induced autophagic lysosmal myopathy, 962–963
Drug-induced hypersensitivity vasculitis, 389

Drugs of abuse, myopathies related to, 975
Duchenne muscular dystrophy (DMD)
 clinical features of, 709, 709f
 dystrophin in, 702
 dystrophin staining in, 89
 exercise studies in, 136
 histopathology of, 710, 710f
 infertility and, 712
 laboratory features of, 709–710
 rehabilitation approaches, 151
Duloxetine
 for diabetic neuropathy, 493
 for neuropathic pain, 591
 for painful sensory neuronopathies, 495t, 510t
Dura, innervation of, 565
Durable medical equipment (DME), 133
Dural arteriovenous fistulas, spinal, 589
Dural vascular malformations, spinal, 586–587
Durvalumab, 461
DUX4 mutations, 741
Dynamin-2 *(DYN2)* mutation, 786
Dynamometry, handheld, 115
Dysarthria
 in ALS, 170
 definition of, 158
 rehabilitation for, 158–159
Dysautonomia
 in botulism, 680
 classification of, 58
 differential diagnosis of, 243
 in Isaacs syndrome, 239
 in Lambert-Eaton myasthenic syndrome, 664
 peripheral neuropathy associated with, 58t
 presentation of, 65
 subacute, 65
 in tetanus, 242–243
Dysferlin, function of, 706
Dysferlin staining, 89
Dysferlinopathies, 723f
Dysmorphic features, 12–13
Dysphagia
 in ALS, 170
 causes of, 156
 classification of, 156
 complications of, 156
 description of, 156
 management of, 186t
 oropharyngeal, 156–157
 in PPMA, 225
 rehabilitation for, 132, 156–157
 secondary, 158
 symptoms of, 156
Dysphagia ophthaloplegia, 847–848
Dystonia, differential diagnosis of, 243
Dystrobrevin, encoding for, 702
Dystroglycan complex, 702
α-Dystroglycan *(DAG1)* mutations, 727, 735
Dystroglycans, muscular dystrophies and, 705–706
Dystrophin
 characteristics of, 702, 712
 mutations, 712
 proteins associated with, 702–706
 staining of, 710f
Dystrophin-associated proteins (DAPs), 702

Dystrophin-glycoprotein complex, 702
Dystrophinopathies
 affected proteins, 703t
 exercise studies in, 136
 molecular genetics of, 712
 pathogenesis of, 712
 treatment of, 713
  corticosteroids, 713
  gene therapies, 713
  supportive therapies, 713–714

E

Eastern Green Mamba (*Dendroaspis* sp.) venom, 688
Echymoses, evaluation of, 13
EcoRI polymorphism, 741
Eculizumab
 adverse effects of, 124
 dosage of, 124
 for juvenile MG, 646
 management of, 124
 mechanism of action, 124
 for myasthenia gravis, 636, 636t, 637
 for neuromuscular disorders
  dosage of, 114t
  monitoring for, 114t
  side effects of, 114t
 uses for, 124
Edaravone in ASL management, 183t, 184
Edema
 imaging of, 71
 limited mobility and, 155–156
 MRI of, 73
Edinburgh Cognitive and Behavioral ALS Screen (ECAS), 174
Edrophonium (Tensilon) testing, 175, 627–628
EEC. *See* El Escorial Criteria (EEC)
Efgartigmod
 adverse effects of, 124
 dosage of, 114t, 124
 for inflammatory myopathies, 927
 management of, 124–125
 mechanism of action for, 124
 monitoring for, 114t
 for myasthenia gravis, 646, 647
 during pregnancy, 647
 side effects of, 114t
 trials of, 639t
 uses of, 124
El Escorial Criteria (EEC), revised, 167t
Elapid venom, 688–689
Elbow
 flexion testing, 13
 neuropathy, 553–554, 553t
 ulnar neuropathy at, 28f
Electrodiagnosis (EDX). *See also* Electromyography (EMG); Nerve conduction studies (NCS)
 basic principles of
  physician skill, 23
  safety considerations, 23
  temperature considerations, 23
 components of examinations, 26
 guide to nerve repair, 56–75
 limitations of, 23, 50–51
 localization of pathology, 52–56, 52t
 nerve injury and, 51

normative data for, 25
 prognosis and, 56
 reporting of results in, 25
 test construction in, 25
 timing considerations in, 26, 525–526
 upper extremities, 525–526
 value of, 50–51
Electrolyte imbalances, 947–948
Electromyography (EMG). *See also* Electrodiagnosis (EDX)
 needle
  arm, 527
  description of, 42
  insertional activity, 42–46
  for Kennedy disease, 175
  serum CK values and, 26
  spontaneous activity, 42–46
  upper extremities, 527
Electron microscopy
 advantages of, 92f
 muscle examination by, 84
Elfabrio for Fabry disease, 300
Elivaldogene autotemcel (Skysona™, eli-cel, Lenti-D™), 302
EMD mutations, 744
Emerin, function of, 707
Emerin staining, 89
Emery-Dreifuss muscular dystrophies (EDMDs), 743–745
 affected proteins, 704t
 clinical features of, 743–744, 743f
 diagnostic approach for, 744–745, 745f
 genetic testing in, 70
 histopathology of, 744
 joint contractures in, 154
 laboratory features of, 744
 molecular genetics of, 744
 pathogenesis of, 744
 subtypes of, 743
 X-linked, 707
Emetine (IPECAC)
 myopathies related to, 959t, 973
Emotional lability in ALS, 171
Encephalitis, poliovirus related, 219–220
Endocrinopathies, neuropathies associated with, 491–503, 492t
Endomysial lipid droplets, 818f
Endoneurium, amyloid disposition in, 107–108
End-plate acetylcholine esterase deficiency, 673
End-plate potentials (EPPs)
 ACh release and, 33
 description of, 33
 prolongation of, 28
Endrophonium, response to, 621
Endurance exercise in ALS, 135–136
Enfortumab vedotin, 461
B-Enolase deficiency, 810–811
Entercept, toxic neuropathies and, 477
Enterovirus D68 A71, 221t
Envenomations, 684–691
Environmental control systems, 150
Eosinophiliic myositis, 98f, 99f, 916f
Eosinophilia-myalgia syndrome, 966–967
Eosinophilic granulomatosis with polyangiitis (EGPA), 387–388, 388f

Eosinophilic myopathy
　clinical features of, 911
　differential diagnosis of, 911
　histopathology of, 911, 911f
　laboratory features of, 911
　pathogenesis of, 911
　prognosis, 912
　treatment, 912
Ephedrine, oral, 678
Epidermylosis bullosa, 727–728
Epidermylosis bullosa simplex (EBS), 673
Epidural injections, polyradiculopathies and, 588
Epon, specimen embedding with, 84
Epoxy resin, specimen embedding with, 84
Epstein-Barr virus
　Guillain-Barré syndrome and, 326–327
　neuropathies and, 421
Equinovarus foot posturing, 16f, 245
Erb palsy, 536
ERG2 protein, 263
Eribulin, toxic neuropathies and, 459
　clinical features of, 456t
　mechanism of, 456t
　nerve histopathology in, 456t
Erlotinib, myopathies related to, 968
Erythema migrans, 416
Erythema nodosum leprosum, 416
Erythromelagia (erythermalgia)
　clinical features of, 284
　histopathological features of, 284
　laboratory features of, 284
　molecular genetics of, 284
　pathogenesis of, 284
　treatment of, 284
Erythromycin
　for autoimmune autonomic neuropathy, 338
　for Lyme disease, 417
　for tetanus, 245
Esophageal atresia, 673
Essential mixed cryoglobulinemia, 389–390
Etanercept for inflammatory myopathies, 926
Ethambutol, toxic neuropathies and
　clinical features of, 473t, 476
　diagnostic testing for, 473t
　laboratory features of, 476
　nerve histopathology in, 473t
Ethylene oxide, toxic neuropathies and
　clinical features of, 479t, 480
　diagnostic testing for, 479t
　laboratory features of, 480
　mechanism of, 479t
　nerve histopathology of, 480
　pathogenesis of, 480
Etoposide (VP-16)
　description of, 458
　toxic neuropathies and, 458
　　clinical features of, 456t
　　mechanism of, 456t
　　nerve histopathology of, 456t
Eulenberg disease, 872–873
Exercise
　aerobic, 134–137, 134t, 139, 924
　for ALS patients, 185
　balance, 134t
　isometric, 34, 35f
　muscle cramps and, 234

　in myasthenia gravis, 648
　recommendations for, 139–140
　rehabilitation, 154
　rehabilitation use of, 133–134
　relevance for NM diseases, 134t
　resistance, 134t, 139–140
　strengthening, 134–137, 134t
　stretching, 154
Exercise tests, 35–41, 38t
　in channelopathies, 864, 866t
　long, 36, 37f, 38t
　　type 4 pattern results, 42f
　　type 5 pattern results, 42f
　short, 35–36, 36f, 38t
　　dominant inheritance pattern, 39f
　　recessive inheritance pattern, 39f
　　type 1 pattern results, 39, 40f
　　type 2 pattern results, 37, 39–40, 39f
　　type 3 pattern results, 40f
　　type 4 pattern results, 41, 41f
　　type 5 pattern results, 41
Exoskeleton devices, 159
Expiratory muscle strength training (EMST), 136
Extensor carpi radialis brevis innervation, 523
Extensor carpi ulnaris innervation, 523
Extensor digiti minimi innervation, 523
Extensor digitorum brevis (EDB) innervation, 574
Extensor digitorum communis (EDC) muscle, 523
　percussion of, 13
Extensor digitorum longus innervation, 574
Extensor hallucis innervation, 574
Extensor hallucis longus weakness, 16
Extensor pollicis brevis innervation, 523
Extensor pollicis longus innervation, 523
Extraocular muscles, evaluation of, 7
Eye examinations, 924
Eye gaze sensing equipment, 150
Eyebrows, evaluation of, 12
Eyelid crutches, 156
Eyelids
　Cogan eyelid twitch, 11–12
　evaluation of, 11
　ptosis, 616–617
Ezetimibe, 957, 960

F

F waves, 26
　arm, 526
　assessment of, 27
　description of, 31–33
　determinations, 30f
　limitations of, 32
　median nerve, 32f
　value of, 31–33, 526
Fabry disease, 299–300
　clinical features of, 299–300
　histopathology of, 300, 301f
　laboratory features of, 300
　molecular genetics of, 300
　nerve biopsy in, 301f
　pathogenesis of, 300
　treatment of, 300
Facet joints, anatomy of, 565
Facial muscles in myasthenia gravis, 619

Facial nerve, conduction studies using, 26
Facial weakness
　causes of, 8, 8t
　ptosis and, 11
Facial-onset sensory and motor neuronopathy (FOSMN), 55, 513
　clinical features of, 513
　features of, 16
　histopathology of, 513
　laboratory features of, 513
　pathogenesis of, 513
Facioscapulohumeral muscular dystrophies (FSHDs), 704t
　clinical features of, 740–741, 740f
　diagnosis of, 741
　histopathology of, 741, 741f
　laboratory features of, 741
　molecular genetics of, 741, 742f
　pathogenesis of, 741
　treatment of, 741–742
F-actin, structure of, 707
Falls
　in neuromuscular diseases, 153–154
　prevention of, 153–154
　questions about, 5–6
Familial amyloid polyneuropathy (FAP), 314–317
　amyloid disposition in, 107–108
　histopathology of, 315f
　nerve biopsy of, 103f
　type III (See Apolipoprotein A1-related amyloidosis)
　type IV (See Gelsolin-related amyloidosis)
　Van Allen type (See Apolipoprotein A1-related amyloidosis)
Familial episodic pain syndrome type 1, 284–285
Familial episodic pain syndrome type 2, 285
Familial episodic pain syndrome type 3, 285
Familial hypokalemic periodic paralysis, 874
Familial myopathy with lysis of myofibrils, 788–789
Family histories, importance of, 10
Fascicular nerve biopsies, 100
Fascicular nerve degeneration, 198
Fasciculation potentials
　in ALS, 175
　discharges, 236f
　spontaneous activity and, 45
Fasciculations
　in ALS, 170–171
　benign, 233–234
　causes of, 235t
　clinical features of, 233–234
Fascioscapulo-humeral muscular dystrophies (FSHDs)
　exercise studies in, 136
　orthotic devices for, 153
　pain in, 155
　pattern of weakness in, 151
　rehabilitation approaches in, 151–152
Fasciotomy in RHB/MGU, 21
Fatigue
　causes of, 225
　myasthenia gravis and, 616–617
　in PPMA, 225
Fatty acid oxidation, 816f

Fazio Lande syndrome, 209
  features of, 204t
Femoral nerve
  anatomy of, 571, 573f
  nerve conduction studies using, 27
Femoral neuropathies, 597
FHL1 mutations, 743, 744
Fiber density, measurement of, 50
Fibric acid derivatives, myopathies related to, 960
Fibric acids, 957
Fibrillation potentials
  in botulism, 56
  in Lambert-Eaton myasthenic syndrome, 664
  positive waves and, 43f, 44
    disorders associated with, 45t
Fibroblast growth factor-3 (FGR-3) antibodies, 67
Fibromyalgia, 952
Fibular nerve, 572–573
  anatomy of, 574f
Fila radicularis, 517
Filamin-C *(FLNC)* mutations, 751
Finasteride, myopathies related to, 959t, 971–972
Finger-nose tests, 15
Fingerprint body myopathy, 787–788
Finkel type SMA
  features of, 204t
Finkelstein test, 988f
Finnish type SMA
  features of, 204t
Fite stain, 101
FKRP mutations, 725, 736–737
Flexibility training
  benefits of, 134t
  rehabilitation using, 134
Flexible Endoscopic Evaluation of Swallowing (FEES), 157
Flexor carpi radialis muscle, 523
Flexor carpi ulnaris innervation, 524
Flexor digitorium profundus, 523
Flexor digitorium superficialis, 523
Flexor digitorum longus innervation, 574
Flexor digitorum profundus innervation, 523, 524
Flexor digitorum superficialis, 523
Flexor hallucis longus innervation, 574
FLNC mutations, 754
Floor reaction orthoses (FROs), 142, 142f, 152
Floppy infants
  congenital myasthenic syndrome and, 676
  differential diagnoses, 3t
  examination of, 15
Fludrocortisone, 338, 495
Fluoroquinolones
  caution in use of, 626t
  in myasthenia gravis, 626t
  toxic neuropathies and, 472, 475
    clinical features of, 473t
    diagnostic testing for, 473t
    nerve histopathology in, 473t
Fluoxetine, 678
Fluvastatin, myopathy and, 957–960
Focal dystonias, features of, 234
Focal mitochondrial depletion, 850

Focal myositis
  clinical features of, 916
  histopathology of, 916–917, 917f
  laboratory features of, 916
Folate
  deficiency of, 433
    clinical features of, 433
    laboratory features of, 433
    pathogenesis of, 433
  dietary sources of, 433
Folic acid deficiency, 63
Fontalis sign, 619, 619t
Foot
  innervation of, 576
  laboratory testing and, 23
  pain in, 155
  peripheral neuropathies and, 154
  temperature of, 23
Foot drop, 742–743
  causes of, 6f
  management of, 186t
  rehabilitation approach in, 152–153
Footwear, foot abnormalities and, 154
Forearm exercise test, 21, 798
Formalin, specimen fixation with, 84
Foscarnet
  for HIV-related mononeuropathies, 421
  for polyradiculoneuropathy, 420
Four and a half LIM *(FHL1)* mutations, 791
Friedreich ataxia
  clinical features of, 305
  differential diagnosis of, 198
  features of, 12–13
  histopathology of, 305–306
  laboratory features of, 305
  molecular genetics of, 306
  treatment of, 306
Frontotemporal dementia (FTD), 166, 168, 173, 179
Frontotemporal dysfunction, 173
Frontotemporal lobar degeneration (FTLD)
  ALS and, 166, 168
  histopathology of, 179–180
Frontotemporal lobe atrophy, 179, 180f
Fukutin, function of, 708
Fukutin *(FKTN)* mutations, 727, 736
Fukuyama congenital muscular dystrophy (FCMD), 708
  clinical features of, 735
  laboratory features of, 735
  molecular genetics of, 736
  pathogenesis of, 736
Functioning, Disability and Health (ICF) model, 132
Furosemide, diuresis with, 21
FUS mutation, 179, 182
  in ALS, 168

G

G ratios, description of, 106
GABA-A receptor antibodies, 249
Gabapentin
  for cramps, 211, 238t
  for diabetic neuropathy, 493
  for fibromyalgia, 952
  for HVZ infections, 422
  for Isaacs syndrome, 242

  for Morvan syndrome, 242
  for myofascial pain syndrome, 952
  for neuropathic pain, 591
  for painful sensory neuronopathies, 495t, 510t
  for stiff person syndrome, 250
GABA-receptor-associated protein (GABARAP), 250
Gag reflex, enhanced, 14
Gait changes, cervical radiculopathies and, 533
Ganciclovir
  for HIV-related mononeuropathies, 421
  for polyradiculoneuropathy, 420
Ganglion cysts, 73f
Ganglionopathies
  HIV-related, 421
  paraneoplastic, 440–443
  Sjögren syndrome and, 397
Gasserian ganglion
  function of, 398
Gastrocnemius muscle
  biopsies of, 83
  innervation of, 574
Gastrostomy
  percutaneous, 211
GBS. *See* Guillain-Barré syndrome (GBS)
GDP-mannose pyrophosphorylase B *(GMPPB)* mutations, 728
Gelsolin-related amyloidosis, 316–317
Gemfibrozil
  myopathies related to, 960
  statin myopathy and, 957
Gender, muscle fiber size and, 93
Genetic testing, approach to, 285–285
Genitals, cutaneous innervation of, 571f
Genitofemoral nerve, 568
Genitofemoral neuropathies, 595–596
Gephyrin (GHPN) antibodies, 249
Gephyrin (GHPN) protein, 250
GFPT1 deficiency, 670t–671t, 671
Giant axonal neuropathy, 107, 310
Giant cell arteritis, 914–915, 915f
  prognosis, 915
  treatment of, 915
Giant cell myositis
  clinical features of, 912–913
  histopathologic features of, 98f
  laboratory features of, 913
  pathogenesis of, 914
  prognosis in, 914
Giant cell vasculitis, 385
Givinostat, 713
GivMohr slings, 141
Givosiran for porphyria, 314
Glaucoma screening, 924
Globoid cell leukodystrophy, 298–299.
  See Krabbe disease
Glucose tolerance testing, 505t
α-Glucosidase deficiency, 799–803
α-Glucosidase replacement, 803
Glutamic acid decarboxylase (GAD), 249–250
Glutamic acid decarboxylase (GAD) antibodies, 244, 247
Glutamic acid decarboxylase-65 (GAD65), 250
Glutamic acid decarboxylase-65 (GAD65) antibodies, 67, 248–249

Glutamine-fructose-6-phosphate transaminase 1 (GFPT1) deficiency, 675, 675f
Glutaraldehyde, 84
Glutaric aciduria type II, 821–822
Gluten, intolerance to, 402
Gluten-induced enteropathy, 402
Gluteus medius innervation, 572
Gluteus minimus innervation, 572
Glycerol kinase (GKD) deficiency, 714
Glyceroluria, 714
Glycine receptor alpha-1 subunit (GLRA1) antibodies, 249
Glycogen metabolism disorders, 800f
Glycogen storage diseases (GSDs), 798–811
  RHB/MGU and, 21
  type IV, 177
  type X, 790
  types of, 798
Glycogen synthase 1 deficiency, 798–799
Glycogen synthase (GYS1) mutations, 799
Glycogenesis type 0, 798–799, 802
Glycogenin 1 deficiency, 811
Glycogenosis type II, 799–803
Glycogenosis type III, 803–804
Glycogenosis type IV, 804–806, 805f, 806
Glycogenosis type V, 806–807
Glycogenosis type VII, 807–808
Glycogenosis type IX, 808
Glycogenosis type X, 809–810, 809f
Glycogenosis type XI, 810
Glycogenosis type XII, 810
Glycogenosis type XIII, 810–811
Glycogenosis type XIV, 811
Glycogenosis type XV, 811
Glycolysis pathways, 800f
Glycoproteins, dystrophin and, 702–706
Glycopyrrolate for myasthenia gravis, 634
GM1 ganglioside titer, 175
GMPPB mutations, 735
GNE myopathy, 750–751
Gold Coast criteria, 167, 167t, 178
Gold toxicity
  clinical features of, 483t, 485
  detection of, 483t
  laboratory features of, 483t, 485
  nerve histopathology in, 485
  pathogenesis of, 485
  treatment of, 485
Golimumab, toxic neuropathies and, 477
Gomori trichrome stains, modified
  benefits of, 84, 87
  muscle fibers on, 85f
  myelin stain by, 101
  for nerve biopsies, 101
  ragged red fibers using, 86f
  target fibers on, 94, 95f
  type 1 fibers on, 93
Gottron papules, 892, 893f
Gout, neuropathies associated with, 405
Gower sign, 709
Graft-*versus*-host disease (GVHD), 454–455
Granulomas, sarcoidosis and, 400
Granulomatosis with polyangiitis (GAN), 388
Granulomatous infiltration, 384t
Granulomatous myositis, 912–913
  histopathologic features of, 98f, 99f, 913, 913f
  laboratory features of, 913

pathogenesis of, 914
prognosis in, 914
Granulomatous uveitis, 400
Graves disease, myopathy and, 940
Gray matter, MRI of, 74f
Gray rami, 517
Greater trochanteric bursitis, 989–991, 991f
Grip myotonia, 13
Groin, cutaneous innervation of, 571f
Growth differentiation factor-15 (GDF-15), 64
Guanidine, side effects of, 690
Guillain-Barré syndrome (GBS)
  antecedent illness and, 326–327
  antiganglioside antibodies associated with, 329f
  clinical features of, 220t
  COVID vaccines and, 423–424
  description of, 326
  diagnosis of, 220t, 221
  differential diagnoses of, 330, 685
  epidemiology of, 326–327
    annual incidence of, 326
    antecedent illnesses and, 326
    vaccinations and, 326
  features of, 221
  histopathology of, 330–331
  immune mechanisms in, 332f
  intravenous immunoglobulin trials, 333t
  IVIGs for, 122
  long-term management of, 333–334
  in malignancies, 229–230
  mortality rate in, 333
  neuromyotonic discharges in, 240, 240t
  plasma exchange for, 125
  plasmapheresis trials, 333t
  prognosis in, 56, 333–334
  rapid EDX support in, 26
  recurrent, 334
  related syndromes and, 327t
  Sjögren syndrome and, 397
  use of steroids in, 118
Gummas, description of, 417
Guyon's canal, 524, 556, 557

H

H reflexes, 26
  absent, 33
  arm, 526
  description of, 32–33, 33f
Hairy cell leukemia, 444
Hammer toes, 196f
Hamstring innervation, 574
Hand
  activities of daily living and, 152
  atrophy of, 170f
  muscle wasting, 220f
  pain in, 155
  rehabilitation approaches in, 152
  temperature of, 23
  weakness in, 152
Hansen disease. *See* Leprosy
Hawkins test, 984f
Head and neck cancers, 176
Head drop
  in ALS, 170f
  in myasthenia gravis, 617
  neck muscle weakness and, 8, 9t
  rehabilitation approach for, 150

Head movement tracking, 150
Headmaster collars, 140, 140f
HeadUp collars, 140
Heart rates
  testing, 505
  variability in, 59, 60f, 508f
Heat shock protein B1 (HSPB1) mutations, 176
Heavy metals
  exposure to, 64
  toxic neuropathies and, 483t
Heel walking, 13
Hematin for porphyria, 314
Hematopoietic stem cell transplantation, 454–455
Hematoxylin and eosin (H&E) stains, 84
  eosinophilic myositis, 99f
  inclusion body myositis on, 99f
  inflammatory cell infiltrates on, 102f
  muscle fibers regeneration on, 86f
  necrotic muscle on, 97f
  for nerve biopsies, 101
  sarcoidosis on, 99f
Hemodialysis, neuropathies associated with, 403
Hemorrhages, retroperitoneal, 591
Hepatitis A vaccines, 117
Hepatitis B vaccines, 117
Hepatitis viruses
  Guillain-Barré syndrome and, 326–327
  HBV, 116–117, 412f, 421
  HVC, 391, 412f, 421, 587
Heptavalent botulinum antitoxin (HBAT), 683–684
Hereditary inclusion body myopathy (h-IBM), 708, 755
Hereditary liability to pressure palsy (HNPP), 55
Hereditary motor and sensory neuropathy type 6 (HMSN VI). *See* Charcot-Marie-Tooth disease, type 2A2
Hereditary motor neuropathies, distal inheritance of, 205t
Hereditary motor neuropathy, distal (dHMN), 175–176. *See also* SMARD1
Hereditary myopathy with early respiratory failure (HMERF), 726
Hereditary neuralgic amyotrophy (HNA)
  clinical features of, 275–276, 540–542
  histopathology of, 276
  laboratory features of, 276
  molecular genetics of, 276
  pathogenesis of, 276
Hereditary neuropathies
  rare, 298f
Hereditary neuropathy with a liability to pressure palsies (HNPP), 261, 263–264
  clinical features of, 263–264
  histopathology of, 264, 265f
  laboratory features of, 264
  molecular genetics of, 264
  pathogenesis of, 264
Hereditary neuropathy with neuromyotonia, 277
Hereditary periodic paralysis
  exercise tests in, 865t
  Fournier electrophysiologic patterns, 865t
  genes involved in, 865t

Hereditary sensory and autonomic
    neuropathies (HSANs), 277
  clinical features of, 278t–279t
  genetics of, 277, 278t–279t
  neurophysiology of, 278t–279t
  pathology of, 278t–279t
  type 1
    clinical features of, 277
    histopathology of, 277, 280, 280f
    laboratory features of, 277
    molecular genetics of, 280–281
    pathogenesis of, 280–281
  type 1A, 280
  type 1B, 280
  type 1C, 280
  type 1D, 280–281
  type 1E, 281
  type 1F, 281
  type 2, 281, 281f
  type 2A, 282
  type 2B, 282
  type 2C, 282
  type 2D, 282
  type 3, 282
  type 4, 282, 283
  type 5, 283
  type 6, 283
  type 7, 283, 284
  type 8, 284
Hereditary spastic paraparesis
  differential diagnosis of, 176
  features of, 12–13
  gene mutations in, 176
Hereditary spastic paraplegia (HSP), 193–201
  clinical features of, 193–198
  differential diagnoses, 197–198
    testing considerations in, 197t
  forms of, 197
  genes involved in, 193, 194t–195t, 198
  histopathology of, 198
  laboratory features of, 198
  management of, 199–200
  morbidity from, 193
  nosology of, 193
  pathogenesis of, 198–199
  treatment options for, 199t
Herniated nucleus pulposus (HNP), 527
Herniorrhaphies, 595
Heroin, myopathies related to, 975
Herpes simplex virus, 587
Herpes varicella-zoster (HVZ)
  neuropathies and, 412f, 421–422
    histopathology of, 422
    laboratory features of, 422
    pathogenesis of, 422
    treatment of, 422
    radicular pain and, 582
Heterogeneous nuclear ribonucleoproteins
    (HNRNPAs), 708
Heterogenous nuclear ribonucleoprotein D-like
    protein (HNRNPDL) mutations, 719
Hexacarbon toxicity
  axonal enlargement in, 107
  clinical features of, 479t, 481
  diagnostic testing for, 479t
  histopathology of, 481, 482f
  laboratory features of, 481

  mechanism of, 479t
  pathogenesis of, 481
Hexoaminidase A deficiency, 177
Highly active antiretroviral therapy (HAART),
    965
Hip girdle weakness, 152
Hip joint
  extension strength of, 13
  external rotation of, 990f
  internal rotation of, 990f
  osteoarthritis of, 989
  weakness of flexion, 7
Hirayama disease, 211–213, 212f
Histocompatibility antigen type 1 (MHC1), 97f
Histone deacetylase inhibitors, 712
Hoffman's sign, 14, 171, 533
Holster sign, 892
Homocysteine (Hcy), 431
Horner syndrome, 447
  ipsilateral, 540
  nerve root injuries and, 517
Hospice care, 133, 185
HSPB1 mutations, 176
HSPB8 mutations, 176
Human immunodeficiency virus (HIV)
  Guillain-Barré syndrome and, 326–327
  myositis associated with, 917–918
  neurological complications of, 418–419, 418t
  neuromuscular disease and, 68
  neuropathies and, 412f
  polyradiculopathies and, 587
  sensory neuropathy in, 57
Human myxovirus resistance protein (MxA),
    424, 424f
Human T lymphocyte virus 1 (HTLV-1)
  neuropathies and, 412f, 421
  progressive myelopathy and, 177
Human T-cell leukemia virus type 1, 918
Human tetanus immune globulin, 245
Humeral cuff slings, 141
Hyaline body myopathy, 788–789, 789f
Hydration in RHB/MGU, 21
3-Hydroxy-3-methyl-glutaryl coenzyme A
    (3-HMG-CoA) reductase
  inhibitors of, 957–960
  pathway for, 959f
Hydroxyacyl-CoA dehydrogenaes deficiency,
    821
Hydroxychloroquine
  caution in use of, 626t
  myopathies related to, 963
  toxic neuropathies and
    clinical features of, 473t, 476
    diagnostic testing for, 473t
    nerve histopathology in, 473t
5-Hydroxytryptophan, 251
Hyoscyamine, 634
Hypercalcemia, myopathic disorders and, 948
HyperCKemia, 64
Hyperekplexia
  clinical features of, 250
  pathogenesis of, 251
  treatment of, 251
Hypereosinophilic syndrome (HES), 403, 911
Hyperglycerolemia, 714
Hyperinsulinemia, neuropathies related to,
    498–499

Hyperkalemia
  myopathies and, 948
  secondary causes of, 870, 870t
Hyperkalemic paralysis, secondary, 947t
Hyperkalemic periodic paralysis (hyperKPP),
    869–872
  chloride channels in, 37
  clinical features of, 869–870
  CMAP amplitudes in, 877
  etiologies of, 870t
  exercise testing in, 39
  histopathology of, 871
  laboratory features of, 870–871
  long-exercise tests in, 871f
  molecular genetics of, 871, 876
  pathogenesis of, 871
  short exercise test results, 41
  sodium channels in, 37
  treatment of, 871–872
Hyperlordosis, impacts of, 152
Hypermagnesemia, 948
Hyperparathyroidism, 942–943
Hyperreflexia
  cervical radiculopathies and, 533
  in hereditary spastic paraplegia, 193
Hypersensitivity vasculitis, 389, 389f
Hypertension, screening for, 924
Hyperuricemia, 806
Hypocalcemia
  myopathic disorders and, 948
  tetany and, 245, 246
Hypoglycemia, 498–499
Hypoglycorrhachia, 221
Hypokalemia
  diagnosis of, 220t
  features of, 220t, 221
  myopathies and, 947–948, 973
Hypokalemic myopathies
  drugs related to, 958t
Hypokalemic paralysis, secondary, 947t
Hypokalemic periodic paralysis (hypoKPP)
  chloride channels in, 37
  etiologies of, 870t
  short exercise test results, 41
  sodium channels in, 37
  type 1, 876–879, 877f
  type 2, 874, 876
Hypomagnesemia, tetany and, 245, 246
Hypoparathyroidism, 943–944
Hypopharyngeal muscles, 225
Hypophosphatemia
  diagnosis of, 220t
  features of, 220t, 221
  myopathies and, 948
  neuropathies related to, 435
Hypothyroid myopathy, 941–942
Hypothyroidism, 499–500, 941–942
Hypoventilation, management of, 186t

I

Ice crystal artifacts, 84
Ice pack test, 618, 619
Ice therapy, 986f
Idiopathic inflammatory myopathies (IIMs),
    887
Idiopathic length-dependent sensorimotor
    polyneuropathy, 504–510

Idiopathic length-dependent sensory
    polyneuropathy, 504–510
  clinical features of, 504
  histopathology in, 507–509, 508f, 509f
  laboratory features of, 504–507
  pathogenesis of, 509–510
Idiopathic perineuritis
  clinical features of, 368
  histopathology of, 370
  laboratory features of, 368, 370
  pathogenesis of, 370
Idiopathic polyneuropathies, 504–516, 505t
Idiopathic sensory neuropathy/ganglionopathy
  clinical features of, 511
  histopathology of, 511–512
  laboratory features of, 511
  pathogenesis of, 512
  treatment of, 512
Idiopathic sensory polyneuropathies,
    443–444
Idiopathic small fiber sensory neuronopathy/
    ganglionopathy
  clinical features of, 512
  histopathology of, 512
  laboratory features of, 512
  pathogenesis of, 512
  treatment of, 513
Ifosfamide, toxic neuropathies and, 460
Iliacus muscle innervation, 571
Iliohypogastric nerve, 568
Iliohypogastric neuropathies, 595
Ilioinguinal nerve, anatomy of, 568
Ilioinguinal neuropathies, 595
Imaging nerve and muscle, 71–76
Imatinib, myopathies related to, 968
Immune checkpoint inhibitors (ICIs)
  caution in use of, 626t
  for Lambert-Eaton myasthenic syndrome,
    667
  myasthenia gravis and, 647–648
  myopathies related to, 966, 966f, 967f
  toxic neuropathies and, 457t, 461–463
    clinical features of, 461–462
    laboratory findings in, 462
    management of, 462–463
    nerve histopathology in, 462, 463f
    pathogenesis of, 462
Immune system homeostasis, 611
Immune tolerance, establishment of, 611
Immune-mediated brachial plexus
    neuropathies (IBPN), 275–276,
    535–536
  clinical features of, 535
  laboratory features of, 536
  pathology of, 536
  treatment of, 536
Immune-mediated necrotizing myopathy
    (IMNM)
  autoantibodies in, 895t
  clinical features of, 908
  diagnostic criteria for, 889t–891t
  histopathology of, 98, 908, 909f
  inheritance of, 887
  laboratory features of, 908
  overlap syndromes, 909–911
  pathogenesis of, 908–909
  rituximab for, 124

  treatment of, 909
  use of steroids for, 118
Immune-mediated neuropathies
  brachial plexus, 536
  diagnosis of, 536
  differential diagnoses for, 384t
Immunoglobulin mu-binding protein 2
    (IGHMBP2) mutations, 176
Immunoglobulins, intravenous (IVIGs),
    122–123
  adverse effects of, 123
  for chronic immune sensory
    polyradiculopathy, 368
  for chronic inflammatory demyelinating
    polyneuropathy, 357t, 358
  dosage of, 113t, 123
  for idiopathic small fiber sensory
    neuronopathy/ganglionopathy, 513
  for inflammatory myopathies, 922t
  for Lambert-Eaton myasthenic syndrome, 667
  management of, 123
  mechanism of action, 122
  monitoring of, 113t
  for multifocal motor neuropathy, 367
  for myasthenia gravis, 634–635, 646–647
  in myositis, 924
  during pregnancy, 646–647
  for radioplexus neuropathies, 591
  side effects of, 113t
  subcutaneous, 122–123
  uses for, 122
Immunoperoxidase stains, 91f, 97f
Immunosuppression
  immunotherapy and, 112
  for sarcoidosis, 402
Immunotherapies
  for autoimmune neuromuscular diseases,
    113t–114t
  general considerations, 112–115
  general principles, 634
  for myasthenia gravis, 634–644
  principles of, 112–130
  risk considerations with, 115–118
  for Satoyoshi syndrome, 247
Impaired glucose tolerance (IGT), 492
Inclusion body myopathy
  autosomal recessive, 750–751
  with central white matter disease, 756
Inclusion body myositis (IBM)
  associated manifestations, 903
  autoantibodies in, 895t
  clinical features of, 891t, 901, 903f, 904f
  diagnosis of, 97–98
  diagnostic criteria, 892t
  differential diagnosis of, 175, 907–908
  electrophysiological studies in, 904
  exercise studies in, 137
  hand exercises in, 152
  histopathologic features of, 99f
  histopathology of, 904–905, 905f, 906f, 907f
  laboratory features of, 891t, 903–904, 904f
  muscle fibers severed in, 96
  pathogenesis of, 905–907
  pathological features of, 891t
  prognosis in, 908
  ultrasound of, 76f
Incontinence, cervical radiculopathies and, 533

Indomethacin for leprosy, 416
Industrial agents, toxic neuropathies related
    to, 479t
Inebilizumab, 640t, 641
Infantile neuroaxonal dystrophy, 310
Infants
  floppy, 3t, 205–206
  head extension by, 15
  muscle fibers in, 93
  vocalization by, 15
  weakness in, 15
Infection-related vasculitis, 389
Infections, neuropathies related to, 411–429
Infectious diseases, immunosuppression and,
    115–117
Infectious neuropathies, 384t
Inferior cervical ganglion, 517
Inferior gluteal neuropathies, 596
Inferior rectal nerve, 576
Inflammation
  imaging of, 71
  MRI of, 73
Inflammatory bowel disease (IBD), 402–403
Inflammatory cells, staining for, 90f
Inflammatory demyelinating
    polyradiculoneuropathy (AIDP). See
    Guillain-Barré syndrome (GBS)
Inflammatory dystrophies, 99f
Inflammatory myopathies, 887–939
  autoantibodies associated with, 895t
  bacteria-associated, 919–920
  categories of, 887
  clinical features of, 888t
  corticosteroids for, 112
  drugs related to, 958t, 965–966
  exercise studies in, 137
  fungus-associated, 920
  immunotherapies for, 922t
  infection-associated, 917–921, 917t
  laboratory features of, 888t
  parasitic infections and, 920–921
  treatment of, 921–927
  virus-associated, 917–919
Inflammatory neuropathies, tacrolimus for, 122
Inflammatory Neuropathy Cause and
    Treatment (INCAT) scores, 115
Inflammatory Rasch Build Overall Disability
    Scale (IRODS), 115
Infliximab, 477, 926
Influenza vaccines, 117, 326–327, 648
Influenza viruses, myositis and, 918–919
Infraspinatus muscle
  innervation of, 544
Inherited neuropathies
  molecular targets of, 260f
  pathogenic targets of, 258t
Instrumental activities of daily living (IADLs),
    146–150
Integrins, function of, 706
Intensive care units (ICUs), critical illness
    neuropathies and, 405–406
Interferon α-2b for WNV treatment, 224
Interferon (IFN) gamma release assay (IGRA),
    116
Interferon-β1 for multifocal motor neuropathy,
    367
Interferonopathy, type 1, 897, 927

Interleukin 6 (IL-6), 642
Intermediate syndrome, 687
Intermedius muscle innervation, 571
Internal oblique muscle innervation, 568
Interpotential intervals, 49
Intervertebral discs, 566, 582
Intervertebral foramina, 517
Intoxications, 684–691
Intraepidermal nerve fiber density (IENFD)
    assessment of, 57, 58
    in idiopathic polyneuropathies, 505, 508–509
Intraepidermal nerve fibers (IENFs), 108–109
Iodine contrast media, 626t
Iontophoresis for pain, 156
IPECAC, myopathies related to, 959t, 973
Isaacs syndrome
    clinical features of, 239
    diagnosis of, 239–240
    histopathology of, 241
    immunotherapy for, 242
    laboratory features of, 240–241
    myotonic discharges in, 236
    pathogenesis of, 241–242
    plasma exchange for, 125
    use of steroids in, 118
Isolated vasculitis, 390
Isometric exercises
    CMAP traces, 35f
    repetitive nerve stimulation versus, 34
Isoniazid (INH), toxic neuropathies and
    clinical features of, 473t, 476
    diagnostic testing for, 473t
    laboratory features of, 476
    mechanism of, 476
    nerve histopathology in, 473t
Isoniazid with pyridoxine, 116
Isoretinoin, myopathies related to, 959t, 973
Ixabepilone, toxic neuropathies and, 456t, 459
Ixazomib, toxic neuropathies and, 460
Ixodes spp.
    I. dammini, 416
    I. holocyclus, 684, 685, 686
    I. pacificus, 684
    I. scapularis, 684
Izazomib, toxic neuropathies and, 457t

J
JAGGED2 *(JAG2)* mutations, 731
Janus kinase (JAK) inhibitors, 125
Japanese encephalitis virus, 221, 221t
Jaw
    strength of, 11
    weakness of, 8
Jaw jerk, 14, 398
Jimmo vs. Kathleen Sebelius, 133
Jitter values, 664
John Cuningham (JC) virus, 116
Joint contractures
    disorders associated with, 12t
    neuromuscular diseases and, 154–155
Jordan anomaly, 817f
Jordan bodies, 64
Juvenile idiopathic arthritis, 125
Juvenile segmental spinal muscular atrophy, 211–213
Juvenile segmental spinal muscular atrophy (JSSMA). *See* Hirayama disease

K
Kaposi sarcoma, 117–118
Karnovsky's fixative, 104f
Kathleen Sebelius, Jimmo vs., 133
KCNJ2 mutations, 880
Kearns-Sayre syndrome (KSS), 834, 844
Kelch-like family member 40 *(KLH40)* mutation, 782
Kelch-like homologue 9 *(KLHL9)* mutations, 752
Kelch repeat and BTB *(KBTBD13)* mutation, 777, 778, 782
Kennedy disease, 55. *See also* X-linked bulbospinal muscular atrophy
    differential diagnosis of, 175, 210
    electrodiagnosis of, 210
    features of, 16, 204t, 209
    histopathology of, 210–211
    labortory features of, 210
    management of, 211
    pathogenesis of, 211
    sensory conductions in, 178
King-Denborough syndrome, 779
Klein-Lisak-Andersen syndrome, 879–880
Klumpke palsy/paralysis, 536–537
Knee extension testing, 13
Knee-ankle-foot orthoses (KAFOs), 143, 143f, 152
Komura-gaeri, 246
Krabbe disease
    clinical features of, 298
    histopathology of, 299
    laboratory features of, 298–299
    molecular genetics of, 299
    pathogenesis of, 299
    treatment of, 299
Krait (*Bungarus* sp.) venom, 688, 689
Kugelberg-Welander syndrome
    features of, 204t
Kyphoscoliosis peptidase *(KY)* mutations, 754

L
Labetalol
    myopathies related to, 961
    for tetanus, 245
Labia, innervation of, 576
Laboratory testing, diagnostic role of, 23–82
Lactate dehydrogenase (LDH) deficiency, 810
Laing distal myopathy, 751
Lambert-Eaton myasthenic syndrome (LEMS)
    azathioprine for, 119
    characteristics of, 56, 68
    clinical features of, 660–662
    congenital, 672
    cranial nerve involvement in, 19
    cyclosporine for, 121
    diagnosis of, 662–665, 663f
    differential diagnoses, 662–665
    histopathology of, 665
    pathogenesis of, 665–666
    response to exercise, 35f
    tacrolimus for, 122
    testing for, 175
    treatment of, 667–668
    weakness and, 6
Lamin β2 deficiency, 673
Lamin-associated protein 1 mutations, 729
Laminin α2-related dystrophies, 731
Laminin deficiency, 678
Laminins
    emerin binding of, 707
    muscular dystrophies and, 705
Lamivudine (3TC), 476
Laryngospasm, 186t, 245
Latent tuberculosis infection (LTBI), 116
Lateral antebrachial cutaneous nerve, 28
Lateral cord lesions, 535
Lateral epicondylitis, 986–987
    diagnosis of, 986
    symptoms of, 986
    treatment of, 986–987
Lateral femoral cutaneous nerve (LFCN), 571, 572f
Lateral femoral cutaneous neuralgia, 596–597
Lateral pectoral nerves
    injury to, 544
    innervation by, 522
Lateral plantar nerves, 28
Latissimus dorsi muscle innervation, 544
A-Latrotoxin, 689
LDP3 mutations, 754
Lead toxicity
    clinical features of, 482, 483t
    detection of, 483t
    laboratory features of, 482, 483t
    nerve histopathology of, 482
    pathogenesis of, 482
    treatment of, 482
Leflunomide toxicity, 477
    clinical features of, 474t
    diagnostic testing for, 474t
    nerve histopathology in, 474t
Leigh syndrome, 834, 849–850
Leisure activities, adaptive equipment for, 149
Lenalidomide, toxic neuropathies and, 457t, 461
Length-dependent polyneuropathy
    EDX localization, 52, 52t
    features of, 17–18
Leomoidin-3 *(LMOD3)* mutation, 782, 788
Leonine facies, 411
Lepromatous leprosy, 411
Lepromatous neuropathy, 108
Leprosy, 594f
    borderline, 411
        features of, 412t, 413, 414f
        histopathology of, 414f, 415f
        treatment of, 413, 416
    clinical features of, 411, 412t
    histopathologic features of, 104f, 412t
    immunological features of, 412t
    laboratory features of, 411–412, 412t
    lepromatous, 411
        features of, 412t
        histopathology of, 415f
    pathogenesis of, 413
    prevention of, 416
    Ridley-Joplin classification, 413
    treatment of, 413, 416
    tuberculoid, 411, 413, 413f
Leprosy, borderline, 108f
    histopathologic features of, 108f
Leucine-rich glioma-inactivated 1 (LGI1) antibodies, 240, 242

Leukapheresis, 926–927
Leukemias, neuropathies associated with, 444
Leuprorelin, 211
Levamisole for leprosy, 416
Levetiracetam
  for cramps, 238t
  for stiff person syndrome, 250
Lewis-Sumner syndrome. *See* Multifocal acquired demyelinating sensory and motor neuropathy (MADSAM)
Lhermitte sign, 431, 455
Lid twitch sign, 619t
Lidocaine for pain, 495t
Lidoderm for pain, 495t, 510t
Ligamentum flavum, 565
LIM domain-binding 3 *(LDB3)* mutations, 750
Limb girdle muscular dystrophies (LGMDs)
  affected proteins, 703t
  autosomal-dominant inherited, 715–716, 715f, 716
  autosomal-recessive inheritance, 719–733, 720f
  description of, 714–719
  diagnosis of, 731–732
  diagnostic approach to, 715f
  LGMD1B/EDMD2, 716–717, 716f, 717
  LGMD1C/crippling muscle disease type 2, 717
  LGMD1D/LGMDD1, 717, 718
  LGMD1E/MFM1, 718
  LGMD1F/LGMDD2, 718
  LGMD1G/LGMDD3, 718–719
  LGMD1H/LGMDD4, 719
  LGMD2A/LGMDR1, 719, 721, 721f
  LGMD2A/LGMDRR1, 720f
  LGMD2B/LGMDR2, 721–722, 721f, 722
  LGMD2C/LGMDR5, 722–724
  LGMD2D/LGMDR3, 722–724
  LGMD2E/LGMDR4, 722–724
  LGMD2F/LGMDR6, 722–724
  LGMD2G/LGMDR7, 726
  LGMD2H/LGMDR8, 726
  LGMD2I/LGMDR9, 91f, 724–725, 725f
  LGMD2J/LGMDR10, 726
  LGMD2K/LGMDR11, 726
  LGMD2L/LGMDR12, 726–727
  LGMD2M/LGMDR13, 727
  LGMD2N/LGMDR14, 727
  LGMD2O/LGMDR15, 727
  LGMD2P/LGMDR16, 727
  LGMD2Q/LGMDR17, 727–728
  LGMD2R/MFM1, 728
  LGMD2S/LGMDR18, 728
  LGMD2T/LGMDR19, 728
  LGMD2U/LGMDR20, 728
  LGMD2V, 729
  LGMD2W/PINCH-related myopathy, 729
  LGMD2X/GLDM25, 729
  LGMD2Y/TOR1AIP1, 729
  LGMD2Z/LGMDR21, 729
  LGMDR22/Bethlem myopathy, 729–731, 730f
  LGMDR23/laminin α2-related dystrophy, 731
  LGMDR24/POMGNT2-related dystrophy, 731
  LGMDR26/Popeye domain-containing protein 3, 731
  LGMDR27, 731
  sarcoglycanopathies, 722
  staining for, 89
  testing for, 175
  titinopathies, 726
  treatment of, 731–732, 732f
Limb stiffness, UMN pathology and, 6
Limbs
  exercise testing and, 35–36
  temperature of, 23, 35–36
  weakness of, 12
LIMS2 mutations, 729
Linezolid
  toxic neuropathies and
    clinical features of, 473t, 475
    diagnostic testing for, 473t
    mechanism of, 475
    nerve histopathology in, 473t
Lipid metabolism, 822f
Lipid metabolism disorders, 815–823
Lipid storage myopathies, stains for, 87
Lipin deficiency, 822–823
Lipin *(LPN1)* mutations, 822–823
Lipofuscin accumulation, 434
Lipopolysaccharide-induced tumor necrosis factor alpha *(LITAF)* mutations, 263
Lipoprotein receptor protein 4 (LPR4)
  antibodies to, 607, 611
  congenital myasthenic syndromes and, 678, 679
  deficiency of, 675
Liquids, swallowing of, 157
Lithium
  toxic neuropathies and, 478
    clinical features of, 474t
    diagnostic testing for, 474t
    nerve histopathology in, 474t
Liver transplantation, 806
LMNA mutations, 744
Long thoracic nerve, 543–544
  anatomy of, 522
  neuropathies, 543–544, 544t
Long-chain acyl-CoA dehydrogenase (LCAD) deficiency, 820
Long-exercise tests (LETs), 864, 866t, 871f
Loperamide, 634
Lou Gehrig disease. *See* Amyotrophic lateral sclerosis (ALS)
Lovastatin, myopathy and, 957–960
Low-density lipoprotein receptor-related protein 4 (LRP4) antibodies, 67
Lower extremities
  embryologic rotation of, 568
  focal neuropathies of, 563–606
  imaging of, 592
  movement of, 570t
  peripheral nerves of, 568–576
  radicular pain, 579
  spasticity of, 193
Lower extremity amyotrophic diplegia (LAD), 172
Lower limb orthoses, 141–143
Lower limb weakness, 152
Lower limbs, neuromuscular mimics, 989–993
Lower motor neurons (LMNs)
  dysfunction of, 167–168
  hereditary spastic paraplegia and, 193
  involvement ALS, 170–174
  paraneoplastic syndromes, 229
  pathology of, 6–7, 7t
Lower motor neurons (LMNs) disease, 158–159
LRIF1 mutations, 741
Lumbar plexus anatomy, 567–568
Lumbar spine
  disc herniation, 581f
  imaging of, 579f
Lumbosacral nerve roots
  anatomy of, 563–566
  compressive radiculopathy, 563–564
Lumbosacral orthoses (LSOs), 140–141
Lumbosacral plexopathies, 447–448, 590t
  etiologies of, 589–591
  evaluation of, 591
  management of, 591–592
  radiation-induced, 448
Lumbosacral plexus, 566–568, 566f, 567f, 568t–569t
Lumbosacral radiculoplexopathy, 496–497, 497f
Lumbosacral spine, imaging of, 577–578
Lumbosacral trunk, anatomy of, 567f
Luxol fast blue stain, 101, 102f
Lyme disease
  clinical features of, 416
  histopathology of, 417
  laboratory features of, 416–417
  management of, 589
  myositis associated with, 920
  neurological disorders and, 416t
  neuromuscular disease and, 68
  pathogenesis of, 417
  polyradiculopathies and, 587
  screening for, 177
  testing for, 686
  treatment of, 417
Lymphomas
  amyloidosis and, 449
  GBS and, 229–230
  motor neuron diseases and, 229
  neuropathies associated with, 444
  sural nerve biopsy, 446f
Lymphomatoid granulomatosis, 444
Lymphomatous polyradiculopathy, 446f
Lymphoproliferative disorders
  amyloidosis and, 449
  immunosuppression and, 117–118
  rituximab for, 123–124
Lyon hypothesis, 712
Lysosomal storage disorders
  neuropathies associated with, 297–305

M

M waves, 31
Macroelectromyography, 50
Macrolides, caution in use of, 626t
Magnesium
  caution in use of, 626t
  for cramps, 211, 236, 238t, 239
  for Lambert-Eaton myasthenic syndrome, 667
  for tetanus, 245
  for tetany, 246

Magnetic resonance imaging (MRI)
　advantages of, 71
　applications in nerve disease, 72–73
　in brachial plexopathy, 527, 528f, 529f
　lumbosacral spine, 578
　muscle selection using
　　for needle biopsies, 83
　in radiculopathies, 527
　short-T1 inversion recovery, 71
Malignancies
　motor neuron disease and, 227–230
　myopathies and, 948–949
　neuropathies associated with, 440–471, 441t
　PET/CT scans for, 64
　in stiff-person syndrome, 248
　tumor infiltration, 444–446
Malignancy-related vasculitis, 389
Malignant hyperthermia, 234, 973–974
Malignant melanomas, risk of, 118
Manual muscle test (MMT), 631–632
Markesbery-Griggs distal myopathy, 750
Massage for spasticity, 155
Masseter reflex, 398, 511
Matrin-3 (MATR3) mutations, 756
Matrin-3 (MATR3) protein, 708
McArdle disease, 806–807
　aerobic training in, 137
　histology of, 88f
　myophophorylase stains for, 88f
MCPs, serum levels of, 63
Meal preparation, adaptive equipment for, 147–148, 147f
Mean consecutive difference (MCD), 49
Mean sorted difference (MSD), 49
Mebendazole for trichinosis, 921
Medial antebrachial cutaneous nerve, 28, 521
Medial cord lesions, 535
Medial cutaneous nerve, 522
Medial pectoral nerves
　injury to, 544
　innervation by, 522
Medial plantar nerves, 28
Medialis muscle innervation, 571
Median nerve
　anatomy of, 523, 549f
　enlarged, 73f
　leprosy and, 411, 415f
　nerve conduction studies using, 26
　sensory conduction studies, 28, 29f
　ultrasound of, 75f
Median neuropathy, 404, 548–553, 548t
Median sternotomy, 540
Median-chain acyl-CoA dehydrogenase (MCAD) deficiency, 820
Medical histories
　diagnosis and, 2
　patient questioning in, 5–6
　sensory, 10
　taking of, 3–10
Medical Research Council (MRC) scale, 14
Mee's lines, 484
MEGF10-related myopathy, 731
Meiosis, 833
Melanoma differentiation-association protein 1 antibodies, 895t
Melphalan for amyloidosis, 451
Membrane attack complex (MAC), 97f

Meningitis, neoplastic, 589
Meningoencephalitis
　differential diagnosis of, 243
　histopathology of, 224
　laboratory features of, 223–224
　WNV and, 223
Meperidine, myopathies related to, 975
Meralgia paresthetica (MP), 578, 596–597
Mercury toxicity
　clinical features of, 482–483, 483t
　detection of, 483t
　histopathology of, 483
　laboratory features of, 483, 483t
　pathogenesis of, 484
　treatment of, 484
Merosin
　deficiency of, 733
　description of, 705
　function of, 734
Merosin staining, 89
Message banking, 159
Messenger RNA (mRNA), 831
Metabolic myopathies, 798–830
Metabolic syndrome, neuropathies associated with, 498
Metachromatic leukodystrophy (MLD), 297–298
　clinical features of, 297
　histopathology of, 297
　juvenile form of, 297
　laboratory features of, 297
　molecular genetics of, 297
　pathogenesis of, 297
　treatment of, 297–298
Metformin, vitamin B12 deficiency and, 431
Methotrexate (MTX)
　adverse effects of, 120
　contraindications for, 646–647
　dosage, 120
　for inflammatory myopathies, 922t, 924–925
　management considerations, 120
　mechanism of action, 120
　monitoring of, 120
　for multifocal motor neuropathy, 367
　for myasthenia gravis, 641–642
　for Satoyoshi syndrome, 247
　uses, 120
　for vasculitis, 391
Methylmalonic acid (MMA), 431
Methylprednisone
　for CIDP, 118
　dosage, 113t
　for inflammatory myopathies, 922t
　monitoring for, 113t
　side effects of, 113t
　steroid myopathy and, 944–945
Metoclopramide, 338, 495
Metronidazole
　neuropathies associated with, 402–403
　for tetanus, 245
　toxic neuropathies and, 472, 473t
Mexiletine
　for Brody disease, 881
　for cramps, 238t, 239
　for Isaacs syndrome, 242
　for Morvan syndrome, 242
　for myotonia fluctuans, 873

　for painful sensory neuronopathies, 510t
　for paramyotonia congenita, 873
　for Schwartz-Jampel syndrome, 881
Mezagitamab/TAK-079, 640t
Miami-J collar, 140
Microscopic polyangiitis, 388
Microvasculitis associated with diabetes mellitus, 389
Middle cervical ganglion, 517
Midodrine, 338
Miller Fisher syndrome (MFS). See also Inflammatory demyelinating polyradiculoneuropathy (AIDP)
　antiganglioside antibodies associated with, 329f
　clinical features of, 336–337
　histopathology of, 337
　laboratory features of, 337
　pathogenesis of, 337
　plasma exchange for, 125
　treatment of, 337
Mirabergron for urinary urgency, 200
Mirvetuximab soravtansine, 461
Mitochondrial DNA mutations, staining for, 89, 90f
Mitochondrial myopathy, 92f
Mitochondria
　disorders of, 831–856
　fatty acid oxidation by, 816f
　function of, 840
　genome of, 831
Mitochondria recessive ataxic syndrome (MIRAS), 846, 848
Mitochondrial disorders
　classification of, 832t
　genes associated with, 834f
　genetics of, 832–837
　inheritance of, 833–834
　testing for, 71
Mitochondrial DNA
　building blocks for, 835
　composition of, 831
　inheritance of, 832–833
　replication of, 835
Mitochondrial DNA depletion syndromes (MDSs), 846
Mitochondrial encephalopathy, 838
Mitochondrial myopathies
　clinical features of, 833t
　drugs related to, 958t, 964–965
　with exercise intolerance, 850
　exercise studies in, 137
　histopathologic alterations in, 96
　histopathology of, 838–840, 838f, 839f, 840f
　inheritance of, 833t
　investigation of, 841f
　laboratory features of, 837–838
　modified Gomori trichrome stain of, 84
　molecular genetics of, 840–842
Mitochondrial myopathy lactic acidosis and strokes (MELAS), 835, 841, 842–844
　clinical features of, 842–843
　histopathology of, 843
　laboratory features of, 843, 843f
　molecular genetics of, 843
　pathogenesis of, 843
　treatment of, 844

Mitochondrial neurogastrointestinal encephalomyopathy (MNGIE), 846–847
Mitochondrial trifunctional protein (MTP) deficiency, 821
Mitofusin 2 protein, 268
Mitosis, 833
Mixed connective tissue disease (MCTD)
  clinical features of, 910–911
  neuropathies and, 400
  secondary vasculitis and, 388–389
Miyoshi myopathy, 721–722, 721f
MMN. See Multifocal motor neuropathy (MMN)
Mobility issues, management of, 186t
Modified barium swallow (MBS), 157
Monoclonal antibodies, immunosuppression by, 112
Monoclonal gammopathy of undetermined significance (MGUS)
  neuropathy associated with, 63, 453–454
    clinical features of, 453–454
    laboratory features of, 454
    pathogenesis of, 454
    treatment of, 454
Monocycline for leprosy, 413
Monomelic polyneuropathies, 592, 600
Mononeuritis multiplex. See Multifocal neuropathy
Mononeuropathies
  axon loss in, 54
  definition of, 53
  demyelinating, 577
  EDX localization, 52, 52t
  etiologies of, 592, 593t
  evaluation of, 592–594
  imaging of, 578
  lower extremities, 577
  management of, 594–595
  multiple, 55
  pathophysiology of, 524
Mononeuropathy syndromes, 17
Monoradiculopathies
  axon loss and, 54
  clinical features of, 578–581
  clinical involvement, 578t
  definition of, 53–54
  EDX localization, 52
  etiologies of, 580t, 582
  evaluation of, 582–583
  features of, 16
  L3-L4, 581
  L5, 581–582
  laboratory features of, 582–583
  management of, 583–584
  motor deficits in, 579–580
  S1, 582
Montréal cognitive assessment (MOCA), 173–174
Morphine, 245, 495t
Morton's neuromas, 155
Morvan syndrome
  clinical features of, 239
  diagnosis of, 239–240
  immunotherapy for, 242
  laboratory features of, 240–241
Mosquitoes, WNV and, 224
Mother's wrist, 987
Motor fibers, course of, 517

Motor nerve conduction studies, 26
Motor neuron diseases (MNDs)
  causes of, 55
  characteristics of, 166
  EDX localization, 52t
  frontotemporal dementia in, 168
  hallmarks of, 15–16
  HIV and, 221
  hyperparathyroidism and, 943
  infectious causes of, 219–227
  symptom management in, 186t
Motor neuronopathies
  causes of, 55
  EDX localization, 52
Motor symptoms
  causes of weakness, 4t
  origin of, 3
  presentation of, 3
Motor unit action potentials (MUAPs), 42
  abnormal, 626, 627f
  analysis of, 46–47
  arm, 527
  configurations of, 46–47, 47f
  enlarged, 175
  enlargement in ALS, 172
  polyphasic, 175
  recruitment of, 47–48
Motor unit number estimation (MUNE) techniques, 41–42
Motor unit potentials (MUPs), age and, 25
Motor units, estimates of, 41–42
Multi-acyl-CoA dehydrogenase deficiency (MADD), 817f, 821–822
Multibacillary leprosy, 411
Multifocal acquired demyelinating sensory and motor neuropathy (MADSAM)
  CIDP and, 346
  clinical features of, 359
  corticosteroids for, 118
  diagnostic algorithm for, 348f
  features of, 347t
  histopathology of, 359–360
  IVIGs for, 122
  laboratory features of, 359
  treatment of, 357t, 360
Multifocal acquired motor axonopathy (MAMA), 367–368
Multifocal motor neuropathy (MMN), 55
  antibodies specific for, 66
  azathioprine for, 119
  clinical features of, 359, 365–366
  cyclophosphamide for, 122
  deep tendon reflexes in, 175
  diagnostic algorithm for, 348f
  differential diagnosis, 174–175
  features of, 347t
  histopathology of, 359–360, 366
  laboratory features of, 359, 366
  pathogenesis of, 366–367
  rituximab for, 123–124
  SCIg for, 123
  treatment of, 357t, 360, 367
  use of steroids in, 118
Multifocal neuropathies
  disorders resulting from, 18
  EDX localization, 52, 52t
  features of, 18
  multiple mononeuropathies versus, 384t

Multi/minicore myopathy, 777–778, 777f, 778f
Multiple acquired demyelinating sensory and motor neuropathy (MADSAM), 55
Multiple EGF-like domains 10 (MEGF10) mutations, 778
Multiple mononeuropathies
  diabetic, 498
  HIV-related
    clinical features of, 420
    histopathology of, 420
    laboratory features of, 420
    pathogenesis of, 421
    treatment of, 421
  multifocal neuropathies versus, 384t
Multiple myeloma (MM)
  amyloidosis and, 449
  clinical features of, 448
  histopathology of, 449
  laboratory features of, 448–449
  pathogenesis of, 449
Multiple sclerosis (MS), natalizumab exposure in, 116
Multisystem proteinopathies, 705t
Multisystem proteinopathies (MSPs)
  MSP1, 755
  MSP2, 755
  MSP3, 755
  MSP4, 755
  MSP5, 755–756
  MSP6, 756
  mutations related to, 708
Muscarinic receptors, 58–59
Muscle atrophy
  in ALS, 171
  cranial nerves and, 11
  evaluation of, 12
  imaging of, 71–72, 72f
Muscle biopsies
  in ALS, 167, 178f
  anesthesia for, 84
  indications for, 83
  needle artifacts, 26
  site selection for, 83–84
  specimen fixation, 84
  specimen handling for, 84
  techniques for, 83–90
Muscle channelopathies, 864–876
Muscle cramps
  in ALS, 170
  benign, 233
  causes of, 235t
  clinical features of, 233
  description of, 233
  diagnosis of, 234–235
  electrodiagnosis of, 235–236
  management of, 186t
  pathologic, 233
  primary, 235
  secondary, 235
  volume depletion and, 235
Muscle fibers
  adult, 93
  atrophic, 94f
  diameter of, 93
  female, 93
  infant, 93
  male, 93

necrosis of, 96–97
random distribution of, 87
reinnervation of, 96
sarcomeres in, 91
size of, 96f
type 1
    atrophy of, 96
    characteristics of, 87f
    distribution of, 93
    hypotrophy of, 96
    myofibrillar ATPase staining, 87, 87f
type 2, atrophy of, 96
type 2A
    characteristics of, 87f
    distribution of, 93
    myofibrillar ATPase staining, 87, 87f
type 2B
    characteristics of, 87f
    distribution of, 93
    myofibrillar ATPase staining, 87, 87f
type 2C, 87
types of, 85f
Muscle infarct, 387f
Muscle-eye-brain disease, 736
Muscles
    abnormal, 93–98
    adventitous movements of, 12
    atrophy of, 11, 12, 71–72, 72f, 171
    biopsies of, 83
    contractures, 12
    histopathology of, 83–105
    hypertrophy of, 12
    isometric testing of, 13
    manual testing of, 11
    necrotic, 96–97, 97f
    pain related to, 10
    provocative testing of, 13
    spasms, 246
    strength of, 14
    syncytial nature of, 96
    ultrasound of, 75
    upper extremities, 521t
    wasting of, 220f
    weakness of, 83
Muscle-specific kinase (MuSK)
    antibodies to, 607, 611
    autoantibodies to, 67
    congenital myasthenic syndromes and, 678, 679
    deficiency of, 673
    testing for, 175
    titers of, 622
Muscular dystrophies, 702–772
    AChR mutations in, 673
    classification of, 709
    endomysial connective tissue in, 97
    molecular defects of, 703t–705t
    NADH-TR stains for, 90f
Muscular dystrophy-dystroglycanopathies, 705–706
Musculocutaneous nerves
    anatomy of, 522
    injury to, 544–545
    nerve conduction studies using, 27
Musculocutaneous neuropathies, 545t
Myalgias
    causes of, 10
    modified Gomori trichrome stain of, 86f
    muscle specimen in, 86f
    in PPMA, 225
Myasthenia
    edrophonium testing for, 175
    overlap syndromes, 915
    presentation of, 18–19
    rituximab for, 123–124
Myasthenia gravis (MG)
    AChR antibodies in, 58, 611–613, 613f
    associated disorders, 628
    autoimmune, 607–659
        epidemiology of, 613–621, 614t
        genetic contributions to, 612–613
        historical events, 607–608
        pathophysiology of, 607–608
    azathioprine for, 119
    clinical characteristics of, 633f
    clinical course of, 615
    clinical presentation of, 615–616
    contraindicated drugs in, 626t
    corticosteroids for, 112, 118
    cyclosporine for, 121
    diagnosis of, 620–621, 620f, 621t
    electrodiagnostic testing in, 622–627
    eosinophilic myositis and, 916f
    examination in, 617, 617t, 619, 619t
    exercise and, 648
    IVIGs for, 122
    laboratory features of, 621
    management of, 632–634, 633t, 635t
    maternal, 15
    MuSK-positive, 112
    natural history of, 614–615, 615t
    neurologic examination in, 617
    ocular muscles in, 617–619, 618f
    outcomes, 630–632, 631t
    pathophysiology of, 609–611
        phenotype and, 613
    plasma exchange for, 125
    pregnancy and, 646–647
    response to repetitive stimulation, 34f
    response to repetitive stimulus, 56
    SCIG for, 123
    serologic testing in, 621–622
    severity of, 630–632, 631t
    subtypes of, 644–646
    symptoms of, 616–617, 633–634
    tacrolimus for, 122
    thymic imaging in, 628–629
    thymoma-associated, 612–613, 615
Myasthenia Gravis Activity of Daily Living (MG-ADL), 115
Myasthenia gravis impairment index (MGII), 632
Myasthenia gravis patient-acceptable symptom state (MG PASS), 632
Myasthenia Gravis Quality of Life (MG-QOL), 115
Myasthenic crisis, 644
Myasthenic sneer, 619
Myasthenics, antibodies detected in, 67–68
Mycobacterium leprae, 411, 412f
Mycobacterium tuberculosis, 116
Mycophenolate monfetil (MMF)
    adverse effects of, 121
    for chronic inflammatory demyelinating polyneuropathy, 358
    dosage of, 121
    for inflammatory myopathies, 922t, 925
    management of, 121
    mechanism of action, 120
    for multifocal motor neuropathy, 367
    for myasthenia gravis, 641–642, 646
    for neuromuscular disorders, 113t
    during pregnancy, 646
    uses, 120–121
Mycophenolate sodium (Myfortic®), 121
Mycophenolic acid, 121
Mycoplasma pneumoniae, 326–327
Myelin
    degeneration of, 297
    growth disturbances, 17
    nerve compression and, 576
    stains for, 101
Myelin protein zero (MPZ), 263
Myelin protein zero *(MPZ)* mutations, 260, 263
Myelin sheaths, damage to, 106
Myelin-associated glycoprotein (MAG)
    antibodies against, 64, 66, 448, 453
    neuropathy and, 63
Myelodysplasia, polyradiculopathies and, 588
Myelopathies, cervical radiculopathies and, 533
Myoadenylate deaminase deficiency (MADD), 814–815, 817f
Myoclonic epilepsy and ragged red fibers (MERRF), 842
Myoclonus, treatment of, 842
Myoedema, definition of, 13
Myofascial pain syndrome (MPS), 952
Myofibrillar myopathies, 705t
Myofibrillar myopathies (MFMs), 752–756
    clinical features of, 752
    histopathology of, 753–754, 753f
    laboratory features of, 752–753
    modified Gomori trichrome stain of, 87
    molecular genetics of, 754–755
    pathogenesis of, 754–755
    treatment of, 755
Myofibrillogenesis, 707
Myofilaments, synthesis of, 93–94
Myoglobinuria, 806
    recurrent, 64
Myokymic discharges, 241, 241f
    disorders associated with, 45–46, 46t
    in Isaacs syndrome, 240
    in Morvan syndrome, 240
    spontaneous activity and, 45
Myonuclei, normal distribution of, 91
Myopathic disorders
    calcium disorders and, 948
    description of, 93
    diagnosis of, 19
    electrolyte imbalance and, 947–948
    features of, 19–21
    hereditary, 19
    histopathologic alterations in, 96
    magnesium disorders and, 948
    malignancies and, 948–949
    muscle cramps and, 234
    muscle fiber loss in, 96
    muscle fiber size and, 96f
    phosphate disorders and, 948
    toxic, 957–982

1018 INDEX

Myopathies
  adrenal disorders and, 944–945
  affected proteins, 704t
  blood testing for, 64
  electrodiagnosis in, 51
  endocrine, 940–945
  necrotizing, 957–963
  pituitary disorders and, 945–946
  systemic diseases and, 940–956
Myopathy with excessive autophagy (XMEA), X-linked, 813–814, 814f
Myopathy with fibrillation and positive waves, 52t
Myopathy with myotonia, 52t
Myopathy without abnormal spontaneous activity, 52t
Myophophorylase *(PYGM)* mutations, 806
Myophophorylase stains, 88f
Myoshi distal myopathy, 751
Myosin heavy chain 2 *(MYH2)* mutations, 755
Myosin heavy chain 7 *(MYH7)* mutations, 743, 751, 777, 778, 789
Myosin light chain 2 *(MYL2)* mutations, 754
Myosin storage myopathy, 788–789
Myositis
  immune checkpoint inhibitors and, 647–648, 647f
  overlap syndromes, 915
Myositis-associated antibodies (MAAs), 68
Myositis-specific antibodies (MSAs), 68
Myotilin *(MYOT)* mutations, 754
Myotilins, 707
Myotonia, eyelid, 11
Myotonia congenita (MC)
  chloride channels and, 28, 868f
  clinical features of, 864, 867
  exercise testing in, 39
  ion channels in, 36–37
  laboratory features of, 867
  molecular genetics of, 867
  pathogenesis of, 867
  screening for, 882f
  treatment of, 867, 869
Myotonia fluctuans, 873
Myotonia permanens, 873–874
Myotonic discharges, 43f, 44–45, 44f
  disorders associated with, 45t
  ion channel disorders and, 44–45
  origin of, 44
Myotonic dystrophies, 857–863
  exercise studies in, 136
  features of, 15
  hand exercises in, 152
  screening for, 882f
  types of, 858t
Myotonic dystrophy 1 (DM1), 857–860
  associated manifestations of, 857–858
  clinical features of, 857, 858f
  electromyography in, 858f
  exercise testing in, 39
  histopathology of, 858–859, 859f
  laboratory features of, 858
  molecular genetics of, 859
  mutations related to, 708
  pathogenesis of, 859
  treatment of, 859–860
Myotonic dystrophy 2 (DM2), 859–860

  associated manifestations in, 860
  clinical features of, 860
  exercise testing in, 39
  histopathology of, 861
  laboratory features of, 860–861
  molecular genetics of, 861
  pathogenesis of, 861
  treatment of, 861
Myotonic syndromes, exercise testing in, 868f
Myotubularin 1 *(MTM1)* mutations, 786f
Mytochondral myopathies
  classification of, 832t
  muscle specimen in, 86f

N

NADH-TR stains
  disorganized filaments on, 94
  for muscular dystrophy, 90f
  target fibers on, 95f
  use of, 89
Naftidrofuryl for cramps, 238t
Nasogastric tubes, 158
Natalizumab exposure in MS, 116
Native American myopathy, 792
Navajo neurohepatopathy, 846, 848
Nebulin, 707
Nebulin *(NEB)* mutations, 751, 777
Neck drop, 186t
Neck extensor myopathy, 779
Neck flexion
  strength of, 15
  testing of, 13
  weakness in, 19
Neck muscles
  strength of, 619–620
  weakness of, 8
Necrosis
  in myopathies, 96
  segmental, 96, 97f
  repair of, 96–97
Necrotizing myopathies, drug-related, 958t
Necrotizing vasculitis, 108f
Needle artifacts, 26
Needle biopsies, 83
Nemaline myopathy
  clinical features of, 779–780
  histopathology of, 780f, 781f
  laboratory features of, 780
  late-onset, 782, 783f
  mitochondria in, 92f
  molecular genetics of, 781–782
Nemaline rod myopathy, 778
Nemaline rods, staining of, 86f
Neonatal Fc receptors (FcRn) antagonists, 638–639, 639t
Neoplastic meningitis, 229–230
Neostigmine, response to, 621
Nerve biopsies, 98–108
  immunohistochemistry of, 101
  indications for, 98–99
  paraffin embedded, 101, 102f
  specimen handling, 100–101
  techniques for, 99–105, 100f
  usefulness of, 98
Nerve conduction studies (NCS). *See also* Electrodiagnosis (EDX)
  in Charcot-Marie-Tooth, 259–261

  motor, 260–261, 525t, 526
  peripheral nerves, 576
  safety considerations in, 23, 25
  sensory, 261, 525t
  Sjögren syndrome and, 397–398
Nerve conduction velocities (NCVs), 256, 260
Nerve fibers
  damage to, 524
  myelinated, 106
  structure of, 106
  teased, 105f
  unmyelinated, 106
Nerve root compression, 16
Nerve sprouts, 107f
Nerve transfers, 56–57
Nerves
  biopsies of, 98–99
  compression of, 548
  entrapment, imaging of, 72–73
  grafting of, 56
  injuries to, 51, 56–75
  ischemic injury to, 108
  reactions to injury, 106–108
  repair of, 56
  structure of, 105–106
Nesprins, location of, 707
Neuralgic amyotrophy. *See* Immune-mediated brachial plexus neuropathies (IBPN)
Neuroendocrine tumors (NETs), 628
Neurofascin 140 (NF140) antibodies, 362, 363
Neurofascin 155 (NF155) antibodies, 67, 363, 364f
Neurofascin 155 (NF155) protein, 364f
Neurofascin 186 (NF186) antibodies, 363
Neurofascin 186 (NF186) protein, 364f
Neurofibromas, 537
  features of, 104f
  plexopathies and, 537
Neurofilament light chain *(NEFL or NFL)* mutations, 263
Neurofilaments, leakage of, 179
Neurogenic atrophy, 93, 94f
Neurogenic claudication, 584, 585f
Neuroleptic malignant syndrome, 234, 243
Neurolymphomatosis
  clinical features of, 444
  definition of, 229
  histopathology of, 445
  laboratory features of, 444, 445f
  treatment of, 445–446
Neuromuscular blocking, 50, 626t
Neuromuscular diseases
  clinician goals in, 2
  differential diagnoses, 2
  energy expenditure in, 153
  exercise recommendations for, 139–140, 139t
  exercise relevant to, 134t
  falls in, 153–154
  genetic testing in, 69–71
  infectious causes of, 68
  plasma exchange for, 125
  rehabilitation for, 155–156
  rehabilitation for people with, 131–164
  risk factors for, 2
  serologic tests for, 68–69
  testing in, 23–82
Neuromuscular disorders

immunosuppression and, 113t–114t
key questions, 3t
Neuromuscular junctions (NMJs)
  AChR antibody positive, 610, 610f
  disorders of, 93
  function of, 608–609
  postsynaptic structures at, 609, 609f
  presynaptic structures at, 608f, 609
  structure of, 608–609
Neuromuscular mimics
  definition of, 983
  lower limb, 984t
  upper limb, 984t
Neuromuscular sclerosis, rehabilitation in, 151
Neuromuscular transmission disorders, 18–19
  features of, 18–19
  postsynaptic, 18–19
  presynaptic, 19
Neuromyelitis optica spectrum disorder (MNOSD), 640
Neuromyotonia, 29f
Neuromyotonic discharges, 44f, 241f
  description of, 27
  disorders associated with, 46, 46t
  Isaacs syndrome and, 240
  secondary causes of, 240t
  spontaneous activity and, 45
Neuronopathies, 52
Neuropathic pain
  management of, 591
  postbiopsy, 99–100
  recognition of, 10
Neuropathies
  immune-mediated, 400–403
  infectious agents associated with, 412f
  inherited, 258t
  painful, 498
  pathogenic targets of, 258t
  systemic disorder-associated, 398t
  treatment-induced, 498
Neuropathy ataxia and retinitis pigmentosa (NARP), 848
Neuropraxia, 524
Neurosaroidosis, 402
Neurosyphilis, 417, 418
Neurotmesis, 524
Neutral lipid storage disease, 822
Niacin
  myopathies related to, 960
  statin myopathy and, 957
Niclosamide for cysticercosis, 921
Nipocalimab, 638, 639t
Nitrofurantoin
  toxic neuropathies and, 473t
Nitrofurantoin, toxic neuropathies and
  clinical features of, 472, 473t
  diagnostic testing for, 473t
  nerve histopathology in, 473t
Nitrofusin 2 (MFN2) mutations, 268
Nitrous oxide, vitamin B12 deficiency and, 433
Nivolumab, 461
NMDA antibodies, 249
Nodes of Ranvier, 106
Nodopathies
  diagnostic algorithm for, 348f
  features of, 347t, 362–363
  histopathology of, 363–364

laboratory features of, 363
pathogenesis of, 363–364
treatment of, 357t, 364–365
Nondiabetic lumbosacral radiculoplexus neuropathy (non0DLRPN), 578
Nondystrophic muscle channelopathies
  electrophysiologic testing of, 35
  exercise tests, 38t, 865t
  Fournier electrophysiologic patterns, 865t, 866f
  genes involved in, 865t
  presentation of, 35
Nondystrophic myotonias
  exercise tests in, 882f
  postexercise myotonic potentials in, 35
  RNS techniques in, 37f
Non-Hodgkin lymphoma, GBS and, 229–230
Noninvasive ventilation (NIV), 185
Non-small cell lung cancer (non-SCLD), 660
Nonspecific/unspecified myositis, 889t–891t
Nonsteroidal immunosuppressive therapies (NSISTs), 641–642
Nonsystemic vasculitis, 390
Nontropical sprue, 402
Notch signaling, muscular dystrophies and, 708
Nucleoside analog neuropathies, 476
Nucleoside reverse transcriptase inhibitors
  toxic neuropathies and, 473t
Nucleus pulposus, discogenic pain and, 566
Numb thumb, 531
Numbness, patient history of, 10
Nurses, rehabilitation and, 131
Nusinersen, 207, 208t
Nutritional deficiencies, neuropathies related to, 430–439
Nystagmus, malignancies and, 440

O

Obinutuzumab, 641
Obstetrically-related plexopathies, 536–537
Obturator nerve anatomy, 571, 572f, 573f
Obturator neuropathies, 597–598
Occupational therapists (OTs), 131
Ocrelizumab for myastenia gravis, 641
OCTN2 mutations, 818
Ocular myasthenia gravis, 644–645
Ocular neuromyotonia, 239
Oculomotor apraxia type 4 (AOA4), 268
Oculopharangeal distal musclar dystrophy (OPDM), 705t
Oculopharyngeal muscular dystrophies (OPMD)
Oculopharyngeal muscular dystrophy (OPMD), 705t, 708, 746–748
Ofatumumab, 641
Oil red O stains, 87, 89f
Okinawa type SMA-LED
  features of, 204t
Oligodendrocytes, 298f
Omeprazole, 959t, 972
Onasemnogene abeparvovev-xioi, 207, 208t
Onion bulbs, 106, 106f
Ophthalmoparesis, 12
Ophthalmoplegia, 7, 8t, 440
Opioids
  myopathies related to, 975
  for painful sensory neuronopathies, 495t

Opisthotonus in tetanus, 243f
Opponens splints, 141
Opsoclonus, malignancies and, 440
Optic atrophy 1 (OA1), 846, 848–849
Optimal neck brace, 140f
Optineurin, 182
ORAI1 mutations, 880
Orai-1 protein, 790
Organophosphate poisoning, 686–688
  clinical features of, 479t, 480–481
  diagnosis of, 687
  diagnostic testing for, 479t
  features of, 686–687
  histopathology of, 481
  laboratory features of, 481, 687
  mechanism of, 479t
  pathogenesis of, 481, 687
  treatment of, 687–688
Oropharyngeal muscles, 619
Orthodromic technique, 28
Orthoses (braces), 140–143, 140f
Orthostatic blood pressure, 15
Orthostatic intolerance, 58
Orthotic devices, disuse atrophy and, 153
Orthotists, rehabilitation and, 131
Osimertinib, myopathies related to, 968
Osteoarthritis (OA)
  carpometacarpal joint, 988–989
  hip joint, 989
  pain in, 155
  thumb, 988f
Osteolysis, multiple myeloma and, 448–449
Osteomalacia, hyperparathyroidism and, 942–943
Osteoporosis, prevention of, 923
Osteosclerotic myeloma
  clinical features of, 451
  histopathology of, 452
  laboratory features of, 451
  pathogenesis of, 452
  treatment of, 452
Out-of-wind phenomena, 808
Oxaliplatin, neuropathies secondary to
  clinical features of, 455
  histopathology of, 455
  laboratory features of, 455
  pathogenesis of, 455
Oxidative enzyme stains, 93
Oxybutynin for urinary urgency, 200
Oxycodone for pain, 495t

P

PABPN1 mutations, 747
Pacemakers, nerve conduction studies and, 25
Paclitaxel (Taxol), 456t, 458–459
Paddling, adaptive, 138f
Paget disease of bone (PDB), 708
Pain
  chronic, 155–156
  management of, 155–156
  neuropathic, 10
  perception of, 10
  radiculopathies and, 16
  weakness and, 6
Palate, weakness of, 156
Palmaris brevis syndrome, 234
Palmaris longus innervation, 523

Pancreatic transplantation, 495
Panhypopituitarism, 946
Paraesthesias, tetany and, 245
Paraffin sections, 84, 96
Paramyotonia, eyelid, 11
Paramyotonia congenita (PMC), 37
    clinical features of, 872
    histopathology of, 873
    laboratory features of, 872–873, 872f
    molecular genetics of, 873
    pathogenesis of, 873
    screening for, 882f
    short exercise testing, 40
    sodium channel mutation in, 40
    treatment of, 873
Paraneoplasia, 228–229
Paraneoplastic antibodies, 65
Paraneoplastic autonomic neuropathy, 443
Paraneoplastic encephalomyelitis (PEM), 440–442
    sensory neuropathy and, 440–442
Paraneoplastic sensorimotor polyneuropathy
    clinical features of, 443
    histopathology of, 443
    laboratory features of, 443
Paranodopathies
    description of, 361–362
    diagnostic algorithm for, 348f
    histopathology of, 363–364
    laboratory features of, 363
    pathogenesis of, 363–364
    treatment of, 364–365
Paraparetic patterns in weakness, 14
Paraproteinemic neuropathies, 448–454
Parathesia, patient history of, 10
Parathyroid disorders, 942–944
Parents, interviews with, 2
Paromomycin for cysticercosis, 921
Paroxysmal extreme pain disorder, 284
Parsonage-Turner syndrome. *See* Immune-mediated brachial plexus neuropathies (IBPN)
PAS stain, 101, 103f
Patients, evaluation of, 2
Paucibacillary leprosy, 411
Pectineus muscle innervation, 571
Pediatric patients. *See also* Infants
    anesthesia for, 100
    causes of weakness in, 4t
    immunotherapies for, 117
    muscle biopsies in, 84
    nerve biopsies, 100
    parent interviews, 2
    plastic hinged ankle-foot orthoses, 142f
Peek sign, 619t
Pegunigalsidase, 300
Pelvic floor innervation, 576
D-Penicillamine
    contraindication for, 626t
    myopathies related to, 968
Penicillin G, 245, 418
Penicillin VK, 637
Penicillins for tetanus, 245
Penis, innervation of, 576
Pentamidine, 115–116
Pentazocine, myopathies related to, 975
Pentoxifylline for leprosy, 416

Percussion myotonia, 13
Percutaneous endoscopic gastrostomy (PEG), 158, 185
Perifascicular atrophy, 896, 896f
Perikaryon, 106
Perineal nerve, 576
Perineum, innervation of, 571f, 576
Periodic acid-Schiff (PAS) stains
    target fibers on, 94
    type 2 fibers on, 93
    use of, 87, 88f, 89
Periodic paralysis
    exercise tests in, 38t
    long-exercise tests in, 871f
Peripheral myelin protein 22 *(PMP22)* mutations, 260–263
Peripheral myelin protein 22 (PMP22) protein, 262–263
Peripheral nerve vasculitis, 384t, 390
Peripheral nerves
    antibodies directed toward, 66–67
    hyperexcitability, 69
    infiltration by lymphomas, 229
    injury to, 576–577
    lesions, 51
    schematic of fibers, 66f
    structure of, 105
    tumors of, 73
Peripheral neuropathies
    blood testing for, 62–64
    causes of, 10
    dysautonomia-associated, 58t
    mitochondrial, 836f–837f
    nutritional deficiencies related to, 431t
    paraneoplastic antibodies in, 65
    rheumatoid arthritis and, 399
    Sjögren syndrome and, 397
Pernicious anemia, 432
Peroneal nerve
    anatomy of, 574f
    leprosy and, 411
Peroneus brevis muscle
    biopsy of, 385f, 386f
    innervation of, 574
Peroneus tertius muscle innervation, 574
Peroxisomal disorders, 300–305
Perseveration, 173
Pes anserine bursitis, 991–992, 991f
PFK deficiency, 807–808
Phalen sign, 550
Phenobarbital, 251, 433
Phenytoin
    for cramps, 238t, 239
    drug interactions with, 433
    for hyperekplexia, 251
    for Isaacs syndrome, 242
    for Morvan syndrome, 242
    myopathies related to, 968
    for painful sensory neuronopathies, 510t
    toxic neuropathies and, 474t, 478
Philadelphia collar, 140
Phosphatidic acid phosphatase deficiency, 822–823
Phosphoglucomutase 1 deficiency, 811
Phosphoglycerate kinase deficiency, 812
Phosphoglycerate mutase (GPAM) deficiency, 92f, 809–810

Phosphoglycerate mutase *(GPAM)* mutations, 790
Phosphorylase B kinase deficiency, 808
Phosphorylated neurofilament heavy chain (pNFH), 179
Phrenic nerve
    anatomy of, 522
    nerve conduction studies using, 27
Physiatrists, rehabilitation and, 131
Physical activities
    adaptive sports and, 138–139
    rehabilitation use of, 133–134
Physical Activity Guidelines for Americans, 135
Physical examinations, 10–15
Physical therapists (PTs), 131
Physical therapy, 924
    for distrophinopathies, 714
    for HSP, 200
Picornaviruses, 227
Pigmentary retinopathy, 434
PINCH-2 related myopathy, 729
Piracetam for hyperekplexia, 251
Piriformis syndrome, 598
Piritramide, myopathies related to, 975
Pironolactone for hypoKPP1, 878–879
Plantar fasciitis
    diagnosis of, 992, 992f, 993f
    pain in, 155
    symptoms of, 992
    treatment of, 992–993
Plasma exchange (PLEX)
    adverse effects of, 125
    for AIDP, 331–333
    for chronic inflammatory demyelinating polyneuropathy, 356–357, 358
    for Lambert-Eaton myasthenic syndrome, 667
    management of, 125
    mechanism of action, 125
    for MuSK ab positive mG, 645
    for myasthenia gravis, 607, 646–647
    for myasthenia gravis management, 634–635
    for neuromuscular disorders, 114t
    for nodopathies, 365
    for paranodopathies, 365
    during pregnancy, 646–647
    for radioplexus neuropathies, 591
    side effects of, 114t, 635
    uses for, 125
    volume of, 125
Plasmacytomas, amyloidosis and, 449
Plasmapheresis, 357t, 926–927
Plastic hinged ankle-foot orthoses, 142f
Plastic posterior leaf spring (PLS) orthoses, 142f
Plastic solid ankle-foot orthoses, 142f
Plectin, 673, 678
Plectin-1 mutations, 727–728
Pleocytosis in poliomyelitis, 221
Plexopathies
    cancer and, 446–448
    definition of, 54
    EDX localization, 52, 52t
    features of, 17
    lower extremities, 577
    neoplasm-related, 537, 540

obstetrically related, 536–537
pathophysiology of, 524
perioperative, 540
radiation-induced, 540
sacral, 589
surgical treatment of, 542
PLIN4 myopathy, 752
Pneumococcus vaccines
in myasthenia gravis, 648
pre-immunotherapies, 117
Pneumocystis jirovecii (PIP), 115–117
Pneumocystis prophylaxis, 923
Pneumonitis pneumonia, 115–117
diagnosis of, 115
presentation of, 115
prophylaxis against, 116
treatment of, 115–116
Pneumothorax, needle electromyography and, 25
Podophylin, toxic neuropathies and, 474t, 478–479
POEMS syndrome
clinical features of, 451
diagnostic algorithm for, 348f
histopathology of, 452
laboratory features of, 451–452
pathogenesis of, 452
presentation of, 63
treatment of, 452
Poliomyelitis
clinical features of, 219–220
description of, 219
electrodiagnosis of, 221
histopathology of, 221
incidence of, 219
pathogenesis of, 221
PCR results in, 221
presentation of, 16
prevention of, 221
spinal cord, 221
treatment of, 221
Poliovirus
motor neuron disease and, 219–222
types of, 221
POLIP syndrome, 846–847
Polyarteritis nodosa (PAN), 387
Polyglucosan bodies, 107f
Polyglucosan body neuropathy, 87, 88f, 103f, 107f, 804
Polyglucosan disease, 177
Polymyalgia rheumatica, 950–951
Polymyositis (PM)
associated manifestations, 899
clinical features of, 898–899
diagnostic criteria for, 889t–891t
differential diagnosis of, 900–901, 901t
electrophysiological features of, 899
exercise studies in, 137
histopathology of, 899–900, 900f
inflammatory cells in, 91f
laboratory features of, 899, 899f
pathogenesis of, 900
prognosis in, 901
use of steroids for, 118
Polyneuropathies
amyloidosis and, 449
discussion of, 54–55

hypoglycemia/hyperinsulinemia and, 498–499
serum MCP levels in, 63
Polynucleotide kinase 3'-phosphatase *(PNKP)* mutations, 268
Polyradiculoneuropathies
EDX localization, 52
electrodiagnostic studies of, 577
etiologies of, 583f
features of, 18
lower extremities, 577
polyradiculopathy *versus*, 54
Polyradiculopathies
axon loss in, 54
definition of, 54
diabetic, 496
EDX localization, 52, 52t
etiologies of, 17, 585–588
evaluation of, 588–589
features of, 16–17
infectious causes of, 587
lower extremities, 577, 584–585
lumbosacral, 420
management of, 589
neoplastic meningitis and, 229
polyradiculoneuropathy *versus*, 54
progressive, 420
sarcoidosis and, 400
Pomalidomide, toxic neuropathies and, 461
POMGNT1 mutations, 727, 735, 736
POMGNT2 mutations, 735
POMK mutations, 735
Pompe disease, 799–803
acid phosphatase stains in, 89f
classification of, 729
clinical features of, 801
histopathology of, 801–801, 802f
infantile, 801, 803
laboratory features of, 801
late-onset, 801
pathogenesis of, 802
screening for, 64
POMT1 mutations, 726
Popeye domain-containing protein 1 *(POPDC1)* mutations, 729
Porphyria, 313–314
clinical features of, 313
diagnosis of, 220t
features of, 220t, 221
laboratory features of, 313
molecular genetics of, 314
pathogenesis of, 314
pathway, 314f
treatment of, 314
Position transfers, adaptive equipment for, 149
Postacute COVID-19 syndrome (PACS), 422
Posterior cord lesions, 534
Posterior cutaneous nerve of the forearm, 28
Posterior cutaneous nerve of the thigh, 571–572, 573–574
Posterior interosseous nerve (PIN), 523
Posterior interosseous neuropathy, 546, 546t
Posterior leaf spring (PLS) ankle-foot orthoses, 142
Posterior longitudinal ligament, 565
Postexercise myotonic potentials (PEMPs), 28

nondystrophic myotonia testing, 35, 37, 38t, 39
in paramyotonia congenita, 872f
periodic paralysis testing, 38t
Postganglionic sudomotor dysfunction, 59
Postpolio progressive muscular atrophy (PPMA)
clinical features of, 224–226, 226f
description of, 224
diagnosis of, 226
electrodiagnosis of, 226
histopathology of, 227, 227f
laboratory features of, 226–227
pain in, 155
pathogenesis of, 227
treatment of, 227
Postpolio syndrome. See Postpolio progressive muscular atrophy (PPMA)
Postsnyptic disorders of neuromuscular transmission, 52t
Postsurgical inflammatory neuropathy, 390
Potassium, serum levels of, 236
Potassium channel *(KCNE3)* mutations, 880
Potassium channel *(KCNJ18)* mutations, 941
Potassium supplementation, 924
Potassium-aggravated myotonia (PAM), 873
chloride channels in, 37
exercise testing in, 39
long exercise testing in, 41
Potassium-sensitive periodic paralysis, 869–872
Power elevation leg rests, 155–156
Power scooters, 145
PPMA. See Postpolio progressive muscular atrophy (PPMA)
Pralidoxime, 688
Praziquantel, 921
Prednisolone, 356, 357t
Prednisone
for amyloidosis, 451
for autoimmune autonomic neuropathy, 338
for chronic inflammatory demyelinating polyneuropathy, 356
for CIDP, 118
in distrophinopathies, 713
dosages, 113t
in Duchenne muscular dystrophy, 713
for giant cell arteritis, 915
for HIV-related mononeuropathies, 421
for inflammatory myopathies, 922t, 923
monitoring of, 113t
for MuSK ab positive MG, 645
for myasthenia gravis management, 634–635
side effects of, 113t, 713
tapering of, 924
for vasculitis, 391
Pregabalin
for diabetic neuropathy, 493
for fibromyalgia, 952
for myofascial pain syndrome, 952
for neuropathic pain, 591
for painful sensory neuronopathies, 495t, 510t
Pregnancy
immunotherapies during, 117
myasthenia gravis and, 646–647
Prembrolizumab, 461

Presnyptic disorders of neuromuscular transmission, 52t
Pressure mapping for wheelchairs, 146
Presynaptic disorders of neuromuscular transmission, 55–56
Priformis muscle, 573
Priformis syndrome, 573
Primary amyloidosis
   clinical features of, 449
   laboratory features of, 449–450
   sural nerve biopsy, 447f
Primary biliary cirrhosis (PBC), 403
Primary carnitine deficiency, 818–819
Primary lateral sclerosis (PLS), 166, 172–173
Primidone for tremor, 211
Probenecid for neurosyphilis, 418
Procainamide
   caution in use of, 626t
   in myathenia gravis, 626t
   myopathies related to, 968
   for Schwartz-Jampel syndrome, 881
Progressive disorders, rehabilitation strategies in, 133
Progressive encephalomyelitis with rigidity (PERM), 247–248
Progressive multifocal leukoencephalopathy (PML), 116
Progressive muscular atrophy (PMA), 166, 175
Progressive external ophthalmoplegia (PEO), 834, 835, 844–845, 845f
Progressive reversible leukoencephalopathy syndrome (PRES), 328
Pronator teres muscle, 523
Propofol, myopathies related to, 961–962
Propranolol for tremor, 211
Proprioception
   balance training and, 137–138
   Romberg test of, 15
Prosaposin *(PSAP)* gene, 297
Prostate cancer, 660
Protein gene product 9.5 (PGP 9.5), 109, 109f
Protein O-glucosyltransferase 1 *(POGLIT1)* mutations, 729–730, 735
Protein synthesis, mitochondria and, 831–832
Protein-O-mannosyltransferase *(POMT)* mutations, 727
Proteosome inhibitors, 457t, 460
Provastatin, myopathy and, 957–960
Proximal diabetic neuropathy, 496–497
Proximal hereditary motor and sensory neuropathy/neuronopathy (HMSN-P)
   clinical features of, 275
   histopathology of, 275
   laboratory features of, 275
   molecular genetics of, 275
   pathogenesis of, 275
Proximal median neuropathy, 548, 548t
Proximal myotonic myopathy, 882f
Proximal radial neuropathy, 546, 546t
Proximal ulnar neuropathy, 553, 553t
Proximal upper limb weakness, rehabilitation in, 151–152
Pseudobulbar affect
   in ALS, 171
   management of, 186t
   UMN signs and, 14

Pseudobulbar palsy, 6
Pseudointernuclear ophthalmoplegia (INO), 619
Pseudomyotonia, 239
Psoas innervation, 571
Psoriatic arthritis, 125
Ptosis
   awareness of, 7
   causes of, 7, 8t, 156
   in congenital myasthenic syndromes, 672f
   facial weakness and, 11
   management of, 156
   in myasthenia gravis, 618
Pudendal nerve, 571, 576
Pudendal neuropathies, 599–600
Pulmonary function testing, 178
Pulse variations, 15
Pupils, examination of, 12
Purine nucleotide metabolism, 814–815
Pyknotic nuclear clumps, 93–94
Pyomyositis, 919
Pyridostigmine
   for congenital myasthenic syndromes, 678
   for diabetic neuropathies, 495
   for juvenile MG, 646
   for Lambert-Eaton myasthenic syndrome, 667
   for myasthenia gravis, 633–634
   response to, 621, 625
Pyridoxine, toxic neuropathies and, 474t, 478
Pyridoxine deficiency, 431
PYROXD1 mutation, 754

Q

Quad canes, 144f
Quadraparetic patterns in weakness, 14
Quadriceps weakness, 186t
Quality of life (QOL) scores, 631–632
QuantiFERON-TB Gold In-Tube assay, 116
Quantitative sensory testing (QST)
   accuracy of, 57
   algorithms for, 57
   measurements provided by, 57–58
   in polyneuropathy, 505
Quantitative sudomotor axon reflex testing (QSART), 57–58, 61, 505, 506f–507f
Quinidine, 239, 678
Quinine, 626t
   for cramps, 211
Quinine sulfate, 237–239, 238t

R

Rabies
   diagnosis of, 220t
   differential diagnosis of, 243
   features of, 220t
Rabies virus, 221, 221t
Radial nerve
   anatomy of, 523
   injuries to, 545–548
   leprosy and, 411
   nerve conduction studies using, 26
   sensory conduction studies, 28
Radial neuropathies, 545–548, 547f
Radiation plexitis, 447, 540

Radiation therapy
   delayed impacts of, 176
   lumbosacral plexopathy induced by, 448
   myelopathy and, 228
   polyradiculopathies and, 588
Radiation-induced motor neuron disease (RIMND)
   electrodiagnosis of, 228
   features of, 228
   pathogenesis of, 228
Radiculopathexitis
   pain in, 155
   use of steroids in, 118
Radiculopathies
   C5, 531
   C6, 531–532
   C7, 532
   C8/T1, 532
   causes of, 531t
   chronic, 16
   lower extremities, 576–577
   lumbar, 579f
   pathophysiology of, 524
   sarcoidosis and, 400
   thoracic, 532–533
   treatment of, 533
Radiculoplexus neuropathies, 590t
   diabetic, 496–498
   etiologies of, 589–591
   evaluation of, 591–592
   lower extremities, 577
   sacral, 589
Radiography, lumbosacral spine, 578
Ragged red fibers, 842
Range of motion exercises, 154
Rapamycin, statin myopathy and, 957
Rapsyn deficiency
   in congenital myasthenic syndromes, 672
   congenital myasthenic syndromes and, 678, 679
   presentation of, 673
Rapsyn mutations, 668
Rattlesnake (*Crotalid* sp.) venom, 688
Ravulizumab for myasthenia gravis, 636t
Rectus femoris innervation, 571
Recurrent myoglobinuria, 850
Red fibers, ragged, 84, 86f, 90f
Reduced cytochrome C oxidase (COX) staining, 89f, 90f
Reducing body myopathy
   clinical features of, 790–791
   histopathology of, 792
   laboratory features of, 791
   molecular genetics of, 792
   pathogenesis of, 792
Reflex loss in polyradiculoneuropathy, 18
Refsum disease (HMSN IV), 302–303
   clinical features of, 302–303
   histopathology of, 303
   laboratory features of, 303
   molecular genetics of, 303
   pathogenesis of, 303
   treatment of, 303
Rehabilitation
   approaches to, 150
   functional challenges in, 132–133
   mobility aids, 143–146

multidisciplinary team for, 131
in neuromuscular diseases, 131–164
patient encounters with, 132
problem orientation of, 132
technological advances in, 159
therapy prescriptions, 133
tools used in, 133–137
uses of, 131
Rehydration for cramps, 239
Reinnervation, changes due to, 96
Renal failure, neuropathies associated with, 403–404
Repetitive nerve stimulation (RNS) techniques, 33–35
in congenital myasthenic syndrome, 677
electrode placement, 33
false-positive decremental responses, 33
in myasthenia gravis, 623–625, 624f
in nondystrophic myotonia, 37f
safety considerations in, 25
Replication factor complex subunit 1 gene, 285
Resistance exercises
benefits of, 134t
guidelines, 139–140
Respiratory chain
genetic control of, 835t
schematic view of, 835f
Respiratory muscles in MG, 620
Respiratory weakness, 156
Rhabdomyolysis
features of, 19
snake venom and, 689
Rhabdomyolysis/myoglobinuria (RHB/MGU)
causes of, 19, 20t
diagnosis of, 20
features of, 19–21
pathology of, 20
symptoms of, 19–20
RHB/GMU. *See* Rhabdomyolysis/myoglobinuria (RHB/MGU)
Rheumatoid arthritis (RA)
clinical features of, 399, 910
histopathology of, 399, 399f
laboratory features of, 399
peripheral neuropathies and, 399
secondary vasculitis and, 388–389
tofacitinib for, 125
treatment of, 399
Rhizotomy for HSP management, 199t
Riboflavin deficiency, 431
Ribosomal RNA (rRNA), 831
Rick's Real Neuromuscular Friends, 116
Rifampin
drug interactions with, 116
for leprosy, 413
TB prophylaxis using, 116
Riluzole, 182, 183t, 184
Rippling muscle disease (RMD), 234
Risdiplam, 207, 208t
Risus sardonicus, 242, 243f
Ritonavir, myopathies related to, 965
Rituximab
adverse effects of, 124
for chronic inflammatory demyelinating polyneuropathy, 357t
dosage of, 113t, 124
HBV reactivation after, 116

for inflammatory myopathies, 922t, 925–926
for Isaacs syndrome, 242
for juvenile MG, 646
management of, 124
mechanism of action, 123
monitoring of, 113t
for Morvan syndrome, 242
for multifocal motor neuropathy, 367
for MuSK ab positive mG, 645
for MuSK-positive MG, 112
for myasthenia gravis, 640t
side effects of, 113t, 640
for stiff person syndrome, 250
uses for, 123–124
RNA-binding proteins, 708
Robotic assistance, 159
Romberg sign, 193, 397, 511
Romberg test, 15
Rose-Bengal test, 64
Rozanolixizumab
function of, 638
for MuSK ab positive mG, 645
for myasthenia gravis, 647
during pregnancy, 647
trials of, 639t
Running, impaired, 6
Ryanodine receptors, 707, 879f
Ryanodine receptors *(RYR1)* mutations, 746, 776–777, 778–779, 880
Rydel-Seiffer tuning forks, 115

S

Sabin vaccine, 219
Sacral plexopathies, 582
Sacral plexus, anatomy of, 568
Safety issues, management of, 186t
Salk vaccine, 219
Saphenous neuropathies, 597
Sapneous nerve, 28
Sarcoglycan complex, 702, 722–724
Sarcoglycan staining, 89
Sarcoglycanopathies, 722–724
Sarcoid myopathy, 914
Sarcoid neuropathy, 118, 121
Sarcoidosis
clinical features of, 400, 401f
histopathology of, 99f, 401, 401f
laboratory features of, 401
management of, 589
pathogenesis of, 401–402
polyradiculopathies and, 587–588
treatment of, 402, 914
use of steroids for, 118
Sarcolemma, satellite cells and, 91
Sarcomeres
connection to sarcolemma, 91
in muscle fibers, 91
normal, 92f
proteins associated with, 706–707
Sarcoplasm, description of, 707
Sarcoplasmic reticulum Ca-ATPase gene *(SERCA1)*, 234, 880, 881
Sarcotubular myopathy, 787
Sartorius muscle innervation, 571
Satellite cells
location of, 91
repair of necrosis and, 96–97

Satoyoshi syndrome
clinical features of, 246
diagnosis of, 246
laboratory features of, 246–247
pathogenesis of, 247
treatment of, 247
Satralizumab, 642
Scanning dysarthria, 440
Scapula
winging, 542, 543f
Scapula, displacement of, 8
Scapular winging
causes of, 8, 9t
evaluation of, 13
Scapuloperoneal dystrophy, 704t
Scapuloperoneal muscular dystrophy/myopathy, 742–743
Scapuloperoneal neuropathy
clinical features of, 276
histopathology of, 276
laboratory features of, 276
molecular genetics of, 276
pathogenesis of, 276
Scapuloperoneal SMA, 215
Schirmer tests, 64
Schistosomiasis, 587
Schmidt-Lanterman incisures, 434
Schwann cells, 298f
damage to, 106
leprosy and, 413, 415f
metachromatic deposits in, 299f
phagocytosis by, 106
structure of, 106
Schwannomas, 537, 539f, 587f
Schwartz-Jampel syndrome (SJS), 881
Sciatic nerve
anatomy of, 567f, 572–573
blood supply to, 573
lesions, 573
Sciatic neuropathies, 598
Sclera, evaluation of, 12
Scleroderma, 400, 909
SCN4A mutations, 675
Scoliosis, 714
Scooters, 200
Scorpion envenomation, 689
Scrotum, innervation of, 576
Sea snake venom, 690
Secondary hypokalemic paralysis, 879
Secretion clearance, 186t
Seipin gene *(SPG17)*, 199
Selenoprotein N1 *(SEPN1)* mutations, 737, 778
Self-care, adaptive equipment for, 147f
Self-feeding, 147–148, 147f
Semimembranosus muscle innervation, 573
Semitendinosus muscle innervation, 573
Semithin sections, 96, 104f
Sensorimotor polyneuropathies, paraneoplastic, 443–444
Sensory ataxia
causes of, 63–64
in dorsal root ganglionopathies, 16
polyradiculopathy and, 54
sarcoidosis and, 400
Sensory ataxia neuropathy dysarthria (SANDO), 847–848

Sensory nerve action potentials (SNAPs), 28–31
　amplitudes, 30
　arms, 525–526
　in Charcot-Marie-Tooth disease, 261
　conduction studies, 28–31
　conduction velocity, 30
　distal latency, 30
　morphologic waveform change, 30–31
　multifocal reductions in, 55
　normal, 31f
　parameters of, 30–31
　pathology localization and, 53
　patient age and, 25
　temperature considerations in, 23
Sensory nerve conduction studies, 28–31
　electrode placement in, 28
Sensory neuronopathies
　causes of, 55
　EDX localization, 52
　HIV-related, 421
　painful, 495t, 510t
　paraneoplastic, 440–443
Sensory neuropathies, 52t
Sensory neuropathy/ganglionopathy
　causes of, 441f
　paraneoplastic, 440–443
Sensory polyneuropathies, 499–500
Sensory symptoms
　examination of, 14–15
　history of, 10
　loss of sensation, 10
　origin of, 3, 5
　patterns of, 11
Sequestome 1 (SQSTM1), 708
Serial casting, 155
Serologic testing, diagnostic value of, 64–65
Serotonin norepinephrine reuptake inhibitors, 591
Serum protein electrophoresis, 62
SETX genotype, 176, 182
Severe acute respiratory syndrome coronavirus 2 (SARS-CoV-2)
　myositis associated with, 919
　neuropathies and, 412f, 422–424, 423f–424f
　organizational impacts of, 6
　vaccines against, 423–424
Shilling test, 432
Shingrix, 648
Short exercise tests (SETs), 864, 866f, 866t
Short-chain acyl-CoA dehydrogenase (SCAD) deficiency, 820–821
Short-T1 inversion recovery (STIR) imaging, 71, 71f, 72f
Shoulder girdle
　examination of, 12
　weakness, 7
Shoulders
　pain in, 6, 151
　subluxation, 151
　support systems for, 141
Shulman syndrome, 967
Sialorrhea (drooling), 157, 186t
Sildenafil, 495
Simvastatin, myopathy and, 957–960
Single fiber electromyography (SFEMG), 48–50
　function of, 48–50

　jitter and blocking, 49f
　in Lambert-Eaton myasthenic syndrome, 664
　in myasthenia gravis, 622–623, 623f, 625
　normal recording, 49f
　normal values for jitter, 49–50
　parameters for, 48–50
　stimulated, 50
Sinusvertebral nerve pain, 566
Sirolumus, statin myopathy and, 957
Sjögren syndrome
　assessment for, 64
　clinical features of, 397, 910
　histopathology of, 398, 398f
　identification of, 69
　laboratory features of, 397–398
　pathogenesis of, 398–399
　secondary vasculitis and, 389
　treatment of, 399
Skiing, adaptive, 138f
Skin biopsies, 108–110
SLC22A5 mutations, 818
Slide boards, 149
Slow-channel syndrome, 672f, 674f, 679
SLUDGE acronym, 686–687
Small cell lung cancer (SCLC), 443–444, 660, 665
Small fiber neuropathies (SFNs), 57, 109f
Small fiber sensory neuropathies, 18
SMARD1. *See* Hereditary motor neuropathy, distal (dHMN)
SMARDI, 208–209
SMCHD1 mutations, 741
SMI-31 stains, 102f
Snake envenomation, 688–689
Snout reflex, presence of, 14
Soccer, adaptive, 138f
SOD1 (superoxide dismutase) gene, 168, 172, 179, 181–182
Sodium channel myotonia (SCM), 37, 882f
Sodium channelopathies, 869, 869f, 875–876
Sodium channels, 28
Sodium phenylbutyrate and taurusodol (PB-TURSO), 183t, 184
Soleus muscle innervation, 574
Solifenacin for urinary urgency, 200
Somatic peripheral neuropathies, 58
Somatosensory-evoked potentials (SSEPs), 261, 526–527
Sorafenib, myopathies related to, 968
Sorbitol dehydrogenase deficiency with peripheral neuropathy (SORD), 276–277
Sorbitol dehydrogenase *(SOD)* gene, 509
SOX-1 autoantibodies, 68
Spasmodic diplopia, 239
Spasms, UMN pathology and, 6
Spasticity
　in ALS, 171
　lower extremity, 193
　management of, 186t
　rehabilitation for, 155
Spastin (SPG1) protein, 198
Specimen handling, 84
Speech and language pathologists (SLPs), 131–132, 157–159
Speech issues, 616–617

Speech patterns, UMN pathology and, 6
Speech synthesizers, 159
Speech-generating devices (SGDs), 159
Speed test, 985f
Spinal abscesses, 220t, 533, 587
Spinal accessory nerve (SAN)
　anatomy of, 521–522
　lesions, 542
Spinal accessory neuropathy, 543f
Spinal canal stenosis, 565
Spinal cord
　ALS histopathology of, 179
　anatomy of, 518f
　cyanocobalamin deficiency, 74f
　intramedullary disorders of, 73
　ischemic disorders of, 586
　lumbosacral, 563–564, 564f
Spinal deformities, rehabilitation in, 150–151
Spinal dural abscesses, 587
Spinal dural arteriovenous fistulas, 589
Spinal epidural abscesses, 220t
Spinal fusion, rehabilitation in, 151
Spinal muscular atrophies (SMAs)
　bulbar symptoms in, 11, 209
　classification of, 204t
　differential diagnosis of, 205–206
　distal, 205t
　distal (dSMA)
　　differential diagnosis of, 175–176
　electrodiagnosis of, 206
　features of, 12–13, 15
　gene mutations in, 176
　histopathology of, 206–207, 207f
　infantile with arthrogryposis, 208–209
　inheritance of, 205t
　laboratory features of, 206
　management of, 207–208, 208t
　non-SMN-related, 208–209
　pathogenesis of, 207
　scapuloperoneal (*See also* Davidenkow disease)
　type I, 16 (*See also* Werdnig-Hoffmann disease)
　type III
　　features of, 204–205
　type IIIb, 204f
Spinal nerves
　anatomy of, 517–518
Spinal stenosis
　L3-L5, 586f
　lumbosacral, 17
　management of, 589
　neurogenic claudication and, 585f
　polyradiculopathies and, 17, 584–585
　spondylosis and, 585
Spine, anatomy of, 565f
Spinocerebellar ataxia type III, 198
Splints
　dynamic, 154–155
　hand, 141
　resting, 154–155
Spondylosis, 565–566, 585
Spurling maneuver, 531
Squamous cell carcinoma (SCC), 118
STAC3 mutations, 792
Stains, 84–85. *See also Specific* stains
Stance control KAFOs, 143f

Standing
    contracture prevention and, 154
    rehabilitation exercises, 154
Statin myopathies, 957–960
    histopathology of, 959, 959f
    laboratory features of, 959
    pathogenesis of, 960
Steatorrhea, vitamin E deficiency and, 434
Stem-cell transplantation
    for adrenoleukodystrophy, 302
Stereognosis testing, 15
Steroid myopathy, 944–945, 945f, 969f
Stiff person syndrome (SPS)
    antineoplastic, 249
    clinical features of, 247–248
    cramp potentials in, 235
    differential diagnosis of, 176
    GAD antibodies in, 244
    histopathology of, 249
    laboratory features of, 248–249
    onset of, 247
    pathogenesis of, 249–250
    plasma exchange for, 125
    rituximab for, 124
    treatment of, 250
    use of steroids in, 118
Stiff-limb syndrome, 248
Strength testing, 115
Strengthening exercises, 134–137, 134t
Stretching
    rehabilitation exercises, 154
    for spasticity, 155
Striated muscle preferentially expressed protein kinase *(SPEG)* mutations, 786
Stromal interaction molecule 1 *(STIM1)* mutations, 790, 880
Strongyloidiasis, 117
Strumpellin gene *(SPG8)*, 199
Strychnine, 243
Subacute motor neuropathy (SMN), 229
Subclavius innervatrion, 522
Subcutaneous immunoglobulins, 357t, 358
Subscapular nerves
    anatomy of, 522
    injury to, 544
Succinate dehydrogenase staining, 89, 89f, 90f
Succinylcholine, side effects of, 690
Sudan black stains, 87
Sudomotor axon density, 110
Sudomotor axon reflex testing, 62f
Sulfasalazine, drug interactions with, 433
Sulfatides
    damage caused by, 298f
Sunitinib, myopathies related to, 968
Superficial fibular nerve, 574
Superficial peroneal nerve biopsy, 99–100, 385f, 386f
Superficial radial nerve, 100
Superficial radial neuropathy, 546, 548, 548t
Superior cervical ganglion, 517
Superior gluteal nerve, 572
Superior gluteal neuropathies, 596
Supervillin *(SVIL)* mutations, 754
Supinator muscles, 523
Suprascapular nerve
    anatomy of, 522
    injury to, 544

Supraspinatus tendinopathy, 983–985, 984f
Sural nerve
    amyloidosis and, 450f
    anatomy of, 576
    biopsy of, 99, 100f
    in diabetic neuropathy, 492f, 493f
    leprosy and, 411, 415f
    lymphoma and, 446f
    primary amyloidosis and, 447f
    sensory conduction studies, 28
    in thiamine deficiency, 430
Sural neuropathies, 599
Suramin, toxic neuropathies and
    clinical features of, 456t, 459
    laboratory features of, 459, 460
    mechanism of, 456t
    nerve histopathology of, 456t, 459, 460
    pathogenesis of, 459, 460
Swallowing
    evaluation of, 157
    of liquids, 157
    phases of, 156
Swine flu vaccine, 326–327
Symptoms
    definitions of, 5–6
    evaluation of, 2, 3t
    questioning patients about, 5–6
SYNE1 mutations, 744
SYNE2 mutations, 744
Synkinesis in ALS, 171
Synthetase, autoantibodies against, 895t
Syntrophin complex, 702
Syphilis
    clinical features of, 417
    histopathology of, 417–418
    laboratory features of, 417
    pathogenesis of, 417–418
    treatment of, 418
Systemic disorders, neuropathies associated with, 398t, 403–405
Systemic lupus erythematosus (SLE)
    clinical features of, 399–400, 910
    histopathology of, 400
    laboratory features of, 400
    pathogenesis of, 400
    secondary vasculitis and, 388–389
    treatment of, 400
Systemic sclerosis, 389, 400

T

T cells, CD4+, 612
Tacrolimus (FK506)
    adverse effects of, 122
    dosage of, 113t, 122
    for inflammatory myopathies, 922t, 926
    management of, 122
    mechanism of action, 121–122
    monitoring of, 113t
    for myasthenia gravis, 642
    myopathies related to, 961
    for Satoyoshi syndrome, 247
    side effects of, 113t
    uses for, 122
Taenia solium, 921
Takayasu arteritis, 385
Tangier disease, 303–305
    clinical features of, 303

    histopathology of, 303, 304f
    laboratory features of, 303
    molecular genetics of, 303–305
    pathogenesis of, 303–305
Tape worms, myositis associated with, 921
TARDBP mutation, 168, 181
TARDNP mutation, 180
Tardy ulnar palsy, 553–554
Target fibers
    denervation and, 94
    reinnervation and, 95f
Targetoid fibers, moth-eaten, 94, 95f
Tarsal tunnel syndrome, 599
Tarui disease, 807–808
Taxane toxicity, 458–459
    clinical features of, 456t, 458
    laboratory features of, 458
    mechanism of, 456t
    nerve histopathology of, 456t, 458
    pathogenesis of, 458–459
T-cell intracellular antigen-1 (TIA1), 708
TDP-43 mutations, 182, 198
TDP-43 protein, 179, 180f
Teased nerve fibers, 105, 105f
Telehealth practice, 6
Telethonin, 707
Telethonin *(TCAP)* mutations, 724
Telithromycin, contraindication for, 626t
Temporal arteritis, 385
Tennis elbow test, 987f
Tenofovir, myopathies related to, 965
TENS
    for pain, 156
    for spasticity, 155
Tensor fascia lata innervation, 572
Teres major innervation, 544
Terminal nerves
    anatomy of, 521, 522–524
    lesions of, 542–550
Testosterone
    replacement therapy, 211
Tetanolysin, 244
Tetanospasmin, 244, 245
Tetanus, 242–243
    cramp potentials in, 235
    incubation period of, 242
    laboratory features of, 243–244
    mortality rate of, 242
    pathogenesis of, 244
    spasms, 242
    treatment of, 244–245
    vaccination programs, 244–245
Tetanus vaccines, 117
Tetany
    clinical features of, 245–246
    diagnosis of, 245–246
    laboratory features of, 246
    pathogenesis of, 246
    treatment of, 246
Tetrahydrofolate, 432
Thalidomide, 416, 457t, 460–461
Thallium toxicity
    clinical features of, 483t, 484
    detection of, 483t
    histopathology of, 484
    laboratory features of, 483t, 484
    treatment of, 484

Thenar eminence, percussion of, 13
Thermal perception thresholds, 504, 505, 506
Thiamine, dietary sources of, 430
Thiamine deficiency, 430–431
    clinical features of, 430
    histopathology of, 430
    laboratory features of, 430
    pathogenesis of, 430
    peripheral neuropathy and, 63
    treatment of, 431
Thigh abduction, 572
Thin filaments, 91, 707
Thiopurine methyltransferase (TPMT) deficiency, 119–120
Thoracic outlet syndrome, 537, 538f
Thoracic radiculopathies, 532–533
Thoracic-lumbar-sacral orthoses (TLSOs), 140–141, 150–151
Thoracodorsal nerve
    anatomy of, 522
    injury to, 544
Thoracoscapular muscle weakness, 151
Thumb osteoarthritis, 988f
Thymectomy
    for inflammatory myopathies, 927
    for juvenile MG, 646
    for myasthenia gravis, 643–644, 646
Thymic carcinomas
    incidence of, 628
    in Lambert-Eaton myasthenic syndrome, 660
    staging of, 628
Thymic epithelial tumors (TETs), 628
Thymic follicular hyperplasia (TFH), 612–613
Thymic imaging, 628–629
Thymidine kinase 2 (TK2) mutations, 846
Thymomas
    autoantibodies linked to, 67
    eosinophiilc myositis and, 916f
    imaging of, 628–629, 629f
    incidence of, 628
    myasthenics with, 67–68, 645–646
    overlap syndromes, 915
Thymus
    hyperplasia of, 629–630
    imaging of, 628–630
    Treg cells and, 611
Thyroid hormone receptor interactor 4 (TRIP4) mutations, 778
Thyroid-stimulating hormone (TSH), 236, 941
Thyrotoxic myopathy, 940–941
Thyrotoxic periodic paralysis (TPP), 879, 940–941
Thyrotoxicosis, 940–941
Thyroxine (T4), 941
Tiagabine, 250
Tibial nerve
    anatomy of, 574–575
    cutaneous, 575f
    nerve conduction studies using, 26
    rastered CMAPs, 237f
Tibial neuropathies, 599
Tibialis anterior muscle innervation, 574
Tibialis muscle, biopsies of issues with, 83
Tibialis posterior muscle innervation, 574
Tick paralysis, 684–686
    clinical features of, 684–685
    diagnosis of, 685
    histopathology of, 685
    laboratory features of, 685
    pathogenesis of, 686
    treatment of, 686
Tick-borne encephalitis, 221t
Tight junctions, formation of, 105
Tilt table testing, 59, 61
Tinel sign, 368, 550
Tissue fixation, 84
Titin, 707
Titin (TTN) mutations, 726, 750, 754, 777, 778, 786
Titinopathies, 726
Tizanidine
    for cramps, 211
    for HSP management, 199t, 200
    for stiff person syndrome, 250
TMEM5 mutations, 735
TMEM43 mutations, 744
Tocainide for cramps, 238t
Tocilizumab, 915, 926
A-Tocopherol deficiency. See Vitamin E deficiency
Tofacitinib, 125
Tofersen, 183t, 184
Toileting, 148–149
Tolterodine, 200
Toluene toxicity, 975
Tongue
    atrophy of, 11, 171f
    myotonia, 11–12
    strength of, 11, 619
    tremulousness of, 11
    weakness of, 8, 11
    wiggling of, 14
Torsin A interacting protein 1 (TPR1AIP1) mutations, 729
Total body irradiation, 927
Toxic myopathies, 957–982
    drugs related to, 958t–959t
Toxic neuropathies
    medication-associated, 472–479, 473t–474t
    screening for, 109
Toxic oil syndrome, 967–968
Toxoplasmosis, 921
Tracheostomy-assisted mechanical ventilation (TAMV), 168, 185
Tramadol, 493, 495t, 510t
Transfer RNA (tRNA), 831
Transfer RNA (tRNA) mutations, 831, 842
Transient receptor vallanoid 4 (TRPV4) mutation, 176
Transport protein particle complex subunit 11 (TRAPPC11) mutations, 728
Transportin-3 (TNP03) mutation, 718
Transthyretin familial amyloid neuropathy (TTR-FAP), 176
Transverse abdominus muscle innervation, 568
Transverse myelitis, 220t
Trapezius hump, 740, 740f
Trapezius muscles, 542
Trastuzumab emtansine, 457t, 461
Treg cells, 611
Tremor
    in infants, 15
    malignancies and, 440
Trendelenburg gait, 617
Treponema pallidum, 412f, 417
Triamcinolone, 969
Triamterene, 878–879
Triazole antibodies, 957
Trichinosis, 920–921
Tricyclic antidepressants
    for HVZ infections, 422
    for neuropathic pain, 591
    for painful sensory neuronopathies, 495t, 510t
Trigeminal neuropathy, 69
Triiodothyronine (T3), 941
Trilaminar myopathy, 788
Trimethoprim-sulfamethoxazole, 115–116, 405
Triosephosphate isomerase deficiency, 811–812
Tripartite motif containing 23(TRIM32) mutations, 724, 787
Tripartite motif-containing protein 32, 708
Triple furrow, 619
Triple Timed-Up-and-Go (Triple TUG) tests, 664
Trismus, 243
Tropheryma whippeli, 404–405
Tropical spastic paraparesis (TSP), 918
Tropomycin, 707
α-Tropomycin (TPM3) mutations, 781–782
Troponin T (TNNT1) mutation, 782
Troponins, structure of, 707
Trospium, 200
Trousseau sign, 239, 245, 948
Trumenba, 637
Trunk
    flexion testing of, 13
    focal processes affecting, 517–562
    lower, 534
    middle, 534
    muscle weakness in, 12
    upper, 533–534
L-Tryptophan, 966–967
T-SPOT.TB assay, 116
TTR-related amyloidosis (FAP types I and II), 315–316
T-tubules, composition of, 93
Tuberculin skin testing (TST), 116
Tuberculosis (TB)
    immunosuppression and, 116
    polyradiculopathies and, 587
    prophylaxis, 116
    screening for, 923
Tubular aggregates, 84, 86f
Tubular aggregates myopathy, 790, 791f
Tumor necrosis factor (TNF) inhibitors
    myopathies related to, 968
    neuropathies associated with, 402–403
    toxic neuropathies and, 477–478
        clinical features of, 474t
        diagnostic testing for, 474t
        nerve histopathology in, 474t
        tuberculosis risk and, 116
Turner syndrome, 712
Tyrosine kinase inhibitors, myopathies related to, 968

U

Ubiquilin 2 mutations, 182
Ubiquitin ligase (RBCK1) deficiency, 812

E3-Ubiquitin ligase *(TRIM32)* mutations, 724
Ublituximab, 641
UBQLN mutation, 180
UDD distal myopathy, 749–750
Ulcerative colitis (UC), 402–403
Ullrich congenital muscular dystrophy
　(UCMD), 730–731
Ullrich disease (UCMD), 734–735
Ulnar nerve
　anatomy of, 523–524, 553–558
　damage to, 557*f*
　leprosy and, 411, 415*f*
　nerve conduction studies using, 26
　sensory conduction studies, 28
Ulnar neuropathies
　at elbow
　　focal demyelination with conduction
　　　block, 28*f*
　at the elbow, 553–554, 553*t*
　at the hand, 554–558
　symptoms of, 17
　at the wrist, 555*t*, 556*f*
Ultrasonography
　diagnostic use of, 75
　for spasticity, 155
Unc-45 myosin chaperone A *(UNC45B)*
　mutations, 778
UNC45B mutations, 754
Upper extremities
　focal processes affecting, 517–562
　innervation of muscles in, 521*t*
　muscle innervation in, 521*t*
Upper limbs
　neuromuscular mimics in, 983–989
　orthoses, 141
　proximal weakness, 151–152
Upper motor neurons (UMNs)
　cranial nerves and, 14
　dysfunction of, 167–168
　involvement ALS, 170–174
　pathology in, 6
　patterns of weakness and, 7*t*
Upper motor neurons (UMNs) disease,
　158–159
Uremic neuropathy
　clinical features of, 403–404
　histopathology of, 404
　pathogenesis of, 404
　treatment of, 404
Urethral sphincter innervation, 576
Urinary urgency
　cervical radiculopathies and, 533
　in HSP, 200
　management of, 186*t*
Utrophin, 706

V

Vaccinations
　GBS and, 423–424
　Guillain-Barré syndrome and, 326–327
　in myasthenia gravis, 648
Vaccines
　caution in use of, 626*t*
　immunosuppression and, 117
Vacuolar cardiomyopathy, X-linked, 812–813
Vacuoles, debris-filled, 86*f*
Valosin-containing protein (VCP), 708

Valproic acid
　for Isaacs syndrome, 242
　for Morvan syndrome, 242
　for stiff person syndrome, 250
Valsalva maneuver, 59, 61*f*
Vamorolone, 713
Varicella zoster, polyradiculopathy and, 230
Vascular endothelial growth factor inhibitors,
　968–969
Vasculitic neuropathies, 383–396
　categories of, 383
　clinical features of, 383
　cyclophosphamide for, 122
　cyclosporine for, 121
　diagnosis of, 99
　histopathology of, 383–385
　identification of, 69
　laboratory findings in, 383
　leukemias and, 444
　lymphomas and, 444
　nerve biopsies for, 98–99
　patterns of involvement, 384*f*
　peripheral neuropathy and, 384*t*
　plasma exchange for, 125
　rheumatoid arthritis and, 399
　rituximab for, 124
　treatment of, 390–392
Vasculitis
　connective tissue associated, 388–389
　histopathology of, 386*f*
　polyradiculopathies and, 588
　sciatic neuropathies and, 573
　Sjögren syndrome and, 397
Vastus lateralis muscle innervation, 571
VCP mutations, 755
Veluzumab, 641
Venlafaxine, 493, 495*t*, 510*t*, 591
Venorelbine, neurotoxicity of, 458
Ventilation
　noninvasive, 211
Ventilation, bedside assessment of, 14
Ventilatory muscle weakness, 8–9, 9*t*
2S-4 Ventral root stimulation, 200
Ventral roots, spinal nerve, 517
Verapamil for cramps, 238*t*
Verbal fluency, tests of, 173
Vercuronium for tetanus, 245
Very long-chain acyl-CoA dehydrogenase
　(VLCAD) deficiency, 819
Vibegron, 200
Vibration testing, timed, 115
Vibratory perception thresholds, 504, 505, 506
Vidarabine, 421
Vigabatrin, 250, 251
Vinca alkaloids
　clinical features of, 455, 456*t*, 458
　laboratory features of, 458
　mechanism of, 456*t*
　nerve histopathology of, 456*t*, 458
　pathogenesis of, 458
Vincristine
　contraindications for, 458
　myopathies related to, 963–964
　toxic neuropathies and, 455, 456*t*, 458
Vinorelbine, 456*t*
Vinyl benzene toxicity, 481
　clinical features of, 479*t*

　diagnostic testing for, 479*t*
　mechanism of, 479*t*
Viper *(Crotalid* sp.*)* venom, 688
Vision, blurred, 616–617
Vital capacity, estimates of, 14, 620
Vitamin B1 complex, 238*t*
Vitamin B1 deficiency. *See* Thiamine deficiency
Vitamin B6, toxic neuropathies and, 478
Vitamin B6 deficiency, 63, 431
Vitamin B9. *See* Folate
Vitamin B12
　deficiency of
　　clinical features of, 431, 432*f*
　　histopathology of, 432
　　laboratory features of, 431–432
　　neuropathies related to, 431
　　pathogenesis of, 432
　　peripheral neuropathy and, 63
　　presentation of, 198
　　secondary to nitrous oxide inhalation,
　　　433
　　treatment of, 433
　malabsorption of, 402
　testing in peripheral neuropathy, 62
Vitamin D, 942
　deficiency of, 246, 943
　for tetany, 246
Vitamin deficiencies, neuropathies and, 63
Vitamin E
　for cramps, 238*t*
　deficiency of, 433–434
　　clinical features of, 306
　　histopathology of, 306
　　laboratory features of, 306
　　molecular genetics of, 306
　　treatment of, 306
　malabsorption of, 402
VMA21 mutations, 813–814
Vocal cord and pharyngeal distal myopathy
　(VCPDM), 755–756
Voltage-dependent sodium channel *(SCN4A)*
　mutations, 871–872, 873, 874, 877
Voltage-gated calcium channels (VGCCs), 875*f*
　antibodies to, 664–666
　types of, 666
Voltage-gated Kv1 potassium channel (VGKC)
　complex antibodies, 67, 240, 242
Voltage-gated sodium channels, 875*f*

W

Waldenström macroglobinemia (WM)
　amyloidosis and, 449
　clinical features of, 452–453
　histopathology of, 453
　laboratory features of, 453
　treatment of, 453
Walkers, 144–145, 144*f*
Walker-Warburg syndrome (WWS), 708
　clinical features of, 736
　laboratory features of, 736
　molecular genetics of, 736
　pathogenetics of, 736
Walking
　contracture prevention and, 154
　rehabilitation exercises, 154
Wallerian degeneration, 26, 105, 107*f*. *See also*
　　Axonal degeneration

Weakness
  acute, 5t
  characteristics of, 6
  chronic progressive proximal, 5t
  in congenital myasthenic syndromes, 672f
  diaphragmatic, 9–10
  differential diagnoses, 5t, 440
  generalized, 5t
  of hip flexion, 7
  jaw, 8
  myasthenia gravis and, 616–617
  neck muscle, 8
  patterns of, 11, 13–14
  presentations of, 4t, 5t
  proximal, 5t
  shoulder girdle, 7
  subacute, 5t
  tongue, 8, 11
Welander distal neuropathy
  clinical features of, 748
  hand exercises in, 152
  histopathology of, 748
  laboratory features of, 748
  molecular genetics of, 748
  pathogenesis of, 748
Werdnig-Hoffmann disease. *See also* Spinal muscular atrophies, type I
  features of, 204t
  laboratory features of, 206
Wernicke-Korsakoff syndrome, 434
West Nile virus (WNV), 221, 221t
  acute flaccid paralysis related to, 221–224
  clinical features of, 223
  diagnosis of, 223
  histopathology of, 224

  laboratory features of, 223–224
  pathogenesis of, 224
  transmission of, 224
  treatment of, 224
Wheelchairs, 145–146
  for HSP, 200
  power controls for, 146f
  pressure mapping for, 146
  ramps for, 150
Whipple disease
  clinical features of, 404
  histopathology of, 404
  laboratory features of, 404
  pathogenesis of, 404–405
Whole exome sequencing (WES), 70
Whole genome sequencing (WGS), 70
Williams distal myopathy, 751
Windsurfing, 138f
Winging
  scapular, 542, 543f
Wolfe-Parkinson-White syndrome, 801
Wrist
  median neuropathy, 550–553, 550t
  weakness of, 7
Wrist extensor stretch, 987f
Writer's cramp, 234

X
Xeroderma pigmentosum (XP), 309–310
  clinical features of, 309
  histopathology of, 309
  laboratory features of, 309
  molecular genetics of, 309–310
  pathogenesis of, 309–310

X-linked bulbospinal disease. *See* Kennedy disease
X-linked bulbospinal muscular atrophy, 209. *See* Kennedy disease
X-linked Charcot-Marie-Tooth disease, 274
X-linked Emery-Dreifuss muscular dystrophy (EDMD), 89, 707
X-linked myopathy with excessive autophagy (XMEA), 813–814, 814f
X-linked vacuolar cardiomyopathy, 812–813

Y
Yawning, forced, 14
Yergason test, 985f

Z
ZAC mutations, 786
Zalcitabine, 476, 965
ZASP, 707
ZASP protein, 754
Z-bands, orientation of, 91
Z-discs
  degeneration of, 96
  sarcomere, 92f
  structure of, 707
Zebra body myopathy, 784
Zidovudine, 964–965
Zika virus, 326–327
Zilucoplan, 636, 636t, 637–638
Zinc, serum levels of, 177
Zoster motor paresis, 582
Zulnar nerve
  ultrasound of, 555f
Zygapophyseal joints, 565